OXFORD MEDICAL PUBLICATIONS

Primary Surgery

Volume One

Non-Trauma

AT LEAST 20 SURGEONS

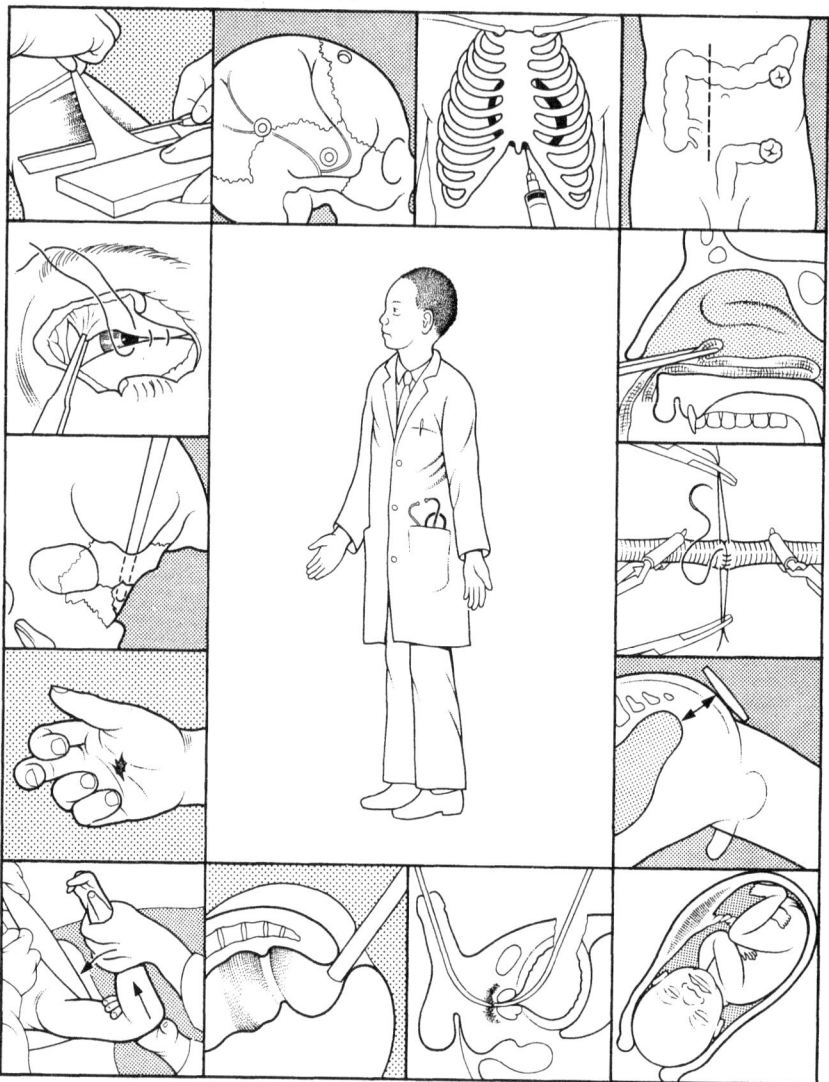

AT LEAST TWENTY SURGEONS IN ONE. Here you are, one of our readers, faced with the difficult problem of knowing what you might do to help a patient in all these fields, and unable to refer him to an expert. Reading from the top left in a clockwise direction you have to be: a plastic surgeon, a neurosurgeon, a thoracic surgeon, a general surgeon, an ear, nose, and throat surgeon, a vascular surgeon, a paediatric surgeon, an obstetrician and gynaecologist, a urologist, a proctologist, an orthopaedic surgeon, a hand surgeon, a maxillofacial surgeon, and a burns surgeon.

This figure does not show your role as a trauma surgeon, an ophthalmic surgeon, a dental surgeon, a leprosy surgeon, a 'tropical surgeon', an oncologist, an anaesthetist, and an 'intensivist'—in addition to doing everything else you have to do in medicine, paediatrics, psychiatry, and management! We hope that these manuals will help you in some of these varied and exacting tasks.

Primary Surgery

Volume One

Non-Trauma

The late NELSON AWORI MB ChB (East Africa), FRCS (Edin), DRCOG (Lond),
Formerly Associate Professor of Urology and Chief Transplant Surgeon, Kenyatta National Hospital; Chairman of the Department of Surgery, University of Nairobi, Kenya.

ANNE BAYLEY, OBE, MB BChir (Cantab), FRCS (Edin), FRCS,
Professor of Surgery, University of Zambia; Sometime Surgeon St Francis Hospital, Katete, Zambia

ALAN BEASLEY, FRCS, DLO,
Consultant Otorhinolaryngologist, Royal Devon and Exeter Hospital, Exeter, England.

JAMES BOLAND MD, ADA,
Professor and Chairman of Surgery, Charleston Division, West Virginia University, USA.

MICHAEL CRAWFORD MD (Liverpool), MRCP,
Director, The Clinical Oncology Unit, University of Bradford, England.

FRITS DRIESSEN MD, DTM&H,
Head of the Department of Obstetrics and Gynaecology, Queen Elizabeth II Hospital, Maseru, Lesotho.

ALLEN FOSTER MD, ChB, FRCS, DO,
Medical Consultant to the Christoffel Blindenmission, West Germany; Senior Lecturer in Preventive Ophthalmology, The Institute of Ophthalmology, Cayton Street, London.

WENDY GRAHAM BSc, DPhil,
Research Fellow, Department of Epidemiology and Population Sciences, London School of Hygiene and Tropical Medicine, London.

BRIAN HANCOCK MD, FRCS,
Consultant General Surgeon, Wythenshawe Hospital, Manchester, England; formerly District Medical Officer, Kamuli Hospital, Uganda.

BRANWEN HANCOCK FRCR,
Consultant Radiotherapist, the Christie Hospital, Manchester; formerly District Medical Officer, Kamuli Hospital, Uganda.

GERALD HANKINS FRCS,
Formerly Honorary Surgeon, The Shanta Bahwan Hospital, Kathmandu, Nepal.

NEVILLE HARRISON MD (Lond), FRCS,
Consultant Urological Surgeon, Brighton, England; formerly Senior Surgical Registrar, Mulago Hospital, Kampala, Uganda.

IAN KENNEDY OBE, MB ChB, FRCS (Edin), DO, DLO,
Medical Superintendent, Bamalete Lutheran Hospital, Ramotswa, Botswana.

JULIUS KYAMBI MD (Heidelberg), FAS (Geissen), FAC (Paed. Köln),
Associate Professor of Paediatric Surgery, Kenyatta National Hospital, Kenya.

SAMIRAN NUNDY, MB BChir (Cantab), FRCS,
Associate Professor, The All India Institute of Medical Sciences, New Delhi, India.

OXFORD
UNIVERSITY PRESS

Great Clarendon Street, Oxford, OX2 6DP,
United Kingdom

Oxford University Press is a department of the University of Oxford.
It furthers the University's objective of excellence in research, scholarship,
and education by publishing worldwide. Oxford is a registered trade mark of
Oxford University Press in the UK and in certain other countries

© GTZ 1990

The moral rights of the author have been asserted

First Edition published in 1990
Reprinted 1993 (with corrections), 2002, 2003,
2007, 2009, 2010, 2012, 2013

All rights reserved. No part of this publication may be reproduced, stored in
a retrieval system, or transmitted, in any form or by any means, without the
prior permission in writing of Oxford University Press, or as expressly permitted
by law, by licence or under terms agreed with the appropriate reprographics
rights organization. Enquiries concerning reproduction outside the scope of the
above should be sent to the Rights Department, Oxford University Press, at the
address above

You must not circulate this work in any other form
and you must impose this same condition on any acquirer

Published in the United States of America by Oxford University Press
198 Madison Avenue, New York, NY 10016, United States of America

British Library Cataloguing in Publication Data

Data available

Library of Congress Cataloging in Publication Data

Data available

ISBN 978-0-19-261694-4

JOE SHEPHERD MD (Monash), FRCS (Edin), FRACS,
Professor of Surgery, Hobart, Tasmania; formerly Senior Lecturer in Surgery, Makerere University, Kampala, Uganda.

JOHN STEWART MD (Harvard), ABOS, AADS,
Clinical Professor Emeritus (Orth), University of Washington School of Medicine; Orthopaedic Consultant, Harborview Trauma Centre, Seattle; formerly Senior Orthopaedic Consultant, Kilimanjaro Christian Medical Centre, Tanzania; Consultant, Rotary International Program, "Malawi Against Polio".

GRACE WARREN AM, Hon MD (Syd), MB, MS, FRCS, FRACS, DTM&H (Syd),
Adviser in Leprosy and Reconstructive Surgery for Asia, The Leprosy Mission (International), The Christian Hospital, Manorom, Chainat, Central Thailand.

The late Sir MICHAEL WOOD CBE, MBBS, FRCS,
Founder and until lately Director of "AMREF". The African Medical Research and Education Foundation, Nairobi, Kenya.

Editors

MAURICE KING MD (Cantab), FRCP, FFPHM
Reader in Community Medicine in the University of Leeds; lately Staff member with the German Agency for Technical Co-operation (GTZ) in Nyeri, Kenya.

PETER C. BEWES MB MChir (Cantab), FRCS, DRCOG
Consultant Surgeon to The Birmingham Accident Hospital; formerly Honorary Surgeon to the Kilimanjaro Christian Medical Centre, Tanzania.

JAMES CAIRNS OGDS (Zambia), OBE, MB BChir (Cantab), FRCS (Edin), DRCOG
Medical Superintendent/Surgeon, St Francis Hospital, Katete, Zambia.

JIM THORNTON MB, ChB, MRCOG, DTM&H
Senior Lecturer in Obstetrics and Gynaecology, St James' Hospital, University of Leeds.

Illustrated by Derek Atherton, Ivanson Kaiyai, Robert Lane (Sir Arthur Keith Medallist of the Royal College of Surgeons), Daphne Paley-Smith, and Terry Collins.

This low-priced edition was funded by the Wellcome Trust.

OXFORD UNIVERSITY PRESS
OXFORD, DELHI, KUALA LUMPUR

FOREWORD

The production of this manual on Surgery was sponsored by the German Federal Ministry for Economic Co-operation within the scope of the Technical Co-operation Agreement with the Republic of Kenya, under project number 78.2048.3-01.100. It was compiled by Maurice King Peter Bewes, James Cairns, and Jim Thornton in close collaboration with Kenyan and other experts.

The manual contains the collective views of an international group of experts. The methods and techniques described correspond to the state of the art with regard to their feasibility in rural hospitals, where sophisticated technical equipment may not be available. These manuals cannot, however, replace personal instruction by a qualified expert. Neither the editors, nor the publisher may be held responsible for any damage resulting from the application of the described methods. Any liability in this respect is excluded.

Dr. R Korte, GTZ
Department of Health,
German Agency for Technical Co-operation
Postfach 5180D
6236 ESCHBORN
West Germany.

While every effort has been made to check the dosages in this book, it is still possible that errors have been missed. Furthermore, dosage schedules are being continually revised and new side-effects recognized. For these reasons the reader is strongly urged to consult the drug companies' printed instructions before administering any of the drugs recommended in these manuals.

These manuals are dedicated by the first editor to his aunt, then Miss Davidona de Winton, who in the hills of Ceylon in 1932, once taught a very small boy unwillingly to read and write.

Contents

Six Prefaces and the Postscript

Chapter 1 The background to surgery 1

1.1 The unmet need for surgical care. 1.2 The surgical scene. 1.3 Twenty surgeons in one. 1.4 Your surgical work. 1.5 Your patients. 1.6 Referral is mostly a myth. 1.7 The limits of this system of surgery. 1.8 Should you operate? 1.9 "Oh, never, let us doubt what nobody is sure about". 1.10 Creating the surgical machine. 1.12 The surgical care of the poor. 1.13 Primary care radiology. 1.14 How to use these manuals.

Chapter 2 Theatres, antiseptics, and antibiotics 15

2.1 The major theatre. 2.2 The minor theatre. 2.2a Health centre surgery. 2.3 Aseptic theatre technique. 2.4 Autoclaving. 2.5 Disinfectants and antiseptics. 2.6 Antiseptic surgery. 2.7 Antibiotics in surgery. 2.8 Particular antibiotics. 2.9 Methods for using antibiotics. 2.10 When prevention fails—wound infection.

Chapter 3 The control of bleeding 29

3.1 Assisting natural mechanisms. 3.2 Arterial bleeding. 3.3 Tying the external carotid artery. 3.4 Tying the third part of the subclavian artery. 3.5 Tying the internal iliac artery. 3.6 Tying the external iliac artery in the groin. 3.7 Tying the femoral artery. 3.8 Tying the popliteal artery. 3.9 Bloodless limb operations with tourniquets. 3.10 Postoperative bleeding.

Chapter 4 Basic methods and instruments 39

4.1 Your instruments. 4.2 Scalpels and dissectors. 4.3 Scissors. 4.4 Forceps. 4.5 Retractors and hooks. 4.6 Suture materials. 4.7 Needles and their holders. 4.8 Suture methods. 4.9 Using tubes in surgery, especially nasogastric tubes. 4.10 Drains and draining. 4.11 Miscellaneous equipment and materials. 4.12 Instrument sets.

Chapter 5 The surgery of sepsis; draining abscesses 52

5.1 'Where there is pus let it out'. 5.2 Abscesses. 5.3 Boils. 5.4 Carbuncles. 5.4a Extradural abscesses. 5.5 Infections of the orbit; cavernous sinus thrombosis. 5.6 Peritonsillar abscesses. 5.7 Retropharyngeal abscesses. 5.8 Dental alveolar abscesses. 5.9 Parotid abscesses. 5.10 Pus in the neck—Ludwig's angina. 5.10a Thyroid abscesses. 5.10b Pancreatic abscesses. 5.11 Axillary abscesses. 5.11a Perinephric abscesses. 5.12 Iliac abscesses. 5.13 Anorectal abscesses. 5.14 Periurethral abscesses. 5.15 Prostatic abscesses. 5.16 Abscesses in the seminal vesicles.

Chapter 6 Pus in the pleura, the pericardium, the peritoneum, and the pelvis 65

6.1 Pus in the pleural cavities—empyema. 6.1a Pus in the pericardium. 6.2 Peritonitis. 6.3 Abscesses in the peritoneal cavity. 6.4 Subphrenic abscesses. 6.5 Pelvic abscesses. 6.6 PID (pelvic inflammatory disease, salpingitis). 6.6a Septic abortions. 6.7 Puerperal sepsis. 6.8 Infection following Caesarean section.

Chapter 7 Pus in the muscles, bones, and joints 83

7.1 Pyomyositis. 7.2 The pathology of osteomyelitis. 7.3 Acute osteomyelitis. 7.4 The general method for osteomyelitis. 7.5 Exploring a bone for pus. 7.6 Chronic osteomyelitis. 7.7 Osteomyelitis of the humerus. 7.8 Osteomyelitis of the radius. 7.9 Osteomyelitis of the ulna. 7.10 Osteomyelitis of the femur. 7.11 Osteomyelitis of the tibia. 7.12 Osteomyelitis of the fibula. 7.13 Osteomyelitis of the calcaneus and the talus. 7.14 Osteitis of the cranium. 7.14a Osteomyelitis of the jaws. 7.15 Osteomyelitis of the spine and pelvis. 7.16 Septic arthritis. 7.17 Methods and positions for particular septic joints. 7.18 Septic arthritis of the hip. 7.19 Girdlestone's operation for an infected hip.

Chapter 8 Pus in the hands and feet 104

8.1 The general method for an infected hand. 8.2 Subcutaneous hand infections. 8.3 Infection of the apical finger spaces. 8.4 Paronychia. 8.5 Infection of the pulp space of the fingers. 8.6 Infection of the spaces over the volar surfaces of the middle and proximal phalanges. 8.7 Web space infections. 8.8 Infection of the superficial palmar space. 8.9 Infection of the middle palmar space. 8.10 Infection of the thenar space. 8.11 Infection on the dorsum of the hand and fingers. 8.12 Infection of the flexor tendon sheaths. 8.13 Infection of the ulnar bursa. 8.14 Infection of the radial bursa. 8.15 Septic arthritis of the fingers. 8.16 Other problems with infected hands. 8.17 Pus in the feet.

Chapter 9 Methods for abdominal surgery 114

9.1 Before a major operation. 9.2 Laparotomy; abdominal incisions. 9.3 Resecting and anastomosing gut, end to end anastomoses. 9.4 End to side and side to side anastomoses. 9.5 Ostomies and bypasses for large gut obstruction. 9.6 Methods for ostomies. 9.7 A feeding jejunostomy. 9.8 Draining and closing the abdomen. 9.9 After an abdominal operation. 9.10 Nonrespiratory postoperative complications. 9.11 Respiratory postoperative complications. 9.11a Respiratory physiotherapy. 9.12 Infected laparotomy wounds. 9.13 Burst abdomen (wound dehiscence). 9.14 Intestinal fistulae.

Chapter 10 The acute abdomen; intestinal obstruction   142

10.1 The general method for an acute abdomen. 10.2 Diagnosing an acute abdomen. 10.3 Intestinal obstruction. 10.4 The diagnosis of intestinal obstruction. 10.5 The management of intestinal obstruction. 10.6 *Ascaris* obstruction. 10.7 Bands and adhesions. 10.8 Intussusception. 10.9 Volvulus of the small gut. 10.10 Volvulus of the sigmoid colon. 10.10a Closing Hartmann's operation. 10.11 Volvulus of the caecum. 10.12 Obstruction following abdominal abscesses. 10.13 Ileus and obstruction following abdominal surgery. 10.14 Other problems with acute abdomens.

Chapter 11 The stomach   170

11.1 Peptic ulcers. 11.2 Perforated peptic ulcers. 11.3 Bleeding from the upper gastrointestinal tract. 11.4 Surgery for a bleeding peptic ulcer. 11.5 Bleeding oesophageal varices. 11.6 Pyloric stenosis. 11.7 Elective surgery for chronic duodenal ulcer. 11.8 Gastrostomy (Stamm).

Chapter 12 The appendix   182

12.1 Appendicitis. 12.2 Difficulties with appendicitis.

Chapter 13 The gall-bladder, pancreas, and spleen   118

13.1 Introduction. 13.2 Gall-bladder symptoms; biliary colic. 13.3 Acute cholecystitis. 13.4 Cholangitis. 13.5 Cholangitis caused by *Ascaris*. 13.6 Primary or recurrent pyogenic cholangitis. 13.7 Cholecystectomy. 13.8 Obstructive jaundice. 13.9 Pancreatitis. 13.10 Pancreatic pseudocysts. 13.11 The surgery of the spleen.

Chapter 14 Hernias   198

14.1 General principles. 14.2 Inguinal hernias. 14.3 Difficulties with inguinal hernias. 14.4 Giant inguinal hernias. 14.5 Inguinal hernias and congenital hydroceles in children. 14.6 Irreducible and strangulated inguinal hernias. 14.7 Femoral hernias. 14.8 Strangulated femoral hernias. 14.9 Hernias of the umbilicus and anterior abdominal wall. 14.10 Umbilical hernias in children. 14.11 Paraumbilical hernias in adults. 14.12 Epigastric hernias. 14.13 Incisional hernias.

Chapter 15 The surgery of conception   220

15.1 Maternal mortality. 15.1a Obstetric aims and priorities. 15.2 Infertility. 15.3 Tubal ligation. 15.4 Using a laprocator. 15.5 Vasectomy.

Chapter 16 The surgery of pregnancy   230

16.1 Surgical problems in pregnancy. 16.2 Evacuating an abortion. 16.4 Fetal death, missed abortion, and intrauterine death. 16.5 Suturing an incompetent cervix for recurrent second trimester abortions. 16.6 'Acute' ectopic pregnancy. 16.7 'Chronic' ectopic pregnancy. 16.8 Angular and cervical ectopic pregnancies. 16.9 Abdominal pregnancies. 16.10 Autotransfusion. 16.11 APH—bleeding after the 28th week. 16.12 Placenta praevia. 16.13 Placental abruption.

Chapter 17 The medicine of pregnancy   246

17.2 Anaemia in pregnancy. 17.3 Diabetes in pregnancy. 17.4 Hypertension in pregnancy. 17.5 Heart failure in pregnancy. 17.6 Urinary infection and chronic renal disease in pregnancy.

Chapter 18 The surgery of labour   257

18.1 The two worlds of obstetrics. 18.1a Obstetric anaesthesia. 18.2 Delay in labour. 18.3 Obstructed labour. 18.4 Managing an obstructed labour. 18.4a Oxytocin. 18.5 Vacuum extraction. 18.6 Symphysiotomy. 18.7 Destructive operations. 18.8 Which kind of Caesarean section? 18.9 Lower segment Caesarean section. 18.10 Difficulties with Caesarean section. 18.12 Classical Caesarean section. 18.13 Extraperitoneal Caesarean section. 18.14 Elective section, 'trial of scar', or section early in labour? 18.15 Injuries of the birth canal. 18.16 Old third-degree tears. 18.17 Rupture of the uterus. 18.18 Vesicovaginal fistulae. 18.19 Rectovaginal fistulae.

Chapter 19 Other obstetric problems   293

19.2 The surfactant test for fetal maturity. 19.3 Inducing labour. 19.4 Preterm labour. 19.5 Preterm rupture of the membranes and intrauterine infection. 19.6 Postmaturity. 19.7 The hopelessly malformed fetus. 19.8 Breech presentation. 19.9 More malpresentations. 19.10 Prolapse and presentation of the cord. 19.11 Multiple pregnancies. 19.11a Primary postpartum haemorrhage. 19.11b Secondary postpartum haemorrhage. 19.12 Resuscitating the neonate. 19.13 Intrauterine growth retardation (IUGR).

Chapter 20 Gynaecology   315

20.1 Some of the simpler operations. 20.2 Abnormal and 'dysfunctional' uterine bleeding (DUB). 20.3 Dilatation and curettage, 'D and C'. 20.4 Bartholin's cyst and abscess. 20.5 Prolapse of the urethra. 20.6 Fibroids. 20.7 Ovarian cysts. 20.9 Prolapse. 20.10 Ventrisuspension. 20.11 Le Fort's operation. 20.11a Anterior and posterior colporrhaphy. 20.12 Hysterectomy. 20.13 The sequelae of female circumcision. 20.14 Other gynaecological problems.

21 The breast and the thyroid   338

21.1 Introduction. *THE BREAST* 21.2 Pus in the breast. 21.3 Lumps in the breast. 21.4 Carcinoma of the breast. 21.5 Simpler operations for tumours of the breast. 21.6 Patey's operation. *THE THYROID* 21.7 The general method for the thyroid. 21.8 Hyperthyroidism. 21.9 Thyroglossal cysts. 21.10 Physiological goitres. 21.11 Colloid goitres. 21.12 Tumours of the thyroid. 21.13 Other problems with the thyroid.

Chapter 22 Proctology   351

22.1 The general method for the anus and rectum. 22.2 Anorectal sinuses and fistulae. 22.3 Rectal bleeding. 22.4 Piles. 22.5 Lord's anal stretch. 22.6 Tying and excising piles. 22.7 Anal fissure. 22.8 Pilonidal infections. 22.9 Rectal prolapse. 22.10 Other anorectal problems.

Chapter 23 Urology   366

23.1 Equipment for urology. 23.2 Catheters and how to pass

them. 23.3 Cystoscopy. 23.4 Haematuria. 23.5 Retention of urine. 23.6 Emergency suprapubic cystostomy. 23.7 Open suprabupic cystostomy. 23.8 Postgonococcal urethral strictures. 23.9 Difficulties with strictures. 23.10 Extravasation of urine complicating a stricture. 23.11 Impassable strictures. 23.12 Stones in the urinary tract. 23.13 Nephrostomy for calculous anuria. 23.14 Ureteric stones. 23.15 Bladder stones in adults. 23.16 Bladder stones in children. 23.17 Urethral stones in children. 23.18 Prostatic obstruction. 23.19 Freyer's transvesical prostatectomy. 23.20 Other causes of urinary obstruction—dyskinesia and bladder-neck fibrosis. 23.21 Ghadvi's lateral perineal prostatectomy. 23.22 The injection method for benign prostatic hypertrophy. 23.22a Epididymo–orchitis and associated conditions. 23.23 Hydroceles in adults. 23.24 Torsion of the testis. 23.25 Orchidectomy. 23.25a Undescended testis. 23.26 Circumcision. 23.27 Paraphimosis. 23.28 Meatal strictures. 23.29 Priapism. 23.30 Other urological problems.

Chapter 24 The Eye 406

24.1 The general method for the eye. 24.2 Operating on an eye. 24.3 The red painful eye. 24.4 Loss of vision in a white eye. 24.5 Uveitis (iritis, iridocyclitis, and choroiditis). 24.6 Glaucoma. 24.7 Onchocerciasis. 24.8 Refractive errors, presbyopia. 24.9 Disease of the neuromuscular system of the eye, squints, and amblyopia. 24.10 Diseases of the lids and nasolachrymal apparatus. 24.11 Proptosis. 24.12 Tarsal cysts. 24.13 Entropion. 24.14 Destructive methods for the eye. 24.15 Other eye problems.

Chapter 25 The ear, nose, and throat 425

25.1 Introduction. 25.2 Deafness. 25.3 Otitis media and externa. 25.4 Acute mastoiditis. 25.5 Foreign bodies in the ear. 25.6 Epistaxis. 25.7 Blocked nose and the general method for sinusitis. 25.8 Frontal sinusitis. 25.9 Maxillary sinusitis. 25.10 Nasal polypi. 25.11 Foreign bodies in the nose. 25.11a Laryngoscopy. 25.12 Bronchoscopy; inhaled foreign bodies. 25.13 Foreign bodies in the 'throat'. 25.14 Oesophagoscopy. 25.15 Corrosive oesophagitis and oesophageal strictures. 25.16 Other problems in the ear, nose, and throat.

Chapter 26 The teeth and the mouth 444

26.1 Introduction. 26.2 Gum disease. 26.3 Extracting teeth. 26.4 Impacted third molars. 26.6 Cancrum oris. 26.7 Jaw swellings. 26.8 Cleft lip and palate. 26.9 Other dental and oral problems.

Chapter 27 Orthopaedics 454

27.1 The scope of primary orthopaedics. 27.2 The general method for contractures. 27.3 Preventing acute and subacute contractures in poliomyelitis. 27.4 Managing chronic polio contractures. 27.5 Appliances for polio. 27.6 Contractures of the hip and knee. 27.7 Equinus deformity of the ankle. 27.8 Back pain and lumbar disc lesions. 27.9 Epicondylitis (tennis elbow). 27.10 Stenosing tenosynovitis. 27.11 Ganglions. 27.11a Carpal tunnel syndrome. 27.12 Congenital dislocation of the hip (CDH). 27.13 The child with a painful hip or a limp. 27.14 Perthes' disease. 27.15 Neonatal talipes equinovarus. 27.16 Ingrowing toenail. 27.17 Other orthopaedic problems.

Chapter 28 Paediatric surgery 475

28.1 Surgery in children. 28.2 Intestinal obstruction in the first few days of life. 28.3 Operating on a neonatal acute abdomen. 28.4 Hypertrophic pyloric stenosis. 28.5 Disorders of the omphalomesenteric duct. 28.6 Anorectal malformations. 28.6a Hirschsprung's disease. 28.7 Congenital abnormalities of the female genital tract. 28.8 Omphalocele (exomphalos). 28.8a The surgery of neonatal jaundice. 28.9 Spina bifida. 28.10 Congenital vascular lesions. 28.11 Other paediatric problems.

Chapter 28a Surgery, AIDS, and hepatitis B 488

28a.1 Introduction. 28a.2 AIDS. 28a.3 AIDS and surgery. 28a.4 Hepatitis B.

Chapter 29 The surgery of tuberculosis 496

29.1 Chemotherapy for tuberculosis. 29.2 Tuberculous lymphadenitis. 29.3 Tuberculous bones and joints. 29.4 Tuberculosis of the spine (and idiopathic kyphoscoliosis). 29.4a Tuberculous paraplegia, costotransversectomy. 29.5 Abdominal tuberculosis. 29.6 The ascitic type of abdominal tuberculosis. 29.7 The plastic type of abdominal tuberculosis. 29.8 The glandular type of abdominal tuberculosis. 29.9 Urogenital tuberculosis.

Chapter 30 The surgery of leprosy 508

30.1 Introduction. 30.1a Managing paralysis, especially during lepra reactions. 30.2 Leprosy of the eye. 30.3 Lagophthalmos. 30.4 Leprosy of the hands. 30.5 The care of anaesthetic feet. 30.6 When the feet have ulcerated. 30.7 Operations on the feet in leprosy. 30.8 Tibialis transfer. 30.9 Other leprosy problems.

Chapter 31 The surgery of 'tropical' diseases 527

31.1 The surgery of neglected infection. 31.2 Tropical ulcers. 31.2a *Mycobacterium ulcerans* infection (Buruli ulcer). 31.3 Mycetoma. 31.4 Gross enlargements of parts of the body (elephantiasis). 31.5 'Podoconiosis' (non-filarial endemic elephantiasis). 31.6 The surgery of filariasis. 31.7 Elephantiasis of the scrotum. 31.8 The surgical complications of typhoid fever. 31.9 Pigbel disease. 31.10 The surgery of intestinal amoebiasis. 31.11 Invasive intestinal amoebiasis. 31.12 Extraintestinal amoebiasis. 31.13 Hydatid disease. 31.14 Other problems in tropical surgery.

Chapter 32 Oncology 546

32.1 Treating cancer in a district hospital. 32.2 Primary cancer chemotherapy. *LYMPHOMAS, BLASTOMAS, AND SARCOMAS* 32.3 Endemic Burkitt's lymphoma. 32.4 Hodgkin's lymphoma. 32.5 Non–Hodgkin's lymphoma. 32.6 Nephroblastoma. 32.7 Retinoblastoma. 32.8 Soft tissue sarcomas. 32.9 Rhabdomyosarcoma. 32.10 Fibrosarcoma. 32.11 Liposarcoma. *TUMOURS OF BONE* 32.12 Malignant tumours of bone. 32.13 Osteosarcoma. 32.14 Chondrosarcoma. 32.15 Giant cell tumours. 32.16 Ewing's tumour. 32.17 Myelomatosis (multiple myeloma). *TUMOURS OF THE SKIN AND SUBCUTANEOUS TISSUE* 32.18 Basal cell carcinoma. 32.19 Squamous cell carcinoma. 32.20 Malignant melanoma. 32.21 Kaposi's sarcoma. *TUMOURS OF THE GUT* 32.22 Carcinoma of the mouth and lips. 32.23 Salivary gland tumours. 32.24 Carcinoma of the oesophagus. 32.25 Carcinoma of the stomach. 32.26 Hepatoma. 32.26a Carcinoma of the pancreas. 32.27 Carcinoma of the colon and rectum. *TUMOURS OF THE RESPIRATORY TRACT* 32.28 Carcinoma of the nasopharnx. 32.29 Carcinoma of the bronchus. *TUMOURS OF THE BLADDER AND THE MALE UROGENITAL TRACT* 32.30 Tumours of the kidney. 32.31 Carcinoma of the bladder. 32.32 Carcinoma of the prostate. 32.33 Carcinoma of the penis. 32.34 Block dissection of the inguinal lymph nodes. 32.34a Tumours of the testis. *TUMOURS OF THE FEMALE GENITAL TRACT AND TROPHOBLAST (other than the breast).* 32.35 Carcinoma of the cervix. 32.35a Carcinoma of the vulva. 32.36 Tumours of the ovary. 32.37 Tumours of the trophoblast. 32.38 Hydatidiform mole and chorion carcinoma. 32.39 Other tumours.

Chapter 33 Terminal care   586

33.1 A task for every district hospital. 33.2 Controlling cancer pain.

Chapter 34 Miscellaneous   590

VASCULAR SURGERY 34.1 Varicose veins. *THE SURGERY OF THE SKIN* 34.1a Hypertrophic scars and keloids. 34.2 Granuloma pyogenicum. 34.3 Sebaceous and dermoid cysts. *SNAKE BITES* 34.4 Snake bites. *RADIOLOGY* 34.5 Some X-ray methods. *EVALUATION* 34.6 Indicators of quality in district hospital surgery. 34.7 Indicators of quality in district hospital obstetrics.

Chapter 35 Appendices   602

Appendix A, equipment. Appendix B, addresses of suppliers.

Stop Press   608

Mass ligation of the uterine arteries. Joel Cohen's method of opening the abdomen for Caesarean section. Measuring the tissue pressure to diagnose the compartment syndrome. Other fragments.

Index   611

Six Prefaces

Any doctor who has worked in a developing country will not easily forget the widespread and pathetic evidence of surgical neglect in the villages. Huge hernias and hydroceles, unsightly lumps on the faces of women and children, and the compound fractures infested with maggots bear testimony to the failure of so many countries to provide even a basic level of surgical care for their people.

Samiran Nundy, All India Institute of Medical Sciences.

No person is so perfect in knowledge and experience that error in opinion or action is impossible. In the art of surgery, error is more likely to occur than in almost any other line of human endeavour; and it is in this field that it should be most carefully guarded against, since incorrect judgement, improper technique, and a lack of knowledge of surgical safeguards may result in a serious handicap for the rest of the life of the patient, or may even result in the sacrifice of that life. For the surgeon, perfection in diagnostic skill is of equal, if not more, importance than operative skill.

Max Thorek, Surgical Errors and Safeguards in Surgery.

Patients should be treated as close to their homes as possible in the smallest, cheapest, most humbly staffed, and most simply equipped unit that is capable of looking after them adequately.

Medical Care in Developing Countries, Makerere, 1966.

First Preface by Kenya's Minister for Health

The Kenyan government has decided to make district the focus for all development activities. This is based on the conviction that people should have an input in their development at local level and they should also decide on their developmental priorities locally.

Traditionally, the district hospital has been referral institution for health centres and dispensaries. The challenges that health workers face at district level are many, and varied and often are of the same magnitude as those at provincial and national level. Different district hospitals face acute surgical emergencies that cannot be safely transferred elsewhere for management. It is intended to develop the necessary expertise at district level to enable the district health work to cope with such problems. Safe anaesthesia during surgery is a prerequisite that is often not available. This is one reason among others that makes this handbook valuable to the medical profession. The handbook, I believe, will go a long way towards assisting them in the problems mentioned above. The style and contents of the handbook make it a valuable companion for reference and a source of practical procedures.

Hon. PCJO Nyakiamo, EBS, MP
Minister for Health

Second Preface by Kenya's Director of Medical Services

Going through this manual, which I recommend to all health workers, one is impressed by the meticulous practical details that are so clearly presented. This is the result of a happy collaboration contributed through many workers in Kenya and elsewhere. The setting of the handbook is based on past experience of many health workers. It was written in an environment of one institution in Kenya which provided the necessary local interaction between the authors, clinicians, and other practitioners. The district hospital will in the very near future cope with the problems that would have otherwise been for the provincial hospitals. The handbook is a good contribution towards this end.

Wilfred Koinange, MBS
Director of Medical Services

Third Preface by the Ambassador in Kenya of the Federal Republic of Germany

Good health is the basis of a joyful and fulfilled life, individually as well as socially. It is one of the most important basic requirements of people and therefore represents a most prominent responsibility on the part of governments all over the world.

The Government of the Federal Republic of Germany considers that finding ways and means towards improving the health of people in the developing countries is one of its major tasks. An integral component of German Development Policy is especially geared towards improving primary health care all over the developing world.

May these four manuals, which are the product of a worldwide team and were jointly sponsored by the Ministry of Health of the Government of Kenya, and the GTZ, the Agency for Technical Co-operation of the Federal Republic of Germany, be a practical and successful guide to the medical profession and help to contribute their share towards a healthier world.

Johannes von Vacano
German Ambassador

Fourth Preface by the Head of the Department for Health, Nutrition, and Population Activities, Deutsche Gesellschaft für Technische Zusammenarbeit (GTZ) GmbH

By the year 2000, 80 per cent of the more than six billion people on our planet will be living in the developing world. Primary Health Care will thus increasingly be the health care for most of mankind. It is however much more than the treatment of the simplest diseases by village health workers, because they need somewhere to refer the patients they cannot treat, who include some with severe injuries or in obstructed labour. The district hospital and particularly its surgical services are therefore essential—hence the importance that we attach to these manuals.

A particular feature of Primary Health Care is its emphasis on 'appropriate technology'. The simplest and most cost-effective technologies, such as oral rehydration, immunization and the use of the weight chart, are now being exploited to their limit. Unfortunately, there are not many technologies which are as useful as these, so what do we do next?

The thinking behind these manuals is that we need to look carefully at *all* the technologies that are practical in particular technical fields, in this case surgery, anaesthesia, and obstetrics in the district hospital, and to promote them intensively. Because there are thousands of of such technologies, far too many to promote individually, they have to be promoted as a systematic, synergistic, practical whole. Tracheal intubation (A 13.2), Perkins traction (74.8), the handbag method for burnt hands (58.29), and symphysiotomy (M 20.7, 18.4) are just a few of the many such technologies which are not applied when they should be, because their details are not known where they ought to be.

There will never be complete agreement on the methods described here. Nevertheless, the reception that has already been given to the manuals that have appeared shows both what a wide degree of consensus can be reached and how valuable this is. Few readers can imagine how difficult it has been to achieve. We should therefore like to thank the editor and his family. To serve the sick he has gone far beyond his original task, and certainly beyond his contract with us. When the project began we knew the task was vast, but we did not know how vast. We expected one book; this is the third of four, which we hope will help you to serve the sick better.

Priv. Doz. Dr. med. Rolf Korte
Head of Department of Health,
Nutrition and Population Activities, GTZ.

Fifth preface by Hugh Dudley, lately Professor of Surgery in St Mary's Hospital, London

These manuals are not a product of the surgical establishment in Africa, India, or Europe, or anywhere else. They are the work of a tiny far-flung band of experienced and highly competent enthusiasts, who work or have worked in the mission hospitals and universities of the developing world. Besides many from Kenya they range from Katete in Zambia (James Cairns) to Kathmandu in Nepal (Gerald Hankins), from Kumasi in Ghana (Josiah Hiadzi) to Kampala in Uganda (the 1983 conference of the Association of Surgeons of East Africa), from Delhi in India (Samiran Nundy) to Durban in South Africa (Hugh Philpott), from Sydney in Australia (Ronald Huckstep) to Seattle in the USA (John Stewart), from Birmingham in England (Peter Bewes) to Beijing in China (Cai Ru Bin), from Hobart in Tasmania (Joe Shepherd) to Laurence Levy in Zimbabwe. All these have given and have not witheld their knowledge.

The contributions of these and many other experts, and they are experts in their own very special approach to surgery, have been woven together into a unified system by an indefatigable editor. Suprisingly, he is a community physician, not a surgeon. As an exercise in 'community surgery', and 'health systems research', he has put himself into your shoes, and during ten years and more than 30,000 hours has asked himself "What should he be able to do, if he had to do what you must do?" These two surgical manuals, together with *Primary Anaesthesia* and *Primary Mother Care,* are his answer. He has tried to describe everything, in complete relevant detail, that he, or you, might reasonably be able to do.

Many people have wondered why such a task should be attempted by a non–surgeon. There are however several good reasons why it should: (1) No practising surgeon has the necessary time to put a million and a half words through at least 25 drafts. He cannot have his scalpel in one hand and his word processor in the other. So it is not surprising that, during the previous 20 years, seven surgeons have started and abandoned this task, most after only a list of contents, one after several years. Paradoxically, it seems that the commitment, skill, and time to weave the knowledge into a system is at as much of a premium as the knowledge itself. (2) As you will have seen from the Frontispiece, surgery is now so specialized that these manuals have had to cover 20 surgical specialities. The alternative, which is to ask each expert to write a chapter, has been tried once and abandoned. (3) The outsider is much closer to the readers for whom the book is intended than the expert, and is thus much more interested in the critical elementary details. (4) As the postscript explains, the interrogation of the expert by the outsider is the standard way of constructing electronic 'expert systems'; this is a close paper equivalent to them.

Most usefully, at a time when surgery seems to be splitting into ever more arcane fragments, this is an attempt to synthesize, to unify our discipline, and to cross specialist boundaries in a way which badly needs doing, and yet to do so practically and in detail. It is far more than a synthesis of existing materials, useful though this is. In many places you will find detailed observations and instructions that are available nowhere else.

To what extent have the contributors and their editor succeeded? This you will have to find out for yourself. I can only say that from the reception given to the experimental editions of these manuals, and to the second volume which has already appeared, you are going to find their completeness, their detail, and their relevance invaluable. You must however use them in the full acceptance of the way in which they were written.

Finally, I hope that this is only the beginning of a great endeavour. How well do these methods work in practice? Can they be improved? What difficulties do you meet in using them? All these questions can only be answered by much fieldwork. That has now to begin.

Hugh Dudley,
Lately Professor of Surgery
St Mary's Hospital, London

Sixth Preface by Maurice King, Reader in Community Medicine, the University of Leeds

After the more useful drugs and vaccines, particularly the antimicrobials, there are no more cost-effective, or death- and disability-preventing methods than the simpler forms of surgery.

Almost none of this essential surgery can be done by community health workers, and little in health centres. This leaves three possibilities for most of the surgery that patients in the developing world need: (1) the district hospitals, (2) the provincial hospitals, and (3) the teaching hospital in the capital city. There is much debate as to how much surgery should be done at level (1) by the general duty medical officers (GDMOs) in the districts, and how much should be sent on to the referral hospitals at levels (2) and (3). On this debate depends the scope and nature of 'primary' or district surgery.

There are two approaches to this problem:

(A) To consider district hospital surgery as a narrow range of procedures only, to assume that patients who need more than these can readily be referred, and to emphasize what should not be done in the districts, rather than what can be and has to be done there.

(B) To accept the fact that the 'referral system' that is supposed to exist in determining what, in an ideal world, should be done by whom and where, is, alas, in large part an abstraction convenient to health planners, a myth to save the consciences of doctors, and a figment in the minds of some of the leaders of the profession, who imagine that it is practicable for each particular condition to be treated only by that particular 'board-certified specialist', into whose narrow field it happens to fall. As we point out in Section 1.7, the prospects for referral from the district to the centre, which were never very good, seem to be getting worse rather than better in many developing countries, particularly those in sub–Saharan Africa.

These manuals take the second view. They assume that, if the villagers of the developing world are ever to be cared for surgically, the vast majority of the care they need must be done in its district hospitals. If this is accepted, 'Primary Surgery' is a large group of procedures. It includes all those which might

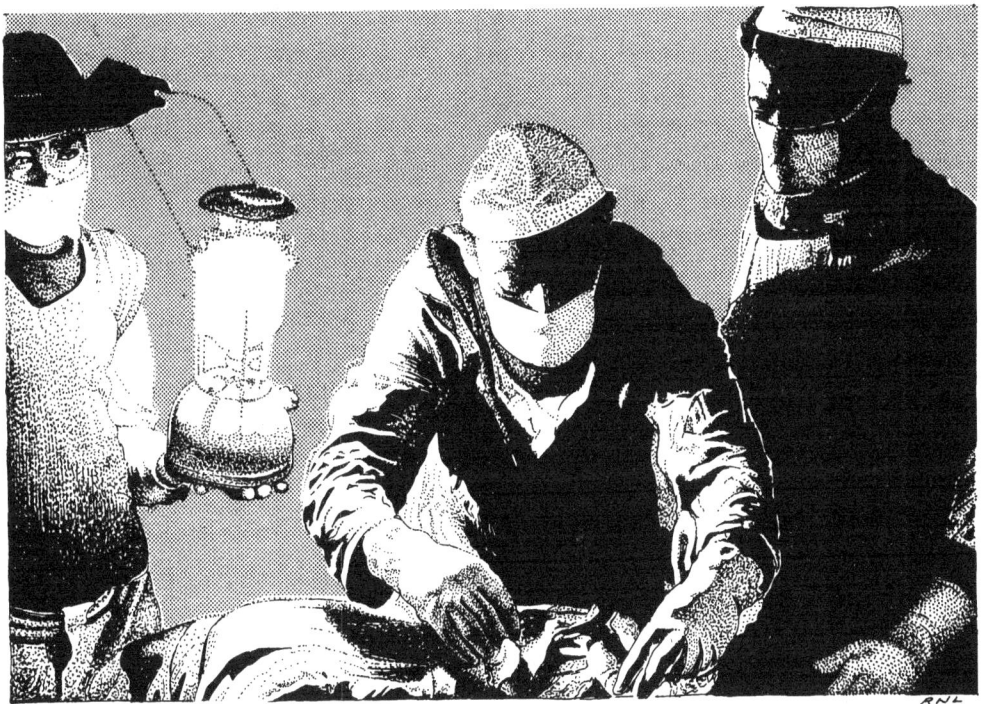

ONE OF OUR READERS. You may have had very little surgical experience and yet have to operate on severely ill patients. In an emergency you may even have to operate by the light of a hurricane lantern. The light will attract insects, and these will fall into the wound, but even so they are unlikely to influence the patient's recovery. *From an illustration kindly contributed by WHO.*

benefit a patient who staggers, or is carried, into such a hospital, who cannot be referred onwards, and who has to be cared for by a general-duty doctor. Such then is the thinking behind them. Their aim is to empower the generalist surgically, to increase the quality, range, and quantity of the surgical, anaesthetic, and obstetric care available to the villager, and to bring these disciplines within the scope of the 'Primary Health Care' movement. The knowledge gathered here is is not oriented towards the systematic training of a certified surgeon, but towards the doctor who has to cope with whatever sick are fortunate enough to reach him.

Very early on, we had to decide whether to write an 'add-on book', that would include only information which is not available somewhere, or to attempt a complete system of methods, regardless of whether or not the information it contains can, with difficulty and expense, be found elsewhere. Boldly, we decided to attempt the latter and assemble a 'total system', because we are sure that this is what you need. For example, most of what is said about hand sepsis is already available, but what is said about osteomyelitis is not. Orthopaedics, particularly fractures, causes great problems, so we have given it particular attention. To make the task manageable we have have confined ourselves to a detailed description of what you need to do, preceded by a general introduction. Inevitably, there is little room for epidemiology, prevention, anatomy, or physiology. If you look closely you will find that almost everything we describe is slightly different in some way or other, from what it is in the industrial world.

We write for: (1) General-duty doctors with only a year or two of surgical experience, responsible for all the patients clamouring for care in a district hospital. We tell you what to do, and what you could do, if there is no real hope of referring a patient to anyone else. We hope that it will be a useful supplement to the 'see one, do one, teach one' method by which many of you have inevitably had to learn most of your surgery, and which is much less well adapted to the uncommon problems, than it is to the common ones. (2) Medical students anywhere in the world, training to be broadly competent doctors. If you want to be real generalists, here is part of your calling. (3) The 23 000 unemployed doctors in India, and indeed those in the world as a whole, who remain wasted and unfulfilled in the face of the pressing surgical needs of the villagers. Perhaps you feel you would like to help them, but realize that your training has not equipped you to know what you could reasonably do. Here it is. (4) 'General surgeons' at the limit of your technical range, particularly those of you who work in the developing world. (5) Specialists in any of the twenty or more surgical specialties who have to do things in a field which is unfamiliar to you—for orthopaedic surgeons coping with ruptured uteri, and gynaecologists treating fractured femurs. Unfortunately, many general surgeons have never done a Caesarean section, and most obstetricians are uncomfortable with an acute abdomen. (6) Any non-specialist 'war surgeon' who has to cope with the casualties from a conventional war under conditions which are usually even more difficult than most of those described here. As this is written there are 12 such wars being fought on any one day, all but one (that in Northern Ireland) in the developing world. This is a wide readership. As you will see in Section 1.6, we have tried to allow for your varying skills. These pages will probably be at their most useful helping a well-grounded doctor to do something he has not done before.

We started with the intention of writing a book of 'basics' for the generalist. As we wrote our scope expanded to include most of the tasks of the general surgeon working in the districts, the 'M. Med. Chir.'s' of East Africa for example.

In the Declaration of Alma Ata, WHO and UNICEF included the care of the common injuries as an essential part of Primary Health Care. In the second of these two manuals we have followed up their concern by describing how all human injuries can be cared for at the 'first referral level', which for the purposes of surgery is the district hospital. About a third of the work of a district hospital is surgical, and of this about half is the surgery of trauma, so it is appropriate that traumatology should occupy so many of our pages.

Everything else that you can do in the other surgical specialties is described here. The methods that you will need to anaesthetize your patients have been described in *Primary Anaesthesia*. We have divided the obstetrics, gynaecology, and family planning into two parts. All the methods which are common to doctors and paramedicals are in *Primary Mother Care* (forthcoming 1990), the rest are here. Between them, this 'corpus' of four manuals comprises an integrated system of surgery, obstetrics, and anaesthesia, that we hope can properly be called 'Primary' in that it should be within the reach of all the world's citizens.

We are keen to support the 'general practice movement' which is, for example, making rapid headway in Nigeria. The true 'general practitioner', or GP, of the developing world is the omnicompetent 'General Duty Medical Officer', or GDMO, in his own way no less an expert than any of his specialist colleagues remote in the centres of tertiary care. It is sometimes thought that the days of the 'VGP'—the 'Very General Practitioner'— are over; but in countries where populations are expanding faster than services, this is far from true. These manuals attempt to define your surgical scope as a 'GDMO' or 'VGP', and to enrich your role, which is surely the broadest and most rewarding one in the whole of medicine.

As a general rule, more harm is done by doctors not operating when they should, than operating when they should not. So, if you have some surgical experience, another of our aims has been to encourage you to operate while carefully following the guidelines in Section 1.8. Paradoxically, theatre time, which is often such a critical constraint in provincial or teaching hospitals, is often abundant in the districts. Paradoxically also, because staff morale is often better there, care may be better too. For a patient with a straightforward condition, a good district hospital may therfore be a better place to be sick in than a central one.

Our final aim is to define a pattern of good practice under the difficult circumstances for which we write, and to improve the quality of this 'peripheral care'—peripheral it may be when looked at from the centre, but from the patient's point of view, the periphery is indeed the centre!

These manuals would never have been written had not GTZ seen fit to support them. Our particular gratitude is due to Dr Klaus Gördel of the BMZ for so graciously and so willingly providing the funds whenever they were required, to Dr Hans Joerg Elshorst, Dr Peter Muller, and to Dr Klaus Jochen Lampe. I should personally like to thank Dr Rolf Korte, a wonderful chief, for having administered the project for ten years with unfailing efficiency, kindness, sympathy, and generosity, together with a remarkable understanding of its technical scope and of the difficulties that had to be overcome in accomplishing it.

Together with two illustrators, Derek Atherton and Ivanson Kaiyai, and two secretaries, Sifolosa Ndabi and Attanasia Mugo, I spent five years in a classroom in the training school at the Provincial General Hospital in Nyeri in Kenya, and the spare moments while doing another job during more than another five in the Department of Community Medicine in Leeds. The project owes everything to Peter Bewes, who gave up a large part of four summer holidays to the task, and without whose initial help I should, very properly, never have started. Many of the trauma methods are his; so in a very real sense are all these manuals. During his holidays over several years James Cairns of St Francis' Hospital at Katete in Zambia contributed greatly to almost every section, and reviewed the final manuscript of this volume before it went to press. Jim Thornton contributed extensively to the obstetrics and gynaecology and reviewed it all. Gerry Hankins of the Shanta Bahwan Hospital in Kathmandu sent us 36 tapes and was indefatigable in his encouragement. John Stewart, formerly of the KCMC hospital in Moshi, Tanzania, contributed much of the orthopaedics and reviewed it all. Samiran Nundy visited us for a final critical week in Kenya and did much to adapt it to the villages of India. The advice, contributions, and support of Professor Anne Bayley of the University of Zambia meant more than she can easily imagine. Brian Hancock did a wonderful job on the proctology; Neville Harrison did the same for the urology. June Brady reviewed the section on neonatal resuscitation. Many kind colleagues here in Leeds reviewed parts of it. Other valuable contributors include Ruediger Finger, John Githiari, John Gower, Martin Hobdel, Naim Janmohammed, John Jellis, Imre Loefler, John Maina, Andrew Pearson, Hugh Roberts, Sam Smith, Mamdur Tahir, Patrick Trevor–Roper, and Adil Keskin. The late Sir Michael Wood was kind enough to hand over his own uncompleted manuscript. There is a real sense in which *all* their contributions were essential.

Richard Jolly, Deputy Executive Director of that paragon among international organizations, UNICEF, was unflinching in his support of these manuals (to him they will always be known as "Cut along the Dotted Line"!). Denis Burkitt called on the project in its first faltering days and was courageous enough to say "So I have seen the place where it *was* written". Gerald Richards, Professor of Community Medicine in the University of Leeds, kindly allowed me to spend a large part of five years completing this task, which is hardly 'community medicine' as this is ordinarily conceived. During this time much of my university work was carried on by my colleagues, Mark Baker, Jenny Green, Rangit Bandaranayake, Martin Schweiger, Elizabeth Kernohan, and Chris Newman, without whose support and forbearance it would never have been completed. Anne Mainwaring's kindness and hard work freed many precious hours for this task.

I gathered a huge pile of books, and have drawn extensively on Hamilton Bailey's 'Emergency Surgery', Farquharson's 'Textbook of Operative Surgery', de Palma's 'Fractures and Dislocations' and Perkins' 'Fractures', to name but a few. My thanks are to the authors and publishers of these and many other books, who have kindly allowed us to redraw some of their most useful illustrations. We are particularly grateful to Mrs Joyce Williams of the W.B. Saunders Company, who let us use many of the illustrations from their medical list, and to Jack Lange. Where I have lost the source of some illustrations, or have overlooked their authors or publishers, I hope that, for the good of the sick of the developing world, I shall be forgiven.

The task of assembling such a quantity of diverse material was made possible by recent developments in information technology. Two years from the end of the project, in the very nick of time, it became possible to service word processors in Kenya. Latterly, we had three Osborne One microcomputers, which also enabled us to code the text for immediate photosetting—'Wordstar' saved the project; so did Nicholas Ouma, who kept our machines running in Kenya, and John Laker, who did the same in England.

'Primary Anaesthesia' and 'Trauma' went through a limited experimental edition before being formally published. Circumstances have prevented 'Non-trauma' doing the same: it is therefore a 'generation' behind them.

Finally, my thanks are due to my wife and two small sons, who, for nine consecutive years, went on holiday and left 'Dad' at these books.

It is my great regret that it is my role to serve the sick with a keyboard rather than with a scalpel. Paradoxically, had I tried to combine practice with writing, I should never have completed the task. I am thus but the scribe and servant of many skilled surgeons. It is they, not me, that speak to you through these pages. Nevertheless, in the theatre and the wards, I share the pain, the anxiety, and the wretchedness of so many of your patients, and your joy in caring for them.

Postscript: On being a 'knowledge engineer'

(1) *"He only listens to what other people have to say and writes it down".* (2) *"He has that peculiar knack of making himself an expert in anything".*
Diverse opinions from the London School of Hygiene and Tropical Medicine.

He only is wise who knows that he knows nothing.

Socrates.

As this book was going through the Press, I was told "You are not an 'editor', nobody sends you completed chapters. You are that scarce and precious species, a knowledge engineer". Although I was aware of expert systems, I had not previously heard this term applied to their creators. Knowledge engineers are people who question experts and express the expertise they obtain in a computer program that can be used by non-experts. These computer-based expert systems do complex inferential reasoning based on a wide knowledge of a limited field, and are finding increasing use in such fields as 'fault-finding on 11GHz radiowave equipment', interpreting mass spectrographs for chemists ('DENDRAL'), and prescribing antibiotics ('MYCIN'). Their role in medicine is limited but is growing.

Although *Primary Surgery* appears on paper rather than on a screen, is less logically sophisticated, and covers a much larger field than do computer-based expert systems, the similarities between them are striking. Like other knowledge engineers, I have had great problems in getting knowledge out of experts. Real ones are hard to find, and when you have found them, they may only be master of a small field, and be so busy that they can spare you little time. If an expert is going to contribute efficiently, he has got to know his field (many do not), he has to to be able to exteriorize his knowledge (many find this difficult), and he must be willing to collaborate (many are not).

An expert often forgets what he does, and may not know what he does. There is indeed no logical reason why anyone should be aware of how a thing is done in order to be able to do it. Even when an expert can describe what he does, he can be wrong. He is more likely to be able to remember actions given conditions, than conditions given actions—expert surgeons know when to operate, but have difficulty listing the indications for doing so. They need cues which a knowledge engineer has to supply. An expert is often better at criticizing someone else's ideas than explaining his own, and may only express his knowledge in response to something he disagrees with. Knowledge engineers have to learn the expert's language: in doing so I became a particular kind of 'theoretical' surgeon, anaesthetist, and obstetrician.

Expert systems require constant refinement and debugging: I worked mostly by asking experts to comment on innumerable drafts assembled from tiny fragments of knowledge. As one expert said when I began, "You will have to build it up comma by comma".

Looking back, it is remarkable that the task was accomplished at all. Only by combing the earth was it possible to find just enough appropriate experts. The task would have been easier had it been possible to start with this postscript, instead of ending with it. Paradoxically, any merit in these manuals lies with the experts ('How could a non-surgeon know this...?'), and any faults with the knowlede engineer—it is his job to spot the fault and patch it with another expert's knowledge. The sixth sense that he needs to develop is to know what knowledge is useful, and when it is likely to be faulty.

From an expert's point of view, working with a 'knowledge engineer' is an efficient way of producing a book. If an expert looks at a draft and passes it with only minor changes, he might have written it. Yet he will have done so in only a fraction of the time that it would have taken to write in the ordinary way.

So, if you are an expert and read this, look kindly on any 'knowledge engineer' who approaches you; understand his difficulties, and do your best for him, since this may be the way in which the more useful knowledge sources of the future will be 'engineered'. As we go to press the EEC is sponsoring the development of a medical computer work-station that will support a variety of expert systems. Perhaps a future edition of *Primary Surgery* will appear on a screen? Meanwhile, there is need for a 'knowledge engineer' to work on *Primary Medicine*. Who would like to give a substantial part of his life to this task?

Here are two books covering the same field, written at the same time in the ordinary manner. How do the two approaches compare? The third, on which this section is based, describes the travails of us knowledge engineers.

Anaesthesia at the District Hospital. Published by WHO. Available in English and French. Price Sw fr 20; US$ 16.00. Order No 1150289. WHO Distribution and Sales, 1211 Geneva, Switzerland, and all WHO sales agents.

General Surgery at the District Hospital. Order No 1150300. Price Sw fr 30; US$ 24.00. Available in English and French. Published by WHO as above.

Welbank, M. 'A Review of Knowledge Acquisition Techniques for Expert Systems. 1983. British Telecom Research Laboratories. Martlesham Heath, Ipswich, England.

Maurice King. MD, FRCP, FFPHM
Reader in
Public Health Medicine.
University of Leeds.

1 The background to surgery

You have just arrived at your hospital and have not yet unpacked, when the ambulance arrives with a note from sister to say that there is a patient with a strangulated hernia waiting for you. You have never done one, because the registrar when you did your internship wanted to do as much operating as he could himself. So you mostly assisted and were occasionally allowed to sew up the skin. All your seniors have left and have gone into private practice, so there is nobody to help you. If you refer this patient, he will die on the way.

These manuals are dedicated to you. This personal reminiscence was contributed by Dr Michael Migue of AMREF, as describing the scene for which these manuals are needed.

1.1 The unmet need for surgical care

Surgically treatable diseases are not as important as the great killers of small children in the developing world—malnutrition, pneumonia, and diarrhoea. However, surveys from the rural areas of Bangladesh, from India and from urban South America indicate that 10% of all deaths, and almost 20% of deaths in young adults are the result of conditions that would be amenable to surgery in the industrial world. If even very simple surgical services were available two-thirds or more of these deaths would not have occurred. One study showed that for every person who died of an accident in the Punjab, there were eight who were permanently disabled.

A study in East Africa estimated that, per 100 000 of the population; 225 mothers needed a Caesarean section, yet only 25 got one, 175 inguinal hernias needed repair each year, but that only 25 were repaired; 30 patients needed operations for strangulation, yet only 4 had them. Since a strangulated hernia is almost always fatal unless it is treated, this is a mortality of nearly 90%.

These are just two examples, one from India, and one from Africa, of the surgery that needs doing and is not done. All this unmet need means that there are many unnecessary deaths in remote villages from strangulated hernias and obstetric disasters, as well as from vesicovaginal fistulae and from cerebral injuries at birth. They illustrate the fact that district hospitals can only care for a fraction of the burden of surgical disease in the communities around them. The result is that millions of people, whom surgery might help, it does not help. Too many people still die from obstructed gut, or are disabled by untreated osteomyelitis, or burns contractures—much as they were in the industrial world a hundred years ago.

Once services are available to prevent the killing diseases of childhood, the simple surgical services described here should surely have the next priority. They can do much to improve the quality of life of the poor. Although much of this manual has a rural orientation, 44% of the people of the developing world are expected to be living in towns by the year 2000, so the surgical care of the urban poor will be almost equally important.

Surgery has an importance in the public mind that medicine does not have. It is also the most technically demanding of the tasks of a district hospital doctor, and is thus a good measure of the quality of his medical education. If this has not been adequate, either because it never was adequate in his medical school, or because the quality of its teaching has fallen, he will be very loath to do much surgery, and may do none. This is why some district hospitals, and many district hospitals in some entire countries, do little surgery. When this happens, patients soon realize that it is no use going to such hospitals, with the result that they soon have empty beds. So if you see a hospital with empty beds, one of the first questions to ask yourself is "What is the quality of the surgery here?" There is thus a qualitative aspect to the unmet need for surgical care as well as a quantitative one.

The constraints on the provision of surgical care are formidable. Here is one very special centre of excellence expressing them: (Nevertheless, over the previous year it had been able to increase its average daily number of patients by 14%, and its major operations by 7%.)

CONSTRAINTS HEROICALLY OVERCOME "It is an anxious time. Costs are rising. The Ministry's manpower resources are scarce, making it well nigh impossible for them to take on the extra responsibility from the Church hospitals. The rural people are very anxious that the Churches continue their health work. It makes sense for both economic and humanitarian points of view. What of our Lord's call for compassion for the sick and identification with the poor? Where is the way forward?" 1981 Annual Report St Francis' Hospital, Katete Zambia.

Burk JF, Gill SG, King TC, McCord C, Rosenfield A, 'Report of a Panel on Emergency Surgery', IOM Committee on International Health 1977 National Academy of Sciences

Nordberg EM, 'The incidence and estimated need for Caesarean section, inguinal hernia repair, and operation for strangulated hernia in rural Africa', British Medical Journal 1984;299:92–3

1.2 The surgical scene

The countries of the third world and the surgical scene within them differ widely. Ethiopia and Brazil, for example, are about as different as two countries could be. Typically, the people of the developing world are poor, hungry, and rural, although they are rapidly migrating to the towns. The population of sub-Saharan Africa, whence these manuals come, is increasing at an inexorable 3% annually. Meanwhile its per capita food production and its already meagre gross national product are falling.

One feature developing countries do have in common. It is that most of the surgery that is done has to be done in their district hospitals. These typically have between 50 and 200 beds and are staffed by two to four doctors, assisted by nurses and auxiliaries. Fortunately, the 'one doctor hospital', which was common until recently, is now unusual. Each hospital serves about 150–250 000 people living in an area which may be as large as 3000 square miles.

Over the world as a whole these hospitals range from the excellent to the indescribable. At one end they provide care which anyone would be fortunate to have, at the other the few patients brave (or foolish) enough to enter them lie largely untended.

If you work in a hospital in the middle or at the lower end of this spectrum, expect to find your wards overcrowded, with more than one patient in a bed. 'Clean' and infected cases will not be separated, so that a patient with an open fracture may lie next to one with a perforated typhoid ulcer. Your maternity ward will be particularly overcrowded, and resist all your attempts to decongest it. Cultural reasons may make it impossible to restrict the number of visitors to the wards. Defects in their construction will make keeping them clean and tidy a major task. Your equipment will be limited and poorly serviced. When it does break down, it may take years to replace. Trees may be so scarce that your staff have to go a long way to collect firewood.

THE SURGICAL SCENE IN AFRICA

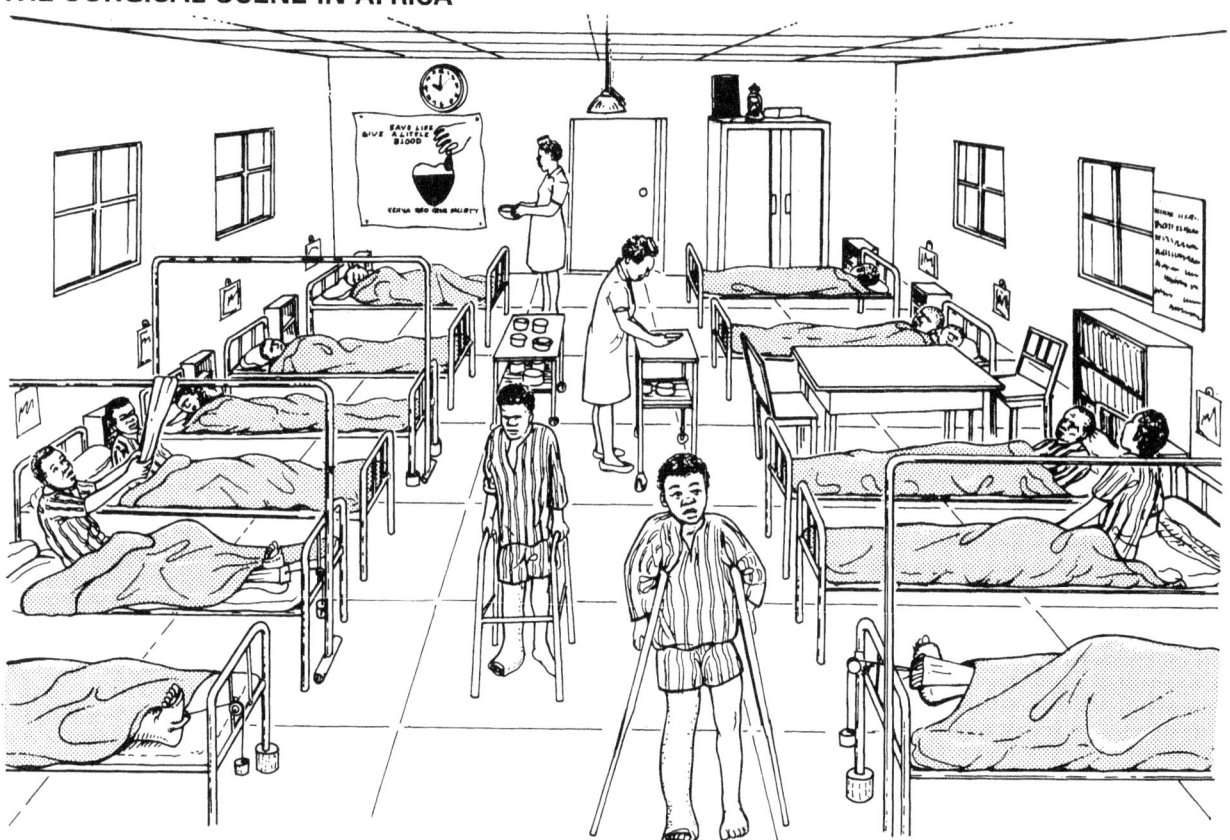

Fig. 1-1 THE SCENE IN AFRICA. Ward 7 in Nyeri Provincial General Hospital. This is somewhat better than the average conditions for sub-Saharan Africa at the time of writing. Note the blood transfusion poster. You will see that there are several patients on traction, two with long leg casts, and that one of the beds contains two patients.

If your hospital is at sea level on the equator, expect to operate at 30°C in 95% humidity, your clothes wet, and everything which can go rusty or mouldy doing so. Only insects enjoy such conditions, and you will find plenty of them.

You may have to rely on locally trained staff with only primary education who find the idea of sterility almost incomprehensible. Most of them will experience considerable hardship, and be so poorly paid that they will have to grow the food they need. Their ability to monitor a patient postoperatively on the wards may be so poor that you may be forced to assume that, once a patient has left the theatre, he is on his own as far as recovery is concerned (A 4.5).

Your anaesthetic facilities will vary greatly. If you are lucky you will have two or three anaesthetic assistants, trained to do most of the methods in *Primary Anaesthesia*. Your laboratory facilities will be minimal. Although AIDS has recently made it much more dangerous in many areas, blood transfusion should always be possible—if you can put enough effort into organizing it. Often, relatives will give blood for a patient, but for nobody else.

So be prepared to find everything—or nothing. On occasion expect to find no water, no steam, no gauze, no bandages, no catgut, no suxamethonium, no gloves (or only gloves with holes in them), no plaster, (or only plaster that does not set)... When you need the autoclave a Caesarean section, expect that there may be no kerosene, and that the patient's relatives may have to go out to the market to buy it. When you go into the maternity ward late one night, don't be surprised if the last sphygmomanometer is missing. Try not to blame your staff too harshly, they may not be responsible—and even if they are, their families may be starving. If you do have electricity, be prepared for it to fail at 3 a.m., just when you are in the middle of a Caesarean section.

Even when you have your 'normal' supplies, you will not have solutions for parenteral nutrition, or plasma, and probably no dextran. Don't be tempted to imagine that the teaching hospital has everything: it too may be without water, spirit, or linen. One teaching hospital is said to have had no temperature charts for 10 years.

You may be cherished, supported, praised, and congratulated by your Ministry of Health, or you may not... You may be in a health service which is steadily improving, or in one which seems to be getting steadily worse, if that were possible. Expect that you may be cut off from the rest of the world for four months of the year. On top of everything else, AIDS may now be endemic in your district... Finally, your greatest blow may be that your predecessor, who was promised that he would be posted to your hospital for only a short time, never ordered any stores, or planted any cabbages...

But you have great blessings. In coping with all this, in creating and caring and leading and serving, you will have done something that your colleagues in the more comfortable circumstances of private practice will never have done. You are an all-rounder, and have one of the last remaining opportunities to practise the totality of medicine, rather than some infinitesimal corner of it. *Sub specie aeternitatis,* in the mirror of eternity, you are a hero and will surely be recognized and remembered as such.

You will need: (1) A willingness to learn from the culture of your patients. This will enrich you greatly, whether you are a a national from the urban elite or a foreigner, and will greatly increase their trust in you. (2) An almost pathological desire for hard work under conditions that are not conducive to it. (3) An unfailing ability to improvise and make the best of things. (4) The capacity to withstand prolonged periods of cultural isolation. If your morale is high, so soon will be that of your staff also. Your patients will be grateful for anything you can do for

AN INDIAN HOSPITAL SCENE

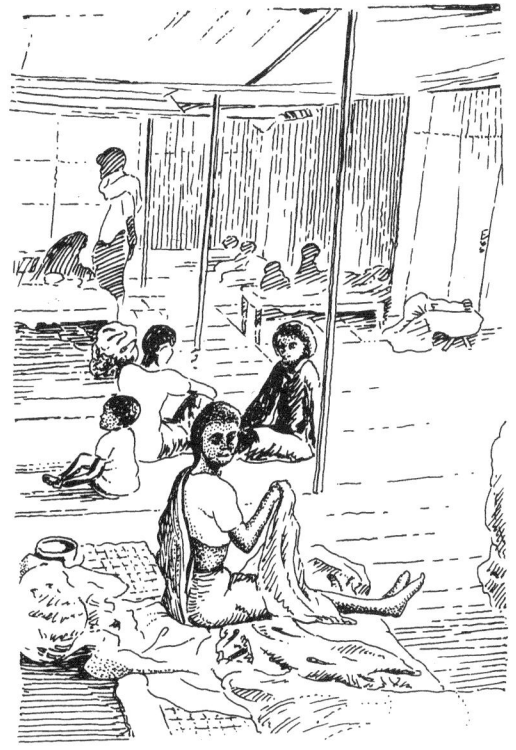

Fig. 1-2 THE SCENE IN INDIA. An improvised ward in a small hospital in Madhya Pradesh. Most patients are accompanied by members of their families or by friends. If they are away from their villages during the planting and harvesting season, they will go hungry. *After GR Howard, with the kind permission of the Editor of Tropical Doctor.*

them, and they will not yet have learnt to litigate against you. If you serve your hospital and the community round it for a lifetime, you will earn a unique place in its affections.

Just to prepare you, here is the kind of thing you may have to cope with.

DIDIMALA (4 years) was severely burnt. You worked for hours to put up a reliable drip and took great care to ring up for a bed in the referral hospital. When you pass by the ward an hour or two later, you find that she has indeed been sent there by ambulance, but the drip has been left behind. You ask "Why was this?" To which you get the reply, "There was no hook in the ambulance".

MARIA (5 months) presented with intermittent vomiting and abdominal swelling and was diagnosed as having intussusception. Unfortunately, the first hospital she went to had run out of anaesthetic gases and so could not operate. Her mother had to take her through three states stopping at four hospitals before she found one which could anaesthetize her (A 18.1). LESSON (1) Anaesthesia is often the limiting factor in surgery. (2) There is no need to have to rely on a supply of nitrous oxide (A 9.1).

Crofts TC, 'Trials and Tribulations of Surgery in Rural Tropical Areas' Tropical Doctor 1980;10:9-14.

1.3 Twenty surgeons in one

As a doctor in one of the hospitals we have just described, you are unlikely to be a fully qualified specialist surgeon with 5 to 8 years of postgraduate training. Instead, you will probably be a 'general duty medical officer' with one or two years of surgical experience or less. But somehow you have to care for the sick in *all* of the 20 specialist fields shown in the frontispiece, into which surgery has fragmented in recent years. The chance of your being able to refer patients to specialists is remote. There may be no maxillofacial surgeon, or hand surgeon, in the country, and if it is a small one, it may not even have a specialist anaesthetist. Even your own teaching hospital may lack the complete range of specialists. Nor, despite present training programs, is the situation in many countries likely to improve much in the near future. Even your nearest regional hospital may only have one or two general surgeons. But surgery will be only part of your work—you will also have to be a physician, and a paediatrician, and manage the district.

So you will have to do your best in *all* these fields simultaneously. To help you we have collected from among the armamentarium of diverse experts: (1) Their easier methods which you could use. Fortunately, many of them, despite the fact that they are normally only part of an expert's expertise, are not too difficult. For example, the position of safety in a hand injury (75-8), or Lord's anal stretch (22-10), are within the competence of any doctor. (2) Those methods, either easy or difficult, which you will have to use to save a patient's life. (3) Those difficult, disability-preventing but non-urgent methods, for which you should refer a patient, but may not be able to, such as sequestrectomy for osteomyelitis (7.6).

Many countries do not even have enough general duty doctors to do all the surgery that needs doing, let alone specialists. Malawi, for example, has recognized that surgery may have to be done by specially trained medical assistants, and Tanzania has trained its AMOs (Assistant Medical Officers) to do emergency surgery. Here is the report of a surgeon (Dr Gunnar Isaksson) on visiting one such AMO trained by the programme at the KCMC (Kilimanjaro Christian Medical Centre) in Tanzania. We quote it to emphasize that, not only may surgery have to be done by non-specialists, but that it is, on occasions, excellently done by non-doctors.

REPORT ON AN AMO 'How nice it was to see how well he was managing his tasks ... he seemed to be well in control, and happily did various operations. He had done several Caesarean sections, two laparotomies for intussusceptions, some hydrocelectomies, and fracture reductions, etc. He was treating three cases of fractured femur with skeletal traction in a very satisfactory way. His management of burns did not give cause for criticism. He had not done a sufficient number of hernia operations to feel confident about them; so he had gathered some and we operated on five of them together, after which he now wants to go on doing them himself. To go to Kiomboi was an inspiration for the work with our AMO training program.

Perhaps there is no AMO teaching program in your country, and yet you are hopelessly overworked. Could you train an auxiliary to do the simpler hernias, Caesarean sections and circumcisions?

Hankins GW, 'Surgery in a Mission Hospital', Annals of the Royal College of Surgeons of England 1980;62:439-44.

Cook J, Loefler IRJ, Gilchrist DS, Bewes PC, 'Surgery in a District Hospital', Journal of the Royal College of Surgeons of Edinburgh 1978;23:151-64.

1.4 Your surgical work

Ten to fifteen per cent of your admissions will probably be surgical, but because operating is time consuming, and some patients remain in bed for a long time, surgery may take 30% of your time, and fill half your beds. How much you will do will depend on how good you are at it. Patients will travel hundreds of kilometres to a doctor with a good surgical reputation. A bad one will soon do little surgery. Look carefully at the ages and sexes of the patients in your wards. When modern medicine first reaches a community, the first patients to present are the men, followed by the women and children. Only when medicine is well established, will you see a proportionate number of older women. If you don't find them in your wards, medicine has not reached this stage in your community. You will see few hypochondriacs, and there will be comparatively few repeat visits to the outpatient department because travel is so difficult.

You will see many of the diseases that are common in the industrial world, but in different proportions, a major difference

SOME OF YOUR PATIENTS

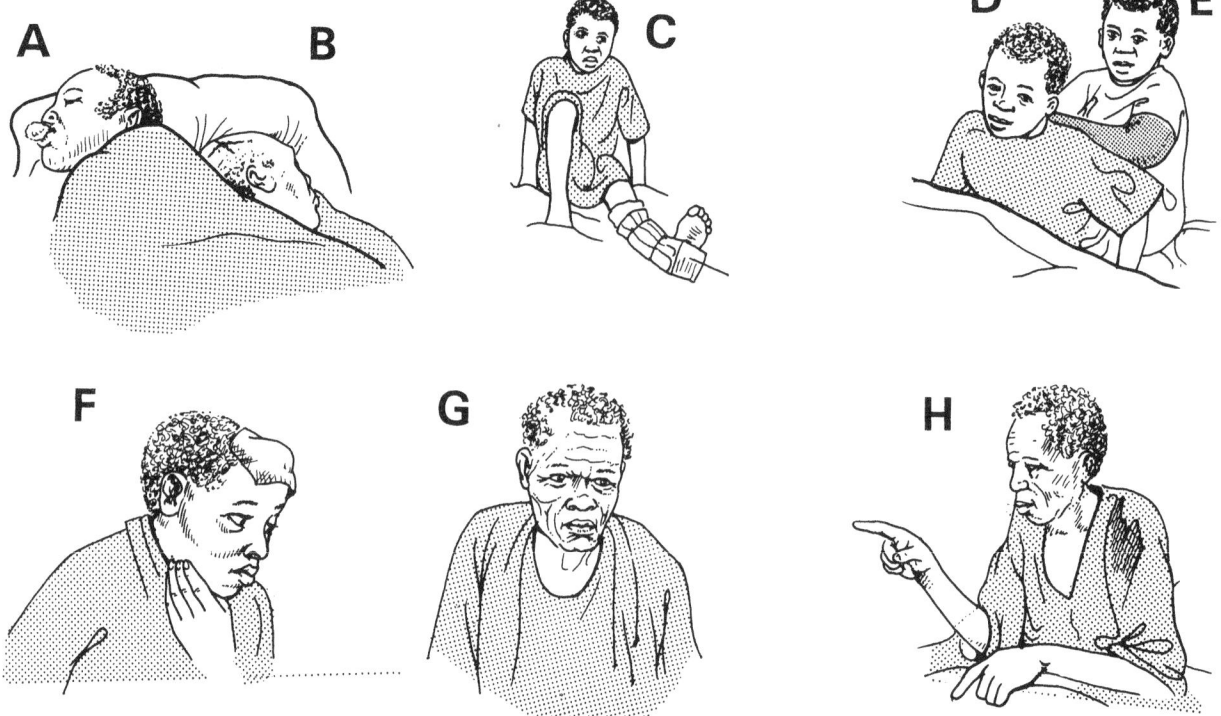

Fig. 1-3 SOME OF YOUR PATIENTS. Here are a random collection of patients who were in the ward when Fig. 1-1 was drawn. Patients A, and B, are sharing the same bed. They were admitted at nearly the same time time with head injuries, having both fallen off different motor cycles, neither wearing helmets (63.1). Child C, has Perthes' disease (27.14). Child D, broke his femur in the playground at school (78.3), and child E, has his fractured forearm in a cast (73.6b). Patient F, was assaulted (63.6). Patient G, a very old man, fell and fractured the neck of his femur (77.7). Patient H, is to have his prostate removed (23.19). We have described the care of all of them. Note also the prevalence of trauma, both from the roads and assault, and the geriatric complaints of patients G, and H.

being that so many of them present late (1.5). 'Western diseases' such as appendicitis, diverticulitis, carcinoma of the colon, haemorrhoids, and varicose veins are rare. Urethral strictures, tubal infections, fibroids and hernias are common, so are some diseases that are almost extinct in the industrial world—osteomyelitis, for example. You will probably see amoebiasis and tuberculosis of the chest, lymph nodes, abdomen, and bones. But you will seldom see carcinoma of the colon, or the thromboembolic complications of surgery that are so common in Europe; you will probably never see diverticulitis. No branch of surgery will differ more starkly from that in the industrial world than orthopaedics, where the cases you see, particularly those with polio contractures, will not have been seen in Europe for thirty years.

You will have to do many kinds of operation. For example, of nearly a thousand patients operated on at Nanyuki district hospital in Kenya, 175 different diagnoses were recorded in the theatre book. Of the patients needing general anaesthesia, only tubal ligations, the evacuation of inevitable abortions, and Caesarean sections came to more than 10% of the whole. Excluding tubal ligations, only about 5% of patients needed a laparotomy. About half the total were obstetric or gynaecological cases of some kind, about 15% were fractures and dislocations, and about 8% a variety of abscesses that needed to be opened under general anaesthesia.

Three-quarters of the bony injuries you will see are likely to be dislocations of the shoulder and elbow, supracondylar fractures in children, extension fractures of the wrist, and fractures of the radius and ulna, or tibia and fibula. All other bony injuries combined will only form the other quarter. Many will be the result of road accidents.

The cases you would like to refer—if you can—will be even more varied. A consecutive list of referrals from Nanyuki were an anaplastic carcinoma for radiotherapy, gas gangrene of the buttock in a diabetic, a brachial plexus injury in a patient with a head injury, rape causing a third degree tear in a girl of 8, and a patient with carcinoma of the stomach. Nanyuki had no instruments for craniotomy, so one referral was a patient with severe headache following a head injury. Another had a burnt scalp followed by osteomyelitis of his parietal bone and cerebral symptoms.

KALPANA (a Nepali aged 46) presented with mild abdominal pain for several days, severe for four days, and diarrhoea with two loose stools tinged with blood daily for a week. She had a tender, fluctuant mass in her right lower quadrant, and a marked leucocytosis. At laparotomy she had a patchy necrosis of her caecum with a localized perforation. A right hemicolectomy was done for suspected necrotizing amoebic colitis (31.11). The operation was a nightmare. Her colon came to pieces in the surgeon's hands and there was gross faecal contamination. She died. LESSONS (1) Expect a different spectrum of disease from that found in the industrial world. There, a fluctuant mass in the right lower quadrant is most likely to be an appendix abscess. (2) Avoid doing a right hemicolectomy for amoebiasis if you can.

1.5 Your patients

In many of the villages of the developing world, the burden of chronic disadvantage, poverty, ignorance, and insanitation are the background to life. A surgical disease on top of this may be the last straw.

As the result, patients often present late. If yours is a really disadvantaged community, tapping a hydrocele may yield litres rather than millilitres of fluid. An elephantoid scrotum may have progressed so far that it hangs to the ground (31-7). If a patient has a urethral stricture, he may leave it until he has multiple fistulae (23-10) or massive extravasation (23.10). If he has carcinoma of his penis (32.33), he may wait until much of it has been eaten away. Most carcinomas of the breast (21.4) and cervix (32.35) present too late for any hope of cure. Too often, patients only present when complications have made their lives unbearable. When even the struggle to keep alive may be a losing battle, the fact that surgical disease is normally treatable is irrelevant.

There are usually good reasons why a patient presents late. His family may have had no money for the operation or for transport, or there may be no transport. Perhaps it is the planting season, or there is nobody to look after his children or his goats? Perhaps his disease is painless, so that he does not realize that he is ill. Perhaps his tolerance to pain, disability, deformity, and misery is so high that he has to be desperate before he seeks help? He may only come to you when he has exhausted local remedies and and the services of traditional practitioners.

Transport, which may have been difficult before the rainy season, can become an insurmountable problem during it, when roads become quagmires, and rivers even more perilous. Acute surgical emergencies, in particular, may only come when patients are in the direst straits.

When a patient does come, you will not be able to send him off for an extensive series of investigations before you start treatment. Instead, you will have to learn to make a firm diagnosis from the history and examination. Expect to find that he has other diseases also. In Nepal, for example, only 15% of operations are in otherwise healthy patients. So expect your surgical patients to be malnourished, anaemic, malarious, tuberculous, or worm-ridden—or all of these things. They help to make a patient weak and wasted and a poor operative risk. Anaemia increases the risks of surgery, and in some communities the average haemoglobin may be only 80 g/l. Some patients may still be walking around with 40 or even only 20 g/l. Apart from a little breathlessness on the hills of Nepal, one 12 year old girl with a haemoglobin of only 20 g/l had no other complaints. So try to prepare your patients for surgery before you operate, especially if the cause is readily treatable.

Pain and disability are unlikely to rate highly when there is rice or maize to be planted, or when there are festivities and holidays. Although the economy may be poor, the culture may be a rich and compelling one. The cultural objections to colostomy, for example, may be so firm that a patient is unlikely to agree to have one, even temporarily, and even after you have explained how it can be managed with colostomy bags. Mastectomy may be similarly abhorrent.

Death is the great enemy of doctors and evidence of our failure. But a patient may have faced up to his own mortality, and may not always share your view. He may have learnt to live with death since childhood, and both his own attitude to it and that of his closest relatives may be very accepting. One of the greatest mistakes you can make is to send him home to die after a useless operation, having used up much of his own resources, and those of the hospital in an unsuccessful attempt to cure him.

1.6 Referral is mostly a myth

A patient with a surgical disease has first to refer himself to you, and if you cannot care for him, you have to refer him to someone else. Referral onwards from a community health worker (CHW) takes place at all the five steps in Figure 1-5. Although surgery is done in other parts of this system, we are concerned with the district hospital, and the critical referral steps from C to D and from D to E.

Although 'referral systems' exist in all health services, the difficulties they put in a patient's way are often insurmountable. Unfortunately, for many patients referral is a myth. In many developing countries the possibilities for referral appear to have got worse during the last decade rather than better, due to their declining economies. Too often, there is just no petrol for the hospital's ambulance to take a patient to a referral hospital, or no money to buy it. Alas, in many countries the future does not seem any more hopeful.

Only too often a patient reaches a referral hospital with great difficulty, only to return no better then he went. Because there are so many uncertainties, assess the chances for each patient individually. Try to find out what happens to each of the patients

A PRIVATE WARD

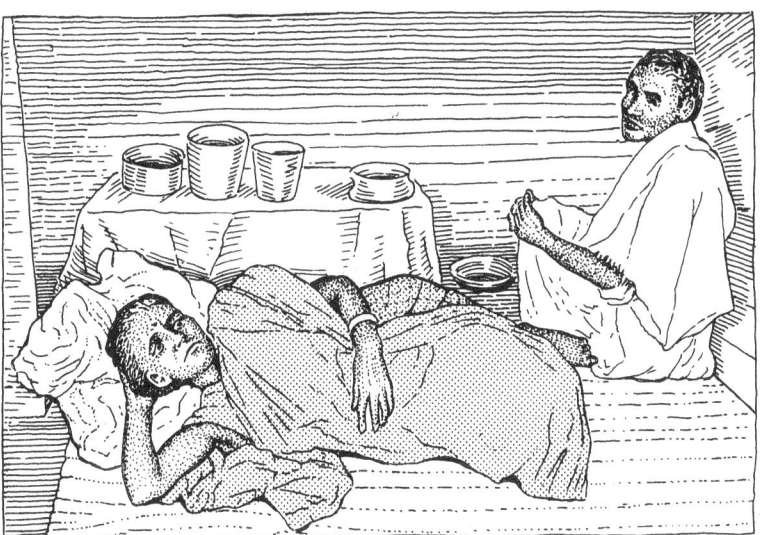

Fig. 1-4 A PRIVATE WARD in an Indian rural hospital. For a village family an illness is more than a biological disorder—it may be a social and economic crisis. *After GR Howard with the kind permission of the editor of Tropical Doctor.*

THE REFERRAL SYSTEM

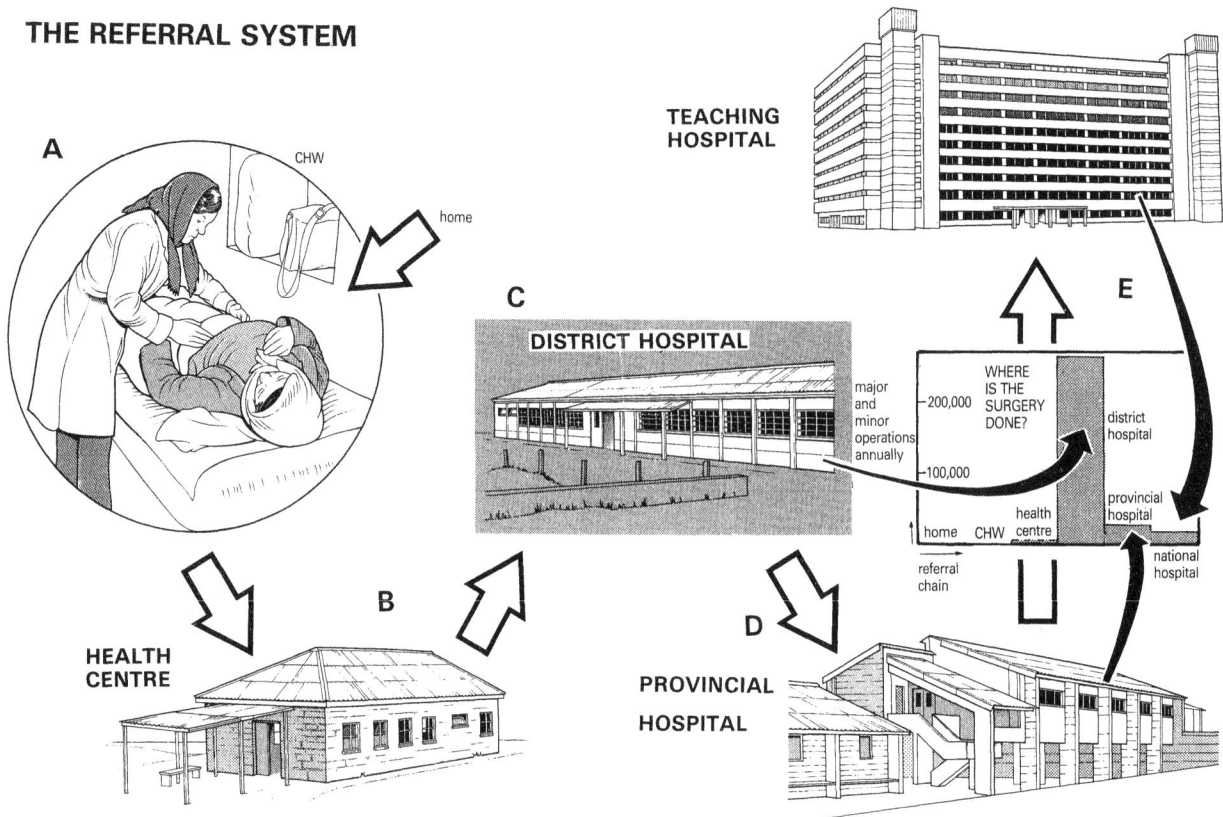

Fig. 1-5 THE REFERRAL SYSTEM. Each of these steps in the referral chain has its difficulties. A, from the patient's home to a community health worker. B, from the community health worker to the health centre. C, from the health centre to the district hospital. D, from the district to the provincial hospital. E, from the provincial to the teaching hospital. The histogram shows the number of major and minor operations combined at each stage in the referral chain in Kenya. Note the overwhelming aggregate importance of district hospital surgery. It is assumed that no surgery is done at home, or by the community health workers, and very little at health centres, for which no data were available. Data are from the Central Province of Kenya in 1983 extrapolated to the whole country. It is also assumed that the Central Province is typical. Kenya's 7 provinces are assumed to have one provincial hospital and 16 district hospitals each. The 6 district hospitals from which data were obtained averaged 2325 operations annually, ranging from 636 in Nyandarong to to 5708 in Muranga. Nyeri provincial hospital did 2,944 operations, and the Kenyatta National Hospital 15,333.

you send. Just what cases is it useful to refer, how, when, and to whom? If there are referral services, be sure to use them, both to refer patients and to learn from yourself.

In the pages that follow we often suggest that you 'refer the patient', but we realize that this is often impossible. So we have done our best to tell you what to do if it is impossible. The urgency, or lack of it with which a patient needs to be referred is critical, and varies with each condition, so we have indicated just how urgent referral is in each case.

Some surgeons working in referral hospitals have a false idea of the practicalities of referral. They see only the tip of the iceberg—the patients who reach them successfully. So they may think that referral is easier than it is. There are however certain cases which referral hospitals should accept without question, and district hospitals should know what they are. They include the closure of intestinal fistulae (9.14), and difficult ankle fractures (82.3).

Referral hospitals have their problems: (1) They may be overcrowded with simple cases that you could care for in your district hospital. One of the purposes of these manuals is *to make sure that any surgery that can be done in a district hospital is done there*, so that referral hospitals can fulfil their proper function. (2) When the time comes to discharge a referred patient who cannot go home unaided, they may be unable to send him there because they cannot contact his rural relatives.

Here is an account of what one patient went through successfully to get himself treated at a referral hospital. It is from the Chairman's address to the 1980 Annual Conference of the Association of Surgeons of East Africa. Fortunately for the patient, he was in the Chairman's care.

Jellis JE, 'Chairman's Address', Proceedings of the Association of Surgeons of East Africa 1981;4:53-56.

PATSON BANDA (49 years) was in a LandRover when it rolled over in deep sand, causing an open fracture of his right humerus and injuring his radial nerve. He was still able to walk, so he eventually reached a district hospital, where his wound was carefully toileted, and left open for delayed primary suture. His radial nerve injury was recognized, his arm was put in a collar-and-cuff sling, and he was asked to return in 48 hours. His wound was clean so it was closed. So far he had received ideal treatment.

It was decided to refer him to the provincial hospital 40 km away, across a river and a flood plain, 20 minutes by air, a day by boat, or two days by LandRover. There was no radio, and the telephone was not working, so there was no way of telling the provincial surgeon that he was coming. He was able to get a seat on a barge and was in the provincial capital 24 hours later. It was dark but he was able to find a relative with whom he could stay the night. The next day he sat in the outpatient queue and handed his slip to the medical assistant. Unfortunately, the provincial surgeon had left the previous day to attend a planning meeting at the Ministry of Health. He would not be back for two days. The provincial surgeon returned and saw him, but decided that his training had not prepared him for posterior exploration of the humerus, plating the fracture and perhaps secondary suture of the radial nerve. Also, he had no 6/0 monofilament. So Patson was given a bus warrant, and a note to the orthopaedic surgeon in the teaching hospital in the capital city.

Unfortunately, he had no money, no food, and no clean clothes for the journey, so he went home. His LandRover had been partly dismantled by thieves, but his partner had towed the wreck back to his village, and hired a lad to help him with the fishing. The family were already deeply in debt. They debated whether he should go 800 km to the capital, but his limp wrist decided them. He started on his long journey with a pack of food, a few clean clothes, and a bus warrant, but very little money.

Four days later he arrived at the orthopaedic clinic on a Friday. He had no appointment, and the surgeon to whom the note was addressed had held his clinic on the previous day. The harassed sister, busy with another clinic, found that he had no relatives in the city, and no money, so she sent him to the orthopaedic ward in the hope that they might have a bed for him over the weekend. They did.

On Monday the surgeon saw him. His wound had healed and he was fit for surgery, and the necessary screws, plates, adhesive drapes, and sutures were in stock. But there was a three months waiting list, so he had to wait 10 days, even for operation as a semi-emergency. A silent cheer went up from the hospital staphylococci, as they began to colonize the skin of this provincial patient.

His radial nerve was freed from compression in its spiral groove, and his fractured humerus was successfully plated. Two weeks later he returned to the provincial hospital with suggestions for physiotherapy (a two day journey for each session) and instructions to return in a year for removal of the plate.

He was lucky. He was one of the minority for whom the referral system worked. His radial nerve palsy recovered. The state paid for nearly 4 weeks in a teaching hospital, and 1600 km in transport. He was in debt, and his family were hungry, but he did not have to sell his boat, or the remains of his LandRover. It could have been much worse.

TOPNO (41 years) fractured his ankle in a bus accident. The very competent doctor who saw him had learnt that difficult ankle fractures should be referred (82.3). He could manipulate fractures, but he thought that an expert would do better, so he sent the patient with a letter to the referral hospital 70 km away. After a long journey, the patient arrived too late at the fracture clinic. He was able to reach the next fracture clinic in time, only to find that the surgeon was away at a conference. So he hung around hopefully for some days, but in the end he was advised to return to his original hospital. Meanwhile, he had had no treatment except the original 'first aid' plaster. When he eventually returned to the doctor who first saw him, his fracture had partly united in a very bad position. It was now too late to manipulate him, so he now has a stiff painful ankle and is waiting to have it fused. LESSON A patient may be better in your hands, if you learn those of the expert's procedures that you can reasonably do.

ASSESS EACH PATIENT'S CHANCES OF EFFECTIVE REFERRAL

REFERRAL

SHOULD YOU SEND HIM? **The chances of being able to refer a patient vary greatly, and are apt to change. They depend on the answers to these questions.**

(1) Is it worth sending him anyway? He may not have a disease for which the referral hospital has any effective treatment. Even if he does reach it, he may not be sure of any better treatment than yours.

(2) Is he prepared to leave his family and his fields or his job?

(3) Can he get himself to the referral centre? In some districts, for example, the roads and airstrips are closed for weeks at a time during the rainy season.

(4) Has he or the hospital got money for transport and for lodging when he gets there? Often, neither of them have.

(5) If he does arrive, will he find his way to the right clinic, wait in the right queue and be seen and admitted? Will there be an empty bed? Will the surgeon you send him to actually be there when he arrives, or will he have gone on holiday, or to a conference in Europe.

AT THE REFERRAL HOSPITAL **a patient you refer will be in competition with ordinary local cases, so try to feed him into its administrative system. Tell him exactly where to go and whom to see. Try to send him personally to a surgeon you know, and who you know will treat a case of this kind. Find out on which days the surgeon has his clinics.**

Inform the surgeon that the patient is coming. Make sure that the patient knows exactly what to do, and where to go when he arrives.

Investigate him first, and state the procedure that you think he needs. If a biopsy is necessary, do it, and refer him with his report. Often a biopsy takes time and may have to be sent to the referral hospital. If referral is urgent, don't wait for the report. Send a careful letter with him, including all necessary information.

If there are any particularly good referral facilities, such as those for artificial limbs, for example, be sure to use them.

Finally, don't refer patients unnecessarily. No surgeon likes to be sent ganglions (27.11)!

1.7 What should we describe? What should you be able to do surgically? The limits of this system of surgery

God is in the details.

Mies van der Rohe

Der teufel (the devil) ist im detail

Old German proverb

In view of the common impossibility of referral, we have tried to describe everything that you, our readers *as a whole might have to do*—if you cannot refer a patient, and which might benefit him; both the 'hot' emergency procdures and the less urgent 'cold' ones. As you will see in the next section, you *individually*, should not necessarily do everything we describe.

Our contributors have varied greatly in what they thought we should include. Some have considered you can do everything that they can do. Others have done their utmost to keep you away from the patient if they possibly can. Many began by considering that most of the procedures that they do themselves would have to be learnt by expert tuition, and could not be learnt from a manual. In the end they came to see that this manual is necessary. That personal tuition from an expert is the best way to learn anything, we take for granted. But, what if there is no expert? A manual is surely better than nothing.

Somehow, we have had to find a balance, so we have considered each procedure on its merits. Our task has been made no easier by the wide range of your abilities. You range from highly trained surgeons doing unfamiliar operations for the first time, to inexperienced doctors doing your first jobs. We have tried to serve all your needs.

Not the least of our difficulties has been your very different ability to use books. One professor of surgery remarked that these manuals would be very useful for mature general duty doctors of the old school, but not for his students. The ability to do anything out of a book varies greatly, whether it is making a cake, mending a car, or treating a fractured femur. For anyone who is not good at doing things out of books, learning to do so is an ability well worth cultivating—over the years it will make a huge difference to your skills.

It has not always been easy to distinguish the tasks which are obviously impossible for you (oesophageal atresia for example), from those which are possibly possible (duodenal or jejunoileal atresia). We have had to balance benefit, risk, and urgency. This has led us to include methods for removing the prostate, for example, but not the thyroid.

Methods have been devised for grading the difficulty of operations. One of them gives the repair of an inguinal hernia a value of one arbitrary unit. On this scale the repair of an episiotomy is given 0.2 units, a clavicle fracture 0.3, a Colles fracture 0.6, an above knee amputation 1.3, the resection of small gut 2.0, and the fusion of a hip (not described here) 3.0 units. Methods of grading were discussed, and this one might be adopted in the second edition. Instead, we have suggested you refer the more difficult cases where you can, and have stressed that some operations are only for the *careful caring operator*. These include vascular repairs (55.6), a groin flap for the back of the hand (75.27), and Girdlestone's operation for fractures of the neck of the femur (77.13).

Although the common conditions may comprise perhaps 60% of your work, the rest will include many rarer ones. *In aggregate the rarities are common.* So we have tried to describe as many of the comparative rarities as we can, in the hope that you will find about 98% of the conditions you could hope to treat surgically described here. The edges of this large collection of appropriate methods are inevitably blurred, and it has not been easy to know how rare, or how difficult we should be. For example, you will find no less than 46 hand fractures, and there is even mention of cystic hygroma. We shall probably be criticized for including oesophagoscopy and bronchoscopy, and some cancer chemotherapy. But it is better to include slightly too much rather than slightly too little—there is no need for you to do things you don't want to! Tibialis transfer (30.8) is our *tour de force*, and the great detail with which we have described it should enable our more experienced and caring readers to do it. Some methods, such as tying the major arteries, are seldom used, but are classical, in that no textbook of surgery would be complete without them. Inevitably, some parts of the 'system' are tidier than others. The trauma methods, for example, seem about as complete as anything could be, but not so those for ophthalmology. Nor is there any sharp distinction between what is medicine and what is surgery, particularly in obstetrics (Chapter 17 on 'The medicine of pregnancy').

We have excluded all procedures which require equipment which you are unlikely to have, and could not reasonably expect to buy. We have assumed that you have an X-ray department, but no X-rays in the theatre and no image intensifiers, ultrasound, diathermy, or equipment for any but the very simplest methods of internal fixation. Although we mostly write for hospitals which are short of both money and skill, there are some, such as those run by mines and plantations, where money is less scarce and who should be able to buy even comparatively expensive drugs for cancer chemotherapy, for example. For them all the equipment we list (even bronchoscopes and oesophagoscopes) should not be a problem. Uncertain sterilizing procedures, and limited nursing care have also guided our selection. AO methods of internal fixation are excluded on all these counts (69.3). If you try it, it is likely to live up to the epithet 'Always Osteomyelitis'!

Overall: (1) We have tried to describe a system of practice which includes all the basics, *but is ahead of of the practice of many district hospitals*, so that even comparatively advanced ones have something to aim for. (2) We have tried to cover most of the range of the 'general surgeon' working in the districts. (3) We have tried to describe this system in complete detail, and in doing so would agree with both the quotations with which this section starts. (4) We have in our mind's eye a concept of 'quality' at the district hospital level; even simple things can and should be done well. Right at the end of this manual there are some indicators to measure this by (34.6).

1.8 Should you operate?

Although the era of 'furor operandi' has passed, one still has almost daily evidence of the disastrous effects of major surgical procedures, attempted lightly by young, or even inexperienced older surgeons. The author would in no way dampen the ardour of the neophyte, or check his ambition to acquire skill. Still, it is well to suppress the feelings of cocksureness and egotistic pride...

Max Thorek, Surgical Errors and Safeguards

Whether or not you should operate on a given patient will be the most important question you will have to answer. Put yourself in his place. What would *you* like to happen if you were him? Several factors will influence your decision. We have already discussed one of them—can you refer him? On the whole we think that for every doctor who operates when he should not, there are many more who don't operate when they should. So one of our aims has been to get more surgery done—on the *correct* indications!

The mature surgeon is one who knows when *not* to operate! On the other hand, if you are always too cautious, you will never learn and some of your patients will never benefit.

So beware of Thorek's *furor operandi*, the furious urge to operate, and ask yourself these questions before you do so.

SHOULD YOU OPERATE?

What will happen if you don't operate? If a patient is likely to die or become disabled if he is not operated on quickly, you will have to operate. We have therefore included all the more practical emergency operations, whether difficult or not. For example, you must drill immediately for acute osteomyelitis, but a patient who needs a sequestrectomy for chronic osteomyelitis can wait. If however you cannot refer him, you may have to operate.

How difficult is the operation? At least three factors determine this: (1) Your technical knowledge, (2) your experience, and (3) your skill. We can provide you with the knowledge, and bring you some of the experience of other people, but only practice will improve your manual skill.

How safe is the operation? What disasters might happen? Little can go wrong with draining most abscesses, or manipulating most fractures, but disaster is only too possible if you decide to close an intestinal fistula or do a block dissection of the groin.

Do you have the necessary instruments, materials, and staff? Even if you don't, you may be able to improvise.

Are you yourself inclined to operate too readily, or not readily enough? Cultural attitudes to operating vary. In India or Indonesia, for exampe, the common failing is to be too timid, and not to operate when necessary. The reverse is true in some parts of Africa, where inexperienced operators are much too bold. So be aware of your own personal and cultural bias and try to correct for it.

What is the known or probable HIV status of the patient? See Chapter 28a.

Finally, if you have difficulty deciding what to do and are able to telephone or radio anyone who might know, don't hesitate do so so.

RULES ABOUT DECIDING WHEN TO OPERATE. (1) You must be certain of the indication to operate, even if it is only exploratory. (2) When life is in danger take risks. (3) If an emergency is hopeless be prepared to say: No! (3) Don't do difficult elective surgery, especially if the expected outcome is likely to be of limited value to the patient.

SEVEN RULES WHEN YOU DECIDE TO OPERATE. (1) You must be familiar with the anatomy; if necessary consult an anatomy book during the operation. (2) You must have someone familiar with anaesthesia giving the anaesthetic. If you are giving it yourself, there must be someone who can monitor its progress and the vital signs. (3) There must be a reliable system of sterilization, preferably an autoclave. (4) You must have a good light, preferably adjustable. (5) You must have the necessary equipment and supplies for resuscitation and homoeostasis (infusions, infusion sets, a laryngoscope, tracheal tubes, adrenalin, calcium etc). (6) Have the highest regard for living tissue and be gentle and circumspect. Operate at your own speed. (7) Finally, don't be too elated over your successes, or too despondent over your failures. If you do fail, forgive yourself—don't 'give up'! A bad spell during which 2 or 3 patients die may be followed by another in which none of them do. Remember that Brock's first 17 mitral valvotomies all died!

CAUTION ! Remember also that with 'cold operations' disasters are more difficult to justify than with 'hot ones', both to the hospital staff and to the general public, and that accusations that the doctor is experimenting on his patients can do much harm.

If you have not done any surgery before, or only very little, start with the easier operations. You should at least be able to open abscesses (Chapter 5).

1.9 'Oh, never, never let us doubt what nobody is sure about'

Inevitably, these manuals contain a huge quantity of didactic detail with few reasons as to 'why' you should do anything, and few references to the original papers. We have tried to select the best methods for your needs. Even so, remember that accepted methods change, that few have been rigorously evaluated by controlled trials, and that some, which were widely accepted only a few years ago have now been completely abandoned or reversed.

Here are some examples of how fallible medical practice can be: (1) A low-fibre diet used to be prescribed for diverticulitis, but is now thought to be one of the causes of it. (2) Complete immobilization was and often still is considered to be the ideal

FOUR SURGEONS
Which are you?

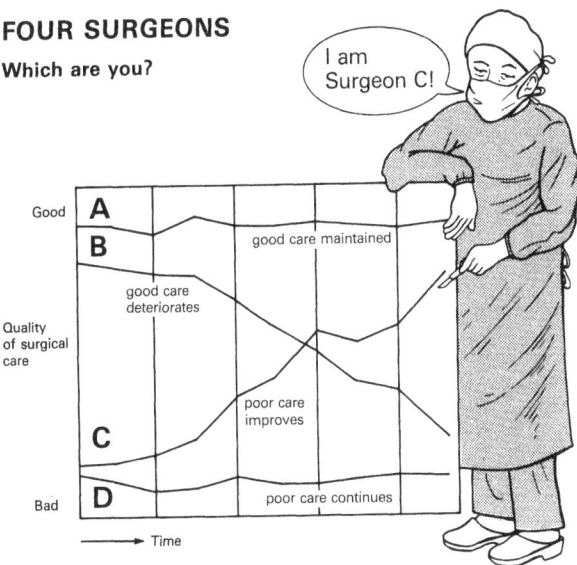

Fig. 1-6 WHICH OF THESE SURGEONS ARE YOU? Doctor A, found a nearly perfect surgical system, and stepped in and out of it without needing to change it. Doctor B, found a moderately functioning system and slowly let it deteriorate. Doctor C, found a poorly functioning system, and with great difficulty was able to improve it considerably. Doctor D, found and left chaos.

treatment for all long bone fractures. It is now increasingly realized that many of them benefit from early controlled movement (69.4). (3) In many centres it has been standard practice to separate mothers from their babies immediately after birth. Now, this is completely reversed and their close contact immediately after delivery is considered essential for bonding. (4) Shaving a patient the day before an operation, which used to be standard practice, has now been shown to increase the incidence of infection...

This list could be expanded. So be prepared to 'doubt what nobody is sure about', even while you follow the didactic instructions we give.

1.10 Creating and maintaining the surgical machine

If you are lucky, you will arrive at a hospital where your colleagues and your predecessors have created a smoothly running surgical system. Or, you may arrive and find almost nothing. More likely, you will arrive and find a system which is working somehow, and which badly needs improvement. As well as actually treating the sick you may have to try to make the hospital as a whole, and particularly its surgical services more efficient. To do this you will have to improve: (1) The morale and training of its staff. Congratulations are likely to be much more effective than reprimands. (2) Its fittings and equipment. (3) Its administrative arrangements. (4) Your own skills. The various options before you are shown in Fig. 1-6. In doing this you must be prepared to do *any* task yourself, no matter how humble and how unfamiliar. There is no place for the attitude "Oh, but it's not my job..." Our jobs, wherever we are, are to create the 'machine' and make it work.

When you arrive inexperienced in a new place, study it carefully and list the things that need changing. Then, cautiously and steadily, try to implement them during the next few months or years. If you don't note them when you first arrive, you will soon take them all for granted, and do nothing. Beware of constant change, because the staff will not accept it. Get to know them and accept their advice before introducing 'improvements'. When you operate, do as best you can on your own to begin with. Then, after two or three months, when you have the feel of the place

TEACHING THE TEAM

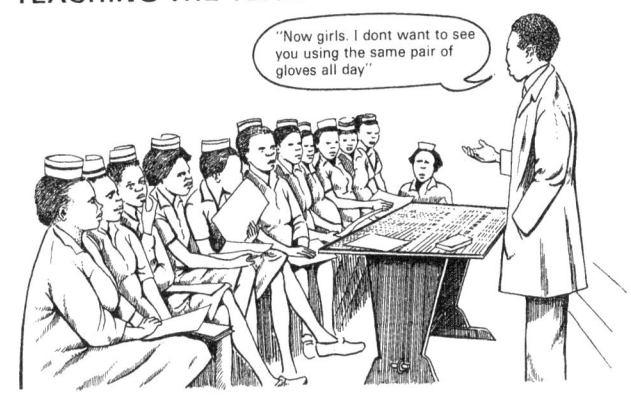

Fig. 1-7 DOCTOR 'C' TEACHING HIS TEAM. When Doctor C from the previous figure first arrived at this hospital he found its obstetric wards in a desperate state, and its beds so overcrowded that mothers ruptured their uteri in the corridors almost unnoticed. He soon got to work, and here you see him correcting some of the sloppy habits of his nurses. Soon, his obstetric services were so efficient that he had empty beds. It has been suggested that this shows a very sexist and authoritarian manner of teaching, and that a round table discussion would have been better.

and its problems, visit the nearest hospital where they do things well, stay a week or two and learn whatever they can teach you in a short time. Then come back and put what you have learnt into practice.

ALL FOR A PIECE OF CHALK There was once a professor of surgery who found to his astonishment that his operating list had been cancelled. When he asked why his houseman replied "Because there is no chalk with which to list the cases". The professor was furious and dismissed his houseman on the spot. The DMS pleaded with him, "...such a nice boy...", even the Minister pleaded, but the professor insisted that he could not have such a person as his houseman. So he continued to clerk his own cases. Finally, weeks later his repentant houseman came to him and said "About that chalk, Sir, I think I made a mistake...". LESSON Failure to improvise, where this is at all possible, is never an adequate reason for not doing something.

1.12 The surgical care of the poor

The purpose of surgery is to heal the sick. What is the use of it if the sick cannot afford it? The rapid growth of the populations of many of our countries requires that we care for ever more people every year, on a health budget which is not only low to begin with, *but is static, or in some countries is even declining in real terms.* Despite this, our patients now know what surgery has to offer, so that their expectations increase steadily.

We easily forget just how poor some of them are. They are about fifty times poorer than patients in Europe or North America. Of the $2 to $5 per head per year that is available in many developing countries for all forms of health care, half or more is spent in the cities, so that only $1 a head, or even only a few cents are available in the rural areas for both hospital and health centre care. The per capita income in India is less than $100 a year, and in the rural areas where 80% of people live, the cash income is even lower than that. Estimates as to how much an Indian villager can spend on health care range from 36 cents to $5 annually. It is however less the cost in cash which devastates his family, than the complete disruption of their earning power.

Fortunately, the kind of surgery we describe is remarkably cheap and cost-effective—compared with the high technology surgery of the industrial world. But it is not so cheap in terms of a villager's income. If you work in a government hospital, such funds as you have will be provided for you. If you work in a voluntary agency hospital, and your patients have to pay, and you really want to care for them, you will have to keep your costs low. Complicated methods can easily lead to rising costs, and so gradually drive the most needy away. Instead, your hospital may fill with richer patients, who could, if they wished, seek care in the towns. Care can indeed be very cheap. For example, one Indian hospital (Herbertpur, Uttar Pradesh, 1977) charges the equivalent of $2.50 a day, which includes everything except food, which the patient's relatives cook. In one district hospital (Chogoria in Kenya) two thirds of the running costs are met from the patient's fees, with charges of only Kshs 20/- ($1.5) a day, no operation costing more than Kshs. 250/- ($20).

PULLING A HOSPITAL 'OUT OF THE RED' Here is some advice from Tumutumu PCEA Hospital in Kenya which was able to turn a substantial deficit in its accounts into a surplus in two years. Try to make the containment of costs, or their reduction, an activity which all your staff share. They and you should know how much everything costs. If you can make your financial decisions by mutual consensus, they will be implemented. Form an action committee consisting of all the spending departments—the medical superintendant, the administrator, the matron, and the senior medical assistant. Meet weekly and pass all decisions involving money through this meeting. A good time to start holding such meetings is after some crisis has occurred, for example, being told to cut your budget by 40%. A crisis atmosphere makes people more co-operative, and more willing to change their ways.

Examine all funds coming into the hospital and all funds going out of it, scrutinize all bills and orders. Discuss demands from each department, and reject any unnecessary ones. Scrutinize all expenditure and expect to make some savings on almost everything. No single item is decisive, but collectively they make the big difference. Look at the large items first—salaries, transport, and food—even small percentage savings here will have a big overall effect. Look at your establishment figures. You may find that your hospital has got fat and that you should let it get a bit leaner by not recruiting after natural staff wastage. You may find that you have to return to the staffing ratios and technologies (such as making your own plaster bandages) of earlier years. For example, you will probably find that most patients with pneumonia can be treated without an X-ray and so can most extension fractures of the wrist.

These meetings will be critical. They will ensure the co-operation of the leaders of all sections of the hospital, who will transmit the sense of urgency to everyone else. They will also help to create an awareness of the economic implications of a decision, to establish priorities, and to ensure the continuation and extension of your economy drive. Follow up your decisions—someone must check that the fire is extinguished once the water is hot, or that the right weight of the right cabbages has been supplied. Make sure that the staff know how much money is running through their hands, and that the viability of the hospital depends on how they use dressing materials, gas, and equipment.

Money coming in is no less important than money going out. So try to keep your beds full. Work out a policy to reduce costs to the patient, and to make your services affordable to as many people as you can. Think about what they can pay, and be prepared to lower some charges.

This manual is mostly derived from experience in Africa, India and Nepal. Valuable contributions to the surgical care of the poor have however been made in South America. Adolpho Velez Gil and others found that in Colombia three quarters of all the operations were simple enough to be done on outpatients with a single anaesthetist supervising two patients simultaneously in the same theatre, mostly using local and epidural methods, and adequately supported by assistants. Operating theatres were only used for 40% of working hours, surgeons only did 120 operations a year and 'physicians' only 18. Gil was therefore concerned to increase the utilization of theatres, and the surgical productivity of both surgeons and 'physicians'. Since most of the operations were simple what was required was more generalists and fewer specialists. Is this true for your situation too?

In most hospitals, services are limited less by resources than by motivation. So expect to be able to do much more, even with what little you think you have. The rest of this section, which is based on the papers listed below, shows what can be done, even when resources seem to be already stretched to their limit. If you think that checking the stores is not your responsibility, remember that it is critically important for the financial viability of the hospital, on which your whole surgical endeavour depends.

Gichero F, Kimunyu E, Kibuyna R, Spellmeier W, 'How we pulled Tumutumu Hospital out of the red'. An article which should have reached Tropical Doctor but never did.

Satow S, 'The Technical Aspects of Small Hospital Surgery', 1977 Proceedings of a Symposium Held at the 19th Meeting of the International Federation of Surgical Colleges.

Gill AV, Galarza MT, Guerrero R, de Velez GP, Peterson OL, and Bloom BL, 'Surgeons and operating rooms: underutilized resources', American Journal of Public Health 1983; 73(12)1361-1364.

ECONOMICAL SURGERY

STAFF Reduce staff to the bare minimum by not replacing unnecessary ones, and make sure they do a full day's work. Keep existing staff busy with additional duties. Junior staff are often willing to have more responsible jobs such as filing and typing, or even preparing intravenous fluids. Try to lay off consistantly dishonest and inefficent staff. Encourage punctuality. Employ inexpensive ungraded staff where you can, to relieve more expensive staff of routine tasks. Employ multipurpose workers, such as a laboratory technician who can take X-rays.

SAVINGS ON CONSUMABLE MATERIALS

Dressings. If necessary, you can treat most wounds without dressings. Most clean closed surgical wounds don't need them. Use gauze and cotton wool economically. Don't make dressings larger than is necessary. Resterilize all dressings which have not been used. Use narrow strapping, and don't allow it to be used anywhere except on the human body. Wash gauze sponges, immerse them in saline to remove stains, dry them and resterilize them. If necessary cut up an old polyurethane foam mattress or cushion into small squares and use these as swabs and sponges. They absorb blood and can be resterilized. Cut up and sterilize old linen. Sterile toilet paper can be used as an alternative to swabs for some purposes.

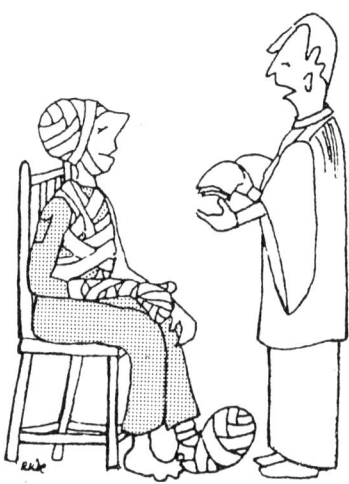

"I pronounce you man and dressing."

Laparotomy pads ('lap pads'). Use a sewing machine to sew enough pieces of gauze 20×25 cm together to make a 5 mm layer; attach a tape to one end, and when you operate attach a haemostat to the tape and leave this hanging out of the wound. Lap pads are a more convenient and economical way of washing and reusing gauze than using it as swabs, and can replace them for some purposes.

Dressing a wound dry uses many more dressings than treating it wet. So keep it wet with saline, which need not be sterile. Make this with ordinary salt and tap water. This is the basis of the saline method for burns (58.16).

If a wound is suitably sited to be immersed, as with the arm, leg, or buttocks, immerse it in saline for 3 hours twice a day. Put a leg in a bucket, an arm in a long arm bath, and let a patient with a buttock wound sit in in a hip bath.

If a wound is not suitably sited for immersion, cover it with a thin layer of gauze or bandage and keep it wet with saline from a jug (58.16). Renew the gauze or bandage once a day. This is more economical in dressings than treating it dry.

Disinfectants. Don't fill gallipots to the brim. Use cotton wool, not gauze for scrubbing the skin. Don't use disinfectant for the preliminary 'scrub' to remove dirt; use soap and water. One gallipot of disinfectant will then be enough to 'prep' the skin. You can use it all day—it is self sterilizing.

Disposable items. Avoid these and replace them by permanent equipment. If you buy plastic equipment which is intended to be thrown away, choose the kind which you can autoclave or boil. Recycle everything you possibly can, and try to throw nothing away. Buy the kind of gloves you can resterilize 3 or 4 times. Resharpen needles and scalpel blades.

Use nylon syringes, such as the French KIGLISS pattern, which you can sterilize indefinitely, and which have a rubber ring to seal the plunger which you can purchase separately. Don't use disposable urine bags; instead, use bottles and tubing from old intravenous sets.

Catheters and cannulae. Use simpler rubber catheters instead of more expensive Foley catheters; if you want to leave them in, secure them with strapping. Use steel intravenous cannulae instead of plastic ones.

Intravenous fluids. Make your own for one fifteenth of the price of the commercial ones (A Appendix A). Where possible, use rectal rather than intravenous fluids (A 15.5). These are not suitable for rehydrating patients, but they may be adequate for maintenance.

If intravenous fluids are scarce, for postoperative patients who have had major gastrointesinal or other surgery, tie two pieces of ordinary intravenous disposable tube together. Insert them as a nasogastric tube with one tube in the stomach for suction, and the other in the distal duodenum or jejunum for feeding. In this way you will greatly reduce your need for intravenous fluid.

Oxygen is only necessary for such indications as pulmonary oedema, asthma and shock, and not for comatose or moribund patients. If it is used for patients with no hope of survival, relatives may come to believe that it is used to kill them!

Drugs. Use cheaper drugs instead of expensive ones. For curettage of the uterus use pethidine with diazepam instead of ketamine; use aminophylline instead of salbutamol, aspirin instead of paracetamol, nitrofurantoin instead of ampicillin for urinary tract infections, and morphine instead of pethidine for many applications. Look carefully at the prices you pay for drugs.

Sutures. Where possible, use surgical suture material bought in bulk on reels, or use nylon fishing line (4.6). Only use atraumatic sutures when they are absolutely necessary. With more expensive suture materials, use continuous sutures rather than interrupted ones. Buy reels instead of packs. The application of warm moist gauze packs to a bleeding surface will halve the number of bleeding vessels that you need to tie. You can tie those that persist with sewing cotton for almost nothing.

Scrubbing up Use ordinary soap not special fluids.

SAVING KITCHEN SUPPLIES

Find the cheapest supplier and buy at the right season. Find out if buying in the market may be better. Watch tenders carefully, change suppliers when necessary, and insist on good quality. Don't let them supply you with old, rotten, or small potatoes. Buy boneless meat. Use powdered milk instead of whole milk. Adjust the number of meals cooked to the bed state. Give high protein diets only on genuine indications. Reduce waste. Fill plates moderately and vary helpings according to the appetites of both patients and staff. Keep pigs and chickens to feed on waste.

ENERGY SAVINGS

Petrol or diesel. Diesel vehicles are cheaper to run. Use the smallest and most economical vehicle for a given job and fill it full. Keep logbooks and use vehicles for hospital journeys only. Drive at economical speeds and use moderate engine revolutions in all gears. Use public transport wherever possible. Encourage a style of driving that is considerate for the vehicle, especially when carrying heavy loads on bad roads.

Gas. Put lids on pots. Reduce the flames when the pot has boiled. Use pressure cookers. Soak beans overnight. Control cooking times.

Electricity. Reduce lighting to the minimum. Use fluorescent tubes instead of bulbs. Reduce hot baths to the minimum. Have one central hot water tap, from which the staff fetch water in buckets—if they do not object too much!

Solar energy. Solar lighting is more practical than solar heating, because of the smaller amount of energy needed.

Washing. Use the timers to set minimum times for washing and spin drying carefully. Avoid tumble dryers unless the climate is very wet; they use much electricity.

OTHER SAVINGS

Use the space fully on all case sheets, use paper on both sides. Make your own forms with a stencil. Minimize the use of paper for internal correspondence. Use scrap paper for messages.

Don't use so much detergent that it causes foaming in the laundry and when scrubbing floors.

Register private calls, and make a 25% surcharge. Avoid long distance calls in favour of letters.

Control all items that could be used in private homes, including torch batteries, soap, matches, pens, toilet paper, female pads, food and medicines.

Keep a pair of tubes of epoxy resin. It is suprising what you will be able to mend.

ECONOMY IS ESSENTIAL TO SURGERY

1.13 Primary care radiology

X-rays are much the most useful method of diagnostic imaging. Next comes ultrasound which you can make good use of, especially in obstetrics where it can replace X-rays for almost all indications, except X-ray pelvimetry (which we do not describe).

WHO has recently made a great advance in the X-ray departments of the world's district hospitals by developing the BRS or Basic Radiological System. The BRS machine is shown in Fig. 1-8, and is made by several manufacturers to WHO's specifications. If you are thinking of buying an X-ray machine, this is the one to get. If you don't have electricity all day, you can run

THE BRS X-RAY SYSTEM

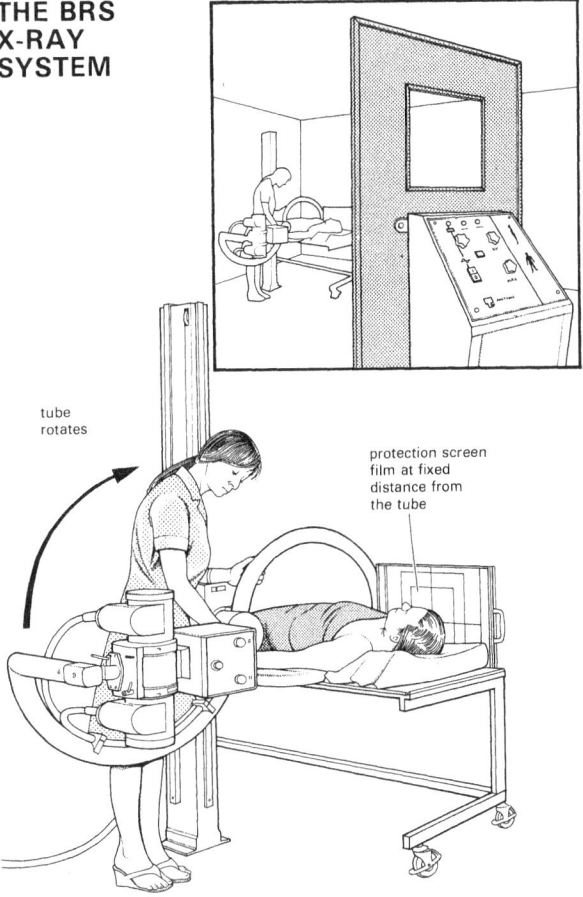

Fig. 1-8 THE BRS X-RAY SYSTEM was developed by WHO to make essential cost-effective radiology available safely and reliably to all the world's people. If you want one of these machines, write to your usual supplier of X-ray equipment and ask if he has a model made to WHO's BRS specifications. Note the screen protecting the operator. *Kindly contributed by Philip Palmer.*

it on a battery which you charge when you turn your generator on. It is so simple that a radiographic assistant can easily work it, but if you have a radiographer who has been trained to use a more sophisticated machine, he will not like this one because it does not give him enough freedom to adjust the settings.

The BRS machine is based on the assumptions that: (1) A good chest film needs a short exposure, and a substantial distance between the patient and the tube. (2) An X-ray of the lumbar spine will be one of the heavier exposures required. It has therefore been designed to produce at least 100 mA at 110 kV, not one or the other, but both simultaneously. It has a fixed tube-to-film distance of 140 cm, which gives satisfactory chest films and is the ideal distance for most other investigations. The tube is fixed so that it can use an accurately focused grid of high quality. The tube and the film are always accurately focused on one another and cannot be angled independently. This makes it easy to position the patient and makes routine views exactly repeatable. The supporting arm of the tube and the film can be rotated through at least 270°, so that horizontal and vertical projections are easy, and angled views are possible. Erect views of the skull, sinuses, shoulders, or abdomen are as easy as routine views of the chest. A radiographer's manual is available; so is a manual of radiography to go with the machine.

Palmer PES, 'Manual of Radiographic Interpretation for General Practitioners',
WHO, Geneva, 1985.

1.14 How to use these manuals

You will notice that after three chapters on 'the basics' there are four on draining pus. Then comes the abdomen and hernias, followed by obstetrics, gynaecology, and the breast. After this there is the surgery of 'special departments' (proctology, urology, etc.) then some specifically tropical surgery, a long chapter on oncology, a short one on terminal care, and finaly a miscellaneous chapter. After dealing with injuries of the various regions the second volume ends with a system of closed methods for virtually all human fractures.

In writing these manuals we have tried to make both language and the typography work for us. You will see that we have divided most sections into an initial introductory, or background part in a Roman type like this paragraph, followed by didactic instructions in another typeface. You will also notice that we use the imperative, and refer to 'the patient' and then to 'he', which does in fact usually mean 'he and she'. Alas, English has no personal pronoun which includes both sexes. Our use of 'he' to include both sexes improves clarity, and shortens the text, but we owe our apologies to our lady readers!

Inevitably, we are mostly concerned with technology—*but behind all this lies the patient himself. That boy with the fractured radius and ulna waiting at the end of the queue might be our own son, that paraplegic our brother, that old lady with the fractured femur, our mother. Tomorrow, we might be that comatose patient with the extradural haematoma in the end bed. These patients are ourselves. Perhaps the thing that we most often miss is any explanation of what is going to happen to us, and any indication that anyone really cares.* One contributor considered that such an outright statement of values has no place in a technical compendium, and suggested it be deleted. Instead, believing the compassionate and devoted care of the sick to be one of the noblest human activities, and something of ultimate value for its own sake, we have put it into italic type!

One reader of one experimental edition commented that it had "...enormously improved the treatment of fractures in St Clair's hospital, Sotik...". We were delighted because that is "our scene". It also shows that these manuals can be put to good use. They contain much detailed factual information, and although we have done our best to make them as easily understandable as we can, if you want to use them to their best advantage, you will have to read them carefully.

SURGEON AND ANAESTHETIST

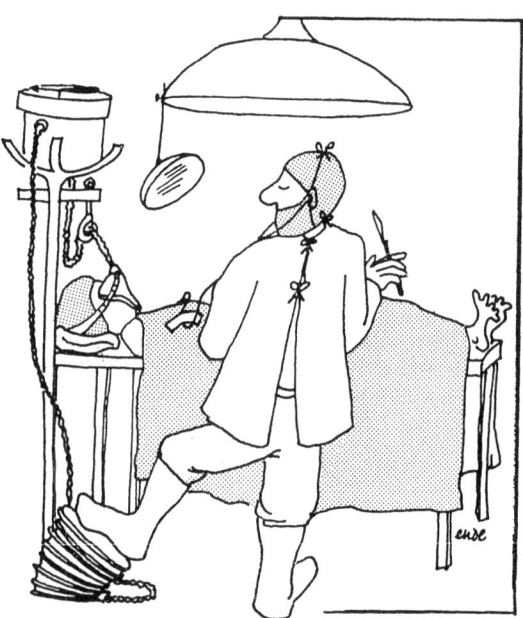

Fig. 1-9 YOU MAY HAVE TO BE SURGEON AND ANAESTHETIST. *Kindly contributed by Nette de Glanville. From the Proceedings of the Association of Surgeons of East Africa.*

A TALE OF FOUR PEOPLE, Everybody, Somebody, Anybody, and Nobody, which was found on the notice board of the Birmingham Accident Hospital. "There was an important job to be done and Everybody agreed that it was a job that could be done by Anybody. It was agreed that Somebody should be detailed off to do it, but although Anybody could have done it, it eventually got done by Nobody. Somebody got angry about it, after all (he said) it was Everybody's job. But, while Everybody thought that Anybody could do it, Nobody realized that Everybody was going to assume that Somebody was going to do it. It ended up that Everybody blamed Somebody when Nobody did what Anybody could have done. LESSON. This book is written to benefit Everybody, so that Anybody who is put in charge of surgical patients will know that Somebody cares enough to write down methods of surgery in a way that a 'Nobody' can find that he or she can do Something even if tucked away in the middle of Nowhere''.

THE PATIENTS ARE OURSELVES

HOW TO USE THESE MANUALS

IF YOU ARE A STUDENT, don't be overwhelmed by the mass of necessary detail you will find here. Don't panic, and don't try to learn it all by heart! These pages *differ enormously in importance.* Try to distinguish between what you should know, and what you can look up when necessary. You must know the emergency procedures, which there will not be time to look up. Study these early in your training. Know your way about these manuals, learn how to use them, keep them and look things up in them.

When you study anatomy, learn the anatomy of the operations we describe, because these are the ones which you will later have to do. Study the anatomical drawings listed below as part of your anatomy course.

Don't sell your dissecting manuals the moment the anatomy exam is over. You know your way about them. So keep them, tainted with the dissecting room though they may be. The ideal textbook of surgical anatomy has yet to be written, and dissecting manuals are the best so far.

Take this book to the wards, clinics, and operating theatre. How does the treatment you see given differ from that described here? The methods of examination we give are summaries only, practise them on a fellow student.

A SUGGESTED INITIAL READING LIST. Start by reading the whole of this chapter. In those which follow, read only the introductory passages in Roman type, and merely glance at the detailed didactic instructions which follow in this typeface—read these carefully later when you need to do something. Start with the common things first. We have used 7 degrees of approximate commonness: Very common, common, not uncommon, uncommon, unusual, rare and very rare. This is based on experience in East and Central Africa, but it is mostly applicable to the developing world as a whole.

Read particularly the first section of each chapter and the following: The major theatre (2.1), aseptic theatre technique (2.3), autoclaving (2.4), antibiotics in surgery (2.7 to 2.9), the control of bleeding (3.1 and 3.2), bloodless limb operations (3.9), the instruments (4.1 to 4.5), suture materials, sutures and needles (4.6 to 4.8), drains (4.9), instrument sets (4.10), 'pus' (5.1 to 5.4), empyemas (6.1), peritonitis (6.2), PID (6.6), pyomyositis (7.1), osteomyelitis (7.2 to 7.5), septic arthritis, especially the positions of rest and function (7.16), hand infections (8.1), abdominal surgery (all Chapter 9), the acute abdomen and intestinal obstruction (10.1 to 10.6), appendicitis (12.1), inguinal and femoral hernias (14.1 and 14.6)...

In Volume Two on trauma, read Chapters 51 to 54, especially Sections 54.1 to 54.3 on wounds. Read the first section in each chapter, and particularly the sections on amputations (56.1), skin grafts (57.1 to 57.5), the entire chapters on burns (Chapter 58) and fractures (Chapter 69) especially 'adequate function with minimum risk' (69.3) and bony injuries in children (69.6 and 69.6a), and catastrophes with casts (70.4). Then read about some of the more common and important injuries: dislocation of the shoulder (71.8), fractures of the humerus (71.17), dislocation of the elbow (72.4), supracondylar fractures in children (72.6), midshaft fractures of the radius and ulna (73.6), the compartment syndrome (73.7), stiffness in hand injuries (75.2), pelvic fractures (76.2), hip and femur injuries (77.2), Perkins traction (78.4), open fractures of the tibia and fibula (81.12), and malleolar fractures (82.6).

THE ABBREVIATIONS you will meet are these: AAFB, acid and alcohol fast bacilli (tubercle bacilli). AAKS, atypical African Kaposi's sarcoma (32.21). AIDS, acquired immune deficiency syndrome. BIPP, bismuth iodoform and paraffin paste (4.11). CPD, cephalopelvic disproportion (18.6). DIP, distal interphalangeal joint. PIP, proximal interphalangeal joint. MP, metacarpophalangeal joint. EIT, examination in the theatre. EUA, examination under anaesthesia. IOP, intraocular pressure. HCG, human chorionic gonadotrophin. HIV, human immunodeficiency virus. IVU, intravenous urogram, also called an intravenous pyelogram (IVP). NSAID nonsteroidal anti-inflammatory drug. PID, pelvic inflammatory disease (6.6). PPNG, penicillinase-producing *Neisseria gonorrhoeae*. PPH, postpartum haemorrhage. STD, sexually transmitted disease. VVF, vesicovaginal fistula. RVF, rectovaginal fistula.

Three capital letters in brackets, for example (TAL), refers to the addresses of the suppliers in Appendix B, in this case Talc, Teaching Aids at Low Cost.

THE MAIN ANATOMICAL DRAWINGS are: the dermatomes (A 6-8, A 7-8, 64-2), the major arteries, (3-5 etc), the scalp (63-12), the orbit (5-4), the optic discs (24-4), the cheek (61-5), the maxillary antrum (25-6), the mandibular region (5-7), the teeth (26-4 etc), the anterior abdominal wall (9-1, 23-17a), the peritoneal cavity (6-3), the biliary tract (13-29), the blood supply of the colon (66-22), the anorectum (22-1), the lower urinary tract (68-1), the relations of the ureter (20-16), the 'ligaments' of the pelvis (20-17), the peritoneal attachments in the region of the bladder (18-10), the uterine blood vessels (18-13a), the inguinal region (14-2, 14-3), the nerve supply of the hand (75-3), the bones of the hand (75-11), the tendon sheaths (8-7).

There are also the following transverse sections: the upper arm (56-8), the forearm (7-8, 73-11), the wrist (27-14a, 75-24), the hand (8-1), the finger (75-6), the thigh (7-9, 56-11), the calf (7-10, 7-11, 81-14), the ankle (27-11).

IF YOU ARE A GENERAL DUTY MEDICAL OFFICER, don't be ashamed to refer to these manuals. A patient will be more grateful for being correctly treated than for being wrongly treated because you could not remember something and had to guess! For example, you cannot possibly remember all the steps in the general method for a spinal injury (64.3), or a hand injury (75.1), so why not refer to them in front of a patient until you have examined so many patients that the necessary clinical routines become automatic? If he is difficult to diagnose, ask him to wait until the end of the clinic, and then use the routines we give here to try to diagnose him.

Keep these manuals in the theatre. If a procedure is long or difficult, sit in an armchair and study it in peace, before you try to do it. Then study it again after you have done it. Don't expect to be able to do everything we describe immediately. *Progressively extend your practice, little by little.*

Don't let things you cannot do, because you do not have the necessary equipment or drugs, prevent you from doing the things you can do.

Whenever you refer a patient, try to learn from the person you refer him to. If possible, be there when he is examined. In the same way, if someone refers a patient to you, he should be there so that you can teach him.

What methods are your staff using? For example, if medical assistants treat fractures in your hospital, study the methods they use and encourage them to use those described here. If they might find this manual useful, see that they have a copy and go through it with them.

If a patient dies and you are not sure of the diagnosis, try to get permission for a post-mortem examination.

Make good use of the endpapers and charts (A 2-4, A 5-1, A 15-4, A 15-6) you find in these manuals. Where convenient photocopy them and stick them up on the wall, or have them printed.

IF YOU ARE A SURGICAL TEACHER, try to integrate these manuals into your teaching, and base your examination questions on them. Aim, less that the students should know these manuals, than that they should know their way around them, and be prepared to use them.

A PATIENT'S RECORDS   John Moshaba ♂ 42

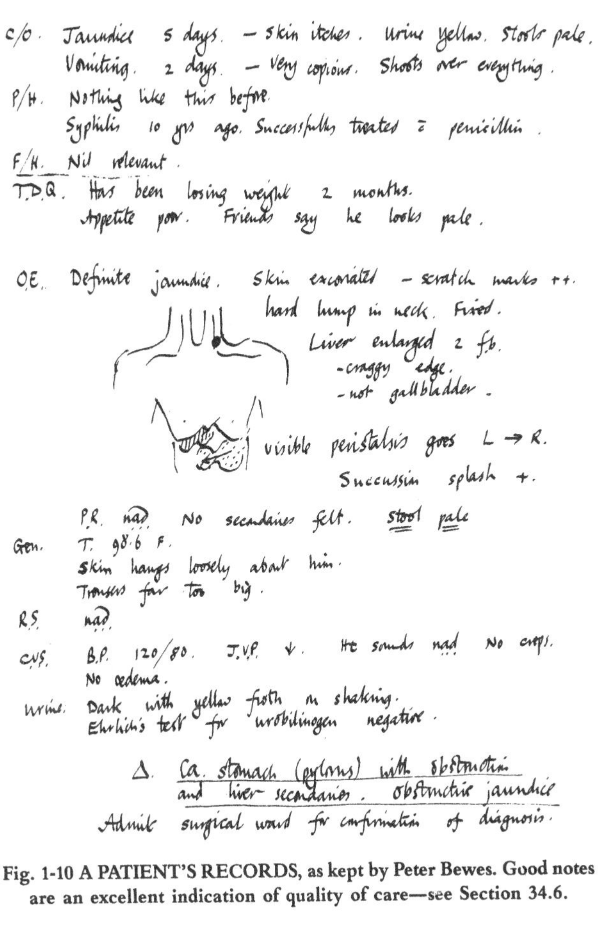

c/o. Jaundice 5 days. — skin itches. urine yellow. stools pale. Vomiting. 2 days. — Very copious. Shoots over everything.

P/H Nothing like this before. Syphilis 10 yrs ago. Successfully treated c̄ penicillin.

F/H Nil relevant.

T.D.Q. Has been losing weight 2 months. Appetite poor. Friends say he looks pale.

O.E. Definite jaundice. Skin excoriated — scratch marks ++. hard lump in neck. Fixed. Liver enlarged 2 fb. — craggy edge. — not gallbladder. visible peristalsis goes L → R. Succussion splash +.

P.R. nad. No secondaries felt. stool pale.

Gen. T. 98·6 F. Skin hangs loosely about him. Trousers far too big.

R.S. nad.

C.V.S. B.P. 120/80. J.V.P. ↓. He sounds nad No crep. No oedema.

Urine. Dark with yellow froth on shaking. Ehrlich's test for urobilinogen negative.

Δ. Ca. stomach (pylorus) with obstruction and liver secondaries. Obstructive jaundice. Admit surgical ward for confirmation of diagnosis.

Fig. 1-10 A PATIENT'S RECORDS, as kept by Peter Bewes. Good notes are an excellent indication of quality of care—see Section 34.6.

YOU TOO ARE PART OF THESE MANUALS HELP TO WRITE FURTHER EDITIONS!

One of the limitations of the project on which these manuals were written was that although it lasted 5 years in Kenya and most of another 5 in Leeds, it was not possible to do all the intensive fieldwork that would have been ideal. The result is that we do not really know what difficulties you will have with the 'handbag method for treating burns', for example, or if there are important disasters which we should have warned you about, and have not. What is missing? What is redundant? We look forward to knowing what your experiences are with the methods we describe, and to getting out the floppy discs to improve them for a second edition. Any contribution, large or small, sent to me (MHK) care of Oxford University Press will be welcome. Ideally, send an annotated copy of this manual, for which we will be happy to return you a clean one, and to include you among the contributors on the cover of the next edition. We look forward to hearing, both from 'experts' and from 'very general practitioners'!

Some TALC (TAL) slide sets on particular surgical conditions would be particularly welcome.

TRANSLATIONS of these manuals or entirely new ones covering the same field are needed in French, Spanish and Portuguese. *Primary Anaesthesia* is available in French as *Eléments d'anesthésie pratique* from Arnette, 2 rue Casimier Delavigne, 75006 Paris, France. If you are insistent enough, they might perhaps translate the other manuals.

DIFFICULTIES WITH THE REFERENCES

If you have TROUBLE LOOKING THINGS UP, this section will probably help you. You will see that section numbers have dots in them (for example, 3.6), while figures have a dash (3-6). Where, for example, we have added a section or sections, say between sections 2.3 and 2.4, we have called them 2.3a, or 2.3b etc. References with an A in them not followed by a comma, as for example (A 2.1), refer to 'Primary Anaesthesia'. An A followed by a comma, as for example (A, 2-7) refers to the first illustration in a particular figure. References to 'Primary Mother Care' have an M (M 2.1).

Some of the sections are long, and many of the problems and difficulties that you may want to look up are at the end of them. So the keywords in the 'Difficulties' are in capital letters (see immediately above), and the section number in the index has a 'D' after it. For example, 'trouble looking things up' is indexed under 1.14D. So, if there is a 'D' in an index entry, go to the 'Difficulties' end of that section.

These paragraphs of 'Difficulties' are also a convenient place for a variety of assorted information that does not fit earlier in the section. Some chapters, such as those on urology and tropical surgery have an entire final section devoted to 'other problems'—see Section 23.30 on 'Other urological problems'.

IF YOU ARE A STUDENT, LEARN THE IMPORTANT THINGS FIRST

STOP PRESS !

As we go to press, a final page of small additions has been included at the end of this manual. The most notable among them is a method for tying the uterine arteries to control bleeding from the uterus, especially in post-partum haemorrhage. They are referred to as 'Stop Press' in various places in the text.

One final word. If you get into difficulties, remember the 'Bewes manoeuvre'. Remain calm, ask an assistant to press a swab firmly on the bleeding area (or deal suitably with whatever is causing trouble). Take off your gloves, 'go and have a cup of tea', and consult these manuals. When you return in 10 minutes you will be better able to cope with the problem. Some problems, especially bleeding, may even have solved themselves meanwhile.

2 Theatres, antiseptics, and antibiotics

"It is one thing to operate with the chief at your elbow on a patient whose vital functions are being monitored by an expert anaesthetist at the head of the table. It is quite another to be almost alone at midnight, struggling with a patient in shock from a ruptured ectopic pregnancy, as the light fades in and out while a superannuated generator tries to function on adulterated diesel oil. Then is the moment of truth when you realize that an excellent theoretical foundation is not the only thing you need..."

Gerald Hankins, The Shanta Bahwan Hospital, Kathmandu, Nepal

2.1 The major theatre

Although aseptic surgery has been done in a tent, under a tree, or on a kitchen table, it is safer if it is done in a room which has been designed to preserve the sterility of the surgical field, to make surgical routines easier, and to prevent mistakes. The difficulty with aseptic methods is that they require an autoclave. If you don't have one, we describe an antiseptic method that you can use instead (2.6). You will need two theatres, a major one and a minor septic one (2.2). We are concerned here with the major one.

When you start work in a theatre, look at it carefully. How many of the desirable features that we are about to describe does it have? Is there anything which you could do to make it safer or more efficient?

THE STERILE ZONE

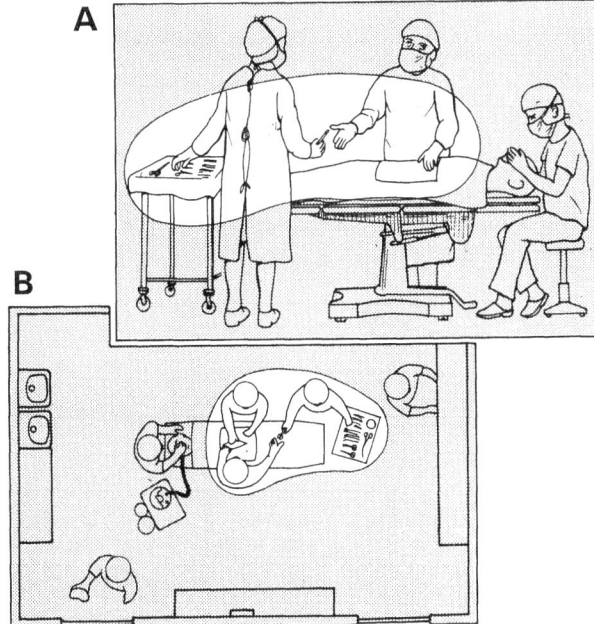

FIG. 2-1 STERILE AND UNSTERILE ZONES IN A THEATRE. A, the sterile zone in a vertical dimension. B, the sterile zone in a horizontal dimension. The sterile zone contains the operation site, the instrument trolley and the three scrubbed up members of the surgical team. The unsterile zone comprises everything else in the theatre. The great danger, when technique is poor, is for the sterile zone to become smaller and smaller as the operation progresses.

The operating team should be as small as possible. It consists of: (1) Yourself the surgeon. (2) Your assistant, when you need one. (3) The scrub nurse responsible for the instruments. (4) The circulating nurse to fetch and carry. (5) The anaesthetist. (6) His assistant, if he has one. Two other people are important: (a) The theatre charge nurse responsible for organizing the theatre, and who in a smaller hospital will take a turn at being on call. And (b) the 'theatre dresser' who is less educated, but, unlike the nurses who come and go, has spent his whole career in the theatre, and so knows its routines and where things are.

In an emergency roles (2) and (3) can be combined in an efficient nurse or medical assistant, and so can roles (4) and (6). The first three members of the team are 'sterile', the last three are not. An important part of the drill is to prevent the last three from compromising the sterility of the first three, and the surgical field.

Two zones in the theatre ensure this. There is : (1) A sterile zone which includes the operation site, the first three members of the team, and that part of the theatre immediately around them. (2) An unsterile zone which usually includes the head end of the patient, and the rest of the theatre. The last three members of the team can move freely in this zone. The patient's entrance and the access to the sluice room are continuous with it. A separate room for scrubbing up is not essential, and it can be done in the theatre in two domestic pattern sinks with draining boards. They should be fitted with elbow taps which are *very highly desirable*, although you can scrub up from a bucket.

Adequate space is essential, so that staff can move freely within their zones, and without touching one another. Space is needed for manoeuvering and parking the patient's stretcher next the operating table, and for parking trolleys without congestion. Twenty-five square metres is the absolute minimum, a room 5×6.5 m (32 m^2) is better, and 42 m^2 is ideal. The more equipment you have in the theatre the more space you need, and in the developed world or in a central hospital 64 m^2 is normal. If the case load is heavy, a second theatre is usually considered more useful than making the first one unduly large.

Straightforward physical cleanliness is important. Sophisticated methods are unnecessary. Sluicing the floor between cases, washing the walls weekly and mobile equipment daily will ensure a high enough standard without using antiseptics on the theatre itself. The floor is important. The most dangerous sources of infection are pus and excreta from the patients, which must be cleared away between every operation, and must not be allowed to contaminate the theatre. To make this easier, it should have a terrazzo floor, but a smooth concrete finish is almost as good and much cheaper. To make it easier to wash down, it should have a 1:1000 slope towards an open channel along the foot of the wall at the unsterile end of the theatre. This channel should have a plugged outlet leading directly outside to an open gulley. Fit a sparge pipe to the wall at the sterile end 150 mm above the floor, so that the whole floor can be flooded by turning a tap. A little dust on trolley wheels or shoes, or from open windows, is less dangerous than is generally believed.

The walls of the theatre should be smooth, but they need not be tiled. A sand and cement backwash application painted with one coat of emulsion and two coats of eggshell gloss is adequate. Gloss paint is satisfactory for the walls, and the fewer the doors, sills, ledges, crevices, mouldings, architraves, and window boards,

THE THEATRE AND ITS TABLE

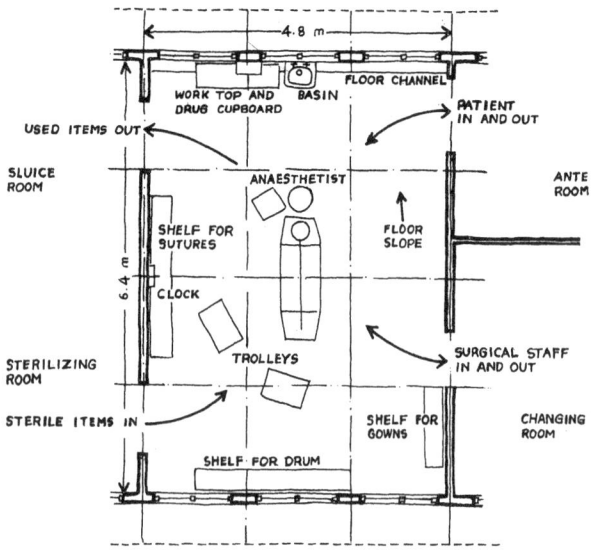

A simple operating table

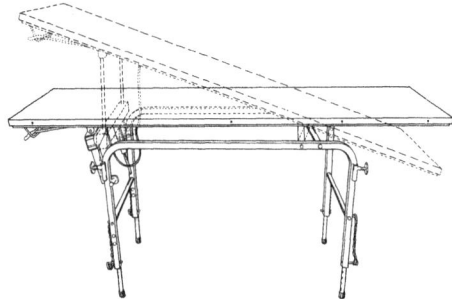

Fig. 2-2 A SIMPLE THEATRE AND ITS TABLE. This is about the smallest practical theatre. Figure 2-3 shows the various ways in which it can be provided with a sterilizing room, an anteroom and changing rooms. B, the simple pattern operating table described in the text. A, adapted from 'Design for Medical Buildings' with the kind permission of the African Medical and Research Foundation (AMREF).

the better. Every time a door is opened, dust from the floor is whirled into the room. There is no need for a door between the changing rooms and the theatre. A door is only needed between the sluice and sterilizing room, if these rooms will be used when the theatre is not.

The ceiling should be at least 3.5 metres high and the roof timbers solid enough to support an operating light. It should also have a pair of 2 metre fluorescent tubes.

The ambient level of illumination should be high, so make the windows big enough. They may enable most operations to be done by daylight. There should be a window of 5 m² at the head and the foot ends, facing north and south shaded by a roof overhang of at least 800 mm. Even better are windows on three sides. Fit ordinary low windows, and frost only the panes below eye level, so that the staff can look out (which improves morale), but that anyone looking in can only see their heads, not the patient. In the tropics avoid windows in the roof.

Don't have more shelves than you need, but keep the things you need daily nearby; use trolleys where you can. When shelves are needed, set them 50 mm away from the wall on metal rods, so that they can be lifted away for ease of cleaning. All shelves should be at least a metre high so that trolleys can be pushed under them. The glove shelf should be at least 1.2 m high, so that you can keep your hands higher than your elbows to prevent water running back down over your now dry hands. The anaesthetist needs a small lockable cupboard, a trolley, and also a worktop near the patient's head. Ideally, he also needs a sink. Electric sockets should be 1.5 m above the floor to minimize the danger of igniting explosive gases.

The preparation room should lead off the theatre. A big one is desirable, because it needs to contain two autoclaves, a big and a small sterilizer, sterile packs, instrument cupboards and space to lay out instrument trolleys. Ideally, it should be 64 m² and serve two theatres. About 25 m² is the absolute minimum, with a terrazzo shelf round most of two walls, a sink, a draining board, a single vertical autoclave (preferably two), a large boiling water sterilizer standing on the floor, and a small one on the bench.

• OPERATING TABLE, simple pattern, (NES) each $240, one only. At the time of writing this table has to be made to order. The minimum requirements of an operating table are that: (1) You must be able to tilt the patient's head down rapidly for the Trendelenburg position, and if he vomits (A 3.1, A 16.2). (2) You should be able to adjust its height. This table does these things at a fraction of the cost of the standard hydraulic ones, which need careful maintenance, and are useless when their hydraulic seals perish. However, if a simple general purpose hydraulic table is well maintained, it lasts a long time. A really sophisticated one can cost as much as the entire building of the theatre. A dirty table is a menace, so make sure yours is kept clean.

If the head of your table does not tilt head down, get one that does. Meanwhile, in an emergency, you can put a low stool under the bar at its foot. If it does not tilt from side to side, make a wooden wedge to fit under the mattress. If it does not have a kidney bridge and you want one (most surgeons don't use them now), use folded plastic covered pillows.

Locally made 'Chogoria' supports (15-3) are a useful addition to a standard table. They are made of two suitably bent pieces of pipe which fit into the holes for ordinary stirrups and keep the patient's hips widely abducted, and his hips and knees moderately flexed, so that his lower legs are horizontal. His legs rest on boards attached to these pipes. These supports are more comfortable than stirrups and are particularly useful for such operations as tubal ligation.

• ALTERNATIVE OPERATING TABLE, as Seward minor (SEW), or equivalent, one only. This is slightly more versatile and considerably more expensive than the table above.

• MATTRESS, for operating table, (a) one only, with (b) three mackintosh covers only. A dirty mattress is a potentially serious source of infection. So swab the cover after each patient, and replace it regularly.

• ARM BOARD, for operating table, locally made, one only. This is simply a piece of hardwood about $20 \times 120 \times 1000$ mm, which you push under the mattress to rest the patient's arm on, when you want to inject it.

• STOOL, operating, adjustable for height, local manufacture, two only. If you do much operating, a chair with a padded seat, wheels, and a back greatly reduces fatigue.

• LIGHT, operating theatre, simple pattern, preferably with sockets to take bayonet or screw fitting domestic pattern light bulbs, in addition to special bulbs, state voltage, one only. Most operating theatre lights take bulbs which are irreplaceable locally, and may cost $70 each, so find out what bulbs your light takes, and try to keep at least three spares. Record their specification and catalogue number somewhere on the lamp casing. When new lights are ordered, they should have fittings that can, if necessary, take ordinary domestic bulbs.

• CLOCK, wall, electric, with second hand, one only. This is essential, you must have a proper awareness of time, especially when you apply a tourniquet (3-11), and without a clock you can readily forget it. The instructions given here for controlling bleeding by applying pressure sometimes tell you to wait 5 minutes by the clock.

• SPOTLIGHT, free standing on the floor, 'Anglepoise' type, to take ordinary domestic pattern bulbs, state voltage, two only. Also, high efficiency internally reflecting bulb to give a parallel beam, five only. This is necessary, both as a standby to the main theatre lamp, and to illuminate positions that the main threatre light cannot reach. A spotlight can direct an undesirable amount of heat into the wound, so, if possible, it needs one of the new high efficiency bulbs which produce little heat, and yet fit ordinary bulb sockets. These are more expensive initially, but have a longer life. You can improvise a spotlight by removing the headlight of a car, especially the sealed beam type, and attaching it to a drip stand in the theatre. Connect it with a long lead to the battery of a car outside. Or use a slide projector held by an assistant. If the level of illumination is not enough, especially for eye surgery, you can increase the contrast by blacking out the theatre.

• SOLAR PANEL, charger, and battery, one only of each. A single solar panel will collect a useful quantity of electricity and enable you to light two wards in the evenings.

• BATTERY CHARGER for the common sizes of rechargeable dry batteries, and five rechargeable batteries of each size, one outfit only. This

IMPROVISED LIGHTING

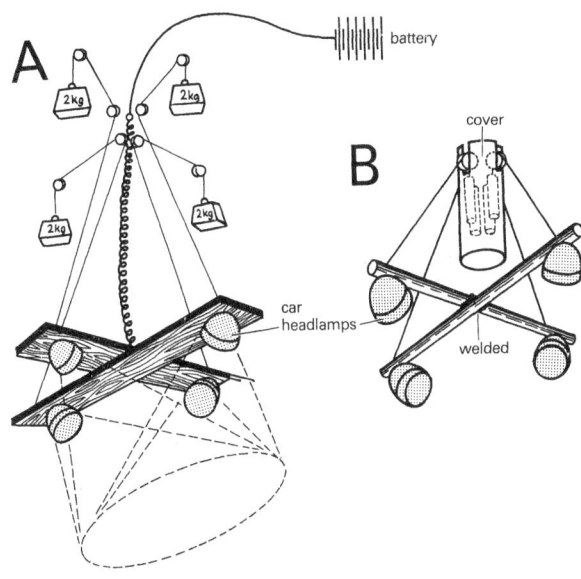

Fig. 2-3 IMPROVISED LIGHTING. A, if you have to make a light locally, suspend 4 car headlights on a cross, and suspend each end of it on a pulley counterbalanced with a weight. B, better, put the counterweights in a metal casing which will be easier to keep clean. Or, less satisfactorily, hang three fluorescent tubes from the ceiling in the form of a triangle.

SOME SURGICAL LAYOUTS

A

The bare minimum with ante-room and changing room

B

The recommended pattern

C

The recommended pattern with a minor theatre

D

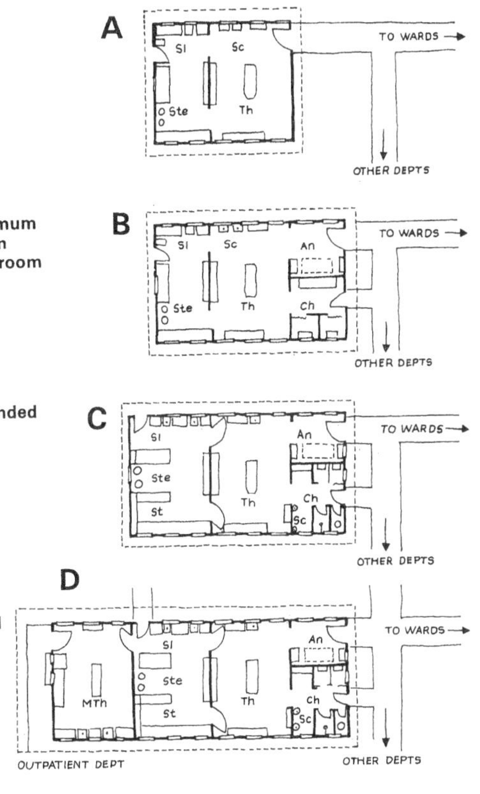

Fig. 2-4 SOME SURGICAL LAYOUTS. This incorporates the theatre in Fig. 2-2 in progressively more developed settings. A, is the absolute minimum. The changing is done in the sterilizing room. B, is similar but has an anteroom and staff changing room. C, is the arrangement recommended, but is 2 or 3 times the cost of A. The sterilizing room is large enough to prepare sterile items for the rest of the hospital. There is also a changing room with shower and toilet. D, shows the further addition of a minor theatre. Th, main theatre. Mth, minor theatre. An, anteroom. Sl, sluice. Ste, sterilizing. *Adapted from 'Design from Medical Buildings' with the kind permission of the African Medical and Research Foundation (AMREF).*

will enable you to recharge batteries for your torches and laryngoscopes etc.

• *INSTRUMENT CABINET glass door, sides and shelves, 1300×600×400 mm, local manufacture, one only.*

• *X-RAY VIEWING BOX, standard pattern, local manufacture, one only.*

• *TROLLEY, instrument, without guard rail, with two stainless steel shelves, antistatic rubber castors, (a) 600×450 mm, three only. (b) 900×450 mm, one only.* Glass shelves ultimately break, so stainless steel ones are better. A larger table will make it easier to lay up for larger cases, especially orthopaedic ones.

• *STAND, solution, with antistatic rubber tyred castors, complete with two 350 mm stainless steel bowls, side by side, one only.* Put water in one bowl, and use the other for spare instruments and the sucker. The bowls can be sterilized in the autoclave or in a boiling water sterilizer.

• *DRIP stands, telescopic, two only* Or, less satisfactorily, use long wire hooks suspended from the ceiling near the head of the table. Hooks for drips sticking out from the wall are useful above some beds in the wards.

Mein P, and Jorgenson T, 'Design for Medical Buildings', AMREF, Box 30125, Nairobi.

2.2 The minor theatre

A minor theatre for septic cases will help to maintain the sterility of the major theatre. Use it for draining all abscesses, for skin grafting and for the closed reduction of fractures. It will need a simple operating table which tips (A 3-1), and a second set of basic anaesthetic equipment, including especially a sucker and the equipment for resuscitation. It will also need two minor sets (4.12), three incision and drainage sets, and a set for drilling for osteomyelitis. If possible the minor theatre should have its own instruments and not be supplied from the main one.

2.2a Health centre theatres

The focus of this system of surgery is the district hospital where, inevitably, most of the surgery that is needed in the developing world has to be done (1-6). There is however some surgery that can and should be done by medical assistants in a health centre. This has been described by Peter Bewes in the manual described below. Surgery can also be done in a health centre by a visiting 'surgeon' and is particularly valuable for tubal ligation (15.4).

Bewes P, 'Surgery', TALC Teaching Aids at Low Cost, The Institute of Child Health, 30 Guilford Street, London WC1N 1EH. Also from AMREF Box 30125 Nairobi.

2.3 Aseptic theatre technique

In order of importance, the most serious sources of infection in a theatre are bacteria from: (1) The pus and excreta left behind by previous patients, especially on its equipment or towels, etc. (3) The clothes, hands, skin, mouths, or perineums of the staff; the bacteria on them may have been derived from other patients. (4) The patient himself.

Minimize the risk of infection by: (1) Following the design rules in the previous section as far as you can. (2) Keeping the theatre as clean as possible, so that the pus and excreta of previous patients are removed. (3) Making sure that the autoclaving is done conscientiously. (4) Following the rules about the indications for operating, the timing of operations, wound closure (54.2), and careful tissue handling. (5) Creating and maintaining the sterile zone in Fig. 2-1.

This sterile zone has to be created anew for each patient in a theatre in which the risk of infection has been reduced as much as possible. Its creation starts when a nurse swabs the top of a trolley with antiseptic, puts two sterile towels on it and lays out sterile gowns and gloves. The sterile zone grows as the surgeon, his assistant and the scrub nurse put on their gowns. The operation site joins the sterile zone as it is prepared with an antiseptic solution and draped. Thereafter, nothing which is contaminated must touch anything in this zone until the end of the operation. If the technique of the team is poor, the sterile zone becomes smaller and smaller as the operation proceeds.

WOUND SEPSIS AND THE ART OF SURGERY Professor IJP Loefler speaks in the reference given below: 'In summary, I believe that regard for tissue is the foremost of our priorities. Let us strive to become first class surgeons, and let us train considerate disciplined theatre staff. Let us have plenty of soap and water, or some not too corrosive detergent. We do need sterilizers and autoclaves. We need well ventilated rooms which are light and easy to clean, and where the number of additional items is kept low. We should don theatre attire, should indeed change frequently, and should certainly change our masks. Gloves are important though not indispensable. Use sharp knives, few instruments and keep things neat and clean. Do not bury undue amounts of biologically irritating material in the tissues. Beware of haematomas and lymph collections. Use suction drains frequently. Use delayed primary closure where this is indicated (54.4). In the wounds you make yourself bring the skin edges together carefully so that the wound is sealed in a few hours. Hydrate your patient, and do not oversedate him. Avoid stasis by elevation and movement. Use dressings sparingly, and observe the wound. If you find a haematoma and evacuate it speedily you will prevent sepsis'.

Loefler IJP, 'Wound sepsis and the art of surgery', Proceedings of the Association of Surgeons of East Africa 1979;2:172-180

- SUITS, *theatre, cotton, with short sleeved shirt, and long trousers, assorted sizes, local manufacture, 30 only.* The purpose of these is to make sure that nobody enters the theatre in his ordinary clothes, or in clothes which he has worn elsewhere in the hospital. Everyone entering a theatre should put on a theatre suit in the changing room. These suits should be laundered, and if possible ironed, but need not normally be sterilized each time they are used, unless they have been used for septic cases.

- CLOGS, *assorted sizes, ten pairs only.* Rubber boots are outmoded; sandals are less easy to keep clean and less comfortable than clogs. Change into them at the barrier between the theatre and the rest of the hospital.

- APRONS, *macintosh, assorted sizes, local manufacture, eight only.* These protect the suits and are worn under a theatre gown. If they are merely hung up in the changing room after use, they become progressively more contaminated and more dangerous. So make sure that they are at least washed and regularly swabbed down with an antiseptic solution, and are always swabbed after septic cases. Keep two for special clean cases only.

- CAPS, *cotton, 30 only.* Put on a cap before you enter the theatre, and make sure it completely covers your hair.

- MASKS, *theatre, 100 only.* Make these from 4 layers of muslin. A mask must cover your nose; if it fogs your glasses, arrange its top edge, so that your breath does not drift upwards, or, rub your glasses with ordinary soap and polish them. Use a new mask for each major case.

- GOWNS, *cotton, 50 only.* These should go right round the wearer and cover his back. Before sterilisation they must always be folded so that the inner surface of the wearer is exposed to the outside in the drum.

- GLOVES, *operating, reusable, (a) Size 6, 20 pairs. (b) Size 6½, 40 pairs. (c) Size 7, 40 pairs. (d) Size 7½, 40 pairs. (e) Size 8, 20 pairs only.* Remember that gloves are designed to protect the surgeon as much as the patient. The type of gloves you buy is critically important, and so is the relative number of the various sizes. They must be capable of being resterilized many times. Most nurses wear size 6½ and most doctors size 7 or 7½. Pack each pair in a cloth or paper envelope, one glove on each side with its cuff turned outwards. Gloves are more useful to protect you and the next patient, than the patient you are actually operating on. If necessary, you can operate without gloves, so don't let the absence of gloves prevent you doing a life-saving operation.

- GLOVES *industrial, three pairs only.* These are useful for picking up hot objects, and used on the correct indications will save many pairs of surgical gloves.

- GLOVE POWDER, *absorbable, 3 kg only.* Don't use starch or talc because it causes granulomas. Put the powder into little gauze bags which can be used as shakers, or use small pieces of paper.

- SOAP, *hexachlorophene, carbolic, 50 tablets only.* If necessary, the cheapest soap that does not irritate the skin will do.

- BRUSHES, *nylon, nesting, autoclavable, 50 only.* Autoclave several of these each operating day and store them between cases in a bowl of antiseptic solution. They will last longer if you merely keep them clean and immerse them in an antiseptic solution.

- TOWELS, *cotton, green, theatre. (a) Hand towels 25 cm square, 100 only. (b) Theatre drapes 100 × 75 cm, 100 only. (c) Abdominal sheets, ten only.* An abdominal sheet covers a patient completely from head to foot and has a slit in it through which the operation is done. The upper end

acts as a guard which keeps the patient's head and the anaesthetist out of the operative field.

- OTHER SUPPLIES, *(1) Pyjamas and pyjama trousers, 20 only. (2) Dresses, 20 only. (3) Macintosh drapes, 75×100 cm, 20 only. (4) Squeegees, two only. (5) Bucket and mop, three only.*

ASEPTIC TECHNIQUE

ENTERING THE THEATRE. Anyone entering the theatre must change, in the changing room, into clogs or sandals and into a suit. Decide which operations need gowns, gloves or masks.

SCRUBBING UP. Adjust the elbow taps to deliver water at a comfortable temperature. In most tropical countries only a cold water tap is necessary. Wet your hands, apply a little soap or detergent, and work up a good lather. Rub your hands and forearms to 5 cm above your elbows for one complete minute. Wash your forearms.

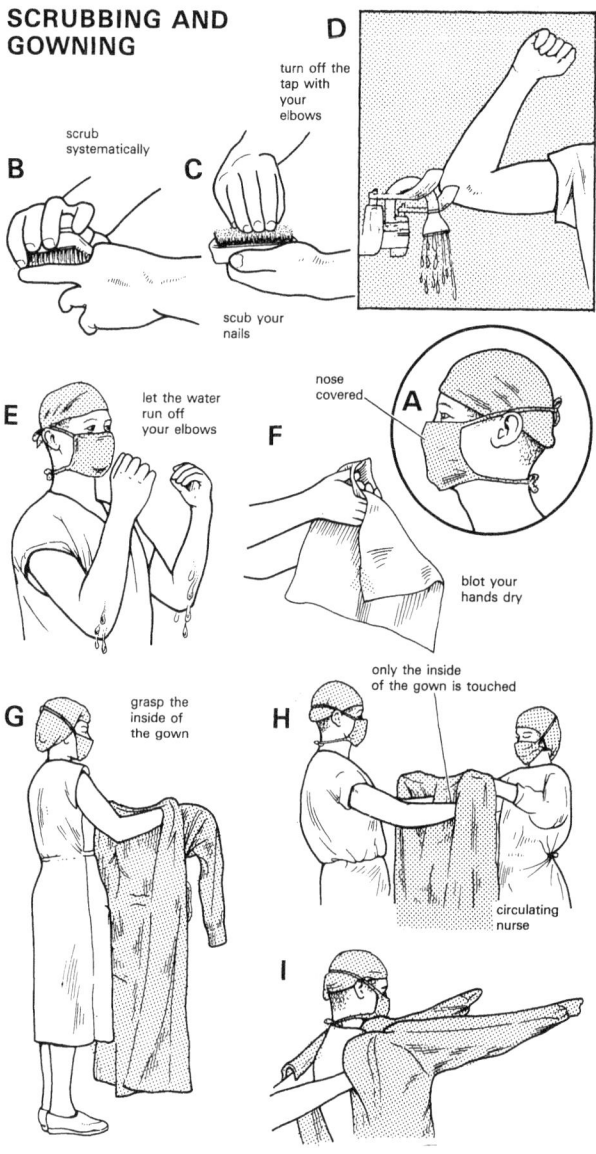

Fig. 2-5 SCRUBBING AND GOWNING. A, make sure your cap covers your nose. B, scrub your hands in a systematic manner. C, scrub your nails. D, turn off the taps with your elbow. E, while your hands are wet, hold them higher than your elbows. F, blot your hands on one corner of the towel, then dry your forearms. G, hold the gown away from your body, high enough not to touch the floor. H, ask the circulating nurse to grasp the inner sides of the gown at each shoulder and pull it over your shoulders (I).

Then take a sterile brush and put soap on it. Scrub the lateral side of your left thumb, then its medial side, then the lateral and medial aspects of each successive finger. Scrub your nails, and then the back and front of your left hand. Do the same with your right hand. Scrub for 5 minutes in all.

Alternatively, some surgeons merely scrub their nails, unless they have got ingrained dirt from some other dirty task, and then thoroughly wash their hands and arms to their elbows.

Rinse the suds from your hands while holding them higher than your elbows. Turn off the taps with your elbows.

Dry your hands with a sterile towel before you put on a sterile gown. Dry your hands first, then your forearms. Grasp the folded towel with the fingers of both hands, then step clear, so that you don't touch anything with the open towel. Blot your hands on one corner, then dry your forearms. Try not to bring a wet (unsterile) part of the towel back to a dry area.

GOWNING. Hold the gown away from your body, high enough to be well above the floor. Allow it to drop open, put your arms into the arm holes while keeping your arms extended. Then flex your elbows and abduct your arms. Wait for the circulating nurse to help you. She will grasp the inner sides of the gown at each shoulder and pull them over your shoulders.

GLOVING. Dust your hands with powder and rub them together to spread it. Be careful to touch only the inner surface of the gloves. Grasp the palmar aspect of the turned down cuff of a glove, and pull it on to your opposite hand. Leave its cuff for the moment.

Put the fingers of your already gloved hand under the inverted cuff of the other glove, and pull it on to your bare hand. It is a good routine to wash your gloved hands in sterile water to remove the powder.

Now help the next person who has gowned on with their gloves.

THE OPERATION SITE

SHAVING. The operation site should be socially clean before the operation, and you may have to check this. There is usually no need to shave a patient. If you shave him, do so on the morning of the operation, or as part of the operation. If you shave him a day or two before, minute abrasions in his skin will become infected and the risk of wound infection will increase. If hair is going to get in the way, all you need to do is to clip it short immediately before the operation.

PREPARATION. Do this as soon as the patient is anaesthetized. Start with a soapy solution, and follow this with spirit. Or, better, if there is a low sensitivity to iodine in the community (as in most of Africa), use alcoholic iodine (2.5). Take a sterile swab on a holder, start in the middle of the operation site, and work outwards. Discard both swab and holder, and repeat the process with a second swab (some surgeons use a third). The spirit will evaporate to leave the skin dry. Some surgeons consider this is over-elaborate, and merely use a single application of iodine.

Be sure to prepare a wide enough area of skin. In an abdominal operation this should extend from the patient's nipple line to below his groin.

DRAPING. Wait until he is anaesthetized. Place the first towel across the lower end of the operation site. Place another across its nearer edge. Apply a towel clip at their intersection. Place another towel across the opposite edge of the site, and finally one across its upper edge. Clip them at their intersections. If necessary, grip his skin with the clips, or secure the towels with a stitch. Alternatively, drape him with two longitudinal towels clipped at each end, with a towel above and below. Then, in an abdominal operation, cover his whole abdomen with an abdominal sheet with a narrow quadrangular hole in it.

If important areas near the surgeon become contaminated, cover them with fresh sterile towels.

SWABS AND PACKS. Use 10 cm gauze squares on spongeholding forceps ('swabs on sticks'). You will also need abdominal packs.

CLEANING THE THEATRE. Clean it thoroughly after each day's list, and completely every week.

CLEANING INSTRUMENTS. Use an old nail brush. Open hinged instruments fully, scrub them, and take special care to clean their jaws and serrations.

DIFFICULTIES WITH ASEPTIC METHODS

If you have NO GLOVES or very few gloves, scrub up and then rinse your hands and arms in alcoholic chlorhexidine (2.6). The alcohol will dehydrate your skin. You can reduce this by adding 1% glycerol to the solution. Unfortunately, although antiseptics may help to protect the patient, they are less effective in protecting you from AIDS (28a.4).

If you have NO DRAPES OR GOWNS or very few of them, use plastic sheets and aprons and soak them in an antiseptic solution (2.6).

If you TEAR OR CONTAMINATE A GLOVE during an operation, remove it. Grasp its cuff from the outside, and pull it down over your palm. Ideally, don't remove the glove yourself, because you will contaminate your other hand. Instead, hold out your hand to the circulating nurse, who will grasp the edge of the cuff and pull it off. In practice most circulating nurses are too nervous to do this, so you will have to do it yourself by touching the outer side of the cuff only.

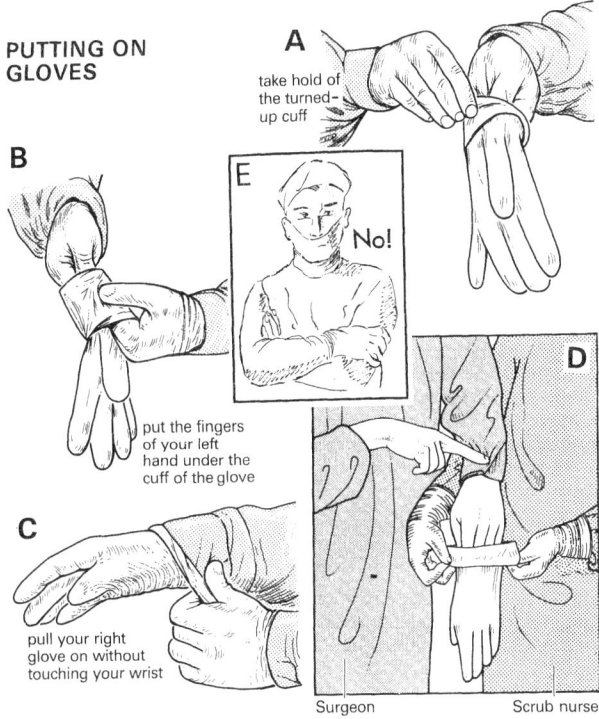

Fig. 2-6 PUTTING ON GLOVES. A, take hold of the inside of the glove with your right hand, and put your left hand into it. B, put the fingers of your left hand under the cuff of the glove. C, pull your right glove on without touching your wrist. D, the first person to glove up (usually the scrub nurse) now gloves the second person (usually the surgeon), by holding out his gloves for him like this. E, How *not* to wear your mask! Don't put your left hand in your axilla—it is not a sterile area, even after gowning. E, *after Ian Donald, 'Practical Obstetric Problems'. Lloyd-Luke, with kind permission.*

2.4 Boiling and autoclaving

Sterilization is the total destruction of all forms of life, including bacterial spores. It is best done with heat, either dry heat in an oven, or steam under pressure in an autoclave. Processes (usually chemical) which do not destroy spores are termed 'disinfection'. Some of the most important agents to be removed by disinfection are HIV and HBV (hepatitis virus B). All the disinfectants described in Section 2.5 will do this if used as directed. The most suitable one for many purposes is hypochlorite, which is described in Chapter 28a.

The basis of aseptic surgery is to kill all micro-organisms on all instruments and dressings, preferably by exposure to steam under pressure. If this is impractical, immersion in boiling water for 10 minutes at sea level will kill all viruses and all vegetative bacteria, but not spores, particularly those of tetanus and gas gangrene. A boiling water 'sterilizer' is therefore badly named. At a height of 3000 metres water boils at 90°C and is much less effective.

Steam is the gaseous form of water. If it is to sterilize effectively, which means killing all spores: (1) It must be at an appropriate temperature (which implies an appropriate pressure). (2) It must be saturated with water. (3) It must not be mixed with air, so it must displace all the air in the chamber of the autoclave. And, (4) it must reach all parts of the load. If it contains droplets of water, it will soak into porous materials. If, on the other hand, it is superheated and therefore too dry, it will be less effective as a sterilizing agent. If air is mixed with steam: (1) the temperature of the mixture at a given pressure will be lower, (2) it will penetrate less well into porous materials, (3) the air may separate as a lower, cooler layer in the bottom of the chamber, so that the contents are not sterilized. If no air is discharged, the bottom of the chamber may be much cooler than the top.

As soon as the chamber of an autoclave is full of steam at the desired temperature and pressure, it must be held there for a critical time—the holding time. The standard holding time is 15 minutes, at 121°C, but you will need to vary it as described below. This temperature is reached at a pressure of about 1 kg/cm^2 (15 pounds per square inch). An easy minimum figure to remember is '1 kg per square cm for 15 minutes' ('15 pounds for 15 minutes'). If your autoclave is rated to 1.3 kgcm^2, you can shorten the sterilizing time to 10 minutes. Here we only discuss the simpler forms of autoclave; high vacuum autoclaves are beyond the scope of this manual.

Single walled autoclaves are strong metal chambers with water in the bottom, like large pressure cookers. They have several disadvantages: (1) The air in the chamber is removed by steam rising from the bottom. This is inefficient, so that an undesirable quantity of air remains. (2) They don't have thermometers at the bottom of the chamber, so you never know what the temperature there is. (3) The load remains moist after sterilization, which can be dangerous, because bacteria can more easily enter through moist wrappings.

Double walled autoclaves can be vertical, but are much better horizontal. They should either have an effective prevacuum, or a pulsing system (neither described here), or rely entirely on gravity to displace the air. A *partial* prevacuum at the start of the sterilizing cycle (which used to be the practice in some older autoclaves) causes turbulence when air is admitted, so that the gravity displacement of air cannot take place satisfactorily.

Steam is generated in, or admitted to, a jacket round the chamber, rather than in the chamber itself. This jacket keeps the walls of the chamber hot, which prevents condensation and helps to dry the load. Steam enters the chamber through a pipe at the top and displaces the air it contains. Air, condensate, and excess steam escape through a pipe at the bottom. This pipe has a thermometer in it to record the temperature in the bottom of the autoclave. In some autoclaves a water pump, which works on the same principle as an ordinary laboratory water pump, sucks out some of the steam afterwards (postvacuum). There is also a means of admitting sterile air to break the vacuum at the end of the cycle.

The drain at the bottom of the chamber should have a 'near-to-steam trap', which will alllow the discharge of condensate and air, and will close automatically when they have been discharged, and the trap meets live steam, thus avoiding the need to close valve 13 in Fig 2-7 manually, which could spoil sterilization.

The thermometer records the temperature in the chamber drain, which is the coolest part of the autoclave. When this reaches the operating temperature, the timing of sterilization can begin.

More sophisticated autoclaves have better pumps, a recording thermometer, a thermocouple to measure the temperature of the load, and an automatic control system.

Inadequate sterilization is an important cause of wound sepsis in poorly maintained theatres. There are many pitfalls. Start by inspecting your equipment and taking an interest in it. Read the maker's instructions carefully, and make sure: (1) That it has been properly fitted and tested. For example, if a water ejector pump is fitted, it is likely to need a water pressure of 1.5 kg/cm^2. (2) That all the staff who use it understand how it works, and how to use it effectively. They must realize the importance of packing the drums loosely, the need to discharge the air, and the correct holding time.

Most of the hospitals for which we write don't have piped steam supplies. If so, you will will have to use a vertical autoclave. You will probably have electricity, but it is likely to be unreliable, so you will want one which can be heated by electricity, or by putting a kerosine pressure heater or a charcoal stove under it. Unfortunately, we have not been able to find such an 'all-fuels' autoclave, but Jacob White (WHI, see Appendix B), will consider making one if the demand is high enough (write to them). If you raise an ordinary vertical electric autoclave on bricks so that you can get a pressure heater under it, you are likely to harm the electric cables to the elements. Unfortunately, there is no WHO specification for a district hospital autoclave, as there is for an X-ray machine (1.13).

• *AUTOCLAVE, horizontal, downward displacement with near-to-steam trap in the chamber drain, post vacuum, six spare gaskets, three spare bellows for the steam trap, and a triple set of other spares, one outfit only.* If you have a steam supply, this is the autoclave you need. Horizontal autoclaves are easier to use, but are more expensive. You will need a standby, in case the electricity fails, so you should have an autoclave that can be heated by kerosene or gas somewhere in the hospital (see below).

• *Alternatively, AUTOCLAVE, vertical, downward displacement, 350 mm, 2½ drum, electric, 6 kw, state voltage, manual operation, with six spare elements, six spare gaskets, and a triple set of other spares as necessary, one outfit only.*

• *AUTOCLAVE, vertical, 350 mm, 2½ drum, for heating by kerosene or gas, manual operation, with six spare gaskets, and a triple set of spares as necessary, one outfit only.* This is for use in emergency, see above.

• *AUTOCLAVE, vertical, 'pressure cooker', 47 l, UNICEF, as (WIS) No.1941, one only (optional).* This is UNICEF's large autoclave which can be heated on a stove and has a machined lid so that it needs no gaskets. It is large enough for 5 litres of intravenous solution, or one laparotomy pack. It is a useful standby. It has an air exhaust tube which leads from the exhaust port to the bottom of the sterilizer. If you use it, you can start timing as soon as steam comes from the exhaust.

• *HEATER, kerosene, pressure, 'Primus' pattern or equivalent, four burners, with 20 spare jets, prickers and washers, two only.* Use this to heat the autoclave, either regularly or in an emergency.

• *TUBES, Browne's, for testing autoclaves, Type one (black spot), for use with ordinary steam sterilizers below 126°C, 100 tubes only.* These change colour on the basis of time and temperature, and are reliable, provided that there is not a long drying cycle, when prolonged heat in a jacketed sterilizer could change their colour.

• *Alternatively, CARDS, autoclave testing, ATI 'Steam-clox' 25 rolls only.* This brand of tape changes colour on the basis of moisture and temperature, to indicate that something has been autoclaved. Most other brands of autoclave tape are only suitable for high pre-vacuum autoclaves, not for the downward displacement ones described here. Another alternative is 'Diack Controls', a pellet in a glass tube which melts at 121 or 126°C.

• *DRUMS, deep, 340×230 mm, ten only.* This is the standard size of drum.

• *DRUMS, shallow, 340×120 mm, ten only.* These are half-size drums. You may have difficulty getting drums because they are no longer used in the developed world. If you are short of drums, sterilize your equipment in packs, covered by two layers of towelling and preferably an outer layer of paper. If you are sterilizing without paper, use all equipment warm straight from the autoclave.

• *DRESSING BOXES, stainless steel, with hinged lid and perforated sliding shutters at front and back, 250×200×150 mm, three only.* Use these for sterilizing gloves and dressings.

AUTOCLAVES

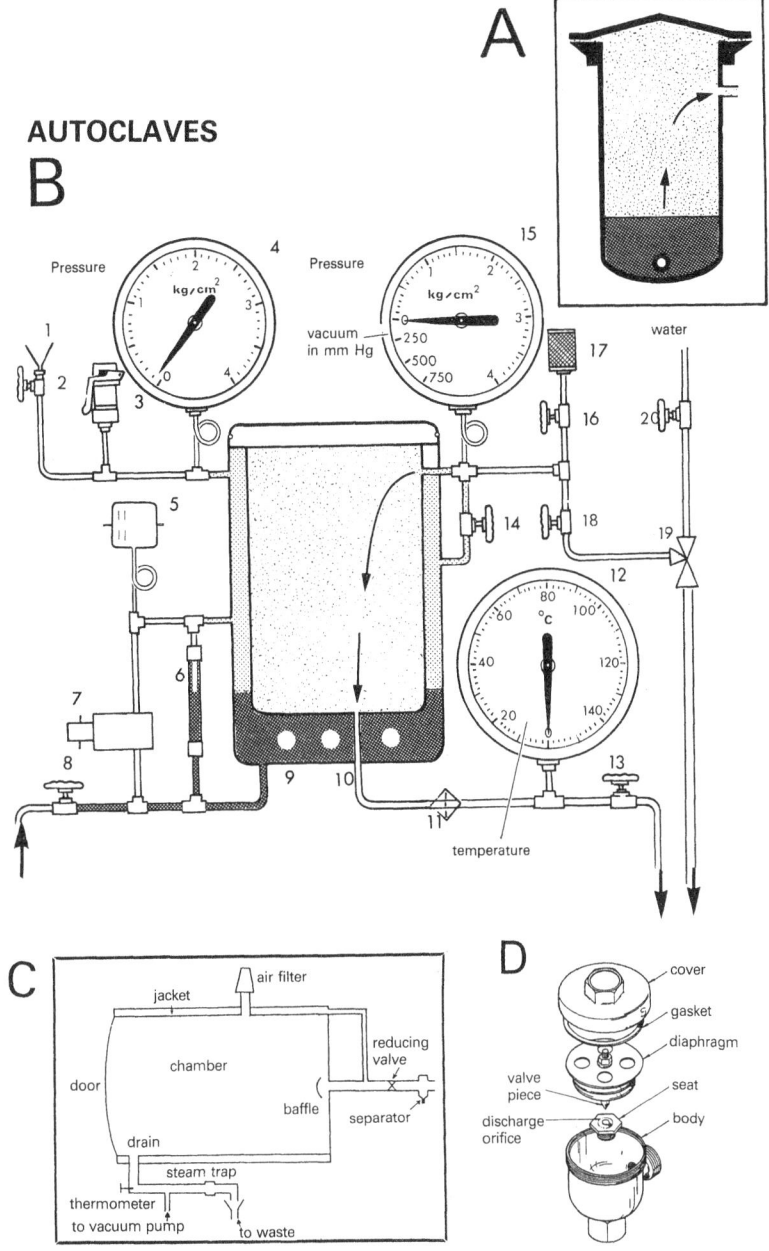

Fig. 2-7 AUTOCLAVES. A, a simple autoclave is a strong metal chamber with water in the bottom, like a large pressure cooker.

B, a jacketed vertical gravity displacement autoclave. This is filled through a tundish (open funnel) (1) and a filling valve (2). On the same pipe there is a safety valve (3) and a pressure gauge (4) to measure the pressure in the jacket. A pressure switch (5) controls the pressure in the jacket and an indicator (6) monitors its water level. A float switch (7) cuts off the power if the water level is too low, and a drain tap (8) lets water out of the jacket. Several heating elements (9) heat it. The chamber is drained through a pipe (10) and a strainer (11). A thermometer (12) and a valve (13) are fitted to the drain pipe (the valve should be an automatic near-to-steam trap, preceded by a non-return valve, to prevent dirty air and some water being sucked up during the vacuum). Steam from the jacket is admitted to the chamber through valve (14). Pressure and vacuum in the chamber are measured by a gauge (15). Air is admitted to the chamber through a valve (16) and an air filter (17). Air and steam are discharged from the chamber through valve (18) by means of the water-operated ejector pump (19) operated by tap (20).

C, a vertical gravity displacement autoclave. Steam is admitted fairly high up the sterilizer. The drain with the thermometer is as near the chamber as possible. There is a near-to-steam trap separated from the drains by a tundish, which prevents dirty water being sucked back up the waste pipe into the autoclave during a vacuum phase.

D, a 'near-to-steam trap' (valve) in the waste line remains open, until steam following the air heats the bellows under the diaphragm and closes the trap automatically. *C, and D, kindly contributed by Dr Ronald Fallon.*

• *TRAYS, dressing, without lids, stainless steel, 275×320×50 mm, 20 only.* Use these to prepare sterile sets for the wards. Boil a tray and the instruments, lay a sterile towel on the tray, put the instruments on it and fold it over them. Better, autoclave the tray.

• *STERILIZER, boiling water, electric: (a) 'Bowl sterilizer', 450×350×380 mm, with counterbalanced lid, 6 kW, with six spare elements, state voltage, one only. (b) Instrument sterilizer, 350×160×120 mm, 1.2 kW, with six spare elements, state voltage, one only.* One of these is for trays and bowls, and the other for instruments. Keep them both in the preparation room. Never try to sterilize anything contaminated with faeces with boiling water in a sterilizer—it does not destroy spores.

• *FORCEPS, sterilizer, Cheatle's, 267 mm, UNIPAC 0735200, two only.*

• *FORCEPS, sterilizer, Cheatle's extra large, 279 mm, complete with can of appropriate size for antiseptic fluid, two only.* These are useful for bowls and utensils, and will also pick up small objects.

• *FORCEPS, bowl sterilizing, Harrison's double jawed, complete with can of appropriate size for antiseptic fluid, one only.* Autoclave these and Cheatle's forceps and their cans after each day's use, then fill them with fresh antiseptic fluid.

STERILIZING WITH MOIST HEAT

BOILING WATER

Microbes are much more easily killed if instruments are clean, so make sure that everything is cleaned before it is sterilized. Remove instruments from boiling water with long-handled Cheatle's forceps which have been in saponated cresol ('Lysol') up to their handles. If you are not wearing sterile gloves, make sure you let the instruments dry. If you use them wet, bacteria from your hands may flow down from your fingers in drops of water.

PACKING ANY AUTOCLAVE

Sterilization is impaired by anything which hinders the removal of air, so: (1) Arrange the contents loosely; a drum which can only be closed with difficulty is grossly overpacked. Place the contents so that air can readily be displaced downwards—the principles are the same in horizontal and vertical autoclaves. To avoid air pockets, interleave sheets of macintosh or jaconet with some permeable fabric, so that no two surfaces of the non-permeable material are in contact.

A SIMPLE AUTOCLAVE (or pressure cooker)

Make sure there is enough water in the bottom of the autoclave. Insert the drums to be sterilized, and turn on the heater. See that the discharge tap is open, and then screw down the lid. As the water boils the steam will rise and carry away the air in the autoclave.

CAUTION ! Let the air and the steam escape freely until there is no more air in the autoclave, usually about 10 minutes. To test this lead a rubber tube from the discharge tap into a bucket of water. When air no longer bubbles to the surface, there is no more air. After some trials you will learn how long to allow for this to happen.

Close the discharge tap. Let the temperature rise until it reaches 121°C. The safety valve will open and allow steam to escape.

Now start to measure the holding period and continue this for 15 minutes. Turn off the heater and allow the autoclave to cool, until the pressure gauge records zero pressure. Then open the discharge tap and allow air to enter the autoclave. Remove the load.

CAUTION ! If anything in the load has paper or cloth wrappings, don't allow them to touch anything unsterile, until they have dried, because microbes can penetrate wet paper.

JACKETED AUTOCLAVE

Keep the jacket full of steam at 121°C all through the working day. Drain the chamber to remove any water that may gather in it.

Load the heated chamber, close the lid, and *open valve (13)*.

STERILIZING. Open valve (14). When the temperature on thermometer (12) has reached the sterilizing temperature (usually 121°C), the holding time can start. Close valve (13). If it is letting much steam through, the temperature will not reach 121°C, until it is closed. So close it as soon as no further air and con-

PACKING AN AUTOCLAVE

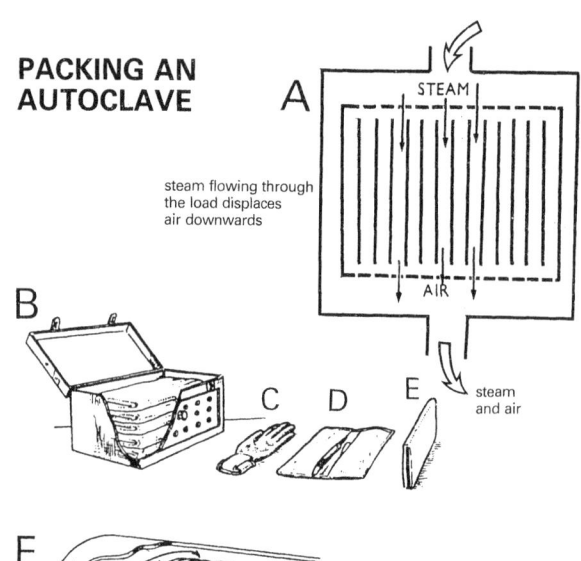

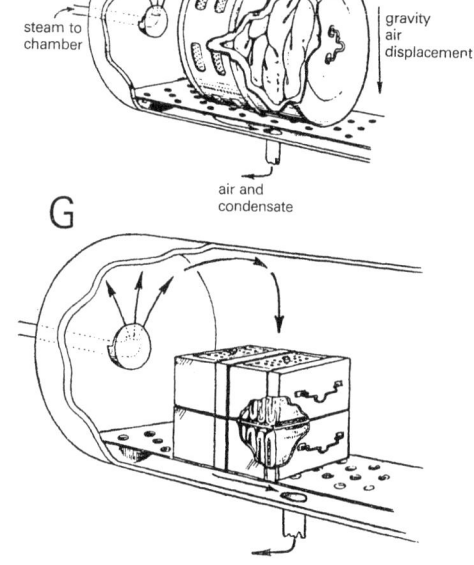

Fig. 2-7a PACKING AN AUTOCLAVE. A, the orientation of a load to facilitate the escape of air in a gravity displacement sterilizer. Steam enters from the top, flows downwards through the load and displaces the air in it. B, a properly packed glove container. C, a folded glove lined with gauze. D, a pair of gloves packed in a fabric envelope. E, a fabric envelope on edge to show its correct position during sterilization. F, a correctly packed drum with open ports positioned to allow air to be displaced by gravity. G, glove containers in an autoclave turned on edge so that steam can displace air through them. *From the Lancet 1959;i:425—435, with kind permission.*

densate come out of the chamber. If you still don't get the temperature you need (usually 121°C), open valve (13) for a minute or two and try again (a near-to-steam trap does this automatically). When the temperature has been reached, start timing.

CAUTION ! Don't infer the temperature from the reading of the pressure gauge. This may give you an inaccurate indication of its temperature and is a common cause of sterilization failure.

POSTVACUUM (drying). Open valve (20), then valve (18). Leave them open for 15 or 20 minutes. Close valve (18) then valve (20).

TO BREAK THE VACUUM. Open valve (16).

TESTING AUTOCLAVES

If you are using Browne's tubes, put a tube in the centre of the load, with, if possible, one on the outside to show that the autoclave has indeed been switched on!

If you don't have Browne's tubes, put some dry earth in an envelope, autoclave this and then culture it in a bottle or tube of nutrient broth. Spores may be slow to grow, so incubate it for a week. If even this is impossible, some theatre sisters have been known to put an egg in the middle of a drum to see if it is hard boiled!

PARTICULAR PROCEDURES FOR AUTOCLAVING

The following figures are guidelines only and vary with the type of autoclave and the size of the load. They apply to a sterilizing temperature of 121°C.

Empty glassware and unwrapped instruments. Sterilizing time 15 minutes, drying 10 minutes.

Wrapped instruments, rubber gloves, tubes and catheters, and sutures being reautoclaved. A common regime is $0.7\ kgcm^2$ (10 lb per square inch) for 20 minutes.

Fabrics and dressings. Sterilizing time 20 minutes, drying 15 minutes.

Liquids in flasks and bottles. Sterilize 100 ml bottles for 20 minutes, 300 ml bottles for 30 minutes, 500 ml bottles for 35 minutes, 1000 ml bottles for 40 minutes, and 3000 ml bottles for 50 minutes. Switch off the heat and let the autoclave cool down. Don't open it until the pressure is zero, or the bottles may burst. See also the Appendix A in *Primary Anaesthesia*.

PREVENTIVE MAINTENANCE Follow the maker's instructions carefully.

DIFFICULTIES WITH DOWNWARD DISPLACEMENT AUTOCLAVES

If the TEMPERATURE FALLS below 121°C, while the pressure remains at 1 $kgcm^2$ (15lb), the outlet from the chamber may be blocked, and the chamber full of air. Check it daily.

If you work at HIGH ALTITUDES, for each 1000 feet you are above sea level, increase the time you immerse things in boiling water by 5 minutes, and increase the pressure of your autoclave by $0.03\ kg/cm^2$ ($0.5\ lb/inch^2$). Water above 80°C will kill all vegetative organisms and viruses; boiling water is still effective at 12 000 feet.

If dressings are WET after autoclaving, the steam is probably wet, due to: (1) inadequate lagging of the steam supply pipe, or (2) inadequate tapping of condensate.

If you have reason to suspect IMPERFECT STERILIZATION, run the tests above. Also check that: (1) The drums are packed properly. (2) The correct temperature and sterilizing times are used. (3) The chamber drain is not blocked. (4) The drums are not being recontaminated after sterilization.

2.5 Disinfectants and antiseptics

Although heat is the best way of killing micro-organisms, you will have to use chemicals to kill them on a patient's skin, or on anything which heat might harm, such as drains or some suture materials. Heat destroys a cutting edge, so store your scissors in a chemical solution which will destroy bacteria. Classically, these chemicals are either antiseptics, which are safe to use on the surfaces of the body, or disinfectants, which are not. In practice, the distinction is not precise, and the only substances in the list below which cannot be applied to the body are saponated cresol ('Lysol'), formalin, and glutaraldehyde. There is an optimum antiseptic for each purpose, so try to use the right one.

Disinfectants have serious limitations and only work when the object they are disinfecting is clean—they are ineffective in the presence of blood or pus. So wash scissors and fine instruments carefully before you store them in an antiseptic solution. If possible, drains and other heavily contaminated pieces of equipment should be boiled or autoclaved after washing and before being immersed in these solutions. Afterwards, wash them well in sterile water before you use them. Catheters and tubes, etc., deteriorate in antiseptic solutions and are better autoclaved before use. Avoid cetrimide; it is mainly a detergent and chlorhexidine is better.

- *IODINE, tincture USP, one litre only.* This is the best skin antiseptic. If necessary, make it by mixing iodine 2 g (if necessary 1 g), sodium iodide 2.4 g, spirit 50 ml and water 50 ml. Tincture of iodine readily evaporates and becomes concentrated; if it does, dilute it. It is still effective and is more economical when it is diluted with spirit until it is a light brown colour.

- *CHLORHEXIDINE gluconate solution BP ('Hibitane'), five litres only.* Both chlorhexidine and cetrimide have so little effect on *Pseudomonas* that cetrimide can be used to select it from mixed cultures. Fortunately, spirit kills *Pseudomonas*, so chlorhexidine should be made up in 70% spirit.

- *GLUTARALDEHYDE concentrate 50% w/w in water, five litres only.* It is related chemically to formaldehyde but is less irritant. It is less stable but more active when buffered to pH 7.5 to 8 as in 'Cidex'. Used as a 2% alkaline buffered solution, glutaraldehyde comes nearest to being a chemical sterilant. It disinfects in 10 minutes, but it needs 10 hours to kill spores. It is very irritant, so keep it away from skin.

- *CRESOL and soap solution BP ('Lysol'), or some other phenolic antiseptic, ten litres only.* Use this for disinfecting the tops of theatre trolleys and the floor, etc. Don't apply it to the skin. The concentration of phenolic antiseptics is important. Use them at a a concentration of 1% w/v active phenols. If solutions are too dilute bacteria grow in them.

- *DRESSING TRAYS, stainless steel, with lids, (a) $250 \times 200 \times 50$ mm, six only. (b) $350mu \times 300 \times 50$ mm, three only.* Fill the smaller trays with chlorhexidine solution or spirit. Use separate trays for sutures and needles, rubber drains, and dental needles and equipment.

- *SODIUM NITRITE TABLETS, 100 g. Alternatively, SODIUM NITRITE powder, 100 g.* This is not an antiseptic, but a 0.4% solution of it in an antiseptic solution will stop steel instruments rusting.

ANTISEPTICS AND DISINFECTANTS

SKIN. Any alcoholic solution will do. Alcoholic iodine is best: use it routinely, except in children, on the scrotum, and in allergic patients. 0.5% chlorhexidine in spirit is a less satisfactory alternative. Apply it to the skin after removing all traces of soap.

WOUNDS. There is no substitute for a scrubbing brush, plenty of water from a jug, and a thorough surgical toilet (54.1). Chlorhexidine is useful for cleaning the skin round a wound.

INSTRUMENTS, SUTURE MATERIALS, AND DRAINS. The following agents are effective against HIV and HBV, in addition to the classical pathogens. (1) 2% alkaline buffered glutaraldehyde is the best. (2) 5% formalin in 70% spirit. (2) A 0.5% solution of chlorhexidine *in 70% spirit* with 0.5% sodium nitrite. (This is in terms of the active agent.) (4) Plain 70% spirit.

Ten minutes is the *absolute* minimum time in these solutions, *provided instruments are scrupulously clean*, 24 hours is safer. Ideally, nothing should be considered 'sterilized' until it has been immersed for 24 hours. Wash all equipment well before using it.

CAUTION ! (1) Except for glutaraldehyde (which can be used for 14 to 28 days depending on the brand) make these solutions up freshly every week, and keep them covered to prevent the alcohol evaporating. (2) A 'wipe' *is not nearly as good* as a soak!

2.6 Antiseptic surgery

This used to be standard practice before aseptic methods made it obsolete. But it may still be useful when power supplies have failed or your autoclave breaks, or an important operation has to be done in some remote place.

Aim to sterilize everything coming into contact with the wound by soaking it for a sufficient time in an antiseptic solution. Unfortunately: (1) An antiseptic solution leaves everything wet. (2) Sterilization is slow so that you may only be able to do one operation at a time. (3) Wide areas of the body are exposed to the antiseptic, which causes much exudation from the wound. Even so, antiseptic surgery is simple, and makes many kinds of operation possible. If necessary, you can combine antiseptic and aseptic methods, and sterilize smaller instruments in a pressure cooker. Chlorhexidine is the most practical antiseptic, but is far from perfect. The methods below are mostly those used by JF Dick working on the slopes of Mount Everest. Here is his account.

ANTISEPTIC SURGERY UNDER ADVERSE CONDITIONS. "The only means of access to our hospital at present is by walking over the mountains for a week. All supplies have to be carried in by porters who take two weeks for the journey. For the first two and a half years, we worked in a traditional Nepali house with a thatched roof and a floor made of mud and cow dung. In it we

OPERATIONS HAVE BEEN DONE UNDER A TREE...

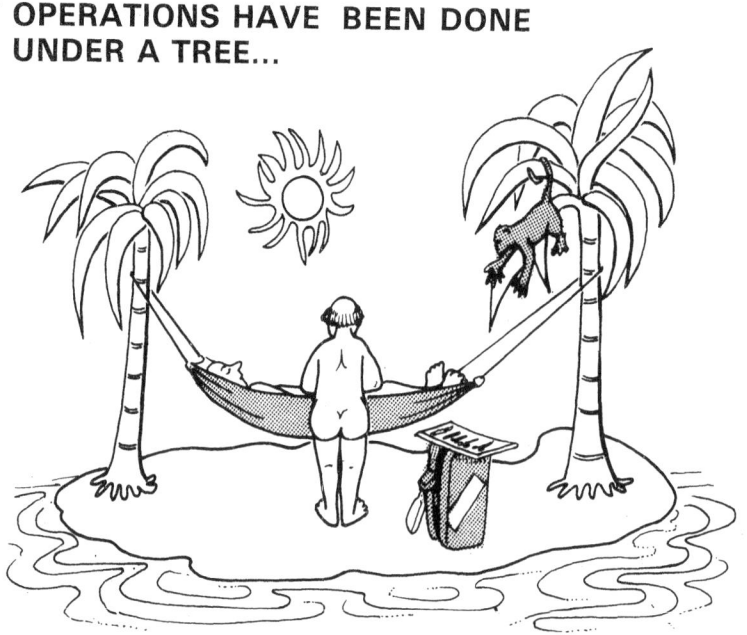

Fig. 2-8 OPERATIONS HAVE BEEN DONE UNDER A TREE. One eminent professor of International Health (Carl Taylor) recalls that during his days as a surgeon he had, on occasion, to release contractures on the steps of a temple! So there *may* be times when you have to operate in a tent or even 'on the kitchen table'. It has been said that a first class surgeon can operate in any theatre in any clothes... *Kindly contributed by Imre Loefler. Drawn by Nette de Glanville, and reproduced with the permission of the Editor of the Transactions of the East African Association of Surgeons.*

did over 100 operations by the antiseptic method, without serious mishap. Later, limited space became available, so that although we enjoyed the advantages of tap water, a concrete floor, a clean ceiling, and adequate window ventilation, we still had to operate on a light outpatient type of table and in the same room in which the outpatients received all their medicines, injections, dressings, incisions, and dental extractions. We almost always used epidural or local anaesthesia".

Dick JF, 'Antiseptic surgery', Lancet 1966;ii:900.

ANTISEPTIC SURGERY

ANTISEPTIC SOLUTIONS. Use chlorhexidine 5% concentrate to make two solutions: (1) A weak solution of 1/2000 of the active agent in water. Use this for soaking towels, etc. (2) A strong solution for instruments, as described above (2.5). Make up small quantities of solutions frequently, make them up hot, and clean out the containers well between batches.

'STERILIZING' EQUIPMENT AND DRAPES. Soak everything which will come into contact with the wound in one of these solutions for at least 30 minutes. Soak sutures and gloves in this solution overnight. Use monofilament (4.6) for ligatures and sutures, and the minimum number of simple instruments.

The most appropriate drape, for a tubal ligation, for example, may be a single solution soaked plastic sheet long enough, and wide enough, to cover the whole patient, with a hole in the middle through which to operate. If you have two such drapes, one can be in use while the other is being soaked in a flat container of solution.

CAUTION ! Don't use syringes and needles soaked in antiseptic to give a subarachnoid or epidural anaesthetic.

PERIOPERATIVE ANTIBIOTICS for routine use in antiseptic surgery. Some operators have given their patients 1 g of chloramphenicol intravenously immediately before the operation. This is questionable practice, but if you are going to try to use antibiotics prophylactically, this is the logical way to use them (2.7).

WHILE OPERATING, Treat the patient's skin with the solution for at least five minutes before the operation.

Wash your hands as usual and put on the wet gloves. If you are not using gloves, soak your hands in solution for five minutes.

Wring out the soaked drapes as dry as you can, and apply them as near as possible to the operation site. Clean the patient's skin with the same solution. If there is a danger that he might get cold, cover him with a dry blanket in a plastic sheet, and put this between his skin and the wet towels above and below the operation site, where it will not get in the way.

Swab the trolley with the solution, or put the instruments on a solution-soaked towel. Keep two bowls near the operating table, one containing water and the other antiseptic solution. When instruments have been used, wash them in water and keep them in the solution until you use them again. Shake off the excess solution before you use them.

Handle the patient's tissues as little as you can, and try to keep the solution out of his wound as much as possible. Don't let it get into his body cavities.

If his wound is well sutured and is not expected to discharge, leave it open to the air. This is better than covering it with a questionably sterile dressing.

AFTER OPERATING rinse everything free of blood. Rinse the instruments, and put them away. If possible, carry nothing over to the next operation.

2.7 Antibiotics in surgery

Antibiotics have two uses in surgery: (1) To treat established infections. (2) In certain circumstances only, and when used in a very particular way, to prevent postoperative infection. They have deliberately been placed last in this chapter, because they are less important than: (1) Careful aseptic theatre routines. (2) A thorough wound toilet (54.1). (3) Delayed primary closure (54.4). (4) Making sure there are no foreign bodies, dead tissue, excessive blood clots, or faeces in the wound. In preventing sepsis, antibiotics give us no licence to neglect the classical rules of good surgery, especially if the patient is diabetic, very old, or very ill, and so less able to overcome any bacteria that may get inside him. So: (1) Handle the tissues gently. (2) Don't leave large pieces of dead tissue in the wound, such as huge, massively ligated pedicles. (3) Where necessary, divert faeces by temporary colostomy.

That said, how can you use antibiotics to the best advantage, when your laboratory staff cannot culture bacteria, or at least not reliably? If they can, do encourage them to examine blood cultures, which are not difficult technically, and, when these are positive, to isolate the organism responsible for septicaemia in pure culture.

If you are fortunate, you will be able to plan a logical antibiotic policy for your district, and keep some antibiotics for hospital use only, in the hope that the arrival of antibiotic-resistant strains from elsewhere in the world will be delayed as long as possible. In such an ideal situation you might decide, for example, that the clinics should use only penicillin and tetracycline, with perhaps a little ampicillin or trimethoprim, and keep streptomycin for tuberculosis only. This will enable you to use chloramphenicol with metronidazole as your main surgical antibiotics, especially when the gut and the genital tract are involved. For other occasions you can use gentamicin (expensive), or a cephalosporin, or a combination of penicillin and streptomycin.

Unfortunately, you are more likely to work in a situation of antibiotic chaos, in which any antibiotic is obtainable over the counter without prescription, and where multiply resistant strains, particularly those resistant to chloramphenicol, are common.

The advice given in later chapters assumes that you are working in an area where chloramphenicol is not freely available in the community, and where organisms resistant to it are uncommon. If they are common, the advice we give may no longer hold, and you had probably better use gentamicin or cephradine.

2.8 Particular antibiotics

Some antibiotics are particularly important in district hospital surgery, either because they are life-saving, or because they are good value for money.

Benzyl penicillin is cheap and safe. For organisms that might possibly be sensitive, it is the antibiotic of choice. There is little point in giving very high doses. If penicillin fails to cure a patient, this will probably be because the β-lactamase of penicillin resistant bacteria is destroying it, not because you are not giving enough. In an adult a megaunit six-hourly is the standard dose for a severe infection, such as spreading hand sepsis, or cellulitis round an infected wound. However, if drugs are scarce, one megaunit given to four people is likely to do more good than four megaunits given to one person. In infants, and in patients with cardiac or renal disease, the sodium or potassium in the penicillin can cause undesirable side effects, so be aware of this.

Metronidazole is effective against anaerobes, and as these are often the most important invaders, it has been a major advance. It is bactericidal to most of them, particularly *Bacteroides fragilis*, and is the drug of choice in the treatment of non-clostridial anaerobic infections and amoebiasis. Resistance to it is unknown, and it has few side effects. It has been expensive, but it is now much cheaper. Give it, blindly if necessary, to all patients who are severely ill with an infection that might be caused by anaerobes, and particularly to patients with intra-abdominal sepsis. Intravenous metronidazole is expensive, but you can achieve adequate blood levels by giving it as suppositories, or as oral tablets rectally. Like this, it is only a tenth the price. Intravenous metronidazole with an aminoglycoside, such as gentamicin, avoids the risk of pseudomembranous colitis (rare). The expensive alternatives, lincomycin and clindamycin, both have this danger. Metronidazole is one of the drugs that no surgeon should be without.

Chloramphenicol is almost outmoded in the industrial world, where expense is less of a constraint. But it is cheap, and has a broad spectrum of activity against aerobic Gram-negative bacilli and Gram-positive cocci. Also, if you don't have metronidazole for anaerobic infections, chloramphenicol is next best. It has good in *vitro* activity against anaerobes from most parts of the world. It also enters the eye (24.3). Its life-saving properties outweigh the small risk of aplastic anaemia. Chloramphenicol with metronidazole is an excellent combination for established or expected peritonitis (6.2).

Cephalosporins (cephradine). If chloramphenicol is freely available in your community, so that it is much used outside hospital, resistant organisms will be common. If so, instead of using chloramphenicol, use whichever cephalosporin you can get most cheaply, such as cephradine. This is active by mouth, but you may need to give it intravenously. Use cephradine and metronidazole as a substitute for chloramphenicol and metronidazole. For infections with intestinal organisms cephradine and metronidazole is a substitute for gentamicin and metronidazole. Remember that 10% of penicillin-sensitive patients are also sensitive to cephalosporins.

Gentamicin is a very valuable broad spectrum aminoglycoside antibiotic for organisms which are likely to be resistant to other antibiotics. It has been expensive, but is now out of patent and is much cheaper. At the time of writing (June 1988) ECHO cost a day's treatment at $0.13 compared with $2.3 for cephradine. For the 'blind' treatment of a serious infection, especially one due to intestinal bacteria, give gentamicin with metronidazole, perhaps with penicillin.

Trimethoprim alone is preferable to cotrimoxazole ('Bactrim', 'Septrin'), which is a combination of trimethoprim and sulphamethoxazole. The latter is rather toxic and not very effective. If you don't have trimethoprim, use cotrimoxazole.

Tetracycline. Oxytetracycline ('Terramycin') is likely to be the cheapest tetracycline.

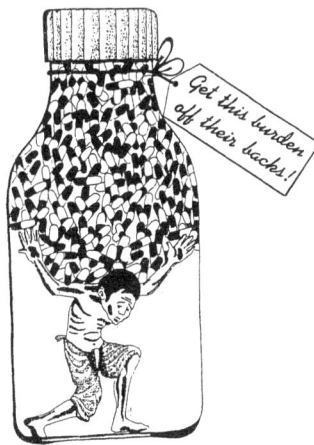

Fig. 2-9 ANTIBIOTICS MUST GET TO THE PATIENTS AND THE DISEASES WHERE THEY CAN DO MOST GOOD. This is a poster from Oxfam's 'Rational Health Campaign' to show the enormous burden many communities bear in misused antibiotics that are bought in the marketplace, or are misprescribed by doctors on the wrong indications for the wrong patients. Some of the most valuable correct uses of antibiotics are the surgical ones described here. *Kindly contributed by Oxfam.*

2.9 Methods for using antibiotics

Antibiotics for treating established infection call for little comment, and are described in many places in these manuals. Antibiotics to prevent infection need to be used wisely, in ways in which their benefits outweigh their risks. An operation site which has no bacteria in it to start with can become contaminated with bacteria from:

(1) Outside the patient, in which case they will probably be staphylococci. Preventing such infection is the purpose of the ordinary aseptic routines, and *prophylactic antibiotics are no substitute for it*. Most surgical patients do not need antibiotic cover for sepsis of this kind. The only absolute indication for it is to cover the implantation of prostheses, which you are unlikely to do.

(2) **Inside a patient,** when you operate on his large gut or his lower urinary tract, or on a woman's genital tract.

When you use antibiotics prophylactically, aim to provide a concentration in the patient's blood that will kill any bacteria introduced into his wound at the time of the operation. If you want to minimize the risk of peritonitis, he will need protection against enterobacteria (mostly *Esch. coli*), as well as aerobic and anaerobic streptococci. He will also need protection against bacterioides, and clostridia.

The accepted ways to give antibiotics are:

(1) To give them perioperatively, so that high concentrations are reached in a patient's wound at the time of surgery. Give them intravenously with the premedication, and for 24 to 48 hours only afterwards, unless there is some good reason for continuing them. Starting them a day or more before the operation, or continuing them unnecessarily afterwards, promotes the selection of resistant organisms and the risk of side-effects.

(2) To instil them into the peritoneum after the pus from peritonitis has been washed out. Tetracycline is very effective in preventing postoperative sepsis in the peritoneum, and in the wound in the abdominal wall.

There are several unacceptable methods: (1) Don't put topical antibiotics into a patient's wound. (2) Don't give them by mouth in the hope of 'sterilizing his large gut'—systemic antibiotics are probably at least as effective, and safer.

As to the antibiotics to use, you will see from the list of indications below that, if chloramphenicol is not much used in the community, chloramphenicol with metronidazole is likely to be the most cost-effective combination. Otherwise, give cephradine (or some other cephalosporin) with metronidazole. These are certainly much better than one commonly used alternative, which is penicillin and streptomycin.

Try to separate prophylaxis from treatment. For prophylaxis give chloramphenicol, or a cephalosporin with metronidazole. For treatment give gentamicin and metronidazole.

Barker EM, 'Rectal adminstration of metronidazole in severely ill patients', British Medical Journal 1983;287:311-313.

Keighley MRB, 'Perioperative antibiotics', British Medical Journal, 1983;286:1844-1846.

**THE DOSE AND THE TIMING ARE CRITICAL
GET ADEQUATE LEVELS AT THE TIME OF SURGERY**

ANTIBIOTICS

PERIOPERATIVE PROHPHYLAXIS

INDICATIONS. (1) Peritonitis. (2) Any operation which is likely to contaminate a patient's peritoneal cavity, especially large bowel surgery. Use a combination of metronidazole with either an aminoglycoside (such as gentamicin), or a cephalosporin, or, to save cost, chloramphenicol. (3) An operation on his urinary tract when his urine is already contaminated, including bouginage, cystoscopy, and Freyer's prostatectomy. Use an aminoglycoside (gentamicin), a cephalosporin (cephradine), or chloramphenicol. (4) Hysterectomy: as (2). (4) Emergency Caesarean section.

Balance cost and benefit. The instillation of tetracycline solution into the peritoneum (see below) may be comparatively expensive; but if it saves another operation for a residual abscess it is cheap.

CAUTION ! Gentamicin and other aminoglycosides may seriously prolong the action of long-acting (non-depolarizing) relaxants (A 14.3), and may prevent the establishment of spontaneous ventilation. Avoid them unless your anaesthetist is experienced.

CONTRAINDICATIONS. Antibiotics are not needed for: (1) Already well localized infections. (2) Hernias, ovarian cysts, etc.

Disputed indications include elective Caesarean section and appendicectomy.

DOSE. Give *two* intravenous doses of *two* suitable antibiotics, one of which is active against aerobic organisms, and the other against anaerobes. Give the first dose *intravenously* with the premedication. You are only giving two doses, so it is safe to use large ones. Give the second dose 6 hours later. If you are using a tourniquet, time the injection to give the maximum concentration about the time that you release it, so that the clot which forms in the wound will be heavily loaded with drug.

For the aerobic organisms, give: chloramphenicol, or gentamicin, or a cephalosporin, or trimethoprim. Gentamicin is the most potent, but also the most expensive.

For anaerobes, particularly bacterioides give metronidazole. Chloramphenicol is also active, but is less effective.

PARTICULAR ANTIBIOTICS

BENZYLPENICILLIN (penicillin G) can be given by several routes. 600 mg is one megaunit (M).

Intramuscularly. Adults, 300 to 600 mg 2 to 4 times in 24 hours. Child up to 12 years 10-20 mg/kg/24 hours. Neonate 30 mg/kg/24 hours.

By intravenous infusion. Adults, up to 24 g in 24 hours. Give it intermittently into a drip. Or give it into an intravenous drip or through a Gordh needle or disposable cannula ('Venflon'), flushed through with 1000 units of heparin.

By intrathecal injection. Adults, 6 to 12 mg in 24 hours.

METRONIDAZOLE, for anaerobic infections Adults, by mouth, 400 mg 8-hourly. By rectum 1 g 8-hourly for 3 days, then 1 g every 12 hours. By intravenous infusion, 500 mg 8-hourly for up to 7 days. Children, any route, give 7.5 mg/kg 8-hourly.

If a patient is seriously ill, give 500 mg (100 ml of 0.5% solution) intravenously as a loading dose over 45 minutes. Preferably give another similar dose 8 hours later. At the same time give a 1 g suppository 8-hourly. For perioperative prophylaxis (as for an emergency Caesarean section or large gut resection) continue for 24 to 48 hours. For peritonitis continue for 5 days.

If you don't have adequate supplies of intravenous metronidazole, you may be able to give it orally, or by suppository, or as an ordinary tablet rectally (1 g 6 to 8-hourly), before and after the operation. Adequate blood levels are not reached for 8 hours after giving a suppository, so start with one, or, better, two intravenous loading doses, and continue with suppositories. Or if you have no intravenous solution, use suppositories only, and start them earlier. It has been suggested that presently accepted doses may be high, and that a 500 mg suppository 12-hourly may be adequate.

CHLORAMPHENICOL. There are several regimes.

Perioperatively. Adults, give 1 g by bolus intravenous injection.

Intravenously. Adults, give an adult 1 g 6-hourly, or 50 mg/kg/24 hours. Child 50 to 100 mg/kg 24 hours in divided doses. Decrease the high dose as soon as clinically indicated. Infant: 50 mg/kg/24 hours in divided doses. Neonate under 2 weeks: 25 mg/kg/24 hours in divided doses. Premature baby: 12.5 to 25 mg/kg/24 hours. In neonates it may cause the 'grey syndrome', but probably not with lower doses.

By mouth. Adults, give 500 mg 6-hourly or 50 mg/kg/24 hours in divided doses for 5 days. Then give 250 mg 4 to 6-hourly for up to 10 days. For children give 25-100 mg/kg/24 hours in divided doses.

In grave emergencies high doses may be justified. Section 31.8 describes a short high dose chloramphenicol regimen for treating typhoid (1 or 2 g 4-hourly for 5 days followed by 250 mg 6-hourly for 14 days). One of the dangers with exceptionally high dosage schemes is that you may come to think of them as normal, and so increase your antibiotic bill unduely.

CAUTION ! (1) Avoid long courses of chloramphenicol. It is among these patients that most cases of aplastic anaemia and leucopenia occur. Their reported incidence in the industrial world is 1:5,000 to 1:10,000 cases. Their incidence is probably lower in non-Caucasians. (2) Avoid intramuscular chloramphenicol; it is poorly absorbed.

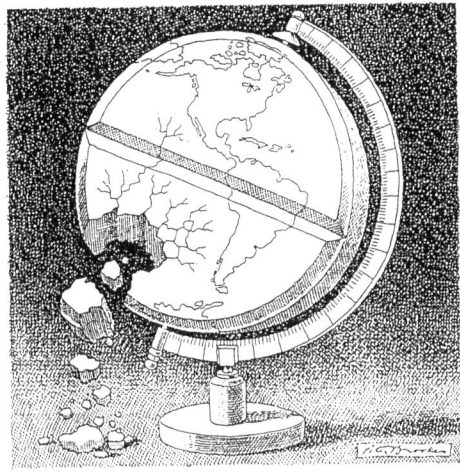

'We may look back on the antibiotic era as a passing phase, an age in which a great natural resource was squandered'

Fig. 2-10 FROM WONDER DRUG TO BITTER PILL. The variety of antibiotics potentially available to treat infections may not be inexhaustible. We should use them wisely.

CEPHRADINE (other cephalosporins have different doses).
By mouth, 250 to 500 mg 6-hourly. Or, 0.5 to 1.0 g 12-hourly. In children 25 to 50 mg/kg in 24 hours in divided doses.
By intramuscular or intravenous injection, 0.5 to 1 g every 6 hours, increased to 8 g in 24 hours in severe infections. Children 50 to 100 mg in 24 hours in 4 divided doses.

GENTAMICIN. By intramuscular injection or slow intravenous injection or infusion, 2 to 5 mg/kg/24 hours, in divided doses every 8 hours. Children up to 2 weeks give 3 mg/kg every 12 hours. 2 weeks to 12 years give 2 mg/kg every 8 hours.
By intrathecal injection 1 mg in 24 hours, with 2 to 4 mg/kg by intramuscular injection in divided doses every 8 hours.
CAUTION ! In renal impairment the interval between successive doses should be increased.

TRIMETHOPRIM. Adults: by mouth in an acute infection 200 mg 12 hourly. Chronic infections and prophylaxis 100 mg at night. Children: twice daily 2 to 5 months 25 mg, 6 months to 5 years 50 mg, 6 to 12 years 100 mg.
By slow intravenous injection or infusion, 150 to 200 mg 12-hourly. Child under 12 years 6 to 9 mg/kg/24 hours in 3 divided doses.

TETRACYCLINE. Oxytetracycline is likely to be the cheapest preparation. For peritonitis, or contamination of the peritoneal cavity with faeces, wash out the pus or faeces with saline until the fluid comes away clear. Then instil 1 g of oxytetracycline in 1000 ml of saline. Close the abdomen without drains.

THE TREATMENT OF SURGICAL SEPSIS

See also particular conditions: peritonitis 6.2, osteomyelitis 7.4, septic arthritis 7.16 etc.
CAUTION ! In any form of sepsis, antibiotics are not a substitute for surgery when this is necessary.

SPREADING PRESUMPTIVE GRAM-POSITIVE SEPSIS when you don't know the sensitivities—give chloramphenicol, cephradine, cloxacillin or methicillin.

SERIOUS PRESUMPTIVE ANAEROBIC SEPSIS, especially intra-abdominal sepsis. Give metronidazole, intravenously or as suppositories with a loading dose intravenously (if available). There may be aerobes also, so give chloramphenicol or gentamicin or cephradine in addition. Continue for not more than 5 days.

PELVIC SEPSIS. Chloramphenicol with metronidazole, or cephradine with metronidazole, or, much less satisfactorily, penicillin with streptomycin.

SEVERE SOFT TISSUE WOUNDS. If there is risk of gas gangrene give benzyl penicillin (or erythromycin if the patient is sensitive to penicillin). And give metronidazole.

INFECTED ABDOMINAL WOUNDS. (1) Chloramphenicol or cephradine as above. Or, (2) a megaunit of benzyl penicillin 8-hourly, and intravenous ampicillin 1 g initially, followed by 0.5 g 8-hourly. AND, give metronidazole 500 mg intravenously initially followed by 1 g 8-hourly by rectum for up to 5 days.

'BLIND THERAPY'. For the severely ill patient presumed to have an infection when the nature and sensitivities of the organism are unknown: give chloramphenicol or cephradine or gentamicin, all with metronidazole. Consider giving benzyl penicillin or ampicillin also if the infection is generalized.

ONLY A FEW HIGH RISK PATIENTS NEED PERIOPERATIVE PROPHYLACTIC ANTIBIOTICS

2.10 When prevention fails—wound infection

If a patient's wound discharges pus, the aseptic routines described earlier in this chapter have broken down. Although this is not the only cause of a wound infection, it is the most unnecessary one.

Keep a record of your wound infections. They are most likely to occur if: (1) You are operating for some infective condition, such as an acute appendix. (2) The operation is long and difficult. (3) You leave dead tissues, foreign bodies, dirt, or clot, or an excessive number of sutures in the wound. (4) You create dead tissue by operating clumsily. (5) You close a wound by immediate primary closure, when delayed primary closure would been have been wiser (54.4).

If more than about 5% of your clean cases become infected, something has gone wrong. Prophylactic antibiotics are *not* the answer! The chances are that the aseptic disciplines in Section 2.2 are not being followed, or you are making the errors 3, 4, and 5 above.

SURGICAL SEPSIS. Here are some of the errors that can be made and the lessons to be learnt from them, mostly from the pre-antibiotic days.
(1) A theatre had extractor fans installed, but the only inlets for fresh air were under the doors, so that dust from the corridor was drawn into the theatre continually. Only when three patients had died of tetanus was the flow of the fans reversed. LESSON Keep dust out of the theatre.
(2) In the days before antibiotics a London teaching hospital had two minor theatres in which many septic operations were done. On two mornings a week the same equipment was used for a list of circumcisions. One circumcised child acquired erysipelas which spread from his umbilicus to his toes and killed him. LESSON Where possible don't do clean cases in a theatre which normally does septic ones.
(3) An eminent professor resected a carcinoma of the pelvic colon and did an end-to-end anastomosis, without doing a preliminary colostomy. The patient's gut obstructed, and when his abdomen was explored there was a huge abscess round a leaking anastomosis. Peritonitis killed him. LESSON If there are surgical procedures which will minimise the risk of infection, use them.
(4) Hamilton Bailey, subsequently a distinguished surgeon, but then a registrar, was deputizing for his chief. Having done a 'cold list' which began at 1.30 p.m. he insisted on continuing with a non-stop flood of emergencies which continued rolling in all the evening. At 3 a.m. the following morning, 'dead on his feet', he pricked himself when operating on a patient with streptococcal peritonitis. Bailey insisted that his finger be amputated, and survived. The patient died. LESSON Accidents, including those which increase the risk of sepsis, are particularly likely if you are overtired. Amputation for this reason should never be necessary, now that antibiotics are available.

Stirling HL, 'The aetiology, prevention, and treatment of surgical sepsis', Tropical Doctor 1979;2:131-134.

WOUND INFECTIONS

For the care of particular wounds, see the appropriate sections, for example, laparotomy wounds (9.12), rectal wounds (66.12), joint wounds (69.8).

THE PREVENTION OF WOUND INFECTIONS

AUTOCLAVING. (1) Check that your autoclave does reach 1 kg/cm^2 (2.4), that the air is being discharged, and that the

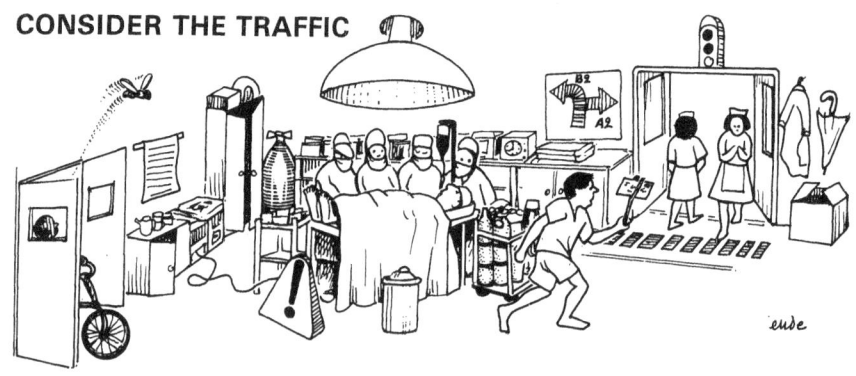

Fig. 2-11 CONSIDER THE TRAFFIC. Wounds are less likely to become infected, if the theatre is not used as a storeroom, and if there is the minimum of traffic in and out of it. So remove the teacups and cartons, the umbrella, and that coat! *Drawn by Nette de Glanville, and reproduced with the permission of the editor of the Transactions of the East African Association of Surgeons.*

holding time is being maintained. (2) Check that the drums are not being overpacked, that they are labelled after autoclaving, and that the label includes the date.

THEATRE DISCIPLINE. Check that you and ALL your staff are following *all* the aseptic disciplines in Section 2.3 carefully. If you set the example, your staff will follow them.

Check that: (1) the theatre table and especially the macintosh cover on its mattress, are being properly cleaned, (2) there is no infected member of staff.

SURGICAL TECHNIQUE. Examine yourself. Are you committing errors 3, 4, or 5 above?

THE TREATMENT OF WOUND INFECTIONS

Sedate the patient with morphine (or pethidine) and diazepam. In infected sutured wounds the pus usually tracks the whole length of the subcutaneous tissues. So remove all sutures and convert the wound into a gutter. Either allow it to granulate or close it by secondary suture. If possible, send a swab for culture.

Establish free drainage, especially in the depths of the wound, keep it open so that it can heal from the bottom, and let it drain into dressings.

If a wound fails to heal, think of HIV (Chapter 28a).

3 The control of bleeding

3.1 Assisting natural mechanisms

If you are going to operate on a patient you have to cut him, and if you cut him he bleeds, so you have to control this bleeding. He can also bleed from an injury (55.1). The body has excellent mechanisms for controlling bleeding, so that your task is mostly to assist them. The main mechanisms are the cascade of enzymic reactions which make his blood clot, and the ability of the muscular walls of his arteries to contract.

If you fail to control bleeding adequately he dies, so watch the blood he loses. The loss of a given volume of blood is much more serious in a child (3-1), than it is in a fit adult, who can usually lose a litre without the need to replace it by blood, whereas a small child can easily bleed to death from what might seem to be a very small loss.

The most generally useful ways of controlling bleeding are pressure and haemostats, but there are also special methods for particular parts of the body, such as the scalp (63.9), the dura (63.9), the gut (9.3) and the liver (66.7).

Pressure is the simplest and most valuable way to control bleeding. If you press on a tissue, the walls of its vessels will come together, and where their edges are cut, clot will start to form. When you release the pressure you will probably find that bleeding has stopped, or that only the arteries will continue to spurt at you, and these you can tie off. Press with a gauze pack. Some surgeons use warm saline packs, but there is no evidence that these are any better than cold or dry ones, and they are certainly less convenient. 'Hot packs' are therefore going out of fashion. If pressure is to succeeed, *you must press for long enough*—this is normally at least 5 minutes by the clock, which is one reason why every theatre should have a method of recording time. If the tissue behind the bleeding area is firm, as when you press a bleeding scalp against the patient's skull (63-19), pressure is even more effective. In an emergency you can control bleeding from a patient's uterus by pressing her aorta against her spine through her abdominal wall (19.11a).

A variation of this method is to pack a wound at the end of an operation and to remove the pack not more than 24 hours later, as with a bleeding liver (66.7), or after a sequestrectomy (7.6). Very occasionally, you may need to pack the uterus (19.11a).

A haemostat (artery forceps) can be used to grasp a bleeding vessel, particularly an artery which is spurting blood at you. You can then tie it.

Raising the bleeding part will lower the pressure in its veins, and and so minimize bleeding. This is valuable if a patient is bleeding from a limb, or the venous sinuses of his brain (a rare and difficult emergency), when the level of his head in relation to the rest of his body is critically important (63.9). But there is a risk of air embolism if a rigid vascular channel, such as a sinus, is raised above the level of the heart.

Adrenalin, added to the local anaesthetic solution, or to saline used to infiltrate the tissues, will minimise capillary and venous bleeding, when scar tissue is dissected for plastic surgery (58.25), or during the repair of a vesicovaginal fistula (18.18). *Never use adrenalin in the penis, or the distal parts of a limb such as a finger or toe, or in an intravenous forearm block,* because it may constrict the vessels so much that the part becomes gangrenous. You can

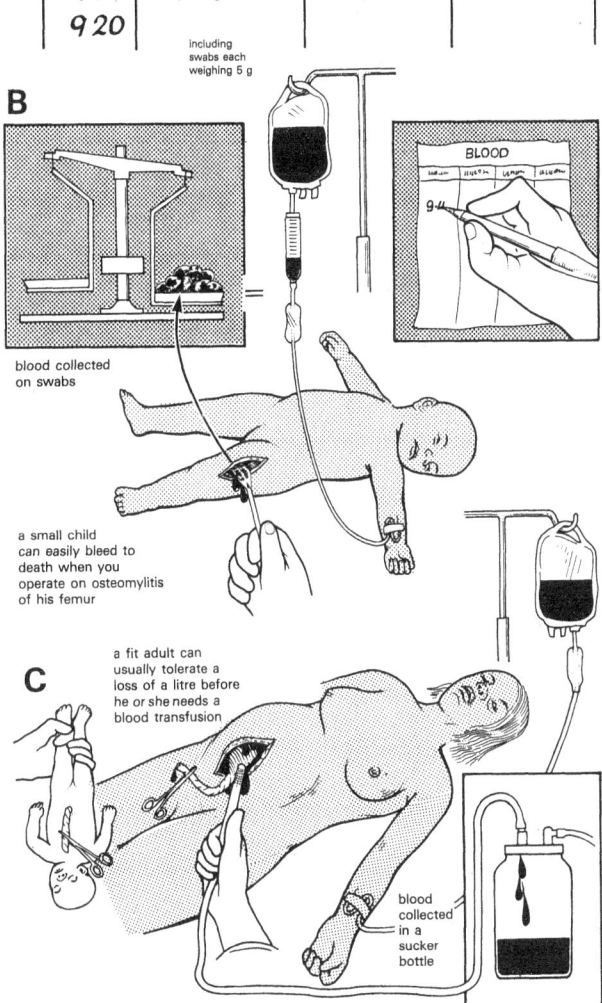

Fig. 3-1 BLOOD LOSS IN ADULTS AND CHILDREN. A, and B, when you operate on a child, make an accurate 'blood balance sheet'. In a major operation measure the blood he loses by weighing the blood-soaked swabs on a balance. Replace blood he has lost with an equal volume of blood as soon as possible. This should be HIV free or from a close relative. C, the balance sheet for an adult need not be nearly so accurate. A fit adult, such as a mother having a Caesarean section, can tolerate a blood loss of up to a litre or even a litre and a half, before you need to give her blood, rather than Ringer's lactate or saline. You can usually measure the blood she loses in a sucker bottle. When an adult needs blood, he needs at least two units. The transfusion of a single unit is useless.

also use an adrenalin soaked pack in a bleeding nose (25.6).

A vessel can be sutured, either to repair a break in its wall, or to anastomose it end-to-end (55.6). If a limb is severely injured, this may save it.

Bone wax can be packed into the bleeding edge of the skull into the diploe (63.9), or into the marrow of a bone, if the bleeding area is not too big.

Haemostatic gauze ('Surgijel') will eventually stop bleeding from the oozing cut surface of the liver (66.7), or the surface of the brain (63.9). Unlike ordinary gauze it is slowly absorbed. It is expensive and rarely indicated. A substitute is to cut a piece of muscle, hammer it flat, and use this (63.9).

The clotting power of the blood can be restored. When you have given a patient many units of blood, the citrate in it will lower his blood calcium and prevent his blood clotting. So don't forget to give him 10 ml of 10% calcium gluconate after every fourth unit of blood. The only other thing you may be able to do when his blood fails to clot is to give him fresh blood, but this may be impractical. You are unlikely to have individual clotting factors to give him, except, if you are fortunate, fibrinogen (19.11a).

Arteries and veins can be formally exposed, clamped and tied high above a bleeding lesion. You will only need to do this on unusual and desperate occasions. The classical sites for doing it are the external carotid (3.3) (rare), the third part of the subclavian (rare, 3.4), the internal iliac (for obstetric haemorrhage, much the most important, 3.5), the external iliac (rare), the femoral (uncommon, 3.7) and the popliteal artery (rare, 3.8).

A tourniquet will control bleeding from the distal part of a limb: (1) You can use a pneumatic tourniquet to control bleeding during an operation as described in Section 3.9. This is very valuable, and for many operations it is essential, because it enables you to operate in a bloodless field (3.9). (2) A tourniquet can be used as a first aid measure. This is so dangerous that many surgeons consider that first aid workers should never use one, but should rely on direct pressure instead (55.1).

The common mistakes are: (1) To panic when there is severe bleeding. (2) Not to apply pressure when this is indicated, or not to apply it for long enough. (3) To grasp wildly with a haemostat in a pool of blood, to fail to grasp the bleeding vessel, and perhaps to injure some important structure. (4) Not to apply the special methods for special sites.

• GAUZE, haemostatic, surgical, 'Surgijel' or equivalent, 5 packs only.

A STORY ABOUT BLEEDING. A surgeon went to an international meeting on prostatectomy. He got bored and said to a friend "I am having a bit of trouble with my waterworks, whom should I see?" "Go to Mr. X" he was told, "he is the best in town". So our surgeon visited Mr. X and said "Could you show me your method of prostatectomy?" The answer was "Yes certainly, but my only secret is, that I drink more tea than the others!". So it proved. At the end of the operation when the prostatic bed was bleeding, Mr. X just put in a monster pack, and had a leisurely cup of tea. When he and his assistant rescrubbed and came back 20 minutes later, the pack was taken out and there were no bleeding points to tie off! LESSONS When you control bleeding by pressure or with a pack sufficient time (5 minutes by the clock) is all important.

SOME USEFUL METHODS
See elsewhere for the special methods described above.

GAUZE PACKS will control oozing. Press dry gauze onto the bleeding area, or wring out gauze or any piece of cloth in hot water, and press this on the wound. If the operation is difficult, and you need a rest, this may be the time to go out to the changing room for a break and a cup of tea, while your assistant applies pressure. This will make sure that pressure is applied for the necessary time.

When you come back, instead of finding the whole area pouring blood, you will probably find one one or two tiny bleeders, which you can pick up in mosquito forceps and tie off. Because fewer ligatures are needed, there will be less chance of sepsis.

DRY FIRM PRESSURE PACKS can be used to compress a large bleeding vessel against something solid such as the spine (18.17).

PACKING A WOUND at the end of an operation is sometimes necessary. If, for example, you remove sequestra under a tourniquet, you can pack the wound tight, and remove the pack 24 or 48 hours later (63.7). Don't leave a pack in longer than 48 hours, or it will promote sepsis, and there may be severe bleeding when you remove it.

LEAVING CLAMPS IN THE WOUND. Very ocasionally, if you are inexperienced and desperate, you may have to clamp a vessel, and send the patient back to the ward with the handle of the haemostat protruding from the wound under a dressing. Remove it cautiously 24 hours later and close the wound. This is indeed a measure of desperation. It may be useful for a bleeding cervix (18.15, 19.11a, M 22.2) and for a bleeding renal pedicle (67.2). Most experienced surgeons have never had to do it.

3.2 Arterial bleeding

If you can see a bleeding vessel, you can grasp it with a haemostat (locking or artery forceps), which is one of the great inventions of surgery. Tie all larger vessels, either immediately or later. Small vessels, especially those in the skin, seldom need tying. Five minutes or more later, when you remove a haemostat you will probably find that bleeding will have stopped. You can encourage it to stop by twisting the haemostat before you remove it, or if the bite of tissue is too large to twist, you can release the jaws and quickly pinch them together again a few times before you remove them. Either of these methods will encourage the blood

HAEMOSTATS

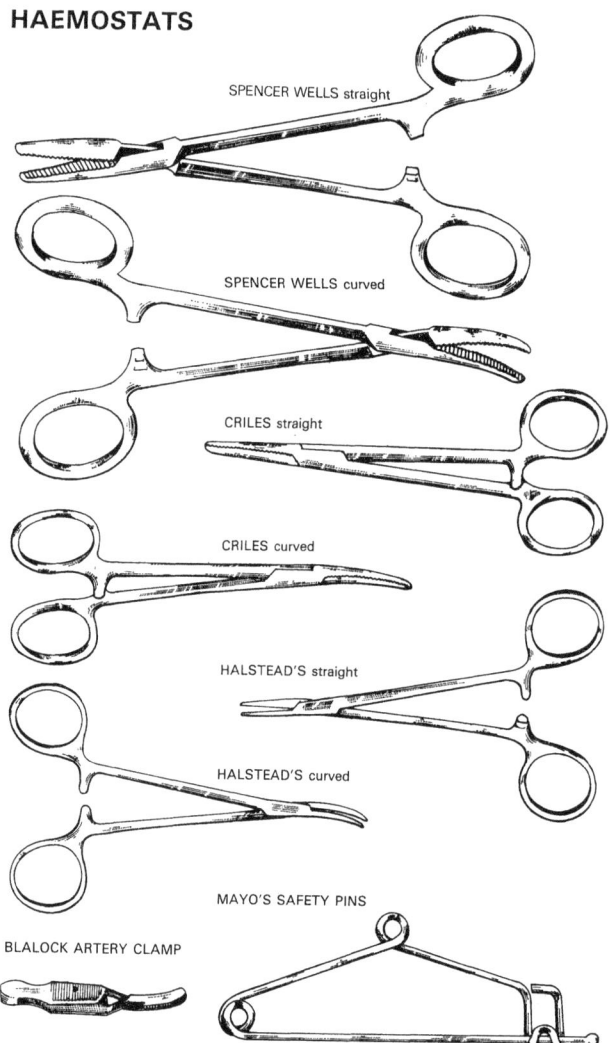

Fig 3-2 HAEMOSTATS. If you can see a bleeding vessel, you can usually grasp it with these locking forceps, which are one of the great inventions of surgery.

in the vessel to clot and will minimize bleeding, so that fewer vessels need tying.

Haemostats can be large or small, straight, or curved, so that they rest over the edge of the wound. An experienced surgeon can go through the skin using few of them or none (pressure from swabs is often enough); a beginner usually needs more.

Haemostats have some disadvantages. Each time you tie off a bleeding vessel you leave some crushed tissue and some suture material in the wound. If this is excessive, it can encourage delayed healing or infection later.

The tips of haemostats, especially small ones, must meet accurately, so good quality instruments are important. Box joints are worth the extra expense. Order them in sixes—you can hardly have too many—because they will enable you to make up several sets (4.12).

- FORCEPS, artery, Spencer Wells, box joint, (a) 200 mm, straight, six only. (b) 150 mm, straight, twelve only. (c) 230 mm, curved, six only. (d) 200 mm, curved, eighteen only. (e) 150 mm, curved, six only. (f) 125 mm, curved, twelve only. These are general purpose haemostats. Fifty-fou in all is a generous number and could be reduced.
- FORCEPS, artery, Crile's, box joint, 140 mm, (a) straight, six only. (b) curved, eighteen only. These are medium sized and are more robust than Halstead's.
- FORCEPS, artery, Halsted's, ultrafine, mosquito, haemostatic, (a) straight, (b) curved, box joint, 120 mm, six only of each type. These are some of the finest and most delicate instruments in the list, so use them with care.
- FORCEPS, artery, Kocher's, (a) straight, (b) curved, box joint, 200 mm, six only of each type. These are large haemostats with a tooth at the end of their jaws. Use them for a wide vascular pedicle when an ordinary haemostat might slip.
- PINS, safety, Mayo's, large, for storing artery forceps, etc., ten only. Use them to keep artery forceps together in bunches during sterilizing.

METHODS FOR ARTERIES

TO TIE AN ARTERY use the following materials in this order of preference—linen thread, cotton thread, or monofilament. Don't use catgut for larger and more important vessels, it slips off too easily.

Grasp the bleeding artery with a haemostat. Either: (1) Tie it with one firm reef knot. (2) Tie it with a surgeon's knot (4.8) followed by two or three more throws. (3) Transfix it, tie it with a reef knot, then pass one ligature through it with a needle, and tie it with another reef knot. This is the method for critically important vessels, such as those of the renal pedicle. For even more security, tie it proximal to a branch, and then cut it distal to this.

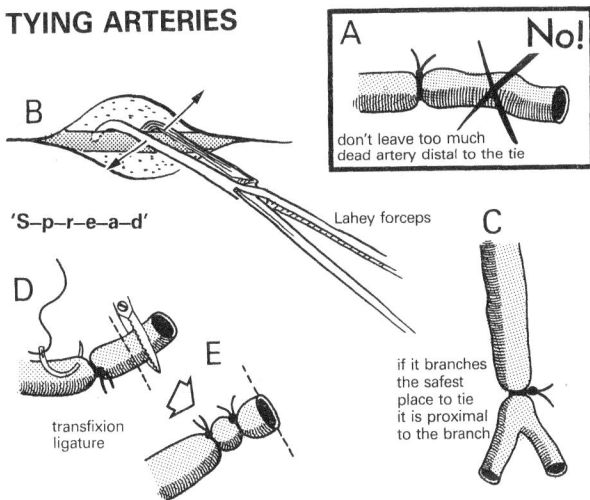

Fig. 3-3 TYING ARTERIES. A, don't leave too long an end; this will leave unnecessary dead tissue in the wound. B, to free a vessel buried in tissue, insert Lahey's forceps and spread the tissues. C, if possible, put the ligature proximal to a branch. D, an artery has been tied and a transfixion ligature is now being inserted; the needle is going through the vessel and its distal end is about to be cut off. E, the completed ligature.

If it is a critically important vessel, ask yourself—"Is what I have done enough?" If it is not, do it again. Put a second tie in a *separate* groove.

If there is a long length of vessel distal to your tie, shorten it, so as not to leave too much dead tissue in the wound, but don't shorten it too much!

If other methods of controlling severe arterial bleeding have failed, you may, very occasionally, have to expose and tie a major vessel, such as the external carotid artery or the subclavian, as described in the methods which follow. Use linen, silk, or cotton thread, and don't divide it after you have tied it.

TO CONTROL BLEEDING FROM A LARGE PEDICLE, such as that of the spleen or uterus, don't try to use a single ligature. Control of the vessels will be safer if you take one or more bites of the pedicle and tie them separately.

TO CONTROL A DIFFICULT BLEEDING ARTERY, try to get into the correct tissue plane. First find the artery by feeling for pulsation. Push the points of a fine haemostat into the connective tissue around it and separate them to open up a plane as in B, Fig. 3-3. Gradually develop this plane until you can see the artery you are looking for. In this way you will avoid tying some important nerve in the ligature.

TO GET A LIGATURE ROUND AN ARTERY, either use an aneurysm needle, or pass a curved haemostat under it, and ask your assistant to pass into your other hand a curved haemostat with a ligature 'bowstrung' across it, as in Fig. 3-4. This is useful in 'deep' surgery.

PASSING A LIGATURE

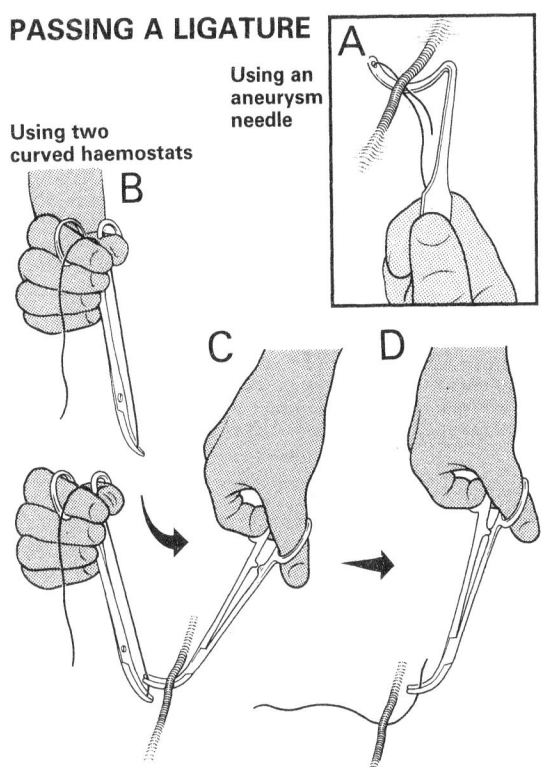

Fig. 3-4 TWO WAYS OF PASSING A LIGATURE UNDER A VESSEL. A, using an aneurysm needle. This is a left-handed needle. B, a length of suture material held in a curved haemostat. C, another curved haemostat is being passed under the vessel to grasp the suture material. D, pulling the suture material under the vessel.

3.3 Tying the external carotid artery

The methods in the sections which follow for exposing and tying major vessels are among the classical methods of surgery. They are very seldom needed, yet no textbook of surgery is quite complete without them.

After a severe maxillofacial injury you may have to tie the external carotid artery. This arises from the common carotid at the upper edge of the thyroid cartilage. It runs upwards behind the neck of the mandible, and ends by dividing into the maxillary and superficial temporal arteries. It lies under the posterior belly of the digastric muscle, and its upper part lies deep to the parotid gland.

3.4 Tying the third part of the subclavian artery

If a fracture of the neck of a patient's humerus tears his axillary artery, it may cause an arterial haematoma which you can only control by tying his subclavian artery. You will find this a desperate procedure, if you ever have to do it.

The subclavian artery crosses the cervical pleura in the root of the neck. It passes over the first rib behind scalenus anterior which divides it into three parts. The first part is medial to this muscle, the second part is behind it. The third part of the artery, lateral to his scalenus anterior, is the part you can most easily tie. The subclavian vein lies in front of the artery and slightly inferior to it. The phrenic nerve runs down the front of scalenus anterior.

Very occasionally, you may have to explore a patient's subclavian artery in his axilla, by removing the middle piece of his clavicle and splitting the fibres of his pectoralis major, so that you can reach it.

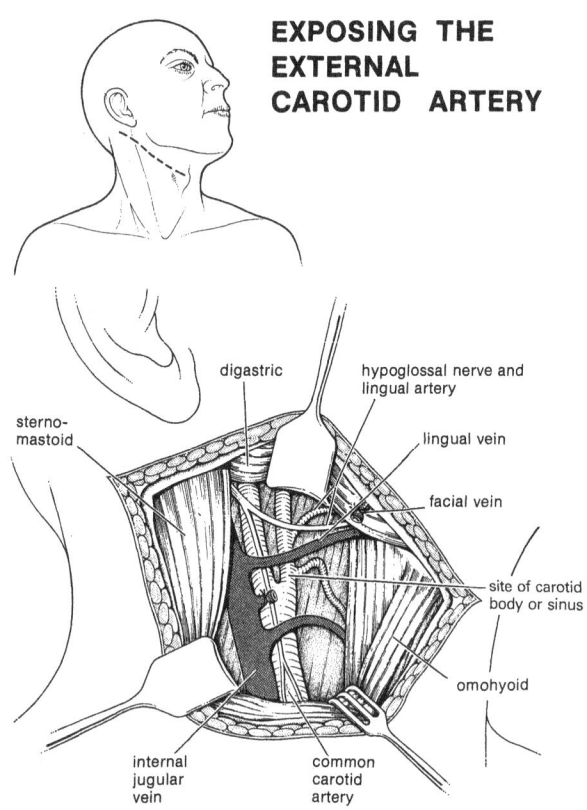

Fig. 3-5 TYING THE RIGHT EXTERNAL CAROTID ARTERY. One of the vessels you may very occasionally have to tie is the external carotid artery after a severe maxillofacial injury. *Adapted from 'Farquharson's Textbook of Operative Surgery', edited by RF Rintoul. Churchill Livingstone, with kind permission.*

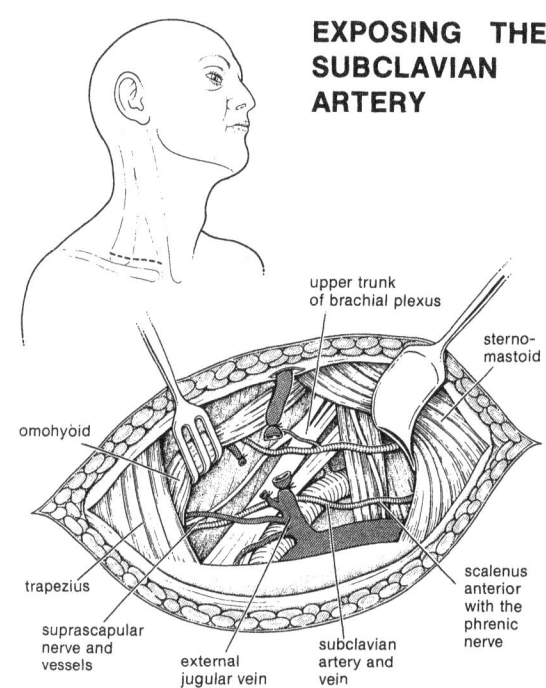

Fig. 3-6 EXPOSING THE THIRD PART OF THE SUBCLAVIAN ARTERY. If a fracture of the neck of the humerus tears the axillary artery (rare), it may cause an arterial haematoma which you can only control by tying the subclavian artery. *Adapted from 'Farquharson's Textbook of Operative Surgery', edited by RF Rintoul. Churchill Livingstone, with kind permission.*

TYING THE EXTERNAL CAROTID ARTERY

Tilt the table 10° head up to minimize venous bleeding; but not more, because this increases the risk of air embolism. Turn the patient's head to the opposite side, and extend it slightly.

Make an oblique incision from just below and in front of his mastoid process, almost to his thyroid cartilage. Divide his platysma and deep fascia in the line of the incision, and dissect flaps upwards and downwards.

Free the anterior border of his sternomastoid and retract it posteriorly. You will see his common facial vein. Divide this between ligatures.

Carefully retract his internal jugular vein backwards, to see his common carotid artery bifurcating to form his internal and external carotid arteries. If you have difficulty in deciding which artery is which, find some branches of the external carotid and follow them backwards to the main stem (the internal carotid artery has no branches in the neck).

Pass an aneurysm needle round it, tie it with zero silk or linen, and don't divide it. Tie it as close to its origin as you can.

CAUTION ! (1) Tie the external carotid just proximal to the origin of the lingual artery. (2) Avoid the patient's hypoglossal nerve which crosses his external and internal carotid vessels and then runs anteriorly to lie on his hyoglossus muscle in company with his lingual vein. (3) Avoid irritating his carotid sinus and body in the bifurcation of his internal and external carotid vessels.

TYING THE THIRD PART OF THE SUBCLAVIAN ARTERY

This is not an easy operation, even for experienced surgeons, so avoid it if you can! If you have to do it, start by tilting the table 10° head up. Put the patient's arm by his side, and draw it downwards to depress his shoulder. Turn his head to the opposite side.

Make an incision 2 cm above his clavicle from the sternal head of his sternomastoid to the anterior border of his trapezius. Incise his superficial fascia, his platysma, and his deep fascia in the line of the incision. If you see his external jugular vein crossing the field, divide this between ligatures.

Retract his omohyoid upwards and you will see the third part of his subclavian artery, with scalenus anterior medially, and the trunks of his brachial plexus laterally. His subclavian vein lies in front of the artery and below it.

Don't cut his transverse cervical artery under his omohyoid muscle, or his suprascapular artery crossing his subclavian artery, because they help to maintain the collateral circulation to his arm.

If necessary, split his clavicle, divide his pectoralis major in the line of its fibres, lay his whole axilla open, and get proximal control of the artery. Pass an aneurysm needle round it, tie it with zero silk or linen, and don't divide it.

3.5 Tying the internal iliac artery

Tying the internal iliac artery is the most common emergency arterial ligation. If a patient has severe and continuing uterine bleeding, after delivery for example, you may have to tie her internal iliac arteries on both sides. When her uterus has ruptured, so that its wall hardly feels any more substantial than blood clot, this is one of the few things you can do. It is not an easy procedure. She is likely to be very ill, your anaesthetist may not be able to give her an adequate anaesthetic, her pelvic wall is difficult to get at, and her pelvic retroperitoneum is difficult to work in. If you are expert, doing a hysterectomy may be easier. So start by getting good exposure, and identify the main trunks clearly before you tie them. The collateral circulation is so good, particularly during pregnancy, that tying both iliac arteries is very unlikely to be harmful. *See also 'Stop Press'.*

TYING THE INTERNAL ILIAC ARTERY

INDICATIONS. (1) Tearing into the lower segment during or base of the broad ligament during a difficult Caesarean section. (2) Severe and persistent PPH when packing fails to control bleeding. (3) Persistent bleeding from an abortion continuing after evacuation. (4) Rupture of the uterus. (5) Trauma to the uterus.

METHOD. If you already have the patient's abdomen open, tying her internal iliac arteries is quickly done. But don't be in too much of a hurry: you must not damage the accompanying vein (see below). Often, you need to tie them when you have not already got the abdomen open. If so make a quick lower median incision.

Hold back her abdominal contents and examine her pelvic brim. You will see her ureter crossing her common iliac artery at the point where it divides into its internal and external iliac branches (A, in Fig. 3-7). Open her peritoneum and lift up her ureter (B). Insert a haemostat under her internal iliac artery (C), and tie it. Do the same thing on the other side.

CAUTION ! (1) Don't tie her internal iliac vein which is closely related to the artery posteriorly. Doing so will increase the venous pressure in her uterus and make bleeding from it worse. (2) Don't damage her internal iliac vein. If you do, bleeding from the tear will be difficult to control and you will have to tie it.

On both sides, if necessary, also tie the anastomotic vessels that connect her ovarian arteries with her uterine arteries. Find them in her broad ligaments under the cornual ends of her tubes.

TYING THE INTERNAL ILIAC ARTERY

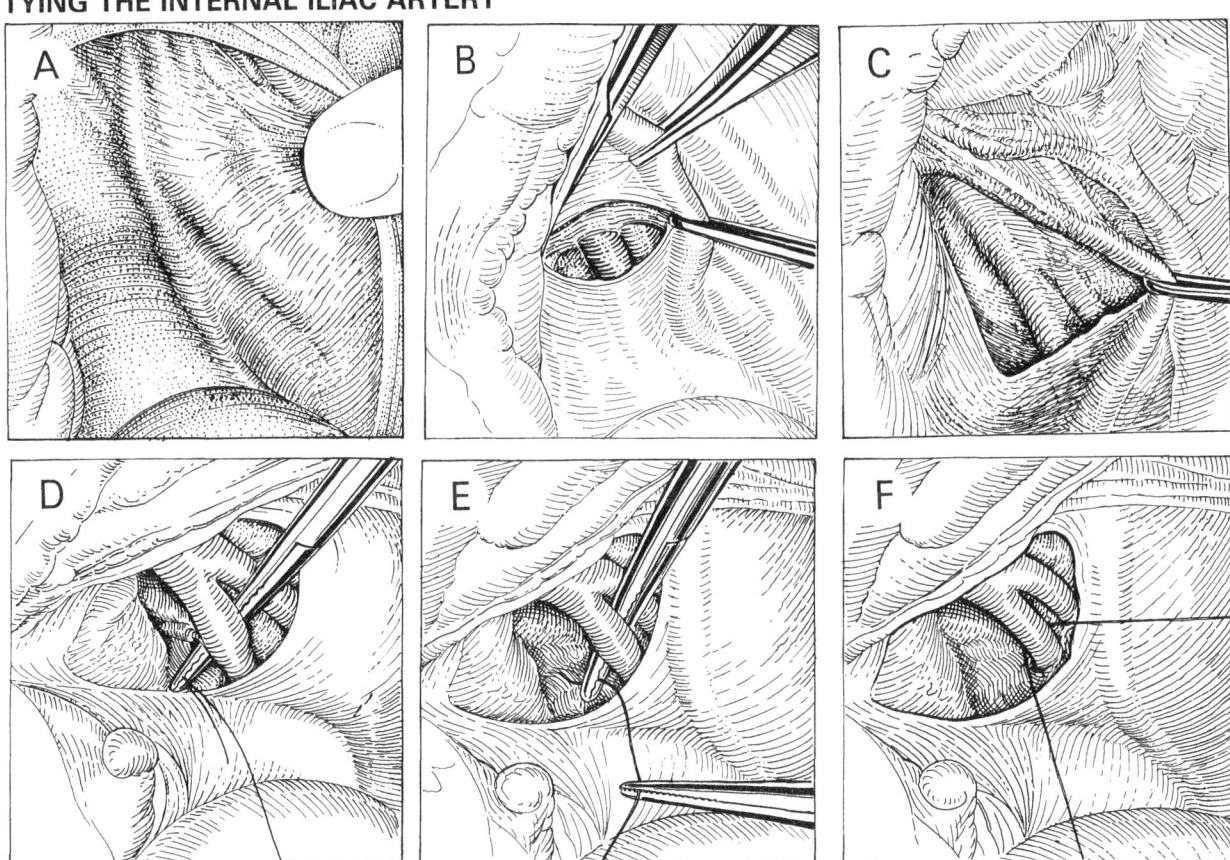

Fig. 3-7 TYING THE LEFT INTERNAL ILIAC ARTERY. A, the ureter crossing the bifurcation of the common iliac artery. B, the ureter retracted and the peritoneum incised. C, the bifurcation exposed. D, a haemostat has been passed under the internal iliac artery. E, grasping the other end of the ligature. F, the ligature ready to tie. *After Lees DH and Singer A, Colour Atlas of Gynaecological Surgery, Vol. 6, p. 108. Wolfe Medical Publications, with kind permission.*

3.6 Tying the external iliac artery in the groin

If a wound is so high up in a patient's thigh that you cannot control bleeding by tying his femoral artery below its profunda branch (which is the main source of his collateral circulation), you may have to tie his external iliac artery instead. Be careful not to injure his external iliac vein and femoral nerve as you do so. This is a difficult procedure, if you are inexperienced.

The external iliac artery arises at the brim of the pelvis from the common iliac artery and runs to the mid inguinal point, where it becomes the femoral artery. The external iliac vein lies medial to it, and the psoas muscle behind it. The femoral nerve lies about a centimetre lateral to it, with the genitofemoral nerve in between them. The peritoneum lies in front of the artery, until the point at which it turns upwards on to the anterior abdominal wall. Below this point, and immediately above the inguinal ligament, the external iliac artery is related from within outwards to: (1) the transversalis muscle, (2) the internal oblique, and (3) the external oblique muscles.

Two branches arise from the external iliac artery : (1) The inferior epigastric artery, which runs upwards into the rectus sheath (23-20). (2) The deep circumflex iliac artery, which runs laterally along the back of the inguinal ligament.

3.7 Tying the femoral artery

If a patient has a penetrating wound of his thigh, you may need to tie his femoral artery. If possible, tie it in his subsartorial canal, below its profunda branch, so that this can supply his leg via the anastomoses that its perforating branches make with the arterial plexus round his knee. If you tie it above its profunda branch, his circulation may be be maintained via the cruciate anastomosis with branches of his internal iliac artery, but this is less reliable.

The femoral artery starts at the mid inguinal point as a continuation of the external iliac artery. It runs down the thigh obliquely, first across the femoral triangle, and then underneath the sartorius muscle. It ends at the junction of the middle and lower thirds of the thigh, by going through a hole in the adductor magnus, and becoming the popliteal artery.

As the femoral artery crosses the femoral triangle, the femoral vein lies medial to it, becoming posterior distally; the femoral nerve lies about a centimetre laterally. Further on, when the femoral artery is in the canal underneath sartorius, the adductor longus and adductor magnus muscles lie behind it; vastus medialis lies anterolaterally. The femoral vein now lies posterolaterally, the nerve to vastus medialis laterally, and the saphenous nerve anteromedially.

The superficial epigastric artery, the superficial circumflex iliac artery, and the superficial and deep external pudendal arteries all arise from the femoral artery close to its origin. The profunda femoris artery arises about 3 cm below the inguinal ligament, runs medially behind the femoral artery, and finally breaks up into branches which run into the adductor muscles.

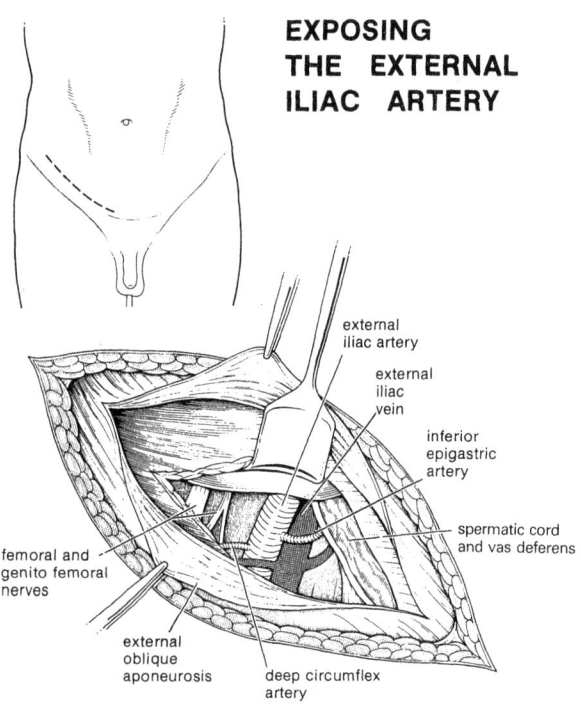

Fig. 3-8. EXPOSING THE EXTERNAL ILIAC ARTERY. If a wound is so high up in a patient's thigh that you cannot control bleeding by tying his femoral artery below its profunda branch, you may have to tie his external iliac artery. *Adapted from 'Farquharson's Textbook of Operative Surgery'. Edited by RF Rintoul. Churchill Livingstone, with kind permission.*

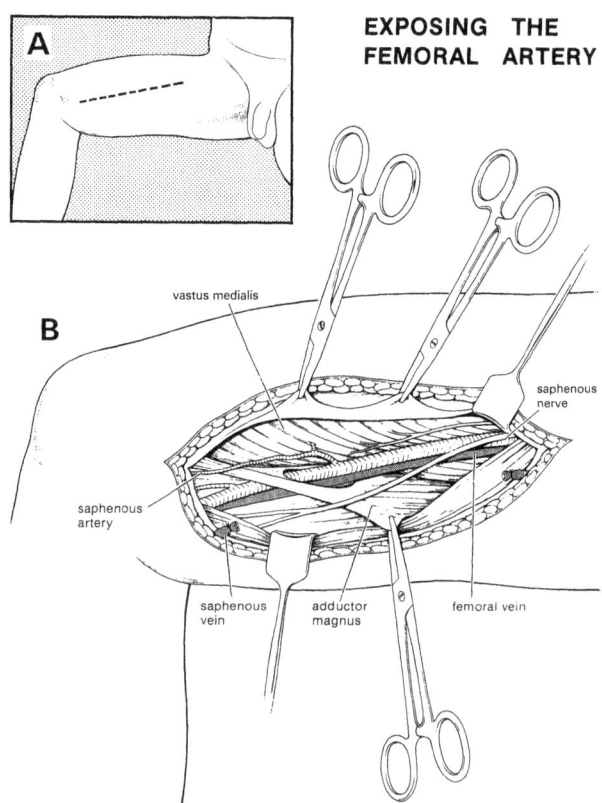

Fig. 3-9 EXPOSING THE FEMORAL ARTERY is one of the more useful of the arterial exposures described here, because you will need it in an above-knee amputation, and you may need it in a penetrating wound of the thigh. *Adapted from 'Farquharson's Textbook of Operative Surgery', edited by RF Rintoul. Churchill Livingstone, with kind permission.*

TYING THE EXTERNAL ILIAC ARTERY

Put the patient into a moderate Trendelenburg position. Make an incision above and parallel to the middle of his inguinal ligament. Open his inguinal canal and divide the muscular fibres of his internal oblique above his inguinal ligament.

Incise his transversalis fascia, and retract his spermatic cord upwards and medially. Gently raise his peritoneum and you will see his external iliac artery and vein. As you do so, try not to cut his inferior epigastric artery and its vein.

Separate the artery carefully from the vein, pass an aneurysm needle round it, tie it with 1 silk or linen, and don't divide it.

TYING THE FEMORAL ARTERY

Flex the patient's thigh slightly, and rotate it laterally. If you plan to tie his femoral artery distal to his mid thigh, apply a tourniquet. Draw a line from his mid inguinal point to his adductor tubercle. His femoral artery lies under the upper two-thirds of this line—palpate it. Make an adequate incision at a suitable place along this line. His long saphenous vein lies in the superficial fascia. Try not to cut it. If by any chance you have to to tie his femoral vein, this will form the main venous collateral.

Incise his deep fascia, mobilize his sartorius muscle, and reflect this laterally to expose the upper part of his femoral and profunda arteries.

To expose the lower part of his femoral artery, reflect his sartorius medially, and divide the bridge of fibrous tissue which roofs his subsartorial canal. His femoral artery may be very difficult to find. If it is, release the proximal tourniquet (if you have applied one), and feel for pulsations.

Separate his femoral artery and vein carefully. Preserve the vein if you can. Proximally, they lie together within the femoral sheath, distally this becomes the femoral fascia. Pass an aneurysm needle round the artery, tie it with zero silk or linen, and don't divide it.

3.8 Tying the popliteal artery

You may need to expose a patient's popliteal artery in wounds of his popliteal fossa. This is difficult. Although the popliteal fossa looks easy in diagrams, in reality all its contents are cramped together. Nerves, arteries, and veins all look much the same until you dissect them out carefully. Unless you have previously exsanguinated the patient's leg with an Esmarch bandage, blood will flood up everywhere, and you can easily injure his common peroneal nerve.

The popliteal artery begins as the continuation of the femoral artery, at the opening in adductor magnus. It then runs downwards in the popliteal fossa until it reaches the lower border of the popliteus muscle, where it divides to form the anterior and posterior tibial arteries, and the peroneal artery. The popliteal vein lies medial to the lower end of the popliteal artery and crosses it posteriorly to lie posterolateral to its upper part. The medial popliteal nerve crosses the popliteal artery and vein posteriorly from the lateral side above, to the medial side below. The lateral popliteal nerve lies more superficially in the lateral part of the fossa.

TYING THE POPLITEAL ARTERY

Lay the patient prone. If he is having a general anaesthetic he must be given a relaxant and intubated, and his respiration controlled. Exsanguinate his leg with an Esmarch bandage and apply a tourniquet.

Make a 15 cm 'lazy S' incision over the centre of his popliteal fossa, with the distal end on the medial side, so as to avoid his superficially placed lateral popliteal nerve. Carefully cut through his superficial fascia. Find his sural nerve and hold it aside. Now incise the fascial roof of his popliteal fossa vertically, and retract his hamstring muscles and the two heads of gastrocnemius.

CAUTION ! Before you tie his popliteal artery, carefully separate it from the vein and nerves which accompany it.

If necessary, you can carry the incision downwards to expose the lower part of his popliteal artery and the origin of his two tibial arteries. Divide the fibrous arch which crosses these vessels and the fibres of his soleus muscle which arise from it.

The popliteal artery has few collateral branches, so preserve as much of its length as you can by by tying it close to the lesion. Pass an aneurysm needle round it, tie it with zero silk or linen, and don't divide it.

3.9 Bloodless limb operations

One of the great advantages of operating on a patient's limb is that you can use a tourniquet to prevent bleeding. This will save blood and enable you to see his tissues more clearly.

You can use any of these:

A special pneumatic tourniquet which resembles the cuff of a sphygmomanometer. The pressure at which a tourniquet is applied is important; this is more easily controlled pneumatically, so a pneumatic tourniquet is much the best. Also you can, if necessary, let it down rapidly during an operation to perfuse the tissues, or to find arteries that need tying.

An Esmarch's bandage which is a strip of red rubber 7 cm wide and 2 metres long. It is satisfactory, provided: (1) You spread it out carefully over an encircling cotton wool pad. (2) You don't put it on too tight, especially on a thin limb.

A reliable sphygmomanometer. You may not have a special pneumatic tourniquet, so this is probably what you will have to use.

Never use a Samway's tourniquet. This is a rubber tube with a hook at one end. It too easily injures the tissues underneath it.

A tourniquet will prevent blood entering a limb, but it will not remove blood which was already there when you applied it. You can remove this blood in two ways: (1) You can raise the patient's limb for at least a minute to help the blood to drain away from it before you apply the tourniquet. This is the only safe thing to do if there is sepsis. It will leave a little blood in his vessels, which can be an advantage, because you can more easily see where they are. (2) You can wind an Esmarch bandage round his limb from its distal to its proximal end to squeeze out the blood. Then you can apply a pneumatic tourniquet (or a sphygmomanometer) round the base of his limb to stop blood entering it. Finally, you can remove the Esmarch bandage. This will provide an almost totally bloodless field, but is only safe if there is no sepsis.

A tourniquet has disadvantages: (1) If you apply too much pressure for too long over too narrow an area, you may injure the nerves to the limb, and cause a paresis; this is usually only temporary, but it may be permanent. A transient radial nerve palsy is common, even if you apply a tourniquet correctly. (2) If you forget to take a tourniquet off, so that it is left on for 6 hours or more, Volkmann's ischaemic contracture, myoglobinaemia, or gangrene may follow. This happens more

EXPOSING THE LEFT POPLITEAL ARTERY

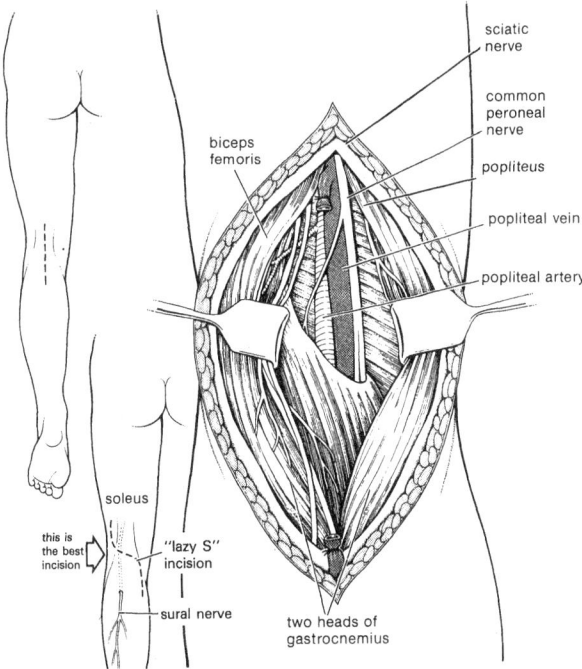

Fig. 3-10 EXPOSING THE POPLITEAL ARTERY is difficult, because, although the popliteal fossa looks easy in a diagram, in real life its contents are cramped together. A vertical incision is shown. A 'lazy S' incision is better. *Adapted from 'Farquharson's Textbook of Operative Surgery', edited by RF Rintoul. Churchill Livingstone, with kind permission.*

easily if a patient has arterial disease. So apply a tourniquet carefully; record the time when you applied it, and don't leave it on too long (arm 1½ hours, leg 2 hours, shorter times and lower pressures in children). (3) If a tourniquet is too loose, it may obstruct only the veins, and increase bleeding.

• TOURNIQUET Conn, improved pneumatic with dial, in case complete, (a) adult, (b) child. One only of each size. A pneumatic tourniquet is one of the most useful surgical instruments, and is almost essential. Alas, few district hospitals have them.

• BANDAGE, rubber, Esmarch 3 m × 75 × 1 mm, fitted with tapes, two only. If you don't have an Esmarch bandage, cut one spirally from the inner tube of a motor cycle tyre, leaving out the elliptical pieces shown as in Fig. 3-12. The tube from an ordinary car tyre is too thick.

HANK (42 years) was to have a bunion removed. The junior resident was asked to apply an Esmarch tourniquet. He had never applied one before, so he just wound the whole bandage round the patient's unpadded leg. 10 days later at the follow up clinic the patient had a numb foot. LESSON Learn how to apply a tourniquet, before you apply one.

**IF YOU APPLIED A TOURNIQUET,
IT IS YOUR RESPONSIBILITY TO REMOVE IT**

TOURNIQUETS

INDICATIONS. (1) A wound toilet in a patient's injured limb, particularly if this has to be followed by the repair of his vessels, nerves, and tendons. (2) Any hand operation, other than a very small one. Hand injuries, and hand sepsis. (3) The exploration and drainage of bones and joints, when this is anatomically possible, as in a patient's lower humerus, his elbow and parts distal to it. Or his lower femur, his knee, and parts distal to that.

CONTRAINDICATIONS. (1) The SS and CS varieties of sickle cell disease, but not AS heterozygotes. (2) Impaired circulation due to arterial disease. Sepsis is not usually considered a contraindication to the use of a tourniquet, but it is to exsanguination with an Esmarch's bandage.
CAUTION! Never use a rubber tube tourniquet (such as Samway's), except on a finger, where you can use a catheter for a few minutes. Anywhere else, a rubber tube may damage the nerves of the limb.

ANAESTHESIA. A tourniquet is painful and a conscious patient will not usually tolerate one for more than 5 minutes. So the practical methods of anaesthesia are: (1) General anaesthesia. (2) Ketamine (A 8.1). (3) Axillary block (A 6.18).

SITES FOR APPLYING A TOURNIQUET There are only four of these: (1) The middle of a patient's upper arm (D, in Fig. 3-11). (2) His finger (F). Use a rubber catheter. This is only safe for a short procedure, such as draining a pulp infection. (3) His upper thigh, a hand's breadth below his groin if he is an adult (E). At this point the femoral artery lies close to the femur and is easily compressed.
CAUTION! (1) Don't apply a tourniquet anywhere else. A tourniquet on the forearm is dangerous, so is one on the lower leg, because you may damage the common peroneal nerve as it winds round the neck of the fibula. (2) Tie a tourniquet to the operating table, to prevent anyone forgetting it, because the patient cannot later be lifted off the table without removing it. A tourniquet hidden under drapes can easily be forgotten.

THE SAFE TIMES for an adult of average build are—the arm 1½ hours, the leg 2 hours. Shorten these times by 60% in a thin adult. Halve them in an 8 year old child. Apply a tourniquet to a finger for a few minutes only. The responsibility for keeping within these times lies with the anaesthetist, who should remind the surgeon every 15 minutes how long a tourniquet has been applied.

ELEVATE THE PATIENT'S LIMB for a few minutes before you apply any kind of tourniquet. If you are going to apply an Esmarch's bandage, now is the time to apply it.

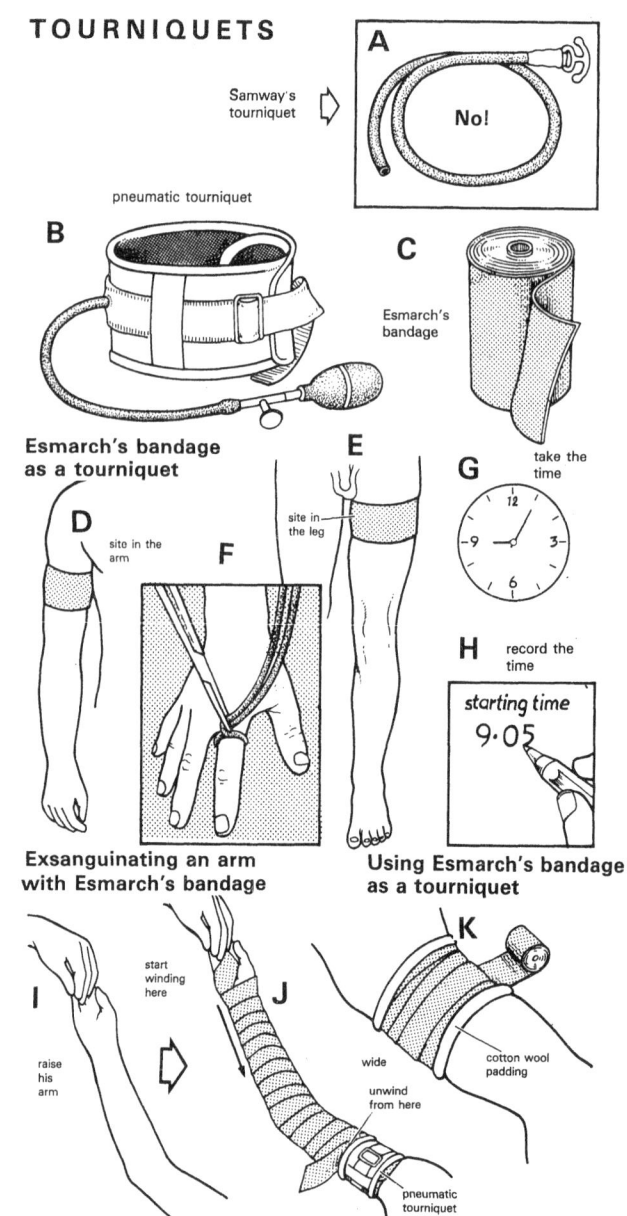

Fig. 3-11 TOURNIQUETS. A, don't use Samway's tourniquet, or you may injure the patient's limb. B, a pneumatic tourniquet is much the best. C, Esmarch's bandage is a roll of red rubber. D, the site to apply it in the arm. E, the site in the leg. F, use a rubber catheter as a finger tourniquet. G, and H, when you apply a tourniquet, take the time and record it. I, if you want to exsanguinate a patient's arm, raise it and then apply Esmarch's bandage, starting in the patient's hand. J, blow up the pneumatic tourniquet, then unwind the bandage, starting proximally in his limb. K, you can use Esmarch's bandage as a tourniquet.

PNEUMATIC TOURNIQUET. Place a folded towel, or a thin layer of cotton wool, around the limb at the site where the tourniquet is to be applied. Wrap this snugly round the patient's limb—it must not be loose. Pump it up to the appropriate reading for 'arm', or 'leg', on the scale. For a child use a lower pressure as indicated out of the way of the operation, but keep the dial where you can read it. If the bag becomes contaminated, autoclave it (2.4).

USING A SPHYGMOMANOMETER AS A TOURNIQUET. On a patient's leg apply the cuff over his femoral artery. On his arm apply it as if you were taking his blood pressure, or if necessary higher up his arm. Bandage it in place with a firm unyielding bandage, and fix this with adhesive strapping.
Blow up the cuff until his distal pulses just disappear. Remember the pressure, and let the cuff down again. When you want to use it, blow it up to 80 or 100 mm above the pressure which just stops the pulses. This is about 200 mm for the arm

MORE TOURNIQUETS

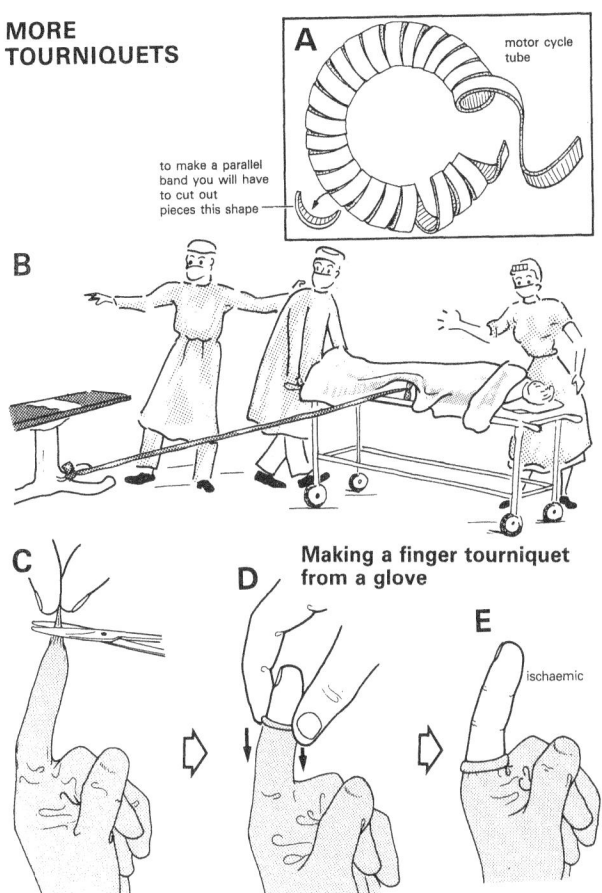

Fig. 3-12 MORE TOURNIQUETS. A, you can cut an Esmarch bandage from the inner tube of a motor cycle tyre (a car inner tube is too thick). B, when you apply a tourniquet, tie it to the operating table, so that you do not leave it on by mistake. C, using a discarded glove as a finger tourniquet. B, after Sally Piper from the British Journal of Anaesthesia.

in an adult and 180 mm in a child. For an adult leg blow it up to 250 mm. Ask an assistant to keep the cuff at this pressure, and to inflate it as necessary.

CAUTION ! Don't inflate any cuff to more than 80 to 100 mm above the pressure that will just obliterate the pulse.

USING AN ESMARCH BANDAGE AS A TOURNIQUET Tape a folded towel or a thin layer of cotton wool in position over his limb. Apply Esmarch's bandage over about 12 cm.

Put on the first two layers of the bandage without pulling. Next, do a trial run to find how many turns are necessary to obliterate the pulse. Pull out the bandage to about three-quarters of its potential expansion length with each wind. Count the number of winds you need to obliterate the pulse.

When you want to apply it, apply five more winds than are necessary to obliterate the pulse. When you have finished, it should feel moderately firm, but not rock hard.

CAUTION ! (1) Don't apply a tourniquet over too narrow a band of muscles. (2) Don't *ever* wind on more than five turns after you have obliterated the pulse. Every turn may add 100 mm more pressure.

AT THE END OF THE OPERATION

There are two ways of controlling bleeding after you have applied a tourniquet. You can release it, either:

(1) Just before you close the patient's wound. Use this method when you do a fine operation on his hand, for example. It will reduce the blood clot in his tissues, and the stiffness and fibrosis that this might cause. Release the tourniquet, raise his limb, apply large swabs to the wound, and press them for five minutes. Lactic acid will have accumulated in his anoxic limb and will make its vessels dilate immediately the tourniquet is released. As this is metabolized, they will contract

again. Remove the swabs and tie any bleeding vessels that remain. Expect him to bleed into his dressings.

Or, (2) at the end of the operation after you have closed his wound. Use this method after operations in which clot in his tissues will be less important, as when you do a sequestrectomy (7.6). Tie any tie major vessels when you come to them during an operation. When the operation is complete, sew up the wound, apply a pressure dressing, and let down the tourniquet. Remove the pressure dressing 48 hours later. Usually, this is all that is necessary. Occasionally, the wound will bleed, so that you have to remove the dressing, open it and tie the bleeding vessel. If you need to immobilize an open fracture, loosely apply a well padded cast.

EXSANGUINATING A LIMB WITH ESMARCH'S BANDAGE

INDICATIONS. Any operation in which you want a completely bloodless field, particularly orthopaedic operations.

CONTRAINDICATIONS. (1) Sepsis. (2) Amputations for malignancy. It may spread both of these.

METHOD. Apply a pneumatic tourniquet round the base of the patient's limb but don't blow it up.

Raise his limb and wind Esmarch's bandage tightly round it from the distal end proximally. As you do so it will squeeze the blood out of his veins. Blow up the tournqiuet. Finally, remove the Esmarch bandage to expose his bloodless limb.

POSTOPERATIVE CARE ALL METHODS

Raise his arm in a roller towel (75-1), for his leg raise the foot of his bed. Observe the circulation in his limb at least hourly; the capillary reflex is important, so pinch his nail beds. If necessary, remove a pressure bandage or split a cast lengthways and open it at least 2 cm.

DIFFICULTIES WITH TOURNIQUETS

If he CANNOT EXTEND HIS WRIST after the operation, he has a tourniquet palsy. The higher the pressure and the thinner he is, the greater the risk. Fortunately, this is usually temporary and recovers within 3 weeks and occasionally up to 6 months; but it can be permanent.

1½ HOURS IN THE ARM AND 2 HOURS IN THE LEG
LESS FOR THIN ADULTS AND CHILDREN

3.10 Postoperative bleeding, reactionary and secondary haemorrhage

When you have closed an operation wound it may start bleeding: (1) During the first 48 hours (reactionary haemorrhage) because a clot in a vessel has been displaced, or a ligature has slipped. Or, (2) 8 to 14 days later (secondary haemorrhage) when the wound has become infected and eroded a vessel, usually quite a small one, sometimes a larger one. One of the purposes of monitoring a patient immediatelay after an operation is to watch for reactionary haemorrhage, so make sure your staff observe him carefully, and take his pulse and blood pressure regularly.

POSTOPERATIVE BLEEDING

See also particular operations, particularly Caesarean section (18.10) and prostatectomy (23.19).

If a patient's WOUND BLEEDS, try firm local pressure and packing. If it bleeds briskly, you may have injured an artery, such as his inferior epigastric. Minor bleeding is probably coming from his subcutaneous tissues, and is unlikely to be serious. If local pressure fails to control bleeding, take him back to the theatre and open his wound. You can usually do this under local anaesthesia. Remove the sutures and tie or coagulate his bleeding vessels. Make sure he is on antibiotics (2.7).

If his BLOOD PRESSURE FALLS POSTOPERATIVELY, he may be hypovolaemic because: (1) The blood he lost at the operation has not been replaced, especially if he was hypovolaemic before it began. (2) The fluid which he lost into his sequestrated gut has not been replaced. (3) He was anaesthetised too deeply and his respiration is still depressed, leading to hypoxaemia and hypotension. (4) He has been given large doses of opioids, such as morphine or pethidine. (5) He has had a high subarachnoid (spinal) anaesthesic (A 7.4). (6) He may be septicaemic. (7) His gut may have been roughly handled. (8) He has been roughly handled on a trolley. If necessary, restore his blood volume, and nurse him with his legs raised. See also A 4.6.

If he goes into SHOCK with a fast pulse, pallor, perhaps with abdominal distension, or bright red blood from a drain incision, he has probably bled into his peritoneum. If two units of blood do not restore his blood pressure, consider reopening his wound to control the bleeding.

If, after a stomach operation, you ASPIRATE QUANTITIES OF FRESH BLOOD from his nasogastric tube he has probably bled from the anastomosis in his stomach. If his blood pressure is only a little depressed, perform gastric lavage every half hour with iced water containing 8 mg of noradrenalin 200 ml. If he has required more than 3 units of blood to maintain his blood pressure above 100 mm, and you are still aspirating fresh blood an hour later, re-explore him and revise his anastomosis. He is unlikely to stop bleeding spontaneously. A complete mucosal layer may have missed getting sutured. See also Section 11.3

If he BLEEDS FROM HIS GUT some days after the operation, the blood may be coming from a stress ulcer, or from a pre-existing duodenal ulcer. It may threaten his life. Monitor his pulse, his blood pressure, and his urine output. Keep a good drip going, and measure his haematocrit 3-hourly. Have at least two units of blood cross-matched for him. Irrigate his stomach with iced saline or tap water containing noradrenalin 8 mg in 200 ml every half hour. See also Section 11.3.

4 Basic methods and instruments

4.1 Appropriate surgical technology—the equipment you need

You may step into a beautifully organized theatre, or you may have to create it from scratch. To help you in this task we have listed everything you might need to do the procedures we describe, down to the last needle and cake of soap. To minimize the tediousness of long lists we have distributed the equipment through the text, and summarized it in Appendix A. We have included everything which you could reasonably have—but may not have at the moment. For example, many district hospitals don't have skin grafting knives, pneumatic tourniquets, simple bone drills, Kirschner wire, or manometers for measuring the central venous pressure (A 19.2)—but you could reasonably have them, so we have included them. Some of the special methods we describe don't need any extra equipment—for example, the plastic bag method for burnt hands (58.29). Learn to recognize the instruments you use and to know them by their names. *When you first arrive at a hospital check the theatre equipment and find out what is missing!*

When you order equipment that is not listed here try to make sure that: (1) It will work reliably without needing to be returned to the makers to be mended. (2) It will work well in your hands. (3) You can afford both its initial and its running costs. (4) Spares are available. (5) You can easily learn how to use it and teach other people to do the same.

If you want to be well supplied, encourage and motivate your storeman. Look at what he has and how he does things. Don't forget to visit your central medical stores; you may find things you need, which the storeman there cannot identify, and you can make good use of. *The equipment we list is the equipment he should stock*, so do your best to see that government does this.

You will certainly have to improvise. If you don't have the standard stainless steel instruments, don't hesitate to use ordinary steel ones, if you can buy, adapt, or make them. Before stainless steel came into routine use in the 1920s, all surgical equipment was made of ordinary steel, and had to be dried and carefully wiped with an oily rag after each operation. For example, you can use an ordinary steel carpenter's drill instead of a bone drill, and a sterile pair of ordinary pliers may be the best way to remove a plate. If you have no Kirschner wires you may be able to use sharpened bicycle spokes. Don't store instruments of ordinary steel sterilized in packs or drums. The interior of these is damp and they will rust rapidly.

STORES AND EQUIPMENT

QUANTITIES OF ITEMS. The quantities of each item we suggest are those appropriate to an initial stock. The quantities of each item we list are sufficient to make all the sets suggested in Section 4.12. You will probably have to make do with less.

CATALOGUE NUMBERS. Where an item is available from UNICEF, we have given its UNIPAC number. We have given the suppliers of a few items which are difficult to get. These have been listed with three letters in brackets, for example, (EVE) for the Everett Needle Company, and the supplier's names are listed in full in Appendix B.

SUPPLY CYCLES. If your supply period for a consumable item is 'X' months, try to keep three times the quantity of it you consume during this period in stock, so that one indent can go astray without causing disaster.

ORDERING EQUIPMENT. When you order equipment, try to include the catalogue number. Where possible write to the supplier and ask for a 'proforma invoice' giving the exact details and costs, etc. This will make ordering much easier.

WHERE THE EQUIPMENT IS DISCUSSED. The anaesthetic equipment is in *Primary Anaesthesia*, the obstetric equipment is in Section 15.1a and in *Primary Mother Care* .

The theatre. Theatre furniture and lighting, gowns, gloves and drapes (2.1 and 2.3), drains and tubing (4.10). Miscellaneous smaller items of theatre equipment (4.11).

Preventing sepsis. Sterilizing equipment (2.3), antiseptics and disinfectants (2.5).

Preventing bleeding. Haemostats and arterial clamps (3.2), tourniquets (3.9).

Cutting and holding tissues. Scalpels and dissectors (4.2), scissors (4.3), forceps (4.4), retractors (4.5), suture materials (4.6), needles and their holders (4.7).

Special procedures Operating on bones and joints (7.4), intestinal surgery (9.3), obstetrics (15.1), proctology (22.1), urology (23.1), eye (24.1), ENT (25.1), dentistry (26.1), first aid equipment (50.3), tracheostomy (52.1), skin grafting (57.1), neurosurgery (63.1), chest aspiration (65.1), plastering (70.1), bone traction (70.9).

4.2 Scalpels and dissectors

A sharp scalpel cuts tissue with less trauma than any other instrument. There are two ways of holding one: (1) If you need force to make a big bold cut, grasp it with your index finger along the back, as in Fig. 4-1. (2) If you want to cut more gently, hold it like a pen. The size of a blade does not change the way you use it, but its shape does. A small blade allows you to make precise turns. Stab the point of a No.11 blade into an abscess and then sweep it upwards in an arc. Experienced surgeons do a lot of knife dissection; beginners find other instruments safer for many purposes.

• *SCALPEL, solid forged, size No.1, 30 mm, and size No.5, 40 mm, two scalpels only of each size.* If your disposable blades are exhausted, you cannot use a solid scalpel and resharpen it (Appendix A), whereas you cannot resharpen a disposable blade. A solid blade is essential for symphysiotomy (18.4).

• *HANDLE, scalpel, Bard Parker, No.4, eight only.* This is the standard handle for blades 20, 21, 22, 23, and 24. Get good quality handles, because poor ones may not fit the blades.

• *HANDLE, scalpel, Swan Morton, No.5, four only.* This long elegant handle fits blades 10, 11, 12, and 15.

• *BLADES, scalpel, disposable, Bard Parker or Swann Morton type, stainless steel in dispenser containing 100 blades. (a) Type 10, ten dispensers only. (b) Type 11, five dispensers only. (c) Type 15, five dispensers only. (d) Type 22, two dispensers only. (e) Type 24, two dispensers only.* The medium-sized curved blade 10, the small curved blade 15, and the pointed blade 11, all fit into the long No.5 blade holder. The big curved blades 22 and 24 fit into the standard No.4 handle. If

SCALPELS

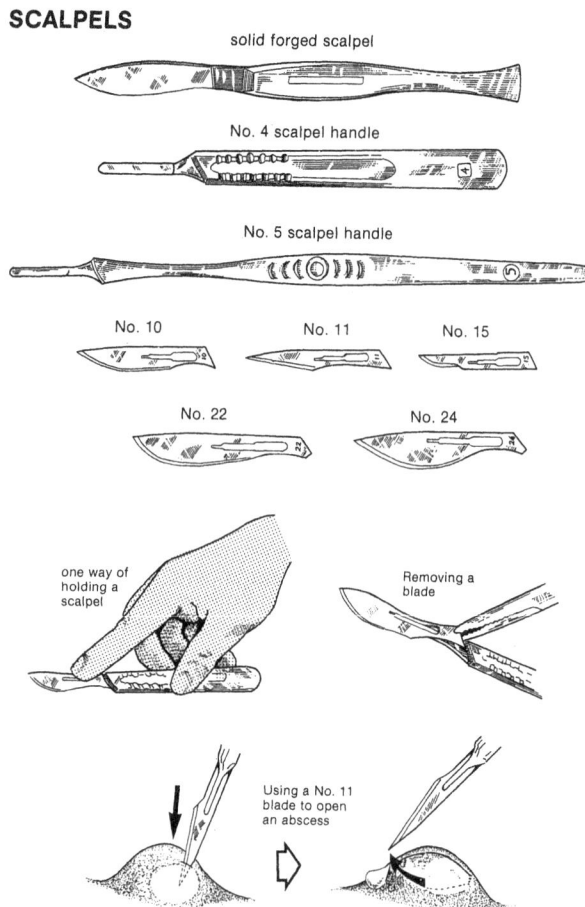

Fig. 4-1 SCALPELS AND HOW TO USE THEM. The advantage of a solid forged scalpel is that you can resharpen it. You also need it for symphysiotomy.

necessary, you can autoclave these blades and use them for 3 or 4 operations.

• OILSTONE, hard Arkansas pattern, 150×70×30 mm, one only. Use this to sharpen scalpels and scissors. A very blunt instrument needs a carborundum stone first.

• DISSECTOR, MacDonald, one only. A blunt dissector is often safer than a scalpel. This is a blunt general purpose dissector, with one straight flat end and one round curved end, neither of which are likely to injure anything.

4.3 Scissors

The tips of a pair of surgical dissecting scissors are usually rounded; scissors in which both tips are pointed are only used for very fine dissection. Look after your scissors carefully. Use straight scissors near the surface and curved ones deeper inside. Hold them with your index finger resting on the blades. Use the tips for cutting.

You can also use scissors for blunt dissection by pushing their blades into tissues and then opening them. This will open the tissues along their natural planes, and push important structures, such as nerves and blood vessels, out of the way. This is the 'push and spread' technique shown in B, Fig. 4-8. If there is something nearby which it would be dangerous to cut, blunt dissection is always safer. But remember that even blunt dissection can injure veins, and that venous bleeding can be very difficult to control.

Remember: (1) Don't use sharp-tipped scissors in dangerous places, or cut what you cannot see. (2) Don't use scissors which are longer than the haemostats you have, or you may find yourself cutting a vessel which you cannot reach to clamp. (3) Mayo's, McIndoe's, and Metzenbaum's scissors are intended for cutting tissues, so don't use them for anything else. Use other scissors for cutting sutures and dressings.

Buy good quality scissors, and don't autoclave them with the other instruments. Instead, keep them in a covered tray of antiseptic (2.5). The very best ones have tungsten carbide inserts, which make their cutting edges last much longer. These are four times more expensive, but justify their extra cost.

• SCISSORS, operating, Mayo, straight, bevelled, 200 mm, one pair only. Use these for cutting sutures.

• SCISSORS, operating, Mayo, curved, bevelled blades, 170 mm, one only. These tissue scissors are curved in the plane of the blades.

• SCISSORS, operating, McIndoe's, curved, with rounded tapering blades, 180 mm, one only. These elegant tapering tissue scissors are curved perpendicular to the plane of the blades.

• SCISSORS, operating, Metzenbaum, curved 275 mm, one pair only. These have long handles and quite narrow blades. Use them for dissecting at the bottom of a deep wound.

• SCISSORS, Aufrecht's, light, curved, 140 mm, one pair only. This pair of scissors is for the set of instruments for hand surgery.

• SCISSORS, straight with fine sharp points, Glasgow pattern, 100 mm, stainless steel, two pairs only. Use these very fine scissors for cutting down on veins.

• SCISSORS, suture cutting, 'assistant's scissors', rounded ends, four pairs only. Keep these in spirit with the other scissors. Your assistant needs a pair; so does the scrub nurse.

• SCISSORS, suture wire cutting, 130 mm, one pair only. If you cut suture wire with ordinary scissors, it will ruin them.

• SCISSORS, bandage, angular, Lister, 180 mm, one only. These have a blunt knob at the end of one blade which goes under the bandage to protect the patient. Insert them away from the wound; if they become soiled or wet, clean and sterilize them before you use them on someone else.

IN DANGEROUS PLACES BLUNT DISSECTION IS SAFER THAN SCISSORS

SCISSORS

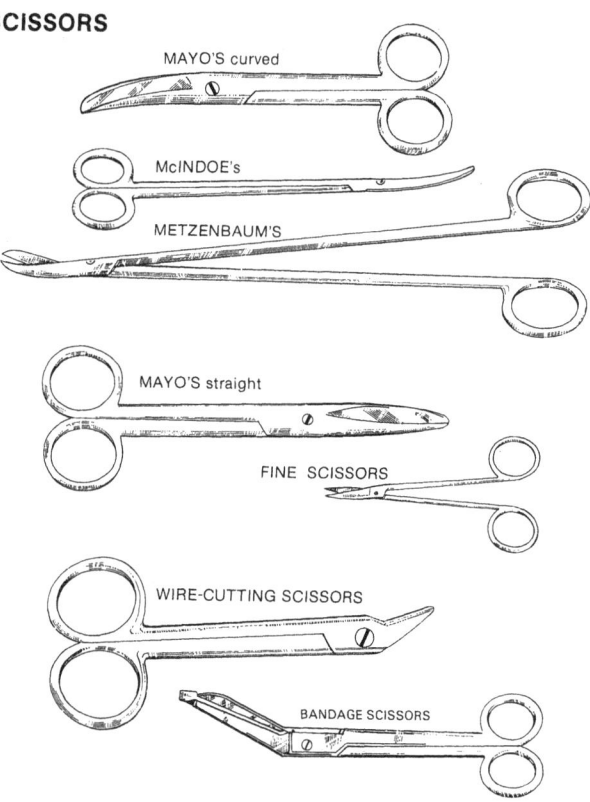

Fig. 4-2 SCISSORS. Mayo's, McIndoe's, and Metzenbaum's scissors are intended for cutting tissues, so don't use them for anything else. Use other scissors for cutting sutures and dressings.

FORCEPS

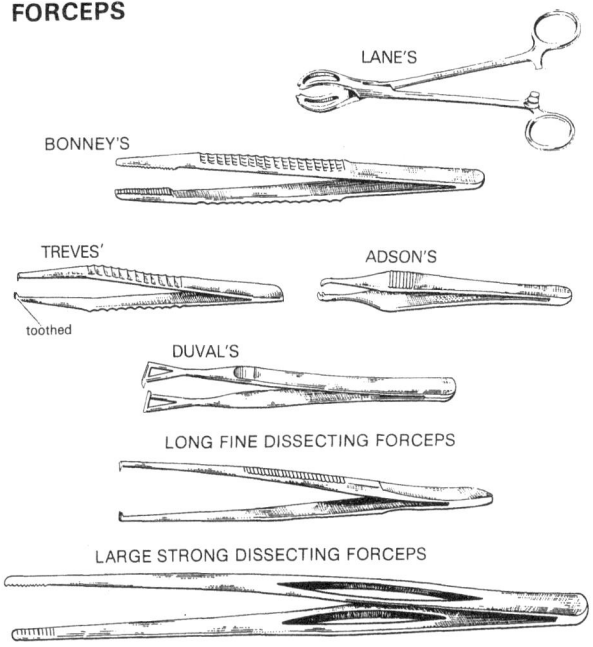

Fig. 4-3 FORCEPS. Dissecting forceps are also called thumb forceps, and can be plain or toothed. Lane's tissue forceps have teeth; Babcock's (not shown) resemble Lane's, but have bars on each blade that come together gently without damaging the tissues.

4.4 Forceps

Dissecting (thumb) forceps can be short for working close to the surface, or longer for working more deeply. They can be plain, or toothed with an odd number of teeth on one jaw, and an even number on the other, either one into two teeth, or three teeth into four, etc. Toothed forceps hold tissue so firmly that only a little pressure is necessary; but they can easily puncture a hollow viscus or a blood vessel. Strong, plain, straight forceps without teeth are even more useful for blunt dissection than they are for holding tissues.

Tissue (locking) forceps have a ratchet which keeps them closed. Some have teeth (Allis') and some have none (Babcock's). The blades of Allis' forceps meet together, and inevitably injure the tissues a little, whereas Babcock's have bowed jaws with a gap between them. This makes them gentler but less secure. When you use Allis' forceps for retracting a skin flap, apply them to the subcutaneous tissue or fascia, and not to the skin itself, which may be injured. Kocher's forceps are stronger, and even more traumatic; they are for clamping wide vascular pedicles, so that the vessels do not slip out (3.2).

- *FORCEPS, dissecting, thumb, blunt, non-toothed, Bonney's, 180 mm, three only.* These are strong dissecting forceps without teeth.
- *FORCEPS, dissecting, thumb, toothed, Treves', 1×2 teeth, 130 mm, five only.* These are the standard toothed dissecting forceps.
- *FORCEPS, dissecting, thumb, fine, Adson's, (a) plain, (b) 1×2 teeth, 120 mm, two only of each.* These have broad handles and fine points and are particularly useful for the eye.
- *FORCEPS, dissecting, thumb, Duval's, 150 mm, with non-traumatic teeth on triangular jaws, two only.* These are thumb forceps for general use.
- *FORCEPS, dissecting, thumb, toothed, 180 mm, one only.* These are long fine dissecting forceps.
- *FORCEPS, dissecting, thumb, Maingot's, 280 mm, one only.* These are large toothed forceps with fenestrated sides that are easy to hold.
- *FORCEPS, dissecting, McIndoe's, plain, 150 mm, one only.* These are for the hand set.
- *FORCEPS, dissecting, ophthalmic, Silcock's, 100 mm, one only.* This is a fine pair of forceps for operating on the eye or the hand.
- *FORCEPS, tissue, locking, Allis', box joint, 150 mm, 5×6 teeth, eight only.*
- *FORCEPS, tissue, locking, Babcock's, box joint, 160 mm, two only.* These have a bar on each blade that comes together gently without damaging the tissues. Use them to hold gut.
- *FORCEPS, tissue, Lane's, 15 cm, two only.* These have curved jaws, teeth and a ratchet.
- *FORCEPS, sinus, Lister, box joint 150 mm, two only.* You can use these for many other purposes besides exploring sinuses. Use them for packing the nose, or putting a drain into an abscess cavity.
- *FORCEPS, cholecystectomy, curved jaws with longitudinal serrations, Lahey's, box joint, 200 mm, one only.* These forceps are useful for other purposes besides dissecting out the cystic duct. If you put them into the tissues and separate them, you can use their rounded ends to define arteries, veins and ducts.
- *FORCEPS, intestinal, Dennis Browne, 180 mm, two only.* Use these to pick up the gut during an abdominal operation, or a hernia repair.
- *FORCEPS, Moynihan, box joint, 220 mm, four only.* Use this massive pair of crushing forceps for wide vascular pedicles, such as those which contain the uterine vessels at hysterectomy.
- *FORCEPS, Desjardin's, screw joint, one only.* Use these for removing stones from the bile duct.
- *FORCEPS (clamps), hysterectomy, curved, box joint, one into two teeth, 23 cm, Hunter or Maingot, four but preferably six only.* Hysterectomy is difficult without several long curved clamps for big vessels, preferably with longitudinal serrations and teeth at their tips.

4.5 Retractors and hooks

You cannot work inside a patient if the rest of him gets in your way. To clear the field, you will have to use retractors. There are two kinds. One has to be held by an assistant, the other holds itself. Any blacksmith should be able to make you the simpler ones from ordinary steel. Strong retraction causes trauma, especially to the edges of the wound. So avoid it by appproaching deep areas through larger incisions.

- *RETRACTOR, Volkmann's rake, sharp, 4 prong, 220 mm, two only.* These have sharp teeth like a cat's paw. Take care that they do not injure anything important.
- *RETRACTOR, Langenbeck, 13×44 mm, two only.* These are fairly small narrow deep retractors.
- *RETRACTOR, Czerny, double ended, four only.* These have a flat blade at one end and two deep prongs at the other. They are thus more versatile than Langenbeck's retractors.
- *RETRACTOR, Lane's modified by Kilner, double ended, 150 mm, two only.* This is a light general-purpose retractor with short shallow hooks at one end and a tongue at the other.
- *RETRACTOR, Gelpie, 170 mm, two only.* A pair of these are very useful as general purpose retractors.
- *RETRACTOR, Morris, double ended, three only.* This is a double ended abdominal retractor. Some surgeons prefer single-ended ones which are easier to hold.
- *RETRACTOR, Deaver's, plain handles, set of five sizes, one set only.* These inexpensive general purpose abdominal retractors nest together, and so are easy to store.
- *RETRACTOR, malleable copper, set of 4 sizes, one set.* These are strips of copper that you can bend into any shape to suit your needs.
- *RETRACTOR, Meydering, 178 mm, two only.* These are for hand surgery and are used as a pair.
- *RETRACTOR, self-retaining, West's, straight, sharp-pronged, one only.* This is a small self retaining general-purpose retractor.
- *RETRACTOR, abdominal, self-retaining, two-blade, adult, Gosset's, one only.* The three blades of this large abdominal retractor can be arranged so that they support one another, and do not have to be held.
- *RETRACTOR, universal, Denis Browne, with (a) one frame 300×240 mm, (b) one frame 300×240 mm, (c) 3 hook-on retractors 50×65 mm, (d) ditto 80×90 mm, (e) ditto 98×50 mm, (f) ditto 105×35 mm, one set only.* This is a useful but expensive retractor. It has a notched ring and hooked prongs, as in Fig. 4-4.
- *HOOKS, tendon, Harlow-Wood, 114 mm.* These are for the hand set (4.12).

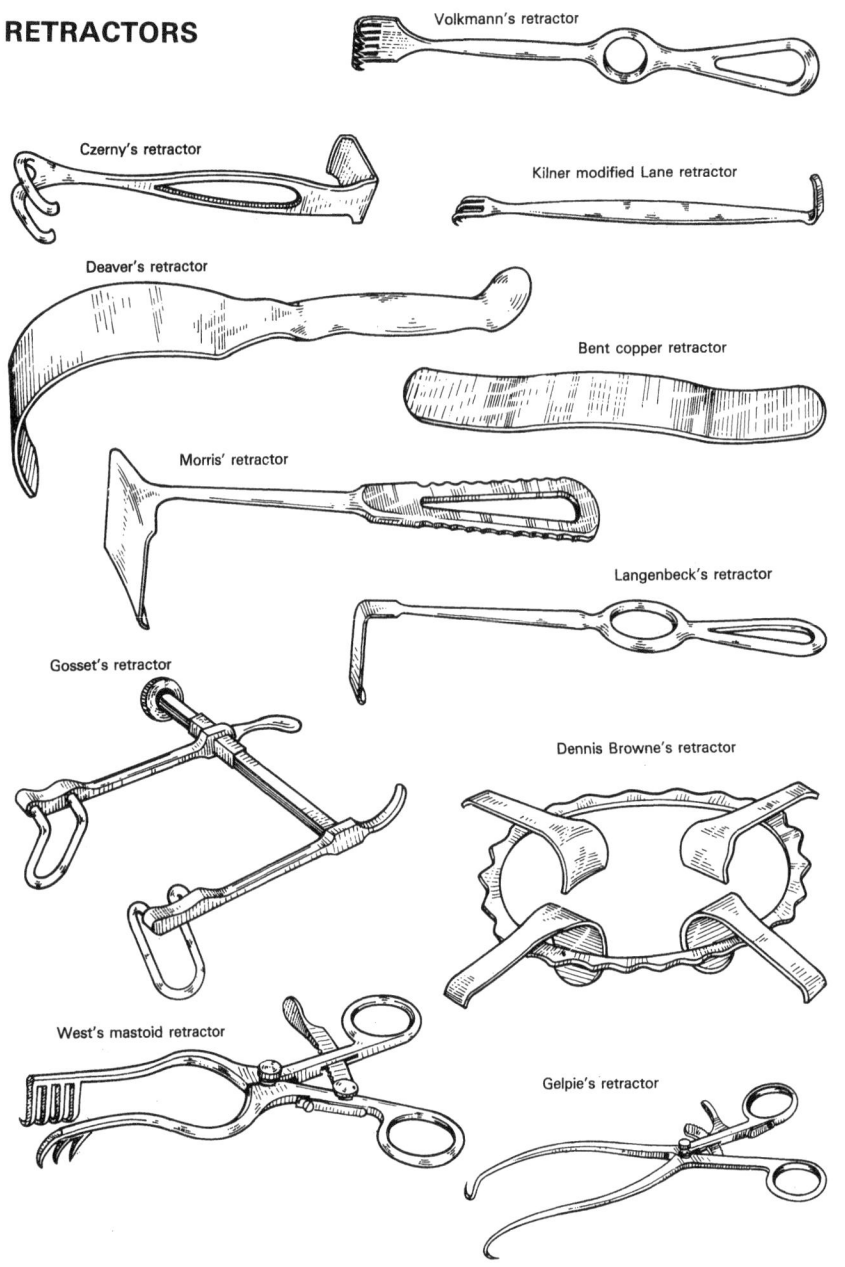

Fig. 4-4 RETRACTORS. You cannot operate on a patient if the surrounding tissues get in your way. These retractors will help to give you a clear field. Some have to be held, others hold themselves.

4.6 Suture materials

If you bring two soft tissues together and hold them there for about 10 days they will join. Most surgery depends on this. The easiest way to hold them is to sew them. You can use: (1) absorbable sutures which are absorbed by the tissues so that you need not remove them. (2) Non-absorbable ones which you leave indefinitely if they are deep, or remove if they are on the skin.

Absorbable sutures can be plain catgut (from the submucosa of sheep, not cats!), which usually holds its strength for about 10 days. Or catgut can be treated with chromic acid (chromic sutures) which slows its absorption and makes it keep its strength for 20 days. Sepsis speeds the dissolution of catgut, especially plain catgut, so that it may dissolve in 2 or 3 days. You can also use absorbable sutures of synthetic material such as polyglycolic acid ('Dexon').

Catgut is soft and holds knots well, but not so well as a non-absorbable multifilament, such as linen or cotton. If a suture material does not hold knots too well, knots made of it need longer ends. So leave knots in catgut with 5 mm ends, unless you are using it for fine superficial vessels. You can cut linen or cotton 2 mm from the knot.

While catgut is being absorbed it makes a good culture medium and may promote sepsis. So don't use more than is necessary, don't leave the ends of ligatures unnecessarily long and avoid thick No. 2 or 3 catgut. Monofilament sutures, especially fine ones, don't have this risk, which is why so many surgeons like them.

If necessary, you can use almost any suture material almost anywhere, especially on the skin. But, *always use use catgut for:* (1) The urinary and the biliary tracts because non-absorbable sutures can act as the focus around which a stone can form. (2) The mucosa of the stomach, where a non-absorbable suture may be the site of an ulcer later. (3) The mucosa of the uterus (less important). (4) Sutures close under the skin, where non-absorbable sutures may work their way to the surface.

Plain catgut does not hold its strength for very long, so *never use plain catgut for:* (1) Tying larger vessels (use linen, cotton or silk). (2) Suturing the gut (use chromic catgut).

One problem with catgut is that it may be of poor quality, and so give way early and perhaps disastrously. This is another reason for using monofilament where you can.

Non-absorbable sutures can be polyamide ('Nylon'), polypropylene ('Prolene'), polyethylene ('Courlene'), linen, cotton, silk, or stainless steel wire. You can use the first three as a single (mono)filament, or as multiple filaments which are braided or twisted together. *Whenever we refer loosely to 'monofilament', we mean a non-absorbable suture of nylon, polyethylene, or polypropylene, or a similar synthetic material as a single filament. It is the most useful general purpose suture material.* Although non-absorbable sutures remain as permanent foreign bodies, monofilament nylon, polyethylene, and steel are less likely to promote infection than catgut, or multifilament cotton, linen, or silk.

Unfortunately, a single thicker filament makes less reliable knots than a many finer ones braided or twisted together, except for steel wire, which is always used as a single filament, and which knots superbly but is difficult to work with. So, always tie monofilament with a surgeon's knot (4.8).

Apart from the indications for catgut given above, you can use monofilament for almost anything, but silk, cotton, or linen threads, are better than monofilament for tying larger vessels. Braided silk may cause troublesome stitch abscesses. Don't use it immediately under the skin, because it may work its way through to the surface, long after healing is complete. If it does become infected, you may have to remove it piece by piece. Even monofilamant can come to the surface, so keep it well buried, and use catgut close under the skin.

The strength of sutures is measured in two systems. In the old system the finest ones are measured in 'zeros' and the thicker ones are numbered. From finest to thickest the sequence is—6/0, 5/0, 4/0, 3/0, 2/0, 0, 1, 2, 3, 4. Although attempts are being made to replace the old system by a metric one from 0 to 8, most surgeons still use the old one. So do we.

Use the thinnest sutures you can—they need only be as strong as the tissues they are holding together. You can do most operations with sutures between 3/0 and 1 on the old scale. Only very occasionally will you need sutures which are thicker or thinner than this, except for fine work such as nerve or tendon repairs, and for eye and plastic surgery. If you do need a thicker suture, you can double up a thinner one.

The cost of sutures can significantly increase the cost of an operation. In the industrial world they are now sold in individual disposable packs, which are expensive to make and waste much suture material each time a pack is opened. This, combined with the use of atraumatic needles, means that the needles and sutures for one operation may cost $20. But if you buy monofilament in rolls, and use ordinary needles, the suture materials for a single operation cost almost nothing. Monofilament suture material in packets is 20,000% more expensive than in reels, and with needles swaged on is 30,000% more!

Never let the lack of suture materials be the reason for not doing an urgent operation. Either use ordinary nylon fishing line, which is exactly the same material as that used for surgical sutures. Or, if necessary, you can use ordinary linen or cotton thread almost anywhere.

- *SUTURES, polyamide ('Nylon'), or polyethylene ('Courlene'), monofilament, strengths 5/0, 4/0, 3/0, 0 and 1, reels of 1000 metres, preferably each size a different colour (PEA), two reels only of No. 1, one reel only of the other sizes.* No. 1 is the most generally useful size. Use 4/0 monofilament as your basic suture material for fine skin sutures.
- *SUTURES, catgut, plain, 3/0, in boxes of 12, five boxes only.* Plain catgut is soft. Use it for suturing the mouth, tongue, and lip.
- *SUTURES, catgut, chromic, strengths 3/0, 2/0, 0, 1 and 2, boxes of 12, ten boxes only of each strength.* This is the most commonly used form of catgut.
- *SUTURES, catgut, chromic, atraumatic, (a) 2/0 on half circle 30 mm needles, ten boxes only. (b) 2/0 on 5/8 circle 30 mm needles, ten boxes only. (c) 4/0 on 16 mm curved needle, ten boxes only.* These sutures have needles swaged on to them. Use them for the gut, the gall-bladder, and the stomach, held in a needle-holder. The smaller needles (c) are for children.

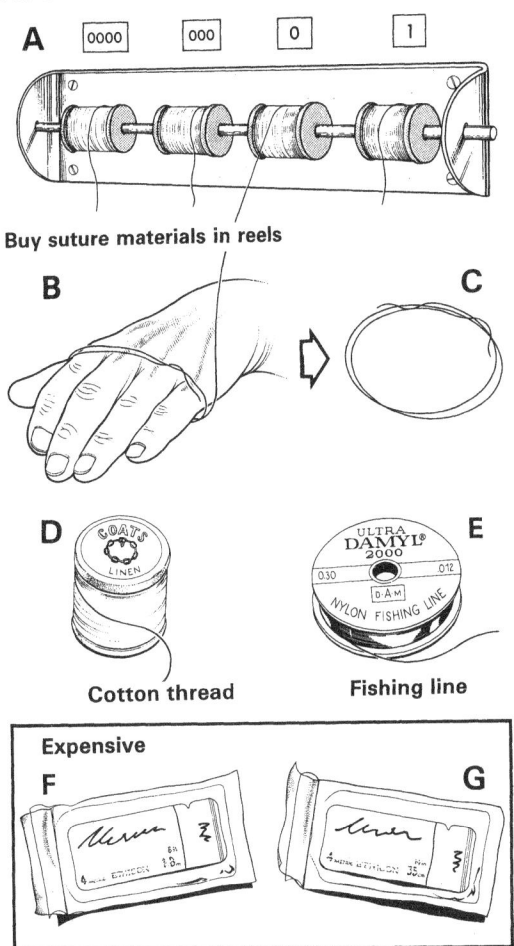

Fig. 4-5 BUY MONOFILAMENT IN REELS. A, hang them from a wall bracket, cut lengths of suture material about a metre long and twist them into loose coils (B, and C) or wind them round the empty spools used for disposable sutures. If funds are scarce, avoid expensive proprietary sutures F, and G. You can also use cotton or linen thread, or colourless fishing line. Match this against surgical monofilament nylon strength for strength. A good strength for abdominal sutures is 5 to 7 kg breaking strength.

- *SUTURES, prolene, atraumatic, (a) 4/0 on 16 mm half circle, round-bodied needles, (b) 8/0 on 3 mm 3/8 circle atraumatic needles, two boxes only of each size.*
- *SUTURES, linen, No. 1, five reels only.* Use linen for tying vessels. It holds knots well and is stronger than cotton.
- *SUTURES, nylon or virgin silk, 8/0, one box only.* These are for suturing the cornea.
- *WIRE, monofilament, soft stainless steel, (a) 5/0, (b) 0.35 mm, (c) 1.0 mm, one reel only of each thickness.* Surgical wire must be soft and malleable because springy wire is difficult to work with. Autoclave the whole reel. (a) Fine 5/0 wire is cheap, and is excellent for the skin, if you can learn to use it efficiently. (b) 0.35 mm wire is for wiring the teeth (62.10) and for hemicirclage (72.18). (c) Tension 1.0 mm wire in a stirrup and use it for exerting traction (70.12). These wires and the equipment to use them (70.9) are essential. One of the advantages of wire is that, unlike more massive pieces of metal, it does not promote infection, so that you can if necessary put it though infected tissues. You can wire tissues in the presence of sepsis; for example, when you repair a burst abdomen (9.13).

Fasten wire by passing its ends through any convenient tube, such as that from a ball pen, and then grasping the ends and twisting them. Finally, cut the twisted ends of the wire short. This will prevent it from coiling up in an inconvenient way.

- *WALL BRACKET, stainless steel, to hold rolls of monofilament, as in Fig. 4-5, one only.* Fix this to the wall, and pull lengths of monofilament from it. If you cannot get one of these brackets, make it.

• *REELS, stainless steel, egg shaped ('eggs'), for holding suture material, five only.* Wind monofilament into these, autoclave them and cut off the length of suture material you require.

Dr JAMES MUKOLAGE was horrified to find in his village a woman with an abdominal wound from which gut was protruding. He was only recently qualified and had not operated on one of these cases before. He had few facilities, but he managed to find some local anaesthetic solution and some linen thread in the shops. A few instruments from the local health centre were boiled up; he washed the wound thoroughly, and anaesthetized the tissues round it with lignocaine. Fortunately, her gut had only a minor cut in it which was easily repaired. When he had returned her gut to her abdomen he was able to close it with linen thread. She survived. LESSON Improvisation can save lives.

**MONOFILAMENT IS THE MOST USEFUL GENERAL PURPOSE SUTURE MATERIAL
TIE IT WITH A SURGEON'S KNOT**

4.7 Needles and their holders

Needles can be round-bodied, or they can have cutting edges. They can be thin or thick, large or small; straight, or curved into 3/8, half, or 5/8 of a circle. Curved needles are for working in confined spaces. The smaller ones have to be held in a needle holder. Use a 3/8 circle needle in a shallow space, and a 5/8 needle in a deep one. The narrower and deeper the hole the smaller and more curved the needle has to be. If necessary, you can try to bend a half curved needle into a 5/8 circle. If you don't have a suture needle, you can bend the wire stylet of an intramuscular needle into a loop, push both ends back into the neeedle, crimp them with a pair of pliers, and then bend the needle into any kind of curve you want, as in K, Fig. 4-6.

A needle can have an eye, or the suture material can be fixed to it to form an atraumatic needle. These are expensive, but they make smaller, neater holes, because the suture material is not doubled through the extra thickness of the eye. Use atraumatic needles to suture gut, the urinary tract, blood vessels, nerves, the cornea and the face, especially the eyelids. For anything else they are unnecessary and wasteful. Unfortunately, because atraumatic needles are so extensively used in the industrial world, needles with eyes may be difficult to get.

Always use a cutting needle for the skin, either a straight one or a large curved one held in your hand, or a smaller curved one held in a needle holder. Use a cutting needle for tough fascia. Mayo's needle is a hybrid—it has a trocar point and a curved round shank. Use it for big wide vascular pedicles and tough tissues, such as ligaments. Use round-bodied needles for most other tissues. If you have difficulty getting needles, we list a supplier in Appendix B (SHO). Resharpen cutting needles on a stone (Appendix A).

You will want a needle-holder to hold small needles and suture in a confined space. Use a holder with a short handle near the surface, and a long one deeper inside. Use big needles in big holders, and small needles in small holders. A large needle can break a fine needle-holder such as Derf's, so treat it with care. Needle-holders can have plain jaws, or tungsten carbide inserts which prevent the hard steel of the needles wearing them away. These cost twice as much, but last more than twice as long. Quality counts in needle-holders, so get good ones.

• *NEEDLES, suture, Keith, triangular straight 64 mm, 25 needles only.* This is the standard straight, hand held needle for stitching skin. It is easy to sharpen and one needle may last you a year.
• *NEEDLES, suture, 3/8 circle, curved, triangular point, sizes 4, 12, and 18, 25 needles of each size.* These are the standard curved needles. Hold the largest ones in your hand and the smaller ones in a holder.
• *NEEDLES, suture, 1/2 circle curved, triangular, sizes 2, 8, 14 and 20, 50 needles of each size only.* Use these strong, triangular cutting needles for the scalp.
• *NEEDLES, suture, round bodied, 3/8 circle curved, sizes 4, 10 and 18, 25 needles of each size only.* Use these for suturing soft tissue such as the peritoneum and broad ligament.

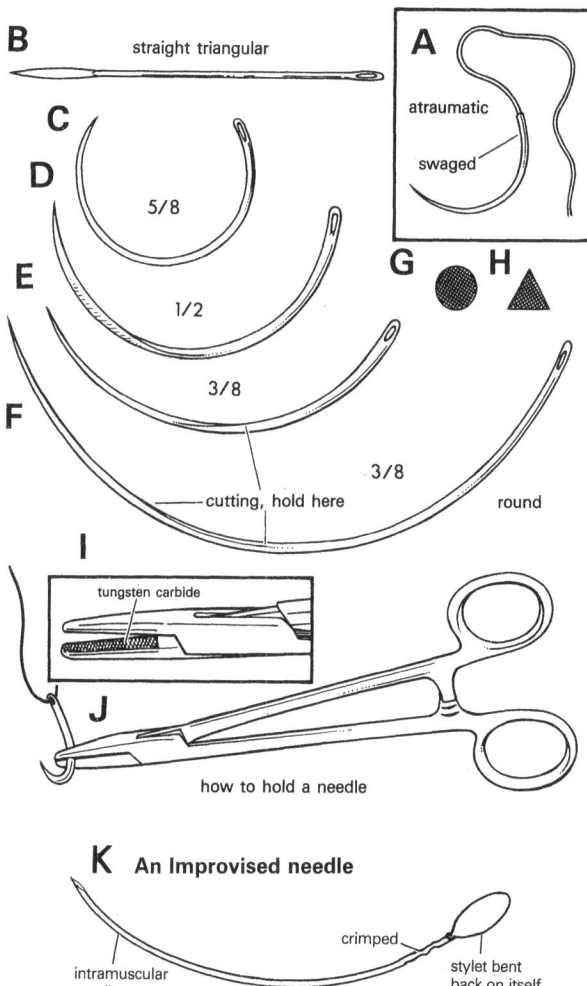

Fig. 4-6 NEEDLES. A, an atraumatic suture with a needle swaged on to it for suturing the gut. B, Keith's straight triangular hand-held needle for suturing the skin. C, a 5/8 circle round-bodied needle for suturing deep in a wound. D, a half circle triangular cutting needle for suturing soft tissues such as the broad ligament. E, a 3/8 circle needle. F, Colt's large curved needle for putting tension sutures in the abdomen. G, and H, needles can be round or triangular. I, the best needle holders have tungsten carbide tips. J, hold a needle where its cutting edge joins the shaft. K, if you don't have a suture needle you can improvise one from an intramuscular needle by bending its wire stylet into a loop, pushing this into the shaft and crimping it tight. *Partly after Robert Remis.*

• *NEEDLES, Moynihan, 5/8 circle curved, round bodied, fine, sizes 1, 4, and 6, 50 needles only of size 1, 25 needles only of sizes 4 and 6.* Hold the larger ones in your fingers for suturing stomach and intestine. Use the small ones in a needle holder for suturing deep in a wound.
• *NEEDLES, Mayo, intestinal, round-bodied, half circle curved with sharp perforating ends, 23 mm, size 20, 100 needles only.* Use this small curved needle in a holder.
• *NEEDLES, suture, round bodied, half circle curved, sizes 1, 4, 10, 15, and 20, 25 needles of each size only.* Hold these in a holder and use them in the depths of a wound.
• *NEEDLES, suture, Moynihan, Lance point, 5/8 circle, 115 mm, twenty five needles only.* Use these large curved needles for sewing up the abdomen as described in Section 9.8.
• *NEEDLES, suture, curved, tension, Colt, 102 mm, five needles.* This is a very large curved needle used for putting tension sutures into the abdomen (9.8).
• *NEEDLES, straight triangular, cutting, 35 mm, 20 needles only.* Hold these in your hand and use them for suturing tendons.
• *NEEDLES, suture, Jameson Evans, triangular, curved, 10 mm, 25 needles only.* These small curved needles have flattened shafts, triangular points and lateral eyes. Use them for delicate sutures, such as repairing the eyelids.

- *NEEDLES, suture, Dennis Brown, round pointed, 5/8 circle, 16 mm, 25 needles only.* Hold these small curved needles in a needle holder, when you are working at the bottom of a narrow deep hole, such as the bottom of a burr hole.
- *NEEDLES, suture, 1/2 circle, catgut, Mayo, sizes 1 and 3, 25 needles of each size only.* These are strong needles for tough tissues. They have short cutting edges, so you can use them to repair an artery.
- *NEEDLE, Deschamps, angled to the right, five only.* This is the only needle (not illustrated) in this list which you can use to thread wire, to close the abdomen (9.8), or to wire the patella (79.12).
- *NEEDLE HOLDER, Boseman, 210 mm, ratchet and box joint, tungsten carbide jaws, two only.* This is the standard needle holder for medium and large needles.
- *NEEDLE HOLDER, Mayo's, with ratchet and box joint, tungsten carbide jaws 185 mm, one only.*
- *NEEDLE HOLDER, Mayo Dunhill, 160 mm, ratchet and box joint, tungsten carbide jaws, three only.*
- *NEEDLE HOLDER, Mayo's with narrow serrated jaws, box joint, tungsten carbide jaws and ratchet, 185 mm, three only.*
- *NEEDLE HOLDER, Derf, box joint and rachet, tungsten carbide jaws, 115 mm, two only.* This is an expensive fine needle holder for tiny needles.

4.8 Suture methods

You will have to suture two kinds of wound: (1) Those caused by trauma, which are described in Chapter 54. (2) Those which you make yourself when you operate. You can sew up both in much the same way. Here, we are mostly concerned with the skin, the special sutures for other structures are described elsewhere—arteries (55.6), nerves (55.9), tendons (55.11), the scalp (63.6), and the gut (9.3).

'Over-and-over' sutures are the most common ones, and can be continuous (A, Fig. 4-7) or interrupted (B). Each interrupted suture needs its own knot; each knot can act as a nidus for infection; and each takes time to tie. So continuous sutures are quicker, but they are also less reliable, because, if the knot on a continuous suture unties, or the suture breaks, the whole wound may open up, whereas the loss of a single interrupted suture matters little. A beginner usually finds interrupted sutures easier. If you wish, you can lock a continuous skin suture to make it more secure; you can lock every stitch (G, Fig. 4-7), or every few stitches.

Vertical mattress sutures (C, Fig. 4-7) take a superficial bite to bring the skin edges together, and a deeper one to close the deeper tissues; so they are useful for deeper wounds, but they leave scars: they are always interrupted. Horizontal mattress sutures may be interrupted (D) or continuous, superficial or buried (E), and are merely alternatives to 'over-and-over' sutures without any special merit, except that they are better at everting the skin edges.

A subcuticular suture brings the skin edges together accurately, and is particularly useful in plastic surgery. It can be interrupted (F, Fig. 4-7) or continuous (I, and J, Fig. 61-2). If it is continuous, both ends have to be anchored, either with a button, or with split lead shot clamped to the suture.

G, and H, in Fig. 4-8 show a simple mattress suture contrasted with a figure of eight suture. Use this to stop bleeding from soft bulky tissue when there is no obvious vessel to tie. This sometimes happens when you have closed the uterus after Caesarean section with the usual two layers of sutures and the wound is still bleeding at one end—put a figure of eight suture through it.

KNOTS AND SUTURES

SUTURING. Hold a straight needle in your hand. Hold a curved one in a holder about 2/5ths of its length from the eye.

You will also have to hold the tissue you are sewing. Hold a hollow viscus, such as stomach or gut, with plain forceps; hold skin or fascia with toothed ones. If the needle is curved, move the holder through an arc, so as to follow its curve.

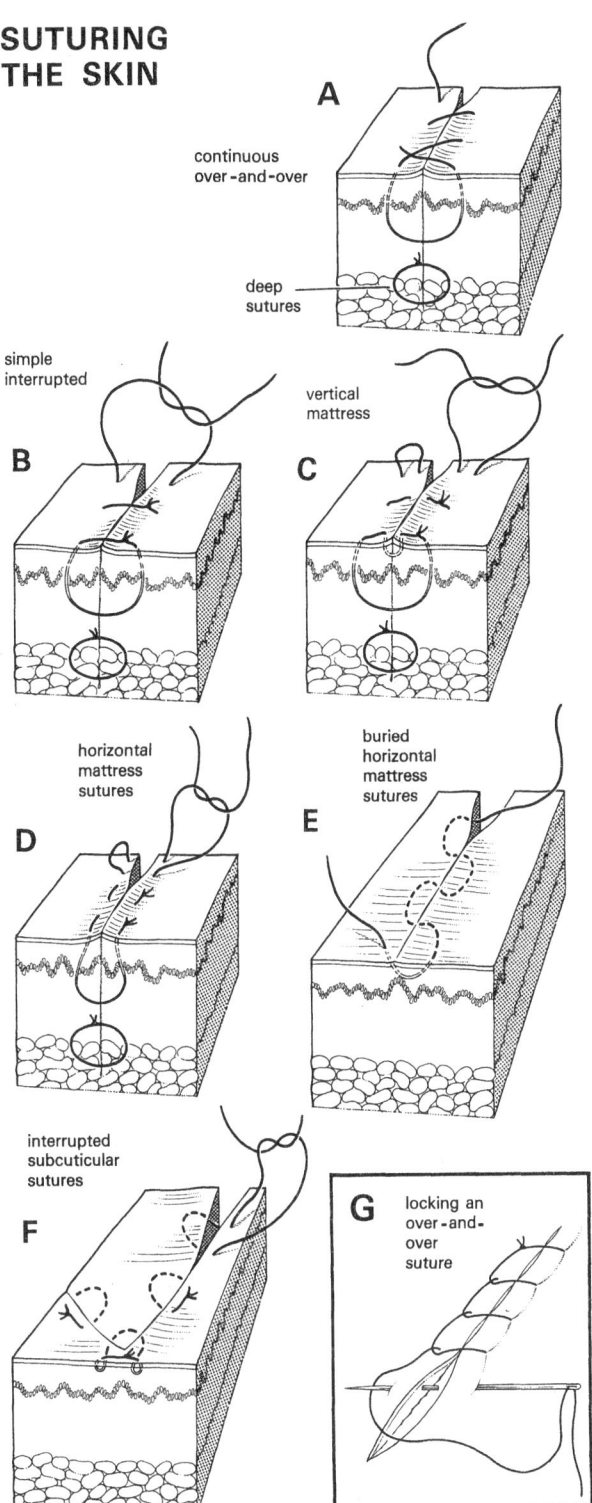

Fig. 4-7 SUTURE METHODS FOR THE SKIN. A, a continuous over-and-over suture. B, simple inturrupted sutures. C, a vertical mattress suture. D, a horizontal mattress suture. E, a buried horizontal mattress suture. F, an interrupted subcuticular suture. G, a continuous over-and-over suture which is being locked. *After Grabb MD and Smith JW, 'Plastic Surgery', Figs. 1-8 and 1-9. Little Brown, with kind permission.*

In the skin, insert the needle about 5 mm from the edge of the wound, and place sutures about 5 mm apart. Include an equal amount of skin on each side of the wound.

Set knots down so that they lie square, and don't tie them too tight—just tight enough to bring the skin edges together. The skin will swell during the following day, and if the knots are already tight, they will become even tighter and impair the circulation, leading to necrosis.

SOME BASIC PROCEDURES

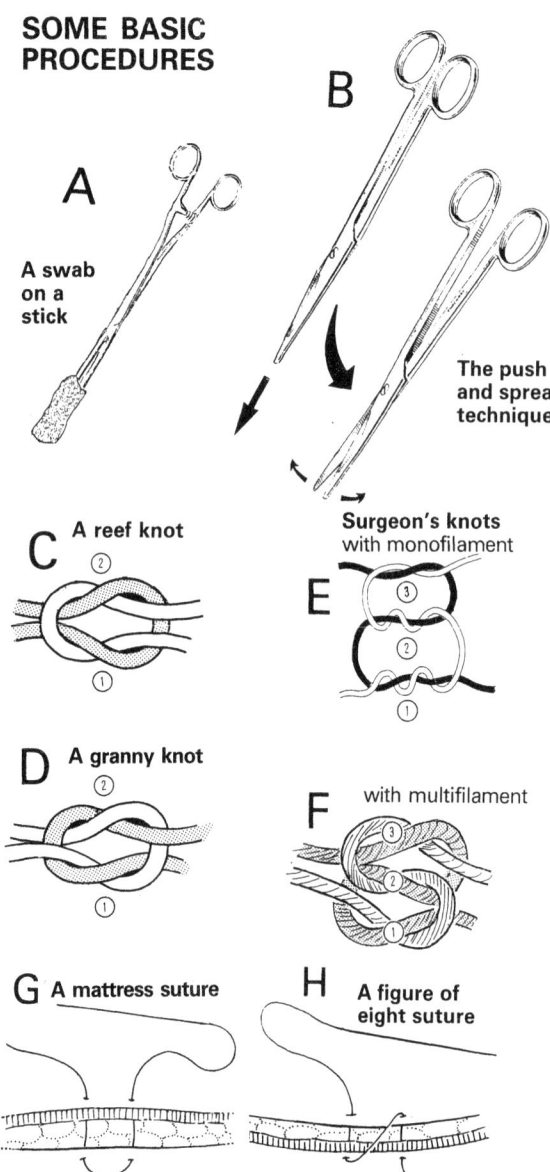

Fig. 4-8 SOME OF THE BASICS. A, a sponge holder grasping a swab ('a swab on a stick') can be a useful instrument for dissecting delicate structures, as when separating the peritoneum from the vagus nerves (Fig. 11-4). B, as well as cutting with scissors you can push them into the tissues and then gently open them to spread structures apart. This is the 'push and spread technique'. Be gentle! It is useful for tissue planes, but forceful spreading can injure thin walled structures, such as veins. C, a 'reef' or 'square' knot. D, a 'granny knot' which does not hold so well. E, a surgeon's knot for monofilament has three hitches (or 'throws') with two turns (or more) on the first two hitches and one turn on the third. F, a surgeon's knot with multifilament is less likely to slip and need only have a single turn on each of the three hitches. Note that each hitch should ideally make a reef knot with the previous one. G, a mattress suture. H, a 'figure of eight' suture, which is like a mattress suture, except that the needle is inserted in the same direction both times.

CAUTION ! (1) Don't insert the needle at different depths, or the edges of the wound will overlap. (2) Don't leave dead spaces, or they will fill with fluid which may become infected. (3) Suture towards you. (3) When you suture two tissues together, one of them may be mobile and the other fixed (because you are holding it). Suture from the mobile tissue towards the fixed one. (4) Continue in the curve of the needle.

KNOTS. Tie reef (square) knots, not 'granny knots'. These are both made from two half hitches—in a reef knot they go in opposite directions, in a granny knot they go in the same direction. Pull equally on both ends, pull horizontally, and watch the knot go down. If one end is tense and the other loose, you will get a slip or sliding knot.

A surgeon's knot is merely a reef knot with a third half hitch in the same direction as the first one. This third half hitch makes the knot less likely to undo. Some surgeons tie three hitches in all suture materials.

Some suture materials undo more easily than others. Non-absorbable multifilament makes the safest knots. Knots in catgut seldom undo, but knots in monofilament undo much more easily. *So always use a surgeon's knot when you tie monofilament. For important knots put two (or more) turns on the first and second hitches.* With multifilament a single turn is enough on each hitch.

Practise these knots with string or your shoelaces, until you can do them quickly, and do them blind. Learn the various ways of doing them in the following order.

REEF KNOTS can be tied in several ways. The first method, as in Fig. 4-9, is the surest way of tying a knot and is the one to use if you want to exert continuous pressure while you tie. In the second method, Fig. 4-10, use forceps in your right hand. The third, Fig. 4-11, is an 'instrument tie' and is useful if one end of a suture is short, or if the knot is in a deep cavity. The

A REEF KNOT (FIRST METHOD)

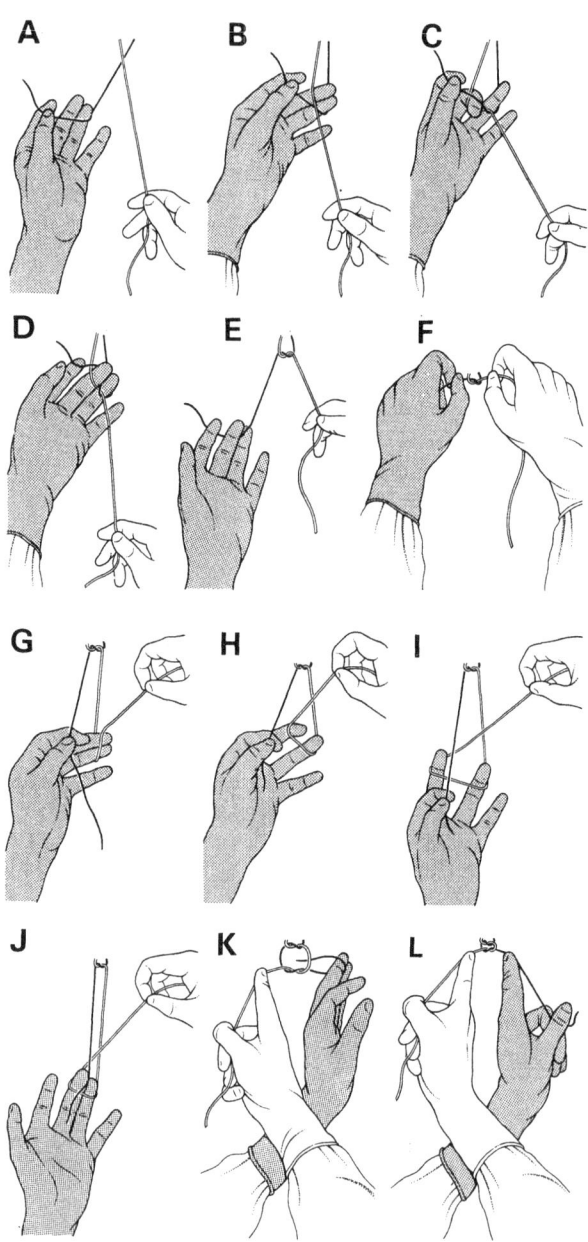

Fig. 4-9 TYING A REEF KNOT—FIRST METHOD. This is the standard method without using instruments. The difficult steps are C, and D, in which you grasp one of the ends between your middle and ring fingers, and I, and J, where you do the same again.

A REEF KNOT (SECOND METHOD)

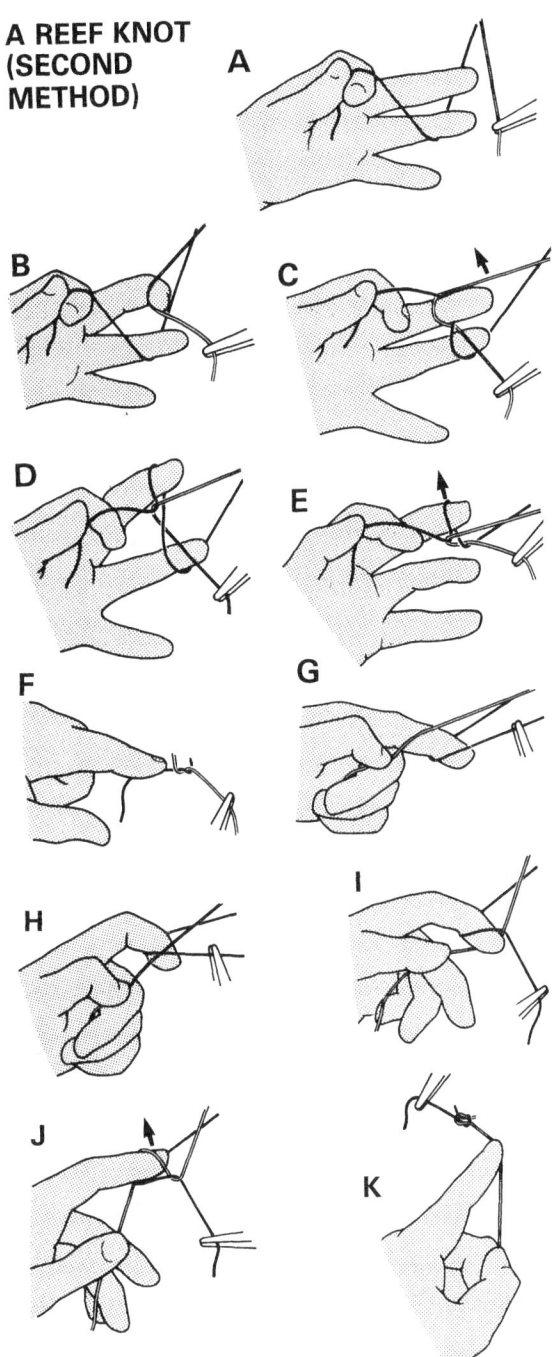

Fig. 4-10 TYING A REEF KNOT—SECOND METHOD. This method is smiliar to the last one except that you are using forceps in your right hand. Use it if you are working in a hole.

short end can be quite short. First, make a loop with the instrument in front of the long end. Grasp the short end and pull it through this loop. Then pull the first half hitch tight in the plane of the knot. To make the second half hitch, start with the instrument behind the long end.

TO CUT A SUTURE almost close the scissors, slip their open ends over the suture material, and move them gently down towards the knot. Twist the tip to give you the length of tail you want, then cut. Cut the tails of interrupted skin sutures short enough to prevent them tangling in the next suture. Leave buried catgut sutures with 5 mm tails. Cut buried sutures close beside the surgeon's knot.

CAUTION ! Keep the tips of the scissors in view, and don't cut unless you can see what you are cutting.

REMOVING SUTURES. Leave them until the wound has healed properly. Some sutures can be removed on the 4th day,

A REEF KNOT (THIRD METHOD)

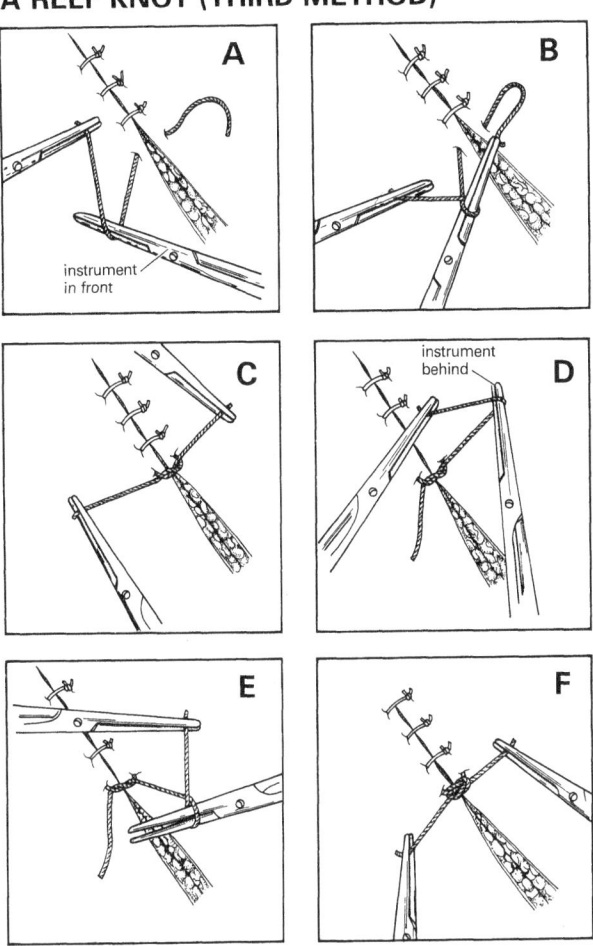

Fig. 4-11 TYING A REEF KNOT—THIRD METHOD. If there is not enough room for your fingers, use forceps in each hand. This is an 'instrument tie'. Notice that for the first half hitch the instrument is in front of the long end (A), and for the second one it is behind (D). In this way you will tie a reef knot, not a granny knot.

others not until the 14th. Here is a guide:
  The tongue 4 days.
  Skin sutures on the face and eyelids 4 days.
  The scalp 6 to 7 days.
  The hand and fingers 7 days.
  The scrotum 5 days.
  The abdomen: transverse incision 7 to 9 days, vertical incision 9 to 11 days.
  The skin of the back over the shoulders 11 to 12 days.
  Retention sutures 10 to 14 days (9.13).
When you remove a suture, try not to pull any part of the suture material which has been on the surface through the tissues, or you may contaminate the wound. Clean the skin, cut the suture where it dips under the skin, and pull it in such a way that it brings the edges of the wound together, as in Fig 54-8.

4.9 Using tubes in surgery, especially nasogastric tubes

Tubes lead fluids from somewhere to somewhere else. Inserting one may be the aim of surgery, as when you drain the pleural cavity (65.2), or it may merely be part of an operation, as in decompressing a patient's stomach when his gut is obstructed (10-9). You can also use tubes to drain pus and exudate. The insertion of a tube for gastrostomy (11.8), jejunostomy (9.7), caecostomy (9.6), and cholecystostomy (13.3) are described elsewhere: here we describe the use of nasogastric tubes, which are of great value, even though they are a burden to nurses and an irritation to patients.

• TUBE, nasogastric, plastic, Ryle's, with several side holes near the tip, 14 Ch, 16 Ch, 18 Ch, ten only of each size. Transparent plastic tubes are better than rubber ones, because they are less irritant, they don't collapse, and you can see what is inside them. Most tubes have markings, the first at 45 cm showing that the tip is about to enter the stomach, and the second that it is in the antrum.

• TUBE, stomach, plastic, adult and child, assorted sizes 8 to 22 Ch, five only of each size. These are critically important for making sure that a patient's stomach is empty before he is anaesthetized (A 16.4), and for washing it out if he has swallowed a corrosive (25.15). Adults need tubes of 16 to 22 Ch, children 10 to 14 Ch, and infants 8 to 10 Ch.

NASOGASTRIC TUBES

Here we are concerned with the use of a tube to keep a patient's stomach empty—for tube-feeding him, see Sections 9.10 and 58.11.

INDICATIONS. (1) To remove fluid from a patient's stomach before anaesthetizing him, so as to reduce the risk of his inhaling it. The solid food from a recent meal will not come up an ordinary nasogastric tube, so if you want to anaesthetize safely a patient who has recently eaten, you will have to empty his stomach with a larger stomach tube (A 16.1), and then pass a nasogastric tube. (2) To decompress the stomach, particularly during upper abdominal surgery when a distended stomach may get in the way of the operation. (3) To empty the stomach during acute intestinal obstruction. (4) To feed a patient (58.10). (5) To monitor gastric bleeding. (6) To minimize abdominal distension postoperatively, so as to reduce tension on the wound, and hence assist respiration. For all these reasons, it is good practice to pass a tube whenever you do a laparotomy.

PASSING A NASOGASTRIC TUBE. Lubricate the tip of the tube with a water-soluble jelly. Sit the patient up and tell him what you are going to do. Choose the nostril which has the widest channel. Pass the tube horizontally through his nose. When the tube touches his posterior pharyngeal wall, he will gag, so give him a little water to sip, as you slowly advance the tube. The act of swallowing will open his cricopharyngeus and allow the tube to enter his oesophagus. Continue to advance it until its second ring reaches his nose; its tip should now be in his stomach.

CAUTION ! If you are only aspirating a tube, you cannot do much harm, but never start tube feeding until you are sure a tube is in the stomach. You can easily pass a tube into the trachea of an elderly, debilitated, or unconscious patient and drown him with feed. To make sure it is in his stomach: (1) Aspirate greenish-grey stomach secretions. (2) Inject a little air down it and listen over his stomach with a stethoscope for a gurgling sound. (3) Listen to the end of the tube. The sound of moving air confirms that the tube is NOT in his stomach, but is in his trachea or bronchi.

When you are satisfied that the tube is in the right place, secure it with two narrow strips of tape, one on the side and the other on the bridge of his nose, extending downwards on to the tube. In this way you will avoid pressure necrosis of his alae nasae.

Connect the tube to a bedside drainage bottle or plastic bag, to let his stomach contents syphon out. Assist this by aspirating. Suck the contents out every hour, or more frequently if there is much aspirate, to prevent the tube blocking. If you cannot aspirate anything, try irrigating the tube with 5 or 10 ml of water; its terminal holes may be plugged.

If the tube fails to decompress his stomach: (1) Its tip may still be in his oesophagus. (2) It may be kinked or blocked. (3) His stomach may be filled with large food particles. Excessive suction may have sucked food or mucosa into the holes in the tube.

Occasional sips (not gulps) of water will help to ease his misery. Keep a fluid balance chart, and as a general rule replace gastric aspirate by normal saline or Ringer's lactate (A 15.5).

CAUTION ! If you don't care for his mouth adequately, his parotid may become infected. So give him 4-hourly mouth care as a routine after major surgery, especially if he has a nasogastric tube in.

REMOVING A TUBE. As a general rule, leave a tube in place until: (1) There are normal bowel sounds. (2) There is no abdominal distension. (3) His bowel has moved normally or he has passed flatus. (4) There are only about 400 ml of gastric aspirate daily. This is the normal volume; if you aspirate 750 ml or more, suspect ileus or gut obstruction.

If his stomach has a suture line in it, remove the tube at 4 to 5 days.

If you are in doubt as to when to remove a tube, clamp it for 24 hours, and if nausea and distension do not return remove it.

CAUTION ! Don't remove a patient's nasogastric tube if he is nauseated, or distended, or he has passed no flatus, or has more than 500 ml of gastric aspirate. If he has any of these, he probably has paralytic ileus (10.13), or obstruction (10.13), or peritonitis (6.2), or an anastomosis that is too narrow.

DIFFICULTIES WITH NASOGASTRIC TUBES

If he is very WEAK, DEHYDRATED OR SHOCKED, the act of passing a tube may cause him to vomit and inhale his vomit. If so, lie him on his side, with his head tilted down, and pass a large stomach tube (30 Ch). If he vomits he will now do so under controlled conditions. Afterwards, pass a nasogastric tube.

If he develops PULMONARY COMPLICATIONS, these may in part be due to the discomfort of the tube: (1) causing ineffective coughing and (2) drying out his mouth by making nose breathing difficult.

If his NASAL CARTILAGES NECROSE (rare), you applied tape unwisely. Pressure is usually caused by an acute angulation of the tube.

If he develops OESOPHAGEAL EROSIONS, you may have been using too hard a tube. A large one may allow regurgitation through the cardiac sphincter and cause an erosive oesophagitis.

4.10 Drains and draining

The purpose of a drain is to let blood, pus, or other fluids escape from a wound while it heals, without letting bacteria get in. Blood or pus will flow through a tubular drain or round a solid one. You will have to use a tube to drain a patient's gut, his bladder, or his pleural cavity (6.1), but when you drain a wound or his peritoneal cavity you have a choice. You can let the exudates flow down a tube, or you can let them seep away round the edge of a corrugated rubber drain. If you have the equipment for suction drainage, you may be able to suck them away. Suction drains are much more effective than corrugated ones, especially if bleeding is expected.

Not all wounds need drains, and drains have their risks: (1) Bacteria may enter from outside, especially if nursing care is poor. The risk of this is small if you use a closed drainage system and your nurses are good. (2) Bacteria may come from inside a patient and infect the tissues through which the drain passes, particularly the abdominal wall. (3) A drain may erode a vessel or a suture line, especially if you leave it in for a week or longer.

If possible, insert a tube drain with a tight seal to the tissues through which it passes, usually the abdominal wall, and lead it into a bag or bottle. There will be less soiling of the dressings and less contamination than with a corrugated rubber drain. Unfortunately, if a tubular drain blocks, it can seal infection in, so that some surgeons prefer corrugated rubber ones.

The modern trend is not to insert a drain unless there is a good reason to do so. So don't drain all wounds routinely—insert a drain when the advantages outweigh the risks, and follow the instructions we give for each procedure: (1) Where possible (see above), try to use a tube which will lead the exudate safely into a bottle, rather than a piece of corrugated rubber which will lead it into dressings. (2) Try to place the drain at the bottom of the cavity to be drained, so that exudate can easily flow out downwards. (3) Make it follow a straight path. (4) If a drain is in any danger of falling out, stitch it in as it passes through the skin. (5) Don't try to drain the whole peritoneum in peritonitis—it is impossible anyway. Instead, wash out the peritoneal cavity and instil tetracycline (6.2). (6) Finally, be sure to explain to the ward staff why you have inserted a drain, how they are to manage it, and when they are to remove it.

- TUBING, red, rubber sterilizable, 2 mm wall, (a) 10 mm bore, (b) 15 mm bore, ten metres only of each size. This is multipurpose tubing, the 10 mm size is for draining air and blood, the 15 mm size is for pus. The firmness of the wall of a drainage tube is important. The tube from a chest drain should be firm enough to ensure an open pathway through the chest wall. The abdominal wall is less likely to pinch a drain closed, so a firm drainage tube is less important. If necessary, use a large bore catheter.

- TUBING, drainage, Penrose, assorted sizes, five metres only. A Penrose drain is a soft latex tube 1 to 2 cm in width and of varying length filled with a wick. Being soft it is unlikely to injure neighbouring structures, but because it is soft, it needs an exit opening of adequate size. Cut these drains in suitable lengths and widths as needed. Don't rely on them for draining deep spaces, such as the subhepatic space. Some surgeons think Penrose drains inefficient because they don't keep the wound open.

- DRAIN, corrugated red rubber, sheets 1×50×300 mm, ten sheets only. Pus drains between the corrugations. Cut the sheets to make drains of various shapes and sizes. Don't discard used sheet rubber drains—wash them, boil them, and store them in antiseptic solution (2.5). For tiny drains, cut up old intravenous sets or gloves.

- SUMP DRAIN, rubber or plastic, five only. In an ordinary drain the holes through which fluid is sucked frequently block. A sump drain overcomes this difficulty by having two tubes, an outer one with many holes in it, and an inner one through which fluid is sucked. Fluid trickles into the outer tube and is then sucked away down the inner one. Ideally, suction down the inner tube needs to be applied with a low pressure pump. There should also be a single hole in the inner tube close to the surface to prevent too high a pressure building up in the sump. There are many kinds, and you may be able to improvise one. A sump drain is particularly useful for draining large quantities of fluid from fistulae or a large localized abscesss in the peritoneal cavity. Alternatively, use a folded catheter. Suck through one end and let air enter through the other (E, Fig. 4-12).

DRAINS AND DRESSINGS

See elsewhere for underwater seal drains (65.2), intercostal drains for empyemas (6.1), and also drains for the abdomen (9.8), the urinary bladder (23.5 to 23.7) and the gall bladder.

If dressings are in short supply, wash the patient's wound with unsterilized salt solution (equal to half or full strength saline) 2 to 4-hourly and cover it with a dressing towel. See also 1.12.

LEAVING WOUNDS OPEN POSTOPERATIVELY, where you can, is a useful economy. Do this if a wound is not going to discharge. If it oozes a little, put a thin dressing of gauze or whatever you have on it for 24 hours.

LAYERS OF GAUZE AND COTTON WOOL will collect the discharges from a wound which is too shallow to let you insert a rubber drain, as in A, Fig. 4-12. Change these dressings frequently. If necessary, place a sheet of plastic or waterproof paper between the outermost layer and the patient's clothes.

INDICATIONS FOR DRAINAGE. (1) To allow the escape of blood when the control of bleeding after an operation has been incomplete. (2) To complete the drainage of an abscess cavity. (3) To drain an abscess or a local area of peritonitis (draining generalized peritonitis is impossible, see above). (4) To permit the escape of secretions from a possibly leaky suture line, for example when you have removed a stone from the ureter (23.14) or anastomosed unprepared large gut which cannot be protected by an ostomy, as when ileum is anastomosed to transverse colon.

HOW TO PLACE DRAINS. Where possible, insert a drain through a separate stab wound; if you drain pus through the main wound, it is more likely to become infected. Make sure the drain lies loosely in the cavity to be drained and follows the shortest path from the site to be drained to the exterior.

To avoid cutting blood vessels, cut only the skin with a scalpel, use a haemostat to poke a hole through the abdominal wall and then use the haemostat to push the drain through the hole.

DRAINS

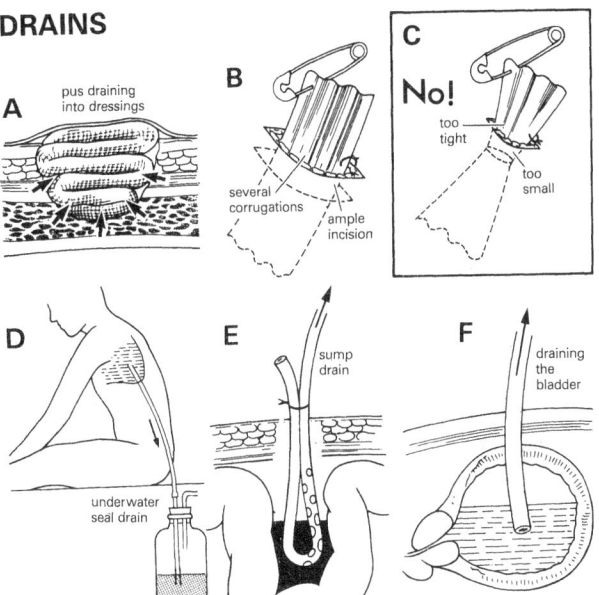

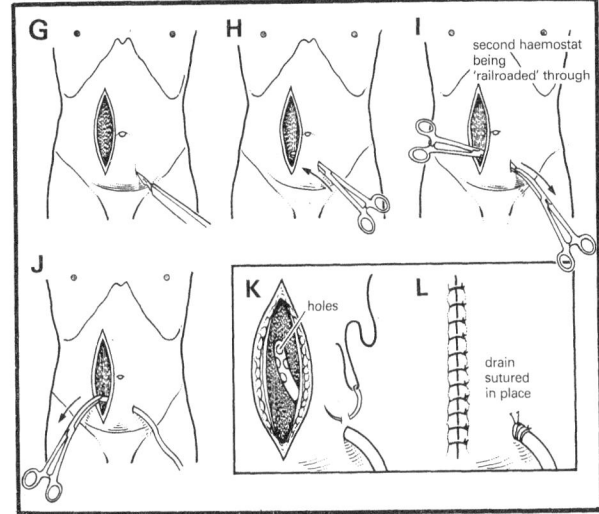

Introducing an abdominal drain

Fig. 4-12 DRAINS. A, in a superficial wound pus can drain into the dressings. B, a corrugated drain should usually consist of several corrugations and fit loosely through an incision in the superficial tissues. C, Don't push a drain tightly through a small incision. D, a chest drain (65-6). E, a sump drain. F, draining the bladder. G, to L, introducing a tube drain into the abdomen. G, making the incision. H, inserting the first haemostat. I, 'railroading' the second haemostat through. J, the second haemostat pulling a drainage tube through. K, holes cut in the end of the drainage tube. L, the drain sutured in place and the abdominal wall closed.

CAUTION ! If you are draining a possibly leaky suture line, place the drain close to it but not actually touching it, or the drain may help to disrupt the sutures. Ideally, there should be no such thing as a 'leaky suture line'—it should not have been made so that it does leak, or if it looks like leaking, it should be made again.

CORRUGATED RUBBER DRAINS are useful for abscesses. Cut more than an adequate hole in the superficial tissues, cut a strip of rubber to fit loosely and push this into the depth of the wound (B, Fig. 4-12). Don't make the hole for the drain so small so that it is tight (C). Use a cutting needle to transfix it with a suture and anchor it to the skin, then tie the ends of the suture several times. When you shorten a drain, you may be able to leave a loop of suture material securing it. A safety pin will prevent it slipping inside the wound, but will not prevent it slipping out.

If there is severe sepsis, as in a septic Caesarean section or a typhoid perforation, make an adequate muscle cutting incision—large enough to take three fingers side by side. Using a scalpel, cut all layers of the abdominal wall in the line of the incision. Control bleeding with a gauze pack. If any bleeding vessels remain after 5 minutes, tie them. Even when the corrugated drain is in place you should still be able to get two fingers into the wound.

TUBE DRAINS are useful in large wounds where you expect much exudate, or in areas of infection or oozing (D). They are especially useful in the abdomen (E). Have two or three sizes of drainage tubes ready sterilized with suitable adaptors. Use silicone rubber or polyethylene, rather than red or latex rubber, which is more irritant.

TO INTRODUCE AN ABDOMINAL TUBE DRAIN try to fit a wide bore tube tightly in a small hole. Make a small incision in the end. Use a 10 mm (30 Ch) tube, and cut side holes in the end. Make a small hole in the tissues and 'railroad' the drain in as in G, to J, Fig. 4-12. Anchor the drain to the skin with a suture. Insert a skin stitch, tie a second reef knot distal to the first one and then tie the ends of the suture round the drain with a surgeon's knot (L). Finally, tape the drain to the skin. Connect it to a sterile bottle.

CAUTION ! (1) Don't put any drain through the main incision. If it is a tube drain you will not be able to make a good seal round it, and it will make an incisional hernia more likely. (2) A tube drain which blocks is useless.

SUCTION DRAINS are ideal, especially the disposable plastic kind. More practical are the reusable 'Redivac' suction bottle type, which have disposable drainage tubes.

SUMP DRAINS (see above) are useful if you have a suction pump and you want to drain fluid, such as urine, or pancreatic juice which is welling up from the depths of a wound.

THE TIME TO REMOVE A DRAIN varies with the fluid to be drained. Here are some guidelines:
Draining blood—48 to 72 hours.
Draining down to a suture line—5 to 7 days.
Draining a septic cavity—until pus ceases to flow, usually in 5 to 7 days.

Don't leave a drain in longer than is necessary, because you run the risk that it may erode a vessel. There is seldom any need to leave a drain more than a week at the most, except in a very large deep abscess, as in the subphrenic space, where you may need to leave one in for 10 days. If you remove a drain too early, pus may build up and seek to discharge itself elsewhere.

If a drain is long, shorten it progressively over several days before you remove it. Shorten it by pulling it out, not by cutting it off. Place a safety pin through it and tape this to the patient's skin.

4.11 Miscellaneous equipment and materials

Some of the humblest equipment is also the most necessary. Here are many of the things which you should not be without.

• *TUBE, rectal, rubber, (a) child's size 8 mm (24 Ch), five only; (b) adult's size 10 mm (30 Ch), five only.* You can also connect these to a large bore funnel and use them to give an enema. Introduce them carefully: you can easily perforate the sigmoid colon.

• *CONNECTOR, end-to-end, polypropylene, external diameter (a) 4 mm, (b) 7 mm, (c) 10 mm, (d) 15 mm, (e) 19 mm, ten only of each size.* Use these to join short lengths of tubing together for suction or drainage etc.

• *CONNECTORS, plastic 3 way 'Y', assorted sizes, 20 only.*

• *CLIP, towel, cross action, 90 mm, 28 only.* These are the simplest towel clips.

• *CLIP, towel, with ratchet, Backhaus, six only.* These are more expensive than the towel clips listed above, but they have several other uses, including holding the sucker tube, and the ribs in chest injuries (65.6).

• *FORCEPS, sponge holding, Rampley, straight, (a) 240 mm, box joint, 22 only. (b) 120 mm, two only.* Use these for swabbing, and for 'swab dissection'.

• *LOUPE, binocular, Bishop Harman, ×2 magnification, one only.* Perch its two lenses on the very tip of your nose, or wear it over your spectacles. Curl its ear pieces, so that it fits your face. This is a twentieth the price of a binocular loupe, and is invaluable for fine operations like repairing nerves (55.9), or arteries (55.6), or 'cut-downs' (A 15.2), or removing splinters. The disadvantage of a loupe is that it focuses close to your nose, so use short-handled instruments.

• *TROCAR AND CANNULA, straight, with nickel silver or stainless steel cannula and metal handle, (a) 4 mm (12 Ch). (b) 8 mm (24 Ch). (c) 12 mm (36 Ch), one only of each size.* The small size is useful for tapping hydroceles, the middle one for suprapubic cystotomy, and the largest one for chest drainage.

• *CANNULA WITH SIDE ARM, one only.* Attach suction to the side arm and use it to aspirate the gall bladder etc. (13-1).

• *PROBE, malleable, with eye, nickel silver, 150 mm, 3 sizes, one only of each size.* Use this to probe perianal fistulae etc.

• *DIRECTOR, hernia, Key's, one only.* Use this for opening the neck of a hernial sac.

• *DIRECTOR, probe-ended, Brodie, 165 mm, one only.* Use this for exploring sinuses.

• *RING CUTTER, one only.* If you don't have this, you may be able to remove a ring with soap and string (75-5).

• *NEEDLE, aneurysm, Dupuytren, (a) one needle curving right, (b) one needle curving left, one only of each kind.* These are curved needles on the end of a handle. Use them for passing a ligature under something (3-4).

• *NEEDLE, aneurysm, small, with blunt point, three only.* Keep these in your 'cut down sets' (A 15.2,) and use them to pass ligatures under a vein.

• *CATHETER, metal female, three only.*

• *BRUSH, for cleaning instrument jaws, ten only.* The jaws and joints of surgical instruments need brushing regularly. You can also use suede brushes with bronze bristles.

• *RAZOR, safety, for preoperative preparation, ten only.* Shaving a patient preoperatively is not the essential ritual that it was once assumed to be (9.1). You can also adapt a safety razor for skin grafting (57.7).

• *BUCKET, stainless steel, with handles, six only.*

• *KIDNEY DISH, stainless steel, with half curled edges, 4 sizes 100 to 300 mm, two dishes of each size only.*

• *GALLIPOT, stainless steel or autoclavable plastic, set of six sizes 40 to 200 mm, two sets only.* Use these for lotions, swabs etc.

• *JAR, stainless steel with dropover lid, 150×150 mm, two only.* Use these for spirit swabs.

• *JUG, plastic, autoclavable, conical, 3 litre, one only.* Stainless steel jugs have become standard, but plastic ones are satisfactory.

• *BIN, soiled, two only.*

• *JELLY, hydroxymethylcellulose, sterile, 'KY jelly' 1 kg only.* This is a sterile non-greasy jelly for catheters etc.

• *'BIPP', bismuth iodoform and paraffin paste BPC, 1 kg only.* This is a mildly antiseptic self-sterilizing anaesthetic packing material. You can leave it in the nose for a week without significant infection, or much smell (25.6). If you don't have any, smear gauze or bandage with any non-adherent antiseptic ointment.

• *CARPENTER'S EQUIPMENT (a) Saw, one only. (b) Twist drill, one only. (c) Hammer, claw head, one only.* If you cannot get the surgical equivalent of these, you will find them very useful.

• *OTHER MATERIALS include gauze, cotton wool, bandages, adhesive tape, and laparotomy pads (1.12).*

4.12 Instrument sets

For most operations you will need about 50 general purpose instruments called 'the general set', with a few special ones when necessary. You can handle additions to the general set in three ways: (1) You can keep special instruments in the cupboard, and sterilize them when needed. (2) You can make them up into incomplete special sets, such as a burr hole set or an orthopaedic set, which you use with the general set when necessary. (3) If you have enough instruments, particularly haemostats, you can make complete special sets. This is the best method, and the one which we follow here, but it requires many more instruments.

You can do an occasional emergency operation with only one general set, but when you have a list of patients to operate on, you will need several general sets—if you are not to wait too long between operations. Boiling a set takes at least 15 minutes, and autoclaving one at least half an hour. A set costs between $750 and $1000, about a third of which is the cost of the haemostats.

If instruments are limited, start by collecting a general set adapted for Caesarean section and laparotomy, and also the more important special instruments. Once you have all these, try to complete a tracheostomy set, and a chest drainage set, three cut down sets, and a second laparotomy set. When you have these your next objective should probably be a minor set for such operations as wound repairs and circumcisions. If you do many uterine evacuations. two or more sets for these would be useful.

A Caesarean section is a particular kind of laparotomy. A set for it differs from a laparotomy set mainly in that it includes four Green Armytage forceps, and that Doyen's retractor, which is specially designed for pelvic operations, replaces Balfour's.

The sets below mostly start with six towel clips and a towel holder, which you can also use to hold the sucker tube. Next come four Rampley's sponge-holders, the first two of which are used for preparing the patient's skin, after which they are discarded. The remaining two are for 'swabs on sticks', and for swab dissection. Then come toothed and plain dissecting forceps, two scalpel handles, and a heavy and a light needle-holder. There are also four pairs of Allis' tissue forceps, and various retractors, depending on the set. The expensive items, because of the large number you need, are the haemostats, straight, curved, big, and small, clipped together in groups of six on Mayo's pins. The more experienced you are, the fewer of these you will need. We list six of each, which is a generous number for a beginner. Finally, there is the Yankauer sucker and its tube; this is an angled suction tube with a handle.

Keep an inventory of equipment and a check list for each set. Nice instruments tend to disappear. One aid to keeping instruments together is to provide them in pairs, or in even-numbered quantities where possible. For example, the nurses will find it useful to remember that haemostats and towel clips should always be in sixes.

The theatre is the best place in the hospital for sterilizing equipment. So try to develop a simple 'central sterile supply' service which can prepare sets for the wards.

INSTRUMENT SETS

You will want the following sets, some of which are described elsewhere—a 'D and C' set (two if possible), a general purpose set (preferably two sets), a Caesar set, a cut down set (preferably two sets or more), an abscess set, a minor set (for hernias, etc.), an orthopaedic set (for drilling for osteomyelitis, etc.), an intestinal clamp set (for resecting gut), a fine instrument set (for hand surgery), an eye set (24.1), a burr hole set (63.1), a chest drain set (65.2), and a tracheostomy set (52.2). The equipment we have listed in all the various sections of these manuals is summarized in Appendix A and should be enough to make up the following sets.

SHARP EQUIPMENT needs to be kept separately, because it gets blunt if it is autoclaved too often. Keep scissors in dishes of antiseptic fluid (2.5). Keep osteotomes and gouges in a cupboard and put them in sterilizing fluid 30 minutes before you use them. Autoclave the bone saw when you want it. Keep the bone drill and the twist drills to go with it in a special sterile pack.

CAUTION ! Re-autoclave the packs and drums regularly. A pack which has not been resterilized for some time is a risk, especially if it is only covered in towels. You may find termites inside it!

THE CONTENTS OF PARTICULAR INSTRUMENT SETS

THE GENERAL SET (including the instruments for laparotomy $800). Six towel clips. One Backhaus towel forceps. Four Rampley's sponge-holders. One toothed dissecting forceps (Treves). One plain dissecting forceps (Bonney's). One No. 4 and one No. 5 scalpel handle. Two needle-holders, a heavy and a light. Two Allis' tissue forceps. Two Lane's tissue forceps. Six 200 mm curved haemostats (Spencer Wells). Six 200 mm curved haemostats (Spencer Wells). Six 120 or 140 mm straight haemostats (Halstead's or Crile's). Six 120 or 140 mm curved haemostats (Halstead's or Crile's). Two Kocher's artery forceps. Two Czerny's (or Langenbeck's) retractors. Two Morris' retractors. Yankauer's sucker tube. One 20 cm receiver and two gallipots.

Desirable additions include Lahey's curved gallbladder forceps.

CAESAR SET ($950). Six towel clips. One Backhaus' towel forceps. Four Rampley's sponge holders. One 18 cm toothed dissecting forceps. One 18 cm plain dissecting forceps. Two No.4 scalpel handles. Two 180 mm needle-holders. Two Allis' tissue forceps. Six Green-Armytage forceps. Twelve 150 mm straight Spencer Wells haemostats. Six 230 mm curved Spencer Wells haemostats. One Morris' retractor. One Doyen's retractor. Yankauer's sucker and tube. One 300 mm bowl (for blood clot), one 200 mm receiver and two gallipots.

Desirable additions include a tenaculum, and a self-retaining retractor.

MINOR SET ($750). Six towel clips. Two Rampley's sponge holders. Four Backhaus' towel forceps. One No. 4 scalpel handle. One No. 5 scalpel handle. One toothed dissecting forceps (Treves). One plain dissecting forceps (Bonney's). Four Allis' tissue forceps. One West's self-retaining retractor. Two Czerny's retractors (or Langenbeck's). Twelve 125 mm curved haemostats (Spencer Wells). Six 200 mm curved haemostats (Spencer Wells). One 20 cm receiver and two gallipots.

Desirable additions include a dissector and a Volkmann's spoon.

ABSCESS SET. Two Rampley's sponge-holding forceps. Four towel clips. One knife handle. One sinus forceps. One Mayo's scissors. One toothed dissecting forceps. One 150 mm receiver, two gallipots and some gauze swabs. Two towels.

'D and C' SET. Four Rampley's sponge-holding forceps. One Sims' vaginal speculum. One Auvard's speculum. Two Teal's vulsellum forceps. One uterine sound. One set of Hegar's dilators. A uterine curette with one sharp and one blunt end. One 200 mm Kocher's forceps. One toothed dissecting forceps.

ORTHOPAEDIC SET. Six towel clips. Four Rampley's sponge holders. Four dissecting forceps (one heavy toothed 180 mm Lane's or Charnley's, one light Adson's 125 mm, one plain 180 mm, one McIndoe's 180 mm). Six curved 150 mm Spencer Wells haemostats. Six curved 200 mm Spencer Wells haemostats. One No. 4 and one No. 5 scalpel handle. Four 220 mm light bone levers, Lane's or Trethowen's. Four 275 mm heavy bone levers. One Faraboef's elevator. One large periosteal elevator (for the femur and humerus) and one small one. One Size C double-ended bone scoop Volkman's. One 350 g mallet. One sequestrum forceps. One 180 mm Read Jensen bone nibbler. One bone file or rasp. One 220 mm Liston's bone cutters. One 200 mm bone hook.

BURR HOLE SET. One Hudson's standard perforator 12 mm. One Hudson's set of conical burrs 13 mm and 16 mm. Hudson's brace. One West's self-retaining retractor. One 60 mm brain sucker. One 14 Ch soft rubber catheter. One 20 ml syringe for washing out with saline.

SMALL (hand) INSTRUMENT SET. Two small sponge holding forceps. One plain 150 mm McIndoe dissecting forceps. One plain 100 mm Silcock's ophthalmic dissecting forceps. One toothed Adson's 120 mm dissecting forceps. Four 165 mm Gilles skin hooks. One light 190 mm McIndoe dissecting scissors. One light 140 mm curved Aufrecht's scissors. Twelve curved Crile's mosquito haemostats. One Bard Parker No. 4 scalpel handle. Two 114 mm Derf needle holders. Two small 178 mm Meydering retractors. Two 114 mm Harlow Wood tendon hooks. One small curette. Two assistant's scissors. One fine probe.

KIRSCHNER WIRE PACK. Six wires of each size 0.75 mm, 1.0 mm, 1.5 mm. One Pulvertaft's Kirschner wire introducer. One pair of Kirschner wire cutters.

5 The surgery of sepsis

5.1 'Where there is pus let it out'

Draining pus is the commonest surgical operation all over the developing world. It is also one of the most useful and is usually one of the simplest. Quite a small district hospital can expect to drain 200 large abscesses each year, some containing up to 3 litres of pus. Although pus can collect almost anywhere, particularly important sites are a patient's pleura (6.1), his peritoneum (6.2), his muscles (7.1), his bones (7.2), and joints (7.16), his hand (8.1), and his eye (endophthalmitis, 24.3). This chapter and the immediately following ones tell you how to drain pus. Pus in the breast (21.2) and the eye (24.3), and the most serious consequence of pyogenic infection—septic shock—are described elsewhere (53.4).

Why septic infections of all kinds are so common here is not altogether clear, but anaemia, malnutrition, and poor hygiene may all play a part in causing them. Abscesses are more common in children and young adults, and a patient may have a dozen or more at the same time. Staphylococci are almost always responsible, except in the perineal and perianal region, which is commonly infected by coliforms and anaerobes. Some abscesses are tuberculous (29.1). AIDS predisposes a patient to infections of many kinds, including abscesses anywhere.

If bacteria are multiplying in a patient's tissues, antibiotics will only be effective in killing them early, when there is cellulitis only, and *before much pus has formed*. At this early stage antibiotics may start to control cellulitis within 24 hours. But once pus has formed, you must drain it. Conversely, before pus has had time to form drainage is useless. Antibiotics and drainage thus both have their proper indications, and one is no substitute for the other. The tighter the space, the more urgent the need for drainage. *If a patient has pus in his bones, joints, tendon sheaths, or the pulp space of his fingers, draining it early is particularly urgent.* Elsewhere, you have more time.

If pus gathers in loose tissues near the surface of the body, you can usually detect fluctuation. But you will not detect fluctuation, or only detect it very late, if pus is under tension in some tight compartment, such as: (1) the pulp spaces of a patient's fingers or toes, (2) the fascial spaces of his hand (8.1) or foot, (3) his ischiorectal fossae, (4) the lobules of a woman's breast (21.2), (5) the neck or iliac region (iliac abscesses, 5.12), (6) the parotid gland (5.9). *Incise abscesses in any of these places without waiting for fluctuation, or for pus to point.* For fluctuation to be a useful sign, a minimum quantity of pus must be present, and it must be near the surface. If you wait for fluctuation in any of these places, you will have to wait until there is a huge bag of pus and much tissue has been destroyed unnecessarily.

WHERE THERE IS PUS, LET IT OUT

5.2 Abscesses

A patient with an abscess has severe throbbing pain. The infected part is tender and swollen, and the skin over it stretched, shiny, and red, although this may not be evident on a dark skin. Moving it is acutely painful. If his abscess is large or he has several abscesses, he may be febrile, weak, toxaemic, and anaemic. The usual signs of inflammation and suppuration suggest the diagnosis, but don't necessarily expect to find fluctuation in the sites listed in the previous section.

Severe pain is a useful sign that an abscess is ripe for incision, but pain may be mild when the tissues are loose. So incise it and let the pus flow out; break down any septa in a large cavity and open up any loculi (smaller cavities off the main one). If diagnosis is difficult, try aspirating it with a syringe and a wide bore (1.5 mm) needle; but remember that this is an unreliable test and that pus may be present even if you fail to aspirate any. Never try to *treat* an abscess by aspiration. There is no need to curette the walls of an abscess, except in the hand where you want inflammation to resolve particularly rapidly and completely.

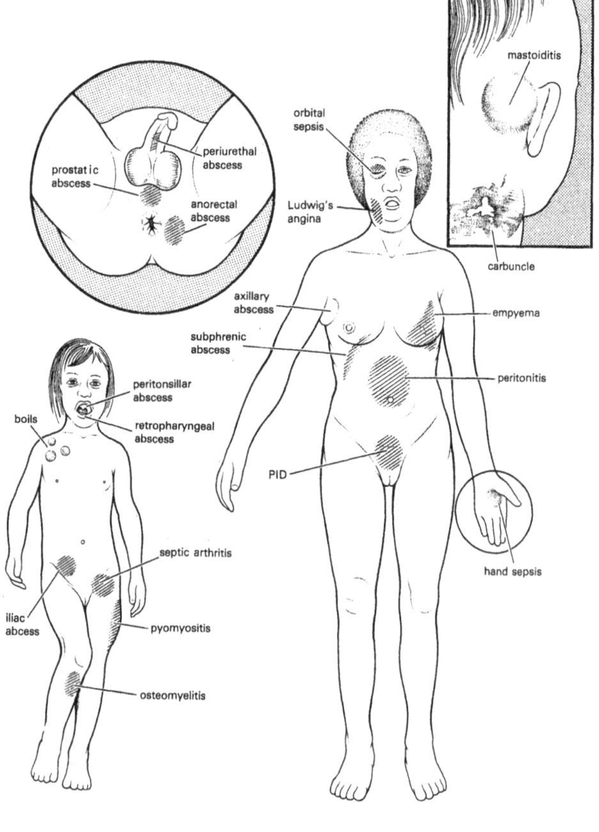

Fig. 5-1 SOME SITES OF SEPSIS. Pus can gather almost anywhere, but here are some of the commoner places where you will find it.

Abscesses are usually placed at the end of a list of otherwise 'clean' cases, and are often left to very junior staff. Nevertheless, be careful: (1) The diagnosis can be difficult, as with an iliac abscess (5.12). (2) Drainage has its risks, especially severe bleeding when a patient has a large abscess or many of them, so watch blood loss carefully (see below). (3) A superficial abscess over the tibia, femur, or humerus may turn out to be pyomyositis (7.1), or, more seriously, osteomyelitis (7.2). (4) A 'chronic abscess' may turn out to be a solid tumour. Some sarcomas are first treated as infections! (32.8).

THE GENERAL METHOD FOR ABSCESSES

EXAMINATION. Assess the patient's general condition carefully, especially if he has many abscesses, or large ones. Look for anaemia.

SPECIAL TESTS. (1) If his infection is severe, take blood cultures. You may be able to isolate the causative organism (this is important in osteomyelitis). (2) Test his urine, he may be diabetic—always do this if he has had more than one septic infection. Your work load will probably be too heavy to test the urines of all patients with abscesses. (3) If he has a particularly large or unusual abscess, or recurrent ones, test for HIV.

ANTIBIOTICS are not usually needed. Give them if: (1) He has a severe constitutional disturbance with high fever and toxaemia. (2) There are signs that his infection is spreading—increasing erythema, cellulitis, lymphangitis, severe lymphadenitis, or fever. (3) Rapid resolution is important, for example, in a deep infection of a hand or finger, or in a woman with a breast abscess where the re-establishment of breast feeding is critical.

If you decide to give him an antibiotic and you can culture the pus, give the first dose in the theatre immediately after drainage. If you cannot culture the pus, give it with the premedication, or an hour before the incision (2.7).

DRAINAGE OF AN ABSCESS

INDICATIONS. A collection of pus anywhere. If you suspect that there is a foreign body in an abscess this is an added reason for exploring it.

If you are not sure if pus is present or not, aspirate the lesion with a needle to see if you can withdraw pus. If pus is present drain it. If you fail to aspirate pus with a needle, this does NOT mean that there is no pus present!

Signs that an infection is spreading are not a contraindication to drainage—if you think pus is present, drain it.

ANAESTHESIA. (1) You don't need muscular relaxation, so ketamine will do (A 8.1). (2) If an abscess is already pointing, you can infiltrate the site of the incision with a local anaesthetic solution (A 5.7). (3) Intravenous thiopentone with pethidine (A 8.8). (4) Morphine. (5) Ethyl chloride local spray is the least satisfactory, but you can use it for very superficial abscesses. It makes the tissues hard and difficult to incise.

INCISION. Drain the abscess at the site of maximum tenderness and try to follow Lange's lines (61-3). This is safer than following any set rule or the dotted line on a diagram. If an abscess is superficial, use a pointed (No. 11) blade, as in Fig. 5-2.

CAUTION ! (1) If the abscess is deep, try to incise parallel to any nerves or vessels, not across them. (2) The common mistake is not to make the incision large enough.

HILTON'S METHOD should always be used if there is anything near the abscess which you might possibly injure. Incise the tissues down to the deep fascia, then push blunt scissors or a haemostat into the softest or most prominent part of the swelling. Open them out inside the abscess. If necessary, enlarge the wound by blunt dissection inside the tissues.

DRAIN THE PUS by putting your finger into the abscess, and breaking down all loculi, so that there is only one cavity. Use your little finger if the abscess is small. If there is much pus, suck it out or clean out the cavity with a swab. Make sure you remove it all.

INCISION AND DRAINAGE

A linear incision

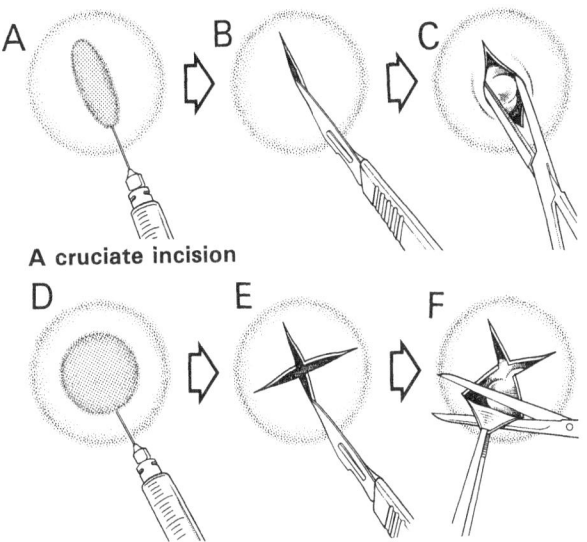

A cruciate incision

Fig. 5-2 INCISION AND DRAINAGE. A, B, and C, show a linear incision being made and its edges spread. D, E and F, show you how to make a cross-shaped incision, cut off the edges of the skin, and so remove the roof of the abscess. *After Hill GJ, 'Outpatient Surgery', Fig. 5.12. WB Saunders, with kind permission.*

PROVIDE FREE DRAINAGE. Make sure that any more pus which forms can drain from the bottom of the cavity.

If the abscess you are draining has a tendency to heal over and leave a cavity, deroof it, as in F, Fig. 5-2. This is especially necessary with perianal abscesses and Bartholin's abscesses. Cut away some skin, particularly any dead skin. Then pack it to make sure that the opening remains wider than the base and allows it to granulate from the bottom up. Gently fill the cavity with gauze. Replace this on the second or third day, and continue renewing it until pus no longer discharges. If the cavity is large, use ribbon gauze or bandage. If you use separate pieces of gauze, tie them together. Small pieces are easily lost in a deep cavity. Even a large one will quickly contract and disappear.

If an abscess is deep, push a corrugated rubber drain down to its deepest extension. This cannot block, and is better than a tube drain.

If pus has to drain downwards, as in the breast, try to incise the lowest part of the abscess. This is better than making a counter incision at its lowest point, and it also avoids making two incisions.

IF AN ABSCESS BLEEDS, pack the cavity (3.1). If necessary, set up a drip and give him 0.9% saline. Blood is seldom needed.

GENERAL MEASURES. If his abscess is in some critical place, such as his lateral pharyngeal space, or his mid palmar space, admit him. Make sure his fluid intake is adequate, and don't forget to give him an analgesic—abscesses are painful!

POSTOPERATIVE CARE. Rest the part, and where possible raise it. For example, put his hand in a St John's sling (71-1), or, if he is an inpatient, raise his hand in a roller towel, as in Fig. 75-1. If his foot is infected, raise the foot of his bed (81-1).

DIFFICULTIES WITH ABSCESSES

If he has NO FEVER BUT IS OBVIOUSLY 'ILL', suspect that his resistance to infection is low and treat him with particular care.

If he has MANY ABSCESSES, he has pyaemia, multiple pyomyositis, or septicaemia. He may bleed much when you drain them. If he is very anaemic, transfuse him first, and, if necessary, again during the operation. Draining multiple abscesses is a major procedure, particularly if a child is

EXPLORING AN ABSCESS

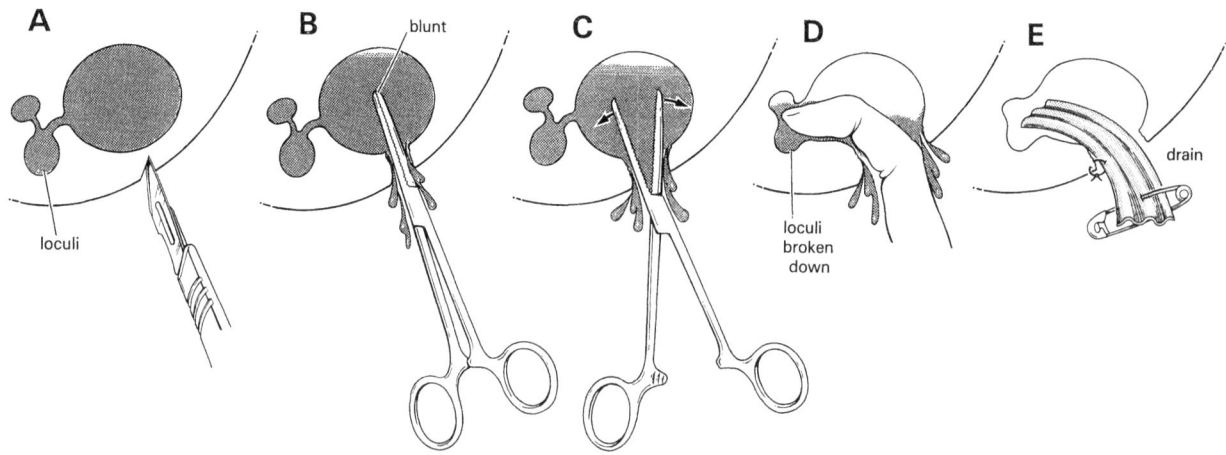

Fig. 5-3 EXPLORING AN ABSCESS BY HILTON'S METHOD. A, incise the abscess at its lowest point, if this is practicable. B, push blunt scissors or a haemostat into it. C, open the haemostat. D, explore the abscess with your finger. E, insert a drain.

anaemic or malnourished, so be careful before you incise too many abscesses at once—children have bled to death!

If he is VERY ILL AND HAS HUGE ABSCESSES, he will not tolerate an extensive procedure. It may occasionally be necessary to take him to the theatre several days in succession and drain a few abscesses at a time.

If an abscess FAILS TO HEAL, don't forget the possibility of tuberculosis (29.1) or HIV (28a.2).

If a child has abscesses, FAILS TO THRIVE, and is miserable, malnourished, and backward with his milestones, suspect HIV and examine his mother for palpable nodes (28a.2).

ALWAYS INCISE AT THE POINT OF MAXIMUM TENDERNESS

5.3 Boils

Boils and carbuncles are contagious skin infections, which are usually caused by penicillin-resistant staphylococci. The patient may have a crop of them, and in a closed community they may become epidemic.

BOILS For the general method, see Section 5.2.

Clean the skin round the a boil with hexachlorophane solution, and cover it with a dry dressing. Let it burst spontaneously. If it is pointing, a small incision will let it discharge and will reduce the pain. Alternatively, aspirate it.

CAUTION ! Never squeeze a boil; especially on the face, never let the patient squeeze it.

If he has many boils, tell him to wash thoroughly with soap and water, and to bath in salt water. Ideally, he should bath with hexochlorophane soap, or 70% spirit, change his underwear daily, and boil it. For very fortunate patients a seaside holiday is one of the best cures.

5.4 Carbuncles

A carbuncle is typically the result of neglected skin infection in a dirty, malnourished, and underprivileged patient, particularly a diabetic. A staphylococcal infection starts in one of his hair follicles, usually at the back of his neck or on the back of a finger (8.1), and then spreads. In doing so the infection lifts the skin above it on a sea of necrotic fat and pus. By the time you see him, pus will probably be discharging. Antibiotics don't cure a carbuncle, although they may stop it spreading. You will probably have to let the slough separate slowly, and then remove it.

CARBUNCLES For the general method, see Section 5.2. Be sure to test the patient's urine for sugar.

If the skin around his carbuncle is hairy, shave it with as little trauma as you can. Wash it with hexachlorophane solution, apply dry gauze, and change this frequently. A large slough will form in the middle of the carbuncle. You may be able to lift the slough off painlessly without an anaesthesic.

If the slough is slow to separate, excise it, and apply a dressing of vaseline gauze.

If the bare area is large, apply a split skin graft, as soon as it is clean and granulating.

If a collection of pus forms, cut down on it and drain it.

5.4a Extradural abscesses

Pus may gather between a patient's skull and his dura as the result of: (1) The spread of infection from sepsis nearby. (2) Exposure of the bone as the result of an injury. (3) Metastatic spread from elsewhere in his body. If his abscess is large, he will be very ill with signs of raised intracranial pressure (impaired consciousness and pupillary changes) and localizing motor signs, usually on the other side of his body, but not always so. Locally, he may have a diffuse inflammatory oedematous swelling of his scalp over the lesion (Pott's puffy tumour). If his abscess is not so large, he will not be so ill, and may have no signs of raised intracranial pressure. Making burr holes should be one of your basic skills (63.5), so draining the pus should not be too difficult. With your limited imaging facilities your problem will be to diagnose that he has an extradural abscess, and to know where it is—Pott's puffy tumour is the most useful sign.

EXTRADURAL ABSCESS X-ray his skull.

If his abscess is secondary to osteitis, and there is a sequestrum, removing it will drain the abscess adequately.

If his extradural abscess is secondary to metastatic spread, drain it through a burr hole. Make this on the edge of the area of swelling on his skull, and nibble away his skull around it until the abscess is well drained.

5.5 Infections of the orbit, cavernous sinus thrombosis

Acute suppurative infection is common near the eye, especially in children. It can occur in front of or behind the orbital septum. This is a sheet of fibrous tissue which stretches from the edges of the orbit into the eyelids, and divides the periorbital region from the orbit. Infections of both these regions usually start acutely with erythema and oedema of the eyelids; distinguish between them as described below. The danger with any infection in this region is that infection may occasionally kill the patient by spreading to his cavernous sinus or his meninges.

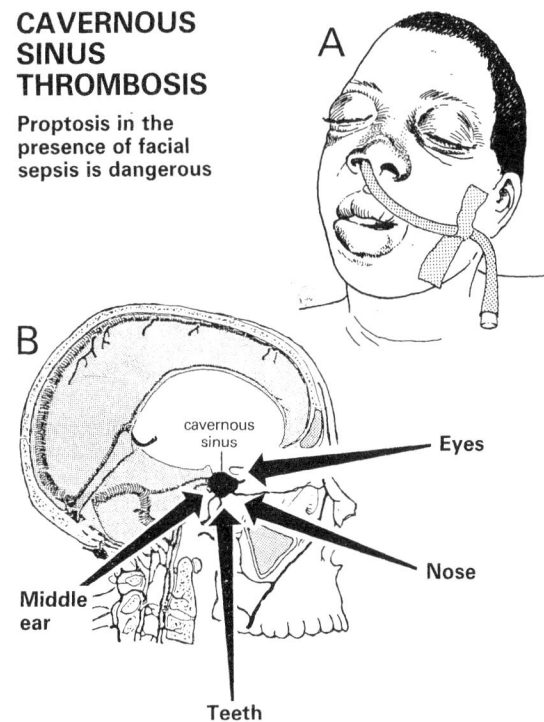

CAVERNOUS SINUS THROMBOSIS

Proptosis in the presence of facial sepsis is dangerous

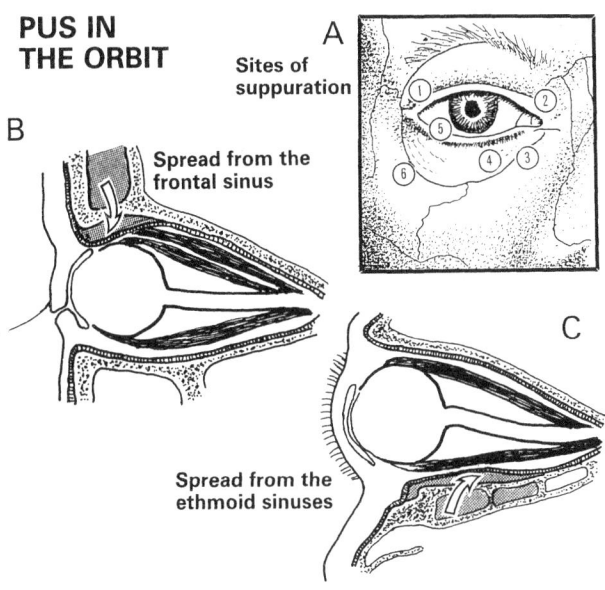

Fig. 5-4 PUS IN THE ORBIT. A, some important infections around a patient's eye. B, pus spreading under his periosteum from his frontal sinus. C, pus spreading under his periosteum from his ethmoid sinus.
1, the lachrymal gland (dacryoadenitis). 2, the frontal sinus and anterior ethmoidal air cells (sinusitis). 3, the tear sac (dacryocystitis). 4, tarsal cysts. 5, styes (hordeola). 6, periostitis of the margin of the orbit. Styes and suppurating tarsal cysts can occur anywhere on the lids, and periostitis anywhere in the orbit. *After Hamilton Bailey's Emergency Surgery, edited by HAF Dudley, Figs 187, 188, and 189. John Wright, with kind permission.*

Fig. 5-5 CAVERNOUS SINUS THROMBOSIS. A, orbital oedema and proptosis may be associated with paralysis of the 3rd, 4th, 6th (commonly), and the first two branches of the 5th cranial nerves, and also with meningeal irritation. B, infection may spread to the cavernous sinus from the eyes, nose, teeth, middle ear, or the paranasal sinuses.

Periorbital cellulitis occurs in front of the orbital septum, is more common than orbital cellulitis and occurs in younger children. It can be primary, or secondary to: (1) Local trauma. (2) Skin sepsis. (3) A recent upper respiratory infection; *H. influenzae* is commonly responsible for the latter, and the child may be bacteraemic.
Orbital cellulitis occurs behind the orbital septum, and is less common but more serious. It is usually due to spread from the paranasal sinuses, commonly from the frontal or ethmoid sinuses
Subperiosteal abscesses may form when bacteria spread from the adjacent sinuses.
Cavernous sinus thrombosis can be: (1) Occasionally, aseptic as result of trauma, tumours, or marasmus. (2) More commonly, it is septic as the result of the spread of infection from the nose (a nasal furuncle is the commonest source), face, mouth, teeth, sphenoid or ethmoid sinuses, the middle ear, or the internal jugular vein. A cord of thrombus spreads from the site of the infection to the cavernous sinus, and sometimes to the cerebral veins and meninges to cause: (1) A rise in pressure in the veins draining the eye, resulting in severe oedema and proptosis. (2) Paralysis of the 3rd, 4th, 6th (commonly) and the first two branches of the 5th cranial nerves. (3) Meningeal irritation. In the days before antibiotics the patient almost always died; now he should not. If you treat him late, he may be left with visual impairment, ocular palsies, and hemiplegia.

Don't be frightened of operating in the orbit. *Because of the danger of cavernous sinus thrombosis you must drain pus early.* A negative exploration will not harm him, and you are very unlikely to damage his globe.

RANGIT (60 years) was admitted with a history of septic teeth for many years. Recently he had had fever, headache, rigors, and gradual swelling of his mandible. He was ill, dehydrated, shocked, jaundiced, and confused. Pus discharged from his mouth, his submental glands were enlarged, his neck was stiff, and Kernig's test was positive. Both his globes were proptosed, particularly the left, which was fixed; his forehead and cheek were oedematous, and his CSF turbid. Despite vigorous penicillin treatment he died. Postmortem examination revealed left dental and mandibular abscesses; his left orbit and cavernous sinus were full of pus. LESSONS (1) This is a very dangerous condition. (2) Proptosis in the presence of facial sepsis is a dangerous sign. (3) The organisms responsible are often penicillin-resistant.

D'arbella PG, Cavernous sinus thrombosis. East African Medical Journal 1964;41:551-9

Anonymous. Orbital cellulitis [Editorial] Lancet 1986;ii:497.

INFECTIONS OF THE ORBIT

For the general method, see Section 5.2. Gently separate the patient's lids. Examine for induration and tenderness of his lids, chemosis (subconjunctival oedema), proptosis (his globe is pushed forwards), limitation of ocular movement, and loss of visual acuity. If you find these, suspect orbital cellulitis, take blood cultures and *start parenteral antibiotics immediately!*
  CAUTION ! (1) Oedema and erythema of the lids are common to both orbital and periorbital cellulitis. (2) If the treatment of orbital cellulitis is delayed or incorrect, cavernous sinus thrombosis may follow.

X-RAYS. Infection may have spread from his paranasal sinuses, so consider X-raying them (if this is possible), to see if you can find a loss of translucency on the affected side. The films will be difficult to interpret, especially in children in whom the sinuses are small.

TREATMENT. Give him penicillin with cloxacillin. Or, give him cephradine alone (2.9). Or, give him penicillin and chloramphenicol.

DIFFICULTIES WITH ORBITAL SEPSIS

If the patient's GLOBE IS DISPLACED BY AN INFLAMMATORY SWELLING, and its movement impaired, perhaps accompanied by loss of visual acuity, suspect that he has a subperiosteal abscess of his orbit. For example, an abscess above his eye will displace it downwards. Try aspirating the pus from the roof of the abscess with a needle. His eye may go back into place. Then incise and evacuate his abscess through a conjunctival fornix—his inferior fornix if swelling is maximal inferiorly, and his superior fornix if it is maximal superiorly. Pus will probably be coming from a paranasal sinus and you may find a track through to it. Insert a drain.

If he has an inflammatory SWELLING IN THE UPPER, OUTER PART OF HIS ORBIT, involving the outer third of his upper lid, suspect that his lachrymal gland is infected (DACRYOADENITIS). Incise the abscess through the upper fornix of his conjunctiva, or through his eyelid.

If he has an inflammatory SWELLING BELOW THE MEDIAL ASPECT OF HIS LOWER LID, suspect that he has an abscess in his lachrymal gland (DACRYOCYSTITIS). Press it, pus may exude through the punctum. If it suppurates, incise it through the skin of his lower lid. When the infection has subsided, refer him for a dacryocystorhinostomy, which will usually re-establish the flow of his tears.

If his conjunctiva becomes increasingly congested, his globes proptose, his OCULAR MOVEMENTS BECOME PROGRESSIVELY IMPAIRED, his accommodation paralysed, his pupil fixed and dilated, and his cornea anaesthetic, he has CAVERNOUS SINUS THROMBOSIS. It will probably involve both his eyes. Early vigorous chemotherapy may save him (2.9). Give him penicillin and cephradine, or chloramphenicol.

5.6 Peritonsillar abscesses

Abscesses round the tonsils are quite common, and follow tonsillitis. The patient, who is usually a child, has a tense swelling above and behind one of his tonsils, displacing it downwards and forwards. Non-operative treatment is almost always successful, and is much safer than draining it, which is a heroic procedure and is seldom necessary, because much of the swelling is inflammatory oedema.

PERITONSILLAR ABSCESSES

For the general method see Section 5.2.

NON-OPERATIVE TREATMENT. Admit the patient, and give him intramuscular benzyl penicillin, or ampicillin, or intravenous chloramphenicol (2.9). He will also need intravenous fluids and morphine or pethidine. He should respond within 24 hours and his abscess will probably burst spontaneously, or the inflammation will subside sufficiently to make drainage much easier.

INCISION. In the unlikely event that he fails to respond to non-operative treatment, sit him upright in a chair with his head supported, and a gag in his mouth. Get a very good headlight.

Spray his pharynx with a local anaesthetic solution, such as 4% lignocaine. If he cannot open his mouth wide enough, you may have to give him a general anaesthetic, intubate him, and place him on his side with his head as low as possible. If intubation is impossible, give him ketamine and keep his head down.

Use a guarded scalpel to incise the abscess over its most prominent part, as in Fig. 5-6. Divide only the mucosa, then use sinus forceps to find pus by Hilton's method (5-3).

CAUTION ! (1) Don't let him inhale pus. (2) Have suction instantly available.

If severe bleeding follows and you cannot control it, try firm compression through his mouth with a tightly rolled swab, or tight mattress sutures. Tying his external carotid artery is a heroic last resort (3.3), and means that you have put your knife too deep.

PUS IN THE THROAT

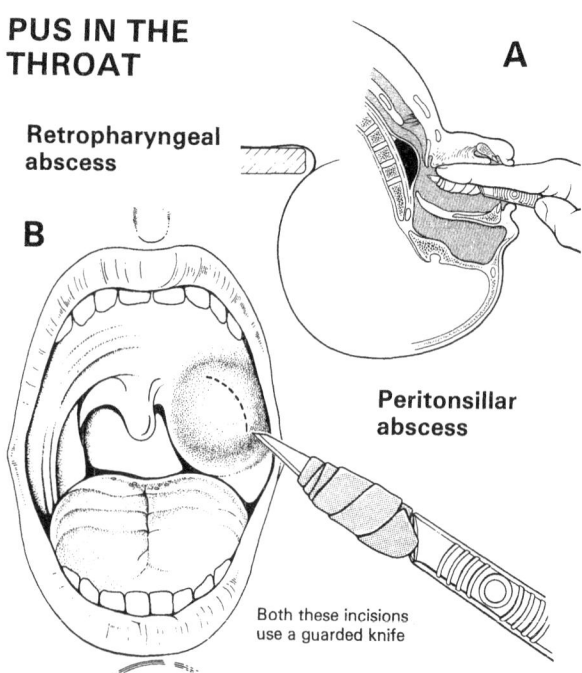

Retropharyngeal abscess

Peritonsillar abscess

Both these incisions use a guarded knife

Fig. 5-6 TWO ABSCESSES IN THE THROAT. A, the danger with a retropharyngeal abscess is that an unconscious child may inhale pus and get bronchopneumonia. Avoid this by incising it while his head is hanging over the end of a table. B, a peritonsillar abscess occasionally follows tonsillitis, and needs draining. Do both these incisions with a guarded knife that cannot cut too deeply.

5.7 Retropharyngeal abscesses

Occasionally, an abscess forms in the lymph nodes behind a child's pharynx which bulges forwards. Sometimes an abscess is the result of infection round an impacted fish bone. If the swelling is large enough, he may asphyxiate. If it bursts, he may get an aspiration pneumonia. The major differential diagnosis is a chronic tuberculous retropharyngeal abscess.

RETROPHARYNGEAL ABSCESSES

For the general method, see Section 5.2. If the patient is dehydrated, give him intravenous fluids.

ACUTE ABSCESS IN A CHILD. The great danger of a general anaesthetic is that the patient will inhale pus. Ketamine is relatively safe because his cough reflex is less suppressed. Give it intravenously, give only just enough, and keep his head down.

Have a tracheostomy set (52.2) and suction ready. Lie him on his back with his head over the end of the table, so that his pharynx is as nearly upside down as possible.

If his abscess is pointing, you may be able to open it with sinus forceps alone. If you can get a really good view, you may be able to aspirate it with a needle. If this is impractical, open his abscess with a guarded knife (5-6). Put your index finger into his mouth, and slide the knife along it. Drain it by Hilton's method (5-3), as for a peritonsillar abscess.

CAUTION ! Don't let him inhale pus—suck immediately you incise.

If severe bleeding follows, and you cannot control it, apply local pressure for 15 minutes. If that fails (rare), be prepared to tie his external carotid artery (3.3).

ACUTE ABSCESS IN AN ADULT. Anaesthetize the mucosa over the abscess with 4% lignocaine, preferably as an aerosol, and incise it with his head down and on one side, as in a child.

TUBERCULOUS RETROPHARYNGEAL ABSCESSES (rare) are usually subacute and follow infection of the body of a vertebra. Refer him if you can. Only consider drainage if obstruction to his airway is a real danger. Drain his abscess through an external incision in front of his sternomastoid down to his prevertebral fascia. Displace his thyroid gland and trachea anteriorly.

5.8 Dental abscesses

If a patient comes to you with a painful, throbbing, swollen, red face (a 'fat face'), perhaps with fever, trismus and lymphadenitis, he is probably suffering from an acute dental or oral infection, most probably an alveolar abscess. He may have:

(1) An alveolar abscess begins as an infection in the bone around a non-vital infected tooth. He has severe pain, which becomes less as pus is released into more superficial tissues and his face starts to swell. After 36 hours of cellulitis he usually has a fluctuant abscess which needs draining. If drainage is delayed, the pus in his abscess discharges spontaneously through a sinus (26-8) in his gum or face, which may become chronic.

First, control infection with antibiotics, and then drain the abscess, either by incising it where it is pointing, or by removing the infected tooth, which acts as a cork to prevent the pus escaping, or by doing both these things. If you remove a tooth before you have controlled the infection with antibiotics, and while his face is still severely swollen, you may spread the infection; your task will also be more difficult.

(2) A periodontal abscess at the side of a tooth, caused by spread from an infected gum.

(3) A pericoronal abscess caused by infection of the gum over the crown of an unerupted and impacted tooth, usually a lower third molar ('an infected wisdom tooth'). Often, an abscess does not form, and the gum round the tooth is merely inflamed.

Pus from all three of these foci of infection, and particularly from an alveolar abscess, can track in various directions, towards his cheek, his tongue, or his palate, or downwards into his neck. It can discharge inside his mouth or outside. It can collect: (1) On any of the surfaces of his gum ('gumboils'). (2) In the buccal sulcus of either jaw on the oral or deeper side of the attachment of his buccinator muscle (common). (3) On the surface of his face superficial to the buccinator attachment. (4) On his palate (less common). (5) In his submasseteric space between his masseter and the ascending ramus of his mandible. (6) In his pterygomandibular space between his medial pterygoid and the ascending ramus of his mandible. (7) In his sublingual space above or below his mylohyoid muscle. (8) In his submandibular space superficial to his mylohyoid. (9) In his submental space in the midline under his jaw. (10) Anywhere down the side of his neck. Don't be daunted by the complexity of this anatomy. Some of these spaces communicate with one another and more than one space may be involved—*incise the abscess where it points*, having due regard, where you can, for the skin lines on his face (61-3).

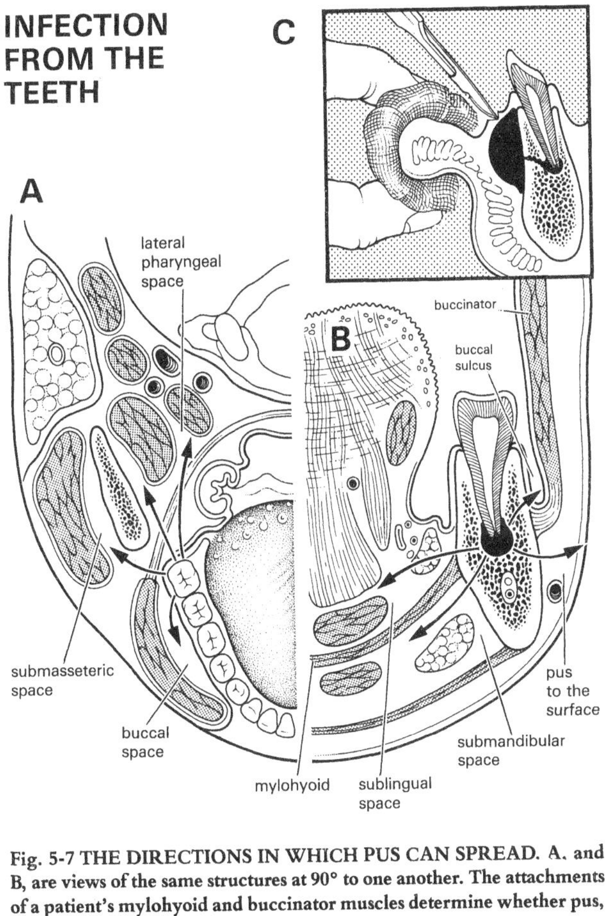

Infection can spread in some particularly dangerous directions: (1) From his upper jaw (or upper lip or nose) to his cavernous sinus, which may thrombose, perhaps fatally (5.5). (2) From his lateral pharyngeal space up towards the base of his skull, down to his glottis or into his mediastinum. Infection of this space is one of the most dangerous conditions in dentistry. He has difficulty swallowing and speaking. (3) From his lower jaw, via his sublingual and submandibular spaces, to the tissues of his neck, where it may cause oedema of his glottis, respiratory obstruction and death. This is Ludwig's angina (5.10).

BEWARE OF CAVERNOUS SINUS THROMBOSIS AND LUDWIG'S ANGINA

DENTAL ABSCESSES

For the general method, see Section 5.2.

HISTORY AND EXAMINATION. A patient of any age over 5 years walks into casualty with a fat face looking ill and distressed. He has usually had toothache in the past, but the pain has gone. Now he tells you that he has had pain for a week. He has fever, trismus, and a unilateral, tender, shiny, warm, indurated swelling. Looking at him will tell you which side of his face and which jaw is involved. Feel for warmth with the back of your index finger and test for fluctuation. A tooth with large holes in it probably has an apical abscess under it. It may be firm, but is usually loose. If he has obvious periodontal disease, or several loose teeth, suspect a periodontal abscess.

If you are in doubt as to which of his teeth is the site of infection, tap them with some metal object or press them with your gloved index finger. A tooth which is much more painful than the others is probably the source of an alveolar infection. It may also be slightly raised in its socket. A tooth with a periodontal abscess is much less tender to percussion.

X-RAYS. If possible, X-ray the offending tooth. You may see: (1) A a radiolucent area at its apex when an apical abscess has been present for 2 or 3 weeks. (2) Caries between two adjacent teeth which may not be visible from his mouth. (3) The impacted tooth which is responsible for a pericoronal abscess. (4) Some other source for the infection, such as an infected cyst, or a fracture.

THE DIFFERENTIAL DIAGNOSIS includes acute inflammation of the salivary glands (5.9), mumps, Burkitt's lymphoma (32.3), lymph node swellings and glandular fever.

GENERAL MEASURES. Admit him and make sure that his fluid intake is adequate; he may find drinking difficult.

CAUTION ! Don't apply poultices or any kind of local heat to his face—they may spread the infection. If an abscess is pointing inside his mouth, hot saline mouth washes may ease his pain.

ANTIBIOTICS are often unnecessary, because many dental infections can be treated by local drainage only. If there is

Fig. 5-7 THE DIRECTIONS IN WHICH PUS CAN SPREAD. A. and B, are views of the same structures at 90° to one another. The attachments of a patient's mylohyoid and buccinator muscles determine whether pus, orginating in his lower jaw, points inside or outside his mouth. A, shows pus from his lower third molar spreading into his buccal space, his submasseteric space, and his lateral pharyngeal space. B, shows the attachments of his mylohyoid and buccinator muscles. The attachments of these muscles determine whether pus spreads into his sublingual space, his submandibular space, his buccal sulcus, or on to the surface of his face. C, shows the incision of an abscess in his buccal sulcus. *Partly after 'Hamilton Bailey's Emergency Surgery', edited by Dudley HAF, Fig. 151. John Wright, with kind permission.*

spreading cellulitis he needs an antibiotic. Procaine penicillin 600,000 units (2 ml) intramuscularly is adequate in most cases. But if his condition is serious give him a megaunit of benzyl penicillin 4 to 6-hourly.

When you have drained an abscess, culture the pus and change the antibiotic if necessary.

CAUTION ! Make sure that he understands that a course of antibiotics is not sufficient treatment for his abscess, and that he must return, even if his swelling improves.

ANAESTHESIA. (1) 2% or 4% lignocaine spray or a swab soaked in lignocaine solution. (2) Inject a local anaesthetic solution into the outer wall of the abscess over the proposed site of the incision. (3) Ethyl chloride local spray is suitable for an abscess which presents on his face or in his labial or buccal sulci. Isolate the infected area with gauze packs, and then spray on ethyl chloride until crusting occurs. Then open the abscess with a No. 11 blade.

CAUTION! Avoid general anaesthesia, if you can, unless it is expert (especially if he is in danger of respiratory obstruction—see A 13.2), and you can intubate him and pack off his throat.

ALVEOLAR ABSCESSES

If you can refer him, a dentist may be able to save his tooth by draining the abscess through it, and later filling its root. If you cannot refer him, remove it. Many abscessed teeth are loose, and you can easily pick them out of their sockets. Removing his tooth to allow pus to drain through the socket, combined with antibiotic treatment may be sufficient. Don't incise a non-fluctuant swelling. If it is not yet fluctuant and ripe for incision, ask him to use hot saline mouth washes, as hot as he can bear without the risk of being scalded, several times a day. Give him an antibiotic and wait. This may control his infection and arrest pus formation.

CAUTION ! (1) Don't pull out his tooth (26.3) before you have controlled his cellulitis. (2) If he has a tense inflammatory swelling of the upper part of his neck, suspect Ludwig's angina and treat him urgently (5.10).

PUS POINTING INSIDE HIS MOUTH can point in several places:

If an abscess is pointing on his alveolus, open it into his mouth.

If it is pointing in his labial sulcus (C, 5-7), make a 1.5 cm incision through his mucous membrane parallel to his alveolar ridge. Push a fine haemostat into it and open the jaws.

If it is pointing in his palate, make an anteroposterior incision, parallel to its nerves and vessels, remove an ellipse of tissue and let the pus flow out.

If he has pus in his pterygomandibular, lateral pharyngeal, or submasseteric spaces, drain it through a vertical incision inside his mouth parallel to the ascending ramus of his mandible, *taking care to avoid his parotid duct (61-5)*. This runs in his cheek under the middle third of a line between the tragus of his ear and the commissure of his lips, and opens in line with his first molar tooth. Push forceps to the lingual or buccal side of his ramus, wherever the pus seems to be pointing. If it is under his masseter, insert a drain deep to this muscle down to his mandible from outside his face. Insert the drain through an incision just below the inferior border of his mandible.

PUS POINTING OUTSIDE HIS MOUTH. Drain it through one of the incisions below, as soon as any cellulitis he may have has stopped spreading. Removing his tooth to let the pus drain is not enough, even if it does drip from his root canal. If his abscess is fluctuant, it needs draining too. If you are not sure if it is ready for drainage or not, insert a wide bore needle under local anaesthesia. If you aspirate pus, incise it by Hilton's method (5.2) where it points at the softest and most tender spot. To minimize scarring, make an incision below the inferior border of his mandible, where possible. If you have to make it on his face, make it in line with the creases in his skin (61-3). These may not always be over the most fluctuant part of the abscess.

CAUTION ! When you plan your incision, consult Figures 5-7a and 61-3 and remember: (1) The extension of the lower pole of his parotid gland into the side of his neck (61-5). (2) The mandibular branches of his facial nerve. These run horizontally and cross the lower border of his mandible, just anterior to his masseter, deep to his platysma muscle in his anterior mandibular region and deep to the fascia posteriorly. (3) His facial artery and vein. These enter his face from between his submandibular salivary gland and the lower border of his mandible; they cross the ramus of his mandible 3 cm from the angle of his jaw and then run obliquely across the lower third of his face superficially on his buccinator muscle. You may have to compromise between chosing the best site for dependent drainage and an inconspicuous scar in the crease lines of his face. Here are some likely sites:

If he has a submental abscess, drain it through a small midline transverse incision under his chin.

If the abscess is under the body of his mandible, drain it through a horizontal incision 1 to 2 cm below the lower border of his mandible, taking care to avoid the mandibular branch of his facial nerve and his facial vessels. Push sinus forceps towards the lingual side of his mandible to drain the pus there.

If the abscess points external to his buccinator, drain it through a small incision over the swelling.

DRAINS. Stitch a corrugated or tubular rubber or plastic drain into the wound for 2 to 5 days, or leave it open with its edges separated by gauze.

PERIODONTAL ABSCESS. If you cannot refer him for a conservative operation, pull out his tooth (26.3).

PERICORONAL INFECTION (infected 'wisdom tooth'). See Section 26.4.

POSTOPERATIVELY, after you have incised any intraoral abscess, give him hot mouth washes to help the incision stay open as long as is necessary.

DIFFICULTIES. **If he CANNOT OPEN HIS MOUTH to let you get at the abscess,** he probably still has cellulitis, and his abscess is not yet fit for incision. So continue antibiotics and try again later.

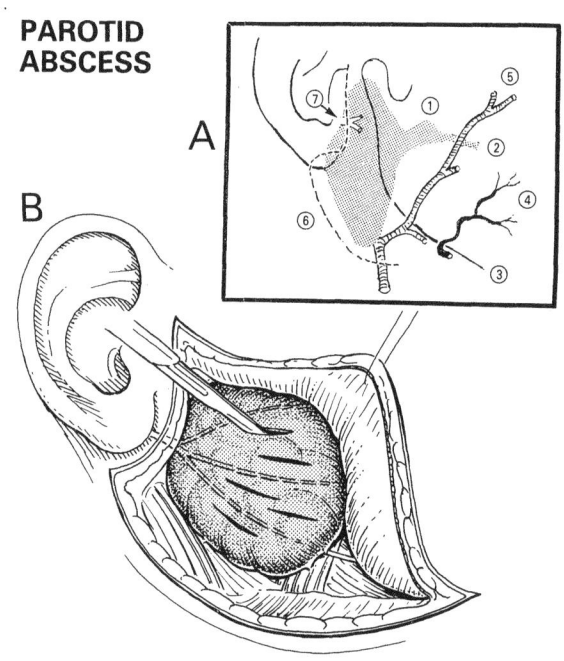

Fig. 5-7a DRAINING A PAROTID ABSCESS. A, the anatomy of the parotid gland. A patient's facial nerve enters the substance of his parotid so that, if you only incise his skin and subcutaneous tissue superficial to the gland when you reflect the flap, you will not injure it. Note that it extends well down into his neck. Incise where his pinna meets the skin of his face and neck and continue on in a skin crease. B, turn back the flap and incise radially to avoid the branches of his facial nerve.

1, the parotid gland. 2, the parotid duct. 3, the border of the mandible. 4, the facial artery crossing the mandible about 3 cm anterior to its angle. 5, the facial vein. 6, the incision. 7, the facial nerve.

5.9 Parotid abscesses

Although parotid abscesses can occur without any obvious cause, you will see them most often in debilitated patients, or after major surgery when mouth care has been neglected. The patient's parotid is painful and is usually much swollen; the skin over it is tight and shiny. You may see pus coming from his parotid duct (inside his cheek level with his first molar tooth). Pus forms in several lobules of the gland between its septa, and does not form a single abscess. This, and the division of his facial nerve into its five branches within his parotid gland, make drainage difficult; it is however essential. Don't wait for fluctuation.

PAROTID ABSCESS

For the general method, see Section 5.2.

THE MAIN DIFFERENTIAL DIAGNOSIS is mumps. There is no pus at the orifice of the parotid duct, mumps is usually bilateral, and the skin over the swelling is less shiny. Mumps parotitis does NOT require surgical drainage, it resolves spontaneously.

INCISION. Start incising anterior to the patient's pinna. Keeping close to it, proceed towards his mastoid and then continue in the angle between his pinna and his neck until you reach a skin crease, then cut along this for up to 10 cm. Raise a flap of skin and subcutaneous tissue, so as to expose his parotid gland. Make multiple incisions into this in line with the branches of his facial nerve. Explore each incision by Hilton's method and clean out each abscess cavity with gauze. Close the wound with continuous or interrupted sutures of 3/0 monofilament, leaving a dependent corrugated drain emerging from the inferior part of the incision.

5.10 Pus in the neck—Ludwig's angina

You may see these acute suppurative infections in a patient's neck:

(1) **Suppuration in a lymph node,** especially a deep cervical one, is common in children, and is much like suppuration in any other lymph node.

(2) **Suppuration arising from an infected tooth (Ludwig's angina)** occurs in children and adults. It is a severe bilateral brawny cellulitis of the sublingual and submandibular regions, and may extend as far as the patient's clavicles. It usually starts as a dental abscess in his mandible, which makes him febrile and very ill. If Ludwig's angina is neglected, it may obstruct his respiration by causing oedema of his glottis, and by pushing his tongue up against the roof of his mouth. Anaerobes and spirochaetes may be responsible. He can also die from septicaemia. He needs intensive antibiotic treatment urgently, and drainage to decompress the tissues at the floor of his mouth.

LUDWIG'S ANGINA

For the general method, see Section 5.2. This is an acute emergency: admit the patient, and give him high doses of antibiotics (2.7). He needs a megaunit of penicillin 4 to 6-hourly, metronidazole and chloramphenicol (2.9).

If his breathing is not significantly obstructed, you may be wiser to wait for 24 hours for the antibiotics to act and the oedema to subside a little, before you drain his lesion.

If it is significantly obstructed, you may be forced to do a tracheostomy (unusual, 52.2). This is difficult, because the tissues of his neck are firm and oedematous.

ANAESTHESIA. (1) Ketamine is acceptable, unless his airway is almost totally obstructed. (2) Don't give him an inhalation anaesthetic. He probably needs the help of his voluntary muscles to maintian his airway, and you will be unable to pass a tracheal tube. (3) You may occasionally have to use local infiltration anaesthesia, but it will be painful and distressing.

INCISION. Make a generous incision below the angle of his mandible, over the point of maximum tenderness, taking care to avoid his facial artery and in the line of a skin crease if possible. The abscess will be surrounded by inflammatory oedema. Cut through his skin and deep fascia, and explore it by Hilton's method (5-3). You may need to do some careful blunt dissection to release a little pus at the centre of the abscess. Leave the wound open, or partly close it and insert a drain. Later, remove the offending tooth (if this is the cause, 26.3).

5.10a Thyroid abscesses (acute bacterial thyroiditis)

Abscesses of the thyroid are rare in the developed world, but are not uncommon here in the developing world. The patient presents with a wide, very painful, oedematous swelling of his neck which is maximal over his thyroid. The pus is too deep for you to be able to detect fluctuation. Inflammatory oedema may be so marked as to cause Ludwig's angina (5.10).

THYROID ABSCESSES

For the general method, see Section 5.2.

DIAGNOSIS. Confirm the presence of pus by needle aspiration.

ANAESTHESIA. Give the patient intravenous ketamine or a general anaesthetic with intubation. Local anaesthesia is not satisfactory, unless the pus is pointing, but if your anaesthetist is not expert, you may have to use it. If he is to have a general anaesthetic the anaesthetist must be experienced.

INCISION. Use a scalpel to make a transverse incision 5 cm or larger over the area of maximal swelling. Insert a haemostat and drain the pus by Hilton's method (5-3). Insert a drain and give him an antibiotic (chloramphenicol or a cephalosporin) for 5 days.

5.10b Pancreatic abscess

This is a dangerous complication of acute pancreatitis (13.9). A collection of pus, necrotic tissue, and clot fills the patient's lesser sac; it enlarges behind his peritoneum, it expands anteriorly to obliterate his lesser sac, and it pushes his stomach and transverse colon forwards.

If his abscess develops during the course of an attack of pancreatitis, the diagnosis is usually obvious, but it may be difficult otherwise. So if ever a severely sick patient has an ill-defined deep-seated epigastric mass, remember that he might perhaps have a pancreatic abscess.

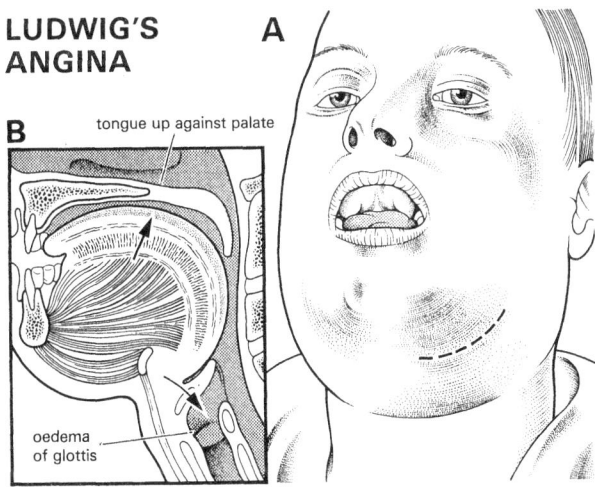

Fig 5-8 LUDWIG'S ANGINA. A, note the massive swelling of the patient's chin. B, his swollen tissues have compressed his tongue against his palate. The infection may spread to cause oedema of his glottis. *Partly after 'Hamilton Bailey's Emergency Surgery', edited by HAF Dudley HAF, Figs. 153 and 154, John Wright, with kind permission.*

PANCREATIC ABSCESS

SPECIAL TESTS. The patient's urinary and serum amylase are high. A plain erect film may show a large cavity with a fluid level, or gas. A barium meal may show a deformity in the outline of his stomach, caused by a mass behind it pushing it forwards. See also Section 13.10.

DRAINAGE. Under general anaesthesia and with adequate relaxation, prepare and drape his upper abdomen. Then feel for the mass again.

Make an upper midline incision from his xiphisternum to his umbilicus. Open his peritoneal cavity with care, because the mass, or his stomach or colon, may have stuck to his abdominal wall.

You may find it difficult to know what you are seeing. Dissection is difficult and dangerous, because his tissues are so vascular and oedematous. Lift and free his abdominal wall from the organs under it, and insert a self-retaining retractor.

Feel for the upper border of the abdominal mass. Try to find a place where you can incise it without injuring anything. This will usually be through his gastrocolic omentuum, or his lesser omentum.

When you have decided where to drain, seal the area from the rest of his peritoneum with large moist packs. Using a syringe and a large needle, aspirate the place where there seems to be the thinnest layer of tissue between the abscess and your finger. Take pus for culture.

If you find pus under pressure, decompress the abscess with a trocar and cannula, to which suction is attached. Enlarge the abscess so that you can insert two fingers, but don't try to dissect further. Wash out floating solid matter.

CAUTION ! At the same time, don't disturb the necrotic pancreatic tissue at the bottom of his abscess—it will bleed!

Place two Malecot catheters in the abscess cavity, and bring them out through stab wounds. Bring one out anteriorly, and the other as far back as possible, in the most 'dependent' position. Use these to irrigate the abscess cavity continuously with saline (about 2 l in 24 hours). Make a feeding jejunostomy (9.7), because he will not be able to eat for 3 weeks, and you will probably be unable to feed him parenterally. Feeding him through a jejunostomy results in less secretion of gastric juice than feeding him through a gastrostomy.

Close his abdomen securely as a single layer (9.8). Leave his skin open, and lay a hypochlorite or saline pack on it.

Continue nasogastric suction, fluids, and antibiotics until his temperature is normal. Don't be in a hurry to remove the drains, even if leaving them in does seem to increase the risk of a fistula. Allowing pus to collect again is a greater risk. If the wound is looking fairly clean, close it by secondary suture in 7 to 10 days.

CAUTION ! A pancreatic abscess carries a 30 to 50% mortality, and often reforms, even with adequate drainage. If so, be prepared to reoperate 3 or 4 times if necessary.

5.11 Axillary abscesses

Suppuration in a patient's axilla can take several forms: (1) Pus can form superficially in his apocrine glands. (2) It can form more deeply in the lymph nodes under his pectoralis major. Open deep abscesses promptly, because pus can track along his nerve trunks into his neck.

AXILLARY ABSCESSES

For the general method, see Section 5.2. Abduct the patient's arm.

If his abscess is superficial (usual), incise over it.

If his abscess is deep (unusual), make a 3 to 5 cm incision just behind the fold of his pectoralis major, so as to avoid his axillary vessels. Push a haemostat upwards into the swelling, open its handles parallel to important structures, and open the abscess. Insert a drain.

If his whole axilla is a bag of pus, incise low in his axilla.

If he has a large subacute or chronic abscess, consider the possibility of tuberculosis, especially if the surrounding tissues are indurated, sinuses are present, and the breast is swollen from lymphoedema, perhaps with peau d'orange.

AXILLARY ABSCESS

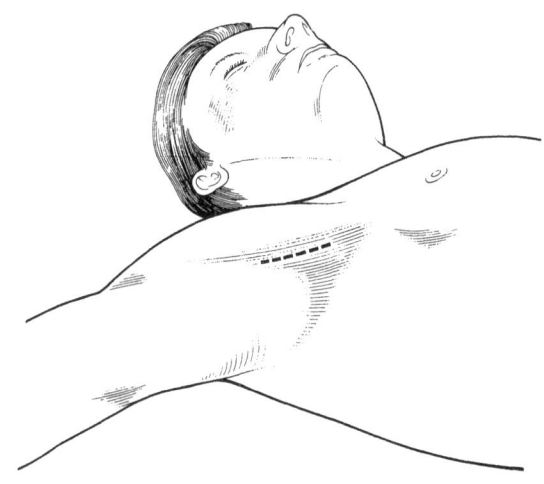

Fig. 5-9 AN AXILLARY ABSCESS can form superficially in a patient's apocrine glands. Pus can also form more deeply in the lymph nodes under his pectoralis major. Open deep the abscesses promptly, because pus can track along his nerve trunks into his neck.

If he has multiple recurrent small abscesses in his skin, they may: (1) Be caused by tuberculosis, so biopsy one. Otherwise do a therapeutic trial with chemotherapy for tuberculosis. (2) Be caused by fungi. (3) Originate in sweat glands (HIRADENITIS SUPPURATIVA, unusual). Incision will not help much and may lead to keloid formation. If you suspect this try metronidazole and regular swabbing with a mild antiseptic, such as cetrimide.

5.11a Perinephric abscesses

Perinephric abscesses are not uncommon; they are usually caused by staphylococci, and arise from a small metastatic abscess in the cortex of the kidney, which may be solitary, or one of many pyaemic abscesses.

The patient, who may be any age, presents with fever and a tender swollen area in his loin or subhepatic area. If his abscess is small and related to the upper pole of his kidney, he may have no localizing signs. The approach to the kidney is the same as that for a nephrostomy, so see Section 23.13, and particularly Fig. 23-16.

PERINEPHRIC ABSCESS

X-RAYS. Take a plain X-ray. Look for obliteration of the patient's psoas shadow, and scoliosis with a concavity towards the abscess. Look also for disease of his spine, especially narrowing of intervertebral discs and erosion of the bodies of his vertebrae nearby, especially anteriorly (osteomyelitis, an important differential diagnosis).

Screen the movement of his diaphragm. This is reduced in most cases of subphrenic abscess, but seldom with perinephric abscesses.

An IVU shows a normally functioning kidney which may be displaced, especially medially or posteriorly.

CAUTION ! An intravenous urogram is essential. Without one you cannot exclude a pyonephros.

DIFFERENTIAL DIAGNOSIS. (1) Pyomyositis of the abdominal wall or paraspinal muscles. (2) Pyonephros. (3) Subphrenic abscess. (4) Osteomyelitis of the spine, with spread to the paraspinal tissues.

MANAGEMENT. His pus must be drained. You may not know for certain if it is perinephric, subphrenic (especially in the posterior or subhepatic spaces), or has spread from osteitis of his spine.

ANTIBIOTICS. Give him an antibiotic (chloramphenicol or a cephalosporin, 2.9).

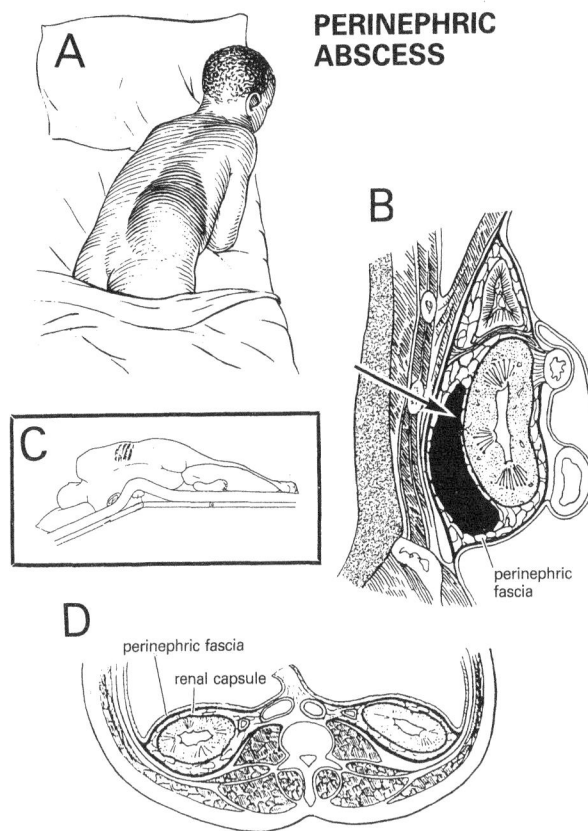

Fig. 5-9a A PERINEPHRIC ABSCESS. A, an unusually large perinephric abscess. B, approach a perinephric abscess through the bed of the 12th rib. C, put the patient into the left lateral position. D, the true renal capsule is closely applied to the surface of the kidney. Outside this, the perinephric fat is surrounded by the perinephric fascia (Gerota's fascia). *After Robert C Flanigan in Rob's 'Operative Surgery'. Figs. 1b, 3, and 12a. With the kind permission of Hugh Dudley.*

ANAESTHETIC. (1) General anaesthesia with intubation. (2) Intravenous ketamine.

POSITION. Lie him in the kidney position as for a nephrostomy—see Section 23.13.

INCISION. Make a 15 to 20 cm incision starting posteriorly over his 12th rib just lateral to his sacrospinalis muscle (about the mid point of the rib). Cut down on the rib, incise and deflect the periosteum, so as to push the nerves and vessels aside. Remove the distal two thirds of his rib and dissect through its bed to expose his perinephric space containing the abscess.

If the pus is in his muscles (pyomyositis), you will discover this before you reach his rib (unless it is in his psoas or quadratus lumborum). If it is spreading from his spine or is subphrenic, you will also find it.

Drain the pus by Hilton's method (5-3). Insert a wide bore tube or corrugated drain and close the wound in layers.

5.12 Iliac abscesses

When you see a child or young adult with a painful flexed hip, and about a week's history of fever, anorexia, pain, and swelling in his inguinal area, think of iliac adenitis. The infection may have reached his iliac nodes from his leg, his perineal area (including his genitalia), or his buttocks. The abscess lies near his psoas muscle; this goes into spasm and sharply flexes his hip, so that he will not let you extend it beyond 90°, and he cannot walk. He has a tense, tender, hard mass in his iliac fossa, which is lower, and closer to his anterior iliac spine, than an appendix mass. You will probably be unable to elicit fluctuation, and only occasionally will you find the site of the primary infection. He has a moderate leucocytosis.

It is useful to distinguish 'periadenitis' without suppuration (common), which resolves on antibiotics and does not need drainage, from an iliac abscess (less common), which needs drainage and which can follow periadenitis, or pyomyositis of the iliopsoas, or be an extension from osteomyelitis of the spine. An appendix abscess is quite different, and is inside the peritoneum, whereas all these other conditions are outside it.

This condition (iliac abscess) is also known as iliac adenitis, deep inguinal adenitis, extraperitoneal iliac abscess, or suppurating deep iliac nodes. It has several important differential diagnoses, and is often misdiagnosed.

ILIAC ABSCESSES

THE DIFFERENTIAL DIAGNOSIS is that of the 'sick child with the painful flexed hip'. It is more difficult if his right hip is flexed, because the diagnosis on this side includes appendicitis.

Suggesting iliac adenitis with periadenitis or an abscess—a septic lesion on the skin which may be minimal and have healed (adenitis may appear 2 weeks after the primary lesion has settled), a markedly flexed hip with a short history, a mass in his groin or right iliac fossa just above his inguinal ligament, no pain when you percuss his greater trochanter; you can flex his hip a bit more, no spasm of his sacrospinalis, and no X-ray changes.

Suggesting pyomyositis of his iliopsoas—the same signs as iliac adenitis. The differential diagnosis may be impossible, and is not important because the treatment is the same.

Suggesting an appendix abscess—a different anatomical site intraperitoneally in his right iliac fossa, nausea and vomiting, less spasm, and only mild flexion of his hip.

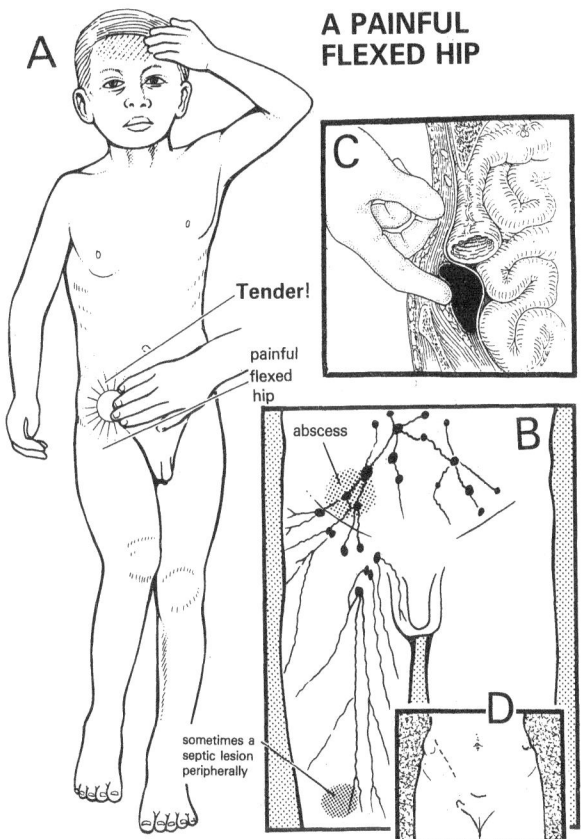

Fig. 5-10 A PAINFUL FLEXED HIP in an ill patient has a variety of differential diagnoses. A, his hip is typically more flexed than is shown here. B, an iliac abscess forms in the iliac nodes. C, exploring extraperitoneally for iliac suppuration. D, the incision for an iliac abscess. *C, and D, after 'Hamilton Bailey's Emergency Surgery', edited by Dudley HAF. John Wright with kind permission.*

Suggesting septic arthritis of his hip—severe joint spasm, acute pain on percussing his greater trochanter, no palpable mass, and an X-ray showing a widened joint space. No movement of his hip due to severe pain. This is also osteomyelitis because the epiphyseal plate is inside the capsule of the hip joint.

Suggesting tuberculosis of his hip—a subacute history and X-ray signs of tuberculosis (29.1).

Suggesting a tuberculous psoas abscess arising from his spine—a subacute history, X-ray changes in his spine. A psoas abscess does not usually need drainage, unless it is very large and causing pain. It will resolve slowly on chemotherapy for tuberculosis; incising it can lead to secondary infection.

Suggesting acute and usually staphylococcal osteomyelitis of his spine (uncommon)—more pain, spasm of his sacrospinalis, X-ray signs in his spine. Drain the lesion as for osteomyelitis (7.2).

Other possibilities include Perthes' disease (27.14), a slipped epiphysis (77.10), and a fracture (77.1).

If the diagnosis is difficult, and you suspect an abscess, you can:

(1) Examine him under anaesthesia, with his abdominal muscles relaxed. Feel the exact site of the mass and its consistency and boundaries, and feel for fluctuation.

(2) Make a 4 cm oblique skin incision, medial to his anterior superior iliac spine, and aspirate the mass with a large-bore needle.

NON-OPERATIVE TREATMENT. Deep inguinal (iliac) adenitis with periadenitis and without pus formation does not require drainage. His hip is flexed as when an abscess is present. You can feel deep tender glands above his inguinal ligament. Give him an antibiotic (penicillin or chloramphenicol). If infection is slow to resolve, use skin traction (1/7th of his bodyweight, 70.10) and raise the foot of his bed.

DRAINAGE. If you have aspirated pus with a needle, you can safely open up the deeper layers. The abscess will have pushed the peritoneal lining of his right iliac fossa medially and superiorly. Make an incision 5 to 10 cm or more over the swelling about 2 cm above his inguinal ligament, starting just medial to his anterosuperior iliac spine (D, 5-10). Take a long haemostat and push this through the muscle over the abscess until you find pus. Then, using your fingers, enlarge the opening until it will take 3 or 4 of them.

Take a specimen, drain the lesion, and continue antibiotics.

If his leg remains in spasm, apply traction as above.

CAUTION ! Draining an iliac abscess is potentially dangerous—you may injure his caecum or his iliac vessels. So follow the method above and aspirate first.

5.13 Anorectal abscesses

Trouble starts when an abscess near a patient's anus bursts through to his skin. It probably originated in an anal gland, and may communicate through a tiny opening with his anal canal, at the pectinate line. A connection betweeen the skin and the anus (a fistula) is the reason why about half of these abscesses recur, or discharge persistently on to the perianal skin as chronic fistulae in ano. Abscesses (with no opening to the skin), sinuses (with an opening to the skin, but not to the anus), and fistulae (with openings to both) are thus part of the same disease process. Most abscesses settle by discharging spontaneously, or being drained, but a serious life-threatening infection can sometimes spread through a patient's perineum, or deeply into his pelvis. For an account of the anatomy of this region and the treatment of fistulae see Section 22.2.

The patient is usually a middle-aged man who says that a severe throbbing pain has kept him awake for several nights. When you examine him, you find a tense tender swelling near his anus. Sometimes, there may be little to see or feel, except mild tenderness at his anal margin, or, his whole perineum may feel tense and tender. If his abscess bursts to the surface, his pain goes. But he may now have a persistently discharging sinus or fistula opening on to the skin near his anus.

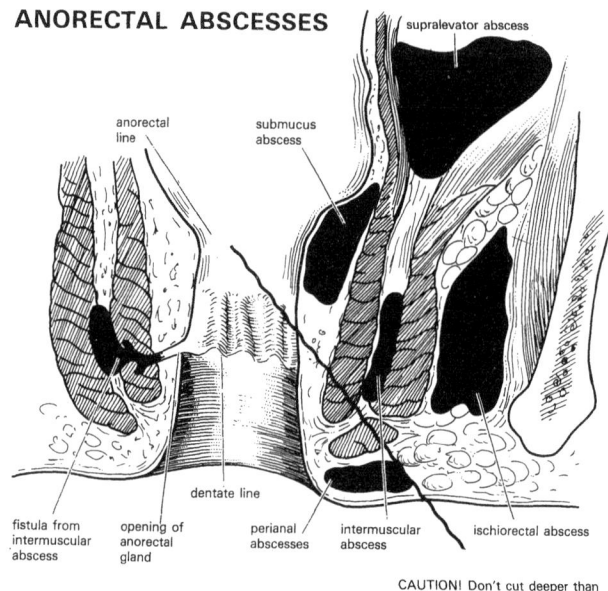

Fig. 5-11 ANORECTAL ABSCESSES form in the anal glands. The pus can track in any of the directions shown here. When an abscess bursts into the anal canal and on to the skin a fistula, may form. *After Macleod JH, 'A Method of Proctology', Fig. 7.9. Harper and Row, with kind permission.*

The anal glands are mostly posterior, so that most abscesses and most fistulae are posterior. These glands also extend into the sphincters, so that pus does too. It can track in various directions: (1) It usually tracks downwards to cause a perianal abscess. (2) It sometimes tracks laterally, through the sphincters, to cause an ischiorectal abscess. The ischiorectal spaces connect with one another behind the anus, so that infection on one side can spread to the other side (horseshoe abscess). (3) Rarely, pus tracks upwards: (a) under the mucosa of the anal canal to form a submucous abscess, or (b) between the sphincter muscles to form a high intermuscular abscess, or (c) above the levator ani muscles to form a supralevator abscess.

Here are the classical types of anorectal abscess, but you may see combinations, and the diagnosis can be difficult. Only the first two are common.

A perianal abscess (common) presents as a red tender swelling close to the patient's anus. On rectal examination, there is little or no tenderness, induration, or bulging in his anal canal. There is usually no fistulous track, but if there is one, it goes straight through or above his subcutaneous external sphincter, and usually through the lowest part of his internal sphincter.

The abscess usually bursts spontaneously (unless it is treated surgically), and may persist as a fistula. Its external opening is surrounded by a button of granulation tissue within 5 cm of his anus. If the track is low, you can feel it through his skin as a cord passing from the external opening towards his anus. You may be able to feel its internal opening as a tender swelling, which is usually below his pectinate line.

An ischiorectal abscess (common) lies deeper than a perianal one, is larger and further from his anus; it forms a deep tender brawny swelling and is not fluctuant until late. He is likely to be toxic, febrile, and debilitated. On rectal examination you may feel a tender induration bulging into his anal canal on the same side. The infection may spread posteriorly and then to the other side as a horseshoe abscess, so that he now has signs on both sides. When an ischiorectal abscess discharges, it does so through an external opening, which is typically more than 5 cm from his anus. If a fistula forms, it almost always opens into his anus in the midline posteriorly below his anorectal line. From there it curves backwards and laterally into one or both of his ischiorectal fossae.

A submucous or high intermuscular abscess (rare) presents with pain in a patient's rectum and no external swelling, unless it is complicated by an ischiorectal or perianal abscess. On rectal examination you may be able to feel a soft, diffuse, tender swelling extending upwards from his pectinate line.

A pelvirectal abscess (rare) presents with fever, but no local anal or rectal signs. Later, it may extend downwards into his ischiorectal fossa. With your finger in his anus, you may be able to feel fluctuation above and lateral to his anorectal ring.

Don't delay treatment in the hope that an anorectal abscess will cure itself—always incise it. Pus will have formed by the time the patient presents, and antibiotics will not make it go away—they are only indicated if he has a high temperature and a spreading infection (rare). If his abscess is large, warn him that it is going to take weeks to heal. Unroof it and let it granulate. Don't try to curette it, and close it by curettage and primary suture. A large incision will not necessarily give a better result—recurrence depends on whether or not there is a tiny communication between the abscess and his anal canal—see Section 22.2.

ZBIG (50 years) complained of painful defaecation and passing pus and blood rectally. He was found to have an anorectal swelling, given a course of antibiotics, and sent home for readmission later for examination under anaesthesia. He returned after three days with severe pain, swollen crepitant buttocks, and a black gangrenous scrotum. His urine was tested and was found to contain sugar. He was referred, but died soon afterwards. LESSONS (1) Bacteria in anorectal abscesses come from the gut and are usually benign, but anaerobic infections can be dangerous. (2) Never treat an anorectal or perineal abscess with antibiotics without also draining it. (3) Spreading anaerobic infections originating in the gut need metronidazole. (4) Always test the urine. Serious infections are particularly common in diabetics.

ANORECTAL ABSCESSES

CAUTION ! (1) If a patient has an acute abscess don't probe around looking for fistulae—wait until his lesion has become chronic. If you probe unwisely, you may create an iatrogenic extrasphincteric fistula which will be very difficult to treat. (2) In the chronic phase, look carefully for the tracks in his skin and rectum that show its presence. If he has a fistula and you fail to diagnose it, he will not be cured. (3) If an abscess lies anteriorly, consider the possibility of a periurethral abscess in a man, and a Bartholin's abscess in a woman.

INDICATIONS FOR INCISION. Operate immediately you can feel a tender swelling. Don't wait for fluctuation. If pain has kept him awake, open his abscess.

ANTIBIOTICS are useless unless there are signs of spreading infection. If so, give him chloramphenicol and metronidazole.

EQUIPMENT. A scalpel and a bivalve speculum. A proctoscope and a sigmoidoscope are not essential; you are unlikely to see anything you cannot feel.

ANAESTHESIA. (1) For a large abscess, use ketamine, or general anaesthesia. (2) Local anaesthesia is unsatisfactory, although you can use it for a perianal abscess; but the patient will not be pain-free. It is even less satisfactory for other abscesses. (3) Intravenous thiopentone with pethidine is not ideal, because you may need more time than they allow you (A 8.8).

A PERIANAL OR ISCHIORECTAL ABSCESS

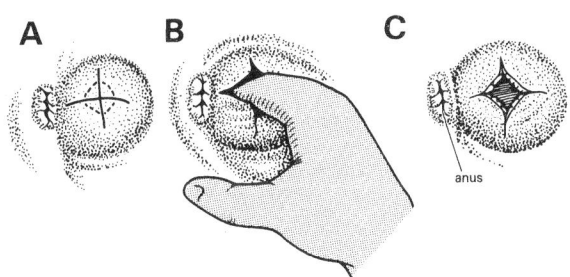

Fig. 5-12 AN ANORECTAL ABSCESS. A, a cruciate incision. B, insert your finger and break down loculi. C, the wound with its edges trimmed, being left to granulate.

EXAMINATION UNDER ANAESTHESIA. Put him into the lithotomy position. Put a finger into his anus and feel its entire wall between two fingers, as in F, Fig. 22-2. Feel if there is an indurated upward extension of the abscess under the mucosa 3 cm or more above his internal sphincter. Feel the extent of the abscess, and for the point of maximum fluctuation.

Insert a bivalve speculum and look for pus coming out of an internal opening in the appropriate segment of his anal canal. You will only find one in about 10% of cases. You may feel the opening as a localized tender depression in his anal canal in the place suggested by Goodsall's rule in Fig. 22-6. Press on the abscess—you may see a bead of pus escape from the internal opening. If you do find a fistula, determine where it is in relation to his pectinate line.

If his abscess is acute, there is no defined wall, so you will not find a track. DON'T probe around, you may make one!

If his abscess is chronic with a well-defined wall, probe carefully to look for a fistula.

INCISION AND DRAINAGE. Support the mass with your finger in his rectum. Make a substantial cross-shaped incision at least twice the depth of the lesion over its most prominent or fluctuant part. This will be externally for a perianal or ischiorectal abscess, and inside his rectum above his anorectal line for a rare submucous or pelvirectal abscess. Make the incision large enough to admit one or two fingers, so that you can explore the abscess fully with your finger and break down all loculi by Hilton's method (5-3). Don't break down any natural barriers to the spread of infection. If possible, send a specimen of the pus for culture.

Now look again—but don't probe—to see if there is a fistulous opening.

If there is no fistula, cut off the corners of the flaps to prevent the edges of the wound coming together and adhering. A linear incision is never adequate. Wrap your finger in gauze and clean the walls of the abscess cavity.

If there is a fistulous opening, you can proceed immediately as follows, or better, wait 4 or 5 days.

If his fistula is low in his anal canal, at or below his pectinate line, lay it open and manage it as a low anal fistula (22.2).

If the opening of the fistula is above his pectinate line, leave it and either refer him, or deal with it later. Some surgeons thread a silk ligature through the fistula and tie it loosely round the sphincter, to mark its internal opening.

POSTOPERATIVELY, pack the cavity *lightly* with gauze—don't pack it too tight, or it won't drain. Tuck the edge of a gauze square into the wound to keep the edges of the skin apart, until the wound cavity has collapsed. Apply a T-bandage. Follow this with daily salt baths and packing, until the abscess cavity has healed from within outwards. It will heal slowly. Discharge him as soon as there is a flat granulating area, and review him regularly.

CAUTION ! (1) Be sure to push a piece of gauze down to the bottom of the cavity, so that it heals from the bottom up, without bridging of the edges. (2) Don't pack it so tightly that the pack interferes with granulation.

If you lack dressings, use salt baths (1.12) and ask a nurse to use her gloved hands to separate the walls of the abscess, which may be sticking together superficially.

DIFFICULTIES WITH ANORECTAL ABSCESSES

If you find AN ABSCESS ON BOTH SIDES, open them both as described above, and incise both his ischiorectal fossae. There is sure to be a track between them, behind his anus; some surgeons would lay this open also at this stage.

If he has SIGNS OF SPREADING INFECTION, such as gross inflammatory swelling, areas of necrosis, or crepitation, he probably has an anaerobic infection, and needs urgent treatment, particularly metronidazole (2.9) and wide drainage.

If A FISTULA DEVELOPS later (common), treat it as in Section 22.2.

If he presents with a RECURRENT ABSCESS (common), there is almost certainly an underlying fistula. The opening may be very small, and you may have overlooked it when you drained his first abscess.

If you find an INTERNAL OPENING which communicates with his ischiorectal fossa above his anorectal ring, (rare) don't cut the muscle superficial to it, or he will become incontinent! Drain the abscess from below. A fistula will probably form.

If THE ABSCESS EXTENDS INTERNALLY under his submucosa, (rare) pass a director along the track and lay it open. It will bleed copiously. Try to tie the vessels. This may be difficult, so don't spend too long trying. If you fail, grasp them with haemostats, and leave these in place for 48 hours.

If he has a SUPRALEVATOR ABSCESS (very rare), refer him—treatment is difficult and controversial.

5.14 Periurethral abscesses

A patient with a periurethal abscess has a tender inflamed area in his perineum, or under his penis. His abscess commonly arises in his bulbar urethra, probably in the paraurethral glands of Cowper, and is usually caused by gonococci to begin with; but these are soon replaced by secondary invaders. The danger is that his urine may leak from the abscess cavity, extravasate widely, and cause extensive cellulitis (23.10), or a fistula. His urine is infected, so this kind of cellulitis is more dangerous than that following traumatic rupture of his urethra. He may or may not have retention of urine due to an inflamed stricture, which will prevent you passing a catheter, so you may have to drain his bladder with a suprapubic cystotomy (23.5).

PERIURETHAL ABSCESSES

DIFFERENTIAL DIAGNOSES. (1) A perianal abscess. (2) A scrotal abscess is in a different place and is not associated with urinary symptoms. (3) Localized penile extravasation of urine.

ANTIBIOTICS. Give the patient ampicillin, or chloramphenicol, until you have the results of culture of his urine and pus—if this is possible.

MANAGING HIS URINE. Most patients have retention of urine.

If he has retention of urine, try passing a soft rubber catheter. If this fails, as it probably will, do a suprapubic cystostomy, preferably a suprapubic puncture with a fine plastic tube (23.6). When the abscess is healing, start to pass bougies. This will be difficult, but take care not to use force.

If you succeed, bougie him every 3 months to start with, and less often later.

If you fail, try again a week later. If you still have difficulty, refer him; he may need a urethroplasty.

If he does not have retention of urine, dilate his stricture later.

THE ABSCESS. If pus is present, and he fails to respond to antibiotics, drain the abscess on to his perineum, and be sure to open it widely. Give him salt baths and pack the wound postoperatively.

DIFFICULTIES WITH A PERIURETHRAL ABSCESS

If his urine EXTRAVASATES, see Section 23.10.

If you CANNOT REFER HIM for urethroplasty, he will have to continue passing his urine through his perineum (32.33), or you will have to attempt a urethroplasty yourself (23.9).

If his ABSCESS RECURS, consider the possibility of tuberculosis or carcinoma of his urethra.

If he develops a FISTULA, see Section 23.9.

5.15 Prostatic abscesses

Gonococci or coliforms can infect a patient's prostate. To begin with they cause a prostatitis, and later a frank abscess. He presents with urgency, frequency, and dysuria, or with retention. He has fever, rigors, and severe rectal or perineal pain, sometimes with tenesmus. His prostate is enlarged, usually more so on one side than the other, and is exquisitely tender. Untreated, his abscess may burst into: (1) his urethra, (2) his perirectal tissues, where it can present as an ischiorectal abscess, (3) his perineum, or (4) his rectum, forming a rectourethral fistula.

PROSTATIC ABSCESSES

DIFFERENTIAL DIAGNOSIS. Extreme prostatic tenderness should make the diagnosis clear. Don't confuse a prostatic abscess with: (1) An ischiorectal abscess—the swelling is to one side of the midline. (2) An abscess in a seminal vesicle—rectally, the site of maximum swelling and tenderness will be higher and more to one side.

SPECIAL TESTS. Test his urine for sugar, and culture it.

ANTIBIOTICS. Give him a broad-spectrum antibiotic, such as ampicillin or chloramphenicol, until you know the results of culture.

MANAGEMENT. If his prostate is not fluctuant, see what antibiotics alone will do in 48 hours.

If antibiotics fail to cause a marked improvement in 48 hours, or his abscess is fluctuant, refer him to an expert urologist, who will drain his abscess into his urethra with a resectoscope.

If you cannot refer him, drain the abscess yourself, as follows. Fortunately, this is very rarely necessary.

DRAINAGE. Anaesthetize him, and put him in an exaggerated lithotomy position. Start by passing a rubber Jacques catheter. If this passes easily, leave it in place. If you cannot pass it, do a suprapubic cystotomy.

To drain his abscess, pass a metal sound, and cut down on to this through a 5 cm midline incision immediately in front of his anus.

Remove the sound and control bleeding. Put your finger through the incision into his prostatic urethra, and then through its posterior wall into the abscess cavity. If this contains several loculi, break down the septa between them.

Pack the wound loosely with a dry dressing and leave it open, or suture the skin edges loosely over it. Remove the catheter about the 7th day.

Alternatively, make an oblique lateral incision, as when removing the prostate by Ghadvi's method (23.21).

5.16 Abscesses in the seminal vesicles (rare)

The symptoms are the same as with an abscess of the prostate, but the warmth, the swelling and the tenderness, instead of being over the patient's prostate, are higher and more to the side, over one, or occasionally both, of his seminal vesicles. He may also have pain suprapubically, in his back, or down the inner side of his thighs.

TREATMENT. Place the patient in an exaggerated lithotomy position, and and make an oblique lateral perineal incision. Dissect bluntly until you feel the swollen vesicle. Push a haemostat into it, drain it, and close the wound lightly round a drain.

6 Pus in the pleura, the pericardium, and the peritoneum

6.1 Pus in the pleural cavities—empyema

Pus usually reaches a patient's pleural cavity from infection of the lung under it. This can be pneumonia, a lung abscess, or the pneumonitis that may follow an inhaled foreign body (usually in a child), or carcinoma of the bronchus (usually in a cigarette smoker). Occasionally, an empyema is tuberculous; rarely it may follow rupture of a liver or subphrenic abscess through the diaphragm.

A common history is that a week or more ago, as the patient was beginning to recover from a chest infection, improvement stopped. He now remains ill, anorexic and febrile, and is starting to lose weight—despite antibiotics.

Many kinds of bacteria can be responsible, but pneumococci are perhaps the most common. Antibiotics are only effective in the earliest stages, and may mask the symptoms of an empyema later. The result is that empyemas can remain undetected for years and are often missed in a busy outpatient department. This is sad because you can treat them, so watch for them, and ask your staff to do so too.

Pus in the pleural cavity, like pus anywhere else, must be removed. To begin with it is thin, like serum; later it thickens and looks like scrambled egg. So adapt your method of removing it to its thickness. While it is still thin, aspirate it with a syringe and needle. When it is too thick for this, but is still fluid enough to flow down a tube into a bottle, use *closed drainage*, as if you were draining blood from an injured chest (65.2). The surfaces of the patient's pleura will not have stuck together at this stage, so you will have to use an underwater seal to prevent air getting into his pleural cavity and letting his lung collapse.

If the pus in his pleural cavity is left undrained, it will soon become too thick to flow down a long thin tube into a bottle. Once his empyema has reached this stage, only thoracotomy and decortication will properly expand his lung, but this is a dangerous operation, even in expert hands. If referral is difficult, you can improve him greatly by draining pus through an open drain. To do this you will have to remove a piece of a rib and push a short wide tube through its bed. The surfaces of his pleura will now have stuck so firmly that air cannot enter his pleural cavity to collapse his lung. When you do this be sure to: (1) Remove the piece of rib from inside its periosteum, so as not to injure the vessels and nerve which run just below it. (2) Place the inner end of the tube where the bottom of the abscess cavity will be while he sits in his usual position in bed.

If the pus in his pleural cavity remains even longer it will be replaced by fibrous tissue which will be very difficult to remove.

Children have special problems. In a child an empyema may follow a post-measles pneumonia, or the rupture of a staphylococcal lung abscess into a pleural cavity. He is likely to be between 1 and 3 years, malnourished, anaemic, and anorexic, with a persistent cough, fever, dyspnoea, diarrhoea, and perhaps vomiting. He may be very sick indeed with a pyopneumothorax under tension. Treat him as you would an adult.

• ASPIRATOR, Martin's, with 3-way tap and needles, one only. This is much the best instrument for draining large quantities of fluid from the chest. It has a tap, so that you can aspirate pus and discharge it through a tube into a receiver, without letting air enter the chest.

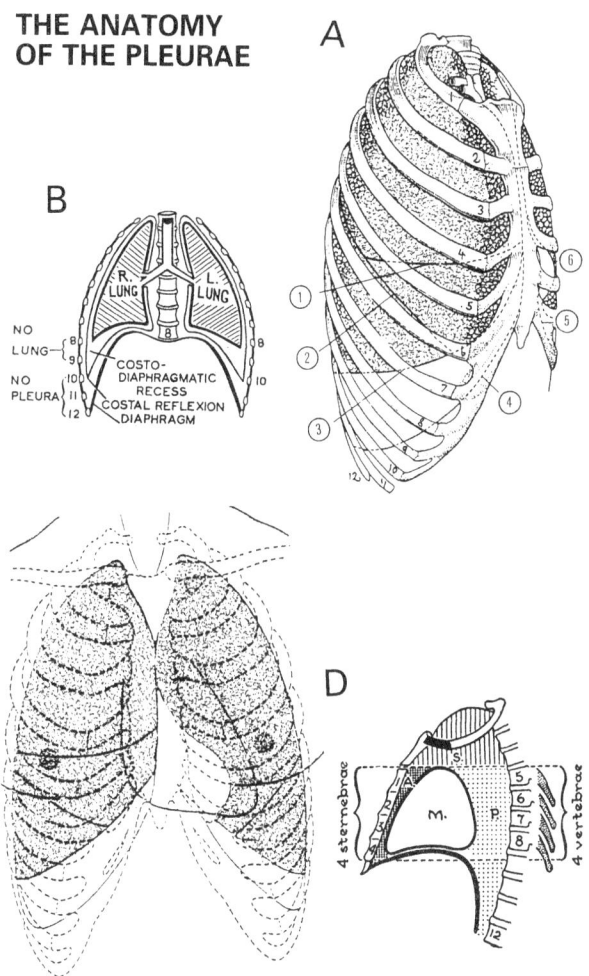

Fig. 6-1 THE ANATOMY OF THE PLEURAE. A, the relation of a patient's pleurae and lungs to his chest wall. B, a coronal section of his thorax (semischematic). C, the ventral aspect of his thorax showing the surface projections of his heart and pleurae. D, the subdivisions of his mediastinum.

1, the horizontal fissure. 2, the oblique fissure. 3, the inferior border of the right lung. 4, the costodiaphragmatic reflexion of the right pleura. 5, the costodiaphragmatic reflexion of the left pleura. 6, the cardiac notch of the left lung. A, Fig. 8.23B and C, Fig. 8.23A from 'Gray's Anatomy' (Churchill Livingstone). B, Fig. 6.6 and D, Fig. 6.8 from Grant's 'Method of Anatomy' (9th edition 1975 edited by JV Basmajian). With kind permission.

EMPYEMA

CLINICAL FEATURES. If an empyema involves the whole of a patient's pleural cavity and contains a litre or more of pus, you should be able to diagnose it clinically. Look for limited movement of his chest on the affected side, shifting of his trachea and apex beat, dullness to percussion, reduced breath sounds and reduced vocal fremitus. Vocal resonance (the sound "99") may be high-pitched at the top of the empyema and absent over its lower part.

X-RAYS. usually show a dense area at one lung base. Take a PA and a lateral to show the site and extent of the empyema.

ANTIBIOTICS. When an empyema is established, antibiotics are ineffective. Pus must be drained. If he has fever or malaise give him chloramphenicol (2.7) until sensitivity tests show the need for change.

ASPIRATING A PLEURAL EFFUSION

INDICATIONS. (1) To confirm the diagnosis. (2) To remove the bulk of the fluid in the early stages while it is still thin.

EQUIPMENT. A Martin's aspirator, with its needles and 3-way tap, a 20 ml syringe, local anaesthetic solution and a receiver. Or, improvise the equipment in Fig. 65-8.

METHOD. Premedicate the patient thoroughly an hour before. If he is not very ill, sit him astride a chair leaning over a pillow on the backrest. If he is very ill, sit him in bed with his arms folded, leaning over a bed table or a pile of pillows.

Aspirate near the lowest point of the empyema, as defined on the PA and lateral X-rays. To establish this, aspirate several sites if necessary, so as to find the lowest site that yields pus, but remember the surface markings of the pleura (9-4a). Commonly, the posterior axillary line is the right vertical line in which to aspirate.

Infiltrate anaesthetic solution into his skin and subcutaneous tissues over the chosen space, and also a space above and below—you may have chosen the wrong one.

Insert the needle, pierce his pleura and aspirate gently; turn the tap and discharge the fluid into a receiver. If you don't have a 3-way tap, and have not improvised the equipment in Fig. 65-8, you can (less desirably) put your finger over the hub of the needle, as you disconnect the syringe to discharge it.

Repeat the aspiration 2 or 3 times a week until pus stops forming, or it becomes too thick to aspirate.

CLOSED DRAINAGE FOR A PLEURAL EFFUSION

Many empyemas do not resolve on aspiration alone. If pus thickens, so that aspiration is even a little difficult, closed drainage is necessary. Insert an underwater seal drain, as for a haemothorax (65.2). Leave it for a least two weeks until firm adhesions have formed between the surfaces of his pleura, which will prevent his lung collapsing when you take the tube out. The instillation of 5 to 10 g of lipiodol before repeat X-rays is a useful way of defining the lowest point of the empyema.

If he improves, and X-rays show disappearance of the empyema and re-expansion of his lung, cut the stitch securing the tube, pull it out and quickly press an airtight dressing over the hole.

If he does not improve, he needs open drainage or referral.

OPEN DRAINAGE FOR AN EMPYEMA, RESECTING A RIB

INDICATIONS. Draining an empyema when closed drainage has failed. *The patient's lung must have stuck to his ribs.* (1) The traditional pre-antibiotic test was to put some of the fluid in a test tube; if the sediment was approximately half the volume of the fluid, it was safe to insert an open drain. Antibiotics make this test less useful, because the fluid is more likely to remain thin. (2) Slowly withdraw the tube of the underwater seal drain from the water. If the column of water does not run up towards the pleura, but stays in the tube, his pleura has stuck to his ribs, so that an an underwater seal is unnecessary and open drainage can start.

CONTRAINDICATIONS. A tuberculous empyema. See below under empyema necessitans.

EMPYEMA

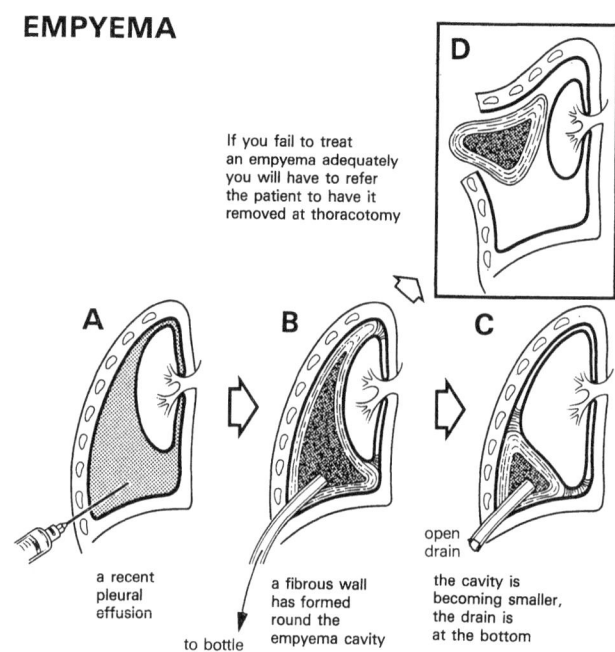

Fig 6-1a STAGES IN THE DRAINAGE OF PUS IN THE PLEURA. A, a very recent pleural effusion can be drained with a syringe and needle. B, if pus becomes too thick for this, you will have to use a rubber tube and an underwater seal drain in a bottle (closed drainage). C, if pus becomes even thicker, resect the patient's rib, and insert a short wide tube (open drainage). Shorten this tube as his empyema drains, and make sure it is in the bottom of the cavity. D, if you fail to drain an empyema, you may have to refer the patient for decortication.

X-RAYS. Examine PA and lateral views with the greatest care to see which rib to resect. If you cannot easily see the lowest point of an empyema, inject 10 ml of oily contrast medium before you take the films.

ANAESTHESIA. Take him to the theatre. Premedicate him well (A 5.2). Use a combination of local infiltration (A 5.4) and intercostal blocks (A 6.7). Block his intercostal nerves at the site of your chosen incision, and also one rib above and one below it as far back as possible.

METHOD. Drain his empyema from its lowest point, in the position he would be in while he sits in bed. Since he lies more supine than prone, choose the lowest point of the empyema posteriorly. Often, his 9th rib in the paravertebral line is the best, but it may be below this.

CAUTION ! Don't make the opening too low, because his diaphragm will rise as the pus drains and block the opening. It should always be at least one space abve his diaphragm.

Sit him on a stool leaning forwards against the operating table. Before incising, confirm by aspiration through more than one intercostal space, that you have chosen the correct rib to remove. Make an 8 cm vertical incision, extending above and below the selected rib, so that you can more easily resect the rib on either side if necessary.

Cut down to the rib, and incise the periosteum along its centre. Use a curved Faraboef rougine to strip the periosteum with its attached intercostal muscles from the outer surface of his rib. Clean its upper and lower borders. Then use Doyen's raspatory (or Faraboef's rougine) to remove the periosteum from its inner surface. Strip its upper and lower borders as in Fig 6-2.

CAUTION ! (1) The intercostal blocks should have anaesthetized his parietal pleura adequately; if they have not, repeat the intercostal blocks and wait. If you fail to anaesthetize him adequately, extreme pain may cause vasovagal shock. (2) His intercostal vessels can bleed severely if you fail to identify them, so be sure to avoid them by keeping inside the periosteum.

Excise a 5–10 cm length of rib with an osteotome, rib shears, or a large pair of bone cutters. Make an incision in the bed of this rib through into his pleural cavity. Open it with a haemostat, explore it it with your finger, and remove what semisolid pus you can with sponge holders. He will probably start coughing.

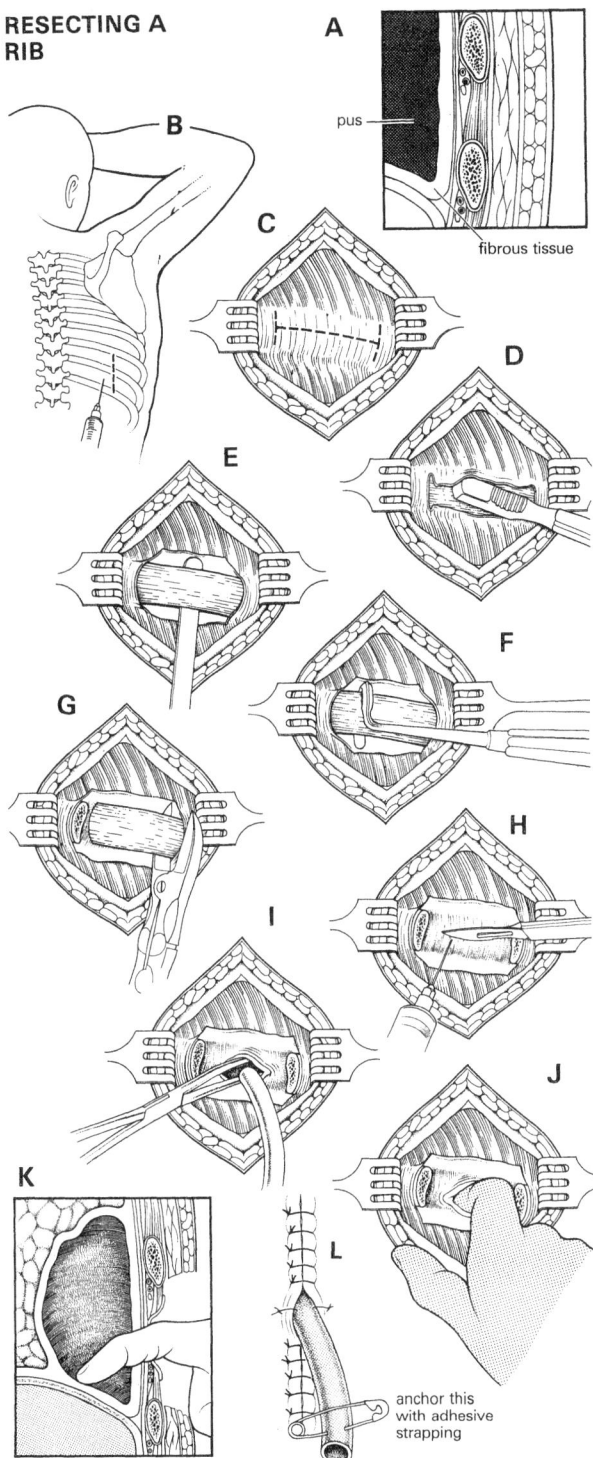

Fig. 6-2 RESECTING A RIB. A, the patient's empyema covered with a thick layer of fibrous tissue. B, a common site for draining an empyema—his 9th rib in his paravertebral line. Vary this as the occasion demands. C, his skin incised, showing the incision over the periosteum. D, reflecting the periosteum with Faraboef's rougine. E, reflecting the periosteum off the inner surface of his rib. F, completing the task with Doyen's raspatory. G, resecting the rib. H, preparing to incise the periosteum in the bed of the rib. I, sucking out the pus. J, and K, putting in a finger to break down the loculi. L, a drainage tube in place.

CAUTION ! (1) If when you explore the cavity with your finger, you find that you have not removed the rib at the bottom of the cavity, remove the rib below. If you don't do this his empyema will not resolve completely. (2) Send pus for smear and culture, it may be tuberculous; tuberculous pus looks different, is more watery, contains particles and should not be drained anyway (see above and below).

Fix a wide tube in the empyema cavity, leaving about 2 cm above the skin surface. Fix it with a suture, a safety pin and adhesive strapping; apply a large gauze and cotton wool dressing.

POSTOPERATIVELY, encourage him to do vigorous breathing exercises. Monitor the size of the cavity by introducing contrast medium and taking X-rays. Alternatively, measure how much sterile saline you can run into it.

When drainage stops or becomes less than 5 ml/day, remove the tube. The residual sinus will heal, provided that there is no bronchopleural fistula. This can take 2 or 3 months.

CHILDREN WITH EMPYEMAS

You cannot drain a small child's pleural cavity adequately by inserting an intercostal drain between two ribs, because the drain will be nipped by his ribs or obstructed by pus. So remove a centimetre or two of rib, using ketamine, to make a hole which is big enough for a tube. Adequate drainage will eventually cure him if: (1) his lung is not immobilized with thick fibrin, (2) he has no bronchopleural fistula, and (3) his empyema is localized.

Start drainage with an underwater seal drainage bottle. This will limit his activity, and may cause the drain to be pulled out; but his lung will expand. If necessary, drain the cavity with another high pleural drain as for a pneumothorax, see Fig. 65-2.

When you are confident that his lung has stuck to his ribs (see above), cut the tube short, fit it with a pin and butterfly strapping, put a colostomy bag over it to collect the pus and allow him up. Increased activity is the best physiotherapy. If he does not settle in 3 or 4 weeks, refer him.

DIFFICULTIES WITH AN EMPYEMA

If his EMPYEMA PRESENTS ON HIS CHEST WALL (EMPYEMA NECESSITANS, unusual), it is almost sure to be tuberculous, perhaps a complication of AIDS. The signs suggestive of a tuberculous empyema are: (1) Swelling of the chest wall, starting first with swelling of its intercostal spaces. (2) Sinuses. (3) X-ray signs of pulmonary tuberculosis. (4) Typically, fluid on aspiration which is not pus, but is thin and watery with small particles of necrotic tissue. You may or may not find AAFB in the smear. *Don't drain it* or it will become secondarily infected. Give him chemotherapy for tuberculosis. If his mediastinum is shifted (unusual), aspirate some fluid.

If AIR COMES OUT WITH THE PUS, he has a BRONCHOPLEURAL FISTULA which is unlikely to close spontaneously. When his condition has improved, refer him to an expert thoracic surgeon, who will find the task of closing the fistula difficult.

If a patient with tuberculosis has an AIR-FLUID LEVEL IN A PLEURAL CAVITY, he has a TUBERCULOUS BRONCHOPLEURAL FISTULA. Give him chemotherapy (29.1). Using careful aseptic precautions, insert an underwater seal drain (65.2) and leave it in until his lung has expanded.

If his INTERCOSTAL VESSELS BLEED, encircle them with a needle and thread. Avoid tying the nerve because this is painful. If you have difficulty, transfix them with a ligature, so that they are compressed against the stump of the rib which remains.

If his EMPYEMA FAILS TO HEAL: (1) You may have put the drainage tube too high or too far forward. (2) You may have removed it too early. (3) You may have put it in too late. (4) There may be a foreign body, such as a piece of drainage tube, in his chest. (5) He may have developed a fistula between his bronchi and his pleura. (6) He may have tuberculosis, carcinoma, actinomycosis, or a ruptured amoebic liver abscess. Further dependent drainage is all that he probably needs for (1), (2) or (3). Instil 5 to 10 ml of contrast medium, repeat the X-ray, and if necessary resect another rib. If this fails, refer him.

6.1a Pus in the pericardium

Fluid sometimes accumulates in a patient's pericardium. If there is only a little, you can leave it there (if indeed you are aware of it at all), unless you need it for diagnosis. But if there is much, it embarrasses the action of his heart (cardiac tamponade) and may kill him, so you may have to remove it *urgently!* The fluid can be blood after a cardiac injury (65.9) or an effusion from many causes, either infected or sterile. Elsewhere in the body, you drain pus to treat an infection. In his pericardium, you are mainly draining it to overcome its mechanical effects.

He is unlikely to present with symptoms that immediately suggest a pericardial effusion. He is more likely to be admitted with a variety of medical diseases and be observed to have some of the following signs: (1) Grossly distended neck veins, (2) pulsus paradoxus (a reduction of arterial pressure of > 10 mm and of pulse pressure on inspiration), (3) pulsus alternans (QRS complexes of alternately varying voltage), and (4) a large cardiac shadow. He is obviously 'ill', and may be febrile. He has signs of a low cardiac output with a poor peripheral circulation; he has a small pulse volume, tachycardia, a low normal or subnormal blood pressure, and soft heart sounds. Early on you may hear a pericardial rub, but the accumulation of fluid soon separates his pericardial surfaces and stops the rub. He has the signs and symptoms of heart failure, and an increased area of cardiac dullness. The severity of the signs of cardiac tamponade are related more to the rate at which fluid accumulates in his pericardium than to the volume of fluid in it. The diagnosis may be obvious, or if fluid has accumulated slowly, it may be difficult.

There are problems: (1) Any cause of cardiac failure may have distended his neck veins. (2) Although pulsus paradoxus strongly suggests a pericardial effusion, not all patients show it. (3) The X-ray finding of a large globular heart can also be due to gross cardiac enlargement without there being any fluid in his pericardium.

The great danger in putting a needle into his pericardial cavity to drain it is that: (1) You can easily penetrate his right ventricle, cause bleeding, increase the fluid in his pericardial cavity, and kill him rapidly. (2) You may cause ventricular fibrillation with the tip of the needle. Even so, in spite of these dangers, not aspirating his pericardium may be more dangerous than aspirating it.

TAPPING THE PERICARDIUM

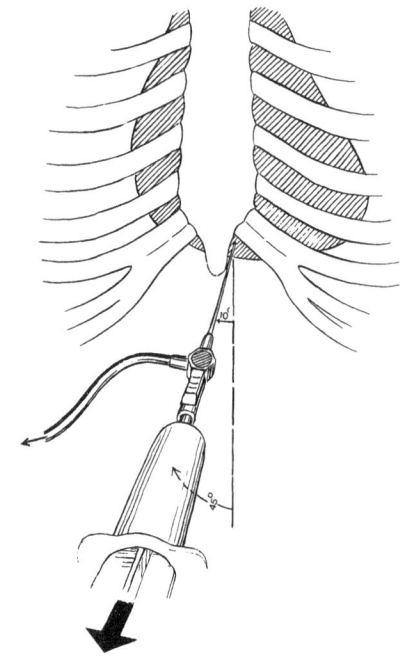

Fig. 6-2a ASPIRATING THE PERICARDIUM. Insert the needle in his epigastrium immediately to the left of his xiphisternum. Incline it 45° to the horizontal and 10° towards the left. In this way, if it does prick his heart it is more likely to meet his thicker left ventricle than his thinner right auricle.

PUS IN THE PERICARDIUM

See also Section 65.9 for cardiac tamponade as the result of trauma.

X-RAYS. A *very large globular heart*, often with venous congestion. Depending on what is causing his pericarditis, you may see basal shadows in his lungs, or pneumonia obscuring his heart.

ECG. Tachycardia, usually sinus rhythm, a raised S-T segment (nonspecific), an inverted T wave (late, nonspecific), low voltage QRS complexes (highly suggestive), pulsus alternans (highly suggestive).

THE DIFFERENTIAL DIAGNOSIS of the causes of pericardial effusion which may lead to tamponade is as follows in probable order of frequency in most of the Third World:

Suggesting tuberculosis—a history of cough, bloody sputum, weight loss and malaise. Patients with AIDS and tuberculosis are particularly likely to develop tuberculous pericarditis and pleural effusions.

Suggesting viral myocarditis—an influenza-like illness with generalized muscle pains. Early, you may hear a pericardial friction rub.

Suggesting a pyogenic bacterial cause—some other site of infection, such as pneumonia, meningitis, or measles with secondary staphylococcal infection. Often, there is some obvious site of infection, but not always (primary pericarditis).

Other causes of pericardial effusion that might cause tamponade include: uraemia, malignant deposits (only if they bleed seriously), collagen diseases, and the rupture of an amoebic abscess into the pericardium (rare).

Here are some causes of a large heart without fluid in the pericardial cavity:

Suggesting rheumatic heart disease (common) —valvular lesions; these are usually easily diagnosed.

Suggesting cardiomyopathy —an enlarged heart clinically and radiologically. The cardiac outline may be globular and closely simulate fluid in the pericardium.

Suggesting endomyocardial fibrosis (EMF) — atrioventricular incompetence left and right is usual. Eosinophilia.

PREPARATION. Find two assistants, one to watch the patient's ECG, or his pulse, and ready to resuscitate him if necessary, and another to fetch anything more that might be needed for resuscitation. Have the full resuscitation equipment available: laryngoscope, tracheal tubes, a sucker, oxygen, and an anaesthetic machine or an Ambu bag. Do an ECG while you are aspirating, or failing this ask someone to feel his pulse continuously.

EQUIPMENT. A needle inside a plastic cannula ('needle-inside-cannula', A 15.2), a 3-way tap (less satisfactorily a 2-way one), and a 20 or 50 ml syringe.

ASPIRATION. Insert the cannula in his epigastrium immediately to the left of his xiphisternum. Incline it 45° to the horizontal and 10° towards the left. In this way, if it does prick his heart, it is more likely to meet his thicker left ventricle than his thinner right auricle.

DRAINAGE. Incise his linea alba and proceed upwards in the extraperitoneal plane until you reach his pericardium. Cautiously incise this and insert a drain.

CAUTION ! If he deteriorates suddenly with a pulse which you cannot feel: (1) Immediately remove the cannula. (2) Start external cardiac massage (A 3.6). (3) While you stop external cardiac massage briefly, ask your assistant to intubate him. Continue to control his ventilation (A 13.1).

6.2 Peritonitis

The area of a patient's peritoneal cavity is three times that of his skin, and is a huge area to become infected. So it is not surprising that the mortality from peritonitis is about 10%, even in good units.

Bacteria, both aerobic and anaerobic, can reach the peritoneum from inside the gut (often), from an outside wound (occasionally), or from the blood-stream (rarely). Peritonitis can also follow a laparotomy if this is carelessly done. It is particularly likely to complicate: a strangulated obstruction of the gut (10.3), appendicitis (12.1), a penetrating abdominal injury (66.2), pelvic sepsis in a female (PID, 6.6), a septic Caesarean section (6.7), a perforated peptic ulcer (11.2) or typhoid ulcer (31.8), the breakdown of an anastomosis, especially of the unprepared large gut, where this has not been protected by a proximal colostomy, amoebic colitis (31.11), the torsion of an ovarian cyst (20.7), acute cholecystitis (13.3), pancreatitis (13.9), or the rupture of a liver abscess (31.12). Sometimes, there is no cause ('primary' peritonitis). The frequency of these causes differs geographically, so find out what the common causes are in your area.

You can reduce the risk of death from peritonitis if you: (1) Operate early—before a patient is very ill. (2) Take the necessary precautions to minimize the infection of his peritoneal cavity, when you do any laparotomy. So handle his tissues gently, anastomose his gut carefully, pack away potentially infected areas, control bleeding meticulously, and give him perioperative antibiotics when these are indicated (2.9).

Peritonitis develops through several stages, which need different treatment:

(1) Disease in an organ before the peritoneum over it is infected. For example, a patient may have the symptoms of peptic ulceration, appendicitis, or of typhoid fever, but no involvement of his peritoneum. At this stage, you may be able to treat the underlying disease and prevent peritonitis.

(2) Localized peritonitis. With proper treatment this localized peritonitis may resolve, and he may recover. A mass may form, but the toxic features of an abscess will not have appeared.

(3) Abscess formation around the organ responsible for the infection. Pus forms, but this is sealed off from the rest of his peritoneal cavity by loops of gut which are stuck to one another by a fibrinous exudate. His abscess may resolve, as an appendix abscess often does, or it may spread, as is common with a perforated duodenal or typhoid ulcer. The mass is bigger than in stage (2) above, and he now has toxic symptoms.

(4) Spreading peritonitis which may become generalized. If spread is incomplete, multiple abscesses form in his peritoneal cavity, particularly in his pelvis and under his diaphragm. If he is unlucky, all his abdominal organs are bathed in pus. If you operate and wash the pus out of his peritoneal cavity, more abscesses may form postoperatively.

Gut which is surrounded by pus usually develops ileus (10.13). If his peritonitis becomes generalized, his abdomen becomes silent and distends, as his gut fills with fluid and dilates. This fluid, and that which is lost into his peritoneal cavity, depletes his circulation, so that his blood volume, his blood pressure, and his urine output all fall, and his pulse rate rises. As peritonitis advances, his peripheral circulation fails, and he may develop septic shock (53.4).

Take a careful history. Ask for the symptoms of any underlying disease which may have caused peritonitis, such as previous dyspepsia, or a fever that may be typhoid. In a woman, enquire for symptoms suggesting PID (6.6).

Ask about pain. The pain of peritonitis is constant and is made worse by deep breathing, by coughing, and by movement. A patient with peritonitis is weak and thirsty, anorexic and nauseated. He vomits, and may have diarrhoea or be constipated.

The signs of peritonitis vary with the state of the disease: (1) An early sign is the failure of his abdomen to move as he breathes. (2) His abdomen is tender. This tenderness is localized at first, then regional, and finally general. It is usually worse where the disease started. (3) Feel for muscle guarding, progressing to rigidity. If peritonitis is advanced, there is no need to test for rebound tenderness—it is painful and unhelpful. But if peritonitis is localized, rebound tenderness is a good indication as to which parts of his peritoneum are involved and which are not. (5) Listen for decreased or absent bowel sounds. (6) Look also for distension, eventually becoming tympanitic, as ileus develops. You will soon find that the intensity of a patient's signs is little guide to the nature of the fluid inside his abdomen. Gastric, bilious, and pancreatic fluids produce the most tenderness; pus, urine, and especially blood are more variable, and may cause almost none. Even faecal contamination produces no peritoneal signs at first.

As his peritonitis advances, he becomes febrile, apprehensive, dehydrated, and hypotensive. His pulse is fast, his breathing is shallow and his facies Hippocratic (pinched, drawn and grey). Finally, he dies in peripheral circulatory failure.

Often, all you will know before you operate is that he has peritonitis, without knowing why. Try to to establish how advanced it is. A laparotomy is usually mandatory but, as you will see below, there are some indications for non-operative treatment. If you are uncertain about these in a particular case, you would be wise to operate.

Aim to: (1) Resuscitate him by treating his dehydration for 2 or 3 hours before you operate (A 15.3). (2) Treat the cause of his peritonitis, for example by closing his perforated peptic ulcer (11.2), by removing his appendix (12.1), or by resecting and anastomosing his gangrenous small gut (9.3). (3) Remove the pus in his peritoneum (if his peritonitis is generalized), by thorough lavage, and then leave some tetracycline solution in his peritoneal cavity. This will reduce the danger of abscesses forming in his peritoneum later, and will increase his chances of recovery.

You are often in a serious dilemma, when you drain an abdomen for peritonitis. If the pus is thin and adhesions few and light, there is no problem. But if loops of his gut are firmly stuck together, how radical should you be? If you don't separate them enough, you will leave pockets of pus behind. If you separate too vigorously, you risk stripping off the muscle layer or opening his gut—a real disaster, because a fistula will probably follow (9.14). This is difficult surgery, and there is no easy answer; only experience will teach you. You feel you cannot win, yet you will have to! Sometimes you will fail, and have to reopen his abdomen.

About 5 days after the operation his tachycardia should subside, his temperature should settle and his bowel sounds should return. When this happens the volume of his nasogastric aspirate will decrease, his abdominal distension will go down and he will start to pass flatus. If he survives the first 10 days, he will probably live.

His postoperative course is likely to be stormy. It may be complicated by paralytic ileus (10.13), the formation of more abscesses (6.3), Gram-negative septicaemia (53.4), intestinal obstruction (10.13), or extreme nutritional deficiency (9.11). One of the greatest dangers is a faecal fistula (9.14). If you separate the adhesions between the loops of his gut too roughly, you may: (1) open it and have to repair it immediately, or (2) strip part or all of its muscular coat and weaken it, so that it breaks down later to form a fistula (9.14).

GENERALIZED PERITONITIS

This extends the general method for a laparotomy in Section 9.2. For tuberculous peritonitis see Section 29.5.

X-RAYS. Take an erect and a supine film. Look for: (1) free air under the patient's diaphragm. (2) Gas and fluid filled adjacent loops which appear to be separated, due to the exudate between them. (3) Distended loops of gut; to recognize the different levels of the gut radiologically, see Section 10.4 and Figs. 10-6 and 10-7.

BLOOD COUNT. He is likely to have a leucocytosis of more than 15,000 µl. If his haematocrit is over 50% he has lost much extracellular fluid and needs Ringer's lactate.

ASPIRATION. If you suspect acute pancreatitis (13.9), confirm it by aspirating his peritoneal cavity with a needle, and if this is negative do a peritoneal lavage (66.1).

RESUSCITATION. The need for this varies:

If his peritonitis is early, and his general signs are minimal, he does not need resuscitation.

If his pulse is rapid and his blood pressure low, delay operation for a few hours (never more than 6) while you resuscitate him (A 15.3). Give him intravenous Ringer's lactate or saline

THE PERITONEAL CAVITY

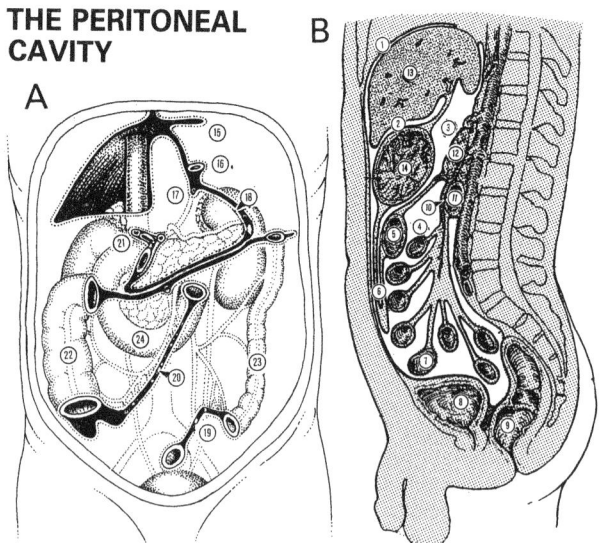

Fig. 6-3 THE PERITONEAL CAVITY. In generalized peritonitis this fills with pus. A, the posterior abdominal wall showing the lines of peritoneal reflection after removal of the liver, spleen, stomach, jejunum, ileum, and the transverse and sigmoid colons. Organs on the back of the abdominal wall are seen through the posterior parietal peritoneum. B, a longitudinal section of the abdomen.

1, the anterior superior subphrenic space. 2, the anterior inferior subphrenic space. 3, the lesser sac. 4, coils of jejunum. 5, the transverse colon. 6, the great omentum. 7, coils of ileum. 8, the bladder. 9, the rectum. 10, the mesenteric artery. 11, the duodenum. 12, the pancreas. 13, the liver. 14, the stomach. 15, the left triangular ligament of the liver. 16, the oesophagus. 17, the upper recess of the omental bursa (lesser sac). 18, the lienorenal ligament. 19, the root of the sigmoid colon. 20, the root of the mesentery. 21, the cut edge of the lesser omentum. 22, the ascending colon. 23, the descending colon. 24, the duodenum.

(an adult may need several litres). If possible, measure his CVP and keep it at 6–8 cm of water (A 19.2). Monitor his hourly urine output (A 15.5) and keep a fluid balance chart. Catheterise his bladder. Operate as soon as his pulse rate falls, his blood pressure rises, and his peripheral circulation improves.

If signs of peripheral circulatory failure do not respond to generous resuscitation, he will probably die, whatever you do. You may be wise not to operate.

If he is confused, severely hypotensive, and hyperventilating, with a fast pulse, and warm pink extremities, or cold clammy ones, he is in septic shock. Treat him as in Section 53.4. If you can, drain the septic focus. Timing is important: he must be fit enough to withstand the operation, so overcome shock, and then do the simplest possible operation.

THE NON-OPERATIVE TREATMENT OF PERITONITIS

INDICATIONS. You have got to be *very* sure about these: (1) Acute pancreatitis. (2) Some cases of typhoid peritonitis (31.8). (3) Peritonitis which is mainly pelvic. You can feel an inflammatory mass vaginally or rectally. Drain this pus vaginally after confirming it by aspiration (16.6), or rectally in a male (uncommon). (4) Pus which is mainly under the diaphragm (6.4). (5) Peritonitis which has been confirmed by aspiration (66.1), but the patient is too ill to withstand laparotomy. Delay operation until he has improved.

METHOD. Start antibiotics and nasogastric aspiration as described below and give him intravenous fluids (A 15.3, 15.5). Give him nothing by mouth. Be sure to correct potassium deficiency (A 15.3). Continue nasogastric suction and intravenous fluids until he shows signs of recovery (his bowel sounds return, there is less aspirate, and he passes flatus).

LAPAROTOMY FOR PERITONITIS

NASOGASTRIC ASPIRATION. Insert a nasogastric tube (4.9).

ANTIBIOTICS are unnecessary if he has: (1) Acute pancreatitis. (2) A perforated gastric or duodenal ulcer (unless you see him late when peritonitis has developed, 11.1). (3) Appendicitis causing only localized peritoneal infection. Otherwise, give them.

If he has generalized peritonitis, take blood cultures (if possible) before you give him antibiotics. You have a good chance of isolating the organisms responsible. When the sensitivity tests come back, adjust his antibiotics accordingly. Meanwhile, give him the perioperative antibiotics, as in Section 2.9. Chloramphenicol or a cephalosporin, and metronidazole are likely to be the practical ones. Give him chloramphenicol 6-hourly, at first intravenously, later orally; and metronidazole 8-hourly, the first two doses intravenously if possible and rectally later. For tetracycline instillation, see below.

CAUTION ! If he is to be given a relaxant, don't give him an aminoglycoside antibiotic unless you have an experienced anaesthetist—it may prolong the paralysis (A.14.2 to 14.4). These include gentamicin (especially), kanamycin, streptomycin, and amikacin.

EQUIPMENT. A general set (4.12). Several litres of *warm* saline or Ringer's lactate. To warm them, see below.

INCISION. As soon as he is draped, and anaesthetized, and his abdomen is relaxed, palpate it (10.1). Unless you have good indication for making another incision, make a median or a right paramedian one, centred on his umbilicus.

For a list of some of the things you might find on opening his abdomen, see Section 10.2. We assume here that he has localized or generalized peritonitis, with pus and fibrinous exudate everywhere. First, take a specimen for culture and sensitivity.

Break down adhesions *with the greatest possible care.* Only break down light ones with your fingers. If they are dense, define them carefullly, and cut them with scissors, or, better (if you are experienced) with a fine scalpel (10-11). If you are rough, you increase the chances of a faecal fistula.

If peritonitis is widespread, search systematically until you can find its cause. Be guided as to where it might be by: (1) His history. (2) The nature of the exudate. (3) The place where pus and exudate are most intense. (4) The density of the adhesions; the densest ones may indicate the origin of the infection.

CAUTION ! (1) Suck out all free pus before you start. (2) You must have good exposure—see Section 9.2. (3) If you find localized pus, try to minimize its spread around his peritoneum! (4) You face the dilemma described above—when to divide adhesions and when not to.

MANAGING THE UNDERLYING CAUSE. First, you will have to find it, and this may not be easy. Look for appendicitis (12.1), PID (6.6), a perforated peptic ulcer (11.2), strangulation obstruction (10.3), and signs of typhoid fever (multiple lesions in his distal small gut, 31.8). In most cases of typhoid, you will probably have decided not to operate. If your search produces something that you can do easily, without breaking down too many protective adhesions, such as removing a gangrenous appendix when the tissues are not too friable, or an infected ovarian cyst, do it. If you cannot find a cause after a full laparotomy, lavage his peritoneum and instil tetracycline. Play safe: he is desperately sick, and you must not risk complications.

If he has a hole in his large gut, repair it and make a proximal defunctioning colostomy (9.5).

If he has a hole in his rectum, do a proximal colostomy or a Hartmann's procedure (9.6).

If a dilated loop of gut 'disappears' into an inflammatory mass that might be tuberculosis, or a sealed-off perforation, don't try to dissect out the mass. Bypass it (29.5). This will keep risk to a minimum, relieve incipient obstruction, and allow the inflammation to subside. If you can easily biopsy the mass, do so. Usually, plan to re-operate and resect the lesion 3 to 6 months later.

If he has a perforated peptic or typhoid ulcer, oversew it and apply an omental graft (11.2).

LAVAGE. If he has *generalized* peritonitis, lavage his peritoneal cavity with saline. If his peritonitis is localized this may only spread the infection, so don't lavage. Sometimes, you can safely wash out only the pelvis.

Tip in several litres of *warm* saline or Ringer's lactate with 1 g of tetracycline (oxytetracycline may be cheaper) to the litre, slosh it around with your hand, and suck it out until the fluid which returns is clear. You may need 8 to 10 litres. Usually 3 or 4 are enough. Wash out his upper abdomen, his paracolic gutters, his infracolic area and his pelvis. Mop his peritoneum dry. Finally, leave a litre of warm tetracycline solution in his peritoneal cavity.

To warm the saline, put the bag or bottle in a basin of hot water and warm it to blood heat, feeling its temperature with your hand. If you have no saline you will have to use water, but the last instillation containing the antibiotic should be saline, or some other isosmotic fluid.

CLOSURE. Close his abdomen with interrupted through-and-through sutures of stout monofilament nylon or steel deep to the skin (9.8). Leave his skin unsutured for delayed closure.

DRAINS. Generalized peritonitis and multiple intra-abdominal abscesses cannot be drained adequately, because the area to be drained is too large: so wash out the pus, instil tetracycline, and don't insert drains.

It may be appropriate to drain a localized abscess—a pelvic abcess (vaginally in a female or rectally in a male), or a single intra-abdominal abscess. Abdominally, use wide bore tube drains; rectally, use corrugated rubber (4.10).

CAUTION ! If you instil tetracycline, don't insert drains, or it will all flow out!

POSTOPERATIVE CARE FOR PERITONITIS

FLUID BALANCE. Continue to 'suck and drip' him (9.9, A 15.5), and keep an accurate fluid balance chart. The common error is not to give him enough fluid.

Nasogastric suction. If he has had generalized peritonitis, he is sure to get ileus; suction will reduce his distension. You may suck out 2 to 6 litres of fluid a day. Replace it with 0.9% saline or Ringer's lactate in addition to his standard requirements (A 15.5).

Intravenous fluids. Manage his fluid balance as in Section A 15.5. For maintenance an adult needs at least a litre of 0.9% saline, or Ringer's lactate, and 2 litres of 5% dextrose in 24 hours. Be sure to monitor his urine output (if possible 2-hourly for the first 48 hours). After the initial period of up to 48 hours, when you expect his urine output to fall, keep his urine output above 1 ml/kg/hour. Replace all losses as appropriate (A 15.5). If his initial resuscitation was inadequate, he may still have a deficit to make up.

Potassium supplements. Don't forget these (A 15.5), especially if there is a large volume of gastric aspirate. Start them when his postoperative diuresis begins.

He may be acidotic. There are several ways you can correct this. You can: (1) Give him 200 ml of 8.4% sodium bicarbonate (200 mmol). Or, give him 500 ml of 4.2% sodium bicarbonate (250 mmol). (2) Give him a litre of 1/6 molar lactate. (3) Give him adequate intravenous fluids and let his kidneys correct his acidosis. If his condition is poor, use (1) or (2), and repeat them daily.

Blood. If he bled during the operation, and this loss was not replaced, replace it now.

POSTOPERATIVE ANTIBIOTICS. If he had generalized peritonitis, continue the same antibiotics you gave him preoperatively for 5 to 7 days. Be guided by his clinical response, rather than by the sensitivities reported by the laboratory. If he has not improved after 3 days change them.

OTHER MEASURES. Examine him carefully each day for complications. Watch his temperature chart, his general state of alertness, his abdominal girth, his bowel sounds, and the volume of his gastric aspirate.

DIFFICULTIES WITH PERITONITIS

These are many, and include septic shock (53.4), which can develop postoperatively.

If you CANNOT FIND A CAUSE FOR PERITONITIS, remember that PRIMARY PERITONITIS without any obvious cause does exist and is not uncommon in Africa. Bacteria may have arrived in the bloodstream as part of a septicaemic or pyaemic process. It is a diagnosis of exclusion, so make sure there is no perforation in *any* part of the gut, no PID or external injury etc.

If he DOES NOT IMPROVE, he may have residual sepsis and need a further laparotomy.

If his ABDOMEN DISTENDS and the volume of his gastric aspirate remains high (or he vomits), either the normal short period of ileus is continuing, or his gut is obstructing, see Section 10.13.

If his WOUND BECOMES INFECTED and breaks down, see Section 9.12. This is rare if you use non-absorbable sutures and close all the layers of his abdomen, except his skin (which should be left open for delayed closure), as a single layer. If you use absorbable sutures and close his abdomen layer by layer, wound breakdown is more likely.

If FEVER CONTINUES he may have a postoperative urinary or chest infection, or any of the abscesses in Section 6.3.

If he has DIARRHOEA, especially with the passage of mucus, suspect a pelvic abscess (6.5).

If FAECES START TO DISCHARGE FROM THE WOUND or a drain, he has a faecal fistula (not uncommon), so see Section 9.14. This is usually due to stripping some of the muscular coat of his gut, as you separate adhesions, and weakening it so that it breaks down later. If the fistula persists, it may produce disastrous fluid losses and severe wasting. Finding and closing it will be very difficult, so manage him non-operatively at first. If his gut is not obstructed distally, his fistula may close spontaneously. If it fails to close, refer him if you can. Try to avoid a fistula by only dividing light adhesions with your fingers. Define all other adhesions clearly, and divide them with scissors or a scalpel. Don't use diathermy close to his gut.

6.3 Abscesses in the peritoneal cavity

Localized abscesses in a patient's peritoneal cavity can be the result of: (1) Generalized peritonitis—they are one of its major complications. (2) Some primary focus of infection, such as appendicitis or salpingitis (PID, 6.6). (3) An abdominal injury in which his gut was perforated or devitalized. (4) Any laparotomy.

If abscesses are going to occur after a laparotomy, a patient's temperature does not fall, or it falls and then rises in a characteristic spiky pattern (Fig. 6-6) which shows that there is pus somewhere inside him. He is not well and does not eat, he loses weight, and his white count is raised. If loops of his gut pass through the abscess, they may become obstructed, acutely or subacutely (10.12).

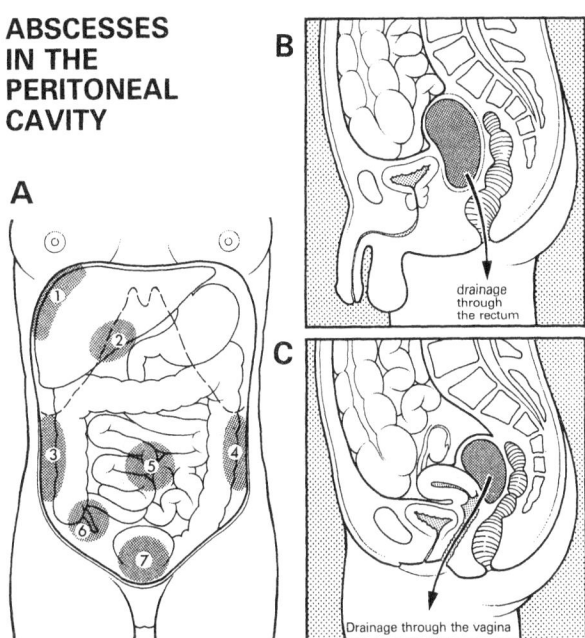

Fig. 6-4 ABSCESSES IN THE PERITONEAL CAVITY. A, the common sites. B, a pelvic abscess pointing into the rectum. C, a pelvic abscess pointing into the vagina.

1, between a patient's diaphragm and his liver. 2, under his liver. 3 and 4 in his right and left paracolic gutters. 5, among coils of his gut. 6, around his appendix. 7, in his pelvis.

Pus can gather: (1) Under his diaphragm or his liver (6.4). (2) Between loops of his small gut in the folds of his mesentery. (3) In his pelvis. If you are wondering where it has got to, remember that pus usually follows recognized paths. For example, in escaping from the appendix, it usually falls into the pelvis or tracks up his right paracolic gutter to his right subphrenic space, so that you are unlikely to find it on the left of his abdomen.

Provided you remember to examine a patient rectally (or vaginally), diagnosing pus in the pelvis should be easy. Diagnosing it under his diaphragm is much more difficult.

If you catch a localized infection early enough, antibiotics alone may possibly cure him; but once pus has formed they will not make it disappear, although they may limit its spread. So be sure to drain residual abscesses on the indications given below.

ABSCESSES IN THE ABDOMEN

If you suspect that a patient has an abdominal abscess, record his temperature 4-hourly, or hourly if he is very ill, especially if he is a young child. Examine him carefully at least once a day. Each time, feel for an abdominal mass, feel under his rib margins anteriorly and posteriorly, do a rectal examination, and in a woman a pelvic examination. The patient's temperature chart and his clinical signs will be of the greatest help, but you may find it helpful to do the following examinations each day: an abdominal X-ray (erect and supine), a chest X-ray, a white count, and blood cultures.

If you feel a mass, mark it out on his abdominal wall. Each day, feel if it has become larger or smaller. If it becomes larger, operate. It may become adherent to his abdominal wall, so you can open it without opening the rest of his peritoneal cavity.

On the appropriate indications, drain pus from his wound (9.12), from between the loops of his gut (see below), from under his diaphragm (6.4), and from his pelvis (6.5). Drainage is paricularly urgent if his general condition is deteriorating, or if he has complete intestinal obstruction which has not responded in 24 hours (10.12).

CAUTION! Don't make a small abdominal incision, his gut will be in less danger if you make a large one.

If you can feel a pelvic abscess vaginally, aspirate it to confirm the presence of pus, then drain it vaginally (6.5). Only drain an abscess abdominally, if you cannot drain it vaginally.

ABSCESSES BETWEEN LOOPS OF GUT. If the swelling is to one side of a patient's abdomen, incise its lateral side. Open the layers of his abdominal wall, then explore his abdomen with your finger until you find pus. If infection is localized, insert a drain.

POSTOPERATIVELY, after you have drained any kind of abscess, watch him carefully, he may have more. Don't neglect his fluid balance or his nutritional state. He will be wasting severely, so do your best to increase his protein and energy intake (9.10). Ideally, he needs feeding parenterally, which is likely to be impossible. Don't try forced feeding, because he will not want to eat. If he will tolerate cautious feeding through a nasogastric tube, he may benefit considerably.

6.4 Subphrenic abscess

Pus under a patient's diaphragm has usually spread there from somewhere else in his abdomen. A subphrenic abscess may be secondary to: (1) Peritonitis, either local or general, following a perforated peptic (11.2) or a typhoid ulcer (31.8), or appendicitis (12.1), or PID (6.6) or infection following Caesarean section (18.11). (2) An injury which has ruptured a hollow viscus and contaminated his peritoneal cavity (66.2). (3) A laparotomy during which his peritoneal cavity was contaminated (9.2). (4) A ruptured amoebic liver abscess (31.12).

Suspect that a patient has a subphrenic abscess if he deteriorates, or recovers and then deteriorates, between the 14th and the 21st day after a laparotomy, with a low, slowly increasing, swinging fever, sweating, and a tachycardia. This, and a leucocytosis, show that he has 'pus somewhere', which is making him anorexic,

SUBPHRENIC ABSCESSES

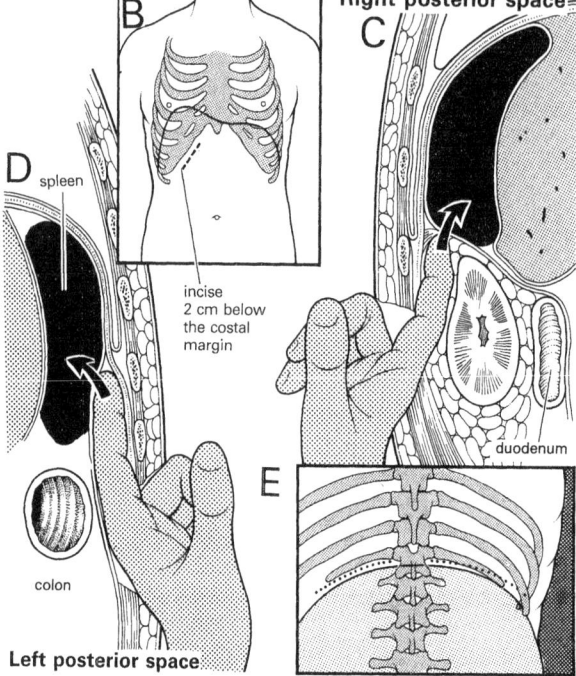

Fig 6-5 SUBPHRENIC ABSCESSES. A, the spaces where pus can collect under a patient's diaphragm. B, make a subcostal incision when you approach a subphrenic abscess anteriorly. C, exploring the right posterior subphrenic abscess. D, exploring the left posterior space. E, exploring the posterior spaces through the ribs.

1, the right anterior subphrenic space. 2, the left anterior subphrenic space, 3, the right subhepatic space. 4, the left subhepatic space (the lesser sac). 5, the right posterior subphrenic space. 6, the left posterior subphrenic space.

wasted, and ultimately cachectic. If he has no sign of a wound infection, a rectal examination is negative, and his abdomen is soft and relaxed, the pus is probably under his diaphragm.

The pus might be between his diaphragm and his liver, in (1) his right or (2) his left subphrenic space, or under his liver in (3) his right or (4) his left subhepatic space in his lesser sac. He may have pus in more than one of these spaces.

Explore him on the *suspicion* that he might have a subphrenic abscess. Exploration is not a major operation; the difficulty is knowing where to explore, so refer him if you can. If you cannot refer him, explore him yourself. If you fail to find pus, you have done him no harm; missing a subphrenic abscess is far worse. If it is anterior, you can drain it by going under his costal margin anteriorly. If it is posterior, you can go through the bed of his 12th rib posteriorly.

KIMANI (15 years) was admitted with abdominal pain and vomiting of sudden onset, about 4 hours previously. He had shoulder-tip pain, but he also said he had pain when he put his tongue out, so it was first thought that he might be hysterical. He had no abdominal signs, so he was admitted for observation. The following day his abdomen started to distend, and aspiration of his peritoneal cavity withdrew greenish fluid. A laparotomy was done, and an ulcer on the greater curve of his stomach was found and repaired. Initially he recovered well, but as he was about to go home 10 days later, he was not well, he ran a fever, he looked toxic, and there was tenderness and induration on the right side of his upper abdomen. He was suspected of having a subphrenic abscess, his abdomen was reopened through his paramedian incision, and a large quantity of foul-smelling pus was evacuated from under the right side of his liver. Several drains were inserted. The drug vote was almost finished and the hospital could not afford intravenous metronidazole, so he was given intravenous chloramphenicol, and metronidazole by mouth, after which he eventually recovered. LESSONS (1) If you are not certain that a patient is hysterical it always pays to observe him. (2) Beware of the 'latent interval' 3 to 6 hours after a perforation, when there may be few abdominal signs. (3) You may be able to drain a subphrenic abscess through the original laparotomy incision, but the incisions described below may be better. (4) When a peptic ulcer causes general peritonitis, a thorough lavage of the peritoneal cavity is as important as the repair.

SUBPHRENIC ABSCESS

This follows from Section 6.3 on abdominal abscesses.

SIGNS AND SYMPTOMS. Thoracic signs are more useful than abdominal ones. Ask or look for: (1) Cough. (2) Shoulder-tip pain on the affected side. (3) An increased respiratory rate, with shallow or grunting respiration. (4) Diminished or absent breath sounds. (5) Dullness to percussion. (6) Dull pain. (7) Hiccup (rare). (8) Tenderness over the 8th to 11th ribs. A subhepatic abscess may cause tenderness under the costal margin anteriorly. A subphrenic abscess, pyelonephritis, a pyonephros or a perinephric abscess can all cause similar tenderness posteriorly. (9) If the patient is thin and the pus is superficial, you may feel a tender indurated mass under his costal margin in front (right subphrenic space), in his right flank (right subhepatic space), or posteriorly.

X-RAYS are essential. Screening is the most important investigation and the cheapest. Look for: (1) The failure of one side of his diaphragm to move. This is a sign of infection, but not necessarily of an abscess. (2) Give him a little contrast medium, and look for downward and forward displacement of his stomach and spleen.

Also take a PA and a lateral view. Look for: (1) a raised diaphragm, (2) a fuzzy upper border to his diaphragm, (3) fluid in his costophrenic angle, (4) collapse or consolidation at one lung base, (5) a fluid level (rare). (6) You may also see gas in his subphrenic space. This can be the residue from a laparotomy, or it can be due to a perforation of his gut, or to an anaerobic infection.

If his first X-ray examination is negative or equivocal, repeat it a few days later.

CAUTION ! (1) His white count is usually raised but may be normal. (2) 10% of patients have no fever. (2) Don't try to diagnose subphrenic abscesses by aspiration—this is dangerous and misleading.

THE DIFFERENTIAL DIAGNOSIS includes a liver abscess (31.12), an empyema (6.1), and pulmonary collapse (9.11).

THE MANAGEMENT OF SUBPHRENIC ABSCESSES

WHICH APPROACH? If you suspect a subphrenic abscess, and a patient's general state does not improve, and his fever does not settle, he needs exploring. Avoid antibiotics which may mask his symptoms.

If he has a swelling, or oedema, or redness or tenderness just below his ribs or in his loin, make the incision there.

If his abscess follows appendicitis, a perforated duodenal ulcer, or cholecystitis, it will probably be on the right. If a high gastric ulcer has perforated, it is more likely to be on the left. If an ulcer in the posterior wall of his stomach has perforated, there will be pus in his lesser sac.

If you don't know which side it is on, there is about a 75% chance that it will be on the right, probably anterior. Approach it anteriorly, if possible through the old laparotomy wound, unless there are very clear signs that it is posterior. If one route fails try another. You cannot reach the posterior surface of his liver through an anterior incision, or vice versa, but if pus extends all the way from front to back, one incision will be enough.

Alternatively, decide if the pus is on the right or left, and then explore all subphrenic abscesses from in front. If you don't find pus, explore posteriorly.

ANAESTHESIA. Take him to the theatre. If he is a poor anaesthetic risk, block his lower 6 intercostal nerves (A 6.7). If he is a better risk, you can give him a general anaesthetic and intubate him.

ANTERIOR APPROACH. Make an incision which is large enough to take your hand. Depending on the signs, make it a finger's breadth below and parallel to his right (usually) or his left costal margin. Cut from the middle of his rectus muscle laterally, as in B, Fig. 6-5. Cut the muscle fibres in the line of the incision. Often, you can open the abscess cavity without entering his general peritoneal cavity, so try to keep outside it until you have found the abscess. His extraperitoneal tissue will probably be oedematous. Push your index finger upwards through it, peeling the peritoneum off his diaphragm as you do so. Sweep your finger under his liver from one side to the other to explore his subhepatic space. If you don't find pus there, sweep it round the lateral edge of his liver, and explore his subphrenic space between his diaphragm and his liver.

Somewhere you will feel an indurated abscess cavity. If you have opened his general peritoneal cavity pack off his gut, and have a sucker ready before you push your finger through it, in case pus squirts out. Explore it with your hand, break down any loculi, and send pus for culture. Insert a drain as described below.

If his liver is not adherent to his diaphragm, there may still be pus posteriorly, pushing his liver forwards.

CAUTION ! (1) Try not to go above his diaphragm. This is more likely to happen with an anterior approach. If you enter his pleura, suture his diaphragm with '1' multifilament or monofilament sutures and insert an under water seal drain (9.2D, 65-6) before you approach the abscess. (2) Be sure that he has only one abscess.

Alternatively, cut everything except his parietal peritoneum in the line of the incision. Burrow upwards with your finger between his peritoneum and his diaphragm, until you feel the induration of the abscess. Peel his peritoneum off his diaphragm as you do so.

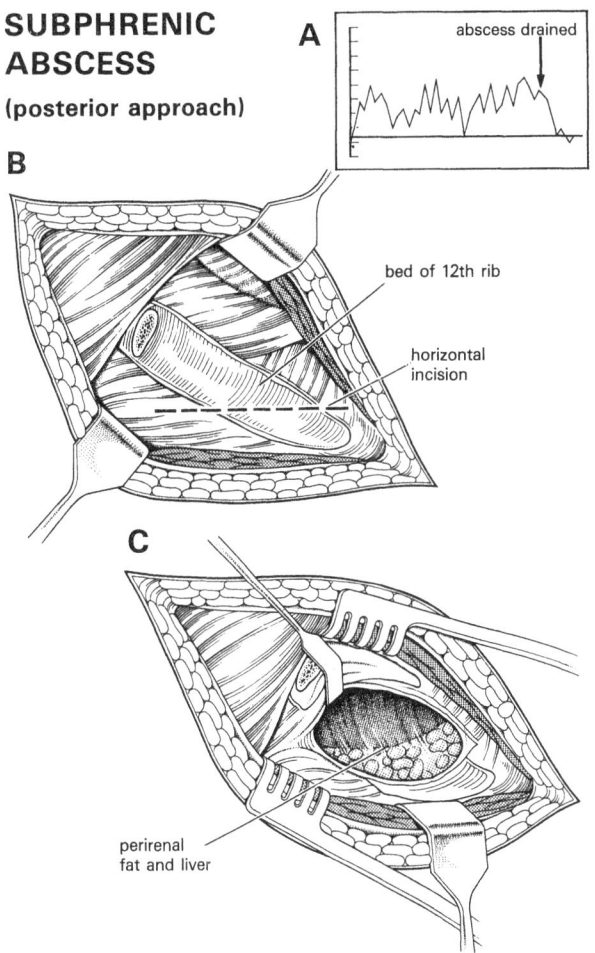

Fig. 6-6 THE POSTERIOR APPROACH TO A SUBPHRENIC ABSCESS. A, a hectic fever subsided as the patient's abscess was drained. B, his 12th rib has been excised and an incision is about to be made in its bed. C, the bed of his 12th rib has been divided, showing his liver and the fat round his kidney. *After Ochsner and Graves.*

POSTERIOR APPROACH. Lay him on his sound side with his lumbar region slightly elevated by breaking up the table or placing pillows under his other side. Make an incision which is big enough to take your hand over his 12th rib posteriorly (E, in Fig. 6-5). Remove the distal 2/3 of his 12th rib; divide it at its angle. Cut through the periosteum, reflect this from the whole circumference of the bone with Faraboef's rougine, as you would when you drain an empyema (6.1).

CAUTION ! Take great care not to damage his diaphragm.

Incise the inner aspect of the periosteum horizontally. Push your finger upwards and forwards above his renal fascia to enter the abscess (C, or D, in Fig. 6-5). Occasionally, you may need to tie his intercostal vessels.

POSTOPERATIVELY (both routes). At the most dependent part of the abscess, insert one or even two 1.5 cm plastic or rubber drainage tubes with several side holes, or a sump drain. Bring the drain out through a stab wound in his flank. Stitch it to his skin. Close his wound as usual, but leave his skin unsutured. If you have left a large space under his diaphragm, connect the drain to an underwater seal, to encourage it to close.

As soon as the discharge is reduced to about 20 ml of pus a day, shorten the drain progressively during a few days and then remove it. Sinograms are unlikely to be helpful.

If there is any rise in his pulse or temperature, or localized pain, suspect that his abscess is not settling. Be sure to leave the drain in. Antibiotics are less important than adequate drainage.

DIFFICULTIES WITH SUBPHRENIC ABSCESSES

If the fluid you aspirated from his chest was a STRAW-COLOURED EFFUSION, and he is not very toxic, X-ray him again in a few days to see what has happened. Is it clearing? Is his diaphragm still raised? If you aspirated frank pus, drain it a day or two later by inserting a chest tube connected to an underwater seal (65.2).

If he is so toxic, weak, and wasted from his subphrenic abscess that SURGERY MIGHT SEEM TO BE TOO MUCH FOR HIM, don't hesitate to explore his abscess. If necessary, drain pus from his pleural space also, it is his only hope.

If you DAMAGE HIS PLEURA ACCIDENTALLY, insert an underwater seal drain.

If pus from below the diaphragm RUPTURES INTO A BRONCHUS, he may drown in a spasm of coughing. The pus is more likely to have spread from an amoebic abscess in his liver than from a subphrenic one.

6.5 Pelvic abscesses

Pus in the pelvis is nearly as dangerous and difficult to manage as pus under the diaphragm. You will see several kinds of pelvic abscess which need managing in different ways:

(1) Following infection of the female genital tract which can be any of the varieties of pelvic inflammatory disease (PID) described in the next section. Those following a septic abortion or puerperal sepsis may be caused by anaerobes, and so are particularly serious and likely to spread. The patient may be very ill; you may have difficulty finding pus, and knowing when and how to drain it. The danger is that pus may build up as a mass above her pelvis, and spread upwards into her peritoneal cavity, perhaps fatally, instead of discharging spontaneously and harmlessly into her rectum. Drain this type of pelvic abscess early, as soon as pus has formed, and don't 'sit on it'.

(2) Following appendicitis. You can treat pelvic abscesses of this type non-operatively with much more safety, as in Section 12.2.

(3) Following generalized peritonitis, such as that caused by a perforated peptic (11.2), or a typhoid ulcer (31.8). If a patient makes good progress from the disease which caused his abscess, the pus in his pelvis is unlikely to kill him.

A pelvic abscess can grow quite large without making a patient very ill, or causing very obvious signs, so that, unless you do frequent rectal or vaginal examinations, you can easily miss one. You will need experience and a sensitive finger. One danger is that a pelvic abscess may obstruct the gut (10.13). Drain a man's abscess rectally, and, if possible, a woman's vaginally. This is easier than doing a laparotomy. If coils of gut lie between the pus and her posterior fornix, it will be more difficult to diagnose, and you will have to drain it suprapubically. Sometimes, an abscess drains into the rectum spontaneously, but incising it speeds recovery.

PELVIC ABSCESSES

This follows from Section 6.3 on abdominal abscesses.

DRAINING A PELVIC ABSCESS

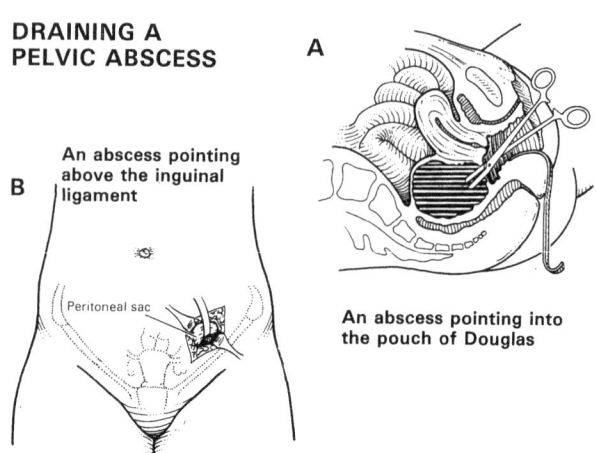

Fig. 6-7 DRAINING PELVIC PUS. A, if you drain pus vaginally, do so with particular care, or you may penetrate coils of gut. B, occasionally, pus presents above the inguinal ligament and has to be drained like this.

DIAGNOSIS. PID is the commonest cause. Watch also for the formation of a pelvic abscess when a patient is recovering from appendicitis (12.1), peritonitis, or an infected Caesarean section (6.8); watch for fever and the passage of frequent stools ('diarrhoea'), with tenesmus and mucus. Feel for: (1) A boggy, tender mass above a man's prostate filling his rectovesical pouch, or a soft bulging swelling in a woman's pouch of Douglas. Sometimes, the mass is almost visible at her vulva. You will not find fluctuation. (2) Tenderness and occasionally an ill-defined mass suprapubically. If you suspect a pelvic abscess in a woman, put one finger into her rectum and another into her vagina. Normally, they should almost touch. If she has an abscess, you will feel it between your fingers.

You can confuse a pelvic abscess bulging into the pouch of Douglas with: (1) A chronic ectopic pregnancy (haematocoele, 16.7). (2) An ovarian cyst (20.7). Some suspected cysts turn out to be post inflammatory collections of fluid (post-inflammatory pelvic pseudocysts).

If there are no signs that the infection is spreading upwards into the peritoneal cavity, operation is not urgent. Give antibiotics as for peritonitis (2.9, 6.2). Carefully monitor the patient's temperature and the mass, and drain the abscess as soon as it is ripe. If you doubt whether it is 'ripe' for drainage or not, wait.

CAUTION ! An abscess which is enlarging suprapubically needs draining urgently.

VAGINAL DRAINAGE OF A PELVIC ABSCESS (posterior colpotomy)

INDICATIONS. A pelvic abscess which extends into the pouch of Douglas.

ANAESTHESIA. (1) General anaesthesia. (2) Ketamine (A 8.1).

PREPARATION. Put her into the lithotomy position and catheterize her bladder. Do a vaginal examination to confirm the diagnosis.

INCISION. Expose the vaginal wall of her posterior fornix (which should be bulging) with a short broad speculum. Ask an assistant to depress her vaginal wall with a Sims speculum, while you raise the posterior lip of her cervix with a vulsellum. Push a large needle into the swelling in the midline and aspirate:

If you aspirate pus, this confirms a pelvic abscess, so proceed as below.

If you aspirate aspirate a pale yellow fluid, you are probably draining a post-inflammatory pseudocyst, so also proceed as below.

If you aspirate blood, either you have punctured a blood vessel (which should not happen if the needle is in the midline; the blood will clot), or she has a haematocoele due to a chronic ectopic pregnancy (if so the blood will not clot), for which you must do a laparotomy (16.7).

If you find an abscess or a post-inflammatory cyst, make a 2–3 cm transverse incision in her vaginal wall in the place where you found pus. Push in a haemostat; pus or fluid should flow. Open the forceps and pull them back to enlarge the opening. Explore the abscess with your finger; feel for loculations in the abscess cavity and gently open them. Insert a large drain and suture it to her perineum or labia. Leave it in for a few days and continue antibiotics. Pus may discharge for up to 2 weeks.

CAUTION ! (1) If pus is pointing laterally, drain it as close to the midline as you can, to avoid injuring her ureters (20-9). (2) Don't push too deeply into the abscess with the haemostat, or its roof may give way and spread the pus into her peritoneal cavity; or you may damage a loop of gut. Be safe, and gently insert your finger through an adequate incision. (2) The effect should be spectacular, and she should improve markedly in a few days. If she does not improve, she has more pus somewhere, and probably needs a laparotomy.

RECTAL DRAINAGE OF A PELVIC ABSCESS

Take the patient to the theatre and anaesthetize him. Put him into the lithotomy position. While his abdomen is relaxed, palpate it *gently*. Then examine him bimanually with one finger in his rectum, and your other hand on his abdomen. If you can ballot the mass, needling is unnecessary —drain it immediately.

To needle it, take a three-ringed 10 ml syringe, as used for injecting piles, and fix a 1 mm needle to it. Place the tip of your gloved right index finger over the place in the anterior wall of his rectum where you feel pus. Slide the point of the needle up alongside your finger, then push it through the wall of his rectum for about 2 cm. Aspirate. If no pus comes, inject a few ml of saline, and aspirate again. The needle may be blocked.

If you aspirate pus, or are sure that his abscess is ripe, drain it. Either push the tip of your index finger into it—pus will burst out. Or take a long curved haemostat, and with your index finger again acting as a guide, push its tip through the anterior wall of his rectum into the abscess. Enlarge the hole by opening and closing the jaws a few times.

CAUTION ! (1) Opening an abscess before it is properly formed is useless and dangerous. (2) Don't use any sharp instrument to penetrate the rectal wall, it may bleed seriously.

SUPRAPUBIC DRAINAGE OF A PELVIC ABSCESS

This is sometimes needed in women (it is almost never necessary in men), particularly after an abortion or a Caesarean section when you can feel a mass suprapubically but not vaginally. Fortunately, you can usually drain an abscess from below, which is easier and safer. Rarely, if more pus collects after vaginal drainage, you may need to drain it suprapubically.

If she is distended and tender, and there is induration behind and above her pubis, especially if she is also severely toxaemic, drain the pus suprapubically.

Catheterize her bladder to make sure it is empty. Make a 10 cm midline incision immediately above her pubis. Incise her linea alba and her peritoneum. If you enter her general abdominal cavity (which you can usually avoid doing), inspect it first, then pack off her upper abdomen with some large moist abdominal packs. Gently feel for the abscess. Look for pus, for loops of gut stuck down in her pelvis, and for oedematous or congested tissues. Insert a self-retaining retractor. Use a 'swab on a stick' to gently mobilize adherent loops of gut, until you have found the pus.

CAUTION ! (1) Don't lower her head to improve exposure; this may spread the infection. (2) Keep manipulation to a minimum.

(3) When you have found pus, do nothing more than is necessary to ensure adequate drainage. Don't break down the outer walls of the abscess cavity, but do break down any loculi. Distinguishing between them may be difficult.

Culture the pus and insert a drain. Remove *all* the packs; suture her abdominal muscles securely, but do not close her skin immediately (9.8).

DIFFICULTIES WITH PELVIC ABSCSSES

If a patient has COLICKY PAIN, VOMITING, AND ABDOMINAL DISTENSION, his small or his large gut is obstructed. Try to treat him non-operatively, with nasogastric suction and intravenous fluids (9.9, 10.13, A 15.5). Draining his abscess will usually cure the obstruction. If it does not, you may have to relieve it operatively (10.12).

6.6 Infection of the female genital tract; pelvic inflammatory disease—PID

PID will probably be the commonest gynaecological disease you will see, and may account for a third your admissions. If it is common in your area, half the women of childbearing age who present with acute abdominal pain may have it. You may admit two or three of them every week, and treat ten times as many as outpatients. The numbers of these patients, their frequent long stay in hospital, their mortality, the surgery they need, and the complications that follow make PID a major public health problem.

Infection elsewhere in the abdominal cavity usually originates in the gut, but infection in a woman's pelvic cavity usually starts in her genital tract. With the rare exception of tuberculosis, it always ascends from her vagina and cervix. PID is thus only a disease of women.

Infection follows two routes:

(A) Infection may spread through her tubes to cause: (1) In her cervix, cervicitis. (2) In her endometrium, endometritis. (3) In her fallopian tubes, salpingitis or pyo- or hydro-salpinx. (4) In her tubes and ovaries, salpingo-oophoritis (acute, subacute, or chronic) or a tubo-ovarian abscess. (4) In her pelvic cavity, pelvic peritonitis or a pelvic abscess. (5) In the rest of her peritoneal cavity, generalized peritonitis or peritoneal abscesses.

(B) Infection may also spread through her uterine wall into her broad ligaments to cause cause pelvic cellulitis (parametritis), a broad ligament abscess, or septic thrombophlebitis of her ovarian or her uterine veins. This is serious and causes septicaemia with few local signs.

Both subacute and chronic PID may cause an inflammatory mass containing her inflamed tubes, her ovaries, her uterus, her omentum, and loops of her gut. Between all these there are collections of pus, and in chronic cases fluid-filled pseudocysts. PID is always bilateral, although it may be dominant on one side.

Although they are similar, it is convenient to discuss: (1) PID unrelated to pregnancy, that is PID which does not obviously follow abortion or delivery. Because this kind of PID typically follows a period, it is sometimes called 'postmenstrual PID'. For want of a better name, this is what we will call it here. It is one of the most serious effects of the three sexually transmitted organisms discussed below (gonococci, chlamydia, and mycoplasma). When 'PID' is referred to it is usually this kind of PID that the speaker has in mind. (2) Post abortal PID (septic abortion, 6.6a). (3) Infected obstructed labour (18.4). (4) Puerperal sepsis ('puerperal PID', 6.7). (5) Sepsis after Caesarean section ('postcaesarean PID', 6.8).

A patient with 'postmenstrual PID' is not pregnant, she has suffered no birth trauma and there are no infected products of conception. She may however have an IUD in her uterus, which increases the risk of serious infection and may delay recovery. This kind of PID is seldom fatal, and never causes septic thrombophlebitis. All the others are dangerous, and commonly kill her. Postabortal peritonitis is particularly deadly and has a mortality of 50%. A girl of 17 may waste away with a bowel fistula like

CAUTION! BEWARE PID (and HIV)

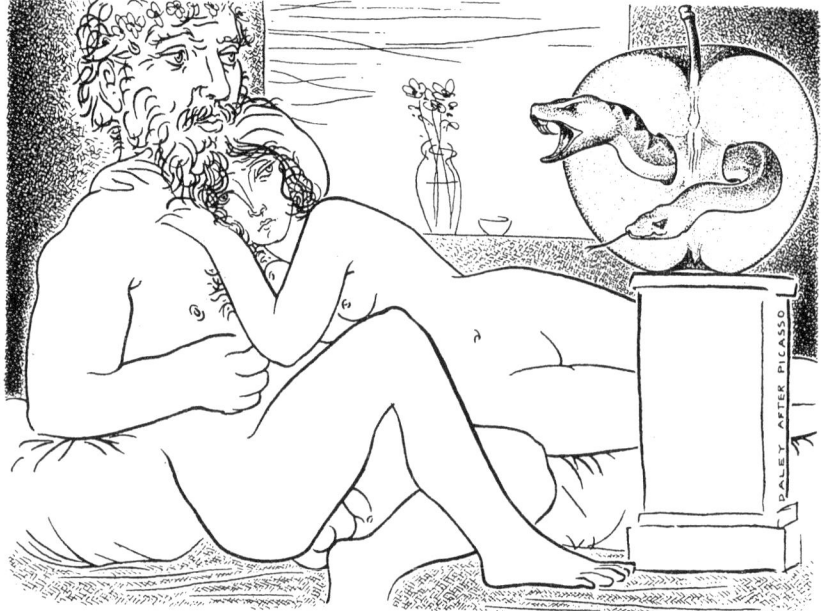

Fig. 6-8 CAUTION! PID AND HIV. The organisms responsible for PID may be: 1, sexually transmitted (gonococci, mycoplasma, or chlamydia). 2, The normal flora of the patient's gut and vagina (coliforms, anaerobes, and, rarely, actinomyces). Both partners are potentially in danger of HIV, see Chapter 28a. *With the kind permission of the Daily Telegraph.*

a terminal cancer patient, as did the patient, 'Grace', described below.

The organisms responsible for PID may be: (1) Sexually transmitted—gonococci (either penicillin-sensitive, or 'PPNG', penicillinase-producing *Neisseria gonorrhoeae*), mycoplasma, or chlamydia (both less common). (2) The normal flora of her gut and vagina—coliforms, various anaerobes, and rarely actinomyces. The latter organisms (and sometimes even the former) live harmlessly in the vagina and cervix, and only cause disease when the barriers to spread are removed by: (a) Abortion or delivery (very common). (b) Menstruation. Or, (c) some medical intervention, such as a 'D and C' (not uncommon), the insertion of an IUD (common but usually mild), or a hysterosalpingogram (rare).

Many gonococci, and typically all chlamydia and mycoplasma are sensitive to tetracycline. But when PID follows pregnancy or an abortion, it is caused by a mixture of organisms, including anaerobes, for which she needs metronidazole with chloramphenicol. By the time you see her, secondary invaders are likely to be present, whatever the primary cause of her infection.

HIV makes a mild genital infection more likely to progress to PID, so if yours is a high AIDS area, test for her HIV if you can.

The clinical manifestations of pelvic sepsis are wide. They range from an otherwise symptomless infertility caused by blocked tubes, to generalized peritonitis, septicaemia and septic shock, with everything between these two extremes. Like a fire, PID can be of any degree of severity, from smouldering to fulminating. Also, like a fire, it can die down, only to light up again later. So you will see: (1) Early acute cases who may not become infertile, if you treat them early and energetically. (2) An occasional fulminating case with peritonitis and shock. This can be an early acute case which is particularly severe, or it can be due to a tubo-ovarian abscess, which has previously caused only minor symptoms, bursting into the peritoneal cavity. (3) Chronic cases. (4) Chronic cases with a flare-up.

The typical acute case of postmenstrual PID has fever, bilateral lower abdominal pain, and tenderness, but seldom any rigidity. She usually also suffers from frequency of urine, dyspareunia, heavy or prolonged periods, and usually also has a vaginal discharge (see below). She may not admit to all these symptoms, especially if she is a young unmarried girl. On pelvic examination, she is usually equally and acutely tender in *both* her vaginal fornices (unlike an ectopic pregnancy, in which she is usually only tender in one of them). Her pain may be so intense that you have to repeat the examination after you have given her an analgesic. She may also have a lower abdominal mass, vomiting, fever and a raised ESR.

Her symptoms are usually mild, but can be severe with signs of peritonitis and occasionally septic shock. Acute cases are often atypical, either because the disease is mild, or because it has been modified by previous treatment.

The typical chronic case complains of infertility, and pelvic pain, often with dyspareunia, poor general health, and much misery. The diagnosis may be difficult, and the differential diagnoses include psychosomatic pain.

You can usually treat a patient non-operatively. Occasionally, you will need to drain pus. Unfortunately, once PID has become chronic, she may have recurrent pain, and if she is educated her threshold to it is likely to be lower. Don't operate on chronic PID unless you have to, because once it has been present for more than a few weeks, her pelvic organs will be so densely stuck to one another that freeing them will be difficult and dangerous— you can easily injure her gut. If you have to operate, do so on the indications given below, and be conservative. Leave her pelvic organs intact unless she has a tubo-ovarian abscess. Removing this can be difficult, so open it and drain it. If necessary, and you are sufficiently skilled, return later to remove her tubes in the chronic phase, or (better) persuade someone else to. If she can be left with her uterus and some ovarian tissue, she will continue to menstruate.

GRACE NYRIENDA (17) was admitted with vaginal bleeding and fever, having attempted to procure an abortion on herself at 16 weeks. Her cervix was wide open, the products of conception were visible, and there was a foul discharge. She was treated with antibiotics and her uterus was evacuated. A few days later she was very ill with a distended abdomen. Three litres of thin pus were washed out of her peritoneal cavity and tetracycline was instilled. There was no perforation in her uterus. She was treated with more antibiotics, intravenous fluids, and nasogastric suction. Two weeks later she was still febrile and very ill. A second laparatomy was done to drain residual abscesses. Chronic sores developed at the sites of the drainage tubes, which continued to discharge pus. She did not eat well, and vomited from episodes of subacute obstruction, but was not well enough for a third laparatomy. Three months after admission she died extremely wasted.
LESSONS (1) This is a typical history; there were no obvious mistakes in her treatment. Often, there is nothing you can do. (2) Any abortion, particularly a procured one, is dangerous at 16 weeks.

PID ('postmenstrual PID')

This is the patient with PID who has not recently aborted (6.6a), or delivered (6.7), or had a Caesarean section (6.8), and who typically has 'postmenstrual PID', commonly either gonococcal, chlamydial, or mycoplasmic. For the drainage of a pelvic abscess, see Section 6.5. For the management of adhesions see also Section 10.7.

ACUTE PID

DIFFERENTIAL DIAGNOSIS. Acute 'postmenstrual PID' has mostly to be distinguished from other causes of acute lower abdominal pain, including appendicitis (12.1) and a urinary infection (10.2). The main gynaecological differential diagnosis is a ruptured ectopic pregnancy (16.6). Fixity of her pelvic organs on vaginal examination is no help in distinguishing between PID (common), tuberculosis (uncommon), and endometriosis (rare), because they all do this.

Suggesting a ruptured ectopic pregnancy—a 'Yes' answer to the following questions: (1) Is she more than slightly anaemic? (2) Has she missed one or more periods by more than a few days? This is often followed by a small loss of dark or brownish blood vaginally. (3) When you examine her vaginally, is she more tender on one side than on the other? (4) Has she a mass on *one* side? In a subacute ectopic pregnancy the Fallopian tube mass is unilateral, but the pelvic haematocele of a chronic ectopic pregnancy usually feels as if it is in the midline. (5) Is she afebrile? An ectopic pregnancy does not usually cause fever, whereas acute or subacute PID usually does.

Suggesting a twisted ovarian cyst: a mass, no fever, and colicky lower abdominal pain, sometimes with vomiting.

If you are not sure of the diagnosis, and have a laparoscope (15.4), look for red, sticky, and oedematous tubes.

CAUTION ! (1) Her vaginal discharge is not proportional to the severity of her PID. *Candida* and *Trichomonas* cause a profuse discharge, but do not usually cause PID. Gonococci and *Chlamydia* cause a less obvious mucopurulent discharge. (2) Expect your diagnosis to be wrong in about 20% of patients.

MANAGEMENT. You can usually treat her as an outpatient. Admit her if: (1) She is too ill to go home, especially if she has: (a) bilateral lower quadrant rebound tenderness (indicating peritonitis), (b) a mass or (c) shock. (2) You cannot exclude an acute surgical condition, especially an ectopic pregnancy. (3) Outpatient treatment has failed. (5) She is unlikely to take her drugs or return for follow up.

ANTIBIOTICS. Cervical smears and cultures are of little help in choosing an antibiotic, because the organisms in her cervix may not be those which are causing the infection elsewhere. The absence of gonococci in a cervical smear does not exclude gonococcal infection. Usually, you will need to treat her blindly with a broad-spectrum antibiotic. If possible follow up and treat her partners.

Give her tetracycline 500 mg and metronidazole 400 mg, both 4 times daily for 7 to 10 days (2.9). Doxycycline 100 mg twice daily is better than tetracycline but is more expensive. Encourage her to complete the course. She is likely to stop if she feels better. Also, give her an analgesic.

If she is very ill with signs of spread outside her uterus, she needs parenteral antibiotics (2.9) in high dose against a wide range of organisms. Give her: (1) Benzyl penicillin 1.2 g 6-hourly. And, (2) give her chloramphenicol 1 g intravenously immediately followed by 500 mg intravenously 6-hourly. And, (3) give her gentamicin 80 mg intravenously 8-hourly. Or, give her intravenous chloramphenicol and metronidazole.

IF SHE FAILS TO RESPOND TO NON-OPERATIVE TREATMENT, as shown by feeling better, a falling temperature, less pain, and a reduction in the size of the mass; and particularly if she gets worse: (1) Have you made the right diagnosis? (2) Is there a collection of pus somewhere which needs draining? (3) Is she on the right antibiotic in the right dose? If you do decide that this is the problem, make sure you have excluded a wrong diagnosis or collections of pus.

Many patients with acute PID have a mass of matted viscera (as distinct from an abscess which needs drainage). This may take 6 weeks to resolve, but there is no point in continuing antibiotics for more than 2 weeks. If she is not well and has a spiking temperature after 6 weeks, she probably has an abscess which needs draining vaginally or suprapubically.

CAUTION ! Don't change antibiotics unless: (1) You have given them for at least 3 days. (2) You have carefully reviewed her. (3) You are sure that your original diagnosis of PID is correct. (4) You are reasonably sure she does not have a collection of pus anywhere.

LAPAROTOMY FOR ACUTE PID

INDICATIONS. Refer her if you can, this is not an easy operation. She has a significant chance of dying. There are three indications for a laparotomy:

(1) The diagnosis is in doubt, and there is a possibility that she might have an ectopic pregnancy or appendicitis, for example.

(2) After 48 hours of antibiotic treatment for PID (particularly after a septic abortion, 6.6a), she is not improving. Instead, her pulse continues to rise, her temperature is maintained, and there are signs that peritonitis is spreading.

(3) She has sudden generalized peritonitis with shock due to rupture of a tubo-ovarian abscess. This may be spontaneous or it may follow a vaginal or rectal examination. If her history is suggestive, resuscitate her and operate immediately. She is in grave danger.

RESUSCITATION. Give her intravenous fluids (A 15.3). She may need 3 or 4 litres of glucose saline during the first 24 hours. She may bleed considerably from the raw surfaces that will form when you free the adhesions between the loops of her gut, so have two units of blood cross-matched. If she is seriously ill, she is in danger of renal failure, so insert an indwelling catheter and monitor her urine output. Pass a nasogastric tube.

PERIOPERATIVE ANTIBIOTICS. If she is not already on tetracycline and metronidazole, start these before the operation. Or, give her chloramphenicol and metronidazole (2.9).

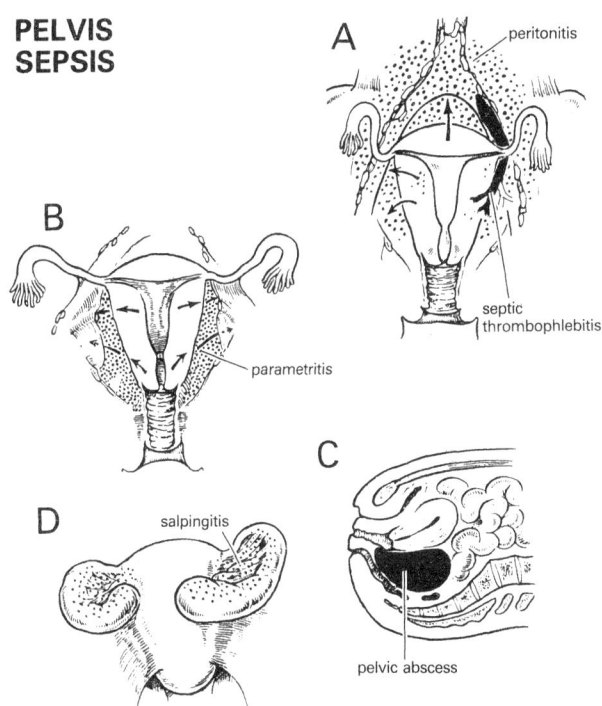

Fig. 6-9 PELVIC SEPSIS. A, infection spreading from the uterus to cause peritonitis. Infection can also spread as an infected thrombus (thrombophlebitis). B, infection of the connective tissue beside the uterus (parametritis). Infection may spread into the broad ligament, round the vagina or uterus, or up into the loin. C, a collection of pelvic pus. D, salpingitis. *After Garry MM et al. 'Obstetrics Illustrated', pp. 319—320. E and S Livingstone. with kind permission.*

ANAESTHESIA. (1) General anaesthesia with intubation (A 10.1). (2) If she is *very* sick, you can if necessary operate under local infiltration anaesthesia (A 6.9) and heavy premedication with pethidine and diazepam (A 5.2), but this will be unpleasant for you and for her. Also, local anaesthetics do not work well in the presence of infection. (3) Ketamine (A 8.1) with local infiltration anaesthesia of her abdominal wall.

INCISION. Make a lower midline incision (9.2) and extend it above her umbilicus if necessary. Here are some of the things you may find. Also be prepared on occasion to find some quite unexpected condition such as a perforated typhoid ulcer (31.8).

If the infection is limited to her pelvis, examine her upper abdominal cavity before you explore her pelvis and disturb the adhesions, which are limiting the spread of infection. Examine her subphrenic and subhepatic spaces, and her paracolic gutters; look for abscesses between the loops of her small gut as far as you can reach them. If you find pus, deal with it as in Sections 6.2, 6.3 and 6.4. If you find dense adhesions, see also Section 10.7.

If you don't find pus in her upper abdomen, carefully protect the upper uninfected part of her abdominal cavity with large abdominal packs. Slowly and methodically divide the adhesions between her gut and her uterus, and look for pus. Divide the adhesions round her tubes and ovaries, and release the pus you find there. Try to get right down into her pouch of Douglas. There is usually no need to remove her tubes or ovaries, however diseased they may look. The tubes have a double blood supply which prevents them becoming gangrenous, and they are not connected to a contaminated viscus like the appendix.

When you find her fundus push your fingers down behind it, between her tubes, which will almost meet in the middle. You need not fear perforating her gut here. Gradually work your fingers down below her tubes. Free them from her gut from below upwards.

Remember her anatomy: it is always the same. Both tubes will be stuck down behind her uterus, over the top of each ovary. Her rectum and colon will be adherent from below upwards to the back of her uterus, and then to both her tubes. Loops of small gut and omentum will have stuck to them on top. If you can find her fundus you will know where you are.

Don't panic when you find a mass of adherent gut and omentum. It will always come clear in the end. First get down to her fundus by lifting off her gut and omentum. Divide all adhesions and release all pockets of pus.

CAUTION ! Don't tear her gut. Avoid doing so by going slowly, and squeezing and pinching the plane of cleavage between your fingers (10.7). Cut dense adhesions with scissors.

If she has generalized peritonitis, suck away as much pus as you can, then suck out her paracolic gutters. Make sure you release any collections of pus under her abdominal wall, between her large gut and her abdominal wall, and under her diaphragm and her liver (subphrenic and subhepatic spaces). Bring out her whole small gut over its full length in stages. Break down adhesions between loops of gut, by careful blunt dissection, to release the many collections of pus between them. Then go to her pelvis, and proceed as above for a localized pelvic infection.

If you find she has a septic abortion, you will have to make the difficult decision as to whether or not to do a hysterectomy. Assess the state of her uterus and adnexa. By the time she has generalized peritonitis, hysterectomy is probably best: (1) The main indication for it is a perforated septic abortion. (2) How many children has she? If she is young and has no children, losing her uterus will be a major disaster. Even if you leave it, she will probably be infertile. (3) How skilled are you? If you are skilled this favours hysterectomy. A subtotal operation will be enough, but it will be dangerous. Occasionally, you may be able to avoid hysterectomy and do a salpingo-oophorectomy if generalized peritonitis seems to originate in an abscess in one of the adnexa (uncommon). Usually, all you need do when this happens is to drain pus and leave a tube in the abscess.

If you find that there is acute inflammation in her pelvis, and perhaps elsewhere without much pus, the infection is very

MANAGING PID

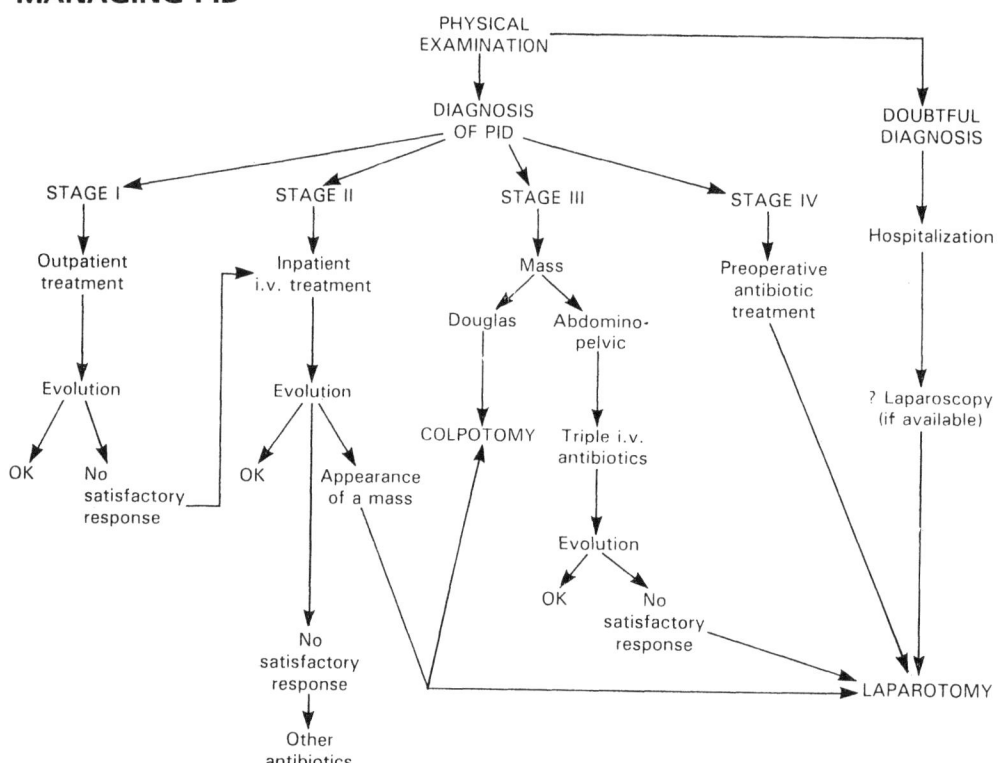

Fig. 6-10 A PLAN FOR MANAGING PID. Stage One: the patient has no peritoneal irritation, and no pelvic mass. Stage Two: she has peritonitis as shown by bilateral lower quadrant rebound tenderness. Stage Three: she has a mass in her adnexa (tubo-ovarian abscess) or pouch of Douglas. Stage Four: she is very ill indeed, as after the rupture of a tubo-ovarian abscess. This regime differs slightly from that in the text. *After De Mulder X, 'Pelvic inflammatory disease in Zimbabwe', Tropical Doctor 1988;2:85.*

early and she is lucky. Wash out what pus there is. Close her abdomen and continue chemotherapy.

If she has a ruptured tubo-ovarian abscess, leave the tube in and insert a drain.

LAVAGE AND DRAINS depend on the extent of the sepsis you found:

If the pus was localized to her pelvis, wash it out of her pelvis only (6.2), before you remove the packs protecting the rest of her peritoneal cavity. Place two tube drains in her pouch of Douglas, and bring them out through stab incisions, lateral to her rectus muscles.

If she had generalized peritonitis, drains do not work well, so wash out her whole peritoneal cavity as in Section 6.2.

CLOSURE. Close her abdomen as a single layer and leave her skin open for secondary closure (9.8). This is better than inserting tension sutures.

DIFFICULTIES WITH ACUTE PID

Be prepared for small gut fistulae (9.14), and a burst abdomen (9.13), especially if abdominal distension persists for some time postoperatively.

If she has a mass and you are not sure if she has a RUPTURED ECTOPIC OR A PELVIC ABSCESS, do a culdocentesis (16-6) under general anaesthesia. If you find pus, drain it through her vagina. If you find blood which fails to clot, do a laparotomy (16.7).

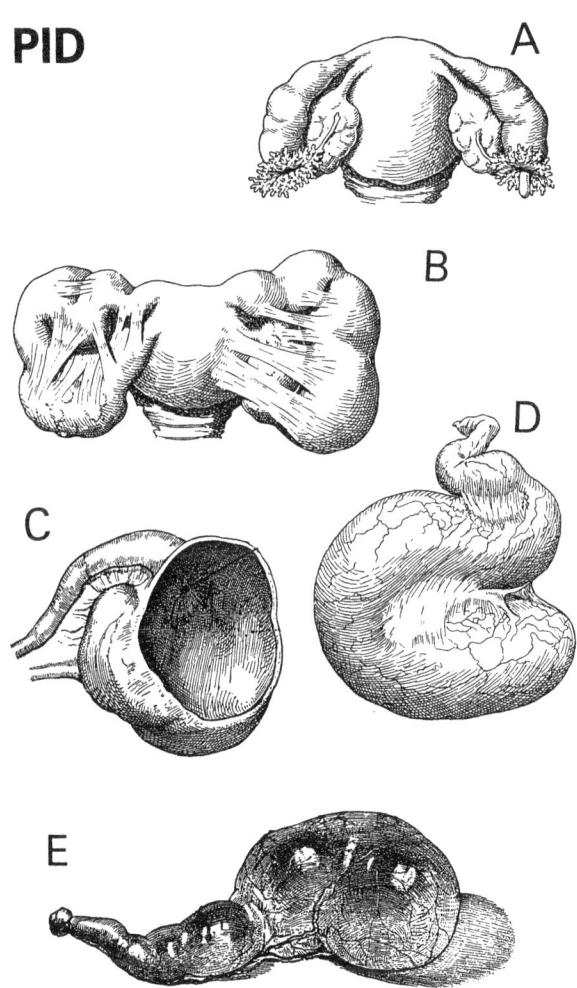

Fig. 6-11 PID AND PELVIC TUBERCULOSIS. A, acute salpingitis with swollen congested tubes and pus leaking from the ostium. B, chronic salpingo-oophoritis with the tubes and ovaries densely bound by adhesions. C, a tubo-ovarian cyst. D, a tuberculous pyosalpinx. E, a hydrosalpinx. *From Young, James, 'A Textbook of Gynaecology' (5th edn, 1939). A and C Black.*

If she HAS AN IUD IN AND PRESENTS WITH WITH PAIN, you will not find it easy to decide if her IUD is causing her pain, or if PID is causing it. If her symptoms are not too severe, and her cervix is merely a little tender, see if she will settle quickly with antibiotics and an analgesic. If she settles, leave her IUD. If you always remove an IUD because it causes a little pain and tenderness, you will remove too many. If she is febrile and very tender, give her antibiotics for 24 hours and then remove her IUD.

CAUTION ! Don't remove her IUD immediately. Removing it from her acutely infected cervix will be very painful.

If you find ACUTELY INFLAMED TUBES (SALPINGITIS), when you expect to find something else, leave them, her infection will settle if you give her an appropriate antibiotic. Do a peritoneal toilet and close her abdomen. Unlike an appendix, which you must remove (12.1), her tubes will not become gangrenous, or form a faecal fistula, or leak faeces into her peritoneal cavity.

If you enter her abdomen, expecting to find pus, but FIND LITTLE PUS OR NONE, and few signs of inflammation, examine her pelvic organs and particularly her infundibulopelvic ligaments (20-17). One or both may be thickened and oedematous, and the thickening may extend under her ovaries to her uterus. If so she has SEPTIC THROMBOPHLEBITIS of her ovarian veins (not uncommon). If you find nothing, the thrombophlebitis is probably in a uterine vein which is not so easily seen. If you don't find anything else, particularly any pus, close her abdomen. Continue with antibiotics in high doses. If possible, 24 hours after the operation start her on intravenous heparin 5000 to 10,000 units by bolus intravenous injection 6-hourly, controlled by estimating her clotting time and lengthening it to about 15 minutes. Continue this for at least 2 weeks. Watch carefully for abnormal bleeding, particularly from the abdominal incision, or her urinary or intestinal tracts. She should improve quite quickly.

If you find DISSEMINATED YELLOWISH-WHITE NODULES throughout her pelvic cavity, or a localized infection in her pelvis with nodules on her tubes and perhaps a CASEOUS ABSCESS, suspect that she has TUBERCULOSIS. Take a biopsy and send this for histology.

If you ACCIDENTALLY TEAR HER PELVIC COLON, what you should do depends on the size of the tear and where it is. If it is small, oversew it. If it is large, either close it and make a defunctioning colostomy (9.5) higher up, or divide her colon, close the distal end, and bring the proximal end out as a terminal colostomy (Hartmann's procedure, 9.5).

If there is PERSISTENT SEPSIS in her peritoneal cavity, in spite of repeated attempts at drainage, she is likely to go steadily down hill and die, after several months of great suffering (see the story of Grace above).

CHRONIC PID

DIAGNOSIS. Feel for tenderness of her uterine adnexa on bimanual examination, and for tender masses.

THE DIFFERENTIAL DIAGNOSIS includes urinary tract infection, endometriosis (rare in the developing world), and pelvic tuberculosis (uncommon).

ANTIBIOTICS. Give these as for acute PID for 10 to 14 days. If she has a recurrent infection, consider giving her three courses starting on the first days of successive menstrual periods.

If she improves, she feels better, her pain is less, and her mass disappears over 1 to 3 months.

If she does not improve, either your diagnosis is wrong, or she has a collection of pus, perhaps a chronic tubo-ovarian abscess or a pyosalpinx. Treatment is difficult. Refer her.

DIFFICULTIES WITH CHRONIC PID

If, on laparoscopy or laparotomy, you see BLUISH OR BROWN NODULES on the surface of her peritoneum and particularly on her uterosacral ligaments, surrounded by puckering, suspect ENDOMETRIOSIS. You are most likely to see such nodules on her uterosacral ligaments, in her pouch of Douglas, on her ovaries, on the posterior surface of her broad ligament, or on the fimbrial ends of her tubes. Refer her. Or, if she has pain give her a non-cyclical progestogen to suppress menstruation, such as norethisterone 10 mg daily starting on the 5th day of the cycle (increased if spotting occurs to 25 mg daily in divided doses to prevent break-through bleeding) for at least 6 months. Or, give her Depo-Provera 50 mg weekly or 100 mg every 2 weeks for 3 months.

If she is a YOUNG WOMAN WHO COMPLAINS OF INFERTILITY, menstrual irregularity, and chronic pelvic discomfort, TUBERCULOSIS (29.5) is a possibility.

If she has an IUD in and presents with UNILATERAL SIGNS and perhaps a HARD TUBO-OVARIAN MASS, suspect ACTINOMYCOSIS (rare) as the result of the introduction of the IUD. Confirm the diagnosis by biopsy at laparotomy. She will recover on treatment, and may possibly become fertile. Give her 2 megaunits of benzyl penicillin 6-hourly for 2 weeks, and then oral penicillin V 250 mg 6-hourly for 8 weeks.

If she has chronic PID and is worried about INFERTILITY, you can assure her that removing masses will not make her fertility better or worse, because she is probably incurably infertile already.

If she has chronic PID and is worried about PAIN but is not worried about having any more children, unilateral or bilateral salpingectomy without hysterectomy is usually possible. This is difficult, so don't attempt it yourself unless referral is impossible and you have considerable operative experience.

6.6a Septic abortions

If a patient with an incomplete abortion has fever and pus discharging from her cervix, the products of conception have become infected. This can follow a neglected spontaneous abortion, or it can follow unskilled interference. Fortunately, the uterus is usually a good barrier to the spread of infection, but it does sometimes spread as pelvic cellulitis or peritonitis. You can usually treat her without a laparotomy, although you will usually need to evacuate her uterus. If she has peritonitis you will have to open her abdomen.

The diagnosis is usually easy—if her history is clear and she is obviously pregnant. Unfortunately, she may be so frightened that she will deny having tried to procure an abortion, even when she is very ill. The only way to avoid a misdiagnosis is to remember that *any* acute pelvic inflammation in a woman of childbearing age may be the result of an abortion.

Try to control both haemorrhage and infection *before* you empty her uterus, usually after about 24 hours on antibiotics. Rarely, a hysterectomy may be the only way to save her life. The great dangers are septic shock (53.4) and renal failure (53.3).

IF SHE IS OF CHILDBEARING AGE, IS HER PELVIC INFLAMMATION THE RESULT OF AN ABORTION?

SEPTIC ABORTION

See also Section 6.6.

THE DIAGNOSIS should not be difficult. A patient becomes ill and febrile (>38°C) after an abortion. She has a foul vaginal discharge, and sometimes frank pus. Examine her vaginally in the ward. If you have the necessary facilities, start by taking an endocervical swab for culture aerobically and anaerobically (if possible). This is better than a high vaginal one. Take it yourself: if you leave it to a junior nurse, it is likely to be a 'low' one. Then use your fingers to remove any of the products of conception, which will come away easily.

Examine her bimanually. Her uterus is tender, there is tenderness on either side, perhaps with a mass. Sometimes she has local or general peritonitis.

Look also for anaemia, jaundice (caused by septicaemia) and chest signs (septic emboli from thrombophlebitis). Measure her haemoglobin, and take blood for grouping and crossmatching. If possible take blood cultures.

Your main concern will be to know how far infection has spread, and if you should open her abdomen.

If her pulse is over 120, the infection has probably spread beyond her uterus.

If moving her cervix causes her great pain and her lateral fornices are hot, thickened, and tender, perhaps with a mass, the infection has spread to her pelvic connective tissue (parametritis, uncommon).

If you are uncertain about the diagnosis and she is very sick, resuscitate her, start her on antibiotics, take her to the theatre and aspirate her posterior fornix. A seriously infected uterus can be silent, apart from a very sick patient.

If her history suggests that her uterus has been perforated with some instrument, her prognosis is worse. If it is leaking pus into her peritoneal cavity, you may ultimately have to do a hysterectomy.

RESUSCITATE HER as in Section 6.6. If she has lost blood, transfuse her as necessary (53.2, 53.4). If you have no blood, give her Ringer's lactate or 0.9% saline, or a plasma substitute.

ANTIBIOTICS. Try to prevent the infection spreading beyond her uterus. This risk is greatest when you evacuate it. So always cover evacuation with perioperative antibiotics. *They will not control the infection, if infected products of conception remain inside her uterus.* So empty it, and don't expect to cure her until you have done so.

If she is not very ill, and there are no signs that infection has spread beyond her uterus, a single broad spectrum antibiotic, such as ampicillin may be enough: (1) Give her ampicillin 500 mg intravenously 4 to 6-hourly. Or, (2) give her benzyl penicillin 600 mg intravenously 6-hourly, with streptomycin 1 g daily intramuscularly. Or, instead of the streptomycin give her gentamicin 80 mg intravenously 8-hourly.

If she is very ill, with signs of spread outside her uterus, she needs parenteral antibiotics—see Section 6.6.

ANALGESICS. Give her pethidine.

CONTROLLING BLEEDING Give her ergometrine with oxytocin ('Syntometrine' 1 ml) intravenously, or ergometrine alone.

EVACUATION. Opinions differ as to when this should be done. We advise that you do it a few hours after starting antibiotics, and never later than 24 hours after. If she is bleeding seriously, do it immediately. Follow the method in Section 16.2. Her uterus will be infected and soft, so be especially careful not to perforate it. Use a blunt curette. Continue antibiotics after evacuation.

POST-EVACUATION MANAGEMENT. Watch her carefully, especially her urine output. Several things may happen during the next few days. If she is seriously ill, an important decision will be whether or not she needs a laparotomy.

If all is well, she should improve dramatically, and her fever should go in 48 to 72 hours.

If she has not started to improve 24 hours after evacuation, but signs of peritonitis are not obvious, she probably has a pelvic abscess. Take her to the theatre and aspirate her posterior fornix (6.5). Avoid her lateral fornices, or you may injure her ureters or her uterine arteries. If you aspirate pus or blood-stained fluid, drain it through her posterior fornix, as in Section 6.5.

If she has not started to improve 24 hours after evacuation, and signs of generalized peritonitis are obvious (pain, tenderness, rigidity, and abdominal distension), she is in serious trouble. Her uterus may have been perforated by an abortionist, or he may have injected some harmful fluid into her peritoneal cavity. She needs a difficult laparotomy. Refer her if you can. Improve her general condition as best you can. Rehydrate her, if necessary, restore her haemoglobin to at least 80 g/l by transfusion, and have at least 2 units of blood available. Then do a laparotomy as in Section 6.6.

DIFFICULTIES WITH SEPTIC ABORTIONS

See also Sections 6.6 and 16.2 (inevitable abortions).

If you are NOT SURE IF SHE HAS PERITONITIS or not, consider waiting 24 hours. If necessary, aspirate her posterior fornix with a needle in the theatre.

If you PERFORATE HER UTERUS when you evacuate a septic abortion, there is no easy answer. If you stop and send her back to the ward incompletely evacuated, she is in danger. If you complete the evacuation, you may spread the infection further. This also is dangerous. As a general rule, if you perforate a *pregnant* uterus, complete the evacuation as best you can, then do a laparotomy and repair her uterus with a single layer of interrupted silk sutures. For the accidental perforation of a *nonpregnant* uterus, see Section 20.3.

If her URINE OUTPUT FALLS below 30 ml/hour, her kidneys are probably failing, so see Section 53.3.

If she has signs of SEPTIC SHOCK, treat it (53.4). The signs to watch for are an alert patient with a blood pressure below 80 mm, and a subnormal temperature.

If you feel CREPITATIONS (bubbles of gas in the tissues), suspect GAS GANGRENE and look for gas shadows radiologically. Treat her as in Section 54.13.

If she has generalized peritonitis without any localizing signs, make a muscle splitting incision as for appendicectomy in an iliac fossa. Open her peritoneum, sweep gently with your finger, and insert a sump sucker. Up to a litre of thin pus will probably escape. If you enter an abscess cavity, gently free any adhesions and open up all loculi. Wash out her peritoneum (6.2), and then instil tetracycline 1 g in a litre of saline.

If her fever recurs after initial improvement, there is more pus somewhere which must be drained, either through the same incision or another one. If you fail to drain a subphrenic abscess (6.4), she will die.

If she recovers from the acute episode, but is left with a mass, she may eventually need a need a full laparotomy, with the separation of adhesions and the removal of a tubo-ovarian mass. Refer her if you can.

6.7 Puerperal sepsis

After childbirth a patient's genital tract has a large bare surface, which can become infected. Infection may be limited to the cavity and wall of her uterus, or it may spread beyond to cause peritonitis (6.2), septicaemia, and death, especially when her resistance has been lowered by a long labour or severe bleeding. If she is more fortunate, her infection may be walled off by her gut and omentum. She may have a pelvic abscess with pus in her pouch of Douglas, or she may have pus high in her pelvis or in her lower abdomen.

If sepsis is localized, only her lower abdomen is distended, she has guarding in both her iliac fossae, and an ill-defined tender mass arising from her pelvis. She may have hyperactive bowel sounds. Vaginally, she shows signs of recent childbirth or abortion, and may have infected lacerations. Her cervix is open and tender, painful on movement, and may be drawn up behind her symphysis. Her pouch of Douglas may be thickened or swollen, but you cannot feel a fluctuant mass vaginally. Her uterus and appendages form a mass which is difficult to define because of their tenderness.

If sepsis is generalized, she is weak, with anorexia, fever (perhaps with rigors), a rapid thready pulse, a low blood pressure and generalized abdominal pain. Her abdomen is uniformly distended, tympanitic, silent, and acutely tender. She may have a visible mass extending up to her umbilicus; you may have to pass a catheter to make sure that it is not merely a distended bladder. She cannot walk. She may have diarrhoea until peritonitis causes ileus and this causes constipation and vomiting.

PUERPERAL SEPSIS

See also Sections 6.6 and 6.6a.

RESUSCITATE HER, if necessary, as in Section 6.6.

GIVE HER ANTIBIOTICS, as in Section 2.9. (1) Give her chloramphenicol and metronidazole. Or, (2) give her: ampicillin 500 mg 6-hourly for 7 days, and metronidazole (2.9). If she is very ill, she must have metronidazole either intravenously, or as suppositories, or tablets rectally (2.7). Too little chloramphenicol will be excreted in her breast milk to harm her baby. Or, give her gentamicin, or kanamycin.

MONITOR HER daily for signs of the spread of infection.

MANAGE HER like this:

If she continues to bleed, she may have retained pieces of placenta. This is a common cause of puerperal sepsis, which will not resolve until her uterus is empty. Give her antibiotics and curette her 24 hours later with *great care!* Use the largest curette which will be less likely to perforate her uterus. Curetting a large, soft, infected uterus is dangerous.

If her uterus is enlarged and tender, with a closed cervix as the result of scarring or carcinoma, it may be full of pus (pyometra, 32-21). This can occur 2 weeks or more after delivery. Drain her cervix with Hegar's dilators, 10 Ch is usually enough.

If she has a definite swelling at one side of her uterus, she has parametritis.

PUERPERAL SEPSIS

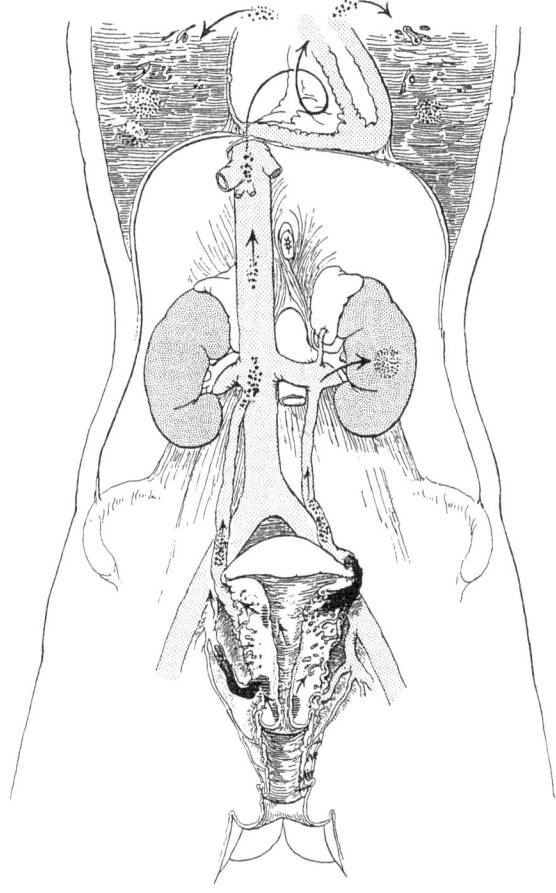

Fig. 6-12 PUERPERAL SEPSIS. There is septic thrombophlebitis. Septic emboli are spreading through the ovarian and internal iliac veins to cause septicaemia and and abscesses in the lungs and kidneys. *Adapted from an unknown source.*

6.8 Infection following Caesarean section

Peritonitis (6.2) may follow any obstructed labour, or an infected Caesarean section, and is common after rupture of the uterus. If a patient dies she will probably do so because you did not anticipate infection, or because you opened her abdomen much too late. She is likely to be infected: (1) If her labour is abnormally long, and the longer it lasts, the greater the risk. (2) If her baby is dead. (3) If her membranes rupture early and her liquor becomes infected. (4) If your sterile procedures are poor. In any of these conditions, anticipate infection and try to prevent it.

INFECTION AFTER CAESAREAN SECTION

See also Section 6.6, 6.6a and 6.7. For vaginal bleeding due to infection (secondary PPH) see Sections 18.10 and 19.11b.

TRY TO ANTICIPATE INFECTION. If you expect that infection will follow Caesarean section: (1) Give the patient the perioperative antibiotic regime in Section 2.9, and (2) consider doing an extraperitoneal Caesarean section (18.13).

If you do not do an extraperitoneal operation, put a pack in each paracolic gutter, and one or two above the incision between her uterus and her abdominal wall. Make a small incision in her uterus first, and suck out her infected liquor and meconium. After delivering the placenta, mop out her uterus, and remove all remnants of membranes and some decidua. After closing her myometrium, and before closing her uterine peritoneum, wash out her pelvis 2 or 3 times with warm saline or water. Repair her peritoneum, control bleeding meticulously, remove the packs and clean up very, very carefully.

Alternatively, and probably less satisfactorily, after doing an ordinary lower segment operation, insert corrugated rubber drains, about 3 fingers width, in each of her paracolic gutters, and lead them out loosely through incisions in her abdominal wall. Cut her peritoneum round these drains, and don't merely stretch it. Insert another good wide drain suprapubically. Make sure there is no remaining amnion in her uterus to prevent free drainage through her cervix. Some surgeons insert insert a fourth drain through her cervix into her vagina.

After you have done the Caesarean section close her peritoneum and rectus sheath with a single layer of interrupted through-and-through sutures of stainless steel wire, or strong monofilament, 1 cm apart, taking 1.5 cm bites each side of the wound (9-21). *Don't close her skin immediately; instead, close it by delayed suture (9.8).*

CAUTION ! Watch carefully for the first signs of infection—fever, and a large soft tender uterus with tenderness deep in her flanks.

IF INFECTION OCCURS, it may take the following forms. It can also cause secondary haemorrhage (3.10), or sterility (15.2). If you left packs or swabs in her abdomen, low-grade peritonitis may follow and obstruct her gut. See also 6.6D.

If pus forms around the wound (9.12), it may discharge through the scar into the cavity of her uterus. Infection may resolve, or you may need to drain pus suprapubically.

If she develops a pelvic abscess, manage it as in Section 6.3.

If pus forms in her peritoneal cavity and spreads upwards, manage her as for peritonitis (6.2, 6.6). Continue intravenous fluids, and gastric suction. Open her abdominal wound, and suck pus from all the cracks and crevices. If her general condition is poor, do this under local anaesthesia. You will probably find that her uterus is totally disrupted, so it is hopeless to try to repair it, and almost certainly fatal to try to remove it. If you do decide to do a hysterectomy, a subtotal operation will usually be enough—commonly with the removal of both adnexa, but retain one if you can.

Wash out her abdomen and instil tetracycline (6.2). Consider inserting four drains, one in each paracolic gutter, one down to the wound, and one through her cervix into her vagina, making sure that this last is not occluded by amnion. Close her abdomen with interrupted wire sutures and leave her skin wound open.

If she has a tender suprapubic mass, make a 5 cm muscle-splitting incision over it, as for appendicectomy. Open her peritoneum, insert a sump sucker, and sweep your finger round the inside of her peritoneum as far as you can reach. A litre of thin pus may escape. Stitch in a large drainage tube.

If she has signs of 'pus somewhere' (a hectic fever, malaise, and anorexia), but there are no obvious signs of it, suspect that she has a subphrenic abscess. This is a common late complication, and is likely to kill her if you don't drain it (6.4); so may multiple abscesses between loops of her gut (6.3).

If her abdominal wall bursts, and exposes her uterus, repair it.

If her fever recurs, and there are signs that more pus is collecting, do another drainage operation.

7 Pus in muscles, bones, and joints

7.1 Pyomyositis

This is a disease of disadvantaged tropical communities in which abscesses form in a patient's muscles. It is common between the ages of 5 and 25, and becomes less common as living conditions improve.

There are several syndromes in which large collections of pus form in the muscles. The first is much the most common. You may see:

Classical pyomyositis in which one or more of a patient's muscles becomes exquisitely painful, tender, and swollen, and the skin over it smooth and shining. A single muscle may be involved, or a group of them, or he may have several abscesses in different parts of his body. His larger muscles, such as those of his thighs, buttocks, shoulders, back, and abdominal wall are more often involved than his smaller ones. Infection makes them hard and indurated, so that movement is painful. Later, the signs of inflammation may subside as the infected muscle is replaced by pus and becomes fluctuant. Infection of the muscle limits the movement of joints nearby. If his abscess is large, he may occasionally be quite ill with fever and rigors. Lymph node involvement is not conspicuous.

Septicaemia associated with pyomyositis may be fatal and is often not diagnosed. He is very ill and drowsy, with a high fever, and multiple tender areas over his muscles. He may have a history of a trivial skin laceration, a blister, or a small sore. The condition rapidly progresses, so that he becomes desperately ill with a swinging fever, weakness, prostration, dehydration and hypotension.

Pyaemia associated with pyomyositis results in a sequence of abscesses in one muscle after another.

Staphylococci are usually responsible. Before pus forms, antibiotics alone may occasionally cure him; but you almost always have to drain it.

SITA (38) presented with fever and a vague, mild pain in her left hip, which was made slightly worse by movement. No malaria parasites were found and no definite diagnosis was made. She was treated with gentamicin and cloxacillin and her fever improved. Ten days later she returned with a huge abscess in her left inguinal region. This was incised and she recovered completely. LESSON Pyomyositis may cause large abscesses in the deeper muscles with few localizing signs.

PYOMYOSITIS

THE DIFFERENTIAL DIAGNOSIS includes osteomyelitis (7.2) and septic arthritis (7.16). The exact site of the tenderness and swelling will usually lead you to the correct diagnosis. There are several other possibilities which depend on the site of the abscess:

In the patient's upper abdomen, think of a kidney swelling, a perinephric abscess (5.11a), an amoebic liver abscess (31.12), a subphrenic abscess (6.4), or an acute abdomen.

In his lower abdomen, think of an appendix abscess, suppuration of his iliac glands (5.12), a psoas abscess, a strangulated inguinal hernia (14.6), or an acute abdomen.

In his loin, an inflammatory mass is more likely to be pyomyositis than a perinephric abscess or a pyonephros.

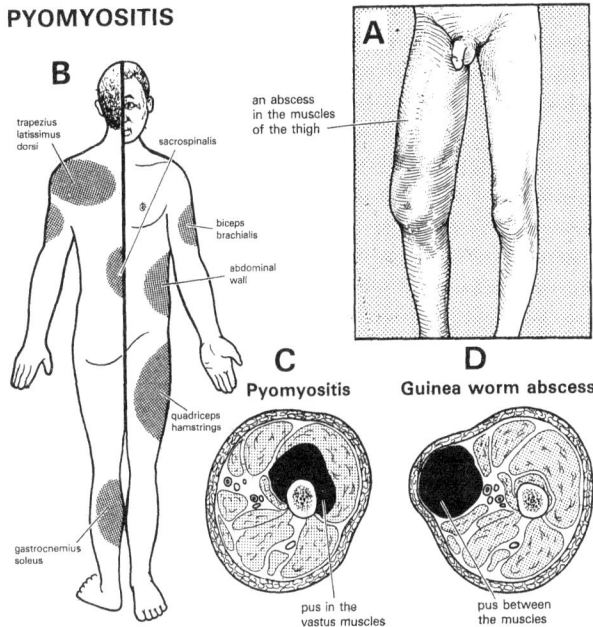

Fig. 7-1 PYOMYOSITIS. A, shows an abscess in one of the muscles of a patient's thigh. B, the common sites. C, the distinction between pus in the muscles (as in pyomyositis), and pus between them, as in an abscess round a dead Guinea worm, which is one of the differential diagnoses. *After Davey WW, 'Companion to Surgery in Africa', Figs. 11.2 and 11.5. Churchill Livingstone, with kind permission.*

If he has an abscess in his iliopsoas, his hip is flexed, and he resists all attempts to straighten it (5.12). Careful comparison with his normal side may show a swelling medial to his anterior superior iliac spine. An iliac abscess (5.12) may be the result of pyomyositis of his iliacus or psoas muscle, suppurating iliac adenitis, osteomyelitis of his spine (7.15), or septic arthritis of his hip (7.18). Lightly banging his greater trochanter with your clenched fist will cause him pain if he has septic arthritis or osteomyelitis, but not in the other conditions. Examining his back should distinguish osteomyelitis. The distinction of pyomyositis from iliac adenitis may be impossible and is not important (5.12).

In his thigh, think of acute osteomyelitis, guinea worm infection, a haematoma, or a sarcoma.

In his calf think of a deep vein thrombosis, or a sickle cell crisis with bone infarction.

INVESTIGATIONS If osteomyelitis is a possibility, X-ray the part, but don't expect any changes for 10 days. Drill it (7.5). Measure his haemoglobin before you operate.

MANAGEMENT depends on the severity of his disease:

If his pyomyositis is early, in that there is merely induration over a small area of muscle, antibiotics alone may cure him. Give him penicillin, or chloramphenicol (2.7).

If he has one or more well localized lesions drain them.

If he has signs of spreading infection, give him antibiotics and drain the lesions.

If he has a succession of abcesses (pyaemia), drain them as they appear, culture the pus, and give him an appropriate antibiotic as soon as you know the results of culture. Give him chloramphenicol meanwhile.

If he is very ill indeed with multiple tender areas over his muscles, give him intravenous chloramphenicol (2.7). Change to oral chloramphenicol as he improves. Drain his abscesses.

If necessary, correct his dehydration with saline or Ringer's lactate. If he is severely anaemic, transfuse him before you drain his abscess.

DRAINAGE. Give him ketamine or a general anaesthetic. If you are not sure if pus is present or not, aspirate it with a needle.

Make a small incision to begin with, if possible in the most dependent position, and open his abscess by Hilton's method (5-3). If it is large, extend the incision, so that you can insert your finger, break down any loculi and explore the whole cavity. Don't curette it. You may find a litre or more of pus.

If the bone feels rough and craggy at the bottom of the abscess cavity, it may be involved; if so, he has osteomyelitis, not pyomyositis.

DIFFICULTIES WITH PYOMYOSITIS

If BLOOD POURS FROM THE ABSCESS, pack the cavity tightly with gauze for 36 hours. If you don't curette an abscess, it is unlikely to bleed much.

If he has very MANY or very SEVERE lesions, you may have to make 20 or more incisions, with repeated visits to the theatre, to evacuate pus and remove dead muscle.

If he has BLACK NECROTIC SKIN, removing it may reveal a huge quantity of avascular greyish-pink, mushy suppurating muscle extending deeply underneath. Remove this, taking care: (1) not to injure vital structures, (2) not to let him lose more blood than he can stand. His life depends on aggressive (but not too aggressive) surgery, intensive antibiotic treatment, and fluid replacement. Even so, he stands a good chance of dying. If you have had to remove much muscle, he will inevitably be left with weakness, deformity, and loss of function—a worthy price to pay for survival.

If he has FEVER and RIGORS after drainage, he is septicaemic, and may form new abscesses.

If he has any tendency to develop CONTRACTURES, apply skin traction (70.10) or a cast, as appropriate.

7.2 The pathology of osteomyelitis

Osteomyelitis is a particularly tragic preventable disease, which has almost disappeared from the industrial world, where it was once common, particularly among the poor. It is now almost entirely a disease of the disadvantaged children of the developing world, whom it often disables for life if it is treated late or inadequately. You can only treat osteomyelitis satisfactorily if you treat it *early*. Later treatment is difficult, expensive, and time-consuming.

There are several kinds: (1) Haematogenous osteomyelitis in which bacteria reach bone through the circulation, and which is the concern of most of this chapter. (2) Traumatic osteomyelitis, particularly following road accidents and war injuries, in which bacteria reach bone through a badly treated open fracture, as the result of: (a) an inadequate wound toilet (54.1), and (b) immediate instead of delayed wound closure (54.4). One of the main purposes of Chapter 54 is to prevent this preventable disaster, so nothing more will be said about it here. (3) Osteomyelitis following unskilled orthopaedic procedures in unsterile theatres, particularly the fixation of femur fractures with Kuntscher nails. The fracture methods described in Volume Two minimize this risk, and about the only possibility of it occurring with the methods described there is the osteomyelitis of the upper tibia that may occasionally follow the insertion of a Steinmann pin for skeletal traction (78.6). Fortunately, this is usually mild and localized.

Acute haematogenous osteomyelitis is a surgical emergency. It is also the supreme example of the axiom—'Where there is pus let it out'. Your challenge is to drill the site of infection and

THE PATHOLOGY OF OSTEOMYELITIS

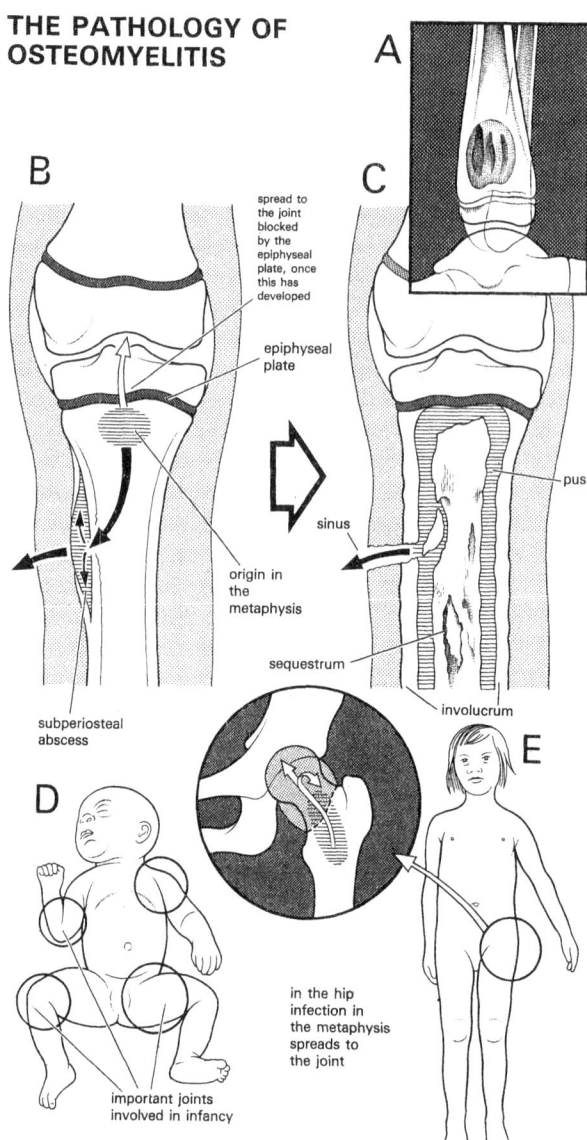

Fig. 7-2 THE PATHOLOGY OF OSTEOMYELITIS. A, Brodie's abscess is an uncommon form of chronic osteomyelitis: the upper end of the tibia or the lower femur are the common sites. B, the initial infection in osteomyelitis is typically in the metaphysis. After the age of 6 months the epiphyseal plates have developed sufficiency to prevent infection spreading to the joints, except in the hip. Before this age infection spreads to the joints. C, chronic osteomyelitis with sequestra and a sinus. D, under the age of 6 months osteomyelitis is always associated with septic arthritis. E, osteomyelitis of the proximal femur is always associated with septic arthritis, regardless of the age of the patient, because the epiphysial line is intracapsular.

to let out the pus *before it causes pressure necrosis of the bone, and to do so with the least possible delay.* If you don't explore an infected bone early enough, or don't explore it at all, the patient may be severely disabled. Drilling is not difficult; but the sequestrectomy that may be necessary later if you fail to drill it will be very difficult.

Staphylococci are usually responsible. But if osteomyelitis complicates sickle-cell disease, or some other haemoglobinopathy, other organisms may cause it, particularly *E. coli* (common) and *S. typhi* (rare). If the patient is a neonate, streptococci or enterobacteria may be infecting him. The metaphysis of a long bone is the usual site. In decreasing order of frequency you are likely to see osteomyelitis in the proximal tibia, the distal femur, the proximal femur, the proximal end of the humerus, the distal radius or ulna, the distal tibia, or the calcaneus. But any bone can be involved, and sometimes several of them at the same time.

Infection thromboses the end arteries of a metaphysis, and so kills the bone that they supply. Pus accumulates under pressure, breaks out through a hole in the bone, and comes to lie under the periosteum. Pus then strips the periosteum off the shaft and deprives part of the bone of its blood supply, so that it dies and forms a sequestrum. The stripped periosteum responds by producing new bone, which is the beginning of the involucrum. Later, this may become so extensive that it forms a new shaft. If the disease progresses, large areas of bone, and perhaps even its entire shaft, become separated from their blood supply, die, and form one or more sequestra. These lie inside the involucrum, bathed in a pool of pus, which discharges through sinuses in the skin.

Occasionally, the disease does not go through this acute stage, and does not form sequestra, or sinuses. Instead, the infected bone becomes sclerotic, and its marrow cavity is obliterated (Brodie's abscess, A, Fig. 7-2).

Before the age of six months an epiphysis offers no barrier to the spread of infection, so that pus in a metaphysis rapidly spreads to a joint. After this age the cartilage of an epiphyseal plate limits the spread of infection, so that a joint is only infected if an infected metaphysis extends inside a joint capsule, as in the proximal femur. Osteomyelitis is uncommon later in life, after the epiphyses have fused.

JOHN (6 years) was admitted late on a Saturday night, in the days before antibiotics, to a London teaching hospital, with the typical symptoms of osteomyelitis. There was no registrar, so the house surgeon consulted his chief (who had gone off for the weekend) over the telephone and was told to 'Keep the boy until Monday morning'. By then it was too late. The boy was ill-nourished and from a poor home; he just went down and down, running pus from his joints, and getting thinner and thinner, until his iliac crests broke out through his skin, and one iliac epiphysis dropped off. He finally died of amyloid disease of his liver. LESSON This boy became a byword and a terrible example throughout the hospital of what can happen if osteomyelitis is 'cooked', and pus under pressure is not drained (a story told by H Leader Stirling).

You will need a bone drill (70.11), and you will find a pneumatic tourniquet useful. Here are the instruments you will need to remove sequestra.

- OSTEOTOME, Swedish model, solid forged stainless steel, (a) 6 mm. (b) 10 mm. One only of each size. Use these for cutting the bones of children. An adult's bones are too hard to be cut by an osteotome alone. Weaken them first with a line of drill holes.

- NIBBLER, bone, Read Jensen, one only.

- GOUGES, Swedish model, solid forged stainless steel, (a) 6 mm, (b) 10 mm. One only of each size. These curved bone chisels must be sharp. If necessary, get them sharpened on a grindstone. Use them for deepening a cavity in a bone.

- MALLET, stainless steel, 350 g, one only. This an adequate size of mallet, there is no need for a larger one.

- BONE FILE or rasp, one only.

- FORCEPS, bone cutting, Liston, angled on flat, 200 mm, one only. These are general-purpose bone cutters. You can also use them instead of special rib cutters.

- FORCEPS, bone-holding, Hey Groves, 210 mm, one only. This is for small bones, such as the radius.

- FORCEPS, bone-holding, Lane's 390 mm, one only. This is a heavier pair of forceps for larger bones such as the tibia.

- FORCEPS, sequestrum, angled, 190 mm, one only. These are slender, angled forceps to remove sequestra.

- CURETTE, or scoop, Volkmann, double ended, size C, four only. Use this to curette infected bone when you operate for osteomyelitis.

- LEVERS, bone, Trethowan, 220 mm, four only. Put these round a bone to expose it.

- LEVERS, bone heavy, 275 mm, four only

- HOOK, bone, 220 mm, one only

- ROUGINE, Faraboef, with curved end, chisel edge, one only. Use this to scrape the periosteum from a bone.

- ELEVATOR, periosteal, large, one only.

7.3 Acute osteomyelitis

Typically, a child from a poor family living under very unhygienic conditions presents with fever and *an exquisitely painful tender bone*

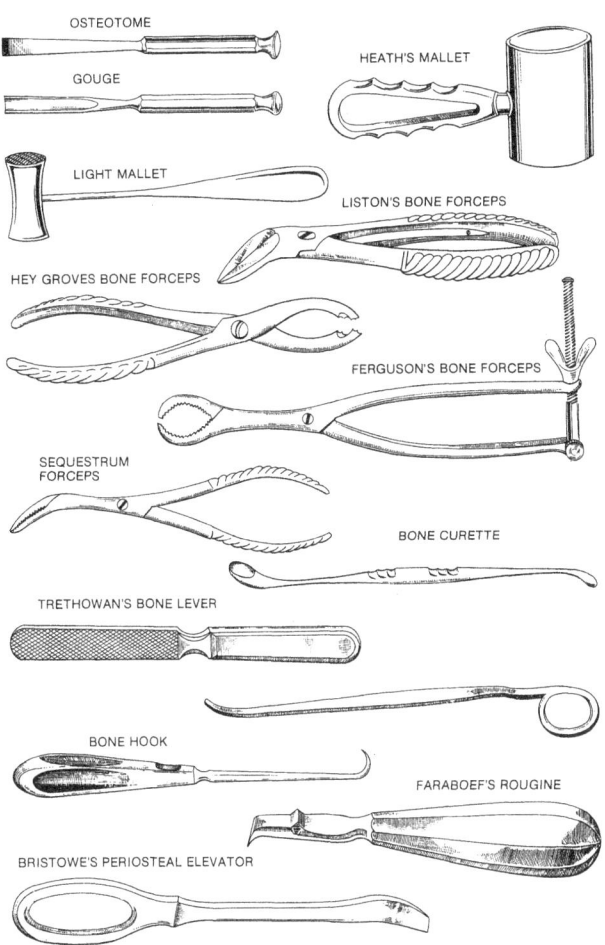

Fig. 7-3 INSTRUMENTS FOR CHRONIC OSTEOMYELITIS. The most important instrument for diagnosing early osteomyelitis—the bone drill—is shown in Fig. 70-12.

near a joint which he is unwilling to move. Or, his mother may bring him to you with fever, pain, and a limp. When you first see him the tender area will probably not yet have started to swell. Soft tissue swellling is a late sign which shows that pus has already started to spread out of the bone.

Unfortunately, many children present late after they have already sought help from traditional practitioners. Often, the history is atypical and may be misleading: (1) There may be no history of an acute illness; the first sign may be a boil-like lesion which discharges spontaneously or is incised, and which is followed by a chronically discharging sinus. (2) If an infant is very ill, he may have no fever and few general signs of infection. (3) He may have signs of a severe general infection, but few local signs. So beware of osteomyelitis *in any ill child who is not using one of his limbs.*

X-rays are of little help in the early stages because periosteal elevation, and bone rarefaction, which are the first signs, do not appear until after infection is established—if the patient is over 15 years *you may not see them for 10 days*. Later, you will see new bone laid down under the periosteum, and patchy rarefaction. In neonates bone changes appear about the 5th day, but even this is too late for diagnosis and treatment at the optimum time.

The only sure way to confirm or exclude osteomyelitis is to *incise the periosteum and drill the bone—urgently*. In an early case fluid under pressure comes out of the hole, but this soon becomes pus. Only if nothing comes out can you be sure that a child has not got osteomyelitis—in that bone. Many doctors are only used to soft tissue surgery—they don't like drilling bone and look upon it as specialized orthopaedics. The main message of this chapter is that *you must drill urgently and early!* If you don't have a surgical drill, use a carpenter's drill. Unlike acute ostemyelitis, operations for chronic osteomyelitis are never urgent, and you may be able to refer the patient.

Do your utmost to drain pus from a patient's infected bone *before it has stripped the periosteum off the shaft*. After this has happened, the bone can only heal by forming a sequestrum and an involucrum, with all the disability that this causes. Early treatment needs early diagnosis, so everyone who provides primary medical care must be aware of osteomyelitis. Make sure that your staff in the clinics know about it, and immediately refer any child with fever and a painful limb which is not obviously pyomyositis. Because of the common practice of giving antibiotics and seeing if the patient improves, osteomyelitis is apt to be one of the worst treated diseases in primary care. One reason why it is such an important disease in the developing world, whereas it has almost disappeared elsewhere, is that patients are so often referred to hospital late, after they have been mismanaged in peripheral units.

Any of the diseases in the list below can cause pain, fever, and inability to move a limb. Local redness and oedema are later signs. The important decision is not what the exact diagnosis is, but whether you should drill or not. The site of the greatest tenderness (at the end of a metaphysis near a joint) is a useful point of differential diagnosis, and so is the young age of the patient. The tenderness is localized and is greatest on direct pressure and percussion.

MURARULAL (9 years) was brought in by his mother with a one-day history of a limp. He was tender over his right fibula and had a mild fever, but no other signs, and no X-ray changes. The diagnosis was uncertain, so his his fibula was explored. It looked normal when it was exposed, but even so it was drilled. Pus came out under pressure. His wound was dressed and left open and he was given an antibiotic. He rapidly improved and his wound healed spontaneously. A month later he had no limp and no discharge, but an X-ray showed periosteal elevation. A year later his X-ray was normal.

BUROO (8 years) was admitted with a swelling over the upper end of her right tibia for 4 days. A small abscess pointed. This was incised and drained. A week later an X-ray was taken and considered normal. After three months of antibiotic treatment, her wound was still discharging, and X-rays showed obvious chronic osteomyelitis. LESSON (1) If osteomyelitis is a possibility, drill the bone, especially the upper tibia. (2) Drill it even if it looks normal when you expose it. If Buroo's bone had been drilled early, she would have been spared many years of disability. (2) When you have found pus, leave the wound open.

FEVER AND A TENDER BONE ARE THE CRITICAL SIGNS

DIAGNOSING OSTEOMYELITIS

If a child is acutely tender over a bone, he has osteomyelitis until you have proved otherwise. If his mother tells you that he has had an injury, remember that she may be wrong, and have invented an injury to explain his symptoms. 50% of patients with osteomyelitis have a history of minor trauma to the affected limb within 14 days of the onset of infection. X-rays don't help in the early diagnosis of osteomyelitis (see above), but they will exclude a fracture.

If she complains that he is ill and is not using a limb, poliomyelitis is a possibility, but there is no swelling and no bony tenderness.

If the tenderness is in his soft tissues, rather than over a bone, he is more likely to have cellulitis or pyomyositis than osteomyelitis.

If his lower leg is swollen, oedematous, tender and warm, but the tenderness is not particularly localized over a bone, should you explore it or not? Its exact site may help you to decide. If you are still in doubt, be safe—drill. You will probably operate on some cases of cellulitis unnecessarily, but if you don't operate, you will miss osteomyelitis.

If the point of maximal tenderness is over a joint, not over the adjacent bone, and all its movements are exquisitely painful, he probably has a primary septic arthritis. Aspirate his joint and if necessary, drain it.

If he has fever and an acutely painful hip which he refuses to move, he has osteomyelitis of the neck of his femur with

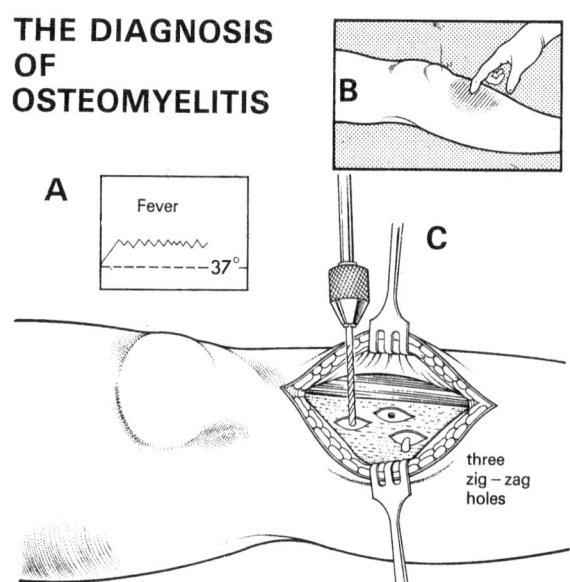

THE DIAGNOSIS OF OSTEOMYELITIS

Fig. 7-4 DIAGNOSING OSTEOMYELITIS. A, and B, the critical signs are fever and a painful tender bone, especially close to an epiphysis. C, the only way to confirm or exclude osteomyelitis is to drill the bone. If a patient comes when pus is already present, he is too late to be easily cured, so try to diagnose osteomyelitis *before* this stage.

septic arthritis (they are in effect the same disease). Aspirate to confirm that pus is present (7.17). Drill his upper femur and its neck, and drain his hip (7.18).

If his muscles are swollen and tender, he probably has pyomyositis—feel the site of tenderness carefully.

If sickle-cell disease is common in your district, suspect that infarction of the bone which is common in this condition may be causing his symptoms if: (1) Several of his bones are involved. (2) An unusual bone is involved, such as his skull, or the small bones of his hands or feet, particularly if he is an infant. Osteomyelitis can complicate avascular necrosis, so he may have both diseases. There is no certain way of distinguishing a sickle-cell crisis from osteomyelitis except by drilling. An SS patient is usually obvious clinically, but SC patients (quite common in West Africa) are not. If he is a sickler, a wait of 24 hours is reasonable, because the pain of an infarct improves rapidly.

If lesions in his hands are causing diagnostic difficulties, remember that: (1) Tuberculous dactylitis is much less painful than sickle-cell dactylitis. (2) Syphilis will probably show abundant new bone-formation elsewhere.

If his disease is some weeks old, but there are no signs of new bone-formation on his X-ray, suspect that he has tuberculosis, or AIDS, or both. This is most likely to be a diagnostic problem in the spine. Tuberculosis usually forms no new bone, whereas chronic pyogenic osteomyelitis is more likely to. Patients with AIDS make very little involucrum.

If there is much swelling, but not much fever, suspect that he may have a sarcoma, which can mimic subacute osteomyelitis and may cause fever. X-rays should distinguish it. Confirm it by biopsy.

If he has pain in many joints, he probably has a rheumatic polyarthritis. Rheumatic fever and parvovirus infections are other acute and subacute causes.

If he has any other septic lesion, such as a carbuncle or middle ear disease, suspect this may be the source of his osteomyelitis.

If the diagnosis is still difficult, consider brucellosis, yaws, syphilis, and leprosy.

7.4 The general method for osteomyelitis

In the developing world osteomyelitis almost never presents early enough for antibiotics to cure it, so drill *all* patients in whom you suspect it—unless they happen to be so privileged that you see them within 24 hours of the start of symptoms.

As soon as you have taken pus for culture, give antibiotics systemically in high doses. Sterilizing a patient's infected bone takes a long time, so continue to give them in adequate doses for 2 weeks in acute cases, or 3 to 6 weeks in chronic ones—if the organisms remain sensitive. Antibiotics are of limited value in chronic osteomyelitis, especially if there is a sequestrum, so don't waste them—they are no use after 6 weeks. Give them again as short-term cover when the patient has a sequestrectomy.

You have three ways to find the organism responsible—from a blood culture, from the pus, and from any septic lesion that might have been the source of his infection. If you cannot culture the organism, at least stain the pus to find out if Gram-positive cocci or Gram-negative bacilli are responsible.

In an area in which antibiotics have not been used, penicillin may be the drug of choice. Unfortunately, the staphylococci of most districts have become resistant to it, so that chloramphenicol is likely to be the most practical drug. Cloxacillin is an alternative, but is usually more expensive. Sensitivities differ from one district to another, so adjust your treatment accordingly. Even if you have no facilities for culture, other hospitals may have, so ask them what organisms they find, and what antibiotics they use.

IF YOU SUSPECT OSTEOMYELITIS—DRILL!

THE GENERAL METHOD FOR ACUTE
OSTEOMYELITIS

EXAMINATION. Look for a septic lesion anywhere, but especially on the child's skin, from which the infection may have spread. If you find one, culture it.

BLOOD CULTURES. If he is febrile, take a blood culture (if you can), and preferably 2 more at 2-hourly intervals, before you start antibiotic treatment. If treatment has already started, they will probably be negative.

X-RAYS should always be taken, because they will give you a baseline against which to assess future changes. Expect no bony changes for 10 days in an older child, or 5 days in an infant. Examine the edge of his bone with care—the earliest sign is the faintest second line of new bone about a millimetre away from the shaft. You will see this more easily if you look at the film obliquely.

TOURNIQUET. A bloodless field will make the operation much easier (3.9). Elevate his limb first. Don't use an exsanguinating bandage, because this may spread the infection.

CAUTION ! Avoid using a tourniquet on an SS or a CS sickler—his diagnosis should be obvious clinically. In practice, no harm follows from using one on an AS sickler. So, if your's is a high sickle-cell district, there is no need to test everyone for sickling before you apply one, even if it is practical, unless haemoglobin C is present in your community.

WHITE COUNT. This will show a polymorph leucocytosis and a shift to the left.

NEEDLE ASPIRATION may be useful in deciding where to drill. Unfortunately, if pus is present under the periosteum the patient has presented late. Good results are obtained by drilling bone earlier than this. Aspiration is also useful for diagnosing septic arthritis, but not for treatment. It is *no substitute for drilling or for draining a joint!*

CAUTION ! (1) Explore his bone, as in Section 7.5, whether or not you find pus. (2) Failure to aspirate pus does NOT exclude osteomyelitis! The indication for drilling is the *suspicion* of osteomyelitis!

SPLINTS. If necessary, splint his limb in the position of function, or use skin traction for a leg.

GENERAL CARE. If necessary, correct his dehydration. Ease his pain with analgesics.

ANTIBIOTICS. Start these immediately after you have taken a swab of pus from the drill hole, and if possible a blood culture also.

If you have been able to drain the lesion early and it is clinically quiescent, and there is no bone necrosis, 2 or 3 weeks' treatment will be enough.

Before you know the results of culture, or if culture is impossible, give him oral chloramphenicol 10 mg/kg 6-hourly, or 50 mg/kg/24 hours. If possible give it intravenously for the first 24 hours. Monitor his white count. Other possibilities are: (1) Intravenous benzyl penicillin, the adult dose being half a megaunit 6-hourly. Give children 25,000—90,000 units/kg/24 hours. Divide the daily dose into 6 and give it 6 times a day. (2) Any antibiotic which is effective against the common staphylococci in your district. This might be cloxacillin or trimethoprim.

CAN AN OPERATION BE AVOIDED? Almost certainly not. If he has had symptoms for less than 24 hours, and, after 24 hours on antibiotics, he is showing obvious local and general signs of improvement, antibiotics alone *may* cure him. Drill all other cases. Although fever and local tenderness may be improving, the infection in his bone may still be continuing, so the lesion needs draining. If he is not obviously improving on antibiotics, don't delay operation more than 24 hours. You are unlikely to see these really early cases.

7.5 Exploring a bone for pus

If you suspect that a patient has osteomyelitis, the critical procedure is to drill his painful tender bone. There is little point in aspirating it first, except sometimes to localise the site, because you will have to drill it anyway, even if aspiration is negative. If you don't find pus, or tissue fluid under pressure when you drill, you can now be sure he has not got osteomyelitis in that part of that bone, and you have done him no harm.

Although a single drill hole will drain a small abscess, it will not drain a large one, so if your drill finds pus, drill a line of at least three staggered holes at least 1 cm apart in the length of his bone. If you find pus under his periosteum, you may find that it has made its own hole in the bone: if this is big enough there is no need to drill.

NEVER HESITATE TO DRILL FOR PUS

EXPLORING ACUTE OSTEOMYELITIS

INDICATIONS. Operate on any patient, particularly a child with a history of 48 hours or more of fever and a painful bone.

EQUIPMENT. A general set (4.12). One light-toothed dissecting forceps. One light plain dissecting forceps. Four light bone levers. Four heavy bone levers. One periosteal elevator. A bone drill, or a carpenter's twist drill with a 4 mm bit: don't use a smaller one.

ANAESTHESIA. Mark the tender area on his skin before you anaesthetize him. Give him ketamine or a general anaesthetic. If he is a sickler, give him 50% oxygen, make sure that he wakes quickly postoperatively, and leave an airway in until he is fully awake.

A TOURNIQUET should always be used, if the site makes it possible—see Section 7.4.

INCISION Expose his bone on either side of the point of greatest tenderness. Try to incise over a bony surface which is covered with muscle, rather than one which is covered only with skin. Make the incision long enough, and start it at the epiphysis. Incise his oedematous subcutaneous tissues.

If you find pus in his muscles away from the bone, don't automatically think that he has pyomyositis. Explore deeper by blunt dissection and make sure that the pus is not arising in his bone, and has escaped into his muscles. If the pus is close to the bone, it is probably coming from a subperiosteal abscess. Use bone levers to retract his soft tissues.

If you don't find pus in his muscles, continue your incision down to the periosteum. Incise it longitudinally.

If pus immediately floods up from under his periosteum, there are three possibilities: (1) If there is no obvious hole, drill; it will help drainage. (2) If there is a big hole, the bone is already adequately decompressed, so there is no point in drilling. (3) If there is a small hole, drilling may help pus to drain.

Drill a minimum of 3 holes into the bone in a lazy zig-zag line, starting about 1 cm from the epiphyseal line and at least 1 cm apart. Make a separate small incision in the periosteum for each drill hole. Drill vertically, not obliquely, because drilling will be easier. If no pus or tissue fluid under pressure comes out, he has probably not got osteomyelitis—provided you really have drilled the tender area.

If pus flows from the first hole, send a specimen for culture. Drill two or more holes 1 cm apart in a lazy zig-zag line down the shaft of his bone until only blood or tissue fluid flows out of the hole from healthy bone.

Close most of the wound loosely with a corrugated drain, in the most dependent part of the wound.

CAUTION ! (1) Don't elevate his periosteum, because the bone under it will die. (2) Don't elevate too much muscle either, because periosteum receives its blood supply from the muscles over it. (3) Don't incise his periosteum beyond his epiphyseal line, or you may spread the infection to his epiphysis. (4) Don't remove any periosteum, because the bone under the raw area will not regenerate. (5) Never drill a row of holes across a bone, because they weaken it. (6) A single drill hole will not drain an abscess sufficiently.

POSTOPERATIVELY, if there is any danger that the bone might break, apply a plaster gutter splint. In his lower femur or upper tibia, apply skin traction. If his limb is painful, elevate it.

If at 2 weeks, the lesion is clinically quiescent, and X-rays show no bone necrosis, stop antibiotics. Otherwise continue them for a maximum of 6 weeks. Follow him up for 3 months; if his X-ray is normal then you need not see him again.

CAUTION ! If the bone is very osteoporotic, apply a cast before he is discharged to prevent a pathological fracture, especially if his leg is involved.

DIFFICULTIES WITH ACUTE OSTEOMYELITIS

If a child has X-RAY CHANGES WHEN YOU FIRST SEE HIM, chronic osteomyelitis will follow. Proceed as above: pus in his tissues or under his periosteum will need draining. If, when you open his periosteum, you cannot see any obvious holes in his bone, drilling it will still be useful.

If he is UNDER 6 MONTHS, osteomylitis arising in the metaphysis is inevitably complicated by septic arthritis. Drain the joint also. Bone necrosis is less likely, because the arteries are not end arteries.

7.6 Chronic osteomyelitis

Try to refer all patients with chronic osteomyelitis—surgery is difficult, bloody, and dangerous. If you have to operate, do so only to relieve persistent pain or remove persistent sinuses, not merely to improve their X-rays. You will see two kinds of disease and some intermediate forms.

(1) The common form of chronic osteomyelitis with an involucrum and sequestra is the result of neglect, or treatment which was too late in the acute stage. At the right moment, when a patient's involucrum is sufficiently formed, he needs his sequestra removed and his sinuses curetted. To do this you will either have to enlarge the existing gap in his involucrum, or you will have to cut a window in it.

If an area of bone is abnormally dense on the X-ray, showing that it is dying or dead, it may be absorbed slowly if it is attached to existing healthy bone. But if it is lying free as a sequestrum it will it act as a foreign body and will not be absorbed, so you will have to remove it. Occasionally, you can remove a small sequestrum through a sinus, but you usually need to operate.

Don't remove a sequestrum until a patient has formed enough involucrum to make a new shaft for his entire bone. Deciding when

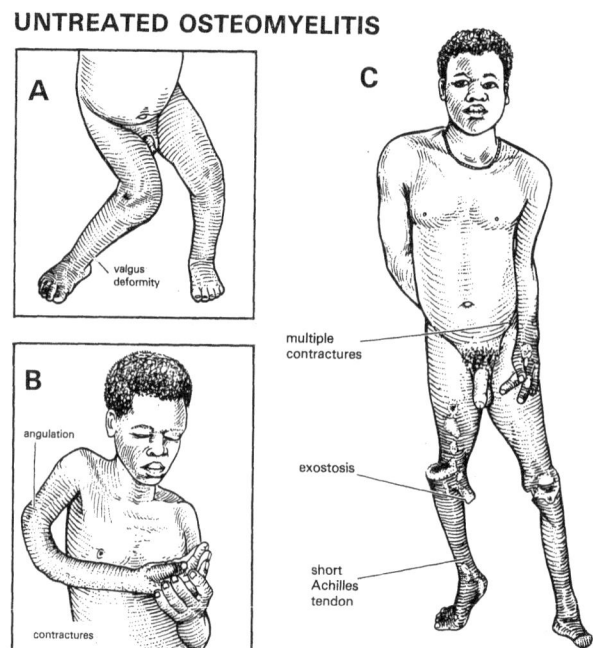

Fig. 7-5 UNTREATED OSTEOMYELITIS. A, late osteomyelitis of the knee with a severe valgus deformity. B, destruction of the humerus causing angulation, combined with contractures of the elbow and wrist. C, osteomyelitis in several joints. This patient could run with simple boots after his exostosis had been excised, and both his Achilles tendons had been lengthened. So save a patient's limb if you possibly can: amputation is almost always avoidable. *Kindly contributed by Ronald Huckstep.*

to operate is critical. Never remove a sequestrum until an X-ray shows that removing it will not leave a gap in his bone. Once you have removed a sequestrum no new involucrum will form. This is an important exception to the general rule that a foreign body should be removed immediately, especially in the presence of infection.

How can you encourage a strong involucrum to form? Encourage him to use his limb so that the newly growing bone of his involucrum is *gently* stressed, without being angulated or shortened. For example, in his femur put him into a hip spica, or a cast from his groin to his knee, give him crutches and allow cautious weight-bearing.

(2) Localized chronic osteitis without an involucrum, and usually with no sequestra (Brodie's abscess), takes the form of a cavity surrounded by dense sclerotic bone, and is much less common. The patient is usually an adult with a long history of localized bone pain, most often in his upper tibia or lower femur, usually without any history of an acute phase. His pain comes and goes, and gradually gets worse. When his infection flares up he has fever and a warm, painful, tender, thickened limb. X-rays show dense sclerotic bone surrounding a translucent abscess cavity. His marrow cavity is obliterated, he has no sinuses, and seldom any sequestra.

Antibiotics are unlikely to cure him. So, if you cannot refer him, explore, curette, and if possible saucerize the cavity. This will relieve his pain dramatically. If possible, leave it open to the outside, and let it granulate from the bottom. If not, leave it open to his soft tissues. If he is unwilling to accept an operation, try antibiotics for 3 weeks only.

Closing the hole in his leg. When you have removed a sequestrum, or cleared an abscess cavity, the hole that you have left behind will have to be filled somehow: (1) If you can, try to saucerize it, which means making a nearly flat surface against which muscle will lie, and eliminate any dead space. This is ideal, but is usually impossible. (2) If saucerizing it would require removing so much involucrum that it would unduly weaken the bone, make a deeper cavity, and accept dead space filled with blood clot, even though it is liable to become infected. Close it loosely with a drain. (3) You can line a gutter you have made in the tibia with a skin graft later. Don't try to make an elaborate flap, this is an expert's task.

An alternative method of closing the wound is said to have advantages under difficult conditions. Pack it with gentamicin-impregnated polymethyl methacrylate (PMMA) beads on a string ('Streptotal' beads, E Merck). Close the wound by primary closure, leave one bead outside, and pull out the string at 10 days. Get the patient up at 24 hours and consider discharging him before the beads are removed. Drains and frequent dressings are unnecessary.

Höök M, Lindberg L, 'The treatment of osteomyelitis with gentamicin-PMMA beads'. Tropical Doctor, 1987;17:157.

OPERATE FOR PAIN AND SINUSES, NOT FOR X-RAY APPEARANCES
DON'T REMOVE A LARGE SEQUESTRUM UNTIL THERE IS A STRONG INVOLUCRUM

SEQUESTRECTOMY

INDICATIONS. If possible refer the patient. If you cannot refer him, consider removing any sequestrum which you cannot remove through a sinus. Don't operate to remove a large sequestrum until: (1) The involucrum extends across the defect that will follow. (2) The involucrum is made of rigid bone. If you remove a sequestrum too early, involucrum will not form to bridge the gap. (3) His limb must be capable of being supported, either by the remaining healthy shaft, or by a sufficiently strong involucrum.

CAUTION ! If you remove the sequestrum too early the involucrum will stop making new bone, and will collapse, so that he has no hope of a sound limb.

SEQUESTRECTOMY

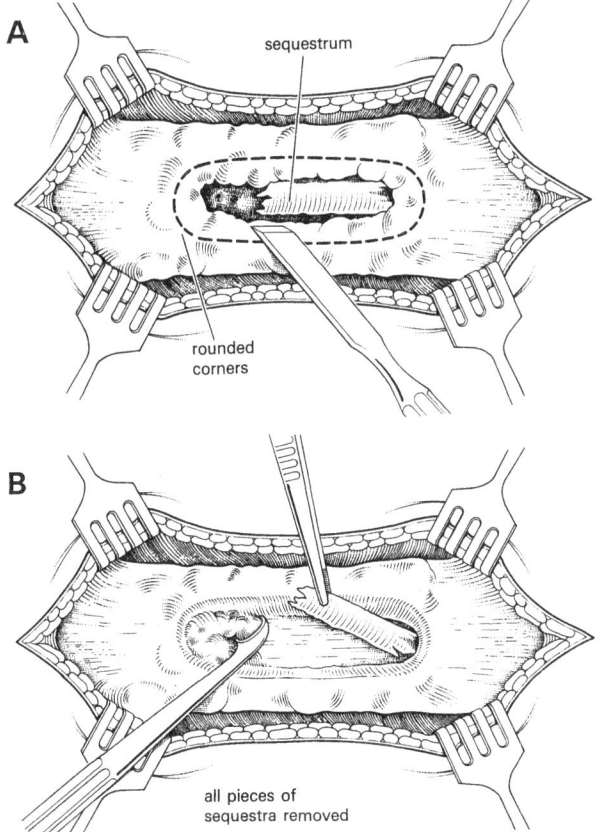

Fig. 7-6 SEQUESTRECTOMY. A, a sequestrum is presenting through a cloaca (hole) in the bone. B, the cloaca has been enlarged and the sequestrum is being removed. *Kindly contributed by John Stewart.*

ANTIBIOTICS. Culture the pus and give the appropriate antibiotic for at least 4 days before you operate, and for at least 2 weeks afterwards.

X-RAYS. Examine AP and lateral films carefully to see where the sequestra are. If ordinary films don't show enough detail inside the bone, take more with greater penetration.

METHYLENE BLUE may help to show up sequestra during an operation. Get it from the laboratory, sterilize a 1% solution, and inject it into the sinus 24 hours beforehand. It will stain everything blue, except the sequestra, which will remain white.

EQUIPMENT. As for acute osteomyelitis (7.5), plus 6 and 10 mm osteotomes and gouges; 10 and 15 mm chisels; a 250 g mallet, a Volkmann's scoop, a curved sequestrum forceps, and a bone nibbler. In the thigh you will need strong retractors, a strong assistant, and a good light. Sterile saline to flood the wound.

ANAESTHETIC. Ketamine (A 8.1) or general anaesthesia (A 10.1). Have blood cross matched, and a drip running.

TOURNIQUET. Bleeding can be alarming, because infected tissues are very vascular, so always use a tourniquet (3.9), unless you are operating on the patient's proximal femur or humerus, or he has sickle-cell disease (7.4). His anatomy may be very distorted, and if you don't use a tourniquet, important structures will be even more difficult to recognize. If you happen to see any vessels as you operate, tie them.

INCISION. Drape everything so as to leave only the operation site exposed. Wrap the distal part of his limb in a towel. Start by probing any sinuses to see where they go. They often go to the same place. Where possible, make one of the standard incisions described later. These are given for the entire length of the bone. *You will usually only need part of an incision.* Very often it will include the draining sinuses. If possible, make the incision over one of the larger gaps in the involucrum. The tissues will be tough, so use a sharp scalpel.

Open his indurated periosteum in the length of the incision, and elevate it on each side. Either: enlarge an existing gap in the involucrum with a gouge. Or: drill holes so as to outline a window, as in Fig. 7-6. Then open it with an osteotome.

CAUTION ! (1) Scar tissue may have disturbed the normal position of the nerves and arteries. (2) Don't break the bone. If you have carefully outlined the window with drill holes, this will be less likely.

Use a hammer and gouges or chisels to cut bits of bone from the involucrum until you get to his marrow cavity. Look for sequestra inside it.

Sequestra move separately from the surrounding involucrum. If they have been covered by tissues they are ivory white and have a brittle texture which is different from ordinary bone. If they have been exposed to the air they may be black or grey.

Use a hammer and gouge to chip away the involucrum around each sequestrum so that you can remove it. To minimize weakening, window the bone longitudinally. Round or taper the ends of the window; these will be stronger and allow it to fill with soft tissue more easily. Pull out sequestra with sequestrectomy forceps. If necessary, remove more involucrum to free a sequestrum. There will be pus, but usually not much.

When you have removed all the sequestra you can find, explore the abscess cavity up and down quite widely with a probe. If necessary, extend the skin incision and enlarge the hole in the involucrum until you have explored the whole cavity. Scrape the granulation tissue in its walls with a bone curette (Volkmann's spoon), until you reach healthy bone. If sinus tracts in the soft tissues are short, excise them. If they are long, curette them.

If bone overhangs the edge of the cavity, chisel it away. When necessary, flood the wound with warm saline and suck it out.

CAUTION ! (1) If the operation is to succeed, you must remove all sequestrated bone. The X-rays will suggest how much there is, but expect to find more.

CLOSURE. If possible, don't close the wound. Instead, leave it open and allow his soft tissue to fall into it, as in Fig. 7-10. Or, close the soft tissues loosely over the bone and keep the most dependent place open with a corrugated drain. Fix the drain to the wound with a stitch, because it may go inside the wound, get lost, and act as a foreign body.

If you leave the wound open, apply vaseline gauze followed by plenty of plain gauze.

If the wound is deep and large, pack it with ribbon gauze or a bandage.

Apply a pressure dressing for the first 48 hours, but watch his circulation distally. After some weeks there will be a floor of healthy granulation tissue, which will either epithelialize spontaneously, or can be grafted. As you change the dressings you will find that fewer are needed as it closes. A large wound takes a long time to close.

CAUTION ! (1) Vaseline gauze is a useful first dressing; thereafter use plain gauze. (2) Remove all the dressings you put into a wound. If any fragments remain, they will act as foreign bodies, and cause infection to persist. If you use pieces of gauze to pack a wound, knot them together, so that you can pull them all out at the same time.

POSTOPERATIVELY, the wound will ooze. If he is anaemic and ill, consider transfusing him, but remember the danger of HIV. Do all you can to improve his nutrition.

He will need quantities of sterile dressings. Change them daily at first, then twice a week, until his wound is small enough for you to treat him as an outpatient. Remove any dead tissue as necessary. Encourage him to use his limb, to walk with crutches without weight-bearing if the lesion was in the leg, and to use his arm as much as he can. In severe cases this active movement will encourage the periosteum to produce a really robust involucrum, which will not happen if he rests his limb completely.

If his involucrum might fracture, apply a cast and window it. Or, in the leg, apply skin traction. If a large area of bone has been destroyed, careful splinting is essential.

X-ray him at a convenient time postoperatively. This is only necessary to assess the strength of his leg for weight bearing, or, if sinuses persist, to look for more sequestra.

LOCALIZED OSTEITIS BRODIE'S ABSCESS

This is the sclerosing type of osteomyelitis. Follow most of the steps above. Use gouges and chisels to remove enough sclerotic bone to reach the abscess cavity. Curette it if you can; failing this, leave it with gently sloping edges. Pack the medulla with sterile gauze as described above.

DIFFICULTIES WITH CHRONIC OSTEOMYELITIS

If he BLEEDS SEVERELY into his dressings, take him back to the theatre, open the wound, tie off any bleeding vessels, repack it tightly, and apply a pressure bandage. Back in the ward raise his limb, and put a cradle over it, so that you can inspect it readily. Don't leave a pressure dressing in place for more than 48 hours, or it will promote infection.

If PUS CONTINUES TO DISCHARGE from his wound it may be due to: (1) Inadequate excision of fibrous tissue and curettage of the granulations. (2) Leaving sequestra behind. (3) Leaving a swab or piece of dressing or vaseline gauze in the wound. (4) Not opening up the cavity in the bone widely enough.

If his leg has united in a DEFORMED POSITION, accept it if you can.

If he has a PATHOLOGICAL FRACTURE, splint his limb in the correct position in a cast until it has healed soundly. While it is healing pay special attention to the alignment of his knee and ankle. Keep the wound open, dress and toilet it regularly. Skin traction is suitable for the femur and upper tibia, especially under the age of 14. Bone traction is contraindicated because you should not put a pin through bone if there is infection nearby. This may be unavoidable if there is significant shortening (unusual).

If you are wondering if AMPUTATION is justified, refer him for a second opinion before you do so. It may be indicated if: (1) The infection is so extensive that antibiotics and surgery have been unable to cure him. (2) So much bone has to be removed that his leg would work better with an amputation and a prosthesis. (3) His life is in danger from infection. (4) He is in constant pain.

If osteomyelitis has followed the ILL-ADVISED APPLICATION OF A PLATE, remove it. The only exception is an AO compression plate. If this is still maintaining compression, leave it. If it is holding a gap open between the fractured ends, remove it.

If he is an INFANT, his bone will probably heal well, even after you have removed a large sequestrum. If an operation is needed, don't hesitate to operate as soon as a satisfactory involucrum has formed.

If he has SICKLE-CELL DISEASE, he is likely to form new bone particularly slowly.

If he has ARC, (he is HIV-positive with weight loss and lymphadenopathy), he may have an unusual type of low-grade slowly progressive and sometimes multiple osteitis, with little sclerosis or involucrum and no large sequestra. Infection may spread from his tibia through his knee to his femur. Antibiotics have little effect, and you will probably have to amputate.

7.7 Osteomyelitis of the humerus

Osteomyelitis usually occurs at the ends of a patient's humerus, more often at the upper than the the lower end. You can expose and drill them through quite limited incisions; the upper end anteriorly and the lower end either anteriorly or posteriorly. If absolutely necessary (rare), and if you cannot refer him, you can expose his humerus from end to end by approaching it from the antero-lateral side.

The main danger is that you may injure his radial nerve, as it winds round his humerus posteriorly. If you are working near it, find it first so that you can avoid it.

Proximally, enter his arm between his pectoralis major and his deltoid. Distally, enter it between his brachioradialis and his biceps. As you do so, retract his radial nerve laterally, and his musculo-cutaneous nerve medially with his biceps.

OSTEOMYELITIS OF THE HUMERUS

Follow the general methods for osteomyelitis, in Sections 7.4 to 7.6. Always apply a tourniquet for operations on the middle (difficult in a young child) or lower third of the humerus.

PROXIMAL END. Approach this in the patient's deltopectoral groove. Find his cephalic vein, and try to displace it medially. If necessary, tie it proximally and distally.

Reflect his deltoid laterally, and expose his humerus by using two pairs of bone levers. Both the heads of biceps, and coracobrachialis lie medial to the insertion of the tendon of pectoralis major.

DISTAL END, POSTERIOR APPROACH. Make a midline incision in the posterior surface of his lower arm, and end it 3 cm above his epicondyles, so as to avoid his olecranon pouch. Don't extend the incision up into the middle third of his arm, or you will injure his radial nerve. Divide the tendon of his triceps and the muscle under it to expose his humerus.

DISTAL END, ANTERIOR APPROACH. Open his arm between his brachioradialis laterally, and his biceps medially, as in B, Fig. 7-7. Separate these muscles by blunt dissection, find his radial nerve and leave it laterally. Incise his brachialis medial to the nerve and expose his humerus. Retract his muscles by placing two pairs of bone levers subperiosteally.

If necessary, you can split his brachialis to within two fingers' breadth of his epicondyles without entering his elbow joint. Don't extend the incision beyond the flexor crease of his elbow, because you may cut his radial artery.

THE SHAFT OF THE HUMERUS. Refer him if you can. If you cannot refer him, put a sandbag under his shoulder on the same side. Drape his whole arm. Extend the approach to his upper humerus distally, or the lower anterior approach proximally.

Distally, divide the deep fascia to expose division between biceps and brachialis. His musculo-cutaneous nerve lies between these muscles. Displace it medially with his biceps. Separate his biceps and his brachialis and find his radial nerve. Above the origin of his brachialis, it lies between biceps and his triceps and winds posteriorly round his humerus in his radial groove.

Postoperatively, put his arm in a sling and encourage active movements within the confines of the sling, or apply a backslab.

EXPOSING THE ENDS OF THE HUMERUS

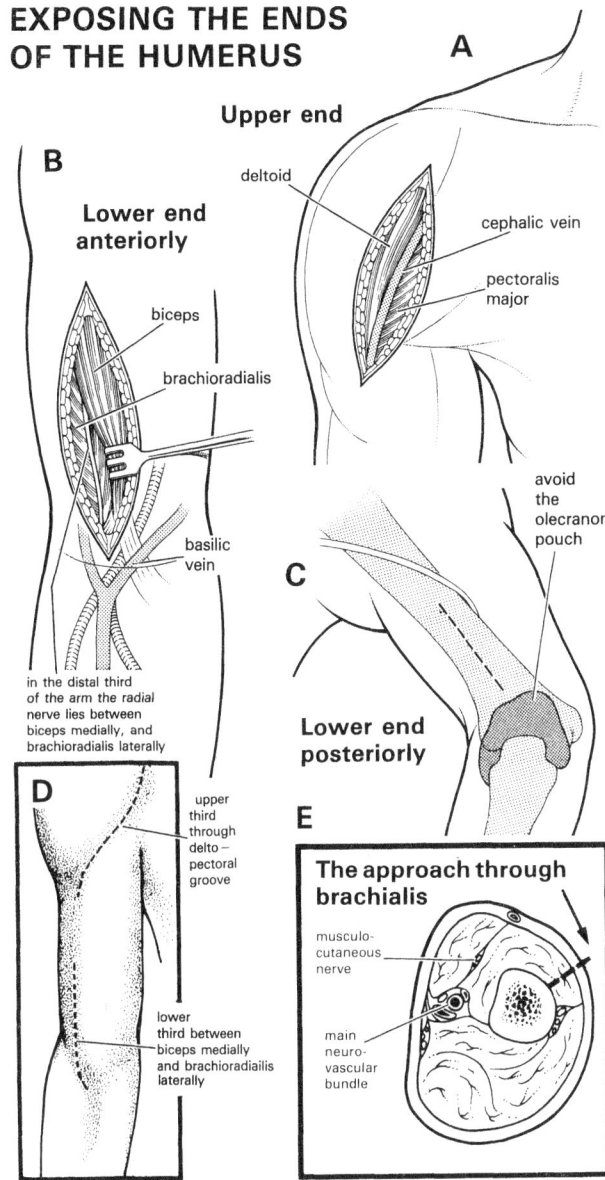

Fig. 7-7 OSTEOMYELITIS OF THE HUMERUS. A, the approach for the upper end. B, the anterior approach to the lower end. C, the posterior approach to the lower end. D, the incisions to approach the ends of the bone. E, a cross section a little below the mid point of the arm above the origin of brachioradialis, to show the approach to the middle of the shaft and the position of the radial nerve.

7.8 Osteomyelitis of the radius

You can expose the distal two-thirds of the shaft of a patient's radius by approaching it from its anterolateral side. The difficult part is its proximal third, which is covered by his supinator muscle, through which his posterior interosseous nerve passes. So avoid operating here if you possibly can. Enter his forearm between his brachioradialis laterally (it has a characteristic flat broad tendon) and his flexor carpi radialis medially. His radial artery lies between these two groups of muscles. Pronator teres is inserted into the middle of the radius. You can approach the bone on either side of this muscle, and displace it medially or laterally. Distally, pronator quadratus covers the radius, so you will have to divide it.

OSTEOMYELITIS OF THE RADIUS

Follow the general methods for osteomyelitis in Sections 7.4 to 7.6. Apply a tourniquet (3.9, 7.4).

Lie the patient on his back with his arm on a side table, and his forearm supinated. Define the line of the incision by identifying the tendons of his palmaris longus and his flexor carpi radialis at his wrist. Incise just lateral to his flexor carpi radialis. Cut here along the dotted line in B, Fig. 7-8. You will probably only need to incise over the distal third of the bone. If necessary, you can continue the incision proximally to include its middle third.

CAUTION ! Don't extend the incision to the proximal third, or you may injure structures on the front of his elbow.

Cut the deep fascia in the line of the skin incision. Tie any vessels you meet. Retract laterally the three muscles that lie along the lateral border of his forearm—brachioradialis, and extensor carpi radialis longus and brevis. When you retract them, his superficial radial nerve will be included with them. This is sensory only.

Find his radial artery and vein, which lie between the lateral group of muscles and flexor carpi radialis. Retract them laterally. You will now have exposed the anterolateral surface of the distal two-thirds of his radius.

Postoperatively, apply plaster only if a fracture threatens or has occurred. If so, apply a tubular forearm cast leaving his wrist and elbow free. The remaining bone will prevent angulation. Encourage him to use his arm.

7.9 Osteomyelitis of the ulna

The ulna is not uncommonly involved by haematogenous osteomyelitis. It has a subcutaneous border throughout its whole length, so it is easy to expose.

OSTEOMYELITIS OF THE ULNA

Follow the general methods for osteomyelitis in Sections 7.4 to 7.6. Apply a tourniquet.

Drape the patient's arm separately from his trunk. Make an incision anywhere from the tip of his olecranon to his ulnar styloid. Use part of the incision in C, Fig. 7-8, not all of it. Cut straight down on to the shaft of the bone and elevate his periosteum. This will carry the muscular origins of his flexor carpi ulnaris anteriorly, and those of his extensor carpi ulnaris posteriorly.

Postoperatively, apply plaster only if a fracture threatens or has occurred. If so, apply a tubular forearm cast leaving his wrist and elbow free. The remaining bone will prevent angulation. Encourage him to use his arm.

7.10 Osteomyelitis of the femur

This is common. If you make the diagnosis early, you need only drill the upper or lower end of a patient's femur, for which you will only need a limited incision. If you make the diagnosis late, osteomyelitis may have involved the entire shaft of the bone. If you approach it laterally, you can expose it from its greater trochanter to its lateral condyle. Cut straight through his vastus lateralis down to the bone. The head and neck of his femur are more difficult to reach. If osteomyelitis has involved the neck, which is partly inside the capsule of his hip joint, it will have also involved the head and his hip joint. This will need draining. You will find the anterior approach easiest for drilling the femoral neck (7.18). Refer him if you can.

Osteomyelitis of the femur commonly involves the hip joint, and occasionally the knee, but seldom both. When a child's knee is involved, his distal femoral epiphysis may slip. When this happens, the shaft of his femur usually slips anteriorly in front of the distal epiphysis—unlike trauma in which it slips posteriorly (79.16). Try to diagnose and treat him early; prevent further slipping by applying skin traction up to his mid thigh. You may need to manipulate him under anaesthesia.

THE SHAFT OF THE FEMUR

Follow the general methods for osteomyelitis in Sections 7.4 to 7.6. Cross-match two units of blood for the patient—this can be a bloody operation, especially if you go too far posteriorly.

EXPOSING THE RADIUS AND ULNA

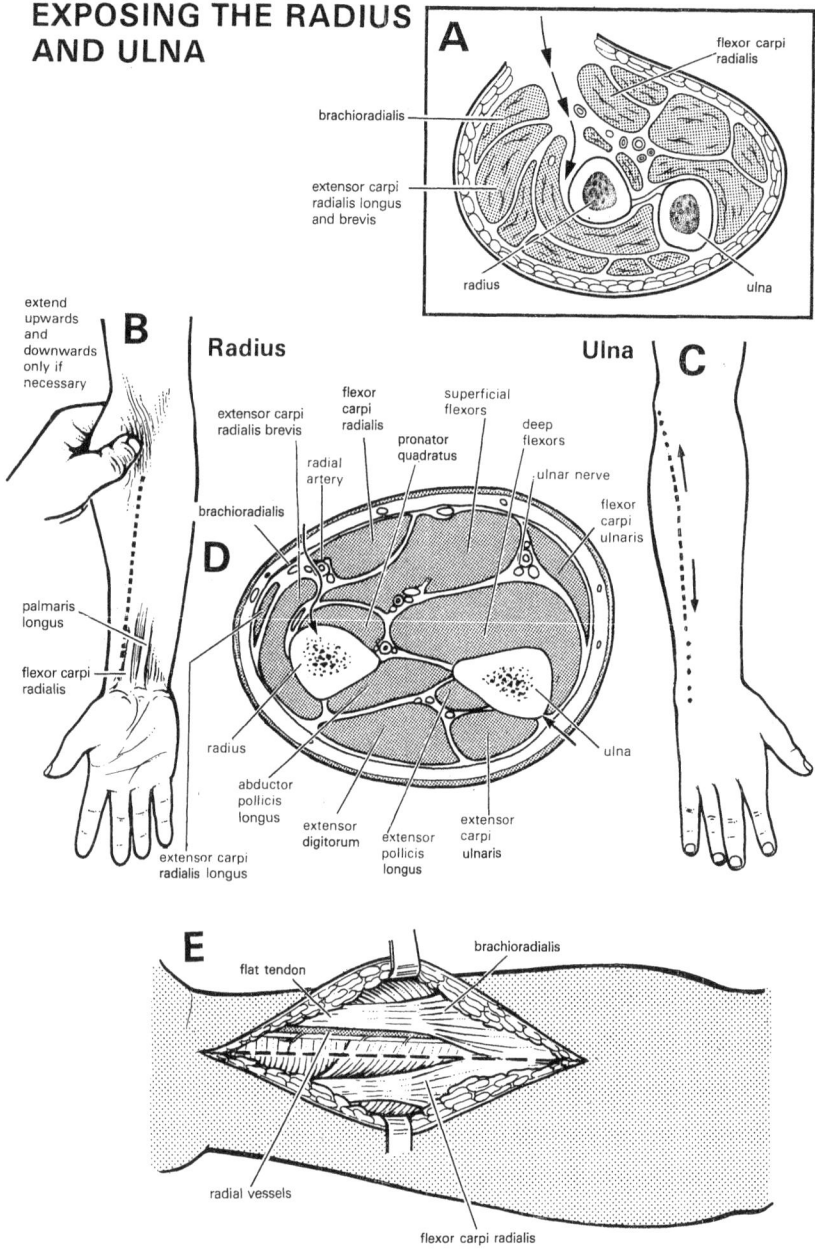

Fig. 7-8 EXPOSING THE RADIUS AND ULNA. A, a cross-section of the arm at the level of the radial tuberosity. A, B, and E, to expose the patient's radius, enter his forearm between his brachioradialis and his two radial wrist extensors laterally, and his flexor carpi radialis medially. Brachioradialis (E) has a long flat tendon, so you can recognize it easily. The ulna is subcutaneous, so you can approach it easily (C). D, a transverse section through the middle of the arm. E, brachioradialis and flexor carpi radialis, showing the incision for the lower part of the radius passing between them. Note: E, is schematic only, both tendons lie much more laterally in the arm. *Partly after Watson Jones, Longman, with kind permission.*

Lay him on his back with a sandbag under his hip on the infected side. Use a tourniquet when you operate on the middle or distal thirds of the bone.

Cut along the relevant part of the dotted line in A, Fig. 7-9. This extends from just distal to his greater trochanter to just above his lateral femoral condyle. Cut through his skin, subcutaneous fat, and fascia lata. Then cut straight through his vastus lateralis, down to the lateral side of the shaft of his femur. There will be some bleeding, but much less than there would be if you cut posteriorly on to his linea aspera.

CAUTION ! (1) Take care to stay on the lateral surface of his femur. (2) Avoid his linea aspera, and the vessels which run close to it. (3) Remember that a small child does not have the blood volume of an adult, and that in him the loss of a given volume of blood is proportionately more serious (53-3).

If you are operating towards the distal end of a patient's femur: (1) Don't enter his knee joint or his suprapatellar bursa. (2) Stay strictly on the lateral side of his knee. (3) Don't go posteriorly, or you may injure his lateral popliteal nerve. (4) Don't go medially because you may injure the main vessels.

If he bleeds from the vessels of his linea aspera, catch them with a haemostat, and transfix them with a ligature on a curved needle. Pass the needle round under the haemostat and the vessels at least twice. Pull the ligatures tight as you release the haemostat. They are usually too deep into the wound to tie on the tip of a haemostat. If you cannot reach a bleeding vessel, pack the wound tightly, raise the foot of the table and wait for the bleeding to stop.

Postoperatively, apply skin traction. This will be easier than applying a medial plaster splint, which is the alternative. Later,

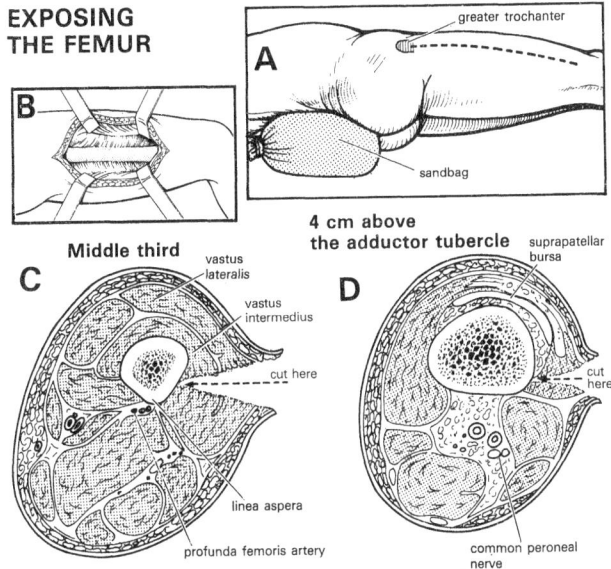

Fig. 7-9 EXPOSING THE FEMUR. You can expose a patient's femur by cutting straight down to it along the lateral side of his thigh. A, prop him up on a sandbag. B, the middle third of his femur exposed. C, a cross-section of the middle of his thigh. D, a cross-section about 4 cm above his adductor tubercle. *Kindly contributed by John Stewart.*

put him in a hip spica or a plaster cylinder from his groin to his knee, give him crutches, and encourage weight-bearing.

7.11 Osteomyelitis of the tibia

The tibia is one of the most common sites for osteomyelitis, which is fortunate, because it is one of the easier bones to approach. If you operate early, drill it through a short incision. If you operate late, don't do so before firm involucrum has formed, or you will leave a gap in the bone which will need extensive reconstructive surgery to repair. A gap is particularly likely in the tibia, because so much of it is subcutaneous.

CHEPESOK was a charming little Pokot girl of about 8 with osteomyelitis of her tibia. The stock of ketamine was finished, so, rather unusually, she was given a subarachnoid (spinal) anaesthetic. Half way through the operation she sat up and said "You will take out all the bad bone, won't you!" LESSONS (1) These can be very rewarding patients. (2) 'Primary Anaesthesia' considers childhood a contraindication to subarachnoid anaesthesia unless you are expert (A 7.4).

OSTEOMYELITIS OF THE TIBIA

Follow the general methods for osteomyelitis in Sections 7.4 to 7.6. Apply a tourniquet.

DRILLING. Make a linear incision 1 cm lateral to the anterior border of the patient's tibia, as in Fig. 7-10.

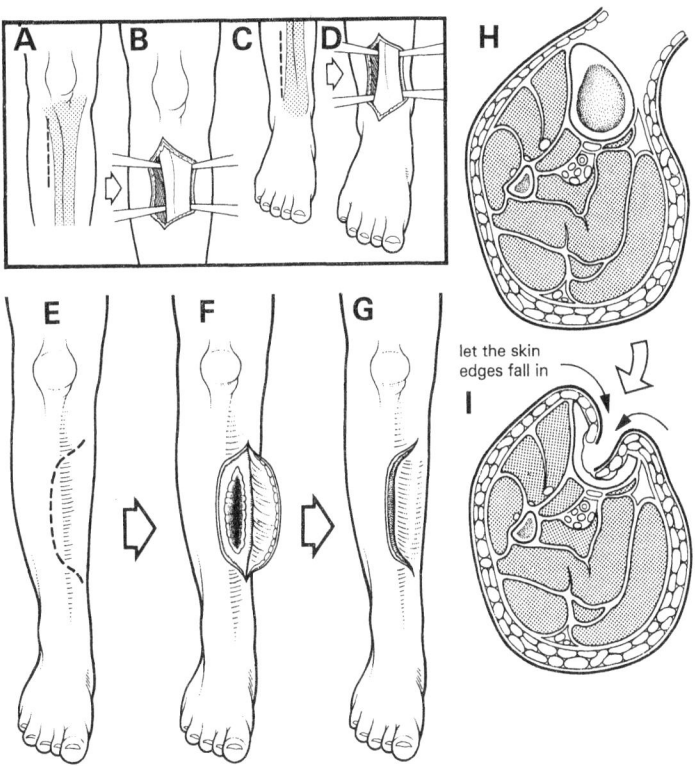

Fig. 7-10 OSTEOMYELITIS OF THE TIBIA. A, and B, exposing the upper end of a patient's tibia. Note that the incision has been made over muscle on the lateral side. C, and D, exposing his lower tibia; again the incision has been made over muscle on the lateral side. E, F, and G, exposing the shaft of his tibia. The main part of the incision has been made on the lateral side and a flap reflected medially. H, and I, allowing the edges of the flap to fall into the wound to close it postoperatively.

SEQUESTRECTOMY. Make the main part of the incision over his muscles rather than his bone. Make the longitudinal part of the incision 1 cm lateral to its anterior border. Proximally, don't extend it higher than his tibial tubercle. If possible, avoid taking it across his tibia where this is infected, because the scar from the incision will stick to the bone and become painful later. If necessary, curve its upper and lower ends to cross the anterior border of the bone.

Reflect his skin with his periosteum. They will probably be so closely bound together that you will be unable to separate them. Hold the skin flap lightly with skin hooks. Incise the periosteum midway between the anterior and posteromedial borders of the bone.

If the position of sinus tracks make it necessary, you can make a medial flap in the same way, with most of the length of the incision over the muscle on the medial side of his tibia.

After you have removed the sequestrum: (1) If the tissues are not too tight, you can close the wound lightly and insert a drain in its lower part. Or, (2) if the tissues are tight, you can let the skin edges fall into the wound and leave it unsutured, as in H, and I, Fig. 7-10. Healing will take longer like this. Apply a posterior slab or a long leg cast with his ankle in neutral, and his knee in 20° of flexion. Mark a window in it while it is still soft, cut out the window with a knife (70.2), or with a plaster saw 2 days later when it is hard. Dress the wound through this window.

If you have left a deep trough in the front of the tibia which is slow to granulate and epithelialize, graft it.

CAUTION! (1) Don't go directly anteriorly through the subcutaneous surface of his tibia. (2) Make sure your assistant retracts the skin flaps gently, because they can easily necrose.

Give him a long leg cast with a walking heel, then encourage early weight bearing with as normal a gait as possible.

DIFFICULTIES WITH OSTEOMYELITIS OF THE TIBIA

If there is a VERY LARGE SKIN DEFECT IN A PATIENT'S TIBIA which is slow to heal consider making relieving incisions about 15 cm long down the medial and lateral sides of his calf, and pushing his tissues forward to cover part of the gap. Hold them in place with sutures or strapping. Graft the gap made by the relieving incisions.

If a LARGE PART OF HIS TIBIA has been destroyed, and inadequate involucrum has formed, try to get this fibula to hypertrophy before referring him. Walk him in a below-knee caliper. Later, refer him for an operation in which a length of his fibula is moved across to form a new tibia. This is done in two steps, moving one end at a time. The transposed piece of his fibula can hypertrophy greatly. Destruction would not have occurred if you had removed the sequestrum at the right time.

If osteomyelitis has COMPLETELY DESTROYED A CHILD'S TIBIA, his fibula may hypertrophy, and push his foot into varus; refer him.

If: (1) you MISTAKENLY REMOVED A SEQUESTRUM before a firm involucrum had formed, or (2) the periosteum in the middle third of the shaft of the tibia is destroyed, keep him in a Sarmiento cast (81.5), to support his leg and prevent his foot going into inversion until such a time as you can refer him to have his fibula moved over under his tibia.

7.12 Osteomyelitis of the fibula

Osteomyelitis of the fibula is uncommon. If the patient's tibia is not involved, you can remove a sequestrum from his fibula as soon as is convenient, without waiting for an involucrum to form, because his tibia will support his leg. You can expose any part of his fibula by approaching it between his peroneal muscles anteriorly and his soleus posteriorly. His posterior tibial nerve and vessels are well out of harm's way; but be careful not to injure his peroneal artery and veins which are close to the posteromedial angle of the shaft of his fibula. If the head of his fibula is involved (rare) be very careful not to injure his common peroneal nerve.

EXPOSING THE FIBULA

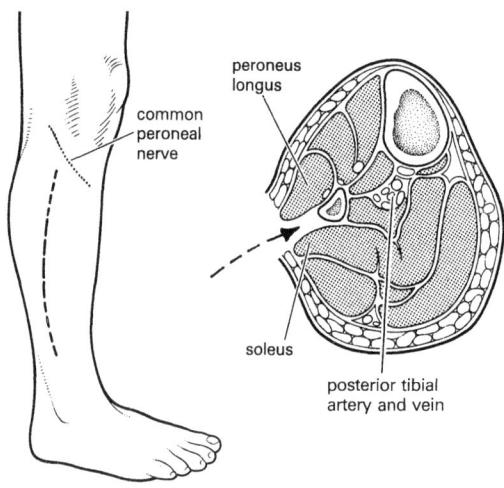

Fig. 7-11 OSTEOMYELITIS OF THE FIBULA. Approach a patient's fibula between his peroneal muscles anteriorly, and his soleus posteriorly.

OSTEOMYELITIS OF THE FIBULA

Follow the general method for osteomyelitis in Sections 7.4 to 7.6. Apply a tourniquet.

INCISION. Lay the patient on his side with his affected leg uppermost, and his knee slightly bent. Use the appropriate part of an incision which starts 5 cm below the head of his fibula, and curves gently posteriorly down towards his lateral malleolus. Reflect short skin flaps anteriorly and posteriorly. Avoid the head and neck of his fibula, because his common peroneal nerve winds round it. If you have to remove sequestra from the head, try to pull them down from below.

If you are working on the middle third of his fibula, incise the periosteum vertically, and separate muscle from bone subperiosteally.

CAUTION! The peroneal vessels are close to the medial side of the fibula, so strip the muscles carefully.

EXCISING THE FIBULA. If necessary, and he is more than 10 years old, you can remove the entire shaft of his fibula, except for its lower 5 cm. Use a Gigli saw, not an osteotome, or bone-cutting forceps, which will splinter it. Be very careful to avoid his common peroneal nerve winding round its upper end.

7.13 Osteomyelitis of the calcaneus and talus

Osteomyelitis of the calcaneus can follow blood spread, a septic infection of the heel, traction with a calcaneal pin, or an open fracture. The calcaneus is a completely cancellous bone which never forms an involucrum and seldom an isolated sequestrum. Pus soon perforates its periosteum without destroying much of its cortex. The most practical operation, and some would say the only one, is to remove the whole of the patient's calcaneus to give him an ugly but surprisingly useful foot.

Fungi sometimes infect the calcaneus and cause multiple sinuses. If chemotherapy fails, as it usually does, try radical excision in early cases, and consider amputation in late ones (31.3, 56.6).

OSTEOMYELITIS OF THE CALCANEUS AND TALUS

THE CALCANEUS

ANAESTHESIA. You will need to lie the patient prone, which makes anaesthesia difficult (16.12). If possible, intubate him and control his ventilation. If this is not possible, give him a general anaesthetic and lie him on his side.

OSTEOMYELITIS OF THE CALCANEUS

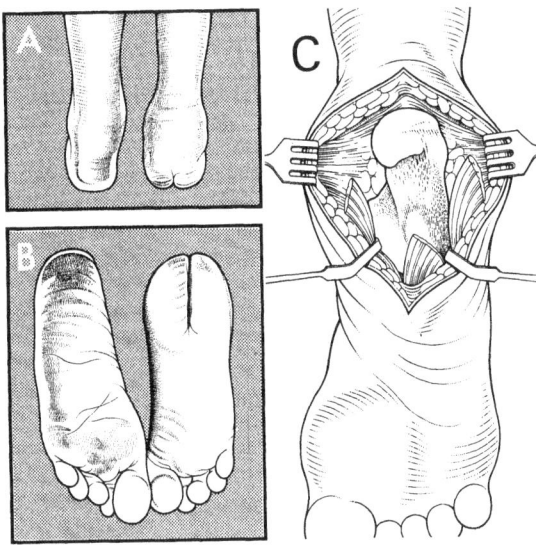

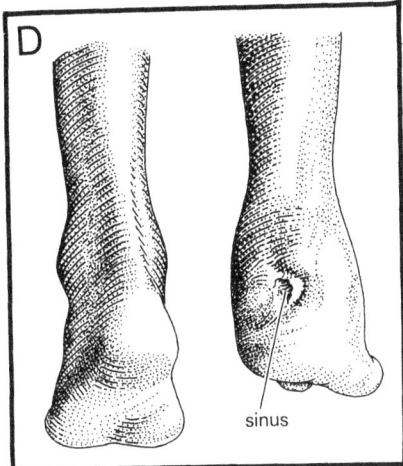

Fig. 7-12 OSTEOMYELITIS OF THE CALCANEUS. Splitting a patient's heel is the easiest approach to his calcaneus; a split heel is no disability. This is the Gaenslen incision. A, and B, after the operation. C, exposing the calcaneus. D, osteomyelitis of the right calcaneus with a sinus. *After Edmondson AS and Crenshaw AH, 'Campbell's Operative Orthopaedics', Fig. 10-18. CV Mosby, with kind permission.*

INCISION. Follow the general methods for osteomyelitis, in Sections 7.4 to 7.6. Apply a tourniquet.

If infection is limited to the pin track, and he is lucky, opening up and scraping out the granulation tissue from around the pin track may occasionally be all that he needs.

If you are draining a soft tissue abscess or want to remove a window from the cortex during the acute stage, you can approach his calcaneus from either side.

If his whole calcaneus is involved, remove it completely. Make a longitudinal incision right down to the bone, and shell it out. You cannot remove it from inside its periosteum, so strip this away from the soft tissues of his heel and remove the bone completely, either as a single piece or in several smaller ones.

Lie him prone with a support under his foot. Make a longitudinal incision exactly in the middle of his heel. Start it in the midline level with the base of his fifth metatarsal. Extend the incision proximally to split the distal end of his Achilles tendon for about 3 cm. Incise his plantar aponeurosis in a plane between his flexor digitorum brevis and his abductor digiti minimi.

CAUTION ! Start in the midline, stay close to bone and reflect everything you meet medially and laterally. In this way you will avoid important structures, especially his plantar nerves entering from the medial side of his foot.

POSTOPERATIVELY, allow the wound edges to collapse together, but don't suture them. Apply much gauze. Hold his ankle in a neutral position with a gutter plaster splint held with a crepe bandage. As his wound heals, start him walking with crutches; later he can progress to full weight-bearing. The edges of the scar will turn deeply inwards and split his heel into two cushions. If its surface is uneven, suggest that he pads his shoe.

THE TALUS

He presents with a painful ankle. X-rays show an irregular dense talus. Sequestra are unusual. If you apply a below knee cast and give him an antibiotic for 3 weeks the infection will probably settle without surgery, but degenerative arthritis may follow. If he has severe persistent disease refer him for the removal of his talus.

7.14 Osteitis of the cranium

Flat bones like those of the skull differ from long ones: (1) They have little marrow between their diploe, so that when they are infected the condition is an osteitis, rather than an osteomyelitis. (2) Unlike long bones, which make much callus when they fracture, and an obvious involucrum and sequestra when they are infected, fractured flat bones make little callus; infected ones seldom sequestrate, and don't form an involucrum. When sequestra do form in the skull, it is usually because a burn has destroyed the blood supply to the outer diploe.

A patient with osteitis of the skull has pain ('headache'), combined with tenderness and swelling over the lesion which may be particularly marked. It may be secondary to:

A burn (common, 58.32), as when an epileptic falls into a fire and burns his head.

A head injury (63.7). Minimize the risk of osteitis by toileting his wound carefully. If it does occur, you may have to remove a dead piece of bone.

Frontal sinusitis (25.8). He presents with a persistent headache. The bone above his orbit is prominent and tender, and he may have a swelling of his scalp which may extend as far as his vertex. X-rays show thickening of his skull and enlargement of his frontal sinus.

Pyaemia causing metastatic lesions in his skull. The skull is very vascular and has no end arteries, so the infection will probably settle without the need for drainage.

An extradural abscess (5.4a). The pus under his skull is more important than the pus in it.

Septic thrombophlebitis of his scalp which has caused it to necrose and expose his underlying skull. This condition is seen in malnourished children, and is related in its pathology to cancrum oris (26.6). It is not a true osteitis, but is rather a loss of the outer periosteum leading to sequestration of the diploe.

OSTEITIS OF THE CRANIUM

When you plan the incision, consider the arteries of the patient's scalp, and incise between them. For example, don't make a transverse incision in his temple which will divide his temporal artery. Split skin grafts will not take on bare skull, but they will take on granulations. So, if necessary, remove dead bone, apply saline dressings for a few days, and wait for granulations to form. See Figure 63-11 and Sections 57.3 and 58.32.

CAUTION ! (1) If a sequestrum is firmly anchored, use an osteotome and light taps from a heavy hammer—don't open his dura or injure his brain.

FOLLOWING FRONTAL SINUSITIS. If you cannot refer him, define the extent of his frontal sinus with X-rays. Shave the anterior 3 cm of his scalp. Make a long incision above his hairline from ear to ear, and reflect the skin of his forehead downwards as a flap, based on his supraorbital vessels.

Remove the anterior wall of his frontal sinus; try to curette away *all* its lining, so that no more fluid will form. If possible, try to establish drainage through into his nose. Insert drains through stab incisions above the outer end of each eyebrow. Lead them horizontally from the frontal region of the sinus

OSTEOMYELITIS OF THE SKULL

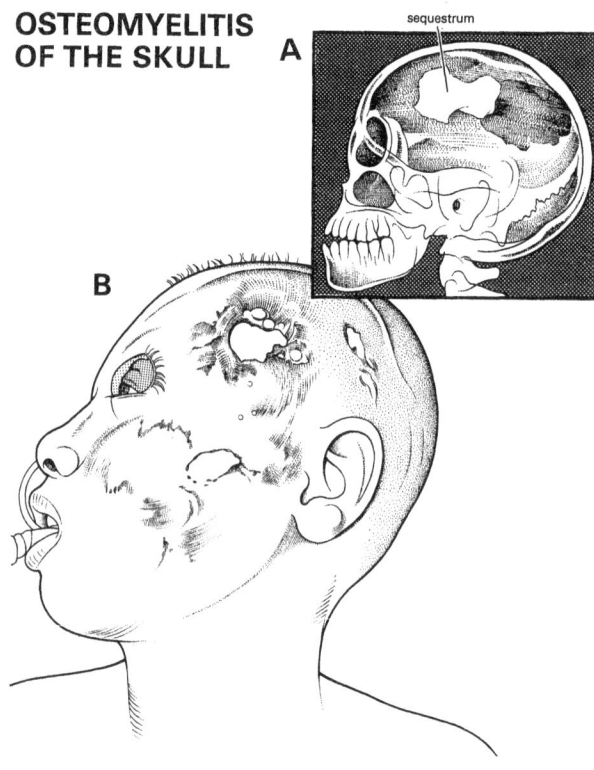

Fig. 7-13 A SEQUESTRUM IN THE SKULL. This patient has a dense white sequestrum in his skull, which has moved forwards. He was reported as having osteomyelitis. Burns of the scalp are however the commonest cause of necrosis of the skull. Another cause is septic thrombophlebitis of the scalp, which causes it to necrose and expose the bone underneath.
Kindly contributed by Gerald Hankins.

through these incisions. Or, insert them below his inner eyebrows. Close the flap.

7.14a Osteomyelitis of the jaws

Osteomyelitis can affect either of a patient's jaws, usually the lower one, and can take various forms:

Osteomyelitis complicating an infected tooth socket in an adult is more common in the mandible (5.8, 26.3). Suspect it if he has pain, swelling, tenderness, trismus, and fever after he has had an infected tooth removed (sometimes months before), or an alveolar abscess drained. If his osteomyelitis becomes chronic he may have sinuses over his lower face, or over the inferior border of his mandible (see Fig. 26-8). Often, he has trismus. His offending teeth are usually loose, and you may see pus discharging around them.

Osteomyelitis complicating an open fracture, (62.7, 69.7), especially a comminuted one of his lower jaw (unusual). A thorough wound toilet should prevent this, provided it is done reasonably early. The mandible has a good blood supply, so that even small pieces of bone may live, if they have some soft tissue connection.

Osteomyelitis in children, especially malnourished ones, may be the result of a subacute necrosis folowing septic thrombophlebitis. This is probably a manifestation of the same process that causes cancrum oris (26.6) and septic thrombophlebitis of the scalp (7.14). Osteomyelitis, particularly of the maxilla, can also be a complication of sickle-cell disease. A child's upper teeth become loose, a sequestrum forms, and pus discharges: (1) inside his mouth, (2) on the surface of his cheek close to his nose, or (3) at his zygomatic process.

OSTEOMYELITIS OF THE JAWS

ACUTE OSTEOMYELITIS

If a patient's osteomyelitis is due to an infected tooth, extract it, and see Section 26.3.

If it is due to an open fracture, it is probably subacute and can be satisfactorily treated by antibiotics. If infection persists, look for a sequestrum and if you find one, remove it.

If it is haematogenous (unusual, and more often in his lower jaw), drilling is not required, treat him with antibiotics. If infection persists, look for a sequestrum and remove it.

CHRONIC OSTEOMYELITIS

X-RAYS. PA and oblique views may show a sequestrum (uncommon), or a patchy osteoporosis accompanied by new bone formation (dense thickened bone).

TREATMENT. Give him antibiotics (penicillin or chloramphenicol, 2.7) for up to 2 weeks. Improve his oral hygiene. Remove any loose teeth in the area.

If no sequestrum is present, extract his tooth or teeth.

If a sequestrum is present, remove it. There is no need to wait for an involucrum to form unless the sequestrum is very large. Involucra form poorly in the mandible, which, in this respect, is intermediate in its behaviour between a long bone and a flat one.

SEQUESTRECTOMY

MAXILLA. As the dead bone separates, it loosens. Wait for the child's nutrition to improve. If the sequestrum is small and loose, remove it under sedation only. If it is larger, remove it under ketamine *in toto* or in pieces. If necessary, chip away a little living bone. Curette the residual defect. If the cavity bleeds, pack it for 5 minutes.

MANDIBLE. To avoid an unsightly scar, incise 1 cm below the inferior border of the ramus of his mandible. Cut through healthy skin and subcutaneous tissue near the sequestrum. Avoid, or clamp and tie, his facial artery and vein, as they cross the the ramus of his mandible 3 cm (in an adult) anterior to its angle. Chisel away the outer bone covering the sequestrum and curette the cavity. Close the wound loosely, leaving a corrugated drain through one end, or through a separate stab wound.

CAUTION! Don't operate on a malnourished child until his general condition is acceptable.

DIFFICULTIES WITH OSTEOMYELITIS OF THE JAWS

If a patient has has a HARD DISCOLOURED SWELLING of the soft tissues of his neck, suspect ACTINOMYCOSIS (rare), especially if it has multiple sinuses (uncommon in osteomyelitis), and persistently negative jaw X-rays rays. Look for 'sulphur granules' in the discharge from them. If the diagnosis is confirmed treat him with large does of penicillin (500 mg 4 times a day), or tetracycline over a period of at least 6 weeks.

7.15 Osteomyelitis of the spine and pelvis (both uncommon)

The spine can be affected by tuberculosis, or by suppurative osteomyelitis due to a variety of pyogenic organisms, especially *Staphylococcus aureus,* streptococci, *Brucella,* and occasionally *S. typhi.* Tuberculosis is always chronic, but pyogenic osteomyelitis can be acute, subacute, or chronic.

A patient with acute osteomyelitis of his spine is usually a very ill child with fever and severe back pain, usually in his lumbar region. There may be some inflammatory oedema over his spine, which is very tender, and may be arched backwards by muscle spasm, as if he had tetanus or meningitis. X-rays may show a paravertebral abscess, usually with normal bones. He may be paraplegic as the result of inflammatory oedema involving his cord. If he is to have any chance of survival the pus must be drained, by removing the transverse processes of some of his vertebrae and part of some of his ribs.

If his osteomyelitis is chronic, he is usually an older child or adult. He is in pain, but has little or no fever, and no arching of his back.

Tuberculosis of the spine is described in Section 29.4, which also gives a detailed description of costotransversectomy for the drainage of a cold abscess. Here we give a short description of the same operation for acute osteomyelitis.

Paraplegia associated with osteitis of the spine, is usually due to inflammatory oedema pressing on the cord. If you can see an abscess on the X-ray, operate; but if there is no X-ray evidence of an abscess, you may still find pus. If he has no spasms, he will probably recover in 3 to 6 months. But if he has extensor, or worse, flexor spasms, his paraplegia is likely to be permanent.

OSTEOMYELITIS OF THE SPINE AND PELVIS

THE SPINE

DIFFERENTIAL DIAGNOSIS. See also Section 29.4a and Fig. 29-3a.

If the bodies of a patient's vertebrae are abnormal, but not his intervertebral discs, suspect malignancy.

If the disc and the adjoining bone are diseased, especially if this is maximal anteriorly, suspect infection. The diseased bone softens, and the vertebral bodies become wedge-shaped.

If there is other evidence of tuberculosis (a positive sputum or suggestive chest X-rays etc), treat him for it.

If there is marked osteoporosis but no osteosclerosis, and tuberculosis is common in your district, treat him for it.

If there is porosis and sclerosis, he may have osteomyelitis or tuberculosis, so:

(1) Refer him for costotransversectomy, or if this is impossible, do it yourself, especially if tuberculosis is uncommon in your district and the condition is acute or subacute.

Or, (2) treat him for both diseases for 3 to 6 weeks. During this time a non-tuberculous lesion should have improved greatly (no pain and little or no tenderness), whereas a tuberculous one will have changed very little.

If you are in doubt as to the diagnosis, treat him for tuberculosis. In most developing countries 90% of cases of osteitis of the spine are tuberculous.

If he is paraplegic, or has a paravertebral abscess (pyogenic or tuberculous) he needs a costotransversectomy. If he has acute osteomyelitis, this is particularly urgent, so refer him or proceed as follows. Aim to drain the pus; there is no need to drill.

METHOD. Give him a general anaesthetic, intubate him, and control his ventilation (A 18.1). Lie him prone with a pillow under his chest to keep his abdomen free. Make a straight longitudinal 10 to 15 cm incision over his spinous processes, or, better, an incision curved towards his left side with its ends over his spinous processes. Use a scalpel and a periosteal elevator to approach the bodies of his vertebrae, by separating his spine from his sacrospinalis muscle on the left. Control bleeding by packing the wound with a large swab and waiting.

In the thoracic area, remove the proximal 3 cm of a rib opposite the middle of the abscess with its transverse process. Cut the rib distally with rib shears or bone cutters, push away the soft tissue deep to the bone, and dissect its proximal end. You will find that it has a small joint with its corresponding vertebral body and another with the transverse process. Cut this transverse process at its base and remove it with the piece of rib. Do the same for one or two neighbouring vertebrae.

Push your finger between the side of the vertebral body and the tissues covering his pleura—recognize this by its movement. If you feel close in front of his spine, you should find pus.

In the lumbar region, when you reach his transverse processes, remove two or three of them with bone nibblers. You will now reach the plane between his quadratus lumborum and the bodies of his vertebrae, where you should find pus.

Clean this out and remove any obviously dead bone. His muscles will fit back snugly next to his spine. Suture his deep fascia. If much pus was present insert a drain. Close his skin. Send pus for culture. For more details see Section 29.4a.

If you don't find pus, nibble away a little bone next to a vertebral disc and send this for histology; it may be tuberculous.

THE PELVIS

Osteomyelitis of the pubis occasionally follows symphysiotomy (18.4). If it involves his innominate bone, try antibiotics for up to 6 weeks. Sequestra are unusual. If pain and or sinuses persist treatment is difficult, so refer him.

7.16 Septic arthritis

This is another disease in which failure to drain pus early is a real disaster—a severe and probably painful disability for the rest of the patient's life. If you don't drain his infected joint *early,* it will be destroyed and may ultimately ankylose. If he is a child, the epiphyses near it may displace, or dislocate. As soon as you have made the diagnosis, drainage is urgent—this is *not* an operation to leave until tomorrow!

Bacteria can reach a joint: (1) Before the age of 6 months from osteomyelitis in the metaphyses of any long bone. After this age the epiphyseal plates prevent spread like this. (2) At any age in the hip, because the proximal metaphysis of the femur is partly within the capsule of the hip joint. This anatomical peculiarity makes septic arthritis of the hip and osteomyelitis of the neck of the femur, virtually the same disease. (3) Through the blood from a distant septic focus. This is haematogenous septic arthritis, which involves the knee, hip, shoulder, and ankle in this order of frequency. (4) Through a penetrating joint wound of a joint, especially of the fingers or knee.

DISASTER WITH AN INFECTED HIP

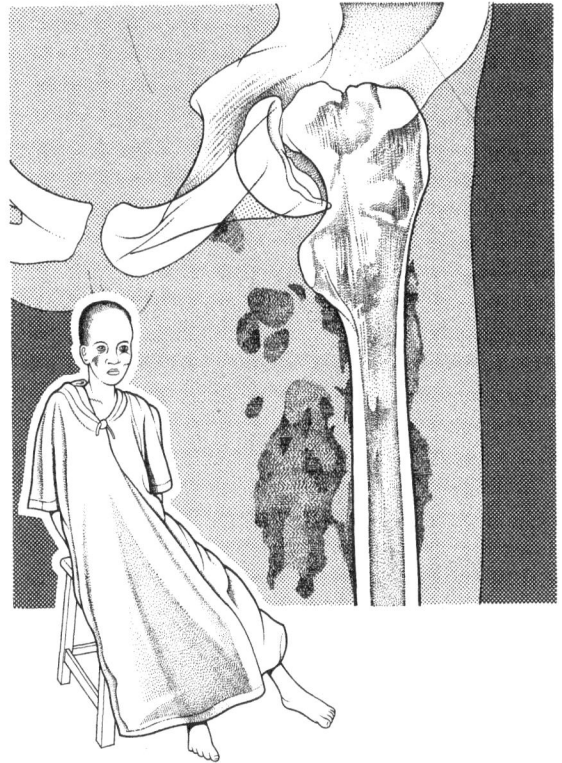

Fig. 7-14 DISASTER WITH AN INFECTED HIP. This is patient Hasina whose story is given in the text. Infection has displaced the epiphysis of her femur, and moved its shaft upwards. The infection in her thigh is producing gas shadows.

The first sign of septic arthritis is that a patient cannot use his limb. One of his joints, commonly his hip or his knee, becomes so painful that moving it even a little in any direction causes him great pain. Sometimes, several of his joints are involved at the same time. He is usually febrile. *The combination of fever and a limb which is too painful to move is either osteomyelitis, or septic arthritis, until you have proved it is not.* Later, if the infected joint is near the surface, you will be able to feel that it is warm and swollen with fluid. Unfortunately, the shoulder and the hip are so deep that you cannot easily detect fluid, so that the *only* local sign is acutely painful limitation of movement.

If septic arthritis always ran a typical course, it would be easier to diagnose. Unfortunately, it often runs a very atypical one. Here are some of the difficulties: (1) If a patient is very old or very young, he may have few general signs of infection, and his effusion may not even appear to be inflammatory. There is only one way to be sure—*aspirate all joint effusions, and examine them.* (2) In the spine, the sacroiliac joints, and the hips, pain may be the only presenting symptom. (3) Only half the patients have a fever or a leucocytosis. (4) You can easily confuse tuberculous arthritis with the subacute type of suppurative arthritis. To distinguish them rely on the X-ray, and your findings on aspiration (pus or caseous tissue). *If you are still in doubt, treat the patient for both diseases.* Review his progress at 3 and 6 weeks, when suppurative arthritis should show much improvement, whereas it is still too early for tuberculosis to show much change.

The diagnosis is particularly difficult in babies as this case shows.

AHMED (1 year) was brought by his mother saying he had fever and was drawing up his left hip in pain. This in itself was unusual, because, if a baby does this, he usually draws up both of them. He was found to have suppurative arthritis of his right hip, which was too painful to move. It was aspirated, chemotherapy was started within 24 hours, and he recovered. LESSON The diagnosis was made early and treatment started immediately.

Remember the risk factors—some patients have several: (1) As with infections of other kinds, septic arthritis is more common in the disadvantaged and malnourished. (2) Infancy and old age. (3) Systemic diseases which affect the body's response such as diabetes, chronic renal failure, liver disease, malignancy, the arthritides, intravenous drug abuse, alcoholism, and immunosuppression, especially by AIDS. (4) Local joint-damage due to earlier earlier surgery or osteoarthritis.

Although *Staphylococcus aureus* is the dominant organism, each risk group has its own characteristic infective organisms, patterns of joint involvement, and clinical response. If the patient has sickle-cell disease, you may find *E. coli* or salmonellae in his joint. *Haemophilus influenzae* is the most frequent organism in newborns, but is seldom seen in older patients. Other organisms include streptococci, brucellae, and gonococci. The gonococcus often affects young healthy adults without any obvious risk factor except sexual activity. With other organisms there is usually a risk factor.

When infection is well established, antibiotics seldom help. Occasionally, if you are fortunate, and are able to give the right one early enough, a patient may be lucky and recover without any other treatment.

The X-ray signs of septic arthritis are: (1) Widening of the joint space. (2) The signs of early osteitis (7.4). You may see the first signs of new bone formation as early as the 5th day in an infant, but it will not appear before the 10th day in an older child, and may take longer.

The critical investigation is *to aspirate the joint as soon as you suspect infection.* Frank pus in the syringe, or even slightly cloudy synovial fluid, confirms the diagnosis. You may get a false negative result, but apart from contaminants in the culture, you will never get a false positive one. *Aspiration alone is not enough; it only tells you that pus is present, so incise the joint and wash out the pus.* Then insert a corrugated drain, or (in the knee) leave the incision open.

Aspirating the more superficial joints is usually easy, but you may fail to aspirate the shoulder, or the hip. If aspiration succeeds or fails, you must incise and drain the infected joint. The results of not doing so are so serious, that the dangers of attempting it are well worthwhile. *If you allow pus to accumulate under pressure in a patient's hip, it may impair the blood supply to the head of his femur within 24 hours,* so that it necroses. Pus can also damage a joint, even if the blood supply is not impaired.

If, when you incise an infected joint and wash out the pus, you feel that its surfaces are smooth, he has a good chance of having a normal or a nearly normal limb. His prognosis is worse if cartilage has been lost, if the joint surfaces are rough, if the bone is soft, or if the X-ray shows severe joint destruction. Even so, he still has some hope of a movable joint, especially if he is young—a child's epiphysis may appear to be largely destroyed on an X-ray, and yet regenerate considerably.

Several things can happen to a severely damaged joint: (1) It can dislocate. (2) An epiphysis can slip, either immediately, or several weeks later, as with the patient Hasina in Fig. 7-14. Prevent this happening by splinting the joint or applying skin traction. (3) A painless stable bony ankylosis can form in the position of function. Provided it really is stable and is in the position of function, this may be only a minor disability. (4) The patient may get a painful unstable fibrous ankylosis, which can be a serious disability. If ankylosis fails, and his symptoms are severe enough, you may be able to refer him to have his joint fused.

If the patient is a child, and is lucky, he will have a painless joint with a useful range of movement. If he is unlucky he will have a painful joint that will ultimately need operative fusion, but meanwhile his limb will have had time to grow. Fusing a joint is difficult in a child, and is rarely necessary; if it is done too early, there will be growth problems. The decision to fuse an adult's painful joint can be taken much earlier.

If movement in a joint is going to be absent or limited, *the position in which it lies is critical.* This is described in the next section.

HASINA (17 years) was admitted with pain in her left hip and inability to walk for 3 days. She was given physiotherapy, nursed on a fracture bed for 3 weeks, and discharged on crutches. Some weeks later she was readmitted, febrile, and with a swelling of her right thigh extending from her knee to her iliac crest. Three litres of yellow-green pus were aspirated. Her X-rays are shown in Fig. 7-14.

MARIAMU (12 years) was admitted with osteomyelitis of her tibia. This was settling nicely when she developed pain in her left hip and became febrile. The X-rays of her hip were normal, septic arthritis was diagnosed, and she was given large doses of the latest broad-spectrum antibiotic. Her pain improved slowly but her fever continued. Later, X-rays showed destruction of the head of her femur. Traction was applied. Sinuses developed, and she was never able to walk again. Two years later her pain was so severe that she had to have her hip disarticulated. All this happened in a 'good' hospital. LESSONS (1) The early diagnosis of septic arthritis of Hasina's hip was not made, although the history and signs were obvious. (2) Rest in bed on traction would have prevented her epiphysis slipping. At best she will have a painful hip, either for life, or until her hip has ankylosed spontaneously, or been fused surgically.(3) Explore a hip on the *suspicion* of septic arthritis.

**ASPIRATE AND EXAMINE ALL JOINT EFFUSIONS
DRAIN ALL INFECTED JOINTS**

SEPTIC ARTHRITIS

If possible take several blood cultures from the patient.

ANAESTHESIA. (1) Ketamine (A 8.1). (2) General anaesthesia (A 10.1). (3) To aspirate his joints sedate him and use local anaesthesia.

ASPIRATION. This is diagnostic only: follow it immediately by operative drainage. Push a *large* (1.2 mm) needle down into the joint, and aspirate as in Fig. 7-15.

SPECIAL TESTS. Culture of the synovial fluid isolates the organism in 30% of cases and blood culture in another 14%. A leucocytosis of <20 000 μl makes the diagnosis unlikely but does not exclude it, especially if the gonococcus is responsible.

ANTIBIOTICS. Give the appropriate antibiotic. If you cannot isolate the organism, chloramphenicol is likely to be the most suitable one (2.9). In acute cases give it for 2 to 3 weeks. In chronic cases give it for up to 6 weeks.

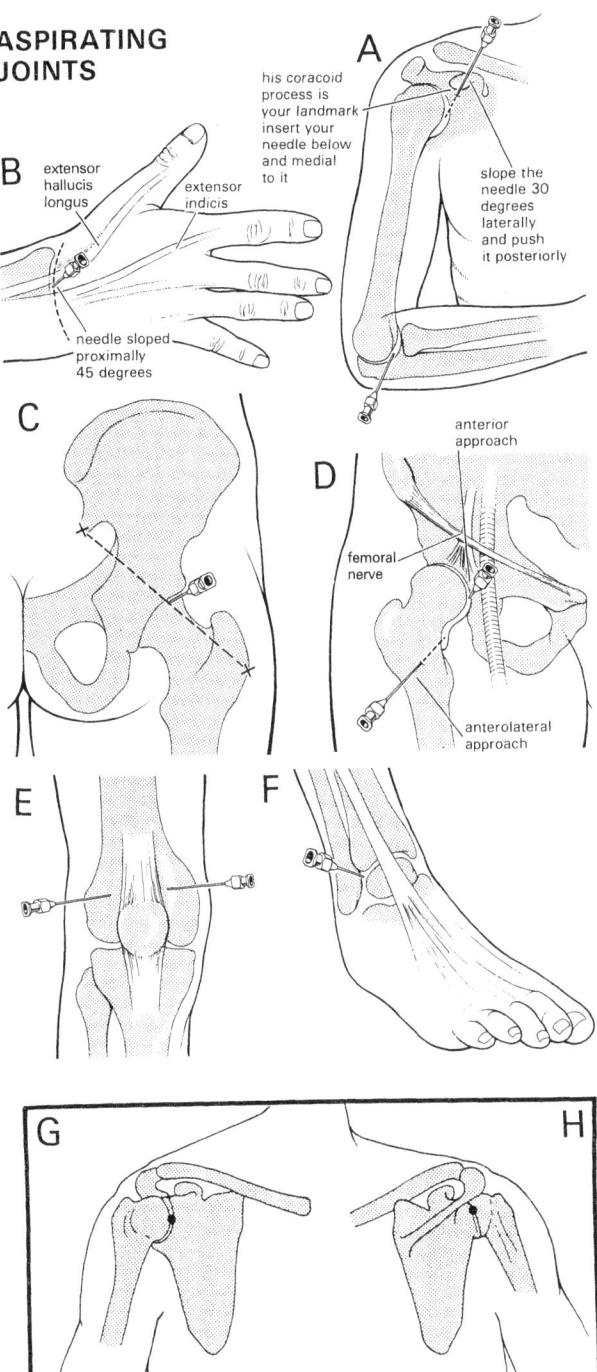

Fig. 7-15 ASPIRATING A JOINT may confirm the diagnosis, if pus is thin enough to come out of the needle. It is not effective treatment because it does not provide enough drainage, and pus may reform. *So always open and drain an infected joint.* A,- the shoulder and elbow. B, the wrist. C, the posterior approach to the hip. D, the anterior and anterolateral approach to the hip. E, the knee, and F, the ankle. G, and H, the anterior and posterior approach to the shoulder. *A, to F, after 'Hamilton Bailey's Emergency Surgery', edited by HAF Dudley. John Wright, with kind permission. G, and H, kindly contributed by Jack Lange.*

EXPLORATION. Open his infected joint by the methods described in the next section. Operate under a tourniquet where possible, and if his hand is involved, watch out for its nerves. Irrigate the interior of the joint forcefully using a syringe and a litre or two of Ringer's lactate or 0.9% saline. Do this until the fluid comes back clear. Feel the surfaces of the joint.

Leave the wound open. The linear incision you have just made will become elliptical, and you will see the cartilage underneath. If the joint is superficial, it needs no drain. If it is deep, as in the hip and shoulder, insert a rubber drain. The wound will heal spontaneously as the infection subsides.

If his joint surfaces feel smooth, his prognosis is good. After 10 days of rest start gradual active movements.

If his joint surfaces feel rough but some cartilage still covers the bones, he may still have useful function in his joint. If all its cartilage has been destroyed, his prognosis is bad. His best hope is a stable ankylosis in the position of function (7-16).

If there is any danger of his joint ankylosing, make sure it does so in the position of function. If his hip or knee are involved, apply temporary skin traction.

If, later, he has a persistently painful joint with limited movement, refer him for operative fusion. In a child, delay this as long as possible.

7.17 Methods and positions for particular joints apart from the hip, most of the methods for which are in the next section

Joints need to be in particular positions for particular purposes, so be sure to use the right one. These positions seldom coincide with one another, and at least one of them, *the position of function is absolutely critical.*

The position of function is the best position for a joint to be in if it is going to be fixed, or if its movement is going to be severely limited. It is also called the position for ankylosis. Any kind of ankylosis, stable or unstable, is a dreadful disability if a patient's joint becomes fixed in the *wrong* position, so make sure that, if it is going to ankylose, it does so in the most useful position for him. The position of function varies from joint to joint, and may depend on what he wants to do with it. You never know for sure when a joint is going to ankylose, so put it into the position of function when you first see a patient with septic arthritis. For example, splint his knee just short of full extension; splint his right (or dominant) elbow flexed. *Make quite sure he is in this position before you discharge him!* Don't leave this task to a physiotherapist in the hope that it will be achieved later!

The position of rest is the most comfortable position for a joint to lie in. Put it into this position if it has to be rested for any reason, but is in no danger of ankylosing.

The neutral position of a joint is that from which its movement is measured. It is for anatomical description only, and is shown in Fig. 69-1.

The position of safety is for the hand only, and is shown in Fig. 75-8. It is the position in which the collateral ligaments of the finger joints are stretched, and in which fingers which are temporarily not going to be moved are least likely to become stiff.

THE POSITION OF A JOINT IS ALL IMPORTANT!

METHODS AND POSITIONS FOR JOINTS

THE SHOULDER

ASPIRATING THE SHOULDER. There are two approaches:

Anteriorly, feel for the patient's coracoid process just below his clavicle in the space between his pectoralis major and his deltoid muscle. Push the needle into the joint slightly below and medial to the tip of his coracoid process. Slope it laterally 30° and push it backwards, until it enters the loose pouch under the lower part of his shoulder joint (A, and G, Fig. 7-15).

Posteriorly, sit him in a chair to face its back, ask him to touch his opposite shoulder with the arm that is to be aspirated, so as to adduct and internally rotate his shoulder. Feel for the head of his humerus. Keeping the needle horizontal, push it it 30° medially into the joint space, from a point just under the posteroinferior border of his acromnion as in H, Fig. 7-15.

POSITIONS OF FUNCTION

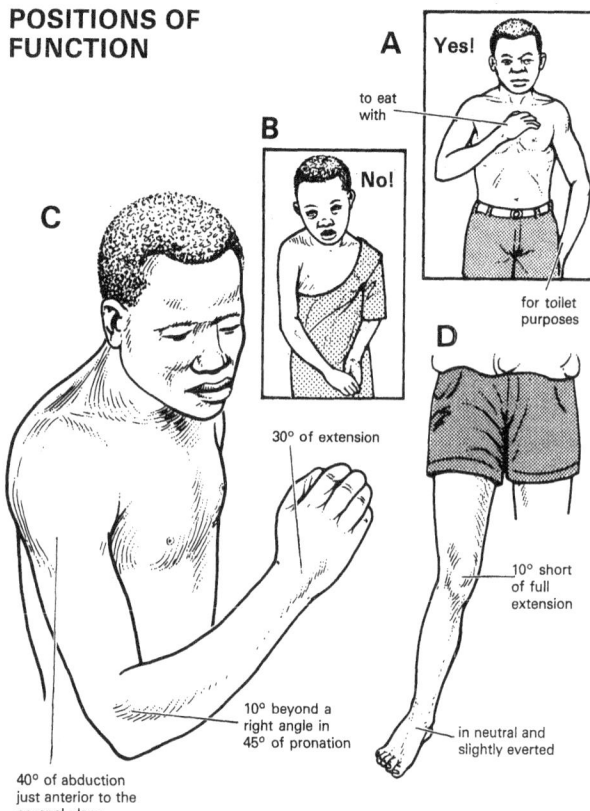

Fig. 7-16 THIS ILLUSTRATION OF THE POSITIONS OF FUNCTION is one of the most important ones in these manuals. If a joint is going to ankylose, the position in which it does so is critical. Notice that this patient's shoulder is abducted, his right elbow is flexed and in mid-pronation, his left elbow is extended (for toilet purposes), his knee is just short of full extension, and his ankle is in neutral and slightly everted.

The girl in box B had an infected burn of her right elbow. The joint became infected. Tragically, it was allowed to ankylose in nearly full extension, so that she cannot eat with it or write! *Kindly contributed by John Stewart.*

EXPLORING THE SHOULDER. Approach his shoulder joint as if you were operating on his upper humerus for osteomyelitis as in Fig. 7-7, and separate his deltoid from his pectoralis major in his deltopectoral groove. Keep the wound open with a drain into the joint.

POSITION OF REST FOR THE SHOULDER. Put his arm in a sling.

POSITION OF FUNCTION FOR THE SHOULDER. If there is gross bone destruction, or you expect that he will have a stiff shoulder, put his shoulder into a spica in 45° of abduction, with his elbow just anterior to the coronal plane, in 70° of medial rotation so that he can get his hand to his mouth.

ELBOW

ASPIRATING THE ELBOW. See also Fig. 72-4. Bend his elbow to 90°. Feel for the head of his radius. Using this as guide, push the needle into the posterolateral aspect of the joint, between the head of his radius and his humerus.

EXPLORING THE ELBOW. Make a 3 cm longitudinal incision posteriorly in the sulcus between his olecranon and the head of his radius. Go through the skin and fascia, insert a haemostat, and open it. Keep the joint open with a drain.

CAUTION ! Stay close to his olecranon, and remember that his posterior interosseous nerve winds round the neck of his radius 2 fingers' breadth distal to its head.

POSITION OF REST FOR THE ELBOW. Keep his arm in a sling in 90° of flexion.

POSITIONS OF FUNCTION FOR THE ELBOW depend on whether one, or both of them, are going to ankylose.

If his major elbow is going to ankylose, consider his needs. For example, Muslims and many other African peoples write and eat with their right hands and use their left hands for toilet purposes. If so, his right elbow should be more flexed than his left.

His major elbow will probably be most useful to him if it is flexed 10° beyond a right angle, with his forearm pronated 45° so that he can feed himself, scratch his nose, and write. Put it into this position by fitting him with a collar and cuff (72-9).

If both his elbows are going to ankylose, arrange their positions so that his major arm can reach his mouth. Let his minor one fuse in 10° short of full extension, so it can reach his anus.

THE WRIST

ASPIRATING THE WRIST. Feel for his radial styloid; it will show you the line of his joint. Feel for the tendons of extensor pollicis longus on the ulnar side of his 'anatomical snuffbox' (74.4). Aspirate on its ulnar aspect, at the level of his wrist joint. Push the needle between extensor pollicis longus and the index tendon of extensor digitorum into the joint inclining it proximally 45° (B, Fig. 7-15).

EXPLORING THE WRIST. Flex and extend his wrist, as you feel for the exact line of the joint. Feel for the hollow between the tendons of extensor pollicis longus and the index tendon of extensor digitorum. Make a 3 cm transverse incision, taking care not to cut the cutaneous branch of his radial nerve which runs in the web space of his thumb.

Retract the skin edges and expose the joint through a longitudinal incision between the two tendons.

POSITIONS OF REST AND FUNCTION FOR THE WRIST. Keep it in 30° of extension with a volar plaster slab.

THE HAND

THE POSITION OF SAFETY (James position) is peculiar to the hand and is the position which will minimize stiffness after an injury (75.2). Keep his MP joints nearly fully flexed, his PIP joints in 15° of flexion, and his DIP joints in 5° of flexion (Fig. 75-8 and many surgeons keep both IP joints fully extended). Keep his thumb well forward of his palm in opposition to his fingers, with its pulp about 4 cm from them. To maintain this position use aluminium finger splints, plaster slabs, or a boxing glove dressing (75.1), as appropriate. *See also Sectiom 75.3.*

THE HIP

See also Section 7.18.

ASPIRATING THE HIP is difficult. The anterior approach is easier than the anterolateral one. His hip lies immediately behind his mid inguinal point. Use a thick lumbar puncture needle. If the anterior approach fails, try the posterior one.

For the anterior approach, feel for his femoral artery 2.5 cm below his inguinal ligament midway between his anterior iliac spine and his pubic tubercle. Insert the needle 1.5 cm lateral to the artery (and thus lateral to the femoral nerve). Push the needle in, inclining it 15° medially and 15° superiorly. This will aim it at the joint directly behind his mid inguinal point. Push it through the capsule into the joint. Aspirate. If you don't find pus, advance it into the cartilage. To prove that the needle is in the cartilage, rotate his thigh internally a little. This should move the adaptor of the needle medially. Withdraw it slightly to remove it from the cartilage, and aspirate. If necessary, alter its position and try again, if need be several times. If you cannot feel his femoral artery, insert the needle 2.5 cm below and 2.5 cm lateral to his mid inguinal point.

For the posterior approach lay him prone. Feel for his posterior inferior iliac spine and the centre of his greater trochanter. Insert your needle midway between these two points into his hip joint.

EXPLORING THE HIP. See Section 7.18.

POSITION OF REST FOR THE HIP. If you are *sure* that his painful hip is only temporary, rest it in moderate flexion and 15° of abduction. In this position his legs are comfortably spread apart. Hold his hip in this position with skin traction. To produce abduction, bring the cord holding the weight to the end of the bar at the foot of his bed. If necessary, make sure it stays there by moulding a plaster pulley on the bar. Or, have a detachable bar with notches at suitable places, which you can tie to the foot of his bed. Or, put both his legs into abduction.

POSITION OF FUNCTION FOR THE HIP. The minimum amount of flexion, and preferably none; 5° of abduction, and no rotation.

If possible, don't make the decision to aim for fusion yourself—refer him. If you cannot refer him, and decide to aim for fusion, don't apply a spica with his hip in the position of function, especially if he is a child. If you do, you will find, when you remove it, that spasm has rotated his pelvis anteriorly, and there is too much flexion. Instead, immobilize his hip in a spica in complete extension and 15° of abduction. When you remove the spica, you will find that it has gone into 15° of flexion, which is where you want it to be.

THE KNEE

See also Section 79.3.

ASPIRATING THE KNEE. Extend the patient's knee. Push the needle into his suprapatellar pouch 2.5 cm above the upper border of his patella, from either the medial or the lateral side.

EXPLORING THE KNEE. With his knee extended, make a 5 cm incision one finger's breadth behind the medial edge of his patella and its tendon. Go through his quadriceps expansion, longitudinally, and put a curved haemostat into his suprapatellar pouch, under the surface of his patella. Put your finger into the joint and use it to remove the pus. Leave the wound open, or sew up the upper part, and leave a corrugated drain in place. Dress his wound and apply skin traction, or a plaster backslab. Without one or other he is likely to have a painful flexion contracture. Leave the drain in for 4 to 7 days.

BIOPSY OF THE KNEE. Make a 5 cm incision a finger's breadth behind the medial margin of his patella. Cut through his quadriceps expansion, and take a piece of diseased joint capsule for biopsy.

POSITION OF REST FOR THE KNEE. Apply skin traction to his lower leg to prevent flexion. Or apply a plaster backslab held on with a crepe bandage.

If he already has a flexion contracture following septic arthritis, put his knee in extension traction until it has been corrected. Then apply a cylindrical cast and encourage him to bear weight. With luck he will develop a painless bony ankylosis. If this does not happen, refer him for a compression arthrodesis of his knee.

POSITION OF FUNCTION FOR THE KNEE. Make sure his knee ankyloses in 10° of flexion, so his foot can just clear the ground when he walks. Do the same when both knees are ankylosed.

THE ANKLE

ASPIRATING THE ANKLE. Find the line of his joint by moving his ankle. Insert the needle into its anterior aspect just medial to his lateral malleolus. Push it backwards and slightly downwards, so that it enters the space in the angle between his tibia and his talus.

EXPLORING THE ANKLE. The following incision will expose both his ankle and his tarsal joints. Start the incision on the anterolateral aspect of his ankle, 5 cm above the joint, and continue it downwards 1 cm in front of his lateral malleolus to the base of his fourth metatarsal, lateral to the extensor tendons of his toes.

Divide his superior and inferior extensor retinaculum as far as is necessary, so as to expose the capsule of his ankle joint. Then divide this and open the joint.

POSITION OF REST FOR THE ANKLE. Keep his ankle in neutral, without any flexion, extension, inversion, or eversion. Apply a plaster gutter splint.

POSITION OF FUNCTION FOR THE ANKLE. Keep it neutral and *slightly* everted. Inversion will produce painful callus under the head of his fifth metatarsal when he walks.

ANKYLOSIS IN THE WRONG POSITION IS A *REAL* DISASTER!

7.18 Septic arthritis of the hip

If a patient has an acutely tender hip in varying degrees of flexion, and fever, suspect that it is infected. The general methods for septic arthritis are described in Section 7.16. An important sign is spasm of his hip muscles. Test for this by rolling his thigh as in Fig. 7-17. If this is acutely painful, suspect that his hip is infected. If he has septic arthritis or osteomyelitis banging his greater trochanter lightly with your clenched fist will be painful; if he has deep inguinal adenitis or pyomyositis it will not, see Sections 5.12 and 7.1. In septic arthritis or osteomyelitis the epiphysis of his femur may become indistinct, or even absent on an X-ray, but it often reappears. This is not an indication for removing it.

Many doctors, and even many general surgeons, are afraid to open the hip joint, and look on this as a specifically 'orthopaedic' procedure. The hip does however require exploring and draining

TWO USEFUL HIP SIGNS

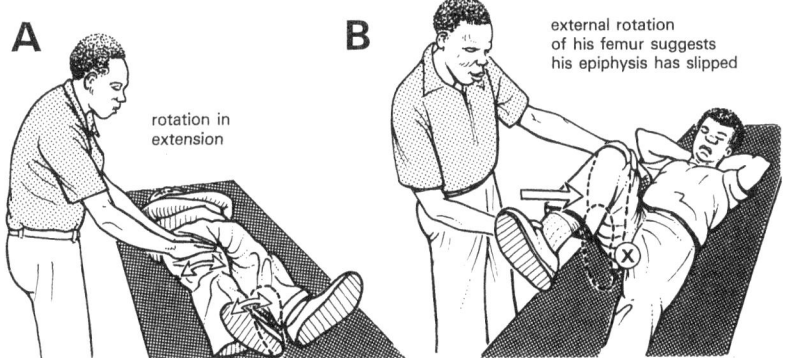

Fig. 7-17 SIGNS IN SEPTIC ARTHRITIS OF THE HIP. A, Lie the patient flat, place your hand on his thighs and try to roll his leg to and fro. A normal hip rolls easily; if it is infected, this will be acutely painful. B, if you flex a normal hip, it will flex without rotation. If it rotates externally into position 'X' as you flex it, his upper femoral epiphysis may have slipped. This can happen spontaneously in teenagers (77.10); it also happens in late septic arthritis. *Kindly contributed by John Stewart.*

just like any other joint. The problem is that it lies a little deeper than the others. There are three operations you may need to do, but only the first is common. Be prepared to: (1) Drain pus in septic arthritis. (2) Remove the head of a patient's femur, when this has been destroyed as the result of infection. (3) Do Girdlestone's operation in chronic septic arthritis to remove the head and neck of his femur.

Here we are only concerned with septic arthritis of the hip. If you don't treat a patient early, any of these things may happen to it:

(1) He may may develop a flexion contracture of his hip, which will be a great disability, if you let it become permanent. You can prevent and treat this in two ways: (a) You can apply extension (skin) traction to his lower leg (70.10). This is very effective prevention, so do it routinely. (b) If a contracture has started to develop, you can extend his leg by laying him on his front for some time each day—if he will tolerate it. Few patients, especially children, will do this for long if their head faces the wall. So make sure his bed faces the centre of the ward.

(2) His upper femoral epiphysis may slip off the shaft of his femur, and become a dead sequestrum in his hip joint, as in Fig. 7-14. Later in the course of the disease there is a useful test to find out if it is slipping. Bend his knee to 90° and then flex his hip, as in B, Fig, 7-17. If his leg goes into external rotation as you do this, the head of his femur may have slipped. Confirm it by taking a frog-leg X-ray view, as in Fig. 77-9. If it has slipped and is forming a sequestrum, you will have to open his hip joint and remove it, as described below.

(3) His hip joint may be destroyed. When this happens, there are two possibilities: (a) Fusion of his hip in the position of function. If you decide that this will be best for him, achieve this position by applying a spica in the position described in Section 7.17, until his hip has fused. (b) If the head and neck of his femur have been partly destroyed, he may benefit if their remains are removed by Girdlestone's operation (7.19). This will give him a much more comfortable joint with some movement.

(4) The infection may extend into his acetabulum and involve the bones of his pelvis. When this has happened, there is little you can do, except drain the pus. His osteitis usually settles.

To explore and drain the hip you can approach it anteriorly or posteriorly. If you can safely anaesthetize a prone patient (A 16.12), the posterior approach is easier, because it allows better drainage. If you cannot do this, use the anterior one, and anaesthetize him in the supine position.

SPECIAL METHODS FOR THE HIP

For the methods of aspiration, and the positions of rest and function, see Section 7.17.

THE RELIEF OF SPASM. If the patient is a child, apply up to 1/7th of his body weight of extension (skin) traction, depending on his weight. This will relieve the spasm of his muscles, and will prevent him developing a flexion contracture.

THE ANTERIOR APPROACH TO THE HIP (really the anterolateral approach, 7-18)

ANAESTHESIA. Ketamine, or general anaesthesia with spontaneous respiration.

POSITION. Lay him supine, but tilt him to the other side by putting a sandbag under his affected hip.

ASPIRATION is useful to check that pus is present. If you don't find it, but think that he probably has got septic arthritis, explore his hip anyway.

INCISION. Cut from the mid-point of his iliac crest to his anterior-superior iliac spine. Extend the incision distally down his leg for 10 or 12 cm. Divide his superficial and deep fascia. Use a periosteal elevator to separate his gluteus medius and tensor fascia lata from his iliac crest. Continue the dissection distally between his tensor fascia lata posterolaterally, and his sartorius and rectus femoris anteromedially. Divide the ascending branch of his lateral circumflex vessels between ligatures.

Insert two bone levers on each side round the upper shaft of his femur and retract his muscles. You will now see the capsule of his hip joint. Check that it is his joint by aspirating. Now open the joint with a cruciate incision. Ask an unsterile assistant to grasp the patient's ankle and externally rotate his hip. You will see the head of his femur moving inside his acetabulum. If you want better access to the joint, insert levers round the neck of his femur. If you suspect osteomyelitis, drill at least 4 holes into the neck and upper shaft of his femur.

Insert a corrugated drain from the joint to the surface, and leave it in for 5 to 7 days. Don't suture the capsule. Bring his muscles together lightly with a few '0' chromic catgut sutures. Close the fascia over his iliac crest. Close his skin with '0' monofilament.

POSTOPERATIVELY, apply 2 to 5 kg of skin traction up to his mid thigh, with his leg in in 1 to 15° of abduction and minimal flexion. Raise the foot of his bed.

THE POSTERIOR APPROACH TO THE HIP (OBER'S APPROACH)

Intubate the patient and control his ventilation. Lie him on his side, slightly inclined towards the prone position. Find the tip of his great trochanter. Cut medially from it for 5 cm in line with the fibres of his gluteus maximus. Cut through his skin and superficial fascia.

Separate the fibres of his gluteus maximus using your index finger and the end of a curved haemostat, until you meet the capsule of his hip joint. Open the incision with retractors.

THE ANTERIOR APPROACH TO THE HIP

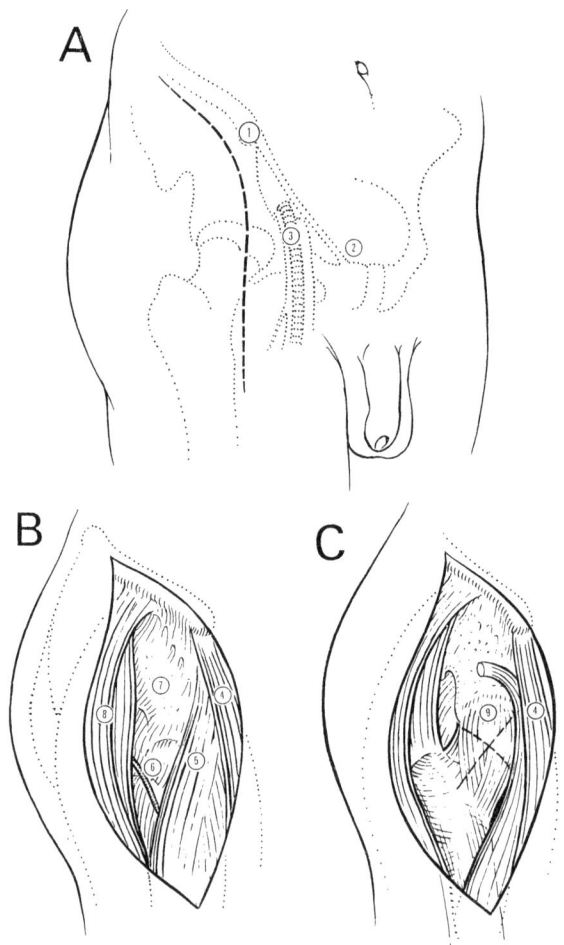

Fig. 7-18 THE ANTERIOR APPROACH TO THE HIP. A, the incision. B, the muscles retracted. C, preparing to incise the capsule.
1, the anterior superior iliac spine. 2, the pubic tubercle. 3, the femoral vein, artery and nerve from medial to lateral in this order. 4, sartorius. 5, rectus femoris. 6, the ascending branch of the lateral circummflex vessels. 7, the exposed surface of the ilium. 8, gluteus medius and tensor fascia lata. 9, the incision in the capsule.

EXPLORING THE HIP THROUGH OBER'S APPROACH

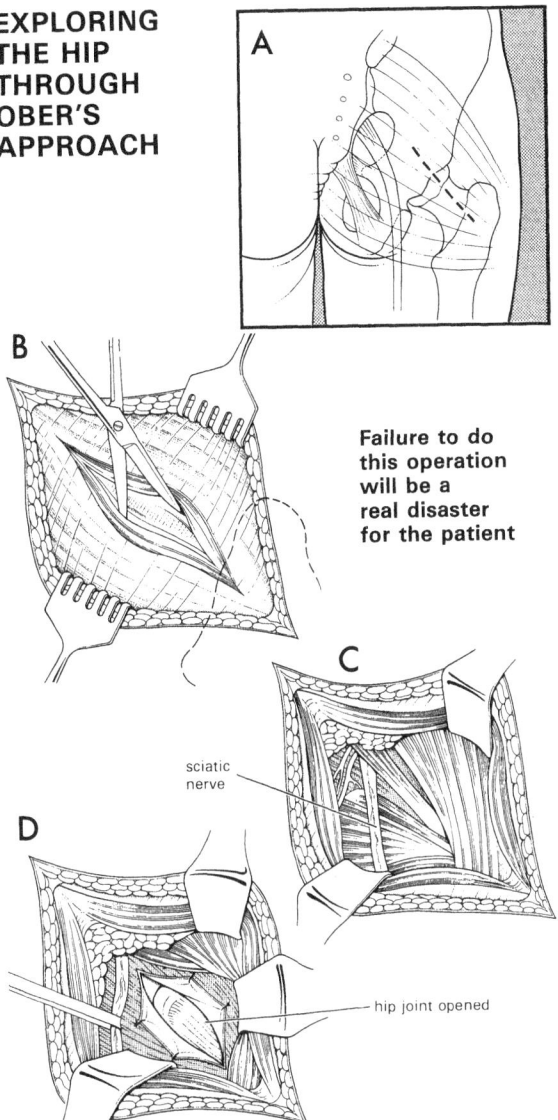

Failure to do this operation will be a real disaster for the patient

Fig. 7-19 EXPLORING THE HIP THROUGH OBER'S POSTERIOR APPROACH. A, incise patient's gluteus maximus. B, separate its fibres. C, be careful not to injure the sciatic nerve. D, incise the hip joint.

If you find pus in the muscles of his buttock, before you reach his hip, stop. He has pyomyositis. If you go further and open a normal hip through an abscess in his muscles, you will probably infect it.

Ask an assistant to take hold of his ankle and rotate his hip internally, so as to increase the space between his trochanter and his acetabulum.

Make a small incision in the distended capsule of his hip joint and widen it with a haemostat.

CAUTION ! (1) His sciatic nerve leaves his buttock half way between his greater trochanter and his ischial tuberosity. There is no need to incise or dissect this far medially. (2) The capsule of the hip joint is only a finger's breadth wide between the posterior aspect of the greater trochanter and the posterior margin of the acetabulum.

If his upper femoral epiphysis has slipped and is forming a sequestrum, remove it. Approach his hip posteriorly as above. Modify this by carrying the incision down his greater trochanter. Remove the loose head of his femur with large bone forceps, and as much of its neck as is necrotic.

POSTOPERATIVELY, reduce the tendency of his hip to slide proximally by putting him into traction for 6 weeks postoperatively, while fibrous tissue forms to limit movement. He will have an unstable hip and will need a crutch, but he should be pain-free and he will be able to walk.

7.19 Girdlestone's operation for an infected hip

The previous hip procedures described in this chapter are mostly needed by children. This one may help an adult whose hip has been partly destroyed by infection, avascular necrosis or a painful ununited femoral neck fracture (77.6). He will walk less painfully, if what is left of the head and neck of his femur is excised, so as to allow the upper end of his femur to bear on scar tissue on the under side of his ilium. A false joint will develop, his leg will be short and he will need a stick, but he will probably have very little pain. This is a difficult procedure and is for more experienced surgeons only, which is why it is in small print. If you are inexperienced: (1) The joint cavity may become infected and seal off. (2) You can injure his sciatic nerve. (3) You may have to abandon the procedure uncompleted, in which case you will feel ashamed, and he will be made worse.

Girdlestone's operation is a salvage procedure to relieve pain when an arthrodesis or, exceptionally, a prosthesis is impractical. It is inelegant and old-fashioned, and is not indicated if you can refer him for an arthrodesis or a hip prosthesis. If this is impossible, *and you are fairly experienced* Girdlestone's operation will be much better than nothing. There are two varieties: (1) For a previously septic or tuberculous hip infection which is now inactive. This is the method which is described below. (2) For an ununited fracture of the neck of the femur, as described in Section 77.13.

Use a posterior approach, like Ober's (7.18), except that you carry the incision further down his femur, for 25 to 40 cm. Make sure that his sciatic nerve is out of the way, and that your assistant does not grasp it with his retractor.

GIRDLESTONE'S OPERATION

INDICATIONS FOR INFECTIVE CONDITIONS. A patient who is walking painfully as the result of: (1) Previous septic arthritis, which is now inactive. (2) Previous tuberculous arthritis, which is now inactive but is still painful. (3) Aseptic necrosis of the head of the femur. (4) A longstanding ununited fracture of the femoral neck. (5) An infected prosthesis.

If you cannot refer him, proceed as follows.

EQUIPMENT. An orthopaedic set (4.12). A Gigli saw. Ideally, two special retractors. Have two units of blood cross-matched.

INCISION. Follow the method in Secction 77.13 until you get to the paragraph 'Cut the neck...' then proceed as follows:

Incise the capsule of the patient's hip joint to expose the head and neck of his femur and the remainder of his greater trochanter. Now open up his exposed hip joint by incising its capsule widely. Ask your assistant to move the patient's leg to help you identify the head of the femur.

If the head of his femur is not necrotic, or his hip is ankylosed, end the operation here.

You will find that removing the head is easier if you excise part of the rim of his acetabulum. Curette all necrotic and infected bone from his acetabulum. Make the excision as complete as possible and leave only the raw surfaces of vascular cancellous bone. Remove the neck down to its base, and smooth it by chiselling away all sharp edges.

Sew back the edges of his incised gluteus maximus. If there is little active infection and you have suction drainage, use it. If you find the bone seriously infected, leave the wound partly open. Insert 2 or 3 rubber drains.

POSTOPERATIVELY, to prevent shortening, apply 3 to 10 kg of skeletal traction through his tibia with his hip in 20 or 30° of flexion for 6 weeks. This will not be necessary if his hip is already fibrotic.

CAUTION ! Try to prevent proximal displacement of his femur. This will prematurely 'seal off' the area and defeat the purpose of the operation, which is to saucerize his acetabulum and allow free drainage when there is active infection.

8 Pus in the hands and feet

8.1 The general method for an infected hand

A badly infected hand can be a real disaster. Some infections arise spontaneously, others follow quite minor injuries, or even a seemingly trivial scratch. They are particularly common in leprosy patients (30.4, 30.6). *The best prevention is an early and thorough toilet of all hand wounds.* If you do this early, it is quite a minor procedure. The great danger of late or inadequate treatment is a stiff finger (75.2), which is a great disability, and may need amputation.

If you treat a patient early enough, antibiotics may be effective, and may prevent a serious lesion spreading. Some hand surgeons make little use of them, and they are certainly much less important than a careful wound toilet and early drainage.

There are many spaces in the hand where pus can collect, each with its own signs and incisions. These spaces are not rigidly defined; some run into one another, and more than one may be infected at the same time, as in Fig. 8-5, so don't be dismayed by the apparent complexity of pus in the hand. The common places for it to collect are in the pulp spaces of the fingers (8.5), and in the web spaces (8.7). Even after pus has formed, he should recover completely—if you treat him correctly, and provided that his tendon sheaths have not been involved.

**PUS IN THE HAND IS COMMON AND SERIOUS!
DON'T BE BOTHERED BY THE NUMBER OF INCISIONS!**

One difficulty is knowing when to incise an infected hand. Pus is so tightly trapped in the spaces of the hand that you cannot use fluctuation as a sign that it is present. A good rule to remember is that, if his hand prevented him sleeping the previous night, it needs incising.

When you operate: (1) Don't cut his digital nerves—remember that they run on the radial and ulnar aspects of his fingers just anterior to the tips of his finger creases, as in D, Fig. 8-6. (2) Don't cut through a more superficial abscess into his flexor sheaths underneath, or you may infect them. These are in the greatest danger where they are nearest to the surface, under the flexor creases of his fingers. So don't incise the palmar surface of a finger proximal to its distal flexion crease, unless you are deliberately draining an infected tendon sheath. (3) When you drain pus, be sure to remove the granulation tissue that surrounds it, so that the wall of the abscess is clean, and antibiotic containing blood can enter it. (4) Use a bloodless field whenever you can, so that you can see the anatomy clearly.

**DON'T WAIT FOR FLUCTUATION
IF PAIN KEPT HIM AWAKE LAST NIGHT, INCISE HIS HAND
USE A TOURNIQUET**

THE GENERAL METHOD FOR HAND (AND FOOT) INFECTIONS

If the patient has leprosy, see Sections 30.4 and 30.6.

WHERE IS THE PUS? Feel carefully for the point of greatest tenderness by probing with a matchstick.

If his terminal phalanx is infected, consult Figure 8-2.

If his whole hand is swollen like an inflated rubber glove, the pus is probably in his mid palmar space, or in a flexor tendon sheath, especially if he cannot move his little and ring fingers.

If the greatest swelling is over the web of his thumb, he probably has pus in his thenar space, especially if his index finger is held flexed, and he cannot move it or his thumb.

If: (1) his whole finger is swollen and tender, (2) there is no obvious sign of the pus pointing, and (3) any movement of the finger is exquisitely painful, he probably has a tendon sheath infection.

If all his fingers, especially the fifth, are held semi-flexed and rigid, suspect that the tendon sheaths in his ulnar bursa are infected.

If he has lymphangitis, lymphadenitis, and fever, his infection is spreading. If pus is present, incise his hand under antibiotic cover, and continue after his temperature and pulse have become normal.

CAUTION ! Pus is much more likely to be present on the palmar surface than on the dorsum, so don't be misled by swelling on the back of his hand. The commonest cause of a swollen dorsum is a web space infection.

SPECIAL TESTS. Test his urine for sugar—diabetes may present as a septic infection.

TREATMENT FOR HAND INFECTIONS

RAISE HIS HAND to make him more comfortable and promote healing. In less severe infections, raise his arm in the St. John's sling. In more severe ones, such as a tendon sheath infection, put him to bed and raise his hand in a roller towel: both are shown in Fig. 75-1.

ANTIBIOTICS are usually unnecessary, but if his infection is spreading (see above) give him penicillin in the dose for a severe infection. If antibiotic resistance is likely, for example if he is working in a hospital, or your local strains are apt not to respond to penicillin, give him chloramphenicol, erythromycin, or, if you can afford it, cloxacillin.

Don't forget to give him an analgesic.

INCISING HAND INFECTIONS

SHOULD YOU INCISE IT? Don't try to treat an infected hand by aspiration only. Base your decision to incise it on: (1) The presence of acute local tenderness. This shows that pus is present and where it is pointing. (2) The length of his history—if symptoms are becoming worse after 48 hours, his hand probably needs incising. (3) The severity of the swelling. (4) The nature of his pain. If throbbing pain kept him awake last night, incise his hand.

ANAESTHESIA must be adequate. For any but the most minor infection, avoid local infiltration close to the infection, because this will only spread it and increase the swelling.

PUS IN THE HAND

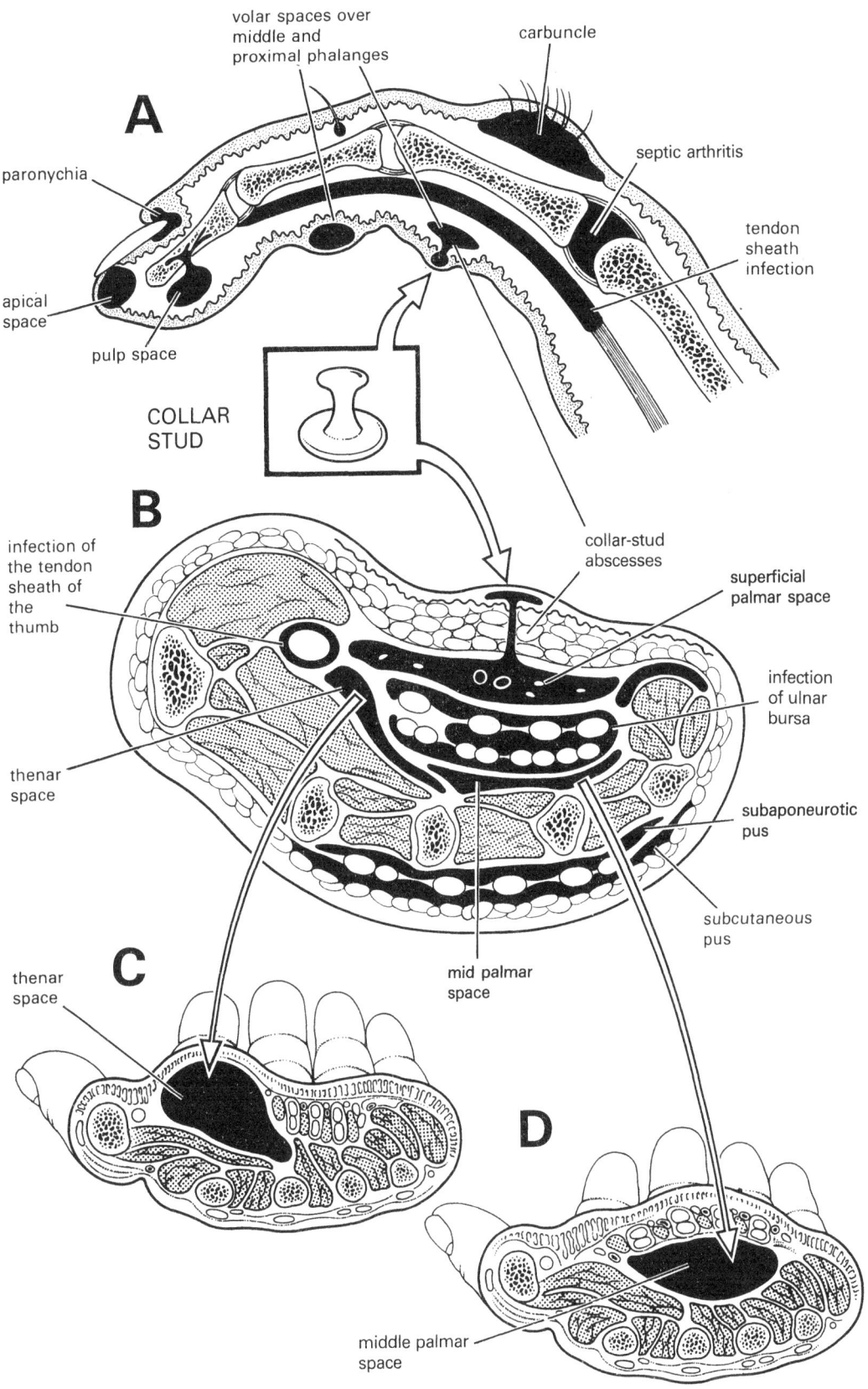

Fig. 8-1 THE MANY PLACES WHERE PUS CAN COLLECT IN THE HAND. There are also three which are not shown here: these are the web spaces in Fig. 8-5. *After 'Farquharson's Textbook of Operative Surgery', edited by Rintoul R.F, Fig. 302 (Churchill Livingstone): and 'Campbell's Operative Orthopaedics', edited by Edmondsen AS and Crenshaw AH—the Chapter on 'Hand Infections' by Lee Milford, Fig. 3-357, (CV Mosby Company). Both with kind permission.*

If the infection is in the distal two thirds of his finger or thumb you can use a finger block *without* adrenalin (A 6.21).

For all other hand infections, use an axillary block (A 6.18), or an intravenous forearm block (A 6.19), or ketamine (A 8.2), or general anaesthesia.

A TOURNIQUET is essential in all but the most superficial infections, because a bloodless field makes the operation easier (3.9). Don't exsanguinate his arm with an Esmarch bandage, because it may spread the infection.

If the pus is in the distal segment, wrap a rubber catheter twice round the base of his finger or thumb, and clamp it with a heavy haemostat.

If the pus is anywhere else, apply a pneumatic tourniquet, or an Esmarch bandage properly applied as a tourniquet (3.9).

EQUIPMENT. Use a small scalpel, fine pointed scissors, skin hooks, fine dissecting forceps, and if necessary Volkmann's spoon.

ASSISTANT. If he has a major infection, you must have an assistant scrubbed up to hold the retractors.

INCISING, DESLOUGHING AND DRAINING. Clean his skin with antiseptic. Incise where pus points, and don't adhere too slavishly to standard incisions, which are described later. We have numbered the incisions that you will need for major hand infections from 1 to 12. Most of them are shown on Fig. 8-6.

When you extend an incision, do so in a skin crease. If necessary jump from one crease to another by making a Z-shaped incision. Remove skin that is already dead. If necessary, extend an incision to explore the whole abscess cavity, and remove deeper dead tissues.

If more than one space is infected, adapt your incision(s) accordingly. For example, if his mid-palmar space, several web spaces and his tendon sheaths are infected, you may need to make several incisions like those in Fig. 8-5.

As soon as you are through his skin, insert a haemostat, open it, and explore the abscess cavity (Hilton's method). Culture the pus.

If there are no vulnerable structures such as periosteum, nerves or tendon sheaths, nearby, scrape away the lining of his abscess with curette or a swab. If there are vulnerable structures nearby, be more cautious, and only use a swab.

Drain the abscess by putting a piece of rubber glove into it. Or, leave a piece of vaseline gauze between the wound edges.

CAUTION ! (1) Don't cut his nerves, see Fig. 8-6. (a) His digital nerves run near the anterolateral margins of his fingers. So either cut near the middle of the palmar surfaces of his fingers, or on their lateral surfaces fairly posteriorly at the apex of his finger creases. (b) The muscular branch of his median nerve comes off the main trunk just distal to the tuberosity of his scaphoid and curves round into his thenar muscles. (2) Don't pack the wound tightly.

TO CONTROL BLEEDING remove the tourniquet, raise his arm and press firmly on the wound *for 5 to 10 minutes without interruption.*

POSTOPERATIVELY, be sure to elevate his hand, until pain and swelling subside—*this is an important way of reducing stiffness.* Rapid resolution of inflammatory oedema is more important than early movement in reducing stiffness. Wrap the wound with plenty of gauze, and use the dressings to splint it in the position of safety (75.8). Leave them on for several days, unless the wound becomes painful, or swells, or there is much discharge. When you change the dressings, use careful aseptic precautions, so as to avoid secondary infection. If they stick, soak them off in saline, and then gently remove them.

If the infection was extensive, check 2 to 4 days later for residual infection or necrotic tissue which may need treatment.

CAUTION ! Start active movements as soon as pain has subsided.

RAISE AN INFECTED HAND
STIFF FINGERS RESULT IN POOR FUNCTION

8.2 Subcutaneous hand infections

A patient's skin and subcutaneous tissue can be infected anywhere in his hand. Pulp infections and paronychia are merely subcutaneous infections at the tip of a finger. If there is pus under the keratinized layers of his epidermis, strip these off, and see if you can find the hole through which it has tracked from a deeper abscess underneath. An abscess near the surface may communicate with pus deep inside his hand through a narrow opening. Pus like this forms a 'collar-stud abscess' as shown in Fig. 8-1. So, whenever you find a superficial abscess, look for the passage which might be joining it to a deeper one.

Carbuncles (5.4) may form in the hair follicles on the back of the fingers and hand. Antibiotics will not cure them, so deslough them.

DON'T BE MISLED BY A COLLAR-STUD ABSCESS

8.3 Infections of the apical finger space

The apical space lies between the distal part of a patient's nail and the bone of his distal phalanx. It may be infected when a splinter runs under his nail. His finger is painful, but there is little swelling. Tenderness is greatest at or just under the free edge of his nail. Cut a small 'V' out of the edge of the nail over the point of greatest tenderness, as in C, and D, Fig. 8-2. Remove the full thickness of the skin as a small wedge, and drain the pus.

8.4 Paronychia

Paronychia is an infection beside or proximal to a patient's nail. Pus may track round it, as in A and B, Fig. 8-2; either superficial to his nail as in E, and F, or deep to it as in G, and H. Early antibiotic treatment may abort the infection, but you usually have to drain pus.

PARONYCHIA For the general method for a hand infection, see Section 8.1.

If the pus is superficial to a patient's nail on one side only, incise it by angling the knife away from his nail to avoid cutting his nail bed, as in E, and F, Fig. 8-2.

If the pus lies under one corner of his nail, reflect a little flap and remove that corner only, as in G, and H.

If pus has tracked to the other side of his finger under his nail, make a second incision there, retract the flap, excise the proximal one third of his nail, pack the wound open and drain it, as in I, to L, in Fig. 8-2.

If the infection fails to resolve, or his nail becomes indurated and red, suspect a fungus infection, and examine scrapings microscopically. If you find fungi, remove his nail and apply wet dressings, or a topical antifungal agent, such as Castellani's paint or gentian violet.

8.5 Infection of the pulp space of the finger

This is the commonest hand infection—pus more often gathers in the finger tips than anywhere else in the hand.

The pulp of a finger is divided into many small fatty compartments by strands of fibrous tissue which run from the skin to the periosteum of the terminal phalanx. A sheet of fibrous tissue runs from the distal flexor crease to the periosteum, and so separates the pulp space from the rest of the finger. There is little room for swelling, so that infection causes a throbbing pain early. Pus from a patient's pulp can track: (1) through to the skin outside, or (2) through the periosteum, causing osteomyelitis of his distal phalanx. Its epiphysis is supplied by a separate artery, so this usually survives the infection.

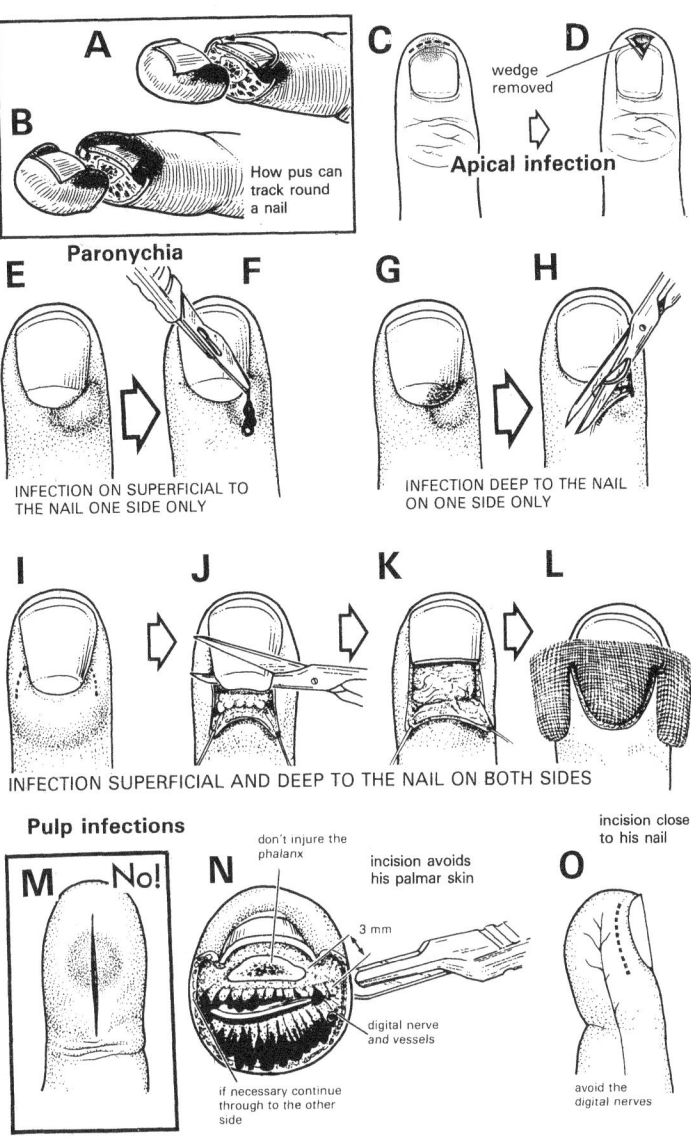

Fig. 8-2 INFECTION AROUND THE NAIL. A patient can have pus on one side of his nail, either superficial (E), or deep (G). It may track all round his nail (A, and B) so that the proximal part of his nail needs excising (I to L). Avoid incising the ball of his finger (M) unless pus is already pointing there. N, and O, if infection is already present in several of the compartments of his pulp, you will have to make a lateral incision. Keep your incision away from his palmar skin, and not more than 3 mm from the edge of his nail. Note: In N, don't cut the end of his finger off; this is a schematic cross-section only! *A, and B, after Flatt AB, 'Functional Anatomy', Fig. 14.2 with kind permission.*

PULP INFECTION

For the general method for hand infections, see Section 8.1. Tenderness is maximal over the ball of the patient's pulp.

If the abscess is in his distal pulp, and is *already pointing to its centre,* drain it by making a cross-shaped incision, or by removing a small circular or elliptical segment of skin over the abscess, as in B, to E, Fig. 8-3. The incision will heal to leave a small punctate scar.

If the abscess is deep, is not pointing, and appears to extend into several compartments, make a J-shaped lateral longitudinal incision close to the bone, and not more than 3 mm in a palmar direction from the free edge of his nail. Keep your knife away from his palmar skin, as in N, and O, Fig. 8-2, and avoid the tip of his finger. Remove pus and slough, and lightly pack the wound with gauze. Don't suture the incision. Change the dressing after two days.

If the infection has been neglected, so that the whole terminal segment of his finger is swollen, continue the incision over the end of his finger and round to the other side. Divide the vertical septa and let the wound gape open. Dress it as above.

CAUTION ! (1) Don't incise the tips of his fingers, or the palmar surfaces of his distal phalanges, unless pus is already pointing there, because pressure on the scar may be painful. (2) Any incision, other than those described, is likely to be painful, especially if you carry it towards the palmar surface. (3) Don't damage his periosteum. (4) Check for a collar-stud abscess (easily seen if you have used a tourniquet to give you a bloodless field).

DIFFICULTIES **If his infected FINGER CONTINUES TO DISCHARGE for some weeks,** suspect osteomyelitis (8.16D). X-ray it. When X-rays show that the sequestrum has separated,

PULP INFECTION

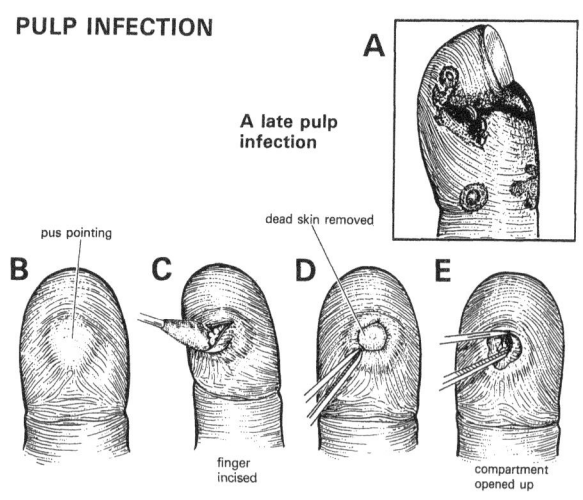

Fig. 8-3 PULP INFECTIONS. A, a neglected pulp infection. Much of the patient's finger tip is already destroyed, and pus is starting to discharge spontaneously. B, *if pus is already pointing*, make a cross-shaped incision. C, swab away the pus. D, remove any dead skin. E, open up the infected pulp compartment. If it is not pointing and several spaces are infected, open up his finger tip from the side as in N in the previous figure.

remove it. If he is a child, his distal phalanx will regenerate under its periosteum. If he is an adult, he will be left with an ugly curved nail and a short terminal phalanx.

8.6 Infections of the spaces over the volar surfaces of the middle and proximal phalanges

Pus sometimes collects on the volar surfaces of a patient's fingers, superficial to his tendon sheaths, as shown in A, Fig. 8-1. The spaces where it forms are separated from one another by the fibrous septa which run dorsally from the flexor creases of his fingers. The proximal space in each finger communicates with the web spaces in his palm. Pus may collect under his epidermis or under his deep fascia, and is less likely to remain localized than in a terminal phalanx.

He holds his swollen, tender, indurated finger semi-flexed. Trying to straighten it is acutely painful. Distinguishing an infection of these spaces from localized infection of a tendon sheath may be so difficult that you will not know which he has, until you have explored his hand.

Drain pus from a volar space through a transverse incision over the point of greatest tenderness. *Take great care not cut into the tendon sheath underneath it or to damage his digital vessels or nerves (G, 8-6)*. Use a tourniquet to give you a bloodless field.

> **DON'T OPEN A TENDON SHEATH OR A JOINT UNLESS IT IS INFECTED**

8.7 Web space infections

Three spaces, filled with loose fat, lie between the bases of a patient's fingers in the distal part of his palm. They lie just proximal to his deep transverse ligaments, near his MP joints. Pus more often gathers here than anywhere else in his hand, except in the pulp spaces of his finger tips. It mostly gathers near the palmar surface, but if it is not drained, it may track: (1) posteriorly towards the dorsum, (2) along a lumbrical canal into his middle palmar space, (3) across the front of a finger into a neighbouring web space, or (4) distally into his finger.

Pain and swelling may be so great that he comes for treatment before much pus has formed. The back of his hand is swollen, as in D, Fig. 8-5. If infection is severe, the fingers on either side of the web separate—*a very useful sign*. The point of maximum tenderness is on the palmar surface of the web, and may extend a short way into his palm. Although you may suspect a web space infection, you may find it difficult to exclude an infected tendon sheath.

WEB SPACE INFECTION. For the general method for an infected hand, see Section 8.1.

Make a V-shaped incision between the patient's fingers, as in incision (1), in Figs. 8-5 and 8-6.

If pus is pointing into his palm, pass a probe proximally from the incision you have just made in his web space up into his palm. Its tip should underlie the place where the pus is pointing. Make a second incision there. Scrape the walls of the abscess cavity free from granulation tissue. If necessary, divide some strands of his palmar fascia.

8.8 Infection of the superficial palmar space

When pus collects in the superficial palmar spaces of a patient's hand, it does so under his palmar fascia. Sometimes, it tracks superficially and forms a collar-stud abscess under the superficial layers of his epidermis, as in B, Fig. 8-1.

SUPERFICIAL PALMAR SPACE. For the general method for a hand infection, see Section 8.1.

If you can see pus under the patient's epidermis, remove it and look for a track leading deeper into his hand.

If you cannot see any pus, make a small transverse incision over the point of maximum tenderness, in the line of the nearest skin crease (not illustrated). Probe the abscess cavity. If you find an opening leading to a deeper collection of pus, enlarge it. Scrape infected granulations from the wall of the cavity.

8.9 Infection of the middle palmar space

This is *the most important space in the hand*, and is frequently infected in leprosy patients (30.4). It lies deep to a patient's flexor tendons and lumbricals, and between them and the fascia covering his interossei and metacarpals. It is separated from his thenar space by a fibrous septum which extends from his middle metacar-

THE THENAR AND THE MIDDLE PALMAR SPACES

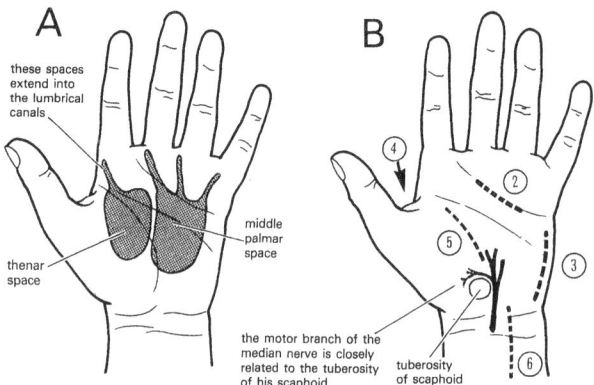

Fig. 8-4 THE THENAR (radial) AND THE MIDDLE PALMAR SPACES lie deep to a patient's flexor tendons, between them and the fascia covering his metacarpals and interossei (see also Fig. 8-1). They communicate with his lumbrical canals. Incise his middle palmar space in the middle third of his distal (or proximal) palmar crease (incision 2), or along the ulnar border of his hand (incision 3). Incise his thenar space in the web between his thumb and his index finger (incision 4), or along his thenar crease in his palm (incision 5). Beware of the motor branch of his median nerve!

pal towards his palmar fascia. Infection reaches this space from a lumbrical canal, or from an infected tendon sheath.

His hand is so grossly swollen that it looks like a blown-up rubber glove. The normal hollow of his palm is obliterated, and the dorsum of his hand is swollen. He cannot move his middle or ring fingers. His interossei are surrounded by pus and paralysed, so that if you ask him to hold a piece of paper between his extended fingers he cannot do so.

The middle palmar space communicates through the carpal tunnel with a space deep to the flexor tendons in the forearm (the space of Parona). If there is pus there you may be able to detect fluctuation between it and the pus in his palm.

MIDDLE PALMAR SPACE. For the general method for a hand infection, see Section 8.1. *Always use a tourniquet.*

Make a transverse incision (incision 2) in the middle third of the patient's distal or proximal palmar creases or wherever fluctuation is maximal. Enter his middle palmar space on either side of the flexor tendon of his ring finger. Or, enter it through an incision along the ulnar border of his hand, passing between his 5th metacarpal and his hypothenar muscles (incision 3). As soon as you are through his skin, use blunt dissection (Hilton's method) in the line of his tendons and nerves. See also under 'ulnar bursa' (8.13).

CAUTION ! (1) Don't make your initial incision deeper than his palmar fascia. Push a blunt instrument through it to free the pus underneath. You can then see clearly to open up the space more by a combination of sharp and gentle blunt dissection. (2) Don't cut his digital nerves or vessels, his flexor tendons, or his lumbrical muscles.

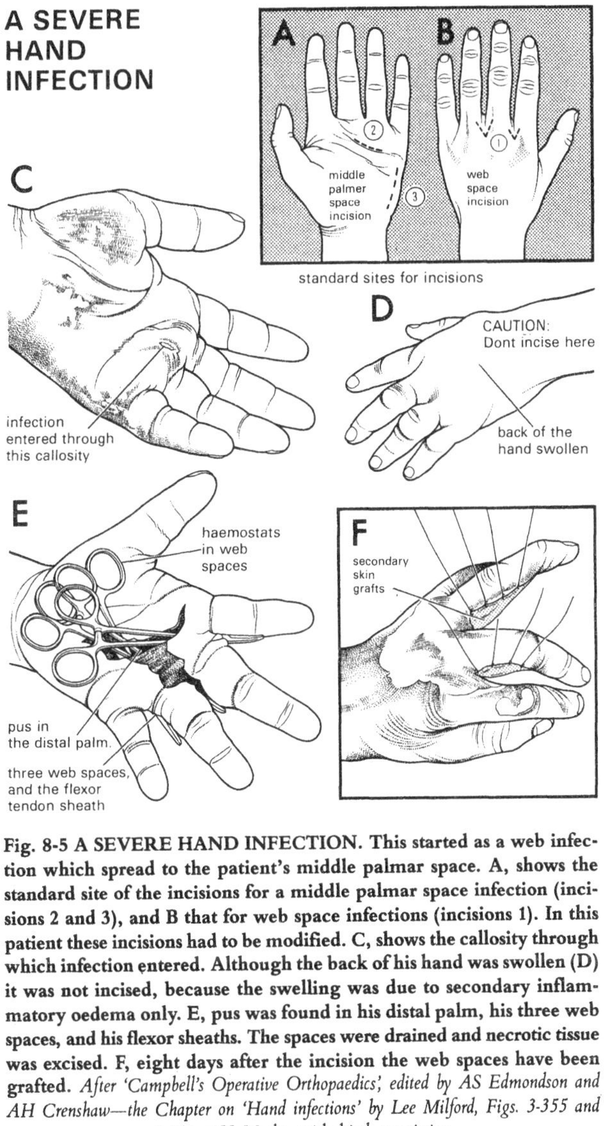

A SEVERE HAND INFECTION

Fig. 8-5 A SEVERE HAND INFECTION. This started as a web infection which spread to the patient's middle palmar space. A, shows the standard site of the incisions for a middle palmar space infection (incisions 2 and 3), and B that for web space infections (incisions 1). In this patient these incisions had to be modified. C, shows the callosity through which infection entered. Although the back of his hand was swollen (D) it was not incised, because the swelling was due to secondary inflammatory oedema only. E, pus was found in his distal palm, his three web spaces, and his flexor sheaths. The spaces were drained and necrotic tissue was excised. F, eight days after the incision the web spaces have been grafted. *After 'Campbell's Operative Orthopaedics', edited by AS Edmondson and AH Crenshaw—the Chapter on 'Hand infections' by Lee Milford, Figs. 3-355 and 3-356. CV Mosby, with kind permission.*

If there is pus in the space of Parona, drain it through a longitudinal incision (incision 6) on one side of his palmaris longus tendon (absent in 5% of people), taking care not to injure his median and ulnar nerves or his radial and ulnar vessels.

8.10 Infection of the thenar space of the hand

A patient's thenar space (B, and C, Fig. 8-1) is sometimes infected by a penetrating wound. It lies underneath his palmar fascia, and is bounded dorsally by the transverse head of his adductor pollicis. On its ulnar side a fibrous septum divides it from his middle palmar space.

His thenar eminence is grossly swollen, and his thumb is abducted.

THENAR SPACE. For the general method for a hand infection, see Section 8.1.

Drain the patient's thenar space over the point of greatest tenderness through a curved incision in the web between his thumb and index finger, parallel to the border of his first dorsal interosseous muscle, on the dorsal edge of his hand (incision 4). Or, drain it in an incision along his thenar crease in his palm (incision 5). Insert a haemostat deep into the abscess, and open it. You will usually find that it is walled off from the muscles of his thumb.

CAUTION ! Remember the course of the sensory and motor branches of his median nerve which lies within his thenar muscles. These are in less danger from incision (4) than from incision (5).

8.11 Infections on the dorsum of the hand and fingers

Infection almost anywhere in a patient's hand makes its back swell, but pus seldom collects there. On the rare occasions when it does collect on the dorsum, it is usually subcutaneous, and only occasionally in the subaponeurotic space under his extensor tendons (B, Fig. 8-1). If localized tenderness persists for more than 48 hours, don't wait for fluctuation. Drain it through a longitudinal incision over the point of greatest tenderness.

THE COMMONEST CAUSE OF SWELLING ON THE DORSUM IS INFECTION IN THE PALM

8.12 Infections of the flexor tendon sheaths of the hand

The sheaths of a patient's flexor tendons come nearest to his skin as they pass under the flexor creases of his fingers. It is here, and particularly over his distal flexor crease, that they are most often punctured and infected. They can also be infected by spread from a pulp infection. The sheaths of his little finger and thumb (and occasionally those of his other fingers also) extend proximally into his palm, and so provide a path through which infection can spread there. If an infected tendon sheath bursts, it does so into the middle palmar space, through one of the lumbrical canals.

There are problems: (1) An infected tendon may later stick to its sheath and make a finger stiff. (2) If pressure inside a sheath exceeds that in its vessels, which can occur if drainage is delayed, the tendon will become ischaemic and slough.

If infection is localized or one area is maximally infected, staphylococci are usually causing it. Only one segment of his finger is swollen, so that distinguishing a localized tendon sheath infection of this kind from an infection of one of his middle palmar and thenar spaces can be difficult (8.9).

If infection is fulminating, streptococci are usually responsible, and his whole finger is swollen, sausage shaped and acutely tender,

SOME INCISIONS FOR HAND INFECTIONS

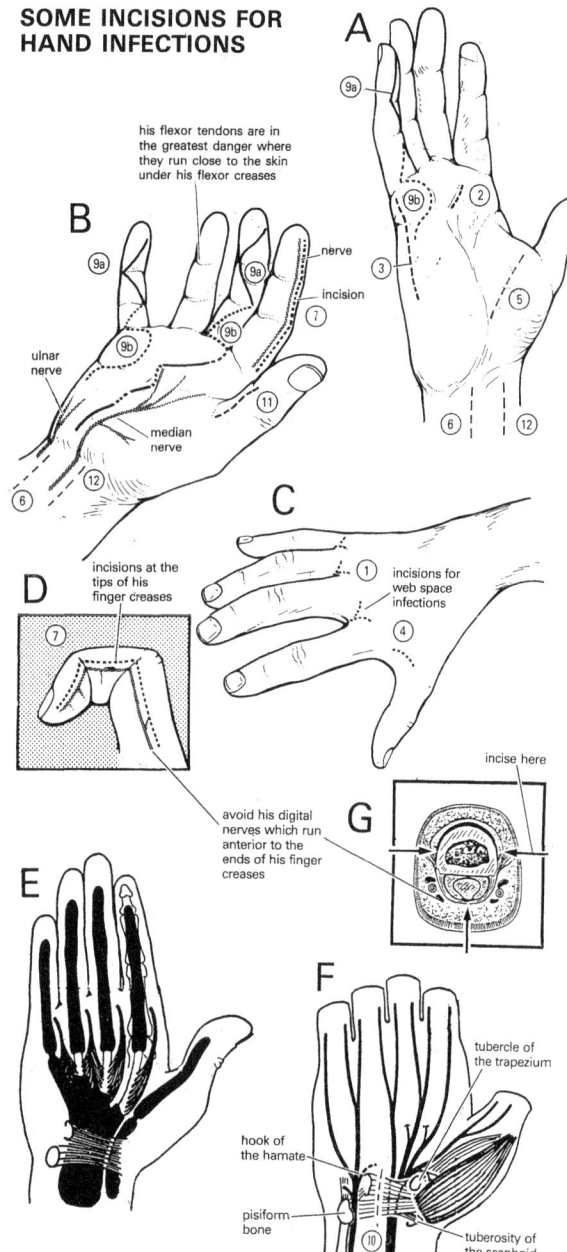

without becoming red. The swelling extends into his distal palm. He holds his finger partly flexed, and cannot bend it, except perhaps for a little movement at its MP joint.

The danger when you open a tendon sheath is that you may cut a patient's digital nerves. So study where these run in the cross-section of the finger shown in G, Fig 8-6. Either approach a tendon laterally, well towards the dorsum, or from the palm. The danger area is the 'palmolateral' region. The other nerve which is in danger is the motor branch of his median nerve as it curves round the distal end of his flexor retinaculum and the tubercle of his trapezium.

Adjust your incisions to the severity of the infection. You can approach an infected tendon sheath: (a) Along the side of a finger towards the dorsum (incision 7). (b) Through several transverse incisions on his palm (incisions 8, see Fig. 8-7). (c) By making zig-zag cuts on his palm (incisions 9); these give the best exposure, but take longer to heal. Incisions 7 and 8 are for less severe infections.

Tendon sheath infections are a common complication of the anaesthetic hands of leprosy (30.4), which allow a patient to neglect an infection until it is so advanced that it has destroyed his tendon sheaths.

FLEXOR SHEATH INFECTIONS

For the general method for a hand infection, see Section 8.1.

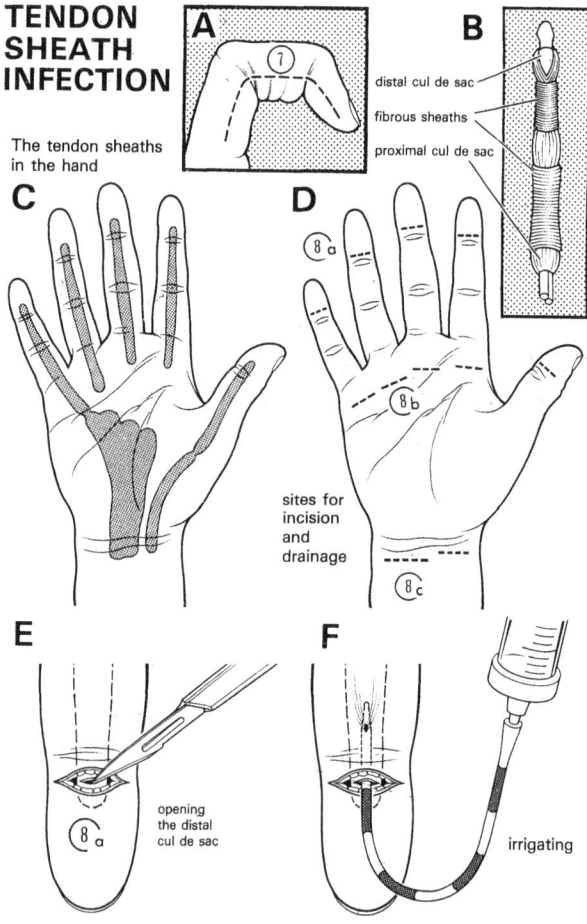

Fig. 8-6 INCISIONS FOR HAND INFECTIONS. Incisions for the finger tips are shown in Figs. 8-2 and 8-3. Some infections don't have fixed incisions (the volar surfaces of the proximal and middle phalanges, the superficial palmar space, and the dorsum of the hand), so these are not illustrated. A, to D, the remaining incisions for more serious hand infections, have been numbered, and most of them are shown here.

Incisions 1 for web space infections. Alternative incisions 2 and 3 for a middle palmar space infection. Alternative incisions 4 and 5 for a thenar space infection. Incision 6 for pus in the space of Parona (proximal to the flexor retinaculum and deep to the flexor tendons).

There are several alternative incisions for tendon sheaths: The lateral ones 7. The transverse palmar ones 8 (shown in Fig. 8-7). The zig-zag palmar ones 9; 9a the first part, and 9b the second part if necessary. Incisions 7 and 8 are for less severe infections, and incisions 9 for more severe ones.

Incision 10 divides the flexor retinaculum. Incisions 11 or 12 drain the radial bursa.

E, the tendon sheaths, the radial and ulnar bursae, the lumbrical muscles, and the flexor retinaculum.

F, the incision for dividing the flexor retinaculum (10). On the ulnar side of the retinaculum the palpable landmarks are the pisiform and the hook of the hamate. On the radial side you can feel the tubercle of the scaphoid and, more deeply, the tuberosity of the trapezium (see also Fig. 27-14a).

G, a cross section of the finger. The digital nerves are at the 'edges' of the palmar surfaces, so don't incise there. Either incise towards the middle of the palmar surfaces or laterally towards the dorsum as shown by the arrows. *E, and F, after Grant's 'Method of Anatomy', (9th edn. 1975 edited by JV Basmajian). Williams and Wilkins, with kind permission.*

Fig. 8-7 INFECTIONS OF THE TENDON SHEATHS. A, lateral incisions for opening an infected tendon sheath (incision 7). B, the anatomy of a tendon sheath, to show the fibrous pulleys opposite the shafts of the phalanges. C, the surface markings of the tendon sheaths. D, transverse incisions for draining tendon sheaths (incisions 8). E, opening the distal cul-de-sac (incision 8a). F, irrigating a tendon sheath. *E, and F, after 'Farquharson's Textbook of Operative Surgery', edited by RF Rintoul, Figs. 317 and 318. Churchill Livingstone, with kind permission.*

EXPOSING THE TENDON SHEATHS

Start by opening the soft tissue over the involved segment through a small lateral incision (incision 7). Examine the synovial sheath. If there is any sign of infection (redness, or thickening) open the sheath itself and look carefully at the fluid. If there is much fluid, it is probably infected; if it is even a little cloudy, it is certainly infected.

If a sheath is infected, make several incisions over the patient's finger(s) and distal palm (incisions 8a, and 8b). Hold the sheath open with hooks and retractors. Using a stiff catheter, syringe the sheath with saline or sterile water (F).

If a sheath is infected in his palm (as is usual with his little finger and thumb), make a further incision (incision 8c) at his wrist, and repeat the irrigation, inserting the catheter through the palmar incision.

If his tendon sheaths are grossly infected, operate urgently. Open the sheath by a zig-zag incision on the volar surface of his finger as in Fig. 8-6. Do this in two stages. First cut along the solid lines (9a), then, if necessary join up these incisions by cutting along the dotted ones (9b). Cut the flaps in the palm larger than those in the fingers, and make them follow his skin creases where possible. Cut through his skin and open the tissues with scissors. Leave bridges of the sheath over the joints to act as pulleys to prevent the tendons prolapsing.

CAUTION ! Don't take the incisions laterally where they may injure his neurovascular bundles.

Wash out the pus with saline. Don't close the incision; the flaps will heal by granulation to leave a linear scar.

If a tendon has become a grey slough, extend the incision, withdraw the dead part into the wound, and excise it. Preserve its sheath and pulley. Allow the wound to heal. If his hand settles well it may be possible to insert a tendon graft later. This will only be worthwhile if the joints of his fingers are mobile. So, as soon as the swelling is starting to settle, he needs intensive physiotherapy, both by himself and a by a physiotherapist—this is vital! If his finger remains stiff, try to persuade him that it should be amputated. A stiff finger can be a severe handicap.

If a tendon and its sheath are extensively disorganized, consider amputating his finger. If you don't do so: (1), infection may spread and cause further damage, (2) when his finger heals, it will be stiff, and cause considerable disability by impairing the grip of his other fingers. It may be better amputated. *But a stiff thumb is much better than no thumb,* so retain it.

If his palm is seriously infected, divide his flexor retinaculum to free his tendons. Either: (a) Approach this through a longitudinal incision 1 cm to the ulnar side of his scaphoid tubercle. Make a 5 cm longitudinal incision over his retinaculum. Keep to the ulnar side of his median nerve and its ulnar branch (incision 10) Or, (b) use the approach shown for the ulnar bursa (incision 3). Both are shown in Fig. 8-6.

AN UNNECESSARY INCISION IS BETTER THAN A LOST FINGER

8.13 Infection of ulnar bursa of the hand

Infection of the ulnar bursa is the most serious hand infection, because it contains all the flexor tendons of a patient's fingers. His whole hand is oedematous, his palm is moderately swollen, and there may a fullness immediately above his flexor retinaculum. His flexed fingers resist extension, particularly his little one, and least of all his index.

The radial and ulnar bursa sometimes communicate with one another. So if one of them has been infected, infection may follow in the other a day or two later.

INFECTION OF THE ULNAR BURSA. For the general method for a hand infection, see Section 8.1.

Open the tendon sheath of the patient's little finger with palmar flaps, using incisions 9a and if necessary 9b.

Incise his skin and deep fascia over the antero-medial side of his fifth metacarpal, using incision 3. Separate his abductor and flexor digiti minimi muscles from the bone. Retract them forwards and you will see his opponens digiti minimi muscle. Divide this close to its attachment to his flexor retinaculum. Divide his flexor retinaculum deep to opponens digiti minimi—you will see his bulging ulnar bursa. Wash this out, as for a tendon sheath infection (8.12)

You can also drain his middle palmar space through this incision, as in Section 8.9.

8.14 Infection of the radial bursa of the hand

A patient's radial bursa is a continuation of the tendon sheath of his flexor pollicis longus, so that any infection inevitably involves both of them. The distal phalanx of his thumb is flexed and rigid. He cannot extend it, although he can extend his other fingers normally. His hand is tender over the sheath of flexor pollicis longus, and you may be able to feel a swelling above his flexor retinaculum. If treatment is delayed, infection may spread to his ulnar bursa, or the tendon of his flexor pollicis longus may slough.

INFECTION OF THE RADIAL BURSA Incise the patient's radial bursa through incision 11 along the proximal phalanx of his thumb. Open it at its distal end; pass a probe proximally towards his wrist, and make a second incision over its proximal end (incision 12). Insert a fine catheter down the sheath and irrigate it with saline.

CAUTION ! (1) Don't incise along the radial border of his first metacarpal. Dissecting among the muscles there may impair the function of opposition, and prevent him bringing his thumb across his palm.

8.15 Septic arthritis of the fingers

A patient's finger joints are easily infected from open wounds, or from nearby infections. A human bite into a joint is particularly dangerous. The infected joint is acutely tender, swollen and painful. Its ligaments, cartilage, and bone are soon involved, so that he inevitably ends up with a stiff joint. A stiff DIP joint is little disability, but if he has a stiff MP or PIP joint, his finger but not his thumb are probably better amputated.

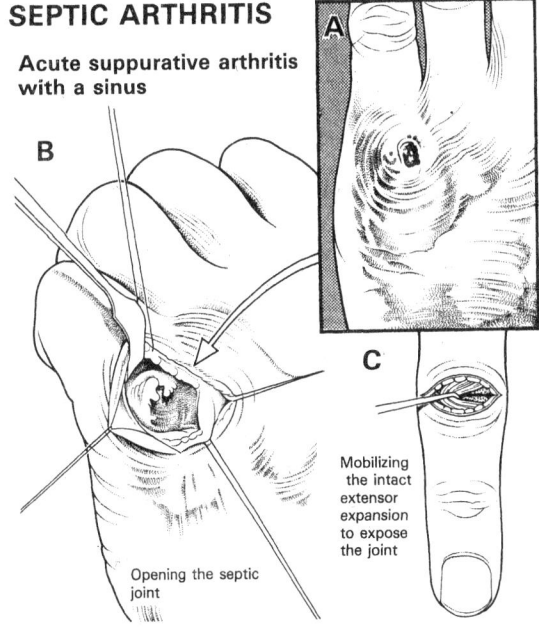

Fig. 8-8 SEPTIC ARTHRITIS. A, acute suppurative arthritis presenting with a sinus. B, exploring the lesion. C, mobilizing an intact extensor tendon to expose a suppurating distal interphalangeal joint. *After Bailey DA, 'The Infected Hand', Figs. 65, 66 and 67. HK Lewis, with kind permission.*

SEPTIC ARTHRITIS OF THE FINGERS

Give the patient an antibiotic (8.1); but this is less important than drainage and an efficient surgical toilet.

Open the joint immediately, especially if there is a wound over it. If the edges of the wound are not obviously infected, excise their extreme margins. Examine his extensor tendon.

If his extensor tendon has not been divided, enter the dorsolateral aspect of the joint and retract it to the opposite side. Look inside the joint. Remove any debris and loose bits of cartilage or bone. Syringe it out with saline. Leave his skin wound open for delayed primary closure. If you had to divide his extensor expansion, repair it at the same time. Immobilize his joint in the position of *function* (7.17), in case it stiffens, *not* the position of safety (75.2).

If his finger (but not his thumb) is stiff, consider amputation if he is an adult—but not if he is a child!

8.16 Other problems with hand infections

Hand infections, particularly if they are not well treated can cause many problems. Here are some of them. For infections in leprosy hands, see Section 30.4.

OTHER PROBLEMS

If, a few hours after a minor scratch, a patient's hand becomes hot and shiny, red lines spread up his arm, and he has rigors, a fast pulse, and severe headaches, he has lymphangitis progressing to streptococcal SEPTICAEMIA. This was common and usually fatal before the antibiotic era. Never incise such an infection, even with antibiotic cover. Give him an antibiotic first (2.9), and if an abscess or gangrene forms later, incise or deslough his hand.

DISASTER WITH AN INFECTED FINGER

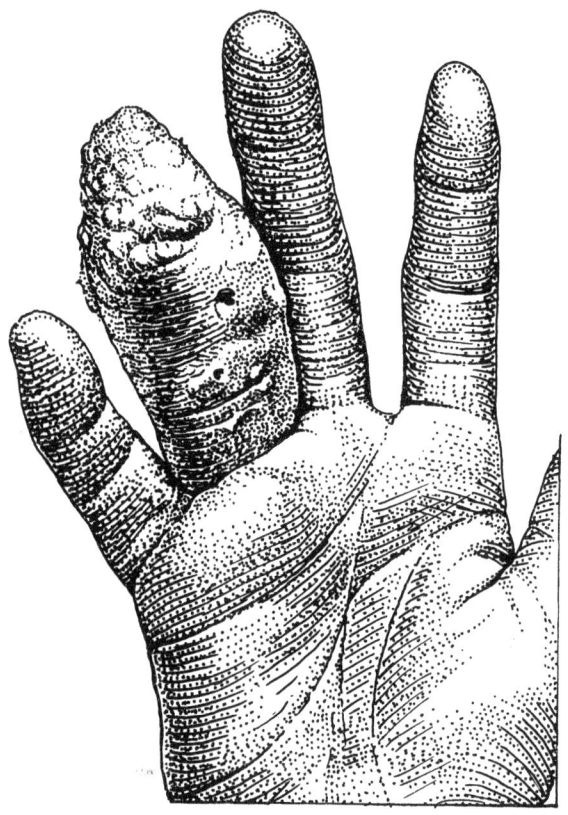

Fig. 8-9 DISASTER WITH A HUMAN FINGER BITE. The wound entered the patient's terminal IP joint which became infected. His finger might have been saved by an efficient wound toilet soon after the injury. Excise all tissue of doubtful viability, leave the wound open, and give him chloramphenicol and metronidazole. *After Charles Bowesman 'Surgery and Clinical Pathology in the Tropics'. E and S Livingstone. Permission requested.*

If his hand has been infected as the result of a HUMAN OR ANIMAL BITE, do an efficient wound toilet under a tourniquet, excise all tissue of doubtful viability, and leave the wound open. Give him chloramphenicol and metronidazole (2.9). He is in great danger of a serious infection, particularly with anaerobes. If you treat him early, he will probably recover and have a useful, mobile hand. If he presents late with a finger like that in Fig. 8-9 it will remain stiff, especially if a joint or a tendon sheath are involved. When his infection is controlled, and if he will allow you, amputate his stiff useless finger.

If SWELLING AND TENDERNESS SPREAD ABOVE HIS WRIST, pus has probably tracked proximally behind his flexor tendons up his arm into the space of Parona, as the result of a neglected palmar infection—see Section 8.9. Drain it through incision 6 in Figs. 8-4 and 8-6.

If he has EXPOSED JOINTS OR TENDONS after a hand infection, leave them open for about a week until infection is controlled. Raise his hand in a roller towel (75-1), and start movements as soon as pain permits. When healthy granulations have appeared, refer him to an expert who will cover his exposed tendons with a flap. If you cannot refer him, close his wound by secondary closure without tension (seldom possible, 54.6), or by secondary split skin grafting unless you have experience in the use of flaps. This will be less satisfactory, because his fingers will not be so mobile.

If OSTEOMYELITIS develops, continue antibiotic treatment, immobilize his hand in the position of function, X-ray it 2 weeks later and remove sequestra through dorsal incisions as necessary. Osteomyelitis of the distal phalanx is common in untreated pulp infections (8.5), and can follow other hand infections. You may eventually have to amputate his infected finger—see below.

If it involves a metacarpal (uncommon), treat this as if it were any other long bone. Approach it through a dorsal incision, and reflect his extensor tendons. Approach his middle and lateral phalanges through midlateral incisions.

If it involves a distal phalanx this will usually present at his finger tip. Bite it off with a bone nibbler.

If DISCHARGE AND PAIN PERSIST, they are probably the result of: (1) Inadequate drainage and desloughing. (2) Osteomyelitis. (3) The spread of a more superficial infection to a tendon sheath, or another fascial space which you did not recognize initially. (4) Sloughing of a tendon. (5) A foreign body.

If an adult's FINGER CONTINUES TO BE PAINFUL AND DISCHARGE because of osteomyelitis or established septic arthritis of an MP or PIP joint, consider AMPUTATION, because the nearby joints may become stiff too. A stiff DIP joint is not a disability. When you amputate, do so at least *through the joint proximal to the involved bone*. Don't merely remove part of the involved bone, because the infection will spread. The thumb is an exception; spare as much bone as you can, and don't amputate if you can avoid doing so, because even a stiff stump of a thumb is better than no thumb. See Section 75.24.

CAUTION! A child is much more likely to regain some useful movement eventually, so don't amputate unless his finger remains stiff after the infection has settled.

8.17 Pus in the foot

Foot infections are common, especially in communities where people don't wear shoes, but they are not as common as hand infections. Fine movements are not so important in the foot as they are in the hand, so that infection of the tendon sheaths of the foot is less of a disaster. You must however drain septic arthritis and osteitis, or persistent sinuses may follow.

Some aspects of foot infections are discussed in other chapters—osteomyelitis of the calcaneus and talus (7.13), and mycetoma (31.3). Leprosy patients are particularly liable to foot infections, and have their own special problems (30.6).

PUS IN THE FOOT

Manage subcutaneous infections (8.2), apical toe space infections (8.3), paronychia (8.4), pulp infections (8.5) and web space infection (8.7) as in the hand. They are all fairly common

ANAESTHESIA. (1) Intravenous ketamine (A 8.1). (2) General anaesthesia (A 10.1). (3) Local anaesthesia is suitable for very localized infections.

For all but the most superficial infections use a tourniquet (3.9), unless the patient's circulation has been impaired by ischaemic disease.

DEEP INFECTION OF THE PLANTAR SURFACE OF THE FOOT is usually due to an injury, such as a thorn, which has penetrated deeply.

If you suspect a foreign body, incise the abscess, search for it and clean out the cavity thoroughly. Leave the wound open sufficiently for it to heal up from below.

If infection is spreading on to his foot and up his leg, explore and drain the lesion, and give him an antibiotic suitable for the staphylococci in your area. As in the hand, rapidly spreading infections are likely to be due to haemolytic streptococci (8.12).

INFECTIONS OF THE DORSUM OF THE FOOT present early, and can usually be drained through a small incision using local anaesthetic infiltration.

INFECTIONS OF THE TENDON SHEATHS are uncommon except in leprosy, and when there is a foreign body involving the tendon sheath. Incise over the infected part, drain, and leave the wound open. In a late case you may need to remove necrotic tendon.

SEPTIC ARTHRITIS can involve any joint.

If an IP joint is involved, open it widely through a longitudinal incision on the dorsal surface to one side of the extensor tendon. Clean it out and leave it open to drain.

If an MP joint is involved, approach it either from the dorsal surface (open it from just to one side of the extensor tendon), or from the plantar surface. Open the wound widely and let it drain. Wounds in the plantar surface heal well.

If other joints are involved, approach them from the side where the bone is nearest to the surface. Clean the joint out well and leave it open.

OSTEITIS. Give him an antibiotic (2.9) and remove necrotic bone as necessary in chronic cases.

If his phalanges are involved, drain the infection and it will probably settle. Osteitis commonly follows infection in the soft tissues, especially infections of the pulp of the distal phalanx.

If his metacarpals are involved (uncommon), he may have: (1) Osteomyelitis following an injury. Approach the bone through a dorsal incision and reflect his extensor tendons. Drain the wound and remove necrotic tissue. Loss of one or two metacarpals is of little functional importance. (2) Acute haematogenous osteomyelitis. If he is under 10 years, an antibiotic alone may be adequate. If he is over 10, his bone will also need drilling. (3) Chronic haematogenous osteomyelitis. He presents with persistent pain and sinuses. Remove necrotic bone, without waiting for the formation of an involucrum.

CAUTION ! If his foot becomes infected without obvious reason look for: (1) A foreign body. (2) Leprosy (30.5). (3) Diabetes. (4) Ischaemia (uncommon in most of the developing world: feel his dorsalis pedis and his posterior tibial pulses).

POSTOPERATIVELY, stop him bearing weight. If he has a severe infection apply a plaster gutter splint to hold his foot in neutral (69-1). This will reduce pain and ensure that his foot is in the best position if it does becomes stiff.

9 Methods for abdominal surgery

9.1 Before a major operation

A patient is much more likely to withstand major surgery successfully if he is as fit as he can be to begin with. So do all you can to get him into the best possible condition first. You will not be able to do a thorough 'workup', but there are things you can do. For example, if you find that he is anaemic, malnourished, or tuberculous, and his operation is not urgent, treat him. Severe malnutrition will greatly reduce his ability to withstand the operation. Above all, don't operate on him while he is still dehydrated—this at least you should be able to correct (A 15.3).

Assess his need for surgery, the best time for it, and the risks it will involve. If a particular procedure would be too much for him, you will have to ask yourself if there is a lesser alternative which you could do under local anaesthesia, and what will happen if you do nothing? If there is a choice of procedures, do the simplest and safest one, for example, the insertion of a drainage tube rather than removing his gall bladder (13.17).

Follow these rules: (1) Don't start an operation without thinking it through step by step before you start. (2) Monitor him closely for 48 hours after any emergency or major operation. (3) Prevent the aspiration of stomach contents (A 16.1), and treat respiratory depression (A 3.4) immediately. (4) The most common postoperative complications are respiratory, and the answer to most of them is vigorous coughing (9.11). (5) Learn the basic principles of fluid therapy (A 15.1 to 15.5). (6) The operation may be routine to you, but it is sure to be a major event in his life, so try to establish a good relationship with him and his family. Tell him why you are operating, and give him some idea of what to expect afterwards—how much pain he will have, and when he will recover. If you might have to make a colostomy, discuss this with him before you operate. If you promise to close it eventually, be sure to do so.

Most of the major operations you do are likely to be abdominal ones, so here is the routine preoperative care for a patient who is to have a laparotomy.

PREOPERATIVE PREPARATION

HISTORY AND EXAMINATION. What previous illnesses has the patient had? Is he taking any drugs? Is he sensitive to anything, particularly to streptomycin, sulphonamides, penicillin, or chloroquin?

Assess his degree of wasting. Ask about a cough, fever, chest pain, dyspnoea, and smoking. How fit is he? Can he climb hills, or do a day's work in the fields? Can he step up and down off a chair for half a minute without becoming short of breath? Or, can he hold his breath for 20 seconds? Look for signs of anaemia. Feel the strength of his grip; this is a good predictor of surgical risk in men, less so in women.

SPECIAL TESTS. Measure his haematocrit or haemoglobin. Test his urine for albumin and sugar, and examine its deposit. This will exclude any serious disease of his urinary tract, and help you to diagnose renal colic, which may present as an acute abdomen. Test his blood group, and if necessary cross-match blood for him. Remember the risk of HIV. If you suspect heart or lung disease, take a chest X-ray.

ASSOCIATED DISEASE. If necessary, and if time allows, try to improve his general health, especially his nutrition and hydration. Look for tuberculosis and chronic renal disease.

If he is malnourished, especially if he is a child, and his disease permits, feed him by mouth or by nasogastric tube, even for as short a period as two weeks before you operate. If he is anorexic, feeding him will be difficult. He may tolerate nasogastric feeding (9.10, 58.11).

If he is febrile, consider the possibility of malaria or typhoid fever, in addition to the possible surgical causes of fever.

If he is anaemic, consider the urgency of the operation in relation to the severity of his anaemia. Most 'routine' operations can be done with a haemoglobin as low as 80 g/l. If it is 60 or 70 g/l, only do urgent procedures. For example, a woman with haemoglobin of 30 g/l who is bleeding slowly from an ectopic pregnancy can be transfused overnight with 20 ml/kg of blood (from her abdominal cavity if necessary) and given 1 mg/kg of frusemide. If an operation is less urgent, for example a hysterectomy for chronic anaemia due to fibroids, transfuse her 2 or 3 days before you operate. For nonurgent surgery you can take a unit of blood 4 weeks and 2 weeks before a planned major operation, and store them.

If a patient has jaundice, it will greatly increase the risks of surgery, but not operating may be even more dangerous. Give him parenteral vitamin K_1 for a few days preoperatively. Exclude hepatitis first, especially the acute stage, when anaesthesia can be dangerous.

If he is producing sputum, give him chest physiotherapy and a course of antibiotics prior to surgery if possible. Anaesthetize him appropriately, using local or regional blocks where possible (A 17.8). If he has a common cold, cancel anything but an emergency operation.

CHEST PHYSIOTHERAPY before and after the operation will reduce the risk of lung complications—see Section 9.11.

SKIN PREPARATION. If he is very dirty, wash the operation site several times. If he has pustules, boils, or eczematous patches near the site of your proposed incision, treat them before you operate. Bacteria from them may infect the wound, so consider delayed primary closure (9.8).

NASOGASTRIC SUCTION. Insert a nasogastric tube before *all* stomach or gut operations. The danger of aspiration pneumonitis is even greater if he has intestinal obstruction or ileus.

PERIOPERATIVE ANTIBIOTICS may be lifesaving—see Section 2.9.

DON'T OPERATE ON A DEHYDRATED PATIENT

9.2 Laparotomy

A laparotomy for an acute abdomen will be the major test of your surgical skill. When you decide to do one, you should usually be sure what you will need to do when you get inside it—so try to make a correct diagnosis first, and try to avoid a purely 'exploratory laparotomy'. Before you start, discuss the procedure

THE ABDOMINAL WALL

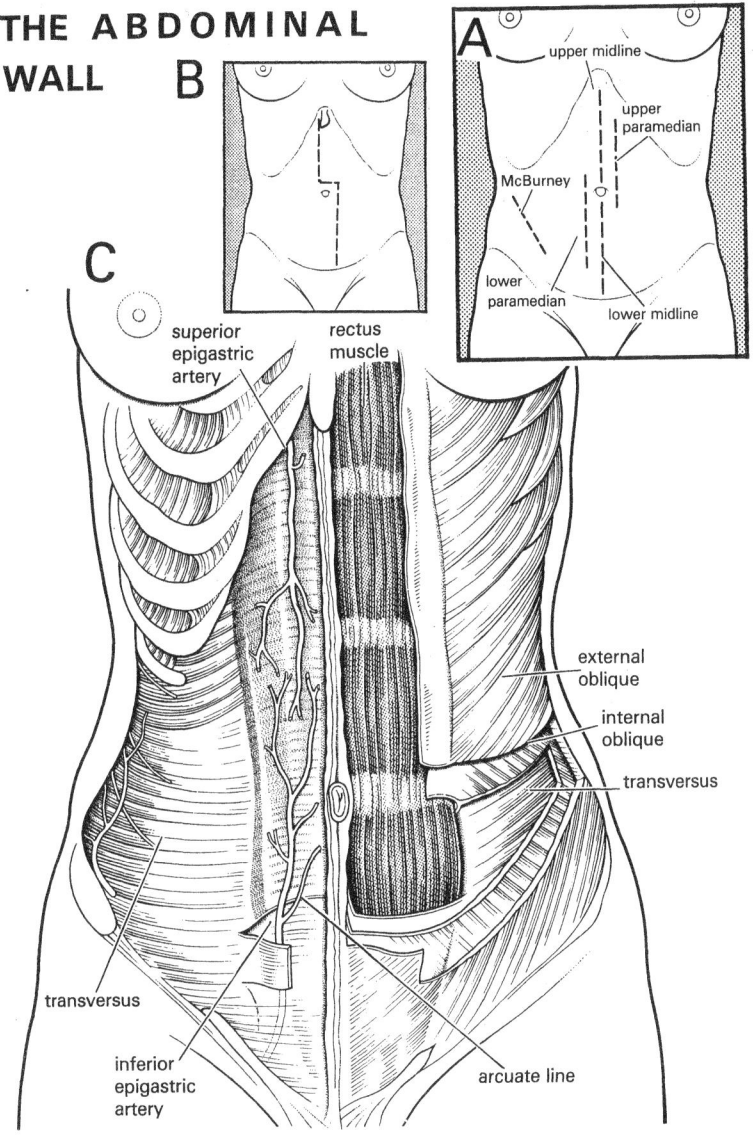

Fig. 9-1 THE ANTERIOR ABDOMINAL WALL. A, common abdominal incisions. B, the 'ultimate incision', if you want an extensive exposure. C, the anatomy of the anterior abdominal wall. *C, after Maingot R, 'Abdominal Operations' (4th edn 1961), Fig. 1, HK Lewis, with kind permission.*

with him and his family, and if he is to have a colostomy, or a T-tube, make sure they understand it.

Try to avoid wound infections and dehiscence ('burst abdomen'), and the incisional hernias that commonly follow them. Make an incision which is big enough to allow you to get at the organs you want to operate on—a common mistake is to make it too short. Incisions heal from side-to-side, not from end-to-end, so don't be afraid of making a long one. The length of an incision has little relation to the incidence of operative shock. If an incision is too small: (1) you will not be able to dissect safely, and (2) your assistant will have to exert excessive traction on its edges, which will kill tissue, and increase the risk of wound sepsis and breakdown. A good surgeon makes incisions that are large enough to ensure safe dissection, and does not exhaust his assistants by requiring them to exert forceful traction.

If you separate muscle fibres instead of cutting across them, you help to make a patient's abdomen as strong afterwards as it was before. Avoid cutting his intercostal nerves, because a paralysed abdominal wall is more likely to herniate. Remember that they take an oblique downwards path between his internal oblique and transversus muscles.

Which incision? If possible, make a transverse incision in an infant because it heals better. In an adult a median or paramedian one will enable you to get at everything in the abdomen if you need to. You can make the middle part to begin with, and extend it from his xiphisternum to his pubis, if necessary. If exposure is particularly difficult, you can extend either incision laterally to make a 'T' incision.

A midline incision above the umbilicus is quick, simple, and bloodless, and is useful for emergency operations. But access to the organs at the sides of a patient's abdomen is not easy, and if you want to extend it around his umbilicus, you have to make a detour which is difficult to sew up nicely. Even so, midline incisions are usually best for trauma, for Caesarean sections, and for most pelvic operations. One contributor felt that they are so much the best, that we should not mention paramedian ones. *If you wish, you can always make a midline incision.* Above the umbilicus they heal well, as they do below it if you repair them with monofilament as a single layer.

The old type of paramedian incision, in which the rectus muscle was retracted laterally, too often dehisced. The newer rectus-splitting type is less likely to do this, especially if you repair it with monofilament in a single layer.

When you get inside, you will have to decide what to do. Here, only experience can tell you what is normal and what is not. For example, some *Ascaris* worms inside a child's gut may feel so abnormal as to convince you that they must be the cause of his symptoms, when in fact they are normal for his community.

Be gentle, gut is highly sensitive. If you handle it roughly, especially if it is obstructed, ileus may follow. Gut does not like being frequently drawn out of a wound. So, if you need to draw it out, do so only once, and hold it with a moist swab. While it rests on the abdominal wall, keep it covered with warm moist packs or towels, or place it in a large sterile plastic bag. If it is grossly distended, even the most gentle handling will burst it, so decompress it (10-9). Break down adhesions gently (10-11).

A COMMON ERROR IS TO MAKE THE INCISION TOO SHORT

LAPAROTOMY

RESUSCITATION. Make sure that the patient has a drip up with a large needle or a cannula. If necessary, splint his arm with an armboard, and tie this to the table. If bleeding is likely to be serious, have some blood cross-matched for him.

X-RAYS. Take these when necessary, and have his films in the theatre.

EQUIPMENT. A general set (4.12). A No. 22 scalpel blade. No. 1 (or 1/0 monofilament used double) for single layer closure. 2/0 monofilament for his skin. 2/0 silk or linen for ligatures. Fine half circle needles with a cutting edge for his skin, and round bodied ones for deeper structures. 2/0 catgut on atraumatic needles for intestinal anastomoses. Gallipots of some soapy solution and alcoholic iodine. Sterile towels and a sheet with a window in it.

ANAESTHESIA. (1) General anaesthesia, preferably with relaxants (A 14.3). (2) Local anaesthesia (6.9). (3) Subarachnoid (spinal) or epidural anaesthesia (A 7.1), provided he is not shocked.

Always pass a nasogastric tube (4.9). Aspirate his stomach contents before you take him to the theatre. If the operation is an emergency, put 30 ml of magnesium trisilicate down the tube to minimize the risk of the acid aspiration syndrome (A 16.3). Spigot it during induction, and aspirate it from time to time during the operation.

If he is gravely ill, from bleeding or infection, local anaesthesia may be safer than a general anaesthetic (A 5.4). Mix 20 ml of 2% lignocaine with 80 ml of saline to give 100 ml of 0.4% solution. To this add 0.5 ml of adrenalin 1:1000. Inject 10 ml of this solution into five sites in his rectus muscle on either side in quantities of 1 ml to block his segmental nerves. Use another 20 ml to infiltrate the midline incision. Use the remaining 10 ml to infiltrate the root of his mesentery if you need to resect his gut. If you have to do some extensive procedure, such as lavaging his abdominal cavity, inject ketamine 1 mg/kg intravenously. Alternatively, and with greater risk, inject pethidine intravenously in *SMALL* quantities of 5 mg. Patients who are old or shocked or sick, especially if they have been previously sedated, are *very* sensitive to even modest doses of pethidine, which may produce coma deep enough to need resuscitation. So be prepared to do this if necessary (A 3.4).

POSITION. For most abdominal operations, lie him on his back. If your table does not rotate from side to side, and you want him turned to one side, place pillows under his back on each side, or use a wedge block under the mattress.

If you are operating on his pelvic organs, you will find the Trendelenburg or head-down position helpful. It will allow his gut to fall towards his diaphragm, so that you get a better view into his pelvis. You will need well-padded shoulder rests to prevent him sliding downwards. Don't tip him too steeply, or the pressure on his diaphragm will impair his breathing. If he is in >10° of Trendelenburg, you must intubate him, keep him on relaxants, and control his ventilation.

Use one arm for a blood pressure cuff and the other for an intravenous line. Keep his hands by his side, or out on arm boards, or folded on his chest with suitable ties; don't place them under his buttocks or under his head.

EXAMINATION. When he is anaesthetized and relaxed, feel his abdomen carefully. You may get a better appreciation of his abdominal pathology than you could when he was awake.

PREPARATION. See elsewhere for shaving and preparation (2.3). Drape his abdomen and fix the drapes with towel clips. Cover these with a large windowed sheet, and add additional sterile towels as necessary.

WHICH INCISION? (also see above) If you are doing a purely exploratory laparotomy, and don't know what you are going to find, make a midline or rectus-splitting incision in the correct half of his abdomen, upper or lower.

If you are reopening his abdomen, go through the old skin incision. Excise and extend it so that you can enter his abdominal cavity *above or below* any adhesions to the under surface of his abdominal wall. Work your way up or down carefully, dividing any adhesions you find, so as not to injure any adherent gut.

CAUTION ! (1) If you are in doubt, make the 'incision of indecision' in the midline 5 cm above and below his umbilicus. Enter his abdomen and then extend it in the most useful direction. (2) Don't make a second incision parallel to an earlier one, because the tissues between them may necrose.

Before you make any abdominal incision, use the back of your scalpel to make some scratches across it. When you come to sew it up afterwards, these scratches will help you to bring the edges of the skin together accurately. Later, as you gain experience, stop doing this, as it may cause keloids.

ENTERING THE PERITONEAL CAVITY

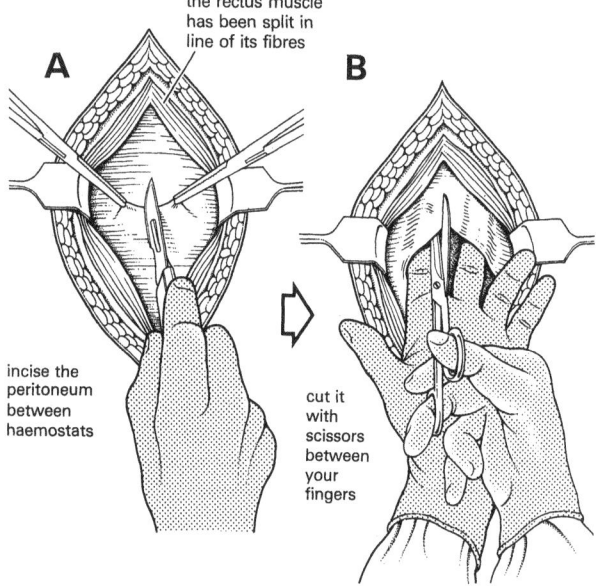

Fig. 9-2 OPENING THE PERITONEAL CAVITY. A, the skin has been incised and the rectus muscle split in the line of its fibres. The posterior rectus sheath and peritoneum form a single layer. Pick this up with a haemostat, and then apply another one 5 mm from it. Release the first haemostat (which might perhaps have picked up gut) and then reapply it. With the peritoneum still tented up, make a small incision between the two haemostats. Air will enter the patient's peritoneal cavity, and his viscera will fall away.

B, put your fingers into the incision to make sure that there are no adhesions to the under surface of his abdominal wall, and then extend it with scissors.

MIDLINE INCISION

UPPER MIDLINE INCISION. Use his xiphoid and umbilicus as landmarks, keep strictly to the midline, and don't cut into his rectus muscle on either side. It does not matter if you do, except that you may have difficulty approximating the wound edges later.

A MIDLINE INCISION

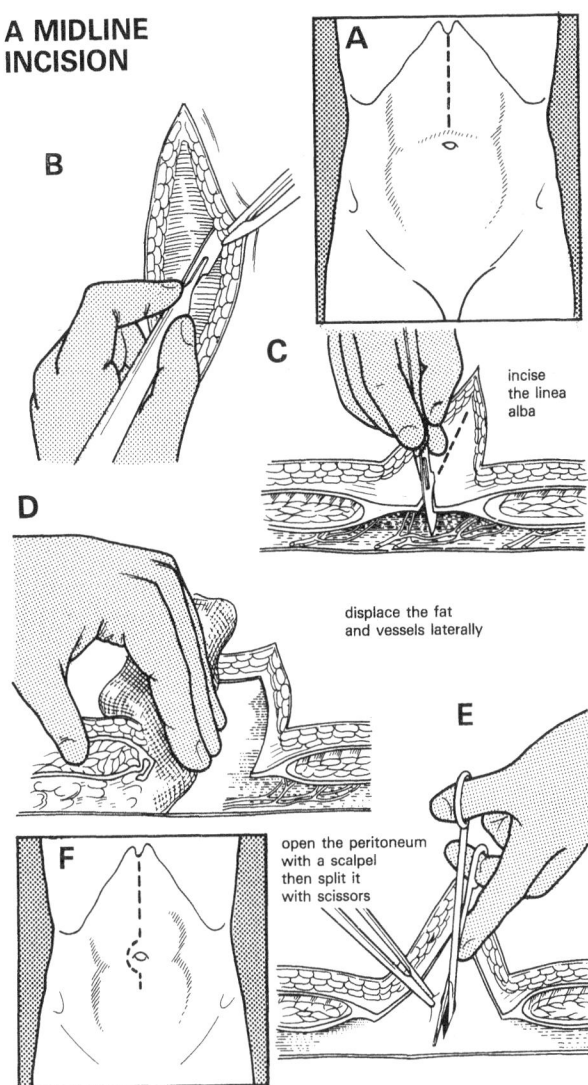

Fig. 9-3 A MIDLINE INCISION. A, the site. B, cut down to the linea alba, and then carefully dissect the fat for a centimetre on either side, using the flat of the knife. C, incise the linea alba to expose the underlying fat and peritoneum. D, displace the fat and vessels laterally by blunt gauze dissection. E, pick up the peritoneum, incise it with a knife and split it with blunt-ended scissors. F, if you want to continue the incision downwards, go round the umbilicus. *After Dudley HAF, 'Operative Sugery—the abdomen.' Butterworth, Permission requested.*

Cut down to his linea alba and then use the flat of the blade to clear 7 mm on either side, ready for closure later. Cut through his linea alba to expose his extraperitoneal fat. Use gauze dissection to move this to one side.

If necessary, extend the incision downwards. Cut 1.5 cm round his umbilicus—don't cut into it—it is full of bacteria! You can also get a little more length by incising between his xiphisternum and his costal cartilage.

LOWER MIDLINE INCISION. Make this in a similar way. You will see his pyramidalis muscle at the lower end of the wound. There is no posterior rectus sheath in the lower two-thirds of the wound, below his umbilicus.

PARAMEDIAN INCISION

Make a paramedian incision 2.5 cm (not more) from the midline on the side where you expect to be working most, in the upper or lower abdomen, as required. If in doubt, centre it on his umbilicus, but carry the incision clear of it. If you expect to be working on a lateral structure, you will need good retraction to get adequate access, so make it at least 20 cm long.

Cut down to his rectus sheath, and then use the flat of the blade to clear 7 mm on either side, ready for closure later.

Divide his anterior rectus sheath, keeping well to its medial side. Above his umbilicus, where there are tendinous intersec-

A PARAMEDIAN INCISION

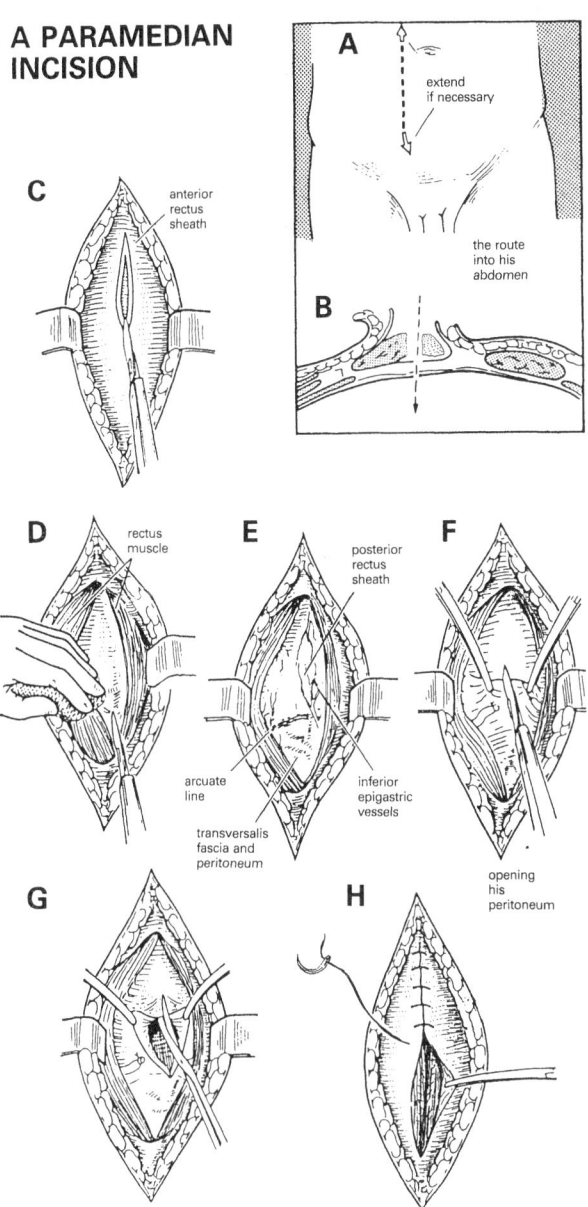

Fig. 9-4 A PARAMEDIAN INCISION. A, the site of the incision, which you can, if necessary, extend up to the inverted 'V' between the patient's xiphisternum and his costal cartilage, or down as far as his pubis. B, the way into his peritoneum. C, incising his anterior rectus sheath. D, incising his posterior rectus sheath after his rectus muscle has been split. E, the anatomy of the vessels to be tied. F, and G, incising his peritoneum. H, closing the muscles of his abdominal wall with a continuous monofilament single layer stitch. Alternatively, close the wound by Everett's method as in Section 9.8.

tions, split it with a scalpel handle. The muscle medial to the split will be deprived of its nerve supply and atrophy, so don't split it more than than 2 cm from its medial edge. Put your two index fingers into the gap, and use them to split the rectus muscle in the length of the incision. Below his umbilicus split his rectus muscle or displace it laterally.

If necessary, tie his deep epigastric vessels before you divide his posterior rectus sheath. You probably won't see them because they lie laterally.

If his abdominal muscles bleed, clamp the bleeding vessels and tie them with catgut. Or, use pressure from a sponge. Or, transfix them with a 'figure of 8' catgut suture.

With his rectus muscle split, or out of the way, open his posterior rectus sheath and peritoneum as in Fig. 9.2, without injuring his gut! You can easily open it by mistake if: (1) it is obstructed, or (2) it has stuck to the a scar from a previous operation.

If you want to extend the incision, you can if necessary: (1) cut from his costal margin to his symphysis pubis, (2) extend the incision upwards between his xiphisternum and his costal cartilage, or (3) make a transverse cut in his left upper quadrant.

PFANNENSTEIL INCISION. See Section 23.15 and Fig. 23-20.

ENTERING THE ABDOMEN

Discovering what is wrong can be easy or very difficult. Be observant, learn to recognise what you see, and search thoroughly.

SMELL can tell you a lot. If a puff of gas greets you as you open his peritoneum, his gut has probably perforated. If there is an abnormal smell, it may be: acrid (a perforated peptic ulcer, or a typhoid perforation), faeculent (a ruptured caecum or sigmoid), the characteristic smell of *E. coli* (appendicitis with abscess formation or peritonitis), putrid (bacterioides or anaerobic streptococci), or urinary, as the result of an intraperitoneal rupture of his bladder.

LOOK FOR FLUID in his abdominal cavity, which may be: blood (an ectopic pregnancy or an injured liver, spleen, or mesentery); bile-tinged small gut contents (a perforated peptic or typhoid ulcer); a foul, turbid brown fluid (peritonitis from appendicitis); a watery, light-brown, odourless fluid (intestinal obstruction without strangulation); a watery, reddish-brown, offensive fluid (strangulation with incipient gangrene); or a pale straw-coloured fluid (ascites).

If there is any exudate, send it for culture, if you can.

If his peritoneum is fiery red with flakes of fibrinous exudate, he has peritonitis—see Section 6.2.

If there is bile-stained fluid in his paracolic gutter, he has probably perforated his gall bladder.

If he has an odourless greenish blood-stained effusion, he probably has pancreatitis (uncommon). Look behind his ileum at the peritoneum over his pancreas. Retroperitoneal oedema will help to confirm the diagnosis. Examine his omentum for flecks of fat necrosis.

If loops of his gut are distended, he has ileus, or his gut is obstructed. First find a loop of undistended gut. If there is one, then trace it proximally and you will find the obstruction. See Section 10.4.

If thickened oedematous omentum is adherent to something, it is a sign of acute inflammation, or strangulation (10.3), or abscess formation (6.3).

EXAMINE THE REST OF HIS ABDOMEN How extensively you should do this will vary. Limit your exploration to what is easily practicable if: (1) there is sepsis, or (2) you are operating for a known problem, or (3) your incision is a small one.

If there is infection, examine the infected area first. When you have dealt with it, consider whether you have done enough. Further exploration may spread the infection.

If there is carcinoma, start with the organs most distal to the diseased area, proceeding 'centripetally' towards the lesion.

If there is no obvious abnormality, search his abdomen in an orderly way. Examine his diaphragm and the upper surface of his liver, then examine his spleen, his stomach, his duodenum, and his intra-abdominal oesophagus. Examine his gall-bladder region. Then examine the whole of his small gut. Draw each loop out of the wound and then return it. Feel his major vessels. Feel his kidneys and look at his ureters. Examine the bladder, rectum, uterus, tubes, and ovaries. Finally look at his hernial orifices from inside. *Don't forget to record your findings.* Even negative ones can be most helpful later.

If you accidentally perforate a distended loop of gut, don't panic. Leave it there while someone gently clamps it with non-crushing clamps, and you surround the injured loop with packs to prevent the contents of his gut flooding into his peritoneal cavity. Have the sucker ready; repair the damage.

GET ADEQUATE EXPOSURE AND A GOOD LIGHT. You cannot do good work if loops of gut are always getting in the way, or if the light is bad, so adjust it as best you can. Make an adequate incision. If necessary extend it in one of the accepted directions. If you are working on a lateral organ through a midline incision, it will have to be a long one. Or, make a lateral T-shaped extension

Get good retraction. A self-retaining retractor will not be enough by itself. Use Deaver's retractor, or any large right-angled retractor, and make sure your assistant knows what you want him to do with it.

Get him into the best position You will never get adequate exposure in the pelvis unless his head is down in the Trendelenburg position. Similarly, if you are working on his upper abdomen (as when doing a vagotomy), tilt his head up a little. Extending his back by breaking the table or by putting a pillow under him will also help. If you want to draw his splenic flexure and small gut towards you, consider rolling him to the right, either by tilting the table or by using sandbags, or a wooden wedge under the mattress. If you are operating on his kidney, a kidney bridge or folded plastic-covered pillows will bring it forwards.

If loops of small gut (or anything else) get in your way, pack them away. This may save you much time, but don't forget to remove the packs afterwards! Anchor each pack by its tape or corner to a large haemostat hanging outside the abdomen.

MINIMIZE THE RISK OF SEPSIS. (1) If you have to open a hollow viscus, or an abscess, pack his abdominal cavity round it with packs or moist towels. Use clamps to prevent the contents of his gut escaping. (2) Handle an inflammatory mass carefully—don't let it burst and discharge pus everywhere. (3) Avoid any manipulation which might spread infection. (4) If an area does become contaminated, wash it out (6.2). (5) Insert drains when indicated (4.10).

BLEEDING can be difficult. You must know how to: (1) tie vessels in the depth of a wound (3.2), (2) tie them in continuity (3.2), (3) use curved and angled forceps, (4) secure temporary tape control over major vessels (55-4).

If a surface is merely oozing, consider applying haemostatic gauze (3.1).

If the bleeding is annoying, rather than brisk, you may be able to suck it away while you go on working.

If you have diathermy, consider applying it to the bleeding point with a fine-tipped dissecting forceps. You can do this with pin-point accuracy.

If bleeding becomes unmanageable, apply packs and pressure (3.1). You can even control bleeding from an avulsed renal artery like this. After 5 to 10 minutes, slowly remove the pack and clamp the bleeding point. If the vessel is a large one or deep, underrun it with a 'figure of 8' or a double mattress transfixion suture.

If there is a constant ooze during the operation: (1) the patient may have an excess of citrate, after the transfusion of many units of blood. This will not happen if you give him 10 ml of 10% calcium gluconate after every 4th (500 ml) unit of blood. (2) He may have DIC (disseminated intravascular coagulation), or some other clotting defect. If possible give him at least 2 units of fresh blood to replace clotting factors.

If you are absolutely desperate, as with bleeding from a ruptured uterus, try compressing the patient's aorta against her spine with your hand, until you have resuscitated her, and then tie her internal iliac arteries (3.5).

CAUTION ! (1) Don't stab blindly with a haemostat in a pool of blood! (2) Similarly, don't apply diathermy through a pool of blood—it won't work!

THE SPECIFIC CONDITIONS you might find when you do a laparotomy are described elsewhere—intestinal obstruction (10.3), peritonitis (6.2), intra-abdominal abscesses (6.3) etc.

THE SPECIMEN. If you have removed tissues from the patient and want to examine them, hand them to someone else and ask him to open them away from the patient, who will then not be contaminated by infection or malignancy.

To close his abdomen, go to Section 9.8. If you have operated for sepsis, delayed closure of his skin may be wiser.

DIFFICULTIES WITH A LAPAROTOMY

If you CANNOT DO AN OPERATION THROUGH ONE INCISION, make another. Keep your original one open until you have finished—it may be useful!

SUTURING GUT

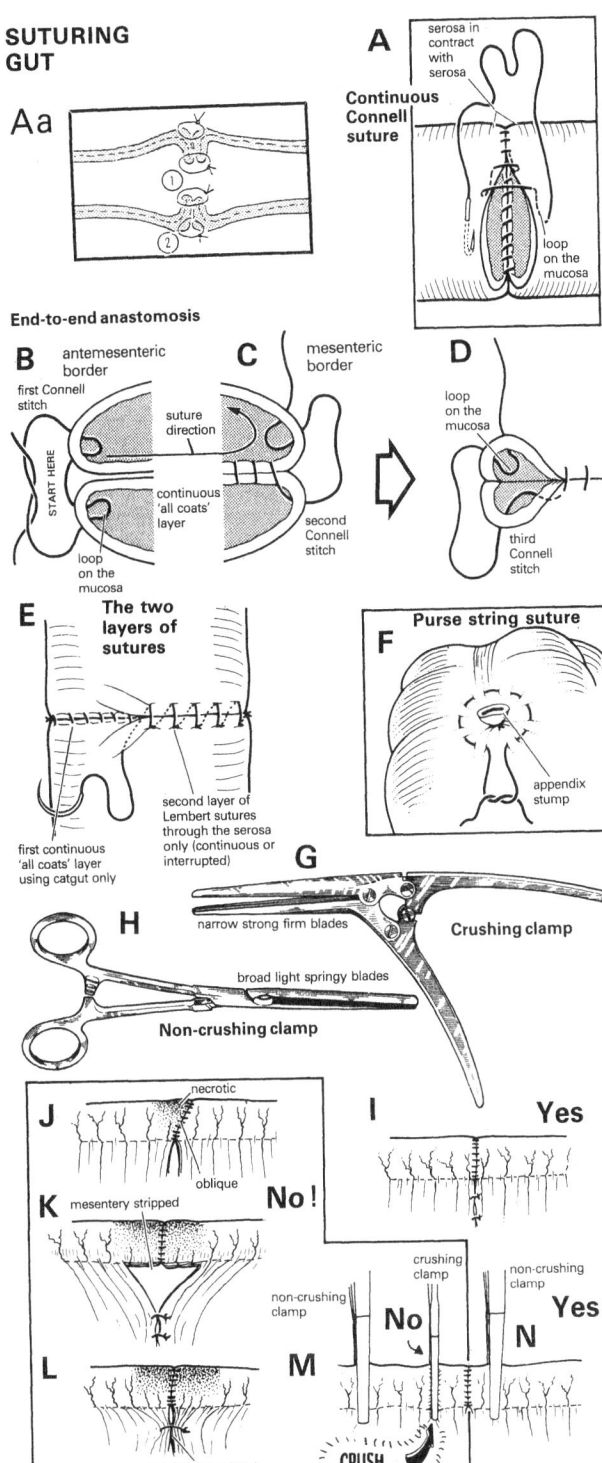

Fig. 9-6 SUTURING GUT. A, suturing gut with continuous Connell sutures, showing the principle of 'the loop on the mucosa' inverting the gut. Continuous Connell sutures like this are only used occasionally in the methods described here. Aa, gut anastomosed end-to-end with two layers of sutures: (1) an 'all coats' layer, (2) a layer of Lembert sutures through the serosa only.

B, the closed method of anastomosing gut end-to-end in Fig. 9-9 uses three Connell stitches. This is the first one on the antemesenteric border of the gut. C, the second Connell stitch, when the suture has reached the mesenteric border, and is about to turn round to close the anterior layer of the gut. D, the third and final Connell stitch closes the gut back at the antemesenteric border again.

E, the two layers of sutures: (1) the first continuous catgut 'all coats' layer and (2) the second or Lembert layer which can be interrupted or continuous; here it is continuous. F, a purse string suture for the appendix. G, Payr's crushing clamp, with firm, narrow blades. H, Lane's non-crushing clamp with springy, broad blades. I, correctly anastomosed gut. J, the gut has been cut obliquely in a way which reduces the blood supply to an area on the antemesenteric border of one loop. K, the gut has been partly deprived of its mesentery, and thus of its blood supply. L, the mesentery has been bunched together with a suture which occludes the vessels supplying the gut. M, gut which has been crushed by a crushing clamp has not been resected. N, the correct method; the gut is being held for suturing by a non-crushing clamp; crushed gut has been excised.

If you want ACCESS TO A HUGE TUMOUR: (1) Start between his xiphisternum and his rib cage, and bring the incision outwards a little to become a standard upper rectus splitting paramedian incision. Continue horizontally just above his umbilicus for 5 cm. Then continue it down the other side of his lower abdomen to the brim of his pelvis as a muscle-splitting paramedian incision, as in B, Fig. 9-1. Or, (2) make a midline incision from top to bottom, skirting his umbilicus.

If you OPEN HIS PLEURA BY MISTAKE, there is a danger that his lung may collapse and cause marked hypoxaemia, not only because only one lung is being ventilated, but also because blood is passing through his collapsed lung unaltered.

If he is not intubated, stop operating to make it easier for the anaesthetist to pass a cuffed tracheal tube using suxamethonium (A 14.2). To do this you may have to move him. As soon as the tube has been inserted, close the hole in his pleura with a continuous multifilament suture. As you insert the last stitch ask the anaesthetist to blow up his lung so that it almost touches his pleura. At the end of the operation insert an intercostal water seal drain (65-5) and leave it in place for at least 48 hours. X-ray his chest, and if his lung is fully expanded, remove the drain, usually at 3 to 5 days.

If you are unable to intubate him, do the same. His lungs will usually expand postoperatively.

9.3 Resecting and anastomosing gut, end-to-end anastomoses

When you do a laparotomy it will often be because you need to resect and anastomose a patient's gut. This is one of the most critical procedures you will have to undertake, and if you are inexperienced, one which will give you much anxiety. *It is one of the few surgical methods which you can usefully practise before you operate on a living human patient.* So go to the butcher's, get some animal gut, and practise anastomosing that. *The penalty for failure will be peritonitis or a fistula!*

Gut is most often anastomosed end-to-end, but there will be occasions when you will have to do it end-to-side, or side-to-side. You may also have to anastomose a patient's stomach to his small gut in a gastroenterostomy.

Don't be worried by the complexity of the methods which follow. The really important points are to: (1) Make sure that you start with two nice viable pink bleeding ends. (2) Get their serosal surfaces together. If you do this, they will soon unite. If only the mucosal surfaces touch one another they are less likely to unite, and more often leak. (3) Close the gut in two layers. You have got to be much more neat and accurate if you only use one. Don't worry about mucosa pouting out after the first layer, it can easily do this at the mesenteric border. Everted mucosa leaks. So if it everts as 'dog ears', push these back when you do the second layer. (3) Do the suturing outside the abdominal cavity on a towel. Contamination will then be less likely and clamps less important. (4) Wash the gut with tetracycline solution after you have done the anastomosis.

If you follow the four points above you won't go far wrong. Now for some of the others: Any sutures which go right through the wall of the gut (and so might leak) are usually infolded by a second layer of sutures which go through serosa and muscle only—*these are called Lembert sutures.* So close gut in two layers. Put the first layer through all its coats—this is the 'all-coats' layer. Make the Lembert sutures of the second layer bring the serosa of one loop into contact with the serosa of the other loop. Only put them through the peritoneum, the muscle, and the submucosa (the strongest layer of the gut), and don't go through the mucosa into the lumen of either loop.

You will need to hold the gut with stay sutures or clamps while you work on it. It is also desirable to hold it shut so that its contents don't leak out. Clamps do this best but you can use a tape.

There are two kinds of clamp: non-crushing ones and crushing ones.

Non-crushing clamps, such as Lane's or Kocher's have thin, wide, flexible blades, and a ratchet with several teeth, so that you can adjust the way you close them to the thickness of the gut. Use non-crushing clamps to hold gut without injuring it; hold them between your fingers and 'milk' the gut contents away from the area you are working on. Apply only as many 'clicks of the ratchet' as you need to stop the contents of the gut from escaping, and blood from flowing from the cut ends.

Crushing clamps have narrower, stiffer blades, a ratchet with fewer teeth, and sometimes interlocking ridges on the blades to grip the gut more firmly. Crushing clamps prevent leaking completely. 'Milk' the contents of the gut away from the area to be crushed, and then apply a crushing clamp with its jaws protruding well beyond the edge of the gut, because gut widens as you crush it. Close the jaws tightly. Crushed gut dies, so *cut the crushed gut away with the clamp.* As you do this, be sure there is a non-crushing clamp nearby to stop the contents of the gut spilling out. Crushing clamps are thus always used with non-crushing ones. You can use crushing clamps in pairs or in sets of four as in Fig. 9-9.

You can use what we describe here as 'the closed method' or you can use 'the open method'. The closed method is usually done with clamps, but it can if necessary be done without them. The open method is usually done without clamps, but it can be done with them. Both the descriptions here assume you are doing an end-to-end anastomosis.

The 'closed method' with clamps is shown in Fig. 9-9 and is the standard one, because it causes the least contamination of the peritoneal cavity. You have first to join the back of the patient's gut (as it lies in front of you) and then the front. The important places for leaks are where the back and the front parts of the anastomosis join one another, at the mesenteric and the antemesenteric borders of the gut. If serosa of one loop is to be in contact with serosa of the other loop at these critical points, the gut here must be inverted. The stitch which does this best is the Connell stitch. You can use Connell stitches all along the front of the gut (A, in Fig. 9-6), but this is not the easiest way of stitching gut. *You should however make three Connell stitches where leaks are most likely.* Make the first one at the antemesenteric border where you start the anastomosis (B, in this figure). Make the second one at the mesenteric border, as you turn over the edge of the gut from suturing its back to suturing its front (C). Make the third one at the antemesenteric border again when you are about to complete the first layer (D).

The principle of the Connell stitch is that the catgut comes out into the mucosa and then goes back into it again, and it comes out of the serosa and goes back into the serosa again. It makes a 'loop on the mucosa'. It is this loop which makes the mucosa invert.

The 'open method' without clamps is shown in Fig. 9-10. The important feature about this is less that it is open without clamps, than that it uses a single layer of mattress sutures (a second Lembert layer is optional, and this method can, if appropriate, be done with clamps). The open method is indicated: (1) In infants and small children, because all clamps crush their delicate gut to some extent. (2) If the two ends of the gut are of widely differing size, as when you need to join large and small gut end-to-end. (3) When you don't have any clamps. (4) When you cannot get clamps on to the gut, as when joining large gut to rectum after a Hartmann's procedure (10.10). The open method does however increase the risk of contaminating the peritoneal cavity. Pick up the gut in stay sutures. Use interrupted mattress sutures for the posterior layer (A, in Fig. 9-10) and continuous ones which pick up the mucosa in a second bite for the anterior layer (B, in this figure). These pick up a tiny bite of mucosa only after going through the whole gut wall. The last two stitches cannot be made too neatly, and have usually to go through all layers.

Some surgeons don't like this method. It is really a single layer method, which is not so safe. Even if you add a second Lembert layer, you cannot cannot continue this across the mesenteric border. Some say it is more difficult.

Which parts of the gut can you safely anastomose to which and when? (1) You can also safely anastomose small gut to small gut, and small gut to stomach. (2) You can safely anastomose the ileum to the colon, because it has a good blood supply, few bacteria, and its diameter matches that of the colon. Both these anastomoses are safe with obstructed gut. Anastomosing large gut to large gut is more dangerous, because it has a poorer blood supply and many bacteria. You *cannot* safely anastomose large gut to large gut when it is obstructed, and instead you have to let its contents escape through an ostomy (see Sections 9.6 and 32.27). When large gut is to be anastomosed, it has to be carefully prepared first with enemas and antibiotics, and even then it is safer if it is protected by a proximal colostomy.

Some other points. If you are not happy that you have made a satisfactory anastomosis (no anastomosis is ever quite 'watertight'), you can bring up a loop of omentum and stitch this loosely over the place which you think will leak. This is optional, and is not even desirable if you think an anastomosis is sound; but there are certain occasions when it is essential—notably the repair of a perforated peptic ulcer, as in Fig. 11-2.

Interrupted sutures use more suture material and take longer, so use continuous ones where you can: (1) In an adult you can use continuous or interrupted sutures for either layer, but, if you use non-absorbable sutures in an infant, they must be interrupted, because continuous sutures will not grow with him, and will eventually constrict his gut. (2) If the cut edges of the gut are not perfectly healthy, the patient very ill, and the risk of peritonitis great, use interrupted non-absorbable Lembert sutures.

In the small gut use whatever suture material you find convenient for either layer. In the stomach use catgut on an atraumatic needle for the first layer—if you use a non-absorbable suture material for this layer, it may be the site of ulcers later. Use whatever you find most convenient for the second (Lembert) layer—catgut, silk, cotton, or monofilament. In the large gut there may be an advantage in using non-absorbable sutures for all layers.

- FORCEPS, intestinal, non-crushing, flexible blades, Kocher's, Doyen's or Lane's, 75 mm, two only. Use these to hold the gut while you anastomose it. Non-crushing clamps have been designed to exert the right pressure without being covered with rubber tubes. If you fit them with rubber, they may crush too tightly.

- CLAMP, Payr's, intestinal crushing, lever action, medium size, 110 mm, two preferably four only. These are the standard crushing clamps.

- CLAMP, Payr, intestinal crushing, lever action, small size for pylorus, 60 mm, two only.

THE ENDS TO BE JOINED MUST BE NICE AND PINK MINIMIZE CONTAMINATION

METHODS FOR GUT

TEN IMPORTANT POINTS. (1) Do the anastomosis on a towel outside the abdomen. (2) Don't contaminate the patient's peritoneal cavity; if you do, wash it out with tetracycline solution (1 g in 1000 ml of saline, 6.2). Be safe and wash any anastomosis with tetracycline solution when you have completed it. (3) Pick up gut with your fingers or Dennis Browne or Babcock's forceps, don't damage it with other forceps. (4) Cut the mesentery square with the gut, and don't undermine it. (5) Don't apply clamps so as to leave the antemesenteric border longer than the mesenteric one, or the tip of the loop will necrose (J, in Fig. 9-6). (6) Don't anastomose gut from which you have removed the mesentery (K, in that figure). (7) Don't occlude blood vessels when you suture the mesentery (L). (8) Don't use a crushing clamp when you should use a non-crushing one. If you do, you will leave crushed gut in the body (M)—excise it (N). (9) Don't use diathermy close to the gut: you may injure it so that it becomes nonviable. (10) *If, when you have completed the anastomosis, the gut is not viable ('purplish'), resect its ends and start again!*

SOME GUT METHODS

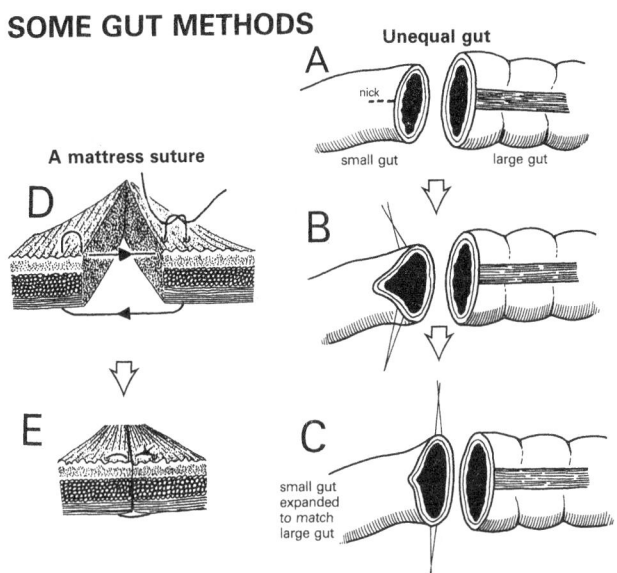

Fig. 9-7 SOME GUT METHODS. If the gut that you want to anastomose end-to-end is unequal in size (A), you can make a nick in the antemesenteric border of the smaller piece (B), so that it enlarges (C). D, and E, the mattress sutures used for the posterior layer of the open method (A, in Fig. 9-10). *After Turnbull R.B. From a publication by Messrs Ethicon, permission requested.*

IS HIS GUT VIABLE?

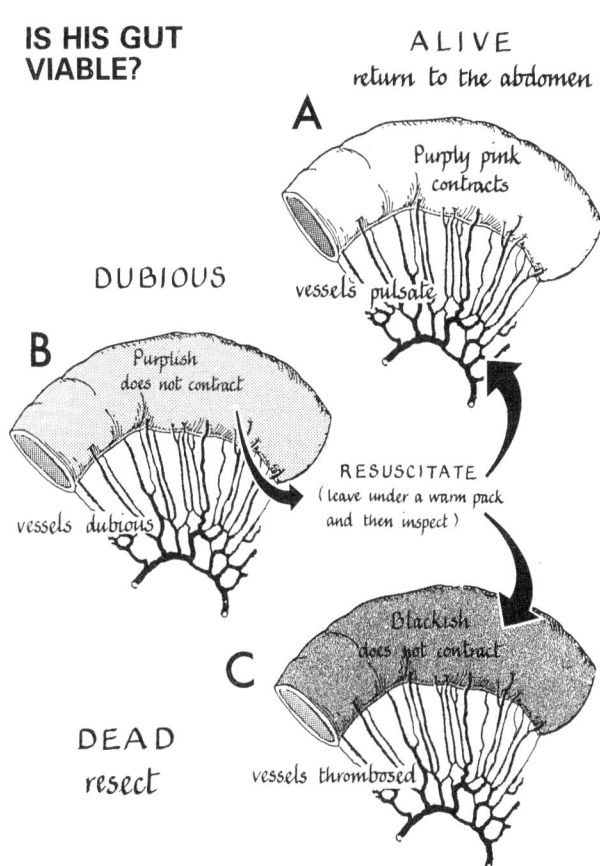

Fig. 9-8 IS THE GUT VIABLE? A, it is viable if: (1) its surface is glistening, (2) its colour is pinkish, or only slightly blue, (3) it feels resilient like normal gut, (4) it contracts sluggishly (like a worm) when you pinch it, and (5) you can see pulsations in the vessels which run over the junction between it and its mesentery.

B, it is dead and not viable if: (1) it tends to dry out and its surface is no longer glistening, (2) it is greyish purple, or a dark purplish red (or even black), (3) it feels like blotting paper, (4) it does not contract when you pinch it, (5) the blood vessels over it are not pulsating or are filled with black clot.

C, if you are in doubt, remove the cause of the strangulation, apply a warm, moist pack to it, and wait 10 minutes. If it is viable, its colour will change from dusky to its normal pink.

THE CHOICE OF THE METHOD depends on the nature of the operation, your skill, and the equipment you have. Commonly, you will need to anastomose small gut end-to-end.

If the loops of gut are equal or only slightly unequal in size, you can use either method. If you use the closed one, apply the clamp on the smaller loop of gut obliquely, but without depriving a tongue of gut of its blood supply. Don't do what has been done in J, Fig. 9-6!

If the loops are very unequal in size (as when anastomosing small to large gut), you will have to use the open method of end-to-end anastomosis, and make a small cut in the *antemesenteric* border of the smaller loop, as in A, to C Fig. 9-7. Or, you can do an end-to-side or a side-to-side anastomosis.

IS HIS GUT VIABLE? TO RESECT, OR NOT TO RESECT?

CAUTION ! For any method of anastomosis the gut must be viable, which also means that its blood supply must be good enough (see below).

Wait to decide if a patient's gut is viable or not until you have removed the cause—divided an obstructing band, or untwisted gut which has twisted on its mesentery. You can usually tell if gut is going to survive or not. Base your decision on several of these signs, not on one only.

Gut is viable if: (1) its surface is glistening, (2) its colour is pinkish, or only slightly blue, (3) it feels resilient like normal gut, (4) it contracts sluggishly (like a worm) when you pinch it, and (5) you can see pulsations in the vessels which run over the junction between it and its mesentery.

Gut is not viable if: (1) it tends to dry out and its surface is no longer glistening, (2) it is greyish purple, or a dark purplish red (or even black), (3) it feels like blotting paper, (4) it does not contract when you pinch it, (5) the blood vessels over it are not pulsating or are filled with black clot.

If you are in doubt, remove the cause of the strangulation, apply a warm, moist pack to it, and wait 10 minutes. If it is viable, its colour will change from dusky to its normal pink. If this happens it is alive, even if you cannot feel the pulsations of the mesenteric vessels. It may be alive if some areas remain purplish because of bruising. But if these areas are large, or do not improve in colour, consider all the discoloured gut nonviable.

If a piece of gut is obviously nonviable, resect it and do an end-to-end anastomosis.

If only part of the wall of the gut is nonviable, as with a Richter's hernia in Fig. 14-1, you may be able to invaginate it.

If you are going to do this, the nonviable gut must: (1) not be perforated, (2) not extend over more than 30% of the circumference of the gut, (3) not extend to the mesenteric border, because suturing here may interfere with its blood supply, (4) be surrounded by a border of healthy gut. Use two layers of catgut to bring the serosal surfaces of the healthy margins together in the *transverse* axis, so as to invaginate the nonviable segment into the lumen of the gut where it can safely necrose (E, and F, 14-1). If it does not satisfy these criteria, resect it. One contributor considers that oversewing with Lembert sutures like this is more difficult and more dangerous than resecting the damaged loop. If this is so, resect it.

If there is a completely encircling narrow band of greyish white necrosis, resect it and do an end-to-end anastomosis: it may turn into a stricture of the gut later (Garré stricture).

If you release a loop of gut from a constriction ring, be especially careful. The loop of gut itself may be viable, but there may be a narrow band of necrosis at both the afferent and the efferent ends. It may slough at these narrow areas. Experts would resect the gut. But, if you are not expert at gut resection, oversewing the necrotic areas with Lembert sutures may be safer. If so, make a note of what you have found and done. A Garré stricture may form, and the obstruction may recur.

IS THE BLOOD SUPPLY GOOD ENOUGH?

If the mesenteric vessels of the gut you are going to anastomose are not pulsating, trim it back boldly until its edge

THE 'CLOSED METHOD' WITH CLAMPS

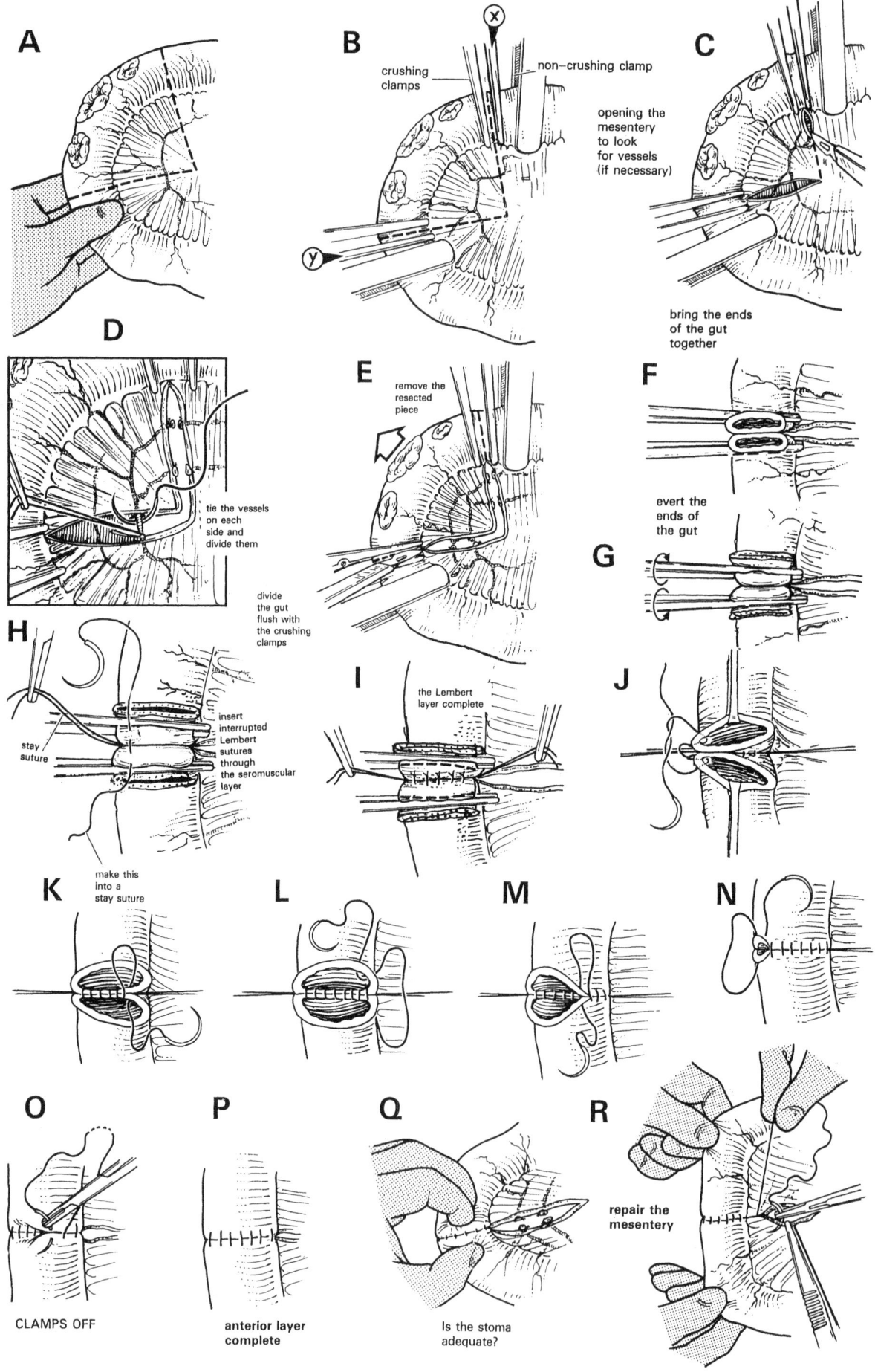

bleeds with healthy red blood. If this does not happen immediately, try waiting a few minutes. If the flow is not pulsatile, it may become so if you wait a few minutes. Pick up the bleeding vessels with 4/0 chromic catgut, and don't rely on your anastomotic sutures to control bleeding.

PURSE STRING SUTURES

A purse string suture is an invaginating suture around a circular opening, and is most often used to bury the stump of a patient's appendix.

Place a continuous Lembert suture through the serosa and muscle only, all round the appendix, as in F, Fig. 9-6. Tie the first hitch of a reef knot, pull the ends of the suture upwards, and push the stump of the appendix downwards. If necessary, ask your assistant to pull up the opposite side of the purse string as you do so. If you happen to penetrate all layers of the gut, reinforce the purse string with some more inverting sutures.

ENTEROTOMY

An enterotomy is an opening in the gut. You may have to make one to make an ostomy (9.5), to inspect the gut to see where bleeding is coming from (11.3), or to remove *Ascaris* worms (10.6) or a foreign body (10.14).

Make an opening in the *antemesenteric border* of the gut and close it transversely in two layers as if you were anastomosing gut. In this way you will not narrow its lumen.

END-TO-END ANASTOMOSIS BY THE 'CLOSED' METHOD

INDICATIONS. Anastomosing small gut, and large gut when there is not too much difference between the sizes of the lumen.

METHOD. This is the method in Figure 9-9. As shown it uses four crushing clamps and two non-crushing ones. You can readily leave out crushing clamps 'X' and 'Y' in B in this figure, and you can use no clamps at all.

Decide the length of gut you want to resect (A). Apply 4 crushing clamps in pairs *close* together at each end of the gut to be resected, and non-crushing ones on the gut to be anastomosed about 2 cm from the crushing ones (B).

If the mesentery is too thick for you to see the vessels clearly through it (as in the sigmoid colon, and the small gut mesentery in moderately fat patients, especially distally), divide the peritoneal layer nearest to you to outline the vessels (C).

Dissect the vessels one by one, pass a suture under each and tie it. Use 2/0 silk or chromic catgut on a mounted atraumatic needle (as shown in D), or an aneurysm needle, or a haemostat.

Divide the gut between each pair of crushing clamps (E).

(Note. From step F until step N each end of the gut is also held by a non-crushing clamp where this is convenient, although these are not always shown.)

Bring the crushing clamps together (F) and evert them (G).

Insert continuous Lembert sutures through the seromuscular coat of the posterior layer of the gut (the one which is furthest from you) starting at the antemesenteric border (H). Leave the ends long to act as stay sutures (I).

Cut the crushing clamps off by dividing the gut flush with them (I).

Start the all coats continuous inner layer at the antemesenteric border as a single all coats inverting Connell stitch (J). This is also shown in B, in Fig. 9-6. Use 2/0 chromic catgut. Continue as a simple over and over suture until you reach the mesenteric end K.

Insert the second all coats inverting Connell stitch on the mesenteric border (L) (also C, Fig. 9-6). Complete the anterior layer as simple over and over sutures (M) (or if you prefer as a continuous Connell suture A, Fig. 9-6). Insert the third Connell inverting stitch as you reach the antemesenteric end again (N) (also D, Fig. 9-6). Tie the two ends of the inner continuous suture together and cut them, leaving 5 mm ends. Now remove the non-crushing clamps.

Insert a continuous layer of Lembert sutures into the anterior seromuscular layer, starting at the mesenteric border and ending at the antemesenteric one. Tie each end to the free ends of the sutures that you have already inserted into the posterior layer and so complete the circle (O, and P). Test the patency of the lumen with your fingers (Q). Push some of the gut contents past the anastomosis to test for leaks. Close the defect in the mesentery with continuous 2/0 catgut or monofilament—*taking great care not to occlude the vessels*.

END-TO-END ANASTOMOSIS BY THE OPEN METHOD

INDICATIONS. (1) Anastomosing small gut to large gut. Or small gut to small gut when there is much difference between the sizes of the gut. (2) The absence of clamps. (3) Children.

END-TO-END ANASTOMOSIS
By the open method

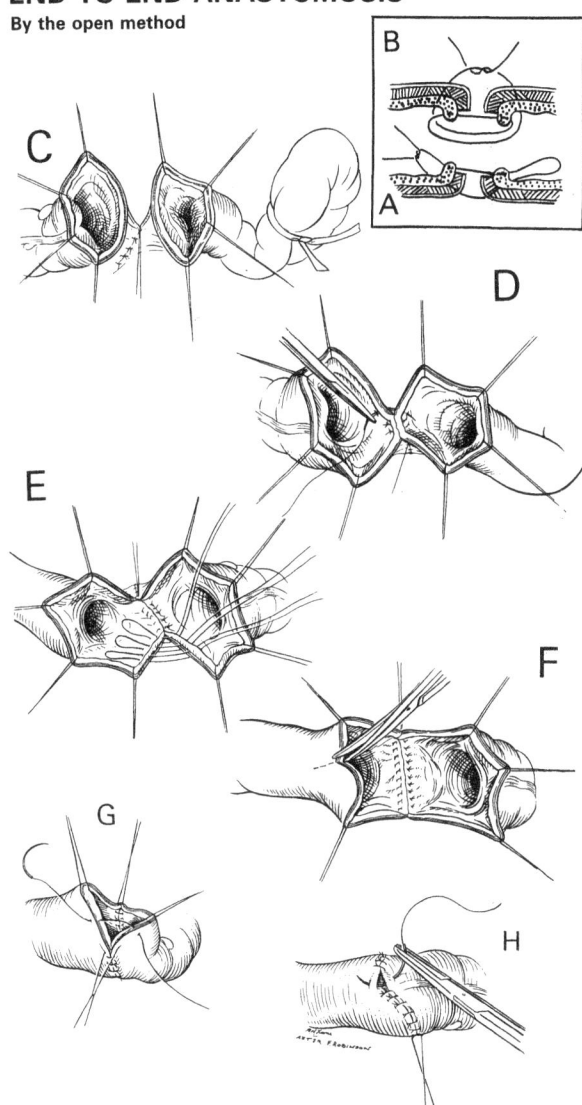

Fig. 9-10 THE END-TO-END ANASTOMOSIS OF UNEQUAL LOOPS OF GUT BY THE OPEN METHOD. Use this method if the ends of of the gut are of very unequal size, or if you don't have clamps. A, the interrupted mattress sutures of the posterior layer. B, the continuous sutures of the anterior layer, which take an extra bite of the mucosa. C, the gut occluded with an umbilical tape, the mesentery united and the ends of the gut held open with stay sutures. D, the first mattress sutures. E, more mattress sutures. F, a nick being made in the smaller loop of gut. G, insert some widely placed sutures to make sure that the circumferences of the two ends of the gut are exactly approximated. H, the final layer of Lembert sutures. *After Turnbull R.B. From a publication by Messrs Ethicon, permission requested.*

Fig. 9-9 END-TO-END ANASTOMOSIS BY THE 'CLOSED' METHOD. This method uses 4 crushing clamps. Clamps 'X' and 'Y' in Step B are optional, and it can be done without any clamps using stay sutures or tapes instead. The first pair of crushing clamps are removed with the loop of gut in Step E. The second pair are cut off in Step I. Non-crushing clamps are applied in Step B and remain on until Step N, although they are not shown after Step E. The critical parts of this anastomosis are the inverting Connell sutures in steps J, L, and N.

END-TO-SIDE ANASTOMOSIS

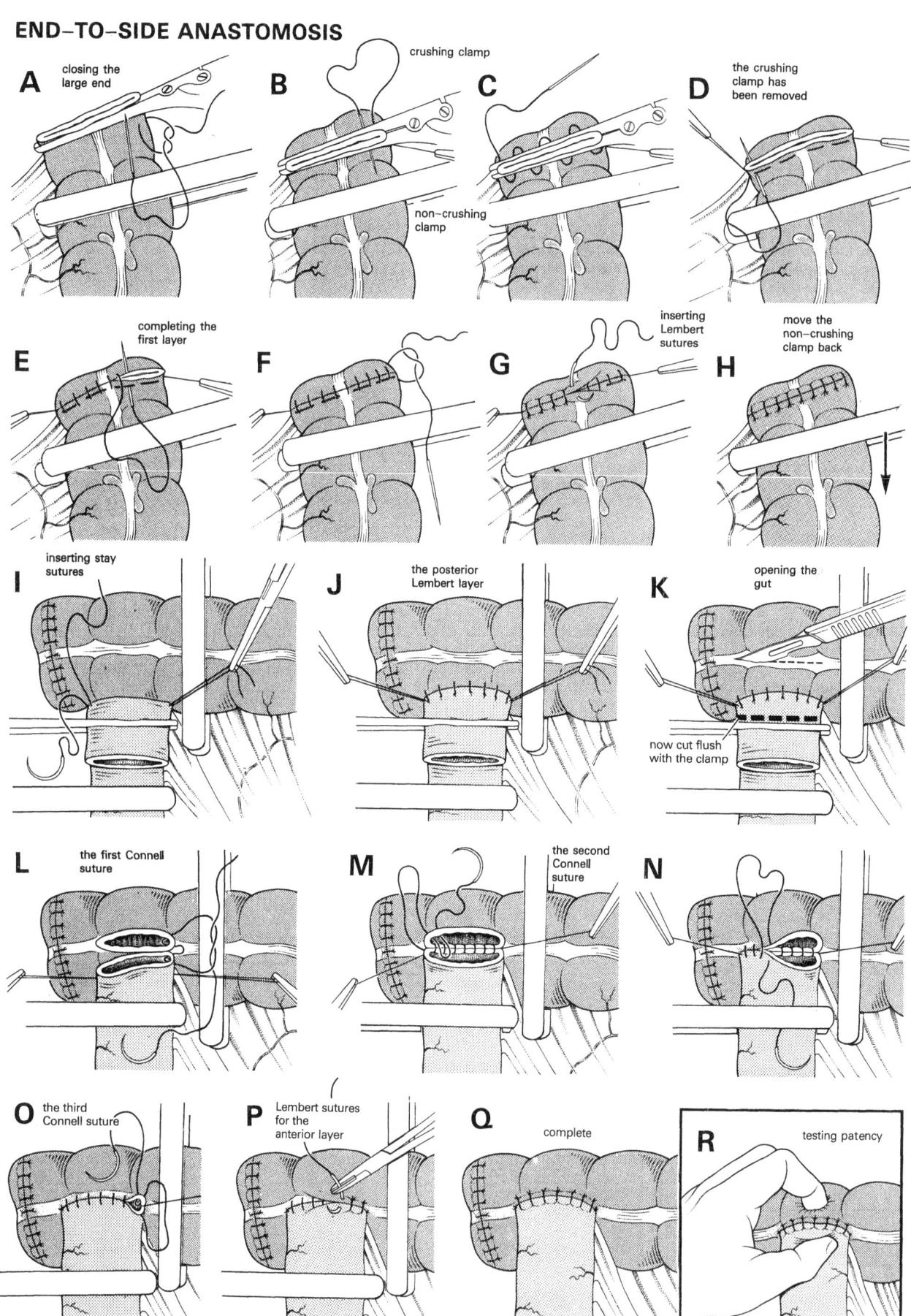

Fig. 9-11 END-TO-SIDE ANASTOMOSIS. A, to H, closing the blind end of the gut. E, to G, inverting the previous layer of sutures. H, moving the non-crushing clamp back. I, to K, the posterior Lembert layer of the anastomosis. L, and M, the posterior all-coats layer. N, and O, the anterior all-coats layer. P, and Q, the anterior Lembert layer. R, testing patency.

METHOD. You can do this in two ways:

(1) You can follow Steps A to E and then J to R in Fig. 9-9, using stay sutures and tapes instead of clamps.

Or, (2) you can use the one-layer mattress suture method in Fig. 9-10. Pack off the peritoneal cavity. Prevent the gut contents from flooding into it by applying umbilical tapes around the gut. Cut the mesentery off square without undermining its cut ends. Apply stay sutures to open the ends of the gut.

To make the posterior layer use interrupted vertical through-and-through mattress sutures of 4/0 chromic catgut as in A, Fig. 9-10, and D, and E, Fig. 9-7.

To make the anterior layer, work from both sides towards the antemesenteric edge, and insert 4/0 chromic catgut sutures through all layers except the mucosa. Make a cut in the antemesenteric border of the smaller loop of gut. Don't trim the corners of the slit. Use continuous sutures which pick up the mucosa in a second bite for the anterior layer (B, Fig. 9-10). If the suture line is snug and inverted, stop at this stage. If not, complete the anastomosis with a final layer of Lembert 4/0 monofilament seromuscular sutures. You should be able to get most of the way round the gut, but you will not be able to suture its mesenteric border. This converts a one-layer method into a partial two-layer method.

9.4 End-to-side and side-to-side anastomoses

When one piece of gut is much larger than the other, an alternative to the open method of end-to-end anastomosis is to join them end-to-side. You can do this when you join the ileum to the colon after a hemicolectomy, or when one loop of small gut is much bigger than the other. Close off one end and make the anastomosis as close to this end as you can, so that there is no 'cul de sac' which might be colonized by bacteria. You can also join gut of differing diameters by joining it side-to-side.

TWO MORE ANASTOMOSES

END-TO-SIDE ANASTOMOSIS

INDICATIONS. Anastomosing small gut to large gut.

METHOD. Mobilize the patient's large gut for 5 or 10 cm, or more if it is very large. Apply a crushing clamp to the end, and cut it off flush. Push away the contents of the distal gut, and apply a non-crushing clamp to it (A, in Fig. 9-11).

Using a straight or curved needle, close the end of the gut with continuous atraumatic sutures working from side-to-side from one end to the other (B, and C). When you have got to the other end, pull the suture tight and remove the crushing clamps. Cut away the crushed tissue. Work back to the end where you started, this time making over and over sutures (D, and E). Tie the ends of the suture and cut them off 5 mm from the knot (F).

Cover the closed end of the gut with a layer of inverting Lembert sutures through the seromuscular coat using 2/0 silk or chromic catgut (G).

Push the contents of his large gut further down and move the non-crushing clamp 6 cm from the end (H). His small gut should have a non-crushing clamp applied 5 cm from its end. Bring it close to his large gut, and insert stay sutures through the seromuscular layers only (I). Complete the layer of interrupted seromuscular sutures (J).

Open his large gut, if possible along a taenia, so as to make a stoma equal in size to his small gut (K).

Start the inner all coats layer with a Connell inverting stitch (L). Continue this as an over-and-over suture to the other end, and use another Connell inverting stitch for that end (M). Return using an over-and-over suture for the anterior layer (N). When you reach the end close it with a third Connell inverting stitch (O). Tie the two ends of the continuous all coats suture together and leave the ends 5 mm long.

Insert a layer of interrupted inverting seromuscular Lembert sutures (P, and Q). Test the patency of the lumen—it should admit two fingers (R). Repair the defect in the mesentery with 2/0 catgut.

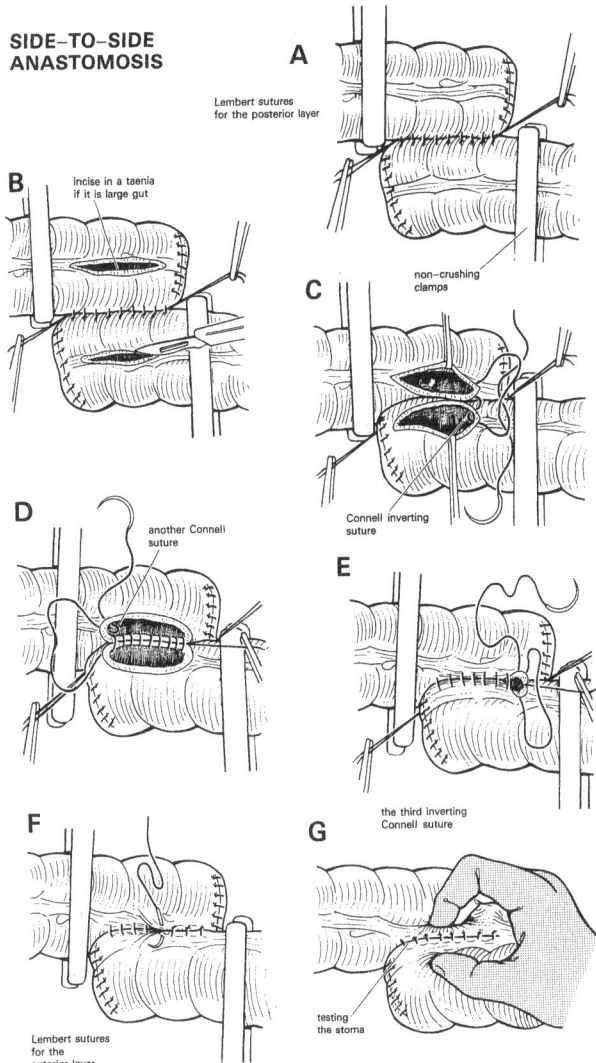

Fig. 9-12 A SIDE-TO-SIDE ANASTOMOSIS is useful for doing a bypass without resecting gut. A, if, as in this figure, gut has been resected, close the ends of the two pieces of gut as in the previous figure. If, as is usually the case, and you are merely doing a bypass operation, no gut has been resected, leave the ends in continuity. Hold them with stay sutures and join them with the Lembert sutures that will form the posterior layer of the anastomosis. B, open both pieces of gut. C, start the posterior all-coats layer with a Connell stitch. D, the posterior all coats layer has reached the other end, so now insert another Connell sitch. E, the third and final Connell stitch. F, insert the anterior Lembert layer. G, test the stoma for patency.

SIDE-TO-SIDE ANASTOMOSIS

INDICATIONS. Anastomosis when the gut is of very different diameter and end to end or end to side anastomosis is difficult, as may happen if it is obstructed: (1) In the new-born when the distal gut is small, because it has never contained anything but meconium. (2) In older patients when end-to-end anastomosis is difficult because of differences in diameter. (3) When gut is difficult to mobilize because of adhesions, as sometimes when anastomosing the ileum to the colon.

METHOD. If gut has to be resected, first close the ends of both loops of the gut to be anastomosed, as for the larger end of an end-to-side anastomosis described above (A, to G, Fig. 9-11). If there is no gut to be resected, leave the ends in continuity.

Expel as much of the contents of both loops as you can, and apply non-crushing clamps about 6 cm from the ends of each. Insert a layer of interrupted Lembert sutures through the seromuscular coats of both of them, starting with stay sutures at each end about 1 cm from the line of your proposed incision (A, in Fig. 9-12).

Incise both pieces of gut for about 3 cm, in the line of a taenia in the case of the colon (B). Starting with a Connell inverting stitch (C), use 2/0 catgut to join the posterior cut edges of the gut with an all coats continuous over-and-over suture (D). When you reach the other end make another Connell inverting stitch. Then continue the over-and-over continuous suture along the anterior layer of the anastomosis. Finally, complete it with another Connell inverting stitch (E) and tie the ends of the catgut together, leaving 5 mm cut ends.

Insert an anterior layer of 2/0 silk or catgut Lembert seromuscular sutures (F). Test the lumen of the stoma with your fingers (G) and move the gut contents over the anastomosis to check for leaks.

9.5 Stomata and bypasses for large gut obstruction

The gut is a tube from the mouth to the anus which can become obstructed in various places. One way of overcoming such an obstruction is to make an opening or stoma or 'ostomy' above or below it, from the lumen of the gut out to the abdominal wall. In the upper part of the gut the purpose of an ostomy (a gastrostomy, or a jejunostomy) is usually to let food and fluid in; in the lower part it is to let the contents of the gut out (an ileostomy, a caecostomy or a colostomy).

An ostomy is seldom necessary in the small gut, because it contains so few bacteria that you can usually resect the obstruction, and anastomose its cut ends quite safely. Ostomies of the small gut cause large losses of water and electrolytes, so try to avoid them if you can. But you cannot so easily anastomose the large gut, which is not only full of dangerous bacteria, but also has a much poorer blood supply, so that anastomoses more easily break down and leak. The standard way to operate safely on the large gut is to wash it out and then to 'sterilize' it with a preoperative course of antibiotics, neither of which are possible in an emergency. So, in an emergency, you have to bring the cut ends of the large gut out to the surface as a colostomy, and close them later. There are two main ways of doing this: (1) You can bring a loop of gut to the surface and make an ostomy at its apex, without resecting any gut. Or, you can bring most of the loop out of the abdominal wall, close it and then resect the loop. This is called *exteriorization*. If you are not skilled, it is useful way of resecting gangrenous or injured gut, and making an ostomy without soiling the abdominal cavity.

Types of ostomy There are several types of ostomy for the large gut, and three standard places in which to make them. First the types. A loop colostomy is the most useful of these. In many cultures a patient would rather die than have any of them. So you may have to do some firm persuasion. Fortunately, ostomies are usually only needed temporarily. You can make any of these:

(1) A loop colostomy brings a loop of gut out of the abdomen over a short length of rubber tube, or a glass rod. This is the easiest ostomy to make and close extraperitoneally, and is suitable for most purposes.

(2) A double-barrelled colostomy, is a loop colostomy modified by stitching the last few centimetres of its limbs together inside the abdomen, so that they resemble a double-barrelled shotgun. The spur (wall) between the two loops is later crushed to make the colostomy easier to close with the special crushing clamp in G, Fig. 9-19. If you are not going to close a colostomy by crushing the spur, there is no point in double-barrelling it.

The advantage of both a loop and a double-barrelled colostomy is that you can close them extraperitoneally.

(3) A 'spectacles colostomy' has limbs that are separated by a small bridge of skin, as in Fig. 9-17. It is useful: (a) if a patient needs a colostomy for a long time, and (b) during the repair of a rectovaginal or vesicovaginal fistula, when work on the rectum and bladder has to be completed before the fistula can be closed. Because the loops of a spectacles colostomy are separated, it has to be closed intraperitoneally with a full anastomosis.

(4) An end (terminal) colostomy forms the 'end' of the gut after excision of the rectum, or in Hartmann's operation (see below).

(5) A mucus fistula (colostomy). A colostomy normally has two openings. The proximal one discharges faeces, and the distal one only mucus. This is the term which is sometimes given to the distal opening.

If you are making a colostomy low in the sigmoid colon, the distal loop may not be long enough to reach the surface as a mucus colostomy, so you have to close it and drop it back into the abdomen—this is Hartmann's operation (G, in Fig. 9-14). If necessary, you can drop a blind loop back into the abdomen anywhere; it will fill with mucus and discharge through the anus.

Some kinds of ostomy 'defunction' the colon better than others. This means that they are better at preventing faeces from entering the distal limb. This may be useful, for example, in protecting a wound in the rectum which you have just sutured. There are several degrees of defunctioning. It is most effective when the two ends of the gut are brought out through separate stab wounds, with the distal one above the proximal one. A 'spectacles colostomy' (9-17) is the next best. Neither a loop, nor a double barrelled colostomy, defunction completely, and a caecostomy is even less effective. Fortunately, a high degree of defunctioning is seldom important.

The sites for ostomies are shown in Fig. 9-14. There are three common places to make them: (1) In the caecum in the right iliac fossa (a caecostomy). (2) In the right side of the transverse colon in the right epigastrium. (3) In the sigmoid colon in the left iliac fossa.

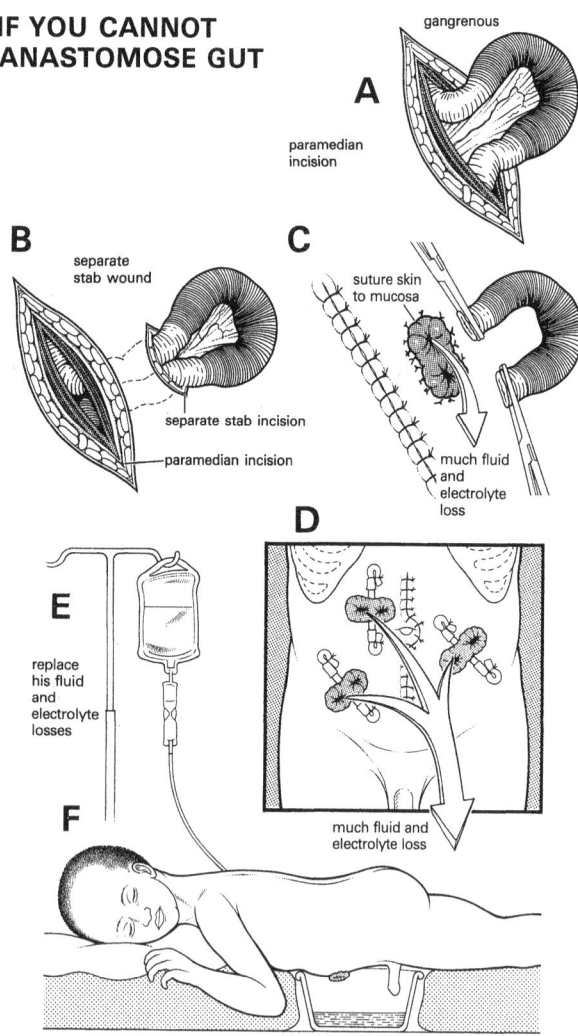

Fig. 9-13 IF YOU CANNOT ANASTOMOSE GUT, for example in a typhoid perforation, bring the gangrenous segment (A) out through a separate incision (B), cut it off so as to make an ileostomy (C), and suture all coats of the patient's gut to the skin of his abdominal wall with interrupted sutures. Refer him quickly, because there will be much fluid and electrolyte loss, which you must replace. D, he may have several stomas.

F, nurse him like this. E, and F, after the late Ian Hulme Moir.

OSTOMIES

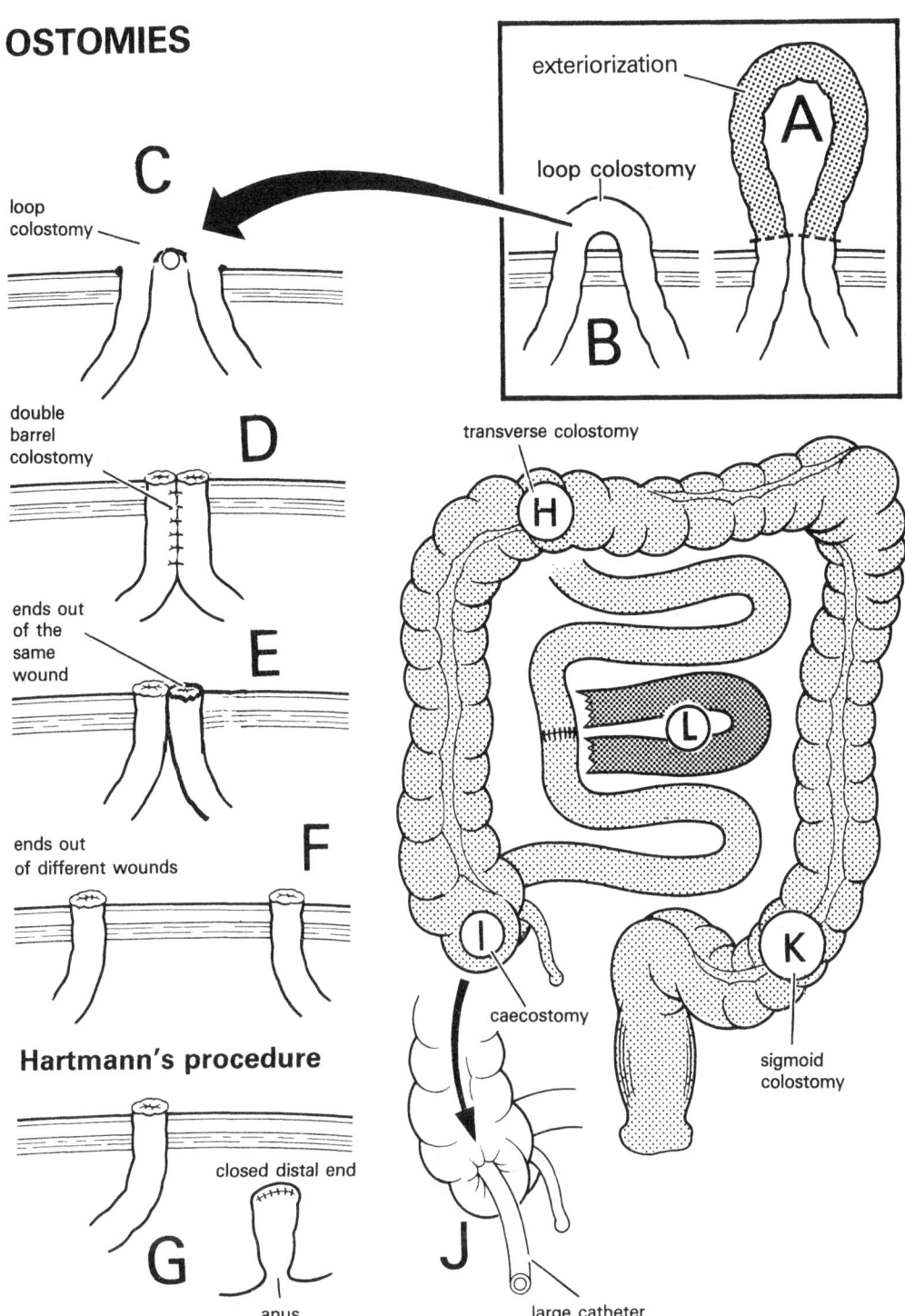

Fig. 9-14 OSTOMIES. A, exteriorization; the gut outside the abdominal wall is later resected to produce a colostomy. B, and C, stages in a loop colostomy. D, a double-barrelled colostomy. E, the ends of a colostomy come out of the same wound. F, they come out of different wounds. G, Hartmann's procedure, in which the distal end of the sigmoid colon is dropped back into the abdomen. H, an ostomy in the transverse colon. I, a caecostomy. J, a caecostomy with a large catheter inserted. K, an ostomy in the sigmoid colon. L, if the small gut is gangrenous, you can excise it and anastomose its ends, you cannot do this safely in an emergency with the large gut, because you do not have time to prepare it first.

A caecostomy can be made by placing a tube in the caecum and letting the liquid faeces drain. This is easier than doing a transverse colostomy, but: (1) The risks of soiling the peritoneum are greater. (2) A caecostomy often does not work well, and needs much washing out, so it is difficult to manage postoperatively. (3) It diverts little of the faecal stream. But, provided the tube is not too small, it may do this adequately. (4) It can only be temporary.

A caecostomy is useful if a patient is desperately ill, and you can, if necessary, do one under local anaesthesia without exploring his abdomen. You will find a caecostomy useful if he has: (a) a caecal injury, or (b) a more distal obstruction, but is too ill for a colostomy.

A transverse colostomy can be made as a loop, or double barrelled, or as a spectacles colostomy. Always make it in the right side of the transverse colon. This should not be difficult unless the colon is very distended, or the mesocolon is short. Use a transverse colostomy as a preliminary to resection of the large gut for a left sided obstruction for carcinoma (32.27), for anal atresia (28.6), and for an injury (66.14).

A sigmoid colostomy is an alternative to a transverse colostomy for obstruction in the rectum or sigmoid colon, such as a sigmoid volvulus. Here again you can make a loop, or double-barrel it.

Closing ostomies can be more difficult than making them. A caecostomy will close by itself, but a transverse or a sigmoid colostomy will have to be carefully closed, unless the patient is to have his colostomy permanently. If you cannot refer him to have it closed, you will have to close it yourself. If possible, try to do this extraperitoneally, so that you avoid the risk of contaminating his peritoneal cavity. You can usually free the ends of a loop colostomy (9-15), or a double-barrelled colostomy (9-19), and sew them together without entering his peritoneal cavity. The ends of the loop may be partly united already, so that you have only to complete the rest of the anastomosis. If you cannot close a colostomy extraperitoneally, you will have to lift out the two loops of gut and close it intraperitoneally as in Fig. 9-18.

There is another way of closing a double-barrelled colostomy extraperitoneally, which is to slowly crush the spur between the two loops of the barrel with a special clamp, as in Fig. 9-19. This makes the barrels join one another, and makes the colostomy easier to close. Some surgeons like this method and others don't. It has the disadvantage of needing a special clamp, although you can use a large haemostat, as described later. Closing Hartmann's operation is much more difficult; if you have to do it, it is decribed in Section 10.10a.

Bypasses. The ostomies above all open a patient's gut to the outside. You can also relieve his obstruction by connecting one part of his gut to another with a bypass. It is often anatomcally difficult and it can be surgically dangerous to bypass one part of his large gut to another, but you can bypass his small gut to his small gut, or his small gut to his large gut. You can: (1) Bypass one part of his small gut to another, when it is obstructed and bound down by septic (10.7) or tuberculous (29-8) adhesions, which are difficult to free. This is an entero-enterostomy, usually an ileo-ileostomy. (2) You can bypass his small gut into his large gut, by anastomosing his terminal ileum to his transverse colon, and closing the free end of his ileum, or leaving it open. This leaves the end of his ileum and his ascending colon as a blind loop. It is useful in amoebiasis (31.11) and carcinoma (32.27). Anastomosing his ileum to his transverse colon is more difficult than doing a caecostomy to relieve his obstruction, but is easier than removing his right colon (right hemicolectomy, 66-20). (3) You can bypass his ileum into his descending colon or rectum. This is major surgery: it will give him diarrhoea and most surgeons prefer a colostomy (32.27). (4) You can bypass his stomach into his small gut when his pylorus is obstructed (11.3).

9.6 Methods for ostomies

There are some important general principles: (1) Always try to bring an ostomy out through a separate smaller incision, and not through a laparotomy incision, unless you have to, because the wound is much more likely to become infected, and perhaps burst. (2) With all colostomies do Lord's procedure (maximal anal dilatation 22.5) before you send the patient back to the ward. This will temporarily paralyse his external sphincter, and allow his distal colon to drain more easily.

Sigmoid volvulus is the commonest cause of obstruction of the large gut in much of the developing world, so it is described elsewhere (10.10), and with it the detailed method for doing a sigmoid colostomy. Here are details of the other methods.

• CLAMP, *enterostomy, crushing, Lloyd Davies parallel action to take apart, one only.* This is for crushing the spur of a double-barrelled colostomy.

OSTOMIES

In most patients you will need to follow the general methods for intestinal obstruction in Section 10.3.

CAECOSTOMY UNDER LOCAL ANAESTHESIA

INDICATIONS. (1) Penetrating injuries of the caecum. (2) An obstruction proximal to the mid transverse colon, if you feel unable to do a right hemicolectomy. (3) Obstruction anywhere in the colon, if the patient is too ill for a colostomy. (3) A minimally skilled operator faced with any large gut obstruction.

X-RAYS. Before you start, make sure exactly where the patient's caecum is. Look for its gas shadow on the X-ray. It can be suprisingly high. Percuss his abdomen to make sure.

EQUIPMENT. A large (30 Ch) Malecot or, less satisfactorily, a large de Pezzer catheter with the top of its bell cut off.

ANAESTHESIA. General or local anaesthesia (A 6.7).

METHOD. Study Figure 66-18. Then, with the greatest possible care, make a small gridiron incision at McBurney's point (12-1) well laterally over his dilated caecum—you can easily nick or burst it. Put packs round the wound inside his abdomen to minimize the consequences of spillage. Have suction instantly available.

Partly deflate his caecum by needle aspiration (10-9), or by decompression (after placing a purse string suture round it), so as to take the tension off it. As soon as you have done this, its walls will become thicker and more vascular.

If his caecum is mobile enough to deliver out of his abdomen, gently bring it out, assisted by Dennis Browne forceps if necessary. In practice this is seldom possible. If you succeed, drain it, and then apply the anchoring sutures described below.

If it is not mobile enough, insert several 3/0 atraumatic chromic catgut sutures from the cut edges of his peritoneum to a 6 cm ring on his caecum. Pick up its seromuscular layer only. Don't penetrate its mucosa. Leave the sutures long, hold them in haemostats and don't tie them yet. Make another 4 cm purse string circle inside this.

With suction immediately handy and the surrounding area carefully packed off, make a small nick in the centre of the purse string. Flatten the end of the catheter in a haemostat. Using a screwing movement, quickly push the haemostat and catheter through the nick in the centre of the purse string. Open the jaws of the haemostat to release the catheter, remove the haemostat, and quickly tighten the purse string to secure the catheter in place.

CAUTION ! Make sure the catheter can drain off to the side, so that it does not flood his abdomen.

Close the muscle layers of his abdominal wall with interrupted catgut, monofilament, or steel wire, but leave his skin unsutured. His wound is sure to become infected, and this will minimize it. Suture the catheter to his skin to prevent it being pulled out. Clamp it and block it with a spigot, until he returns to the ward. Then connect it to a bag or bottle. Flush it out with one or two litres of saline, which need not be sterile, at least twice a day.

DIFFICULTIES WITH A CAECOSTOMY

If his CAECUM BURSTS with a puff of gas as you open it, suck vigorously. This will not be a major disaster if you have previously sutured the cut edges of his peritoneum to his caecum, and so isolated his peritoneal cavity. Deliver his burst caecum, and extend the incision if necessary. Apply a soft clamp and repair the perforation, invaginating it as you do so. Then do a standard caecostomy away from the site of the perforation. Alternatively, exteriorize his caecum. If necessary, you can sew the caecostomy tube into the tear in his burst caecum, provided it is not necrotic or gangrenous.

If, when you open his peritoneum, you find that his CAECUM IS GANGRENOUS but has not yet perforated, exteriorize it. Make a bigger wound and deliver his caecum through it. Resect it. You now have two choices; (1) You can do an end-to-side anastomosis of his ileum to his terminal colon (9-11). Or, (2) you can close his colon, exteriorize the gangrenous area, do an ileostomy and then close this 3 weeks later. Meanwhile, he will lose much fluid and many electrolytes.

A LOOP COLOSTOMY

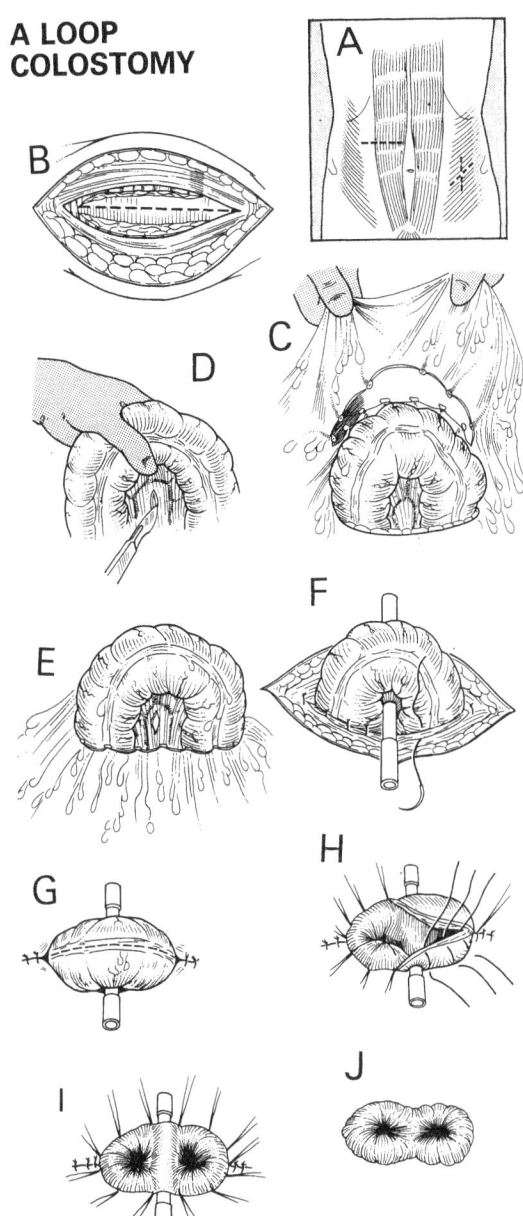

Fig. 9-15 A LOOP COLOSTOMY IN THE TRANSVERSE OR SIGMOID COLON. A, make these incisions for a transverse or a sigmoid colostomy. B, incise the rectus muscle for a transverse colostomy. C, incise the greater omentum and bring a loop of transverse colon through it. D, incise the mesentery. E, bring the transverse colon through the greater omentum. F, push a piece of tube or a glass rod through the hole, and suture the colon to the peritoneum. G, close the wound. H, open the colon and suture it to the edges of the skin wound. I, the completed colostomy. J, after healing of the wound. *After Goligher JC, 'The Surgery of the Anus, Rectum and Colon', Figs 347 to 361. Baillière Tindall, with kind permission.*

If you DON'T HAVE A SUITABLE CATHETER, you can stitch the wall of his caecum to his parietal peritoneum before you open his caecum. Then apply a colostomy bag over the opening. The difficulty with this is that it tends to close spontaneously.

TRANSVERSE COLOSTOMY

INDICATIONS. (1) Obstruction distal to the middle of a patient's transverse colon. (2) A penetrating injury of his transverse colon. (3) Gangrene of part of his transverse colon due to strangulation or interference with its blood supply. (4) A rectovaginal fistula prior to repair. (5) Protecting an anastomosis for sigmoid volvulus after resection.

A transverse colostomy is not difficult, and is better than a caecostomy. There are 3 types: (1) A plain loop. (2) A double-barrel colostomy. (3) A 'spectacles colostomy' as in Fig. 9-17.

METHOD. Make a right (or left) paramedian incision centered on his umbilicus. Open his peritoneum with the greatest care, as for any gut obstruction (9-2).

Try to find his transverse colon without allowing loops of his small gut to protrude from his wound. They will probably bulge into the wound, covered by omentum.

Lift his omentum upwards and forwards, so that you can see his transverse colon. Is it very distended? If it is not distended, his large gut is probably not obstructed and you will have to look for some other pathology. If it is very distended, you may need to deflate it first (10-9). Is it mobile enough to lift forward to skin level? If he is very obese, this may be difficult.

Make a 4 cm separate *transverse* skin incision above and to the right of the laparotomy incision, as in A Fig. 9-15. Divide his anterior rectus sheath in the same line as his skin. Cut his rectus muscle transversely. Your index and middle finger should be able to lie comfortably in the wound, but should not allow another finger to enter it.

CAUTION ! (1) Make the incision well to the right. (2) It must be high enough to avoid his umbilicus, and not so high that his transverse colon cannot reach it. (3) Make it just large enough to take the loop comfortably. (4) Make sure you have got his transverse colon and not his stomach or his sigmoid colon! The transverse colon has taenae (unlike the stomach), and is attached by a short omentum to the greater curvature of the stomach.

Choose an area of his transverse colon to the right of the midline. Trim off the omentum attached to 7 to 10 cm of its anterior surface so as to make a gap in it (C, Fig. 9-15, B, Fig. 9-19). Try to avoid tying any small vessels that may be present. Deliver a loop of his transverse colon through this gap.

Make a small window in his transverse mesocolon next to the mesenteric border of his colon (D, Fig. 9-15, C in Fig. 9-19). Do this by pushing a large blunt haemostat through it close to the wall of his gut, while you open and close its jaws. Avoid injuring the branches of his middle colic artery as you do so.

Pass a rubber catheter through the window you have made, and grasp both its ends with a haemostat (D, Fig. 9-19). Test the colon for mobility again. If it is very tense and distended, decompress it.

If you want to double-barrel it, insert a few interrupted catgut sutures between its loops, biting only its seromuscular coat as in D, Fig. 9-19.

CAUTION ! You must be able to deliver the loop of colon you have isolated through the transverse incision comfortably.

Push a second haemostat through the smaller transverse incision that is to be the site of the colostomy, and grasp the catheter you have placed round his colon. Release the first haemostat, and by pulling with one hand and pushing with the other, withdraw the loop of colon, so that it comes out through the colostomy incision and rests on his abdominal wall.

If the wound is loose enough to let you insert a finger alongside the loop of colon, there will be no risk of the lumen occluding, and the colostomy should function satisfactorily. If his colon is not loose enough, extend the incision.

Close his abdomen so as to withstand a high intra-abdominal tension, as in Section 9.8.

Pass a short piece of thick rubber tube, or a short glass rod attached to a piece of rubber tube, through the window occupied by the catheter(F, Fig. 9-15), and keep it there with two stitches anchored to his skin. Pass a few interrupted sutures between the fascia of his abdominal wall and the seromuscular layer of his gut, and between his skin and the free margin of his gut.

CAUTION ! Before you place these sutures, make sure his colon is not twisted, and that it runs transversely, as a transverse colon should.

Open his colostomy immediately. If you delay, his obstruction is not relieved. Apply a substantial dressing to the laparotomy wound. Make a 3 cm incision (as in E, Fig. 9-19) through both coats of his colon across its axis (in line with the rubber tube), or better, longitudinally along a taenia (G, and H, Fig. 9-15). It will open to form two stomata (I, Fig. 9-15). You will have to close the opening transversely to avoid obstruction: opening it longitudinally ensures a wider lumen. Suture his skin to his mucosa, as in H and I, Fig. 9-15. Push a finger down the afferent loop to make sure that it is patent—a gush of gas and faeces is an encouraging sign. If possible, apply

A COLOSTOMY BAG

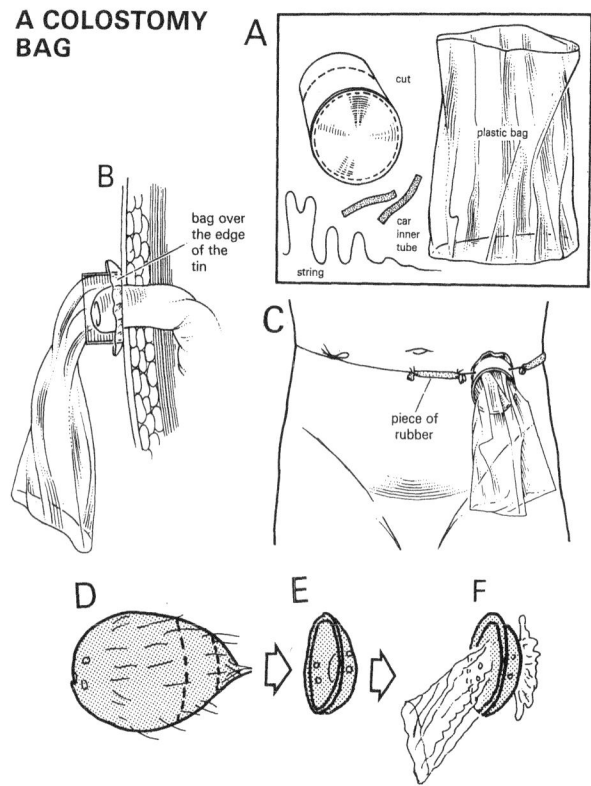

Fig. 9-16 IF YOU DON'T HAVE A COLOSTOMY BAG, you can make one from an ordinary plastic bag, a tin, a piece of rubber, such as that from the inner tube of a car tyre, and a piece of string. The tin should be a small one and should fit comfortably over the patient's colostomy. A small 'Carnation milk' tin works well, provided it has no sharp edges. Make holes for the string in the side of the tin, and make sure it has no sharp edges. You can also use a pessary ring to hold the bag. If you are using disposable bags be sure to give the patient enough. A washable non-disposable bag may be more practical. He needs at least two. Make sure that he or his relatives know how to wash and use them. D, E, and F, an ostomy appliance made from a coconut and a plastic bag. A, B, and C, kindly contributed by John Tarpley.

a commercial colostomy bag. If not, improvise one as in Fig. 9-16.

SIGMOID COLOSTOMY

INDICATIONS. (1) Wounds of the rectum. (2) Chronic obstructive rectal lesions including carcinoma. (3) Following resection for sigmoid volvulus.

CONTRAINDICATIONS. Situations in which a sigmoid colostomy wound would interfere with subsequent operations, for example the repair of a rectovaginal fistula.

METHOD. This is described under volvulus of the sigmoid colon as part of Hartmann's operation in Section 10.10 and Fig. 10-16. It also closely resembles a transverse colostomy. You can 'double-barrel' and 'spectacle' it as with a transverse colostomy, as described above, or leave a blind distal end.

Draw a line from the patient's umbilicus to his left iliac spine (A, in Fig. 9-19). Site the mid point of the incision at the junction of the medial two-thirds and the lateral one third. This is the same as McBurney's point but is in the left iliac fossa. Site the incision carefully. Choose a site for the stoma in the upper part of the mobile loop of the sigmoid colon, to prevent the colostomy prolapsing later.

END (TERMINAL) COLOSTOMY

INDICATIONS. (1) As part of Hartmann's procedure when this is done for sigmoid volvulus or for any other reason. (2) Severe damage to the pelvirectal colon complicating surgery for PID (6.6). (3) A permanent colostomy, as after resection of a low carcinoma of the rectum.

The disadvantage with the method which follows is that it leaves a lateral space through which gut can herniate internally. The alternative, which is to lead the sigmoid colon through an extraperitoneal tunnel round the left paracolic gutter, is too difficult to be described here.

METHOD. Make an appropriate incision in the patient's abdominal wall, as in A, Fig. 9-15. Insert a crushing clamp through it and draw out the end of his gut. Before you close his abdomen, put in a few catgut sutures between the seromuscular coat of his gut, and the peritoneum of his abdominal wall. Place them so that there will be 1.5 cm of healthy gut protruding beyond the skin, then close his abdomen.

To open the colostomy, cut off the crushing clamp with a sharp scalpel. Control bleeding. Suture mucosa to skin all round with interrupted 2/0 or 3/0 monofilament.

Ideally, use the method in F, and G, Fig. 9-17. Use stitches which take a bite of: (1) his anterior rectus sheath without going through his skin, (2) the seromuscular coat of his gut about 8 mm proximal to its tip, (3) the mucosa and seromuscular coat of the tip of his gut. When you eventually tighten these sutures, you will find his colostomy will evert itself beautifully.

BYPASSES

AN ILEO-TRANSVERSE COLOSTOMY takes the end of his ileum about 15 cm from his ileocaecal valve, and anastomoses it to his transverse colon, leaving the stump of his ileum, his caecum and his ascending colon in place. Use it to provide temporary relief for obstruction of his caecum or ascending colon, by ileocaecal tuberculosis (29.5) or carcinoma.

Make an end-to-side anastomosis, as in Section 9.4, Fig. 9-11. Use the second part of the method of end-to-side anastomosis in Fig. 66-20. Close the stump of his ileum with an all-coats layer, and then invert this with Lembert sutures

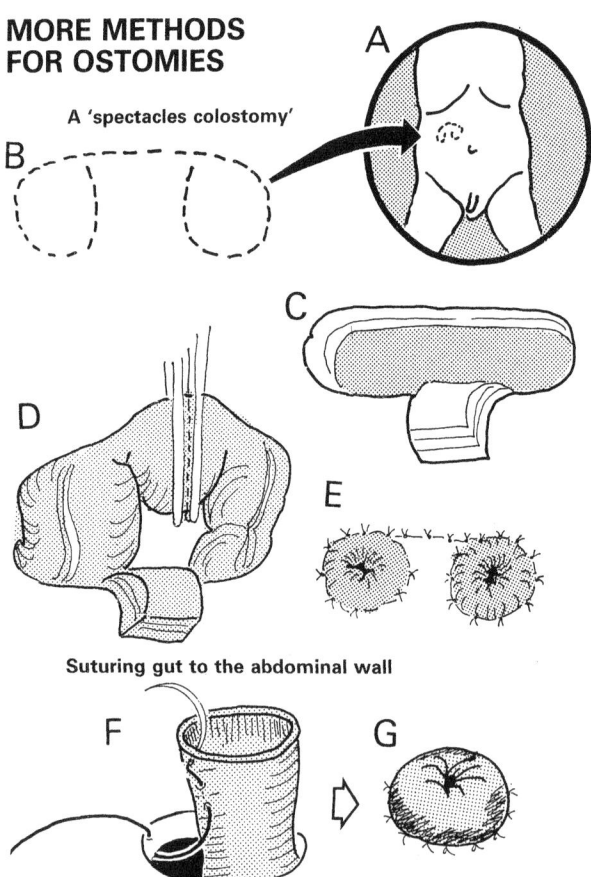

Fig. 9-17 MORE METHODS FOR OSTOMIES. A, the site of the incision for a spectacles colostomy. B, the spectacles incision. Remove the skin inside each loop. C, turning back the flap. D, the transverse colon exteriorized and clamped with two crushing clamps. E, the completed colostomy. F, and G, a secure method of suturing a patient's colon to his abdominal wall.

CLOSING A COLOSTOMY INTRAPERITONEALLY

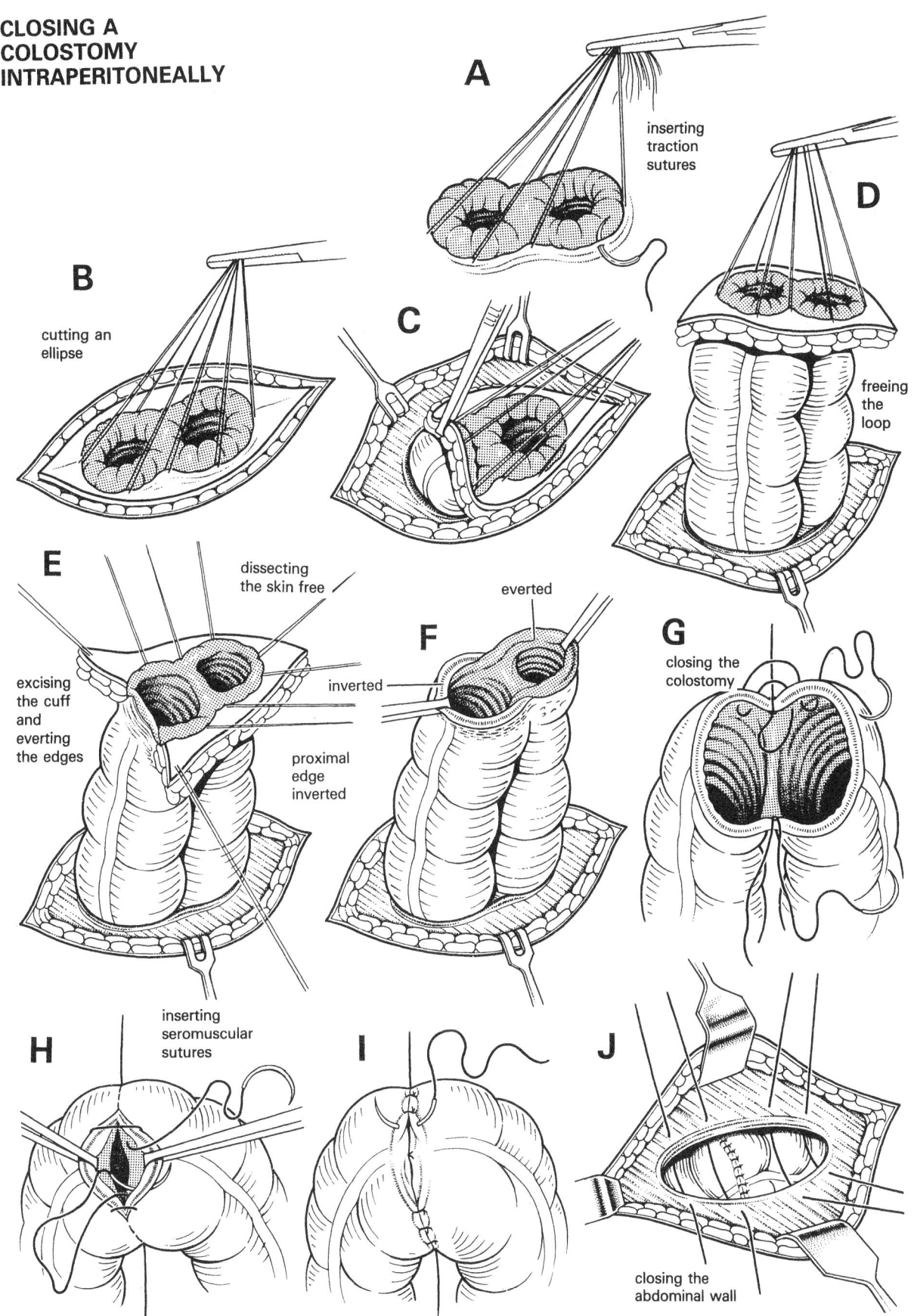

Fig. 9-18 CLOSING A LOOP COLOSTOMY INTRAPERITONEALLY. Only do this if you cannot close it extraperitoneally, as in the next figure, which is safer. A, insert traction sutures. B, raise an ellipse of skin round the colostomy. C, dissect the ellipse of skin free from the rectus sheath. D, free the colostomy loop. E, excise a cuff of skin and evert the gut edges. F, the proximal gut edge is everted, the distal gut edge is still inverted. G, and H, closing the colostomy with Connell loop-on-mucosa stitches. I, inserting a second layer of seromuscular Lembert sutures. J, closing the muscles of the abdominal wall in one layer. *After Maingot R, 'The Management of Abdominal Operations', Figs. 396 to 404. HK Lewis, with kind permission.*

(one contributor leaves the stump open, it will not leak into the peritoneal cavity). Leave his right colon and the stump of his ileum in place to be joined up later.

AN ENTERO-ENTEROSTOMY. Make a side-to-side anastomosis as in Fig 9-12. This figure shows the ends of the gut resected: you usually need to leave them in continuity. Make it between adjacent loops of his small gut (for obstruction of his small gut by adhesions or tuberculous peritonitis), or between his small gut and his large gut (G, Fig. 32-15b) for obstruction of his ascending colon, usually by ileocaecal tuberculosis or carcinoma.

SPECTACLES COLOSTOMY

INDICATIONS. A moderately defunctioning colostomy, as in preparing a child with an imperforate anus for definitive surgery later.

METHOD. Site the spectacles colostomy in his right hypochondrium, as in A, Fig. 9-17. Make a spectacles-shaped incision (B), and remove the skin inside each loop. Turn back the flap (C). Exteriorize and clamp the transverse colon with two crushing clamps (D), to make the colostomy (E).

CLOSING A COLOSTOMY INTRAPERITONEALLY

If you cannot refer him, do this *4 to 6 weeks later,* when his wound is healthy and he has recovered from his original operation.

CAUTION ! (1) He will be hoping for this as soon as possible. Don't let him persuade you to do it too early. (2) It is not an easy operation, so refer him if you can.

Wash out his gut proximally, and distally through his rectum. Repeat this daily for 2 or 3 days before the operation. Some surgeons give him magnesium sulphate to help empty his proximal gut and to make sure that the next faeces he passes will be soft. Give him neomycin 500 mg 6-hourly for 2 days, then give him oral perioperative chloramphenicol and rectal metronidazole (2.9).

To minimize bleeding infiltrate the skin and subcutaneous tissues around his colostomy with a local anaesthetic solution containing adrenalin 1:200,000 (A 5.4). Wait to allow the anaesthetic to act. Or, use general anaesthesia. The infiltration is valuable in demonstrating tissue planes.

Insert traction sutures round the colostomy (A, in Fig. 9-18). Make an elliptical incision round it (B). Use a fine knife and sharp scissors to dissect it free from the surrounding skin and fascia, and from the muscle of his abdominal wall (C). Keep a finger in the lumen to tell you when you are getting dangerously close to it.

Raise the ellipse of skin from his abdominal wall (D). Using sharp dissection, clean the sheath of his rectus muscle until you reach the edge of the opening through which his gut is passing.

If, at this stage you think you can unite the two loops of his gut *extraperitoneally,* do so (see below).

If this is difficult, you will have to enter his peritoneal cavity. Free the parietal peritoneum round the circumference of the opening. Divide any adhesions that may be present. Draw his colon out of the incision, and place packs over the wound. Trim away the everted edges of his gut (E). Close it transversely with Connell stitches (G, and H; see also A, Fig. 9-6). Start by placing two atraumatic sutures through all the coats of the gut where his proximal and distal colon meet. Tie the knot in the lumen, and work from each side.

Check, by pinching with your fingers, that, when you cut off the skin remnants and closed the colostomy, you left plenty of room for faeces to go through.

If there is enough room for his faeces to go through, add a second layer of interrupted Lembert inverting sutures through the seromuscular layer (I), and tuck it into his abdomen.

If there is not enough room, resect the colostomy and do a new end-to-end anastomosis.

Close his abdominal wall with interrupted sutures. Now do a Lord's procedure (maximal anal dilatation) before he goes back to the ward.

CLOSING A COLOSTOMY EXTRAPERITONEALLY

This mostly applies to a loop colostomy and a double-barrelled colostomy with a spur that can be crushed. The description that follows is for the double-barrelled colostomy in Fig. 9-19, but you can do it with the loop colostomy in Fig. 9-15.

As soon as the patient no longer needs his colostomy, crush the spur, as in G, Fig. 9-19. When you are ready, put one finger into each lumen to check that no tissue has been caught between the loops. This should not happen if you have double-barrelled it satisfactorily. If you mistakenly crush his small gut, he will get an ileo-colic fistula. Put the crushing clamp on the spur and tighten the clamp a little. Each day, tighten it a bit more, until it falls free.

When the crushing clamp has fallen off, put your finger into the stoma. The spur should have gone, so that the contents of his gut can pass easily along his colon. Insert your index finger to check that there is a nice big opening between the two loops of colostomy. If there is, close the colostomy extraperitoneally.

Under appropriate anaesthesia (which can be local), infiltrate round his colostomy with adrenalin 1:200,000; wait 5 minutes, make an elliptical incision close to the edge of the colostomy, and prolong it along Lange's lines as shown. With a finger in the colostomy, and with Allis' forceps applied to the skin round the edge of the colostomy, dissect with a No. 11 scalpel blade, or fine scissors, in the plane between his gut and his abdominal wall. Try to avoid entering his peritoneal cavity; but if you do it is unimportant. Lift the cuff clear. Check that the spur is sufficiently deep to allow the faecal stream to pass over the top of it easily. A colostomy is rather bulky, so you may have to sweep his peritoneum away from his abdominal wall a little with your finger to make space for it.

Complete the closure in two layers in the same way as for an intraperitoneal anastomosis, first with an all-coats layer of continuous catgut, and then with a layer of interrupted inverting seromuscular Lembert sutures. The suture line may leak, so put a rubber drain down to it.

If you don't have a proper crushing clamp, either don't use this method, or use a large rubber covered straight haemostat, or Kocher's forceps. Apply them for 15 minutes the first day, half an hour on the second day, and an hour on the third day. By 5–7 days you should be able to leave them on continuously, until they fall off by themselves 2–4 days later. If the stoma bleeds, stop the process for a day.

CLOSING HARTMANN'S OPERATION. See Section 10.10a.

DIFFICULTIES WITH COLOSTOMIES

If his COLOSTOMY 'RUNS LIKE A RIVER', this is likely to be a good sign in the early stages, because it means that his obstructed gut is emptying itself. If it happens later, give him kaolin mixture with 1 to 2 tablets of codein phosphate 3 times a day. If it happens after you have crushed the spur of a double-barrelled colostomy, you may have crushed a loop of small gut at the apex of the spur and made an ileostomy in error. Refer him to an expert immediately.

If his COLOSTOMY DOES NOT WORK at all, this is likely to be serious. Put a finger into the afferent loop to make sure that it has not become occluded. If this fails to start it, put a glycerine suppository or an enema solution into the afferent loop. If it is still not working after 3 days, he may have a proximal obstruction or ileus.

If the GUT FORMING HIS COLOSTOMY NECROSES (rare), you probably damaged its mesentery by stretching or compressing it into too small a hole. Take him back to the theatre, enlarge the opening in his abdominal wall, and make a fresh colostomy by bringing out more gut.

Fig. 9-19 A DOUBLE-BARRELLED COLOSTOMY. MAKING IT AND CLOSING IT EXTRAPERITONEALLY. A, the incisions. B, the site in patient's mesentery through which to pass the loop of bowel. C, the site in his mesocolon through which to pass the rubber tube. D, the loop double-barrelled and brought out through the transverse colostomy incision using a rubber tube. E, opening his colostomy (in this case transversely), and anchoring it in place with a short rubber tube. F, skin-to-mucosa sutures have been inserted all round. G, applying the crushing clamp when his colostomy is ready for closure. H, the two stomas are now one. After checking that loops have united in the depths of the wound, infiltrate around the colostomy and use the skin incision shown. I, excising the skin. J, the gut sutured and about to be returned to his abdomen with a drain. K, a cross-section of the finished colostomy.

A DOUBLE-BARRELLED COLOSTOMY CLOSED EXTRAPERITONEALLY

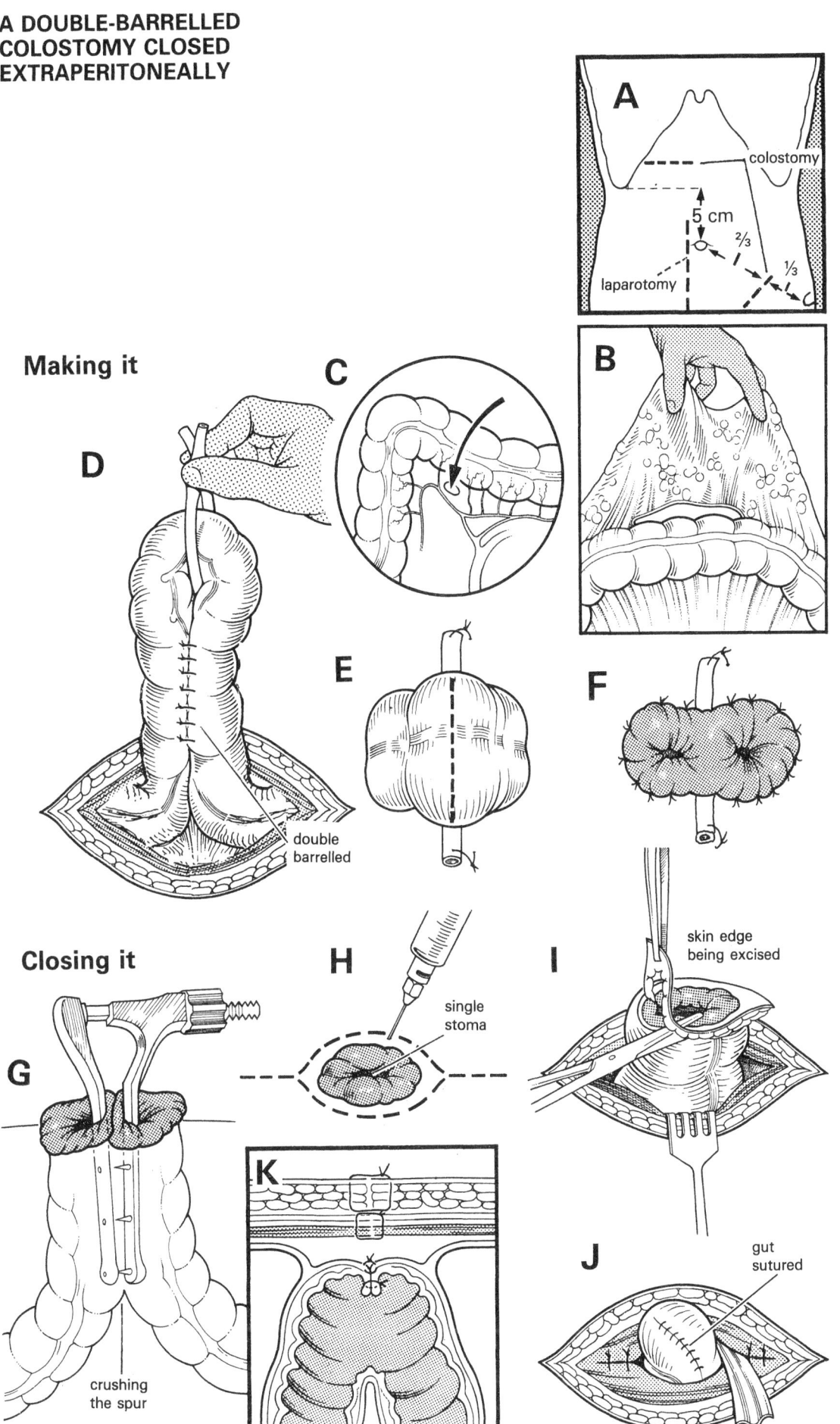

Making it

Closing it

If his COLOSTOMY WITHDRAWS BACK INTO ITS HOLE, it will contaminate his peritoneum and cause faecal peritonitis, which may be fatal. A glass rod or rubber tube through a loop colostomy should prevent it doing this. To be even more certain, put 6 interrupted sutures between the seromuscular coat of his colon and his anterior rectus sheath (F, and G, Fig. 9-17). When it has withdrawn, you may need to operate to put it right.

If A HERNIA FORMS round his colostomy, it will probably only be a little bulge, and is unlikely to grow big. Prevent it by: (1) not making the opening for the colostomy too big, (2) stitching the seromuscular layer of the gut to the anterior layer of the fascia of his abdominal wall (F, and G. Fig. 9-17).

If his COLOSTOMY PROLAPSES, it will look just like a prolapse of his rectum. Gut spouts out, but you can usually push it back. This is quite common and embarrassing. Prevention is difficult, but the deep sutures mentioned above are some help (F, and G, Fig. 9-17). Reduce it as necessary

If he develops signs of INTESTINAL OBSTRUCTION, adhesions may be forming inside his abdomen at the site where his colostomy emerges, or from the original disease process. They are no different from the adhesions developing after any other abdominal operation. Explore him if he does not improve.

9.7 A feeding jejunostomy

The common purpose of an ostomy is to let a patient's intestinal contents get out past an obstruction in his large gut. Occasionally, you may need to make an ostomy in his small gut to let food and drink get in past an obstruction in his oesophagus. Alternatively, you can make an ostomy in his stomach (gastrostomy, 11.8), unless his problem happens to be there.

If he cannot feed himself by mouth, and needs building up, an alternative to total parenteral nutrition (which will probably be impossibly expensive) is to put a tube into his jejunum and feed him through that. Feeding jejunostomies are seldom needed, but they can be life-saving: for example, when a suture line in an injured duodenum needs protecting. To reduce the danger of a leak, introduce the tube into his gut through a long oblique track.

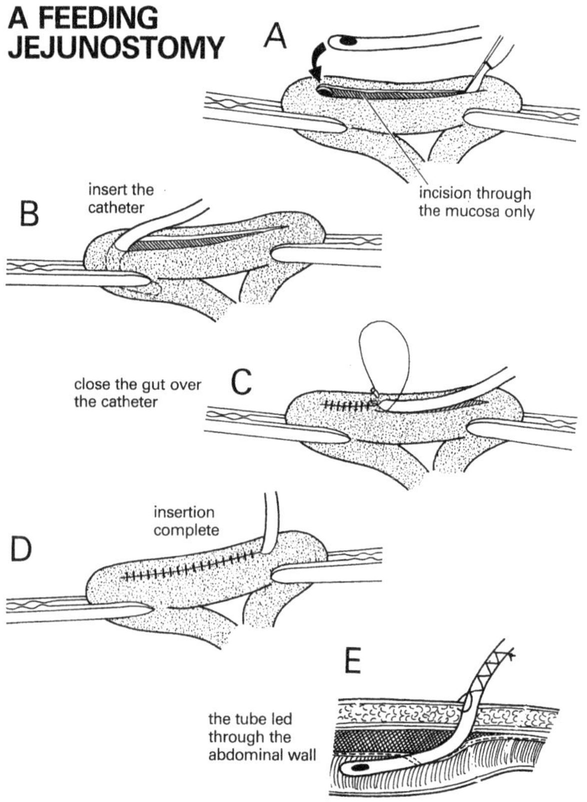

FEEDING JEJUNOSTOMY

INDICATIONS. (1) An oesophageal obstruction which is correctable. (2) To protect a suture line in the duodenum following an injury. (3) To protect a suture line in the stomach which has leaked. (4) A pancreatic abscess.

METHOD. Make a small laparotomy in the patient's upper abdomen under local or general anaesthesia.

Find his upper jejunum by following it downwards from his duodenojejunal flexure. Confirm that it is his duodenojejunal junction by finding his inferior mesenteric vein along its left border and feeling it emerge from its fixed position behind his peritoneum. Take a loop about 25 cm from his duodenojejunal junction, and make an incision on its antemesenteric border through the longitudinal muscle layer for about 8 cm. At the distal end of this make a hole through into the lumen. Insert a feeeding catheter (18 Ch for an adult), or a long Ryle's tube, through this hole for about 10 cm. Close his gut around it with continuous catgut, as if you were doing the Lembert suture of a bowel closure (9-6).

Make a second incision in his abdominal wall above where this loop of jejunum will comfortably lie. Draw the end of the tube back through his abdominal wall, as you would with a caecostomy (66-18). Draw his jejunum and the interior of his abdominal wall together with a purse string suture, as for a caecostomy. Close his abdomen and anchor the tube to his abdominal wall with a 'Saxon stocking' type of anchoring stitch, or with tape (D, to G, Fig. 65-8).

To remove the tube, snip the ligature anchoring it to the skin, and pull. The long oblique tunnel through the mucosa and submucosa will seal rapidly. The purse string anchoring it to his peritoneal wall will prevent his jejunal contents soiling his peritoneal cavity.

9.8 Draining and closing the abdomen

After a laparotomy a patient's skin has always to be closed separately, either at the operation or a few days later. There are two other layers to be closed: (1) His peritoneum, which is fused to his posterior rectus sheath. (2) His anterior rectus sheath. These layers can either be closed separately in a classical three-layer closure (the skin is the third layer). Or they can be closed together in a two-layer closure (the skin is the second layer) by Everett's or Goligher's methods. These two-layer methods: (1) Are much better at preventing a burst abdomen than the classical three-layer method. (2) Are cheaper: (a) because they are quicker and so save in anaesthetic and staff time, and (b) because they use no catgut. They use monofilament or stainless steel and take big bites which are not too tight, instead of many smaller ones. Everett's method leaves knots on the peritoneal side of the wound where they cause no discomfort.

Delayed primary skin suture will reduce the risk of wound infection in high-risk cases in the same way as in wounds of other kinds (54.1). Antibiotics help, but they are less effective than leaving the skin wound open for a few days.

DRAINING AND CLOSING THE ABDOMEN

Before you close a patient's abdomen, make quite sure that, if it is contaminated, you wash it out and instil tetracycline 1 g in 1000 ml of saline or Ringer's lactate, as in Section 6.2 on peritonitis. Drains are not useful, except for localized abscesses, bleeding, or leaks of bile or urine.

SWAB COUNT, etc. Check the operation site thoroughly before you close his abdomen to make sure that you have restored his anatomy as you wish, that there is no bleeding, and no

Fig. 9-20 MAKING A FEEDING JEJUNOSTOMY. A, making the incision. B, inserting the tube. C, closing the jejunum over the tube with continuous catgut. D, the tube fixed in the gut. E, leading the tube out through the abdominal wall. The inner suture between the jejunum and the parietal peritoneum is not shown.

CLOSING THE ABDOMINAL WALL

Everett's method

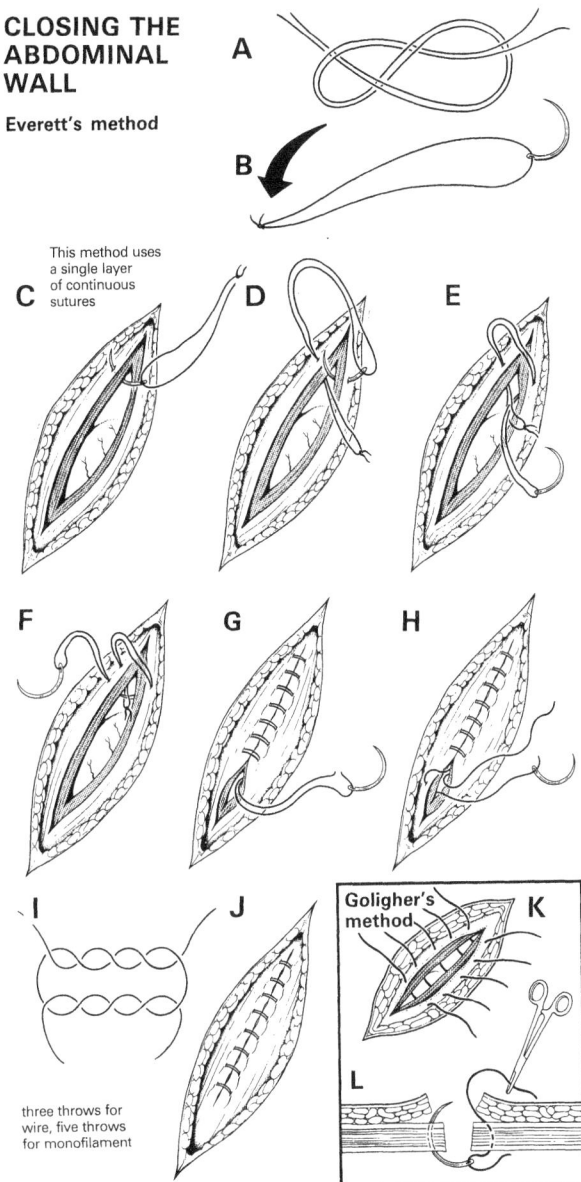

Fig. 9-21 EVERETT'S AND GOLIGHER'S METHODS OF CLOSING THE ABDOMEN. Everett's method A, to J. A, and B, take a long length of No. 1 monofilament, double it and knot it. C, D, and E, catch the end of the loop in the first bite. F, and G, make large continuous stitches. H, and I, open the loop and tie it with a surgeon's knot inside. J, the muscle sutured, and the skin left for delayed primary closure.

Goligher's method, K, and L, is an almost infallible method of closing the abdomen in high-risk cases. Use interrupted wire sutures through all layers of the abdominal wall except the skin. Take big bites and don't tie them too tight. Place all the sutures first and then tie them.

leakage from hollow viscera. Make sure that you have left no instruments, swabs, or packs behind. It is reckless to rely only on a swab count!

ABDOMINAL DRAINS are described in Section 4.10. Read this carefully!

PREVENTING ADHESIONS. Bring his greater omentum down so that it underlies the incision. This will help to prevent adhesions forming between his viscera and his abdominal wall.

EVERETT'S MASS CLOSURE METHOD *should be your standard way of closing the abdomen.* Take a piece of No.1 monofilament 8 times the length of the incision, fold it in half, and tie a 'figure-of-8' knot (A, and B, Fig. 9-21).

Pass the needle from the deep surface of his peritoneum, then go from the outer surface of his abdominal muscle inwards on the opposite side of the wound. Thread the needle through the loop, so as to bury the knot.

Go all the way along the wound like this taking deep bites and not pulling too tightly. Place the stitches 1 cm from the edge of the incision and 1 cm apart. At the end of the wound come out from the deep surface, and cut the needle out of the loop. Rethread one end and pass it from outside inwards. Tie the two ends together with a double surgeon's knot, and cut them short. Now either close his skin with monofilament now, or leave it open for a few days for delayed primary skin suture. This method does not require tension sutures.

CAUTION ! (1) Don't take the bites too close to the wound edges. (2) Don't make the sutures too far apart. (3) Don't make them too tight.

GOLIGHER'S METHOD is for preventing a burst abdomen in the ultimate poor risk case. It differs from Everett's method, mainly in that it preferably uses steel instead of monofilament and the sutures are preferably interrupted instead of continuous.

Gather everything except the patient's skin together with *large* bites of 28 SWG steel wire. If you don't have wire, use No. 0 monofilament or thicker. Insert the sutures 1.5 cm from the wound edge, and 1 cm apart. Use interrupted sutures only. Tie them with three throws (turns) for steel, and five for monofilament. If you are using continuous sutures (you are advised not to), keep them fairly loose. Close his skin with monofilament now, or leave it open for a few days for delayed primary skin suture.

CLOSURE IN THREE LAYERS is traditional, and is included for completeness. You will find the above methods safer. (1) Use a continuous suture of No. 1 catgut to close the patient's peritoneum together with his posterior rectus sheath. (2) Use continuous or interrupted sutures of '0' monofilament or 28 SWG stainless steel to bring the fascia of his rectus sheath together. (3) Use No. 2/0 monofilament to close his skin and subcutaneous tissues.

TENSION SUTURES are controversial, uncomfortable, and leave ugly scars. Some surgeons never use them, even for burst abdomens, when they use Goligher's method. Others use them when a patient's abdomen has already burst, and no other closure is possible because of oedema and infection.

Place haemostats at each end of the wound, and at 2.5 cm intervals all down the wound before you suture the abdomen. Use them to bring the edges of his abdominal wall together when you tie the sutures. Load up a long curved cutting needle with No. 1 monofilament. Thread a 3 cm length of fine rubber tubing on to this to prevent the monofilament biting into the skin. Insert the sutures through all layers of the abdominal wall, including the skin, taking bites at least 2.5 cm deep on each side of the wound (B, and C, Fig. 9-24). Hold each end in a haemostat. Now suture the wound in the usual way. When you have closed the skin, tie the tension sutures with triple throw surgeon's knots, making sure the rubber tubes lie over the wound itself.

Alternatively, insert the tension sutures as in D, to G, Fig. 9-24. Pass them through all coats including the skin, as is usual for tension sutures, then hold them out on artery forceps ready for tying (D, and E). Put rubber tubes on each alternate suture (F), rather than on each one (as with the usual method). G, instead of tying them across the wound, tie them to their next door neighbours.

Remove the skin sutures first at 9 days, and the deep tension sutures at 12 to 14 days.

DELAYED PRIMARY SUTURE FOR POTENTIALLY INFECTED ABDOMINAL WOUNDS

INDICATIONS. Any kind of sepsis which contaminates a patient's abdominal wound puts him at risk, especially: (1) Caesarean section in the presence of infected liquor. (2) Appendicitis. (3) Perforated typhoid ulcers of the ileum. (4) Perforations of his large gut. (5) The excision of gangrenous gut. (6) Generalized peritonitis.

METHOD. Close the muscles of his abdomen with steel wire, or monofilament. Make the sutures *just* tight enough to bring the muscles of his abdominal wall together and prevent his gut escaping. Test this as you go along by feeling the inside of the wound with your finger, as if it were a loop of gut trying to escape. Then put a dry gauze pack on his wound, and return him to the ward. If the condition you are operating for demands antibiotics, give them.

At 3 to 5 days, examine the wound. If it is clean, close it by delayed primary closure. If it is infected, apply hypochlorite or saline dressings regularly until it is fit for secondary suture, or secondary skin grafting. Occasionally, you will find the wound already healing so well, that it will close spontaneously. If so, let it do so.

CAUTION ! (1) NEVER close the fascia or muscle of his abdominal wall with catgut. It will be absorbed too soon, and increase the risk of early bursting and later herniation. (2) Don't use braided silk, which increases the risk of sinuses. (3) Make the sutures just tight enough to bring the edges of the muscles together—don't strangle them. (4) Don't try to close the abdominal wall *and skin* in a single layer, except when a burst has already occurred, and you decide to insert deep tension sutures.

DIFFICULTIES CLOSING THE ABDOMEN

If you have DIFFICULTY GETTING HIS GUT BACK INTO HIS ABDOMEN, (1)Ask the anaesthetist keep him well relaxed. (2) Use a 'fish' as in I, Fig. 10-9. This is a piece of stiff rubber sheet (such as that from a car inner tube) with a tail on it. Place this under the incision to hold his gut down; just as you are closing the incision, pull it out by its tail.

9.9 After an abdominal operation

If you have struggled hard to save a patient in the theatre, it is tragic to lose him in the ward afterwards. If you are working under difficult conditions, postoperative care can be at least as difficult as surgery. You will find an ICU (intensive care unit), like that in *Primary Anaesthesia,* very useful for any ill patient, and particularly for someone who is recovering from a severe operation (A 19.1). The staff of even the simplest ICU should be able to check his vital signs, keep an accurate fluid balance, and watch for postoperative bleeding. If he is recovering from a major operation, he will need need very careful monitoring, and frequent visits from you. If the nurses there are not yet fully trained, you will need to do much of this monitoring yourself. If you don't have an ICU, gather critically ill patients near the nurse's station in an ordinary ward, so that the senior nurse can watch them. The list below of the things she should check is a long one, but most of the checks are quick. Postoperative care is also discussed in *Primary Anaesthesia* (A 4.6). Above all, try to anticipate complications before they occur.

POSTOPERATIVE CARE

THE RECOVERY POSITION. Nurse the patient on his side in the recovery position (A 4-5), with the foot of his bed raised if his blood pressure is low. Turn him 2-hourly.

MONITORING. All patients should be carefully watched, but only a few need careful measurement of their vital signs. The most useful observations are those of the pulse rate, blood pressure, consciousness, skin temperature, peripheral perfusion, and urinary output. If a patient is critically ill, make sure that, during the first few hours, some competent person checks: (1) His level of consciousness. (2) The pattern of his respiration. (3) His peripheral circulation—the warmth of his extremities. (4) The capillary circulation in his nail beds, and (5) his pulse. (6) His temperature. (7) His urine output. (8) His degree of pain, and any changes in it. (9) Any bleeding and discharge from his wound. (10) Abdominal distension. His blood pressure need only be measured if these other signs indicate that it might be abnormal, or if he is old, very ill, or has had major surgery.

The nurses in the ICU must be on the look out for: (1) a falling blood pressure and a rising pulse rate, (2) respiratory depression and arrest (A 3.4 and 4.5), (3) bronchospasm (A 3.3), (4) failure of the nasogastric suction to work properly, and (5) the aspiration of gastric contents (A 16.3).

Later, as he recovers, their attention can change to: (1) Maintaining nasogastric suction. (2) Coughing and breathing exercises.

INTRAVENOUS FLUIDS should be managed as in A 15.5. If there is any doubt about the adequacy of fluid replacement, be sure to monitor his urine output. Only a very ill patient needs an indwelling catheter; remove it when it is not absolutely necessary. A Paul's tube is often adequate in men.

If you did not adequately replace the blood he lost at the operation, he will have diluted his blood by the first day, so measure his haemoglobin or his haematocrit, and transfuse him if he is in danger.

NASOGASTRIC SUCTION will prevent the aspiration of vomit; it will remove gas and fluid and relieve distension. Manage it as in Section 4.9.

BOWELS. If he is on a traditional high-residue diet, he will probably have no difficuty with his bowels once any ileus he may have had has subsided. He is more likely to have difficulty if he is on a on a 'Western' type of low-residue diet. If he has passed flatus, but no stool by the fifth day, consider giving him a rectal suppository.

PAIN. If he is in severe pain, give him half the standard dose of intravenous pethidine or morphine (A 2-4) initially. Give the other half ten minutes later if the first was not enough. A useful method is to add further doses to his intravenous fluids 4 hourly (A 8.9). Or, better, run it in continuously with his intravenous fluids. This makes sure that he gets it all the time without having to call the nurses. Intramuscular drugs are not absorbed rapidly enough. 20 mg of morphine 8 hourly is an average dose for a fit adult. Give half or a quarter of this if he is very sick, thin or malnourished. By 3 to 5 days he should have no need of injectable opioids, so taper them off, and occasionally, if necessary, replace them by an oral opioid.

OTHER DRUGS. (1) Don't give him a hypnotic for 5–7 days, it will not help him while he is in pain. (2) Don't give him an antiemetic without looking for a cause. It may help him if he has an inoperable carcinoma. (3) Continue his perioperative antibiotics only if necessary (2.9). Otherwise, don't give him an antibiotic, unless he has an established infection.

AMBULATION. Encourage him to move his legs in bed. If possible, get him up and about early. Dependent immobile legs have a higher incidence of deep vein thrombosis (rare in the developing world) than raised ones. This is more likely to occur sitting still in a chair than sitting still in bed.

9.10 Non-respiratory postoperative complications

Many complications can interrupt a patient's recovery, but you can prevent most of them. Some important ones involve his lungs; these are in the next section. Infections are more likely if he is HIV positive (Chapter 28a).

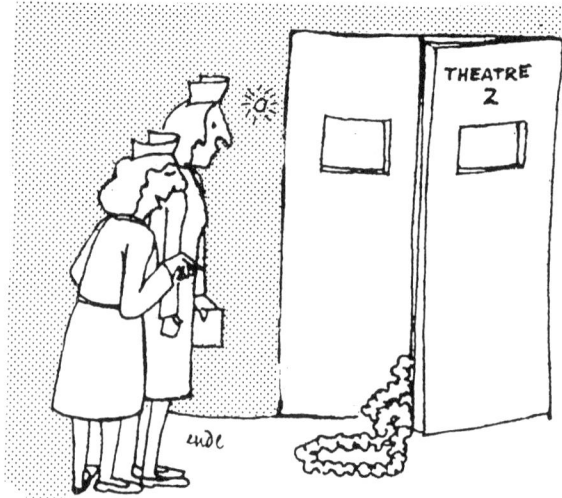

'That must be the new surgeon again.'

If he is to recover uneventfully from an abdominal operation, his gut must start to work soon. The passage of flatus and bowel sounds show that his small gut is starting to work; his large gut starts a day or two later. If all goes well, he should start eating in 2–3 days. But eating will be delayed if he is recovering from peritonitis, from an anastomosis of his stomach or upper small gut, or from ileus (10.13), or if he is anorexic from any other cause, such as burns or severe sepsis. If he does not eat he starves, and although he may be able to live for several weeks without eating, he will waste severely. Unfortunately, the common intravenous fluids provide little energy and no protein, and you are unlikely to have the necessary solutions of proteins and amino acids for parenteral nutrition. But if you can get some food into him, as described below, it may save his life.

You are fortunate in that deep venous thrombosis and pulmonary embolism are uncommon in the developing world.

NON-RESPIRATORY POSTOPERATIVE COMPLICATIONS

For postoperative bleeding and shock, see Section 3.10. For the anaesthetic complications see A 4.5 and 4.6.

VOMITING

If a patient VOMITS IMMEDIATELY AFTER THE OPERATION turn him on his side. It may be due to the anaesthetic, especially ether, or to morphine or pethidine. He is likely to recover quickly. If he vomits for more than 8 hours or copiously at any time, start gastric aspiration.

If he VOMITS AFTER 48 HOURS, this is likely to be more serious, and may be due to ileus, postoperative gut obstruction, or rarely to acute gastric dilatation. If you don't replace his fluids and electrolytes, he will become severely hypovolaemic. He may lose much potassium if he continues to vomit, so replace this (A 15.5).

If he is VOMITING WITH A DISTENDED, SILENT ABDOMEN, he has ileus (10.13). This may be due to postoperative peritonitis (6.2, 10.13) which also causes pain, fever, and toxaemia. The nature of his previous operation, such as a pelvic abscess or an injury to his large gut, usually suggests its site. Later, watch for an abdominal (6.3) or subphrenic (6.4) abscess.

URINE OUTPUT POSTOPERATIVELY

If he passes NO URINE, or only a little, and his bladder is not distended: (1) He may be dehydrated. (2) He may be hypovolaemic. (3) He may have suffered a period of low blood pressure during the operation, which has caused tubular necrosis and renal failure. (4) He may have retention due to an enlarged prostate or a stricture. Some degree of urinary suppression is normal for 24 to 60 hours after major surgery, as a normal response to stress.

If he passes a little urine of high specific gravity, and is obviously dehydrated, give him 1000—2000 ml of saline as rapidly as you can. If his urinary output does not improve, give him 500 to 1000 ml of intravenous mannitol, or 40 to 80 mg of intravenous frusemide. If this produces a diuresis, he was severely dehydrated. If it produces no flow, he may have tubular necrosis and renal failure. If so, go to Section 53.3.

CAUTION ! (1) If he is a child, don't overhydrate him. Give him about 30 ml/kg of fluid for the first 2 hours, and repeat it over the next 3–4 hours if necessary. (2) Before you diagnose anuria, make sure that his Foley catheter is not blocked!

If he passes NO URINE, and he has a bladder which is distended and dull to percussion, he has retention. This is common after perineal operations especially in an old man. Stand him by the edge of his bed, and run a tap. The sound of running water may make him urinate. If this fails, aspirate his bladder suprapubically (entrust this task to the nurses, 23.6). Often it is only needed once. If the problem recurs and provided he has not had an intestinal anastomosis, try carbachol 250μg subcutaneously, if necessary repeated twice at 30 minute intervals. If this fails, catheterize him.

FEVER POSTOPERATIVELY

Most patients have a mild fever for 1–4 days after a major abdominal operation.

If he has more than minimal FEVER postoperatively, suspect pulmonary collapse (9.11), streptococcal wound sepsis (2.10, 9.12), a urinary tract infection (especially if he has been catheterized), a drug reaction, malaria, an abscess either under his diaphragm or somewhere else (6.3), Gram-negative or anaerobic wound infection (54.13), pneumonia, peritonitis (6.2), septicaemia or septic shock (53.4), a subphrenic (6.4) or a pelvic abscess (6.5), or deep vein thrombosis.

If he has PERSISTENT FEVER, and a raised white count, and is not improving, suspect that he has an abscess somewhere in his peritoneum, especially if you operated on him for peritonitis, or infected his peritoneum during the operation. Examine him carefully every day. If he also has a raised diaphragm and fluid in his costophrenic angle, he has a subphrenic abscess until you have proved otherwise—see Section 6.4. If he also has diarrhoea with the passage of mucus, he probably has a pelvic abscess. The passage of mucus is a particularly valuable sign. Avoid 'blind' antibiotic treatment unless his condition is critical. It may merely mask the problem which will become worse later.

FEEDING DIFFICULTIES POSTOPERATIVELY

If his RETURN TO NORMAL EATING IS MUCH DELAYED, he will waste considerably. Here is a variation of the instructions in Section 58.11. Let him eat what he can of his usual staple, such as rice, maize, or potatoes, and supplement this with nasogastric feeding (4.9), using the high-energy milk feed that you usually give to malnourished children. A convenient mix for a litre of feed is: dried skim milk 86 g, sugar 67 g, oil 86 ml, water 811 ml. Or, evaporated milk 443 ml, sugar 67 g, oil 52 ml, water 448 ml. Or, 'Nespray' 118 g, sugar 65 g, oil 54 ml, water 813 ml. This provides 1370 kcal/l. If he is to recover on this alone he needs at least 2 and preferably 3 litres of it daily. Watch his fluid balance (A 15.5), and give him 10 mmol/day of potassium, which is 10 ml of the commonly used solution (58.11, A 15.1).

If he cannot take fluids by mouth, pass a small plastic tube and start by feeding him 200 ml of a quarter-strength feed every 3 hours. Increase this to the limit of nausea and diarrhoea, until he is having 2 to 2.5 l of full-strength feed in 24 hours.

If he is VERY WASTED , and you have done an operation on his stomach or duodenum, consider feeding him through a jejunostomy (9.7). This is seldom necessary if he can be fed by mouth or by nasogastric tube.

9.11 Respiratory postoperative complications

If a patient's respiratory tract is to function normally, it must be kept clear of secretions. After some operations and in some patients this clearing mechanism fails, with the result that secretions accumulate, become infected and infect the lung, perhaps fatally. So you must get him to cough, and bring up the sputum that might otherwise block his smaller bronchi and cause atelectasis. Getting him to cough is most of the purpose of the physiotherapy in the next section.

Anything which will get him moving will help his chest. This may not be easy, but any activity is better than lying in bed. Antibiotics are less important, but he may need ampicillin, chloramphenicol, or tetracycline if his chest infection does not resolve with physiotherapy, or is very severe initially.

If he will not cough, there are various ways in which you can suck out his sputum for him. The last three in the list below—cricothyroid irrigation, tracheobronchial suction, and tracheostomy—are heroic measures of last resort.

POSTOPERATIVE RESPIRATORY COMPLICATIONS

See also 'Primary Anasthesia' Section 4.6 and Section 9.11a.

RISK FACTORS. A patient is more likely to have respiratory difficulties if: (1) He has emphysema or chronic bronchitis. (2) He has a painful operation site, particularly an upper abdominal or thoracic one, which makes coughing painful, and so prevents him bringing up sputum. (3) He was given excessive opioids or barbiturates. (4) He only recovered slowly from the anaesthetic. (5) He had a high subarachnoid block. (6) He smokes. (7) He is dehydrated, which makes his sputum thick and more difficult to cough up. (8) He is immobile postoperatively as with a fractured femur or paraplegia. (9) He has any other reason for poor breathing postoperatively, such as multiple injuries or a head injury. (10) He is severely ill, debilitated, immobile, or had a prolonged general anaesthetic.

COMPLICATIONS. Here are some of the complications you may have to manage:

If his RESPIRATION IS DEPRESSED, and a tracheal tube is still in place, he should remain in the recovery room until he is breathing normally. Anaesthesia may have been very deep, or he may be very ill. Attach a self-inflating bag to the tube and inflate his lungs. Don't remove the tube until he is breathing adequately on his own. If the tube has been withdrawn, pull his tongue forward and insert an oropharyngeal airway. If this does not restore normal breathing, inflate him with a mask and a self-inflating bag. If necessary, reintubate him, and continue ventilation. If you treat postoperative respiratory depression vigorously, as in Section A 3.4, his lungs are less likely to collapse. If you have a ventilator (A 19.3), use it.

If he is CYANOTIC, WHEEZING, or has an EXPIRATORY STRIDOR; if he is breathing rapidly, with a fast pulse, or if he has vomit on his lips, suspect that he has INHALED HIS VOMIT. Put him in the head-down position. Immediately insert a laryngoscope, and intubate him. Pass a sterile suction catheter into his trachea and bronchi. Fill a 10 ml syringe with 0.9% saline or 1% sodium bicarbonate and inject 5 ml down the tube. Turn him to one side, then the other, and then suck the fluid out again. Repeat this until he is breathing easily and quietly. Or, better, bronchoscope him, and suck him out through this (25.12). Give him oxygen. If his respiration is still poor, keep him in the recovery room or the ICU. See also A 16.2 and A 16.3.

If he has BRONCHOSPASM, give him aminophylline 250 mg by slow intravenous injection (A 3.3). This can also be due to the inhalation of vomit, see above.

If he has RESPIRATORY FAILURE with cyanosis, give him oxygen through a face mask with two side holes for his nostrils. If he has a tracheal tube down, give it to him through this.

CLEARING HIS RESPIRATORY TRACT

In the following three situations a patient needs an antibiotic and physiotherapy to clear the secretions from his chest. Tracheobronchial suction, cricothyroid irrigation, and tracheotomy or 'minitracheotomy' may also be useful.

(1) If he has a cough, confusion, restlessness, fever, tachycardia, cyanosis, rapid or irregular or grunting breathing, with flaring of his alae nasi he has a postoperative lung complication.

(2) If, in addition, he is dull to percussion over the bases of his lungs, usually on the right, with decreased breath sounds and bronchial breathing, low-pitched rhonchi, and X-rays show basal segmental areas of increased density, thick mucus has plugged his smaller bronchi, and caused his lung distal to them to collapse (atelectasis).

(3) If, in addition to the above signs of atelectasis, he has mucuopurulent sputum, rales, and toxaemia, he has bronchitis, bronchiolitis, or pneumonia.

TRACHEOBRONCHIAL SUCTION is useful if he has a 'bad chest' and you think that he is going to get chest complications after surgery. Consider leaving his tracheal tube in for 24–48 hours, so that you can suck out his chest through it. He will not be able to cough forcefully, but you will be able to aspirate his chest frequently. Before you aspirate, turn him to one side and inject 5–10 ml of saline. This will help to liquefy his sputum and will make suction easier. Turn him on to the other side and repeat it. Be sure there is a Y-connection on the suction tube. Release your thumb from the side arm intermittently to prevent you aspirating too much air, and making his bronchi collapse.

If you have already removed the tracheal tube that he had during the operation, and have done everything you can to make him cough, consider passing a nasotracheal tube (A 13.4), and sucking out his chest through that.

CRICOTHYROID IRRIGATION will usually make a patient cough when he is not inclined to do so. Under local anaesthesia, push a needle and cannula combination ('Intracath') on a syringe through his cricothyroid membrane in the midline. Aspirate to make sure that you withdraw air, and then remove the syringe and push the catheter in another 2 cm to be sure it is well inside his trachea. Suture it in place, and plug the opening to make sure that air does not go in or out. Instil 2-3 ml of saline several times a day to make him cough.

TRACHEOTOMY. If other methods of aspiration, including bronchoscopy (25.13) fail; or you need to intubate him for more than 72 hours, consider doing a tracheostomy (52.2), and sucking out his chest through this. If you have bypassed his nose with anything but a minitracheotomy tube (see below), humidify the air he breathes (19.3), if necessary with a steam kettle. It will help him to cough. If you have a steam room put him in it for the first week.

A **'minitracheotomy'** is the most practical way to suck out a patient's trachea. Use a *small* (4 mm) tube (preferably a disposable 'Portex' one). Using local anaesthesia with adrenalin in the solution, insert it through his cricothyroid membrane using a guarded scalpel and an introducer. Failing this use a 4 mm paediatric tracheotomy tube and pass a 10 Ch suction catheter down it. A tube of this size is not large enough to obstruct his respiratory tract, there is little bleeding, and the traditional complications of the cricothyroid approach using a large tube (particularly stenosis) are avoided. He can speak, cough, eat, and drink, and humidify his inspired air normally without the need for sedation or anaesthesia. His wound heals quickly with little scarring.

9. 11a Respiratory physiotherapy

Some simple physiotherapy will often prevent the complications described in the previous section. If an at-risk patient (9.11) is to have an elective operation this physiotherapy should start *before* the operation. You will probably have no physiotherapist, so you will have to learn these skills yourself, and teach them to your nurses and to his relatives.

PHYSIOTHERAPY CAN BE LIFE-SAVING

RESPIRATORY PHYSIOTHERAPY

INDICATIONS. These are the 'at-risk' patients in the previous section.

PREOPERATIVELY, take the patient through the motions of breathing in deeply through his nose and mouth. Either, sit him up at 70° well supported from behind by a back support, and with a bolster to prevent his knees slipping down. Or, lay him on his back with his knees bent.

Put your hands on his chest as he tries to breathe. Give him about 6 breaths only at a time, or he may become dizzy.

CAUTION ! Be sure to explain to him *why* these exercises are so necessary.

POSTOPERATIVELY, adequate analgesia is a *big* help. Try to get him to breathe properly, to move about in bed, and to get up *as soon as he can.*

His position is important; he must avoid the semirecumbent 'slumped' position, because this restricts the movement of his diaphragm, and promotes the collapse of his lower lobes. Encourage him to sit up with a back support, or lay him on his side sitting up and rolled well forward to 'free' his abdomen. Get him out of bed and walking on the second day, if you can— even if he has a catheter or a drip.

Ask him to do the exercises he has already learnt. An 'incentive spirometer' is very useful.

'Cough him' and 'huff him' as described below, and ask him to do the same every hour. Start on the day of the operation, visit him twice on the following day, and thereafter once daily.

PHYSIOTHERAPY

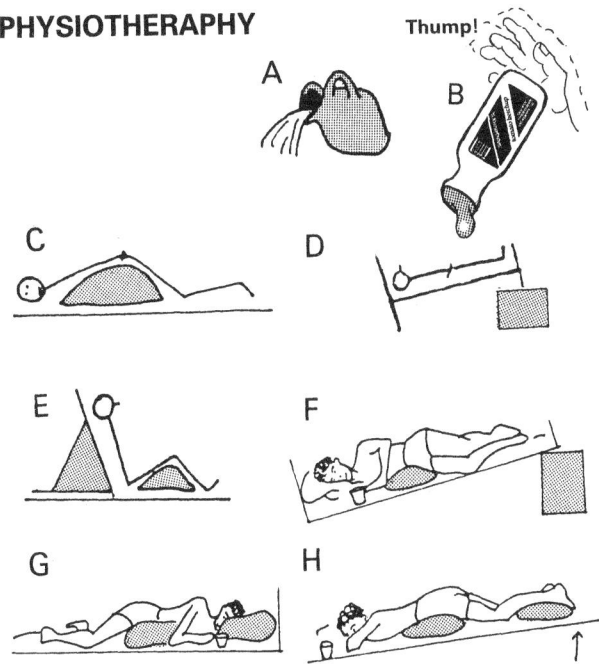

Fig. 9-22 CHEST PHYSIOTHERAPY. A, if secretions are sufficiently liquid you can pour them out of a patient's chest. B, if they are viscid, you may have to shake them out of his bronchi by percussing his chest in the same way that you can percuss tomato ketchup out of a bottle! C, you can lay him with his hips on pillows, so that his hips are higher than his shoulders. D, you can raise the foot of his bed. E, you can sit him up against a back-rest with pillows under his knees. F, you can raise the foot of his bed and put a pillow under his hips. G, if he is too weak to sit up you can rest him against a pillow and lay him on his side. H, you can lay him on his abdomen with a pillow under his hips and the foot of his bed raised. *After Hardinge E, and Wilson PMP, 'A Manual of Basic Physiotherapy', published by TEAR Fund.*

POSTURAL DRAINAGE

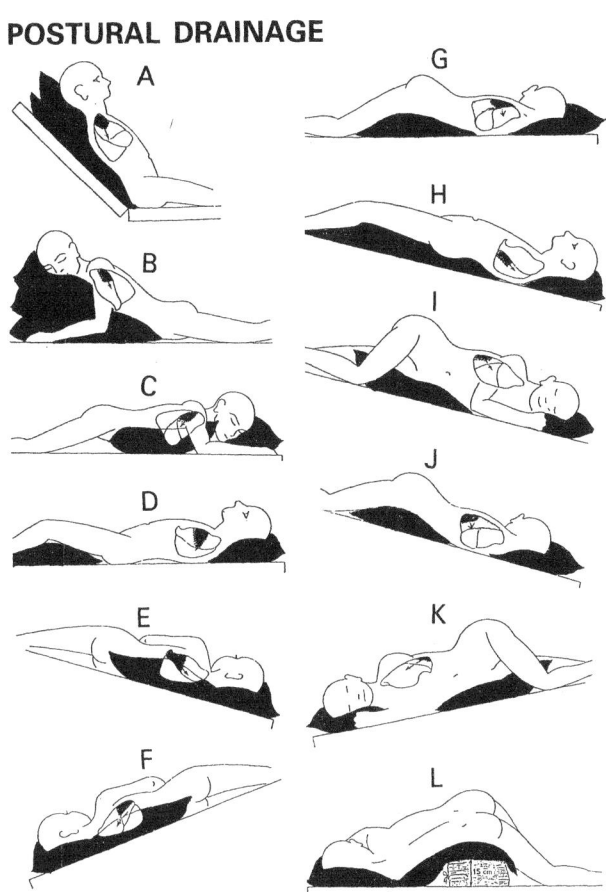

Fig 9-23 POSTURAL DRAINAGE. The positions which allow gravity to promote the drainage of secretions from particular parts of a patient's lung. Study his chest X-ray, and decide which position will be best. *Kindly contributed by Lynne Wilson of Killingbeck Hospital, Leeds.*

'COUGH HIM'. Distinguish between an effective *deep* productive cough (which is what you want) and a noise in his throat, which is useless. Several short expiratory 'huffs' before coughing will help to loosen his secretions. Ask him to take a deep breath after each cough, and not to cough continually without pausing.

If he has an abdominal wound, ask him to bend his knees, to hold the wound, and then to take a deep breath and cough. Or, he can hold a pillow against the wound while he coughs. Reassure him that his stitches will not split. If you wish, you can vibrate him while he coughs.

'HUFF HIM'. A 'huff' is a rapid forced expiration without a cough. If he 'huffs' when his lungs are full, he will dislodge secretions from his larger airways. If he 'huffs' when they are half full, he will dislodge them from his smaller airways. So 'huff him' in both, with periods of relaxation and abdominal breathing between them.

CAUTION ! To be effective a 'huff' must be long and controlled and not spasmodic. He must use his abdominal wall. The noisiest 'huff' is not necessarily the best.

PERCUSSION AND VIBRATION. Percuss his thorax over a towel or blanket with your cupped hands for periods of about a minute. Then rapidly shake his chest during expiration. Relax while he inspires, and follow this with some deep breathing. Repeat this two or three times.

POSTURAL DRAINAGE will be useful if there is much fluid in his bronchi. Listen carefully to his chest, and if possible examine his chest X-ray. Decide where his secretions are worst, and arrange him so that this part of him is uppermost, using any of the positions in Fig. 9-23. Ask him to breathe deeply for 10 minutes, vibrate and slap his chest for 10 minutes, then repeat the breathing. If he has established collapse or infection repeat this two or three times a day.

If he is too ill for his hips to be raised, lay him on his side.

If his secretions are viscid, ideally he needs inhalation therapy to 'loosen' them prior to physiotherapy—steam with Friar's balsam, or saline with mucolytics from a nebulizer.

9.12 If a laparotomy wound becomes infected

A laparotomy wound usually remains tender for 7 to 10 days after an operation. If it is abnormally tender and indurated, and the patient is also febrile, and does not feel well, he has pus somewhere. His abdominal wall and his peritoneal cavity are two of the places where it can be. Finding it may not be easy, and you can easily overlook an intraperitoneal abscess under a healing incision. Be guided by the severity of his symptoms. More than a little anorexia, fever, and malaise, should make you suspect an abdominal abscess. Antibiotics alone will not cure it. If many of your wounds become infected, try delayed primary closure! (9.8)

POSTOPERATIVE WOUND INFECTION

If a patient's wound is red, painful, and tender, and discharges pus, it is infected. Take a Gram stain of the pus, and give him a broad-spectrum antibiotic while you wait for the result of culture, if this is possible. If it is not draining, sedate him with pethidine and diazepam, and start by removing one to three skin sutures on the ward. This will show you the extent of the infection. If it seems to be deeper, but is still extraperitoneal, press the sides of the wound, and probe suspicious areas with sinus forceps. Don't open up the deeper layers of all infected wounds from top to bottom, or remove the deeper stitches. His peritoneum will probably have healed in spite of the infection, but the sutures in the fascial layers will probably pull away. If pus flows adequately, drainage should be adequate. Irrigate his wound with saline or 1/4 strength hydrogen peroxide, or hypochlorite solution. Pack it with dry gauze, or gauze soaked in a mild antiseptic or half strength saline, and change this 1 to 3 times daily.

CAUTION ! (1) Be sure to make a wide enough opening to release the pus. (2) If possible test his HIV status (Chapter 28a).

If his wound SMELLS PUTRID, or you see NECROTIC MUSCLE or fascia, when you remove skin sutures, suspect an ANAEROBIC INFECTION. Give him metronidazole and chloramphenicol.

If his wound is TENSE, SWOLLEN, and BRUISED, with old blood exuding from between the sutures, suspect a haematoma. Sedate him, remove a few of his skin sutures, and wash out old blood and clot with a syringe of saline. Lift out more clots with a swab. Irrigate the wound with saline or hydrogen peroxide, and leave it open for a few days.

If his wound discharges a LITTLE BROWNISH FLUID WHICH SMELLS MOUSEY, suspect GAS GANGRENE (54.13). This is commoner than you probably think. *Obvious gas in the tissues is uncommon,* so that gas gangrene is often missed. Remove most or all of his skin sutures, make a Gram film of the exudate, and look for Gram-positive bacilli (you are unlikely to have the facilities for anaerobic culture). *Treat him thoroughly.* Give him benzyl penicillin 10 megaunits daily as four 6-hourly doses for 5 days. And give him metronidazole 400 mg orally *and* 1 g rectally 8-hourly. Clean his wound with iodine, remove any dead tissue, and isolate him from the other patients.

9.13 Burst abdomen (wound dehiscence)

An abdomen which bursts some days after you have sewn it up is a tragedy, because it is preventable, and because the patient has a 30% chance of death. His abdomen is likely to burst if: (1) It is swollen for any reason, such as ileus, intestinal obstruction, or a large tumour. (2) He has severe intra-abdominal sepsis, such as an infected Caesarean section, typhoid peritonitis, or a perforation of his large gut. (3) You have sutured his abdomen with catgut or some other absorbable suture, especially if this is of low quality or out of date, or if his abdominal wound becomes infected. (4) You have sutured it in layers, taking bites of tissue that are too small. (5) He has carcinomatosis, uraemia, or obstructive jaundice.

An abdomen will almost never burst if: (1) You suture it with a non-absorbable sutures, such as steel, nylon, or polyethylene. (2) You close its muscles with one layer of through-and-through sutures, which are not too tight and take wide bites of tissue (9.8). (3) You use delayed skin suture (9.8) if the wound is infected or potentially so.

BURST ABDOMEN

DIAGNOSIS. **If a patient's wound is painful about a week after the operation, and he has a thin reddish-brown discharge,** his abdomen is probably going to burst. Treat him *before* it bursts!

TREATMENT. Take him to the theatre, prepared for general anaesthesia. If his abdomen has actually burst, give him a general anaesthetic. Only repair him under local anaesthesia if he is very unfit. If it is a long wound, have blood available. Prepare him for a laparotomy.

Remove the skin sutures in the area where you suspect the burst. Remove the dressings and gently explore the depths of his wound with a sterile gloved finger. Open it down its whole length by removing all the skin sutures. You will soon find out what has happened. If you confirm a burst abdomen, remove all sutures from the fascial layers. Try to insert your finger between his parietal peritoneum and his underlying gut and omentum. In this way you should be able to mobilize enough of his abdominal wall to take some more sutures.

Resuture his abdominal wall with interrupted steel or monofilament sutures, either intermittent or continuous (see Everett's method 9.8). Suture from within outwards through his peritoneum, posterior rectus sheath, rectus muscle, and anterior rectus sheath—but not through his skin. Hold all the sutures out on haemostats until you have placed the last one.

Some surgeons also insert tension sutures (9.8), and consider that this is the only indication for them.

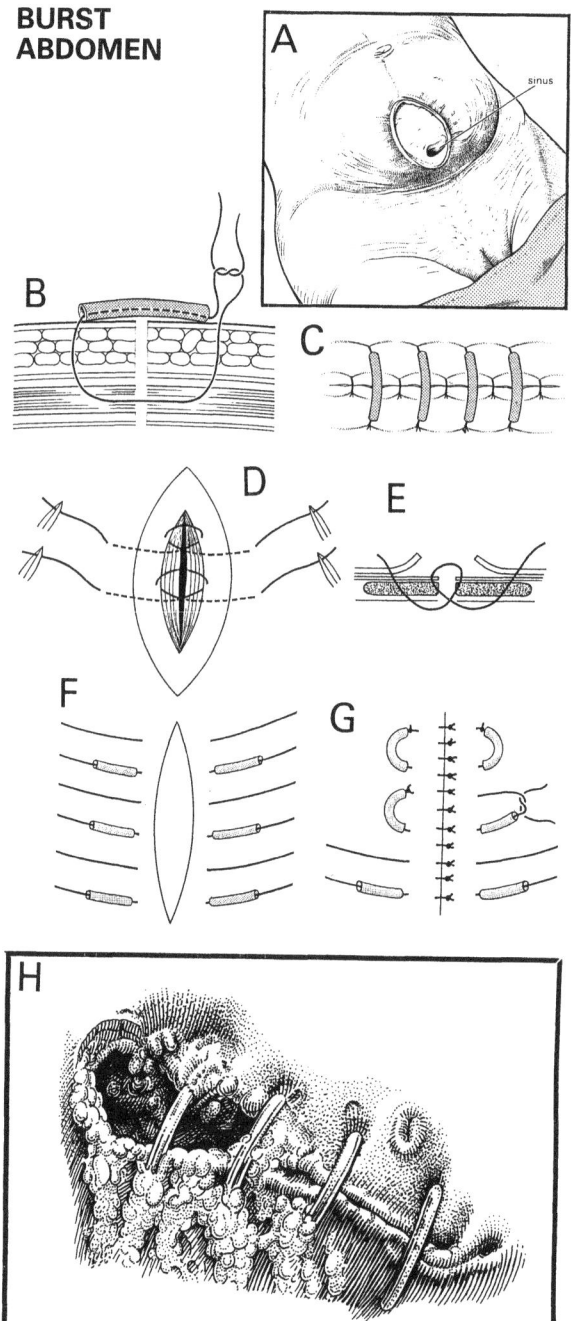

Fig. 9-24 BURST ABDOMEN. A, a burst abdomen after Caesarean section. B, and C, the usual way of inserting the tension sutures that are sometimes used to prevent this tragedy. A better way of preventing it would have been to use the method of single-layer closure with monofilament shown in Fig. 9-21. D, to G, an alternative way of inserting tension sutures. See Section 9.8. H, a burst abdomen and an intestinal fistula. The tension sutures have broken down. This is a detail from Fig. 9-25.

The alternative method was kindly contributed by Mr Brian Sterry Ashby.

If his skin is already infected, **use delayed closure (9.8), and graft it later if necessary.**

9.14 Intestinal fistulae

An intestinal fistula is an abnormal track, usually lined by granulation tissue, between the gut and the skin. Fistulae are unusual but serious complications of abdominal surgery, and occasionally arise spontaneously as the result of disease. Beware of postoperative fistulae: (1) After you have divided adhesions for

AN INTESTINAL FISTULA

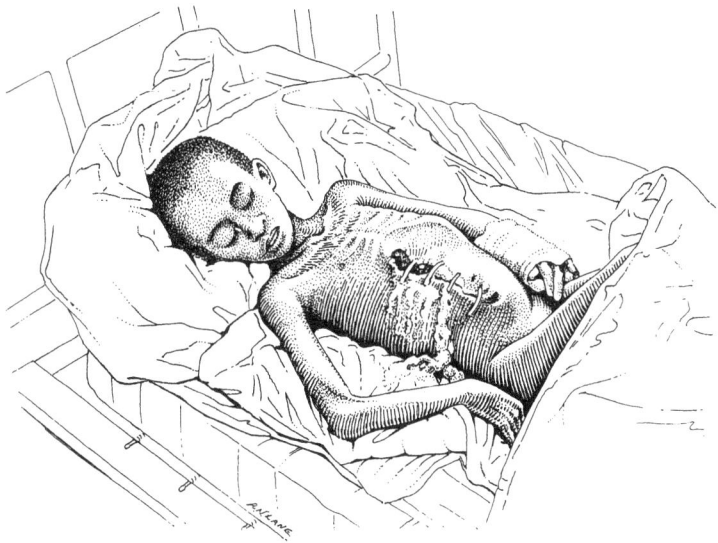

Fig. 9-25 AN INTESTINAL FISTULA. This patient was operated on for obstruction of his small gut by *Ascaris* worms, and a length of it was resected. The anastomosis broke down; a fistula developed. He died a few hours later.

intestinal obstruction, especially if you have opened the gut by mistake, and closed it inadequately, or if it is obstructed distally. (2) When you have anastomosed it inaccurately, or in the presence of tension, a poor blood supply, or local disease. (3) If gut is caught in the sutures, especially tension sutures, when you close the abdomen. (4) After appendicectomy (a caecal fistula). (5) After crushing the spur of a double-barrelled colostomy.

Don't try to operate yourself. Even in good hands the mortality rate of a high output fistula (>1500 ml/24 hours) is 70%, and a low output one 30%. The repair of a fistula is one of the most difficult operations in surgery.

SUDHA (25 years), a young housewife had an operation in a district hospital for 'appendicitis' through a McBurney incision. Five days after the operation the wound discharged large quantities of pus, and then liquid faeces and gas. She was fed on a low-residue diet, and the skin round the fistulous opening was painted and protected with zinc oxide paste. Absorbent dressings were changed 3 times a day and her distal colonic obstruction due to constipated faeces was treated with glycerine suppositories and a plain water enema. The fistula healed in 2 weeks and she went home. LESSON Some fistulae will close on nonoperative treatment. They are more likely to do so if there is no obstruction distal to the internal opening of the fistula.

INTESTINAL FISTULAE

If pus or intestinal contents discharge from the main wound, or the site of a drain postoperatively, suspect that a fistula is forming. If the patient says that gas comes out, this confirms it; so does charcoal, given orally, appearing in the wound, or an X-ray with contrast medium (a fistulogram).

If necessary, insert a plastic tube into the track and inject 10 to 20 ml of water-soluble contrast medium.

TREATMENT is supportive.

Replace fluid and electrolytes, orally, intravenously (15.5), or by jejunostomy (9.7). He may need large quantities of electrolytes.

Maintain his nutrition, orally, or by jejunostomy. You are unlikely to have the protein and energy-rich fluids to give him intravenously.

Care for his skin, by keeping the contents of his gut away from it, with adequate drainage, if necessary with a sump drain (4-11), by nursing him prone, as in Fig. 9-13, and by applying karaya gum or zinc oxide to his skin.

Control infection with antibiotics and drainage, when necessary.

Keep his distal colon empty, with saline enemas and glycerine suppositories on alternate days.

REFER HIM if: (1) His fistula discharges >1500 ml/day for >3 days. (2) It has not closed after 3 weeks of non-operative management. (4) He is very ill. (5) It is high—oral charcoal appears within 15 minutes. (6) A fistulogram shows communication with his duodenum or jejunum. (7) He does not pass faeces or flatus for 5 days.

THE INDICATIONS FOR OPERATION are: (1) A high output fistula >1500 ml/24 hours. (2) Distal obstruction. (3) A drain abscess. (4) Failure to close after 3 weeks of non-operative treatment. (5) Disease of the fistula track, as with tuberculosis or a foreign body. (6) Intestinal mucosa pouting on to the skin.

10 The acute abdomen: intestinal obstruction

10.1 The general method for an acute abdomen

Unlike the chest, which seldom needs surgery, the abdomen often does. It does so because the gut it contains can obstruct, perforate, or strangulate, and so allow the organisms inside it to infect the peritoneal cavity. Infection can also reach the peritoneum from the gall-bladder or the female genital tract. These events are the common causes of an 'acute abdomen'. Unless you operate on a patient within a few hours of admission he stands a good chance of dying.

Pain is the main symptom of an acute abdomen. If he was previously well, and has had an abdominal pain for more than 6 hours which is not accompanied by severe diarrhoea or urinary symptoms, the chances are that he has an acute abdomen. If peritonitis is the cause, his abdomen will become tender and rigid early, and distend late. If his large gut is obstructed, his abdomen will distend early, and become tender late. If his gut is obstructed high up, frequent vomiting predominates.

Although the frequency of the many causes of an acute abdomen differs from one developing country to another, their pattern is similar, and differs from that of the industrial world: (1) Small gut obstruction is more common (10.3). (2) Large gut obstruction is much more likely to be due to sigmoid volvulus than to carcinoma of the colon. (3) Tenderness in the right lower quadrant can be caused by amoebiasis, by caecal tuberculosis, or by a 'helminthoma', as well as by appendicitis. (4) Generalized peritonitis can be caused by a typhoid perforation, a leaking liver abscess, or perforation of the gut by *Ascaris*. (4) You are unlikely to see diverticulitis, Crohn's disease, or acute abdomens due to vascular disease.

As always, but particularly with an acute abdomen, *there is no substitute for a careful history and a full examination*—the commonest mistake is to leave out some of the essential parts of both. A patient's history should suggest the diagnosis, and examining him should merely confirm or refute it. When you decide to operate, don't do so merely on the diagnosis of an 'acute abdomen', but on its most likely cause, with a list of possible alternatives, based on as much evidence as you can find. His early symptoms and signs will be more distinctive than his later ones, when he has deteriorated towards the common pattern of generalized peritonitis.

Abdominal pain is usually his presenting symptom, and if only you can interpret this, you have gone a long way towards finding its cause. It can be of at least three kinds: (1) A colicky pain due to obstruction at various levels in his gut, which he feels in the positions shown in Fig. 10-1. His colic comes in waves or spasms. Often, he moves about restlessly. (2) A sharp continuous pain due to inflammation of his parietal peritoneum. (3) An agonizing continuous pain due to ischaemia of his gut. Pain may also be referred from the diseased area to the other parts of the body that are derived from the same segment. For example, he may refer pain from his gall-bladder to below his right scapula; pus or blood under his diaphragm may give him a pain

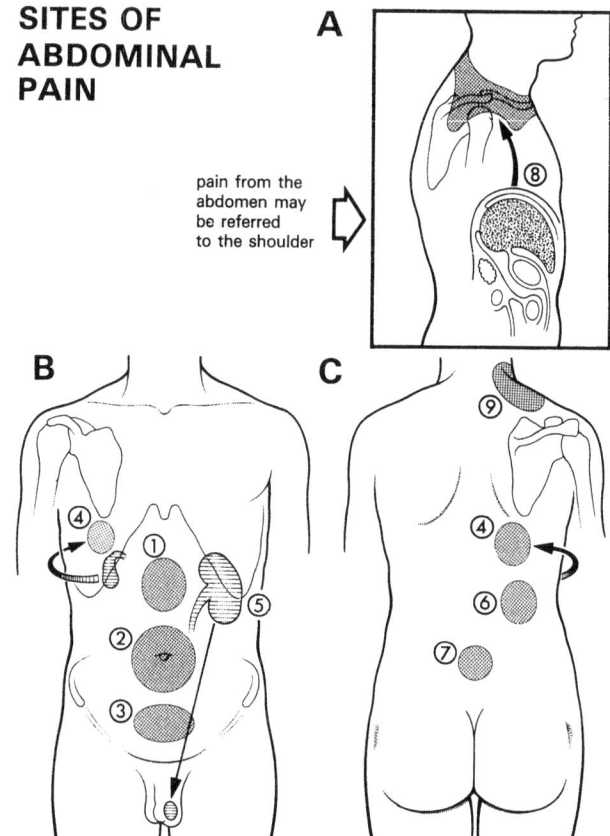

Fig. 10-1 THE SITES OF ABDOMINAL PAIN. (1) Lesions in a patient's stomach, duodenum, gall-bladder, and pancreas cause pain in his epigastrium. (2) Lesions from his duodenum down to the middle of his transverse colon cause pain in the middle of his abdomen. (3) Lesions from that point onwards cause pain in his lower abdomen. (4) The pain of biliary colic is primarily epigastric or in his right hypochondrium, but may be referred under the angle of his right scapula. (5) Ureteric colic is frequently referred to the testicle on the same side. (6) Pain from his kidney and pancreas may be referred to his back. (7) Pain from the uterus and rectum may be referred to the sacral area. (8) Pain from the diaphragm is frequently referred to the shoulder. *After Silen S, 'Cope's Early Diagnosis of the Acute Abdomen', (15th edn, 1979) Figs. 2 and 3, OUP, with kind permission.*

in his shoulder. He can have pain of more than one kind. For example, when the lumen of his appendix is obstructed, he has central abdominal pain of type (1), but as soon as the peritoneum over it becomes inflamed, he has pain of type (2) in his right iliac fossa. If it becomes gangrenous, he has ischaemic pain of type (3).

Vomiting in the form of a single initial vomit, is usual in most kinds of acute abdomen, so it is little help in diagnosis. It has few special features, except in intestinal obstruction, when its nature will give you some indication of the level of the obstruction (10.3). He vomits most frequently and profusely when his small gut is obstructed, but he may not vomit at all if the obstruction involves his large gut, especially if it is not strangulated. If his vomit is faeculent (smelling like faeces), his small gut has been obstructed for some time.

Constipation varies according to the level of the obstruction. If he has large gut obstruction (or ileus) he has absolute constipation, and passes no faeces or flatus. Obstruction high in his small gut does not cause constipation.

Abdominal tenderness is a sign that the peritoneum underneath the tender area is inflamed or irritated. The tenderness may be localized, as in early appendicitis, or generalized, and is not easy to evaluate, because his tolerance to your examining hand depends so much on how stoical he is. The parietal peritoneum of the pelvis does not share a common innervation with the abdominal wall, so he, or more usually she, can have pus in the pelvis with little abdominal tenderness or rigidity.

Rebound tenderness is tested for by pressing firmly and steadily on a patient's abdomen for a minute or two, and then releasing your hand suddenly. If he finds this agonizingly painful, the sign is positive. It is an uncomfortable and not a very reliable sign, and is most useful when pressure applied in one place causes rebound pain in another. For example, if pressure in his left lower abdomen causes pain in his right lower abdomen, it suggests appendicitis (Rovsing's sign). Many surgeons use light percussion, which is more accurate and much less cruel than rebound tenderness.

Guarding is another sign that a patient's peritoneum is inflamed, but you must examine him gently, so that the contraction of his muscles is involuntary rather than voluntary.

Rigidity of the abdominal wall can be of any degree, from none to 'boardlike'. Gastric and duodenal exudates produce the most marked rigidity, pus is more variable, and blood may produce almost none, especially when it seeps up from the pelvis.

If he is in very severe pain, a judicious dose of morphine will: (1) improve his shock, (2) reduce his pain, (3) make him more comfortable and better able to give a history, and (4) prevent him immediately guarding his abdomen whenever you touch it, so that his physical signs become more localized.

The common mistakes are: (1) Not to ask the right questions properly and methodically. (2) Not to examine him carefully and systematically. (3) Not to make and record a diagnosis and a differential diagnosis. (4) Not to admit him and monitor him carefully, if there is any chance that he *might* have an acute abdomen. (5) To forget that many medical conditions, especially pneumonia (by causing diaphragmatic pain), can mimic an acute abdomen. (6) To forget that age and sex can profoundly influence the probability of a particular diagnosis. Children for example are more likely to have intussusception, or a gut obstruction by *Ascaris*. (7) To fail to make adequate allowance for the late case whose history is obscured, whose mind is clouded, and whose signs are altered. (8) To forget the 'silent interval' between the immediate chemical peritonitis of a perforated peptic ulcer and the delayed onset of bacterial peritonitis (11.2). (9) To forget that in advanced peritonitis 'septic shock' (53.4) may prevent a patient from showing the signs you expect. (10) Finally, worst of all, not to go and see a patient with a suspected abdominal emergency immediately.

KOFI, a little boy of 6 months, was taken to hospital with vomiting, abdominal pain and some blood and mucus in his stools. After several days treatment for gastroenteritis he was becoming steadily worse, so his parents took him in the bus many miles to the teaching hospital. There he was found to have intussusception, and eventually recovered after a long illness. LESSON In children the occasional acute abdomen is easily missed among many cases of gastroenteritis. Vomiting and pain with no diarrhoea, or only perhaps some blood and mucus, should make you suspicious.

THE GENERAL METHOD FOR AN ACUTE ABDOMEN—ONE

Base your diagnosis on as many items of information as possible. The explanations given for a particular sign or symptom are suggestions only.

HISTORY

ONSET. **"How did your pain start?"** (if it woke the patient at night it is probably serious). "Did it start with an injury?" (quite a minor one can rupture the spleen). "Was it so severe that you collapsed or fainted?" (a perforated peptic ulcer, a ruptured ectopic pregnancy, and acute pancreatitis can all present like this).

PAIN. Form a detailed picture of this, and expect it to have more than one component.

"Did the pain start suddenly or slowly?" (suddenly, suggests a perforated duodenal ulcer).

"Where is the pain and where did it start?" If it is epigastric or subumbilical, it is probably from his small gut or appendix. If it is hypogastric, it is probably from his large gut. If it started "all over" his abdomen, think of a perforated peptic ulcer, or a ruptured ectopic pregnancy, or a pyosalpinx in a woman. If it is his loin and is referred to his testis, it is probably ureteric pain, perhaps caused by a stone.

"What is it like?" (a throbbing pain or a constant ache suggests an inflammatory process, such as an appendix abscess). Burning or boring? (peptic ulcer, pancreatitis). Coming and going in waves or spasms? (colic). If it is colicky, how long do the spasms last, and is there complete relief between them?

"How long did it last?" A patient with biliary colic may be free of pain between attacks.

"Has it moved?" (if it started in his umbilical region and moved to his right iliac fossa, suspect appendicitis).

"Does your pain spread anywhere?" To the testis of the same side? (ureteric colic). To the top of the shoulder? (a perforated peptic ulcer, a subphrenic or liver abscess, diaphragmatic pleurisy, gall-stones, a ruptured spleen, sometimes peritonitis). To the middle of the back? (peritonitis).

"What makes your pain better?" Lying absolutely still? (peritonitis). Walking bent forwards? (appendicitis). Lying with your knees flexed? (inflammation in contact with the psoas muscle, such as appendicitis, or a psoas abscess).

"What makes it worse? Breathing, coughing, moving, drinking, eating, opening your bowels, or passing urine?" Breathing aggravates the pain of pleurisy, peritonitis, a peritoneal abscess, abdominal distension due to intestinal obstruction, cholecystitis, etc. Dysuria may be caused by pyelitis, a stone, acute hydronephros, a pelvic abscess close to the bladder, or an appendix abscess irritating the right ureter. Dysuria and fever? (pyelonephritis).

VOMITING. **"Tell me about the vomiting"** It started with the pain but is now less? (perforated peptic ulcer: persistent vomiting is rare in patients who have perforated a peptic ulcer). Severe and persistent? (strangulation of the small gut, acute pancreatitis). At the height of the pain? (intestinal or renal colic).

"What is the association between the pain and the vomiting?" In an acute abdomen the vomiting almost always comes after the pain. Vomiting *before* the pain suggests gastroenteritis. Vomiting sudden and soon after the pain? (strangulation or obstruction of the upper small gut, a stone in the ureter or bile duct). Vomiting about 4 hours after the pain? (obstruction of the ileum, appendicitis). Vomiting many hours after the onset of the pain, or no vomiting? (large gut obstruction).

"How frequent is the vomiting?" It usually varies directly with the acuteness of the condition. Vomiting mild, absent, or late? (many acute abdomens, including large gut obstruction and a ruptured ectopic).

If he has pain but no vomiting, suspect that: (1) The cause is outside his gut, as in salpingitis, a tubo-ovarian abscess, or a haemoperitoneum. (2) He may have a high threshold to vomiting—if so anorexia and nausea are important.

"What is his vomit like?" Stomach contents, perhaps mixed with bile? (acute gastritis). Greenish jejunal contents (the colics). Frequent retching but little vomiting? (torsion of a viscus). First his gastric contents, then bilious, then greenish-yellow, then faeculent? (small gut obstruction).

PREVIOUS HISTORY. "**Have you ever had a pain like this before?**" Minor attacks of pain like the present one but less severe? (intussusception, obstruction, appendicitis, etc). Pain when hungry relieved by food? (duodenal ulcer). Pain in the epigastrium or right hypochondrium irregularly related to meals? (gall-stones).

BOWELS. "**Have you noticed any change in your bowels, have they been normal?**" If they are usually regular, constipation for several days is important. Hypogastric pain and diarrhoea with mucus, followed by hypogastric tenderness and constipation? (pelvic abscess). Diarrhoea, colic, fever? (gastroenteritis). 'Red currant jelly' stools? (intussusception). Frequent bloody stools? (amoebic colitis). Worms? (Ascaris obstruction).

"**When did you last pass a motion, and what was it like?**" He may pass two or more stools after the onset of a complete small gut obstruction. In complete low large gut obstruction, he passes no flatus or stools.

PERIODS. (1) "When was your last period?" (2) "Was it before or after the normal time?" (3) "Was the loss more or less than usual?" (4) "Has there been any slight loss since your last period?" Last period late or scanty? (ectopic pregnancy). One to three periods missed, followed by a small dark loss? (subacute bleed from an ectopic). Last period painful, and not accustomed to dysmenorrhoea? (threatened abortion, salpingitis).

CAUTION! (1) Always ask the four questions above with care. The question "Are your periods normal" is not enough. (2) Occasionally, a patient's periods may be normal in an ectopic pregnancy.

OTHER SYMPTOMS. Enquire about appetite, swallowing, weight loss, fever, and changes in girth. Weight loss or general deterioration in health? (abdominal tuberculosis, etc). Severe illness with fever? (typhoid perforation). Increase in abdominal girth, or change in the fit of his clothes? (ascites).

THE GENERAL EXAMINATION OF AN ACUTE ABDOMEN

GENERAL CONDITION. His general condition may be surprisingly normal, even though he has an acute abdomen. Is he well or badly nourished, bright and moving about? If he is limp, lethargic, and slow to respond, suspect toxaemia, septicaemia, or shock. If he is both lethargic and restless, suspect cerebral hypoxia, due to hypovolaemia. Look at his tongue and his conjunctivae, and smell his breath.

His face may be characteristic later on when his disease is advanced. If the face of a a Caucasian is pale and livid and his brow sweating, or an African or Indian goes mildly grey, suspect a perforated peptic ulcer, acute pancreatitis, or a strangulated gut. Deathly pale with gasping respiration? (ectopic pregnancy with severe bleeding). Gaze dull and face ashen? (severe toxaemia). Eyes sunken, tongue and lips dry, and skin elasticity reduced? (dehydration, intestinal obstruction). Nose and hands cold? (hypovolaemia, peripheral circulatory failure).

His pulse may be *normal* early on, even if he has an acute abdomen. The *trend* in his pulse is important in deciding if he has some serious abdominal condition, especially an abdominal injury (66.1). Tachycardia? (late peritonitis, strangulation of the gut). The pulse of typhoid fever is no longer slow after the ileum has perforated.

His attitude in bed may be characteristic. Restless? (severe colic or haemorrhage). Knees drawn up to relax the tension on his abdomen? (extensive peritonitis). Only changes his position in bed with pain and difficulty? (peritonitis, perforated gastric ulcer). Lies still with his hips and knees flexed? (generalized peritonitis). Right knee flexed (appendix or psoas abscess). Constantly moving around? (ureteric colic). Straight one minute and doubled up the next? (intestinal or biliary colic).

His respiration rate will help you to decide if his condition is abdominal or thoracic. If his respiration rate is twice normal, he probably has pneumonia. Shallow and occasionally grunting respiration? (peritonitis, especially of his upper abdomen). Rapid and shallow? (shock). Look at a child's nose; if his alae nasi are moving, he has pneumonia. Listen to his chest.

His temperature may be normal, especially in intestinal obstruction. Severe fever from the onset? (typhoid, basal pneumonia, pyelonephritis).

SIGNS OF DEHYDRATION. If his small gut is obstructed he will become dehydrated rapidly.

ABDOMEN. Ask him to point to where the pain started, to where it is now, and to where it is worst.

Look at his abdomen. Is its contour normal? If it is severely distended, is this due to gas, fluid, or a tumour? If necessary, test for shifting dullness.

Does his abdomen move freely as he breathes? Peritonitis anywhere may splint all or part of it, and stops the normal movement that accompanies breathing. Reduced or no movement in the lower abdomen? (PID, appendicitis).

Can you see visible peristaltic waves? Watch for at least one measured minute in a good light from a low angle. If so, he is either very thin or a neonate, in which case they are normal, or he has pyloric stenosis, or small gut obstruction.

Look at his groins—his central abdominal pain may be due to an obstructed hernia. Are there any old operation scars? If so, adhesions may be causing his symptoms.

Feel his abdomen. First relax it by flexing his hips. If necessary, ask an assistant to support his flexed knees. Your hand must be warm, *gentle,* patient, and sensitive. Use light palpation first to test for muscle rigidity and spasm, and localize the tenderness. Then, if necessary use deep palpation.

Lay your hand flat on his abdomen, and keep your fingers fully extended as you feel for tenderness. Avoid the painful area, and start feeling his abdomen as far from it as you can (Don't worry if he tells you it is the wrong place!). Move towards this slowly. Where is the area of greatest tenderness? It will be easier to find if there is no guarding, and is a useful clue to the organ involved. In his right iliac fossa? (appendicitis). In his flank? (renal suppuration). Suprapubically in a woman? (PID). Superficial induration and tenderness? (pyomyositis of the abdominal wall).

Can you feel any masses? In his right iliac fossa? (appendix mass, amoebiasis, a mass of Ascaris worms)

Is his abdomen soft, or firm and rigid, or do his muscles only contract when you move your fingers towards them? Abdomen rigid like a board? (generalized peritonitis, especially that due to perforated peptic ulcer). How widely distributed is this rigidity? If rigidity is due to pleural pain, you can overcome it by continuous pressure on his abdomen, and the pain is not usually increased. But if he has disease in his abdomen, his pain gets worse as you press (confirm pneumonia by listening to his chest).

CAUTION ! A patient may show very little rigidity if: (1) His perforation occurred about 6 hours ago, so that his immediate rigidity has had time to go, and secondary bacterial peritonitis has not yet had time to develop. (2) He is very fat and flabby, and his muscles are thin and weak. (3) He is very toxaemic and ill. (4) He is very old or immunosuppressed. (5) A woman is pregnant.

Feel his loins. Press your fingers forwards under his ribs. Resistance and tenderness without swelling? (an inflammatory focus). Now put your other hand in front of his loin, ask him to take a deep breath, and feel for an abnormal swelling moving between your two hands as he breathes (pyo- or hydronephros).

The iliopsoas test is only indicated if he is not very ill, and does not have generalized peritonitis. Lie him on the opposite side, and extend his thigh on the affected side to its fullest extent. If this is painful, there is some inflammatory lesion near his psoas muscle (appendix abscess, iliac abscess, pyomyositis of his iliopsoas). This test is less useful if his anterior abdominal wall is rigid.

The obturator test. If rotating his flexed thigh so as to stretch this muscle causes pain, there is pus or perhaps a haematocoele (in a woman) in contact with the surface of the patient's obturator internus.

The fist percussion test. Percuss gently with your fist over his chest wall. On the right a sharp pain indicates an inflammatory lesion of his diaphragm or liver; on the left one of his diaphragm, spleen, or stomach. This sign is often positive in acute hepatitis.

Percuss for liver dullness in his right nipple line from his 5th rib to below his costal margin. If he is resonant here, or in his axillary line (and his abdomen is not distended, and his

THREE SIGNS

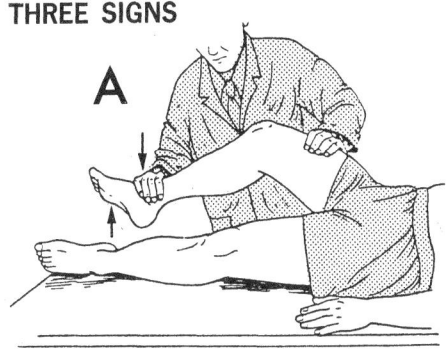
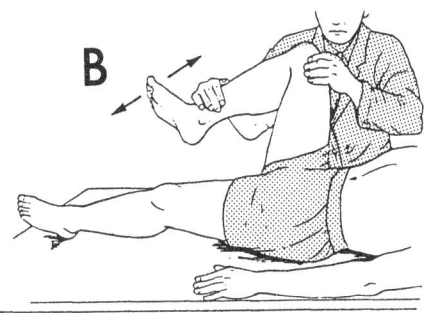
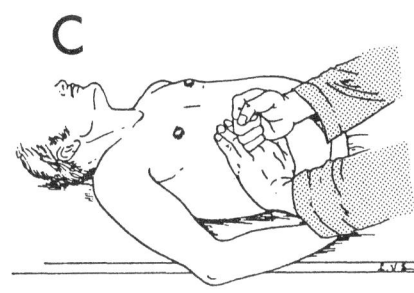

Fig. 10-2 THREE TESTS. A, the iliopsoas test. Ask the patient to flex his hip against the resistance of your hand. If he feels pain, there is inflammation in relation to his psoas muscle. B, the obturator test. Flex his hip to 90° and gently rotate it internally and externally. If this causes pain, there is inflammation in relation to his obturator muscle. C, the fist percussion test. Percuss gently with your fist over his chest wall. On the right a sharp pain indicates an inflammatory lesion of his diaphragm or liver; on the left one of his diaphragm, spleen, or stomach. *Kindly contributed by Jack Lange.*

liver is not atrophic), there is probably free gas in his peritoneal cavity.

Listen to his abdomen. Decreased or absent bowel sounds? (peritonitis or ileus from some other cause). Loud peristaltic rushes? (gastroenteritis). A rush of high-pitched tinkling bowel sounds, coinciding with worsening of his abdominal pain? (obstruction—this is a very important sign, see Section 10.3).

THE HERNIAL SITES. Feel both his femoral and inguinal openings, his umbilicus, and any old incisions.

CAUTION ! (1) A hernia does not have to be tense, tender, or painful to be obstructed. (2) It may be small, especially if it is a femoral hernia—only a centimetre or two. (3) He may be quite unaware of it. (4) Femoral hernias are very easy to miss in fat patients. (5) Don't overlook a small umbilical hernia lying deep in fat, or think a lump is not a hernia because his symptoms are not very acute. (6) Has he 'pushed back a hernia recently'—he may have obstruction from 'reduction en masse'. (7) In a baby, it is not the bulging inguinal hernia which will strangulate, but the small slim one one containing only a thin loop of his tiny gut. It may feel like slightly thickened cord and testicle, with reddening and oedema of his scrotal skin.

THE PELVIC CAVITY is just as important as the abdomen. You will find a vaginal examination more useful than a rectal one (except in a child). If necessary, do both.

Feel and percuss suprapubically, press deeply behind the patient's inguinal ligament and pubis. Feel for tenderness, muscular resistance, the mass of a pelvic abscess, a full bladder, or an enlarged uterus.

Never forget to examine the rectum. Lay him on his side or back. Press a well-lubricated finger as far up his anal canal as it will go. Feel for tenderness in all directions. *Feel forwards,* in a man for an enlarged prostate, a distended bladder, or enlarged seminal vesicles; and in a woman for swellings in her pouch of Douglas or displacements of her uterus. *Feel upwards* for a stricture, the ballooning of the anal canal below an obstruction, the apex of an intussusception, or the bulging of an abscess against the rectal wall. *Feel laterally* for the tenderness of an inflamed swollen appendix. *Feel bimanually* for a pelvic tumour or swelling, or for any fullness in the pouch of Douglas. Is there blood or mucus on your glove afterwards?

CAUTION ! It has been well said that "If you don't put your finger in a patient's rectum, you will put your foot in it!"

OTHER SYSTEMS. Don't forget to listen to his chest, he might have a basal pneumonia. Examine his spine (spinal tuberculosis or a tumour can cause root pain felt in the abdomen). Feel for a stiff neck (meningitis can cause vomiting and abdominal pain).

SPECIAL METHODS. If you suspect intraperitoneal bleeding, do a four quadrant tap (66.1) or peritoneal lavage.

If the diagnosis of an acute abdomen is uncertain or examination is difficult, examining him under anaesthesia may help, especially to assess a mass in the pelvis. Be prepared to follow this by laparotomy, depending on your findings.

LABORATORY TESTS. Don't diagnose an acute abdomen until you have examined his urine. Red cells, pus cells, or sugar in it may alter your management completely. Also remember that uraemia can present as abdominal distension and vomiting, and diabetes as vomiting and abdominal pain.

CAUTION ! A normal white count never excludes any of the diseases that cause an acute abdomen.

X-RAYS must be good, because you are interested in gas shadows. Be selective, and look at the films yourself. Ask for: (1) A PA film of his chest to check his diaphragm and subphrenic area. (2) An erect and a supine film of his abdomen. If he cannot sit up (he usually can if you support him), take a left lateral decubitus film.

An erect normal film may show a gastric air bubble, perhaps a fluid level, gas in his colon, but none in his small gut except under the age of 2 years. His psoas shadows should be clear and his renal shadows well outlined.

Abnormal signs include: (1) A shadow caused by free air under his diaphragm (or his anterior abdominal wall in a decubitus film). If you see it, a hollow viscus has perforated. Free gas under the diaphragm is often better seen on an erect chest X-ray than on an abdominal one. (2) Fluid levels (usually multiple) due to intestinal obstruction (10-6). (3) Air in the small gut is always abnormal, except in a child under 2 years. (4) Displacement of normal gas shadows. A ruptured spleen may displace the shadow of a patient's splenic flexure downwards and medially. (5) Obliteration of his psoas shadow can be caused by bleeding from an injured kidney, pyomyositis of his psoas, a psoas abscess from a tuberulous spine, or a retroperitoneal abscess. (6) Look for the shadows of renal calculi along the lines joining the tips of the transverse processes of his vertebrae to his sacroiliac joints.

CAUTION ! The absence of free gas does not exclude a perforation, nor does the absence of fluid levels exclude an obstruction.

10.2 Diagnosing an acute abdomen

How are you going to diagnose all the many causes of an acute abdomen, if the pattern of the symptoms they produce is so similar? Here is a check list of the more important features of each to help you sort them out, together with an indication of their frequency, and whether they are seen all over the developing world, or in some areas only. As is usual in medicine, a patient is more likely to have a rare presentation of a common disease, than a common presentation of a rare one. *Don't be alarmed by the complexity of the check lists that follow!* Take a careful history and examine him; consult the list, and then if necessary, extend your history and examination.

Be familiar with the pattern in your own area. For example, the causes of acute abdomens in Uganda in 1960 were: intestinal obstruction 93%, appendicitis 3%, and perforated peptic ulcer 2%. Cholecystitis, renal calculi, and pancreatitis together accounted for about 1%. The causes of intestinal obstruction were: external hernias 71%, volvulus 13%, intussusception 4%, bands and adhesions 4%. Adult pyloric stenosis, congenital anomalies and malignant disease each comprised about 1%. In another area (Kilimanjaro) intussusception was a more common cause of obstruction than hernias.

If you think that diagnosis is difficult, you can comfort yourself with the thought that, in a developing country, few of your patients will be hysterical, and that you are most unlikely to see the Munchausen syndrome (a clever group of patients who persistently fake their symptoms). When it does happen, you will be lost!

THE GENERAL METHOD FOR AN ACUTE ABDOMEN—TWO

CAUTION ! (1) Don't be frightened by this list. It is more important to decide when to operate and when not to operate, than the exact diagnosis. (2) "If in doubt, it is better to look and see than to wait and see". (3) The terms 'common' and 'uncommon' in the list below are relative only, because incidence varies geographically. (4) Read the list and refer to it, but don't try to learn it.

SHOULD YOU OPERATE ?

THE INDICATIONS FOR OPERATION after adequate resuscitation are: (1) Diagnosis made and condition needing operation, for example, appendicitis or perforated ulcer. (2) Diagnosis not made, and no improvement in spite of 4 hours of conservative treatment (fluids, nasogastric suction, morphine).

CAUTION ! Always operate if there are signs of peritoneal irritation, unless the patient has: (1) A typhoid perforation of slow onset (31.8). (2) Acute pancreatitis (13.9).

THE INDICATIONS FOR NON-OPERATIVE TREATMENT are: (1) Diagnosis made, condition not needing operation: for example, acute cholecystitis, pancreatitis, uraemia. (2) Diagnosis not made, but patient improving.

THE DIAGNOSIS OF AN ACUTE ABDOMEN

If a patient has CENTRAL ABDOMINAL PAIN, consider the the early stages of small gut obstruction (10.3), or appendicitis (12.1), or acute pancreatitis (uncommon in much of the developing world, but not so in urban areas where the alcohol intake is high). Examine him in a few hours, when you will probably find some other sign, such as vomiting, fever, or local abdominal (or rectal) tenderness, which will point to the diagnosis.

If he has SEVERE CENTRAL ABDOMINAL PAIN AND SHOCK, consider volvulus of the small gut (10.9), rupture of an ectopic pregnancy (16.6), acute pancreatitis, coronary thrombosis (rare), mesenteric thrombosis (rare), or a dissecting aneurysm (very rare).

If he has severe central abdominal pain and shock, as above, AND RIGIDITY, consider a perforated peptic ulcer (11.2), or a perforated gall-bladder (uncommon in most areas).

If he has PAIN, VOMITING, AND INCREASING DISTENSION, BUT NO RIGIDITY, he probably has small gut obstruction (10.3). Most acute abdomens cause a single initial vomit, but persistent vomiting indicates mechanical obstruction or ileus, or, if there is also rigidity, peritonitis.

If he has ABDOMINAL PAIN, with CONSTIPATION, increasing DISTENSION, and little or NO VOMITING his large gut is probably obstructed, probably by sigmoid volvulus (10.10) if he is an adult, or intussusception, if he is a child.

If he has LOCALIZED PAIN, TENDERNESS, and RIGIDITY, the causes depend on where they are:

In his right hypochondrium, **consider a leaking duodenal ulcer**

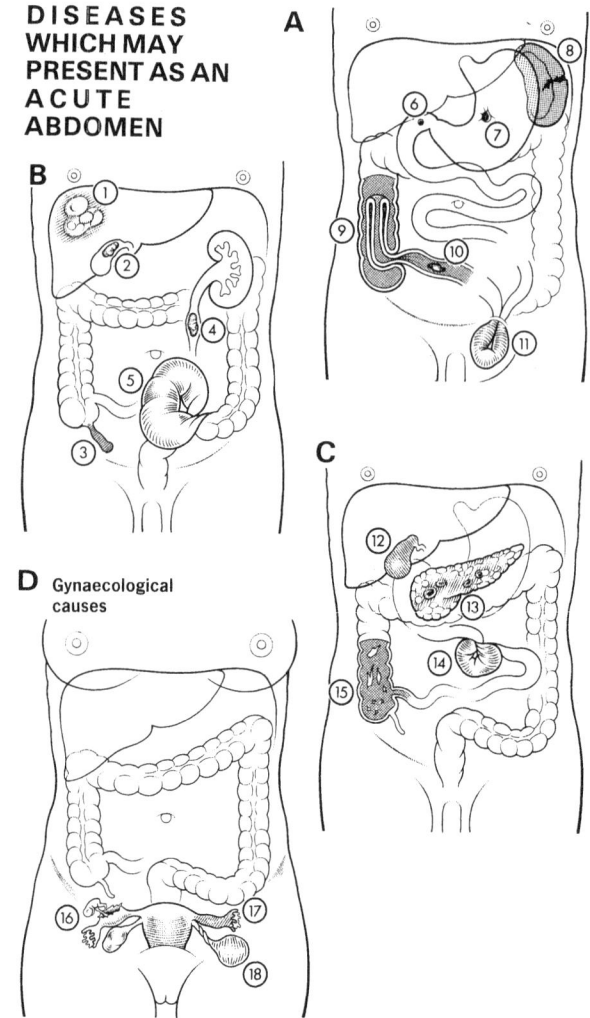

Fig. 10-3 DISEASES WHICH MAY PRESENT AS AN ACUTE ABDOMEN. 1, a liver abscess. 2, biliary colic. 3, appendicitis. 4, renal colic (very rare in some countries, but not uncommon in others). 5, sigmoid volvulus. 6, a perforated peptic ulcer. 7, a perforated gastric ulcer. 8, a ruptured spleen. 9, intussusception. 10, perforation of a typhoid ulcer. 11, a strangulated hernia. 12, acute cholecystitis. 13, acute pancreatitis. 14, volvulus of the small gut. 15, amoebic colitis. 16, rupture of an ectopic pregnancy. 17, PID. 18, torsion of an ovarian cyst.

(11.2), a liver abscess (31.12), or acute cholecystitis (13.3).

In his left hypochondrium (rare), **consider a splenic infarct** (if sickle-cell disease is endemic in your area), bleeding from an injured spleen, a leaking gastric ulcer (11.2), or acute pancreatitis (13.9).

In his right iliac fossa (very common), **consider acute appendicitis** (12.1) and most of its differential diagnoses.

In his left iliac fossa, **consider diverticulitis** (very rare in Africa).

In his, or her, hypogastrium, **consider appendicitis, or PID** (6.6).

A CHECK-LIST OF THE CAUSES OF AN ACUTE ABDOMEN

INTESTINAL OBSTRUCTION is the commonest cause of an acute abdomen in most parts of the developing world.

Small gut obstruction (everywhere, common)—colicky central or upper abdominal pain, severe early vomiting, distension, characteristic high-pitched bowel sounds, commonly a tender, tense, hard lump at a hernial orifice.

Volvulus of the small gut (everywhere, uncommon)—short history, sudden onset, constant acute pain, vomiting, a tender central abdominal mass increasing in size, collapse.

Intussusception (everywhere, fairly common)—children, previous episodes, colicky pain with vomiting, a mobile mass, usually on the right but moves around, 'red currant jelly stools' (10.8), usually described by the child's mother as bloody diarrhoea. This blood is often found on a rectal examination.

Large gut obstruction (everywhere, common)—moderate colicky pain, little vomiting, much distension, no flatus, obstructive bowel sounds (10.3). In sigmoid volvulus, which is the common cause, the patient will probably have had previous subacute episodes, and may have extreme distension and a large tender tympanitic swelling (10.10). If his gut is strangulated he will be in severe pain and ill.

PERFORATIONS all of which need surgery, include:

A perforated peptic ulcer (everywhere, common)—the sudden onset of rapidly spreading abdominal pain, with diffuse abdominal tenderness, boardlike rigidity, and a previous history of dyspepsia (11.2). After 6–8 hours his symptoms improve temporarily.

A perforated typhoid ulcer of the ileum (fairly common everywhere in the developing world, very common in West Africa)—headache, fever, and malaise for 2 weeks, followed by a dull pain suddenly getting worse and spreading, moderate tenderness, and guarding (31.8). The association of intestinal obstruction with protracted fever.

TROPICAL DISEASES. Here are the specifically tropical causes of an acute abdomen. Amoebiasis and its complications are uncommon except in certain areas, mainly humid low-lying ones, where they may be very common.

Amoebic colitis—cramps, diarrhoea with blood and mucus, slight tenderness over his colon, perhaps pain and a tender mass in his right hypochondrium (31.10).

Amoebic perforation of the gut—an acute abdominal catastrophe in a patient complaining of fever, pain, and diarrhoea (typically bloody), with a large tender mass in his right iliac fossa.

Amoebic liver abscess—fever, diffuse pain and tenderness in his right hypochondrium, a large diffusely tender liver, a rapid response to amoebicides, right iliac and shoulder pain (31.12).

Ileocaecal tuberculosis with subacute obstruction (common in some areas)—wasting, mild colic getting worse week by week, fever, distension, perhaps a mass in his right lower quadrant, or periumbilical area, ascites sometimes (29.5).

'Pigbel' disease (common in some areas, 31.9)—he presents with severe colicky pain, vomiting, and foul flatus.

Pyomyositis—an alert patient with a painful, warm, tender abdominal wall, fever, and no nausea, vomiting, anorexia, diarrhoea or constipation. He usually has normal bowel sounds and no rebound tenderness (7.1).

THE APPENDIX is only beginning to cause trouble in the developing world.

Acute appendicitis—anorexia, nausea, low-grade fever, central pain settling in the right lower quadrant, localized tenderness (12.1).

ABSCESSES in the abdominal wall and the iliac glands can mimic an acute abdomen.

Pyomyositis—local tenderness in the abdominal wall, perhaps abscesses elsewhere (7.1).

Extraperitoneal abscess, suppurating iliac adenitis—swinging fever, acute lower abdominal pain, hip flexed, tender induration of the abdominal wall extending upwards from the groin, minimal gastrointestinal disturbances (5.12).

TRAUMA. A ruptured spleen and a bowel perforation can both present as an acute abdomen.

Ruptured spleen—fainting, pallor, shock, a tender mass in the left hypochondrium, peritoneal irritation, the signs of hypovolaemia, shoulder pain, and a history of an injury (66.6).

Gut perforation—signs of peritonitis following a history of a blunt injury (66.9).

CAUTION! Remember that signs of a large gut perforation are minor for several hours.

GYNAECOLOGICAL CAUSES. A ruptured ectopic pregnancy is the most important of these.

Ruptured ectopic pregnancy (everywhere, common)—missed or scanty periods, sometimes followed by a small dark vaginal loss, moderate lower abdominal pain suddenly getting worse and spreading, pallor, tachycardia, perhaps shock. Occasionally, symptoms are chronic (16.7).

Intermenstrual ovarian bleeding ('mittelschmertz')—mid-cycle sharp lower abdominal pain, variable abdominal tenderness, normal periods.

PID—fever, vaginal discharge, pain in one or both suprapubic areas, tender adnexae on vaginal examination (6.6).

Tubo-ovarian abscess with pelvic peritonitis—recent abortion or delivery or neglected salpingitis, followed by fever, toxaemia, lower abdominal pain, perhaps a suprapubic mass, a tender mass on vaginal examination. Induration and tenderness are usually such that fluctuation is not felt.

Torsion of an ovarian cyst—sometimes a pre-existing mass, sudden pain and vomiting, a tense, tender, firm mass palpable bimanually on pelvic examination (20.7).

RENAL CONDITIONS can sometimes present as an acute abdomen.

Renal colic (occasionally everywhere but common or very common in some regions)—a sharp severe colicky pain spreading from the patient's loin down to his groin, vomiting, a vague diffuse tenderness in his flank. Reflex intestinal ileus is not uncommon (23.12).

Pyonephros (everywhere, uncommon)—a high fever, pain in his costovertebral angle, often toxaemia, a tender enlarged renal mass.

THE GALL-BLADDER commonly causes trouble in the industrial world, and in North India but seldom does so in Africa.

Biliary colic—dyspepsia, colicky pain in the epigastrium or right hypochondrium, and below the right scapula, slight tenderness (13.2).

Acute cholecystitis—a history of dyspepsia, acute constant pain and narrowly localized tenderness in the right hypochondrium or epigastrium, Murphy's sign is positive, fever (13.3).

Empyema of the gall bladder (uncommon)—as for acute cholecystitis, but the pain is more intense, he is more ill, and you may be able to feel the fundus of his gall bladder (13.3).

THE PANCREAS is an occasional cause of an acute abdomen in the developing world.

Acute pancreatitis—a history of alcohol ingestion, acute deep epigastric pain penetrating to the back, prostration, vomiting, diffuse tenderness in the epigastrium and left hypochondrium (13.9).

Pancreatic abscess (rare)—earlier like acute pancreatitis, later swinging fever, toxaemia, an ill-defined tender deep-seated mass in the upper abdomen (13.11).

Pancreatic pseudocyst (uncommon)—a history of acute pancreatitis or earlier trauma, a large deep-seated tense fluctuant mass in the upper abdomen, anorexia, fever, sometimes jaundice (13.10).

SOME MEDICAL DISEASES commonly mimic acute abdomens everywhere in the world. In most of them the fever is higher, the general symptoms worse, and the abdominal ones less than in acute abdomens. But beware of peritonitis when the patient is so ill that the general signs predominate over the local surgical ones.

Acute gastroenteritis (everywhere, very common)—diarrhoea, vomiting and fever, colicky pains, minimal abdominal tenderness, hyperactive (but not obstructive) bowel sounds, fever early, perhaps with rigors.

Basal pneumonia and pleurisy (everywhere, common)—early high fever, cough, rapid breathing, spasm of the upper abdominal muscles, and tenderness. Abdominal pain and rigidity may be very marked in a child, and involve the whole of the upper half of his abdomen, or the whole of one side. Signs of consolidation in his chest, usually in his right lower lobe.

Virus infections causing muscular pain (common)—sudden onset with high fever, local or general abdominal and chest pain; marked superficial muscle tenderness and rigidity of variable intensity, quickly changing its position; tender intercostal muscles on one or both sides; lateral compression of his chest is painful; nausea but seldom vomiting, no chest signs. During an epidemic of 'influenza' it is easy for an occasional patient with an acute abdomen to be misdiagnosed.

Diabetic precoma (uncommon)—the slow onset of abdominal pain and vomiting, dehydration, sugar and ketone bodies in his urine and breath.

SOME MEDICAL DISEASES MIMICKING AN ACUTE ABDOMEN

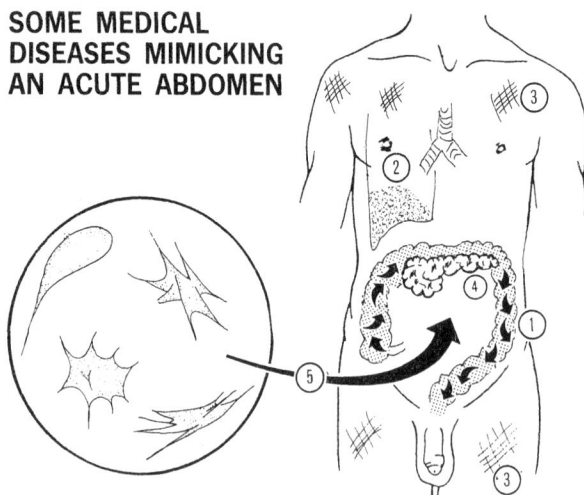

Fig. 10-4. SOME MEDICAL DISEASES MIMICKING AN ACUTE ABDOMEN. 1, acute gastroenteritis. 2, basal pneumonia and pleurisy. 3, virus infections causing muscle pain or simulating peritoneal irritation. 4, diabetic precoma. 5, a sickle-cell crisis.

Sickle-cell crisis (common in some areas)—vomiting, central abdominal pain, guarding frequently, rigidity sometimes, sickle test positive. Headache, a high fever, and pains in his limbs and back.

Uraemia (uncommon)—may simulate ileus by causing abdominal distension and vomiting. The signs and the history are vague and variable.

DIFFICULTIES DIAGNOSING AN ACUTE ABDOMEN

If you are in any doubt about the diagnosis when you first see a patient, admit him, re-examine him, and monitor him carefully, if necessary every hour for the first few hours. If he deteriorates, operate. He will be easier to assess in the ward than in the outpatient or casualty department, so examine him again there. You are also likely to get a truer reading of his pulse and temperature. This is especially important if you suspect him of having a strangulated gut, appendicitis, or a peptic ulcer.

If you are worried that he might be hysterical, and he is vomiting enough to be clinically dehydrated, he probably has an organic disease.

If he is is mentally 'odd' in any way—'aggressive', 'violent', 'dim', 'stupid', 'apathetic', or 'uncooperative', don't forget the possibility of an organic, and particularly a metabolic cause. He may be alkalotic, anaemic, hypovolaemic, toxaemic, uraemic, alcoholic, drugged, or febrile.

If a patient happens to be on steroids, pregnant, or aged, any of the symptoms of an acute abdomen may be masked, so be prepared to do a laparotomy on minimal signs.

If he is on antibiotics, they will not seal a perforated peptic ulcer, but they may diminish the signs of a perforated appendix.

10.3 Intestinal obstruction

Abdominal obstruction will be one of your major challenges. It is a common abdominal emergency, and in some communities the most common one. Some patients with simple obstruction resolve spontaneously, for example those with ascariasis (often) or tuberculous peritonitis (often) or non-specific adhesions (less often). When you operate, you may only need to divide adhesions, or massage a ball of *Ascaris* from a child's ileum on into his colon. But if you find that his small gut is gangrenous, you will have to excise it and anastomose its ends. You cannot safely do this with the large gut, because an unprotected anastomosis of the large gut is dangerous. So you will have bring its ends to the surface temporarily in some form of ostomy (9.6). Or, you can resect the gangrenous part, join cut ends of his large gut, and protect the anastomosis you have made with a proximal colostomy (9.6).

Unfortunately, a patient with intestinal obstruction often presents late, so that by the time you see him he may be severely dehydrated, hypovolaemic, oliguric, and shocked. You will have little difficulty deciding that he is obstructed, but will he withstand an operation? Deciding why he is obstructed may have to wait until you do a laparotomy. When you look inside his abdomen, it may not be easy to recognize what has happened, to decide what to do, or to do it.

One of the many ways in which the industrial and the developing worlds differ is the way in which the guts of their inhabitants obstruct. In the industrial world intestinal obstruction is caused about equally by adhesions, hernias, and carcinoma of the colon. In the developing world adhesions and carcinoma of the colon are unusual. Their place is taken by ascariasis, volvulus of the sigmoid colon or small intestine, and by intussusception. Although developing countries differ, their similarities are more striking than their differences.

THE CAUSES OF INTESTINAL OBSTRUCTION vary geographically. Find out the common causes in your area.
Common causes. Incarcerated or irreducible external hernias (inguinal and femoral). Volvulus of the sigmoid colon. Ascariasis. Intussusception. Obstruction due to ileus due to sepsis; for example, when a patient presents late with sepsis resulting from a perforated typhoid ulcer, a tubo-ovarian abscess, appendicitis, or a perforated duodenal ulcer. Adhesions or bands following previous surgery, or abdominal sepsis. Adhesions or fibrosis due to abdominal tuberculosis.
Uncommon causes. Volvulus of the small gut. Carcinoma of the colon. Carcinomatosis of the peritoneum. Amoebic granuloma or stenosis.
Rare causes. Primary tumours of the small gut. Congenital bands. Crohn's disease. Mesenteric vascular occlusion. Gallstone ileus. Diverticulitis. Lymphogranuloma.

WHAT IS THE PATTERN OF INTESTINAL OBSTRUCTION IN YOUR AREA?

10.4 The diagnosis of intestinal obstruction

You will see several patterns of intestinal obstruction. They are determined by how a patient's gut is obstructed, and where it obstructs. Firstly, the obstruction can be simple or strangulated.

(1) Simple obstruction is caused by a mechanical block or ileus, without impairment of the blood supply of the gut. The causes include obstruction by a ball of *Ascaris* worms, or adhesions. Simple obstruction may resolve spontaneously. Operation is usually not urgent, and may be unnecessary.

An obstructed gut dilates above the obstruction, so that it fills with several litres of fluid and gas. Bacteria grow in this pool of fluid, which becomes faeculent and highly infectious for the peritoneal cavity, should it get there. The patient's dilated gut makes his abdomen swell. Initially, the peristaltic activity of his dilating gut increases to overcome the obstruction. This causes rushes of hyperperistaltic bowel sounds, or high-pitched tinkling sounds, or both, which you can hear if you listen to his abdomen. Later, as ileus develops, his gut becomes silent. Inadequate fluid intake combined with the loss of fluid, by repeated vomiting, and into the lumen of his gut, depletes his extracellular fluid, so that he becomes dehydrated, hypovolaemic, shocked, and acidotic. An adult secretes 7 litres of gastrointestinal juice in 24 hours, so his fluid loss can be considerable.

(2) Strangulation obstruction occurs when there is is a mechanical block and the blood supply to the gut is impaired. Strangulated hernias and sigmoid volvulus are common causes. About 6 hours after the interruption of its blood supply the gut becomes gangrenous and may perforate. If it perforates into his peritoneal cavity it causes generalized peritonitis which may end

INTESTINAL OBSTRUCTION

Small gut obstruction

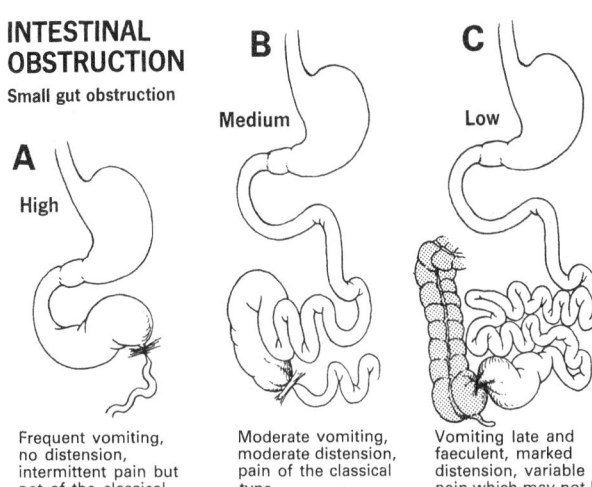

The role of the ileocaecal valve

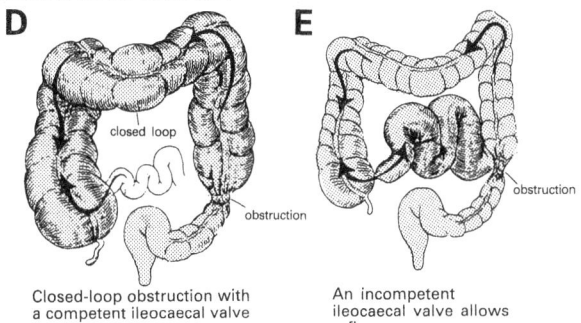

Fig. 10-5 INTESTINAL OBSTRUCTION. A, B, and C, small gut obstruction. In A, the obstruction is high, there is frequent vomiting, no distension, and intermittent pain, which is not of the classical type. In B, the obstruction is in the middle of the small gut. There is moderate vomiting, moderate distension, and intermittent pain of the classical, colicky, crescendo type with free intervals. In C, obstruction is low in the small gut. Vomiting is late and faeculent, and distension is marked. Pain may or may not be classical.

In D, and E, the large gut is obstructed. In D, the ileocaecal valve is competent, and prevents distension spreading to the small gut, so that there is a closed loop. In E, the valve is incompetent, so that there is reflux into the small gut which distends. *After Dunphy and Way, 'Current Surgical Diagnosis and Treatment' Figs, 33-5 and 34-5. With the kind permission of Jack Lange.*

in septic shock; if it perforates into a hernial sac the infection may be more localized. He is very ill and will probably die if you don't operate immediately. If you think that peritoneal irritation might be due to strangulation obstruction *operate soon!*

Now for the levels at which gut obstructs:

Small gut obstruction produces effects which differ according to the level at which it occurs. The higher the obstruction the earlier and the worse the patient's vomiting, and the greater the threat to his life from electrolyte imbalance—but the less his distension. Conversely, the lower the obstruction the greater his distension, the greater his pain, and the later he starts to vomit.

Large gut obstruction follows a slower course. Because there is more gut to dilate, there is more abdominal distension, which may be so severe as to interfere with his breathing by pushing up his diaphragm. To begin with, only his colon dilates, but his ileocaecal valve usually becomes incompetent (two-thirds of patients), and allows the dilatation to progress proximally into his small gut. The symptoms of dehydration are less severe, because his colon can still absorb fluid above the obstruction.

'Closed-loop obstruction' (unusual) is the result of his ileocaecal valve remaining competent. It is a double obstruction which shuts off a loop (D, 10-5). It can occur in volvulus, and in neglected obstruction of the large gut. Dilatation of the closed loop may obstruct its blood supply and cause gangrene and peritonitis.

The common mistakes are: (1) Not spending enough time, both taking his history and sitting beside him watching, palpating, and listening to his abdomen. (2) Forgetting the possibility that obstructed gut may strangulate, even when the signs of peritoneal irritation are minimal, for example when the strangulated gut of an intussusception is inside viable gut. (3) Not making proper use of X-rays. (4) Operating too early, before you have rehydrated him, or too late, after you have allowed his gut to strangulate. (5) Not emptying his stomach and giving magnesium trisilicate before you operate. (7) Doing a complicated operation when a simpler one would have saved his life. (8) Poor surgical technique—open his abdomen with care, dissect dense adhesions gently, make anastomoses carefully, and don't soil his peritoneum with the contents of his obstructed gut—the organisms inside it are particularly virulent. (9) Not washing out his peritoneal cavity and instilling tetracycline, when you have spilt the contents of his gut into his peritoneal cavity, or he has peritonitis. Not closing his abdomen sufficiently securely to prevent it bursting (9.9, 9.13). (10) Not replacing fluid and electrolytes before he is able to take fluids by mouth.

SITA (8 years) presented with vague abdominal tenderness and few other signs. She was not well, and the only striking sign was a a pulse of 148 per minute. 12 hours were wasted while she was observed, before a laparotomy was done and a metre of gangrenous gut was resected.

Mrs PATEL presented with abdominal distension, colicky pain, and vomiting. She was examined by a medical assistant who noted pain in her right lower quadrant and a 'lymph node' in her right groin, and diagnosed appendicitis. He rang up the doctor, who came in, made a cursory examination, and proceeded with an appendicectomy, using a 'gridiron' incision. Her appendix was normal. Later, she had to have an emergency operation for a strangulated femoral hernia. LESSONS (1) Strangulation can be difficult to diagnose. Tachycardia is a useful sign. (2) "When acute abdominal pain presents, one maxim I enjoin, pray do not miss that tiny lump, in one or other groin." (Zachary Cope)

THE DIAGNOSIS OF INTESTINAL OBSTRUCTION

Here are the typical features of a patient with intestinal obstruction—they are often atypical. Follow the steps of inspection, palpation, percussion, and auscultation.

HISTORY

PAIN differs in large and small gut obstruction.

If his pain is periumbilical and colicky, comes in spasms, builds up to a crescendo, and then tapers off, his small gut is obstructed. Vomiting may relieve it temporarily. Sometimes he has regular pain-free periods at intervals of 2 to 5 minutes. This is the classical pain of small gut obstruction. If peristalsis stops, colic stops—so its disappearance may be a bad sign.

If his pain is below his umbilicus and comes at intervals of 6 to 10 minutes, his large gut is likely to be obstructed.

If he has no pain, but only 'gurgling and bloating' his obstruction is subacute in his large gut or his distal small gut.

If his pain is severe and continuous, this suggests strangulation obstruction. He may have continuous and colicky pain. For example, he may have continuous pain from a strangulated hernia at a hernial site, and colicky central abdominal pain.

If pain and fever preceded his symptoms of obstruction, suspect that it may be secondary to abdominal sepsis.

VOMITING. The higher his obstruction, the worse this is. If it is high in his small gut, he vomits profusely and frequently; if it is low in his large gut, he may not vomit at all. After about 3 days of complete obstruction, his vomit becomes faeculent. If paralytic ileus develops, it becomes 'effortless'.

CAUTION ! Look at his vomit. If it is faeculent, his large gut or lower small gut are almost certainly obstructed. Vomiting never becomes faeculent if his upper small gut is obstructed.

ABDOMINAL FULLNESS. The more distal his obstruction, the more he swells. If large gut obstruction has come on slowly, he may say that his "clothes fit tightly" or that he "feels filled up with gas".

CONSTIPATION. If his small gut is obstructed, his colon may take a day or two to empty, after which "nothing comes". The absence of flatus confirms the diagnosis. Constipation may be his major concern in a culture where regular bowel movements occur two or three tims a day. Pain may be tolerable, but the absence of a decent bowel movement may not.

PREVIOUS OPERATIONS OR PERITONEAL SEPSIS. Adhesions and bands can follow any operation or septic process in the abdomen. In a woman enquire especially for symptoms suggesting PID (6.6).

THE EXAMINATION FOR INTESTINAL OBSTRUCTION

DISTENSION AND HYPER-RESONANCE. If he has colic and is vomiting, his gut is obstructed until you have proved otherwise. Distension is not an essential part of the clinical picture. The earliest signs of it are a little fullness in his flanks, or an increased resonance to percussion.

If the percussion note over his abdomen is 'tympanitic', he has distended gas-filled loops of gut, and is obstructed.

If distension is conspicuous and other signs are minimal, suspect large gut obstruction. If it is extreme, suspect sigmoid volvulus.

If you are not sure if his distension is caused by gut obstruction or ascites, examine him for shifting dullness. Remember that fluid and gas in a distended gut can cause shifting dullness, but that it is less obvious than with ascites.

If you are not sure if he is distended or not, measure his girth at some fixed place, and see if it increases.

OBSTRUCTIVE GUT SOUNDS. Listen for these at any time he appears to be in pain, while you are taking his history. This is essential if you are going to pick up the critical sign of intestinal obstruction—the half minute during which peristaltic waves make a ladder pattern on his abdominal wall, accompanied by a rush of high pitched tinkles and splashes. If you miss this opportunity it may not return for 15 minutes. So, if he loses interest in the conversation, and grimaces with pain—listen quickly. If you hear: (1) runs of borborygmi, or (2) a chorus of tinkling high-pitched musical sounds *at the same time that he grimaces with colic,* he is almost certainly obstructed. *These are very useful early signs.* Don't mistake them for: (1) the peristaltic rushes of gastroenteritis, or (2) normal hyperactive bowel sounds.

VISIBLE PERISTALSIS. If he is thin, look for waves of peristalsis passing across his abdomen. If he is very thin this may be normal, especially in a young child.

A TENDER MASS AT ONE OF HIS HERNIAL ORIFICES. Examine his inguinal and femoral canals. If you find a painful tender mass, he has an incarcerated or strangulated hernia.

CAUTION ! (1) You can easily miss a strangulated femoral hernia—it may not be tender or painful—see the story of Mrs Patel, above. (2) Rarely, a hernia becomes reduced 'en masse' (14.1), so that there is no mass, tender or otherwise.

ABDOMINAL TENDERNESS is not a prominent feature of uncomplicated obstruction. Obvious tenderness over part of the abdomen suggests strangulation.

AN OLD LAPAROTOMY SCAR suggests that the cause of an obstruction may well be a band, an adhesion, or an area of stenosis.

A PALPABLE ABDOMINAL MASS is unusual, apart from a mass at a hernial orifice. Feel carefully, here are some of the masses you might find.

If, in a child, you feel an ill-defined mobile mass (or masses), usually in his umbilical region, sometimes in his iliac fossae, it is probably a mass of Ascaris worms.

If you feel an ill defined lump or lumps in a patient's right lower quadrant, he may have ileocaecal tuberculosis. You may also feel more central lumps caused by caseating tuberculous lymph nodes.

If he has a large, slightly tender, mobile abdominal mass, some of his gut may have infarcted due to torsion or intussusception.

If his mass changes its position from one day to another, and is accompanied by colicky pain, he probably has recurrent intussusception or a mass of Ascaris worms.

If he has a tender indurated mass, suspect that his obstruction is due to an intraperitoneal abscess (6.3).

If you feel hard impacted masses in his colon and rectally, they are masses of faeces, and may be causing his obstruction (not uncommon in the old and debilitated).

If he has one or more masses and also ascites, and is thin and debilitated, he probably has disseminated carcinoma.

RECTAL EXAMINATION must not be forgotten!

If you find fresh blood and mucus on your finger, or he passes these, he probably has a strangulating lesion higher up, or carcinoma of his large gut, or an intussusception. Occasionally, you may feel its tip.

If you feel a hard mass of faeces, suspect that constipation may be causing his obstruction.

If his rectum is empty and even 'ballooned', this is an additional sign of intestinal obstruction, but the reason for it is not clear.

If there is a tense, feeling in his pelvis, as you feel through his rectal wall, it may be caused by tense loops of obstructed gut.

If you feel a tense tender, possibly fluctuant mass bulging into the pouch of Douglas, it is probably a pelvic abscess. You may feel it more easily bimanually, with your other hand exerting pressure suprapubically (6.5).

If you find a hard mass in the rectovesical pouch (a 'rectal shelf'), it is probably malignant. Tumour deposits here may be well-defined hard lumps, or a 'shelf' caused by tumour growing into the surrounding tissue.

HAS HIS GUT STRANGULATED?

You may not be certain about this until you do a laparotomy. Strangulation is easy to diagnose when it is advanced, unless it is so advanced that he is in septic shock. Try to diagnose it early. Individually, the features below are not diagnostic, but his gut has probably strangulated if he shows several of them.

(1) The sudden onset of symptoms.

(2) Severe continuous pain. This is the result of irritation of his parietal peritoneum. If he is fairly comfortable and pain-free between waves of hyperperistalsis, his gut is probably not strangulated, but only obstructed (unless it is sealed off in a hernial sac or is an intussusception).

(3) A fast pulse. This is perhaps the most reliable sign; if his pulse is only 88, he is unlikely to have strangulated his gut.

(4) Fever. Simple obstruction does not cause fever. If he is febrile, suspect strangulation, or sepsis.

(5) A low or falling blood pressure.

(6) Localized tenderness, or rebound tenderness. This is a sign of peritoneal irritation, and can be caused by inflammation, blood in the peritoneal cavity, or strangulation. Tenderness may be masked by loops of normal gut over the strangulated area, so its absence is not significant.

(7) The passage of blood or blood and mucus rectally. This is typical of intussusception, but you may see it whenever the blood supply of the gut is impaired.

(8) Signs of peritonitis, (tenderness, guarding, and absent bowel sounds), prostration, and shock are late signs.

X-RAYS IN INTESTINAL OBSTRUCTION

Take films while he is erect and supine. They can usually tell you: (1) That he is obstructed. (2) The site of the obstruction. (3) Its severity. (4) Sometimes its cause, for example, intussusception. See also 10.1.

While he is lying down, take a supine AP film. If he is not well enough to sit up by himself, support him in the sitting position while you take an erect film. This will be more useful than the alternative, which is a lateral decubitus film, taken from the side while he is lying down. Its purpose is to show fluid levels, and gas under his diaphragm.

CAUTION ! Never give contrast media by mouth in intestinal obstruction. A barium enema is occasionally useful in communities where carcinoma of the colon is common, but is seldom needed in the developing world.

When you examine the films, first see if the patient has a distended large gut shadow, and especially a caecal shadow. If he has, his large gut is obstructed. To distinguish large and small gut shadows, remember that: (1) Fine folds or partitions, (valvulae conniventes) extend right across a distended jejunum which is more central in the abdomen. (2) The ileum has no folds distally, and few proximally. (3) His caecum is a rounded

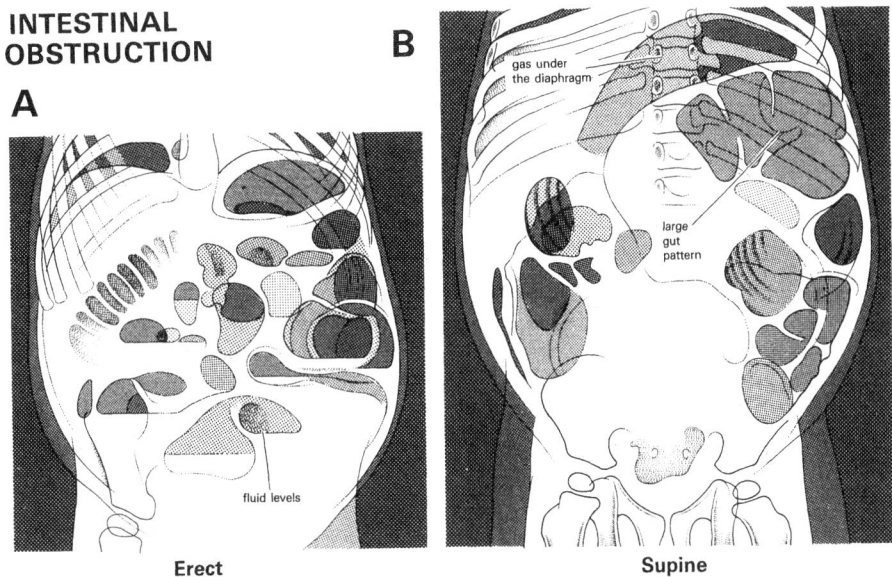

Fig. 10-6 OBSTRUCTED GUT—ONE. A, an erect film showing the multiple fluid levels of small gut obstruction. B, a supine film showing small and large gut shadows, and gas under the diaphragm.

mass of gas. (4) The haustral markings of obstructed large gut are rounded and much further apart than the valvulae conniventes of the jejunum, and do not cross its full diameter. The large gut is more peripheral in the abdomen, whereas the small gut is more central.

Gas in his peritoneum, is the only certain sign of gangrene and perforation. You may see it under his diaphragm in an erect chest film, and under his abdominal wall in a lateral supine one.

Gas in the small gut is always abnormal, except: (1) in the duodenal cap, (2) in the terminal ileum (rare), (3) in children under 2 years.

Fluid levels in the small gut, are always abnormal except where gas is normal (see just above). Elsewhere, fluid levels in the small gut indicate: (1) mechanical obstruction, (2) ileus, or (3) gastroenteritis. Look for them in erect films. The larger and more numerous they are, the lower and the more advanced the obstruction.

Gas in the large gut is normal.

Fluid levels in the large gut: (1) may be normal (if there are only a few), or (2) may be caused by gastroenteritis. If the large gut is also distended there is: (1) a mechanical obstruction, (2) ileus, or (3) some other cause for the dilatation, such as amoebic colitis.

CAUTION ! The gas shadows may be far away from the site of the obstruction.

If the films show distended loops of large and small gut irregularly distributed with gas in his rectum, suspect ileus.

If he has no gas shadow in his caecum (which normally contains some gas), suspect that his small gut is obstructed.

If he has a large caecal shadow (which may be huge), his large gut is obstructed. As the pressure builds up, his small gut often starts to distend, because his ileocaecal valve is incompetent (2/3rds of patients).

If you see a really massive gas shadow, his stomach may be dilated, or he may have volvulus of his sigmoid (common, 10.10) or of his caecum and ascending colon (rare, 10.11).

If there is a gas shadow in his rectum and rectal examination is normal clinically, he is unlikely to be obstructed.

If his large gut is relatively empty, and the fluid levels in his erect film pass obliquely upwards from his right iliac fossa to his left hypochondrium, like a stepladder, they suggest volvulus of his small gut (rare but characteristic).

If signs are uncertain, take more films a few hours later.

OTHER INVESTIGATIONS A high haemoglobin or haematocrit are some indication of the severity of his dehydration.

DIFFICULTIES IN DIAGNOSING INTESTINAL OBSTRUCTION

If he has EXCRUCIATING ABDOMINAL PAIN, MASSIVE ABDOMINAL DISTENSION, and CIRCULATORY COLLAPSE, the possibilities include: (1) Volvulus of his sigmoid with gangrene. (2) Volvulus of his sigmoid with secondary volvulus of his small gut (compound volvulus 10-17). (3) Volvulus of his small gut. (4) Perforation of a peptic ulcer presenting late. (5) Generalized peritonitis leading to ileus. (6) Typhoid fever with perforation. (7) Acute pancreatitis. You may not be able to diagnose which of these he has until you operate. He needs rapid resuscitation and urgent surgery, but try to exclude pancreatitis first.

If he has OBVIOUS ABDOMINAL SIGNS, BUT LOOKS COMPARATIVELY WELL, (because he has not been vomiting), suspect large gut or incomplete small gut obstruction.

If he presents with a HISTORY OF SEVERAL DAYS OF FEVER, anorexia and localized abdominal pain, followed by colicky pain and the other symptoms of obstruction, suspect that obstruction has followed intraperitoneal sepsis. Distension may mask the abdominal findings, but you may be able to elicit deep tenderness and induration in his right lower quadrant, suprapubically, rectally, or, in a woman, vaginally.

If he is DISTENDED AND VOMITS but does NOT HAVE THE TYPICAL COLICKY PAIN of obstruction, suspect ileus rather than obstruction, especially if he is toxic and dehydrated. Obstruction appears spontaneously, whereas ileus usually follows some good reason for it, such as local or general peritonitis, a previous operation, or an intraperitoneal injury or haemorrhage.

If he has the other SIGNS OF OBSTRUCTION, but PASSES LOOSE STOOLS with or without flatus, he may have: (1) An incomplete large gut obstruction. (2) A pelvic abscess. (3) A Richter's hernia—part of the circumference of his gut may be trapped in a tight inguinal ring, leaving enough lumen for its contents to pass through and cause diarrhoea (14.1).

If SIGNS OF OBSTRUCTION DEVELOP AFTER SURGERY, you will find it difficult to know if his obstruction is mechanical or due to the paralysis caused by ileus—see Section 10.13.

The general method is continued in the next section.

10.5 The management of intestinal obstruction

The treatment of strangulation obstruction is always operative. The treatment of simple mechanical obstruction may be non-operative or operative. If it fails to improve after 48 hours of non-operative treatment, operate. The detailed indications for

INTESTINAL OBSTRUCTION

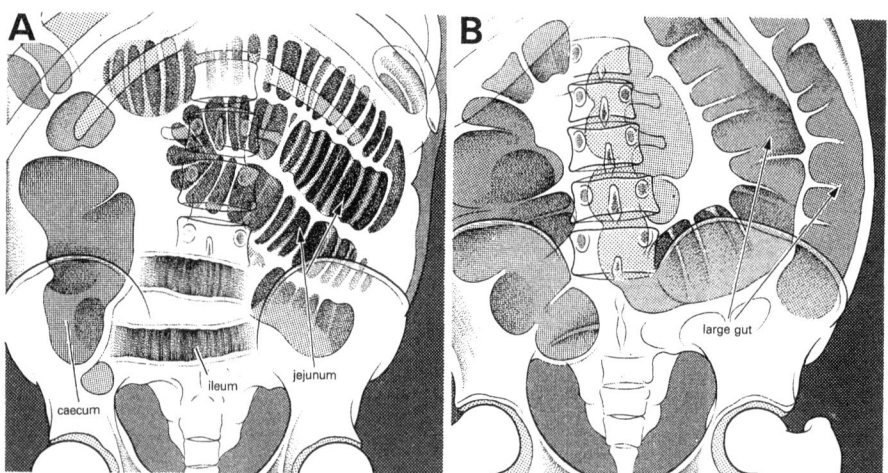

Both these are supine films

Fig. 10-7 OBSTRUCTED GUT—TW0. Patient A has distended loops of small gut. Note the different patterns of his jejunum and ileum, The jejunum has 'valvulae conniventes' (transverse bands across it), whereas the ileum is more featureless. His caecum and ascending colon are distended, but there are no signs of his transverse colon or rectum. A barium enema showed a carcinoma just beyond his splenic flexure.

Patient B's large gut is distended down to his sigmoid colon, but he has no rectal bubble. This is typical of distal large gut obstruction; he had a carcinoma of his sigmoid colon. These are supine films, so there are no fluid levels, but the valvulae and haustra are shown well.

operating are listed below. Operate at the optimum moment after you have rehydrated a patient, but don't operate if his condition is hopeless.

Rehydrate him rapidly over a few hours, as in Section 15.3. of *Primary Anaesthesia*. If you rehydrate him energetically, you should be able to operate within 4 hours, and certainly within 6 hours. If you suspect strangulation obstruction, try to operate within one hour, and rehydrate him as best you can before doing so. If he is conscious with a normal blood pressure and is passing urine, he is probably fit for operation.

At the same time suck the fluid and gas from his dilated stomach and upper small gut. This will stop him vomiting, and may reduce his distension. Most importantly, it will reduce the danger that he will aspirate his stomach contents when he is anaesthetized.

When you have resuscitated him, he may improve so much that you may wonder if he really needs a laparotomy. *So, decide if he wants one or not, before you resuscitate him!* If he has improved so much after resuscitation that you really do wonder if he needs a laparotomy, try clamping his nasogastric tube to see if he distends again.

Your first task is to save his life, so do an operation which will achieve this. In desperate cases, removing the underlying cause is a secondary consideration, and may have to wait until later. Sometimes, you can remove the cause quite easily: for example, you may be able to cut some easier adhesions. Don't do complicated operations which need much dissection.

Open his abdomen with the greatest possible care—you can so easily perforate his gut, and flood his abdomen with faeces. Distended loops of gut will bulge through the incision. Deliver them on to the surface, and don't go pawing around in the depths of his wound—they will continually obscure your field.

Because distended loops of gut are so difficult to work with, you will have to decide if you are going to decompress them. Doing so makes distended gut much easier to handle, and makes the abdomen easier to close. The danger of decompression is that it inevitably contaminates the peritoneum a little, unless you use the retrograde method. But carefully opening distended gut with the proper precautions causes much less contamination than an uncontrolled burst—which is the probable alternative. So, if gut is greatly distended, decompress it. If it is only moderately distended, don't.

There are four ways to decompress a patient's gut; surgeons vary as to which they like:

(1) You can push the fluid and air back up his gut into his stomach, between your fingers, starting distally. The anaesthetist then removes it through the nasogastric tube. This may be the best method, *but be sure that the suction through the nasogastric tube is working properly, or your patient may aspirate the fluid!* Only use other methods if this fails.

(2) You can use a specially prepared spinal needle. This will remove gas, but is soon blocked by food particles when you try to remove liquid. A spinal needle is especially useful for the sigmoid colon and the caecum, which are often distended with gas. Its advantage is that there is no need to insert a purse string round it.

(3) You can use a Savage decompressor, which is a long tube with a trocar, which you push into the patient's gut through a purse string suture, and then suck out fluid and gas through a side tube. If it blocks, leave it in and clear it with its trocar. You can decompress a long length of gut by 'skewering' it over the decompressor.

(4) You can insert a Yankauer sucker through a purse string suture. This has a nozzle with several holes. It blocks less easily than a needle, but the risks of a spill are greater. It always blocks eventually. Removing it, unblocking it, and reinserting it may be necessary, but is likely to cause a spill.

When you have decompressed a patient's obstructed and distended gut, you will have to: (1) Find the obstruction. (2) Decide if his gut is strangulated or not. (3) Resect strangulated gut, if you find it. Having resected it, what you should do next will depend on whether it is large or small gut: (a) If it is his small gut you can anastomose its ends. (b) If it is his large gut you can: (i) Anastomose its ends and do a proximal protective colostomy (9.5). (ii) Exteriorize its ends and do a double-barrel colostomy. (iii) Bring the proximal end to the surface as a colostomy, and close the distal end (Hartmann's operation).

If you cannot anastomose gut, you can bring both ends to the surface as a colostomy, as in Figure 9-13, and refer him. This is more practical with the large gut; if you do it with small gut, his fluid losses will be so high that you will have to refer him within a few hours.

If you fail to resect and anastomose (or exteriorize) gut when it is not viable, he will certainly die of peritonitis.

DON'T OPERATE IF HE IS MORIBUND

THE MANAGEMENT OF INTESTINAL
OBSTRUCTION

PREOPERATIVE PREPARATION

NASOGASTRIC SUCTION. Pass a nasogastric tube of a suitable size, and aspirate it regularly (4.9). Make sure it reaches the patient's stomach, and be sure it is draining properly. Suck efficiently to remove air and fluid before operating. Suck by syphoning the fluid into a bag, and sucking every 15 to 30 minutes with a syringe. Empty his stomach thoroughly, and then instil 30 ml of magnesium trisilicate mixture before induction.

INSERT AN INDWELLING CATHETER if he is very ill, and measure his urine volume hourly. If he is not very ill, its risks may outweigh its advantages. If an adult passes 35 to 60 ml per hour, his kidneys are being adequately perfused, and his blood volume is becoming normal. For a man Paul's tubing is acceptable.

SET UP A CVP LINE, if you can do so (A 19.2).

RESUSCITATION FOR INTESTINAL OBSTRUCTION
This is critical. If he is severely dehydrated, and you fail to resuscitate him, he will probably die. If his obstruction has lasted longer than 24 hours, he is sure to be dehydrated, especially if he has been vomiting profusely, and his abdominal signs are unimpressive, indicating that his obstruction is probably high in his small gut. Start a fluid balance chart (A 15.5), and rehydrate him as in (A 15.3). Here are some rough rules, which give him rather more fluid than is given in *Primary Anaesthesia* (A 15.3). They assume that he is a 60 kg adult—modify them according to his actual weight.

Either: (1) Give him the first half of his deficit as Ringer's lactate or saline and the second half as alternate bottles of this and 5% dextrose. Fluid replacement is more important than potassium replacement (except in pyloric stenosis, which produces a specific metabolic defect, see Section 11.6). In late cases add 10 mmol of potassium to each 500 ml bottle after the first two. Or, (2) if you don't trust your nurses with strong potassium solutions, give him half-strength Darrow's solution (K 17 mmol/litre) every second bottle.

If he is thirsty, and his lips and tongue are dry, he is mildly dehydrated, and needs at least 4 litres of fluid.

If he also has sunken eyes and loss of skin elasticity, he is moderately dehydrated and needs about 6 litres.

If he also has oliguria, anuria, hypotension, and clammy extremities, he is severely dehydrated and needs about 8 litres.

If he is also weak and disorientated, he has probably lost more than 8 litres. Don't be afraid to give him up to 4 litres over one hour.

If he is elderly or has cardiac problems, watch his lung bases for crepitations, and his jugular venous pressure or his CVP.

If his gut strangulates, its veins block before its arteries, so that he loses blood into the lumen. He may need blood, about 2 units per metre of strangulated gut. If he was anaemic before he became obstructed, he also needs blood; but his main need is for water and electrolytes. Remember the danger of HIV. If an adult is sufficiently ill to need blood he needs at least 2 units.

If you have corrected his hypovolaemia as shown by an adequate urine output, or a normal CVP, but he is still hypotensive, he is probably in septic shock (53.4).

ANTIBIOTICS. Give him perioperative antibiotics (2.9). Give him chloramphenicol 500 mg intravenously, followed by an equal dose 6-hourly; and give him metronidazole 7.5 mg/kg 8-hourly. If you give it rectally give 1000 mg.

Or, give him gentamicin 2–5 mg/kg daily in divided doses 8-hourly. Or, give him penicillin 1 megaunit 6 hourly, and streptomycin 0.5 g 12-hourly, and metronidazole 8-hourly. If he is to have a long-acting relaxant, start the gentamicin or the streptomycin postoperatively, before he leaves the theatre (A 14.3). Much better, give him something else that can be started preoperatively.

THE NON-OPERATIVE TREATMENT OF INTESTINAL OBSTRUCTION

INDICATIONS. Obstruction due to: (1) A mass of Ascaris worms. (2) Plastic tuberculous peritonitis. (3) A localized inflammatory mass, such as an appendix mass, a pyosalpinx, or PID. (4) A pelvic abscess which can be drained rectally or vaginally. (5) Some patients with adhesions—see Section 10.7. (6) Typhoid fever causing partial mechanical obstruction or ileus (not uncommon).

CAUTION ! Non-operative treatment is never indicated if there is even a suspicion of strangulation obstruction.

METHOD. Continue nasogastric suction and intravenous infusions. Observe him carefully. Measure his girth. If you 'suck and drip him' for more than a few days, try to add at least 8.5 MJ (about 2000 kcal) of energy to his daily intake. If possible, give this as 50% dextrose into a central vein (A 19.2).

Signs of improvement are: (1) Reduction in the gastric aspirate. The normal minimum is 500 ml of clear light-green fluid, which is the volume excreted into an unobstructed stomach. (2) A reduction in his girth. (3) Return of his bowel sounds to normal. (5) Less pain. (6) Finally, he passes flatus and stools.

THE OPERATIVE TREATMENT FOR INTESTINAL OBSTRUCTION

EQUIPMENT. A general set (4.12). A large (2 mm) spinal needle attached to a glass connector with a piece of rubber tubing, as in Fig 10-9. A Savage decompressor.

ANAESTHESIA. The aspiration of stomach contents is his major risk. Nasogastric suction reduces it, but does not remove

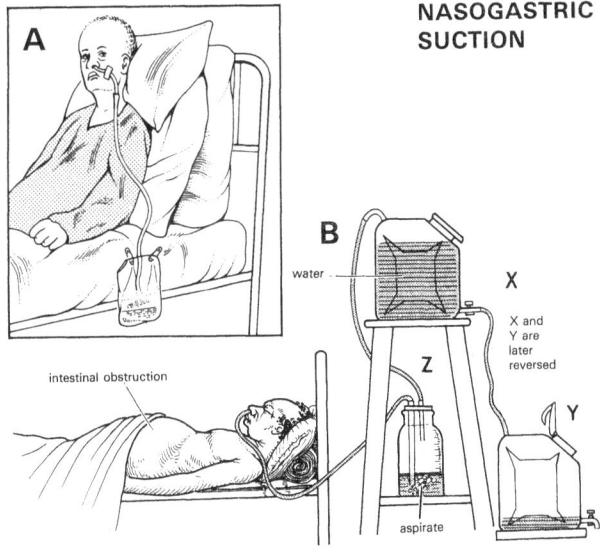

Fig. 10-8 NASOGASTRIC SUCTION. A, pass a large (16 Ch) nasogastric tube and aspirate it with a 20 or 50 ml syringe half-hourly. Meanwhile, let it syphon freely into a drip bag beside the patient's bed. Cut off the corner of the drip bag to let the air out. B, if you don't have an electric sucker, you may find this apparatus useful. X and Y are two jerricans with pipes and taps soldered in. Water flows from X to Y creating a negative pressure in X. When X is empty, X and Y are reversed. Z collects the fluid and measures the flow. *After Les Agreges du Pharo, 'Techniques Elementaires pour Medecins Isoles', Fig. 168. Diffusion Maloine, with kind permission.*

it. Intubate him using cricoid pressure (A 16.5). Make sure that repeated attempts are made to empty his stomach every 15 minutes before the operation. Even aspirating air reduces the risk. Instil 30 ml of magnesium trisilicate mixture into his stomach before you induce him.

INCISION. A right paramedian or a midline incision is usually best, one-third above his umbilicus and two-thirds below it. Start with a 10 cm incision and enlarge it up or down as necessary. You will probably find that his posterior rectus sheath and his peritoneum will appear as two distinct layers, now that his abdominal wall is distended. Have moist packs (laparotomy pads) ready. Put them into warm water and then wring out most of the fluid. Use them: (1) to cover any gut that bulges out of the wound, (2) to wall off any fluid that spills.

If he has an old scar, a loop of gut may have stuck to its under side, so open his abdomen at one end of it, as in Section 9.2. This is safer than making a parallel incision, which may lead to necrosis of the abdominal wall between the two incisions.

If he has a strangulated external hernia, make the appropriate incision (Chapter 14).

CAUTION ! (1) Open his abdomen with the greatest care as in Figure 9-2. Distended loops of gut will be pressing up against it, and the smallest nick of a scalpel will go straight through them. You can so easily cut the thin wall of his distended colon and cause a fatal peritonitis. (2) Note which parts of his gut are distended; you will need to know this later, to decide where the obstruction is.

HANDLING HIS GUT. If it is very distended, decompress it before you do anything else. If it is less distended, use a moist swab to lift the dilated loops gently out on to the surface of his abdomen.

CAUTION ! (1) Handle them with the greatest care. They can easily tear. If you handle them roughly you will prolong the period of postoperative ileus. Be especially careful of his caecum. It is often greatly thinned, and if it does burst, soiling will be particularly dangerous. (2) Don't let loops of his gut get dry—cover them with moist packs. (3) If they are heavily laden with fluid, ask your assistant to support them.

If you nick only the seromuscular wall of a loop of gut, leave it alone. Close a deeper injury with a purse string suture, or by sewing it up transversely in two layers, while trying to keep spills to a minimum. If you do soil his gut with faeces, suck them out immediately. Irrigate his peritoneal cavity thoroughly two or three times with liberal amounts of warm saline, preferably with tetracycline (2.9), and then suck this out.

DECOMPRESSION FOR INTESTINAL OBSTRUCTION

Be safe, and decompress a patient's gut if there is any risk of rupturing it, if gets in your way unduly, or if it prevents your closing his abdomen. Decompress it after you have brought it out of the wound, and closed it off well with packs, so that fluid will not soil his peritoneal cavity if it bursts.

If his caecum is distended, needle it, or decompress his transverse colon.

If his distension is mainly gaseous, as in the colon, needle that. You can also needle loops of small gut containing gas and fluid, provided you do it 'above the water line'.

RETROGRADE DECOMPRESSION is the method of choice, provided his gut is not too oedematous and friable. It is useful for his entire small gut and for much of his large gut, if his ileocaecal valve is incompetent. Start at his jejuno-ileal junction, and milk the contents proximally between your straight index and middle fingers. You may need some firm pressure on his proximal jejunum. When you have emptied enough fluid out of his jejunum, strip the fluid from his ileum into it and repeat the process. *As you decompress, ask the anaesthetist to keep aspirating fluid from his stomach.*

A SPINAL NEEDLE is only useful in the colon. Pack this off well. Push the needle through a taenia coli, and advance it longitudinally between the muscle coats for 3 cm. Then angle it inwards through the circular muscle to reach the lumen. Keep its point in the gas and clear of the fluid. If it blocks, pinch the rubber tube, then pinch it again distally. This should provide enough pressure in the needle to free it. If you insert the needle obliquely, there is no need to close the hole, which should not leak.

A YANKAUER SUCKER does not have a trocar, so it is difficult to use without spilling. Insert a purse string suture round the

DECOMPRESSING OBSTRUCTED GUT

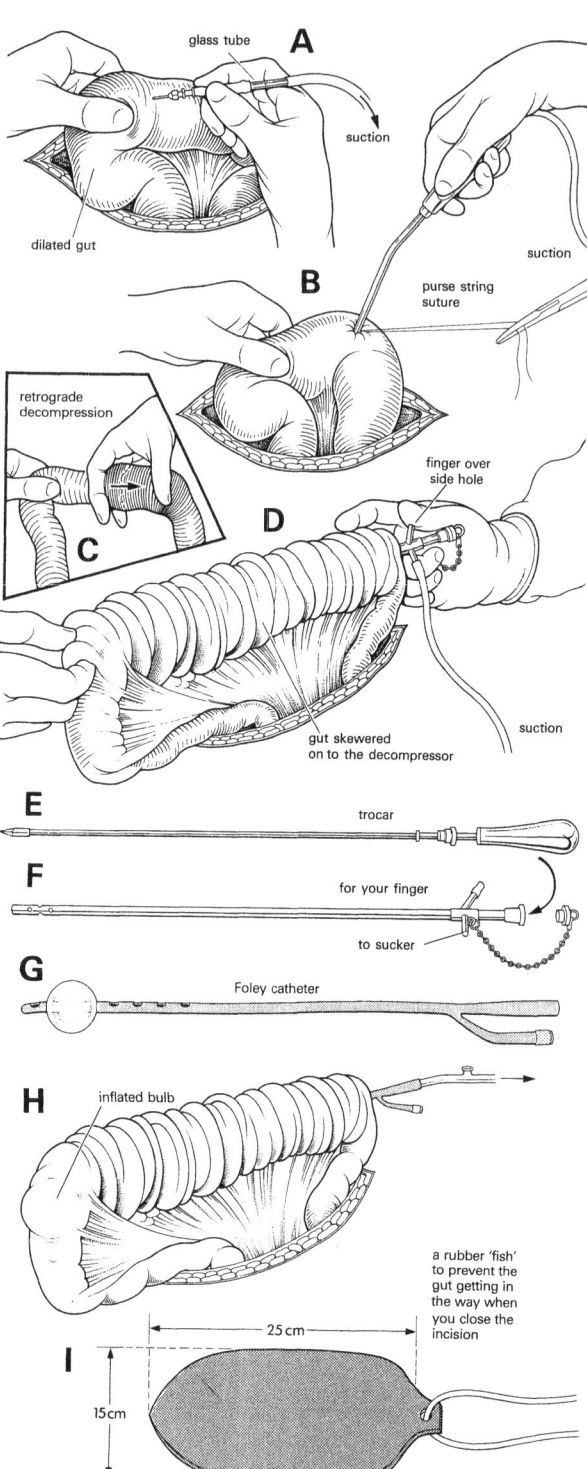

Fig. 10-9 DECOMPRESSING OBSTRUCTED GUT. A, using a needle. Note the glass tube, so that you can see what you are sucking. B, using a Yankauer sucker held in with a purse string suture. C, by retrograde stripping between your index and middle finger. D, E, and F, Savage's decompressor. G, and H, using a Foley catheter. Blow up its bulb after introducing it. Then milk the bulb along the gut. I, a rubber 'fish' to prevent gut getting in the way of an abdominal incision while you close it. Many surgeons think that C, if it works, is the best, and if C fails they use D. *The idea of the Foley catheter was kindly contributed by Georg Kamm.*

chosen site. Nick the seromuscular layer with a scalpel, raise it up and make the final incision through the mucosa. Then rapidly plunge the sucker through into the patient's gut, and close the purse string. Manipulate the sucker within his gut; eventually, the holes will plug up and you will have to withdraw it.

CAUTION ! When you have inserted a sucker, don't remove it unless you have to. If you have to remove it to clear it, pack off the peritoneal cavity to avoid spillage, and discard any contaminated 'lap pads'.

TO USE A SAVAGE DECOMPRESSOR insert a purse string suture on the antemesenteric border of his gut. Make an enterotomy incision in the centre of this, and push the decompressor with its trocar through. Withdraw the trocar and close the proximal opening of the decompressor with its threaded cap. With your thumb on the vent to control the degree of suction, start sucking out gas and fluid.

Pass the decompressor proximally and distally, carefully threading the distended loops of gut over it as you suck. To minimize clogging the holes, remove your finger from the vent from time to time. This will reduce the suction and let the food particles fall away. Or, more effectively, reintroduce the trocar.

When you have decompreessed enough gut (there is no need to decompress it all), remove the decompressor, close the purse string, and put it in the 'dirty basin'. Reinforce the purse string with a second layer of sutures, 3 mm beyond the first, going through the seromuscular layer only.

Alternatively, use a standard abdominal sucker. This is not so good, because it does not have a side tube, and blocks more easily.

TO USE A FOLEY CATHETER make a purse string suture and an enterotomy incision as above. Insert the catheter (with its side holes cut close to the balloon) connected to the sucker. Suck his gut empty. Then blow up the balloon and 'milk' it along his gut, sucking as you go. If it blocks, inject some saline and start again. Withdraw it, sucking as you go, then close the purse string.

Measure the fluid you have aspirated to see how much he has lost.

ON OPENING THE ABDOMEN IN INTESTINAL OBSTRUCTION

Here are some of the many things you might find, either immediately, or after a careful search.

If there is straw-coloured fluid in his abdomen, he has probably only got a simple obstruction.

If the fluid is very dark and foul-smelling, his gut has probably necrosed and strangulated, or recently perforated.

If pus is present, he has an inflammatory lesion somewhere.

If loops of his gut are red and congested, peritonitis is present.

If they are dusky and plum-coloured, they are strangulated—see below.

If a huge purple mass fills his abdomen, it is likely to be a strangulated sigmoid volvulus.

If most of his small gut is deeply congested and haemorrhagic, it has probably undergone volvulus.

FINDING THE CAUSE OF INTESTINAL OBSTRUCTION

First decide if the obstruction is proximal or distal to his caecum. In the developing world obstruction is more common proximal to the caecum than distal to it. Your task will be easier if you decompress his gut and then lift as many of its loops on to his abdominal wall as you can. Protect them by wrapping them in a moist 'lap pad' or in a sterile plastic bag.

If his caecum was distended when you opened his abdomen, the obstruction is distal to it, so feel his upper rectum and sigmoid. Then raise the left side of the incision and feel his descending colon. Then feel his splenic flexure, his transverse colon, his hepatic flexure, and his ascending colon.

If his caecum was collapsed, the obstruction must be in his small gut. First look for a strangulated hernia by palpating his hernial orifices from inside his abdomen—you should have examined them earlier from outside. If these are clear, ask your assistant to retract the right side of the lower end of the wound. Pick up the last loop of his ileum, start at his ilio-caecal junction, and run his small gut through your fingers, loop by loop, and then return it to his abdomen. Try to handle only collapsed gut distal to the obstruction, and not fragile distended gut proximal to it. *The place where collapsed gut meets distended gut is the site of the obstruction.*

If you find a loop which feels 'tethered', and you cannot lift it into view, it is probably the site of the obstruction. Expose this area well, by appropriate retraction, by packing gut away, and by lengthening the incision.

If you cannot find a collapsed loop, withdraw the distended loops and explore his pelvis and right iliac fossa.

If the obstruction is be difficult to find, remember that it is more likely to be in his small gut.

If you are not sure if a piece of gut is large or small, remember that large gut has taenia coli running over its surface.

If you don't know which piece of gut is proximal and which is distal, pass your hand down to the root of his mesentery, and remember that it runs obliquely downwards from left to right.

If you really are lost as to which way the gut goes, you have no alternative except to deliver the obstructed loops until you reach his duodenum proximally, or the obstructed focus distally.

CAUTION ! Don't try to rely on the standard differences between ileum and jejunum. Obstructed gut loses some of its characteristic features.

If you cannot find the cause of the obstruction, and yet his gut is grossly distended, decompress it—if you have not already done so—and search its length again.

IS HIS GUT VIABLE? Decide this by the criteria in Section 9.3 and Figure 9-8.

SPECIAL METHODS. See elsewhere for: obstruction due to bands and adhesions (10.7), inguinal hernias (14.6), femoral hernias (14.7), other hernias (Chapter 14), ascariasis (10.6), intussusception (10.8), volvulus of his small gut (10.9), sigmoid volvulus (10.10), volvulus of his caecum (10.11), and abdominal tuberculosis (29.5).

CLOSING THE ABDOMEN AFTER INTESTINAL OBSTRUCTION

Do this with particular care—a 'burst abdomen' is a major risk (9.13). Distension may also recur, hopefully only temporarily. Remember to bring his omentum down over his gut to separate it from his abdominal wall—this will often prevent adhesions, and is especially important if you have done an anastomosis.

Close his abdomen by Everett's or Goligher's methods in Section 9.8.

If his abdomen is difficult to close, decompress his small gut into his stomach, and again empty it by aspiration through his nasogastric tube. If necessary use the 'fish' in Fig. 10-9; and see Section 9.8.

If you have had to resect gut, or his peritoneum has been soiled, wash out his peritoneal cavity with warm saline or Ringer lactate, and instil tetracycline (6.2).

If there has been significant soiling, leave the skin edges unsutured for delayed primary closure (9.8).

POSTOPERATIVE CARE FOR INTESTINAL OBSTRUCTION

Continue nasogastric suction until he is passing flatus, his distension is becoming less, his bowel sounds are returning, and you are aspirating 400 ml or less of light-green fluid, which is his normal gastric secretion. Continue to keep an accurate fluid balance chart. Measure his urine output, and when necessary his CVP.

An adult *in the tropics* loses at least 3 litres of fluid a day (skin 1000 ml, lungs 500 ml, urine 1500 ml). Replace this with one litre of 0.9% saline and 2 litres of 5% dextrose. In a hot humid environment increase these volumes by 50% after the first 24–48 hours. Monitor his urine output: he should be passing at least 1500 ml by the third postoperative day.

Replace the fluid you aspirate from his stomach as in Section A 15.5. You can usually replace it with 0.9% saline or Ringer's lactate.

As soon as his postoperative diuresis starts (at 24–60 hours) replace the potassium he loses. His basic needs are about 40 mmol/24 hours. But if he still needs intravenous fluids after

48 hours, he may need up to 80 mmol of potassium a day, depending on the volume of secretions he has lost (A 15.1). Give it to him, either as a solution of 1 mmol/ml added to his intravenous fluids, or as Darrow's solution (K 34 mmol/litre) or as half-strength Darrow's.

If he has been very ill he may have a postoperative diuresis—see Section 53.3.

DIFFICULTIES WITH INTESTINAL OBSTRUCTION

If he is obstructed clinically, and yet you CANNOT FIND ANY CAUSE FOR THE OBSTRUCTION, the only useful thing to do may be to decompress his gut. He may have one of three kinds of pseudo-obstruction. (1) You may see many short (2 cm) intense spasms of his ileum, making it narrow like string, with gross dilatation in between. Try giving him pethidine. (2) His ileum may be distended down to its last metre or so, after which it gradually returns to its normal size. (3) You may see his colon hugely distended without any cause. Look for a retroperitoneal carcinomatous mass in the region of his pancreas, and remember the possibility of uraemia and Hirschprung's disease. Dilate his anus by Lord's procedure (22.5).

If you DON'T KNOW WHAT TO DO about an obstruction, and the situation looks very complex, one contributor advises you to consider bypassing the obstruction by anastomosing a distended to a collapsed loop. Or, if you cannot do this, to bring out the proximal loop of gut as an ileostomy, and then to refer him rapidly.

If his large or small gut is not viable, but you CANNOT DO AN ANASTOMOSIS, exteriorize it. Bring it out through a stab wound which is big enough to accommodate it. Stitch its margins, at a point where it is healthy, to the skin of his wound, so that it won't slip back inside. Close your laparotomy wound carefully. He now has an ileostomy of rather generous proportions, sticking out of a short wound in his flank. Either, cut off the non-viable bowel about 3 cm from his skin to form a double barrelled ileostomy, or refer him to an expert, as soon as you see he is going to survive the procedure. He will loose large volumes of small gut contents, which will have to be replaced—so referral is urgent! See Fig. 9-13.

If his BOWEL SOUNDS DO NOT RETURN, the fluid you aspirate does not decrease, and he becomes more distended, paralytic ileus is developing—see Section 10.13.

If he has DIARRHOEA postoperatively, don't be alarmed. This is common after any operation to relieve intestinal obstruction: it is a sign of recovery and usually clears up spontaneously. Measure his stools and replace them litre for litre with Ringer's lactate or normal saline with added potassium (A 15.5).

10.6 The surgery of ascariasis

Obstruction of the gut by *Ascaris* worms is the classical indication for non-operative treatment. Heavy infestations can obstruct a child's gut, partly or completely. The children of impoverished shanty-towns are most heavily infected, but in only a few of them is the infection so heavy that it obstructs their guts. The number of worms a child has is directly proportional to the number of ova he has swallowed. So the prevalence of Ascaris obstruction is a sensitive indicator of very poor hygienic conditions indeed. Sadly, the environment of many cities is deteriorating, and Ascaris obstruction is becoming more common.

A child between the ages of 2 and 14, or occasionally a young adult, usually has several mild attacks of central abdominal pain and vomiting, before his small gut finally obstructs. Often, he vomits worms, or they may come out of his nose, but this by itself is unimportant. If obstruction is partial, as it usually is when it is caused by a bolus of living worms, non-operative treatment commonly succeeds. Even if a solid mass of tightly-packed dead worms obstructs his gut completely, you can usually treat him nonoperatively.

Complete obstruction commonly follows an attempt to deworm a heavily infested child. It paralyses the worms, and so makes them even more likely to form a ball and obstruct his gut. *So wait to deworm a child until his obstruction has passed.* Don't operate if you can avoid it. If you have to operate, try not to open or resect gut. This is a particularly dirty and contaminating procedure in Ascaris obstruction, because an obstructed small gut contains bacteria that are normally only found in the large one. Instead, try to milk the worms through the small gut into the large one, whence they will be expelled naturally. The danger of opening the small gut or resecting it is that a fistula may follow—the patient with the fistula in Fig. 9-25 had his gut resected for Ascaris obstruction.

Ascaris worms occasionally obstruct a child's biliary tract and cause jaundice, or his appendix and cause appendicitis. Sometimes, they block drainage tubes. They can also penetrate a recent suture line, or the site of an injury, and cause peritonitis.

OBSTRUCTION DUE TO ASCARIS

For the general method for gut obstruction see Sections 10.1 and 10.3.

HISTORY. Enquire for: (1) Recent attacks of colicky abdominal pain. (2) Vomiting worms, or passing them rectally or nasally.

INTESTINAL OBSTRUCTION
caused by Ascaris

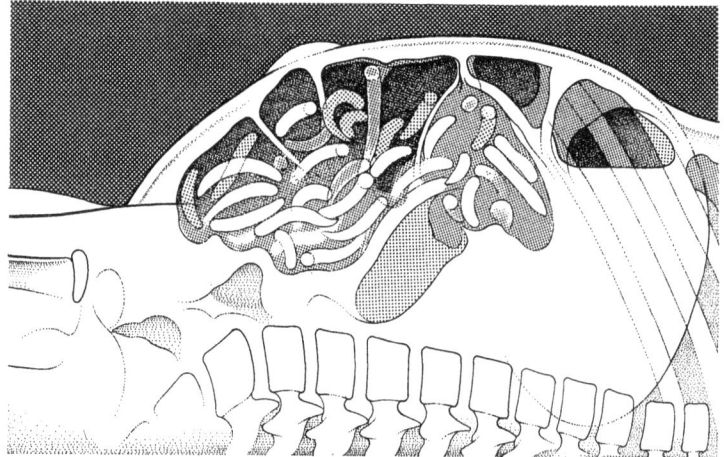

Fig. 10-10 INTESTINAL OBSTRUCTION caused by *Ascaris* worms. This is a lateral X-ray in the supine position. Note the fluid levels and gas-filled coils of gut. In the film from which this was drawn worms could easily be seen, but not quite as clearly as this! Typically, they are coiled in a mass, like 'Medusa's head'. *Kindly contributed by John Maina.*

EXAMINATION. The child is unwell and vomits. Distension is mild to moderate. There may be visible peristalsis. Feel for a mobile irregular mass in the centre of his abdomen, 5 to 10 cm in diameter, firm but not hard, and only moderately tender. This feels like a mass of worms, and he may have more than one mass. It may change in position and you may be able to feel the worms wriggling under your hand. If his abdomen is very distended the mass will be difficult to feel. Signs of peritoneal irritation are absent.

Examining stools for ova is of no help in a community where most children have worms.

X-RAYS show multiple fluid levels, and you may see the worms, as in Fig. 10-10. If you do see them, they are not necessarily the cause of his symptoms. Often, X-rays are not necessary, because you can make the diagnosis clinically.

THE DIFFERENTIAL DIAGNOSIS includes the other common causes of intestinal obstruction in childhood.

Suggesting intussusception—a more regular sausage-shaped mass, the passage of blood and mucus rectally, and tenderness which is more acute.

Suggesting an appendix abscess causing obstruction—the mass is not mobile, tenderness is more acute; a swinging temperature and toxaemia.

Suggesting an abdominal injury—tenderness and guarding are more prominent than the symptoms of obstruction and a mass; a bruise on the abdomen.

Suggesting congenital (Ladd's) bands—no characteristic mass, a very young child (28.3).

NON-OPERATIVE TREATMENT FOR ASCARIS OBSTRUCTION

INDICATIONS. The child's general condition is good, his colic is intermittent, and his vomiting is mild. There are no signs of peritoneal irritation.

METHOD. Give him nothing by mouth. Continue nasogastric suction until his obstruction resolves, or you decide to operate (rare). Give him intravenous fluids, as in Section A 15.5.

CAUTION ! (1) Don't try to deworm a child with partial or complete obstruction. Wait until the obstruction has gone—see below. (2) Don't give him purgatives—they may precipitate intussusception or volvulus.

LAPAROTOMY FOR ASCARIS OBSTRUCTION

INDICATIONS. A laparotomy is not often needed. The absolute indications for one are: (1) signs of perforation, which is usually caused by: (a) perforation of the gut by a worm (uncommon), or (b) by associated intussusception or volvulus (both uncommon). (2) Jaundice which you think might be caused by a worm in his bile duct.

The relative indications are less important, and are: (a) failure of the obstruction to resolve, (b) failure of the mass of worms to disappear.

INCISION. Make a right paramedian incision and inspect his gut. You will find a ball of worms blocking it.

If possible, try to break up the ball and milk the worms through to his caecum, where they will be safely expelled. If they are in his terminal ileum, this should be easy. If they are more proximal, try to milk them up into his stomach. This is less satisfactory, but it will relieve his obstruction.

If you cannot milk his worms upwards or downwards, and the wall of his gut is healthy, isolate the mass carefully with abdominal packs. Make a 2 cm *longitudinal* incision through the *antemesenteric border* of his healthy gut over the mass, and then remove the worms from the lumen with sponge forceps. Telescoping his gut over the forceps will help you to remove them proximally and distally.

Try to remove as many worms as you can by milking them down to and through the opening you have made. Most of them will probably be in his upper small gut. If you can remove most of them, there will be less chance of them working their way through the suture line later. If you have difficulty milking them out of his retroperitoneal duodenum—leave them. Close the enterotomy *transversely* in two layers, just as you would if you were doing a gut anastomosis (9.3). One contributor advises you to use non-absorbable sutures of silk, cotton, or nylon, on the grounds that the enzymes produced by the worms dissolve catgut, so that the wound is likely to fall open, leading to abscesses and fistulae. Make sure your nonabsorbable sutures are interrupted, so that they don't constrict his gut as he grows (9.3).

If the mass of worms has thinned, devitalized, or eroded his gut, resect it and do an end-to-end anastomosis (9-9 or 9-10). Some surgeons prefer this to an enterotomy, which is apt to be a septic process, even if the gut wall is healthy.

CAUTION ! If you have difficulty, don't be tempted to do an ileotransverse colostomy (9.6) above the level of the worms.

If you have done an enterotomy, his wound may become infected, so close his abdominal muscles as a single layer and leave his skin unsutured (9.8).

POSTOPERATIVE DEWORMING. Don't deworm him until 48 to 72 hours after all signs of obstruction have gone, and he has no palpable masses of worms. Then give him a single dose of piperazine citrate 4 g, which will paralyse his worms so that he passes them rectally. Or, give him mebendazole 100 mg twice daily for 3 days.

10.7 Obstruction by bands and adhesions

Bands and adhesions sometimes form outside a patient's gut and obstruct it. They are the result of some focus of infection being slowly converted into fibrous tissue, and can follow: (1) A previous abdominal operation, which may be followed by obstruction soon afterwards, as in Section 10.13, or later, as described below. You can reduce the probability of this happening by pulling his omentum down over his gut, and particularly the site of an anastomosis, before you close his abdomen after a laparotomy. This will reduce the chances of his gut sticking to his abdominal wall. (2) Abdominal sepsis of any kind, such as local or general peritonitis, an appendix abscess, a perforated peptic ulcer and especially PID (6.6). In communities where there is much PID, obstruction due to adhesions is common, and is apt to recur, so that a woman who has had one attack is likely to have another. (3) A congenital anomaly—congenital bands are unusual.

If a loop of gut has stuck to the parietal peritoneum at the site of an old scar, you can usually free it without too much difficulty, but even this can be dangerous because you can easily damage it. If PID has caused massive adhesions that have stuck loops of her gut firmly into her pelvis, releasing them may be very difficult. As you will soon learn, freeing them is an art.

Obstruction due to adhesions is less likely to strangulate than some other kinds of obstruction, and is more likely to be subacute, self-limiting, and recurrent, so you *may* be able to treat it non-operatively—if you are sure of the diagnosis!

BANDS AND ADHESIONS OBSTRUCTING THE GUT

For the general method for gut obstruction see Sections 10.1. and 10.3. For non-operative treatment, see Section 10.5. See also PID in Section 6.6.

INCISION. Open the patient's abdomen *with great care.* Always dissect under direct vision: so get good exposure, and keep the field dry. Don't use diathermy close to the gut wall: it too easily causes necrosis.

If he has had a previous paramedian incision, reopen his abdomen through it, unless this is difficult. Start above or below it in an area which is free of adhesions. Put a finger into the incision and explore the deep surface of the old scar. Work slowly with a sharp scalpel and detach the adherent gut from under it.

If he had a transverse or oblique incision previously, make a median or paramedian one now.

If he had a vertical midline incision, reopen that instead of making a parallel paramedian incision, because the intervening skin may necrose. Start in normal skin at one end where, hopefully, there will be no adhesions.

SEPARATING ADHESIONS

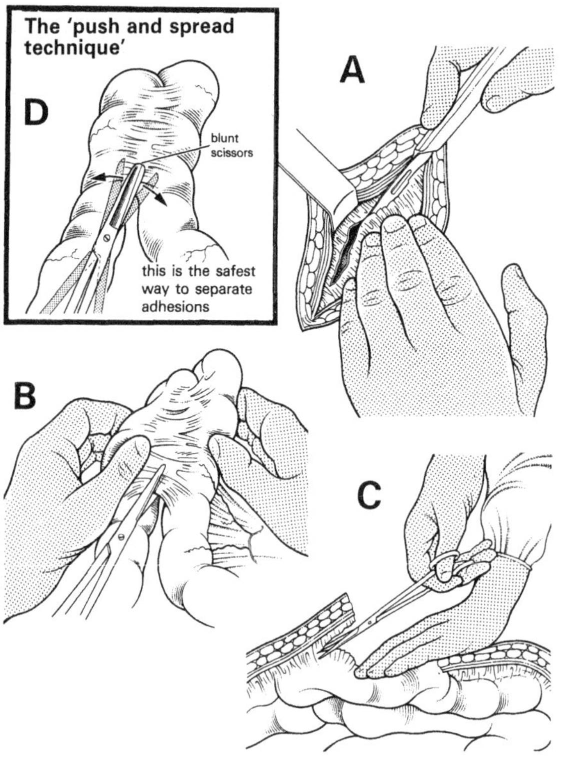

Fig. 10-11 SEPARATING ADHESIONS. The great danger is that you may perforate the patient's gut: A, on entering his abdomen. B, on cutting adhesions between two loops of gut. C, when freeing adhesions between his gut and his abdominal wall, or (not shown) when closing his abdomen in the presence of obstructed gut. D, the safest way to separate adhesions is to use the 'push and spread technique' (4-8; preferably use Metzenbaum's or McIndoe's scissors, which are not so blunt as those shown here).

If you have to enter his abdomen through the site of multiple adhesions, dissect them away with the utmost care and patience.

If his gut has completely stuck to his abdominal wall, be prepared to excise a piece of the adherent peritoneum when necessary, rather than damage his gut.

FREEING THE ADHESIONS. Look for the site of the obstruction, which may be a band with a knuckle or loop of gut caught under it. This has a 95% chance of being in his small gut and a 75% chance of being in his ileum. Use the 'push and spread technique' with blunt tipped Metzenbaum's or McIndoe's scissors (D, 10-11 and B, 4-8). Use the outer sides of the blades to spread the tissues. If you work carefully, you can define tissues when they are matted together, by opening up tissue planes, and without injuring anything. You will see what is gut, and what is an adhesion, and will be able to cut in greater safety. Work away at one site and then at another until the adherent loops unravel.

Alternatively, use the 'pinching technique'. Pinch your index finger and thumb together between two loops of adherent gut.

Gentle traction will help you to dissect the loops of his gut free from one another. Grip them firmly with moist gauze, and release it periodically, to help you to identify what you are cutting, and to control bleeding.

When you have divided a band, you will want to know if the trapped gut is viable or not—do this using the criteria in Section 9.3 and Fig. 9-8.

If you can squeeze gut contents past a kink in the gut, you can probably leave it safely. Don't try to cut every adhesion you see. Freeing them can go on indefinitely, and can be dangerous. If there are adhesions between loops which are not causing obstruction, leave them.

CAUTION ! Work slowly and carefully. Making a hole in the gut wall increases greatly the postoperative morbidity, especially the risk of a fistula (9.14).

DIFFICULTIES WITH INTESTINAL ADHESIONS

If BLEEDING OBSTRUCTS YOUR WORK, apply gentle pressure with a warm moist pack. Leave it alone for a few minutes, and dissect somewhere else.

If you STRIP UP THE SEROSA WITH SOME OF THE MUSCLE layer, leave it. But, if you open his gut, close it carefully in two layers. If the edges of the defect are ragged, trim them neatly, so that you only use full-thickness gut for closure—*make sure that there is no obstruction distal to the point of repair!* If there is, a fistula is sure to form.

If COILS OF GUT ARE FIRMLY STUCK down in the pelvis, try to carefully pinch them off the pelvic wall. If you fail, bypass them with an entero-enterostomy (29-8). This is a safe way out of a difficult problem, provided that a long length of small gut is not bypassed. Choose an easily accessible loop of gut proximal to the obstruction, and anastomose it side-to-side with a collapsed loop distally. Some of the absorptive surface of the patient's gut will be lost, but you will have saved her life (she is usually female). If necessary, another operation can be done later when she is in better condition. This is a common and difficult gynaecological problem.

10.8 Intussusception

This takes several forms—you will see the first one in children, and the others in adults: (1) All over the world a child's ileum may telescope into his caecum and colon and cause an ileocaecal or ileo-colic intussusception. These are the common types, and there is no point in trying to make a fine distinction between them. In some areas this also happens in adults (Uganda, and Natal). (2) An adult's caecum can intussuscept into his ascending colon. This is the caeco-colic variety, which is common in the Ibadan area of Nigeria. (3) Amoebiasis or a tumour of the colon at any age can cause it to intussuscept into itself (colo-colic, rare). (4) Rarely also a tumour of the ileum can cause it to intussuscept into itself (ileo-ileal). The relative frequency of these varieties differs considerably from one area to another. In the industrial world intussusception of any kind is rare in adults.

The danger of any intussusception is that the patient's gut may strangulate—usually the inner part (intussusceptum), but occasionally also the outer one (intussuscipiens). Intussusception is thus always a strangulation obstruction, or is potentially so. But remember that: (1) The signs of peritoneal irritation are initially absent, because the gangrenous intussusceptum is covered by the initially normal intussuscipiens. (2) Intussusception may occur backwards, because gut contractions may be reversed (unusual).

The childhood type of intussusception presents with symptoms of intestinal obstruction and can take two forms: (1) Primary intussusception has a shorter history and is less likely to present with abdominal distension and a palpable mass. (2) Secondary intussusception follows diarrhoea, with or without vomiting and dehydration; it has a longer history and is more likely to present with a mass and distension. Blood and mucus are commonly passed rectally in both types, with the result that intussusception is often misdiagnosed as 'diarrhoea'.

In the developed world the child is usually between 6 months and 2½ years; in the developing world he may be as old as 7 or 8. He draws up his knees in spasms of colicky pain. He vomits, and may pass 'red currant jelly' stools. You can usually feel a sausage-shaped abdominal mass in the line of his transverse and descending colons, above and to the left of his umbilicus, with its concavity directed towards his umbilicus. His right lower quadrant feels rather empty. His abdomen is seldom much distended, so that the mass is usually quite easy to feel. Rarely, it is hidden under his right costal margin, or is in his pelvis, where you may be able to feel it bimanually. Sometimes, the apex of the intussusceptum presents at his anus, or you may feel it rectally, and see blood and mucus on your finger afterwards. If you do see a mass at his anus, be careful to distinguish an intussusception from a rectal prolapse (22.9).

The clue is to find a shifting mass, which moves as his intussusceptum forces its way down his gut, and then returns to its starting point. Occasionally, a child's intussusception reduces itself, so that his symptoms come and go spontaneously.

The adult type of intussusception may be ileo-colic, caeco-colic or colo-colic. In the caeco-colic type the apex of the intussusception is that part of the patient's caecum which is opposite his ileo-caecal valve. His ileum is drawn up into his caecum, and with it, his appendix, but they seldom strangulate.

Colicky pain usually starts suddenly, but its onset may be gradual. At first, the obstruction is not complete, his abdomen is not markedly distended, and he may have diarrhoea, with or without the passage of bloody mucus. Feel for a sausage-shaped mass in his epigastrium in the line of his colon. During an episode of colic the lump hardens, and you may be able to hear a chorus of obstructive bowel sounds as it does so.

At operation, you should be able to reduce about 80% of intussusceptions by *gentle* manual reduction. If you fail you can: (1) Do a resection and anastomosis; often this need only involve part of the lesion. The danger, when you do it, is that he may die from peritonitis if you fail to remove all nonviable gut. (2) You can exteriorize the lesion, close the abdominal incision, and then resect his gangrenous gut to make an ostomy, which will have to be closed later, hopefully by an expert. By doing this, you may avoid contaminating his peritoneal cavity and improve his chances of survival. Don't try to reduce an intussusception with a barium enema.

Exteriorization is is a messy but life-saving procedure. In the ileo-colic type of childhood intussusception, you have first to mobilize the child's gut, so that you can bring his strangulated terminal ileum, his caecum, and his ascending colon out to the surface (his ileum has a mesentery, so that it is already more or less 'mobilized'). To do this you have to free up his ascending colon, and carefully tie off the vessels which supply the part you are going to exteriorize. When you have done this, he will find himself with a temporary ileostomy, but you will have saved his life. You will however have to replace the quantities of fluid he loses from his stoma, and, if possible, refer him to have this closed. Or, you will have to close it yourself by crushing the spur between the two loops of his gut (9.5).

COLIC, AN ABDOMINAL MASS, AND DIARRHOEA?—
THINK OF INTUSSUSCEPTION!

Hulme-Moir I, 'Paediatric Intussusception in Moshi'. Tropical Doctor 1979;2:114-118.

INTUSSUSCEPTION

Follow the general method for gut obstruction in Section 10.4. Correct the patient's fluid and electrolyte deficit, and pass a nasogastric tube. Treat any medical complications vigorously—pneumonia, malaria, measles, gastroenteritis, and convulsions.

CHILDHOOD ILEO-CAECAL INTUSSUSCEPTION

X-RAYS. You will see the ordinary signs of any small gut obstruction—a dilatated gut with fluid levels. There are also some other more specific but rather difficult ones: (1) An empty right iliac fossa with no caecal gas shadow. (2) A soft tissue mass. (3) A 'ground glass' appearance to the child's abdomen, especially on the right, due to exudate.

MANUAL REDUCTION. Make a short right paramedian incision, insert two fingers, and feel for the mass. Retract the edges of the wound and try to lift out the mass. Look at it to see which way the intussusception goes, backwards or forwards.

If the outer layer of the intussusception looks viable, try to reduce it by manipulation. If it is not viable proceed immediately to exteriorize it, as described below, or to resection and anastomosis, if you have had some experience of bowel surgery.

If the intussusception has not gone beyond his splenic flex-

INTUSSUSCEPTIONS

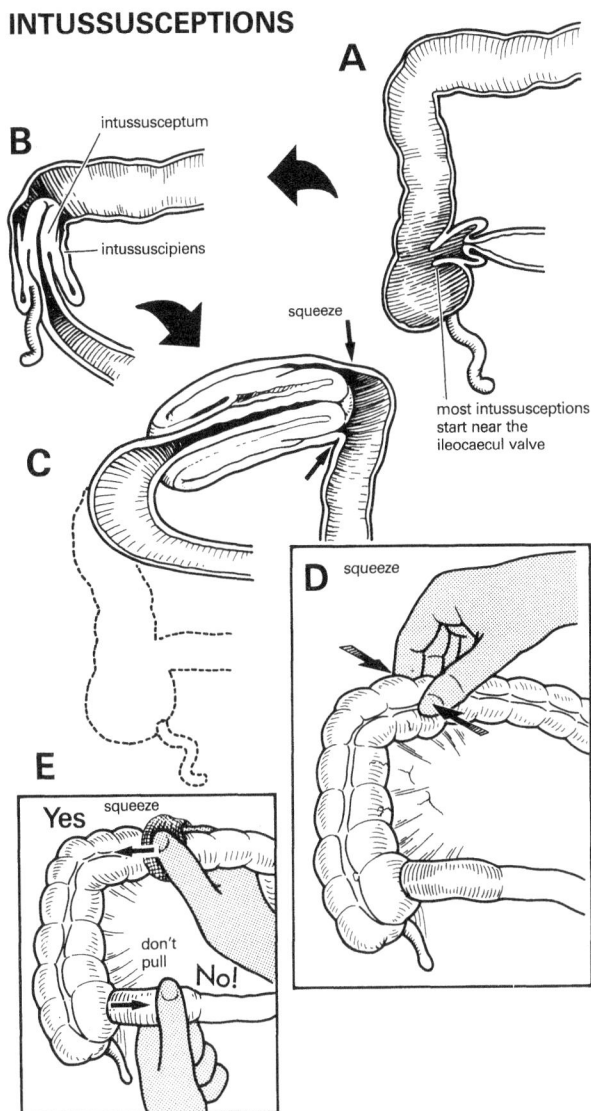

Fig. 10-12 INTUSSUSCEPTION. A, B, and C, stages in the development of the common ileo-colic intussusception in children. D, squeeze the colon that contains the leading edge of the intussusception. In practice the caecum does not move quite as far as is shown in C, because it is fixed to the posterior abdominal wall. E, don't try to reduce an intussusception by pulling. *Partly after Ravitch et al., 'Paediatric Surgery', Fig 93-3. Yearbook Medical, with kind permission.*

ure, manual reduction should not be too difficult. But if it has reached his sigmoid colon, or if it has lasted more than 24 hours, you may have trouble.

Using a thick, moist gauze 'lap pad' between the thumb and index finger of your right hand, apply gentle pressure to the part of his colon which contains the leading edge of the intussusception. Reduce it from its apex proximally. Use the gauze to transmit the pressure to as wide an area of his gut as you can. Squeeze it gently, so as to make the mass go proximally. Be patient, and change the position of your squeezing hand as necessary. The intussusception will usually reduce itself quickly.

Manual reduction will be most difficult near the end, and the seromuscular layers of his gut usually split. Persist up to a point. Abandon reduction if: (1) Splitting becomes deep. (2) You cannot reduce his intussusception any further. (3) You see a necrotic area of gut (the intussusceptum) emerging proximally.

If you split the serous and muscular coats of the last few centimetres of the child's gut as you reduce it, don't worry. This usually happens. Provided his mucosa is intact and his gut is not gangrenous, it will heal.

CAUTION ! (1) Do all the reduction by squeezing. (2) Don't

pull the proximal end. (3) Try to reduce the last dimple, or the intussusception may recur. (4) Make sure the apex is viable, because this is the part which is most likely to become gangrenous.

If, after manual reduction, any part of his terminal ileum, caecum, or ascending colon is gangrenous, exteriorize them. If you are inexperienced, this is probably safer than trying to do an end-to-side anastomosis—you will probably contaminate the peritoneal cavity if you try, and the tissue will probably not hold your stitches.

EXTERIORIZATION FOR INTUSSUSCEPTION

Examine the proximal and distal ends of his strangulated gut to find parts which you are sure are healthy. Protect the area with carefully applied towels. Apply Babcock forceps or a silk ligature to healthy gut at least 3 cm away from either end of the gangrenous area.

TO MOBILIZE THE CHILD'S ASCENDING COLON stand on his left side and ask an assistant to retract the right side of the wound, so as to expose his caecum and ascending colon. Use a pair of long blunt-tipped dissecting scissors to incise the peritoneal layer 2 cm lateral to his ascending colon. Free his colon as in Fig. 66-20 using the 'push and spread technique' (4-8). Put a moist pack over his colon and draw it towards you, so as to stretch his peritoneum in his right paracolic gutter.

As you incise his peritoneum, draw his entire colon medially, from his caecum to his hepatic flexure. Use a 'swab on a stick' to push away any structure which sticks to its posterior surface—especially his duodenum and his ureter, which runs downwards about 5 cm medially to his colon, and which you should identify and preserve.

As you lift his caecum and ascending colon medially, you will see his ileocolic vessels which supply them. Hold up his colon and try to see them against the light.

Make windows in his peritoneum on the medial side of his colon, and clamp the branches of these vessels, one by one, 3 cm medial to the wall of his colon. Insert two haemostats through each window and cut between them, leaving a cuff of tissue distal to the proximal hamostat. Then tie the vessels held in each haemostat with No. 1/0, 2/0 or 3/0 chromic catgut or silk, depending on the size of the child. Tie them twice on the proximal side for safety.

If you cannot find the blood vessels because strangulation has altered his anatomy, lift up his colon and apply haemostats to the mesentery close to the wall of his colon. Cut between them and his colon, until it is completely free.

Apply haemostats to the mesentery of his ileum 2 cm from his gut, and cut between them until you reach healthy gut supplied by a visibly pulsating vessel. Raise his greater omentum towards his head, and use scissors to separate the filmy adhesions between it and his hepatic flexure.

Mobilize his hepatic flexure under direct vision. Cut peritoneum only and draw the flexure downwards and medially. Free his colon from his duodenum with 'a swab on a stick'.

You should now be able to lift his strangulated gut out of the wound, free of all its peritoneal, mesenteric, and vascular attachments. As you lift it up, make sure that there is healthy gut above skin level at both ends.

TO MAKE THE COLOSTOMY if possible, use a separate incision for the bowel and thread it through, as in Fig. 9-19. This is much better than exteriorizing his gut through the paramedian incision, which is an alternative.

Make a transverse colostomy incision, as in Fig. 9-19. Bring the healthy parts of his ileum and colon together, and thread them through this incision.

Alternatively (and less satisfactorily), bring them out at the top of his paramedian incision.

In either case, bring his ileum and colon together to form a double-barrelled colostomy-cum-ileostomy. Apply a series of seromuscular sutures for about 5 cm. Attach the joined parts of his ileum and his colon to the cut edges of his peritoneum. Three sutures on each side will probably be enough.

CAUTION ! (1) Check again that viable gut extends 2 cm above his skin. (2) Make sure that there is no tension on his ileum or colon inside his abdomen.

Close his abdominal wound including his skin. Make sure you have not closed it too tightly round his gut. Can you easily slide a finger down beside it?

Place two clamps across each end of his exteriorized gut. Cut between the two clamps and leave the two proximal clamps on. Secure them in place with strapping, or suture the mucosa to the skin at this stage.

POSTOPERATIVELY, remove the two clamps on his abdominal wall 24 hours later. By this time the two ends of his gut should have sealed to his skin enough to prevent contamination.

There are several ways you can manage his ileostomy, either alone or in combination: (1) You can fit him with a standard ileostomy bag. (2) You can use the makeshift bag in Fig. 9-16. (3) You can protect his skin with zinc oxide cream, barrier cream, or karya gum powder, which will help to protect his skin. Change his dressings frequently. (4) You can give him codeine to slow down peristalsis, so that he forms a semisolid stool. (4) You can nurse him in a prone position with his hips and chest supported on several pillows so as to allow the contents of his ileum to discharge by gravity, as in Fig. 9-13.

Refer him rapidly—if possible within 48 hours—for careful electrolyte control, and for elective surgery to restore the continuity of his gut. Manage his fluid losses as best you can meanwhile (A 15.5).

If you cannot refer him, wait 2 to 3 weeks—if he survives this long— and apply a clamp to the spur between the two loops of gut, as in G, Fig. 9-19. This will cause pressure necrosis, so that the contents of his gut can pass from his ileum to his colon.

RESECTION AND ANASTOMOSIS FOR INTUSSUSCEPTION

The most suitable kind of anastomosis depends on the type of intussusception.

For an ileo-colic lesion, do an end-to-side anastomosis (9.4).
For an ileo-ileal lesion do an end-to-end anastomosis (9.3).
For a colo-colic lesion do an end-to-end anastomosis (9.3), with a proximal colostomy (9.5).

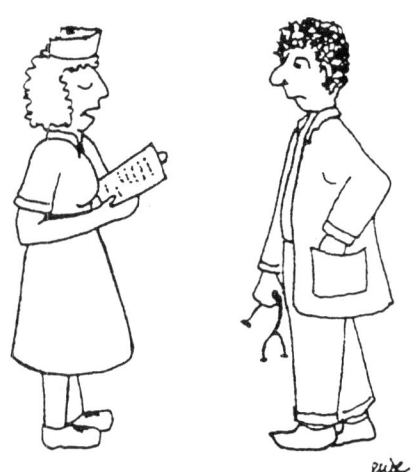

'Mr Y is asking to have his whole-gut irrigation with beer, Doctor.'

10.9 Volvulus of the small gut

In the industrial world volvulus of the small gut is rare, except in babies and small children, but in much of the developing world it is seen at all ages, particularly in young men. The small gut rotates on its mesentery, or on a band 5–10 cm from the ileocaecal valve, which tethers it to the posterior abdominal wall. As it rotates it traps large volumes of blood and fluid. Most of the small gut may rotate, apart from its top and bottom ends, or only a smaller part. Sometimes, an adhesion to a loop of small gut starts the twist, or the patient may have a primary sigmoid volvulus, and loops of his small gut may twist around this (10-17).

Volvulus of the small gut is a sudden deadly illness in which the symptoms of acute obstruction rapidly become those of strangulation. As his mesenteric vessels occlude, and his gut strangulates, he has a sudden severe diffuse abdominal pain and vomits copiously. A typical history is of sudden abdominal colic, distension and vomiting, coming on after a large evening meal. Early on, he looks ill and has a fast pulse and a low blood pressure—his abdomen may be fairly relaxed and not particularly tender at this stage. You may feel an ill-defined mass, but high pitched bowel sounds and a few loops with a fluid level may be the only signs of a dangerous volvulus. A notable feature is the speed with which his abdomen distends. He is in severe pain, and is always shocked. Later, his abdominal muscles become rigid. If his strangulation is not relieved, his gut eventually becomes gangrenous. You will also see: (1) Mild cases with a typical history, but no signs other than mild abdominal distension, who recover spontaneously. (2) Cases which progress slowly and which are difficult to distinguish from other forms of ileal obstruction.

In theory, treatment is easy—untwist his gut. One of your difficulties will be to make the diagnosis, when all you see at laparotomy are distended loops of small gut. Manipulating them is dangerous, whether or not they are strangulated. If a loop ruptures, he will be lucky to survive the flooding of his abdomen that results. He has about a 30% chance of death, but if he lives his volvulus will not recur.

VOLVULUS OF THE SMALL GUT

For the general method for gut obstruction see Sections 10.1 and 10.3. Resuscitate the patient vigorously.

X-RAYS show distended small gut, sometimes with a regular horizontal step-ladder pattern, and many fluid levels in the erect film.

CAUTION ! When a strangulated closed loop is distended with blood, there may be no fluid levels, so that the X-rays look normal.

INCISION. Make a midline or a right paramedian incision. You will find purple, congested, haemorrhagic, distended small gut full of food and fluid. A collapsed caecum shows that the obstruction is in his small gut.

Try to reach the base of his mesentery. Approach this by first putting your hand down into his pelvis, and then up along the posterior border of his abdominal wall. Usually, the whole of his small gut is twisted, except the first few centimetres of his jejunum and his terminal ileum. Rotate the whole mass until his volvulus is undone. If you find a band near his ileo-caecal valve, dividing it may help you to reduce the volvulus.

Deliver his gut, untwist it, pack it with moist towels, *and decompress it.* Do this before you assess its viability. Push fluid proximally (10-9), or distally into his caecum through his ileo-caecal valve. This will probably be more satisfactory than doing an enterotomy and using Savage's decompressor. If you decide to use one, do so through an incision *in healthy gut* distal to the point of torsion.

If you have difficulty untwisting his gut before you decompress it, decompress it first. Introduce the decompressor into a distended loop through a single or double purse string suture, and decompress it proximally and distally.

If his gut is viable (usual), leave it. If it is not viable, resect and anastomose it (9.3). If you are not sure if his gut is viable or not, assess it as in Fig. 9-8. Wait for at least 10 minutes before you decide that it is gangrenous.

If the gangrenous section ends above his ileo-caecal valve, resect it and do an end-to-end anastomosis

If his gut is gangrenous down to his caecum (unusual), do an ileo-colic anastomosis.

CAUTION ! Be sure to select healthy gut for the anastomosis, with obviously visible pulsations in the vessels that supply it—a serious and sometimes fatal complication is a fistula due to necrosis of the gut at the site of the anastomosis.

Continue nasogastric suction and intravenous fluids postoperatively. He may need blood.

10.10 Volvulus of the sigmoid colon

A high-fibre diet has many advantages, which are said to include the low incidence of appendicitis, and a much lower incidence of carcinoma and diverticula of the colon. But it may have at least one disadvantage. A large sigmoid colon distended with the gas of a high-fibre diet is more liable to twist on its mesentery. This is the commonest cause of large gut obstruction in most communities in the developing world, particularly in Africa, and is sufficiently characteristic to allow you to diagnose it before you do a laparotomy. If an obstructed sigmoid colon strangulates, its wall will become gangrenous, and may perforate. Sigmoid volvulus is however less dangerous and more common than volvulus of the small gut.

There are several kinds of sigmoid volvulus: (1) The common volvulus of the large thick-walled pelvic colon that is usual in people who eat a high-fibre diet, and which usually presents subacutely. (2) The less common volvulus of the thin-walled type of pelvic colon which usually presents acutely. (3) A rare compound volvulus in which the small gut twists around a volvulus of the sigmoid (see under 'Difficulties' at the end of this section).

The common subacute volvulus typically occurs in an adult man (it is rare in women) whose first symptom is difficulty passing flatus. This is followed over a few days by increasing abdominal distension, so that by the time you see him his abdomen is hugely distended and tympanitic ('like a drum'), but is not very painful or tender. He may be so distended, especially on the left, that he is hardly able to breathe. Despite the distension, his abdomen is usually soft enough for you to be able to feel his sigmoid as an enormous loop rising out of his pelvis, like a motor cycle tyre, towards one or other costal margin. Vomiting is unusual, except perhaps once at the start of the attack. His general condition is usually good: he can drink and is not dehydrated. The contrast between his satisfactory general state, and his huge abdomen is striking—unless he presents late, in severe shock.

He may have had several previous milder attacks, during which twisting and subsequent release of his colon caused abdominal pain and constipation, followed by diarrhoea with much flatus.

The uncommon acute volvulus seems to occur more frequently in areas where sigmoid volvulus is relatively uncommon. Of the few women who do have volvulus, most have the acute form. A patient's first symptom is colicky, central lower abdominal pain, which is severe enough to make him seek early treatment. At the onset he may have an urge to defaecate, but only passes a small stool, perhaps followed by a little blood. He may vomit at the onset, and frequently later.

He is anxious and in pain, his pulse is rapid, his temperature raised, and his blood pressure low. His abdomen is only moderately distended, but it is tense and tender, and the individual loops

VOLVULUS OF THE SMALL GUT

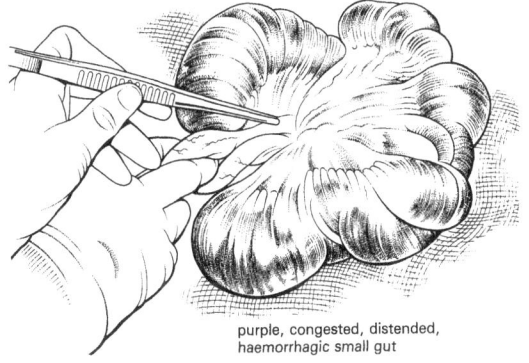

Fig. 10-13 VOLVULUS OF THE SMALL GUT is a sudden deadly illness in which the symptoms of obstruction progress rapidly to those of strangulation. *Kindly contributed by Gerald Hankins.*

of his colon are difficult to feel. He has nearly a 50% chance of developing gangrene, peritonitis, and shock within 24 hours.

Some patients fall midway between these two extremes. Remember also that gangrene may occur after many days of subacute volvulus.

X-rays are useful—an erect abdominal film is usually diagnostic: (1) In the subacute form there is a huge gas shadow like an inverted 'U' reaching from his pelvis to his upper abdomen, inclining right or left, often with smaller fluid levels proximal to the loop (A, 10-14). (2) A supine film may show three dense curved lines converging on his left sacroiliac joint. The middle line is the most constant one, and is caused by two walls of the distended loop lying pressed together (B, 10-14).

Management. Subacute volvulus is an obstruction to the passage of flatus, usually without damage to a patient's gut or its blood supply. You can usually relieve it without operation. (1) Try to deflate his dilated sigmoid colon with a sigmoidoscope. You have a 50% to 90% chance of success, depending on the area. (2) If you fail do a laparotomy: (a) If his sigmoid is gangrenous, he has a 50% chance of death. You will have to resect it urgently, either by exteriorization or by Hartmann's procedure (10-16), depending on how much of it is gangrenous, and whether or not you can bring the distal end of his gut to the surface. (b) If his sigmoid is not gangrenous you can untwist it. This will relieve his immediate symptoms, but it is not sufficient treatment, because his volvulus has at least a 30% chance of recurring (some say 90%). After a second attack it has a 60% chance of doing so. To avoid this: (i) You can close his abdomen and ask him to return later for an interval resection of his colon, or you can refer him to have this done. Unfortunately, he will probably think himself cured, and so be unlikely to return. (ii) You can resect his colon and leave him with a temporary pelvic colostomy—which will certainly make him return! (iii) You can resect and anastomose his colon, and protect it with a transverse colostomy. Whatever you decide to do, don't just do a resection and anastomosis, without doing a protective transverse colostomy also—the risk of peritonitis is too great.

If you are unskilled, (i) is best. If you have some experience do (ii) or (iii). An interval resection of the sigmoid colon involves excising his sigmoid and joining its ends. This is a moderately difficult elective procedure, so it is not described here.

The main danger in deflating a patient with a sigmoidoscope is that you may miss gangrene, and not operate when you should. But this should be rare, if you follow the method described below. An intussusception usually shows you that gut is gangrenous by the passage of blood and mucus rectally. Unfortunately, a gangrenous sigmoid colon rarely produces these clues, so that finding out if it is gangrenous or not is more difficult.

If you have to resect a sigmoid colon, you can always mobilize enough healthy descending colon proximally to reach the surface of the patient's skin and make a colostomy. If he has enough healthy colon distally, you can exteriorize his gangrenous sigmoid, and make a double-barrelled colostomy out of both ends (9-19 and 10-16). But, if his sigmoid is gangrenous right down to his rectosigmoid junction, he will not have not enough healthy colon distally to reach his abdominal wall. So you will have to do close his rectum and drop it back into his pelvis (Hartmann's operation).

If he has enough healthy colon distal to the the diseased segment to reach the skin of his abdominal wall (there is always enough proximally), you can, if you wish, exteriorize (9.6) the gangrenous area. Take it out of his abdominal cavity, close the wound round it, and then cut off the gangrenous part. This reduces the risk of contaminating his peritoneal cavity. If his abdomen is very distended, you may have to do this through the main wound, rather than a stab wound, which is preferable.

If possible, refer him to have his colostomy or Hartmann's procedure closed. If not, close his colostomy as in Section 9.5 and Hartmann's procedure as in Section 10.10a. He will not like being left with a colostomy.

Temporary colostomy as a permanent treatment for sigmoid volvulus. As we go to press an account has just reached us of simple one-stage method of treating non-gangrenous cases of sigmoid volvulus. If his sigmoid is viable you can pass a Foley catheter into it through his abdominal wall. When you withdraw the catheter the stoma will close spontaneously, and enough adhesions will have formed to make recurrence unusual. This appears to be a useful method for the inexperienced operator who does not want to attempt elective sigmoid resection (the best method).

Odonga AM, 'Varieties of intestinal volvuli seen at Mulago Hospital Kampala' (1966—1975), East African Medical Journal 1982;59:711-7.

Mout P, 'Temporary colostomy as a permanent treatment for sigmoid volvulus: a simple and safe one-stage procedure'. Tropical Doctor 1989;19:28-30.

IF YOU SUSPECT GANGRENE, OPERATE

SIGMOID VOLVULUS

For the general method for gut obstruction see Sections 10.3 and 10.4.

DIFFERENTIAL DIAGNOSIS. Carcinomatous obstruction of the left colon or rectum is the main one (a rectal examination should exclude the latter). The enormous gastric distension of pyloric obstruction can confuse you; so can caecal volvulus.

Suggesting carcinoma of the colon—a change from a normal bowel habit to constipation over a much longer period; a smoothly distended abdomen without obvious coils of colon; X-rays showing caecal distension, and not the characteristic signs of sigmoid volvulus.

CAUTION ! Be on your guard if the patient is a woman. In Uganda volvulus in a woman is likely to be acute or compound.

MANAGEMENT. Suspect that a patient's gut has strangulated if: (1) His symptoms started abruptly, with severe pain, especially radiating to his back. (2) He is ill, with a raised pulse, fever, or a low blood pressure. (3) He has signs of peritonism—tenderness, guarding, and absent bowel sounds. (4) His mucosa is discoloured at the limit of sigmoidoscopy. (5) A rectal tube yields blood-stained fluid. (6) X-rays show gas in his peritoneal cavity. This is likely to be a late sign and mean that an operation is almost hopeless.

If you suspect strangulation do an immediate laparotomy.

If he presents in a subacute attack, and you are fairly sure of the diagnosis, and do not suspect gangrene, deflate him at sigmoidoscopy.

DEFLATION AT SIGMOIDOSCOPY. A sigmoidoscope, a well lubricated rectal tube—and a sense of humour! If you don't have a sigmoidoscope, or its light does not work, you may succeed in deflating him with a soft rubber tube while he is in the knee-elbow position. Take blood for cross-matching.

Take him to the theatre, prepared for a laparotomy, in case sigmoidoscopy fails, or you perforate his gut. Put him into the knee-elbow position, as in G, Fig. 10-14. The weight of fluid in the loop will pull the apex out straight. You will also be less likely to get an eyeful of faeces when an explosive burst from the rectal tube splatters you in the face. Pass the sigmoidoscope (22.1). It usually travels 15 cm before it reaches a point where the lumen is narrowed and the colon is twisted, but you may have to pass it to 30 cm. When you reach the twist, look at the mucosa carefully.

CAUTION ! (1) Don't anaesthetize him or give him a heavy sedative. Pain during or after sigmoidoscopy is a useful indication of trauma or gangrene. (2) If his sigmoid is gangrenous, deflating it is dangerous; you may perforate it. (3) Insufflating air is undesirable, because escaping air mimics successful decompression. (4) Don't pass a sigmoidoscope more than 5 cm without seeing where you are going. (5) Don't use too much force—you may push it through his colon. (6) Wear suitable clothes and shoes, because a huge quantity of flatus and fluid will rush out.

If you see any discoloration through the sigmoidoscope, or any blood-stained fluid, or there is recurrent pain,

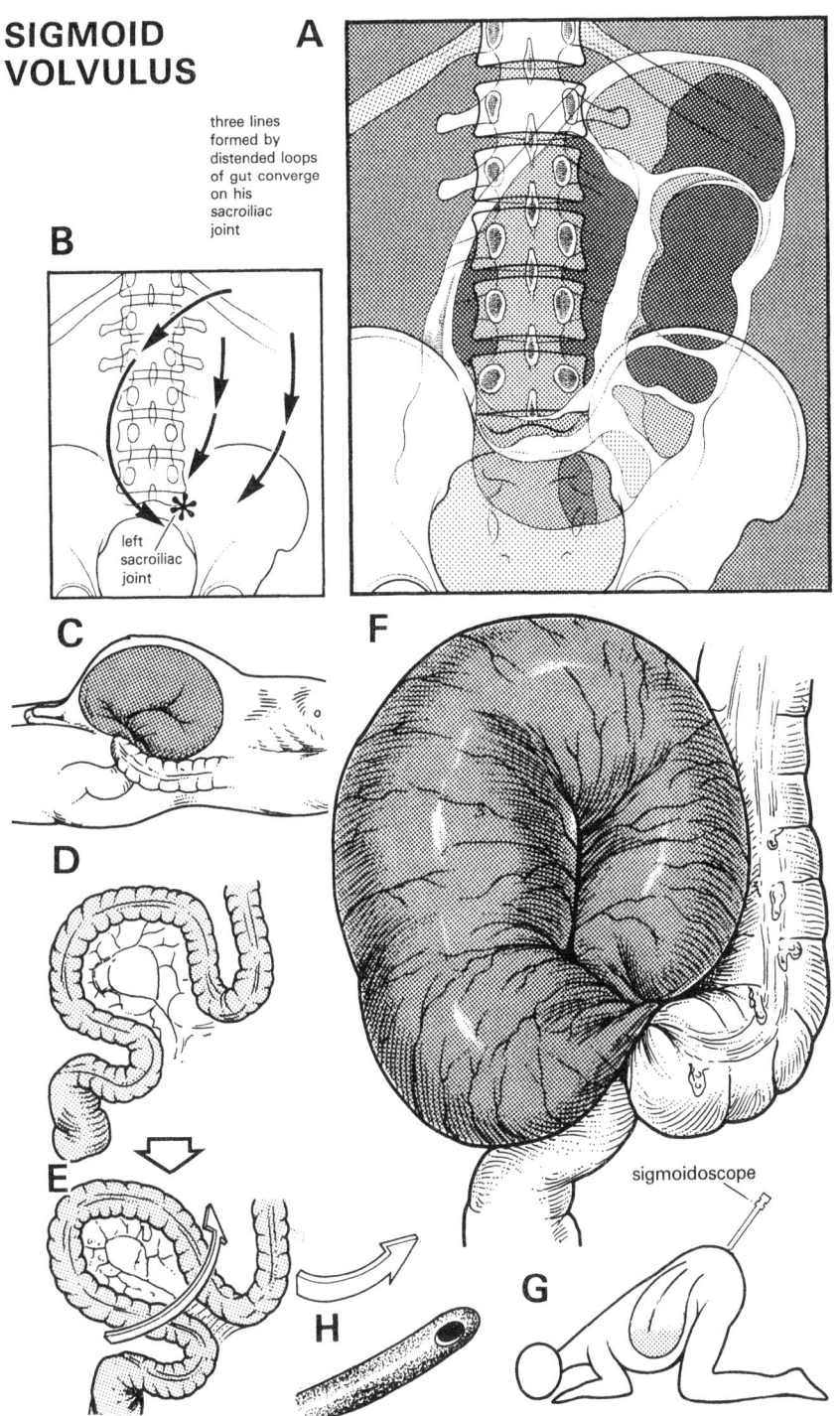

Fig. 10-14 SIGMOID VOLVULUS. A, a supine X-ray showing a huge distended inverted loop of sigmoid. B, is a diagrammatic version of A, to show three lines formed by the walls of the patient's sigmoid converging on his left sacroiliac joint. C, the abdominal distension caused by sigmoid volvulus. D, E, and F, show the mechanism of sigmoid volvulus. G, sigmoidoscopy in the knee-elbow position. H, a large rectal or stomach tube for sigmoidoscopic reduction. *Partly adapted from drawings by Frank Netter, with the kind permission of CIBA-GEIGY Ltd, Basle (Switzerland).*

tenderness, or shock, suspect strangulation, and do an immediate laparotomy.

If the mucosa looks normal through the sigmoidoscope, hold its distal end firmly, so that it lies immediately at the twist. Pass a large (36 Ch or about 12 mm) well-lubricated rectal (or stomach) tube along it. With a gentle rotatory movement, ease the tube past the twist into the high-pressure area of his dilated sigmoid. If you succeed, you will be rewarded by much flatus and some loose faeces. You and he will recognize that you have relieved his obstruction.

Withdraw the sigmoidoscope, taking care to to avoid displacing the tube (D, E, and F, 10-15).

Using a local anaesthetic, stitch the flatus tube to his anal margin, and leave it in place for 2 days. It may continue to discharge liquid faeces, so attach an extension tube to it, and lead this into a bucket beside his bed. If drainage stops wash out the tube. Don't leave the tube in for more than 72 hours, or it may cause pressure necrosis.

SIGMOIDOSCOPY

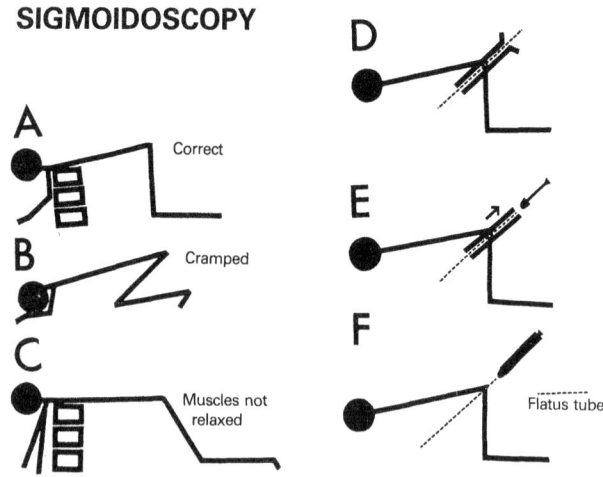

Fig. 10-15 SIGMOIDOSCOPY FOR SIGMOID VOLVULUS. A, the correct position for sigmoidoscopy. B, and C, two incorrect positions. The patient is not anaesthetized. The danger is that you may withdraw the tube with the sigmoidoscope, so D, E, and F, show you how to withdraw the sigmoidoscope on to its obturator and leave the flatus tube undisturbed as you do so. *After Joe Shepherd, with the kind permission of the editor of Tropical Doctor.*

If the fluid which runs out is bloody, assume that his sigmoid has an area which is non-viable. Operate immediately. A smear of blood is not a sufficient indication for laparotomy.

If you succeed in relieving his volvulus, either refer him to have his sigmoid colon resected as soon as possible, or prepare to do it yourself. It may recur if he waits too long—so warn him. If you are going to resect it yourself, keep the flatus tube in, give him preparatory bowel washouts on the 3rd and 4th day, and start oral chloramphenicol or neomycin with metronidazole on the 2nd day. Give the latter rectally with the premedication (2.9). On the 5th day do a laparotomy (see below) to resect his colon, and do a transverse colostomy to protect your anastomosis. You can now do an elective operation on viable deflated gut.

If you fail to relieve his volvulus at sigmoidoscopy, operate immediately.

LAPAROTOMY FOR SIGMOID VOLVULUS

INDICATIONS. (1) Failure to reduce a patient's volvulus with a sigmoidoscope. (2) Signs of strangulation and gangrene.

RESUSCITATION. If necessary, resuscitate him vigorously (A 15.3). He may have lost large volumes of fluid into his sigmoid. If he has a compound volvulus, he may need 3 or even 5 units of blood.

ANAESTHESIA. You will need good abdominal relaxation (A 14.3).

EQUIPMENT. This includes a sigmoidoscope, a 36 Ch rectal or stomach tube, and two Payr's clamps or stout Kocher's clamps. A sterile spinal needle for decompressing the colon.

Have an assistant under the towels ready to insert a rectal tube up the patient's anus from below.

METHOD. Lie the patient on his back, head down, with his legs up and spread apart (LLoyd-Davies Trendelenburg position). You can sigmoidoscope him in this position, and do a laparotomy.

Pass a Foley catheter, and attach it to a sterile drainage bag. Pass a thick 36 Ch stomach tube up his anus, but don't try to pass it through the twist in his colon.

Make a generous lower left paramedian incision. You will see an enormously distended loop of colon. Gently draw it out of his abdomen.

CAUTION ! Open his tensely distended abdomen with the greatest care: you can easily nick or perforate his bloated sigmoid.

If feeling his colon and percussing it shows that it contains much gas, decompress it 'above the water line', using the spinal needle Fig. 10-9, or any 2 mm needle attached to the sucker. Pack his sigmoid off well. Push the needle through a taenia coli, and advance it longitudinally between the muscle coats for 3 cm. Then angle it inwards through the circular muscle to reach the lumen.

WHAT NEXT? AT LAPAROTOMY FOR SIGMOID VOLVULUS

If the sigmoid loop is of normal colour, gently introduce the rectal tube into it. Ask your (suitably clothed) assistant to get under the drapes and pass it further up the patient's rectum. As he does this, guide it manually past the twist. The loop will deflate and allow you to untwist it. Suture the tube to his anus so that it acts as an internal splint.

Alternatively, find the pedicle and see which way it is twisted. Using both hands, try to untwist it. This will be safe provided it is not gangrenous. The loop seldom rotates by more than 360°. If you succeed in untwisting it, he will discharge flatus through the rectal tube. If you cannot find the pedicle and don't know which way it is twisted, twist it first one way and then the other.

What you should do next depends on your experience: (1) If you are very inexperienced, deflation alone without resection will be wiser. The problem of the patient returning to have an interval resection is a very real one—see above. (2) If you are very experienced, resect the viable loop and do an end-to-end anastomosis, protected by a proximal colostomy.

If you are not sure if his colon is viable or not, apply warm moist packs to it, wait 10 minutes, and then assess it by the criteria in Fig. 9-8. The large gut has a poor blood supply, so don't be too conservative, and resect if necessary.

If the loop is obviously gangrenous, assume that the area of the twist is likely to be even more unhealthy. Pack it off (it may pop like a balloon). Very cautiously decompress it by passing a spinal needle obliquely through a taenia as described above. Then untwist it.

If you are experienced, consider doing a resection and an end-to-end anastomosis protected by a transverse proximal colostomy.

If you are inexperienced: (1) If he has enough healthy gut to reach his skin, exteriorize his sigmoid colon, resect it, and do a double-barrelled colostomy (9-19, 10-16). (2) If there is not enough healthy gut for this, do Hartmann's operation.

In all these operations you will have to mobilize some of his descending colon by incising the peritoneum 2 cm lateral to it, followed by blunt dissection.

EXTERIORIZATION FOR SIGMOID VOLVULUS

INDICATIONS. Sigmoid volvulus, or wounds of the sigmoid colon, in which there is enough healthy gut distally to reach the surface of the skin.

METHOD. If you think you can get the patient's sigmoid colon through a separate smaller wound, do so (see below for details as to how to do it). If not bring it out through the main wound, and make the colostomy in this.

Start by mobilizing enough of his descending colon to bring healthy gut out to the surface as a double-barrelled colostomy. You may have to go higher than you think initially. If so, ask your assistant to retract the left side of the patient's abdominal wall, so as to expose the junction of his descending and sigmoid colon. If you need more length, incise the peritoneum in his left paracolic gutter, as in B, Fig. 10-16, and carefully displace his mobilized colon medially and upwards. Draw the whole loop of sigmoid colon out of his abdomen, so that his mesocolon is transilluminated.

CAUTION ! Remember that his inferior mesenteric vessels and ureter may take a looping course near his sigmoid colon, as in C, in Fig. 10-16. Shine a laterally placed light behind the gut to reveal the mesenteric vessels, and divide them well out towards the gut wall, so that you avoid injuring his left ureter or his superior rectal vessels.

Carry the dissection back to the point where his descending colon and rectum are viable.

Bring his sigmoid colon outside his abdomen, either through the main wound or, better, through a separate small incision (see below).

If you have made this second wound, close the main one now.

Place a small crushing clamp across the lower end of his *healthy* colon at the point you are going to resect it. Apply a larger one immediately proximal to this.

OPERATIONS FOR SIGMOID VOLVULUS

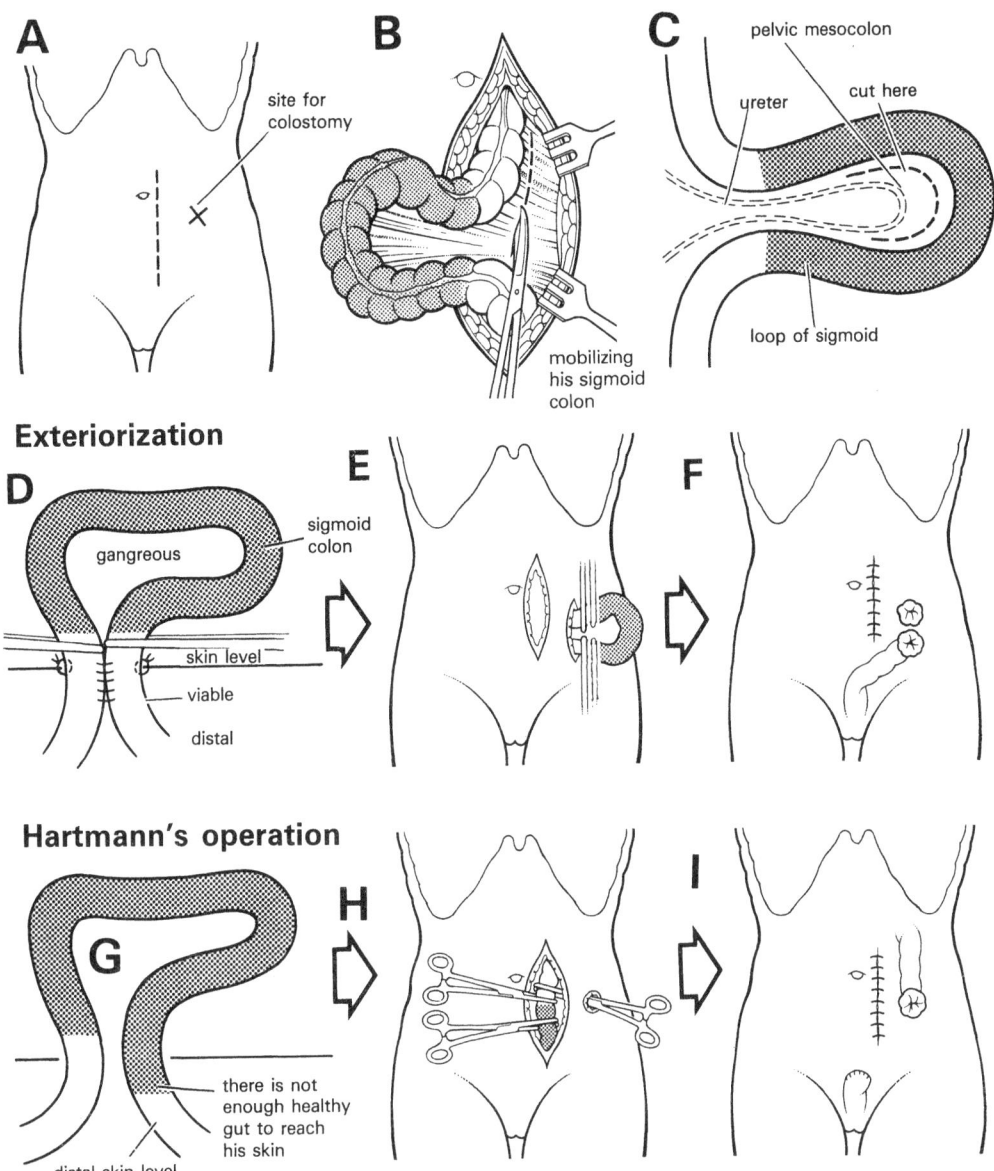

Fig. 10-16 OPERATIONS FOR SIGMOID VOLVULUS. A, the site for a pelvic colostomy through a small wound midway between the patient's umbilicus and his left iliac spine. B, if the proximal end of his sigmoid colon is too short, you may have to mobilize his descending colon. C, his ureter is usually on his posterior abdominal wall, but it may run close to his sigmoid, so avoid it by dividing his sigmoid mesocolon close to his gut. If there is enough healthy gut distally to reach skin level, you can excise it (D, E, and F), or you can do a Hartmann's operation. If there is not enough healthy gut distally to reach skin level, you will have to do Hartmann's operation (G, H, and I). D, healthy gut reaches his abdominal wall. E, his sigmoid exteriorized. F, the completed colostomy. G, there is not enough healthy gut distally to reach his abdominal wall. H, preparing to bring out healthy gut on to the abdominal wall. I, Hartmann's operation completed.

Place two more clamps side by side where you are going to divide his recto-sigmoid junction. Divide his sigmoid through healthy gut between both sets of clamps, and remove the gangrenous loop.

If possible, make a double-barrelled colostomy by sewing the ends of the proximal and distal loops together, as in Fig. 9-19. If you have misjudged the length of gut you need for this, proceed to do Hartmann's procedure, and close the distal end, as described below.

HARTMANN'S OPERATION FOR SIGMOID VOLVULUS etc.

INDICATIONS. Sigmoid volvulus, or wounds of the sigmoid colon, in which there is not enough healthy gut distally to reach the surface of the skin.

METHOD. Mobilize enough of the patient's descending colon to bring healthy gut to the surface as a terminal colostomy, as described above.

Excise a 3 cm circle of his skin and external oblique muscle at a point in his left iliac fossa which is equidistant from his ribs, his umbilicus, and his antero-superior iliac spine. Open the jaws of a large haemostat repeatedly, to split the muscles of his abdominal wall in the direction of their fibres. When you reach the peritoneum, nick it with a scalpel, and push the haemostat right through. Put both your index fingers through the hole, and enlarge it to accept 3 fingers without compression. Push a clamp through the incision and apply it to the patient's colon at a point which is viable enough to resect.

CAUTION ! (1) Cut and clamp the mesentery of his sigmoid colon less than 5 cm from the wall of his gut, so as to avoid his ureter. Better, find and avoid his ureter first: it may lie close to his sigmoid colon, as in C, Fig. 10-16. (2) Make sure that there is enough gut to come to the surface without tension, by mobilizing his descending colon first.

From within his abdomen, apply a second clamp immediately distal to the first one. Cut between the two clamps.

Withdraw the first clamp, and gently pull his colon through the hole in his abdominal wall. Leave the clamped end of his colon on his abdominal wall for the time being. Lift his sigmoid out of the wound, and wrap a towel round it.

TO DIVIDE HIS RECTUM AND REMOVE HIS SIGMOID COLON, select a point at or near his recto-sigmoid junction, where his gut appears normal, clamp it with a crushing clump (or a large haemostat or Kocher's forceps), and apply a second one just proximal to this.

Divide his gut between these clamps (having previously withdrawn the rectal tube!).

Irrigate the operation site liberally with saline, especially the pelvis, and aspirate it dry.

TO CLOSE HIS RECTAL STUMP, start at one end with a continuous suture of 2/0 chromic catgut on a curved atraumatic needle. Run a suture through all layers and pass it around the crushing clamp, as in A to H, Fig. 9-11. Place the bites 4 mm apart, and don't pull the suture tight.

When you have reached the free end of his colon, ask your assistant to open the jaws of the clamp, and slowly pull it out. As he withdraws it, pull the loops tightly, using a haemostat and non-toothed forceps together. With the clamp removed, take another bite and tie it.

Insert a reinforcing layer of interrupted or continuous Lembert sutures, to invert the stump of his rectum (Fig. 9-11 shows the end of the colon being closed by a slightly different method).

Leave a '2' mono- or multifilament non-absorbable suture to mark the closed end of the distal loop. This will make finding it easier, when it has to be closed.

CLOSE HIS ABDOMEN. While your assistant retracts his abdominal wall, close the space between his colostomy and his parietal peritoneum, because this is a space into which loops of gut can herniate and obstruct. Do this with 3 or more interrupted catgut sutures between his parietal peritoneum and the seromuscular layer (only) of his colon.

Apply a non-crushing clamp to the proximal gut inside his abdomen. Remove the crushing clamp from his proximal colon. Open it out and excise the crushed bowl. Pass interrupted sutures of 2/0 catgut through all coats of the cut end of his colon, and then through his skin at 4 mm intervals all round his colostomy. Place them so that there will be 1.5 cm of healthy bowel protruding beyond the skin. Better, secure the colostomy as in Fig. 9-17. Remove the non-crushing clamp holding his proximal gut inside his abdomen. Finally, put your finger through the stoma, to make sure it is not too tight.

Have a final look at his colostomy from within, to make sure his gut looks pink and healthy. Then close his abdomen, taking the precautions for secure closure (9.8) and sepsis (wash out any contamination with saline, and instil tetracycline, 6.2).

If possible, apply a colostomy bag. If not, apply vaseline gauze, plain gauze, and a dressing pad, and tape it in place. He will probably not pass faeces for 3 days.

Finally, do an anal stretch (22.15), and insert a rectal tube for 5 cm. Suture it to his anal verge. This will prevent mucus or exudate collecting in his rectal stump.

ALTERNATIVE: TEMPORARY COLOSTOMY AS PERMANENT TREATMENT

Insert a rectal tube without using a proctoscope and without intending to decompress his gut (if you happen to decompress it, consider resection 2 weeks later). Make a long left parmedian incision.

If his sigmoid is not viable, treat him as described above.

If it is viable, untwist it and decompress it through the rectal tube handled by an assistant. Insert a large Foley catheter through a small incision 50 mm above his anterior superior iliac spine. Place a purse string at the apex of his sigmoid. If necessary complete decompression by making a hole in its centre and sucking. Push the catheter through the purse string and inflate the ballon. Tie the purse string and insert a second one for safety. Pull gently on the catheter and anchor it to bring his sigmoid into contact with his lateral abdominal wall. Insert some sutures between his sigmoid near the catheter and his parietal peritoeum. To prevent internal herniation stitch his sigmid to his abdominal wall. If his distal sigmoid is very long put a few seromuscular sutures between adjacent loops.

Close his abdomen without a drain; fix the rectal tube in place and leave it for 48 hours. Attach the catheter to a collecting bottle and give him postoperative antibiotics. Remove the catheter in 10-14 days. The stoma will close spontaneously in 2 weeks.

COMPOUND VOLVULUS

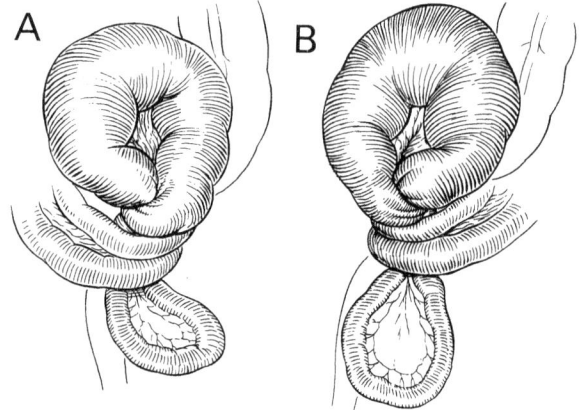

Fig. 10-17 COMPOUND VOLVULUS complicates about 10% of cases of sigmoid volvulus in Uganda. A loop of the patient's ileum is twisted in with his sigmoid colon. The twist in his gut may be left-handed (A) or right-handed (B). If you cannot untwist it, you will have to deflate it and resect it. Don't try to untwist it if its circulation is impaired.

DIFFICULTIES WITH SIGMOID VOLVULUS

If a LOOP OF ILEUM IS TWISTED IN WITH HIS SIGMOID COLON (COMPOUND VOLVULUS or ileosigmoid knotting, unusual), you may not be able to untwist it. Puncture and deflate it, and then clamp and resect it before you untie the knot. Anastomose his small gut end-to-end, and bring his large gut out as a temporary colostomy. If the lower limit of the gangrene on his ileum is close to his ileocaecal valve, consider closing his ileal stump and anastomosing viable small gut to his caecum.

10.10a Closing Hartmann's operation

This is one of the more difficult operations in this manual, so refer the patient if you can. Hartmann's operation will have left the proximal end of his gut blind, and his anal canal open. You will have to mobilize his proximal colon, open his distal colon, and bring his proximal colon down to meet it. The key step is to place all the sutures on the posterior ('Lembert', 9.3) layer of his gut, before you close any of them.

CLOSING HARTMANN'S OPERATION

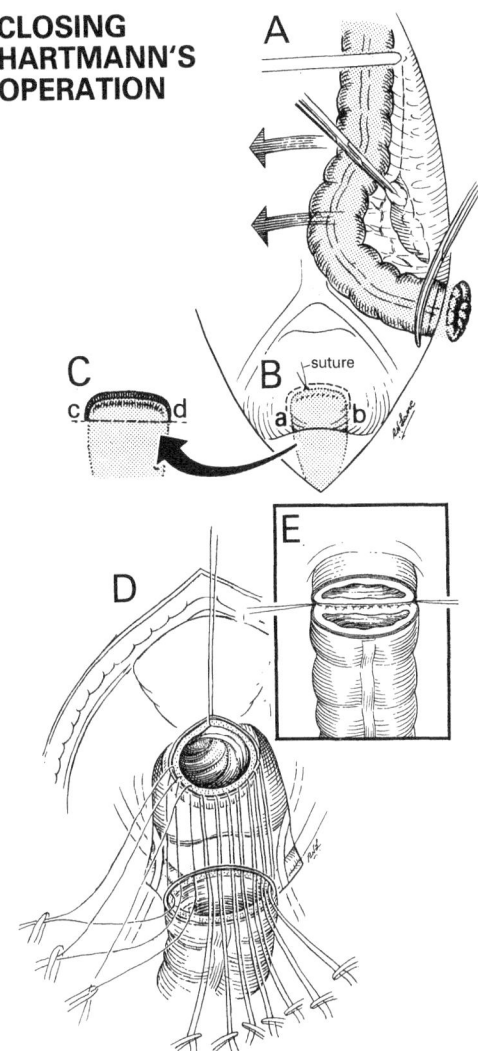

Fig. 10-17a CLOSING HARTMANN'S OPERATION. If you cannot refer a patient and have to close his colostomy, do it like this—his distal gut is usually deeper in his pelvis, even than shown here. A, mobilizing his colon. B, freeing his rectal stump. C, cutting off the top of his rectal stump. D, placing the seromuscular (Lembert) sutures that will draw the two ends of his gut together. You can use simple sutures like the three on the left, or the mattress sutures shown on right which are slightly more difficult. E, the sutures placed in D, have been pulled tight. Note that the two end ones have been left long.

CLOSING HARTMANN'S OPERATION

TIMING. Do it 6 to 12 weeks after the first stage.

PREPARATION. Give him fluids only for the first two days preoperatively. On the day before the operation wash out the proximal loop, and give the rectosigmoid stump an enema.

ANAESTHESIA. Subarachnoid anaesthesia, or general anaesthesia, intubation, and relaxants. Insert an intravenous line.

METHOD. Lay the patient supine, and raise the foot of his bed to give you better access to his pelvis. If you are right-handed, stand on his left. Open the previous wound (midline or paramedian). Using scissors and gentle blunt dissection, carefully separate the adhesions between his gut and his abdominal wall. If you operate at the best time (6 to 12 weeks) these should be light.

Find the proximal end and free it for 15 cm, without damaging its mesentery. To do this, incise the peritoneum covering his posterior abdominal wall 1 cm lateral to his descending colon. Then mobilize his colon medially by blunt dissection (as shown by the arrows in Fig. 10-17a). Mobilize it well, so that it reaches the distal stump without tension.

Apply a crushing clamp 2 cm from the exit of the proximal end through his abdominal wall. Apply a non-crushing clamp well proximally to prevent contamination (his gut should be empty). Mobilize the proximal end, so that it can reach the distal end easily.

Dissect out the distal end (the suture you placed earlier will make this easier to find). Dissect across the top and about 2 cm down each side (Diagram B, line a-b). Cut it across 5 to 10 mm from its blind end (C, line c-d).

Insert about 10 atraumatic 2/0 multifilament sutures through the musculoserosal layer of the posterior aspect of both ends of his gut about 3 mm apart, leaving their ends long, and held in haemostats (D). Avoid the mucosa by turning this inwards. When these are complete draw them all together to approximate the bowel ends. Leave one suture at each end long (E). Insert a continuous 'all coats' layer of 2/0 chromic catgut or 'Vicryl' or 'Dexon', starting at one end and leaving the end long.

Continue the 'all coats' layer to close his gut anteriorly, and tie the ends of the suture together to complete it. Then insert Lembert sutures for the anterior musculo-serosal layer in the usual way. Use a long needle-holder and small (16–25 mm needle) atraumatic sutures. Check the soundness of the anastomosis and the size of the lumen by pinching it between your thumb and finger (Q, 9-9).

Close any hole through which a loop of small gut might prolapse (see Section 10.10). Close his abdomen as a single layer (9.8), and manage him postoperatively as for any other gut anastomosis (9.9) and do Lord's procedure.

DIFFICULTIES CLOSING HARTMANN'S OPERATION

If you CANNOT BRING THE ENDS OF HIS GUT TOGETHER easily, remove the non-crushing clamp, and mobilize more descending colon, by cutting his peritoneum further up his paracolic gutter, and raising more descending colon and mesentery. You can always bring the gut ends together if you mobilize enough mesentery.

If the ENDS OF HIS GUT ARE DIFFERENT SIZES (the proximal end is usually bigger), place the sutures for the wider end further apart.

If the LUMEN IS TOO NARROW, or there is a DOG EAR OF SPARE GUT, undo the anastomosis and start again. This may harm him, and should trouble your conscience.

If the ENDS OF THE GUT BLEED, press them firmly for up to 5 minutes. If there is a bleeding vessel beside the gut, clamp and tie it.

10.11 Volvulus of the caecum (rare)

Rarely, a patient's caecum, his ascending colon and his ileum, may all twist. This can only happen if they are all free to rotate as the result of a rare anomaly of his mesentery, which seems to be more common here in the developing world than it is elsewhere. Twisting causes him sudden severe pain, vomiting, and prostration. His abdomen distends and becomes tender centrally and in his right lower quadrant. Signs of strangulation develop (10.3). X-rays show a huge gas shadow which is not where his caecum should be, but is central, or even in his left upper quadrant where it may mimic his stomach. Unlike a torsion of his sigmoid colon (B, 10-14), this gas shadow does not have two limbs descending into his pelvis. At laparotomy, a huge drum-like structure seems fill his entire abdominal cavity.

VOLVULUS OF THE CAECUM. For the general method for gut obstruction see Sections 10.3 and 10.4.

At laparotomy you will see a tense, blue dilated volvulus. Decompress it (10-9). When you inspect his right lower quadrant, you will find that his caecum is not in its normal place.

Untwist his caecum.

If it is viable, ask your assistant to retract the right side of the abdominal incision. Anchor the patient's caecum to the peritoneum to the right of it with a few seromuscular sutures of 2/0 chromic catgut, passed through one of its taenia. This is of temporary value only, so refer him for a right hemicolectomy later. Or, do a temporary caecostomy, the fibrosis that

VOLVULUS OF THE CAECUM

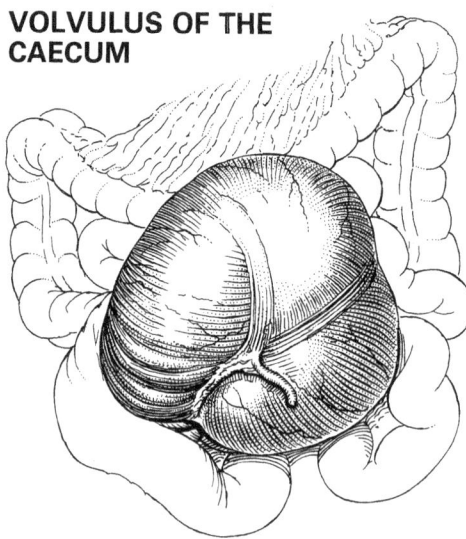

Fig. 10-18 VOLVULUS OF THE CAECUM can only happen if a patient's caecum, his ascending colon and his ileum are all free to rotate, as the result of a rare anomaly of his mesentery, which seems to be more common in the developing world than it is elsewhere. *Adapted from a drawing by Frank Netter, with the kind permission of GIBA-GEIGY Ltd, Basle (Switzerland).*

will follow will keep his caecum anchored. To do this make a small incision over his caecum, insert a Foley catheter, blow it up, draw it back to his abdominal wall and anchor it with some catgut stitches, as in Fig. 66-18.

If it is not viable, and you are skilled, do a right hemicolectomy (66-20). If you are less skilled, exteriorise it, as for an ileocolic intussusception (10.8).

10.12 Obstruction following abdominal abscesses

Peritoneal pus sometimes obstructs the gut. The patient presents with the symptoms of obstruction, and you have to take a careful history to find out that they started with some form of sepsis, such as an appendicitis, a pelvic abscess, or a tubo–ovarian abscess. Suspect that this has happened: (1) If pain and fever preceeded the obstructive symptoms, or, (2) you can feel a tender indurated area abdominally, vaginally, or rectally. The patient has no signs of general peritonitis, and his bowel sounds are exaggerated. A raised white count is suggestive. Treat him with nasogastric suction, intravenous fluids, and antibiotics, and drain his abscess as necessary (6.3). His obstruction will usually be relieved as you drain it. If not, you will have to operate and try to free the obstruction.

10.13 Ileus and obstruction follow abdominal surgery

After a laparatomy the normal muscular action of a patient's gut is usually absent for 6 to 72 hours. The return of his bowel sounds is a sign that his gut is starting to work normally again, and that it is time to remove his nasogastric tube. His gut may fail to work as the result of: (1) Paralytic ileus, which is a prolongation of the normal postoperative inactivity of the gut. This is the commonest cause, especially after an operation for abdominal sepsis. (2) Obstruction due to sepsis which has caused loops of small gut to mat together and obstruct. (3) Mechanical obstruction due to adhesions. Distinguishing between these three causes is difficult because: (a) postoperative obstruction may cause little or no pain, and (b) a recent abdominal incision makes careful abdominal palpation more difficult. (c) Organising pus eventually becomes fibrous adhesions so there is no sharp distinction between (2) and (3). Postoperative intussusception is a rare cause of obstruction, but it must be operated on.

If a patient's abdomen is silent and steadily distends after an abdominal operation, how long can you wait before you decide that his distension is caused by some mechanical obstruction that you should try to relieve? Perhaps his gut is being kinked by a fibrinous adhesion or an inflammatory mass? A way out of this problem is to treat him symptomatically for ileus and obstruction, and not to operate for 7 to 10 days, or until you are forced to. This will give an inflammatory mass time to resolve. You may however be forced to operate earlier, if there are signs of peritoneal irritation (which could be due to a leaking anastomosis or to new infection), or some mechanical obstruction unrelated to the original operation (see below).

NJOROGE aged 10 had a splenectomy for a ruptured spleen. On the 3rd postoperative day he was clearly not well. He had obstructive bowel sounds, some colicky pain, and a moderate amount of fluid was coming up his nasogastric tube. He was immediately operated on and an intussusception was found. LESSON Don't wait too long before you reopen an abdomen, be guided by the whole clinical picture. Early mechanical obstruction like this is rare; ileus is more usual early.

POSTOPERATIVE GUT OBSTRUCTION OR ILEUS?

This is the patient whose bowel sounds do not return after an operation.

DIAGNOSIS. After a messy operation with much pus and spillage, expect ileus. After a clean one severe ileus is unlikely; if his gut obstructs the cause is more likely to be mechanical. Ileus tends to occur earlier and mechanical obstruction later.

Examine him twice a day asking these questions: Has he any pain? Is his girth increasing or decreasing? How much fluid is being aspirated? Have his bowel sounds returned? Is he passing any flatus? Does he have signs of peritonitis? Is his general condition deteriorating?

The signs of mechanical obstruction requiring surgery are—colicky abdominal pain, an increasing girth, a large volume of gastric aspirate, no flatus, and X-rays showing fluid levels. Typically, absent bowel sounds indicate ileus, and 'tinkling' ones indicate mechanical obstruction. If he has little pain, and X-rays show gas filled loops with fluid levels all through his large and small gut, he is more likely to have ileus.

If he distended progressively from Day 1 and is still distended on Day 5, he probably has ileus. The normal postoperative musclar inactivity usually starts to resolve after 72 hours, but may last 7 to 14 days or more in the presence of infection, metabolic imbalance, impaired renal function or severe general illness.

If he was all right until Day 5, and then started distending, he probably has a mechanical obstruction, especially if he has colic, 'tinkling' bowel sounds, distension, vomiting, no fever and a normal white count. The tinkling bowel sounds may be intermittent, so you may have to listen for a long time.

If at Day 5 his abdomen is silent and painless, he is febrile and he has a raised white count, he probably has ileus. If he has no fever, a normal white count, and tinkling bowel sounds, suspect a mechanical obstruction.

If he does not pass flatus when he has had bowel sounds or gas pains for some hours, or he has colicky pain, or X-rays show distended small gut and collapsed large gut, suspect mechanical obstruction.

If normal bowel function starts, and then stops again, or he vomits or distends, or you aspirate progressively more fluid, even several litres a day, suspect mechanical obstruction. If at the same time he has diarrhoea, he may have a pelvic abscess, or uncommonly staphylococcal enterocolitis, or he may have a partial obstruction, which allows some fluid to pass and obstructs the rest. Maintaining his fluid balance will be difficult. If you have excluded enterocolitis, you may have to operate.

NONOPERATIVE TREATMENT. 'Suck and drip' him diligently (9.9). Hypokalaemia aggravates ileus, so take care to give him potassium supplements to replace the potassium he loses in

INTESTINAL OBSTRUCTION AND PARALYTIC ILEUS

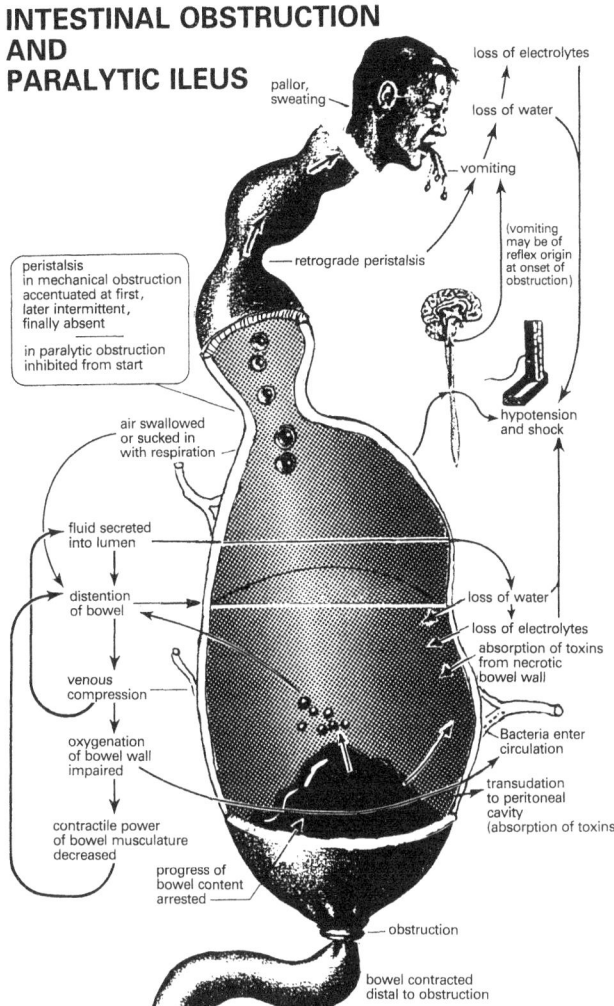

Fig. 10-19 INTESTINAL OBSTRUCTION AND PARALYTIC ILEUS. The passage of intestinal contents down the gut can be prevented by a mechanical obstruction, or by a functional disturbance of the motility of the gut (paralytic ileus). The physiological effects are much the same in both and are shown here. *Adapted from a drawing by Frank Netter, with the kind permission of GIBA-GEIGY Ltd, Basle (Switzerland).*

the intestinal secretions that you suck up his nasogastric tube—see A 15.5. He needs about 40 mmol/day plus any extra potassium he loses through the tube.

OPERATION. Proceed as for obstruction due to adhesions in Section 10.7. Take great care not to exert traction on previous anastomoses. Decompress his upper small gut before you close his abdomen.

10.14 Other problems with intestinal obstruction

Don't forget constipation as a cause of intestinal obstruction in elderly sedentary people, especially if they are taking codeine derivatives for arthritis. It is less common in communities of the developing world with their soft bulky stools from high fibre diets. Here are some more causes of obstruction. Most of them are rare.

OTHER PROBLEMS WITH INTESTINAL OBSTRUCTION

CONSTIPATION CAUSING INTESTINAL OBSTRUCTION

If a patient's **COLON IS OBSTRUCTED BY A MASS OF FAECES,** try a soap suds enema. If this fails, try an oil retention enema left in for an hour, and washed out by a soap suds enema. If this too fails, remove his faeces manually.

INTERNAL HERNIAS CAUSING INTESTINAL OBSTRUCTION

If an **INTERNAL HERNIA is obstructing his gut (rare),** it will probably be of the closed loop variety. You can usually divide the obstructing structure quite safely, but be careful with a hernia into the recess formed by the paraduodenal fold at his duodenojejunal flexure, because you can easily cut his inferior mesenteric vein.

If gut is **STRANGULATING THROUGH A HOLE IN THE MESENTERY,** don't cut the neck of the constricting ring, or it will probably bleed severely. Instead, decompress the distended loop (10-9), withdraw it, and suture the hole in the mesentery, carefully avoiding its blood vessels.

FOREIGN BODIES CAUSING INTESTINAL OBSTRUCTION

If you feel a **SOLID OBJECT at the point where the distended loops join the collapsed ones,** decompress his obstructed gut proximally and apply noncrushing clamps to the empty segment. If you can easily move the solid object to another site in the gut where the mucosa will not have been ulcerated, do so. Isolate the segment with packs and make a longitudinal incision in its antemesenteric border. Remove the foreign body and repair the gut transversely.

If a **FOOD BOLUS has impacted in his small gut,** try to break it up and massage down into his caecum. If you fail, do an enterotomy as above.

STRICTURES CAUSING INTESTINAL OBSTRUCTION

If he has a **TIGHT STRICTURE of his small gut,** consider the possibility of tuberculosis (29.7). Resect it and do an end-to-end anastomosis.

TUMOURS CAUSING INTESTINAL OBSTRUCTION

If he has a localized **CARCINOMA of his sigmoid colon (rare in the developing world),** see section 32.27.

If he has a **TUMOUR OF HIS SMALL GUT (carcinoma, carcinoid, or a benign mesenchymal tumour),** resect it if you can, and do an end-to-end anastomosis. If this is impossible (unusual), make a bypass (29-8) to relieve the obstruction.

If he has **CARCINOMATOSIS of his peritoneum,** don't do a colostomy, or an ileostomy. If his gut is obstructed, do a bypass procedure, because intestinal obstruction is one of the most horrible ways to die. For further management, see Chapter 33.

11 The surgery of the stomach

11.1 Peptic ulcer

The surgery you can do on a patient's stomach or duodenum is limited to: (1) Treating his peptic ulcer if it perforates. (2) Doing a gastroenterostomy or pyloroplasty if his pylorus stenoses. (3) Treating him if his ulcer bleeds. (4) Perhaps doing an elective truncal vagotomy and gastroenterostomy if he has a chronic disabling duodenal ulcer which has resisted medical treatment.

Duodenal ulcers are a common cause of epigastric pain in most parts of the world. You will need to take a careful history to diagnose and manage them. This can be difficult in a villager, so enquire how the patients in your community express their ulcer symptoms. They are unlikely to give you a clear history that their pain is relieved by food, or by antacids, for example, and their physical signs may be minimal. So, in spite of the limitations of the history, it is likely to be the only way you have of making the diagnosis. When a patient presents with the surgical complications of peptic ulcer disease, you may have to enquire carefully to find out that he has had any previous ulcer symptoms.

In India, antacids may be as expensive as cimetidine from a cheap secondary source. The decision to abandon medical for surgical treatment will often depend on how poor he is. If he is rich, he can afford surgery, or cimetidine and antacids; if he is poor, these drugs may cost more than his salary, so you may have to operate. Peptic ulcers, in India in particular, behave differently from those in the West. Operate early, and don't wait to be pressed to do so by the patient.

PEPTIC ULCER DISEASE

HISTORY. Has the patient had heartburn, dyspepsia, or epigastric pain? If, so, how long for, and has it recently got worse? Does it have the features of peptic ulcer pain—epigastric, dull, boring, worse at night and when his stomach is empty; relieved by food, milk, antacids, vomiting, and belching; and aggravated by coffee, alcohol, and smoking? The periodicity of the symptoms is important at first. Has he any reason for stress, in his family or at work? Has he been drinking? Weight loss? Black stools?

EXAMINATION. Tenderness in his epigastrium will be his only physical sign?

MEDICAL TREATMENT. No smoking, no spices, and frequent small meals help his symptoms. Four weeks treatment with cimetidine 200 mg three times daily, with 400 mg at night will cure 70% of cases temporarily. If this can be followed by 400 mg at night, there will be less chance of recurrence.

11.2 Perforated gastric or duodenal ulcer

Classically, when a patient's peptic ulcer perforates, it floods his peritoneum with the acid contents of his stomach, and gives him a sudden agonizing pain. He may be able to tell you the moment the pain began; it is constant, it spreads across his entire upper abdomen and later all over, and is made worse by deep breathing or movement. Usually, he lies still in excruciating pain, and breathes shallowly without moving his abdomen. Occasionally, he writhes about in agony. He is pale, sweating, and hypotensive, with a fast pulse (usually), a normal temperature, and a stomach which is not distended. Typically, his abdomen has a board-like rigidity, unlike that in any other disease, which may be so complete that you cannot elicit tenderness, except when you examine him rectally.

After 3 to 6 hours his pain and rigidity lessen, he feels better and a 'silent interval' begins. Then, at about 6 hours, signs of diffuse peritonitis develop, accompanied by abdominal distension and absent bowel sounds.

There are difficulties: (1) So many patients have dyspepsia, that a previous dyspeptic history is not much help. (2) You may have difficulty in distinguishing the exacerbation of a peptic ulcer from a subacute perforation (a small sealed leak)—so remember this possibility and watch him carefully. (3) Fluid may track down his right paracolic gutter and cause pain and tenderness in his right iliac fossa, simulating appendicitis. (4) If he perforates in bed while he is suffering from something else, which is not uncommon, the dramatic onset may be absent. Instead, he may merely 'take a turn for the worse', his pulse rate rises, and you find that he has upper abdominal guarding.

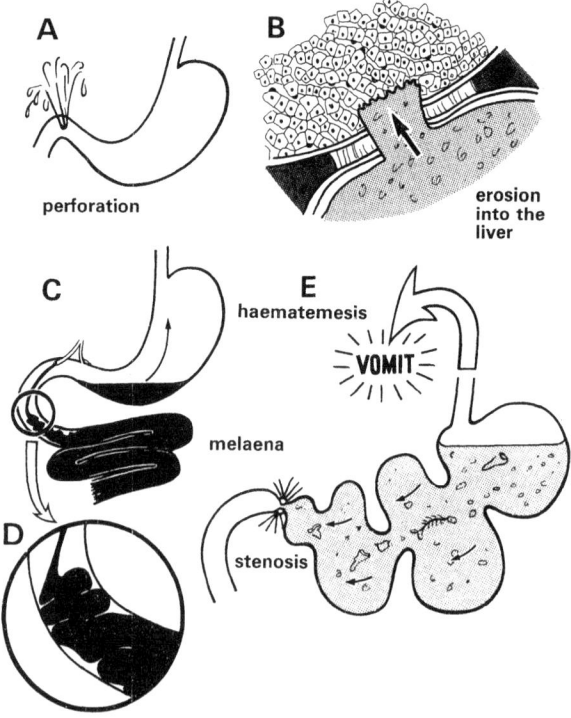

Fig. 11-1 SOME COMPLICATIONS OF PEPTIC ULCERATION. A, anterior perforation of a duodenal ulcer. B, penetration into the liver (penetration into the pancreas is more common). C, and D, haematemesis and melaena. E, pyloric obstruction. Note the hyperperistalsis and the old food in the stomach.

If he has perforated, he needs an urgent laparotomy. If he is fit, and you operate within 8 hours, the result will be good. If you delay 12 hours, his chances of survival fall greatly. If you can suture his perforation, he has a 50% chance of having no more symptoms, and a 25% chance of having dyspepsia which will not be severe enough to need major surgery.

Although the standard treatment is an urgent laparotomy, to close the hole in his duodenum or stomach, and to wash out his peritoneal cavity, there are some indications for treating him non-operatively, as described below. This is less demanding technically, but it needs more time, and you will need good judgement to know: (1) When you have made a wrong diagnosis, and (2) when non-operative treatment is failing, so that you need to operate.

The rule in all emergency surgery is to do only what is necessary. Closing the perforation is not difficult, *but be sure to wash out his peritoneum when it has been contaminated.* For this you will need plenty of warm saline.

PERFORATED PEPTIC ULCER

DIFFERENTIAL DIAGNOSIS. The main diagnostic difficulty is appendicitis, which is important because it needs a different incision. Find out the relative frequency of these two diseases in your community.

Suggesting perforation—referred shoulder pain, usually on the patient's right, the absence of fever—this develops late in a perforation—shock (when generalized rigidity is the result of appendicitis, he is not usually shocked), and a litre or more of stomach aspirate.

Suggesting appendicitis (12.1)—a colicky onset, fever, a small stomach aspirate of mucoid or bile-stained fluid.

X-RAYS. If the diagnosis is clear, these are unnecessary and unkind. If you take them, give him some intravenous morphine and aspirate his stomach first. Take an erect AP chest film. Make sure he is upright and the tube is horizontal. Look for a thin linear gas shadow between his diaphragm and his liver or stomach. If he cannot sit or stand, take a lateral decubitus film and look for air under his anterior abdominal wall.

If his ulcer has perforated into his lesser sac, you may see a large irregular gas shadow in the centre of his upper abdomen, with an outline which is different from that of a loop of gut.

CAUTION ! (1) An ulcer can perforate almost silently in the very old, or in the course of another disease. (2) The absence of gas does not exclude the presence of a perforated ulcer. (3) Gas can also come from a ruptured diverticulum or an appendix (uncommon).

NON-OPERATIVE TREATMENT FOR A PERFORATED PEPTIC ULCER

INDICATIONS. (1) A perforation which appears to have sealed itself already, as shown by diminished pain and improved abdominal signs. (2) Heart or lung disease, which increases the surgical and anaesthetic risks. (3) The patient who is admitted after a day or two and is almost moribund with diffuse peritonitis. Non-operative treatment may be best, because it is unlikely that he would have survived so long with an open perforation.

CONTRAINDICATIONS. (1) An uncertain diagnosis. (2) The absence of really good nursing by day and night. (3) The seriously ill patient, *with a short history,* whose only hope is vigorous resuscitation and an urgent laparotomy. If you do decide that such a patient is 'not fit for surgery', wait to do so until vigorous resuscitation has failed—don't make the decision when he is first admitted.

METHOD. Give him morphine 5 to 10 mg intravenously. As soon as this has had time to act, pass a large tube and empty his stomach. When it is empty, pass as wide a radio-opaque nasogastric tube as he will tolerate. Take him to the X-ray department and take AP erect films of his chest and lower abdomen. These should show that there are no fluid levels in his stomach, and that the tube is well placed. If not, adjust it and take more films. Look for subdiaphragmatic gas to confirm the diagnosis.

Back in the ward, ask a nurse to aspirate his stomach every 15 minutes initially. Set up an intravenous drip, and monitor his pulse and blood pressure hourly.

He is progressing well if: (1) His pain eases, so that he does not need more analgesics, and (2) another erect film 12 hours later (optional) shows no fluid level, and no increase in the gas under his diaphragm. Continue to 'suck and drip him' for 4 or 5 days, until his abdomen is no longer tender and rigid, and his bowel sounds return.

If pain persists, or the gas under his diaphragm increases, operate.

LAPAROTOMY FOR A PERFORATED PEPTIC ULCER

EQUIPMENT. A general set. Several litres of warm saline. Two assistants make upper abdominal surgery easier.

PREPARATION. Pass a nasogastric tube and aspirate his stomach (4.9). He will have lost much fluid into his peritoneal cavity, so correct at least part of his fluid loss before you operate, as in Section A 15.3. If he is dehydrated or hypotensive, give him 1 to 3 litres of fluid rapidly. If more than 12 hours have elapsed since he perforated, he will need even more. Operate soon, but not before you have resuscitated him. He has not bled, so he does not need blood.

PERIOPERATIVE ANTIBIOTICS. (2.9) are only indicated in late cases with peritonitis.

ANAESTHESIA. (1) General anaesthesia with good relaxation. (2) If this is contraindicated because of lung disease, do an intercostal block (A 6.7), from T6 to T11.

Premedicate him with intravenous morphine, and palpate his abdomen when this has taken effect. If his rigidity is generalized, morphine will make little difference if he has a perforation, but if he has appendicitis, rigidity will now be localized to his right iliac fossa.

INCISION. Make a midline or upper right paramedian incision (9.2). The escape of gas as you incise his peritoneum confirms the diagnosis.

Initial examination will probably show a pool of exudate under his liver, with food and fluid everywhere, and an inflamed peritoneum. The fluid may be odourless and colourless with yellowish flecks, or bile-stained—if it is pure bile, he has biliary peritonitis. If you see patches of fat necrosis, he has acute pancreatitis. If there is no fluid or little fluid, push a swab on a holder beside his ascending colon towards his caecum. If you withdraw it soaked with fluid, this suggests a perforation. Draw his stomach and transverse colon downwards: you may see flecks of fibrin, and perhaps pieces of food.

To expose his stomach and duodenum place a self-retaining retractor in the wound. Place a moist abdominal pack on the greater curvature of his stomach. Draw this downwards, and ask your assistant to hold it; at the same time ask him to hold the patient's liver upwards with a deep retractor. Put an abdominal pack between the retractor and his liver to protect it. If necessary, get the help of a second assistant.

Suck away any fluid, looking carefully to see where it is coming from.

Search for a small (1 to 10 mm or more) circular hole on the anterior surface of his duodenum, looking as if it has just been drilled out. Feel it. The tissues around it will be oedematous, thickened, scarred, and friable. If his duodenum is normal, look at his stomach, especially its lesser curve. If the hole is small, there may be more to feel than to see. Sometimes, a gastric ulcer is sealed off by adhesions to the liver. Remember that a gastric ulcer may be malignant: consider biopsy.

If his stomach is adherent to his liver, separate it.

Open his lesser sac through his lesser omentum. Feel the posterior surface of his stomach. An ulcer high up posteriorly may be difficult to find. Feel carefully.

If his stomach and duodenum are normal, feel gently downwards towards his appendix. If there is a mass or it is obviously inflamed, close the midline incision and make a gridiron one. Two smaller incisions are better than one huge one.

To close the perforation, use 2/0 chromic catgut on an atraumatic needle to bring its edges together with 1 to 3 deep stitches. If the tissue is so rigid that the stitches cut out, you may be able to reduce the size of the hole with loose sutures, or by using a purse string suture. Always sew omentum over

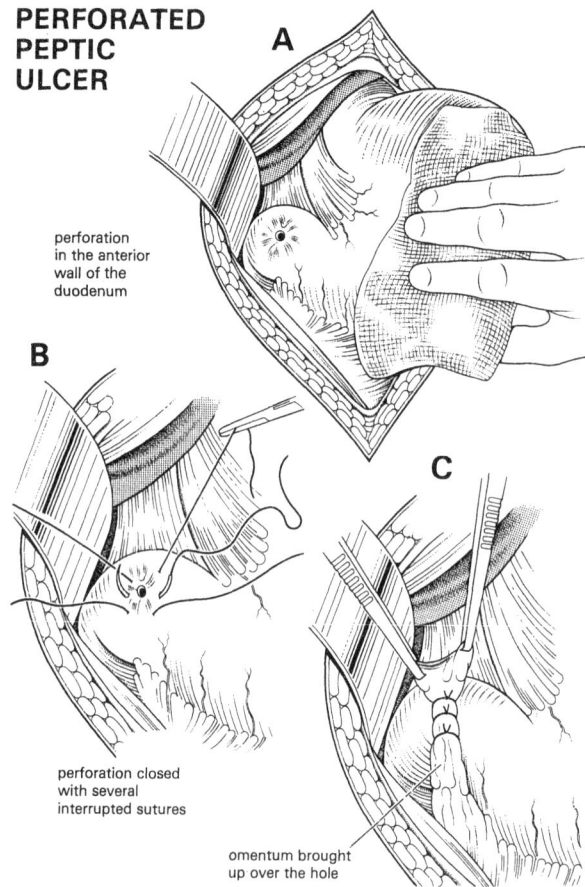

Fig. 11-2 CLOSING A PERFORATED PEPTIC ULCER. A, the stomach retracted and a perforation on the anterior of the duodenum exposed. B, the perforation being closed with several interrupted sutures of 2/0 catgut on an atraumatic needle. C, a fold of omentum being sewn over the hole. *Kindly contributed by Gerald Hankins.*

the perforation, by bringing up a fold of greater omentum. A hole so plugged is unlikely to leak.

Wash out his peritoneal cavity. This *is absolutely critical*, and may be more important than closing the hole. Tip a litre of warm saline into his peritoneal cavity, spread it well, and then suck it out again. Repeat this several times, and try to wash out every possible recess in his upper abdomen. Mop the upper surface of his liver. Instil tetracycline 1 g in a litre of of saline and leave it in. This may be unnecessary if you operate within 6 hours of the perforation.

FURTHER PROCEDURES. If: (1) his general condition is good, and you are operating early (within 6 to 8 hours of a duodenal, or particularly a gastric perforation), and (2) he has severe ulcer disease (uncontrollable symptoms, or a previous bleed or perforation), and (3) *you are experienced,* consider doing a vagotomy and gastroenterostomy (11-4). Otherwise, proceed to close his abdomen.

CLOSURE. Close his abdomen securely with non-absorbable sutures in a single layer (9.8), because it is particularly likely to burst (9.13). Don't insert drains.

POSTOPERATIVELY. Nurse him sitting up in a high Fowler's position. He will breathe more easily, he will be less likely to have chest complications, and any exudate will gravitate downwards. Continue with nasogastric suction and intravenous fluids, as in Sections 9.9 and A 15.5. Replace gastric aspirate with 0.9% saline. If he is likely to get lung complications (9.11), chest physiotherapy *is vital*.

DIFFICULTIES WITH A PERFORATED PEPTIC UCER

If a patient who is VOMITING for any reason suddenly feels a severe pain in his epigastrium and behind his lower sternum, or spreading between his shoulders, suspect that he has a RUPTURED OESOPHAGUS, and see Section 25.16.

If his ulcer is BURROWING INTO HIS LIVER, separate his stomach or his duodenum from his liver by pinching between them with your finger and thumb. If this is difficult, or it is leaking into his peritoneal cavity, cut around it, and leave its base fixed to his liver. If you have been able to separate it from his liver, deal with it as usual. If you are experienced and he is fit, partial gastrectomy (not described here) is appropriate.

CAUTION ! Don't put your finger through his ulcer into his liver, it will bleed severely.

If he runs a FEVER in the second week, suspect that he has a subphrenic abscess (6.4).

If you continue to obtain MUCH GASTRIC ASPIRATE, he probably has pyloric stenosis aggravated by the suture. If it continues for more than 10 days, and you are competent to do so, do a gastroenterostomy and truncal vagotomy (a gastroenterostomy alone has a high incidence of anastomotic ulcers, except in women over 50).

11.3 Bleeding from the upper gastrointestinal tract

In South and Central Africa, and in most of the developing world, a bleeding peptic ulcer is the commonest cause of bleeding from the upper intestinal tract, but there are parts of East Africa and India where bleeding varices as the result of portal hypertension are more common. They may be the result of cirrhosis of the liver, schistosomiasis causing noncirrhotic periportal fibrosis, or extrahepatic portal vein obstruction. Other causes of bleeding include stress ulcers, hiatus hernia, uraemia, gastric carcinoma, a tear in the lower oesophagus following a forceful vomit (the Mallory–Weiss syndrome, 25.16), and multiple shallow erosions following aspirin or some other drugs. In all these conditions the patient vomits bright blood or 'coffee grounds', or he passes melaena stools, or occasionally bright blood, from his rectum.

Aim to: (1) Resuscitate him, (2) make the diagnosis, (3) assess his risk status, and (4) control bleeding.

Try to make the diagnosis epidemiologically and clinically, because you are unlikely to have a fibre-optic gastroscope, although you may be able to do barium studies (34.5). The important distinction is whether or not he has oesophageal varices, because you will not want to operate on these, whereas you may need to operate for most of the other causes. A large spleen is the most useful sign. Fortunately, in contrast to the situation in Western countries, if a patient in India has portal hypertension and oesophageal varices, he is unlikely to be bleeding from an ulcer. Even the best surgical centres cannot find a cause for the bleeding in about 10% of cases. You will need plenty of blood.

UPPER GASTROINTESTINAL BLEEDING

HISTORY. A history of peptic ulceration is suggestive only. There is at least a 25% chance that the patient has a peptic ulcer and no symptoms. Has he been taking aspirin, phenylbutazone, indomethacin, or steroids? All these can cause ulcers.

EXAMINATION. Look for signs of anaemia. A pulse of 120 or more is a reliable sign of recent blood loss. Take his blood pressure. If you are not sure if he is hypovolaemic or not, do the 'pulse test' for orthostatic hypotension (66.1). Examine him for epigastric tenderness. Examine him rectally to make sure that a history of black tarry stools is correct. Look for malignant deposits. Measure his blood urea.

DIAGNOSIS. The following three conditions account for 90% of cases. Other causes, such as hiatus hernia, gastric carcinoma, or the Mallory–Weiss syndrome are rare (25.16).

Suggesting bleeding oesophageal varices—a large spleen, a firm enlarged irregular liver, or a small hard one; anastomotic vessels on his abdomen, ankle oedema. Ascites is common in cirrhosis, less common and often not marked in periportal fibrosis, and very uncommon in extrahepatic obstruction. Spider naevi, and palmar erythema are uncommon in India and Africa. He may be drowsy or in coma from hepatic encephalopathy (made worse by the digestion of the blood in his gut). His liver function tests are abnormal in cirrhosis, but are often normal in the other causes of bleeding varices.

Suggesting a duodenal or gastric ulcer—a history of epigastric pain.

Suggesting gastric mucosal erosions—the recent ingestion of alcohol or analgesic tablets.

Suggesting Schistosomiasis mansoni causing periportal fibrosis—he is from an endemic area and has a large liver, and blood in his stools. There is little point in looking for ova in a rectal snip, because in an endemic area everyone has them.

Suggesting non-cirrhotic portal fibrosis or a thrombosed portal vein—his only abnormal sign is an enlarged spleen.

Use his history and physical signs to form some estimate of how much blood he has lost, and over how long. Decide if his blood loss has been mild, moderate, or severe.

RESUSCITATION. Group and cross-match blood for him. Sedate him heavily 4-hourly with diazepam 5 to 10 mg intravenously, or chlorpromazine 25 mg. Avoid morphine. Cimetidine is of no value, because it does not affect bleeding.

Depending on his condition, set up 1 or 2 intravenous drips of 0.9% saline or Ringer's lactate, with large-bore needles. If he has bled severely, give him 1 to 4 litres of fluid, or more, until his blood pressure returns to 100 mm Hg. He may need at least 3 units of blood and possibly many more. If you have a colloid plasma expander, give him a litre or two while you wait for blood, or even continue with it, if HIV is a high risk in your area.

If you don't have blood, or enough blood, don't hesitate to give him large quantities of saline or Ringer's lactate—his great need is for fluid to fill his vessels.

Pass a large nasogastric tube. This will tell you if he is continuing to bleed, and whether the blood is fresh or altered. If you aspirate clots, irrigate his stomach to wash them out. Then wash out his stomach with ice-cold saline containing noradrenalin every half hour until bleeding stops, as described below. Consider putting 500 mEq of sodium bicarbonate (A 15.1) down the tube 12-hourly. Or, give him magnesium trisilicate mixture 30 ml every 2 hours.

MONITORING. Measure and chart his pulse, his blood pressure, and his peripheral circulation half-hourly. A rising pulse or a sustained tachycardia are more important than isolated readings. Monitor his urine output, and, if possible, his central venous pressure if he is very ill (A 19.2). Early measurements of his haemoglobin and haematocrit will be of little value, except as a baseline with which to compare later ones, because his blood will not yet have had time to dilute. Continued bleeding is suggested by: persistent nausea, tachycardia, pallor, restlessness, very active bowel sounds, and the failure of his haemoglobin to rise in spite of transfusion (a useful sign).

THE OUTCOME. Several things can happen. A gastric ulcer or oesophageal varices are more likely to continue to bleed than a duodenal ulcer. Melaena alone is not as serious as haematemesis, but beware of continuing melaena and unaltered blood in the stools, which indicate continued bleeding.

(1) He may stop bleeding either before he is admitted, or with the above treatment, and not bleed again (75% chance).

(2) He may continue to bleed severely, and vomit up kidney-basin after kidney-basin of fresh or clotted blood, each bleed being accompanied by a wave of weakness and sweating. Or, he may continue to pass large tarry stools. He looks pale, his pulse is rapid (>100), and his blood pressure low (<90 mm), showing that you have been unable to make up for the blood that he has lost.

(3) He may continue to bleed moderately, and respond to the transfusion, but continue to pass small melaena stools, or have small haematemeses, so that his haematocrit drifts downwards. His resting pulse may only be 90, but the least exertion may send it up to 120 or more. Non-operative treatment is dangerous if he stays like this for more than 72 hours.

(4) Bleeding may stop completely and start again in a few hours, or a day or two later. This also is dangerous.

The indicators of low risk and a favourable outcome are: melaena alone, no loss of consciousness, aged <45, BP >100 mm Hg, pulse <120/min.

The indicators of high risk and an unfavourable outcome are: haematemesis, loss of consciousness, aged >45, BP <100 mmHg, pulse >120/min, bleeding varices.

MANAGEMENT depends on his risk status. The following regime comes from India.

If he is at low risk put him to bed for a week, give him 30 ml or more of antacids 2 hourly. He may need 500 mEq of sodium bicarbonate 12-hourly. Later, if possible, refer him for a barium meal and endoscopy.

If he is at high risk management depends on whether or not you suspect varices.

If you suspect varices, insert a Sengstaken tube for 48 hours, then deflate the balloon. If bleeding recurs, reinflate the balloon and refer him.

If you don't suspect varices, continue conservative treatment. If this fails, operate on the indications given below.

INDICATIONS FOR SURGERY. Situations (2), (3) and (4) above and blood shortage are the main indications for surgery. *If you are going to operate do so immediately.* If he is more than 45, he needs surgery all the more urgently, unless he has some other disease, such as cardiac failure.

If he is not suitable for surgery, or for some reason you decide not to operate, there are two things that *may* help—cold noradrenalin lavage and, if you suspect varices, vasopressin.

COLD NORADRENALIN LAVAGE. Over 10 min run 200 ml of ice-cold saline containing noradrenalin 8 mg into his stomach. Half an hour later, aspirate it and replace it. It will lower the temperature in his stomach, and may cause a bleeding vessel to constrict.

A gastric ulcer has stopped bleeding when the fluid that comes out is no longer bloody. If this has not happened after 4 hours, abandon this method. If he has a duodenal ulcer, blood may not be returned in the effluent, so you will have to rely on his pulse and blood pressure to know when he has stopped bleeding.

VASOPRESSIN. ('Pitressin') constricts the sphlanchnic blood vessels, and is more useful for varices than for an ulcer. Dilute 20 units in 500 ml and and give it over 2–3 hours. Warn him about its side-effects—abdominal cramps, headache, and palpitations. It will also raise his blood pressure for a short time. Vasopressin loses its activity in the heat, so, if he does not get abdominal cramps, it is likely to be inactive.

11.4 Surgery for a bleeding peptic ulcer

If a patient has a bleeding peptic ulcer, there is about a 75% chance that it will stop bleeding spontaneously, if you treat him non-operatively by replacing the blood he loses, as in the previous section. If he does not bleed again after his admission to hospital, his chances of living are good. If non-operative treatment succeeds, he can, if necessary, have an elective operation for his ulcer later. There is however about a 25% chance that the time will come, when it looks as if transfusion alone is going to fail. At this point you will have to decide whether or not to operate in the hope of saving his life. If he needs surgery, on the indications in the previous section, and he does not get it, he has about a 50% chance of death, especially if he is over 45. If you operate skillfully, his chances of death are only about 10%. In spite of the limitations of your services, about 90% of your patients with severe bleeding should live, most of them as the result of your efforts. One of your main difficulties will be to get enough blood.

The purpose of emergency surgery is to save his life, so you will have to decide when he is more likely to die if you don't operate than if you do. Try, especially, to judge the best time to operate. When you operate, try to find where the blood is coming from, and stop it. Doing an operation which will prevent it recurring is a lesser priority, because you may be able to refer him to someone else for a definitive operation later.

If you decide to operate, you will have to open his stomach and duodenum. If you find a bleeding duodenal or gastric ulcer, the simplest way to stop it bleeding is to underrun it. At the same time, you can—if you feel competent enough, and he is fit enough—take the opportunity to do a vagotomy and a pyloroplasty or gastroentrostomy, which will reduce the chances of recurrent ulceration afterwards. Cutting his vagus will reduce the acid his stomach secretes, but it will also hinder its emptying. A pyloroplasty will correct this by making a wide opening into his duodenum, through which his stomach can empty more easily. A pyloroplasty also helps a duodenal ulcer, but it should be combined with a vagotomy.

Surgery for gastrointestinal bleeding is difficult. The two common mistakes are: (1) To choose the wrong patients to operate on. (2) To operate at the wrong time—if you wait too long, you risk the patient's life, but if you operate too soon, the risk may be equally great, especially if you operate before you have restored his blood volume. Be much more ready to operate if he is over 45, and if he is bleeding moderately or severely.

The bleeding point may be difficult to find, and when you have found it, blood may obscure it, so that controlling it will be difficult. You will need a large opening in his stomach (gastrotomy), a good assistant, a good light, and good suction.

ANATOMY. The oesophagus continues inside the abdominal cavity for about 2 cm before it joins the stomach. One vagus nerve lies under the peritoneum in front of the oesophagus, and one behind it, not quite so close to it. Both of them lie slightly towards the right, and both usually divide into several branches at the point where the oesophagus joins the stomach. Sometimes the anterior vagus, and less often the posterior one, divide into branches before they pierce the diaphragm. So don't be content with only finding a single trunk. These nerves are more easily felt than seen.

SURGERY FOR A BLEEDING PEPTIC ULCER

INDICATIONS. If a patient is in group (3) or (4) in the 'Indications for Surgery' in Section 11.3, you should be able to prepare him adequately for surgery. Blood will surely be scarce, and HIV may be a problem, but you should try to restore his haematocrit to 30% before you operate, and have 2 or 3 units of blood ready for the operation. A patient in group (2) requires so much blood that providing it will be a severe strain on your blood bank; even so, you should try.

ANAESTHETIC. Intubate him and give him a general anasthetic. Leave a nasogastric tube in place. The anaesthetist must realize that there may still be clots in his stomach. Find two assistants in addition to the trolley nurse.

WHERE IS HE BLEEDING FROM? Make a high midline incision extending up to his xiphisternum. Open his abdomen, and insert a self-retaining retractor in his abdominal wall. Insert a deep retractor under his liver, so that your assistant can retract it upwards. Gently draw the greater curve of his stomach downwards.

Suggesting peptic ulceration—a scarred, deformed first part of his duodenum; a puckered, thickened, hyperaemic area on his stomach, especially on the lesser curve. There may be nothing to feel if a posterior ulcer is eroding into his pancreas.

Suggesting bleeding oesophageal varices—a firm or hard, shrunken, irregular liver, and dilated veins on his stomach. If you find this, and there are no signs of an ulcer also, close his abdomen, and treat him as in Section 11.5. Sometimes a patient has varices *and* an ulcer.

IF THERE IS NO OBVIOUS BLEEDING SITE, feel every part of his stomach between your thumb and forefinger, and go right up to his gastro-oesophageal junction. Open his lesser sac by dividing his greater omentum between the lower edge of his stomach and his colon. Feel the whole posterior surface of his stomach. You may fail to find the source of the bleeding, or to control it, but unless you try, the chances of his surviving are small.

If you still cannot find the source of his bleeding, and he has been having melaena stools, check his small gut first. Blood might be coming from anywhere from his duodenojejunal flexure to his caecum. If you are not sure if the contents of his gut are blood or bile insert a needle obliquely and aspirate them. Look for a bleeding leiomyoma of the stomach or small intestine, or a bleeding Meckel's diverticulum. Then check his colon for ileocaecal tuberculosis, carcinoma, amoebic colitis, and intussusception, etc.

If, even after you have done this, you cannot find the source of the bleeding, and he has vomited blood, open his stomach and duodenum. There is no substitute for having a good look.

Alternatively, if you have a cystoscope, consider inserting this into his stomach through a purse string suture. You can see into the second part of his duodenum, and up into his oesophagus. You may have to wash out his stomach to get a clear view.

OPENING THE STOMACH AND DUODENUM IN GASTROINTESTINAL BLEEDING

Insert moist packs to seal off his abdominal cavity. You have a choice of two incisions, depending on the degree of fibrosis of his duodenum.

If the scarring and fibrosis of his duodenum is mild or absent, make a linear incision as in A, Fig. 11-3 with 3/5 of it in his stomach, and 2/5 in his duodenum.

If the scarring and fibrosis of his duodenum is severe, make a Y-shaped incision as in E, Fig. 11-3.

Make your linear or Y-shaped incision through the serous and muscular coats of the anterior wall of his stomach, starting 4 cm proximal to his pylorus, and extending over the front of the first and second parts of his duodenum for 3 cm beyond his pylorus. If he has an ulcer, centre the linear incision on this, and make it about 1 cm above the lower border of his stomach and duodenum, as in (A).

Use tissue forceps and a scalpel to make a nick through the mucosa of the gastric end of the incision, so as to open his stomach. Enlarge the opening a little with scissors. Slowly cut through the remaining mucosa with scissors. Pick up bleeding points as you reach them, or bleeding from the incision will obscure everything. If there are too many haemostats, run a continuous layer of catgut along each side of the incision, and tie the bleeding points.

Inspect the inside of his stomach and duodenum. Mop out clots, and suck out fresh blood, trying to see where it is coming from. Evert the mucosal layer with Babcock forceps. Place a deep retractor in the upper end of the opening in his stomach and ask your assistant to expose as much of its interior as he can. If necessary, extend the incision 2 to 5 cm proximally. Is there blood trickling down from anywhere? Feel the inside of his stomach. You may see or feel: (1) An artery spurting from an ulcer on the posterior wall of the first part of his duodenum (the common site), or round the corner in its second part. (2) An ulcer anywhere in his stomach. (3) Shallow erosions, high on the lesser curve.

If he has had a haematemesis and you cannot find any abnormality: (1) Try to look at his gastro-oesophageal junction from inside his stomach. Make a high longitudinal gastrotomy up to the cardia. You may see oesophageal varices, or forceful vomiting may have produced a Mallory–Weiss tear of his lower oesophagus (see below and 25.16). (2) Put the tip of the sucker, or a swab on a holder, into the second part of his duodenum, to make sure that he is not bleeding from a post-bulbar ulcer.

If you still cannot find any cause for the bleeding, close the incisions in his stomach and his abdomen. Some surgeons would do a truncal vagotomy and a gastroenterostomy, or a pyloroplasty.

If you find an acute ulcer, a solitary erosion, or multiple small bleeding erosions, do a truncal vagotomy and gastroenterostomy, or a pyloroplasty. Postoperatively, warn him not to take drugs containing aspirin.

A CHRONIC BLEEDING ULCER AT LAPAROTOMY

Control bleeding from a chronic duodenal ulcer by underrunning it. Retract the edges of the V-shaped pyloroplasty incision. Using chromic catgut in the stomach and silk in the duodenum on a curved needle, pass 2 or 3 stitches deep to the ulcer, as in B, Fig. 11-3. Tie the sutures so that you stop the bleeding. Ask your assistant to keep the area dry, and be sure to go deep enough to include the walls and base of the ulcer, but not so deep that you catch important structures, such as the common bile duct. Tie the sutures tight, but not so tight that they cut out.

If you don't feel happy about doing a vagotomy, do a pyloroplasty, and refer him for a definitive vagotomy later.

PYLOROPLASTY

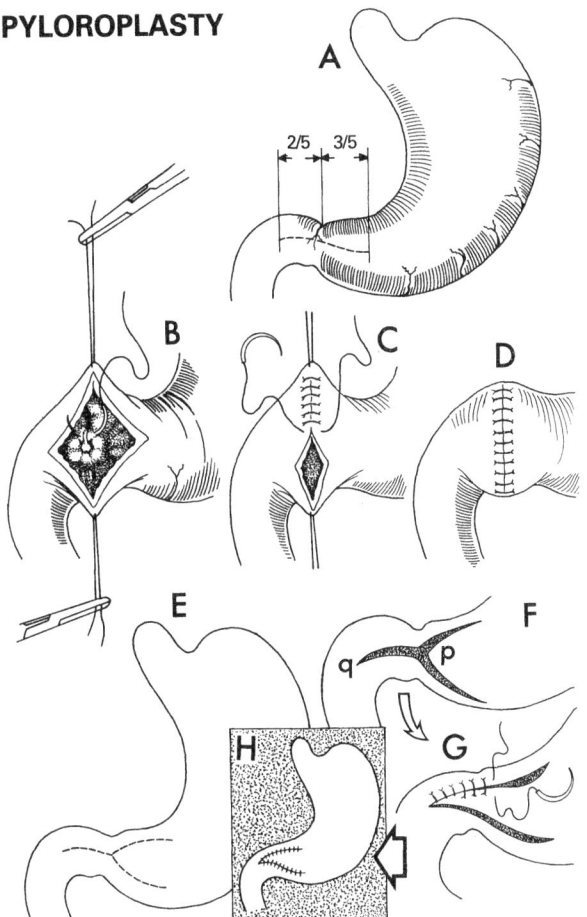

Fig. 11-3 PYLOROPLASTY (Heinicke–Miculicz). A, the incision when there is only moderate fibrosis. The incision into the stomach is slightly longer than that into the duodenum. B, the incision held open with stay sutures, held in haemostats, while a bleeding ulcer is being undersewn. C, the stay sutures have been pulled, so as to elongate the incision transversely. It is being closed with close sutures of 2/0 chromic catgut through all coats. D, the completed pyloroplasty. E, if there is severe pyloric stenosis, which makes suturing in the transverse direction impossible, make a Y-shaped incision. F, the flap of the incision ('p') is going to be sutured into the duodenum ('q') so as to make a 'V'. G, suturing has begun. H, the finished pyloroplasty.

PYLOROPLASTY (Heinicke–Miculicz)

INDICATIONS. (1) A bleeding duodenal ulcer. (2) For other complications of a duodenal ulcer, see 11.2.

METHOD. First make sure bleeding is controlled as described above. The kind of pyloroplasty you should make will depend on the kind of incision you made, which in turn depended on the severity of the fibrosis you found.

If you made a linear incision, because there was only mild fibrosis, hold it open with stay sutures. Pull on these so as to elongate it transversely, and close it with close 2/0 chromic catgut sutures through the mucosa and serosa.

If you made a Y-shaped incision, because there was much fibrosis, either: (1) Close it as you found it, and do a gastroenterostomy. Or, (2) sew it up as a 'V', as in G, and H, Fig. 11-3.

Finally, with both incisions, bring up a tag of omentum and fix this across the suture line with a few sutures which pick up only the seromuscular layer (C, 11-2).

VAGOTOMY FOR PEPTIC ULCERATION

Postpone this if his condition does not permit it—you have already done the life saving part of the operation. You must get adequate access. This may be difficult if he is fat, or has a deep chest, or if the left lobe of his liver is large.

Extend the abdominal incision right up into the notch between his costal margin and his xiphisternum. Ask your assistant to lift up his left costal margin with a deep gauze-covered retractor. With your right hand draw his stomach and colon downwards and keep them packed down with 2 or 3 large moist abdominal packs. Feel for the short abdominal part of his oesophagus, and for the nasogastric tube running through it. Or slide your hand upwards over the fundus and body of his stomach, until you reach his diaphragm, and then feel for his oesophagus.

You have now to free the left lobe of his liver from his diaphragm. Grasp its free edge between the index and middle finger of your pronated left hand, and pull it downwards and medially. This will reveal his left triangular ligament attaching this part of his liver to his diaphragm. Under good vision and with a long pair of scissors cut about 4 to 6 cm of this bloodless attachment from left to right, making sure that you do not go too far medially (B, in Fig. 11-4), because his inferior vena cava is there. Then reflect the left lobe of his liver medially and to the right, and hold it there with a deep (Deaver's) retractor over a large pack (C).

Pick up the peritoneum over his oesophagus with a long (25 cm) haemostat, and use scissors, or a long-handled scalpel with a small blade, to make a very superficial 2 cm transverse or longitudinal incision in it, just above its junction with his stomach.

CAUTION ! (1) Cut his *peritoneum only*. This is a thin layer. Don't cut the muscle of his oesophagus. (2) Don't cut any of the branches of his left gastric vein, on the right margin of his stomach.

Using gauze on a sponge holder (D), gently push away the peritoneum from the site of the incision, so exposing the front of his oesophagus (E). Dissecting with your right index, and repeatedly spreading your index and middle finger to open up tissue planes, free his oesophagus from the areolar tissue holding it to the right crus of his diaphragm and his aorta. If you dissect like this there is little chance of your tearing blood vessels, or damaging his oesophagus. But, don't 'finger dissect' too close to his oesophagus posteriorly, or you will push his posterior vagus nerve away from it, so that finding it will be difficult. Stay close to the crus, especially as you dissect towards the right side of his oesophagus. On the right your finger may be arrested by peritoneal folds and small vessels. Persist with blunt dissection, and resist the urge to cut anything, until you have gone all round his oesophagus with your finger.

Gently draw his oesophagus downwards until you can feel 4–5 cm of it. Pass a long curved clamp, such as a Lahey, behind his mobilized oesophagus, and use it to draw a soft catheter, or nasogastric tube, through and around it, so that you can pull on it (F). This will help to expose the site better, and will hold the vagus taut, so you can feel it.

Feel for his anterior vagus nerve. You may see it as a fine white strand running down in front of the central part of his oesophagus, but it is usually easier to feel (G). Run your right index finger across his oesophagus—feel for a taut thread or fine cord, quite different from anything else. Follow it up to where it emerges from under the crus of his diaphragm. Place a long O'Shaughnessy or Lahey haemostat on the nerve and draw it down slightly, to make sure that it does not have any branches. Apply another long clamp just distal to the first, and cut the vagus between them. Draw the second clamp and the vagus downwards, and cut off a 1 cm segment of the nerve (H and I). Search the anterior aspect of his oesophagus for other branches of his vagus—incomplete vagotomy is the commonest reason why the operation fails.

Look for his posterior vagus nerve—it is harder to find, but is larger. If your dissection has been adequate, you should find it. Pass a finger of your right hand round the back of his oesophagus, and feel for the thick cord of his posterior vagus, just behind the right edge of his oesophagus. Try lifting it forwards over the tip of your finger (J); then clean away any obscuring strands of tissue with a pledget of gauze on the end of a sponge forceps. You should be able to expose a short section of it without rupturing any of the small veins. Remove a piece of his posterior vagus as you did his anterior one (K), and look for accessory branches. Control minor bleeding by packing his subphrenic area with warm moist packs for a few minutes. Control any more active bleeding by ligation.

CAUTION ! Feel for these nerves, pull them up on a finger, see them, and then cut them.

VAGOTOMY

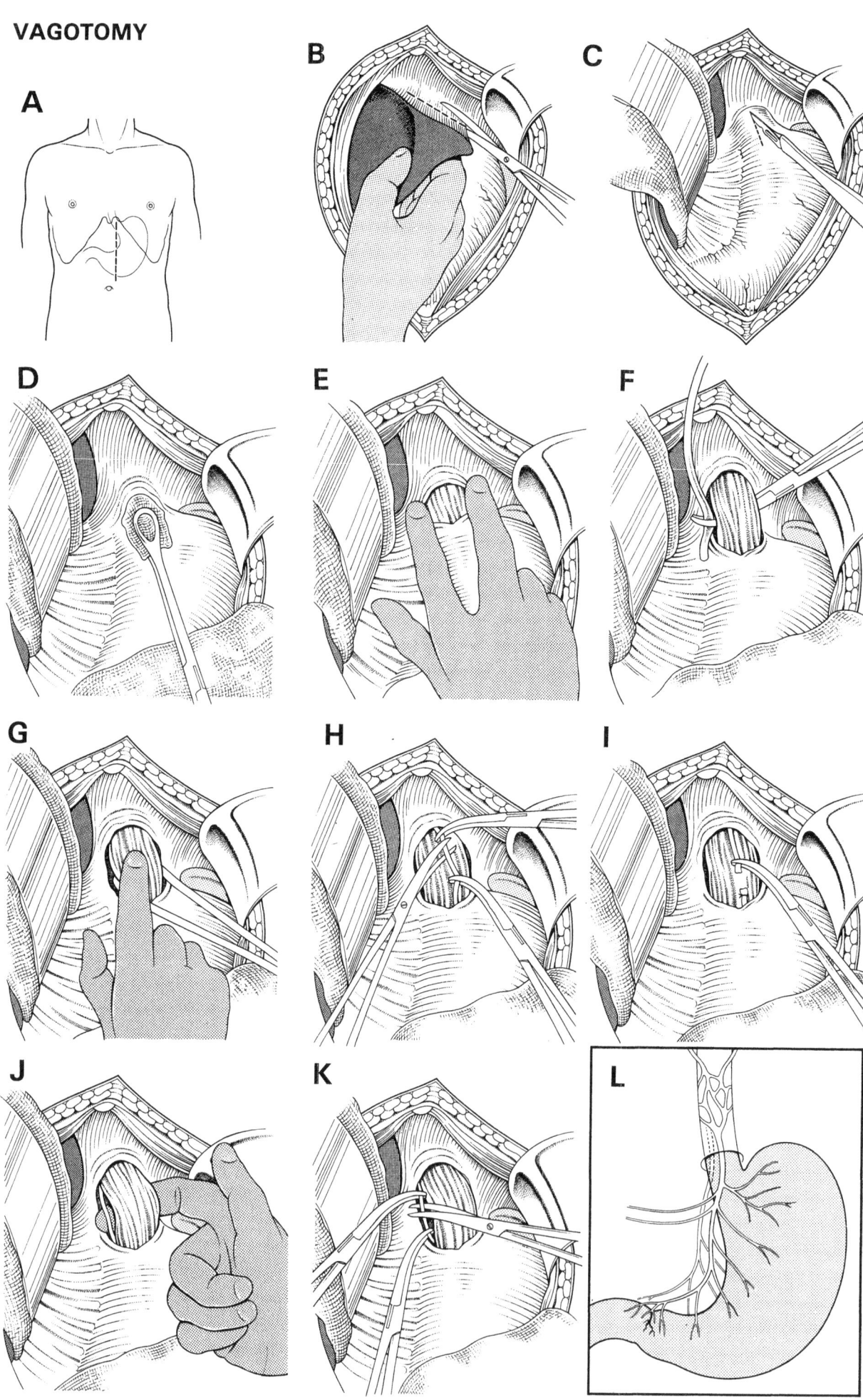

Remove the sling round his oesophagus. Close his abdomen, preferably in a single layer by Everett's or Goligher's methods (9.8). Don't insert a drain, unless you are worried about the safety of the anastomosis of his pyloroplasty. He has bled severely, and his wound is likely to heal poorly. If it breaks down, he will be in danger.

'Suck and drip him', and replace his gastric aspirate, as usual (9.9, A 15.5). If his postoperative haematocrit is less than 35%, transfuse him.

DIFFICULTIES WITH GASTROINTESTINAL BLEEDING

Expect respiratory complications (9.11), and wound breakdown (9.13).

If the BLEEDING POINT IN HIS DUODENUM IS OBSCURED BY BLOOD, apply warm packs and pressure, and wait 10 minutes.

If BLEEDING RESTARTS after the operation, manage him non-operatively, or refer him; don't try to explore him again.

If you find what looks like a MALIGNANT GASTRIC ULCER, adapt what you do to the size of the lesion:

If the lesion is small, do a local excision with a 2 cm margin, and repair the defect in two layers.

If the lesion is advanced, take a biopsy, and if it has metastasized to lymph nodes or his liver, refer him for more radical surgery later if you can.

If he BLED AFTER A SEVERE INJURY, or a burn, a head injury, or a major surgical operation, or he is an alcoholic or takes drugs, such as aspirin, indomethacin, or phenylbutazone, suspect STRESS ULCERS (superficial erosions in the stomach or typically in the second or third parts of the duodenum). These are usually multiple, shallow, and irregular. He will have had little pain, and severe bleeding is likely to have been the first sign. Minor harmless gastric bleeding is common after an alcoholic bout. Ulceration of this kind may ooze severely, so that he has melaena stools for several days. Give him antacids half-hourly, and try a noradrenalin in saline lavage (11.3) and, if possible, intravenous cimetidine. Don't operate if you can avoid doing so. If you have to operate, do a vagotomy and gastroenterostomy. His chances of dying are high, whatever you do.

If you are giving him cimetidine intravenously, **give him 100-200 mg/hour for 2 hours repeated after an interval of 4-6 hours. Or, 400 mg in 100 ml of 0.9% sodium chloride infused over half to one hour, repeated after 4-6 hours. Or, by continuous infusion at an average rate of 50-100 mg/hour over 24 hours, maximum 2.4 g daily.**

If he started to BLEED AFTER A SEVERE EPISODE OF VOMITING from some other cause, such as a drinking bout, suspect that he has a tear in his oesophagus at, or just above, his gastro-oesophageal junction (the Mallory-Weiss syndrome). See Section 25.16.

If you ENTER HIS OESOPHAGUS DURING A VAGOTOMY (which should never happen!), repair the tear as in Section 25.16 and Fig 25-12.

11.5 Bleeding oesophageal varices

A patient who is bleeding from the rupture of his oesophageal varices will be such a formidable challenge to you, that stopping it may be impossible. You will not be able to do a portacaval shunt, or to suture them with an automatic stapling instrument, so you will have to rely on plenty of blood and a Sengstaken tube to compress them. If he has cirrhosis, his prognosis outside a major centre will be so bad, and he will need so much blood, that you may not feel justified in treating him.

Fig. 11-4 VAGOTOMY. A, make a high midline or left paramedian incision. B, free the attachment of the left lobe of the patient's liver from his diaphragm. C, incise the peritoneum—*only*—over the anterior of his oesophagus. D, gently push the peritoneum away from the incision. E, open up the tissue planes with your index and middle finger. F, draw a catheter round his oesophagus. G, pull his oesophagus down and feel for his anterior vagus. H, and I, cut out a length of vagus. J, feel for his posterior vagus. K, cut his posterior vagus. L, the anatomy of the vagus nerves.

Dilated varices are the result of a high pressure in his portal venous system—more than 18 cm of saline. The common causes are: (1) cirrhosis of his liver, (2) periportal fibrosis due to *S. mansoni* infection, (3) noncirrhotic portal fibrosis, and (4) thrombosis of his portal vein. He dies from loss of blood and loss of liver function. The final cause of his death may be hepatic encephalopathy, due to the failure of his liver to detoxify the breakdown products from the blood in his gut, either because its cells have failed, or because blood has been shunted from his liver. Liver failure commonly complicates cirrhosis, but not the other causes.

Aim to: (1) stop him bleeding, (2) restore his blood volume, and (3) prevent encephalopathy.

• TUBE Sengstaken, 18 and 21 Ch, two only of each size. This has 3 channels and two balloons. You will need this tube if bleeding oesophageal varices are common in your area. It will usually control bleeding while the tube is in place, and bleeding may stop after it is removed. One danger is that a balloon may displace into the patient's glottis and obstruct his respiration. If you don't have a Sengstaken tube, you may be able to use a Foley catheter with a 30 ml balloon.

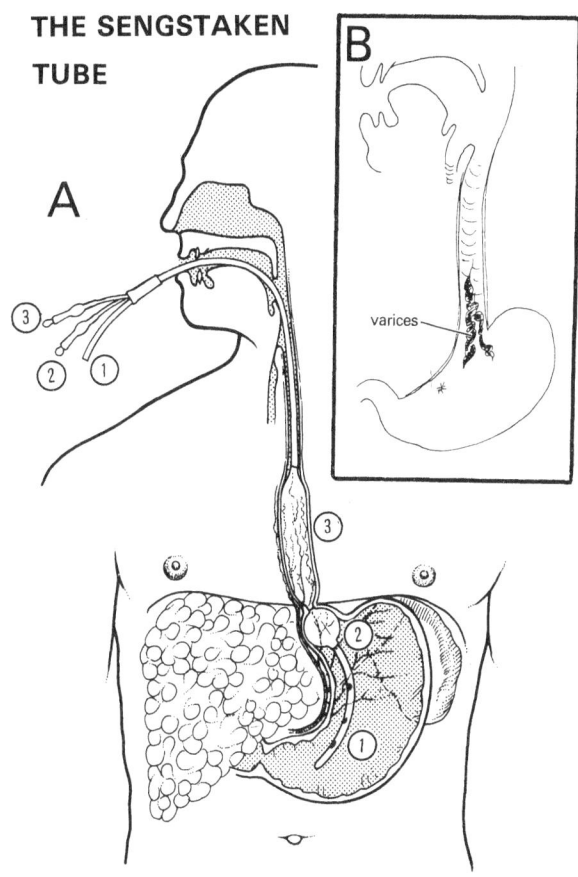

Fig. 11-5 A SENGSTAKEN TUBE. A, this has three channels: 1, to aspirate blood from the patient's stomach. 2, to inflate a balloon in his stomach to anchor the tube. 3, to inflate another balloon in his oesophagus to compress his varices. B, the varices that the balloon tries to compress.

BLEEDING VARICES

WHEN THE PATIENT IS NOT BLEEDING

If you see him between bleeds, do his liver function tests. Do a barium swallow with a thick suspension of barium to demonstrate the varices. If necessary, examine a rectal snip. Give him 3 injections of vitamin K_1 10 mg daily for 5 days.

WHEN HE IS BLEEDING

PREVENT ENCEPHALOPATHY. Give him a saline purge through the Sengstaken tube. Empty his large gut with an enema, and give him oral neomycin 1 g 4 to 6-hourly to reduce the bacterial activity in his gut. Don't give him any protein by mouth.

DRUG CONTROL OF BLEEDING. Vasopressin ('Pitressin') will reduce his portal venous pressure by constricting his sphlanchnic arterioles. See Section 11.3.

SENGSTAKEN TUBE. Measure the capacity of the two balloons, and check that neither of them leak. The distal gastric balloon of a large tube holds about 120 ml. Inflate the oesophageal one to 30 mm Hg, checked against an ordinary sphygmomanometer. Add the contents of 2 ampoules of 45% 'Hypaque' (or a similar contrast medium) to 250 ml of saline.

Have a sucker available. Local anaesthesia of his mouth and pharynx may be helpful. Lay him on his side, and pass the tube quickly through his mouth into his stomach. Inflate the gastric balloon with the saline/hypaque mixture. Withdraw it until it impacts against his cardia, and take an X-ray film to check its position. Inflate the oesophageal balloon to 30 mm Hg. Tie a thread round the tube opposite his lips to mark the correct position of the balloons.

Aspirating the tube will show you if he has stopped bleeding. Use it to give him a mixture of magnesium hydroxide, neomycin, and glucose. He will be unable to swallow his saliva, so lay him on his side to let it dribble frm his lips, and have a nurse always available to suck out his mouth, if necessary.

After 24 hours deflate the oesophageal balloon, then the gastric one, and continue to aspirate his stomach. If he starts bleeding again, you can apply the tube for a further 12 hours, but this is a sign that he should have surgery—if this is possible.

CAUTION ! (1) If the tube displaces upwards, it may obstruct his glottis. Warn the nurses about this, and tell them to remove it quickly if it does so. (2) Deflate the tube after 48 hours. Don't leave it in any longer, because his mucosa will necrose. (3) If you continue to aspirate fresh blood, reconsider your diagnosis. (4) Don't take a needle biopsy of his liver while he is in the acute bleeding stage.

A FOLEY CATHETER is less satisfactory. Pass this through his mouth, inflate the balloon, and draw it upwards so that it presses against the varices at his gastro-oesophageal junction. Either tape the catheter to his cheek, or, better, tie it to a weight suspended from a pulley.

DIFFICULTIES WITH BLEEDING VARICES

If he BLEEDS AGAIN after you have removed the tube, his prognosis is not good, but varies with the cause of his varices. If he is cirrhotic, his prognosis is bad.

If his RECTAL SNIP IS POSITIVE for *Schistosoma mansoni,* or he is excreting ova in his stools, this may be the cause of his symptoms. Unfortunately, in an endemic area most of the population will have ova in their stools. Live ova, detected by a concentration test if necessary, are more significant than dead ones. If however he does have periportal cirrhosis due to this worm, his liver function is likely to be good, and his prognosis will not be so bad—if you can refer him to a centre where he can have a portosystemic shunt, or a course of sclerotherapy. This is probably only justified if he is under 50, has no jaundice or ascites, and his serum albumen is above 3 g/dl.

If his PORTAL VEIN HAS THROMBOSED, or he has NON-CIRRHOTIC PORTAL FIBROSIS, he will probably have a normal liver, and his bleeding will eventually stop. Refer him if you can.

11.6 Pyloric stenosis

The scarring around a patient's duodenal ulcer sometimes obstructs his pylorus, especially if he does not have his earlier ulcer symptoms treated. He may come to you saying that he has been vomiting for days or weeks. He may only vomit once a day, or he may say that he vomits "everything he eats". His vomit may contain food that he ate days before. Or, he may not actually vomit, but merely feel abnormally full and bloated after only small amounts of food. He may have eructations, and he may have taught himself to vomit to relieve his symptoms. He loses weight. Continued vomiting depletes his extracellular fluid, and causes hypoclhoraemic alkalosis, and hypokalaemia; eventually he becomes dehydrated and oliguric.

Occasionally, he may improve with a few days of conservative treatment, so that he is able to eat without feeling nauseated. If he does, don't press him to let you operate. He is unlikely to improve permanently. But if he has been vomiting for many days, and is starved and dehydrated with a huge dilated stomach, operate as soon as you have corrected his fluid and electrolyte deficit.

When you operate, do a vagotomy and a gastrojejunostomy, which is a side-to-side anastomosis between the antrum of his stomach and his jejunum. This will be easier than doing a pyloroplasty (11.4) when his duodenum is very scarred, as it usually is in the developing world. In India and Africa a gastroenterostomy may be better than a pyloroplasty, even if his duodenum is not much scarred at the time of surgery, because it may scar later. A retrocolic gastroenterostomy is better than an antecolic one, because the loop of jejunum to be brought up to the stomach is shorter, and there is no abnormal hole in his mesentery, through which loops of gut can herniate and twist. Make the stoma vertical so that it drains more easily.

His duodenal ulcer may be anterior or posterior. The other important cause of stenosis of his distal stomach is carcinoma, see Section 32.25.

PYLORIC STENOSIS

EXAMINATION. Lay the patient down and look for visible peristalsis, as his stomach struggles to empty itself through his narrowed pylorus. Look for slow waves moving from his left hypochondrium towards and beyond his umbilicus. Rock him from side to side. You may hear hear a succussion splash. You may also hear it if you depress his epigastrium sharply with your hand (a splash may be normal after a large meal).

WASHOUTS will empty his stomach, remove debris, and rest it. With luck, his inflamed and oedematous pylorus will open up. Washouts, as in Fig. 25-11, will also reduce the risk of postoperative infection.

Find a funnel, a *large* (36 Ch, about 1 cm diameter) stomach tube or a catheter, and a longer piece of rubber connecting tube the same size. Lay him supine with his head supported over the end of the bed, as in Fig. 25-11. Pass the well-lubricated stomach tube through his mouth and encourage him to swallow it. Connect the stomach tube via the other tube to the funnel. Hold the funnel and pour in 500 ml of water. Before the last drop has left the funnel, lower it over a bucket (to prevent air entering). His stomach contents will run out. Repeat the process, this time using a litre of water. Go on doing this until the fluid returns clear. Finally, leave 500 ml inside him.

Repeat this daily, for 3 days, or until he is fit for surgery, whichever is later. Don't wash him out on the day of the operation.

FOOD. Give him any convenient fluid diet, such as milk with added sugar, but don't give him anything to eat.

X-RAYS are useful if the diagnosis is in doubt. Take an erect abdominal film, and look for a large fluid level in his left upper quadrant. A drink of barium will produce a mottled shadow showing that his gastric outline is much enlarged. Little or no

---

Fig. 11-6 GASTROENTEROSTOMY. A, reflecting the patient's colon upwards, so as to expose the back of his stomach. Incising his mesentery. B, bringing his stomach and jejunum together through his transverse mesocolon. Notice the position of his middle colic vessels. C, applying a non-crushing clamp to his jejunum. D, stay sutures and the posterior seromuscular (Lembert) layer. E, tying the vessels in the muscle of his stomach. F, opening his jejunum, G, the posterior all–coats layer. H, the second Connell inverting stitch. I, the anterior layer. J, the final Connell stitch. K, the anterior seromuscular layer of sutures. L, testing the stoma.

GASTROENTEROSTOMY

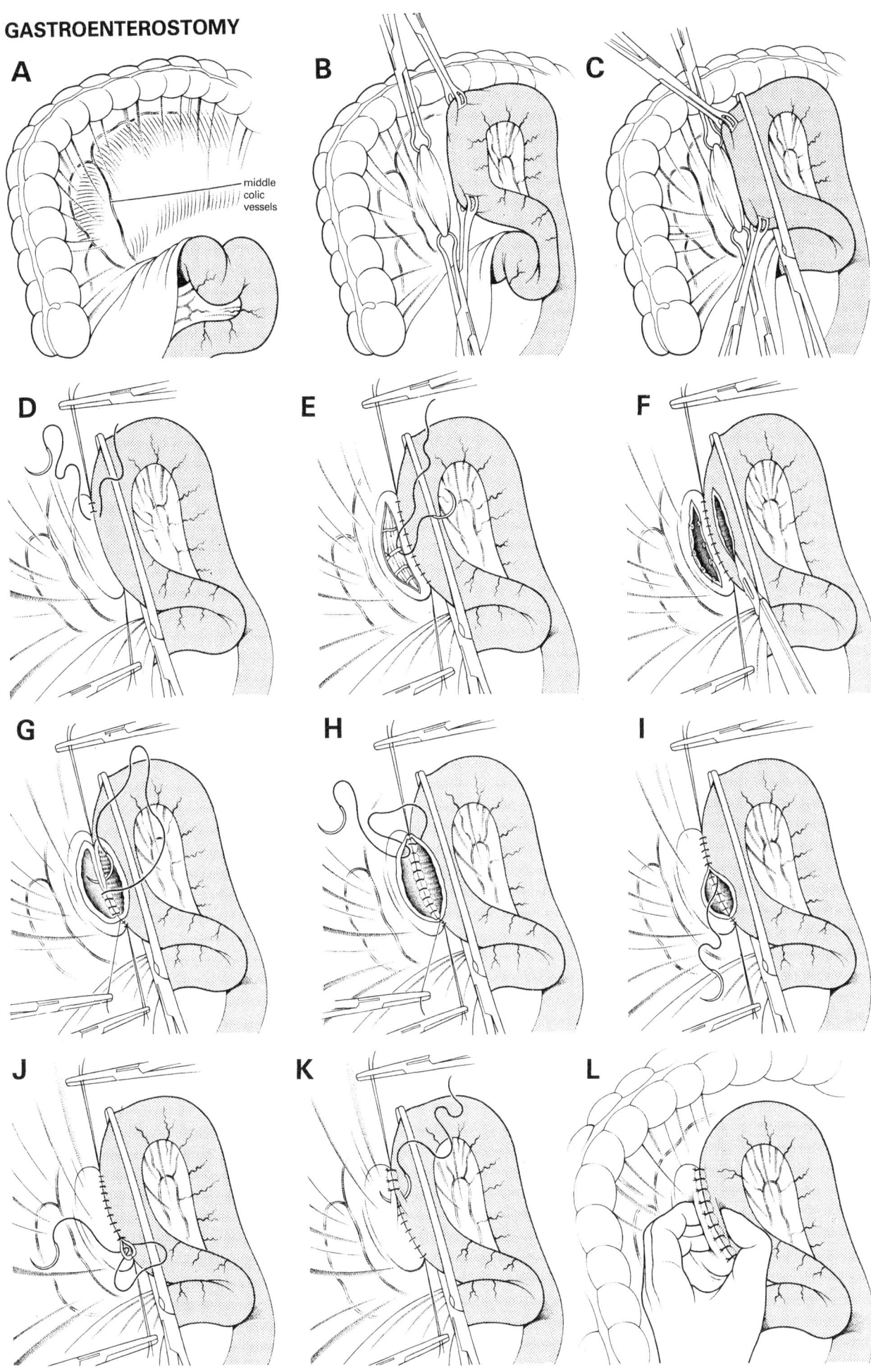

barium passes his pylorus. Don't give him a large quantity, because it may be difficult to wash out.

NON-OPERATIVE TREATMENT FOR PYLORIC STENOSIS

REHYDRATION, may be necessary over several days to restore his extracellular fluid volume. Use the methods in A 15.3. Give him 0.9% saline or Ringer's lactate. If necessary, correct his potassium loss with up to 80 mmol of potassium daily, or use Darrow's solution (K 34 mmol/litre). Be guided by the volume and specific gravity of his urine output.

GASTROENTEROSTOMY FOR PYLORIC STENOSIS

INDICATIONS. (1) Pyloric obstruction causing dehydration and weight loss, or other long-standing obstructive symptoms as described above. (2) Duodenal ulceration with sufficient scarring to contraindicate pyloroplasty; combine it with a truncal vagotomy. (3) As a palliative procedure for stenosis caused by an antral carcinoma. (4) For a duodenal ulcer in a woman of over 60.

ANAESTHESIA. Give him a general anaesthetic with a muscle relaxant (A 14.3).

POSITION. Lay him supine with his upper abdomen pushed forward by 'breaking the table', or by putting a pillow under his back.

INCISION. Make an upper midline incision, or, if he has well developed muscles, a right upper paramedian one.

If you find a large thick walled stomach, the diagnosis of pyloric stenosis is confirmed. Ask your assistant to retract his liver upwards with a deep retractor, and to draw his stomach downwards at the same time.

Is the obstruction malignant? First, try to make sure that he has not got a carcinoma of his pylorus. If he has lumps and nodules, enlarged hard lymph nodes, and perhaps an ulcer crater, *just proximal to his pylorus*, suspect a carcinoma. Biopsy a node. He has probably got a chronic duodenal ulcer if he has: (1) Puckered scarring on the front of the first part of his duodenum, perhaps with adhesions to surrounding structures. (2) An indentation on the posterior wall of his stomach extending into his pancreas to which it is fixed. Carcinoma does not attack the first part of the duodenum, so that lesions there are almost certainly benign.

If you are not sure what is obstructing the outlet of his stomach, do a gastroenterostomy and biopsy a regional node. Don't biopsy his stomach itself unless you intend to resect it. If you find a carcinoma, you can refer him for definitive surgery later—if the tumour is resectable (no spread to his liver or to nodes beyond those on the greater and lesser curves of his stomach). See Section 32.25.

METHOD FOR GASTROENTEROSTOMY. Start by doing a vagotomy (11.4), if this is indicated.

Ask your assistant to lift up the patients's transverse colon with both his hands, so as to expose the posterior layer of his transverse mesocolon. Find his middle colic vessels. You will see the posterior wall of his stomach through his mesocolon (A, in Fig. 11-6). If he is thin, you will see it easily; if he is fat, it will be easier to feel.

Apply Babcock's forceps to the posterior aspect of his stomach about 6 cm apart (B). Take up his mesocolon in the bite in an area well to the left of his middle colic vesels, leaving enough rooom for his jejunum to be brought alongside. Using the Babcock's as markers, push his stomach through his mesocolon from above.

CAUTION ! Make sure that the Babcock forceps are not too near any lesion he may have on the greater curve of his stomach.

Find his upper jejunum and apply Babcock forceps to that. The first should be about 8 cm from his duodeno-jejunal flexure, and the second about 6 cm distal to that (B). Apply a non-crushing clamp as shown (C), to hold two-thirds of the width of the gut.

Insert stay sutures through the seromuscular coats of his stomach and jejunum at each end, going through his mesocolon. His stomach wall is likely to be thick, perhaps very thick, if his pyloric stenosis is long-standing.

Continue the layer of interrupted seromuscular sutures using 2/0 multifilament silk (D).

Carefully incise the muscle of his stomach. This will reveal some blood vessels. Doubly tie these with 2/0 silk or smaller (E), and divide them between the ties.

Open his stomach by cutting its mucosa, for about 3 fingers length (5 cm). Then, open his jejunum for an equal length, half way between the suture line and the clamp (F).

Use 2/0 atraumatic catgut for the 'all coats' layer (G), starting at one end with an inverting Connell stitch, in the same way as for a side-to-side anastomosis. See Fig. 9-12.

CAUTION ! (1) Be sure to include all layers of his stomach wall in the anastomosis. If it is hypertrophied, the cut edges of its mucosa will curl away. If you fail to include them in your sutures, they may bleed, or the suture line may leak. (2) Take care not to rupture his spleen, or his gastrosplenic vessels by pulling on his stomach too much—make sure you have adequate exposure.

Continue the suture along the posterior layer of the anastomosis, and do an inverting suture at the end (H). Then do the anterior layer (I), using a simple over-and-over suture and ending with a Connell inverting stitch (J). Tie the ends of the suture together and and cut them 0.5 cm distal to the knot.

Insert a layer of interrupted sutures through the seromuscular coats of his stomach and jejunum, picking up his mesocolon with them (K). Remove the clamp, and feel the size of the stoma: it should admit 2 or 3 fingers (L). Replace his transverse colon in his abdomen.

DIFFICULTIES WITH A GASTROENTEROSTOMY

If his PEPTIC ULCER SYMPTOMS recur, you have not been successful in cutting all the branches of his vagus. An incomplete vagotomy is the main reason why this operation fails. If possible, give him a course of cimetidine, 200 mg three times a day and 400 mg at night for 4 weeks. If not try medical treatment with antacids (11.1). If his pain is not relieved, or he bleeds sigificantly, refer him.

If you CONTINUE TO ASPIRATE A LITRE OR MORE OF FLUID after the operation, the stoma is not functioning, or he has paralytic ileus. Bowel sounds and the absence of abdominal distension will exclude the latter. The stoma will be less likely to obstruct, if you make it big enough to take three fingers. It may remain obstructed for 2 weeks. Continue nasogastric suction, unless there is an indication to reoperate (10.13), and give him parenteral fluids. His stoma is almost certain to open eventually.

If, some time after the operation, he STARTS TO VOMIT BILE, reassure him. Bile and pancreatic juice are accumulating in the afferent loop, and when they are suddenly released into his stomach, he vomits. His symptoms will probably improve with time. If they don't improve in 2 years, consider referring him for a revision procedure.

11.7 Elective surgery for chronic duodenal ulcer

If a patient has 'peptic ulcer disease', you can usually treat him by medical treatment with diet and antacids, and by persuading him to abandon alcohol and cigarettes. Unfortunately, you are unlikely to be able to give him the expensive H_2 receptor antagonists, cimetidine or ranitidine, because he cannot afford them. So, if inexpensive medical treatment fails, the only way you can help a poor patient may be to operate. If he has uncontrollable pain and dyspepsia, or if his quality of life has been spoilt over the years by nagging pain, heartburn, and indigestion, do a truncal vagotomy and gastroenterostomy or pyloroplasty (11.4), as an elective procedure, especially if he is older and has atypical symptoms. He may have a gastric ulcer, with its higher rate of complications and recurrence. Don't wait until he has a severe bleed, or the overwhelming vomiting of pyloric obstruction. You will not have an endoscope, and may not be able to do barium studies, so you will only be able to confirm the diagnosis at laparotomy.

The absolute indications for operation are: (1) perforation, (2) a continuing or recurrent haematemesis, (3) pyloric stenosis, (4) suspicions of carcinoma—if he is fit enough. Otherwise, he is

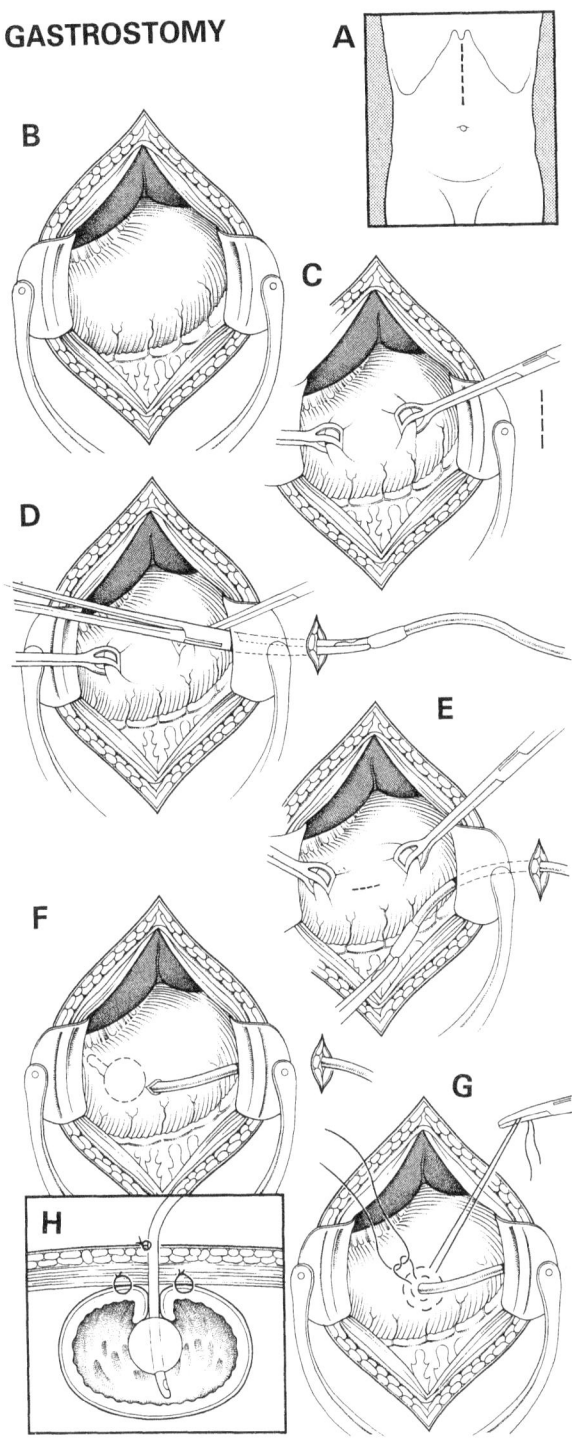

Fig. 11-7 GASTROSTOMY. A, the incision. B, the patient's stomach exposed. C, picking up his stomach in Allis forceps. D, introducing the catheter through his abdominal wall. E, the incision in his stomach. F, the catheter introduced. G, the purse string sutures. H, how his stomach wall is invaginated.

likely to be the best judge as to whether he should undergo surgery or not—provided he is not neurotic!

Your methods for investigating him will be limited, so when you do a laparotomy, expect to find that your preoperative diagnosis was wrong. What you thought was a duodenal ulcer may be chronic cholecystitis, carcinoma of his stomach, chronic pancreatitis, or some other abdominal condition.

11.8 Gastrostomy (Stamm)

If a patient's oesophagus is obstructed, he cannot swallow food, so he starves. He cannot swallow saliva, so it drips from his mouth. You can feed him through an opening in his stomach, but this will not help him to swallow his saliva. This is such a disabling symptom, that there is little to be gained by prolonging his life merely to endure it. There is thus seldom any indication for doing a gastrostomy for inoperable carcinoma of the oesophagus or pharynx. The possible indications for it are given below. For many of them a jejunostomy is an alternative.

GASTROSTOMY

INDICATIONS. (1) Strictures of a patient's oesophagus following corrosive poisoning, prior to referral for reconstruction. (2) A malignant stricture of his oesophagus or gastro-oesophageal junction, with no signs of advanced disease, and when you plan to insert a Celestin tube. (3) Operable oesophageal carcinoma to 'build him up' before referring him for resection. (4) Diseases of his pharynx or larynx which make swallowing impossible, but which can be cured (for example, retropharyngeal abscess or perforation from a fish bone). (5) Temporary postoperative drainage of his stomach, when a nasogastric tube is impractical. (6) Inoperable carcinoma of the oesophagus is seldom considered a suitable indication, see above and Section 32.24.

METHOD. Under local or general anaesthesia make a small upper median incision (9.2). Pick up the cut edges of his peritoneum and draw them apart. You will probably find that his stomach is small and tubular, so that the first thing that you see is is his great omentum or transverse colon. Pull this downwards and deliver the upper part of his stomach into the wound.

CAUTION ! Check that you really have found his stomach, and not his transverse colon by mistake!

Make a small stab wound beside the median incision and use a haemostat to pull a 12 or 14 Ch Foley catheter through it. Make the gastrostomy high on the anterior wall of his stomach, midway between its greater and lesser curves, and as far from his pylorus as you can. Hold his stomach with two pairs of Babcock's forceps, and draw it upwards and forwards into a cone. Make a small incision between the forceps, and push the catheter through this. Encircle it with 2 purse string sutures, and invaginate his stomach wall as you tie them.

CAUTION ! (1) Take the bites of the inner purse string suture through the full thickness of his stomach wall, so as to control bleeding. (2) The main dangers are haemorrhage and leaking. His gastrostomy must be as leak-proof as possible, so that his gastric juice does not enter his peritoneal cavity.

Anchor his stomach above and below the tube to his parietal peritoneum. Spigot the tube, and fix it to his skin with an encircling stitch.

Before he leaves the theatre instil some fluid (milk if possible) through it, to make sure it is patent, and to start giving him the food he so badly needs.

12 The appendix

12.1 Appendicitis

Appendicitis is the commonest abdominal surgical emergency in the industrial world, and the one with the most variable symptoms. It is unusual in Indians or in African peoples living in their traditional way, but it has started to become more common as they discard their high-fibre diets. It can occur at any age, but is rare under five.

The disease starts as a localized infection of a patient's appendix, which either resolves, or proceeds further—perhaps to suppurate, or even to go gangrenous and perforate, or maybe only to quieten down and fibrose. If peritonitis does develop, it can either remain localized, or it can spread. If it remains localized, it does so by forming an 'appendix mass' of adherent coils of gut. This may then resolve, or pus may gather, so that an abscess forms. The distinction between: (1) a 'mass' which is not tender, or is only minimally tender, and over which there is no guarding or rigidity, and (2) an obviously tender 'abscess' is important, because an abscess may need draining, but a mass can be treated nonoperatively.

An abscess may resolve, or it may enlarge until it drains spontaneously to the surface, or into the patient's gut, or into his peritoneal cavity, where it causes generalized peritonitis.

The stages in the development of appendicitis merge into one another, they take time to develop, and a patient may present in any of them. So keep a picture of the evolution of the disease in your mind, and ask yourself "What stage would his disease be in if he had appendicitis?". If he has had time to develop a mass, an abscess, or peritonitis (several days), and he has not done so, he is unlikely to have appendicitis, or if he has it has resolved.

Peritoneal inflammation is responsible for the most important sign of appendicitis—tenderness in the right iliac fossa. Significant rigidity is a sign that peritonitis is spreading.

Central abdominal pain is usually his first symptom, and it may be severe enough to wake him from sleep. He feels it in the midline at or above his umbilicus, as a dull ache, or as central midline colic. Some hours later it moves to his right iliac fossa, and he may be able to point to it with one finger. Here it increases gradually, and is constant. It is now seldom severe or colicky, and is worse when he moves, as when he coughs, strains, or walks and so irritates his parietal peritoneum. He moves with caution, and may find it easier to stoop forwards. When he lies in bed, he is more comfortable with his right leg flexed.

He is almost always anorexic and nauseated. He usually vomits once or twice only, soon after pain starts; at this stage vomiting is never as severe as in cholecystitis, pancreatitis, or gut obstruction.

He may present at various stages:

(1) **When the infection is localizing as an appendix mass.** His history is likely to be that his symptoms began as above, then he began to feel better, his pain improved, and his appetite has begun to return. He now looks fairly well and he has only mild fever (37.5°C). The mass in his right iliac fossa is only mildly tender, with no guarding or rigidity.

(2) **When infection has failed to localize, so that the mass has become an abscess.** In this stage he is very unwell, anorexic and toxic; he has pain in his right iliac fossa, and his temperature has started to swing. The mass in his right iliac fossa has now become an abscess: (a) it may be only just palpable, (b) it may be bulging, tender, and fluctuant, (c) it may be in his pelvis, so that you cannot feel it abdominally, (d) it may bulge into the rectum, or (e) into the vagina (unusual), or (f) it may be palpable above the pubis. (g) It may even track along the right paracolic gutter to present in the right flank. (h) It may stretch and obstruct coils of gut.

(3) **Just after perforation,** when the colic and bursting pain of his distended appendix are suddenly relieved, so that he thinks he is much better, before peritonitis has had time to spread.

(4) **When infection is spreading to cause local or generalized peritonitis.** He now has generalized abdominal pain, tenderness, guarding, and rigidity. If he presents very late, he may be dehydrated, cachectic, oliguric, and hypotensive with a silent, distended abdomen. All you will know is that he has peritonitis—appendicitis is merely one of its possible causes. If he presents very late, he may be moribund.

Try to recognize appendicitis early, before it is allowed to reach the stage of peritonitis or an abscess. The delay of even a few hours can be critical. Experience will teach you when to operate. If you always wait until you are absolutely certain, an appendix may rupture while you wait. So be prepared to operate on the strong suspicion that a patient may have appendicitis. If you find a normal appendix on about 15% of occasions, your criteria for operating will be about right. Some of the alternative diagnoses require operation anyway, and some of those that might be harmed by operation, such as basal pneumonia, *Ascaris* infestation, or gastroenteritis, should be easy to exclude.

In spite of the long list of differential diagnoses that follows, the diagnosis is usually easy. But, remember that: (1) He may have no tenderness in his right iliac fossa if his appendix is deep in his pelvis. His pain may be central, but he may only be tender rectally—so always do a rectal examination. (2) He may have no central abdominal pain, so that pain first appears in his right iliac fossa. (3) The diagnosis is particularly difficult, but no less important, if he (or she) is very young, or very old, or pregnant.

Removing an appendix is sometimes easy, but is sometimes very difficult. Divide it between crushing clamps. Some surgeons invert the stump through a purse string suture. You may have difficulty: (1) His appendix may be difficult to find. (2) It may be difficult to deliver, if it is stuck deep in the wound and is obscured by bleeding. When this happens, you will find the procedure of retrograde removal described below very useful. (3) His caecum may be fragile—so take great care not to injure it. (4) If he has peritonitis, postoperative wound infection is common, so be prepared to leave his skin wound open.

Finally: Don't give him an antibiotic in the hope of 'cutting short early appendicitis'. It will only give you and him a false sense of security.

APPENDICITIS

HISTORY

EARLY HISTORY. Ask carefully how the symptoms began—

"Where did the pain start?" How do the other symptoms fit into the story? *Most importantly,* where in the natural history of the disease is the patient now? Remember that a retrocaecal or pelvic appendix may cause diarrhoea or frequency of micturition.

EXAMINATION

PULSE AND TEMPERATURE. In the early stages his pulse is normal, and his temperature nearly so. If his pulse is raised, his appendix has possibly perforated. *A steadily rising pulse is always serious.* If he has a rigor or a high fever within 24 hours of the onset of symptoms, appendicitis is most unlikely.

INSPECTION. Typically, his lower abdomen moves little, but there is otherwise nothing else on inspection.

TENDERNESS on deep palpation in his right lower quadrant over McBurney's point is *the single most useful sign,* but: (1) You must examine his whole abdomen systematically *with the flat of your hand. Examine his left hypochondrium first.* Compare both sides, and his upper and lower quadrants on the right. Don't dig your fingers into his right lower quadrant. (2) If his appendix is behind his caecum, he may be tender in his flank. If it is in his pelvis, he may only be tender in his rectum, or above his pubis. (3) If he has spreading peritonitis, he may be tender well beyond McBurney's point, over much of his abdomen.

If you press gently but firmly in his right iliac fossa, and then quickly release your hand, he may feel a sudden pain. This is rebound tenderness, and is a sign of peritoneal irritation. A kinder way of eliciting this sign it to test for tenderness to light percussion. This is not so painful and is a better sign as to where the disease began.

Pain felt in the right iliac fossa when you press deeply in his left iliac fossa (Rovsing's sign) is another suggestive feature of appendicitis.

GUARDING is a sign of local peritonitis. Lay your hand flat on his abdomen, and gently flex your MP joints. If there is complete painless relaxation over his left inguinal fossa, and any tightening over his right fossa, the sign is positive. *Gently* compare both sides, testing the left one first and and distracting his attention while you do so.

RIGIDITY is a comparatively late sign, and shows that infection has reached his anterior abdominal wall. Generalized rigidity is a sign of generalized peritonitis. It is less marked if he is obese, emaciated, very old, or very young.

AN APPENDIX MASS may be palpable if his symptoms have lasted more than 2 or 3 days. If he is obese, or has a very low pain threshold, it will be difficult to feel. Distract his attention while you feel it. The mass is ill-defined and is probably an abscess if: (1) it is tender, (2) he has a high fever, or (3) there are features of intestinal obstruction.

RECTAL (or vaginal) EXAMINATION for a mass or tenderness must *never* be forgotten—the patient's inflamed appendix may be dangling into the pelvis. A rectal examination will often distinguish salpingitis, and a right-sided ectopic pregnancy. Slowly pass your half-flexed, well-lubricated index finger into his rectum (use your little finger in a child under 10). When it is completely inside, keep it still for a moment. Wait for him to relax, then gently press forwards, posteriorly, and on each side on his pelvic peritoneum with the tip of your finger.

CAUTION! Don't let him confuse the discomfort of you putting your finger into his anus, with the pain of you pressing on his pelvic appendix. Wait with your finger in his rectum until his initial discomfort has settled, then flex the tip of your finger and note the response.

SPECIAL TESTS. Do the psoas and iliacus tests (10.2).

THE DIFFERENTIAL DIAGNOSIS OF APPENDICITIS

IN EITHER SEX. This is long list, but the most important possibilities are the first two.

Suggesting an UPPER RESPIRATORY INFECTION, a viral infection, or tonsillitis—upper respiratory symptoms, generalized muscle aches. All these can cause central abdominal pain in a child. Watch him, especially his pulse, and if this does not settle, and his abdomen remains painful and resistant to palpation, he probably has appendicitis.

Suggesting GASTROENTERITIS—diarrhoea, perhaps with vomiting. His pain will be colicky, his tenderness poorly localized, and there will be pus cells in his stool. Be sure to do a pelvic examination, if necessary several times, because he may be developing a pelvic appendix abscess.

Suggesting AMOEBIASIS—a history of diarrhoea with blood and especially mucus: look for amoebae in his stools (31.10).

Suggesting TYPHOID with involvement of his terminal ileum or a perforation—a history of fever, diarrhoea, and diffuse abdominal pain for about 3 weeks, suddenly becoming acute (31.8).

Suggesting ILEOCAECAL TUBERCULOSIS—chronic pain which is sometimes colicky, and general deterioration in his health (29.5).

Suggesting a PERFORATED PEPTIC ULCER—the pain, which he now has in his right iliac fossa, started suddenly in his upper abdomen, and he has a history of chronic dyspepsia. Enquire for shoulder tip pain (10.1).

Suggesting ILIAC ADENITIS—a tender fluctuant mass in his lower quadrant, and a marked flexion contracture of his hip (5-10). Look for the primary source of the infection in his legs or perineum (5.12).

Suggesting a URINARY INFECTION—frequency and dysuria. These symptoms can also be caused by appendicitis.

Suggesting HYDRONEPHROSIS—a nagging pain in his costovertebral angle.

Suggesting RENAL COLIC—severe intermittent pain radiating into his groin. No fever. Test his urine for red cells.

If he has adopted a western life style, carcinoma of his caecum and diverticulitis are other possibilities.

IN WOMEN there are several more possibilities.

Suggesting PID—pain on both sides of the patient's lower abdomen for 3 days or more (rather than 12 to 36 hours, as is usual with appendicitis), a history of infertility, and previous pelvic infection. A tender fixed, or occasionally fluctuant, adnexal mass on her right side. If she has advanced signs of pelvic peritonitis with a short history, the mass (a tubo-ovarian abscess) may have ruptured. Examine her cervix for a purulent discharge (6.6). PID may be impossible to distinguish from a pelvic appendix (12.1).

Suggesting TORSION OF AN OVARIAN CYST—a brief history of acute pain localized to her suprapubic area (20.7). A mass palpable vaginally or bimanually. Her temperature will not be high.

Suggesting a right-sided ECTOPIC PREGNANCY—signs of hypovolaemia, signs on pelvic examination (16.6), and the aspiration of blood on a 4 quadrant tap (66.1). If her ruptured ectopic pregnancy bleeds more slowly (16.7), diagnosis may be more difficult.

Suggesting OVULATORY BLEEDING—the pain started in the middle of a menstrual cycle; mild abdominal tenderess without fever. It will settle in a few hours.

MANAGEMENT OF APPENDICITIS
Treatment is usually straightforward.

(1) If you see a patient early, with appendicitis or suspected appendicitis, remove his appendix.

(2) If you see him later, with a satisfactorily localizing condition (an appendix mass), and nothing suggesting peritonitis, an abscess or obstruction, treat him non-operatively, and delay the appendicectomy until 6 weeks later. Adhesions will not be much of a problem.

(3) If his history has lasted more than 3 days, and he has signs of an abscess which is enlarging, drain it through his abdominal wall, or else into the rectum or posterior fornix of the vagina. If, when you drain an abscess abdominally, you find an appendix which is not friable, remove it; otherwise leave this part of the treatment for 2 months, when the infection will have settled. See below.

(4) If he presents with local or general peritonitis, resuscitate him and treat him for peritonitis (6.2). If his appendix is friable, or requires much dissection from the neighbouring tissues, leave it, otherwise remove it.

(5) If he appears to be moribund with severe toxaemia,

hypotension, oliguria, and a tense, tender, silent, abdomen, his outlook is poor. Resuscitate him as best you can, 'suck and drip him' (9.9), give him antibiotics (chloramphenicol and metronidazole, 2.9), and operate as soon as he is fit.

CAUTION ! (1) Infection is less likely to localize at the extremes of life, so don't be too non-operative if he is very young or very old, or in pregnancy. (2) Don't try to remove an appendix if infection is arrested or resolving. You can safely do an interval appendicectomy 6 weeks later. If you leave it, it will probably resolve.

NON-OPERATIVE TREATMENT FOR APPENDICITIS

INDICATIONS. A patient who is satisfactorily localizing his infection—an appendix mass, with no signs of spread. It is seldom advisable in children under 10 or in the elderly.

METHOD. Monitor him with the greatest care. Give him no antibiotics. Rely on his own assessment of himself, especially on such questions as "Is your pain still subsiding?" "Can you move about more freely?" "Has your appetite improved?". Monitor his temperature, his pulse, and his white blood count. Palpate his mass gently, and mark its outline on his abdominal wall daily with a felt pen. Examine and manipulate it as little as possible. Give him fluids only by mouth at first, then after a day or two a light diet. If he continues to improve, and his mass continues to shrink—good. He can start to eat quite normally in 4 days and treatment can be relaxed. Ask him to return for an interval appendicectomy in 6–12 weeks.

If any of the following occur, abandon non-operative treatment: (1) His pain gets worse, or he begins to feel generally worse. (2) His mass enlarges. (3) His abdominal tenderness increases or guarding develops (peritonitis). (4) He develops signs of intestinal obstruction (due to an abscess). (4) His pulse rate increases. *This is a very important sign.* A slightly raised temperature is of less importance in the early stages, provided that his pulse is steady or falling. A persistently high or swinging temperature shows an abscess that needs drainage. Any or all of these things show that infection is spreading, so operate for an enlarging abscess, peritonitis, or obstruction. Remember the danger signs as 4 'Ps'—'pain, pulse, pyrexia, and palpable mass'.

If his general condition improves, but the mass shows little sign of shrinking, it may be a sterile abscess—wait until it is dull to percussion, showing that it is extraperitoneal, and then drain it extraperitoneally.

CAUTION ! (1) Non-operative treatment is only applicable in hospital. (2) Be particularly careful when you apply it to the very old and the very young. (3) Don't give him antibiotics (unless he has generalized peritonitis): they may mask the symptoms which show that non-operative treatment is failing.

ACUTE APPENDICETOMY

EQUIPMENT. A general set (4.12). Suction.

PREPARATION. Start nasogastric suction (4.9). If he is dehydrated, resuscitate him for an hour or two before you operate. Give him intravenous Ringer's lactate or saline. If an adult looks dehydrated, he may have a fluid deficit of up to 4 litres (A 15.3). If he has generalized peritonitis, insert an indwelling catheter, and monitor his urine output. He should pass 1 ml/kg/hour (A 15.5).

ANTIBIOTICS. If he has peritonitis, give him perioperative antibiotics (2.9). Some surgeons give rectal metronidazole routinely.

ANAESTHESIA. Aspirate his stomach and put 30 ml of magnesium trisilicate down the tube. (1) Thiopentone, suxamethonium, and intubation under cricoid pressure, followed by ether from a vapouriser. (2) Ketamine drip with relaxants. (3) Plain ether (A 11.1). (4) A general anaesthetic from a Boyle's machine. You will need good relaxation. In the early stages, anorexia and vomiting may have kept his stomach empty, but you cannot rely on this—if there is ileus it may be full.

WHICH INCISION? Prepare and drape his abdominal wall, so that you can see his anterior superior iliac spine and his umbilicus. As soon as it is relaxed under anaesthesia, palpate it carefully. You may be able to feel a mass whereas previously you could not. This may help you to site the incision.

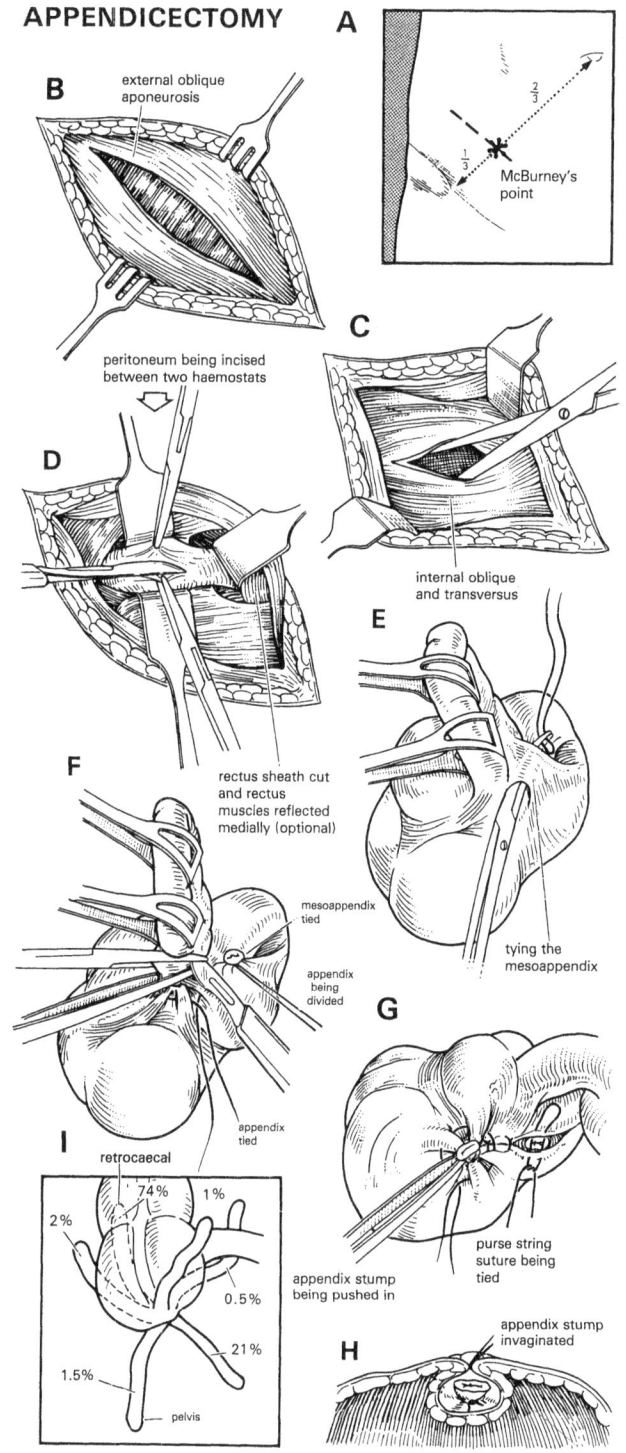

Fig. 12-1 REMOVING AN APPENDIX through McBurney's gridiron incision (if the diagnosis is in doubt a low midline or paramedian incision is easier). A, McBurney's point and the position of the incision. B, splitting the patient's external oblique aponeurosis. C, splitting his internal oblique and transversus muscles. D, opening his peritoneum between two haemostats. This drawing also shows how you can, if necessary, extend the incision medially by incising his anterior rectus sheath, and retracting his rectus muscle. E, passing a ligature through his mesoappendix. F, the purse string suture is in place, but is not pulled tight. His appendix has been tied, and is now being grasped between two haemostats and divided. G, the stump of his appendix is about to be pushed into his caecum, as the purse string is pulled tight. H, the stump of his appendix invaginated into his caecum by the purse string. I, the various positions in which you may find his appendix. About 3/4 of the time it is behind his caecum, and 1/4 of the time it is in his pelvis. It is seldom anywhere else. *Partly after Maingot R, "Abdominal Operations", (4th edn. 1961), p.811 Figs. 2 and 3. HK Lewis, with kind permission.*

If the diagnosis is not in doubt, and the symptoms have not lasted long, make a gridiron incision.

If he presented late, and you suspect that adhesions may make dissection difficult, make the same skin incision as for a gridiron, but cut through the muscles in the same line as the skin incision. This incision has the advantage of being easily extended in either direction. If you have just palpated a mass, centre your muscle-cutting incision on the mass.

If the diagnosis is in doubt, and a gynaecological condition or a perforated peptic ulcer is a possibility, or he has generalized peritonitis (especially if he is a child), make a median or right paramedian incision (9.2). You can explore more widely, and you will also be better able to wash out his peritoneal cavity afterwards if necessary.

TO MAKE A GRIDIRON INCISION draw a line from his umbilicus to his anterior superior iliac spine. McBurney's point lies at the junction of its outer and middle thirds. Centre a 7 to 10 cm skin incision on this point. Alternatively, site it over the mass or at the point of maximum tenderness and resistance.

Split his external oblique muscle aponeurosis in the line of its fibres, which is the same as that of the skin incision, over its whole length. Resist the temptation to extend the incision too far medially.

Hold the edges of his oblique aponeurosis aside with haemostats, and you will see the fleshy fibres of his internal oblique running transversely, and a little upwards. Insert a closed pair of blunt scissors between them and use the 'push and spread technique' (4-8) to separate them. Then extend the incision with your fingers. Replace these by retractors, to expose his transversalis fascia and peritoneum. Pick these up as a single layer and separate them in the same way. Open his peritoneum between haemostats by the method in Fig. 9-2.

EXPLORING THE ABDOMEN FOR ACUTE APPENDICITIS

Raise the edges of his peritoneum with retractors and look inside. Some exudate may escape. It does not indicate peritonitis, unless it is obviously purulent and foul-smelling. Suck it away. If his caecum is covered by small gut, look for it by sliding a finger into his paracolic gutter. If there is much fluid, suck it away.

If you have difficulty finding his appendix: (1) Look for his pink to grey-blue caecum first. It is often higher than you expect, and it may lie under his liver (unusual). The three taenia coli of the caecum converge on the appendix, which lies on its posteromedial side. Follow the anterior taenia to its base. The tip of his appendix may lie under his caecum, or in his pelvis. With your index finger, feel for something tense and rigid. (2) Retract the wound edges a bit more. (3) Extend the incision as described below.

CAUTION ! (1) If he has localized peritonitis, take particular care not to spread the infection. (2) Don't mistake his caecum for his transverse colon—this has greater omentum attached along its anterior surface. (3) Try to break down as few fibrinous adhesions as you can.

Put your finger under the anterior taenia and test the mobility of his caecum. If the tip of his caecum is free, it and his appendix should come to the surface easily. Grasp his caecum with a moist pack, and gently drag its lower end into the wound. His appendix should follow it. Don't rupture it, and use the minimum of force. If omentum is folded round his appendix, try not to separate it. Instead, tie it, and remove the adherent part with his appendix.

If you need to extend a gridiron incision: (1) Extend the muscle splits. Or, (2) cut across his muscles superolaterally. Or, (3) cut into his rectus sheath medially (D, 12-1), taking great care not to cut his inferior epigastric artery, which runs vertically on the deep surface of his rectus muscle.

CAUTION ! (1) Don't try to work through too small a hole. (2) The only common differential diagnoses which you cannot treat through a gridiron incision are a perforated peptic ulcer and cholecystitis, in which case, close the gridiron incision and make a paramedian one.

If you have been able to deliver his caecum and appendix into the wound, the next step is to tie the vessels in his mesoappendix. Hold this up to the light, and look for a 'window' close to the base of his appendix, clear of blood vessels, in which to make a small incision. Pass an aneurysm needle through

RETROGRADE APPENDICECTOMY

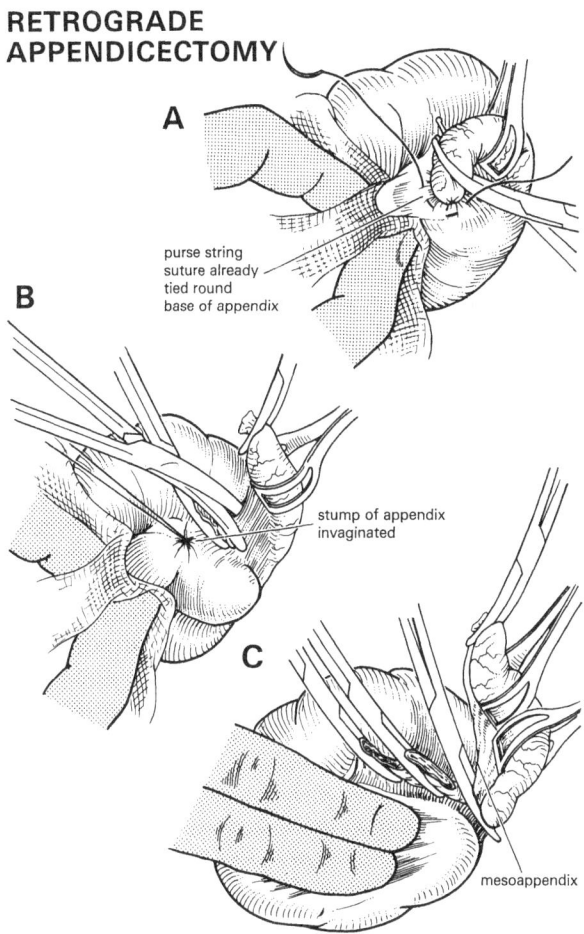

Fig. 12-2 RETROGRADE APPENDICECTOMY. A, the proximal end of the patient's appendix has been freed from his caecum and tied. B, it has been divided proximally and is being released distally from his caecum. C, it is very nearly free. *Partly after Maingot R, 'Abdominal Operations', (4th edn. 1961), p.816 Fig. 7. HK Lewis, with kind permission.*

it, and tie the vessels with 2/0 chromic catgut. If they are friable, tie them several times.

Apply two clamps to the base of his appendix, and divide it between them. Tie its base with chromic catgut, as close to his caecum as you can.

Inversion of the stump (optional). Use an atraumatic suture of 2/0 or 3/0 chromic catgut to apply a purse string suture, about 1 cm away from his appendix, through the seromuscular layer only (F, 9-6). Leave this loose for the moment. Invert the stump with fine forceps, and then close the purse string snugly over it.

If his caecum is very oedematous, tie his appendix, but don't invaginate it—drain it instead.

If his appendix has stuck in his pelvis, or behind his ileum, and is surrounded by a small abscess, improve exposure by retraction, and by extending the wound downwards. Pack the area off with swabs, and cautiously free it by sharp or blunt dissection.

CAUTION ! (1) Don't apply artery forceps to his mesoappendix. If they fall off, there will be brisk bleeding. (2) Be patient and gentle when you try to remove a tense, unruptured, gangrenous appendix. (3) If it is on the point of bursting, try to deliver it intact. If it bursts, you will greatly increase the chances of peritonitis.

If his appendix is stuck down behind his caecum or colon, it will be held by fibrous tissue, so that you will not be able to free it with your finger. Extend the incision upwards and laterally by an oblique cut through all layers of the abdominal wall to get better access. Now expose the lateral side of his caecum where there is a gutter. Using MacIndoe scissors, carefully divide the peritoneal reflection on the lateral side of his caecum, using the 'push and spread' technique. Using a swab on a sponge-holding forceps, mobilize his caecum medially. Grasp it with a swab, and gently draw it up and out of the wound. If it will not come, work your finger in the plane between it and his posterior abdominal wall. If convenient, do a retrograde appendicectomy, by tying off the base of his appendix first, and then freeing it towards its tip.

If his appendix has perforated, there is a 90% chance that there is a faecolith somewhere, either in his abdomen or his appendix. Faecoliths are calcified, and may show on a plain X-ray.

CLOSING HIS ABDOMEN. If he had a 'cold' or early acute appendicitis, close his peritoneum with a running suture, and tie its ends together. Bring the edges of his transversus and internal oblique muscles together with a few stitches. If necessary, bring his peritoneum, transversus, and internal oblique together as a single layer, taking care not to strangulate them. If you have had to cut muscle, bring its edges together with one or two sutures. Close his external oblique with continuous catgut, and his skin with interrupted monofilament.

If you have removed a dirty contaminated appendix, leave his wound open. Close his peritoneum in the usual way, and close his muscles with interrupted monofilament, but don't put any sutures in his skin. Insert some gauze to keep the fascial layers a little open. If there is no significant discharge, suture his wound on the 5th day.

DRAINS are not usually indicated. They are much less important than sucking out and washing out the infected area at the time of surgery. Consider inserting an intraperitoneal drain if: (1) You have had to leave his appendix behind. (2) You are worried that there may be bleeding from any cause. (3) His caecum has been involved in the inflammatory process. (4) A gangrenous appendix has caused severe local contamination of his peritoneum.

If he does need a drain, insert a corrugated rubber one down to his appendix stump, or insert a 6 mm rubber tube. Remove one-third of its wall in the area which is to be drained, bring it out through a short incision in his flank, and suture it in place. Remove it as soon as it stops discharging.

DRAINING AN APPENDIX ABSCESS

INDICATIONS. A tender mass which is increasing in size in a patient with a history of appendicitis, or more rarely following appendicectomy 3 or 4 days previously, especially if he has increasing pain, pyrexia, and toxaemia.

THE EXTRAPERITONEAL APPROACH is best. If his abscess is dull to percussion, there is no gut between it and his abdominal wall. It has probably stuck to his abdominal wall, so that you can easily drain it under local anaesthesia.

Try to enter the abscess, but not his peritoneal cavity. Mark the point of maximum tenderness and fluctuation with a felt pen. Anaesthetize and incise his skin and muscles at this point. Try to enter the abscess as far laterally as you can. His muscles will be soggy and oedematous, but you can split them in the usual way, by pushing in a haemostat and opening it. Push a finger in laterally and backwards to make sure that the drainage track is big enough. Suck out pus, break down any loculi, and feel for and remove any faecoliths. Then push a large corrugated rubber drain well in. Suture this to his skin and shorten it gradually after the 5th day. Remove it completely at the 8th or 9th day. He does not need an antibiotic unless there are signs of peritonitis. Ask him to return in 8 weeks to have his appendix removed.

CAUTION ! (1) Don't try to remove an appendix from the bottom of a large abscess cavity with much friable tissue that bleeds easily. Drain the abscess and leave his appendix in place. Do an interval appendicectomy later. (2) Avoid the intraperitoneal approach, unless it happens by accident, as when laparotomy unexpectedly reveals an appendix abscess.

INTERVAL APPENDICECTOMY

If you have treated an appendix mass or abscess conservatively or by drainage, and left the appendix in, and he lives far from hospital, advise him to return for an interval appendicectomy at 8 weeks.

If he has any symptoms while he is waiting for it, ask him to report immediately. If you have allowed 6 to 12 weeks to elapse since his attack of appendicitis, you can usually remove his appendix quite easily. If you leave too long an interval (say three months), there is an increasing risk that he will get another attack of appendicitis meanwhile.

12.2 Difficulties with appendicitis

This is a substantial list. Fortunately most of them are rare. We have divided them into those involved in diagnosing appendicitis, those you will meet while you are removing an appendix, and those which occur afterwards.

DIFFICULTIES DIAGNOSING APPENDICITIS

If the patient is VERY YOUNG beware, because: (1) a good history will be difficult to get in a child, (2) his abdomen will be difficult to examine, (3) gastroenteritis may cause tenderness and cramps. If he does have appendicitis, he needs early surgery. Don't leave him overnight. The most common mistake is to misdiagnose lobar pneumonia as appendicitis, so count his respirations and see if his alae nasi move as he breathes.

If he is asleep, try to feel his abdomen, even for a few seconds, before he wakes up yelling. If he resents any attempt to examine it, there is probably something serious inside it. Examine him repeatedly at intervals of a few hours, until you have enough evidence to justify a laparotomy. If abdominal pain, vomiting, and fever persist, and he is tender in his right iliac fossa, he has appendicitis.

If he is OLD or FAT beware, because infection is poorly localized, complications are frequent and he may present atypically: (1) Tenderness and rigidity may be minimal. If you wait for them to become marked, he may develop ileus and distension while you wait. (2) He may have no fever. As with a child, examine him at intervals of a few hours.

If she is PREGNANT don't be afraid to operate if you think she may have appendicitis. Early in pregnancy, hyperemesis may confuse her symptoms. Narrowly localized tenderness will

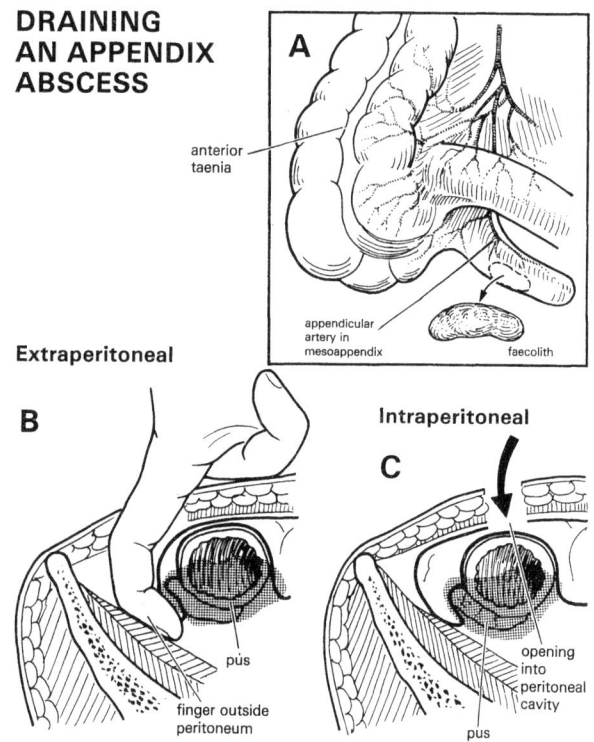

Fig. 12-3 DRAINING AN APPENDIX ABSCESS. A, the anatomy of the appendix. If you cannot find a patient's appendix, follow the anterior taenia of his caecum down to it. Sometimes, a faecolith forms in his appendix. If this escapes into his peritoneal cavity, it may be the cause of a persistent abscess. B, approaching an abscess extraperitoneally. C, avoid the intraperitoneal approach, unless you happen to come across an appendix abscess unexpectedly during laparotomy.

often provide the diagnosis. Later, her caecum and appendix move upwards, and so does the tenderness of appendicitis. Appendicectomy is unlikely to upset her pregnancy in the first two trimesters. The third is the dangerous one; she is more likely to die from peritonitis (which increases the risk of premature labour) than from having her appendix out.

DIFFICULTIES AT APPENDICECTOMY

If you find GREENISH FLUID in his peritoneal cavity, it has probably escaped through a perforated duodenal ulcer, and tracked down his right paracolic gutter. Remove his appendix if appendicitis is fairly common in your area, close the wound, and repair the perforation through a paramedian incision.

If his APPENDIX LOOKS NORMAL, and appendicitis is common in your area, excise it and look for other pathology, as listed above under 'Differential diagnosis': (1) If he has enlarged mesenteric nodes, and a clear yellowish serous exudate, suspect mesenteric adenitis (common). (2) If you find a purulent exudate, suspect PID in a woman (common) and other causes of peritonitis. These include Meckel's diverticulitis (rare). Look for an inflamed diverticulum about a metre from the ileocaecal junction (28-4). If it is inflamed, excise it with a wedge of tissue on either side; if it is normal, leave it. Another possibility is primary peritonitis (rare, 6.2). (3) If you can feel a tensely distended gall bladder when you pass your finger up through the incision, he has cholecystitis. (4) If he has a tensely distended caecum, he has some large gut obstruction. Enlarge the incision and feel for its cause. (5) If there is pure blood in the abdominal cavity, the possibilities include ectopic pregnancy, a leaking ovarian follicle, and trauma—see below. (6) If there is blood-stained fluid, consider pancreatitis, or intestinal infarction. (7) If you find distended small gut, consider strangulation of a hernia—perhaps an internal one, or a femoral or an obturator hernia.

If his CAECUM IS MUCH THICKENED, suspect amoebiasis.

If his appendix is inflamed, but is so TIED DOWN BY ADHESIONS that it is difficult to remove safely, insert a drain and close the wound. Do an interval appendicectomy.

If the BASE OF HIS APPENDIX IS NECROTIC, you cannot tie it. If his caecum is healthy, insert a purse string suture. If it is unhealthy, and will not take a suture, infold it with some Lembert sutures, and tack some omentum over it. Put a drain down to it, close the muscles of his abdominal wall, but leave his skin open.

If his APPENDIX IS BURIED in a mass of adhesions and pockets of pus, avoid spreading the infection. Enlarge the incision, lift its medial side forwards, isolate the mass with warm packs, suck out the pus, and remove his appendix if this is not too difficult. Otherwise, leave it and do an interval appendicectomy.

If he has GENERALIZED PERITONITIS, remove his appendix as above if this is not too difficult, and manage his peritonitis as in Section 6.2.

DIFFICULTIES FOLLOWING APPENDICECTOMY

These include ileus (10.13), respiratory complications (9.11), and acute dilatation of his stomach (very rare).

If he goes into SHOCK some hours after the operation, suspect that he is bleeding from his appendicular artery (rare). Transfuse him, reopen his wound and tie it.

If he VOMITS, his ABDOMEN DISTENDS, and he becomes constipated, suspect: (1) intestinal obstruction (10.12) due to an abcess or to kinking of his gut. If necessary, drain the abscess, otherwise manage him as in Section 10.13. (2) Intussusception (10.8). (3) Gram-negative septicaemia and septic shock (53.4).

If he develops a FAECAL FISTULA, it will probably heal spontanously in 2 or 3 weeks-provided there is no distal obstruction (9.14). If it persists, suspect obstruction, or amoebic colitis or actinomycosis (rare). Give him amoebecides. Wait several weeks before referring him.

If his TEMPERATURE RISES IN THE SECOND WEEK, accompanied by malaise and local symptoms, there is probably pus somewhere. (1) He may have a metastatic abscess in his liver, or a subphrenic abscess. (2) If he has a mucous rectal discharge or diarrhoea, suspect that there is pus in his rectovesical pouch. Feel for a hard inflammatory mass above his prostate, or in a woman's rectovaginal pouch. (3) Feel also for an inflammatory mass in the abdomen.

If a PELVIC ABSCESS FORMS, monitor him carefully, do a daily rectal examination, and, if he is not very toxic, wait until it drains into his rectum or into an adjacent loop of gut. 95% of pelvic abscesses drain spontaneously, and do not need surgery. If he is no better after a week of non-operative treatment, drain the abscess rectally or vaginally. This applies only to abscesses following appendicitis, *not* those following PID, which should be drained vaginally as soon as they form (6.6).

If his wound CONTINUES TO DISCHARGE, you may have left a faecolith behind. Explore the track and remove it. He may have: (1) amoebiasis, (2) actinomycosis (rare), or (3) Crohn's disease (rare).

13 The gall-bladder, pancreas, and spleen

13.1 Introduction

Most disease of the gall-bladder is due to stones, apart from the uncommon occasions when *Ascaris* invades it. Such is the lifestyle of most of your patients that you probably won't see it very often. In Africa it is unusual, but it is commoner in Northern India and Tibet. Disease of the pancreas is also uncommon in much of Africa, but calcified chronic pancreatitis and carcinoma of the pancreas are not uncommon in India.

Many patients are found at postmortem to have gall-stones which have caused no symptoms. Stones may however obstruct the common bile-duct and cause biliary colic, or obstructive jaundice. They can promote infection of the gall-bladder and cause acute or chronic cholecystitis. They can also promote infection of the pancreas and cause pancreatitis. You can treat acute cholecystitis non-operatively, or if this fails, you can drain a patient's gall-bladder by doing a cholecystostomy. If he has chronic cholecystitis, you may sometimes be able to remove his gall-bladder. But if he has obstructive jaundice due to stones in his common duct, you should refer him to an expert. If he has obstructive jaundice due to carcinoma of the head of his pancreas, you may be able to relieve his symptoms by making an opening between his gall-bladder and his jejunum—a cholecysto-jejunostomy (13-6).

You can treat acute pancreatitis (13.9), a pancreatic abscess (5.10b), and drain a pancreatic pseudocyst (13.10). There are also a few occasions when splenectomy is indicated, other than for trauma (13.11).

13.2 Biliary colic

Biliary colic is due to a stone passing through the cystic duct or impacted in it. The patient has a severe colicky epigastric pain which radiates to his right subcostal region and right scapula. He wants to bend himself double, he rolls around, and rarely keeps still. Intense pain comes in waves against a background of severe pain, typically in attacks lasting about half an hour, one to three hours after a fatty meal. Pain makes his breathing difficult and may be accompanied by nausea and vomiting. Attacks occasionally last as long as 6 hours. If they last 24 hours, he has cholecystitis, not uncomplicated biliary colic. He may be tender in his hypochondrium or his right epigastrium, and have a positive Murphy's sign (see below).

BILIARY COLIC

MURPHY'S SIGN. Put your hand under the patient's ribs on the right side, and ask him to take a deep breath. If he feels pain as his gall-bladder moves down on to your hand, the sign is positive and indicates cholecystitis.

X-RAYS. Most gallstones don't show on an X-ray, so a plain film is unlikely to help. An oral cholecystogram will show 90% of stones, provided he is not jaundiced; if he is clinically jaundiced you won't get good X-rays. Look for: (1) the negative shadows of gallstones floating in the contrast medium, (2) no outline to his gall-bladder, showing that his cystic duct is blocked, or his gall-bladder is severely diseased. If his symptoms are suggestive, repeat the test with a double dose of contrast medium.

ULTRASOUND is a simple, cheap and accurate way of finding stones in the gall-bladder, whether or not he is jaundiced; it is better than a cholecystogram, but it needs skill.

SPECIAL TESTS. A slightly raised serum bilirubin may indicate subclinical jaundice. Occasionally, only his serum alkaline phosphatase is raised when his bile duct is obstructed.

THE DIFFERENTIAL DIAGNOSIS OF BILIARY COLIC includes a perforated peptic ulcer (11.2), an amoebic liver abscess (31.12), and upper small gut obstruction (10.3).

Suggesting ureteric colic—pain radiating towards the genitalia. Blood in the patient's urine on microscopic examination. Radio-opaque shadows along the line of his ureter.

Suggesting right basal pneumonia—cough, fever, and lung signs at his right base.

THE NON-OPERATIVE TREATMENT OF BILIARY COLIC. If necessary, give him pethidine 50 to 100 mg 4-hourly intravenously or intramuscularly, for 24 to 48 hours. An anticholinergic drug is optional.

Give him only clear fluids by mouth. If he vomits, give him fluids intravenously.

If he is fortunate, his pain will stop in 24 to 48 hours, and you can start to feed him cautiously, avoiding oily or fatty foods. Start to investigate him as soon as he has recovered from his pain. Advise him to take a low-fat diet.

13.3 Acute cholecystitis

The patient's symptoms are those of biliary colic (13.2), but they last more than 24 hours. To begin with they are due to a chemical inflammation caused by concentrated bile under pressure, but bacterial infection may follow. He has a 95% chance of recovering in 10 days, even without treatment. There is a 5% chance that the infection will spread to his smaller bile-ducts (cholangitis), or that he will develop peritonitis from a perforation of his gall-bladder.

Operate if: (1) he has cholangitis which is threatening his life, or (2) his gall-bladder forms a gradually enlarging acute inflammatory mass. It will be acutely inflamed, oedematous, and perhaps gangrenous, so don't try to remove it. Instead, drain it (cholecystostomy). This may save his life and is simple and safe, but it will seldom cure him permanently, so you will probably have to refer him for cholecystectomy later.

Acute on chronic cholecystitis (relapsing cholecystitis, recurrent biliary colic) is usually less severe than a typical acute attack, and is one of the more common kinds of gall-bladder disease. His symptoms may subside without infection and leave his gall-bladder distended with mucus (mucocoele of the gall-bladder), or it may distend with pus and perhaps burst (empyema of the gall-bladder).

• FORCEPS, gallstone, Desjardin's, one only. Use these long slender forceps for removing stones from the biliary system.

ACUTE CHOLECYSTITIS

SIGNS. The patient is febrile, looks sick, and lies still. Tenderness is well localized in his right upper quadrant. He may be exquisitely tender (unlike biliary colic), and show guarding and rigidity. Murphy's sign is usually positive (13.2). A well-localized mass usually forms a few days after the start of his attack, just below his right costal margin. Mild jaundice does not always mean that his common duct is obstructed by a stone.

If he has jaundice, swinging fever, chills and rigors, suspect that his cholecystitis is complicated by cholangitis.

SPECIAL TESTS. His serum bilirubin and alkaline phosphatase will probably be slightly raised, and his total white count markedly so.

X-RAYS are less useful than ultrasound. Vomiting will make it impossible for him to take contrast medium by mouth.

THE DIFFERENTIAL DIAGNOSIS includes amoebic liver abscess (31.12), perforated peptic ulcer (11.2), acute pancreatitis (13.9), acute pyelonephritis, and volvulus of his small gut with strangulation (10.9).

NON-OPERATIVE TREATMENT FOR ACUTE CHOLECYSTITIS

This is only safe if you are sure of the diagnosis.

Analgesics are needed, because his pain is severe. So give him enough pethidine (avoid morphine because it may increase the pain of biliary colic), if necessary 4-hourly for 24 hours.

Nasogastric suction is not essential, but it will keep his stomach empty and so relieve his nausea and vomiting.

Rehydration may be necessary. Correct his initial fluid loss with saline, and then give him his daily fluid requirements (A 15.3).

Antibiotics are less necessary than you might expect, because the inflammation in his gall-bladder is predominantly chemical. Give him chloramphenicol, ampicillin, or tetracycline.

Continue this treatment for 3 or 4 days, and then start to feed him. His symptoms should start to improve in 24 hours, and he should be symptom free in 3 weeks. Advise him to take a low-fat diet, and refer him for an interval cholecystectomy after about two months.

CHOLECYSTOSTOMY FOR ACUTE CHOLECYSTITIS

INDICATIONS. Drain his gall-bladder if: (1) intense pain persists, (2) swinging fever continues with tachycardia, (3) his abdominal tenderness gets worse, the area of guarding extends, or the mass increases in size, or (4) he has rigors and deepening jaundice, indicating cholangitis.

EQUIPMENT. If you don't have Desjardin's stone forceps, a Fogarty balloon catheter, pushed past the stone, inflated, and withdrawn is often effective. You may possibly be able to use a tiny Foley catheter. Sponge forceps are much less satisfactory. Find two assistants in addition to the trolley nurse.

ANAESTHETIC. (1) General anaesthesia, intubation, and relaxants. If he is very sick or very old you can operate under local anaesthesia.

INCISION. Feel for the area of maximum tenderness, an ill-defined mass, or both (A, in Fig. 13-1). Centre the incision over this area, and cut through all layers of his abdominal wall. Or, do an upper median or paramedian incision. You will probably find his gall-bladder easily. If you don't find it, carefully separate the adherent omentum and transverse colon by pushing them away with your finger. Pack large swabs ('lap pads') round his gall-bladder carefully; it easily ruptures and spills infected bile into his peritoneal cavity.

If the structures below the right lobe of his liver are matted together in an oedematous haemorrhagic mass, so that his gall bladder is difficult to find, insert your hand over the upper surface of his liver, and draw your fingers down until you reach its edge. Then move your hand medially over the convex surface of his liver until you reach his falciform ligament, joining his liver to his diaphragm. At its lower edge is his ligamentum teres. About 5 cm to the right of this, you should be able to feel the tense, turgid, elongated mass of his fiery-red, acutely

CHOLECYSTOSTOMY

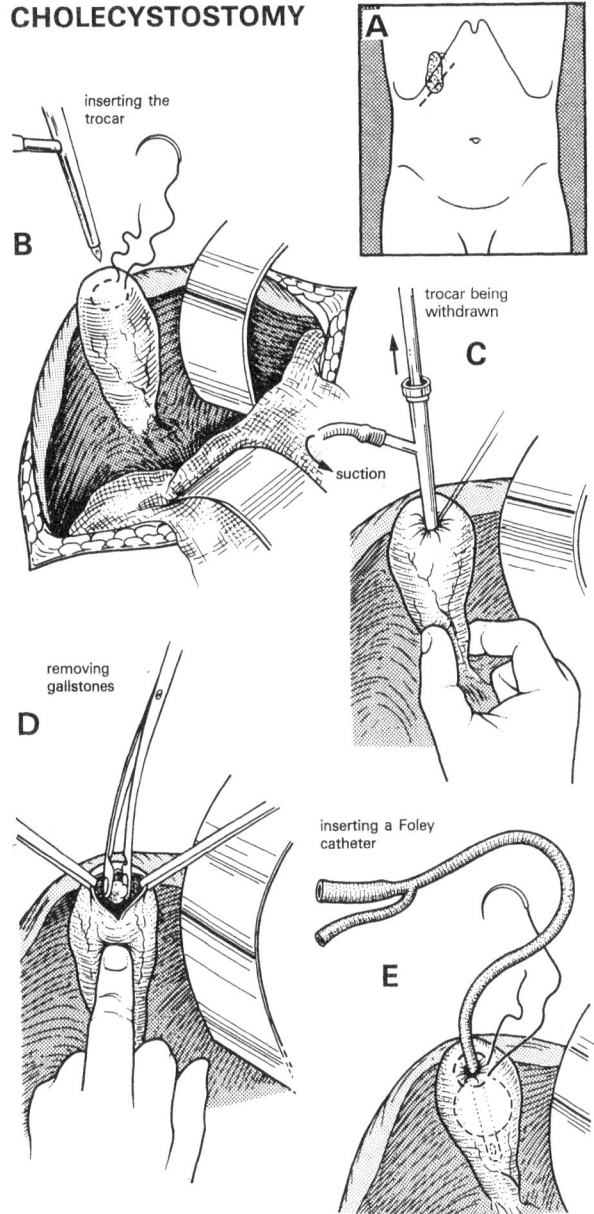

Fig 13-1 CHOLECYSTOSTOMY. A, the incision. B, the purse string suture inserted. C, aspirating the gall-bladder. D, removing stones. E, inserting a Foley catheter. *Kindly contributed by Gerald Hankins.*

inflamed, oedematous, and perhaps partly necrotic gall-bladder.

Try to expose enough of the fundus of his gall-bladder to allow you to drain it. Use your finger, or a 'swab on a stick' (4-8), to carefully 'peel' away his omentum, the hepatic flexure of his colon, and his transverse mesocolon. Avoid sharp dissection. If he bleeds, control it with packs.

If you don't find a tense inflamed gall-bladder when you operate, look for acute pancreatitis (13.9), a liver abscess (31.12) or a localised perforation of a peptic ulcer (11.2) etc.

Surround the exposed area of his gall-bladder to minimize spillage. Insert a purse string suture of 2/0 chromic catgut (B). Plunge a trocar and cannula, attached (if you have the kind with a side tube) to a sucker, through the purse string (C). Withdraw the trocar far enough to allow you to aspirate his gall-bladder, milking any remaining exudate up towards the suction. When you have sucked his gall-bladder empty, take a swab from the wall for culture. Feel for gallstones. Expect to find them in Hartmann's pouch (13-3), near the point where his gall-bladder joins his cystic duct. Gently try to get your hand into a position where it can palpate this area comfortably, taking care not to tear his gall-bladder.

Use scissors to enlarge the opening to 1.5 cm. Feel for stones with a pair of Desjardin's stone forceps or sponge-holding forceps. Guide the stones into the jaws of the forceps (D) with your fingers outside his gall-bladder.

CAUTION! Don't try to remove stones which are too tightly wedged lower down. You may do much damage. Leave them. They may free themselves later: if they don't they can be removed later at an interval cholecystectomy.

Insert a 20 to 26 Ch Malecot, de Pezzer, or Foley catheter, into his gall-bladder. Tie the purse string snugly around it (E), and apply a second one 5 mm away from the first. Bring the tube out through a separate stab incision. Irrigate the wound with saline, close it in a single layer (9.8), and leave his skin unsutured for delayed primary closure.

Pass a piece of silk around the catheter at least twice, and suture it to his skin. Attach it to a bottle for drainage.

POSTOPERATIVELY, expect bile to start draining in a day or two. Remove the tube in 10 to 15 days. If it is still discharging, he can go home for a few weeks with it in place. The fistula will slowly close unless a stone has been left in Hartmann's pouch (when a small mucous fistula will result). Warn him that his underlying disease has been relieved, not cured. Refer him to an expert for cholecystectomy about 2 months later.

13.4 Cholangitis

If a patient has a stone in his common bile-duct, it may promote ascending cholangitis. Untreated, this may be followed by multiple abscesses in his liver, or by septicaemia. Antibiotics are useful, but surgery may be necessary. Ideally, his common bile-duct should be explored, and any stones removed. This is difficult and needs special instruments and X-rays. If it is impractical, you may be able to save his life by decompressing his common duct and inserting a T-tube (choledochostomy). This will be easier than trying to anastomose his gall-bladder to his jejunum (choledochojejunostomy), which will be difficult because his gall-bladder is diseased, and there may be a stone in his cystic duct.

A patient with cholangitis usually has a history of gall-bladder symptoms. Typically, an attack of colic is followed the next day by fluctuating jaundice, dark urine, pale stools, nausea and vomiting, fever and rigors, and a leucocytosis. His gall-bladder and liver are tender, but his gall-bladder is not palpable.

CHOLEDOCHOSTOMY

ANTIBIOTICS. in order of preference give the patient: (1) Mezlocillin, piperacillin, or azlocillin (all reach high concentrations in bile). (2) Ampicillin with gentamicin or another aminoglycoside or a cephalosporin.

INDICATIONS. Cholangitis, as described above. If he is jaundiced, with rigors and spiking fever which fails to respond to antibiotics in 24 hours, operate. If you delay he will probably die.

PREPARATION. If he has circulatory failure, give him 2 litres of 0.9% saline rapidly. If this does not soon improve him, give him blood. If he still does not improve, operate urgently; it is his only chance. Give him 10 mg of vitamin K_1 twice daily intramuscularly. Insert a nasogastric tube.

EQUIPMENT. Desjardin's stone forceps. A T-tube or a 14 Ch urethral catheter.

INCISION. Make an upper median or paramedian incision and follow the initial steps for a cholecystostomy, as in Section 13.3, until you have exposed his subhepatic area and found his gall-bladder, cystic-duct, and common bile-duct. The incision will have to be longer than that for a cholecystostomy, so extend that incision, cutting the muscles in line with the skin incision, parallel to his costal margin and about 3 cm below it.

Place two large moist packs under his liver to get good exposure. Place another one deep in his right subhepatic space (Morrison's pouch), to absorb any of the infected bile which will later come gushing out.

Use a small gauze swab on the end of a large curved haemostat to dissect in the triangle between his common bile-duct, his cystic duct, and his common hepatic duct. Feel for his hepatic artery; his bile-duct is the tube lying immediately to its right in the free edge of his lesser omentum. His portal vein lies behind both of them. As Fig. 13-3 shows, there is considerable anatomical variation in this region. Make sure you have found his bile-ducts before proceeding further. Palpate them to be sure none of them pulsates! Then expose 2 cm of his common duct, which will probably be dilated—even to 5 cm or more (A, Fig. 13-2).

If in doubt, aspirate his common duct to make sure it contains bile and not blood. Now place two 3/0 catgut stay sutures on its anterior surface about 4 mm apart (B).

With the tip of the sucker close by, make a 2 cm longitudinal incision between the stay sutures (C). Suck out all the bile and exudate, and take a swab for culture and sensitivity. Using Desjardin's stone forceps, gently remove any stones that you easily can (D). The curve on the forceps may help you—the stones are probably well down his common duct at its lower end, where it enters his duodenum. Don't prolong this stage of the operation if it is difficult—you can do much harm. If there is much 'sludge', wash out his common duct by irrigating it with plenty of saline using a plain rubber catheter and a 20 ml glass syringe.

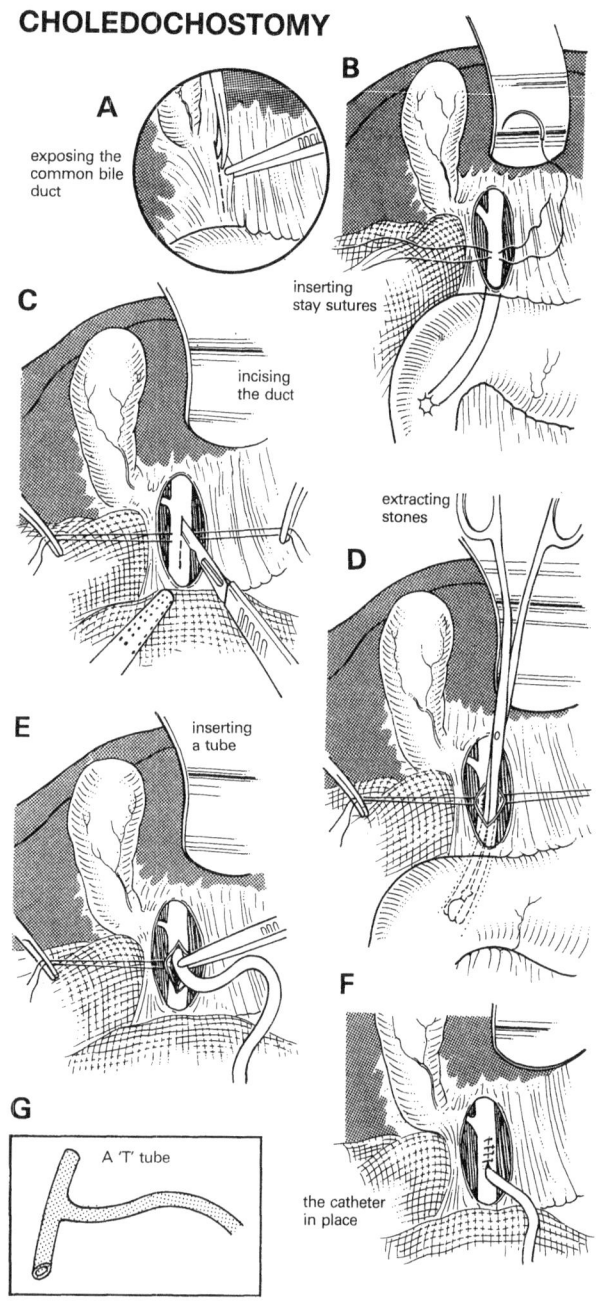

Fig. 13-2 CHOLEDOCHOSTOMY. A, expose the patient's common bile-duct. B, insert stay sutures. C, incise his common bile-duct. D, remove stones. E, insert a catheter. F, the catheter sewn in place. G, insert a T-tube.

Insert a T-tube. Failing this, insert a 14 Ch urethral catheter in his common bile-duct for about 4 cm (E), and suture it to the upper end of the incision in the duct with 3/0 chromic catgut (F). Close the opening in the duct snugly round the drainage tube with the same material.

Bring the tube out through a stab incision, leaving some slack inside, in case it is pulled on. Anchor it securely to his skin with a non-absorbable suture.

Close his abdominal wall carefully—his wound is likely to become infected, so don't close his skin (9.8).

POSTOPERATIVELY, connect the tube to a bedside bottle, and allow it to drain freely until his jaundice and fever subside. Refer him. If you cannot refer him, do a tube cholangiogram 7 to 10 days postoperatively using 'Hypaque' or similar aqueous contrast medium diluted one part to two parts of 0.9% saline. This will help in further management. It should show any residual stones. If you find any, try again to refer him. The stones can be removed by an expert through the T-tube tract by passing a fibre-optic endoscope into his duodenum and slitting his sphincter of Oddi, or by opening his duodenum at operation. This is very difficult surgery. Only a few patients need it.

If you see no stones, and the medium flows nicely into his duodenum, try clamping the tube. Provided that he has no pain, fever, or jaundice, remove the tube.

If you cannot do a tube cholangiogram, connect the tube to a vertical length of plastic tubing (as when measuring the CVP, A 19.2) to see what pressure builds up. It should not be higher than 8 to 10 cm of bile. If after 24 hours no higher pressure develops, try clamping the tube. Remove it after two weeks if no discomfort develops. If pressure does build up in the tube, don't remove it. He may need it for months, but try to refer him. If fever and jaundice reappear, unspigot the tube— he will need further surgery to remove his remaining stones.

13.5 Cholangitis caused by *Ascaris*

Ascaris worms sometimes crawl up into a patient's common bile-duct and gall-bladder, where they can cause biliary colic, acute cholecystitis, obstructive jaundice, and cholangitis. This most often happens when a child has been given an antihelminthic. So, if a child has cholangitis, or if an adult does not fit the usual clinical picture for biliary disease, suspect Ascariasis. Finding *Ascaris* ova should arouse your suspicion, but does not confirm the diagnosis. Do an intravenous cholangiogram when the jaundice is ebbing—it may outline the worms. Don't operate, except on the indications below.

ASCARIS CHOLANGITIS

Nasogastric suction will rest the child's upper intestinal tract. Systemic antibiotics will help to control his cholangitis. Later, give him piperazine or mebendazole.

INDICATIONS FOR SURGERY. Deepening jaundice, spiking fever, chills and rigors which do not respond to antibiotics; nausea and vomiting, toxaemia, dehydration, tachycardia, and perhaps hypotension; together with a leucocytosis. If he has these symptoms, explore and drain his bile-ducts (choledochostomy), as in Section 13.4. Remove any worms you find.

13.6 Primary or recurrent pyogenic cholangitis

This differs from 'secondary cholangitis' in that: (1) It has no known cause; it is not secondary to stones, strictures, carcinoma, or worms. (2) The primary pathology is not in the gall-bladder, but in the bile-ducts (intra- or extrahepatic), which contain sludge and pigment stones. (3) Treatment involves drainage of the bile-ducts, not removal of the gall-bladder, unless it is very distended and gangrenous. (5) Symptoms commonly recur (unusual in secondary cholangitis). This was one of the most common abdominal emergencies in East Asia—China, Korea, Taiwan, Hong Kong and Malaysia, but its incidence is now declining.

The patient, who is usually between 30 and 40 years (the sexes are affected equally) presents with a high swinging fever, chills, and rigors, a gnawing right upper abdominal pain, and mild jaundice (Charcot's triad), usually with a history of previous attacks. His liver is tender and enlarged and his gall-bladder may be palpable. His urine is dark, but his stools are seldom clay-coloured—complete obstruction of the common bile-duct is rare.

PRIMARY PYOGENIC CHOLANGITIS

SPECIAL TESTS. The patient's white count is raised, so is his serum bilirubin (3 mg/dl or more). If infection is severe and his liver cells are involved, his transaminases are raised. Measure his serum amylase, because there is a 10% chance that he also has pancreatitis.

X-RAYS. A plain X-ray may show air in his biliary tract due to an incompetent sphincter of Oddi.

During an acute attack neither an oral nor an intravenous cholangiogram will demonstrate his biliary system. Four weeks later an intravenous cholangiogram may show filling defects in his common bile-duct.

NON-OPERATIVE TREATMENT. If the disease is mild, take blood cultures and give him antibiotics (cephradine or gentamicin, 2.9). Give him 10 mg of vitamin K_1. Give him intravenous fluids, and aspirate his stomach through a nasogastric tube.

INDICATIONS FOR OPERATION. (1) the failure of non-operative treatment. (2) A palpable, tender, enlarged gall-bladder. (3) Septicaemia. (4) Peritonitis.

LAPAROTOMY. Aim to remove all biliary grit and mud by washing out his extra- and intrahepatic bile-ducts with copious amounts of saline. If this is impossible, do a wide (>2.5 cm) choledochoduodenostomy so that stones that are left behind can pass into his gut without totally obstructing his biliary tree.

If he is very ill with septicaemia or peritonitis, do a cholecystostomy if his gall-bladder is enlarged. If it is shrunken and his common duct dilated, do a choledochostomy, and insert a T-tube. Refer him for a choledochoenterostomy or cholecystectomy 6 weeks later.

If you cannot refer him and you are sufficiently skilled, do a choledochoduodenostomy, or a choledochojejunostomy (13.8) at that time.

13.7 Cholecystectomy

Removing a patient's gall-bladder is the standard method of treating chronic gall-bladder disease, but it is not an operation for the occasional surgeon, so if you do see a patient with cholecystitis, or gallstones, try to treat him non-operatively as in Sections 13.2 and 13.3.

If his symptoms persist, and you are experienced, you may feel justified in removing more normal-looking, easier gall-bladders on the indications given below. This is something which district hospitals in areas where gall-bladder disease is common, should be able to do. Even so, it is right at the edge of this particular system of surgery. *Whatever you do, don't try to remove the more difficult fibrotic, contracted gall-bladders.* These really are for the experts. Unfortunately, you will not know if a patient's gall-bladder is going to be easy or difficult, until you are inside his abdomen. So, be prepared to close it, or do a cholecystostomy, if you find that he has a difficult one. We describe the retrograde method of removing the gall-bladder in which you first dissect and tie its neck. An alternative method is to start at the fundus.

The main danger is injuring his common bile or hepatic ducts. *But, provided you don't operate when chronic inflammation has scarred his gall-bladder and porta hepatis severely,* you should be able to avoid this.

A patient's symptoms and your findings, when you operate, are likely to bear little relation to one another. A few small stones may give him severe colic, while a gangrenous gallbladder may cause him little distress. So don't let moderate symptoms lead you to expect an 'easy gall-bladder', and don't operate in a hurry.

The commonest cause of an injured bile-duct or hepatic artery is an 'easy' gall-bladder done quickly. Another cause is the anatomical variability shown in Fig. 13-3.

ELECTIVE CHOLECYSTECTOMY

INDICATIONS. (1) You must be fairly experienced. (2) You must be sure of the diagnosis. (3) The patient must have symptoms which justify the operation. (4) He must not be too fat. (5) There must be no complicating factors. (6) You must be unable to refer him. (7) You must be prepared to back out, or do a cholecystostomy, if you find that he has a difficult gall-bladder.

ANTIBIOTICS. The main cause of death in gall-bladder surgery is postoperative sepsis. Give him a perioperative antibiotic (2.9) if he is: (1) Over 50. (2) Actively infected. (3) Jaundiced. Or, (4) when you are likely to have to explore his bile-ducts.

ANAESTHESIA. (1) A general anaesthetic with good muscle relaxation. (2) Subarachnoid (spinal) anaesthesia.

EQUIPMENT. A general set. A self-retaining and a Deaver's retractor. You will need two assistants and a trolley nurse.

INCISION. Make a midline or upper right paramedian incision extending up to his costal margin (A, in Fig. 13-4).

Feel for his gall-bladder. Feel for stones. Feel both lobes of his liver to be sure they are smooth and normal. If his gall-bladder seems far up under his rib cage, run your hand over its right lobe, divide his falciform ligament across the dome of his liver, and draw it down. Put some large packs between his diaphragm and his liver—don't forget to remove them afterwards!

Insert a self-retaining retractor, and try to see his gall-bladder. Use long tissue forceps to place large moist abdominal packs over the hepatic flexure of his colon, his duodenum, and his stomach. Ask your first assistant to draw these downwards and medially. You should now be able to see under his liver clearly.

Protect his liver with a pack, and ask your second assistant to retract it upwards and laterally with a large Deaver's retractor (B). Look at his gall-bladder.

If his gall-bladder is acutely inflamed, do a cholecystostomy (13-1).

If it is very small, shrunken, thick-walled, contains stones, and is firmly stuck to nearby structures, leave it alone, or take out the stones and do a cholecystostomy and close the wound. Removing such a gall-bladder will be very difficult.

If it looks and feels reasonably normal, apart from a few stones, and is attached by fine adhesions only, it should be safe to proceed.

Find his cystic duct, his common bile-duct, and his hepatic artery, in the free edge of his lesser omentum. His epiploic foramen (of Winslow) lies behind it; you should be able to pass one or two fingers through it into his lesser sac.

Place a gall-bladder clamp, or sponge-holding forceps on Hartmann's pouch (C). This is a widened area in the lower part of the patient's gall-bladder, just before it tapers off into his cystic duct. Pull gently upwards on these forceps, so as to stretch the tissues and make dissection easier.

Incise the triangle of peritoneum between Hartmann's pouch and the common bile-duct. This will appear when you apply traction to the sponge-holding forceps on Hartmann's pouch. *It is a most important step.* Start by making a small nick in the peritoneum with a long pair of Metzenbaum scissors. Carefully insert the tips of the scissors, then, using 'the push and spread technique' (4-8), or a Lahey dissecting swab, open up enough of the patient's peritoneum to expose the deeper structures.

CAUTION! Be careful not to cut any small blood vessels. Bleeding will make the operation difficult. By spreading the blades of the scissors (but not too far!) before you cut, or using a Lahey dissecting swab, you should be able to separate peritoneum only.

Take a pledget of gauze in the beak of a pair of curved artery forceps (a 'peanut' or Lahey swab, as shown in C, and E, Fig. 13-4), and gently push apart the peritoneum, so that you see his common bile-duct.

Now, use your left hand to try to feel his cystic duct as it leaves his gall-bladder to join his common bile-duct. It may be helpful to lift up the clamp on his gall-bladder while you do this, so as to stretch the ducts.

BILIARY ANATOMY

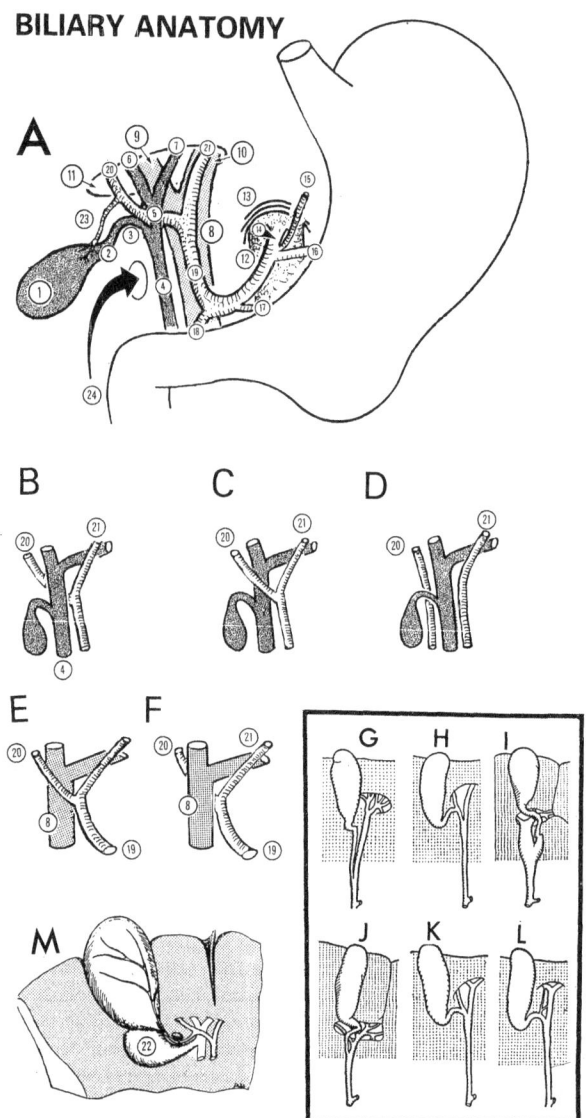

Fig. 13-3 THE ANATOMY OF THE BILIARY SYSTEM. A, the normal relationships of structures in this region.

B, to F, the relations of the right hepatic artery. In B, (and A) it runs posteriorly to the common hepatic duct (64%). In C, it runs anteriorly (24%), and in D, it arises from the superior mesenteric artery (9%). In E, it runs anteriorly to the portal vein (91%) and in F, posteriorly (9%).

G, to L, variations in the bile passages. Note the accessory hepatic ducts in positions of surgical danger. M, a small pouch (Hartmann's pouch) may project from the right wall of the neck of a diseased gall-bladder downwards and backwards towards the duodenum. When it is well marked the cystic duct arises from its upper left wall and not from what appears to be the apex of the gall-bladder.

1, the fundus of the gall-bladder. 2, the neck of the gall-bladder. 3, the cystic duct. 4, the common bile-duct. 5, the common hepatic duct. 6, the right hepatic duct. 7, the left hepatic duct. 8, the portal vein. 9, the right branch of the portal vein. 10, the left branch of the portal vein. 11, the porta hepatis. 12, the aorta. 13, some fibres of the diaphragm. 14, the coeliac artery. 15, the left gastric artery. 16, the splenic artery. 17, the right gastric artery. 18, the gastroduodenal artery. 19, the hepatic artery. 20, the right hepatic artery. 21, the left hepatic artery. 22, Hartmann's pouch. 23, the cystic artery. 24, the epiploic foramen (entrance to the lesser sac). *After "Grant's Method of Anatomy", (9th edn 1975 edited by JV Basmajian). Williams and Wilkins, with kind permission.*

CAUTION! There are some important anatomical variations: (1) The common bile-duct and the cystic duct may join high or low, as in G, to L in Fig. 13-3. (2) The right hepatic artery may pass behind the common hepatic duct (A, and B, more common) or in front of it (C, less common). (3) The cystic duct may be closely bound to the common hepatic duct. (4) The cystic artery usually (64%) arises from the right hepatic artery. It may cross behind (usually) or in front of (unusually) the common

CHOLECYSTECTOMY

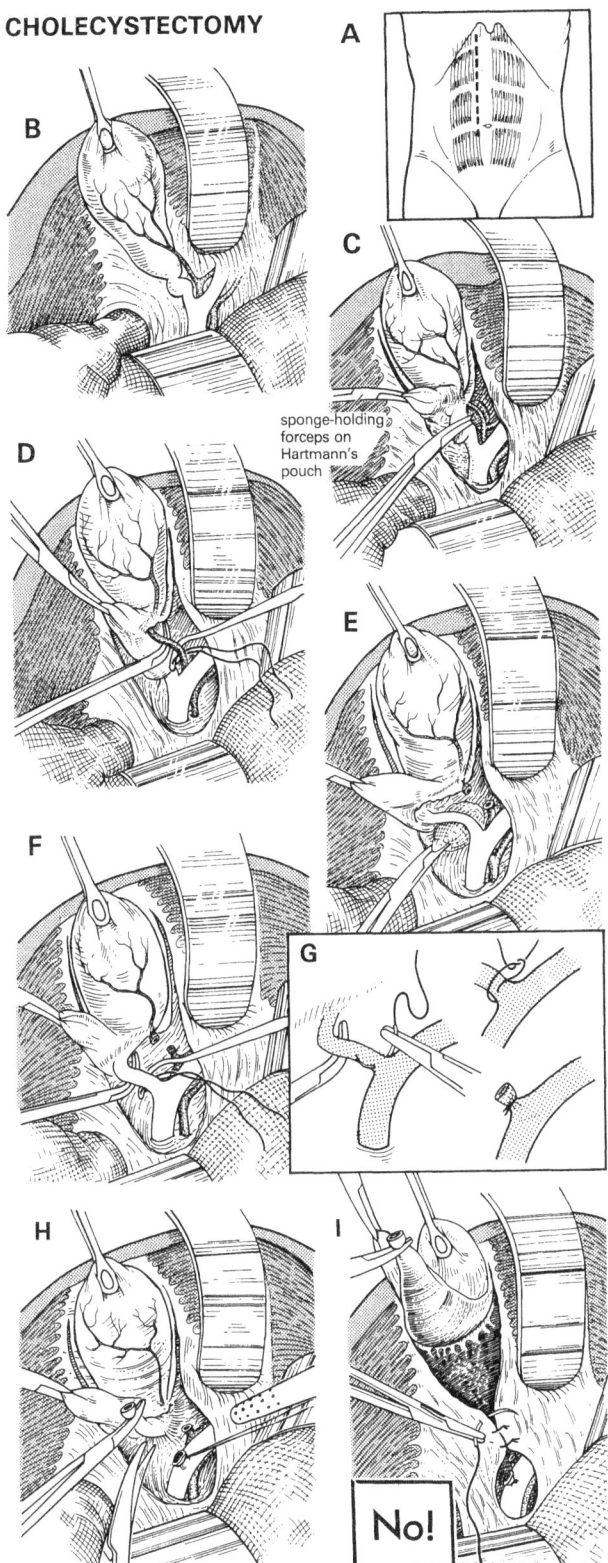

Fig. 13-4 REMOVING THE GALL-BLADDER. A, the incision. B, exposing the gall-bladder. C, exposing the cystic duct. Note that the second forceps holds a Lahey swab. D, tying the cystic artery. E, freeing the cystic duct. F, tying the cystic duct. G, if the cystic duct is very large and thickened, transfix and tie it like this. H, separating the gall-bladder from the liver. I, a further possible stage in removing the gall-bladder. Don't close its bed like this, it is unnecessary and may cause damage. *After Rob C and Smith R, "Operative Surgery," (2nd edn 1969), Vol. 4 p. 404. Butterworths, with kind permission.*

hepatic and cystic ducts to reach the gall-bladder. Sometimes, it arises from the common hepatic (27%) or the left hepatic artery (5%), or from other arteries in the region (rare). (5) Be sure of your landmarks before you start to divide anything. (6) Use a Lahey swab and dissect by the 'push and spread' method.

Find the junction of the patient's cystic and common bile ducts, as described above. Be sure to identify 2 cm of his common duct, both proximal and distal to the junction. This will give you an idea of its course and direction. The common bile-duct lies to the right of the structures going to the porta hepatis, and is a greenish colour—*identifying it is one of the keys to safe gall-bladder surgery.*

If you have found the junction of his cystic and common bile ducts, and you are sure that what you presume is his cystic duct is going to his gall-bladder, and nowhere else, define it further, using blunt dissection. Then tie it off, by the following method, close to his common bile-duct, but not too close.

Using a long pair of Lahey forceps, gently open up the cleft between his cystic and common hepatic ducts. Pass a tie of '0' chromic catgut through this cleft, and around his cystic duct, and tie it (F). Place another Lahey clamp on his cystic duct just above the tie close to his gall-bladder. Cut his cystic duct between the two ties close to the gall-bladder.

CAUTION ! Only divide and tie structures that are passing to his gall-bladder. A long stump to the cystic duct is not important, unless it contained an obvious stone.

If his cystic artery runs posterior to his common hepatic and cystic ducts (usual), take extra care. Using Lahey's forceps on his divided cystic duct, and traction with your left hand, feel carefully with your right thumb and index finger for any bands or structures that are still tethering his gall-bladder. One of these is probably his cystic artery, or a branch of it. Don't cut these structures; isolate them with finger dissection. Don't expect to feel any pulsation in such a small vessel. If a strand of tissue runs to his gall-bladder, assume it is his cystic artery, tie, and divide it. Expect to find other branches and deal with them in the same way.

If his cystic artery runs anterior to his common hepatic and cystic ducts (unusual), define it by blunt dissection, and make sure that it is indeed going to his gall-bladder.

CAUTION ! Don't tie his right hepatic artery by mistake.

If you are sure you have found his cystic artery, tie it close to his gall-bladder with 2/0 black silk, leaving a long tail, so that you can easily find it if it bleeds. Leave a short cuff of tissue, distal to the tie.

You should now be able to strip his gall-bladder from its bed by pulling it gently upwards on the clamps. Cut any peritoneal bands that join it to his liver, but tie off anything else—there may be a vessel or an anomalous bile-duct inside a band.

If the bed of his gall-bladder oozes, press a warm pack into it. If small veins continue to bleed, cauterize them. It is unnecessary and dangerous to close the peritoneum over the bed of the gall-bladder as in I, Fig. 13-4.

CAUTION ! Check to make sure that the stump of his cystic duct is secure and that no bile is leaking.

CLOSING THE WOUND. Either leave no drain, or place a soft rubber drain through a stab wound down to his porta hepatis. Close his abdominal wound as in Section 9.8.

DIFFICULTIES REMOVING THE GALL-BLADDER

If, when you open his abdomen, you find an INFLAMMATORY MASS or an unrecognizable mass of tissue, withdraw and close the wound. If you cannot refer him, consider operating later, when the inflammation has subsided.

If you INJURE HIS CYSTIC DUCT early on, tie it between ligatures and divide it. If you injure it very near its union with the common bile-duct, divide it carefully, tie it, and close the common duct opening with interrupted 3/0 catgut sutures.

If you find that you have DAMAGED HIS COMMON BILE-DUCT you will have done so in one of three ways: (1) By ligature; undo the ligature. (2) By clamp; take off the clamp and inspect the damage. Do a choledochostomy higher up, and pass a fine catheter through the damaged area. Proceed as for a choledochostomy (13-2). (3) By partly dividing it. Leave a T-tube threaded up and down the duct and proceed as for choledochostomy. Refer him. If this is impossible, keep the T-tube in for 3 months, and then do a T-tube cholangiogram and remove it. Learn from your mistakes, learn to be able to forgive yourself, and carry on.

If his CYSTIC ARTERY BLEEDS from the depths of his wound, this can be alarming. *Don't clamp blindly.* (1) Insert warm moist packs, apply pressure and wait 5 minutes by the clock. The spurting vessel will then be easier to find and control. Or, (2) put your index finger into the epiploic foramen (of Winslow) and squeeze the structures (portal vein, bile-ducts, and hepatic artery) in the free edge of the lesser omentum between your index finger and your thumb. This will control bleeding from the stump of the cystic artery. Transfix it carefully with 3/0 silk.

If FRESH BLOOD DISCHARGES from the drain, his pulse rises, his blood pressure falls, and he has signs of a haemoperitoneum, his cystic artery is probably bleeding. Reopen his abdomen and control it.

If BILE COMES FROM THE DRAIN, his temperature and white count rise, and he has pain, suspect that infected bile and exudate are pooling under his liver. Give him an antibiotic. If he does not improve reopen his abdomen and make sure the area is adequately drained.

13.8 Obstructive jaundice

When jaundice is due to an obstruction in the flow of bile: (1) The patient's stools are pale. (2) His urine is dark, and contains little or no urobilinogen. (3) His skin itches. These features are most marked in complete obstruction, as when carcinoma blocks the common duct. Stones typically cause an intermittent obstruction, and a less characteristic picture.

If a stone impacts in Hartmann's pouch or in the cystic duct, it causes pain but does not impede the flow of bile down the common duct, so jaundice is absent or is mild (due to associated cholangitis).

If a an older patient has a steadily deepening and usually painless obstructive jaundice, and his gall-bladder is palpably enlarged, some tumour is probably obstructing his common duct. He is probably incurable, but a cholecystojejunostomy to decompress his gall-bladder, by diverting his bile into his jejunum, may make his last days more bearable. So make the best of such means of diagnosing him as you may have, and don't necessarily give him up as hopeless. In East and Central Africa, for example, obstructive jaundice is most commonly caused by: (1) Secondary carcinoma of the liver. (2) A secondary tumour in the porta hepatis, usually from a primary in the stomach. (3) Carcinoma of the head of the pancreas. (4) Gall-stones. (5) Hepatoma; although this is a common disease, presentation as obstructive jaundice is unusual. (6) Carcinoma of the extrahepatic bile-ducts. (7) Carcinoma of the gall-bladder. This is rare in Africa, but is the most common cause of malignant obstructive jaundice in India.

With the exception of gallstones, in which the jaundice may be intermittent, all these diseases present with progressively deepening jaundice over weeks or months, usually without the fever and rigors of cholangitis that so often complicate the jaundice of gallstones. The patient may have no pain, but if he has, it is usually not severe; it is deep, penetrating, and present most of the time—quite unlike the agonizing episodic biliary colic that gallstones cause. He is anorexic, and nauseated, and may lose so much weight that he becomes severely emaciated, with no other symptoms than jaundice.

First exclude hepatocellular jaundice, which has 'obstructive' features at first, although these diminish later. Then, if you decide that his jaundice is obstructive, weigh the evidence for malignancy or stones. If his jaundice continues to deepen, he needs surgery, if he is fit enough.

OBSTRUCTIVE JAUNDICE

DIFFERENTIAL DIAGNOSIS. First try to decide what kind of jaundice the patient has.

Haemolytic jaundice. His stools are dark. There is no bilirubin in his urine, but his urinary urobilinogen is increased. His blood shows increased levels of unconjugated prehepatic bilirubin (leading to high readings on the indirect van den Bergh test). His transaminases (GPT and GOT) are normal, and so is his alkaline phosphatase.

Obstructive jaundice. His stools are pale (clay-coloured if obstruction is complete), and *show no improvement in colour in 10 days*. There is bilirubin in his urine, but little or no urobilinogen. He has high blood levels of conjugated (posthepatic) bilirubin (giving high readings on the direct van den Bergh test). His alkaline phosphatase is very high. His transaminases are normal.

Hepatocellular jaundice This is commonly viral hepatitis with an obstructive phase lasting 7–10 days, but sometimes much longer. At this stage his stools are pale. His urine contains bilirubin but little urobilinogen. His serum bilirubin is moderately increased (mostly conjugated). His alkaline phosphatase is usually only moderately increased, but if cholestasis is a prominent feature it can rise to levels seen in obstructive jaundice. His transaminases are increased.

As the oedema of his cells settles, his stools become normal or even dark, his serum bilirubin falls, his urinary urobilinogen rises or reappears, and his transaminases fall gradually. *The return of stool colour is the most important sign.* This form of jaundice is not common in most developing countries after the age of 35.

CAUTION ! You may have difficulty distinguishing the obstructive phase of hepatocellular jaundice from surgical obstructive jaundice. Do try to make the distinction. A laparotomy for stone may be life saving, but anaesthesia and the trauma of surgery may cause hepatocellular jaundice to deteriorate, perhaps fatally.

Ultrasound is very useful. An intravenous cholangiogram is not helpful in the presence of jaundice. The ducts will not be outlined.

Suggesting malignancy—(1) Relentlessly progressive steadily deepening obstructive jaundice, weight loss. (2) A palpable gall-bladder which you can feel as an elongated, smooth, non-tender mass, normal in contour, and slightly mobile, which may extend to the patient's umbilicus or even below it. If you can feel his distended gall-bladder, it strongly suggests a malignant obstruction at the lower end of his common bile-duct, but its absence does not exclude this.

Suggesting secondary deposits in his liver—a large, knobbly liver.

Suggesting a carcinoma of his stomach with secondaries in his porta hepatis—pain, anorexia, vomiting, an upper abdominal mass, and the visible peristalsis of pyloric stenosis. Anaemia is common.

Suggesting carcinoma of the head of his pancreas—vague epigastric pain, and weight loss.

Suggesting gallstones—a long history of intermittent varying jaundice, severe intermittent colicky pain, a non-palpable gall-bladder, fever, chills, and rigors (suggesting cholangitis), little or no weight loss, flatulent dyspepsia. A raised white count suggests cholecystitis.

Suggesting hepatoma—a large, hard, irregular liver. A bruit is often present, ascites is common, and is often bloodstained.

Suggesting stenosis of his bile-ducts, either malignant or benign—a tender, enlarged liver. His gall-bladder may or may not be palpable.

Suggesting carcinoma of the gall-bladder—the patient is a woman with an enlarged liver and a hard, irregular mass in her right hypochondrium.

MANAGEMENT. If the patient has gall-stones, try to refer him to an expert. If he has malignant disease with obstruction at the lower end of his common bile-duct, a cholecystojejunostomy may help.

CHOLECYSTOJEJUNOSTOMY FOR OBSTRUCTIVE JAUNDICE

INDICATIONS. In practice the presence of a smooth enlarged gall-bladder is the only clear indication to operate. Its absence does not exclude the possibility of doing the operation.

CONTRAINDICATIONS. Cachexia, debility, a hard irregular gall-bladder mass, a hard, craggy liver due to secondary deposits, hepatoma, a large gastric tumour, ascites etc.

PREPARATION. Give him vitamin K_1 (water-soluble) 10 mg intramuscularly daily for 3 days preoperatively. This will reduce his tendency to bleed.

CHOLECYSTO-JEJUNOSTOMY

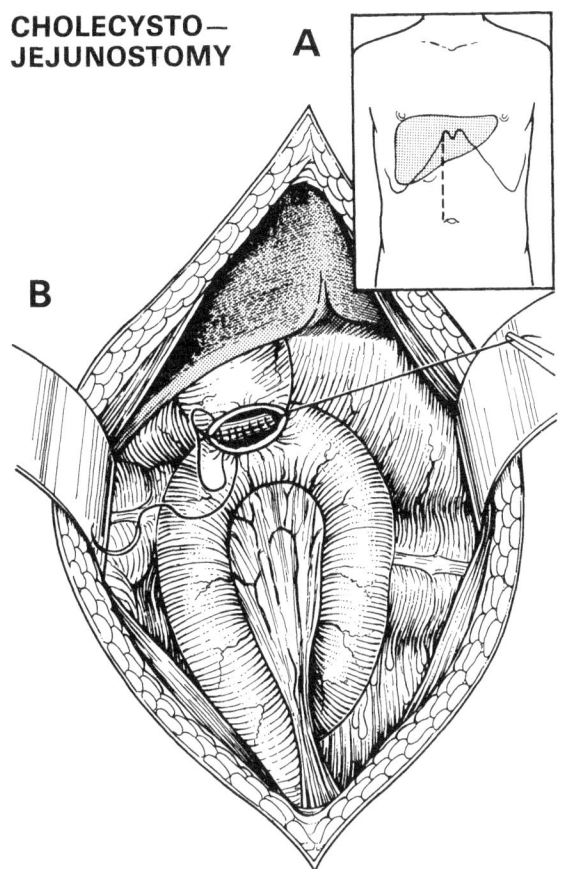

Fig. 13-5 CHOLECYSTOJEJUNOSTOMY. A, the incision. B, the first layer of the anastomosis.

HYDRATION. Patients with jaundice are prone to acute renal failure if their glomerular filtration rate falls. So make sure he is well-hydrated preoperatively. Give him plenty of saline during the operation, catheterize his bladder, and leave the catheter in. Also give him frusemide.

INCISION. Open his abdomen through an upper midline or an upper right paramedian incision. Expose his liver and subhepatic area as in Section 13.7. Good exposure is essential.

Inspect and feel his upper abdominal viscera carefully. Is his gall-bladder normal in size and appearance? If it is a hard, irregular mass which is fixed to the surounding organs, it is probably malignant.

Feel his pancreas, especially its head. (1) Lift his transverse colon upwards and forwards out of the wound with your left hand, while you feel his pancreas at the base of his transverse mesocolon. Its head lies to the right of his vertebral column at this level. A hard, knobbly, craggy mass suggests a tumour. (2) You can also feel the head of his pancreas from above. Stand on the left side of the table and feel with your right hand while you pull the hepatic flexure of his colon medially. Place your thumb anteriorly and your fingers posteriorly. Feel the head of his pancreas lying in the concavity of his duodenum. If necessary, Kocherize it (66.16), so that you can feel it properly.

CAUTION ! Don't biopsy his pancreas. Unless you use special methods you will cause pancreatitis and a fistula.

Feel his porta hepatis and the structures lying in the free edge of his lesser omentum. Can you feel any craggy, fixed, indurated masses, suggesting primary carcinomas of his bile-ducts or secondary deposits? Feel his stomach.

THE INDICATIONS FOR PROCEEDING FURTHER can only be decided at this stage.

A bypass is indicated if he has an enlarged and distended but otherwise normal gall-bladder, showing that he has an obstruction in his common bile-duct, proximal to or within the head of his pancreas, with no obstruction to his cystic duct. If you find any gallstones, remove them. Then make sure that his jaundice is not caused by stones. If it is, do a choledochostomy as in Fig. 13-2.

A bypass is contraindicated if: (1) He has multiple liver secondaries, a hepatoma, or a carcinoma of his gall-bladder. (2) The tumour involves his gall-bladder or porta hepatis. (3) He has an advanced tumour of his stomach, or colon, etc. Most of these conditions make the operation impossible.

CAUTION ! (2) If his gall-bladder is diseased, or contains many stones, abandon the operation. Don't try to anastomose a thick walled, inflamed, oedematous gall-bladder.

METHOD. Decompress his distended gall-bladder as for a cholecystostomy in Figure 13-1. Remove the purse string suture, and extend the opening with scissors to a length of 1.5 cm. Apply Babcock clamps to the fundus of his gall-bladder about 1 cm from each end of the incision. Lift his transverse colon upwards and look for the ligament of Treitz. This is the point where the retroperitoneal 4th part of his duodenum emerges to become his jejunum slightly to the left of his vertebral column, and distal to the attachment of the mesentery of his transverse colon. Choose a loop of jejunum 30 cm distal to the ligament of Treitz, and draw it up towards his open gall-bladder.

Apply two Babcock clamps 3 cm apart on the antimesenteric border of his jejunum, to match those on the fundus of his gall-bladder. Bring these clamps alongside one another, making sure that there is no tension on the jejunal loop. Aim to make a 1.5 cm stoma.

CAUTION ! Make the anastomosis neatly and carefully: it must not leak, because bile easily escapes, and a pool of bile is a serious complication.

The anastomosis is similar to that for a gastroenterostomy (11.6) or ileotransversostomy. Make the seromuscular first layer of interrupted sutures of 3/0 silk on an atraumatic needle. Insert five sutures, which should ideally pick up only the seromuscular layer of his jejunum, but which will probably be of full thickness, in the wall of his gall-bladder. Place them about 2 mm away from the cut edge of the incision, and on the gut side about 2 cm back from the antemesenteric border of his jejunum.

Incise his jejunum 3 mm back from the suture line. Trim away redundant mucosa with fine scissors. Apply Babcock's forceps temporarily over any bleeding points.

Insert a continuous 'all coats' posterior layer of 3/0 atraumatic chromic catgut sutures, starting at one end; then continue to close the anterior layer with the same sutures. Finally, use 3/0 silk to insert an anterior layer of seromuscular interrupted Lembert sutures.

Close his abdominal wall as soundly as you can, as in Section 9.8.

13.9 Pancreatitis

Both acute and chronic pancreatitis are not uncommon in India, but are seldom seen in Africa. You you may have to treat them, or to drain a pancreatic abscess (5.10b), or a pancreatic pseudocyst.

Pathologically, acute pancreatitis varies from oedema and congestion of a patient's pancreas to its complete autodigestion, with necrosis, haemorrhage, and suppuration. Less severe forms may go on to form a tender, ill-defined mass in his epigastrium.

His main symptom is pain, which can vary from moderate epigastric discomfort to an excruciating, penetrating agony, which bores through to his back, and needs high doses of pethidine to relieve it. He is tender in his epigastrium, perhaps with guarding. Later, his abdomen distends, and he vomits. Vomiting, and the outpouring of fluid into his retroperitoneum, sends him into shock and his gut into ileus.

You may diagnose pancreatitis clinically, or you may only find it when you do a laparotomy for an acute abdomen. Estimating the serum amylase is not difficult, and your laboratory should be able to do it.

Chronic relapsing or recurrent pancreatitis is one of the causes of a severe chronic upper abdominal pain. It is quite common in the states of Kerala and Orissa in India, and in alcoholics anywhere. It only needs surgery if the pain is debilitating, or if it constricts the common bile-duct, so that it causes jaundice and produces a syndrome which resembles carcinoma (13.8). A bypass (cholecystojejunostomy) will relieve a patient's jaundice, but this is not common.

ACUTE PANCREATITIS

THE DIFFERENTIAL DIAGNOSIS includes perforated peptic ulcer (11.2), acute cholecystitis (13.3), biliary colic (13.2), rupture of an amoebic abscess (31.12), and strangulating upper small gut obstruction (10.3).

SPECIAL TESTS. The patient's serum amylase rises within a few hours of the start of his pain, and remains high for about 2 days. A level of more than 1000 Somogyi units is almost diagnostic. A peritoneal tap in his right lower quadrant will confirm the diagnosis—the aspirate may be straw-coloured, or reddish-brown, but its amylase is always high. In the severest haemorrhagic form of the disease the serum calcium is low.

X-RAYS may show pancreatic calcification, if he has had previous attacks; gallstones, a left pleural effusion, or distended loops of gut (ileus).

TREATMENT. Treat his shock energetically with large volumes of 0.9% saline, Ringer's lactate, or a plasma expander. Monitor his urinary output, his haematocrit, and if posssible, his central venous pressure (A 19.2).

His pain may be overwhelming. Give him large doses of pethidine, supplemented by diazepam or promethazine. Keep his stomach empty with nasogastric suction. Antibiotics are useless.

If you are reasonably sure of the diagnosis, don't operate; but it is better to operate unnecessarily, than not to operate on a case of strangulated gut, for example.

If you do open his peritoneum, you will know that he has pancreatitis, because you will see areas of whitish-red fat necrosis on his transverse mesocolon, or omentum, and the exudate described above. His pancreas feels swollen and oedematous, and may contain greenish-grey necrotic areas.

Don't insert drains: there is no evidence that they help.

DIFFICULTIES WITH ACUTE PANCREATITIS

If you find that he also has GALLSTONES, consider doing a choledochostomy (13-2). Don't be tempted to remove his gallbladder, or a stone in his common bile duct, which may have precipitated the attack. Theoretically, this might be beneficial; but practically it is very difficult.

If, during the course of 2 or 3 weeks, he develops the signs of SEPTICAEMIA, suspect that he is developing a pancreatic abscess.

If his pancreatitis has progressed to form an ABSCESS (uncommon, 5.10b), you will need to do a laparotomy to drain it, and a jejunostomy (9.7) to feed him while 'resting' his pancreas.

If he develops RESPIRATORY OR RENAL FAILURE, usually in the first 48 hours (5-10% chance), he will probably die. There is little you can do except give him oxygen, plenty of intravenous fluids, and plasma expanders, together with frusemide to stimulate his urine flow. If necessary, ventilate him (A 19.4).

13.10 Pancreatic pseudocyst

A large watery pancreatic exudate sometimes collects in a patient's lesser sac. This has no epithelial lining, hence the term '*pseudo*'cyst.

He usually presents some weeks after an abdominal injury, or an attack of acute pancreatitis, with a mass in his abdomen and epigastric discomfort or pain. He may be toxic with fever and tachycardia, but he is not nearly as ill as he would be if he had acute pancreatitis, or a pancreatic abscess. The mass usually distends his abdomen: it may extend right across his epigastrium, and reach down to his umbilicus or beyond it. It is tender, tense, immobile, and is often not fluctuant. Sometimes, he has symptoms of pancreatic insufficiency, with steatorrhoea.

If you make an opening between the cyst and his stomach, it will drain, without, surprisingly, the food in his stomach causing problems inside the cyst. You will have to open the anterior wall of his stomach, and then make another opening through its posterior wall into the cyst (cystogastrostomy). The correct timing of this is important (see below). Draining it is less urgent than operating on a pancreatic abscess (5.10b), and there is less chance of complications.

PANCREATIC PSEUDOCYST

SPECIAL TESTS. The patient's serum amylase is usually raised. If he is jaundiced (unusual), liver function tests will show the changes of obstructive jaundice.

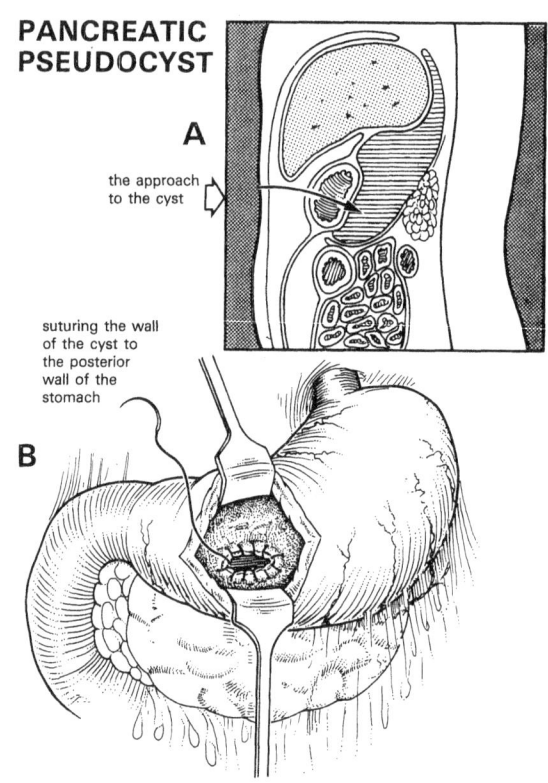

Fig. 13-6 A PANCREATIC PSEUDOCYST. A, the approach to the cyst through the anterior and posterior walls of the stomach. B, the wall of the cyst sutured to the posterior wall of the stomach to control bleeding. *After Cattell and Warren in Maingot R, "Abdominal Operations", (4th edn 1961) p. 557 Fig. 26. HK Lewis, permission requested.*

IMAGING. Ultrasound is much better than X-rays. If you are using X-rays: (1) Give him some barium. A lateral film of his stomach will show a mass bulging into the barium shadow from behind. A barium meal shows gross widening of the normal contour of his duodenum. You may see patches of calcification in his pancreas. Or, (2) insert a nasogastric tube. Inject 200 ml of air into his stomach and take a lateral supine view of his abdomen. In a pancreatic pseudocyst the stomach is displaced forwards, in an amoebic liver abscess, backwards.

THE DIFFERENTIAL DIAGNOSIS includes an amoebic abscess (31.12), hepatoma (32.26), an infected hydatid cyst (31.13), a hydronephrosis, pyloric stenosis (11.6), Burkitt's lymphoma (32.3), abdominal tuberculosis (29.5), gastric carcinoma (32.25), and an aortic aneurysm.

CYSTOGASTROSTOMY FOR A PANCREATIC PSEUDOCYST

WHEN TO OPERATE. Don't operate until 6 weeks after an attack of pancreatitis, by which time the cyst wall will be mature enough to take sutures. Once a pancreatic pseudocyst is palpable it rarely disappears spontaneously. Operate as soon as possible after 6 weeks; if you leave it too long it may bleed, rupture, become infected, or destroy much of his pancreas.

However, if after an attack of pancreatitis the cyst is enlarging rapidly, and rupture is imminent (rare), drain the cyst to the exterior with a large Malecot catheter—even before 6 weeks have elapsed. Don't try to do an anastomosis. Some surgeons consider external drainage disastrous.

RESUSCITATION. If he is dehydrated, wasted, or toxic, prepare him suitably. He may need parenteral fluids for a few days. Insert a nasogastric tube the previous evening, and wash out his stomach thoroughly.

INCISION. Make a median or paramedian incision (9.2).

Choose an area on the anterior wall of his stomach that is overlying the cyst. Use a knife to start a 6 cm incision in the long axis of his stomach between 2 Babcock forceps. Enlarge it with scissors. Clamp any briskly bleeding vessels, and retract the edges of the incision, so that you can inspect the posterior wall of his stomach. Suck it empty.

After opening his stomach, cautiously insert a needle connected to a syringe through its posterior wall into the mass (this is your last chance if you find it is an aortic aneurysm!). Expect to find a mildly opaque straw-coloured, or murky brownish fluid. If so, insert a small haemostat through the hole in his stomach into the cyst, and open it so as to enlarge the opening. Then insert forceps to enlarge the opening gently a bit more to 5 cm. Suck out the fluid, expect to aspirate up to 4 litres.

CAUTION ! Don't incise the cyst, it may bleed severely.

Lift up the cyst wall on sponge forceps and enlarge the incision until it is 6 cm long. There is no need to suture the stomach wall to the cyst, because they are already tightly stuck together. You will need to control brisk bleeding, so quickly oversew the opening all round with a continuous interlocking haemostatic stitch of 2/0 silk. Lock it (G, 4-7) because if one bite goes the whole must not collapse. Use silk, because pancreatic juice digests catgut. Reinforce the continuous suture with four interrupted 1/0 silk sutures at the ends and the middle of the elliptical incision.

When you are sure the posterior opening in the stomach is no longer bleeding, close the anterior one in two layers, the first a full-thickness haemostatic continuous layer of 3/0 chromic catgut sutures, and the second one a seromuscular Lembert layer of continuous catgut, silk, or cotton. Close his abdominal wall in the usual way.

POSTOPERATIVELY, 'suck and drip' him for 4 to 5 days (9.9, A 15.5), until his suture lines are well-healed, and he has bowel sounds. Then start a fluid diet. Postoperative complications are unusual.

13.11 The surgery of the spleen

One of the few things you can do to a spleen surgically is to remove it. The indications for doing so (apart from trauma, 66.6) must be good, because the spleen of a tropical patient is commonly large, and is so firmly stuck to his diaphragm that: (1) Exposing it is difficult. (2) If he has portal hypertension he is likely to bleed from the vascular adhesions that join it to his diaphragm, and through which high pressure venous blood will be escaping into his systemic circulation. A further danger is the increased risk of subsequent infection (see below).

A Splenic abscess occurs occasionally. It starts acutely, it may become chronic, and it shows up radiologically as a fluid level in an irregular space. The pus is sterile, and he may have sickle cell disease. Drain it, don't try to remove his spleen.

Torsion of the spleen occurs when it has an exceptionally long pedicle, and is one of the rare indications for splenectomy. You are unlikely to make the diagnosis before you operate.

The tropical splenomegaly syndrome, which is an immune response to recurrent attacks of malaria, is responsible for nearly all large spleens in malarious areas. It responds to long courses of antimalarials—pyrimethamine or chloroquine weekly, or paludrine daily. Don't remove such spleens. This is only indicated if hypersplenism is a complication.

Sickle-cell anaemia in children sometimes benefits from splenectomy. This is rarely necessary, it is not urgent, and it is dangerous in an SS patient. If you really think it is indicated refer him.

KASHY (20 years) complained of a swelling in his right iliac fossa. Ordinarily, it was painless but during attacks of 'fever' it became painful and tender. At laparotomy, his whole spleen was found to be in his right iliac fossa, but his splenic vessels crossed his abdomen to their normal position. His 'wandering spleen' was removed easily. LESSON Some rare conditions have easy solutions.

SPLENECTOMY OTHER THAN FOR TRAUMA

INDICATIONS. The strong indications are conditions in a patient's spleen itself, as: (1) Spontaneous rupture. (2) Torsion. (3) Wandering spleen. (4) Hydatid disease (31.13). (5) Tumours (very rare).

Splenectomy may also be indicated in: (6) Hypersplenism. (7) Idiopathic thrombocytopenia. (8) Myeloid leukaemia. (9) Congenital spherocytosis. (10) Sickle-cell disease (rarely). (11) As part of surgical operations which you are unlikely to do.

CAUTION ! (1) Don't operate lightly, your only definite indications for doing so are the first four. (2) If a patient's spleen is huge, think seriously about referring him: it may need a thoracoabdominal approach.

METHOD. Follow the method for the removal of the spleen for trauma in Section 66.6.

SPLENIC IMPLANTATION. Depending on the indications for splenectomy, consider the advisability of a splenic implant. Unless, there is: (1) an obvious accessory spleen, (2) malignant disease, or (3) hypersplenism. Keep some slices of spleen, say $5 \times 3 \times 0.5$ cm, and implant them under the peritoneum in the side wall of his abdomen, or in his anterior abdominal wall (66.6). Or, place some 1 cm cubes of spleen on his omentum. They will usually take, and will reduce the severity of attacks of malaria and the danger of septicaemia, especially that due to pneumococci. In a malarious area, he must take prophylaxis against malaria for the rest of his life.

14 Hernias

14.1 General principles

An external abdominal hernia is the protrusion of the contents of a patient's abdomen (some abdominal organ, part of his omentum, or his abdominal fat) through an abnormal opening in his abdominal wall. The swelling varies in size from time to time, but tends to become larger. He may learn to reduce it himself. The only way to repair it is to excise the sac, and usually to repair his abdominal wall also; so you will need to operate on most hernias.

If you or he can easily return the contents of his hernia to his abdomen, it is reducible, and you can operate at your convenience. A reducible hernia expands as he coughs, the gut in it may gurgle as you reduce it, and if it contains omentum, it feels doughy.

Several things can happen to a hernia:

(1) It may become irreducible. Coughing or straining may push the omentum, or a loop of gut, through the neck of the sac, after which oedema may prevent them slipping back. Sometimes, you may be able to reduce an otherwise irreducible *inguinal* hernia manually by taxis (14.6). This is dangerous in all other hernias. If you attempt it for an inguinal hernia, be sure to observe him carefully, and operate urgently if it fails, or if he develops signs of obstruction or strangulation.

(2) The gut in a hernia can obstruct, so that food and faeces cannot pass along it. Hernias are one of the commonest causes of intestinal obstruction (10.4). His symptoms depend on the level of the obstruction. If his upper small gut is obstructed, he has colicky central abdominal pain and vomits early. If his distal small gut is involved (common), he vomits late. If his large gut is obstructed (very uncommon in a hernia), he also vomits late.

(3) Blood may be unable to enter or leave the organs in a hernia, so that they strangulate. This is more likely to happen in a hernia with a narrow neck. Most strangulated hernias are therefore either inguinal or femoral, because these hernias have narrow necks.

(4) If strangulation persists for more than a few hours, the organs in a hernial sac become gangrenous. If this happpens to the omentum or Fallopian tube, the risk to a patient's life is small. But if his gut becomes gangrenous, the bacteria inside it can escape, so that peritonitis, cellulitis, or a fistula follow. If more than a little of the gut strangulates, it cannot propel its contents onwards normally, so it obstructs. Most strangulated gut is therefore obstructed also. The important exception is a Richter's hernia (see below).

The term 'incarceration' is a bad one and is not used here. The terms reducible, and irreducible, obstructed, and strangulated describe everything that can happen to a hernia.

When a hernia strangulates, it suddenly becomes painful, tense, and tender, and loses its cough impulse. Even so, you will often find it difficult to know if a hernia is merely irreducible and obstructed, or whether it is strangulated, because pain and constipation are present in both. Pain usually remains colicky until ileus and peritonitis develop, so the change from colicky to continuous pain is a bad sign. Occasionally, a strangulated hernia causes so little pain that a patient does not call your attention to it. Usually, however, his pain, his general condition, and the signs at the hernial site are reliable indicators.

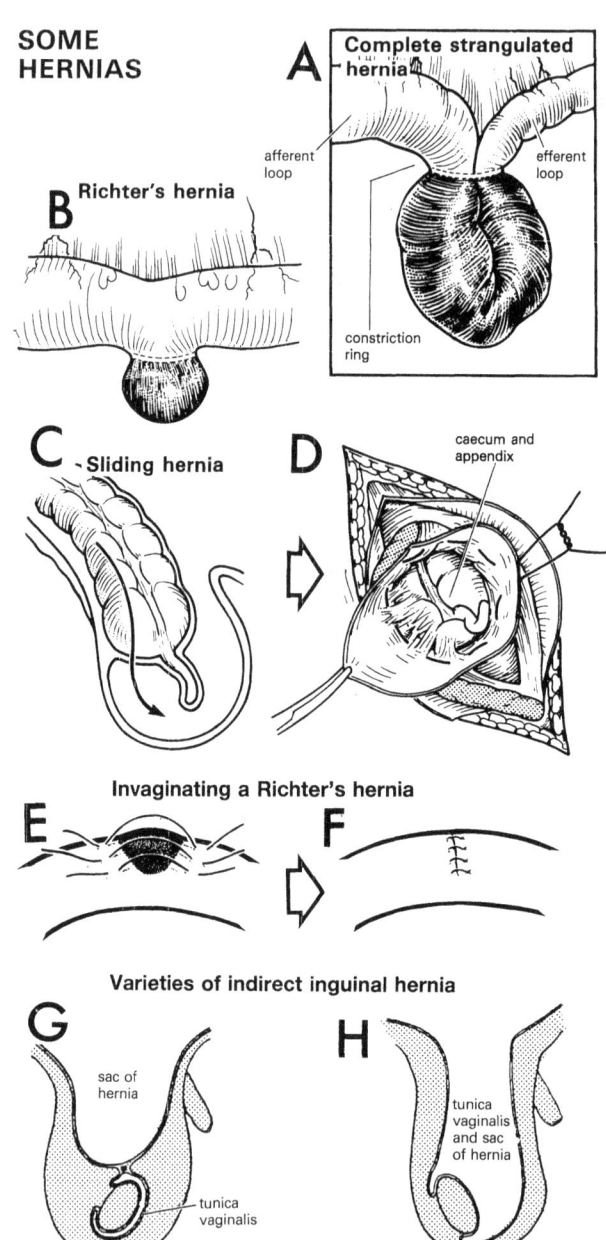

Fig. 14-1 THE PATHOLOGY OF SOME HERNIAS. A, a loop of gut has been caught in a hernial sac. The contents of the gut cannot enter or leave it, so it is obstructed. Blood cannot enter or leave it, so it is also strangulated. Note the afferent and the efferent loops, and the constriction ring. B, Richter's hernia. C, a sliding hernia. D, a sliding hernia opened. E, and F, invaginating a Richter's hernia is safe, if the gangrenous segment does not extend across more than half the circumference of the gut, and its margins are clearly healthy. G, an incomplete inguinal hernia; the sac of the hernia and the tunica vaginalis remain separate. H, a complete inguinal hernia; the sac and the tunica vaginalis are in continuity. E, and F, kindly contributed by Brian Hancock.

Unfortunately, you have no way of being certain what has been caught in a hernial sac, and you can never be sure that whatever has caught has not strangulated. Obstruction is ultimately as dangerous as strangulation, because, if you leave it, strangulation usually follows. So, *be safe,* and treat all painful, tense hernias as if they were strangulated.

If only part of the wall of a patient's gut is involved, he has a *Richter's hernia* (not very common). This is particularly dangerous because: (1) His gut may strangulate without being obstructed, so that he may not vomit, or be constipated. Instead, he may have diarrhoea until he finally develops peritonitis. (2) Occasionally, the local signs of strangulation may not be obvious.

If only his omentum strangulates, he has local abdominal pain, but his attacks of general abdominal pain may stop, and he may not vomit or be constipated. Gangrene is delayed, but after days or weeks his necrotic omentum may become infected, so that a local abscess or general peritonitis follows.

If the peritoneal lining of his hernial sac is incomplete, an abdominal organ (commonly his caecum), may slide into it, partly behind his peritoneum. When this happens he has a *sliding hernia.*

The common mistakes are: (1) To forget to examine the hernial sites of anyone with an abdominal pain or vomiting. (2) To forget the possibility of a Richter's hernia, which may confuse the diagnosis by causing diarrhoea instead of constipation. (3) To persist in using taxis (14.6) when an inguinal hernia should be operated on.

Here we only describe the more common hernias—indirect and direct inguinal hernias (14.2), femoral hernias (14.7), umbilical hernias in children (14.10) and adults (14.11), and epigastric (14.12) and incisional hernias (14.13). You will have many inguinal hernias to repair, so let them provide you with an unhurried opportunity to increase your surgical skills. If they are very common, it may be worth teaching an assistant to do them. This chapter partly follows from the sections on the acute abdomen (10.1), and on intestinal obstruction (10.3).

TREAT ALL PAINFUL HERNIAS AS IF THEY WERE STRANGULATED

14.2 Inguinal hernias

You will see many *indirect inguinal hernias* in which a patient's abdominal viscera slide down his inguinal canal, from his deep to his superficial inguinal ring, and sometimes down to his scrotum. The hernial sac is closely related to his spermatic cord, and lies in the same fascial planes. You will also see a few *direct inguinal hernias* which bulge through a weakness in the posterior wall of his inguinal canal. They do not present through his internal ring, they lack any special relation to his cord, and they do not have the coverings from his cord that an indirect hernia has. Because of the way they arise, *the spermatic cord lies behind an indirect hernia, and in front of a direct one.* Occasionally, a patient has a hernia of both kinds.

Indirect inguinal hernias are common in males. Women less often have indirect hernias, and seldom have direct ones. If the sac of an indirect inguinal hernia and the tunica vaginalis are continuous with one another, it is complete. If they remain separate, it is incomplete. Treat complete and incomplete hernias in the same way.

A patient with an indirect hernia has a bulge in his groin, sometimes with a dragging feeling. He may say that he felt something 'give' in his groin during severe exertion, just before his hernia appeared. He is almost sure to need an operation, which will remove the risk of strangulation, and possibly death. Don't advise him to wear a truss. He will find it expensive and difficult to get; he is unlikely to understand that his hernia must be completely reduced before he applies it, and he is likely to find it very uncomfortable in a hot climate. Instead, treat him like this:

(1) If he has an indirect hernia, find the sac, isolate it, tie it as high as you can, and then excise it (herniotomy). Having done this, restore his anatomy exactly, without damaging it. Finding the sac may be the most difficult step. Remember to: (a) tie it *high,* so as to obliterate the sac completely, and, (b) transfix the neck of the sac with a ligature, so that the tie does not slip off. In children under 10 this is all you need do. You can do it at the external ring of an infant, or at the internal ring of an adult or older child (14.5).

Having tied and excised the sac, you may need to repair his inguinal canal (herniorrhaphy), which you can do in several ways:

(2) If he has had an indirect hernia for some time, it may have enlarged his internal ring. If this is only moderately enlarged, you can narrow it with a few stitches, as in A, Fig. 14-5.

(3) If the posterior wall of his inguinal canal is weak, you can reinforce it by suturing his conjoint tendon (which is formed by the fibres of his internal oblique and transversus) to his inguinal ligament *behind* his cord. This is a modified Bassini repair. Having done this, you then suture his external oblique aponeurosis in front of his cord.

(4) If, when you are about to do a Bassini repair, you think that there is going to be unacceptable tension in the suture line, you can relieve it by first making a long incision in the fused aponeurosis of his internal oblique and transversus muscles superiorly, as in Fig. 14-7. This will allow part of the aponeurosis to slide down, and will relieve the tension on the suture line considerably. This is often known as a 'Tanner slide'.

(5) If he has a very large indirect inguinal hernia, or a recurrent direct one, and you cannot refer him, you can take a reef in the posterior wall of his inguinal canal and darn it, as in Fig. 14-14.

Direct inguinal hernias are of two kinds: (1) Ordinary direct hernias, which are rare in Africa and seldom strangulate (14-8). They may cause no symptoms, and remain the same size for long periods, so that they may not need surgery. (2) A special variety of direct hernia in which the patient has a narrow defect in his conjoint tendon, or in his transversalis fascia (14-9). In Europe this kind of direct hernia is called a Gill–Ogilvie hernia, and is rare. But it is common in the Busoga area of Uganda, and in some other parts of Africa (including Ghana, where it is not uncommonly seen in women), so that it is sometimes known as the Busoga hernia. Gut readily strangulates through the Busoga type of direct hernia. The neck of the sac is small, so that when strangulation occurs, it often does so in only part of the circumference of the gut, to cause a Richter's hernia (14-1).

You can usually repair direct hernias by much the same methods as indirect ones, unless they are very large. But there are differences, and a direct hernia does have problems: (1) The sac may have no obvious neck (unless it is a Busoga hernia), so that you cannot excise it; instead, you have to tuck it in, as in Fig. 14-8. (2) The weak area in a direct hernia is ill-defined, and tends to involve all or most of the posterior wall of the inguinal canal. You can strengthen this by suturing the external oblique aponeurosis *behind the cord* —something you should never do with an indirect hernia. (3) A patient with a direct hernia is likely to be older with poor tissues, and perhaps prostatism, a stricture, dyspnoea, a cough, or constipation, all of which will stress his hernia repair. (4) His bladder may enter the hernia, and is easily injured. (5) A direct hernia is twice as likely to recur as an indirect one.

Recurrence is a problem with any inguinal hernia, especially if the patient is old and has weak muscles. Preventing recurrence needs care and skill, but curing a hernia that has recurred needs even more skill. Recurrence is less likely if you: (1) Repair a hernia early, before it has grown too large. Alas, many patients in the developing world do not present until their hernias are already huge. (2) Tie off the neck of the sac close to the inguinal ring. If you leave the neck, a hernia is much more likely to recur. (3) Narrow a patient's dilated internal ring by bringing the edges of his transversalis fascia together (A, 14-5). (4) Look to see if he has a coexisting direct hernia when he has an indirect one,

SOME INGUINAL ANATOMY

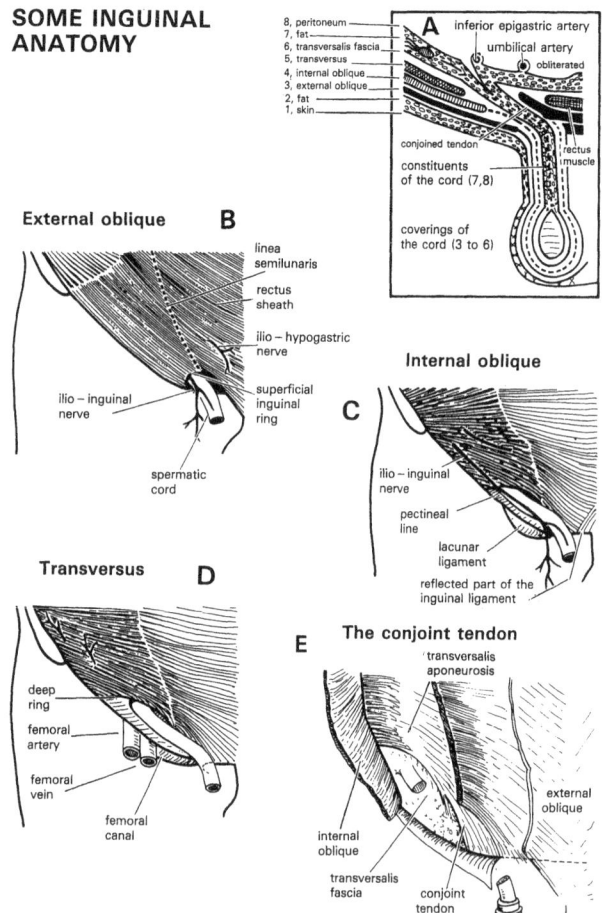

Fig. 14-2 SOME INGUINAL ANATOMY. A, shows the coverings of a patient's spermatic cord, which also become the coverings of an inguinal hernia. B, his external oblique muscle. C, his internal oblique. D, his transversus abdominis. E, his conjoint tendon is formed from the aponeurosis of his internal oblique and transversus muscles as they arch over his spermatic cord.

1, his skin. 2, his fat. 3, his external oblique aponeurosis. 4, his internal oblique aponeurosis. 5, his transversus muscle. 6, his transversalis fascia. 7, his extraperitoneal fatty tissue. 8, his peritoneum. *After "Grant's Method of Anatomy", (9th edn 1975 edited by JV Basmajian), p.183 Figs. 217 and 219. Williams and Wilkins, with kind permission.*

or vice versa. (5) Put the sutures in a Bassini repair through the aponeurosis of his internal oblique, rather than through its muscle. (6) Do a Tanner slide when the sutures of a Bassini repair would otherwise be too tight. (7) Try to control any factors which might increase his intra-abdominal pressure for at least three months after the repair.

ANATOMY. The internal inguinal ring is a gap in the transversalis fascia, about a finger's breadth above the mid-inguinal point, midway between a patient's anterior superior iliac spine and his pubic tubercle. His external inguinal ring is an opening in his external oblique aponeurosis just above and lateral to his pubic spine. This aponeurosis forms the anterior wall of his inguinal canal: its posterior wall is formed by his transversalis fascia. As his cord passes down his inguinal canal, the muscle and tendon of his internal oblique and transversus arch over it, to form his conjoined tendon.

Divide the inguinal canal into thirds: in the lateral third, the internal oblique forms its lateral wall; in the middle third it forms its roof; in the medial third (as part of the conjoined tendon), it forms its floor. A hernia deforms this normal anatomy, but you can always see that this was its original state.

The inferior epigastric vessels leave the femoral artery and vein, and run vertically on the medial side of the internal inguinal ring. Direct hernias bulge medial to them, through the posterior wall of the inguinal canal, while indirect ones pass lateral to them through the internal ring.

The inguinal ligament is attached to the antero-superior iliac spine laterally, and to the pubic tubercle medially. At its medial end a small curved ligament, called the *lacunar ligament*, joins it to the pubic bone. The lacunar ligament forms the medial boundary of the femoral canal. A few of its fibres continue laterally along the upper border of the pubic bone to form the *pectineal ligament* (Cooper's ligament). You can pass sutures through this when you repair a femoral hernia.

In the infant the two inguinal rings overlie one another; in the adult they separate. In many West African people the inguinal canal remains short into adult life, with the two rings widened and almost on top of one another. Inside the inguinal canal you will meet two very constant vessels, but you can easily control bleeding from them: they are the cremasteric artery, and the pubic branch of the inferior epigastric artery.

TREAT INGUINAL HERNIAS WHILE THEY ARE STILL SMALL

UNSTRANGULATED INGUINAL HERNIAS
IN ADULTS

DIAGNOSIS. Examine the patient lying down. If he has no swelling, his hernia is reducible. Ask him to stand, cough or strain to make the bulge return. Insert your little finger into his external ring; direct it laterally, and ask him to cough. You will feel 'a cough impulse'.

CAUTION! Sometimes in a muscular young man, when the neck of the sac is narrow, there is no cough impulse, even in an uncomplicated hernia.

Does the hernia extend into his scrotum? Are both his testes present? Testicular atrophy is one of the complications of herniorrhaphy, and if one testis is already atrophic, you will have to be particularly careful. In children, inguinal hernias are occasionally associated with cryptorchidism.

If a hernia is irreducible, can you reduce it by manipulation?

If he has a history of a lump that comes and goes, but he has no physical signs, ask him to stand, strain, and cough. This will often demonstrate it. If it does not appear, don't operate. See him again later, and wait until you have actually seen it.

THE DIFFERENTIAL DIAGNOSIS usually causes few problems.

Suggesting a hydrocele—a translucent swelling with no cough impulse. A hernia in a young child also transmits light, but not one in an adult. A hydrocele is the main differential diagnosis. If, with your finger and thumb, you can get above the swelling, no matter how large it is, it cannot be an inguinal hernia, because it cannot have come down through his external inguinal ring.

Suggesting a femoral hernia—the bulge is more globular, is below the inguinal ligament, and is just medial to the femoral vessels.

Suggesting inguinal lymphadenitis—the swelling is constant, and below the inguinal ligament. Distinguishing adenitis from a strangulated femoral hernia may be difficult.

Suggesting funiculitis—a thickened oedematous spermatic cord, with no cough impulse (31.6).

Suggesting torsion of the testis, epididymis, or both—there is no normal testis in addition to the hernial sac.

DIRECT OR INDIRECT? You can usually make a firm preoperative diagnosis; but if you cannot it is unimportant. In a direct hernia: (1) The patient is older, (2) the bulge is globular rather than elongated, (3) the sac does not extend into the scrotum, (4) your finger, when you put it into the external ring, feels as if it is going straight into the patient's peritoneal cavity, (5) irreducibility and strangulation are almost unknown (the Busoga type of direct hernia is an exception to some of these rules).

Lie the patient supine and reduce the hernia completely. Press your thumb firmly over his deep inguinal ring. Ask him to stand up and cough. If his hernia is controlled, it is indirect, otherwise it is direct.

THE MANAGEMENT OF AN INGUINAL HERNIA

Always operate on an indirect hernia, unless a patient is very old and frail. You can use local anaesthesia, so his poor general condition is not a bar to operation. If he has a simple hernia, you can treat him as an outpatient.

AN INDIRECT INGUINAL HERNIA

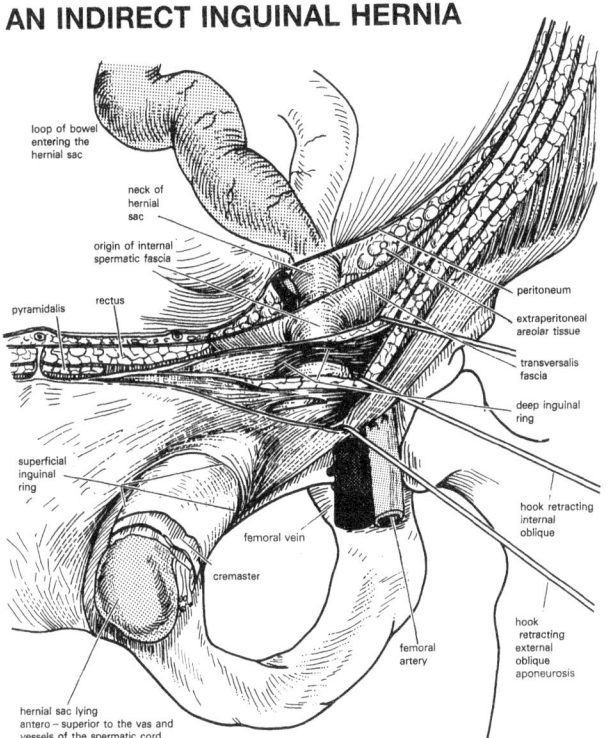

Fig. 14-3 AN INDIRECT INGUINAL HERNIA, showing the patient's hernial sac passing through his internal and external rings, and lying anterosuperior to the vessels of his cord. The narrow part is the neck and the distal part is the fundus. The sac takes a covering from each layer of his abdominal wall. *Adapted from a drawing by Frank Netter, with the kind permission of CIBA-GEIGY Ltd, Basle (Switzerland).*

If he is an infant only a few days old, do nothing until he is at least 3 months old. Strangulation is unlikely in infancy, because the neck of the canal is fairly wide and the canal is so short. Then, dissect out the sac and transfix and divide its neck distally at his *external* ring. Excise the sac without opening up the canal. See Section 14.5.

If he is a child under 5, open up his canal, dissect out the sac, define its neck well, transfix it, tie it at his *internal* ring, and excise it.

CAUTION ! (1) In a child, in particular, dissect carefully to ensure that his cord, which lies posteriorly, but close to the sac, is not injured. (2) Simple herniotomy is all that he needs, if a hernial sac is his only abnormality. This is only so in infants and children. In all other patients you will have to narrow the internal ring. In some of them you will also have to do a Bassini repair, if necessary with a Tanner slide.

If he is a teenager, or young adult with a small indirect hernia and good tissues, excise the sac and narrow his internal ring.

If he is an older patient, do a Bassini repair, with a Tanner slide when necessary.

If he is an old man and has a difficult recurrent hernia, you can remove his testis (with his permission, which is seldom given) and close his inguinal canal completely, with a modified Bassini repair, and a Tanner slide if necessary.

If he has the standard type of direct hernia, which is a bulge in the posterior wall of his inguinal canal, do a Bassini repair, with a Tanner slide.

If he has a Busoga hernia, excise the sac and close the defect.

If the patient is a woman, excise her round ligament with the sac, and anchor them to her abdominal wall.

If he has a small recurrent indirect hernia, treat it as if it were a primary hernia.

If he has a very large primary hernia, or any but the smallest recurrent one, and you cannot refer him, you may have to operate as described in Section 14.4, but you will need skill. In a recurrent hernia the tissues may be tough and fibrotic, so that you will find monofilament or wire helpful in repairing them.

If his inguinal hernia is irreducible, but is not yet strangulated (he has no generalized abdominal pain or vomiting), you may be able to treat him conservatively by taxis (14.6).

If his hernia has strangulated, see Section 14.6.

SIMPLE HERNIOTOMY

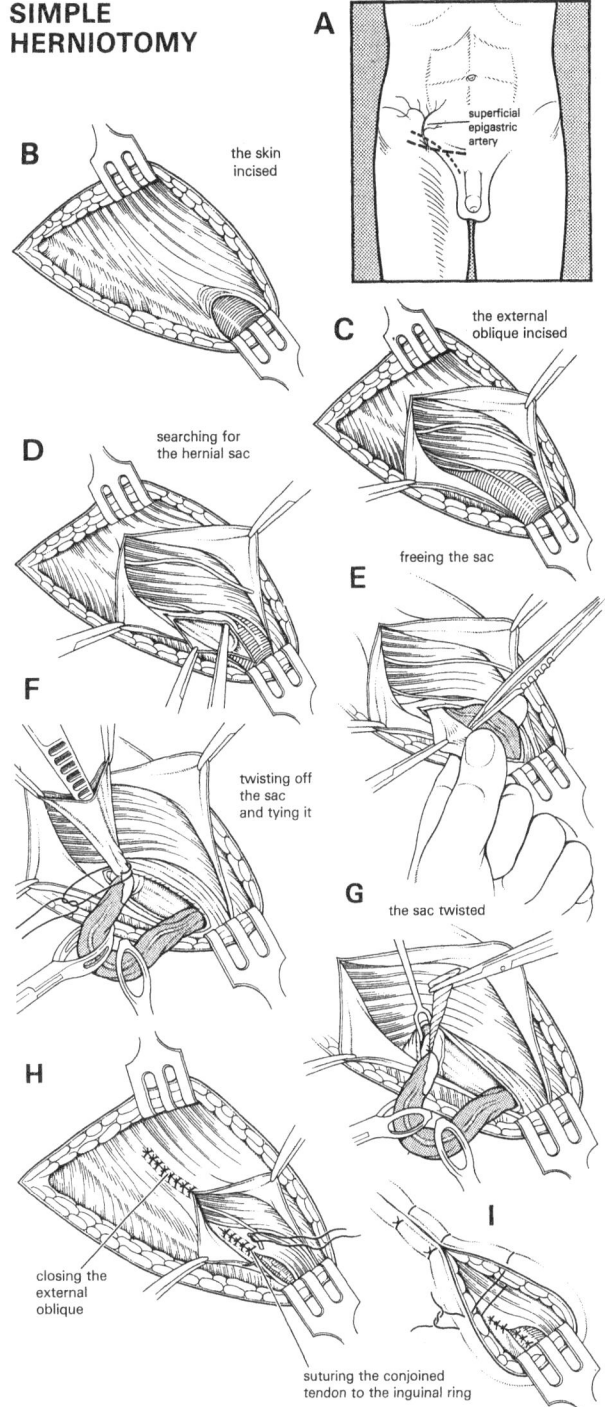

Fig. 14-4 SIMPLE HERNIOTOMY. The text does not follow this figure exactly, and does some steps in a different order. A, the site of the incision. B, the patient's skin has been incised and the aponeurosis of his external oblique is exposed. C, his external oblique aponeurosis has been opened, from his external ring laterally, to expose his internal oblique with his ilio-hypogastric and ilio-inguinal nerves. D, his cord is being opened to search for the sac. E, his cord is being freed. F, the sac of his hernia is being opened. G, the sac is being twisted off. If a Bassini repair is needed, it would be done at this point. H, his external oblique aponeurosis is being sutured. I, the operation complete. *After Maingot R, 'Abdominal Operations', (4th edn 1961), pp. 874 and 876, Figs. 1 and 3. HK Lewis, with kind permission.*

A REDUCIBLE INGUINAL HERNIA IN AN ADULT

PREPARATION. If a patient suffers from a chronic cough, treat him for a few days before the operation, in the hope of reducing the risk of recurrence. Use postural drainage, chest physiotherapy, and antibiotics as necessary. If he has a stricture, treat that first.

ANAESTHESIA. (1) Local infiltration anaesthesia (A 6.12) is excellent for ordinary small and medium hernias. It will show up the tissue planes beautifully. It is also useful if he is is old and feeble. It is less satisfactory if his hernia is strangulated. Don't use it in children, or if he is tense and anxious. (2) Epidural or subarachnoid (spinal) anaesthesia is excellent for all sizes of hernia, because relaxation is so good. (3) Intravenous ketamine with relaxants (A 8.1). (3) General anaesthesia, preferably with relaxants.

If you use local anaesthesia you can operate on all inguinal hernias as day cases, except for those which are complicated by an obstructive uropathy. If your surgical wards are overcrowded, this will relieve the pressure on them.

EQUIPMENT. A minor instrument set (14.2), plus McIndoe's dissecting scissors, sterile tape or a catheter to place round the cord, and curved needles and monofilament for the repair.

CAUTION ! Don't use silk; if it becomes infected, it will cause sinuses, and you will later have to pick out every piece.

PREPARATION. On the side of the operation, prepare his skin from his umbilicus to a third of the way down his thigh and across to the midline. Drape his groin, and use towel clips to mark two critical anatomical landmarks: (1) His anterosuperior iliac spine, and (2) the midline over the superior border of his symphysis pubis. Between them lies his inguinal ligament. With towel clips on these markers, you are less likely to cut too high or too low.

INCISION. Find his mid-inguinal point by palpating his femoral artery, where it pases under his inguinal ligament, midway between his anterior superior iliac spine, and his pubic tubercle. Make the incision in a skin crease, or parallel to and 1 to 2 cm above his inguinal ligament, from just lateral to his mid-inguinal point to just medial to his pubic tubercle. For small hernias it can be a little shorter, and for large ones a little longer (A, Fig. 14-4). Find and tie securely his superficial epigastric and superficial external pudendal vessels. If they bleed later, he may get a postoperative haematoma.

Apply straight haemostats to all bleeding points, and tie them. Cut through the two layers of his superficial fascia down to the shining fibres of his external oblique aponeurosis (B).

Clear the upper skin flap from the underlying aponeurosis by swab dissection, to expose a wide area of aponeurosis above his internal ring.

Free the lower flap in a similar way to display his inguinal ligament, and its attachment to his pubic spine. Display his external ring, and insert a self-retaining retractor (not shown).

OPENING THE INGUINAL CANAL. Incise the aponeurosis of his external oblique in the length of its fibres over his inguinal canal, and about 1.5 cm above his inguinal ligament (C).

Open his inguinal canal right to its lateral end, starting at his external ring. Free the upper edge of his external oblique aponeurosis, including its extension as his cremaster muscle, from his underlying internal oblique, as far as the outer border of his rectus sheath.

Clip the upper border of his external oblique aponeurosis with straight haemostats. If you do this, you will not mistake them later for the curved haemostats you have used to control bleeding.

Use gauze or sharp dissection to free and clean the lower flap of his external oblique, as far as his inguinal ligament inferiorly, which is the lower border of this aponeurosis. You will now see his internal oblique muscle, leading medially to his conjoined tendon.

Look for his ilio-hypogastric nerve, and, a little below it, for his ilio-inguinal nerve on the surface of his cremaster, in front of and slightly below his spermatic cord. Mobilize his ilio-inguinal nerve, and retract it behind the haemostat on the lower flap. Try not to crush or overstretch either of these nerves, or include them in a stitch, because you may cause persistent pain.

Pick up his cremaster covering the sac and and cautiously split it with the points of scissors. You should see the white areolar tissue around the hernial sac and his spermatic cord. Free the cut edges of the cremaster, and separate them from structures of his cord.

Find his cord, dissect it out enough to put a sling or rubber catheter round it (kinder than the forceps shown in the figure), and retract it (F).

CAUTION ! Don't try blunt dissection high up where landmarks are hard to distinguish, especially if there is much extraperitoneal fat.

At this point you may be able to confirm which kind of hernia he has (direct or indirect), by observing the relationship of his inferior epigastric vessels to the neck of the sac. Examine the posterior wall of his inguinal canal for signs of a direct hernia. Examine also his conjoint tendon, where the Busoga type of direct hernia occurs.

If you have difficulty outlining a hernial sac, open it and insert the index finger of your left hand. Use this to help you define the rest of the sac for further dissection.

In a DIRECT HERNIA, the posterior wall of his inguinal canal is weak and flabby and provides little resistance to your fingers as you press. There usually an obvious bulge medial to his epigastric vessels. His cord almost always lies anterior to it. If its medial wall feels thick and fleshy, suspect that there is bladder in it (see below). If he has a direct hernia, go to near the end of this section.

In a BUSOGA HERNIA, the opening may be quite narrow, and is in the transversus or the conjoined tendon. Go to the end of this section.

In an INDIRECT HERNIA the neck of the sac is lateral to his epigastric vessels, and is intimately attached to his cord which is almost always posterior. You will see the white wall of the sac lying close to and in front of his spermatic cord, which contains his vas and his spermatic vessels. Continue as described immediately below.

CAUTION ! Make quite sure that he has not got the unusual combination of a direct *and* an indirect hernia (saddle hernia). A few minutes looking for an indirect sac is time well spent.

INDIRECT HERNIA

FINDING AND FREEING THE SAC. If you are using local or subarachnoid (spinal) anaesthesia, ask him to cough. The sac will swell slightly. It may be easy to find, or difficult if fibrous tissue has formed round it. Catch an edge with forceps, and retract it upwards and outwards (F). Dissect the sac carefully, hold it with a haemostat, and keep close to its edge. Hold it at extra places as necessary. Usually, sharp dissection with a knife or scissors is better than using gauze, unless the tissues are very loose, because there will be less oozing. Free the sac from strands of his cremaster at their origin from his inferior oblique. If you don't do this, they may obscure his internal ring. Separate it from his cord with non-toothed forceps by working transversely to its long axis, using a mixture of sharp knife and gauze-on-finger dissection (E). If there is extraperitoneal fat round the sac, consider removing it.

CAUTION ! Be sure to find and define clearly: (1) his vas, (2) his spermatic artery, and (3) his spermatic veins (there is usually more than one). All these may separate during dissection. Avoid injuring them by keeping close to the sac.

If the sac descends into his scrotum, pull it into the wound, and dissect it free from the white tissue of his scrotal wall.

If, however, this is too difficult, divide the sac (but not his cord !) and drop the distal part back into his scrotum, while you continue to dissect out the proximal part.

Dissect the sac free from areolar tissue right down to its neck. You may see his inferior epigastric vessels running medial to its neck. Avoid them. If necessary, tie any small branches.

You will know that you have dissected it up as far as you should when you find: (1) His deep epigastric artery and veins on its medial side. (2) The constriction that forms its neck. (3) A collar of extraperitoneal fat around it. (4) Its wider junction with his peritoneal cavity. You can see this when you pull it.

OPENING THE SAC. Open its fundus (if you have not already done so) between haemostats, as if you were opening his peritoneal cavity. Pass a finger or forceps (F) through its neck into his peritoneal cavity to make sure it is empty, and no bowel or omentum remains inside. It has a moist shiny inside.

CAUTION! (1) If his hernia is irreducible, you can very easily open his gut as you open the sac. (2) If one side of the neck is thick, there may be bladder or gut in its wall. This is more likely in a sliding hernia, either direct or indirect, see under 'Difficulties' below.

CLOSING THE SAC. Twist its neck until the turns reach his internal ring (G). If there is any gut or omentum in the sac, this will force it back into his peritoneal cavity. Transfix the neck as far proximally as you can. Tie it twice with monofilament or chromic catgut, leave the ends of the knot long, and hold them with haemostats.

If the neck of the sac is wide, place haemostats round it from outside, divide it distally, and close it with a continuous suture, as if you were closing the peritoneum of an abdominal wound.

Divide the stump 1 cm distal to the ligature. Examine it. When you are sure that the ligature is not going to slip, or ooze, cut its threads. If it is loose, apply another ligature or a continuous suture. When you release the stump, it will quickly disappear from view under the arched fibres of his internal oblique.

CAUTION! (1) If you tie the sac distal to his deep ring it is more likely to recur. (2) Don't include his vas in your ligature. (3) If you divide the sac, don't tie it off and drop the distal part back into his scrotum. If you do, he may develop a hydrocele. Leave it open. (4) Try to avoid damaging small vessels; good haemostasis is important to prevent a haematoma forming.

TWO METHODS FOR HERNIAS

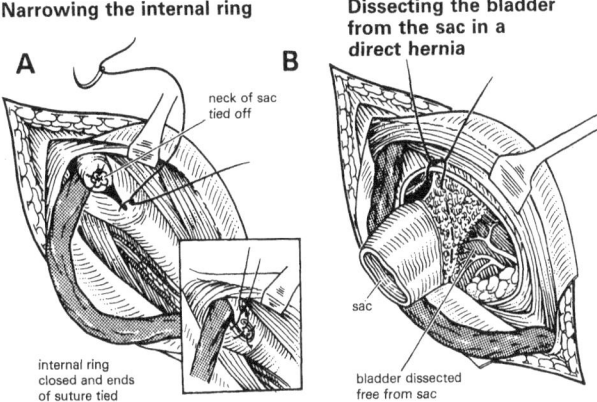

Fig. 14-5 TWO METHODS FOR HERNIAS. A, narrowing the internal ring. In an adult a normal internal ring just admits the tip of your little finger. If it is larger than this, "snug it up". Start medially and work laterally. Tie the two ends of the suture together to prevent the inner end of the suture line from pouching forwards. B, the bladder occasionally bulges forwards extraperitoneally on the inner side of a direct hernia, and you can easily injure it. *From Rob C and Smith R, "Operative Surgery", (2nd edn 1969), Vol. 4, Part 1, p. 223 Fig. 8 and p. 229 Fig. 25. Butterworths, with kind permission.*

NARROWING THE INTERNAL RING. Feel the size of the patient's internal ring. In an adult, a normal internal ring just admits the last joint of your little finger. If it is wider than this, it is dilated. If it is only a little dilated, narrowing it will be enough.

If his internal ring is only moderately dilated, stitch it with monofilament or catgut, starting medially, and stitching laterally, until the ring fits snugly around his cord. Tie the inner and outer ends of the suture together to prevent the inner end of the suture line pouching forwards.

CAUTION! (1) If you don't narrow his internal ring when you should, his hernia will be more likely to recur. (2) Don't constrict his internal ring too much, or his testis may atrophy.

If necessary, proceed with a Bassini repair, as described below.

IN A WOMAN an inguinal hernia is probably caused by a congenital sac which is firmly stuck to her round ligament. This is narrower and less vascular than a man's spermatic cord. Her inguinal canal is smaller and you will hardly see anything to represent cremaster. Her hernial sac can extend only to her labia majora. Proceed as above until you come to reflect her cremaster from her round ligament. Pick up the sac, her round ligament, and the nearby vessels. Use sharp dissection to free them from her labium, or blunt dissection if her tissues are very loose.

Clamp, tie, and divide her round ligament close to its insertion. Then clean it and the sac as far as her internal ring. Open the sac, inspect its inside, and then probe it to make sure it is empty.

Grasp the sac, her round ligament and their vessels. Crush, transfix, and tie them, leaving the ends of the ligature long. Then divide these tissues 1 cm beyond the ligature. Use the long ends of the ligature to anchor the stump to the aponeurosis of her external ring above and lateral to her internal ring.

Obliterate her now empty inguinal canal with a few sutures joining her conjoined tendon and her transversalis fascia to her inguinal ligament. You will probably be able to make a Bassini repair without any tension on the suture line, so that she is unlikely to need a Tanner slide. Close her internal inguinal ring completely. There is nothing to strangulate.

If her muscles are weak, draw the edges of her external oblique aponeurosis together with interrupted monofilament sutures.

MODIFIED BASSINI REPAIR FOR INGUINAL HERNIAS

INDICATIONS. A weak internal ring, or a weak posterior wall to the patient's inguinal canal.

If a Bassini repair looks as if it is going to be unacceptably tight, you can do a Tanner slide before or afterwards.

A BASSINI REPAIR

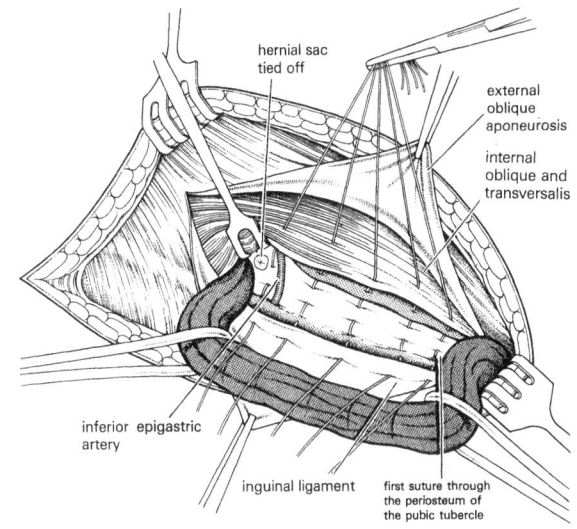

Fig. 14-6 A BASSINI REPAIR. Interrupted sutures are being used to join the arching fibres of a patient's internal oblique and conjoined tendon to his inguinal ligament. The first suture goes through the periosteum of his pubic tubercle. *After Maingot R "Abdominal Operations", (4th edn 1961) p.879 Fig. 4 drawing 1. HK Lewis, with kind permission.*

REPAIR. Release the curved haemostats that you originally inserted on the lower flap of the patient's external oblique, and replace them *in front of his cord* while you repair the posterior wall of his inguinal canal. This will keep his cord out of the way while you proceed with the repair. Alternatively, hold his cord with gentle traction using the slings you have placed round it, as in Fig. 14-6.

Clean away all the areolar tissue from the upper shelving surface of his inguinal ligament. Retract his fleshy arching internal oblique muscle upwards, to expose the aponeurotic part of his transversus muscle, and his conjoined tendon. Use this layer for reconstruction, not the overlying muscle layer. You may have to use muscle if the aponeurosis is poorly developed.

Use 1/0 or 2/0 monofilament, or steel, on a round-bodied half-circle needle, to apply interrupted simple or mattress sutures 8 mm apart, from the arching fibres of his conjoined tendon above, to the inner shelving margin of his inguinal ligament below. Put a narrow retractor at the medial end of the wound, and take the first bite through the periosteum over his pubic tubercle. Proceed from the medial side laterally taking substantial (6-8 mm) bites of the aponeurosis. To avoid splitting his inguinal ligament, take bites which are alternately large and small. Space the sutures evenly, and don't go too deep, or you may puncture his underlying femoral vessels. Hold the interrupted sutures in haemostats, until you have inserted them all, and then tie them all together. Proceed from medial to lateral.

CAUTION ! (1) Beware of his femoral artery, which lies just behind his inguinal ligament under his mid-inguinal point. *Injuring the femoral vessels is the most serious potential complication of hernia surgery* (see below). (2) Don't strangulate his cord with your last suture. Make sure you can still insert the tip of your forceps through his internal ring, alongside his emerging cord. (3) If you have had to use tension to bring the structures together, do a Tanner slide. (4) Use non-absorbable sutures only.

If you are not going to do a Tanner slide, close the wound as described below.

THE TANNER SLIDE FOR INGUINAL HERNIAS

INDICATIONS. (1) A Bassini repair that requires unacceptably tight sutures. (2) Large direct inguinal hernias. (3) Old indirect inguinal hernias, where the internal ring is so large, and the inferior epigastric vessels displaced so far medially, that they resemble a direct hernia. (2) Recurrent and strangulated hernias, provided there is no infected or gangrenous gut.

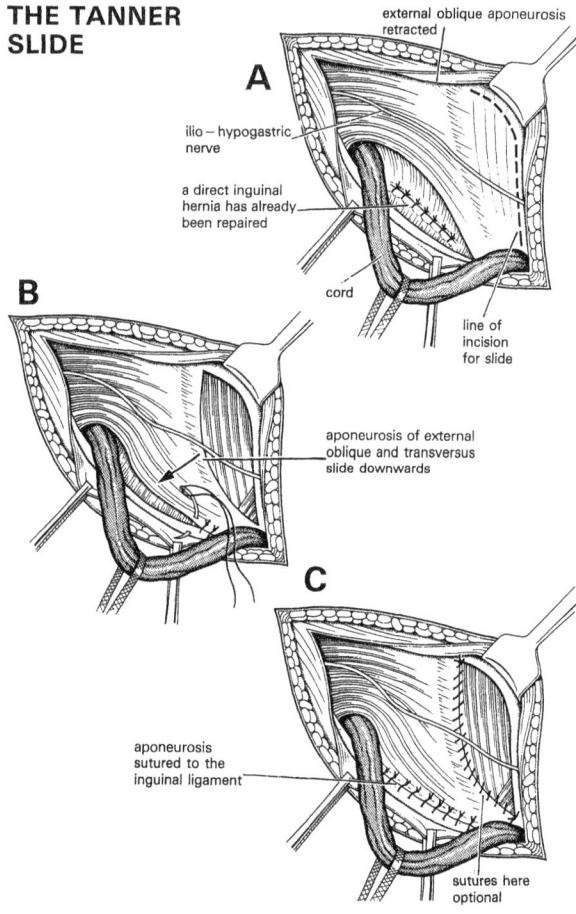

Fig 14-7 THE TANNER SLIDE for larger inguinal hernias. A, retract the patient's external oblique aponeurosis and excise the sac. B, incise the fused aponeurosis of his internal oblique and transversus, slide it downwards, and suture his conjoined tendon to his inguinal ligament (Bassini repair). C, the slide complete. The lateral cut edge of his aponeurosis has been sutured to his rectus muscle. This is an optional step. *After Tanner.*

CONTRAINDICATIONS. (1) A patient in whom it is unnecessary: (a) an indirect inguinal hernia, where the inguinal ring is not dilated. Or, (b) where you can narrow it with a few sutures. Or, (c) a Busoga hernia. (2) A hernia containing infected or gangrenous gut. If you find a hernia like this, postpone repair to a second operation, or do a Bassini repair if this requires little extra dissection. (3) Damage to the lower rectus sheath and muscle, by a previous operation, for example prostatectomy.

Extreme age, feebleness, or a very large hernia are *not* contraindications to a Tanner slide.

METHOD. In doing a Bassini repair as described above, you found that you needed unacceptably tight sutures to complete it. If so, gently retract the superomedial leaf of the patient's external oblique aponeurosis. You may have to use sharp and blunt dissection to undermine his skin and superficial fascia a bit more first. Separate his external oblique from his underlying internal oblique, and burrow under it until you have exposed his rectus sheath, as in A, Fig. 14-7.

Continue to dissect medially using blunt dissection, and a few careful strokes of the scalpel. Dissection is easy, because at this point his external oblique is only loosely attached to the fused aponeurosis of the two muscles under it.

CAUTION ! Try not to damage his ilio-hypogastric nerve, which either: (1) leaves his internal oblique muscle lateral to his rectus sheath and runs medially to perforate his external oblique. Or, (2) runs straight forwards through his anterior rectus sheath.

Continue to separate the two layers medially to the junction of the inner one-third with the lateral two-thirds of his rectus muscle. Extend your separation to below his pubic crest inferiorly, and a hand's breadth above it superiorly.

Incise the fused aponeurosis of his internal oblique and transversus (B). Make a curved incision starting at or below his pubic crest as far medially as you can. Carry the incision upwards and then laterally to end a hand's breadth above his pubis, and 2 cm medial to the lateral edge of his rectus muscle. Again, try not to damage his ilio-hypogastric nerve.

As soon as you have made this incision, its lateral edge will start to slide downwards, especially if he strains. Help this sliding movement by catching the lateral part of his rectus sheath with Allis forceps, or a retractor, and gently pull it downwards and laterally.

The insertion of pyramidalis to the sheath will prevent you completing the slide. Free this from his rectus sheath by sharp dissection.

Continue the slide until his pyramidalis and his rectus muscles are widely exposed. Provided you have not cut too near to the lateral edge of his rectus muscle, its edge will not be exposed by the incision, even when he strains. Even if it is exposed, this is not important.

An optional step is to use fine sutures of continuous monofilament to join the lateral cut edge of the aponeurosis to his adjacent rectus and pyramidalis muscles, taking wide, deep bites of these muscles (C). This will prevent overslide. This can happen if you have taken the incision too close to the lateral edge of his rectus muscle.

ORDINARY DIRECT HERNIAS

Don't try to open, tie, or excise the sac of a direct hernia, unless it is very obvious. Push it inwards with a sponge dissector, and while you keep it pushed in, bring its edges together with interrupted monofilament sutures. Apply 2 or 3 layers of sutures to close the defect. If these sutures are tight, do a Tanner slide.

It may help to bring the layers of the patient's external oblique aponeurosis together *behind* his cord (an anterior transposition of the cord), to strengthen his inguinal region. If it is convenient, overlap the flaps, suture the upper one to his inguinal ligament, and bring the lower one on top of it so as to overlap it about 2 cm.

If his hernia is very large, see sections 14.3 and 14.4.

BUSOGA DIRECT HERNIAS (Gill-Ogilvie hernias)

You will see a tight bulge of gut coming through a patient's conjoint tendon medially.

Hold the bulging gut lightly with Babcock forceps to prevent it slipping back (A, Fig. 14-9). Cut the edge of the tight ring in the conjoint tendon with a scalpel cautiously (B). Dilate it with

A LARGE DIRECT HERNIA

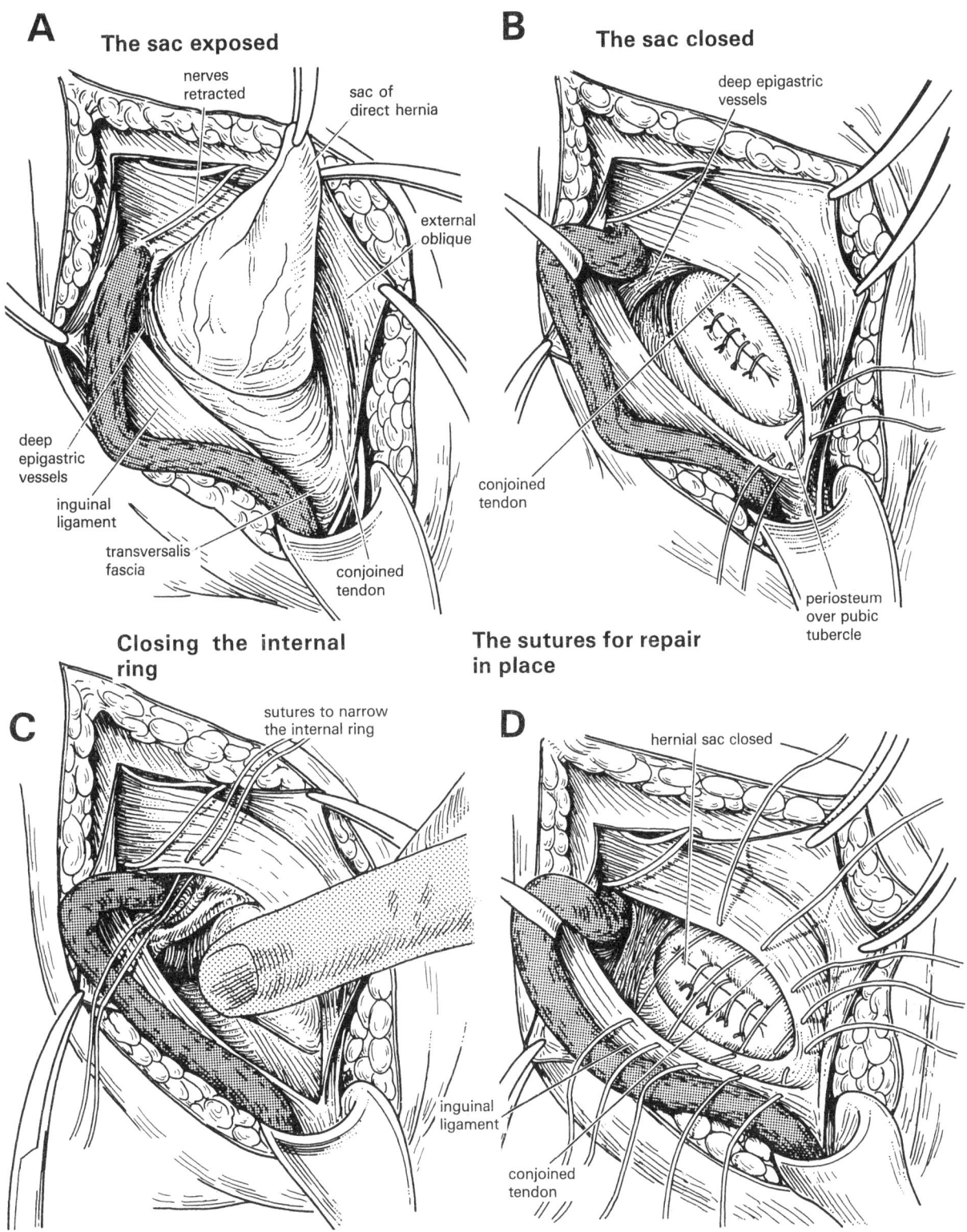

Fig. 14-8 REPAIRING A LARGE DIRECT HERNIA of the ordinary kind.

A, a large direct hernia protrudes through most of the posterior wall of the patient's inguinal canal.

B, having reduced the large direct hernia in A, close the orifice in his transversalis fascia with interrupted sutures. Insert the first suture in his conjoint tendon.

C, close his internal ring snugly round his cord, taking care not to compress it. To do this place interrupted sutures in his internal oblique and transversalis.

D, insert more sutures. Put the three medial ones through his conjoined tendon, his pectineal ligament, and his inguinal ligament. Put those that go lateral to his femoral vessels through his conjoined tendon and his inguinal ligament only. This is the Estes rather than the Bassini procedure, and shows the sutures going through the pectineal ligament, which is rather more difficult than putting them through the inguinal ligament only, and is optional. *After Estes, as reproduced in Maingot R, "Abdominal Operations", (4th edn 1961), p.890 Figs. 17 to 20. HK Lewis, with kind permission.*

A BUSOGA HERNIA—ONE

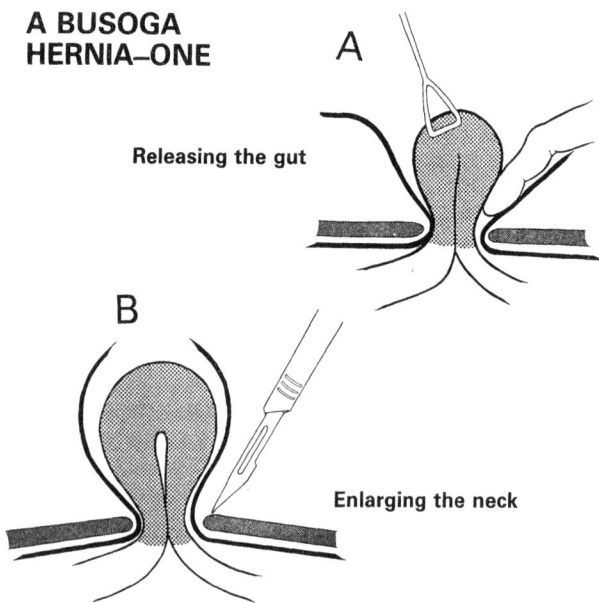

Fig. 14-9 A BUSOGA (Gill–Ogilvie) HERNIA—ONE. A, releasing a strangulated Busoga hernia. As soon as the sac is opened, grasp a loop of trapped gut gently with Babcock forceps. As you do so, gently but firmly stretch the neck of the sac with the tip of your little finger. B, sometimes you have to make a small nick in the fibrous edge of the ring. You can release a femoral hernia in much the same way. *Kindly contributed by Brian Hancock.*

your finger alongside the sac. Open the sac. Withdraw his gut and assess it by the criteria in Section 9.3 and Fig. 9-8.

If it is viable, return it to his abdomen.

If it is dubiously viable, leave it for 10 minutes covered with a warm, wet swab.

If it is not viable, you will have to decide whether to invaginate or resect it:

Invaginate the necrotic area of gut if it is: (1) A typical Richter-type strangulation which has produced a 'coin like' area of necrosis with a sharp margin, as in E, and F, Fig. 14-1. (2) The necrotic area has not yet perforated, so that it has been able to prevent the contents of the gut spilling into the peritoneal cavity. (3) It does not extend over more than 50% of the circumference of the gut. (4) It does not extend on to the mesenteric border of the gut, because invaginating it may interfere with its blood supply. (5) The gut at the edge of the necrotic area is healthy and pliable. If *any* of these criteria are not fulfilled, resect the necrotic segment of gut and do an end-to-end anastomosis (9-9).

To invaginate the necrotic area, use two layers of 2/0 or 3/0 catgut to bring its healthy borders together in their transverse axis, so as to invaginate the ischaemic segment into the lumen, where it can safely necrose (14-1).

If you need to enlarge the defect to get better access, extend the incision in his skin a little more laterally, and then split his internal oblique and transversus abdominis about 5 cm above his internal ring, level with his iliac spine, exactly as in the standard approach for appendicectomy. Open his peritoneal cavity, and withdraw his gut for inspection, invagination, or resection.

Alternatively, do a formal laparotomy through a low paramedian incision.

Finally, excise the sac, and close his transversalis fascia with a few monofilament sutures.

SLIDING HERNIAS (not uncommon)

If you find a boggy thickening in the wall of a hernial sac, suspect that some viscus has slid into it partly behind his peritoneum as in C, and D, Fig. 14-1. On the right his caecum and appendix can slide into an inguinal hernia. On the left his pelvic colon can do the same (unusual). His bladder can do so on either side, more commonly in a direct hernia. You may feel something irreducible in the sac which you cannot return to his abdomen. When you open it you find that the internal margins of the sac are impossible to identify along one side, because there is some viscus in the way. Dealing with a hernia like this can be difficult.

CAUTION ! If you cut through a thick part of the wall of the sac, you may enter the viscus.

Dissect the sac free from his cord and the surrounding tissues, without damaging the viscus which forms part of the wall of the sac. Continue dissection until you have defined the sac clearly. Then pinch a fold of its wall where there is no viscus (usually anteriorly in an indirect hernia), and open it there. Remove redundant sac wall from around the viscus, leaving a margin of 1 or 2 cm all round. Free the viscus from the extraperitoneal tissue next to it by a combination of sharp and blunt disection. If the defect in the wall of the sac is small, close it with a transfixion suture. If it is larger, close it with continuous 2/0 chromic catgut sutures. Push the viscus with the stump of the sac into his abdominal cavity. Proceed with the herniorrhaphy.

Narrow his internal ring as usual (14-5). This may be sufficient; if not proceed to do a Bassini repair (14-6), with a Tanner slide (14-7) if necessary.

CLOSING THE WOUND AFTER ANY INGUINAL HERNIA

Now that you have narrowed his internal ring, and done a Bassini repair, with perhaps a Tanner slide, you can replace his cord. Put it back in his inguinal canal, and tuck its distal end down into his scrotum. Close the gap in his cremaster (if you can identify it) with fine catgut.

Use continuous monofilament, or chromic catgut, to repair his external oblique in front of his cord (unless he has a direct hernia), starting from the lateral side and working medially. When you reach his external ring, reduce it to a size that will transmit his cord comfortably.

Repair the well-defined layer of superficial fascia with 4/0 continuous monofilament, or catgut, and his skin with 2/0 interrupted or continuous monofilament.

A BUSOGA HERNIA—TWO

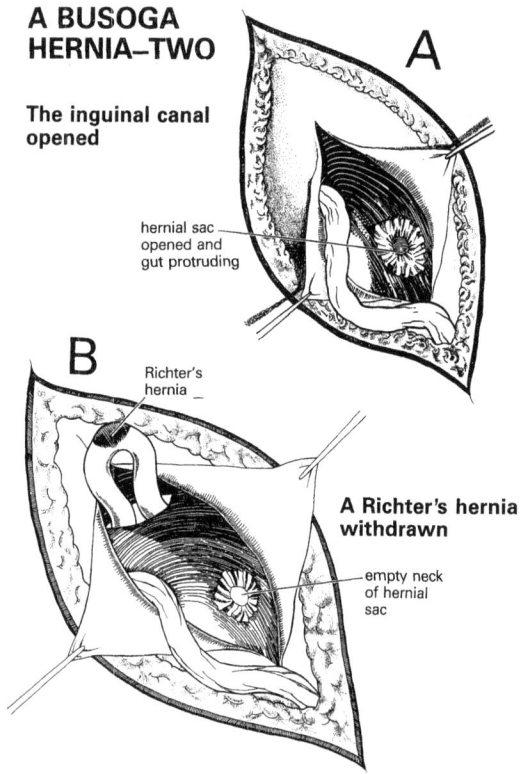

Fig. 14-10 A BUSOGA HERNIA—TWO. A, the patient's inguinal canal has been opened to show a small defect in his conjoined tendon and a hernia bulging through it; the sac has been opened. B, if his gut slips back while you are operating, extend the incision in his external oblique laterally, then split his internal oblique and transversus, as if you were doing an appendicectomy. Withdraw his gut. In this way you avoid enlarging the neck of the sac and weakening his conjoined tendon. *Kindly contributed by Brian Hancock.*

CAUTION! Postoperative bleeding is particularly likely to occur in the inguinoscrotal region. So control all bleeding vessels carefully. Any hernia repair can be spoilt by a haematoma, especially if it becomes infected.

POSTOPERATIVELY, get him up and walking on the next day. Give him a laxative to prevent him straining at stool. If he is bronchitic, give him an antibiotic and breathing exercises.

If he smokes, persuade him to stop. If he is a manual worker, he should avoid lifting or straining for 3 months, and if possible, give up heavy work.

14.3 Difficulties with inguinal hernias see also 14.4–6

These are not quite as bad as they look—fortunately, many of them are rare. As with so many other diseases, one of your difficulties will be the fact that patients commonly present so late. Giant inguinal hernias are described in the next section.

DIFFICULTIES WITH INGUINAL HERNIAS

DIAGNOSTIC DIFFICULTIES WITH INGUINAL HERNIAS

If you work in an area where ONCHOCERCIASIS is endemic, expect to see ADENOLYMPHOCELES in advanced cases (14-11). These are masses of oedematous fibrous tissue which hang from the groins and arise from enlarged inguinal nodes as the result of progressive lymphatic obstruction. Look for microfilariae in skin snips. Treat the disease medically before you operate. Although adenolymphoceles are easy to remove, the wound heals badly because so many lymph vessels are severed.

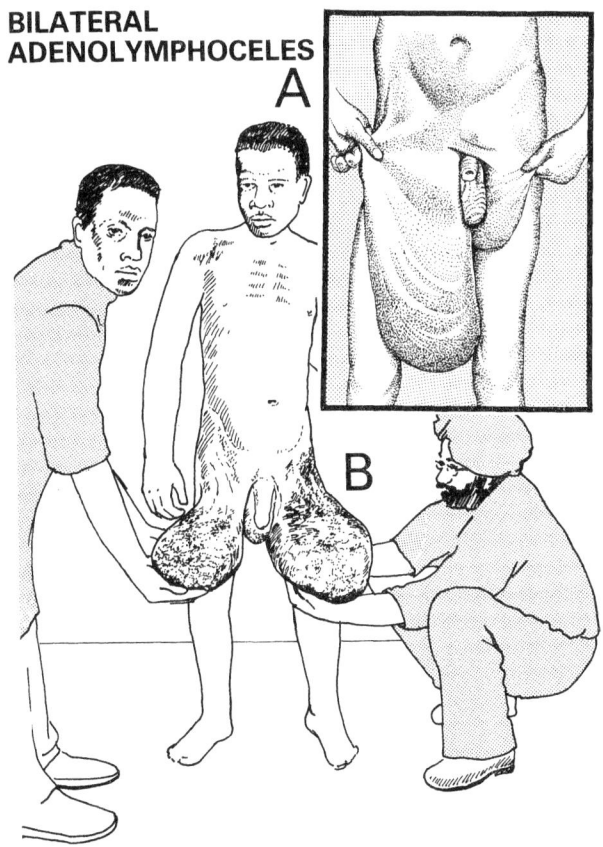

Fig. 14-11 ADENOLYMPHOCELES or "hanging groins" can occur in severe onchocerciasis. Don't confuse them with inguinal hernias. A, bilateral adenolymphoceles of unequal size. B, two very large symmetrical ones in a Ugandan patient. *Dr KT Cherry's patient. Tropical Doctor 1959;36:229.*

PREOPERATIVE DIFFICULTIES WITH INGUINAL HERNIAS

If a patient presents with a HYDROCELE AND A HERNIA, deal with the hernia as usual. Either open the hydrocele and leave its top end open, or dissect and excise it, as in Section 23.23.

If he also has an UNDESCENDED TESTIS, see Section 23.25a.

PERIOPERATIVE DIFFICULTIES WITH INGUINAL HERNIAS

If you CANNOT FIND THE SAC, and you are operating under local anaesthesia, ask him to cough. If that does not demonstrate the hernia, lift his cord and dissect it out carefully, using scissors to spread it proximally. Examine it carefully between your finger and thumb. Look for something like the finger of a glove, but made of tisssue like amnion. That's it. If you still cannot find it, confess to this in his notes, and narrow his internal ring. Refer him if his hernia recurs. Next time, consider operating under subarachnoid or local anaesthesia.

If the SAC IS LARGE and goes into his scrotum, dissecting it out distally will be difficult. Dissect it out proximally as usual, and clamp and transfix its proximal end. Divide it and leave its distal end open. If you leave its distal end closed, a hydrocele may form.

If the POSTERIOR WALL OF HIS INGUINAL CANAL WILL BE WEAK, if you do a Bassini repair, even with a Tanner slide, darn it with slings of No. 1 monofilament, as in Fig. 14-14.

If you have mistakenly passed the NEEDLE THROUGH INTO HIS FEMORAL VEIN, remove it and press the bleeding area for 5 minutes until the puncture seals itself. If it does not, you have a major problem. Press hard for another 10 minutes. If this fails, open up his inguinal area about 2 cm distal to his inguinal ligament. Use an aneurysm needle to encircle it with '0' silk, and tie it off. His leg will be oedematous postoperatively, but this is usually only temporary. Don't tie his saphenous or femoral veins distal to the profunda branch, because this will not control bleeding.

If you think that you have INJURED HIS BLADDER, repair its mucosa with plain catgut, and its muscle with chromic catgut. Tuck it back and continue with the repair. Drain the wound and leave an indwelling catheter in for 2 weeks.

If a hernial SAC CONTAINS PUS, which has drained from the peritoneal cavity, do a laparotomy (9.2).

If you find an inflamed or GANGRENOUS APPENDIX in a hernial sac, excise it. Close the wound by delayed primary closure (9.8).

If a piece of gut has a WHITE RING on it and you return it to his abdomen, a stricture may develop later at the site of the ring. Record this in his notes.

If a LOOP OF GUT ESCAPES into his peritoneal cavity, and you are not sure if it is viable or not, make a paramedian incision and examine it. This will be much safer than leaving it.

If his TESTIS IS TWISTED, see Section 23.24.

If a woman's OVARY AND TUBE appear in the sac (rare), untwist them. If they are viable, return them. If they are gangrenous, tie the pedicle and excise them.

POSTOPERATIVE DIFFICULTIES WITH INGUINAL HERNIAS

If a HAEMATOMA forms, you probably failed to tie his superficial vessels adequately, or used blunt dissection forcefully. Next time, prevent this by delicate technique and carefully controlling bleeding at every stage. Release blood from the haematoma by removing 1 or 2 skin sutures, and ease the wound open with sinus forceps.

If a FAECAL FISTULA forms, you have injured his gut. This is a serious problem. If it is not obstructed distally, wait; it will probably close, see Section 9.14.

If his SCROTUM SWELLS postoperatively (common), you can reassure him that the swelling will probably only be transient, provided you have not tied off the lower end of the sac of an inguinoscrotal hernia. Swelling often follows the repair of such a hernia, and may be due to venous obstruction.

If his TESTIS SWELLS POSTOPERATIVELY (not uncommon after a difficult hernia repair), this is usually due to thrombosis of his spermatic veins. This usually settles and leaves a normal testis.

BOTH KINDS OF INGUINAL HERNIA
in the same patient

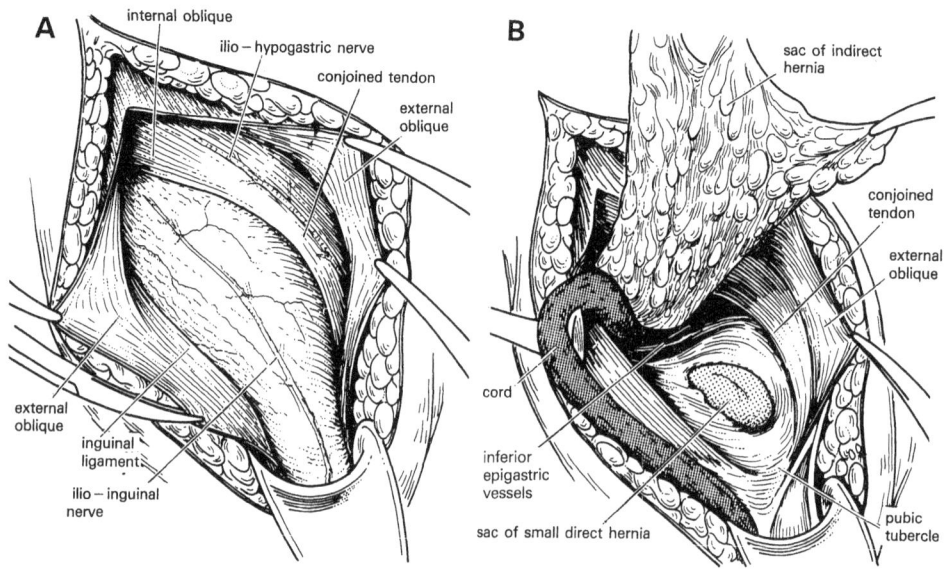

Fig. 14-12 YOU MAY FIND A DIRECT AND AN INDIRECT HERNIA in the same patient. A, the patient's external oblique has been split in the line of its fibres. His cord is exposed with his ilio-inguinal nerve on its surface. The aponeurosis of his external oblique has been freed, medially to its fusion with his internal oblique, and laterally to his inguinal ligament.

B, his cord has been freed and retracted. The sac of a large indirect hernia, with some fat attached to it, has been freed from his cord up to his inguinal ring. His pubic tubercle has been exposed. A small direct hernia protrudes through his transversalis fascia. Few of your patients will be as fat as this. *After Estes, as reproduced in Maingot R, "Abdominal Operations", (4th edn 1961), p. 889 Figs. 15 and 16. HK Lewis, with kind permission.*

If his TESTIS ATROPHIES, you have probably interrupted the circulation in his spermatic artery by handling it roughly, or strangulated it with sutures at his internal ring.

If his SYMPTOMS OF INTESTINAL OBSTRUCTION PERSIST after you have reduced a hernia, you may have reduced it 'en masse'—his hernial sac has slipped back into his abdomen with its constriction ring, so that it is not properly reduced. This is unusual, but is more likely to happen after a strangulated hernia. Do a laparotomy. You will find a loop of gut trapped in a constriction ring. Isolate the part with packs, divide the neck of the sac, and dissect out the loop(s) of gut. If it is not viable, or is very fibrosed, a resection is necessary. Repair his internal ring with 2 or 3 monofilament sutures from inside his abdomen.

CAREFUL TECHNIQUE WILL REDUCE THE RISK OF RECURRENCE

14.4 Giant inguinal hernias

It has been said that there are two kinds of inguinal hernias in the tropics—those above the knee and those below it! This section deals mainly with those below it, which may have been present for as long as 50 years.

If a patient has a very large indirect inguinal hernia, or a recurrent direct one, the posterior wall of his inguinal canal will be very weak and its anatomy deformed. It will be difficult to repair, and much more likely to recur. Repair will be more secure if you can divide and transfix his spermatic cord just below his deep inguinal ring, so that you can close it and reinforce the posterior wall of his inguinal canal more securely. If he will allow it, you can excise his cord and his testis completely. He will probably be old, so that he may well let you do this. If not, you can divide his cord and leave his testis in place, in the hope that collateral vessels will nourish it.

GIANT INGUINAL HERNIAS

If possible, refer the patient. Even if the journey is difficult, the swelling will be such that he is likely to agree to travel. If his hernia is reducible, you may be justified in operating on him.

ANAESTHESIA. Good anaesthesia is essential; use subarachnoid or general anaesthesia with long-acting muscle relaxants (A 14.3).

METHOD. Proceed as in Section 14.2. You will almost certainly have to do a Tanner slide. If the posterior wall of his inguinal canal is weak, which is likely, reinforce it as in Fig. 14-14.

If he will let you remove his testis, do so, and tie and divide his cord at his internal inguinal ring.

If he wishes to retain his testis, but will let you divide his cord, tie, transfix, and divide it as near his internal ring as you can. Leave its distal part untouched, so that you do not disturb the collateral vessels. Be gentle, or you will destroy them, so that his testis will atrophy.

If he wishes to retain his testis and will not let you divide his cord, close his external oblique aponeurosis behind his cord.

SOME SCROTAL SWELLINGS

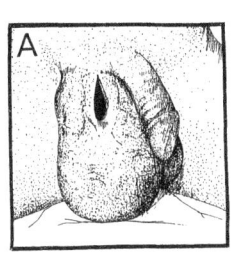
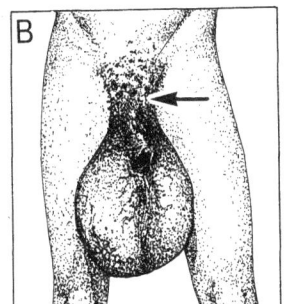
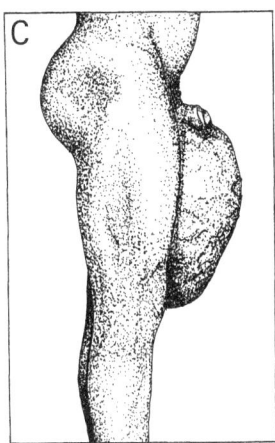
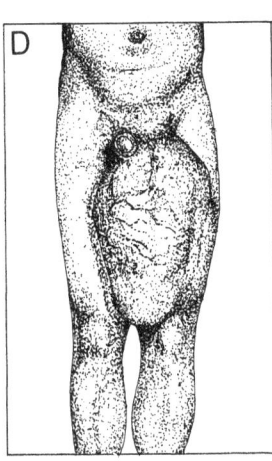

Fig. 14-13 SOME SCROTAL SWELLINGS. A, if a strangulated hernia presents so late that the scrotum is oedematous, you may be justified in puncturing the mass to form a faecal fistula, as has been done here. B, bilateral giant hydroceles. If, with a finger and thumb you can get above a scrotal swelling, as you can here, as shown by the arrow, it cannot be a hernia. C, and D, a giant indirect inguinoscrotal hernia. Repair will be more secure and recurrence less likely if the patient will allow you to excise his testis. B, C, and D, after Lade Worsornu, by kind permission of the Editor of Tropical Doctor. D, after Charles Bowesman. "Surgery and Pathology in the Tropics". E and S Livingstone, with kind permission.

REINFORCING THE POSTERIOR WALL

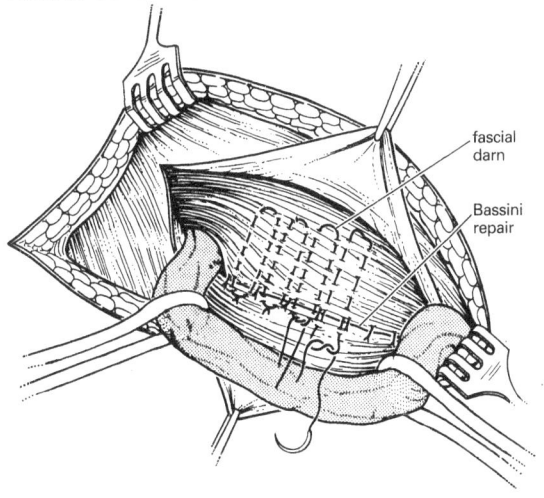

Fig. 14-14 REINFORCING THE POSTERIOR WALL of a weak inguinal canal. Do this if you think that it is going to be weak, after you have done a Bassini repair, perhaps with a Tanner slide. Use No.1 monofilament to make the darn.

14.5 Inguinal hernias and congenital hydroceles in infants and children

A baby's processus vaginalis is usually open at birth, and closes before he is two. If it is not completely obliterated it can have any of the abnormalities in Fig 14-15.

When you see him, his hernia may be present, or it may have reduced itself, so you have to depend on his mother's history that he has a lump which comes and goes, and gets larger when he cries. If you want to see it, find some way to make him cry.

Inguinal hernias in a child are always indirect. Unlike umbilical ones, they do not become smaller spontaneously as he grows older. They seldom strangulate, but they often become obstructed, especially in the first year. The smallest ones strangulate most easily and are most easily missed. You can usually reduce an inguinal hernia by taxis, as described below. Repairing them is one of the most common operations in paediatric surgery, but it is not easy. The sac is thin, delicate, and difficult to find, and a baby's vas is small and easily injured.

At birth the canal is short, and if his hernia is large, his external ring may lie directly over his internal one, which is convenient, because it allows you to dissect out the sac, without opening his external oblique aponeurosis. In young children, simply excise the sac.

Wait to operate until a baby is 3 or preferably 6 months old, when anaesthesia will be easier. All you usually need to do is to dissect out the sac carefully (making sure that you do not damage his spermatic vessels or his vas), to transfix its neck at his external ring, and to excise it. There is no need to open the inguinal canal of a young child, but if he is more than five years old, you will have to open it. You may occasionally need to narrow the internal ring of an older child. Don't try to shift any muscles, and don't apply a truss.

In principle, the repair of an inguinal hernia in a child is the same as in an adult, as described in Section 14.2. Only the differences are described here. You may find a sliding hernia of his bladder or colon, or of a girl's adnexae. If you operate in the morning, a child can be up and about in the afternoon, as soon as he has recovered from the anaesthetic.

Hydroceles in children are formed in a different way from those in adults, and need different treatment: (1) In adults fluid is secreted by the tunica vaginalis, so this has to be excised or inverted as in Section 23.23. (2) In a child they are the result of fluid passing from his peritoneal cavity to his tunica vaginalis, through a narrow (2 to 10 mm) connection between them (a persistent processus vaginalis, C, in Fig. 14-15). If you divide this, fluid will not reform. So, find the processus vaginalis, dissect it out, and divide it between ligatures.

INGUINAL HERNIAS AND CONGENITAL HYDROCELES IN CHILDREN

DIFFERENTIAL DIAGNOSIS. A hydrocele in a child is difficult to distinguish from a hernia, because they both transmit the light of a torch, so they are both considered together here. The distinction is not critical, because most hydroceles need to be operated on.

Suggesting a hydrocele—a swelling which cannot be reduced and does not have a cough impulse. Its size varies, but much less so than a hernia.

TAXIS FOR INGUINAL HERNIAS IN CHILDREN

If a child's hernia is irreducible, so that its contents will not return to his abdomen, sedate him, and put him into gallows traction (78.2). There is a 50% chance that it will reduce spontaneously, or with a little help. If taxis succeeds, put him on the waiting list, and operate as soon as it is convenient. If it fails, operate without delay.

HERNIOTOMY IN YOUNG CHILDREN

INDICATIONS. (1) If he is a neonate, or very young, don't operate

ABNORMALITIES OF THE PROCESSUS VAGINALIS

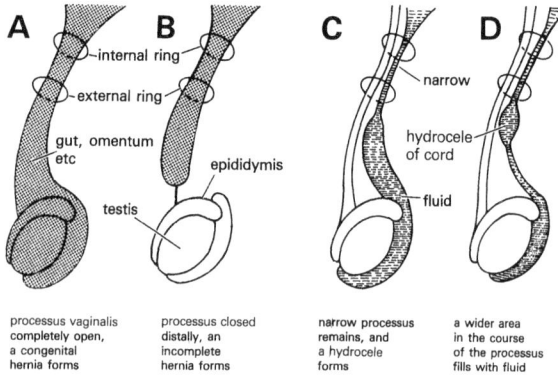

Fig. 14-15 ABNORMALITIES OF THE PROCESSUS VAGINALIS. A, when it remains completely open, a complete inguinal hernia forms. B, if it closes distally, and leaves the tunica vaginalis covering the testis, an incomplete inguinal hernia forms. C, when the processus vaginalis becomes narrow, but does not disappear, fluid passes down it from the peritoneal cavity and forms a hydrocele around the testis. D, if there is a wider area in the course of the processus vaginalis, it may form a hydrocele of the cord. Operate on a congenital hernia and and on a congenital hydrocele—tie and divide the processus vaginalis. *After Bailey and Love.*

until he is 3 to 6 months old, when anaesthesia will be easier. If he is fortunate, his hernia may occasionally resolve spontaneously while he is waiting. (2) All inguinal hernias in children over 6 months old.

ANAESTHESIA. (1) Ketamine (A 8.1). (2) General anaesthesia. Don't use local anaesthesia.

INCISION Make a 5 cm incision in the skin crease above his inguinal ligament, from above his mid-inguinal point (found by palpating his femoral artery) to the medial aspect of the swelling of his hernia.

Cut through his subcutaneous tissues, and pick up his small superficial epigastric and external pudendal vessels with 3/0 plain catgut or monofilament. Expose his external oblique aponeurosis, and his external ring, which lies above and lateral to his pubic tubercle.

Find the hernial sac, which should be anterior to his cord, and apply haemostats to its edge. Dissect it away with scissors from his spermatic vessels and vas. Use blunt gauze dissection to separate any light connective tissue. In this way separate his cord from the sac.

Open the sac between haemostats, as if you were opening the peritoneum for an abdominal operation. Enlarge the opening and apply 4 haemostats conveniently placed on its circumference. If it is big enough, insert the index finger of your left hand as you dissect down to its neck.

CAUTION ! (1) Free the sac completely before you open it. In this way you are less likely to split it. (2) A girl's Fallopian tube and ovary may slide into the sac—don't remove them as part of it. (3) If you meet the appendix, don't remove it. (5) A boy's vas is very small, don't mistake it for a piece of fibrous tissue.

Transfix the neck of the sac with 3/0 chromic catgut, and tie it off. If the sac does not continue into his scrotum excise it. If it continues to become the tunica vaginalis of his testis (common), cut this across about 1 cm above his testis and tie it. In doing so you restore its normal anatomy. A hydrocele does not reform in a child, as it does in an adult.

CAUTION ! (1) Make sure you are cutting the sac only. You can easily cut his vas, because it is adherent to the posterior surface of the sac. (2) Don't split the sac. (3) Don't use blunt dissection, except on very light connective tissue. It may lead to the formation of a haematoma.

If he is older than five years, assess the size of his internal ring. Try to put your finger though it into his peritoneal cavity. If it is big enough to take the tip of your little finger, it probably needs repair. If his internal ring is more than 1.5 cm across, close it as described below.

INGUINAL HERNIAS IN OLDER CHILDREN
First do a herniotomy as described above.

The internal ring of an older child is no longer under his external one. It will have started to migrate laterally, as in an adult. Open his inguinal canal for about 2 cm. Cut upwards and laterally from his external ring, in the direction of the fibres of his external oblique aponeurosis. Then isolate and tie the sac as above, but do it at his internal ring.

REPAIR OF THE INTERNAL RING. If his internal ring is more than 1.5 cm across, repair it. Retract his cord laterally. Put the tip of your finger through the hole in which the stump of the sac has retracted. Feel the margins of the hole, put a haemostat on its medial margin, and lift it forwards. Bring the fine upper and lower edges together with 2 to 4 sutures of 3/0 chromic catgut or monofilament, so as to 'snug' his transversalis fascia round his cord. You should still be able to pass the tip of your forceps through the ring alongside his cord. Close his inguinal canal with 3/0 catgut or monfilament.

CONGENITAL HYDROCELES IN INFANTS AND CHILDREN

Proceed as above for a congenital hernia. At operation it will be obvious that a child has a hydrocele rather than an inguinal hernia, because his tunica vaginalis will be swollen with fluid, and there is no obvious neck to the swelling. Confirm it by aspirating a little fluid.

When you follow his hydrocele proximally it will finally disappear into his processus vaginalis. Find it in close relation to his spermatic vessels and his vas, and divide it between ligatures. There is no need to open his tunica vaginalis.

CAUTION ! His vas is very small (2 mm in diameter) and is thin-walled.

If you have difficulty, aspirate more of the contents of the hydrocele, and instil some Bonney's blue or gentian violet. Massage the fluid and it may demonstrate his patent processus vaginalis.

Close his subcutaneous tissue with 3/0 plain catgut and his skin with 3/0 monofilament.

DIFFICULTIES WITH INGUINAL HERNIAS IN CHILDREN

If he has a HERNIA and a HYDROCELE, gently draw the mass upwards, and dissect off its outer coverings down to the hydrocoele sac, so as to expose it. Don't disturb his testis. Do a herniotomy for the hernia. To do this you will have to divide his processus vaginalis. If you can find it, tie it; if you cannot find it, this is not important.

If his SAC SPLITS up to and perhaps through his inguinal ring, this is inconvenient. Be specially careful, as you search for something to sew together, that you don't tie his vas.

If his TESTIS ATROPHIES later, you have probably interfered with its blood supply. This is one of the commonest complications. His parents, who may have difficulty accepting that one testis can function as efficiently as two, will not be pleased. His other testis should however be normal, so reassure them.

If his hernia RECURS (unusual), try to refer him. If you are inexperienced, re-operation can be difficult.

14.6 Irreducible and strangulated inguinal hernias

You can relieve a strangulated inguinal hernia and resect gut through the ordinary incision for an inguinal hernia. Unlike a femoral hernia, there is no need to open a patient's abdomen through a separate incision to get better access.

• *BISTOURY, guarded, one only.* This is a curved probe with a cutting edge on its concave surface near the tip (B, in Fig. 14-18). It is the safest instrument for enlarging the inguinal ring.

IRREDUCIBLE OR STRANGLATED INGUINAL HERNIAS

THE DIFFERENTIAL DIAGNOSIS. is seldom difficult.

Suggesting torsion or inflammation of an inguinal testis
—absence of the testis from the scrotum. A retained testis is often associated with an interstitial hernia.

Suggesting inflamed inguinal nodes—the swelling is more diffuse, there is sometimes redness and oedema of the overlying tissues. Vomiting and abdominal pain are minimal or absent.

TAXIS FOR IRREDUCIBLE INGUINAL HERNIAS

INDICATIONS. An inguinal hernia which has only been caught in its sac for an hour or two. Taxis is dangerous in all other hernias, besides being painful, and usually impossible.

CONTRAINDICATIONS. The patient is suspected to have had a an irreducible hernia for more than 3 hours. Any obvious signs of strangulation.

METHOD. **If the patient is a child** see Section 14.5. If he is an adult, give him morphine and put him to bed in a steep Trendelenburg position. Wait for at least half an hour, or even up to one hour. Often, a hernia reduces spontaneously. If it does not, use *gentle* sustained pressure to push the contents of his hernial sac back into his peritoneal cavity.

CAUTION ! Don't do anything which may rupture it, or risk reducing it 'en masse'.

The inguinal canal passes obliquely through the abdominal wall, so try to push his hernia back in an oblique direction. Try pressing the fundus of the sac with one hand, and gently manipulating his internal ring with the other. If you succeed, he can have an operation later in the next elective list. About a quarter of otherwise irreducible hernias will reduce spontaneously like this. If you fail after an hour in a steep Trendelenburg position, proceed as follows.

CAUTION ! Watch him carefully for signs that any nonviable tissue has been reduced. This is unlikely to have happened, and if it has, the tissue is more likely to be omentum than gut. If you are in any doubt treat him as a strangulated hernia.

OPERATION FOR IRREDUCIBLE OR STRANGULATED INGUINAL HERNIAS

PERIOPERATIVE ANTIBIOTICS. Give these as in Section 2.9.

ANAESTHESIA. (1) Local anaesthesia is satisfactory and safe (A 6.12). Infiltrate the medial aspect of the sac, and his cord, as you reach them. (2) Subarachnoid, or, (3) epidural anaesthesia. (4) General anaesthesia with tracheal intubation.

INCISION. Incise his skin 2 cm above his inguinal ligament, and open his inguinal canal as in Section 14.2.

CAUTION ! When necessary surround the operation site with large swabs ('lap pads') to prevent the soiling of his peritoneal cavity by the contents of the hernial sac, which is likely to contain virulent aerobic and anaerobic organisms.

OPENING THE SAC. You will see a tense mass emerging from his internal ring and passing towards his scrotum. If oedema and congestion make identifying the overlying structures difficult, use blunt-tipped scissors and the 'push and spread technique' (4-8) to incise the first two layers—his external spermatic fascia and his cremaster muscle. If they dissect off easily, good, if they don't, leave them, except for a small area near the fundus. Incise this between a pair of fine haemostats, just as you would if you were opening his peritoneum for a laparotomy.

Pick up each layer in forceps, and carefully incise it. When you reach his peritoneum fluid will run out, and you will see gut or omentum.

RELEASING THE CONSTRICTION RING. Use scissors or a bistoury (14-18) to slit his external oblique, and open his inguinal canal towards his internal ring. Feel for the constriction with your finger. If you can insert an instrument through it and nick its *lateral* margin, good. If not, retract its the upper edge with a retractor, and cut down on it from outside.

Alternatively, push your little finger into the ring. While your assistant holds the contents of the sac out of the way, push a large haemostat into the ring lateral to the neck (unless you suspect a direct hernia, rare) and open it so that its jaws push the sides of the ring apart and dilate it. Divide the *lateral* side of the ring with scissors or a bistoury.

When you have opened the sac, apply several haemostats to its peritoneal margins to prevent them retracting into his abdomen.

Gently deliver the contents of the sac. If it extends to his scrotum, it may be easier to deliver his testis also. His gut or omentum may be blue, purple, or black.

CAUTION ! (1) Don't damage his spermatic cord as you open the sac. (2) Don't nick the medial side, or you may cut his inferior epigastric artery. Don't cut his gut!

Examine the contents of his hernia. If his gut has been trapped, withdraw a few centimetres of the afferent and efferent loops. Assess its viability by the methods in Fig. 9-8 and Section 9.3.

If viable gut or omentum are present, replace them.

If you are wondering whether to invaginate or resect gut, see the end of Section 14.2 on Busoga hernias. Invagination, if it is indicated, reduces mortality, especially if you are not skilled.

If gut is strangulated, resect it.

If omentum is strangulated, pass long haemostats across the healthy part, cut off the gangrenous part distal to them, transfix the healthy omentum with a needle, and then tie it off. You may need more than one haemostat and transfixion suture.

CAUTION ! Be sure to control all bleeding before you return anything to the peritoneal cavity.

CLOSURE. Depends on what you have done.

If he has had an obstructed hernia or a short term strangulation with viable gut, do a herniorrhaphy, preferably only a Bassini repair; a Tanner slide will open up new tissue planes to possible infection.

If you have had to resect gut: (1) If his strangulation is recent, continue with herniorrhaphy. (2) If his strangulation is late, for example with peritonitis present, do a herniotomy at this stage and advise him to return for a formal repair later. Close his skin by delayed primary closure (9.8). If he has had an obvious perforation, drain the canal.

DIFFICULTIES WITH IRREDUCIBLE OR STRANGULATED INGUINAL HERNIAS

If he PRESENTS LATE with oedema of his abdominal wall, or scrotum, over the gangrenous contents of a strangulated inguinal hernia, a faecal fistula is about to form. Expect this if he lives beyond the 4th day. It can form: (1) In his inguinal region, where his prognosis is better, especially if his hernia is of the Richter type (14-1) and the obstruction to his gut incomplete. (2) In his scrotum, where his prognosis is worse.

If a fistula is going to form, encouraging it to do so may be safer than immediately resecting gut in the usual way. Open the gangrenous gut in his hernia, as in Fig. 14-13. If faeces do not immediately discharge, probe the tissues until they do and pass a catheter proximally. Observe him carefully.

If he improves, defer further surgery for the moment.

If he deteriorates, operate immediately. Make an abdominal incision somewhat higher than a normal hernia incision and open his peritoneum. Make a side-to-side anastomosis between loops of gut above and below the hernia. Do the minimum of surgery, and avoid disturbing the gut in the hernial sac. If he recovers, reconstruct his gut later and do an end-to-end anastomosis.

If he presents very late with an ESTABLISHED FAECAL FISTULA, following a strangulated hernia weeks or months ago, don't attempt local repair. Do a laparotomy and resect the involved loop of his gut. Make the incision well away from the discharging area, and resect enough gut (about 30 cm) to let you apply clamps outside the abdomen, where they will be less likely to slip off. Pack off the area of his internal inguinal ring, and remove the gut from the fistula. Curette the fistula track, taking care not to damage any local structures. Leave the skin opening unsutured to allow it to drain; it will close itself.

If, in an indirect inguinal hernia, you CANNOT BRING DOWN ENOUGH GUT through his internal ring, enlarge the opening by cutting the fibres of his internal oblique upwards and laterally.

If, in a Busoga hernia, you CANNOT BRING DOWN

ENOUGH GUT through the narrow opening in his conjoined tendon, extend the incision in his external oblique a little more laterally, and then split his internal oblique and transversus muscles about 5 cm above his internal ring level with his iliac spine, as in the muscle splitting approach for an appendicectomy (C, 12-1). Open his peritoneal cavity, withdraw his gut, and if necessary, invaginate or resect it. This approach is useful in a strangulated Busoga hernia and avoids enlarging the opening in the conjoined tendon and weakening it.

If, when you operate on a strangulated Busoga hernia, you find STRANGULATION OF THE SAC, but no gut in it, there is probably no need to open his abdomen and examine his gut. If it has slipped back, it is unlikely to be seriously nonviable. Postoperatively, observe him carefully for signs of peritoneal irritation and general deterioration.

If you CANNOT RETURN HIS GUT to his abdominal cavity, (1) tilt the table head downwards, (2) put a retractor under the anterior lip of the wound to raise it, (3) gently return his gut to his abdomen, a little at a time, starting at one end and gently squeezing it between your finger and thumb. (4) Decompress it as in Fig. 10-9.

See also the 'Difficulties' at the end of Section 14.3.

14.7 Femoral hernias

Femoral hernias are more likely to strangulate than inguinal ones, and are much less common. They are rare in India and Africa and in children everywhere. Whereas inguinal hernias are almost entirely a male disease, the sex incidence of femoral hernias is more nearly equal, with femoral hernias only marginally more common in men than in women in most communities.

A patient with a femoral hernia complains of a painful spherical 3 cm mass in the subcutaneous tissues of his or her upper thigh. Sometimes, a femoral hernia turns upwards, and may come to lie over the inguinal ligament, where you can mistake it for an inguinal one, or it can turn outwards or downwards. Repair is not difficult, and recurrence is rare. So always operate; a truss cannot control a femoral hernia. There are several ways of approaching a femoral hernia: use the low one described here, unless you need to resect gut.

ANATOMY. A femoral hernia comes through the femoral canal. This is about 2 cm long and is filled with fat and a lymph node (Cloquet's). Anteriorly, it is bounded by the inguinal ligament, and posteriorly by the pectineal ligament (Cooper's ligament) which is a thickened part of the pectineal fascia, and overlies the pectineal ridge of the pubic bone. The femoral vein lies *laterally,* and the sharp edge of the lacunar ligament lies medially. A femoral hernia extends forwards through the fossa ovalis where the long saphenous vein joins the femoral vein.

FEMORAL HERNIA UNSTRANGULATED

DIAGNOSIS. The patient has a tense, slightly tender, spherical mass *below* his inguinal ligament, 2 cm inferolateral to his pubic tubercle. Usually, you cannot reduce it. If you can reduce it, you may be able to pass your finger upwards through his dilated femoral canal. There is usually no cough impulse.

THE DIFFERENTIAL DIAGNOSIS given here applies to unstrangulated femoral hernias, and to strangulated ones.

Suggesting an indirect inguinal hernia—an elongated swelling arising above the inguinal ligament, and perhaps extending to his scrotum.

Suggesting a direct inguinal hernia—a bulge above his inguinal ligament, which is usually easily reducible, and has a cough impulse.

Suggesting enlarged lymph nodes, from either a pyogenic infection, or tuberculosis—perhaps a septic focus on his leg, his lower abdomen, or his buttock. Evidence of tuberculosis elsewhere. An enlarged deep inguinal lymph node may be almost impossible to distinguish from a femoral hernia. If you have difficulty distinguishing between a hernia and lymphadenitis, put him to bed, give him antibiotics and see if the mass becomes smaller. Or make a careful incision over the mass, and see if you can get underneath it. If you think it *might* be a strangulated hernia, operate without delay.

Suggesting a varix of his long saphenous vein—a soft, easily compressible swelling (unless it is thrombosed), which fills up again when you release the pressure.

Other rare differential diagnoses incude: an inflamed appendix in a hernial sac, an obturator hernia, and a tense painful pointing psoas abscess (much larger).

ANAESTHESIA. (1) Local infiltration, especially if his general condition is poor. Use the same method as for an inguinal hernia (A 6.12). Infiltrate a wide subcutaneous area, and infiltrate the neck of the sac as you dissect deeper. (2) Subarachnoid or epidural anaesthesia (A 7.6). (3) General anaesthesia with relaxants.

INCISION. Make a 6 cm incision directly over the hernia below his groin crease. Deepen the wound through his subcutaneous tissue to expose the sac (A, in Fig. 14-16). Tie the tributaries of his long saphenous vein.

Use blunt dissection to mobilize the sac free from the tissues around it (B). Trace it to its neck, where it disappears into his femoral canal.

Carefully incise the fundus of the sac. Cut through fat until you find the much smaller peritoneal sac. Expect to cut through many layers. Inspect its contents. This will usually be omentum, except in long-standing hernias. Reduce the contents completely, and divide any adhesions.

When the sac and its contents are cleanly exposed, and you are quite sure that you have completely reduced its contents, twist it. Transfix its neck with thread as high up as you can, and excise it, leaving a generous neck distal to the transfixing suture. The stump will disappear up into his femoral canal.

Then insert a few monofilament stitches, so as to approximate his inguinal ligament to the thickened part of his pectineal fascia, on the floor of his femoral canal. This is his pectineal ligament (Cooper's ligament) (C). Protect his femoral vein laterally with your finger, while you are inserting these stitches. Close his skin unless his hernia was strangulated.

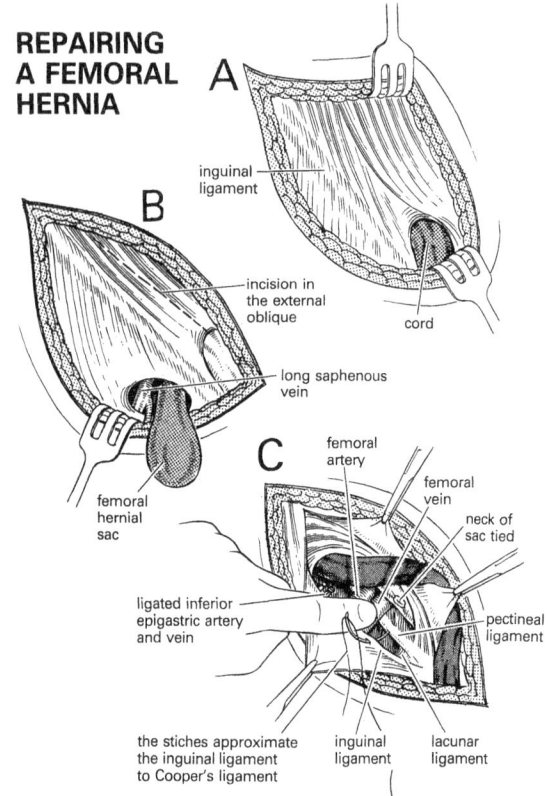

Fig. 14-16 REPAIRING A FEMORAL HERNIA. A, the external inguinal ring exposed. B, the sac mobilized. C, the inguinal ligament being stitched to the pectineal ligament (Cooper's ligament).

INGUINAL AND FEMORAL HERNIAS

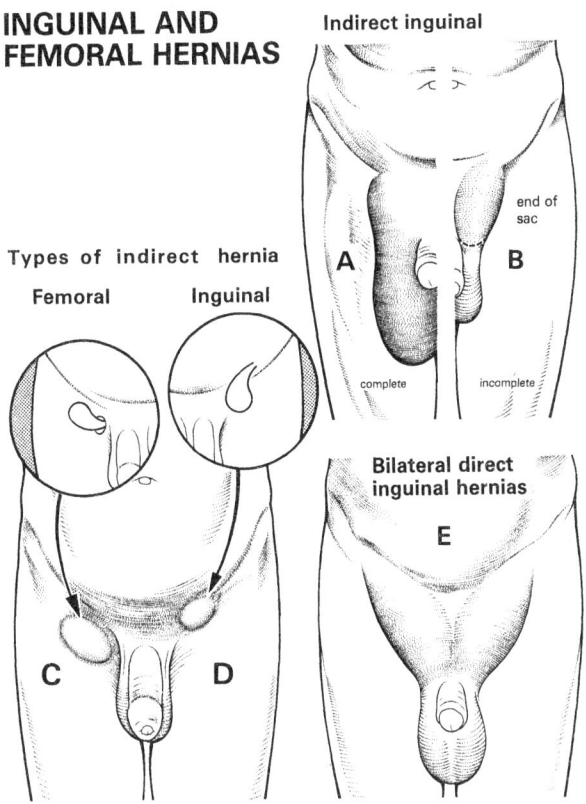

Fig. 14-17 INGUINAL AND FEMORAL HERNIAS. A, a complete indirect inguinal hernia reaching right down into the patient's scrotum. B, an incomplete indirect hernia in which the processus vaginalis ends just above his testis. C, a femoral hernia, showing how the sac extends upwards. D, a small indirect inguinal hernia showing the sac extending downwards. E, bilateral direct inguinal hernias. *After Bailey and Love.*

DIFFICULTIES WITH A FEMORAL HERNIA

If you injure his femoral vein see 14.3. See also the 'difficulties' in Section 14.8.

If you CANNOT RETURN THE CONTENTS OF THE SAC easily pass your finger gently upwards outside it and dilate his femoral ring. If this fails, stretch the ring by putting a haemostat into it and opening it. Or, carefully enlarge the *superomedial* side of his femoral canal, but be careful of an abnormal obturator artery, (A, 14-18, also see below).

If you CANNOT GET GOOD BITES OF HIS PECTINEAL LIGAMENT as it lies on his pectineal fascia, get a short curved needle, or a fish-hook needle, and set it in a needleholder in such a way that it points back at you. Insert this into his femoral canal, and try to hook the ligament on your way out.

If there is ARTERIAL BLEEDING as you enlarge his femoral canal, you have injured his abnormal obturator artery. Normally, the obturator artery arises from the anterior trunk of the internal iliac artery. In about 25% of people the pubic branch of the inferior epigastric artery takes its place. This abnormal obturator artery may occasionally pass over the internal aspect of the femoral canal, or run in the edge of the lacunar ligament—where you can easily cut it (A, 14-18).

If so, open up his inguinal canal, open up its posterior wall between his inguinal ligament inferiorly and his conjoined tendon superiorly. This will expose his peritoneum. Push this up and you will find his abnormal obturator artery crossing the internal aspect of his femoral canal. Grasp it with a haemostat and tie it.

14.8 Strangulated femoral hernias

A strangulated femoral hernia causes more mistakes in diagnosis than a strangulated inguinal one: (1) It may be small, and lost in the thick fat of a patient's groin. (2) Only the circumference of his gut may be caught (Richter's hernia), so that you can hardly feel anything in his thigh. (3) When it is large, it may have a rounded fundus and a narrow neck, which allows the fundal part to move painlessly, so you may think there is no strangulation. This makes it very important to explore any doubtful lump in the femoral region, when a patient has abdominal symptoms, especially if femoral hernias are not uncommon in your area.

The femoral canal is so small that you cannot easily bring gut out through it for resection and anastomosis. Explore the canal from below, and if you have to resect and anastomose gut, do this through a lower abdominal incision, either a lower midline, or a Pfannensteil incision.

There are two approaches to a strangulated femoral hernia, with some doubt as to which is best: (1) the standard approach, which requires two incisions, one over the hernia and another in the lower abdomen, and (2) the Lotheissen approach through a single incision in the posterior wall of the inguinal canal.

In the standard approach, cut down over the patient's inguinal ligament and aim to: (1) Expose and isolate the sac. (2) Open and inspect its contents. If his gut is viable, you can do the whole operation from below. (3) If it is not viable, open his abdomen through a lower midline or Pfannensteil incision. Expose and if necessary enlarge his femoral ring from above. (4) Return the contents to his abdomen through the ring. (5) Resect gut if necessary. (5) Excise the sac and repair the wound.

If you have difficulty reducing the sac: (1) You can incise the lacunar ligament on the medial side of the sac. The danger in doing this is that abnormal obturator vessels may pass close to its lateral (or medial) sides, and be cut by mistake (14-18). (2) You can divide and then repair his inguinal ligament. The danger with this is that, if his wound becomes infected, a hernia may form later which will be difficult to repair. Whatever you do, remember that the femoral vein lies on the *lateral* side of his femoral canal!

IF THERE ARE ABDOMINAL SYMPTOMS, EXPLORE ANY TENDER FEMORAL LUMP

STRANGULATED FEMORAL HERNIA

For the general method for intestinal obstruction, see Section 10.3.

DIFFERENTIAL DIAGNOSIS. See Sections 14.2 and 14.7. You can easily overlook a strangulated femoral hernia in a fat patient.

ANAESTHESIA. (1) Local anaesthesia is particularly suitable if the patient is old or sick (A 6.12). (2) Ketamine (A 8.1). If you are using local anaesthesia, infiltrate the field widely as in A 5.4. Inject more solution into the deeper tissues as you get to them. (3) Subarachnoid or epidural anaesthesia if the patient is fairly fit. (4) General anaesthesia and tracheal intubation with relaxants.

PREPARATION. Pass a catheter and empty his bladder.

STANDARD APPROACH

INCISION. Make a transverse incision in the skin crease over the hernia itself. Divide the covering layers, including his deep fascia, and dissect them off the sac. Sweep your finger round the hernia to mobilize it, and define its neck. Clean it by dissection with your finger, and a swab and not-too-sharp-nosed scissors.

TO OPEN THE SAC insert retractors and pack off the sac while you carefully cut down on it. Like an onion, it will have more layers than you expect. As soon as you are inside it, there will be a warning spurt of turbid blood-stained fluid. If his gut is gangrenous, this will be faeculent.

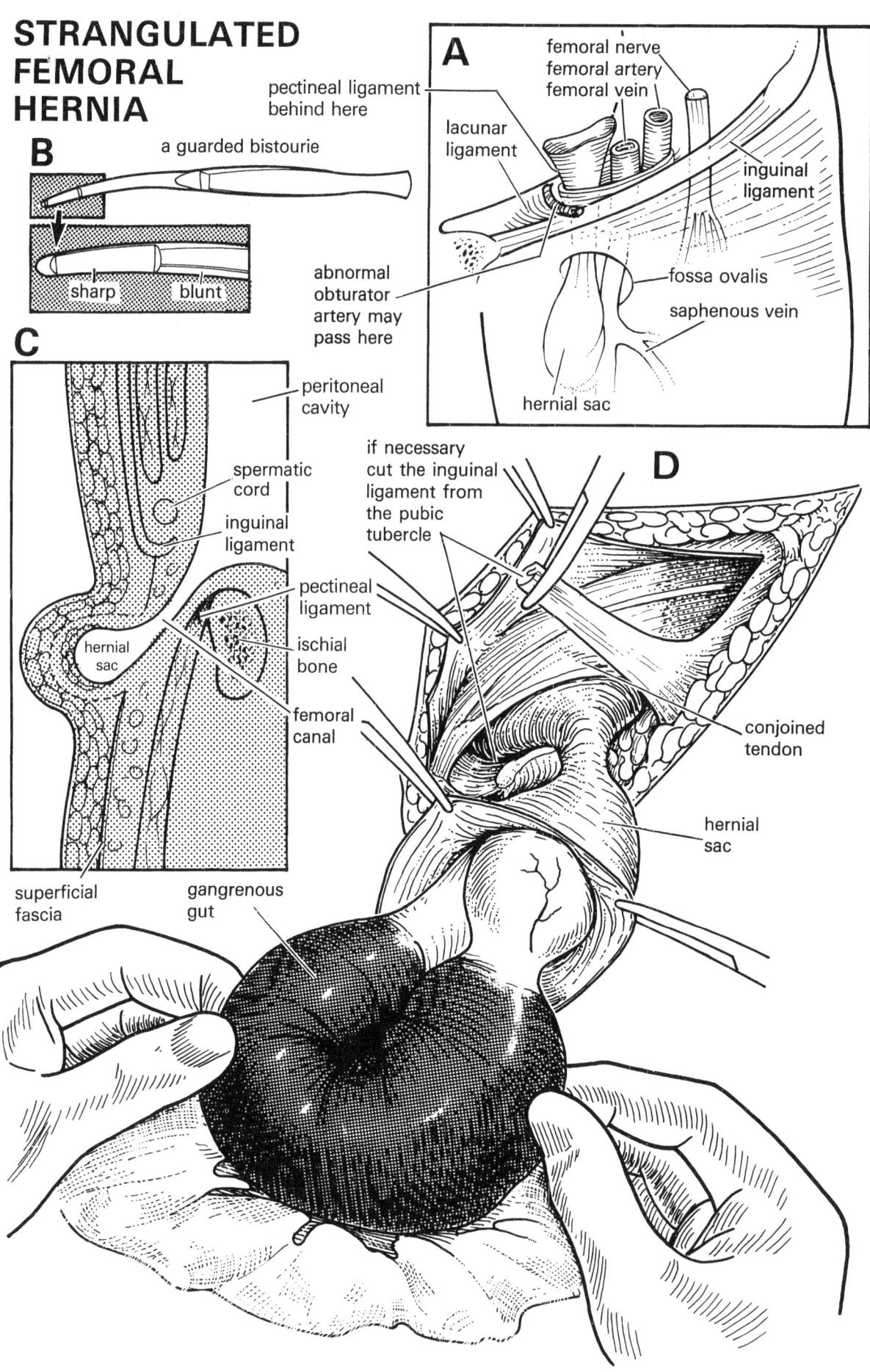

TO RELEASE THE STRANGULATION hold his gut in a swab between the finger and thumb of one hand. Meanwhile, try to widen his femoral canal by inserting the very tip of your finger into his hernia, *just outside the sac itself.* With your finger inside his femoral canal, move it around the neck of the sac and try to free it.

CAUTION ! Don't let go of his gut at this point. You may find that you have to do a laparotomy to retrieve it.

Now draw the gut down into the sac a bit more. If it does not quite come, repeat the dilating manoeuvre, but this time with your finger inside the sac, between it and his gut.

If you still cannot deliver his gut into the wound, clear the neck of fatty tissue. Enlarge the ring on its *medial* side by dividing his lacunar ligament, and the fibrous tissue in front of the ring. Protect the contents of the sac while you divide the ligament by passing a grooved director up the medial side of its neck. Then carefully cut down on the director with one or two nicks of a scalpel. Or, use a guarded bistoury. Watch out for an abnormal obturator artery.

With his gut drawn down into the sac, wrap it in a warm wet swab, to see if it is viable (9-8).

If it is viable, let it slip back into his abdominal cavity, and repair his hernia from below.

If it is not viable, do a lower midline (or Pfannensteil) incision, and resect and anastomose his gut from above.

If his omentum looks as if it might not be viable, transfix it, tie it, and excise it.

If an area of necrosis only involves part of the wall of his gut (Richter's hernia), bury it with invaginating seromuscular catgut sutures, as in Fig. 14-1. You need not resect it, provided it follows the criteria for safe invagination. These are described for a Busoga hernia near the end of Section 14.2 and in Section 9.3.

If you are in any doubt about the viability of his gut, (including a Richter's hernia), excise the damaged portion and do an end-to-end anastomosis (9-9).

CAUTION ! (1) Always open the sac and inspect its contents before you return them to his abdomen. They may be gangrenous. If he has a Richter's hernia, be especially careful not to let it escape back into his abdomen. (2) Take great care not to contaminate his peritoneal cavity.

REPAIR. If you have opened his abdomen, you can repair his hernia from above or below, as you wish. You may find it convenient to repair it from below and to add a few stitches from above, if necessary. Transfix, tie, and excise the sac, as in Section 14.7.

CAUTION ! Take care to clean it free of surrounding tissues before you excise it, or you may pass sutures into a protrusion of his bladder or colon.

Close his femoral canal by passing three interrupted monofilament sutures between his inguinal ligament and his pectineal ligament (C, 14-16). Don't go too far laterally with them, or you may constrict his femoral vein.

ALTERNATIVE LOTHEISSEN APPROACH THROUGH THE POSTERIOR WALL OF HIS INGUINAL CANAL

Strangulated gut and omentum may be more easily dealt with by this method, than by the 'standard approach' described above.

Make an incision 1 to 2 cm above his inguinal ligament, as for a strangulated inguinal hernia (14.6). Sweep away the superficial fatty tissue from his external oblique in the lower wound flap, until you come to the bulging femoral hernia below his inguinal ligament.

Fig. 14-18 A STRANGULATED FEMORAL HERNIA. A, the anatomy of the femoral canal. Note that the femoral vein lies laterally and the lacunar ligament (reflected part of the inguinal ligament) lies medially. An abnormal obturator artery may run in the edge of this ligament. B, a guarded bistoury can be used to open up the femoral canal on its medial side. In view of the risk of cutting an abnormal obturator artery, this is best used only in inguinal hernias. C, a side view of the femoral canal showing how a femoral hernia forms. D, a strangulated femoral hernia opened from below. Most femoral hernias are smaller than this. The inguinal ligament has been divided—this is very rarely necessary. D, adapted from a drawing by Frank Netter, with the kind permission of CIBA-GEIGY Ltd, Basle (Switzerland).

Deal with the hernial sac as above.

Open up his inguinal canal as for an inguinal hernia. Hold his cord out of the way, and incise its posterior wall (his conjoint tendon and transversalis fascia medially and his transversalis fascia only laterally). Make a 2.5 cm incision 5 mm above and parallel to his inguinal ligament. Tie and divide his inferior epigastric artery and vein, that lie deep to his inguinal ligament in the medial border of his internal inguinal ring; then extend the incision laterally to 4 cm. Apply haemostats to its upper and lower edges to hold them apart.

Look for the neck of the hernia from above by gauze dissection. You will find a tongue of peritoneum disappearing into his femoral canal. Working from above and below, and using the methods described above, reduce the hernia and the sac. Be careful to clear the sac from his bladder medially. Deal with strangulated gut or omentum as above.

Transfix, tie, and excise the sac. Use interrupted monofilament to close his femoral canal, by passing sutures between his inguinal ligament and his pectineal ligament. Protect his femoral vein laterally with your finger while you place these sutures. Close the posterior wall of his external oblique aponeurosis as for an inguinal hernia.

DIFFICULTIES WITH STRANGULATED FEMORAL HERNIAS

See also the 'difficulties' at the end of Sections 14.7 and 14.3.

If you CANNOT DILATE UP HIS FEMORAL CANAL ENOUGH to mobilize his strangulated gut, approach it from above. Use blunt dissection to expose the the neck of the sac medial to his femoral vessels.

If this is not successful, cut the medial boundary of his femoral ring under direct vision. Be careful—you may meet an abnormal obturator artery (A, Fig 14-18)!

If you still cannot dilate up his femoral canal enough, **divide his inguinal ligament**—this is very rarely necessary. At the end of the operation, suture its free end against his pectineal line, so as to obliterate his femoral canal.

14.9 Hernias of the umbilicus and anterior abdominal wall

There are several hernias in this region, and you must not confuse them. You will see: (1) The common true umbilical hernias of children, which rarely need surgery. (2) The much rarer paraumbilical hernias of adults through or beside the umbilicus, which usually need surgery. (3) Small and usually harmless epigastric hernias of the linea alba between the xiphoid and the umbilicus, which usually do not need surgery, but which are easy to repair if they do. (4) Hernias which follow incisions, particularly Caesarean sections.

14.10 Umbilical hernias in children

In many areas of the developing world a child commonly has a defect in his linea alba at his umbilicus through which a hernia forms. These hernias rarely obstruct or strangulate, usually heal themselves without treatment, and seldom need repair. In areas where they are common, and accepted as being merely a variant of the normal, there will be little demand for surgery. Accept this and don't operate without good reason.

If you do have to operate, repair is usually straightforward. The patient's umbilical scar is weak and the neck of the sac wide; it has one compartment, and is covered by skin, to which it may be closely adherent. It may contain small gut, omentum, or large gut, and rarely strangulates. Strapping it is useless.

KAKAZI, a 14 year old Munyankole girl, who had just received a letter admitting her to a secondary school, presented at a remote rural hospital (Stojo) with an obstructed, infected, ulcerated, gangrenous umbilical hernia the size of a small fist. She was vomiting and her abdomen was was distended. There were no sterile drums, and no diesel with which to run the generator and operate the electrical sterilizer. There was no petrol for the ambulance, so she could not be referred. Equipment was sterilized on a charcoal stove. She was given the hospital's last bottle of intravenous fluid and anaesthetized with ether from an EMO. There was no hernial sac to isolate, because infection had destroyed it. Gangrenous small gut was resected and anastomosed, her abdomen was closed, and she recovered completely. LESSON Never give up! Dr Bosco Rwakimari's patient.

UMBILICAL HERNIAS IN CHILDREN

For exomphalos, see Section 28.8.

MANAGEMENT. If a child is born with a small hernia, reassure his mother that it will become a little larger up to 4 or 5 years, then it will become relatively smaller as he grows, before it finally disappears. If she blames a hernia for recurrent bouts of periumbilical pain, make sure that this is not due to hookworms or sickle-cell crises.

OPERATIVE TREATMENT for an uncomplicated hernia is only indicated if a child has reached the age of 6, and his hernia is more than 5 cm across at its neck (rare).

INCISION. Preserve his umbilicus if you can; if his hernia is large you may have to excise it.

Make a curved transverse incision, below the hernia (A, in Fig. 14-19). Dissect down to his anterior rectus sheath and around his umbilicus, so as to reflect an upper flap to include his umbilicus. If dissecting the fundus of the sac free from his umbilicus is difficult, leave it. Find and define the sac back to his linea alba (B).

Reduce the contents of the sac, if it is not already empty, and open it between haemostats, as usual when entering the peritoneal cavity (9-2). Enlarge the opening with small lateral incisions. Transfix the sac with a purse string suture, or, transfix, tie, and excise it (C).

Drop the stump back into his abdomen. Overlap the edges of his rectus with interrupted sutures (D). Close his skin, and apply a firm dressing (E).

If an umbilical hernia does become irreducible, or strangulates (rare), you may have to operate. The same principles apply as in any other strangulated hernia. See the story of Kakazi above.

14.11 Paraumbilical hernias in adults

In adults most hernias in the umbilical region occur above or below a patient's umbilicus, through a weak place in his linea alba, rather than directly through the umbilicus itself. In Africa, a few of these may be true umbilical ones, which may be so huge that they can accommodate a pregnant uterus.

The patient is usually an obese multiparous woman, with a large multilocular hernia in the upper part of her umbilicus. Its

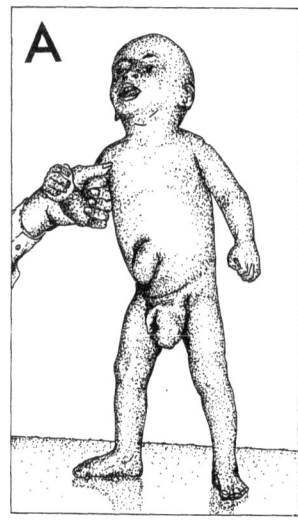

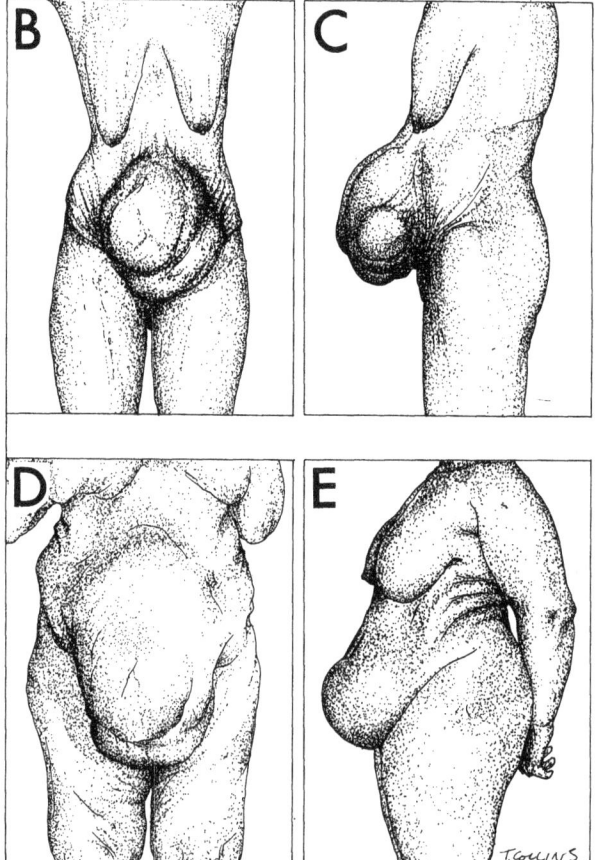

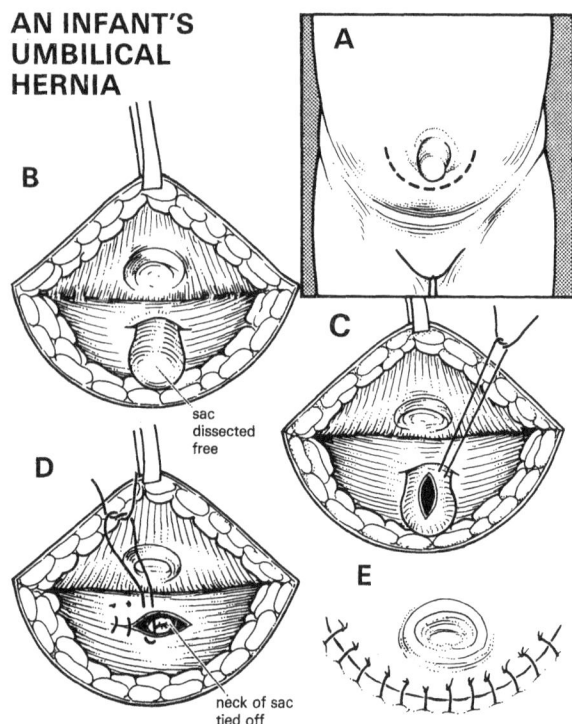

Fig. 14-19 THE INFANTILE TYPE OF UMBILICAL HERNIA. A, make a curved incision below the child's umbilicus. B, reflect a skin flap which includes it. C, open the sac at its neck, and close it with a purse string suture. D, close the opening in his linea alba with a few interrupted sutures. E, the operation complete. *After Rob C and Smith R, "Operative Surgery: Part I: Abdomen, Rectum and Anus (2nd edn 1969) p.208 Figs. 1 to 4. Butterworths, with kind permission.*

Fig. 14-20 SOME MORE HERNIAS. A, an umbilical and an inguinal hernia in boy of 3 years. His inguinal hernia will need repairing, but his umbilical one will not. B, and C, a paraumbilical hernia containing most of the patient's gut and omentum. Note the healed ulcer on the fundus. The mass is knobbly because of visible peristalsis. D, and E, incisional hernias following Caesarean section. *After Lade Worsunu, with the kind permission of the Editor of Tropical Doctor.*

margins are firm, so that obstruction and strangulation, particularly Richter type strangulations of the large gut (14-1), are common.

If a paraumbilical hernia is small, you should be able to repair it quite easily. Repairing a large one is difficult, because: (1) The viscera in the sac stick to its wall, and in freeing them you may damage gut. (2) There are usually several loculi, divided by fibrous septa. (3) The sac often extends to the skin. (4) You have to raise flaps, under which blood and exudate can collect and become infected postoperatively. Minimize this risk by closing the dead spaces under any flaps you make, as best you can.

PARAUMBILICAL HERNIAS IN ADULTS

PREPARATION. If the patient is very fat, encourage him to lose weight before you operate. Obesity makes surgery difficult. Clean his umbilicus carefully to remove all debris that might contaminate the wound.

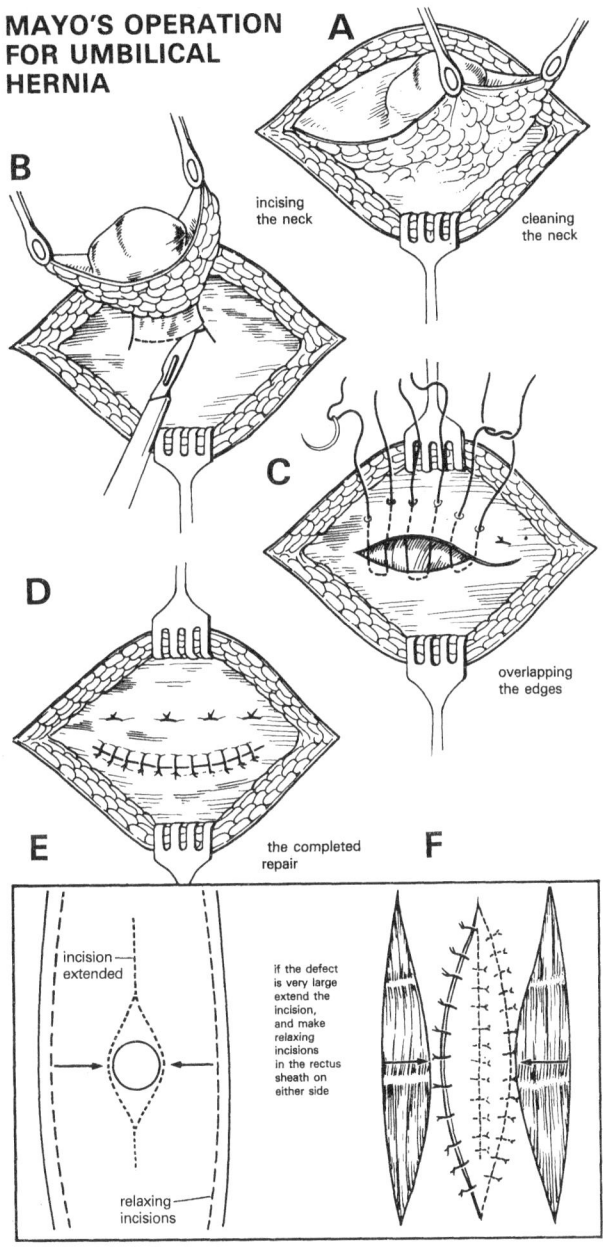

Fig. 14-21 MAYO'S OPERATION FOR A PARAUMBILICAL HERNIA. A, clearing the tissues towards the neck of the sac. B, cutting round the neck. C, inserting mattress sutures, so as to pull one flap under the other. D, the complete repair. E, and F, if the defect is very large, you may have to extend it longitudinally, make relaxing incisions in the rectus sheath on either side, and then overlap the aponeurosis laterally.

SMALL PARAUMBILICAL HERNIAS

These are hernias in which the lump (not the ring) is less than 5 cm in diameter. Preserve his umbilicus if you can.

INCISION. Put a plastic-covered pillow under his knees to help relax his abdomen. Make a curved transverse incision 1 cm above or below his umbilicus (A, Fig. 14-21). Above, make the incision concave downwards; below, make it concave upwards. Extend it so that it goes 5 cm beyond the lump on either side.

Deepen the incision down to his linea alba and his rectus sheath on either side. Reflect flaps above and below, so that you can see all round under his umbilicus. Control bleeding carefully.

Define the margins of the neck of the hernia. This is seldom as neat as in other hernias. You will not be able to grasp the fundus because of its attached umbilical skin, so define the neck on all sides, and ignore the fundus initially. *Open the sac close to its neck,* because this will be free of adhesions. Do this between haemostats, as if you were opening the peritoneum (9-2).

Continue to open the sac with blunt-tipped scissors, working from the neck towards the fundus. As soon as you have made a sufficient opening, put your finger into it and feel for adhesions. Cut round the circumference of the sac with scissors (B). The ellipse of skin containing the umbilicus will then only be attached to the patient by any viscera that are adherent to it. Carefully examine the contents of the sac.

If a loop of gut has stuck to the sac, pass your finger up beside it. Find a part of the sac wall which is free of adhesions, and open this up as best you can—it is better to leave a piece of sac adherent to the gut than to injure it.

If his omentum has stuck to the sac, clamp, transfix, tie, and divide small sections of it at a time, and return it to his abdomen.

Turn the sac inside out, so that you can see its contents and peel them away. Remove adherent omentum along with the sac, and separate adhesions between loops of gut. Finally, cut the ellipse of skin with his umbilicus free.

Enlarge the opening in his abdominal wall laterally, without trying to separate the peritoneum as a separate layer. His rectus muscles will probably be so widely separated, that you will not need to open their sheaths. If necessary, incise his anterior rectus sheath at the ends of these incisions, but don't injure his rectus muscle.

You will probably be unable to separate his peritoneum as a separate layer, so suture it with his linea alba, which is likely to be broad. Overlap the upper and lower edges of the defect. Clear the under surface of the superficial flap free of as much fat as you can. Then insert several mattress sutures of No.1 monofilament (C). When these have drawn one flap under the other, insert some simple interrupted sutures (D).

Apply two corrugated rubber drains under the skin through separate stab wounds. Close his skin incision, and apply a pressure bandage over the wound.

LARGE PARAUMBILICAL HERNIAS

Under general anaesthesia, proceed as above, making a transverse elliptical incision to include and excise his umbilicus. Dissect down to the fascia above and below his umbilicus on either side. Open the sac at its neck. Expect it to have several locules, and be prepared to find firmly adherent transverse colon. Evert the sac, and carefully free his viscera from the loculated pockets of the sac.

You may be able to overlap the edges of the sac longitudinally. Make a long midline incision and lateral relaxing incisions in his rectus sheath, as E, and F, in Fig. 14-21. Overlap them and suture them with No.1 monofilament.

Suture his superficial fascia to his anterior rectus sheath. If possible, insert suction drains. Apply pressure dressings, and hold them in place with an abdominal binder, or plenty of adhesive strapping.

DIFFICULTIES WITH PARAUMBILICAL HERNIAS

If a paraumbilical hernia DISCHARGES PUS OR FAECES, or both, a loop of gut has strangulated and perforated, and caused a faecal fistula (rare). General peritonitis is usually prevented by the tight fit of the neck of the sac, which seals off the rest of his peritoneal cavity. The differential diagnosis includes other causes of a discharging umbilicus, carcinoma of the transverse colon or stomach, and a persistent urachus, etc. Treat him as if a faecal fistula had formed in a strangulated inguinal hernia, and see 14.6D.

14.12 Epigastric hernias

A patient with an epigastric hernia complains of attacks of pain and a lump, or occasionally more than one lump, which may be surprisingly painful. You find a small, soft, rubbery, globular, and sometimes lobulated lump, somewhere along his linea alba, between his xiphoid process and his umbilicus. Extraperitoneal fat has bulged through a small (10 mm or less) cleanly punched-out hole. It may be so close to his umbilicus as to resemble an umbilical hernia. Because the fat in it is tightly wedged, it has no cough impulse, and you cannot reduce it. You can easily mistake it for a lipoma, although it is more firmly fixed. The key to the diagnosis is its position. Repair is usually straightforward.

EPIGASTRIC HERNIAS

If the patient's hernia is small, and his symptoms mild, leave it. If the lump is more then 3 or 4 cm, or is causing symptoms, consider repairing it.

ANAESTHESIA. Infiltrate the tissues with 0.5% lignocaine with adrenalin (A 6.7).

INCISION. Make a small horizontal skin-crease incision, reflect upper and lower flaps, and dissect out the mass. Clean and mobilize the sac. It will probably shell out. The contents are usually omentum or transverse colon or both, and rarely small gut. Reduce the mass by poking it back inside his abdomen with tissue forceps. Repair the hole with a monofilament purse string suture.

If you cannot reduce his hernia, enlarge the defect in his linea alba by extending it at the 3 and 9 o'clock positions. Replace the mass, and repair the hole with interrupted monofilament sutures on a cutting needle. Overlapping the linea alba is rarely necessary.

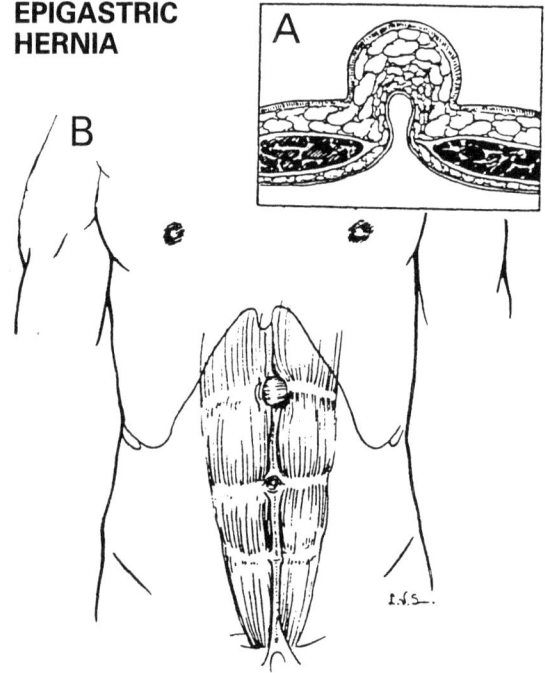

Fig. 14-22 AN EPIGASTRIC HERNIA. Note that it has occurred through the linea alba above the umbilicus. *After Dunphy and Way, "Current Surgical Diagnosis and Treatment", Fig. 36-7. With the kind permission of Jack Lange.*

14.13 Incisional hernias

These range from a small bulge at the site of a stab drain, to the huge multiloculated swelling that follows the breakdown of a major incision, usually a lower median one. Incisional hernias are more likely to occur when a patient's wound has been poorly sutured, particularly with catgut (9.8), or has become infected, or if he has a chronic cough, constipation, or some serious systemic disease, such as advanced malignancy, or a typhoid perforation of his gut. Hernias are much less common if you follow the methods of closing the abdominal wall in Section 9.8.

He presents with a lump, or a bulge, under the scar of a previous abdominal incision. If he allows it to grow large, his gut may only be covered by peritoneum and skin, which may be paper-thin and adherent to his gut. If it is very large and long-standing, his rectus muscles may have separated widely round it, so that you are quite unable to reduce it. It may reach from one of his flanks to the other, from his xiphoid to his symphysis pubis, and contain almost any of his abdominal organs.

In the developing world the commonest incisional hernias follow lower midline incisions for Caesarean section. Fortunately, they are not too difficult to repair. Other incisional hernias may be very difficult. Although recurrence is common, strangulation is not, so don't operate on these other hernias unless you have to, especially if a hernia is large, and above a patient's umbilicus. Fortunately, he unlikely to be fat, because this makes repair even more difficult.

INCISIONAL HERNIAS

EXAMINATION. Lay the patient down, and put your hand through the weakened area in his abdominal wall to feel the size and shape of his hernia. It may be elliptical, or irregular, and he may have more than one. Ask him to raise his head and shoulders off the couch without using his arms. This will fill the sac and show you its true size.

If the hernia followed Caesarean Section, ask the patient to contract her abdominal muscles. If her recti become taut, almost meet in the midline, and grip your fingers, you should be able to repair her hernia without too much difficulty.

MANAGEMENT. Don't operate on difficult incisional hernias if you can avoid it.

If a patient's hernia is very large, and long-standing, and he is obese, refer him. Surgery will be very difficult; advise him to wear a corset.

If you have to operate yourself, prepare for a difficult procedure.

If his hernia is above his umbilicus, it will be harder to repair than one below it, because his ribs will prevent you bringing the edges of the opening together. Refer him.

If he is elderly, sick, or sedentary, and his hernia is completely reducible, consider fitting him with an abdominal belt or corset. This will be dangerous if you cannot reduce it completely. A corset is not ideal, but he may tolerate it. If necessary, improvise one.

If his hernia is not too large, say 8×4 cm, is in his lower abdomen, and you can use standard methods, consider operating. If it is in his upper abdomen, it should be smaller than this before you decide to operate.

PREPARATION. If he is obese, encourage him to lose weight. He may have infected intertrigo, so prepare his skin with special care.

ANAESTHESIA. You will need good relaxation (A 14.1), so use subarachnoid (spinal) anaesthesia, or general anaesthesia with relaxants. While his abdomen is relaxed under anaesthesia, feel the margins of the defect carefully.

LOWER MIDLINE HERNIA PARTICULARLY FOLLOWING CAESAREAN SECTION

INCISION. Under general, low subarachnoid, or epidural anaesthesia, make an elliptical incision in the long axis of the patient's hernia, wide enough to include a third to a half of her

AN INCISIONAL HERNIA

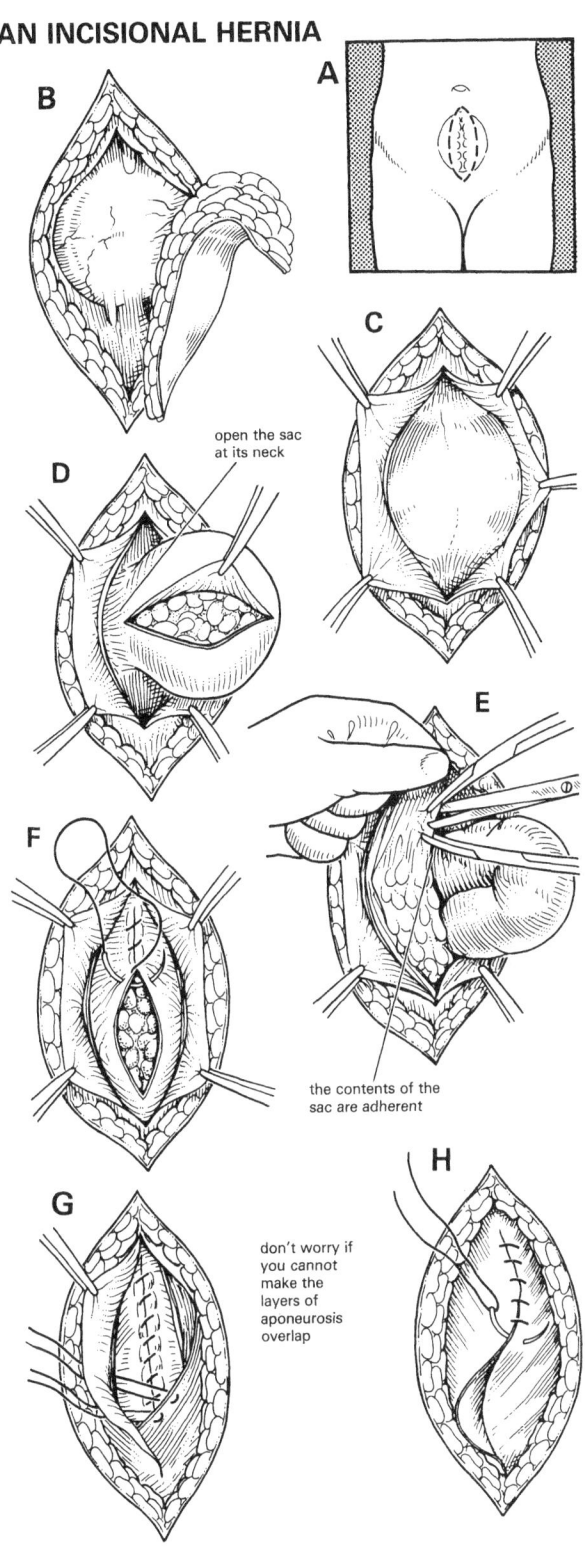

Fig. 14-23 AN INCISIONAL HERNIA. A, the hernia with the ellipse of swelling to be removed. B, removing redundant tissue over it. C, dissecting flaps of stretched aponeurotic tissue from the sac. D, opening the hernial sac at its neck. E, freeing adherent contents of the sac. F, closing the peritoneum. G, and H, overlapping the aponeurotic layer. *After Rob C and Smith R, 'Operative Surgery: Part I: Abdomen, Rectum and Anus', (2nd edn 1969), p.212 Figs. 1 to 9. Butterworths, with kind permission.*

bulging skin, and extending 4 cm beyond the defect at each end. Design the ellipse so as to remove the original scar and to produce a new one, without redundant skin or a tense suture line.

Define the margins of the defect, and free her adherent small gut and omentum from the fundus and sides of the sac. Use sharp dissection to free her peritoneum, and her anterior rectus sheath, from the fleshy fibres of her rectus muscles, which are sandwiched between them.

Control bleeding, which may be troublesome, and try to repair her lower abdominal wall, layer by layer. Before starting the repair insert 6 or 8 tension sutures of No. 1 monofilament.

Make flaps at either side, so that her skin and subcutaneous tissue (if there is any) are undermined for at least 4 cm (not shown in the Fig. 14-23). Try to find a plane of cleavage between her peritoneum and her skin, without button-holing either of them. Undermining will be easier if you insert 4 or 5 interrupted sutures near the skin edge, and ask your assistant to exert traction on them, while you dissect them free from the underlying sac.

If freeing the ellipse of skin from her underlying hernial sac is difficult, because her hernia is subcutaneous in the centre of the sac, leave the ellipse attached to the sac. Proceed to raise flaps of scar tissue as described below, and excise the ellipse and part of the sac together. Control bleeding carefully.

Raise flaps of aponeurotic scar tissue from the covering of the sac on either side (C).

The neck of the sac will probably be diffuse, and not easy to define. Open it between haemostats near its neck, as for a laparotomy (D), and incise her peritoneum far enough to see if there are adherent loops of gut. Free these adhesions (E), and return her gut and omentum to her abdomen.

If you cannot easily free her gut and omentum from the fundus of the sac, leave them attached to it; free it from her skin, if you have not already done so, and fold the sac inwards into her abdomen.

Excise the redundant part of the sac, and suture its edges with continuous catgut (F).

Dissect and trim the scarred flaps of aponeurosis, to expose the edges of her rectus muscles on either side. Trim these flaps away to leave a broad strip on one side, and a narrow strip on the other. Overlap these strips so as to bring her rectus muscles to the midline (G). Using interrupted No. 1 monofilament, make mattress sutures on one side, and simple ones on the other. Take good-sized bites, and don't tie the sutures so tightly that they strangle her tissues. In this way, a double-thickness layer of fibro-fascia will replace her linea alba.

Insert a few catgut sutures between her superficial and her deep fascia, so as to obliterate any potential spaces where blood might collect.

If you can use suction drainage, insert a multiholed catheter through a stab wound, let it lie under the flap, and attach it to the suction. Or insert two corrugated drains subcutaneously, and bring them out through stab wounds.

Suture her skin edges, apply a firm pressure dressing, and don't disturb it until the stitches are to be removed. A many-tailed bandage will provide physical and psychological support.

Alternatively, don't open, or remove, the hernial sac. Instead, dissect off the skin and scar tissue, pleat and infold the sac, and bring the skin edges together.

CAUTION ! If she develops a cough postoperatively, it is likely to disrupt the repair. Teach her to support the wound as she coughs by pressing her hands to the sides of her abdomen.

DIFFICULTIES WITH INCISIONAL HERNIAS

If she has such a large incisional hernia that her PREGNANT UTERUS COMES THROUGH THE INCISION and falls into her lap, consider doing the repair immediately after delivery, and tying her tubes.

If she has a RECURRENT incisional hernia, repair is likely to be very difficult indeed. If she is comfortable in a corset treat her nonoperatively. Otherwise, refer her.

15 The surgery of conception

15.1 Maternal mortality

The next few chapters describe the diseases peculiar to women. Women produce more than half the food in the non-Muslim parts of India and Nepal, and up to 80% of it in Africa. Yet their health has been much neglected. Half a million of them die in childbirth each year, 99 per cent in the developing world. The chances of this happening depend on how often a woman becomes pregnant (the concern of this chapter), and how dangerous each pregnancy is, as measured by the maternal mortality *ratio* (MMR). This is the number of maternal deaths expressed per 100,000 live births. A maternal death is: 'The death of a woman while she is pregnant, or within 42 days of the termination of pregnancy, irrespective of the duration and site of her pregnancy, from any cause related to, or aggravated by her pregnancy, or its management, but not from any accidental or incidental causes'. (ICD–9) In the Maternal Mortality *Rate*, which is not discussed here, the denominator is 10,000 women in the 15–49 reproductive age group.

The MMR varies widely. It used to be high all over the world. In some communities in Africa it is still 1000 or more, which means that a mother has a 1 per cent chance of dying from pregnancy-related causes, or a 10 per cent chance if she has 10 pregnancies in her lifetime. In the developing world as a whole it is about 450, but in the developed world it has fallen to 30. The result is that a mother who delivers in Bangladesh has a 400 times greater chance of dying than a mother in Scandinavia.

The deaths of mothers are more difficult to prevent than those of their children. Apart from family planning, there are no simple ways of preventing a mother's death in the way that oral rehydration and immunization can save a child. Mothers die from abortions and ectopic pregnancies, eclampsia, anaemia, haemorrhage, obstructed labour, ruptured uteri, or sepsis, and often from more than one of these causes. Mostly, they either die at home, or present late in hospital as unbooked emergencies who have had no antenatal care. Tragically, those who most need care are least likely to get it. Saving their lives requires improved education for women and services at three levels: (1) In the community. (2) In clinics and health centres. (3) In adequately equipped and staffed district hospitals. Especially, it needs plenty of well-trained midwives. Establishing all this needs political will. To raise this you will need to know your local MMR. Here is a simple new way of measuring it. Ask adults what happened to their adult sisters and whether or not they died in childbirth. Their mortality experience will be a measure of that of the community as a whole.

SAMPLE SIZE is important, and depends on the expected level of maternal mortality, the average number of 15+ sisters respondents will have, and the amount of error you are willing to tolerate. If the expected level of maternal mortality is high (an MMR of about 1000), and most respondents come from large families, you will probably be able to get a reasonable estimate from 2000 respondents, which is the absolute minimum, and is only applicable for least developed rural areas. 4000–6000 is suitable for most other situations, but you will need at least 8000 for urban populations in more advanced developing countries. In the developing world, each household often has three adults who can be interviewed, so that to find 2000 respondents, you may only need to visit 667 households (2000/3).

TOTAL FERTILITY RATE (TFR). You will need this to calculate the MMR. It is the average number of live births that a mother could expect to have in her lifetime if she experienced the same age-specific fertility rates as mothers now living. You can get it from the UN Demographic Yearbook, or from your Central Statistical Office. Or, much less satisfactorily, you can work it out. You can ask women aged 15–49 how many live births they have had in the last 12 months, and work out the TFR as described below. Alternatively, you can use a range of TFRs, from 4 to 7, which will cover most developing-country populations, and see what answers you get.

PRESENT AND PAST FATALITY AND FERTILITY. The older your respondents, the longer ago their sisters will have died, the longer ago they will have had babies, and the less 'up to date' your estimate. By using the information from all your respondents aged 15–45, you will get an estimate which reflects the level of maternal mortality over the last 10–12 years. This estimate is likely to be similar to the current one, because in the populations in which this method is used, the MMR is unlikely to have changed much over the previous decade.

THE SISTERHOOD METHOD FOR
DETERMINING THE LEVEL OF MATERNAL MORTALITY

You will need some interviewers and a calculator. Carefully translate the questions into the local language, and stencil them with separate answer boxes for each respondent. You should be able to get all the answers for each household on a sheet of A4 paper.

Use interviewers with a reasonable level of literacy and numeracy. Pupil nurses are ideal; make the survey an educational project for them. They will need to question at least 2000 respondents (see above), so it will take them several days. Take them into a classroom and explain the method. Then, ask them to visit a reasonably random selection of households, which you think will reflect the population in your district. In each house ask the head of the household to list all adults aged 15+; then question each in turn. Try to talk directly to all adults over 15, rather than using another household member to respond on his or her behalf.

(a) "How old are you?" Or, "What is your date of birth?" Interviewer: check that the respondent is over 15 years old.

(b) Interviewer: What is the sex of the respondent? If the respondent is female, and you are going to calculate the TFR, ask question (c):

(c) "How many live births have you had in the last 12 months, even if the baby is no longer alive?"

(d) For all respondents, male and female ask: "How many sisters have you ever had who were born to your mother?"

(e) "How many of these sisters ever reached the age of 15, including those who are now dead?"

(f) "How many of these sisters, who reached the age of 15, are alive now?"

(g) "How many of these sisters are dead?"

Interviewer: Check that the sum of (f) + (g) = (e), and sort out any discrepancies. (e) should be equal to or less than (d), it cannot be greater than (d).

(h) "How many of these dead sisters died while they were pregnant, or during childbirth, or in the 6 weeks after the end of pregnancy?"

For practice, do a pilot study on about 10 households, and adjust your questions as necessary.

THE TFR based on question (c) above, can be derived from the age-specific fertility like this:

(1) Group the female respondents aged 15–49 by 5-year age-group, that is 15–19, 20–24, ..., 45–49.

(2) For each 5-year age-group, divide the number of live births in the last 12 months by the number of all women for that age

MATERNAL MORTALITY

AGE GROUP (1)	NUMBER OF RESPONDENTS (2)	SISTERS REACHING AGE 15 (3)	MATERNAL DEATHS (4)	ADJUSTMENT FACTOR (5)	SISTER UNITS OF RISK EXPOSURE (6)
15-19	320	493*	4	0.107	53
20-24	263	405*	6	0.206	83
25-29	275	427	11	0.343	146
30-34	265	414	11	0.503	208
35-39	214	334	12	0.664	222
40-44	157	238	11	0.802	191
45-49	158	233	10	0.900	210
50-54	140	202	2	0.958	194
55-59	133	215	9	0.986	212
60+	238	373	15	1.0000	373
TOTAL	2163	3334	91		1892

The TFR (total fertility rate) for the population was 6

Divide the total maternal deaths by the sister units of risk exposure

$$91 \div 1892 = 0.048$$

Divide 0.048 by the TFR and multiply by 100,000

$$0.048 \div 6 \times 100,000 = 800$$

The MMR is 800 per 100,000

Fig. 15-1 MATERNAL MORTALITY BY THE THE SISTERHOOD METHOD, as determined for the Gambia in 1987. *Kindly contributed by Wendy Graham.*

(not just those giving birth). This will give you an estimate of the age-specific fertility rate for each age-group as a proportion.

(3) Add the proportions together and multiply the total by 5 (for the 5 years in each age-group) to get the TFR, which will probably be between 4 and 7.

MMR. Work out a table like that in Table 15-1. You will need to make two corrections:

(A) Respondents in the age-groups 15-19, and 20-24, can expect some more sisters to reach the age of 15. So work out the average number of sisters reaching age 15 for the respondents over 25. In Fig. 15-1 this was 1.54, that is each respondent above the age of 25 had 1.54 sisters reaching age 15. Multiply the number of respondents in the age-groups 15-19 and 20-24 by this figure to fill in the first two entries in column (3). These have been marked with a star. For example, in Fig. 15-1 there were 320 respondents aged 15-19. When questioned they said they had 325 sisters who reached age 15. They could however expect some more, so 320 was multiplied by 1.54 to give 493, the first figure in Column (3).

(B) Column (5) is an adjustment factor based on a typical developing-country population model. Respondents aged 50, or more, will be referring to sisters who will have been subjected to the full risks of a lifetime of childbirth. Younger respondents will be referring to sisters who have only been exposed to part of that risk, so a correction has to be made to the reported number of sisters reaching the age of 15 to calculate 'sister units of risk exposure' in column (6). To get column (6), multiply column (3) by column (5). Column (5) is 'given' and is always the same.

Sum column (4), which is the total number of maternal deaths reported by your respondents, and sum column (6).

Divide the sum of (4), by the sum of (6), to give you the total lifetime risk of maternal death. It was 0.048 in Fig. 15-1, which means that a woman reaching the age of 15 has nearly a 5%, or about a 1 in 21 (1÷21 = 0.048) chance of dying of pregnancy-related causes during her reproductive life.

To calculate the MMR divide the estimate of the total lifetime risk of maternal death by your estimate of the TFR, and multiply by 100,000.

For example, the TFR for the population in Fig. 15-1 was 6. So, 0.048/100,000 = 800. The MMR calculated by this method is therefore about 800. As noted above, strictly speaking, this figure refers to period 10-12 years before the data were collected. However, in situations where this method is used, it is unlikely to have altered significantly.

Try to publish your findings somewhere. Inform the appropriate government office about your results, and include details of your study design, sample size, the questions you used, and any problems you found.

DIFFICULTIES IN MEASURING THE LEVEL OF MATERNAL MORTALITY

If a RESPONDENT IS UNAVAILABLE, ask the household member who is most likely to know about the respondent's sisters.

Alternatively, omit missing respondents, and visit more households to collect the number of respondents you need. But make sure that the time of day you call would not exclude certain groups, such as women working in the fields.

If for any reason you CANNOT GET AN ADEQUATE SAMPLE, consider carrying out the study jointly with a neighbouring health unit.

If a HOUSEHOLD SURVEY IS IMPRACTICAL, consider questioning all adults attending a fixed health facility, such as mothers attending an immunization clinic. They will be a selected group, but their sisters will probably be less so.

If questions on pregnancy-related matters are CULTURALLY SENSITIVE, confine your questions to female respondents aged 15+.

If you are worried about the RELIABILITY of your data: (1) Calculate the MMR separately for males and female respondents. It should be similar. If it is not, the sample may be too small, or the responses may be biased between the sexes. Women may be better informed about the circumstances of the death of their sisters than men. (2) Compare the MMR for the 15-49 age group (who will be younger and better able to remember past deaths) with that for all 15+ respondents. The figures should not be very different. The higher of the two is likely to be nearer the truth. The figure from the 15-49 age group will probably be the most reliable, provided more than ¾ of your respondents are in this age group. Try to get at least half your sample between 25-49, without too many <25 or >50.

Graham W, Brass W, Snow R, 'Estimating maternal mortality in developing countries', Lancet 1988;i:416-7.

Graham W, et al. 'Indirect Estimation of Maternal Mortality; the Sisterhood Method'. Centre for Population Studies. The London School of Hygiene and Tropical Medicine. London WC1E 6AZ.

Graham W, and Airey P, 'Measuring the maternal mortality, sense and sensitivity'; Health Policy and Planning 1987 (2);4:323-333.

15.1a Obstetric aims and priorities

Mothers die from the diseases listed in the previous section. Between 5 and 10 per cent of their babies die in the perinatal period (from 28 weeks of pregnancy to 7 days after delivery). When they die *in utero* their deaths are often unexplained, but preventable causes include malaria, syphilis, and obstructed labour. Most perinatal deaths in Africa are of normally formed, normal weight babies who die avoidably from trauma, asphyxia, or infection. Many neonatal deaths occur in babies whose low birthweight is due to their being born too soon (prematurity), or to not having grown normally before birth (intrauterine growth retardation, or IUGR). The deaths of both mothers and babies are mostly due to the material and social conditions under which they live. Here we are concerned with the obstetric causes of their deaths.

Obstetrics differs from surgery in that there is no surgical equivalent of the midwife. This is because birth is usually sufficiently routine for most obstetrics to be done by non–doctors, whereas all but the the most minor surgery has to be done by doctors. The surgery in these manuals is therefore for doctors.

Obstetrics, on the other hand can be divided into: (1) The more difficult and less commonly needed procedures, which are normally only done by doctors, and which are assembled here. (2) The easier, common procedures which can be done by doctors, or by midwives. These are in the fourth volume in this series—*Primary Mother Care*, which is a manual of 'paramedical obstetrics and gynaecology', rather than traditional midwifery (In preparation 1989). The distinction between what only doctors can do, and what both doctors and midwives can do, is however somewhat arbitrary. There are, for example, some midwives and many medical assistants who can do a Caesarean section. The next few chapters and *Primary Mother Care* form a whole, so that unless you can refer to *Primary Mother Care*, what you read here will be incomplete. For example, you may wish to look up the selection of cases for hospital delivery (M 5.3), the management of normal labour (M 18.11), vacuum extraction (M 22.3), outlet forceps (M 22.6), or the closed method of symphysiotomy (M 22.7). Some conditions, such as postpartum haemorrhage, are managed differently by a midwife in a clinic and by a doctor in a hospital, so these are described twice, but from different perspectives. *Primary Mother Care* describes methods of terminating pregnancy early, including menstrual regulation. Following the wishes of one of our contributors we have not included methods of termination later in pregnancy here.

THE NEXT FEW CHAPTERS ARE NOT COMPLETE WITHOUT 'PRIMARY MOTHER CARE'

Despite the challenges of pregnancy and childbirth, the most important task in many communities is to reduce the frequency with which pregnancy occurs. The priority of priorities is likely to be a national population policy—most countries in sub-Saharan Africa don't yet have one. Populations there, and to a lesser extent those elsewhere, are growing so fast that they are causing acute pressure on land, on food, on the wood to cook it with, on jobs, on education, and on the health and other social services. In some areas this population pressure is already finding its expression in desertification and starvation, in abject poverty and in civil disorder. Your own community may not have reached this point yet, but is it already exerting such pressure on its environment that 'ecological collapse' is not far away? If it occurs your community may become 'ecological refugees', if indeed there is anywhere to flee to. If birth rates don't fall, death rates may rise to their old values or higher, with a much larger population in a much impoverished environment ('the demographic trap'). Part of the answer is to make sure that family planning services are available at all health units. *Many families who would like to use them still don't have access to them.*

Because so much obstetrics has to be delegated, the instruction and supervision of those to whom you delegate it is critical. Some mothers will be delivered in hospital, and some by midwives in health centres. Most of them will probably be delivered at home, attended either by their families, or by traditional birth attendants (TBAs), such as the *dais* of India. One way to reduce the maternal and perinatal mortality in your district may therefor be to start with the TBAs, to concern yourself with what they do, and to retrain them where you can. If a specialist group of TBAs are at work in your area, each of whom delivers several mothers every year, try to run retraining courses for them.

• *STETHOSCOPE fetal, plastic, three only.* These don't bend so easily as aluminium stethoscopes.

• *DOPPLER FETAL HEART DETECTOR, 'Sonicaid' pattern or equivalent, one only.* This is comparatively inexpensive (about $250) and very useful.

• *SPECULUM, vaginal, Sims', double-ended, medium size, 27.30 mm, three only.* This is the most generally useful vaginal speculum.

• *SPECULUM, vaginal, Cusco's, duckbill, small and large, stainless steel, three of each size only.* These specula open like the beak of a duck, and in doing so enable you to examine the cervix.

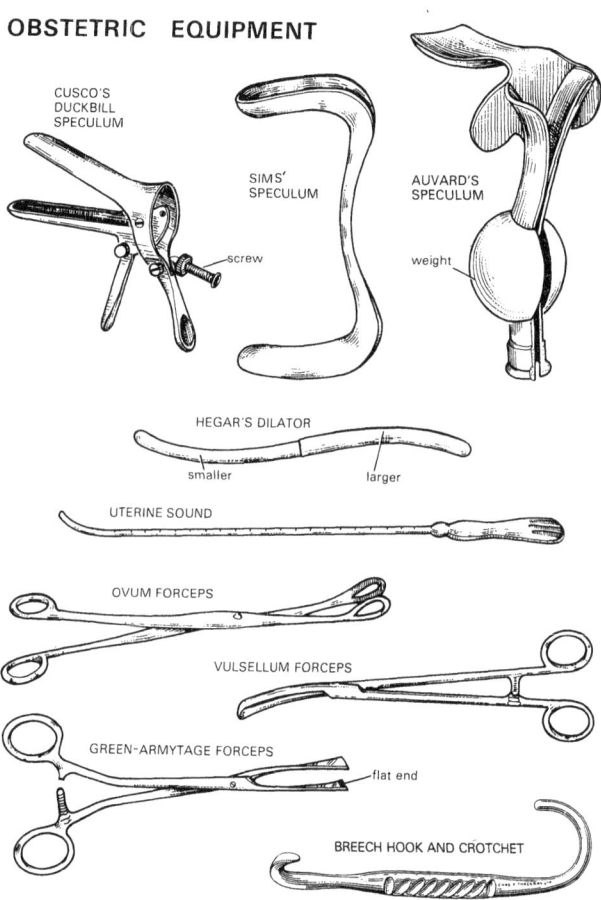

Fig. 15-2 SOME OF THE EQUIPMENT you will need.

• *SPECULUM, vaginal, weighted, Auvard's, chromium-plated, one only.* The weight on this speculum presses it downwards, and so keeps the vagina open.

• *FORCEPS, uterine vulsellum, curved, 1×2 teeth and 3×4 teeth, box joint, 230 mm, one only of each size.* Use these to grasp the non–pregnant cervix when you curette it. In pregnancy, ring (sponge) forceps are better.

• *SOUND, uterine, malleable, metric, graduated shaft, two only.* Use this to measure the depth of the uterus before inserting dilators. A sound is a dangerous instrument in a pregnant uterus, because you can easily perforate it.

• *DILATORS, cervix, double-ended, Hegar's, 222 mm, set of 12 sizes, 1/2 mm to 23/24 mm, one, or preferably two sets only.* Use these to dilate the cervix before curetting it. You are likely to have several patients needing dilatation and curettage on the same list, so two sets of dilators will be useful.

• *MANIPULATOR, uterine, one only.* Use this to bring the uterine fundus up against the abdominal wall when you do a minilaparotomy.

• *FORCEPS, ovum, curved, screw joint, McClintock 250 mm, one only.* Use this to remove the products of conception from an incomplete abortion, after you have dilated the cervix. If you don't have them, use sponge-holding forceps.

• *CURETTE, uterine, double-ended, blunt and sharp, 8 mm and 5 mm, two only of each size.* The great danger with a curette is that you may push it through the wall of the uterus, especially a pregnant uterus. Opinions differ as to whether a blunt curette is more dangerous than a sharp one. Let a curette lie gently in your fingers, so that you can 'feel' the wall of the uterus—don't grasp it firmly.

• *CURETTE, suction, stainless steel, reusable, sizes 8 and 10 Hegar, one only of each size.* Use this for evacuating moles (it causes much less bleeding than dilatation and curettage), and for terminating a pregnancy which has lasted less than 12 weeks.

• *CURETTE AND SYRINGE for menstrual regulation, sterile, plastic, disposable, five hundred only.* You will only need these if you intend to introduce menstrual regulation as part of your family planning activities.

- *CATHETER, Drew-Smythe, one only.* This is useful for rupturing the membranes if the head is high, especially if there is polyhydramnios, to control the gush of fluid and to prevent prolapse of the cord (19.13).
- *CANNULA, cervical, Leech Wilkinson or Miller, one only.* This is for doing a salpingogram.
- *SCISSORS, episiotomy, Vant, one only.* These have straight blades and round points.
- *VACUUM EXTRACTOR, Bird's modification of Malmstrom's, complete with 3 suction cups 40, 50, 60 mm, one posterior cup, traction handle, vacuum hand pump, chain, spare vacuum bottle and spare baskets, one only.* Bird's modification is better than the original Malmstrom extractor, and is quicker and easier to assemble. The anterior and posterior cups are not really necessary. Some workers advise the 50 mm cup only.
- *FORCEPS, outlet, Wrigley, one only.* Outlet forceps are the only safe ones for anyone but an experienced obstetrician.
- *FORCEPS, obstetric, Neville Barnes, one only.* You will need these for the aftercoming head of a breech delivery, for which Wrigley's forceps do not have long enough handles. For the uses and dangers of forceps, see Section 18.1.
- *FORCEPS, haemostatic, straight, Green-Armytage, 203 mm, six only.* Optional. Use these for clamping the cut edges of the uterus during a Caesarean section, and for repairing a ruptured uterus.
- *BREECH HOOK and CROTCHET combined, one only.* Use this to deliver a dead baby presenting by his breech.
- *PERFORATOR, Simpson's, one only.* This is the standard instrument for opening the skull when doing a destructive operation.
- *RETRACTOR, Doyen's, one only.* Use this for Caesarean section, it has a curved lip which fits over the lower end of the wound and keeps the bladder out of the way of the operation.
- *RETRACTOR, Kirschner, one only.* This gives an excellent exposure for laparotomy, with a good view for operating in the pelvis.
- *SCISSORS, embryotomy, Queen Charlotte's pattern, one only.* These scissors were specifically designed for destructive operations.
- *SAW, decapitation, Blond-Heidler, complete with ring, thimble and blades, one only.* Use this for decapitating a dead baby when labour is obstructed by a transverse lie. It is a piece of wire with teeth on it, hooks at each end to fit handles, and pieces of tubing to prevent it from cutting his mother. It also has a thimble you can push round his neck to fix the saw to. Alternatively, you can use large scissors, preferably the embryotomy scissors described above.

15.2 Infertility

Infertility causes much distress, particularly in those districts of Africa where as many as 30 per cent of families are childless. *Primary Mother Care* describes what health centres can do for it (2.3), and if they have done their job properly, there is little more that you can do in a district hospital. You may decide that you have other priorities, and that infertility is so unrewarding that you are not going to try to treat it. If you do decide to do so, *make it part of your family planning activities* and promote an integrated 'fertility service', which is concerned with both too much and too little fertility.

Typically, about 60 per cent of infertility is caused by the adhesions that follow PID (pelvic inflammatory disease). Repairing tubes that PID has blocked is an expert's task, and even then the success rate is low, so you may decide that there is little point in investigating or referring these patients. If you decide to do so, you can: (1) Do a hysterosalpingogram which will tell you where a block is. Many district hospitals find these too expensive and time-consuming. (2) Insufflate the tubes, which is cheaper, but gives less reliable information. Also, the instrument often leaks, and you can make mistakes. (3) Do a laparoscopy which again is expensive and time-consuming.

Some couples will be childless because the wife is not ovulating. You can find this out by: (1) Taking her history. If she has regular cycles, she is almost certainly ovulating. Failure to ovulate is typically associated with irregular cycles or amenorrhoea. (2) Dilating and curetting her during the second half of the cycle, and sending the scrapings for histology. (3) Asking her to keep a temperature chart, as described in *Primary Mother Care*. She may be sufficiently intelligent and motivated to do this, particularly if she is a member of the hospital staff or a teacher. A regular 0.5°C temperature rise 14 days before the start of menstruation is good evidence that she is ovulating. Lack of this rise, especially if her periods are irregular or scanty, is strong evidence that she is not doing so. (4) If you are fortunate enough to have a laparoscope or laprocator, you can examine her ovaries (15.4), to see if they are scarred, showing that she has ovulated. At the same time you can test the patency of her tubes, by injecting a blue dye though her cervix, and seeing if it appears in her peritoneal cavity.

If she is not ovulating, refer her. If you cannot refer her, you *may* be justified in inducing ovulation with clomiphene, which is comparatively safe, if she can afford it. One contributor considers it has no place in this manual. Only an expert should give her bromocriptine or the gonadotrophins. Use a temperature chart to monitor your success.

A very occasional patient is sterile as the result of tuberculous endometritis; sterility is its most common presentation. Treating tuberculosis is not difficult, but it is unlikely to make her fertile—she has about an 8 per cent chance of conception, but only a 2 per cent chance of a live child. She also runs an increased chance of an ectopic pregnancy.

INFERTILITY

The health centre staff should have taken a history, examined both partners, and sent the husband's semen for examination. If their workup is incomplete, complete it (M 2.3).

HUSBAND. His seminal fluid must be examined within 2 hours. It is normal if: it has a volume of 2 ml to 6 ml, it is liquid after 30 minutes, it has 60% of motile sperms, and if it has 20 million sperms or more per ml, less than 15% of them being abnormal.

If he has a low sperm-count, suggest they abstain from sex until the 12th to 14th day of the cycle, to increase his sperm-count at the time of ovulation. If he has pus cells in his ejaculate, treat his infection.

WIFE. Curette her late in the second half of her cycle. Either: (1) Use a microcurette of the Novak or similar type, as an outpatient. Or, (2) dilate and curette her under anaesthesia. Put half the curettings into formol saline for histology, and the other half into a sterile bottle for culture and, if possible, for guinea pig inoculation for tuberculosis. Indicate on the request form for histology that you want to know if she is ovulating. Remember not to overload a pathology service which is overloaded already.

HYSTEROSALPINGOGRAM

CAUTION ! (1) Before you start, do a pelvic examination to exclude pregnancy and active pelvic infection. (2) Do a hysterosalpingogram within 10 days of the patient's last period, and not in the premenstrual or active menstrual phases of the cycle. (2) Wear a lead apron.

EQUIPMENT. An intracervical cannula, preferably of the Leech Wilkinson screw-in type. A Miller cannula causes less trauma to the cervix, but does not make such a good seal with it, unless she is under general anaesthesia, which allows you to use more force. A 20 ml syringe filled with a water-soluble contrast medium such as 'Urografin'. Avoid oily contrast media.

ANAESTHESIA. No anaesthesia is usually needed, but if she is very anxious, premedicate her with diazepam 30 minutes beforehand and do a cervical block.

METHOD. You can do a salpingogram in the X-ray department. If possible, screen her during injection of the dye. If not, lie her on her back on the X-ray table with her hips and knees flexed, and the plate under her pelvis. A tube–plate distance of a metre is satisfactory and no grid is needed.

Insert Cusco's speculum and clean her cervix with cetrimide. Hold her cervix gently with a single-toothed tenaculum, lightly closed to the first ratchet; she should feel little pain.

Expel all air from the syringe and cannula, inject 20 ml of contrast medium firmly into her cervix, and take a film. If she has a cornual block, 20 ml will not go in. If possible, take a second film some hours later. The dye should have spread into her peritoneal cavity. If it remains loculated, this suggests adhesions and impaired fertility.

TUBAL INSUFFLATION

INDICATIONS. Although theoretically simple, false results are not uncommon. If insufflation is the only method of investigation you have, this suggests that expert tubal surgery is unlikely to be available, which should make you question the value of insufflation.

EQUIPMENT. An insufflator, a source of a carbon dioxide, and preferably a device for recording the pressure graphically. If necessary you can use air.

METHOD. Give her a general anaesthetic and put her into the lithotomy position. Insert a Sims' speculum. Insert the insufflator into her cervix and fill her vaginal canal with fluid, so that the cannula is submerged, and you can see if there is a leak. Discharge some carbon dioxide, and listen over her lower abdomen for the sound of it bubbling out of her tubes. Measure the rise in pressure of CO_2 before free flow occurs. If her tubes are patent, pressure will peak, and flow occur below 40 mm Hg. If they are blocked it may rise as high as 160 mm.

If you are using air, use a maximum of 250 ml, and don't go above 100 mm Hg, because of the risk of air embolism.

LAPAROSCOPY AND DYE INJECTION

Under general anaesthesia insert a Miller cannula into her cervix. Insert a laparoscope, as for tubal ligation (15.4), and tilt her head down until you see a good view of her pelvis. If you cannot see clearly, insert the Verres needle (with the valve closed) in the midline suprapubically, and use this to manipulate her tubes. Inject 10–20 ml of methylene blue dye diluted 1:10 in sterile water, and look for dye spilling from the ends of her tubes.

Normal tubes Her fimbriae look healthy and the dye spills through easily. It may spill on one side only, but if both tubes look healthy, they are probably both patent.

Cornual block No dye enters her tubes. As your assistant injects the dye, the region of their insertion into her uterus blanches slightly.

Fimbrial block Her tubes are often distended; their fimbriae are clubbed and sealed over the ostia, and may be adherent to her ovaries. As you inject the dye, the thin walls of her tubes allow you to see it entering them. Usually, no dye spills out. Sometimes the fimbrial block is partial, so that only a little spills.

ANOVULATORY INFERTILITY

CLOMIPHENE is only indicated for anovulatory infertility. If you cannot refer her and can afford it, consider giving her clomiphene. Warn her of the increased incidence of multiple pregnancies. Unless she is also receiving gonadotrophins, this risk is small. Give her 50 mg daily from the second to the sixth day of her menstrual cycle, or at any time if cycles have stopped, to a maximum of 6 courses. Monitor ovulation with a temperature chart. If she does not ovulate increase the dose by 50 mg amounts each month, to a maximum of 200 mg daily for 5 days.

CAUTION ! (1) Only give clomiphene to adequately investigated patients with patent tubes and fertile husbands. *Don't use it randomly on all infertile patients.* (2) It is contraindicated in hepatic disease, ovarian cysts, pregnancy, and abnormal uterine bleeding. (3) Side-effects include visual disturbances, ovarian hyperstimulation (very rare unless it is used with gonadotrophins; if it occurs stop treatment), hot flushes, nausea, vomiting, depression, insomnia, breast tenderness, weight gain, rashes, dizziness and hair loss. It may make her ovaries tender, and simulate an acute abdomen.

15.3 Tubal ligation

This should be the most common operation you do, and the most important one. It is chosen after careful consideration of the alternatives, so it must be as safe and as painless as it can be. Try not to keep a mother waiting too long for surgery, or she may become pregnant meanwhile!

Large numbers of mothers need their tubes tying, and if you take the trouble to encourage them, many will be willing to accept it. But however many ligations you do, you will probably be only able to satisfy a small fraction of the community's need. You can: (1) Tie a mother's tubes at the same time that you do a Caesarean section (18.9). (2) Do a 'minilap', which is a laparotomy through a very small incision. (3) Do a standard laparotomy—but this should seldom if ever be necessary. (4) Tie her tubes through a laparoscope, or a laprocator (15.4).

Tying a mother's tubes immediately after delivery has several advantages: (1) They are easier to get at when her uterus is still enlarged. (2) You already have her in hospital, whereas if you send her out and ask her to come back, she may never return. (3) Immediately after a normal delivery she will tolerate the minimal additional trauma of sterilization particularly well. (4) If you have already opened her abdomen for some other reason, such as Caesarean section, tying her tubes is easy. But there are some minor disadvantages in doing it at this time: (a) She is more likely to change her mind later. (b) You have little time to examine the baby and exclude any abnormality before you tie them.

Local anaesthesia has many advantages, and if you follow the methods described here carefully, complications should be few and easily managed. Finding a tube and bringing it painlessly up into a small incision needs gentleness, skill, and practice. Carefully trained theatre sisters and assistants can tie tubes, but you should examine all patients first, and be at hand in case there are difficulties. Tubes can also be tied on a large scale in special 'camps'.

OPERATING IN A HEALTH CENTRE. Grand multips with large families don't like going to a remote hospital to have their tubes tied, but they may be pleased to have this done at their local health centre, if you can visit it and do a list there. Operating in a health centre is not easy, but it extends the benefits of this most necessary operation to those who need it most—if the health centre has a theatre (2.2a).

Ask the staff to prepare a list of all the mothers in the district who want their tubes tying. Often only a few will come the first time, but more will come later. If you plan ahead, you can work without an autoclave on the site, or you can combine antiseptic methods (2.6) with aseptic ones. Bring sterile packs of drapes and gowns, and use the same gown for several patients; for gloves see Section 2.3. Use a single square drape with a 12×12 cm opening for each patient. If necessary, this can be a plastic sheet sterilized between patients in an antiseptic fluid. Boil instruments between cases. Some workers give each patient a gram of chloramphenicol intravenously at the start of the operation (2.6).

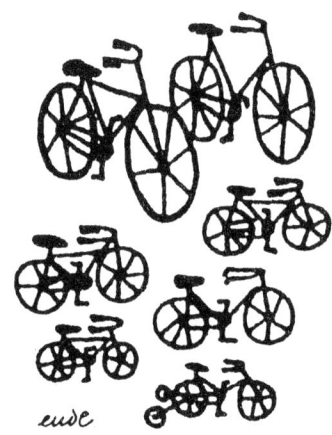

Fertile cycles

Barss P. 'Tubal ligation with local anaesthesia', Tropical Doctor 1985;175-178.

MINILAP

CAUTION ! (1) Before you tie anyone's tubes, make sure you know what the local cultural attitudes to it are. (2) Always get consent from the patient and her husband, and if necessary her mother. (3) Don't try to press for consent during labour. (4) This operation has a mortality of the order of 5/100,000 from

TUBAL LIGATION

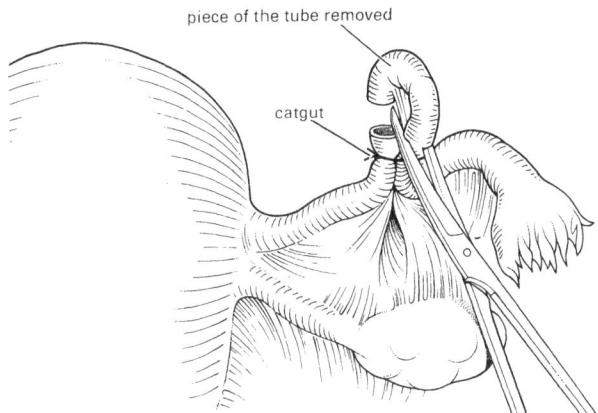

Fig. 15-3 TUBAL LIGATION. A loop of tube has been tied with catgut and is being excised. The catgut will later be absorbed, and allow the ends of the tube to separate. This will make them less likely to recanalize.

CHOGORIA SUPPORTS

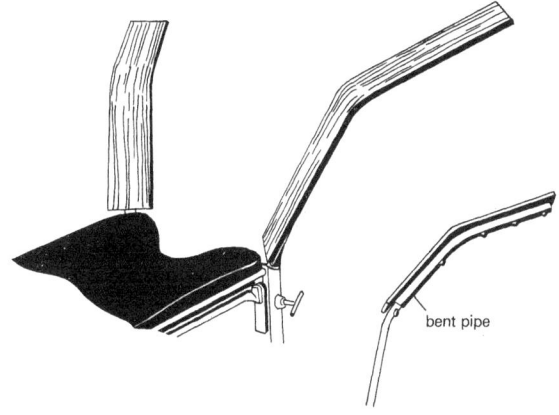

Fig. 15-4 CHOGORIA SUPPORTS hold a patient's legs only partly flexed, so that you can have simultaneous access to her abdomen and her perineum. They are from a mission hospital of this name in Kenya, and are a cheaper locally-made alternative to Lloyd Davies stirrups, or to an attachment for an operating table that enables you to angle its lithotomy poles.

anaesthesia (the major risk), tetanus and haemorrhage, so take the appropriate precautions.

INDICATIONS. (1) Mothers who are sure they want no more babies. (2) Medical diseases contraindicating pregnancy, particularly severe heart disease, renal failure or severe diabetes.

CONTRAINDICATIONS. (1) Extreme obesity (see below). (2) Excessive anxiety. (3) A history of pelvic sepsis (PID) immobilizing the uterus of a non-postpartum patient make a minilap under local anaesthesia difficult. She needs subarachnoid or general anaesthesia, and she will probably be infertile anyway. Dense adhesions are unusual immediately postpartum in multips. (4) A chronic cough will increase the risk of an incisional hernia later. (5) Pregnancy. (6) Refusal of the patient *or her husband* to sign a consent form.

ARRANGEMENTS. You can do a minilap as a day case, but if you admit her the night before, she is more likely to be present when the list starts.

THE EQUIPMENT includes two long narrow, 13×44 mm Langenbeck retractors, a scalpel, a needle-holder, ovum (ring) forceps, a circular cutting needle, chromic catgut, and monofilament.

A special manipulator is listed above, which you can use to press a patient's fundus against her abdominal wall, and bring it into a small minilap incision. This is unnecessary immediately postpartum, but if you are inexperienced, it makes the tubes easier to find in a non-postpartum patient.

ANAESTHESIA. Take all the precautions for an abdominal operation (9.1), and be sure to *starve her*. There are several alternatives:

(1) A method of local anaesthesia is described below with the surgery. Use 100 ml of 0.5% lignocaine *with* adrenalin. This is the maximum dose (A 5-1). Premedicate her with pethidine 25 mg and diazepam 5 mg intravenously. Double this premedication if she is large or anxious. The minimum intravenous premedication will enable her to get up and walk away immediately afterwards.

(2) Local infiltration as in A 6.7, with a paracervical block (A 6.14) for the dilatation and curettage, if you do one (see below). (3) Ketamine (A 8.1). (4) Pethidine with diazepam (A 8.8). (5) Subarachnoid or epidural anaesthesia are convenient. (6) If she is obese, you may need general anaesthesia with muscle relaxation.

CAUTION ! (1) Local anaesthesia, properly used, is the only safe anaesthetic for a national sterilization programme. (2) Avoid large intramuscular doses of pethidine. Instead, use small intravenous doses, followed by intravenous diazepam as in A 8.8.

METHOD. *Immediately* before the operation ask her to pass her urine, or catheterize her, to prevent you cutting into her distended bladder. Do a careful bimanual examination to make sure that she is not already pregnant. Put her into the semilithotomy position, with her thighs flexed to 45° and moderately abducted, her knees flexed, and her lower legs horizontal. Use Lloyd Davis stirrups, or, cheaper, 'Chogoria supports' (15-4).

Clean her abdomen, perineum, and vagina, empty her bladder with a catheter, and cover her with an abdominal sheet. Pass a Sims' or Auvard's speculum.

If more than 10 days have elapsed since the first day of her last period, consider doing a 'D and C' (20.3), to prevent implantation in this cycle. If you are operating under local anaesthesia, you will have to do this under a paracervical block (A 6.14). Many surgeons consider this unnecessary interference, and point out that it is not sure to prevent implantation.

THE INCISION depends on the position of her fundus.

If she has delivered within the last few days, and her uterus is at her umbilicus or can easily be pushed there, make a 2 cm horizontal incision in its inferior fold. This is good cosmetically, and avoids the need to shave her.

If her uterus has involuted, or she is not postpartum, make a short transverse incision just above her pubic hair. One contributor always makes a suprapubic incision, even if her uterus is enlarged; you can always find her tubes down beside it.

MINILAPAROTOMY

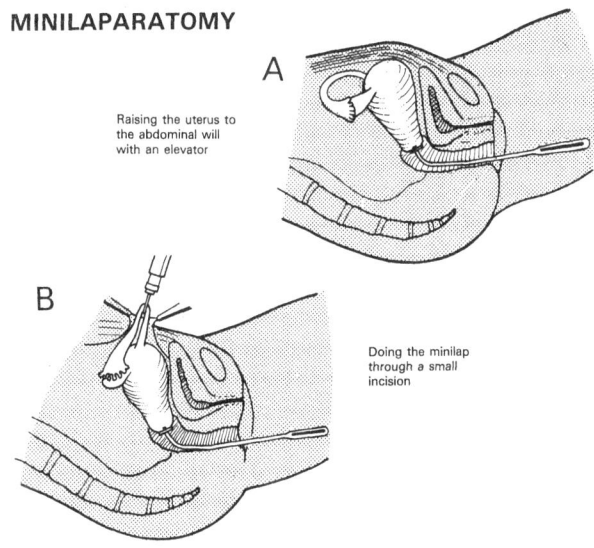

Fig. 15-5 MINILAPAROTOMY. If you wish, you can use a special manipulator to push a patient's fundus up against her abdominal wall, so that a very small incision can be made in her abdomen. If she is immediately postpartum, a manipulator is unnecessary.

If you are using a uterine manipulator, insert it and move to her abdomen. Ask your assistant to raise her fundus against her abdominal wall until you see and feel a bulge. Make a 5 cm midline incision over this.

Tilt the table moderately head down to let her gut fall away from her uterus. Prepare her skin widely with iodine. Drape her abdomen, leaving a large area exposed. Use a 0.4 mm needle to raise bilateral skin wheals, just lateral to her rectus sheath and about 4 cm above the proposed incision. Push a long 1 mm subarachnoid (spinal) needle through the wheal, and inject a track of anaesthetic along either side of the proposed incision, extending well above and below it. Inject 10 ml on each side. These injections just lateral to the rectus sheath block a wide area.

Use a shorter 0.7 mm needle to inject another 10–15 ml into her skin and subcutaneous tissue at the site of the incision.

Inject each rectus muscle through its anterior sheath about 2 cm from the midline. Inject 5 ml at three levels on each side, above, at the level of, and below the planned incision. Expect to find the rectus muscles further apart in multips. A total of 30 ml gives good muscle relaxation.

If you are going through her umbilicus, inject above and below it on both sides so as to infiltrate it completely. Stretch it and make a 2 cm horizontal incision in its inferior fold. Spread the subcutaneous tissue vertically with scissors until you see the fascia. Insert two small narrow right-angled retractors, one towards her head and the other towards her feet, and pull them apart. Pick up the fascia between two haemostats, and inject another 10 ml of lignocaine at a few points just beneath the fascia to anaesthetize her peritoneum. Open the fascia vertically with a knife. You will find it and and her peritoneum almost fused, and will enter her peritoneal cavity bloodlessly. Enlarge the incision in the fascia to admit your index finger. Her skin will stretch, so you can make the skin incision shorter than the fascial one.

If you go through her suprapubic area, do so in the *exact* midline between her rectus muscles. Spread them carefully to avoid bleeding. Spread the fat with scissors until you see her peritoneum. Pick it up, open it, and secure it with haemostats. Optionally, inject 10–20 ml of lignocaine over her pelvic organs for a topical effect.

Feel for her fundus with your index finger. Feel behind it laterally to the point where each ovary is attached. Her tubes lie just anterior to them. As you hook a tube towards the incision with your finger, rotate her uterus to bring its cornua close underneath it. Next, insert two long Langenbeck retractors at right angles to one another. Use the upper one to pull gut and omentum away, and the other to pull laterally, so that you can see the tube. Grasp it with ovum forceps. If it is difficult to find, go to the cornua of her uterus, and follow the tube from there to its fimbriated end.

Deliver a tube into the wound. If it is difficult to deliver, try lowering the head of the table. Look for its fimbrial end, to make sure that it is her Fallopian tube, and not her round or ovarian ligament. Either, (1) apply two clamps, 2 cm apart, cut out a piece of tube between them, and tie each end. Or, (2), alternatively, tie catgut (not monofilament, you want to cause a mild inflammatory reaction) round a loop of tube, and excise it as in Fig. 15-3 (Pomeroy tubal ligation). Does the tube you cut have a lumen? If not, it is her round ligament! There is no need to bury the stumps. Do the same thing on the other side.

CAUTION ! Be sure to use catgut, which is more reliable for this particular purpose than other materials.

Check carefully that there is no bleeding, cut the sutures on the tube, and then operate on the other tube in the same way.

CLOSING HER ABDOMEN. Close her peritoneum and fascia with a suture of 2/0 monofilament. Close all dead space to minimize oozing when the vasoconstrictor effect of the adrenalin wears off.

Sit her up, dress her, and let her walk back to the ward. If you have had to give her extra sedation, she will need help. If she lives close she can go home the same day. If she comes from a remote village, don't discharge her until her sutures have been removed, and her wound has been carefully inspected and palpated—she must not develop a wound infection at home.

DIFFICULTIES WITH A MINILAP

CAUTION ! If you are not operating in a hospital, and there are any complications, treat her as best you can and immediately refer her for admission.

If she complains of PAIN when you are injecting the local anaesthetic, give her intravenous pethidine. A wide area of local anaesthesia should prevent this. She is starved, and if you have great difficulty pulling her tubes into the wound, give her ketamine 2 mg/kg and atropine 0.6 mg intravenously.

If she is OBESE, it will be difficult to pull her tubes into view through a layer of fat. Enlarge the incision and apply more head-down tilt. An umbilical incision may be easier than you expect, because there is less fat around it.

If you CANNOT FIND HER TUBES, (1) the incision may be too far above her fundus; it should be slightly below it. Turning her uterus with your finger behind it helps. If she is is postpartum, and her uterus is large, try manipulating it through her abdominal wall. You may find it helpful not to release the first tube, until you have moved across her fundus and found the other one. Try passing Cusco's speculum through the incision to help you look around. (2) Her uterus may be stuck down with adhesions. A careful initial pelvic examination should have excluded this.

If you find ADHESIONS, you may be able to divide fine ones. Dense ones need general anaesthesia. If her tubes are adherent to her uterus or her pelvis, you may have to make a standard incision, or abandon the operation. This is particularly likely to happen if she has adhesions following Caesarean section.

If you find any CYSTS on her ovaries, leave them if they are small (<5cm). All normal ovaries have some physiological cysts. If a cyst is larger, collapse it by draining it with a syringe and needle, pull it into the wound, and if you don't think it is malignant (20.7), excise it.

If you OPEN HER BLADDER (rare), close it with 2/0 absorbable sutures in two layers, and leave a catheter in for 10 days. Prevent a full bladder by having her empty it *just before she enters the theatre.* If you find it full at surgery, empty it with a needle and syringe.

If you OPEN HER GUT (rare), close it in two layers transversely, 'suck and drip' her for a few days, and observe her closely.

15.4 Using a laprocator

A standard laparoscope is a 1 cm tube, which you insert through a tiny incision near a patient's umbilicus, and which you can use to inspect her abdomen. You can also do a variety of minor operations through it, including tying her tubes. Because a standard laparascope with its associated equipment costs about $3000, and is fragile, a simpler and more robust instrument, the 'Laprocator', has been extensively used by the JHPIEGO programme (Johns Hopkins Program of International Education in Gynaecology and Obstetrics), and is specially adapted for use under the difficult conditions of the developing world. It is only suitable for tubal ligation and diagnostic inspection of the peritoneal cavity, and not for the other procedures which are possible with a standard laparoscope. Unfortunately, like a standard laparoscope, it also needs special training, which is usually given at the JHPIEGO courses, a laprocator being given free to all those who pass the course, and who can demonstrate that they have adequate facilities. It is described here, so that it becomes more widely known. One contributor comments that a standard laparoscope with a separate ring applicator is smaller, safer, and easier to use than a laprocator, the only advantage of which is that JHPIEGO provides it free!

A laprocator is robust, reliable, and relatively inexpensive, and is popular with patients. It has a bulb, not a fibreoptic light source; and you can use it with local anaesthesia, but you will find it more convenient with general anaesthesia. You will need a cylinder of carbon dioxide, but if you can get oxygen, you should be able to get this too.

If you are skilled and have a good team, laparoscopic ligation is quick, and safe, and can be done on outpatients. The incision is so small that it soon becomes almost invisible. If you use carbon dioxide and not air, there is no risk of air embolism. If you use rings or clips instead of diathermy, you will not injure the gut.

THE JHPIEGO LAPROCATOR

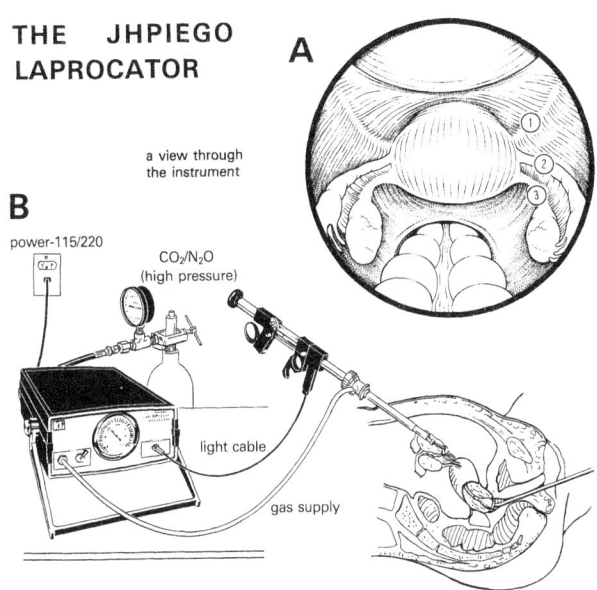

Fig 15-6 THE JHPIEGO LAPROCATOR. A, a view through the eyepiece. B, the instrument in use. 1, the patient's round ligaments. 2, her tubes. 3, her ovarian ligaments. See also Fig. 20-17.

There are disadvantages. A laprocator is delicate, and the possible complications include burns, air embolism, and bleeding, and if you don't sterilize it properly, peritonitis.

You can introduce the laprocator through a small laparotomy incision, or you can use a special trocar called the Verres needle. If you are a beginner, start with the open laparoscopy method described below, which is safer and does not need a CO_2 supply. The only disadvantage of the open method is that the skin incision is slightly longer, and needs two sutures instead of one.

Laparoscopy has caught the imagination of doctors and patients. Illogically perhaps, possessing one is likely to increase your interest in sterilization. If you demonstrate it at at health education talks (M 7.1), you can be sure that some mothers will come forward afterwards to have their tubes tied.

• LAPROCATOR, JHPIEGO pattern (JHP), with Verres gas needle, and carbon dioxide supply, in case complete, one only.

USING THE LAPROCATOR

INDICATIONS. (1) For sterilization. (2) For the diagnosis of PID, endometriosis, and the exclusion of ectopic pregnancy.

CONTRAINDICATIONS. (1) Most lower abdominal scars. If you are experienced you can do a laparoscopy, if the scar was for a lower-segment Caesarean section, because it seldom causes adhesions between the gut and the abdominal wall. (2) A history of chronic PID with possible adhesions. (3) Extreme obesity. *Mild* obesity is an indication for laparoscopy, because the incision does not have to be larger if a patient is mildly obese, as it does in a minilap.

EQUIPMENT. A laprocator, with its carbon dioxide supply; a uterine manipulator. If possible sterilize it in 'Cydex', otherwise immerse it in aqueous 0.5% chlorhexidine changed weekly.

ANAESTHESIA. (1) General anaesthesia. (2) Pethidine with diazepam (A 8.8). (3) Ketamine (A 8.1). (4) Local infiltration (A 6.7).

PREPARATION. Put the patient into the semilithotomy position, as for a minilap. Clean her abdomen, perineum, and vagina. Empty her bladder. Pass a uterine manipulator and attach it to her cervix. Move up to her abdomen. Wait until she is relaxed and not coughing. Tilt her head downwards.

LAPAROSCOPY WITH THE VERRES GAS NEEDLE

If you are right-handed, stand on her left. Move your mask down your nose to prevent your breath clouding the lens. Hold her abdominal wall with your left hand, and insert the needle with your right hand. Hold it by the barrel, so that the blunt trocar is free to slide up and allow the cutting needle to enter. Make a nick in the lower border of her umbilicus, and insert the Verres needle through it almost at right angles to her skin, pointing it slightly towards her feet. Insert it firmly and feel it penetrate her rectus sheath and peritoneum.

Use the following methods to check that the end of the Verres needle is indeed in her peritoneal cavity: (1) You are able to move its point freely from side to side. Be careful as you do this, and don't use force, because you may tear adhesions. (2) When you lift up her abdominal wall, the pressure shown on the gauge falls, and a drop of saline, placed over the hub of the needle, is sucked in. (3) CO_2 flows into her peritoneal cavity with little resistance. There will be a normal range of insufflation pressures for your machine, shown in green on the dial. If the pointer moves to the red area, the needle is probably in the wrong place. (4) A small volume of CO_2 obliterates the normal dullness to percussion over her liver.

Let the CO_2 flow into her peritoneal cavity. A multip who is being sterilized needs up to 4 litres (2 are usually enough). A nullip who is having a laparoscopy for diagnosis needs 2 or 3 litres. The insufflator does not measure volume, but carbon dioxide flows at the rate of a litre a minute, so allow it to flow for 2 minutes.

Remove the Verres needle, and enlarge the skin incision with a scalpel, until you have a 1.5 cm horizontal incision at the lower border of her umbilicus. Insert the trocar and cannula. Push it in almost at right angles to her skin, pointing slightly towards her feet. You will have to push quite hard, so keep the trocar sharp. *A blunt trocar is dangerous, and much more difficult to control.* Prevent it from going in too far by placing one finger alongside the cannula as a guard. When it is through her peritoneum, withdraw the trocar into the cannula, and insert the cannula fully. Withdraw the trocar fully and insert the laparoscope. Touch her gut to clear the objective lens.

Look for her tubes. Recognize them because: (1) They join her uterus at the cornua, whereas her round and ovarian ligaments join it below the cornua. (2) They are in the middle behind her round ligaments and in front of her ovarian ligaments. (3) They end in fimbriae. (3) You can pull them up to form a loop, much more easily than you can pull up a loop of her round or ovarian ligaments.

If you have difficulty manipulating her tubes, try inserting the gas needle in the midline 5 cm below her umbilicus. Turn the knob on it to prevent gas leaking. Use it to help you manipulate her tubes.

Apply one ring or two clips to each tube. Withdraw the laparoscope. Open the valve to expel the CO_2 and remove the cannula. Close her skin with one catgut suture or a skin clip.

OPEN LAPAROSCOPY WITH THE LAPROCATOR

INDICATIONS. (1) Beginners. (2) The absence of a CO_2 supply.

METHOD. Apply two tenaculum forceps to the floor of her umbilicus, one towards her head and the other towards her feet. Pull on them to lift her umbilicus away from her gut.

Make a horizontal incision with a scalpel through her umbilicus, her abdominal wall, and her peritoneum into her abdomen. All the layers of her abdomen are adherent here, so you will go through them as a single layer. Make the incision at least 2 cm long, and if necessary longer. When your are in her abdominal cavity, insert the laparoscope with its cannula, but without its trocar. Use two towel clips to tighten the skin around it and prevent gas leaking.

Fill her peritoneum with two litres of gas. If necessary, you can safely use air instead of CO_2, because there is now no danger of air embolism.

Proceed as if you were using a laprocator by the closed method above. The skin incision is a bit longer, and you may need two sutures.

Using air for the pneumoperitoneum. The laprocator control box has a small air reservoir which is filled by a rubber pump. Switch the gas tube to the patient from the carbon dioxide output to the air output, and fill her abdomen with air through the cannula. Air is only slowly absorbed, so take care to let it all out when you have finished.

If you use air through the Verres needle for closed laparoscopy, remember the possibility of air embolism (uncommon). Also, if you allow air to get into the wrong place, for example into the extraperitoneal tissues, you will not be able to wait a few minutes and try again, because it takes hours to be reabsorbed.

DIFFICULTIES WITH THE LAPROCATOR

If CO_2 GOES INTO THE EXTRAPERITONEAL TISSUES, it will take a minute or two to be absorbed. Wait until it has gone and then try again.

If there is EXTENSIVE BLEEDING, because you have damaged her mesenteric vessels (rare), do a laparotomy and tie them, taking the precautions listed in Section 66.10.

If you have DAMAGED HER AORTA OR VENA CAVA, do a laparotomy. This should never happen if you go in below her umbilicus and keep in the midline. But it has happened!

If you CANNOT SEE HER TUBES, abandon the procedure, or do a laparotomy.

If you mistakenly put a RING ON AN IMPORTANT WRONG STRUCTURE, you can usually pull it off again by catching its edge with one prong of the laprocator forceps. If this fails do a laparotomy.

If you PERFORATE HER GUT with the trocar, do a laparotomy, oversew the perforation with two layers of 2/0 catgut, and give her antibiotics (2.9). There is no need for a proximal colostomy, unless her gut is diseased.

If you PERFORATE HER GUT with the insufflation needle, give her antibiotics and observe her closely. *Don't* do a laparotomy unless she develops signs of peritonitis.

15.5 Vasectomy

Primary Mother Care explains what a couple should know about vasectomy (3.18). Although it is a simple operation, it must be done well, because its success as a family planning procedure depends on there being very few side-effects.

The normal vas is about 2.5 mm in diameter. When you pinch it between your finger and thumb, it has a characteristic firm feel, like partly cooked spaghetti. It is difficult to feel immediately behind a patient's testis, but between the upper pole of his testis and his inguinal ring you can feel it quite easily, and deliver several centimetres of it through a small incision in his scrotum. Rarely, it is double, which is one reason why vasectomy occasionally fails.

After you have incised his skin, you will meet his superficial fascia containing his dartos muscle. Deep to this lies the connective tissue which sheaths his spermatic cord. When you reach his vas, you will find that this also has a sheath of its own. Take care: (1) Don't injure the veins of his spermatic cord (the pampiniform plexus), which will bleed during the operation, and possibly afterwards also. (2) Don't tie his testicular artery, or his testis will atrophy.

• FORCEPS, *vasectomy, two only.* If you are going to do many vasectomies, get these.

VASECTOMY

THE CONTRAINDICATIONS to vasectomy as an outpatient include: a varicocele, a large hydrocele, a local scar, an inguinal hernia, genital tract infection, diabetes, recent coronary heart disease, and filariasis.

EQUIPMENT. Ideally use the special vasectomy forceps shown in Fig. 15-6. A No. 15 scalpel and blade, mosquito forceps, equipment for local anaesthesia, No. 0 plain catgut, 1% lignocaine.

PREPARATION. Ask the patient to shave his scrotum before the operation, and bring with him a tight-fitting undergarment to support it afterwards. Take careful aseptic precautions, scrub up, and wear a mask. There is no need for a gown. Either shave the relevant part of his scrotum just before you operate, or clip it. Prepare the skin of his scrotum.

CAUTION ! Don't use iodine—it is painful on the scrotum.

FINDING AND ANCHORING HIS VAS. Stand on his right. Find his vas where it is easily palpable in his scrotum. Pull on his spermatic cord just above his testis, with the thumb and index finger of your right hand.

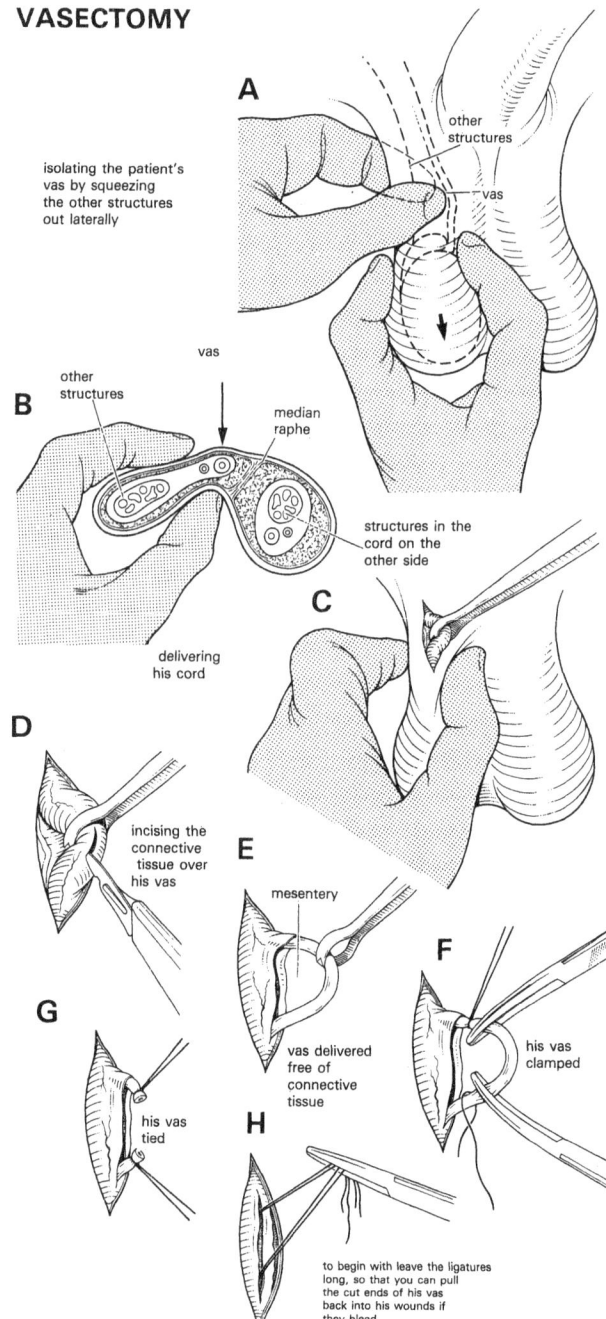

Fig. 15-7 VASECTOMY. A, and B, isolating a patient's vas from the other structures in his cord. C, delivering his vas with vasectomy forceps. D, incising the connective tissue over it. E, freeing it from its mesentery. F, clamping it. G, a piece of vas excised. H, the ligatures left long initially, in case the cut ends bleed.

Use the thumb and fingers of your left hand to manipulate his cord, so as to push his vas upwards and medially into the anterior part of his scrotum close to its median raphe. Isolate his vas from the other structures, by squeezing them out laterally (A, in Fig. 15-7).

Hold his vas well above his testis with your thumb over it and two fingers underneath it. If his skin is thin you will be able to see it. Pulling on it will cause him some discomfort, and pain referred to his abdomen. This is a useful sign that you have indeed found it (B).

CAUTION ! Make sure you have isolated and anchored it in the manner described. This is the critical step. Doing it without causing discomfort needs practice.

ANAESTHESIA. With his vas now anchored, find an area in his skin which is free of cutaneous blood vessels, and use 1% lignocaine to raise a small wheal. Then push the needle deeper and inject 1 or 2 ml of solution as close to it as you can, while holding it away from the other structures in his cord. If he has persistent discomfort while you are handling it, inject more solution into its sheath.

CAUTION ! Don't infiltrate the other structures in his cord. This is unnecessary and dangerous, because you may injure his pampiniform plexus. If there is adrenalin in the anaesthetic solution, it will constrict the vessels, and make his testis temporarily ischaemic and painful.

Pull his testis downwards, so as to tighten his spermatic cord. Carefully feel for his vas.

If you cannot feel his vas (rare), don't give up too soon. If you still cannot feel it, leave it *don't explore his cord*. Proceed to operate on the other side. Very occasionally the vas is absent. If you have not been able to find it, you will know whether it is indeed absent, by examining his ejaculate later.

DELIVERING HIS VAS. While still firmly anchoring it, incise the skin over it vertically. Push the tip of mosquito forceps, or blunt dissecting forceps through the incision, and split his dartos vertically. Then push vasectomy forceps into the incision. Confirm that his vas has not slipped away by feeling it with these forceps. Open them just wide enough to grip it. Release your fingers, which are holding his testis and cord, and pull his cord gently into the incision (C).

CAUTION ! Don't mistake his vas for thickened bands of cremaster muscle, thrombosed veins, thickened lymphatics, or calcified worms.

TO ISOLATE HIS VAS FROM ITS SHEATH lever the tip of the forceps upwards by lowering their handle. Use a No. 15 blade to incise the connective tissue over his vas vertically in line with it. Make sure that the connective tissue is completely divided by continuing the incision into the vas itself (D).

Hold a segment of his exposed vas with a second pair of vas forceps, or with a special vasectomy hook. Meanwhile, release the first forceps. If you have judged the site and depth of your incision correctly, you can now easily pull out his vas, leaving only a thin mesentery on its medial surface (E).

Use mosquito forceps to make a small window in a piece of the mesentery of his vas which is free of blood vessels. Isolate a 1 to 5 cm segment of vas between clamps. Tie its clamped ends with catgut, placing your ties beyond the clamped area (F). Excise the isolated segment (G).

CAUTION ! (1) Don't put the ligatures over the crushed area. (2) Don't tie them too tight, or they will cut out. (4) To begin with, leave the ends of the sutures long, so that, if the cut ends of his vas bleed, you can pull them back into the wound. (5) Leave a reasonable length of vas above his epididymis. If a reanastomosis has to be done later, this will make it easier. Keep the ligatures away from his epididymis.

Pull on his testis to separate the ends of his vas. Inspect the wound. If it bleeds, pull out the ends of his vas, and tie any bleeders with plain catgut. Then cut the ends of the ligatures short and drop them back.

CAUTION ! (1) Don't damage his pampiniform plexus. (2) Control all bleeding carefully. A small vessel can form a big haematoma later. He can also bleed from the skin edges, from the fascial sheath covering his vas, or from his pampiniform plexus.

If the incision is less than 1 cm, the skin edges may come together without any sutures. If necessary, suture them with catgut, using a mattress suture if they need to be everted. Place a swab on the wound, and hold it with strapping.

Repeat the same procedure on the other side of his scrotum through a separate incision.

Alternatively it is not obligatory to wears gloves. If you choose not to wear them, handle his vas only with sterile instruments, using a strict no-touch technique.

POSTOPERATIVELY, the sutures will fall out by themselves. Ask him to rest after the operation, and not to do any heavy manual work for a day or two.

CHECKUP. Warn him that he may not become sterile for up to 3 weeks. He should continue to use a contraceptive: (1) until two examinations of his ejaculate have shown no sperm, or (2) until he has had 15 ejaculations after vasectomy.

To examine his ejaculate, ask him to produce a specimen by masturbation, or from a condom after intercourse. Put several loopfuls under a microscope, and examine them for sperm under the low power. There should be none.

DIFFICULTIES WITH VASECTOMY

If you CANNOT FIND HIS VAS, don't continue the operation under local anaesthesia as an outpatient.

If YOU LOSE THE CUT ENDS of his vas after sectioning them, try to recover them by systematically palpating his vas, and feeling for them with forceps. The ligature may have slipped, or you may have released the forceps holding his vas too soon, and let them be drawn quite a distance into his scrotum. Don't injure any blood vessels. If you cannot find the cut ends, the operation will still probably succeed. Tell him that you have had difficulty, and watch for haematoma formation. Check to see that his ejaculate becomes sperm-free.

If a HAEMATOMA FORMS, it may spread into his scrotum, his thighs, or his abdominal wall. If it is small, it will disappear spontaneously. If it is larger, you may have to admit him and evacuate it.

If his WIFE BECOMES PREGNANT, either vasectomy has failed, or he is not the father. If sperms are present in his ejaculate, you can re-explore his vas under general anaesthesia, and divide it again. Consider carefully what you should tell him! A more diplomatic alternative than testing his sperm count is to tell the couple that his vasectomy has presumably not worked, and to offer the wife sterilization.

HAEMOSTASIS MUST BE ABSOLUTE

---

16 The surgery of pregnancy

16.1 Surgical problems in pregnancy

The staff in your clinics should be able to manage most of the minor complications of pregnancy. In early pregnancy they will need to refer incomplete abortions, especially septic ones (6.6a). McDonald's suture (16.5) will prevent some second-trimester abortions. They will also need to refer acute ectopic pregnancies (16.6), and, if they are well-trained, an occasional chronic one (16.7). Rarely, you may have to treat an abdominal pregnancy (16.9), a missed abortion (16.4), or a hydatidiform mole (32.38).

Late in pregnancy, after the 28th week, your main concerns will be antepartum haemorrhage, from *placenta praevia* (16.12) or placental abruption (16.13). Both of these need differentiation from incidental bleeding from lower in the birth canal. Another problem will be the dead baby, whose management before 18 weeks differs from that later on (16.4).

16.2 Evacuating an abortion

Primary Mother Care tells midwives how to evacuate an incomplete abortion, if they have to, using their fingers and sponge forceps. Here we describe the hospital procedure for doing the same thing. For septic abortions see Section 6.6a.

Many abortions don't need evacuating (see below), but those that do need evacuating soon, so don't let incomplete abortions wait unnecessarily. Evacuating a pregnant uterus differs from curetting a non-pregnant one (20.3) in two important ways: (1) After an abortion the cervix is open, so there is rarely any need to dilate it. (2) The wall of an infected uterus is so soft that you can perforate it much more easily with a curette.

SOME TERMINOLOGY An abortion is the expulsion of a pregnancy from the uterus before 28 weeks. An early (first trimester) abortion occurs before 14 weeks, a late one (second trimester) from 14 to 28 weeks. A septic abortion is an incomplete abortion with signs of intrauterine infection. Postabortal sepsis is pelvic infection after a complete abortion. A missed abortion is an intrauterine death during the first trimester or early in the second, after which the pregnancy is not expelled for at least another month. A carneous mole is a continuation of a missed abortion, in which the dead fetus is surrounded by shells of organized blood clot. Habitual abortion is a sequence of three successive first trimester abortions, or two successive second trimester ones.

An abortion goes through these stages: (1) threatened (bleeding and perhaps cramps, but the cervix is still closed), (2) inevitable (the cervix is open but no products of conception have been expelled), (3) incomplete (part of the products have been expelled), and (4) complete (all the products have been expelled, bleeding has stopped, the cervix is closed, and the uterus is now much too small for the duration of the pregnancy). In the first trimester the distinction between an inevitable and an incomplete abortion is pointless, because you can manage them both in the same way. In the second trimester the distinction is important, because an inevitable abortion is not ready for evacuation, whereas an incomplete one must be evacuated. Before 14–16 weeks it is difficult to tell if an abortion is complete or not; because to make sure it is complete you have to identify the fetus and the whole of the placenta, with the membranes, as fully formed structures. Before 14–16 weeks they are not sufficiently well formed for you to be sure about this.

SITI (27 years) was admitted with a threatened 16-week abortion. It seemed to settle, and she was discharged, but she bled in the bus on the way home and was readmitted. Fetal parts were extracted through a dilated cervix, and traumatized pieces of gut were seen through it. A laparotomy showed a tear in her descending colon, old clots and pus in her peritoneal cavity, and a rupture of her uterus. The tear in her descending colon was sutured and her abdomen closed. Some days later she passed faeces through her cervix. She was re-explored, and a proximal defunctioning colostomy was done, after which she eventually recovered. LESSONS This true story is an extreme case. It shows the magnitude of the disasters that can follow the mismanagement of what might seem to be quite a minor condition. She was fortunate to escape with her life. The many lessons include: (1) An abortionist had tried to abort a 16-week pregnancy, which is dangerously late. (2) If an abortion is incomplete, evacuation is mandatory. She should not have been discharged before her uterus had been emptied. (3) Whenever the large gut has to be repaired, a proximal defunctioning colostomy must be done immediately. Had this been done at her first laparotomy, she would not have required another one.

BLEEDING BEFORE THE 28TH WEEK

THE DIFFERENTIAL DIAGNOSIS includes the various stages of abortion, ectopic pregnancy (16.6), and hydatidiform mole (32.38). In late pregnancy consider also *placenta praevia* (16.12), and abruption (16.13). There are also gynaecological causes of bleeding: trichomoniasis, candidiasis, venereal warts, cervical polypi, cervical erosions, and cervicitis. These can all cause a bloody vaginal discharge. Also, a patient may not be pregnant, and have DUB (dysfunctional uterine bleeding, 20.2). Much bleeding remains unexplained.

THREATENED ABORTION. Ask her to rest in bed at home and give her a sedative (although neither are of proven value). Admit her if: (1) She has bled much (regardless of her gestational age). (2) She is more than 14 weeks pregnant. (3) She has a bad obstetric history (admit her for psychological reasons), or she lives far away and cannot get help if bleeding becomes much worse, especially during the night.

UNCOMPLICATED INEVITABLE ABORTIONS. Here are the instructions for an uninfected abortion. If a patient is febrile, has a foul discharge, and perhaps signs of peritonitis, her abortion is septic, so see Section 6.6a. Management also depends on the duration of her pregnancy.

If she is less than 14 weeks, monitor her pulse, blood pressure, and temperature, her peripheral circulation, and the amount of bleeding. Measure her haemoglobin, and take a specimen for grouping and cross-matching. Give her 0.25 or 0.5 mg of ergometrine intramuscularly on admission. If she has bled much, set up a drip. Starve her, and prepare to evacuate her uterus as soon as possible. If it is the custom of the hospital to shave her labia and perineum, do so.

If you have plenty of theatre time, you will save time and morbidity if you take all abortions less than 14 weeks, other than threatened ones, to the theatre for formal evacuation.

If theatre time is scarce the mandatory indications for evacuation are: (1) Considerable bleeding (evacuation is urgent). (2) Bleeding which continues for more than 24 hours. (3) Patients in whom the retained products of conception are obviously still present on vaginal examination. Together, these cases form about a quarter of the total; treating the others non-operatively will considerably reduce your workload and is less expensive. Some obstetricians think that all abortions less than 14 weeks, except threatened ones, should be evacuated.

If she is more than 14 weeks, with an inevitable abortion (her cervix is open at least one finger, but the products of conception, especially the fetus, have not been expelled), assess and monitor her as above. *Don't evacuate her uterus until the fetus has been expelled.* When it has been expelled, and there is even a possibility that evacuation is incomplete, complete it. If however the fetus and placenta are expelled together, and the membranes are complete, there will be nothing left to evacuate.

Opinions differ on on the use of a curette after 14 weeks: (1) One contributor considers than an instrument should never be used on an abortion which is more than 14 weeks (except perhaps occasionally ovum forceps). Her cervix will always be open enough for your finger. Fishing around with any instrument in a large flabby uterus for a few fragments of tissue is likely to do more harm than good, especially if you use a standard curette. If she has stopped bleeding, do nothing. If she continues to bleed, put up an oxytocin drip, and give her intravenous ergometrine. This will probably complete her abortion. If these measures fail, and she continues to bleed, explore her uterus as if you were removing her placenta manually (19.11a). (2) Another contributor reminds you that these patients can bleed severely, and cannot always be evacuated with a finger. He advises you to use a large curette carefully!

EVACUATING AN INCOMPLETE ABORTION

ERGOMETRINE may make evacuation unnecessary, so try it first. Give her ergometrine 0.25 mg intravenously or 0.5 mg intramuscularly (0.5 mg intravenously will cause nausea and vomiting, and is unnecessary). The products of conception may be discharged, and she may stop bleeding. If it fails, it will not prevent you dilating her cervix. Alternatively, use ergometrine with oxytocin. Even 0.25 mg will often make her sick, so if there is little bleeding, you can omit it.

RESUSCITATION may be necessary. Do it at the same time as the evacuation.

EQUIPMENT. A catheter. Three ovum forceps or sponge-holding forceps without rachets (one for swabbing the vagina and the other for removing the contents of the uterus), uterine curettes blunt and sharp, preferably a few sizes of each. A vaginal speculum (Sims' or Auvard's). Don't use a sound, because this can readily perforate her uterus. A set of Hegar's dilators (only occasionally necessary).

ANAESTHESIA. (1) Intravenous pethidine with diazepam (A 8.8). (2) Intravenous ketamine (A 8.2). (3) Thiopentone with pethidine (A 8.8), provided she is not shocked and anaemic. Thiopentone alone is adequate, unless you need to dilate her cervix. (4) A saddle block (A 7.7), or a caudal block (A 7.3). (5) Light ether (A 11.3).

CAUTION ! Don't operate until: (1) She has a drip up, if this is necessary. It is necessary if there is: (a) much bleeding, or (b) hypovolaemia or anaemia. Some contributors consider it is mandatory always. It may be unnecessary if she is in vasovagal shock because the placenta is distending her cervix (see below).

METHOD. Put her into the lithotomy position with her buttocks over the end of the table, so that you can insert your instruments comfortably in any direction. Clean her suprapubic area, vulva, and perineum with chlorhexidine, and put a drape under her and on her abdomen. If you cannot drape her, clean her abdomen and thighs. *Take careful aseptic precautions.* Catheterize her bladder. An empty bladder will make it easier for you to check that her uterus is contracting well after evacuation. Use a swab in a sponge-holder to swab out her vagina.

Do a bimanual examination with two fingers in her vagina and your other hand on her abdomen. Check: (1) The state of her cervix and its degree of dilatation. (2) The size of her uterus and the products of conception palpable inside it. (3) Any adnexal masses (don't miss an ectopic pregnancy, but don't use an examination under anaesthesia to diagnose one! 16.6).

If you can get your finger into her cervix, use it to empty her uterus (finger curettage). A finger is much safer than a curette, because you can feel where you are, so avoid using a curette if you can. Put half your hand into her vagina and use your right index or middle finger. *At the same time push down the fundus of her uterus with your left hand on her abdomen,* so that your finger can reach right into it. Ideally this requires good muscular relaxation. If you are using a local block, be gentle, talk to her kindly, and persuade her to relax. Loosen all the retained tissue with your finger. If you can empty her uterus with your finger, there is no need to curette it.

If you cannot get your finger into her cervix, insert a speculum and grasp her cervix with a sponge-holder, as in B, Fig. 16-1. Give her 0.25 mg of ergometrine intravenously, and wait a minute for it to make her uterus contract, harden it, and reduce the risk of perforation. With your left hand pull her cervix well down with the sponge-holder to straighten her uterine cavity. *Keep pulling during the rest of the procedure.* Introduce the second pair of sponge-forceps into her uterus with your right hand. Slide them in gently until you can lightly feel the top of her fundus. Open them, turn them through 90°, close them, and remove them (C). Do this several times, to remove pieces of placenta hanging from her uterine wall, until her uterus is empty.

If you cannot insert your finger or a curette, as occasionally happens in the first trimester when her cervix is not sufficiently dilated but her uterus seems enlarged, dilate it to size 9 Hegar. First insert a small dilator, and then progressively larger ones, until you have reached size 9. You can easily make a cervix incompetent. So don't dilate a cervix beyond Hegar 9.

CAUTION ! (1) Don't put a sound into a pregnant uterus. If you want to know how long it is, insert a large Hegar dilator or sponge-holder and mark how far it goes in with your finger. (2) Be gentle, or you will perforate her fundus. Your exploring finger will have shown you how deep it is. (3) Don't try to put large ovum forceps into an undilated cervix, and don't explore it with other instruments.

With your left hand on her abdomen, explore her uterus again with your finger to make sure it is empty.

If it is not empty, use a blunt curette to remove the remaining pieces of placenta. While it is still hard under the influence of the ergometrine, *very gently* scrape the inside of her uterus with a blunt curette (E). Let it almost rest in your hand as you use it. Leaving the retained products of conception behind is serious, but perforating it (F) is more so. You will know that her uterus is empty by: (1) A characteristic grating feeling (difficult to detect on the anterior surface). If part of its wall feels a little rough, this is probably the placental bed. (2) Your failure to remove any more tissue.

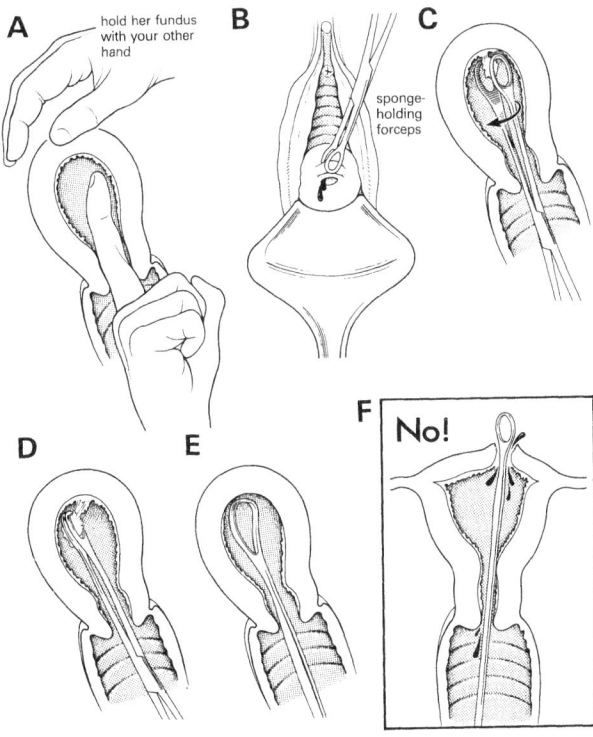

Fig. 16-1 EVACUATING AN INCOMPLETE ABORTION. A, explore the patient's uterus with your finger while your other hand is holding her fundus. You may find it easier to use two fingers or your middle finger. B, grasp her cervix with sponge forceps and use them to pull it down. C, and D, while holding her uterus with your other hand, introduce ring forceps, turn them through 90°, grasp and remove any products of conception, reinsert the forceps and do the same thing again. E, *gently* curette her uterus. F, this is the disaster you are trying to avoid!

CAUTION ! Don't curette a uterus which has not been hardened by ergometrine. An intravenous dose will keep it contracted for about half an hour, and an intramuscular one for somewhat longer.

Finally, do a bimanual compression (19-9) to encourage contraction and expel clots from her uterus. Put two fingers into her anterior vaginal fornix, and your other hand on to her abdominal wall. Compress her uterus between them.

Send her back to the ward with a vulval pad. Inspect this from time to time during the first hour or two after the evacuation. If bleeding recurs, give her another dose of ergometrine 0.5 mg intramuscularly.

POSTOPERATIVELY, monitor her for further bleeding and check her vital signs. If she is well send her home the next day, and advise her on contraception, which should be part of the ward routine. If there has been a suspicion of interference or venereal infection, consider giving her the appropriate broad-spectrum antibiotic (for example, tetracycline) for a few days.

DIFFICULTIES EVACUATING A UTERUS

See also Sections 6.6aD and 20.3 (dilatation and curettage).

If she is admitted apparently VERY SHOCKED, and is hypotensive and semiconscious, she may be having a VASOVAGAL ATTACK because the placenta has stuck in her cervix (common). Her external os may be tight, while her internal os and cervical canal dilate to accommodate the pregnancy. This is quite different from a cervical pregnancy (rare, 16.8). Don't wait to put up a drip. Remove the placenta with a gloved finger on the ward without anaesthesia. If this fails (unusual), pass a Sims' or Cusco's speculum. If you see products of conception in her cervix, remove them with sponge forceps. She will recover miraculously.

If she is ADMITTED WITH HEAVY BLEEDING, resuscitate her, give her ergometrine, and at the same time evacuate her uterus with a finger on the ward. Even if evacuation is not complete, it will help to stop bleeding.

If she is or becomes SERIOUSLY ANAEMIC, are you going to transfuse her? If yours is a high-HIV area, you will hardly transfuse anybody. In a low-HIV area, if her haemoglobin is >100 g/l, transfusion is unnecessary; between 80 and 100 g/l transfuse her only if she is symptomatic; if it is below 80 g/l transfuse her. Always give her iron.

If you find INJURIES to her vagina, cervix or uterus, and there is a possibility that an instrument has entered her abdominal cavity, do a laparotomy immediately, and inspect it.

If SHE DOES NOT IMPROVE after evacuation, reconsider the diagnosis. She may have an ectopic pregnancy, or be severely anaemic, or have a collection of pus. If you find an abscess in her pouch of Douglas, drain it (6.5).

If you think you have PERFORATED HER UTERUS, console yourself with the thought that experts sometimes also do this, perhaps more often than they admit.

If you perforate her uterus after you have emptied it, and you don't think you have damaged her gut or omentum (they don't appear in her vagina), send her back to the ward. Starve her, set up a drip, give her antibiotics (2.9), and observe her pulse, temperature, and blood pressure carefully. Her perforation will probably heal. If there are increasing signs of infection or bleeding (unusual), do a laparotomy to sew up the wound in her uterus.

If you perforate her uterus before you empty it, you have the difficult task of completing the evacuation in the presence of a perforation. If you can do a laparoscopy (unlikely, 15.4), you can observe her uterus while you curette it. If not, accept that evacuation is incomplete, give her antibiotics, set up a drip, and observe her very carefully.

If she collapses, and OMENTUM OR GUT APPEAR IN HER VAGINA (very rare), you have certainly perforated her uterus. If this happens, do an immediate laparotomy, and sew up the tear. If her large gut is perforated, do a diversionary colostomy (9.5). If there is severe bleeding or an extensive tear, tie her internal iliac arteries (3.5). If this fails a hysterectomy may be necessary. If you have sewn up a tear, warn her that her uterus is in danger of rupturing in later pregnancies. She will need an elective Caesarean section (18.9).

If you FEEL A FIBROID in her uterus (uncommon), it may have been the cause of her abortion (unusual). Leave it for 3 months before you treat it. If it is pedunculated and submucous with a narrow neck, *don't be tempted to to twist it off vaginally*. This can cause severe bleeding. Leave it for 3 months. See Section 20.6.

If BLEEDING DOES NOT STOP after the evacuation, it is probably due to poor contraction of her uterus, or there may still be products of conception in her uterus. Often there is no obvious reason. (1) Make sure her uterus is empty. (2) Give her a second dose of intravenous ergometrine, rub up her uterus to stop it bleeding, and repeat bimanual compression. *Be patient at this stage,* 5 or 10 minutes of bimanual compression may be necessary, but it will usually succeed. (3) If this fails, give her an oxytocin drip (40 units per litre), and run this in fast.

If the above measures fail to control bleeding (rare), curette her again if you have not already done so. Don't try packing her uterus, it will not remove the cause of the bleeding.

If even this fails to control bleeding (very rare), tie both her internal iliac arteries (for a discussion as to the feasibility of doing this see Section 3.5). If even this fails (very rare indeed), a hysterectomy is necessary. See also cervical ectopic pregnancies (very rare) in Section 16.8.

If you think you are evacuating an incomplete abortion, and yet there are VERY FEW CURETTINGS, her abortion is probably complete. There is however a possibility that your diagnosis may be wrong, and that she has a CHRONIC ECTOPIC. Read the story of Theresa in Section 16.7.

If you feel that she has a UTERINE SEPTUM, clean out each side of her uterine cavity.

BE CAREFUL WITH THE CURETTE!

16.4 Fetal death, missed abortion, and intrauterine death

A baby can die at any time during pregnancy. What you can do about it depends on whether he dies before or after 18 weeks. Before this time his death is termed a missed abortion, after it he is an intrauterine death.

Before 18 weeks a dead baby is usually aborted without his mother knowing that he is dead. Occasionally however, the abortion is delayed for several weeks (a missed abortion). When this happens the only sign of fetal death is that her uterus fails to grow. Or, she may have a threatened abortion which stops bleeding, and is followed by a brown discharge and no further periods. Although the loss of a baby may be tragic, a missed abortion has few risks, there is little risk of a clotting defect this early in pregnancy, and provided nobody interferes, she runs no risk of infection.

After about 18 weeks: (1) a mother is aware of the death of her baby (intrauterine death) because the fetal movements stop, or do not occur when they should (18 to 22 weeks in a primip, 16 to 20 weeks in a multip). (2) The fetal heart cannot be heard when it should be (28 weeks), but remember that this is an unreliable sign, especially if she is fat, or has polyhydramnios. Listen to it electronically if you can. (3) The height of her fundus, as found by palpation, fails to match that expected from her dates. Instead, it either remains stationary or falls (M 6.4). For this sign to be useful, the height of her fundus above her *symphysis pubis* must be measured accurately with a tape measure. So, when fetal death is suspected, impress this on your midwives. (4) There are radiological signs of fetal death, but they are not easy before 28 weeks. The most reliable ones are overlapping of the bones of the baby's skull (Spalding's sign), hyperflexion of his spine, and gas in his great vessels. Endocrine tests for pregnancy take 4 or even 8 weeks to become negative, so they are of little value.

If you do nothing, there is a ninety per cent chance that she will deliver her baby in 4 weeks, whatever the duration of her pregnancy. But, as long as he remains inside her, she runs the remote but serious risk of a serious coagulation defect, and catastrophic bleeding. This risk is low initially, but increases with time, particularly after he has been dead 4 to 6 weeks. Rupturing the membranes to induce labour is dangerous, because the dead fetal tissues are easily infected by anaerobes. The following regime attempts to balance these risks. Use oxytocin and/or prostaglandins. The sensitivity of her uterus to prostaglandins remains constant, but its sensitivity to oxytocin increases with each gestational week.

Prostaglandins are expensive. The most commonly used one is PGE_2 or dinoprostone ('Prostin' E_2 Upjohn). You can use: (1) A solution of prostaglandin instilled into the extra-amniotic space through a Foley catheter. (2) Pessaries or tablets in the posterior fornix (19.3).

THE DEAD BABY

DEATH BEFORE 18 WEEKS (missed abortion)

If a mother's uterus is small for her gestational age, perhaps with a brownish vaginal discharge, suspect the death of her baby. Monitor the growth of her uterus carefully. If he is dead, it will not grow, and may even become smaller. Pregnancy tests become negative. Methods of detecting the fetal heartbeat vary in their sensitivity: ultrasound scanning detects it at 8 weeks, Doppler ultrasound at 10–16 weeks, and an ordinary stethoscope at 20–28 weeks.

THE DIFFERENTIAL DIAGNOSIS includes a normal pregnancy of shorter duration (wrong dates), a slow-leaking ectopic pregnancy, a false pregnancy, and fibroids.

MANAGEMENT. You can, if you wish do nothing for several weeks. Spontaneous abortion will inevitably follow. Alternatively:

If her uterus is smaller than 10 weeks (a *small* orange), you can do a 'D and C', either using the ordinary method (16.2) or a Karman curette. Give her perioperative chloramphenicol and metronidazole (2.9) when you do this (one contributor considers this unnecessary). Dilate her cervix up to at least Hegar 10. If possible, 'prime' her cervix with prostaglandins beforehand. Either, (1) put a 0.5 mg tablet of prostaglandin E_2 in her cervix, and repeat this 6-hourly for 24 hours. Or, (2) place 3 mg prostaglandin E_2 vaginal tablets in her vagina 6 hourly. Or, (3) use a newer preparation, gemeprost ('Cervagem').

If you are using a Karman curette, dilate her cervix to 8 Hegar and then use a Number 8 Karman curette with a vacuum of up to 500 mm Hg. Continue until her uterus is empty, and you can feel her uterus tight round the curette.

If her uterus is larger than 10 weeks, don't attempt an ordinary 'D and C'. Instead, either use oxytocin and/or prostaglandins, see below. Or, dilate her uterus to 11 Hegar, and use a No 10 Karman curette, which is safe up to 12 weeks—*but not beyond!*.

CAUTION ! Attempting to do a 'D and C' on a uterus larger than this can cause disastrous bleeding, and perhaps infection. We have advised a 10-week threshold rather than the more normal 12 weeks, to allow for a margin of error.

DEATH AFTER 18 WEEKS (intrauterine death)

A mother notices that fetal movements stop, or do not occur when they should (at 18 weeks). Or, a midwife fails to hear the fetal heart after 24 weeks. If possible, confirm the absence of the fetal heartbeat with Doppler ultrasound. During 2 to 4 weeks observe if her uterus fails to grow or gets smaller.

CAUTION ! A pregnancy test is no use at this stage. It may be positive when the baby is dead.

THE DIFFERENTIAL DIAGNOSIS includes: (1) A normal pregnancy of shorter duration (wrong dates). (2) A hydatidiform mole. (3) Polyhydramnios (her uterus will be large for her dates). (4) Multiple gestation with small fetuses. (5) An abdominal pregnancy. (6) Ascites, an ovarian tumour, fibroids, or a false pregnancy.

MANAGEMENT. Do nothing for a month after the fetal movements have stopped. Explain carefully why you are doing nothing. She may find this difficult to understand and her husband may try to persuade you to act prematurely. Explain that, if you attempt induction by the method below, it may fail and she may need a few days rest before you try again.

If she is still undelivered a month after fetal movements have stopped, consider induction. Before you induce her, check her clotting time (16.13).

AN ESCALATING OXYTOCIN DRIP. Use this regime from about 10 (before which it is unnecessary), until about 28 weeks when the method in Section 19.3 is indicated. See also Section 18.4a on oxytocin. Her uterus is less likely to rupture in early pregnancy, so start with 5 units of oxytocin in 500 ml of Ringer's lactate or saline, at 25 drops a minute. You may find that labour does not start until the following day. If this fails, repeat the drip the next day with 25 units in 500 ml. If necessary, wait and repeat it in another week. If this does not work, wait and try a third time. You may have to give her up to 100 units in 500 ml (the absolute maximum). Usually, much less is necessary.

EXTRA SPECIAL CAUTION ! is necessary when you use oxytocin at this stage of pregnancy! (1) You may have to use large doses. Oxytocin has an antidiuretic effect, so you can overload her with fluid, so that she develops water intoxication (rare). So: (a) increase the strength of the infusion, rather than the volume you give, (b) give it in Ringer's lactate or saline, rather than 5% dextrose, and (c) give it for a day and then stop. (d) Don't give more than 3 litres of fluid in 24 hours. (e) Keep a fluid-balance chart; if she has a positive fluid-balance of more than 2 litres stop the drip. Because of these dangers some obstetricians wait to let nature take its course between 14 and 28 weeks. (2) Oxytocin can rupture the uterus as early as 18 weeks, so don't give more oxytocin than you need.

If she becomes drowsy or has convulsions while on an oxytocin drip, she has probably developed water intoxication. Stop the drip and let her kidneys excrete the water. Give her a slow infusion of 5% sodium chloride (if you have it).

If an escalating oxytocin drip fails, and the products of conception have not been expelled within 2 to 4 weeks of presention, refer her to an expert. If you cannot refer her, see below.

EXTRA–AMNIOTIC PROSTAGLANDINS. The indications are: (1) The termination of pregnancy after 14 weeks. (2) Missed abortion (intrauterine death) after 14 weeks. (3) The evacuation of a hydatidiform mole.

CAUTION ! With both methods follow the manufacturer's instructions carefully.

Using a Foley catheter (the preferred method). Using a Cusco's speculum and sponge forceps pass a sterile 12 to 14 Ch Foley catheter with a 30 ml balloon gently through her cervix into her extra-amniotic space. A Foley catheter of this size will always enter a pregnant cervix.

Now inject prostaglandin E_2 in the following regime.

Prepare a solution containing 100 micrograms in 1 ml (add 0.5 ml of a 10 mg/ml solution to 50 ml of diluent). Fill the dead space in the catheter system with the dilute drug solution. Then inject 1 ml of solution through the catheter initially, followed by 1 or 2 ml 2-hourly to maintain regular contractions. Go on until the catheter falls out.

Alternatively, cut the tip off the Foley catheter, pass an infant feeding-tube through it, and push the catheter through her cervix, so that the balloon lies just above her internal os. Through the feeding tube instil PG F_2alpha (dinoprost) 5 mg diluted with 4 ml of sterile isotonic saline. Repeat this 2-hourly until she has adequate contractions.

The Foley catheter will always be expelled eventually. Most obstetricians would give her an oxytocin drip at the same time; a few consider this dangerous, and only give oxytocin if prostaglandins fail to establish contractions in 6 hours.

Using dinoprostone (PGE_2) vaginal tablets. The standard tablets are 3 mg ('Prostin' Upjohn, expensive). To terminate her pregnancy, insert 3 mg vaginal tablets in her posterior fornix 4-hourly up to a total of 6 tablets in 24 hours. This will usually evacuate her uterus within 12 hours. If it has not succeeded in 24 hours, try another method, or wait for 2–3 days and try again.

CAUTION ! Don't rupture her membranes. It may hasten delivery, but it is not worth the risk. See also 'Stop Press'.

THE DEAD BABY at term or during labour

See also Sections 18.4 and 18.7.

A dead baby is usually easy to deliver when he has died as the result of gestational hypertension or abruption, because he is usually small and is often macerated. But if he died because labour was obstructed, delivery is more difficult.

Caesarean section might seem to be the obvious answer. Unfortunately, if his head is impacted deep in her pelvis, removing it from her uterus at Caesarean section is difficult. She also runs the serious immediate risk of septic shock and peritonitis, and the later one of a scar in her uterus. Provided his head is well down in her pelvis, an operative vaginal delivery, if necessary a destructive one, will be safer. If it is high, you will have to section her.

DIFFICULTIES with a dead baby before about 30 weeks

If you are NOT SURE IF A BABY IS DEAD OR NOT, wait, and see her again in 2 weeks. If necessary, wait 4 weeks. By this time it should be clear if he is dead or not.

If delivering a dead baby late in pregnancy or at term is complicated by SEVERE BLEEDING, disseminated intravascular coagulation (DIC) is a possibility, so see Section 19.11a. Maintain her blood volume, and try to give her fresh blood. If bleeding is not controlled by two doses of ergometrine with oxytocin ('Syntometrine'), or by ergometrine alone, intravenously or intramuscularly, give her a prostaglandin such as dinoprost ('Prostin $F_2\alpha$') 250 to 500 µg directly into the myometrium through her abdominal wall. Try compressing her uterus, pack it for 24 hours, and then remove the pack. This is a useful temporary measure for any bleeding uterus, and may save the need to do a laparotomy. If this fails to control bleeding, tie her internal iliac arteries (3.5). If this too fails, remove her uterus (20.12). Give her fresh blood.

If oxytocin and prostaglandins FAIL TO EXPEL A DEAD BABY (rare), suspect an extrauterine pregnancy (16.6).

If she has FEVER and GASTROINTESTINAL SYMPTOMS while she is having prostaglandins, these are probably side-effects. They are much less likely when lower doses are instilled through a Foley catheter.

16.5 Suturing an incompetent cervix for recurrent second-trimester abortions

Mothers with a history of repeated first-trimester abortions are not easy to help. These are often the result of of some fetal abnormality for which nothing can be done. The best advice for them is to: "Keep trying". Most of them will eventually achieve a sucessful pregnancy.

Second-trimester abortions are different. They are not usually caused by recognizable fetal abnormalities. Some are due to maternal illness (syphilis, hypertension, diabetes, etc.), or to a congenital malformation of the uterine cavity. Others are caused by a somewhat mysterious condition called 'cervical incompetence'. As in the first trimester, often no cause can be found. The prognosis of a mother with repeated second-trimester abortions depends on the cause, and is excellent if syphilis can be treated, or cervical incompetence corrected surgically. Hypertension and diabetes are more difficult to treat, and the outcome of the pregnancy is less certain. Mothers in whom no cause can be found have a reasonable prognosis: about 70 per cent of their pregnancies go to term.

Here we are concerned with the management of patients with 'suspected cervical incompetence'. This means that the cervix opens spontaneously during the second trimester, without the uterus contracting. Sometimes this is due to a too-forceful dilatation during a 'D and C', or to a previous traumatic delivery. Usually, there is no obvious cause.

The diagnosis is difficult. It is usually made by the history alone. A typical patient gives a history of two or more spontaneous second-trimester abortions, without uterine contractions (until the membranes have ruptured), or bleeding. Her first symptom is a watery vaginal discharge, often followed by a sudden loss of amniotic fluid. Soon afterwards the fetus is delivered, sometimes still alive. The diagnosis is only certain in the present pregnancy if the uterus is found to be effacing and dilating, without any uterine contractions. When this is happening it is too late to insert a cervical suture—in this pregnancy.

Doctors differ greatly in the frequency with which they diagnose 'cervical incompetence'. True cervical incompetence is probably quite rare. If you make this diagnosis too often, you will suture many patients without cervical incompetence unnecessarily. This is undesirable, because inserting them is time-consuming, and they can cause complications. So only suture those patients with a highly suggestive history. Cervical incompetence never causes first-trimester abortions.

The simplest method is McDonald's, and is a variation of the original Shirodkar suture. If you do it on the right indications, it has a good chance of succeeding. Timing is critical. If you do it too early (<14 weeks), the patient may get a first-trimester abortion due to a fetal abnormality, and the suture is wasted. If you do it too late (>24 weeks), she may abort before you place it. Don't insert a suture between pregnancies. This will cause more trouble than it is worth. As we go to press, Chalmers has reported that this method prevents one delivery before 33 weeks about every 20 times it is used, so its benefit is minimal.

SIFLOSA (20 years) had a McDonald suture inserted at 14 weeks, following three second-trimester abortions. Her pregnancy continued uneventfully until term, when she was admitted for delivery. Unfortunately, the consultant who inserted the suture was on leave, and it was not noticed by the duty team. She complained of severe pain during the second stage, but this was ignored. Labour proceeded normally, and she delivered a live baby without help. Immediately after delivery she complained of urinary incontinence and collapsed. No notice was taken of this, and she was discharged after 2 days. On examination 2 months later in another hospital she was found to have a high juxta-cervical 1 cm vesicovaginal fistula, which was contiguous with her cervix, which was torn and ragged. This was successfully repaired abdominally. LESSON (1) Always explain clearly to the patient that she must have the suture removed at 38 weeks or in labour. (2) Take her complaints seriously. Reported by Timothy Goodacre in 'Tropical Doctor'.

McDONALD'S CERVICAL SUTURE

INDICATIONS. Two or more painless abortions between 16 and 28 weeks. The patient may have a scarred patulous cervix. Exclude syphilis, hypertension, and diabetes. If you see her between pregnancies, exclude abnormalities such as uterine septa (for which she needs a hysterosalpingogram) and fibroids, which can also cause second-trimester abortions.

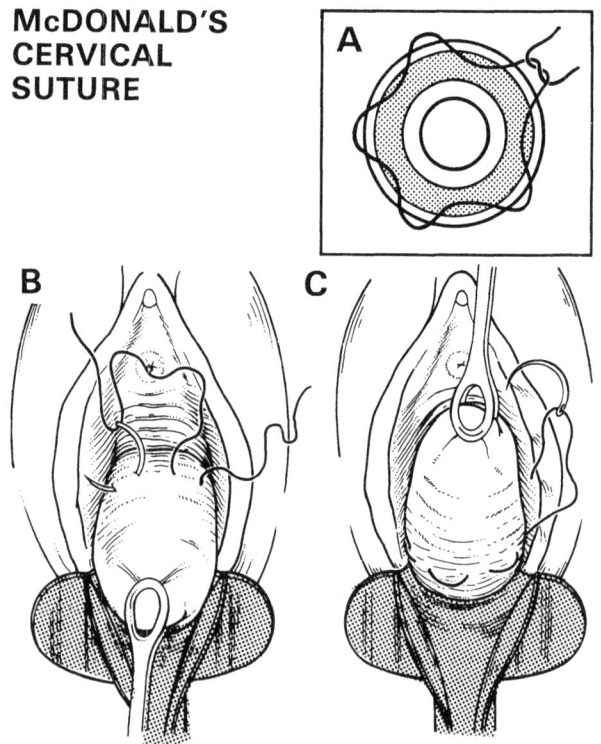

Fig. 16-2 McDONALD'S CERVICAL SUTURE. A, the position of the suture. B, inserting it anteriorly. C, inserting it posteriorly. *Partly from Bonney's 'Gynaecological Surgery'. Baillière Tindall with kind permission.*

CONTRAINDICATIONS. (1) Drainage of amniotic fluid or rupture of the membranes. (2) Vaginal bleeding. (3) Established premature labour. (4) Local infection. (5) Fetal anomalies if you can detect them. (6) An IUD or a missed abortion.

CAUTION ! Don't insert these sutures unless: (1) She has access to hospital. (2) It can guarantee that at all hours of the day and night there will be someone who will see her, who is competent to remove her suture. (3) You have explained to her what you are going to do, and that she must have her suture removed at 38 weeks, or when she goes into labour. (4) If she does go into labour with her suture in, it may cause a severe cervical tear, even worse cervical incompetence, a vesico-vaginal fistula or rupture of her uterus.

Preferably insert the suture at 14 weeks, when the danger of an early abortion is passed. Experts insert them up to 26 weeks, but never after 28 weeks. Check the fetal heart with Doppler ultrasound if you can. If you have an ultrasound scan, check that the fetus is alive, and confirm the gestational age.

ANAESTHESIA. (1) General anaesthesia is preferable. You must be able to retract her cervix and dilate her vagina widely to insert the sutures. (2) Ketamine.

METHOD. Insert a speculum. Grasp her cervix with sponge forceps. Insert a suture of No. 2 monofilament superiorly in the *outer surface* of her cervix, near the level of her internal os. Continue to place sutures in her cervix at regular intervals as shown, so as to encircle it. Then tighten the suture round it, so as to reduce its diameter to a few mm. The canal must be just patent as the suture is tied. If she is pregnant, don't insert a dilator. Admit her for 8 days; most failures occur in the first week.

Write on her notes in large red letters 'For removal of suture' at 36 weeks. See her every 2 weeks, and insert a speculum to check that the suture is still in place. Occasionally a stitch comes out and has to be reinserted.

At 36 weeks, or better, at 38 weeks (to avoid the respiratory distress syndrome in the baby) remove the suture, or remove it in early labour if she does not come in until then.

CAUTION ! Remove the suture immediately (rare) if: (1) The operation fails, and signs of imminent abortion develop. If you don't, her cervix may tear. (2) Her membranes rupture in the absence of labour. If you leave it in place, the risk of infection to both her and the baby may be increased.

If she has a tear at the side of her cervix, don't try to repair it. If she has signs of cervical incompetence, insert a McDonald's suture as above.

REMEMBER TO RECORD 'FOR REMOVAL OF STITCH AT 36 WEEKS'!

16.6 'Acute' ectopic pregnancy

In many parts of the world one in every 50 to 200 pregnancies is ectopic. Ninety-nine per cent of them implant somewhere along the Fallopian tube. An occasional one implants in the abdominal cavity (16.9), or in the cervix (even rarer). Trouble occurs either because the tube ruptures, or because the pregnancy aborts through the abdominal end of the tube, into the abdominal cavity. How soon there is trouble depends on where the fetus embeds. It can embed: In the distal two-thirds of the tube, sites (1) and (2) in Fig. 16-3. These are the common places for an ectopic pregnancy. Here, it may cause either: (a) An acute or subacute rupture 6 to 10 weeks after the last period. Or, (b) a tubal abortion at 8 to 14 weeks, in which the fetus aborts into the peritoneal cavity out of the free end of the tube, which is not ruptured. Instead, chronic bleeding continues slowly into the pelvis, to cause a pelvic haematoma (haematocele). (3) In the isthmus (unusual), where it ruptures at 4 to 6 weeks. (4) In the uterine part of the tube (unusual) where it ruptures early. (5) In an angle of the uterus (cornu, unusual) where it may proceed to 20 weeks (see 16.8). (6) In the body of the uterus, which is the normal place. (7) Close to the internal os, leading to placenta praevia. (8) In the cervix (rare). (9) On the ovary (rare). Or, (10) elsewhere in the abdomen

SITES OF IMPLANTATION

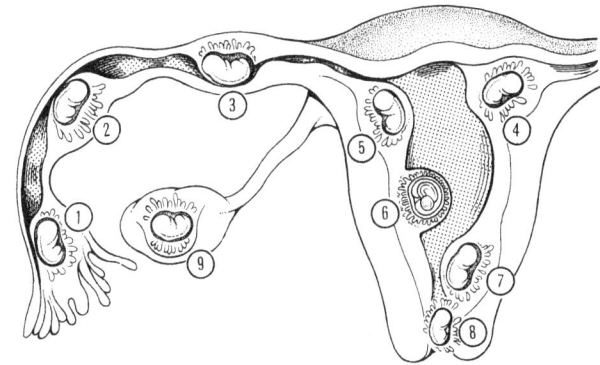

Fig. 16-3 SITES OF IMPLANTATION. 1, the fimbria. 2, the ampulla (with the fimbria, the most common abnormal site). 3, the isthmus. 4, the uterine part of the tube. 5, the angle. 6, the body of the uterus, which is the normal site for implantation. 7, close to the internal os, leading to placenta praevia. 8, the cervix. 9, the ovary. 10, elsewhere in the abdominal cavity.

(rare), where it may rupture after the end of the first trimester (16.9). If an ectopic pregnancy survives to 20 weeks without causing serious symptoms, it is probably in one of the less common sites, perhaps in an angle.

Patients with an ectopic pregnancy form two groups: (1) Those who have had a massive bleed into the abdominal cavity. These are the acute and subacute cases described below. (2) Those with little abdominal bleeding. A few of these will have a massive bleed later, but many will never lose more than a few hundred millilitres of blood into their abdominal cavities. These are the 'chronic ectopics' in Section 16.7. There are also various intermediate forms.

Symptoms start when an ectopic pregnancy grows so large that it ruptures out of the tube that contains it. The patient's periods are usually a few days to a few months late, and she may rightly think she is pregnant. Or, she may not think she is pregnant because: (1) Her tube may rupture before she has missed a period. (2) Vaginal bleeding due to the ectopic pregnancy may begin at about the time of the expected period. (3) She may have an IUD in, or be on the minipill, and assume she cannot be pregnant. If her period of amenorrhoea is short, before her symptoms start, her pregnancy is likely to be in the isthmus, and the effects of rupture worse.

An acute rupture presents as a sudden severe lower abdominal pain, with signs of hypovolaemia. Her pain and internal bleeding may be severe enough to make her vomit and faint. Her pulse rises as she starts to bleed. Her blood pressure falls and she becomes shocked. Some mild dark red or brown vaginal bleeding usually follows 24 hours after the onset of the pain, as the decidua are shed (if she has had a very severe rupture and has not been treated, she may have died from internal bleeding before this happens). A 'four quadrant tap' (66.1) confirms the presence of blood in her abdomen. The blood that remains in her circulation may not have had time to dilute, so she may not yet be anaemic. Surgery is urgent.

A subacute rupture typically presents with a history of 3 to 7 days of weakness, anaemia and abdominal swelling, usually with little pain. Her lower abdomen may be tender, with rebound tenderness and guarding, but these signs are often minimal. Blood irritating her diaphragm may cause referred pain at the tip of her shoulder. She should give a history of a small dark vaginal bleed, but you may need to question her carefully to find this. A four quadrant tap confirms the presence of blood. Treatment is fairly urgent, but transfuse her first.

A chronic ectopic pregnancy presents as a vague lower abdominal pain, that is easily confused with PID (pelvic inflammatory disease) and does not require urgent treatment—see Section 16.7.

The diagnosis is easy when she has bled massively into her abdominal cavity, and is either shocked or grossly anaemic. But it can be very difficult, and if there is only a little bleeding, even the expert may be misled. Remember that any woman with a menstrual irregularity (a period or more missed or periods which have been lighter than usual), combined with abdominal pain and adnexal tenderness on one side probably has an ectopic pregnancy. Anaemia, dizziness, shoulder pain, and a tender mass are all extras which encourage the diagnosis, but are not necessary for it.

Ectopic pregnancies can be fatal, so if you are in doubt do a laparotomy soon. Even if your diagnosis is wrong, and she has salpingitis or appendicitis, you have done no harm. Don't let anyone who *might* have an ectopic pregnancy go home—admit her. If you decide to observe her on the ward rather than operate immediately, you must: (1) monitor her carefully, and (2) be able to operate at very short notice. As so often, 'look and see' is better than 'wait and see'.

These are rewarding patients, because they seldom die, if you treat them correctly, even if they have bled severely. So be watchful.

DON'T FORGET ECTOPIC PREGNANCY IN A WOMAN OF CHILDBEARING AGE

ECTOPIC PREGNANCY ACUTE AND SUBACUTE

EXAMINATION. Look for signs of blood loss (shock and anaemia), and for signs of bleeding into the patient's abdomen. If she has generalized tenderness (which may be mild), distension, a thrill, and shifting dullness, bleeding has been severe. Rebound tenderness and guarding are variable, and may be absent. If she has a large tender mass in her lower abdomen, bleeding has been confined there by adhesions.

Gently examine her vaginally. The important signs are pain on moving her cervix, tenderness in her posterior fornix and pouch of Douglas, and perhaps acute adnexal tenderness, which is worse on one side (highly suggestive).

CAUTION ! (1) *Don't do a vigorous vaginal or bimanual examination, or an examination under anaesthesia.* You may squash the ectopic and may make bleeding worse. (2) Most patients are afebrile, but some have a low fever.

HER HAEMOGLOBIN is normal to begin with, falls as her blood dilutes, and shows no change for at least 24 hours, unless she has been given intravenous fluids which will dilute her blood faster. A few days after a severe bleed it may fall to as little as 30 g/l.

THE TEST FOR ORTHOSTATIC HYPOTENSION is sensitive to much milder degrees of hypovolaemia than a change in her blood pressure, which may not fall until she is quite severely hypovolaemic. If her pulse taken when she is sitting up is more than 25 beats faster than when she is lying down, she is hypovolaemic (see 66.1).

OTHER TESTS. A raised temperature and white blood count, favour a diagnosis of appendicitis, salpingitis, or torsion of an ovarian cyst, but do not exclude an ectopic pregnancy.

PERITONEAL ASPIRATION. Culdocentesis (16-6) is not very reliable. If the diagnosis is in doubt, aspirate her peritoneum. Empty her bladder, and push a syringe attached to a large needle into one of her iliac fossae pointing towards her pelvis. If you aspirate blood which does not clot, she has internal bleeding, probably from an ectopic pregnancy. If necessary, repeat this in the other four quadrants of her abdomen (66.1). You can do this in the ward.

CAUTION ! A negative test does not exclude an ectopic pregnancy.

PREGNANCY TESTS Routine tests become positive at 2000 iu/l HCG and are only positive in 50% of ectopic pregnancies, so they are not helpful. However, there are more sensitive pregnancy tests which become positive at 75 iu/l, and are positive in 90-95 per cent of cases. A negative test of this kind is very useful.

THE DIFFERENTIAL DIAGNOSIS includes many of the causes of an acute abdomen in Section 10.2, especially PID (6.6), appendicitis (12.1), urinary tract infection, and torsion of an ovarian cyst (20.7). The degeneration of a uterine fibroid in early pregnancy can also cause acute abdominal pain, but there are no systemic signs of bleeding. Other causes of anaemia, especially hookworm anaemia.

If shock and anaemia parallel the blood that she has lost vaginally (which they do not in an ectopic pregnancy), suspect an abortion. If she has ascites and anaemia, suspect an ectopic until you have proved otherwise.

LAPAROTOMY FOR ECTOPIC PREGNANCY

EQUIPMENT. A general laparotomy set, equipment for autotransfusion (16-8).

RESUSCITATION. Set up a drip immediately with saline or dextran. Take blood for grouping and cross-matching. If possible, try to replace most of the blood she has lost. Contributors differ on the value of the vacuum bottle autotransfusion method (16.10) preoperatively. Some consider it very valuable.

If she is shocked and blood is scarce, restore her blood volume with saline. After you have operated and controlled the bleeding, give her whatever compatible blood you have.

CAUTION ! Operate as soon as you have started resuscitation, especially if blood and fluids are scarce. If she is bleeding severely, you may never be able to resuscitate her until you tie the bleeding vessel; large volumes of fluids will only wash her last red cells into her abdomen.

PREPARATION. Catheterize her and leave the catheter in. One ectopic pregnancy is often followed by another, so, if she has had all the children she wants, ask her permission to tie her normal tube. However, it is common for a patient with an ectopic pregnancy to have few children and want more. One contributor dislikes asking for permission for sterilization in an acute crisis, and would only do it with a 'super-grand multip'.

ANAESTHESIA. If she is shocked, or very anaemic, follow the general precautions for anaesthesia in hypovolaemic shock (A 16.7). Give her pethidine 25 mg intravenously as premedication. (1) Ether, tracheal intubation, relaxants, and controlled ventilation. Keep anaesthesia light. Give her the minimum of ether, or use nitrous oxide and a Boyle's machine. (2) Ketamine, preferably with a relaxant (A 8.4). You do not need much muscle relaxation, and most cases can be done under ketamine alone. (3) Infiltration anaesthesia (A 6.9). *Subarachnoid (spinal) anaesthesia is contraindicated!*

PINCH HER BROAD LIGAMENT

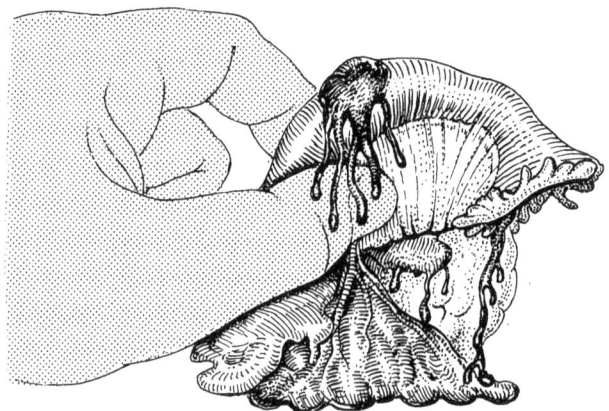

Fig. 16-4 PINCH THE PATIENT'S BROAD LIGAMENT TO STOP HER BLEEDING. As soon as you open her abdomen and have cleared away the blood (for autotransfusion if necessary), find her burst Fallopian tube. If it is still bleeding significantly, grasp its broad ligament between your finger and thumb, so as to compress the vessels and stop bleeding.

INCISION. Make a subumbilical midline incision (9.2). There will be blood in her abdominal cavity. Put your hand into her pelvis and feel for her uterus. Find her burst Fallopian tube, and if it is still actively bleeding, grasp its broad ligament between your finger and thumb, so as to compress the vessels in it, as in Fig. 16-4.

If there is much free blood in her peritoneal cavity, ladle it out into a sterile container, and filter it through gauze as you do so. Return it to her circulation by autotransfusion (16.10). It will have the same HIV status as she has, and is therefore safer than donor blood.

Examine both her tubes to make sure that she has not got two ectopic pregnancies (rare). The other tube may contain a little blood, but this is not an indication to remove it. The fetus will probably only be about 1 cm long, so you don't usually find it. Or, you may find quite a large unruptured amniotic sac containing it.

If she has a subacute ectopic, her ruptured tube will be covered with blood clot and adherent to the surrounding structures. Free it from them with scissors or a finger.

Apply two haemostats, one from the lateral and one from the medial side, as in Fig. 16-5. Let them meet in the middle with their points in contact, so that no part of her broad ligament is unclamped. Try to preserve her ovary.

Contributors disagree about positions 'X' and 'Y' for the second clamp in Fig. 16-5. Position 'X', is easier for beginners, and preserves the fimbrial end for a possible repair later (difficult, seldom successful, and unlikely to be practical). It has the disadvantage that an ovum may be fertilized by sperm which have swum up the other tube, so that a second ectopic pregnancy may occur in the same tube. Position 'Y' avoids this.

Remove the burst part of the tube by cutting along the free side of the clamps. Put two ligatures of chromic catgut under the joints of each clamp. Tie them with a sliding knot (4.8). Leave the ends of these ligatures long, and hold them in haemostats.

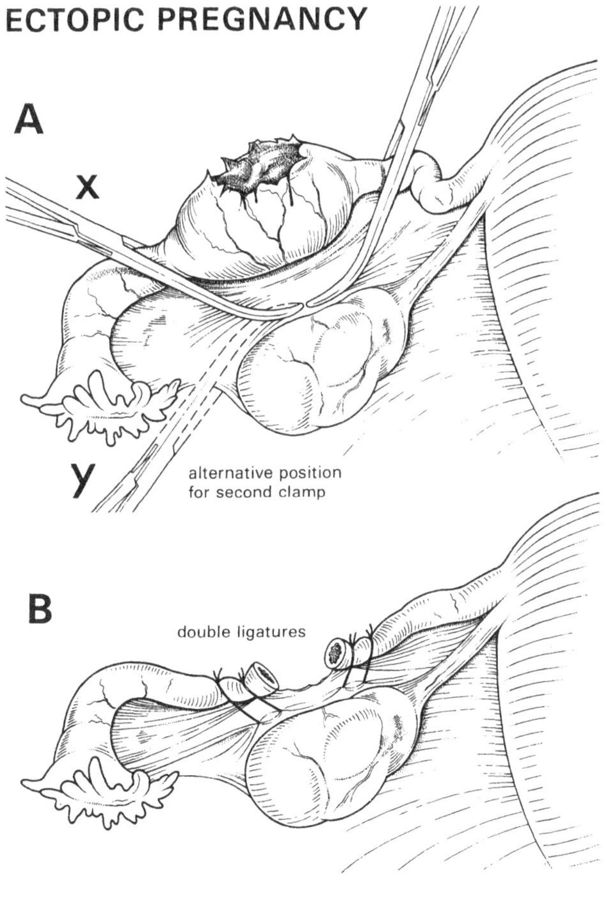

ECTOPIC PREGNANCY

Fig. 16-5 ECTOPIC PREGNANCY. A, put clamps on either side of the patient's ruptured tube. Try to preserve its fimbrial end if you can (position 'X'). If necessary, you can put the second clamp in the position 'Y'. B, cut out the ectopic pregnancy, and put two ligatures round the clamps.

Make double ligatures on both sides, to make sure that no arteries are missed.

CAUTION ! (1) If you don't tie these ligatures carefully, she will bleed postoperatively. (2) If she continues to bleed when you have applied two ligatures, apply more. (3) Don't do anything else which is not essential.

Clean her peritoneal cavity thoroughly. Close her abdomen without drainage. If she has previously consented, tie her other tube.

Examine the specimen. In the middle of an ill-defined placenta and blood clot you will see the amniotic sac. If there is evidence of a hydatidiform mole (rare, 32.38), send it for histology.

POSTOPERATIVELY, monitor her urine output until she is out of danger (A 15.5). Treat her anaemia, she may need further transfusions: folic acid by mouth, or iron.

DIFFICULTIES WITH ACUTE AND SUBACUTE ECTOPIC PREGNANCIES

See also Sections 16.7 (chronic ectopic pregnancy), 16.8 (angular and cervical pregnancy) and 16.9 (abdominal pregnancy).

If you CANNOT FIND THE TUBE with the ectopic in it, don't panic. Allow yourself time to scoop out blood and clots. Tip the head of the table down (the Trendelenburg position), so as to make the blood and her gut move away from her pelvis. Feel for her uterus in the midline in the hollow of her sacrum. Pull it into the wound. If it is stuck down by adhesions, tear them with traction, or cut them with scissors. Having found her uterus, feel for the affected tube. If this is stuck down by adhesions to her omentum or gut, separate them (usually not too difficult). If her tube is stuck to her broad ligament on the same side (more difficult), try to get your fingers under it and her ovary, and lift them into the wound, by scraping the tip of your fingers along the back of her broad ligament. If necessary, cut adhesions between her tube and her rectum.

If her ovary is stuck to her tube, or you have torn it as you mobilized it, remove it.

CAUTION ! Before you remove her ovary (if you have to), make sure you separate adhesions between it and her broad ligament. If you don't do this, you may clamp her broad ligament too low down, and so include her ureter.

If adhesions obscure everything, **search for:** (1) her uterus, or (2) her infundibulopelvic ligament (20-17). On the right this comes away from under her caecum and appendix, and on the left side from under her mesosigmoid.

The blood supply to the tube and ovary comes from: (1) the ovarian vessels in the infundibulopelvic ligament. (2) The ascending branches of the uterine vessels. If you can put a clamp across her infundibulopelvic ligament, and another one across her tube and broad ligament next to her uterus, you will interrupt the blood supply to the ectopic.

If there is a RAW AREA IN HER PERITONEUM which oozes, after you have removed her ectopic pregnancy, it will usually stop spontaneously, if there are no obviously bleeding vessels. Try compressing if firmly for 5 minutes with a warm pack. If is continues to ooze, insert a drain for 24 hours, and monitor her carefully.

If you find that she has INFLAMED TUBES with pus pouring from their fimbriated ends, she has salpingitis (6.6), not an ectopic pregnancy. Don't excise them; close her abdomen and give her antibiotics.

If she has a TUBO-OVARIAN abscess (6.6), drain it.

If she has a CHRONIC PYOSALPINX, excising it will be very risky if it has stuck to her gut, but this may be possible if it is not too friable and adherent.

If you find her APPENDIX STUCK TO HER TUBE, peel it off. If you damage it, do an appendicectomy (12.1).

If there is no ectopic, and you find a BLEEDING CORPUS LUTEUM, control bleeding with sutures. If this is difficult, excise the corpus luteum from her ovary and suture the gap. Or, less satisfactorily, remove her ovary. If she is less than 8 weeks pregnant, she will probably abort. After 8 weeks the placenta makes enough progesterone to keep the pregnancy going.

If there is a SECOND PREGNANCY in her uterus (very rare), removing the ectopic pregnancy may not disturb it. If she continues to have amenorrhoea its presence will soon be obvious.

If she has a LARGE PURPLE HAEMATOMA in her broad ligament (rare), her ectopic pregnancy has ruptured into it, and not into her peritoneum, and may be quite large (12- to 16-week size or larger).

CAUTION ! (1) Don't burrow into the lower part of her broad ligament. You may damage the large venous plexuses there, or her ureter. (2) Don't try to control bleeding by suturing deeply, unless this is absolutely essential. You may tie her ureter.

Here are two ways of treating her:

First method. Clamp and divide her round ligament on the same side 2 or 3 cm from her uterus. Clamp her tube and ovarian ligament close to her uterus, but don't divide them yet (if her anatomy is confused, leave this and do it later). Cut the peritoneum from her round ligament in the direction of her infundibulopelvic ligament. This will open the top of her broad ligament. As you approach her infundibulopelvic ligament, find, clamp and divide her ovarian vessels *without including her ureter!* For the anatomy of her ureter and pelvic ligaments see Figs. 15-6, 20-16, and 20-17.

This will have isolated both blood supplies to her ectopic pregnancy. Now you can clamp and divide her tube and ovarian ligament. If the ectopic is not already free, a little blunt dissection should free it from the base of her broad ligament. If oozing from the base of her broad ligament does not stop spontaneously, clamp and tie the bleeding vessels.

Second method. Mobilize her uterus by removing blood clot and dividing light adhesions. Apply two large artery forceps to her tube as shown in Fig. 16-5, but don't excise the ectopic pregnancy yet.

Cut a half a centimetre opening in the back of her broad ligament, and squeeze out the haematoma by pressing it from below.

Watch her; several things can happen after either method.

If the haematoma does not reform (usual), you are lucky, the artery forceps have controlled the bleeding. Excise the ectopic pregnancy, complete the operation in the usual way, and then suture the hole in her broad ligament.

If the haematoma reforms (unusual), open her broad ligament more widely, look for a bleeding point, and tie it.

If there is no bleeding point, but only a general ooze, press a warm pack against the oozing area, and wait 10 minutes by the clock. If this controls bleeding, complete the operation.

If a pack fails to control the bleeding, tie or undersew as many bleeding vessels as you can. Be careful to feel for her ureter to avoid including it in a ligature. Trace it from where it enters her pelvis over her sacroiliac joint (20-16). It has a characteristic firm feeling, and you can roll it between your fingers.

16.7 'Chronic' ectopic pregnancy, (ectopic pregnancy without massive abdominal bleeding)

Two kinds of ectopic pregnancy do not cause massive bleeding: (1) An acute ectopic which has, so far, only caused a small bleed, and a massive bleed is to follow later. (2) A 'chronic ectopic' in which repeated small bleeds have caused a haematoma (pelvic haematocele) containing 100 to 500 ml of blood and clot. Some of these chronic cases resolve without treatment, but don't wait for this to happen. You can never be sure that the patient will not have another larger bleed, and they can cause much trouble.

A patient with a chronic ectopic may present with varying combinations of the following: (1) Lower abdominal pain, perhaps combined with pain on micturition, defaecation, or sex. (2) A small dark vaginal blood-loss (less than a normal period), perhaps preceded by amenorrhoea, and sometimes with the passage of a decidual cast. (3) A mass in her lower abdomen, at the side of her uterus, or in her pouch of Douglas. Occasionally, if her adnexae have a long pedicle, this mass is entirely outside her pelvis. Moving her cervix is painful, but this is not such a reliable sign as in an acute rupture. Her uterus is usually slightly enlarged.

The diagnosis of a chronic ectopic can be difficult, and is often missed. Its symptoms are like those of PID; if she has had several similar attacks without any missed periods, she probably does have PID.

THERESA (24 years) was seen in hospital complaining of heavy prolonged bleeding for 5 days. She had missed two periods and said that she had passed clots. She was anaemic, her uterus was slightly enlarged, and her cervix was closed and still bleeding. A doctor diagnosed her as having an incomplete abortion, and did a 'D and C'. There were few curettings, so he thought "she must have had a complete abortion". He gave her iron tablets and discharged her, but she continued to bleed and have low abdominal pain. So she went to another hospital where the doctor there felt a tender mass on the left side of her uterus. He thought at first that she had an ectopic, but he read the discharge card from the first hospital, which said that she had had an incomplete abortion, and a 'D and C'. So he was misled and diagnosed PID with a tubo-ovarian abscess. He gave her antibiotics, and she went home. Nearly a month later she went to a private clinic run by a medical assistant. He correctly diagnosed an ectopic pregnancy, before even doing a vaginal examination, and referred her. Her haemoglobin was 40 g/l. She had had 5 children, so at laparotomy her tubes were tied. LESSONS (1) Don't be misled by other people's clinical opinions. (2) 'Abortions' may be ectopics. (2) PID can produce symptoms which are very like those of a chronic ectopic pregnancy. (3) This patient has some of the features of a subacute ectopic (severe anaemia), and some of those of a typical chronic ectopic pregnancy (a history of chronic pain); this shows that there is no sharp borderline between these two conditions. (4) Before you diagnose PID, stop and think—'Could this be a chronic ectopic?'.

DON'T FORGET THE POSSIBILITY OF AN ECTOPIC PREGNANCY IN A WOMAN OF CHILDBEARING AGE

CHRONIC ECTOPIC PREGNANCY

DIAGNOSIS. You will only make the diagnosis if you think of a chronic ectopic pregnancy whenever you see a patient with irregular, missed, or prolonged periods. Ask her if she has low abdominal pain, and examine her for tenderness. Examine her vaginally and look for slight vaginal bleeding. Move her cervix and feel for tenderness on either side. If you can feel a mass, or tenderness which is greater on one side than on the other, she may have an ectopic.

The diagnosis may be difficult to confirm. She has no evidence of blood loss (except perhaps one or more episodes of fainting). She may be anaemic. A pregnancy test may or may not be positive.

CULDOCENTESIS is the confirmatory test for rupture of a chronic ectopic pregnancy, or a pelvic abscess. *It is only positive if the haematocele is in her pouch of Douglas,* and not if it is elsewhere (unusual). You can do a culdocentesis in the ward without an anaesthetic. But do it in the theatre after induction if: (1) she has a pelvic mass which could be a chronic ectopic pregnancy for which she will need a laparotomy. Or, (2) she has a pelvic abscess which needs drainage.

CULDOCENTESIS

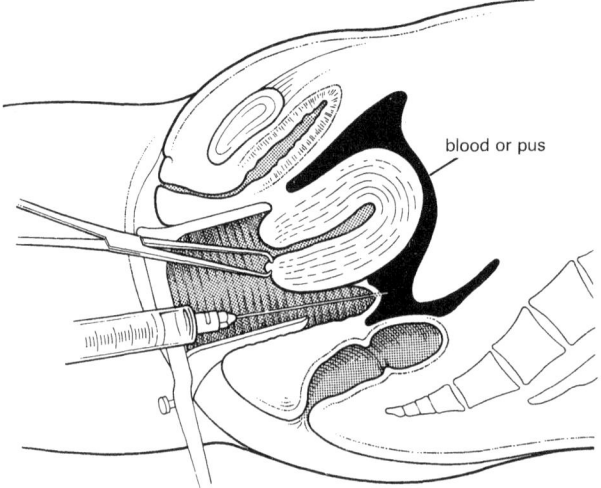

Fig. 16-6 CULDOCENTESIS can be used to confirm the presence of blood or pus in the pelvic peritoneum, and to distinguish between PID and a pelvic heamatocele (chronic ectopic pregnancy) as the cause of a pelvic mass.

Put her into the lithotomy position, Clean her vulva and do a careful bimanual examination, feeling for a mass. Insert a sterile bivalve speculum. Clean her vagina with 1% chlorhexidine. Stab a 1.2 mm needle on a 20 ml syringe through her posterior fornix 1 cm behind her cervix. Withdraw the plunger.

If you withdraw more than 2 ml of dark or free-flowing fresh blood, often with bits of clot in it, she has blood in her peritoneal cavity, probably from an ectopic pregnancy.

If you aspirate a little fresh blood which clots easily, you have punctured a blood vessel.

If you aspirate nothing, or only a little fresh blood which clots easily, there is either no ectopic pregnancy, or her pouch of Douglas is obliterated by adhesions.

If you aspirate pus, she has pelvic peritonitis or a pelvic abscess.

CAUTION ! A negative test makes an ectopic pregnancy unlikely, but does not exclude it. (2) The test is only positive if you aspirate blood which does not clot when you leave it in a tube for 10 minutes. If it clots after removal, it is probably venous.

DIFFERENTIAL DIAGNOSIS. The main one is PID, see also Section 6.6. The important features are the volume, appearance, and timing of the blood loss, the history of missed periods (in an ectopic) and of fever (in PID). Culdocentesis should distinguish them.

A LARGE PELVIC HAEMATOCELE

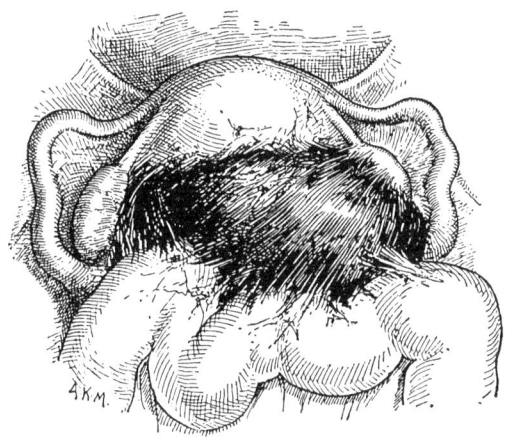

Fig. 16-6a A LARGE PELVIC HAEMATOCELE (chronic ectopic pregnancy). You will only make the diagnosis if you think of this whenever you see a patient with irregular, missed, or prolonged periods. *From Young, James, 'A Textbook of Gynaecology; (5th edn. 1939), Fig. 101. A and C Black.*

Suggesting a chronic ectopic—one or more missed periods. Anaemia, which may be severe. No fever. Little vaginal bleeding not defined into periods. No obvious relationship between low abdominal pain and 'periods'. Sometimes a history of faintness when the pain started.

Suggesting PID—no missed periods. No obvious anaemia. Fever, which may be severe. Low abdominal pain which is often worse during and after periods, and which usually begins after the bleeding starts. A vaginal discharge, which may only be mild. No history of faintness.

Other pitfalls: (1) If she believes she is pregnant, and bleeds vaginally, you may think that she has a threatened abortion, especially if the haematocele surrounds a normal-sized uterus, and makes it appear to be enlarged to that of a 10- or 12-week pregnancy. (2) If she has passed a decidual cast, you may think she has a complete or incomplete abortion. (3) If you feel what you think is an enlarged uterus (a uterus surrounded by haematocele) in the presence of abnormal bleeding, you may think she has fibroids. (4) If the mass is difficult to feel you may think she has DUB (dysfunctional uterine bleeding, 20.2).

LAPAROTOMY. Proceed as in Section 16.6 where relevant.

You will find blood in her pelvis, mostly in her pouch of Douglas and mostly clotted. Clean it out. Find the tube which has the ectopic and do a salpingectomy, as in Fig. 16-5 and Section 16.6.

DIFFICULTIES WITH A CHRONIC ECTOPIC PREGNANCY
See also Section 16.6.

If there are MANY DENSE ADHESIONS between the ectopic pregnancy and her surrounding organs, scoop out as much blood clot as will easily come out without tearing and pulling. If you try to remove firmly adherent clot, there will be much oozing. Don't try to remove the whole 'wall' of the haematoma cavity, or you may injure her gut.

If the surfaces of her pelvic organs are congested and OOZE BLOOD, as may happen when blood has been present in her pelvic cavity for some days, control bleeding with warm abdominal packs.

If you INJURE HER RECTUM or sigmoid colon (this should be rare), suture the injury, and do a transverse colostomy (9.5). Pass a drain down to the site of the repair, and close her abdomen. Close the colostomy at a convenient time later.

If you INJURE HER SMALL GUT (this should also be rare), and the injured area is healthy, anastomose it. If the injured area is inflamed, resect a length of gut and do an end to end, or side to side, anastomosis. If this is not possible, exteriorize (9.5) a loop of gut proximal to the lesion, and make an ileostomy. Later, refer her for expert repair.

16.8 Angular and cervical ectopic pregnancies

An ectopic pregnancy occasionally implants itself towards the medial end of a patient's Fallopian tube. If it implants itself at the point where her tube enters her uterus, it ruptures early, but if it implants in the intramural part of the tube near her uterine cavity (angular or cornual pregnancy), it may not rupture until 20 weeks (see Fig. 16-3). In either case the whole angle of her uterus becomes a bleeding mass. When this happens, you can usually resect part of her uterus (a wedge resection).

If an ectopic pregnancy implants itself in her cervix (a cervical pregnancy, rare) this will be open and contain a thin-walled cavity in which you can feel fragments of chorionic tissue. This cavity bleeds massively, and may resemble an abortion, but whereas there is little bleeding after an abortion has been evacuated, a cervical ectopic pregnancy continues to bleed. You are most likely to be aware of it as an abortion which continues to bleed after evacuation (16.2).

ANGULAR AND CERVICAL ECTOPIC PREGNANCIES

ANGULAR PREGNANCY. At laparotomy for an ectopic pregnancy you find a purple bleeding mass arising from one angle of the patient's uterus. Bleeding can be torrential. If the only way to control it is to clamp her broad ligaments, clamp both of them and do a subtotal hysterectomy (20.12). Usually, a wedge resection is possible. Plan for Caesarean section in her next pregnancy.

CAUTION ! In some societies a woman who does not menstruate is not acceptable as a wife, and if this is so in your community, don't sacrifice her uterus unless her life is in danger.

To do a wedge resection, aim to remove the mass by cutting her uterus from around it, so as to leave a wedge-shaped gap.

If there are not too many dense adhesions between her uterus and her pelvis, tie a rubber tourniquet around the lower part of her uterus. Or ask your assistant to compress the angle as firmly as he can while you insert the sutures. Bring the two sides of the gap together firmly, and suture them with two layers of No. 2 chromic catgut, the inner layer being mattress sutures, and the outer layer simple ones (difficult, because the tissue is friable and vascular). When you have done this, you will probably find that the bleeding has stopped.

Alternatively, repair her uterus with a single layer of silk through the full thickness of its wall. Place as many sutures as necessary before you tie any. Then, as your assistant pulls all but one tight, tie the remaining one. This will minimize the risk of them cutting out.

Alternatively, remove the tube and ovary on the same side. This has the advantage of avoiding the possibility of a further ectopic pregnancy on that side.

If she already has several children, consider tying her tubes, because the risk of rupture of the scar is considerable.

CERVICAL PREGNANCY (rare). She either presents as an abortion which continues to bleed, or you may suspect that she has a cervical pregnancy, when you find a bleeding thin-walled cavity in her cervix. The important differential diagnosis is an ordinary abortion which has stuck in her cervix, because her external os is too tight to let it out (16.2).

Pack the cavity tightly to stop bleeding, and let you resuscitate her. She will bleed severely.

If her ectopic pregnancy is early, packing may be all she needs. Bleeding may have stopped when you remove the pack 24 hours later.

If a pack does not control bleeding, there are two more manoeuvres you can do before hysterectomy: (1) Suture the descending cervical branches of her uterine arteries. Pull her cervix firmly down and insert catgut sutures at the 3 o'clock and 9 o'clock positions, as high as you can at the level of her cervicovaginal junction. Provided you do not go above this level her ureters will be safe. Don't do any dissection. (2) Insert a large (50 ml or more) Foley catheter into the bleeding cavity in her cervix, blow it up, and leave it for 24 hours. Fluid from her uterus will be able to drain through the tube. If this fails, tie her internal iliac arteries (3.5); if this too fails do a hysterectomy (20.12).

16.9 Abdominal pregnancies

An ectopic pregnancy occasionally aborts backwards down a tube, or bursts out of it without killing the patient, and embeds itself elsewhere in her abdominal cavity. Sometimes, an ovum is fertilized outside a tube on the surface of an ovary, and then implants itself in the abdominal cavity. Such an ectopic may die at any stage, or proceed to term. An abdominal pregnancy is thus a rare complication of an ordinary ectopic pregnancy, so that in areas where ectopic pregnancies are common, the incidence of abdominal pregnancies is increased also. An abdominal pregnancy causes comparatively few symptoms. None of them are individually diagnostic, so the diagnosis depends on the sum of many clues, none of which is enough by itself.

A patient with an abdominal pregnancy may present with: (1) Persistent abdominal pain from about 26 to 28 weeks onwards of variable severity, which is not well localized. (2) Her 'uterus' (in reality the gestational sac) is ill-defined, and feels 'odd', when you palpate it. The fetal parts may be abnormally easy or abnormally difficult to feel. The lie of the baby is often abnormal, and may be persistently transverse or oblique. (3) The features of (1 and 2) accompanied by the failure of her 'uterus' to enlarge, typically at 32 weeks, and a dead baby. (4) The features of (1 and 2) combined with a 'uterus' that distends more than it should, so that you suspect polyhydramnios. (5) Postmaturity (>40 weeks). (6) A dead baby which she does not expel, either spontaneously or with oxytocin (16.4).

Less commonly, she may present with: (7) An abdominal mass after 26 weeks adjacent to an empty uterus (or a uterus enlarged to the size of a 12- to 16-week pregnancy), which is quite separate from it. (8) A distended abdomen which is like a full term pregnancy, and a mass which is less cystic and rubbery than a normal pregnancy. She says she is pregnant but is having normal periods. On questioning she admits having missed some periods, possibly nine, in the past. (9) Loss of weight and general ill health.

The diagnosis depends on recognizing (a) that she is pregnant and (b) that her pregnancy is not in her uterus. Her history is seldom helpful, but: (1) She may have had episodes of pain in early pregnancy. (2) She may have a history of a previous ectopic pregnancy. (3) If she is an experienced multip, she may say that her pregnancy 'feels different'.

The fetus can implant itself anywhere, but because the placenta is so large, it is always attached to gut or omentum somewhere. The common sites are: (1) In her pouch of Douglas. (2) In her broad ligament, where it is attached to her uterus, or the wall of her pelvis. (3) On an ovary.

MARY (19 years) was observed to have a transverse lie at 7 months. External version failed, so she was allowed to go to term. At 40 weeks she had abdominal pains, but the lie was still oblique. On pelvic examination her cervix was in a curious position in front of the fetal head. At Caesarean section she did not seem to have a uterus, instead her membranes were close against her abdominal wall. After a live baby girl had been delivered, the placenta was found to be attached to her left Fallopian tube. It was left in place and as many of the membranes as possible removed. She recovered uneventfully. LESSONS (1) If something rather unusual happens, think of the possibility of an extrauterine pregnancy. (2) If you cannot easily remove the placenta, leave it.

ABDOMINAL PREGNANCY

X-RAYS. (1) The fetus may be in an abnormal attitude and remain in it over a long period. (2) In a standing lateral film the fetal parts may overlap the shadow of the patient's spine. This is rare in a normal pregnancy. Ultrasound in the hands of an experienced operator is very helpful, so refer her for it if you can.

MANAGEMENT. If you make the diagnosis before 24 weeks, a laparotomy is usually indicated. This is difficult, so try to refer her.

If the pregnancy is more than 24 weeks and the baby is still alive, consider leaving him until 34 to 36 weeks, so as to improve his chances of survival. Often, she has few children or

ADVANCED EXTRAUTERINE GESTATION

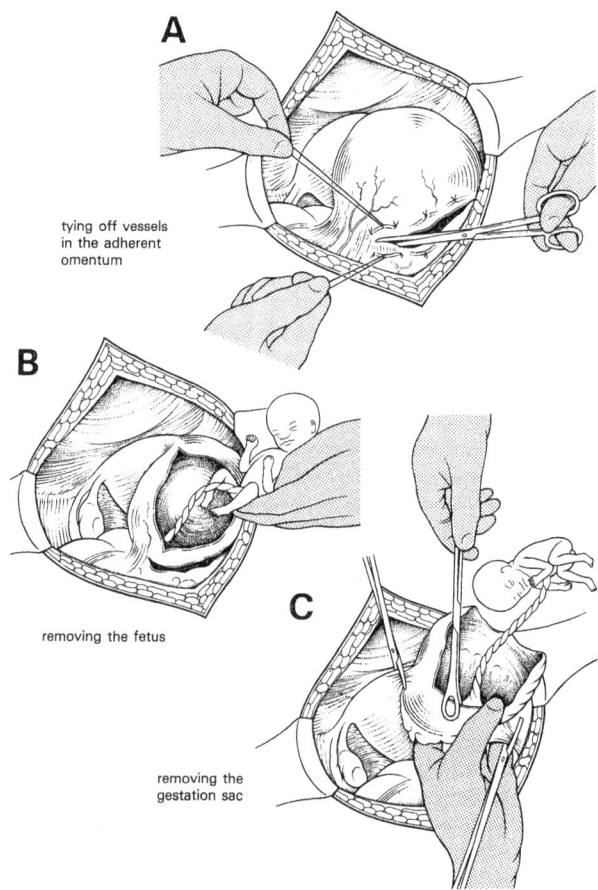

Fig. 16-7 AN ADVANCED EXTRAUTERINE PREGNANCY in the omentum. A, tying off the vessels in the omentum. B, removing the fetus. C, in this patient the entire sac is being removed; if it is not easy to remove, leave it. *From Bonney's 'Gynaecological Surgery'. Ballière Tindall, with kind permission.*

none, and is grateful for a live child. If you decide to do this she may bleed before term (uncommon), so keep her in hospital to wait.

If the pregnancy is more than 24 weeks but the baby is dead, postpone the operation for 3 or 4 weeks after the fetal movements have stopped, so that the vascularity of the placental bed is reduced. If he has been dead for more than 4 to 6 weeks, check her clotting time before you operate, because of the possibility of DIC (19.11b).

If he has been dead for more than a month, book her for the next operating list, whatever the duration of pregnancy. There is always a danger that he may become infected. Check her clotting time.

If she has sudden pain at any time, it may indicate rupture of the membranes or haemorrhage, so operate immediately.

REMOVING AN ABDOMINAL PREGNANCY

This is an expert's task, so refer her if you can. If you have to operate yourself, prepare for much bleeding. You will need at least 2 units of blood and preferably more.

ANAESTHESIA. General anaesthesia with tracheal intubation.

INCISION. Listen over her abdominal wall for a vascular bruit (sound). This may tell you where the placenta is getting its blood from. If you hear one, place your abdominal incision over some other part of her abdominal wall. If you can feel the baby close under it, this may be a good site to incise. If there is no obvious site to be preferred or avoided, make a paramedian or midline incision, if necessary above the umbilicus. Open her abdomen with care, because her gut may have stuck to her abdominal wall.

Search for the amniotic sac and placenta. Open the sac through a thin area where there is no placenta. If necessary, remove any gut and omentum from the front of the sac. Dissect away the sac and remove the baby. Clamp and tie his cord firmly.

If he was alive when he was removed, leave the placenta.

If he was dead, and: (1) the placenta is not fixed to her gut, or some other essential structure, and (2) you think you could shell it out quite easily, then remove it. But if it is fixed to the gut or some other vital structure, or to her mesentery or to her parietal peritoneum over a large area, leave it. Disturbing it will cause severe bleeding.

If the pregnancy has arisen in a tube or ovary, and the sac has a vascular pedicle which you can clamp, divide the pedicle and remove the sac completely with the placenta.

CAUTION ! (1) Don't dissect in the region of the placenta. This may cause catastrophic bleeding, especially if he is still alive. (2) Take care not to injure the mesentery, or its blood supply, or part of her gut will necrose, and she will die from peritonitis. (3) Take special care not to injure her large gut!

If you decide to leave the placenta, cut and tie the cord as short as possible. Then remove as much of the sac as you safely can. Don't insert a drain, the placenta is going to be absorbed anyway, and a drain might only introduce infection. Close her abdomen (9.8).

DIFFICULTIES WITH ABDOMINAL PREGNANCIES

If you CANNOT CONTROL BLEEDING in any other way (rare), you may have to send her back to the ward with clamps in place protruding from the wound, and then cautiously remove them later (3.1). Or, pack the bleeding area, and then gently withdraw the pack later (3.1).

If she presents with an ABDOMINAL MASS and a SINUS on her abdominal wall (rare), the sinus may be arising in an ectopic pregnancy. Probe it, you may feel fetal bones. Open it with great care not to injure her gut.

16.10 Autotransfusion

Blood from the peritoneal cavity can be life-saving, especially when it comes from a ruptured ectopic pregnancy or a ruptured spleen. Also, it carries no risk of hepatitis or HIV, and it will be perfectly cross-matched. Autotransfusion is thus very useful.

AUTOTRANSFUSION

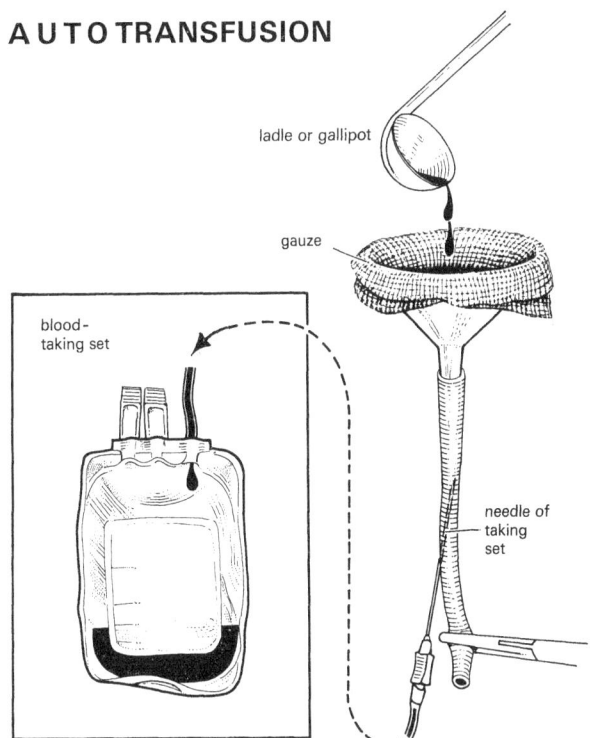

Fig. 16-8 AUTOTRANSFUSION using a funnel and a blood-taking set. This is also useful if the patient has a ruptured spleen (66.6). Use large pieces of gauze, and collect the blood in a taking set. *Kindly contributed by Stephen Whitehead of Maua Hospital, Kenya.*

AUTOTRANSFUSION

INDICATIONS. (1) Ectopic pregnancy. (2) Rupture of the spleen (66.6).

CONTRAINDICATIONS. Don't attempt autotransfusion if: (1) There is an offensive smell when you open the patient's abdomen. (2) Her gut has been injured. (3) The blood is obviously haemolysed. (4) She is more than 14 weeks pregnant with a ruptured amniotic sac. Her blood will be contaminated with amniotic fluid containing large quantities of thromboplastin. If you transfuse this, it could theoretically cause DIC (disseminated intravascular coagulation).

CAUTION ! The presence of fresh clots is not a contraindication to autotransfusion.

THE VACUUM BOTTLE METHOD is the best one and allows you to transfuse her before induction (not usually desirable). Buy vacuum bottles, or prepare them by closing blood-taking bottles containing a citrate solution immediately they have been sterilized, before the steam in them has had time to condense (Primary Anaesthesia, Appendix A). Clamp a taking set, introduce one of its needles into her abdomen, as if you were doing a four quadrant tap (66.1), and then put the other needle into the bottle and remove the clamp. To fill the bottle insert another sterile needle connected to a vacuum pump into the bung. You may be able to collect up to 3 litres of blood this way. If the vacuum is imperfect, and does not fill the bottle, apply suction with a vacuum (water) pump connected to a sterile needle inserted through the bung.

THE SOUP LADLE METHOD is less satisfactory, but is useful when you cannot use a vacuum bottle because there are too many clots. Keep the equipment shown in Fig. 16-8 ready sterilized. Put her into a slight Trendelenburg position, make a small opening in her peritoneal cavity to begin with, and be prepared to catch the blood, as it escapes, with a sterilized stainless steel soup ladle or gallipot. Then complete the incision and ladle out the rest of the blood. Her right hypochondrium may be the easiest place to collect it. Pour it through a filter made of 2 or 3 thicknesses of gauze, and collect it in a blood-taking set. The filter in the drip set will remove smaller clots.

Alternatively, you will find a sump useful. This is a conical vessel with a handle and holes towards its tip. Insert it deep in the abdomen; blood will flow in through the holes and can be sucked out.

CAUTION ! (1) Either transfuse the blood immediately, or throw it away. (2) Don't give it to someone else.

16.11 APH—bleeding after the 28th week

In about half the patients who bleed antenatally you never find a cause. When you do find one it may be: (1) Obvious placental abruption (mild, moderate, or severe). (2) *Placenta praevia* (Grades One, Two, Three, or Four). (3) A variety of usually harmless lesions of the lower genital tract. The first two causes are much the most dangerous ones, but fortunately they are both about equally uncommon. An important problem in the antenatal clinic is the patient with a small bleed: "Has she got *placenta praevia*, or is it going to remain unexplained?"

BLEEDING AFTER THE 28TH WEEK

Admit her, keep her in bed, and observe her carefully. Record all the blood she loses. Measure and record her pulse, blood pressure, and haemoglobin.

Decide how much blood she has lost. She may be: (1) An emergency with severe bleeding (500 ml or more), or in shock, or in labour. (2) A non-emergency with none of these things.

Resuscitation may need to start immediately. Take blood for grouping and cross-matching, and make sure that there are always 2 units of blood cross-matched for her.

Examine her, but *don't do a vaginal examination with your fingers!* Ask yourself three questions: (1) Has her uterus ruptured (18.17) due to obstructed labour? (2) Has she ruptured the scar (18.14) from a previous Caesarean section? Both these are uncommon causes of vaginal bleeding during pregnancy or labour. (2) How likely is she to have placenta praevia? (see below)

Decide the probable duration of her pregnancy (don't use the surfactant test (19.2), because the amniocentesis needle may go through a low-lying placenta). Record the position, presentation, and lie of the baby. Feel for rhythmical contractions. Listen to his heart.

CAUTION! If you find an abnormal lie, don't try to correct it.

Test her urine for protein. This is worth doing even though interpreting the result may be difficult.

DIAGNOSIS. Assess the probabilities like this:

Suggesting placenta praevia—(1) Bright red painless bleeding which can be anything from mild to severe, especially after 32 weeks, and tends to stop and start again. (2) A soft non-tender uterus that relaxes between contractions. (3) The fetal heart can be heard. (4) Shock is proportional to the blood she has lost. (5) The presenting part is higher than expected, and an unstable lie or an abnormal one are common. Suspect placenta praevia if you find a high head or a breech, a head or breech overlapping her symphysis by more than two finger widths, or a transverse lie. Placenta praevia is unlikely (but not impossible), if the head or breech are in easy contact with her symphysis, and do not overlap it. You can only be sure that she has not got placenta praevia, if the head or the breech are deeply engaged in her pelvis. If placenta praevia is likely, see Section 16.12.

Suggesting abruption—(1) Painful bleeding which is slight to moderate. (2) The presenting part is not higher than you expect, and the lie is usually stable. (3) A tense, tender, woody-hard uterus with poorly defined fetal parts. (4) An absent fetal heart. (5) Shock which is worse than you would expect from the blood she has lost vaginally. (6) Constant lower abdominal pain. (7) Loss of fetal movements. If abruption is likely, see Section 16.13.

CAUTION ! Beware of diagnosing abruption in a patient who has had a previous Caesarean section; rupture of her uterus is much more likely, even if she has not been in labour for long.

Suggesting a heavy show—(1) There is less than 10 ml of blood. (2) She bleeds with contractions. (3) Blood is usually mixed with mucus. (4) Bleeding stops when her membranes rupture.

Suggesting rupture of her uterus—See Section 18.17.

If she does not have an obvious abruption or placenta praevia, and is not in labour, do a speculum examination.

SPECULUM EXAMINATION. Do this to see where the blood is coming from, and to diagnose the incidental causes of bleeding. Do it in the labour ward in the lithotomy position in a good light. It is not easy, and can precipitate bleeding if you do it roughly. Even poking around to find the cervix can cause bleeding if she has placenta praevia. Pass a sterile speculum.

CAUTION ! Don't examine her vaginally with your fingers. If she does have a placenta praevia, you may cause massive bleeding. Use gentle speculum examination only.

Look for: (1) Cervical erosions. (2) Cervical polypi. (3) Vaginitis. (4) Carcinoma of her cervix. (5) Varicose veins (rare). (6) Decidua in her upper endocervix.

If she has placenta praevia (hopefully most unlikely, since you are examining her in the labour ward), you may see—a normal cervix, a haemorrhagic mucous plug, a blood clot in her external os, active bleeding from her cervix, or an open cervix with placental tissue peeping out of it. If you mistakenly do a digital examination, there will be a boggy feeling of placenta in front of the baby's head, followed by torrential bleeding as you remove your finger!

If she has abruption, you will see blood coming out of her cervix (if you mistakenly do a digital examination, you don't feel placenta).

If she has trichomoniasis (red vaginal wall and a pale green frothy discharge), treat her and her sexual partner at the same time (M 29.6).

If she has cervical erosions, they will usually heal after delivery and need no specific treatment. Treat any associated trichomoniasis. They seldom cause more than staining of her underwear or spotting, which may be related to sex.

If she has vulval varicosities, local pressure will probably stop it. If necessary, insert a suture. Varicosities sometimes occur at the vulva or introitus of older multips and occasionally bleed.

If she has a cervical polyp, don't twist it off during pregnancy: it may bleed severely. Leave it alone, and deal with it after delivery (20-5).

If she has carcinoma of her cervix, and is in labour, section her. If the lesion is large, the classical operation is better.

If you find an incidental cause of bleeding, she can get up and go home, if appropriate, depending on the cause. *However, finding an incidental cause (such as a small polyp) does not prevent her from also having a placenta praevia, so beware!* Does the incidental cause look as if it could have caused the bleeding she describes?

If you are not sure what she has, she will probably only have mild bleeding, but you will be wise to assume that she might have placenta praevia.

16.12 Placenta praevia

In the last trimester of pregnancy the isthmus of the uterus unfolds to form the lower segment. Normally, the placenta does not overlie it, so there is no bleeding. If however the placenta does overlie the lower segment, it may shear off over a small area and bleed.

Most patients with placenta praevia bleed before labour starts. They bleed painlessly and pass bright red blood. The first bleed may be slight, and subsequent ones increasingly severe, as the area of placental separation increases. You are unlikely to have ultrasound, or any other test to confirm the position of a patient's placenta, so you will have to find out where it is by examining her *in the theatre,* when you are fully prepared for an elective or emergency delivery. The correct timing of this is vital. You can do it early, soon after she presents. Or, if she is not bleeding severely, you can postpone it, and manage her non-operatively in hospital until she reaches 36 weeks, by which time her baby's chances of survival are almost as good as they would be at term. Most of your patients with *placenta praevia* will present before the 36th week, so non-operative treatment will improve your perinatal mortality—but it is only justified if Caesarean section is instantly available 24 hours a day, 7 days a week!

Unfortunately, the worst type of *placenta praevia* (Type Four) often does not bleed until labour starts. Even so, a high presenting part, or a persistent transverse lie, should lead a smart midwife to suspect it in the antenatal clinic.

There are several ways in which you can deliver a patient with *placenta praevia:*

(1) Caesarean section is the safest method in 95 per cent of cases. Its various risks and difficulties are described in Sections 18.8 and 18.10.

(2) You can deliver her vaginally. This may be necessary in health centres, if she cannot be referred, so it is described in *Primary Mother Care*. There are two ways of doing this. (a) The baby's head can be brought down on to the placental site, if necessary with Willet's forceps or a vulsellum, and a weight attached to his scalp. (b) A leg can be brought down and his buttocks used to compress the placental site. These methods almost always kill him, so it is desirable that he be already dead, or so small as to be unlikely to survive. They are both ancient methods, and are no longer done when Caesarean section is available, unless he is dead, and her cervix well dilated (>5 cm) and not too thick.

The main risks of vaginal delivery are that, in trying to bring down the head or a leg, you separate more of the placenta and increase bleeding. If you fail, and the task is not easy, you worsen her prognosis. You may also be tempted to force delivery before adequate dilatation, and so tear her cervix.

Placenta praevia increases the risk of puerperal sepsis, and of postpartum haemorrhage, because the lower segment, to which the placenta was attached, contracts less well after delivery.

MRS X died in hospital during labour. The doctor who treated her certified her death as being due to *placenta praevia*. The specialist obstetrician said that haemorrhage might not have been fatal, if she had not been anaemic due to parasitic infection and malnutrition. There was also concern because she had only been given 500 ml of blood, and because she died on the table while being sectioned by a trainee. The hospital administrator noted that she had not arrived at the hospital until 4 hours after the onset of severe bleeding, and that she had bled several times during the previous month, for which she did not seek treatment. A sociologist observed that she was 39 years old, with seven previous pregnancies and 5 living children. She had never used contraceptives, and her last pregnancy was unwanted. She was also poor, illiterate, and lived in a rural area. LESSONS Here we are concerned with the technology of treatment, but the critical factors are often the social ones.

PLACENTA PRAEVIA

This is the patient with a probable placenta praevia diagnosed in the last section.

If she continues to bleed, and the the presentation is cephalic do an EIT (examination in theatre). If it is not cephalic, section her.

If she is no longer bleeding, her baby is alive and she is not in labour, admit her to the labour ward for observation and non-operative treatment. If she has not bled for 6 hours transfer to the antenatal ward and ask her to do a kick count (M 28.3). Keep her in bed in the antenatal ward for 5 days. If she does not bleed during this time, she can get up to go to the toilet. Abandon non-operative treatment at any time if she goes into labour, or she bleeds seriously, or her baby dies. If none of these things happen, allow her to continue to 36 weeks if you can confirm lung maturity with a surfactant test (19.1). Otherwise, 38 weeks is safer for the baby. If you don't know her dates, wait until her baby has reached a reasonable size.

CAUTION ! This non-operative management is only indicated if: (1) Her baby is alive. (2) She is not in labour. (3) She is in hospital. (4) You have plenty of blood to transfuse her, if necessary. (5) You can section her at any moment.

If her baby is dead, don't section her unless her placenta praevia requires it. Encourage her to go into labour. See Section 16.4 on the 'dead baby'.

AN EXAMINATION IN THE THEATRE ('EIT') FOR PLACENTA PRAEVIA

The purpose of a vaginal examination at this stage is to find whether she has a placenta praevia or not, and what type it is. If it is Type One or Two, she should be able to deliver vaginally, unless she has other problems. For Types Three or Four she needs Caesarean section.

ANTEPARTUM BLEEDING

Types of abruption

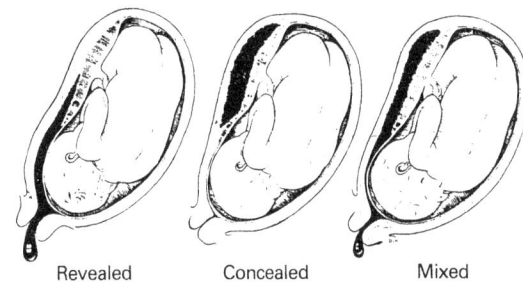

Revealed   Concealed   Mixed

Types of placenta praevia

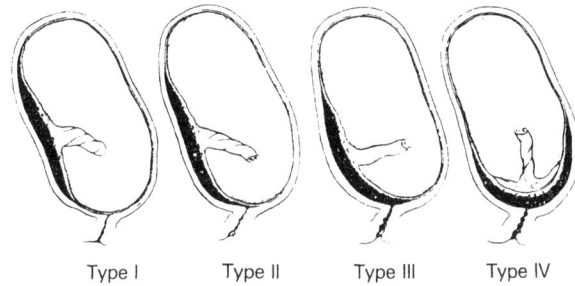

Type I   Type II   Type III   Type IV

Fig. 16-9 ANTEPARTUM BLEEDING. The three types of abruption, revealed, concealed, and mixed, and the four types of placenta praevia. *From Munro Kerr's 'Operative obstetrics' (7th edn. edited by Chassar Moir), Figs. 30,1 and 30,2. Ballière Tindall, with kind permission.*

INDICATIONS. A patient with suspected placenta praevia and a cephalic presentation who has (1) reached 36 weeks, or (2) bled heavily before reaching 36 weeks.

PREPARATION. Take her to the theatre and have everything absolutely ready for a Caesarean section, with the trolley laid, the trolley nurse scrubbed up, and your assistant also scrubbed up ready for a Caesar. Have two units of blood crossmatched for her ready in the theatre.

ANAESTHESIA. If she is very likely to have a placenta praevia, give her a general anaesthetic and intubate her. There may not be time for a local one. If she is unlikely to have placenta praevia, *and your anaesthetist is good* have everything ready to give her a general anaesthetic, if necessary, but don't actually start to give it. If there is time, starve her.

CAUTION ! If your anaesthetist is unskilled, anaesthetize all patients having an EIT. She may bleed suddenly, and an unskilled anaesthetist may panic.

Don't pass a stomach tube, because gagging may precipitate bleeding. Set up a drip. Catheterize her bladder.

VAGINAL EXAMINATION. Start by doing a vaginal examination with one or two Sims' specula to confirm that blood is actually coming from her cervix. Occasionally, you find that it is coming from a varicosity on her vulva or in her vagina.

Then ask an assistant to press the baby's head into the brim of her pelvis. Explore her vaginal fornices with your finger.

Can you feel any abnormal thickness in her lower uterine segment between your finger and the presenting part? Is the thickening all round her os, or only related to part of it? You should be able to get a fairly good idea of what type of placenta praevia she has: One, Two, Three, or Four (Fig. 16-9). If necessary, put your whole hand into her vagina.

If you can feel an abnormal thickening, she probably does have a placenta praevia. The type pf placenta she has is all important. Feel very carefully where the thickening is in relation to her os. If there is abnormal thickening all round it (probably Type Four), *don't put your finger through her os*. Section her.

If: (1) you cannot feel any abnormal thickening, or (2) the thickening you can feel does not suggest a Type Four placenta praevia, put your index finger *very gently* through her os, and explore all round it. Sweep it in gently widening circles, until you have examined all round as far as you can reach with your finger. *Stop, as soon as you feel any placenta!* Remove your finger from time to time to see if she has started to bleed. If you feel placenta over her os, or if she bleeds, section her.

If you cannot feel the placenta anywhere, when you put your finger through her os, and she does not bleed much, she is probably a case of abruption, or Type One placenta praevia. Rupture her membranes. Avoid oxytocin to begin with, because its use in a case of abruption can cause nasty cervical tears, rupture of the uterus, and occasionally amniotic fluid embolus. If, however, she does not go quickly into labour, set up an oxytocin drip (2.5 units in 500 ml of dextrose 5%). If you are giving her oxytocin, watch the fetal heart carefully. If fetal distress develops in the first stage, section her.

If she bleeds so severely that it cannot be controlled by rupturing her membranes, and pressing his head into her pelvis, section her.

PLACENTA PRAEVIA DURING LABOUR

IF SHE IS IN LABOUR AND IS BLEEDING SEVERELY, she is usually an emergency admission. Take her to the theatre, give her a general anaesthetic, and do an EIT as above. Section her, unless her cervix is fully dilated or almost so, and her membranes are presenting at the os.

If you can feel the vertex is presenting through the membranes, rupture them, so as to bring her baby's head down on to her placenta. This is possible for a Type One and an anteriorly placed Type Two placenta, and usually stops bleeding in a multip when it begins during labour.

If bleeding continues, section her, unless you expect her to deliver soon.

If the placenta is fully detached or nearly so, and is sitting on top of the baby's head (rare), **remove it and deliver him.**

If any other part is presenting, management depends on where the placenta is.

If the breech is presenting, the placenta does not cover her internal os, and her cervix is sufficiently dilated, **consider bringing down a leg and delivering her vaginally** (M 12.2). This is always satisfactory for a dead fetus; but only consider it for a live one, if her cervix is more than 5 cm dilated and the baby is very small. Improvise a string of gauze swabs, tie this to his leg, tie a weight of 500 g to the other end, and hang this over the end of her bed. CAUTION ! Don't pull the baby through an inadequately dilated cervix (it need not necessarily be fully dilated, depending on the size of the baby).

If the placenta covers her internal os and she bleeds, **section her** and transfuse her if necessary.

OTHER TREATMENT

Finally, don't hurry labour, take careful aseptic precautions, and restore her blood volume. Monitor the fetal heart carefully. If there are signs of fetal distress, consider Caesarean section.

Give her ergometrine with oxytocin at the completion of the second stage. Watch carefully for further bleeding for at least 24 hours.

16.13 Placental abruption

Abruption is not common, and is not easy to treat. The longer you leave a patient undelivered, the worse her prognosis. If she has severe abruption, she has at least a 25% chance of DIC (disseminated intravascular coagulation), if you leave her more than 48 hours. So try to deliver her vaginally well within this time. She will usually go into labour spontaneously within 24 hours. Only section her on the uncommon indications given below. If she has severe abruption, DIC will make it dangerous. Her baby is often dead, and is usually growth-retarded and premature, so CPD (cephalopelvic disproportion) is seldom a problem.

The principles of management are: (1) Correct hypovolaemia. (2) Deliver her quickly, preferably vaginally. (3) Prevent the complications—postpartum haemorrhage, DIC, and renal failure.

If she has DIC, try to: (1) Empty her uterus. (2) Give her fresh blood. You can manage most cases with 2 or 3 units, but you may occasionally need much more. Stored blood is less useful, but is much better than no blood. You are unlikely to have fresh frozen plasma, or cryoprecipitate. If you have fibrinogen give it, she will need 3 g (19.11a).

There is no practical way of diagnosing mild abruption, so the account below refers to severe abruption only.

SEVERE ABRUPTION

Make the diagnosis, as in Section 16.11. This account applies to revealed and concealed abruption (more common), and combinations of the two. If you are going to rupture a patient's membranes, and you will probably have to, do this EARLY, before you do anything else—see below.

THE CLOTTING TIME.

If you want to know if her blood will clot normally or not, take 5 ml into a dry glass tube. Invert it every 30 seconds, and see when it clots. It should clot in 5 to 8 minutes. If it takes longer than this, she has a clotting defect. If it clots in 2.5 minutes or less, it is hypercoagulable. Then put the tube in your pocket. If the clot lyses in 30 minutes (fibrinolysis), fibrin degradation products are present, and she needs fibrinogen and an antifibrinolytic agent (aprotinin)—if you have it!

RESUSCITATION. Start a rapid transfusion of 0.9% saline, or Ringer's lactate, through a wide needle or cannula. Take a sample to determine her blood group. Ask for an emergency (30 minutes) crossmatch of 4 to 6 units of *fresh* blood. Measure her clotting time. Give her pethidine 25 to 50 mg by slow intravenous injection.

As soon as blood is ready, transfuse her rapidly. Give her calcium gluconate (10 ml of 10% solution) with every third unit. If you don't have blood, give her Ringer's lactate or saline. Try to correct her hypovolaemia and anaemia within 2 hours of admission. You want her to deliver soon, and you don't want to let her go into labour while she is shocked.

Insert an indwelling catheter and measure her hourly urine output: it should be more than 60 ml. If possible, and you are experienced, insert a central venous catheter (A 19.2). Keep her CVP between 8 and 12 cm of water. Ideally, her haemoglobin should be not less than 110 g/l, and her haematocrit above 30.

If you cannot measure the CVP, here is a guide as to how much blood she needs.

Transfuse her until her systolic blood pressure is at least 100 mm Hg. If it is below this, she needs at least 1000 ml. If it is below 80 mm she needs 1500 to 2000 ml.

If she is dehydrated, correct her dehydration with 0.9% saline or Ringer's lactate.

If the above measures fail, try correcting her acidosis, with 50 to 100 mmol of sodium bicarbonate (A 15.1).

CAUTION ! (1) Heparin is contraindicated. (2) Don't give plasma expanders, such as dextran, because these may precipitate DIC, and cause uncontrollable haemorrhage.

MONITORING. Start a partogram (M 18.2). All through labour check her pulse, her blood pressure, and her central venous pressure half-hourly. Every 2 hours check her urine output, her clotting time and her haemoglobin, and do a vaginal examination. Note the size of her uterus, and repeatedly check it. An increase in height shows that she is continuing to bleed.

THE DELIVERY OF A PATIENT WITH ABRUPTION

If her baby is alive (unusual), and weighs more than 1.5 kg, consider section, as soon as she is resuscitated. If you are going to section her, you MUST do so immediately, before a clotting defect develops. Waiting a few hours and then sectioning her is a recipe for disaster.

If he is dead and she is not in labour, rupture her membranes (M 19.3) and give her an oxytocin drip (M 22.2). Labour is usually fast. Try to deliver her in 6 to 8 hours. Once she is in the active phase, labour should progress rapidly. You may decide to rupture her membranes, regardless of his condition, and give give her life precedence over his. Besides inducing labour, rupturing her membranes will reduce her intra-amniotic pressure. This will slow the abruptive process, and may also release retroplacental clot. Her tense, tender, woody-hard uterus will make her contractions difficult to monitor, and the dose of oxytocin difficult to adjust. If she is obese and highly parous, with an unfavourable cervix, she is particularly at risk; so try to feel for uterine contractions as best you can, and assess the progress of her labour by careful vaginal examination.

If active labour has not started after a further 6 to 8 hours and her clotting time is normal, consider section. If it is abnormal, Caesarean section will probably kill her.

LATER STAGES. **The second stage** is usually rapid. Her dead baby, the placenta, and clot may all be expelled suddenly, and tear her perineum, cervix, or uterus.

The third stage causes problems, because of the clotting defect, and because she may have an atonic uterus. She runs a serious risk of postpartum haemorrhage, so be sure to manage this actively. As he is delivered, give her an ampoule of intravenous ergometrine with oxytocin ('Syntometrine'). Add 15 units of oxytocin to 500 ml of Ringer's lactate or saline, and run this in fast to keep her uterus well contracted.

CAESAREAN SECTION should rarely be necessary. Either do it immediately, or don't do it at all. Late section (after 24 hours) is dangerous if she has an abnormal clotting time, unless you have plenty of blood and plenty of experience. At section her uterus will look bruised ('Couvelaire' uterus), but will contract normally.

The absolute indications for Caesarean section include: (1) A previously scarred uterus. Avoid a 'trial of a Caesarean scar' (18.14), because you will not know if she is rupturing—vaginal bleeding, tachycardia, and pain can all be caused by abruption, or by a uterus which is rupturing. (2) Failure to progress, despite artificial rupture of her membranes and oxytocin. (3) A patient who is bleeding to death before having a chance to deliver. Caesarean section is a desperate step and may save her life. (4) A live baby at term, with signs of fetal distress. (5) The transverse lie of a baby at term for whom vaginal delivery is impossible.

If you have fibrinogen, give it just before you operate. Have hot packs ready when you operate, and empty her uterus quickly. Bleeding usually stops, but if she bleeds severely, deliver her uterus into the wound, surround it with hot packs, grasp it firmly, and give her ergometrine with oxytocin. If this fails to control bleeding, tie her internal iliac arteries (3.5); if this too fails proceed to hysterectomy (20.12).

DIFFICULTIES WITH PLACENTAL ABRUPTION

If her URINE OUTPUT FALLS to below 30 ml an hour in spite of adequate fluid replacement, as observed by her CVP, give her at least a litre of Ringer's lactate, and then give her frusemide 40 mg intravenously as a bolus injection. If she develops renal failure, see Section 53.3.

If her UTERUS DOES NOT CONTRACT after vaginal delivery (atonic uterus), manage her in the usual way by giving her oxytocin, making sure that her bladder is empty and all blood clot expressed from her uterus. Give her an oxytocin drip as above, and a repeat dose of ergometrine with oxytocin, provided this is not contraindicated, either because she is hypertensive, or because you have already given her two 0.5 mg doses. Compress her uterus bimanually (19-3). If her bleeding fails to stop, you may have to open her abdomen and tie her internal iliac arteries, or do a hysterectomy as a last resort. If possible, give her an ampoule of prostaglandin F_2alpha, either intravenously, or through her abdominal wall directly into her myometrium.

If she CONTINUES TO BLEED AFTER DELIVERY from multiple small tears, she may have: (1) DIC. (2) An atonic uterus (see above). (3) Multiple lacerations in her cervix. Correct (1) and (2). Examine her vaginally, and you may see many small lacerations and bleeding points. Carefully pack her genital tract as in section 19.11a. Give her an oxytocin drip to make sure her uterus is well contracted. Remove the pack in 24 to 48 hours.

If you diagnose ABRUPTION IN A PATIENT WITH A CAESAREAN SCAR, it is probably a ruptured uterus. Section her immediately.

17 The medicine of pregnancy

17.2 Anaemia in pregnancy

Severe anaemia in pregnancy makes a mother sick, and in some parts of the world it commonly kills her as the result of congestive heart failure, before, during, and after labour. Anaemia impairs her resistance to genital and respiratory infection, and the cerebral anoxia it causes can lead to mental confusion and coma. How ill she is depends on how rapidly her anaemia developed. If it developed slowly, she may have suprisingly few symptoms. Even so, a traumatic delivery or a small blood-loss can kill her. Severe anaemia can also harm her baby by causing late abortion, prematurity, low birthweight (IUGR, 19.13), and perinatal deaths. Even moderate anaemia harms him, and severe anaemia can cause a perinatal mortality of thirty per cent.

Mild anaemia (down to 100 g/l) is physiological and is the result of the plasma volume expanding during pregnancy. More severe anaemia is caused by: (1) *P. falciparum* malaria, especially in primips. (2) Iron deficiency, especially in grand multips, and in patients with hookworms. (4) Folate deficiency, especially if they also have malaria, malnutrition, or twins. (3) Sickle-cell disease and other haemoglobinopathies. (4) AIDS. Fortunately, anaemia is also cheaply preventable, and fairly easily treated; if this is done promptly, it will remove most of its risks to her and her baby. *So find out what the causes are in your area and adapt the regime below to them.* You will need to measure her haemoglobin. The most practical instruments for doing this at the present time are the Spencer haemoglobinometer (AOC) and the microhaematocrit centrifuge.

Unfortunately, you may see her for the first time late in pregnancy, when she may need blood. The risk of transfusion is that it will increase her blood volume, and may precipitate cardiac failure. You can minimize this risk by giving her packed cells only, by transfusing her slowly, and by giving her a rapidly acting diuretic.

The prevention of anaemia in pregnancy is a community problem. Births must be spaced, parasites controlled, nutrition improved, and prophylactic treatment given to all mothers from the beginning of pregnancy.

Malaria especially *falciparum* malaria: (1) Destroys red cells and so causes anaemia, which may be megaloblastic if she also has a secondary folate deficiency. (2) Causes abortions, perinatal deaths, premature labour, and low birthweight (IUGR, 19.13). If she is non-immune, her placenta may be so heavily parasitized that it is black with malarial pigment. Malaria may be more serious in areas where it is unstable, than in those in which it is stable. In an area of stable malaria, she may only get attacks when she is pregnant, especially during the second trimester, and while she is a primip.

Antimalarials have their risks. In a village mother in an endemic area the risks lie strongly with the parasite—she needs prophylaxis, either from the antenatal clinic, or through PHC workers—if you can get them the drugs. For a minimally exposed visitor to an endemic area, you will have to balance the risk of malaria against those of the drugs to prevent it.

Chloroquine gives the best and safest protection against sensitive strains of *P. falciparum,* and all the other malaria parasites. Proguanil is safe in pregnancy. Although the antifolate pyrimethamine is theoretically embryopathic, it seems to be safe in practice. One contributor considers it should be supplemented with folic acid, especially during the first trimester. Avoid 'Fansidar' (pyrimethamine/sulphadoxine) except for the treatment of chloroquine-resistant strains (see below). 'Maloprim' (dapsone/pyrimethamine) is controversial; one tablet a week gives fairly good protection if there is little resistance locally to pyrimethamine, and is said not to be embryopathic. One contributor considers it should be supplemented with with folic acid.

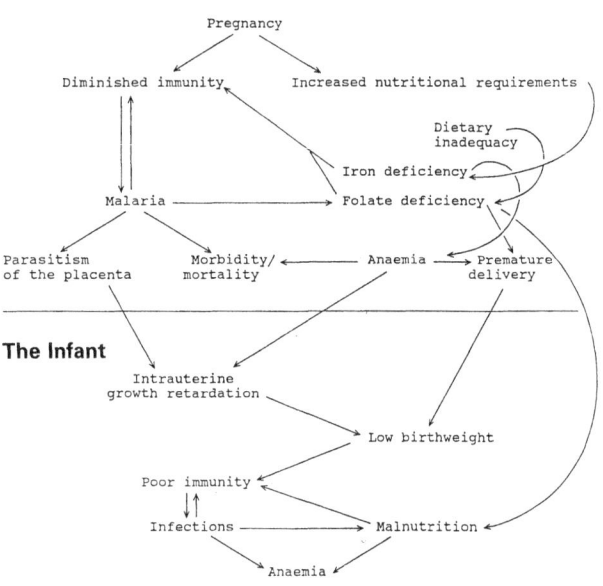

Fig. 17-1 THE PATHOPHYSIOLOGY OF ANAEMIA, malaria, iron- and-folate deficiency in pregnancy. *Kindly contributed by Alan Fleming, from a Distance Learning Module prepared by the Wellcome Tropical Institute.*

SEVERE ANAEMIA

PREVENTION

DEFICIENCY ANAEMIA. If anaemia is common, give all mothers ferrous sulphate 200 mg with folate 50 µg once daily throughout pregnancy. This is the standard UNICEF tablet. There is no need for other more expensive preparations. If anaemia is not common, treat only those with anaemia. Healthy well-nourished non-anaemic mothers do not need extra iron in pregnancy.

MALARIA. In highly malarious areas give all mothers, especially all primips, a curative dose of the appropriate antimalarial (usually chloroquine 600 mg base once and 300 mg twice a day for two days), on first coming to the antenatal clinic, and then give them weekly prophylaxis until 4 weeks after delivery.

If the local strains are completely or partly chloroquine-sensitive, give her 5 mg/kg chloroquine base once a week. In some areas a higher dose may be necessary.

If there is chloroquine resistance locally, the choice of drugs is difficult. Proguanil ('Paludrine') 100 mg daily may be suitable. One contributor advises proguanil in all circumstances and *never* gives chloroquine prophylactically, on the grounds that its routine use for prophylaxis in the community promotes chloroquine resistance.

If she is normally immune, and gets a clinical attack during pregnancy, give her a full curative dose of chloroquine as above. If she is not normally immune, she needs speedy and effective treatment by the most effective drugs available.

If she is non-immune, she must have regular chemoprophylaxis throughout pregnancy, especially in the last trimester.

CAUTION ! (1) No chemoprophylactic regime is completely effective. If you think she is having a modified attack, treat her. (2) *Falciparum* infection is especially dangerous during the last trimester.

THE MANAGEMENT OF ANAEMIA

Screen all antenatal mothers clinically by examining their conjunctivae and their tongues. If a mother seems anaemic, measure her haemoglobin, and diagnose her as having 'anaemia' if it is <100 g/l. The important symptom is progressive dyspnoea on exertion. Look for: pallor, warm hands, dyspnoea at rest, a collapsing pulse, a large pulse pressure, pulsation of her retinal veins, tachycardia, an ejection systolic murmur (all signs of severe anaemia).

If she is moderately anaemic (60 to 100 g/l), before 34 weeks, investigate her as best you can, and examine a thin blood film. Routine tests for malaria and hookworms are of little value. If sickle-cell disease is common in your area, test for it. Give her tablets of ferrous sulphate three times a day, and folic acid 5 mg daily (this is a larger dose than that in the UNICEF ferrous sulphate/folate tablet) for 3 weeks. This will replace her body folate. Don't give more, and don't give it parenterally. Continue it until delivery. In malarious areas give her a therapeutic antimalarial course, followed by a prophylactic one. If necessary, treat her for hookworms. See her every two weeks in the high-risk clinic, and measure her haemoglobin.

If she is moderately anaemic after 34 weeks, proceed as above, but consider admitting her for parenteral iron and a blood transfusion.

If she is severely anaemic (<60 g/l), admit her, treat as above, and transfuse her if you can.

If she is very severely anaemic (45 g/l or less), or her haemoglobin has has fallen rapidly, watch for these danger signs: Cardiovascular: pulse >120, respirations >24, dyspnoea at rest. Cerebral: mental confusion or coma. Signs that the haemoglobin is falling due to bleeding or haemolysis: bleeding, jaundice, and fever. If she has any of these admit her to the labour ward or an ICU. Nurse her in the half-sitting position. Give her at least 2 units of packed cells and medical treatment as above.

PARENTERAL IRON FOR ANAEMIA

This will not make her haemoglobin rise any faster; it is more expensive, more painful, and may cause reactions. Its only advantage is that it avoids the oral route and the need for her co-operation.

INDICATIONS. Proven iron deficiency anaemia (haemoglobin <60 g/l), in which: (1) oral treatment is unlikely to succeed, or (2) there is not time for it to succeed because she is in the last trimester of pregnancy. And there are no contraindications such as sickle-cell anaemia or some other haemolytic anaemia.

AS A COURSE OF INJECTIONS. Calculate her iron need from her haemoglobin. Give her 150 mg of elemental iron parenterally for every 5 g/l that her haemoglobin needs raising. This will correct the iron deficit in her circulating red cells, with 50% extra to correct her iron stores. A typical dose is 1800 mg. Give her 1 ml (50 mg) the first day, then 2 ml (100 mg) daily or at longer intervals; the maximum daily dose is 5 ml (250 mg). Also give her a 20-day course of 5 mg folic acid tablets by mouth at the same time.

TOTAL DOSE IRON INFUSION (TDI) can supply a patient with all the iron she needs in half a day. But it has risks and can be fatal. A typical indication is the patient who lives far from hospital, can make few antenatal visits, and cannot be admitted. It is contraindicated if she is asthmatic. Give her the iron she needs, calculated as above, in a litre of dextrose slowly over 6 to 8 hours. Give her an antihistamine (promethazine 50 mg) 30 minutes before. For the first 15 minutes, give her 10 drops a minute, then, if all is well, give her the rest of the dose at not more than 1 ml/minute. Expect the maximum effect in 4 to 6 weeks.

CAUTION ! (1) Stop the drip if she has rashes, if her blood pressure falls, her pulse rises, or she has giddiness or rigors. (2) Have adrenalin, aminophylline, and an injectable glucocorticosteroid immediately available. (3) Don't give intravenous iron by bolus intravenous injection. (4) There is some evidence that TDI can make iron available for the metabolism of invading pathogens, increase her susceptibility to infection, and increase the incidence of postnatal malarial parasitaemia, so watch her carefully, and treat her if necessary.

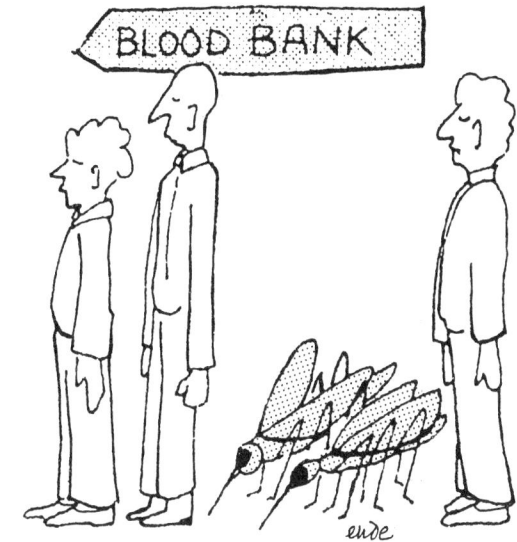

TRANSFUSION FOR ANAEMIA

INDICATIONS. These vary with the risk of HIV:

If there is little or no risk of HIV transfuse her if: (1) She is in incipient cardiac failure with a Hb <40 g/l. (2) She is breathless at rest or needs an operative delivery with a Hb of <60 g/l. One contributor would transfuse all women with a haemoglobin of <60 g/l who are >36 weeks. (3) She has sickle-cell disease and needs an operative delivery with a Hb <80 g/l (transfusion may prevent a sickle-cell crisis). (4) You expect her to lose >1000 ml of blood at operation and her Hb is <80 g/l (500 ml is commonly lost at a normal delivery). (5) She bleeds severely and loses >30% of her blood volume.

If HIV is a risk, only transfuse her to save her life. See Chapter 28a. She is at particular risk if her Hb is <40 g/l, she has twins, or a large spleen, or heart disease, or she needs an operative delivery.

TRANSFUSING RED CELLS. If she has a haemoglobin of less than 60 g/l, give her repeated small transfusions of cells only over several days. You will not be able to centrifuge bottles of blood, so: (1) decant the plasma and transfuse only the packed cells. Or, (2) slowly invert a bottle after you have inserted a giving set. Or, (3) if the blood is in bags, so that decantation is difficult, let them hang upright in a refrigerator to allow the cells fall to the bottom. Open the vent at the top of a bag, squeeze out the plasma by hand, or use a home-made instrument made of two sprung boards. You can then transfuse the packed cells without transfusing most of the plasma.

Don't give her more than 500 ml of packed cells at a time. Add 20 mg of frusemide to 500 ml of packed cells, and transfuse them slowly over 6 hours. Or, precede the transfusion by frusemide 40 mg intravenously. It will cause an intense diuresis, which will reduce her plasma volume, and make room for the packed cells.

If she has rigors or a rise in temperature, stop the drip immediately.

If her pulse pressure or her heart rate rise, they are the earliest signs of cardiac failure, so stop the drip—before a rise in her jugular venous pressure and pulmonary oedema make failure obvious. Give her frusemide 40 mg intravenously. Don't repeat it for at least 12 hours.

THE DELIVERY OF A SEVERELY ANAEMIC PATIENT

Premature labour is a common complication of severe anaemia, and may cause heart failure. If her haemoglobin is less than 50 g/l at term, she is an obstetric emergency. A blood transfusion at any stage is often life-saving.

Deliver her sitting up, and give her oxygen if necessary. Don't put up a routine drip—it will overload her circulation unnecessarily. Shorten the second stage with a vacuum extractor. Take great care to reduce blood loss. Do an episiotomy only if it is important. Give her ergometrine, or oxytocin, with the third stage. Deliver the placenta actively, using ergometrine and controlled cord traction. Manage any operative procedure with scrupulous asepsis, because she runs an increased risk of puerperal infection. If she loses more than 500 ml transfuse her.

If she is clearly in heart failure, avoid ergometrine and oxytocin ('Syntometrine').

Keep her in the labour ward or the ICU for at least 24 hours after her condition has stabilized. Before you discharge her, warn her to come for antenatal care in her next pregnancy, because she may become anaemic again.

CAUTION ! She can easily go into failure after delivery.

DIFFICULTIES WITH SEVERE ANAEMIA

If, during pregnancy, her ANAEMIA FAILS TO RESPOND to conventional treatment: (1) Is your diagnosis correct? For example, are you really dealing with iron-deficiency anaemia? (2) Is she taking her drugs? (3) Is she continuing to bleed (perhaps hookworms) or to haemolyse (perhaps malaria)?

If she becomes SEVERELY ANAEMIC IN EARLY PREGNANCY, consider the possibility of an ectopic pregnancy.

If she presents with GROSS ANAEMIA DURING THE PUERPERIUM, consider a retained placenta and puerperal sepsis, correct her anaemia, and control infection before you try to remove it.

If she has chloroquine-resistant falciparum malaria (RII), try three tablets of pyrimethamine 25 mg with sufladoxine 500 mg ('Fansidar'). Or, amodiaquine base 600 mg orally once and 400–600 mg daily for two days. If this fails, give her oral quinine 600 mg three times daily for 7 days. If necessary give quinine intravenously 10 mg/kg base over 2–4 hours. Quinine occasionally provokes uterine activity, slows the fetal heart, and causes hypoglycaemia.

17.3 Diabetes in pregnancy

Diabetes is one of the more difficult conditions to manage, under the conditions for which we write, especially in pregnancy. Insulin supplies are likely to be a major problem, with patients dying when their supplies are interrupted. Even where care is good, it may only be the teachers and health workers who are sufficiently motivated and educated to manage their diabetes well enough to survive for long. Here is what you should do, with some advice as to what you can do, if your facilities are so limited that you can only measure the blood glucose exceptionally, if at all. If so, you will not be able to control a patient's diabetes well enough to prevent its adverse effects on her or her baby, but you should be able to keep her out of coma.

Pregnancy and diabetes adversely affect one another, and the more complicated or long-standing the diabetes, the stronger the effect. Diabetes increases maternal mortality 10 times, as the result of ketoacidosis, hypoglycaemia, and infection. A mother is also at increased risk from polyhydramnios ($\times 50$), gestational hypertension ($\times 3$), and infection (especially pyelonephritis). Fortunately, pregnancy will not usually harm her health in the long term. If however she has retinopathy, this may get worse during pregnancy, although it may improve afterwards; uropathy on the other hand may worsen irreversibly. Her baby is at increased risk from sudden intrauterine death (usually at 36 to 38 weeks), fetal macrosomia (excessive size), neonatal hypoglycaemia (19.12), prematurity (particularly hyaline membrane disease), and congenital malformations ($\times 3$). Careful diabetic management reduces these risks.

At the start of pregnancy she can have: (1) Type One diabetes (IDDM, insulin-dependent diabetes mellitus). (2) Type Two diabetes (NIDDM non-insulin-dependent diabetes mellitus). This is uncommon in women of childbearing age in Africa, and is more common in obese mothers in India and the Middle East. We shall not make any further reference to Types One and Two diabetics; it is the insulin-dependent Type One patients who are important. (3) Impaired glucose tolerance. However, following Chalmers, who concluded that: 'Except for research purposes, all forms of glucose tolerance testing should be stopped (in pregnancy)', we say nothing more about it here. (4) Renal glycosuria, which is a lowered renal threshold to glucose, and is harmless. If diabetes resolves after pregnancy, it is said to have been 'gestational'.

About 1% of women have glucose in their urine when they are fasting. Most of them have renal glycosuria, and a few have diabetes.

Although testing the urine for glucose in early pregnancy picks up all cases of diabetes, it is an imperfect screening method because it picks up many harmless cases of renal glycosuria. Glucose in the urine may vary greatly from day to day during pregnancy, so that a patient may have glycosuria on one visit and not on the next. Also, testing the urine is a poor way of monitoring the insulin requirements of a pregnant diabetic, especially after 16 weeks.

Unfortunately, testing the urine for glucose is the only practical screening test, so test the urine of all mothers, and investigate them as best you can.

Diabetic babies tend to be large, so don't let a mother become overdue. Ideally, she should deliver at 36 to 38 weeks. If she is a multip, you can usually induce her fairly easily.

Chalmers I, Enkin M, Keirse MJNC, 'Effective Care in Pregnancy and Childbirth', 1989 OUP.

DIABETES DURING PREGNANCY

DIAGNOSIS

Test the urine of all pregnant mothers.

If a mother has obvious symptoms (polyuria, thirst, pruritus, etc.), and heavy glycosuria, the diagnosis of diabetes is almost certain; but confirm it, if you can, by measuring her blood glucose and consulting Fig. 17-1a.

If she has glycosuria and no symptoms, do a random blood glucose, or a fasting blood glucose. She has renal glycosuria if she has glucose in her urine when her blood glucose is <6.7 mmol/l.

RANDOM BLOOD GLUCOSE. She is diabetic if, when she is not fasting, this is >10.0 mmol/l venous, or >11.1 mmol/l, (200 mg/dl) capillary (both whole blood). If she has no diabetic symptoms (polyuria or polydipsia, etc.), two abnormal levels are preferable for diagnosis.

A FASTING BLOOD GLUCOSE tells you more than a random blood glucose, but it is less convenient, because she does have to fast for 8 hours, and this is likely to mean another visit. If it is <6.7, she has not got diabetes.

THE MANAGEMENT OF DIABETES

A baby's survival and welfare depend absolutely on strict 'normoglycaemia' (his mother's fasting blood glucose should be <4 mmol/l and her postprandial peaks 2 hours after meals <7.5 mmol/l). Ideally, this requires careful blood glucose monitoring, if possible at home also.

If she is a diabetic on oral hypoglycaemic agents she will be better controlled if you can change her to soluble insulin,

DIAGNOSING DIABETES

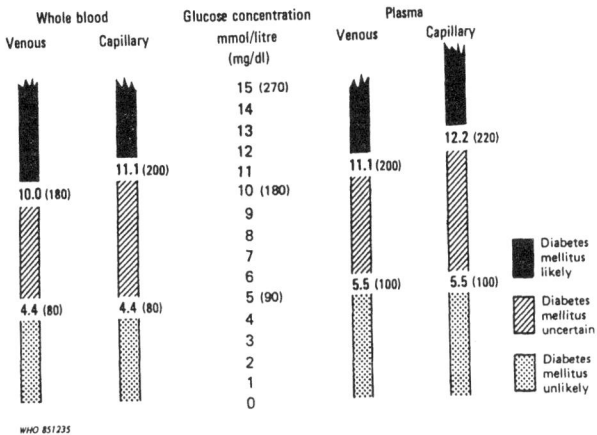

Fig. 17-1a DIAGNOSING DIABETES. Note that the significance of a particular value varies, depending on whether the sample is whole blood or plasma, venous or capillary. 'Diabetes'. 1985. WHO Technical Report Series 227.

and manage her as below. These agents are not recommended in pregnancy, although they have not been proved to be teratogenic. They cause neonatal hypoglycaemia, so be sure to stop them by 28 weeks and change to insulin. Stop them at least a week before a planned delivery.

If she is a known diabetic on insulin, she should, ideally, have a planned pregnancy, and be carefully stabilized for 3 months before she becomes pregnant, so that she conceives when she is normoglycaemic, because this reduces the risk of a congenital abnormality.

If she is a known diabetic on insulin, or has been diagnosed as diabetic by the criteria above, try to check her diabetic stability every 2 weeks during pregnancy, and if necessary admit her for the day. Adjust her diet so that it is steady in terms of content and timing, and put her on twice- daily injections of short- and medium-acting insulins ('soluble and isophane', 'soluble and lente', 'Actrapid and Monotard', or regular and NPH). If she is sophisticated, she may be able to adjust her food intake to match this regime; if not, adjust her injections to fit her meals. In early pregnancy, her insulin needs may fall (unusual), so that if she has previously been well controlled, she may become hypoglycaemic. You may have to reduce her dose by about 25% until 16 weeks. After 16 weeks her insulin needs rise again (usual), so that near term she needs 1.5-2 times as much as she did before pregnancy. She is therefore most likely to become ketotic late in pregnancy. Her insulin needs fall immediately the placenta is delivered.

If she is well-motivated and co-operative, aim for a fasting blood glucose of <4.5 mmol/l, and a postprandial level of <8 mmol/l. In achieving this she may be hypoglycaemic sometimes, so make sure she takes a glucose or sugar drink with the first signs of hypoglycaemia, and is prepared for them.

If she is sufficiently frightened by hypoglycaemia to stop taking her insulin, or fears harming herself or her baby, accept less strict control, but aim for a blood glucose of <6 mmol/l, and a postprandial level of <10 mmol/l.

DETERMINING HER GLUCOSE ('sugar') PROFILE. **Give her insulin half an hour before breakfast and half an hour before her evening meal. Measure her blood glucose 4 times: at 0600 hrs (reflecting her evening isophane insulin); at 1000 hrs (reflecting her morning soluble insulin; at 1500 hrs (reflecting her morning isophane insulin); and at 2000 hrs, reflecting her evening soluble insulin. Adjust her dose by 2-5 units, increasing it by one unit for each mmol/l (20 mg/dl). If any value is >4 mmol/l higher than you want, or if more than 2 doses need adjusting, keep her for another day and repeat the profile.**

Starvation ketosis is bad for a baby, so test her urine for ketones after an overnight fast. If she has ketones, give her a late-night snack.

If only 1 or 2 insulin doses needed changing by <4 units each, repeat the profile in 2 weeks. Otherwise, or if she has had any ketones, check her in one week.

DIABETES IN LATE PREGNANCY. Admit her and adjust her insulin dose on the basis of her blood glucose, or, failing that, her glycosuria. Estimate fetal maturity clinically; if her dates are uncertain, withdraw some amniotic fluid and do a surfactant test (unfortunately, this is less reliable in diabetes). Repeat this weekly and, provided she has no complications, especially no hypertension or gross hydramnios (girth more than 100 cm), induce her as soon as her surfactant test is positive (19.2). Do kick counts (M 28.3), and try to bring her to at least 36 weeks.

THE DELIVERY OF A DIABETIC MOTHER

If her diabetes has been well controlled, and her baby is of average size, and she has no CPD (cephalopelvic disproportion), and she has a positive surfactant test, induce her at 37 weeks.

If she has serious hypertension or polyhydramnios, deliver her earlier, whatever the maturity of her baby.

Section her, if control has been poor, or there is CPD, or she has a malpresentation, or severe gestational hypertension, or a history of a previous difficult delivery, or polyhydramnios or a previous section, or if she is elderly. Your threshold for section should be lower in a diabetic, especially if she wants her tubes tied.

DIABETES DURING DELIVERY. Aim to provide her with glucose, insulin, and fluid, to prevent ketosis, and to keep her normoglycaemic. Don't worry if her blood glucose rises moderately during labour; hypoglycaemia is much more dangerous.

Ideally, give her a continuous constant glucose infusion at a fixed rate using a drip counter, and insulin by a syringe driver, adjusted according to her hourly blood-glucose levels.

Alternatively, give her a continuous glucose, potassium, and insulin ('GKI') infusion: 500 ml of 5% dextrose, with 8 units of soluble insulin (any kind), and 10 mmol of potassium chloride, at 120 ml/hour or 20 drops/min (if you use 10% dextrose give her 15 units of insulin). A 500 ml bottle will then last 4 hours, which will coincide with her 4-hourly urine tests. Test her blood glucose hourly with 'BMstix', or less satisfactorily 'Dextrostix', accepting a range of 4 to 10 mmol/l. If it is >10 mmol/l, take the present bag down and put 12 units in the next one. If it is <4 mmol/l, put 4 units in the next one.

If you cannot measure her blood glucose, test her urine, but make sure that she empties her bladder half an hour beforehand. At 0700 hrs on the morning of delivery (whether for induction or section) give her no food. Instead, start a drip of 5% dextrose in water and run it at 20 drops a minute. If she is having soluble insulin, give her half her normal dose.

Measure and chart her urine glucose 4-hourly, and give her soluble isulin intramuscularly on the scale below. If you find ketones, add 8 units. If you give insulin intramuscularly, it is active for longer, and hypoglycaemia is less common.

Urine glucose nil, add no soluble insulin (blood glucose <6.2 mmol/l, 120 mg/dl).

Urine glucose +, soluble insulin 8 units (blood glucose 6.2-8.4 mmol/l, 120-150 mg/dl).

Urine glucose ++, add soluble insulin 16 units (blood glucose 8.4-11.2 mmol/l, 150-200 mg/dl).

Urine glucose +++, add soluble insulin 24 units (blood glucose 11.2-14 mmol/l 200-250 mg/dl).

Urine glucose ++++, add soluble insulin 32 units (blood glucose >14 mmol/l, 250 mg/dl).

CAUTION ! While she is in the labour ward, test her urine for ketones routinely. If you find them, she needs extra glucose. This is best given with insulin.

INDUCTION. If she is to be induced, rupture her membranes (19.3), and give her an oxytocin drip (M 22.2) in a separate bottle from the dextrose.

If she is not in established labour within 4 to 6 hours of induction, or if delivery is not imminent 10 to 12 hours after induction, section her. In a diabetic there is no place for a 'trial of labour', or a long labour. If necessary, assist vaginal delivery with a vacuum extractor, or outlet forceps.

CAUTION ! In communities where CPD is common shoulder

dystocia can be a problem in delivering diabetic babies. You can avoid it by sectioning her, but if you deliver her vaginally, be prepared for it—see below.

A DIABETIC BABY should be normal if his mother's diabetes has been well controlled. If it has not been well controlled, see above and Section 19.12.

CAESAREAN SECTION. Give her a 'GKI' infusion or the alternative method, as described above. Put her first on the list and continue the drip through the operation and afterwards until she can take oral fluids.

AFTER DELIVERY of the placenta, her insulin requirements fall sharply (less sharply if she gets an infection). Give her subcutaneous insulin with the next meal. If she has been sectioned, do the same, but she will need the drip up for longer. She should need about a third or half the insulin she needed before delivery, and about the same amount as she needed before she became pregnant. She can start to eat and drink as soon as she wishes, but if this is delayed continue to give her 2 litres of 5% dextrose and one litre of 5% dextrose in 0.9% saline daily (her glucose infusion must be continuous).

If she needed insulin before she became pregnant, she will still need it and can return to her original dose.

If her diabetes disappears after pregnancy, it was only gestational. If so, her blood glucose will usually have fallen to normal 48 hours after delivery, without any risk of ketosis.

DIFFICULTIES WITH DIABETES IN PREGNANCY

If you CANNOT MEASURE HER BLOOD GLUCOSE, you will have to rely on testing her urine. Make sure she empties her bladder half an hour before producing the next specimen for testing. Aim to make her urine specimens negative without causing hypoglycaemia. If she has hypoglycaemic episodes with glucose in her urine, she probably has renal glycosuria.

If she has SEVERE NAUSEA AND VOMITING OF PREGNANCY, and is receiving insulin, admit her and give her a glucose/insulin infusion.

If her INSULIN REQUIREMENTS FALL ABRUPTLY AT 36 WEEKS, it is probably a sign of impending placental failure, and delivery is indicated.

If her baby's head delivers but his SHOULDERS HAVE STUCK, there is SHOULDER DYSTOCIA, which can be serious (see M 21.4). An episiotomy will not help the dystocia, but it will reduce the risk of perineal or anterior vaginal injury. Ask your assistant to apply firm fundal pressure. Strong traction on his head may disimpact his shoulders, but injure his brachial plexus. Symphysiotomy is safer, so infiltrate local anaesthetic solution round her symphysis at the same time as you do an episiotomy and insert a catheter. If you are very skilled, wait for his head to deliver and then decide if a symphysiotomy is necessary. If so, do it quickly. If you are less confident, do it as the head crowns in any patient in whom you anticipate difficulty. As always, never do a symphysiotomy without also doing an episiotomy.

If he is alive, you can push his head back into her pelvis and do a Caesarean section (the Zavanelli manoeuvre). For example, if his head was born occipito-anterior, and has turned (restituted) to the side, turn his occiput anterior again. Then flex his head. It will probably go back into her uterus easily. Section her without delay.

17.4 Hypertension in pregnancy

The hypertensive disorders of pregnancy cause many of the developing world's maternal deaths. They kill mothers by causing cerebrovascular accidents: heart failure, respiratory failure and kidney failure, postpartum haemorrhage, DIC (disseminated intravascular coagulation), and abruption of the placenta.

When you find that a mother's blood pressure is high during pregnancy, she is likely to have one of four conditions:

(A) She might have had essential hypertension before she became pregnant.

(B) She might have had renal hypertension before she became pregnant (uncommon, see Section 17.6).

(C) She might have developed essential hypertension during pregnancy. This typically happens to an older multip who doesn't get much, if any, proteinuria with her hypertension. Her blood pressure is usually raised before 28 weeks, so that she may need antihypertensive treatment early in pregnancy. Her long-term risks are those normally associated with essential hypertension.

(D) She might have developed the disease that has been traditionally known as 'pre-eclampsia', and which is more common than hypertension developing during pregnancy. 'Pre-eclampsia'

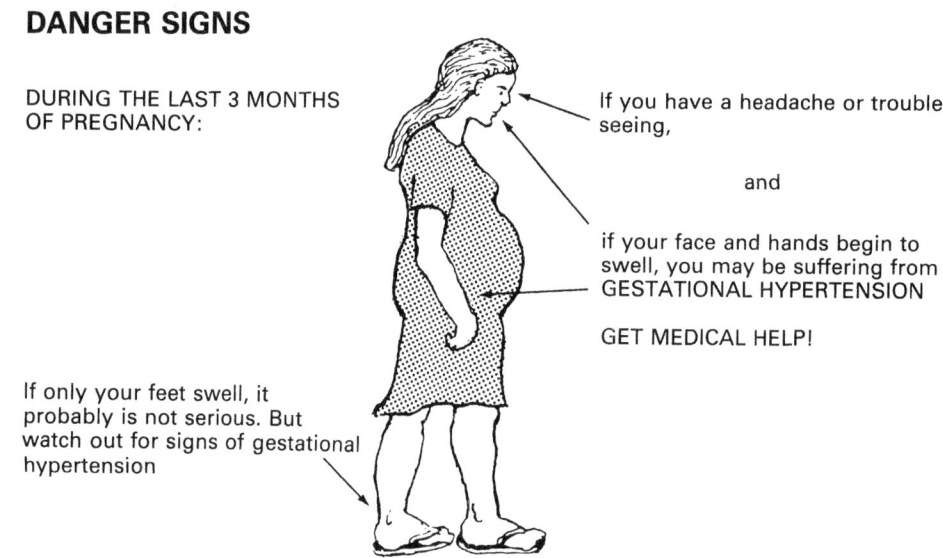

Fig. 17-1b DANGER SIGNS in gestational hypertension, as seen by a community health worker. From David Werner's 'Where there is no doctor'.

AN ECLAMPTIC FIT

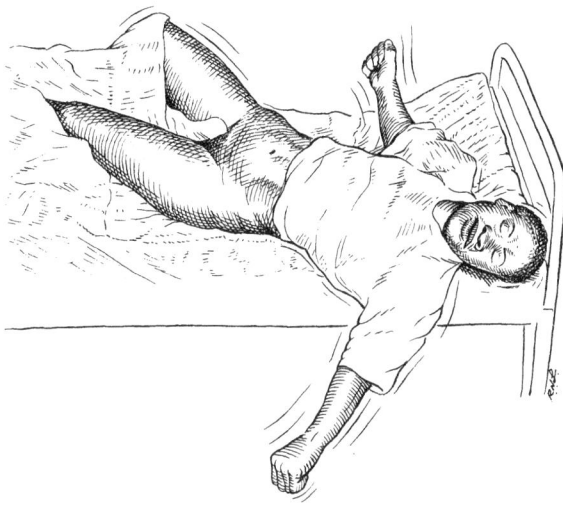

Fig. 17-2 AN ECLAMPTIC FIT is a *grand mal* epileptic convulsion. This is what you must try to prevent. A tonic phase in which all the muscles of the body contract, so that it becomes rigid, is followed by a clonic phase of rhythmic muscular contractions, as shown here.

typically happens to a young primigravida whose blood pressure rises after 28 weeks, and who has a significant proteinuria. Her blood pressure is normal when she is not pregnant, and her long term prognosis is normal in respect of her blood pressure.

So far so good. But: (1) You are unlikely to know what a mother's blood pressure was before she became pregnant. (2) What about the hypertensive primigravida without proteinuria, and the hypertensive multip with it? (3) (C) and (D), have many features in common, and babies in both of them are at increased risk from IUGR. (4) Two rival international societies dispute the classification and terminology of hypertension in pregnancy, so it is in great confusion. In practice, however, (C) and (D) are inseparable, so we have put them together and called all hypertension arising during pregnancy 'gestational hypertension'. This is WHO's term, which strictly refers only to (D). Other terms include 'pregnancy-induced hypertension', or 'PIH'.

Detecting gestational hypertension early is one of the main aims of antenatal care. If the staff of your clinics are hard pressed, the most important occasion on which to measure a mother's blood pressure is when she first attends early in pregnancy. If it is normal then, the risks of it rising are small until the second half of pregnancy, when she may develop gestational hypertension.

If a mother has gestational hypertension, aim to monitor her blood pressure, to test her urine for protein, and to bring her as near to term as you can. The value of bed-rest, and particularly phenobarbitone, are disputed. We don't use the latter for treating mild hypertension.

If her gestational hypertension is severe enough to cause eclampsia (fits), or severe pre-eclampsia (signs or symptoms which indicate that fits are imminent), aim to: (1) Deliver her baby; this is the definitive cure. (2) Prevent or treat her fits *as soon as possible* with magnesium sulphate, or one of the forms of sedation described below. (3) Control her blood pressure with hydralazine.

Magnesium sulphate: (1) Has a curariform action on the neuromuscular junction which stops convulsions. (2) Has no central action, so it does not sedate her, with the result that she remains fully alert, and can co-operate better during labour. (4) Does not sedate her baby, although it can affect him. (5) Is cheap. (6) Will depress her respiration, perhaps fatally, if you give her too much. However, although the margin of safety of magnesium sulphate is small, you can assess its anticonvulsant effect quite easily by testing her knee-jerks—it will abolish these before it depresses her respiration. You will not overdose her if you are very careful and if: (a) you test her knee jerks before each intramuscular dose, and (b) you keep her urinary output above 25 ml per hour—her kidneys are the only way she can excrete it.

If you are going to use sedation instead of magnesium sulphate, it has to be deep enough to control her convulsions. She should be semiconscious, so that she can only just be aroused, but not unconscious. You can produce this deep sedation with:

(1) Chlormethiazole ('Heminevrin'). This is a sedative and anticonvulsant; it has a wide margin of safety and controls eclampsia rapidly. It normally requires an intravenous drip, but you can give it without one; it is also comparatively expensive. Chlormethiazole is available as a powder for adding to a drip, as tablets, and as capsules in arachis oil.

(2) An intramuscular 'lytic cocktail' of pethidine, chlorpromazine, and promethazine, which has the advantage of not needing a drip.

(3) Diazepam has two uses: (a) As a bolus intravenous injection to control fits urgently at the start of any anticonvulsant regime. (b) Orally, or with an intravenous drip, to maintain constant sedation and a constant anticonvulsive effect. But: (i) the intravenous infusion of diazepam ideally needs an infusion pump; (ii) if you give diazepam for more than 36 hours before delivery, the baby will be 'floppy', and liable to neonatal cyanotic attacks. Diazepam is thus best avoided, except to control fits urgently.

(4) You can use phenytoin ('Epanutin'), which is widely used for epilepsy.

(5) Sodium amytal and (6) paraldehyde can be used but are not so effective. (7) Thiopentone will control fits, but has all the risks associated with its use as an anaesthetic (A 12.1).

There is no agreement as to which is the best method, especially under difficult circumstances like yours. Magnesium sulphate gives good results in centres of excellence, but needs particularly careful monitoring. An alert patient on magnesium sulphate is easier to nurse than a heavily sedated one. However, if your midwives cannot be relied on to monitor the administration of magnesium sulphate, their patients *may* be safer sedated, even if nursing them is more difficult. Under difficult conditions, chlormethiazole is probably the best of the sedative methods.

The methods above may fail to control a mother's blood pressure, so after you have controlled her fits with magnesium sulphate or sedation, you may have to use hydralazine to bring her systolic blood pressure down to less than 170 mm. If it is less than this, and she is also sedated, she should have no more fits. But if she is unsedated on magnesium sulphate, they can occur at systolic pressures of less than 160 mm.

If she has imminent eclampsia (visual disturbances, and exaggerated reflexes, etc., or severe proteinuria), deliver her baby early, whatever the duration of pregnancy.

If she has mild or moderate proteinuria, and no symptoms of imminent eclampsia, management depends on the duration of pregnancy: (1) If her baby is more than 36 weeks deliver him, regardless of the quality of your neonatal care, because he will probably survive. (2) If he is less than 36 weeks, balance the risk of death *in utero* with that of induction followed by death in your neonatal nursery. If your nursery is very good (unlikely), consider delivering him at 32 weeks. If it is poor, continue to 36 weeks.

Induce her on the above indications, or if this is impractical, section her. Provided you don't section her too late, it will improve her chances. If however, she is already *in extremis* (unusual), a Caesarean section will speed her death.

She will usually improve rapidly after delivery. Unfortunately, delivery sometimes fails to control gestational hypertension, and fits may occur for the first time during labour, or soon afterwards. Occasionally, her blood pressure starts to rise for the first time after delivery. She will not be out of danger from eclampsia until at least 48 hours after her baby is born.

There are problems: some patients have a high blood pressure and no eclamptic symptoms; a few have eclampsia with a normal blood pressure.

Some common errors: (1) Don't use thiazides or other diuretics in the attempt to treat her oedema. (2) Don't use morphine unless you have no other way of treating her. Don't use heparin. (3) Don't nurse her in the dark—this is old-fashioned, unnecessary,

TREATING ECLAMPSIA

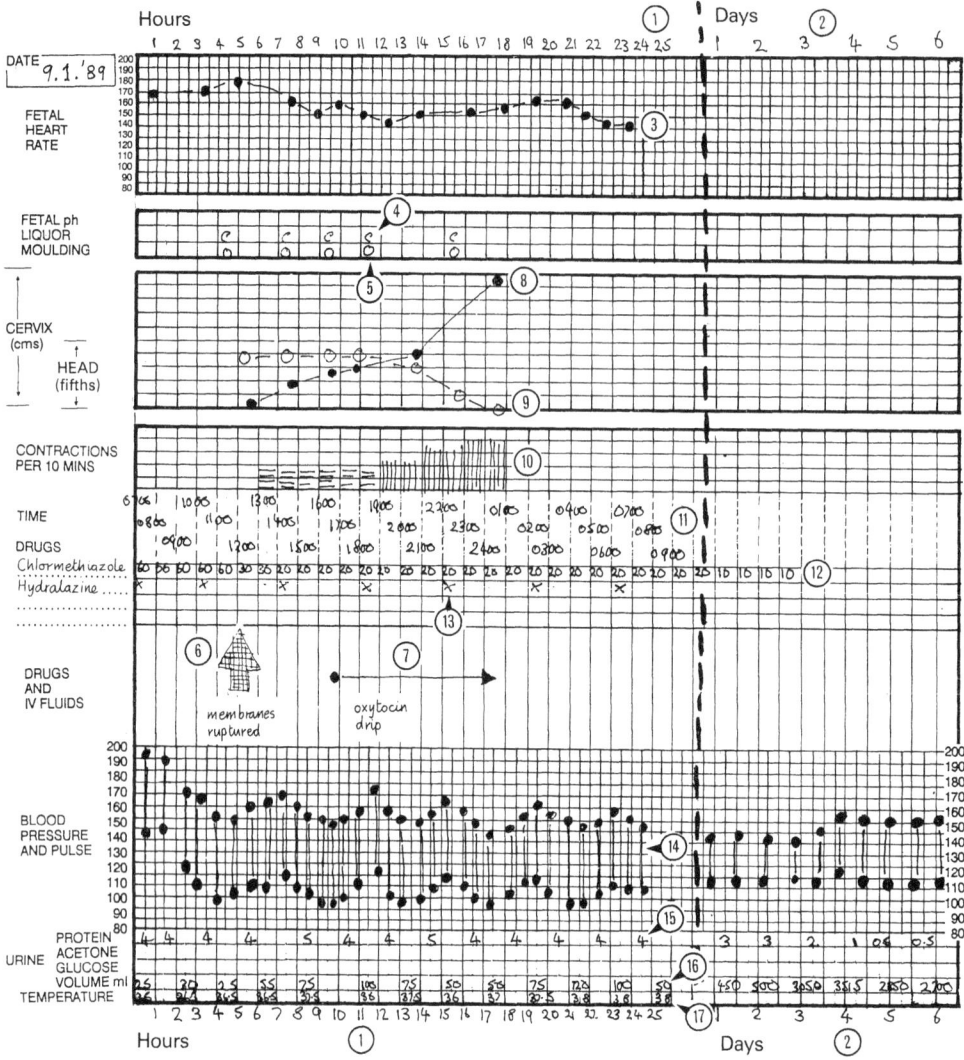

Fig. 17-3 THE PARTOGRAM of a primigravida admitted in labour after having had three eclamptic convulsions (schematic).

1, the first part of the partogram shows her course during the first 24 hours after admission. 2, the second part shows the days after delivery. 3, the fetal heart fell to normal levels as she improved. 4, her liquor was clear. 5, there was no moulding. 6, rupture of her membranes induced labour. 7, she was given an oxytocin drip of 2.5 units in 500 ml starting at 10 drops a minute (18.4a). This was sufficient, and there was no need to increase the dose. The drip speeded the dilatation of her cervix (8) and the descent of the head (9) in response to increased contractions of her uterus (10). 11, the time of day. 12, a chlormethiazole drip has been recorded in drops per minute (a slightly different regime was used from that described here). 13, 10 mg intramuscular doses of hydralazine were given whenever her blood pressure rose above 160/110 mm. 14, her blood pressure. 15, the protein in her urine in g/l. 16, her urine volume. 17, her temperature. *Modified from a figure by Ian MacGillivray.*

and may lead to lack of attention.

'The Hypertensive Disorders of Pregnancy'. 1987. WHO Technical Report Series No. 758.

HYPERTENSION IN PREGNANCY

Check the sphygmomanometers and make sure that your staff know how to use them. If the circumference of a patient's arm is >30 cm, use a wide long cuff. Don't diagnose a high blood pressure on one measurement alone. Use the fourth sound of Korotkoff to measure her diastolic blood pressure. This is the point at which they become muffled, rather than when they disappear (the fifth sound).

ESSENTIAL HYPERTENSION

Suspect essential hypertension if her blood pressure is raised before 28 weeks. If her diastolic blood pressure is consistently >90 mm Hg before 28 weeks, she ideally needs treatment with methyldopa ('Aldomet'), but this is not essential.

MILD AND MODERATE GESTATIONAL HYPERTENSION

This is the patient with a blood pressure of <160/100 mm Hg and no proteinuria. Risk factors which suggest that her gestational hypertension may progress are: (1) A history of previous IUGR, a previous intrauterine death, or a low birth-weight baby. (2) Signs of IUGR in this pregnancy.

Rest her. She need not be in bed all the time, but when she is in bed, she should be *lying on her side*, not on her back. Watch for the signs and symptoms of impending eclampsia. Record her blood pressure 4-hourly, and test her urine for protein daily. If her blood pressure settles, and she has no danger signs (proteinuria, headache) she can go home.

Ideally, induce her at 38 weeks, or as soon as her surfactant test (19.2) is positive. If you are in doubt about the maturity of her baby, it is probably safe to wait until term.

CAUTION! (1) Primigravidae 18 years old or less are at special risk, so treat them in a grade higher than their symptoms suggest. For example, consider a primigravida aged 16 with a blood pressure of 140/90 and no protein in her urine as having moderate hypertension. Consider a primigravida of 15 with a blood pressure of 150/100 as having severe hypertension. (2) Mild gestational hypertension can progress to eclampsia in a few days. (3) A primigravida can go into labour at term with no signs of gestational hypertension. Her blood pressure can rise rapidly during labour, and fits appear before she has any protein in her urine (unusual).

SEVERE GESTATIONAL HYPERTENSION (pre-eclampsia)

LESS THAN 35 WEEKS. She has a blood pressure of >160/110 mm Hg, and/or proteinuria of '2+' (0.45–1 g/l) or more, on more than one occasion, but she has no symptoms—headaches, visual disturbances, epigastric pain, or fits. If she does have them, treat her as for eclampsia (see below).

Admit her, and sedate her heavily with oral phenobarbitone (60 mg 6 hourly, or 30 to 60 mg twice daily), or sodium phenobarbitone 200 mg intramuscularly. If her blood pressure settles, treat her with phenobarbitone by mouth, until her baby is mature.

If her blood pressure does not settle, give her methyldopa, starting with 250 mg 3 times daily, and gradually increasing; maximum dose 3 g daily. It works slowly, and will not have much effect for 2 days.

Maternal indications for terminating pregnancy: (1) Her blood pressure is uncontrollable (>160/110 mm Hg) in spite of 2 g of methyldopa daily. (2) Imminent signs of eclampsia (see below). (3) Signs of renal failure, with a rising blood urea and a falling urine output.

Fetal indications for terminating pregnancy: (1) Severe IUGR (19.13) after 32 weeks with a viable baby. (2) The decision to terminate pregnancy is also dependent on its duration, and the severity of her proteinuria. For example, proteinuria of <0.5 g/l at 28 weeks does not demand termination. Once it reaches 0.5 g/l, whatever the duration of pregnancy, it is a general rule that eclampsia will probably follow within 2 weeks, unless she is delivered sooner.

If her baby is alive, induce her; this is usually easy. Section her if there are difficulties (CPD, a breech, or a cervix which you are not able to ripen, etc.).

If he is dead, spontaneous labour is likely in a few days, but induce her if necessary.

CAUTION ! (1) Always admit her for antihypertensive treatment. (2) It does not invariably prevent eclampsia and abruption.

MORE THAN 35 WEEKS. Lower her blood pressure by one of the methods below, and terminate her pregancy if her cervix is favourable for induction.

ECLAMPSIA OR IMPENDING ECLAMPSIA

If she has fits, she has eclampsia. The signs of impending eclampsia are: a blood pressure of >160/110 mm Hg or a rapidly increasing blood pressure, proteinuria >2+, oliguria (<400 ml daily), headaches, visual disturbances, and epigastric pain. Muscle twitches and exaggerated reflexes indicate that fits are about to begin. Aim to deliver the baby. Give her magnesium sulphate, or sedate her heavily.

CAUTION ! (1) Before you diagnose gestational hypertension as the cause of fits or coma, don't forget that they can be caused by cerebral malaria, meningitis, or epilepsy, and also by less common causes. Be especially careful if her blood pressure is normal and she has little proteinuria. If her fits really are unexplained, treat her as if she had eclampsia. (2) Eclampsia is rare before 26 weeks, or more than two days after delivery. (3) Meningitis may produce fits and little neck stiffness in a pregnant patient. (4) The intensive treatment of cerebral malaria is not the same as the 'routine' treatment of ordinary malaria (17.2). (3) Record her blood pressure not less than 4-hourly, and if necessary half-hourly.

An eclamptic fit is a *grand mal* epileptic convulsion. A tonic phase in which all the muscles of the body contract, so that it becomes rigid, is followed by a clonic phase of rhythmic muscular contractions. She becomes unconscious with the fit, and remains so for a variable time afterwards. When she has a fit, clear her airway and insert an oral airway. Give her diazepam 10 to 20 mg intravenously slowly by bolus injection (or give her chlormethiazole, see below). Then give her: (1) magnesium sulphate. Or (2) phenytoin. Or (3) heavy sedation with chlormethiazole. Or (4) the lytic cocktail. Or (5) diazepam as an infusion.

IF YOU ARE USING MAGNESIUM SULPHATE, you will need 20% and 50% sterile solutions, calcium gluconate 10%, and a tendon hammer. If you have no sterile magnesium sulphate, make it. Most brands of magnesium sulphate, including magnesium sulphate BP, are satisfactory. Be sure to monitor her carefully, because an overdose can cause respiratory failure. Inject 4 g of magnesium sulphate (20 ml of a 20% solution) intravenously over a period of 3 to 5 minutes. Then immediately give her 10 g intramuscularly (10 ml of a 50% solution deeply into each buttock). This loading dose of 14 g will usually control her fits immediately. If they don't stop, give her diazepam 10 to 20 mg by bolus intravenous injection in addition.

As a maintenance dose, every 4 hours afterwards, give her 5 g of magnesium sulphate into alternate buttocks, but only provided that: (1) her respirations are more than 16 per minute, (2) her knee-jerks are present, and (3) she has excreted at least 100 ml of urine since the last dose. Alternatively, give her a drip of 1 g/hour. Continue this regime until 48 hours after delivery.

CAUTION ! (1) If her respiration becomes depressed while she is having magnesium sulphate, give her 10 ml of 10% calcium gluconate intravenously slowly over not less than 10 minutes. This is an instant antidote, *so it must be available.* (2) Stick to one anticonvulsant regime and don't mix them. (2) If you are giving her magnesium sulphate (or phenytoin), there is no need to sedate her.

IF YOU ARE USING PHENYTOIN, give an initial dose of 10 mg/kg slowly intravenously, followed 2 hours later by 5 mg/kg intravenously. Maintain her on oral or intravenous doses of 200 mg 8-hourly for 3 or 4 days.

CAUTION ! There is a small risk of inducing cardiac arrhythmias with intravenous phenytoin, so give it very slowly over 5 minutes.

IF YOU ARE SEDATING HER, adjust the level of sedation carefully. She should sleep, but just be able to respond to her name if you rouse her. If she talks coherently when roused, she is too light. If she does not respond at all, she is too deep. Provided she does not become too deep, her laryngeal reflexes will be adequately preserved. She usually needs to be sedated for about 4 days, and often for less. This includes 24 hours for control, time to induce labour and deliver her, and 48 hours afterwards (see below).

CAUTION ! (1) If with any of the sedative methods, particularly it is said chlormethiazole, she becomes restless and perhaps uncontrollable, she may be 'too deep' rather than 'too light', and may be in the excitement stage of anaesthesia (equivalent to Stage Two with ether, A 11.2). If this happens, give her less not more sedation. (2) You are giving agents which can produce anaesthesia in higher doses. So if she gets too deep be prepared to intubate her.

If you are using chlormethiazole ('Heminevrin'), in severe cases, give it as a rapid infusion of 8 g/l until she is asleep and her jaw sags. Pass a (Ryle's) stomach tube, and give her 2 g intragastrically (aspirate the oily capsules, and pass the contents down the tube). Insert an oral airway to prevent her tongue falling back. Give her pethidine as necessary for analgesia also. Regulate the intravenous drip so that she can just be roused. Use the intragastric route as the main one, and the intravenous one for fine adjustment. This will economize in intravenous fluids, and avoid overloading her. She may need 24 g of chlormethiazole or more each 24 hours.

If you are using the lytic cocktail, give her pethidine 50 mg, chlorpromazine 50 mg, and promethazine 50 mg intramuscularly 4 to 6-hourly. This is easy, effective, and cheap, but they are poor anticonvulsants. Alternatively, give the first dose by bolus intravenous injection and then give the drugs intramuscularly. Don't exceed chlorpromazine 300 mg in 24 hours.

If you are using diazepam for continued sedation, give her 40 mg in 500 ml of 5% dextrose (for the use of intravenous diazepam see A 2.8). Start at 30 drops a minute, and maintain heavy sedation as for chlormethiazole. Unfortunately, it is difficult to maintain the drip at a constant speed, and you may find other methods easier.

CAUTION ! Give her diazepam intravenously or orally. Don't try to give it intramuscularly: its absorption is unpredictable, and it acts more slowly than oral diazepam. If she is unconscious and cannot swallow, give it down a tube.

BLOOD PRESSURE. If, when you have controlled her fits, her blood pressure is more than 170/110 mm Hg, give her hydralazine ('Apresoline'); this is the most suitable drug, but it may cause tachycardia. Give her 10 mg intramuscularly. Measure her blood pressure after an hour, and if it is >160/110, give her another 10 mg. Continue to monitor her blood pressure hourly, and whenever it is >160/110 give her another 10 mg. Explain this regime to the midwives, and let them continue. This is much easier than giving it intravenously.

CAUTION ! (1) Don't use methyldopa, it is too slow-acting to control hypertension in an emergency. (4) Don't try to induce her if she has a blood pressure of more than 170/110 mm, without first lowering it, or she may have fits during labour.

FLUID BALANCE. Monitor her carefully, and keep a chart like that in Fig. A 15-5. Keep the fluid balance part of it accurately, and pass an indwelling catheter. Take care not to overload her circulation. You can easily cause pulmonary oedema by giving her too much fluid. As soon as she is delivered she will shift the oedema fluid into her circulation. There are two regimes:

The 'dry regime' Give her a litre of fluid in 24 hours and don't worry too much about oliguria: she will eventually get a diuresis.

The 'wet regime' is sometimes advised to maintain renal perfusion and a good urine output. There is however a danger of fluid overload and pulmonary oedema. It is probably safer to err on the side of undertransfusion. Give her plasma expanders (dextran or albumen 2 l/24 hours) or 2 litres of intravenous fluid in 24 hours. Give her her normal requirement of one litre of Ringer's lactate or saline, and 1 litre of 5% dextrose intravenously in 24 hours. Add to this a volume of Ringer's lactate, or saline, equal to any vomit or diarrhoea, etc., that she may have. Aim for a minimum urine output of 30 ml/hour. There is a danger of causing pulmonary oedema with this regime, especially if nursing is poor. So watch her central venous pressure, (preferably with a CVP line), and maintain her urine output >30 ml/hr. If it falls below this, give her intravenous mannitol (A 15.1), or frusemide 20 to 40 mg at a rate not exceeding 4 mg/minute.

HYPERPYREXIA is a serious risk, especially in hot climates. Record her rectal temperature 4-hourly, and if necessary hourly. If it rises over 39°C, use tepid sponging. If it reaches 41°C, remove all clothing, cool her with a wet sheet in contact with as much of her skin as possible, and turn a fan on her. This will cool her 0.5°C in 10 minutes. An irreversible hyperpyrexia of >43°C indicates brain damage.

NURSING is critical and needs to be expert and continuous. Nurse her in a side room, or in the labour ward. A patient with severe gestational hypertension ideally needs a nurse to herself day and night, with no other duties except to turn her every 1–2 hours, to aspirate her pharynx, and to measure and chart her blood pressure and her urine output. She may die from the aspiration of secretions or vomit, so lay her in the recovery position (51-2), and keep a sucker handy. Protect her corneae: keep her eyes closed, if necessary with tape across her eyelids. Watch and treat her pressure areas (64.15).

VAGINAL DELIVERY. Provided there are no contraindications to vaginal delivery, induce her (19.3) and deliver her vaginally as soon as you can, when her fits and her blood pressure are controlled, and her general condition is stable. Don't delay. To induce her, rupture her membranes, and then give her an oxytocin drip (M 22.2). (Watch the volume of intravenous fluid you are giving her.) If you give her >1 l/24 hours, keep her urine flow >30 ml/hour. If you cannot insert a finger to rupture her membranes, you can insert a Foley catheter to ripen her cervix (19.3), but section may be wiser. Alternatively, if there is less urgency for delivery, and the condition of her cervix is unfavourable, insert prostaglandin gel (2 mg) in a diaphragm to induce contractions and soften her cervix. Or proceed immediately to section her.

CAESAREAN SECTION is indicated if she has: (1) an unfavourable cervix, (2) a breech, (3) CPD, or (4) the scar from a previous Caesarean section. (5) If induction is not followed by active labour in 8 hours. (6) If she does not progress in labour.

AFTER DELIVERY, continue her hypotensive, anticonvulsive, and sedative drugs for 48 hours, after which the risk of fits is very low. Don't discharge her until her diastolic blood pressure is <100 mm Hg.

DIFFICULTIES WITH GESTATIONAL HYPERTENSION

If your CIRCUMSTANCES ARE VERY DIFFICULT, such that you may not even have a sphygmomanometer, so that the routine monitoring of patients described above is impractical: (1) Encourage them to come into hospital early if they have the warning symptoms of eclampsia (headaches, visual disturbances and epigastric pain). (2) Test their urine for protein, and encourage them to do it at home with test papers. A urine protein of >0.25 g is likely to indicate gestational hypertension.

If a patient has GENERALIZED OEDEMA during pregnancy, she is at increased risk of gestational hypertension, so monitor her blood pressure and urine for protein with extra care.

If she is not pregnant and has ESSENTIAL HYPERTENSION with a diastolic pressure of >110 mm Hg (uncommon), counsel her about the possible problems of hypertension during pregnancy. If you treat her hypertension before and during pregnancy (methyldopa or propanolol are suitable), her baby's prognosis is quite good, and her own risks are very small unless she has renal failure. She runs a higher risk of gestational hypertension, but renal problems seldom develop for the first time, although they may get worse. She can expect more problems in pregnancy (eclampsia and abruption), but the long-term prognosis of the disease, including her life-expectancy is not affected.

If you have had to give her MORE THAN 30 mg OF DIAZEPAM within 15 hours of delivery, her baby may have APNOEIC ATTACKS (a major problem), hypotonia, reluctance to suck, or an impaired metabolic response to cold. So manage him with particular care (19.12). At the time of writing there is no specific 'antidiazepam' licensed, although one is under development.

If her URINE VOLUME FALLS to less than 500 ml in 24 hours: (1) She may be dehydrated. Provided that her lung fields are clear and there is no chance of cardiac failure, give her a litre of 5% glucose during about an hour. She is in more danger of pulmonary oedema from too much fluid than of renal failure from too little fluid. If you cannot be certain that she has not got a raised central venous pressure, don't push fluids. (2) If this does not produce a diuresis, she has renal failure. Give her 100 ml of 20% mannitol over 10 minutes (A 15.1). If this fails, try frusemide 80 mg intravenously, repeated in 2 to 4 hours if it is not effective. If this too fails to restore her urine output, limit her intake to 500 ml in 24 hours plus a volume equal to her urine output. See also 53.3. If she has renal impairment and subsequently has a diuresis, she will need extra sodium and potassium (53.3).

If she starts HYPERVENTILATING or is CYANOSED, (1) She may be developing pulmonary oedema, so sit her up and give a diuretic and oxygen. Or, (2) she may be acidotic (uncommon). If so, correct her acidosis cautiously with 50 to 150 mmol (50 to 150 ml of an 8.4% solution) of sodium bicarbonate intravenously (A 15.1).

If her UTERUS BECOMES TENDER, her blood pressure and urinary output fall, and the fetal heartbeat disappears (uncommon), suspect abruption. Restore her blood volume with Ringer's lactate, or saline, and blood in appropriate proportions. For this to be safe, monitor her CVP (A 19.2). Hasten delivery.

If she becomes cyanosed or develops PULMONARY OEDEMA, give her continuous oxygen and frusemide 20 to 40 mg intravenously. The need to observe cyanosis is one reason why she must not be nursed in a dark room.

If her FITS CONTINUE despite heavy sedation and adequate doses of magnesium sulphate, make sure the diagnosis of eclampsia is correct (see above), that her blood pressure is adequately controlled, and that she is not in pain. Try another sedative, for example paraldehyde 10 ml intramuscularly. If even this fails, paralyse her with a muscle-relaxant and ventilate her with IPPV (A 13.2, A 19.4), using a cuffed tracheal tube (rarely necessary).

If she goes into prolonged deep COMA, make sure you have not oversedated her. Keep her adequately oxygenated. Intubate her to maintain a clear airway, and suck out her trachea. Start IPPV when necessary (rare). She has probably had a cerebrovascular accident.

If her BLOOD PRESSURE STAYS HIGH 48 HOURS AFTER DELIVERY, treatment depends on how high it is. If it is >160/120, acute complications (a cerebrovascular accident or renal failure) are likely. Lower it actively. If it is <160/120, maintain mild sedation for a few days. It will probably fall spontaneously. See her in 6 weeks. If it remains high (diastolic pressure >110 mmHg), consider long-term medical treatment with all its problems and complications, which she will be unlikely to accept. In most countries of the world the cost and inconvenience of long-term antihypertensive treatment probably outweighs its benefits.

If her blood pressure is noticed to be HIGH FOR THE FIRST TIME AFTER DELIVERY, or she has FITS AFTER DELIVERY, it may have been high before delivery, or it may have risen for the first time afterwards. She may develop eclampsia, especially within 48 hours of delivery; after this time the risks of a first fit are minimal. If she has signs of severe gestational hypertension, treat her for it with magnesium sulphate or sedation as above. If her blood pressure remains high, see above.

If she has ALREADY ASPIRATED secretions before she was admitted, suck her out as best you can (9.11), raise the foot of her bed, and give her antibiotics.

17.5 Heart failure in pregnancy

Where obstetric care is good, and the more easily preventable causes of maternal mortality have been eliminated, death from heart disease is one of the important remaining reasons why mothers die. *Primary Mother Care* warns staff in the antenatal clinic to be on the look out for mothers with heart disease, which usually presents as a cough, dyspnoea on exertion or at rest, malaise, oedema, or palpitations. Only rarely will a mother know that she has heart disease. It is most commonly due to anaemia, rheumatic carditis, or congenital heart disease. Fortunately, provided she is properly cared for, pregnancy does not influence the long-term outcome of her heart disease. One of the dangers is that she may suddenly go into failure, with little warning, in the last weeks of pregnancy, while in labour, or in the puerperium; so watch her carefully and treat her early.

Obstetrically, mothers with heart disease fall into these four groups:

Group One Mothers with heart disease, but no limitation of their physical activity.

Group Two Mothers with slight limitation of physical activity. They are comfortable at rest, but ordinary activity fatigues them and makes them short of breath.

Group Three Mothers who have marked limitation of their physical activity and are comfortable at rest, but less than ordinary activity gives them symptoms. They may show signs of heart failure.

Group Four Mothers who cannot do any physical activity without discomfort. They have symptoms at rest, obvious signs of heart failure, and any activity makes them worse. They are less likely to become pregnant, but if they do, delivery by any method may kill them.

The diagnosis of heart disease can be difficult, because systolic murmurs, oedema, and dyspnoea are common in normal pregnancy. Base your diagnosis of significant heart disease on: (1) Obvious cardiac enlargement. (2) Diastolic, presystolic, or continuous heart murmurs. (3) A harsh, loud, systolic murmur, especially if there is also a thrill. (4) Serious arrhythmia. (5) Signs of congestive failure—a raised jugular venous pressure, basal crepitations, ankle oedema, and an enlarged liver.

HEART DISEASE

GENERAL MEASURES. Try to ensure that a mother has as much rest as possible and avoids undue weight gain, fluid retention, infection, and anaemia. Keep her haemoglobin above 100 g/l. If necessary, transfuse her with packed red cells, and give her frusemide.

GROUPS ONE AND TWO. Allow her to go through pregnancy; see her regularly in the antenatal clinic: she is unlikely to go into failure.

GROUPS THREE AND FOUR. If possible, try to prevent her from becoming pregnant.

If pregnancy has not progressed beyond 12 weeks, opinions vary. (1) If she is well cared for, death from heart failure in pregnancy or labour is rare, so avoid termination. Some obstetricians working under ideal conditions never terminate a pregnancy for heart disease. (2) If care is less good, a therapeutic abortion might be indicated.

If she goes into failure during pregnancy, admit her for bedrest and control it. Give her frusemide. If possible restrict the sodium in her diet. Digoxin is indicated if she has auricular fibrillation, otherwise its value is disputed. If failure is controlled, she can go home, provided you can keep in touch with her, and she and her family realize that she must rest.

DELIVERING A MOTHER IN HEART FAILURE

Admit a mother with heart disease at 34 weeks, or earlier, if she goes into failure before then. For all degrees of heart disease vaginal delivery is likely to be safer than Caesarean section. Avoid section late in labour. If you expect complications, do it electively under general anaesthesia. Beware of cardiac failure developing after delivery as oedema fluid returns to her circulation.

If she has valvular disease, prevent endocarditis. Give her 3 doses at 8-hour intervals of: (1) ampicillin 500 mg orally or intramuscularly; and (2) gentamicin 80 mg intramuscularly. Or give her any other broad-spectrum antibiotic which is safe in pregnancy. Give the first dose when her membranes rupture, or you will encourage the growth of resistant organisms.

EQUIPMENT. Prepare for a cardiac emergency, and have digoxin, frusemide, aminophylline, and morphine ready. Also, a venesection set (M 13.4), tracheal tubes, a laryngoscope, and oxygen.

FIRST STAGE. Deliver her sitting up. Adequate analgesia is essential. Epidural anaesthesia is ideal, if you are skilled,

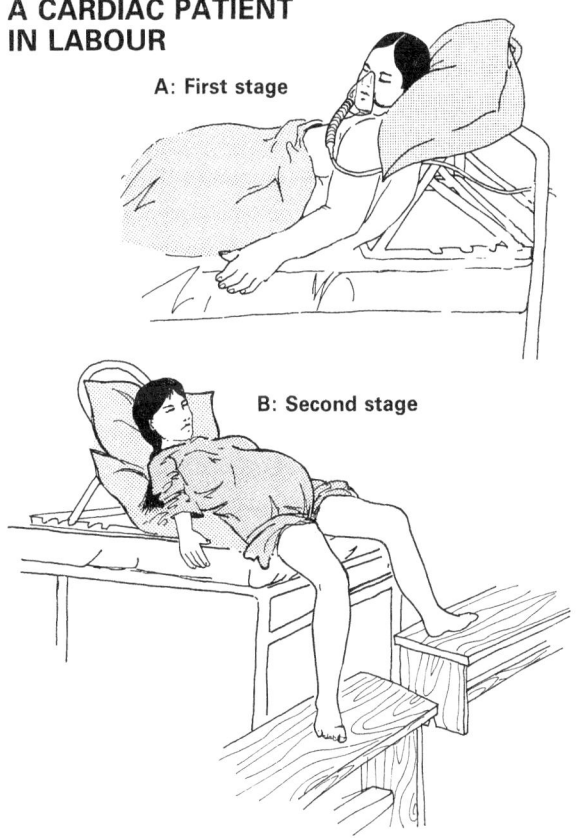

Fig. 17-4 A CARDIAC PATIENT IN LABOUR. A, during the first stage deliver her sitting up. B, during the second stage avoid the lithotomy position. Sit her up with her buttocks over the end of the bed. Ask two assistants (not shown) to support her with her legs resting on chairs. Discourage her from bearing down as much as you can.

because it decreases cardiac output. If this is impractical, give her morphine rather than pethidine.

Count her pulse and respiration rate every 30 minutes. If her pulse rises above 100 and her respirations above 24, and she is obviously dyspnoeic, she is in failure.

SECOND STAGE. Avoid the lithotomy position. Sit her up with her buttocks over the end of the bed. Ask two assistants to support her with her legs resting on chairs. Discourage her from bearing down as much as you can.

If she progresses quickly, allow her to deliver spontaneously. If her progress is slow, shorten this stage with outlet forceps or a vacuum extractor, or a generous episiotomy. Use enough local anaesthetic to prevent her feeling pain, and sit her up when you suture it.

Give her frusemide 40 mg intravenously, as soon as she is delivered.

THIRD STAGE. A small bleed is likely to benefit cardiac failure. So only give her ergometrine with oxytocin ('Syntometrine'), if she has lost more than 500 ml. If you give it when she has not bled, the sudden return of blood to her circulation from her contracting uterus may precipitate failure.

Watch her carefully for the next 24 hours, because this is the time when she is most likely to go into failure.

CAUTION ! (1) Don't overload her circulation, and avoid transfusion, especially after delivery. (2) Don't use local anaesthetics with adrenalin in them.

If you have used morphine, have nalorphine or naloxone ready for the baby. After delivery watch her pulse, temperature, and respiration carefully, and watch for puerperal infection. Advise her not to become pregnant again, and give her family-planning advice—preferably tie her tubes.

DIFFICULTIES DELIVERING A PATIENT WITH CARDIAC DISEASE

If she goes into CARDIAC FAILURE which was not previously diagnosed or treated, give her intravenous morphine 10 to 15 mg, intravenous frusemide 40 to 80 mg, and if necessary apply rotating tourniquets (M 13.4). Give her oxygen through a nasal tube, and aminophylline 250 mg during 10 minutes timed by the clock. If she is fibrillating give her intravenous digoxin.

If her cervix is partly dilated and she is NOT IN SEVERE FAILURE, allow delivery to proceed vaginally. Interference of any kind is likely to make her worse.

If she is in SEVERE FAILURE AFTER FULL DILATATION, and you don't expect delivery in the next few minutes, deliver her with the vacuum extractor, or outlet forceps.

17.6 Urinary infection and chronic renal disease in pregnancy

Urinary infection. Minor urinary symptoms (frequency and stress or urge incontinence) are common in pregnancy. Cystitis (bladder infection) is not more common during pregnancy than it is at other times, but because the ureters dilate during pregnancy, infection is more likely to spread proximally and cause acute pyelonephritis.

One pregnant woman in 20 has an asymptomatic bacteriuria, but because you can only diagnose this by routine screening, it will not be a problem you notice. A quarter of patients with bacteriuria have an acute attack of pyelonephritis, which affects 1–2 per cent of pregnant women. Bacteriuria is associated with an increased risk of prematurity, but there is no evidence that treatment reduces this risk. Treatment does however reduce the risk of pyelonephritis, so it is worth doing.

Chronic renal disease is not adversely affected by pregnancy unless a patient is already in renal failure, or has pyelonephritis. Advise her as described below. Chronic renal disease can also cause severe hypertension (17.4).

URINARY DISEASE IN PREGNANCY

URINARY INFECTION can usually be treated without difficulty. If you cannot culture a patient's urine, use '>10 white cells in one high-power microscope field' as evidence of infection.

If she has no symptoms and you find bacteria on screening, only treat her if she has >100,000 bacteria/ml.

If she has symptoms suggestive of cystitis (dysuria and frequency), manage her like this:

If you can examine her urine, treat her if you find any bacteria in her urine.

If you cannot examine her urine and she does not have the symptoms of pyelitis (see below), her symptoms may be due to: (1) Bacterial cystitis. (2) Schistosomiasis (in endemic areas). (3) Pressure of her pregnant uterus on her bladder. (4) Vaginitis.

Exclude vaginitis by examining her with a speculum. Meanwhile, try sulphadimidine 500 mg three times a day for a week. This small dose is often effective, and will not harm the fetus. Nitrofurantoin in therapeutic doses (100 mg 6-hourly) often causes nausea, and is less suitable. Or give her ampicillin, if you can spare it for such a comparatively minor problem.

If she has fever, rigors, frequency dysuria, and loin tenderness, she has pyelonephritis. Admit her, and give her a broad-spectrum antibiotic (2.8), such as chloramphenicol, ampicillin, trimethoprim, or gentamicin, intravenously if possible for the first 12 hours, and continued orally for at least a week and preferably longer. When she has recovered, give her a prophylactic antibiotic, such as a low dose of nitrofurantoin (100 mg daily) until delivery.

CAUTION ! If a pregnant mother has a fever without any obvious symptoms (a 'PUO'), the causes include malaria, typhoid, miliary tuberculosis, and infection of her urinary tract. Culture her urine, and if possible her blood.

CHRONIC RENAL DISEASE during pregnancy (uncommon).

If her blood urea (normal in pregnancy <6 mmol/l), or her creatinine (<100 μmol/l) are normal or nearly so, her prognosis is good.

If her blood urea is 6–10 mmol/l or her creatinine is 100–250 μmol/l, she is likely to have a hectic pregnancy complicated by severe hypertension, and perhaps by progressive renal failure, which will probably require early delivery. Risks to her and her baby are increased. At the upper limit of this range she is at risk from DIC. Some obstetricians advise against pregnancy at creatinine levels >180 μmol/l.

If her urea is >10 mmol/l or her creatinine is >250 μmol/l, the outlook for a successful pregnancy without dialysis or transplantation is very poor, so advise termination strongly.

If she has an attack of acute renal failure on top of chronic renal failure, she is unlikely to recover.

18 The surgery of labour

18.1 The two worlds of obstetrics

If labour does not proceed normally, you will have to intervene and help a mother. How best you should do this, and what methods you should use, depends greatly on where in the scale of advantage and disadvantage she is. This has been beautifully described by John Lawson:

> Obstetrically, there are now two worlds, with pockets of one world in the other, and every gradation between the two. In the advantaged industrial world Caesarean section is now so safe that it has done much to change the whole pattern of obstetrics there. In that world obstetric services are good, and theatres and blood banks well organised. If a mother needs a Caesarean section, it is done by a skilled obstetrician and an experienced anaesthetist. Antenatal care is available everywhere, transport is easy, and most mothers are sufficiently educated to understand why they should have a hospital delivery if they need one. Most of them only plan to have two or three children anyway, and are not frightened by the possibility that Caesarean section might reduce their chances of having any more. Just because it is so safe, it is used electively for between 5 and 10% of mothers as a means of anticipating difficulty, rather than dealing with disaster. It is done so efficiently that traumatic vaginal deliveries and perinatal deaths from birth injury have almost disappeared.
>
> Most mothers in the developing world are less fortunate. A really disadvantaged one must have six or seven children, so that three or four will survive. If she has an obstructed labour in a distant village, she may arrive in your hospital after a long journey, dehydrated, ketotic, shocked, anaemic, or infected, or all of these things. If you have to do a Caesarean section, you may have to do it through infected tissues, so that it may be followed by peritonitis, which antibiotics may fail to control.
>
> When she has recovered, she may remember only a frightening operation followed by a difficult puerperium, and deliberately not seek hospital care when she becomes pregnant again. If her baby died, she may blame the hospital for his death, and decide to have her next one at home. Unfortunately, Caesarean section seldom removes the factor which caused it, so that her narrow pelvis, which may have been the reason for her Caesarean section, is probably still there. But the scar in her uterus is now its weakest part, so that the chances of it rupturing are great.

How can you help a mother like this? She may have no antenatal care in her next pregnancy, and be unable to reach hospital for her next delivery. How can obstetrics be adapted to her needs, without being dominated by the practice of the industrial world? One answer is to make good use of the alternatives to Caesarean section, and one of the main purposes of this chapter is to describe them.

Unfortunately, in many hospitals the methods used to assist a mother who is delayed or obstructed in labour are unnecessarily limited. If an oxytocin drip and a vacuum extractor fail, Caesarean section is automatic, and other possibilities are not considered. If her CPD (cephalopelvic disproportion) is mild, she can have a symphysiotomy (18.6, M 22.7). If her baby is dead, she can have a destructive operation (18.7).

An alternative, which is not practical, except in the hands of an expert obstetrician, is the standard type of mid-cavity rotational forceps, such as those of Kielland. In the hands of anyone else, these forceps are so dangerous that a mother and her baby will be safer if you do a Caesarean section, which you will have to learn to do anyway. So you will find that the only forceps mentioned here are Wrigley's pattern of outlet forceps ('low forceps', M 22.6). The only acceptable use of the standard mid-cavity forceps by non-experts is their application to the aftercoming head during a breech delivery. For this purpose outlet forceps can however usually be used instead.

Your first priority should be to see that, when a mother is admitted, she is examined by the most experienced person available. She must be carefully observed not less than four-hourly thereafter, and the observations that are made accurately recorded on her partogram. Unless this happens, the whole process of labour management breaks down.

The team will need guidelines to know when to call you. For the most part, they are the same as those for which a health centre refers her to hospital (M 18.11). Make sure you are called too often, rather than not often enough.

Besides the methods described here, you will also find the following useful: an oxytocin drip (M 22.2), vacuum extraction (M 22.3), symphysiotomy (M 22.7), and outlet forceps (M 22.6).

(1) When you start any operative delivery make sure that the midwife who is assisting you knows how to resuscitate the baby, and has the equipment ready for doing this (19.12). In some hospitals, the results of not doing so are seen only too tragically, in the numbers of handicapped children who attend their paediatric clinics. (2) Don't forget to relieve pain when you can, so make proper use of pethidine (M 18.15), pudendal blocks (18.1a), and trichloroethylene (A 11.7).

Lawson J. 'Embryotomy for obstructed labour'. Tropical Doctor. 1974;188-91.

18.1a Obstetric anaesthesia

Anaesthesia is often the most dangerous part of a difficult delivery. In most district hospitals general anaesthesia is best avoided in obstetrics, except for Caesarean section, when the patient is bleeding, or is already hypovolaemic, or is very ill. It should be expert, and she *must* be intubated. It is dangerous in the circumstances of most labour wards, and the theatre may take dangerously long to get ready.

Most Caesarean sections can be done under subarachnoid (spinal) anaesthesia, *provided you take the necessary precautions* (A 16.6). You can also use local anaesthesia (A 6.9). For a vacuum extraction and outlet forceps, use a pudendal block, with local infiltration anaesthesia for the episiotomy. For a destructive operation, other than a transverse lie, use a pudendal block combined with intravenous pethidine and diazepam (A 8.8). For a transverse lie, she must have a general anaesthetic. For manual removal of the placenta, use intravenous pethidine and diazepam. Epidural anasthesia is excellent, but is probably impractical, except in specialized well-staffed obstetric units. The routine aseptic prcedures in your wards may not be reliable enough to justify its routine use, and you will probably not have the staff to monitor it.

LOCAL ANAESTHESIA FOR AN OPERATIVE VAGINAL DELIVERY

Primary Anaesthesia describes transvaginal pudendal block, but not the alternative perineal pudendal block, nor any method of local infiltration. These are described here. Use a total of 50 ml of 0.5% lignocaine or 1% procaine, both with adrenalin (A 5-1).

LOCAL ANAESTHESIA FOR AN OPERATIVE VAGINAL DELIVERY

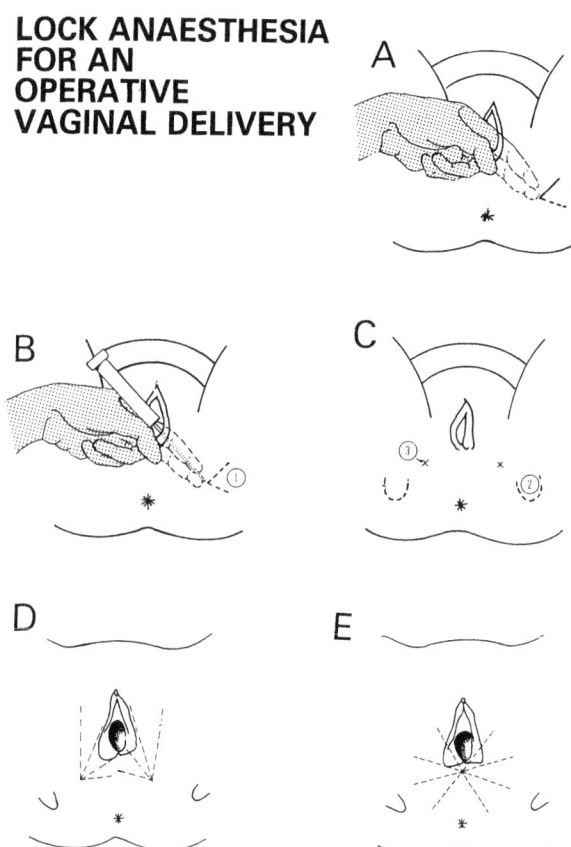

Fig. 18-1 LOCAL ANAESTHESIA FOR AN OPERATIVE VAGINAL DELIVERY. A, feeling for a patient's ischial spine for a transvaginal pudendal block. B, injecting for a transvaginal pudendal block. C, the injection site for doing a pudendal block through her perineal skin. D, local anaesthesia after a pudendal block. E, local infiltration alone from a single central puncture site.

1, her ischial spine. 2, her ischial tuberosity. 3, the site of injection for pudendal block through her perineum and for local infiltration anaesthesia after a pudendal block. *After Howie, Beryl. 'High Risk Obstetrics' Fig. 14-6 and 14-7. Macmillan Publishers, with kind permission.*

Transvaginal pudendal block: see Section A 6.13.

Perineal pudendal block: raise a skin wheal half way between the patient's vaginal opening and her ischial tuberosities, as in C, Fig. 18-1. Use a 12 cm × 1 mm needle to reach her ischial spines. Inject about 12.5 ml of solution on each side.

Local infiltration anaesthesia is needed to supplement a pudendal block for most operative vaginal deliveries. For a low forceps delivery or episiotomy local infiltration alone may be enough. *Keep the needle moving* while you inject 25 ml of solution.

After a perineal pudendal block, use the same needle to puncture and infiltrate, as in D, 18-1. After a transvaginal one make fresh punctures.

For local infiltration alone, inject radially from a single central puncture site (E).

CAUTION ! (1) Premedicate her with pethidine and diazepam. (2) Distinguish her ischial spines from her ischial tuberosities. (3) ALWAYS withdraw the plunger before you inject. If you withdraw blood, move the needle, or you will inject the anaesthetic solution intravenously. (4) Give the anaesthetic enough time to act (at least 3 minutes).

18.2 Delay in labour

Labour is seldom any problem if it goes at its proper pace. Most trouble starts when it is delayed. If you are going to manage delay, you must know as early as possible that it has occurred. To know this you will need an effective method of monitoring labour—the partogram (or in WHO's terminology, the 'partograph') which *Primary Mother Care* describes in detail (M 18.2). The most important part of this is the 'cervicograph' which plots the dilation of the cervix in centimetres, and the descent of the head in fifths above the brim, against the duration of labour in hours.

The purpose of the partogram is: (1) To prevent obstructed labour and ruptured uterus (which cause 70% of maternal deaths in some areas) by enabling *peripheral health workers* to monitor labour, so as to detect deviations from the normal more effectively, and thus to refer mothers at the optimum moment—before it is too late. This is the purpose of the 'alert line'. Ideally, the partogram should only be used to monitor those labours which are expected to be normal; mothers with 'risk factors' should have already been referred. (2) To monitor *all labours in hospital*, so that you know when to intervene. This is the purpose of the 'action line'. If the 'progress line' of a mother's cervical dilatation moves to the right of the alert line, be extra vigilant. If she reaches the action line you must do something, if you have not already done it (see below).

The partogram depends on the principles that: (1) The latent phase of labour should not last longer than 8 hours, hence the thick vertical line at this point. (2) The latent phase ends and the active phase starts when her cervix is 3 cm dilated (4 cm is sometimes used). (3) During the active phase her cervix should dilate at not less than 1 cm per hour. (4) A lag time of 4 hours is *usually* acceptable between the slowing of labour and the need to intervene; this is the distance between the alert and the action lines. The WHO partogram uses fixed alert and action lines and transfers her to the alert line as soon as she reaches 3 cm, as has been done for Mother C, in Fig. 18-2a.

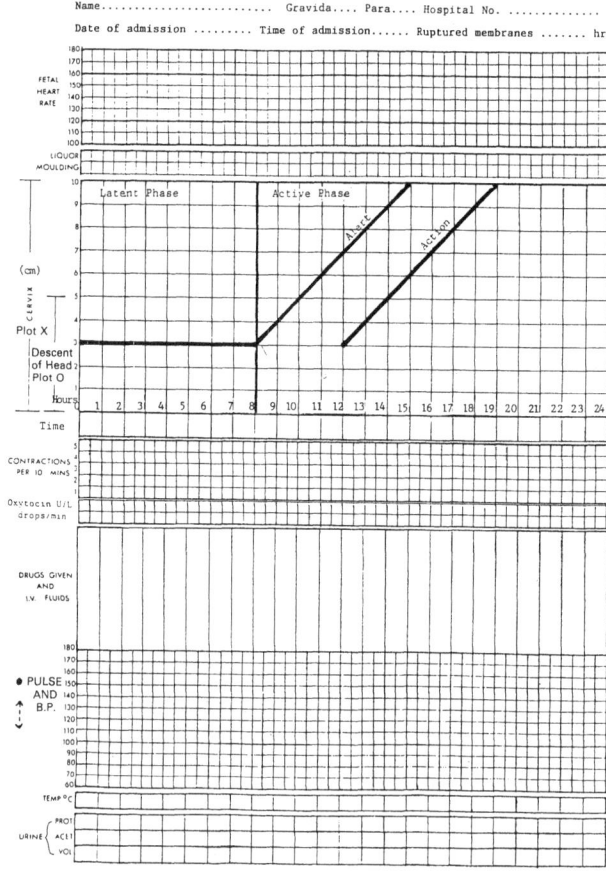

Fig. 18-2 THE PARTOGRAM is a very useful tool for managing labour, but it will not help you to identify risk factors that may have been present before labour started. The vertical scale on the left measures the dilatation of the cervix in centimetres and the descent of the head in fifths above the brim.

SOME CERVICOGRAPHS

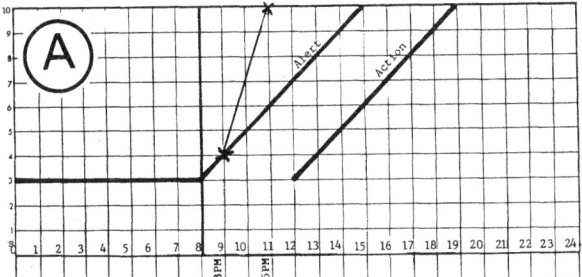

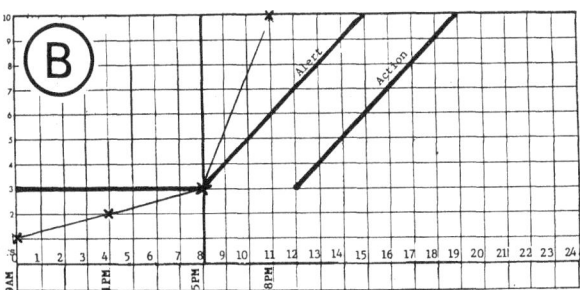

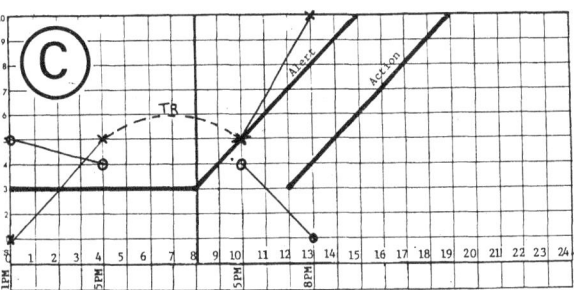

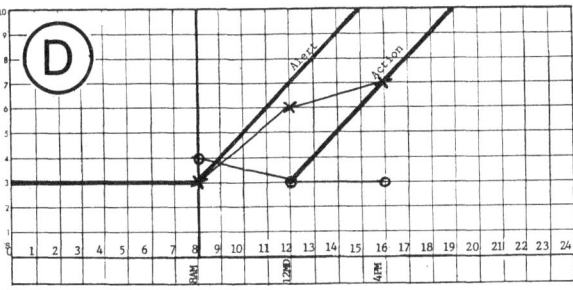

Fig. 18-2a SOME PARTOGRAMS. If you don't have enough partograms for every mother, put a clean sheet of X-ray film over one of them, write on this with a marker pencil, and then wash the film clean for the next patient.

Mother A, was admitted at 3 p.m. 4 cm dilated in the active phase of labour; her progress line remained to the left of the alert line and she delivered normally.

Mother B, was admitted at 9 a.m. 1 cm dilated; her latent phase lasted 8 hours and her active phase 3 hours.

Mother C, was admitted at 1 p.m. 1 cm dilated with her baby's head head 5/5 above the pelvic brim. At the next vaginal examination (5 p.m.) his head was 4/5 above the brim and she was 5 cm dilated. She was therefor transferred to the 'alert line'; her cervix continued to dilate, his head descended, and she delivered normally.

Mother D, was admitted to a health centre with her baby's head 4/5 above the brim and her cervix 3 cm dilated, so she was put on the alert line. At 12 midday she was only 6 cm dilated and had moved to the right of the alert line, so she was transferred to hospital. When she arrived at 4 p.m. she was still only 7 cm dilated and had reached the action line. His head was 3/5 above the brim, with a moulding score of 3; it was not possible to put a finger between his head and her pelvic wall, so, following the indications in Section 18.4, she was sectioned.

THE CRITICAL AREA IN A CERVICOGRAPH

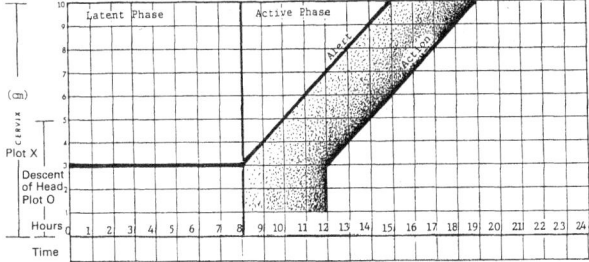

Fig. 18-2b THE CRITICAL AREA IN A PARTOGRAM. In a peripheral unit, if a mother's progress line reaches this area, she should be referred. In hospital, it is the area in which you should consider intervening; the darker the shading the more important this is. Don't let her cross the action line!

Dilatation of the cervix and its relation to the action line is only one of the factors measuring the progress of labour, and the necessity to intervene. It and the descent of the baby's head are the only two factors plotted on the cervicograph. Although they are the most useful and the most easily plotted ones, there are others which determine what you should do and when you should do it, they include: his presentation, his moulding score, his condition (fetal distress), his mother's condition, and the strength and frequency of her contractions. Consider all these factors, and don't be guided only by the dilatation of her cervix in relation to the action line and by the descent of his head, critical though these are.

The position of the action line is to some extent arbitrary, and some obstetricians like the alert and action lines closer together. Intervention needs to be earlier in a multip than in a primip, so some partograms have two action lines, one at 3 hours for multips and one at 4 hours for primips. Some hospital partograms leave out the action line altogether and take the alert line as the action line. The important point is that *the further the progress line is from the alert line, the greater should be your vigilance,* and usually the greater your need to intervene. When, later, we say "If she approaches the action line, do..." what we really mean is that she has already crossed the alert line and is getting progressively nearer the action line (if your partogram has one). When this is happening, assess all the factors listed above (and others) and decide what to do next, using the guidelines below and in Section 18.4.

Some hospitals consider that 1 cm per hour is 'too active', and leads to an unnecessarily high Caesarean section rate, which is not suitable for populations with an average of perhaps 8 children, and when Caesarean section has to be done under less than ideal circumstances in small hospitals, so they give the alert line a flatter slope.

Partograms have proved so useful in reducing both maternal and perinatal mortality, that not to introduce them might almost be considered criminal neglect. If you don't already use them, *you must!* There is full-size copy on an endpaper, and also an interim version of the the other side. A further version of this will be included in *Primary Mother Care*.

'Obstetrics Handbook', Faculty of Medicine, University of Natal, 1984.

Philpott RH, 'Obstetric Problems in the Developing World', Clinics in Obstetrics and Gynaecology 1982;9:3.

'The Partograph'. Section One, 'The Principle and Strategy'. Section Two, 'A user's manual'. 1988 Maternal and Child Health Unit, Division of Family Health. WHO Geneva.

ARE YOU AND YOUR CLINICS USING PARTOGRAMS?

THE GENERAL METHOD FOR DELAY IN LABOUR

Here is the general method for delay in labour. If the presenting part has not only failed to descend, but there have also been these signs, labour is not only delayed, it is also obstructed: severe moulding and caput, fetal distress, a stretched lower segment, bloody urine, etc. If so, see Section 18.3.

DELAY IN THE LATENT PHASE (primips and multips)

The latent phase is prolonged, if a patient who was 'admitted in labour' has not reached the active phase after 8 hours. First distinguish 'false labour' and a truly prolonged latent phase.

False labour: her membranes are still intact, a nullip's cervix remains long and closed (or just admits a finger tip), a multip's cervix is not effaced (even though it may be 1 or 2 cm dilated). Explain that she is not in labour, and send her home if she wishes. If she insists that she feels painful contractions give her pethidine 100 mg, let her sleep, and then discharge or review her.

Truly prolonged latent phase: Her cervix is completely effaced, but remains stationary at about 2 cm. Or it effaces and dilates very slowly. Either, (1) Sedate her with pethidine 100 mg, repeated if necessary, and wait. Or, (2) let her walk about. Or, (3) rupture her membranes and give her an oxytocin drip.

DELAY IN THE ACTIVE PHASE primips

If a primip's progress line approaches the action line, she may have primary uterine inertia, or there may be some mechanical reason for it. Section her if: (1) She has gross CPD (head 4/5 above the brim and marked moulding). (2) A malpresentation (breech, transverse lie, face, or brow, etc.). (3) Fetal distress (M 20.4, M 21.3). If she has none of these things, manage her actively to decide if she has doubtful CPD, or no CPD. Manage her like this.

(1) Correct her dehydration and ketosis. Give her a drip of 5% dextrose.

(2) Provide adequate analgesia (A 2.9, M 18.15). Either give her a lumbar epidural block (A 7.2), or give her pethidine 100 mg and promethazine 25 mg, both intramuscularly.

(3) If you are sure she is in labour (that is her cervix is dilated 3 cm or more) and her membranes are not already ruptured, rupture them.

(4) Stimulate her uterus with oxytocin. Add 5 units of oxytocin to 500 ml of 5% dextrose, and start at 10 drops a minute. Increase the rate of the drip by 10 drops a minute at half-hourly intervals, until she is having contractions lasting 45 to 60 seconds at a frequency of 3 to 4 in 10 minutes. Make the first increment to 20 drops a minute, and half an hour later to 30 drops a minute. As soon as she has good contractions, don't increase the speed of the drip any more.

(5) Monitor her progress and her baby's condition carefully. Monitor his heart and watch for signs of fetal distress, especially slowing of the fetal heart (meconium staining of the liquor is common, and is an unreliable sign, M 20.5).

Decide how you are going to deliver her within 6 hours of starting the oxytocin drip. Section her if any of these things happen, they are probably all signs of severe CPD: (1) There is fetal distress. (2) At the end of 6 hours she is still dilating less than 1 cm per hour, and the head is not descending. (3) It remains high, with moulding.

DELAY IN THE ACTIVE PHASE multips

If a multip's progress line approaches the action line, this is serious, and you will need to assess her carefully. Don't try to stimulate her uterus with oxytocin, unless you are absolutely sure there is no CPD (see Section 18.4a). This is difficult to be sure about, and if you are wrong, and there is CPD, her uterus may rupture. *One contributor advises no oxytocin for multips!*

If she is in definite labour (her cervix is 3 cm or more) and her membranes have not already ruptured, **rupture them**.

If you are in doubt, **observe her for 2 more hours** with adequate analgesia, and then reassess her. Feel her contractions yourself. She may progress to full dilation even when there is major CPD. You can only detect this by finding severe moulding and caput, with failure of the head to descend, and delay (more than 20 minutes in the second stage).

CAUTION! Some mothers have 6 or 8 normal labours, and then need section for CPD with their next pregnancy.

DIFFICULTIES WITH DELAY IN LABOUR

If a patient is referred because of DELAY IN THE LATENT STAGE (M 20.7), look carefully for hidden CPD. If there is no CPD, rupture her membranes, and give her an oxytocin drip. Clinics should refer these cases, because CPD is not easy to recognize. Provided there is a vertex presentation, it is always worth rupturing the membranes and waiting a little to see what happens. CPD is almost impossible to diagnose when the membranes are intact.

18.3 Obstructed labour

The exact point at which the 'delay' discussed in the previous section becomes the 'obstruction' discussed in this one is arguable. Obstruction is 'the failure of the presenting part to descend in spite of uterine contractions' (M 23.1). What really distinguishes delay from obstruction is the secondary signs and complications that follow: severe moulding and caput, foetal distress, a stretched lower segment, bloody urine, fistulae and rupture of the uterus, etc. Whereas delay in labour is usually inevitable and readily treatable, and is comparatively harmless, obstructed labour is none of these things. It should never happen where care is adequate.

Obstruction may be due to: (1) An abnormality in a mother's pelvis (a contracted pelvis). (2) An abnormality in her baby (hydrocephaly, etc.). (3) An abnormality in the relationship between them. This can either be: (a) an abnormal lie or presentation (a breech, a brow, or a face, or a shoulder presentation, or a prolapsed arm in a transverse lie), or (b) an unfortunate coincidence of their relative sizes (CPD, cephalopelvic disproportion, he may be too big for her, or she may be too small for him). (4) Rarer causes, such as stenosis of the vagina, locked twins, or a pelvic tumour, particularly fibroids or an ovarian cyst. CPD is the most important cause (two-thirds of cases), and an impacted transverse lie is the next. This is much less readily anticipated antenatally, especially when it complicates the delivery of a second twin. Much of the purpose of antenatal care is to screen mothers who are at risk from obstructed labour. The purpose of the partogram is to detect it early.

In practice, when the presenting part stops moving through the birth canal, you may not be able to tell if this is because: (1) the uterine contractions are weak (uterine inertia), or (2) because the baby and the pelvis are such that one will not go through the other (CPD). Often, there is a combination of inertia and CPD.

Preventing obstruction depends on: (1) Good nutrition starting in childhood, so that mothers reach their genetically determined height, and their pelves their genetically determined size. (2) Universal antenatal care, so that obstructed labour can be anticipated from a mother's history, and any risk factors for it identified. (2) The monitoring of labour by skilled staff, so that she can be referred at the first sign of danger, before she obstructs. The detailed preventive measures are: (a) Screening for risk factors, especially short stature (M 5.3). (b) A pelvic assessment at 36 weeks (M 6.6). (c) The routine use of the partogram. When adequate antenatal care is impossible, and where health centre and hospital beds are limited, the establishment of a 'mother's waiting area' or a 'mother's village' is a useful alternative.

Obstructed labour is a major failure of obstetric care. Unfortunately, it still happens, even in some hospitals. How often you will see it will depend on the prevalence of CPD in your area, and the quality of your antenatal and obstetric care. Alas, the poorest communities with the worst health services are usually those with the most CPD.

In a labour that is going to obstruct, the first stage is often prolonged, but it can be normal or even short. A mother's membranes rupture, and her liquor escapes. Her uterus contracts and retracts, and forces her baby into its lower segment, which gradually becomes overstretched. Obstruction prevents his escape, so her lower segment moulds closely round him and thins. The contractions of her uterus become hypertonic, and relaxation between them poor. The placenta is poorly perfused, there is fetal distress, and he dies.

Obstructed labour has two main dangers: (1) Her vagina, bladder, and rectum are trapped between his head and her pelvis, so that they become necrotic, slough, and develop fistulae. (2) Her uterus ruptures. Primips usually develop fistulae, and multips usually rupture their uteri, but both can do either, and rupture and fistulae can occur in the same patient.

A **primip** begins to have trouble when her cervix fails to dilate normally. An oxytocin drip (M 22.2) may speed it up if her CPD is minimal, but cannot do so if it is gross. The result is that her labour usually obstructs before she is fully dilated, although she will usually reach full dilatation eventually. If her obstruction is not rapidly relieved: (1) It produces asphyxia in her baby, due to prolonged uterine contractions reducing the placental blood flow. (2) It may injure his head, so that he is born with a birth injury. (3) It causes a pressure necrosis, and sloughing of her anterior vaginal wall. As this slough separates, she develops a fistula between her bladder and her vagina (18.18), which may involve the proximal half of her urethra and/or the neck of her bladder, up to its ureteric orifices. Later, as the ring of necrosis in her vagina heals and contracts, it stenoses. Or, she may develop a fistula between her rectum and her vagina (18.19). If she does not die herslf, she delivers an injured, severely moulded dead baby.

She is also at risk from septic shock (53.4), peritonitis, peritoneal abscesses, atonic postpartum haemorrhage (19.11a), and foot drop from the pressure of his head on her sciatic nerves. Even if her fistula can be repaired, and there is at best only about an 80% chance of this, she may be infertile, and her vagina may be so stenosed that sex is difficult. If it is repaired, and she becomes pregnant again, she must be sectioned to prevent the repair breaking down. If it is not repaired (in which case she is less likely to become pregnant), stenosis of her vagina is likely to prevent vaginal delivery. Here is one such primip.

MPHO MOKETE (14 years, para 0, gravida 1) became pregnant after her first period. She hid her pregnancy from her parents, and so received no antenatal care. She arrived tired, exhausted, anxious, and febrile, with a fast pulse. Her contractions were strong and painful, with little relaxation between them. The head of her baby, who showed signs of fetal distress, was high, and overlapped the brim of her pelvis. Her liquor had drained, so that her uterus was moulded around him.
Her vulva and cervix were oedematous, and although his head could be felt just inside her cervix, this was not because it had descended, but because his head was severely elongated. Abdominal examination showed that most of it was still above her pelvic brim. Her vagina was dry and 'hot', and her cervix not fully dilated.
Her bladder was distended. Catheterizing her was difficult, and his head had to be dislodged by putting two fingers into her vagina, and pushing it up. Her bladder was drawn up so high that the catheter had to be passed a long way before any urine flowed; when it did so, it was blood-stained. Her baby was alive, and his head was 4/5 above the brim, so she was not suitable for symphysiotomy or vacuum delivery. She was therefore resuscitated with intravenous fluids, given antibiotics, and delivered by Caesarean section. He survived, but her wound became infected, and she developed a pelvic abscess, which was drained. She was in hospital a month, and was lucky not to develop a fistula. LESSONS (1) The decision to section her was correct, but it should have been done extraperitoneally (18.13). (2) She is only 14, so her pelvis will continue to grow. (3) She is at risk of a ruptured uterus in future, so she must deliver in hospital.

A **multip** may show the same failure to dilate as a primip, or her cervix may dilate normally to begin with, and then slow during the active phase, only to dilate finally if she is left untreated. Meanwhile, the presenting part fails to descend. Here is one such multip.

MAPULESA (35, para 8 gravida 10) arrived just before her uterus ruptured. She too was anxious, distressed, and febrile. Her cervix however was fully dilated. Her lower segment had continued to retract and thin, so that the junction between her upper and lower segments had risen in her uterus as far as her umbilicus. She had a 'three-tumour abdomen'—an oedematous distended bladder, a distended, tender lower segment, and a tonically contracted upper segment. A ring (Bandl's ring) could be felt through her abdominal wall between her upper and lower segments (G, Fig. 18-3). Her round ligaments stood out on either side of her ballooned lower segment, like the guy ropes of a tent. Vaginal examination revealed a brow presentation. She was resuscitated with intravenous fluids, and sectioned. At operation her uterus was found to have ruptured into her abdominal cavity. Her baby was alive, but was asphyxiated, and died in an hour. Her uterus was repaired, her tubes were tied, and she recovered uneventfully. LESSONS (1) Even a patient who has had many normal deliveries may

OBSTRUCTED LABOUR

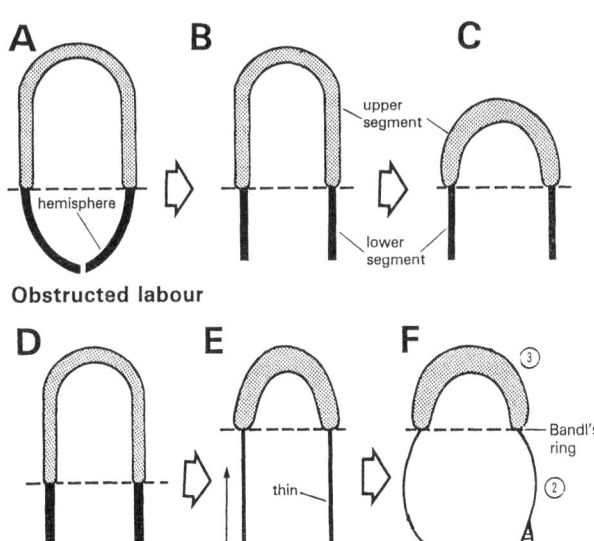

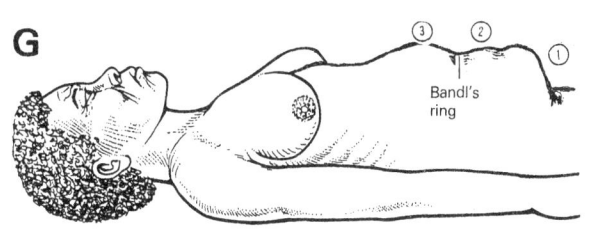

Fig. 18-3 OBSTRUCTED LABOUR. A, B, and C, during a normal labour the hemispherical lower segment is converted into a cylinder: it thins but does not elongate. During the second stage the uterus shortens itself by contraction of the upper segment. During an obstructed labour the uterus cannot empty, so the thinned lower segment elongates (D, and E). F, sometimes a palpable ring (Bandl's ring) forms between the upper and lower segments. G, you may sometimes see or feel three distinct abdominal swellings: (1) the bladder, (2) the lower segment, (3) the upper segment. Bandl's ring separates the lower and the upper segments. *After Lawson JB and Stewart DB, 'Obstetrics and Gynaecology in the Tropics', Fig. 11.2. Edward Arnold (1967), with kind permission.*

get an obstructed labour from a malpresentation or malposition. (2) A partogram would have given earlier warning of her impending obstruction.

The critical event in a patient like this is rupture of her uterus. This usually starts in her thin lower segment, and extends downwards on one side into her vagina, as well as upwards towards her fundus. Several things can then happen: (1) The presenting part may remain jammed in her pelvis. (2) Her baby may be expelled through the rupture into her peritoneal cavity. (3) She may bleed from the rupture into her vagina. (4) Occasionally, her bladder also ruptures, especially if it has stuck to the scar of a previous lower-segment Caesarean section.

Before rupture the signs that it is imminent are: (1) The failure of labour to progress. Lack of progress should therefore alert you to the possibility that rupture might be imminent. (2) Bandl's ring. (3) A distended bladder which is difficult to catheterize. (4) Frequent strong uterine contractions, with little or no pause between them. If a patient is brought in on the verge of rupture, you may perhaps see it occurring, before you can treat her.

After rupture, a mother may have little or no pain. If you ask her, she will tell you that contractions were strong, but then suddenly stopped, and were replaced by a lesser continuous pain, or no pain. She may be in severe hypovolaemic shock, with cold, sweaty skin, and a weak or absent radial pulse. She may be quite obviously collapsed, or alert and even talkative. You can feel no uterine contractions, but you can usually feel her baby through her abdominal wall lying free in her abdomen.

For the management of a ruptured uterus, see Section 18.17.

To summarize: (1) A primip's uterus seldom ruptures, but she often develops fistulae. (2) A grand multip's uterus often ruptures, but she seldom develops fistulae. (3) Failure to dilate is a useful warning signal in a primip, and in most multips. In a multip the first sign of obstruction may be failure of the presenting part to descend at full dilatation, in spite of strong and frequent contractions, and increased moulding of her baby's head. A multip who has not delivered after 20 minutes in the second stage is in great danger.

18.4 Managing an obstructed labour

If a patient with obstructed labour is admitted from home, she may have been in labour for days, and tried many home remedies. Her stomach is likely to be full, and she can inhale its contents only too easily. She is thus a major anaesthetic risk. There are several ways in which you can deliver her, but the standard midcavity or rotational forceps, such as Kielland's, should never be one of them (18.1).

Vaginal delivery is often possible, but try to avoid a difficult one. Learn to predict when it is going to be difficult, so that you can avoid a 'failed vacuum', and do a Caesarean section or a symphysiotomy (18.6, M 22.7) to begin with, especially when there is fetal distress. *An operative vaginal delivery is absolutely contraindicated if her uterus has already ruptured*—do a laparotomy. Often, you will not know if it has ruptured or not, so do all vaginal operations for the relief of obstructed labour in the theatre, with a set of laparotomy instruments ready for instant use.

Caesarean section has a limited role, and is likely to be a serious risk, so don't do it lightly. It is mainly indicated: (1) when a baby is alive and his mother is in reasonable condition. (2) When a destructive operation on a dead baby would be dangerous, because his head is mobile 3/5, or more, high above her pelvic brim (rare). Try not to section her, if she cannot be sure of adequate care in her next delivery, or if your skills and facilities for doing so safely are not good. If you have to section her, Section 18.8 will help you to decide on the most suitable method.

A destructive operation (M 22.10) is indicated when her baby is dead, her cervix is fully dilated or nearly so, the presenting part is fixed in her pelvis, and her uterus has not ruptured, and is in no danger of doing so. Usually, you can be fairly sure that a uterus is not going to rupture. If you are in any doubt, the only way to find out is to do a laparotomy, and see if there is a rupture. If you don't find one, close her abdomen and deliver her vaginally.

OBSTRUCTED LABOUR

A mother in obstructed labour is in great pain, anxiety, and distress. In the bustle of treating her, don't forget to comfort and reassure her. If her baby is already dead, tell her. If you don't, she may blame you for his death, and not come to hospital when she is pregnant next time. Many of the steps and complications are the same as for rupture of the uterus, so see Section 18.17.

THE DIAGNOSIS. Suspect obstructed labour when: (1) Her cervix does not dilate in spite of good contractions. (2) Moulding and caput increase, but her baby's head does not descend. (3) She becomes anxious and restless. (4) She develops hypertonic uterine contractions, with poor relaxation between them. Other signs are: (5) A stretched lower segment. (6) Bloody urine. (7) A cervix which is not well applied to the head (variable).

An important differential diagnosis is a prolonged latent phase without obstruction. If she was made to push during the latent phase, she may be distressed and dehydrated, and her vulva and cervix may be oedematous. Her cervix will however not be dilated, or only slightly so, her membranes are likely to be intact, and there will be no Bandl's ring. Reassurance, analgesics, and fluids may be all she needs.

The diagnosis of obstruction is certain if: (1) Bandl's ring (18-3) is present, or (2) she has a bladder fistula or necrosis. This takes 2 or 3 days to develop, so it is rare for her to present with one.

When you diagnose obstructed labour, the next critical question is: *has her uterus already ruptured?* To answer this, see Section 18.17 on rupture of the uterus. If it has not ruptured, proceed as follows:

HYPOVOLAEMIC SHOCK (very common). **Resuscitation must be rapid**, because delivery is urgent. Admit her directly to whatever high-risk area you have, usually the labour ward or the theatre, and resuscitate her there. This will allow you to operate as soon as she is in an optimal condition.

Correct her dehydration, her electrolyte deficit, and her acidosis (A 17.2). Rehydrate her with 0.9% saline or Ringer's lactate, and continue with dextrose 5%; there is usually no need to give her bicarbonate. She may need blood, preferably the red cells only. If her haematocrit is raised as the result of dehydration, a transfusion, even of safe blood, may be harmful—she needs fluids.

If possible, set up a central venous line and measure her CVP (A 19.2). If this is within the range of 5 to 8 cm of water, and she is still shocked, at least part of her problem is likely to be septic shock exacerbated by ketosis.

Record her pulse, her blood pressure, and her CVP every five minutes during the operation. Monitor her urine output regularly. If it falls to less than 30 ml/hour, see Section 53.3.

SEPTIC SHOCK (less common). If she is ill and weak, but not actually in septic shock (53.4), she probably soon will be, if you don't prevent it. So start the following regime prophylactically.

Give her intravenous chloramphenicol and intravenous or rectal metronidazole (2.9). If, in spite of this, her blood pressure remains low, her urinary output is poor, and her vessels remain constricted, she needs a titrated infusion of dopamine (53.4). This will cause peripheral dilatation, and a fall in her CVP. Correct it immediately with more intravenous fluids.

ANAESTHESIA. If she is to have a Caesarean section, see Section A 16.6. If she is to be delivered vaginally, use a pudendal block (18.2, A 6.13), a saddle block (A 7.7), or an epidural block (A 7.3). Remember to insert a nasogastric tube.

METHODS OF DELIVERY WHEN THE PRESENTING PART HAS STOPPED DESCENDING

You will probably find the following summary one of the most useful sections in this manual, since it is the key to this chapter. It covers a variety of situations in which the presenting part no longer descends in the birth canal. In some of them, the classical signs of obstructed labour (severe moulding, etc.) have yet to occur, *so it is a combination of methods for the management of delay and obstruction*. First the various methods are considered (episiotomy, etc.), and then the various clinical situations you might meet. Before you continue, you will need to:

Assess the height of the baby's head (M 18.4). Don't assess the height of his head by vaginal examination only. There will be much caput, and this will mislead you. It is the descent of his skull that matters, not the descent of his caput!

Assess his moulding score (18.6). Feel where his parietal and occipital bones touch one another. Bones still separate, score 0. Bones touching, score 1. Bones overlapping, but separate when you press with a finger, score 2. Bones overlapping but not separable, score 3. Overlapping at both the sagittal and the lambdoid sutures, is more serious than overlapping at the lambdoid suture only (this is the suture between the parietal and the occipital bones).

Watch for fetal distress. Count his heart rate for 30 seconds, before, during and after a contraction. Fetal distress is shown by: (1) A rate of < 120 or > 160. (2) Slowing which persists after a contraction (slowing during it is normal).

CAUTION ! (1) Don't use an oxytocin drip if there are signs of obstruction. On the correct indications, you can use it for delay (18.4a). (2) If there is obstruction or delay, don't use Kielland's forceps, or try internal version. (3) *Never do an operative vaginal delivery if her uterus has already ruptured*—do a laparotomy. You may not know if it is ruptured or not, so do all vaginal opera-

CHOOSING THE BEST METHOD TO DELIVER A MOTHER WITH A LONG SECOND STAGE AND A LIVE BABY

	Amount of baby's head above the brim.	Contractions of the uterus	Is the baby distressed?	Lower abdomen	Moulding score	Does the head move down to the ischial spines?	Treatment
1	1–2/5	Weak	No	No bulge	2	Yes	Oxytocin drip
2	1/5	Good	No	No bulge	2–3	Yes	Vacuum extractor or Forceps.
3	1–2/5	Good	Yes	No bulge	4–6	No movement	Symphysiotomy
4	3/5	Good	No	No bulge	1–2	Yes	Trial of Vacuum or Symphysiotomy
5	3/5	Good	Yes	No bulge	4–6	No	Transfer for Caesarean section.
6	3–4/5	Weak	Yes or No	Bulging	4–6	No	Transfer for Caesarean section.
7	4/5	Good	No	No bulge	4–6	No	Transfer for Caesarean section.

Fig. 18-4 CHOOSING THE BEST METHOD TO DELIVER A MOTHER WITH A LONG SECOND STAGE AND A LIVE BABY. This is a table from 'Primary Mother Care' which advises midwives what they should do in health centres. You may also find it useful. It differs slightly from the instructions for similar situations given here. *Kindly contributed by Hugh Philpott.*

tions for the relief of obstructed labour in the theatre, with a set of laparotomy instruments ready for instant use.

EPISIOTOMY M 18.16

This is sometimes all that a primigravida needs, especially if her baby's vertex is in an occipito–posterior position. Putting her into the lithotomy position may make delivery easier.

VACUUM EXTRACTION 18.5, M 22.3

INDICATIONS. (1) A live baby with less than 2/5 of his head above the brim. And, (2) only moderate moulding. Vacuum extraction may be very suitable, if obstruction is due to an occipito-transverse or an occipito-posterior position, without CPD, or with only mild CPD.

CONTRAINDICATIONS. (1) A dead baby, unless delivery by vacuum extraction is very easy. (2) A live baby with more than 2/5 of his head above the brim. (3) Severe moulding. (4) Definite CPD contraindicates any kind of forceps or vacuum extraction.

CAUTION ! (1) Delivery with a vacuum extractor or outlet forceps should never be a difficult operation. If fetal asphyxia is already present, it should merely be a 'lift-out'. (2) If you use the vacuum extractor, be sure to follow the rule of the 'Three pulls' (M 22.3). The first pull must dislodge his head from its arrested position, the second must bring his head to the pelvic floor, and the third must deliver, or at least crown it. If any one of these three pulls does not achieve its purpose, stop, and try another method of delivery. This will have to be symphysiotomy or section, and not forceps, which are too dangerous for a baby after a failed vacuum. If possible, try to predict difficulty, and choose the right method in the first place. (3) If (a) she was >3 hrs dilating from 7 to 10 cm on the partogram, or (b) her fundal height is >40 cm, suggesting a large baby, expect difficulty. Do the vacuum extraction in the theatre, and prepare for section.

OUTLET FORCEPS M 22.6

INDICATIONS. (1) In mento–anterior (face) presentations, because vacuum extraction is impossible (M 22.6). One contributor considers section safer. (2) When there is fetal distress, because outlet forceps are quicker than vacuum extraction.

SYMPHYSIOTOMY 18.6, M 20.7

INDICATIONS. Symphysiotomy may be indicated if a baby is alive in a cephalic presentation, with not more than 2/5, or in some cases (see Section 18.6) 3/5, of his head above the brim. He should not be too big, or too small (2.5 to 4 kg), and his moulding score should be less than 3. An indication of his maximum size is that her fundal height should be <40 cm.

DESTRUCTIVE OPERATIONS 18.7, 18.10

INDICATIONS FOR CRANIOTOMY. All the following conditions must hold: (1) He must be dead. (2) 2/5 or less of his head must be above the brim (if it is higher than this, Caesarean section is usually safer, although if you are expert you may be able to do a craniotomy at 3/5). (3) His head must be impacted. (4) His mother's cervix must be at least 7 cm dilated, and preferably fully dilated. (5) Her uterus must be unruptured, and not in imminent danger of rupturing. If she is a multip, and has been in labour for a long time, her lower segment will be very thin. If it is tender and distended, it is certainly very thin. She can only be saved by Caesarean section; any destructive operation, except pushing a needle into a hydrocephalic head, will rupture it.

INDICATIONS FOR DESTRUCTIVE OPERATIONS FOR A TRANSVERSE LIE. The baby is dead and is lying transversely, her cervix is 8 cm or more dilated, and her uterus is not ruptured.

CAESAREAN SECTION 18.9

INDICATIONS. (1) A live baby whose head is too high for vacuum extraction or symphysiotomy. (2) A dead baby who is too high to be delivered by a destructive operation (rare).

CONTRAINDICATIONS. (1) A head which is deeply engaged in the pelvis (2/5 or less above the brim). A vaginal delivery by vacuum extraction or symphysiotomy is safer. (2) A dead baby who can be delivered by a destructive operation.

CLINICAL SITUATIONS WHEN THE PRESENTING PART HAS STOPPED DESCENDING

Here we are mostly concerned with a vertex presentation, and a few curiosities. See elsewhere for a breech presentation (19.8), a transverse lie, and a brow or a face presentation (19.9).

VERTEX PRESENTATION. Follow this scheme.

If rupture is suspected but uncertain, section her.

If her baby is alive and her cervix is not fully dilated, section her.

If he is alive and it is fully dilated, management depends on: (1) the height of his head, (2) the degree of moulding, and (3) signs of fetal distress.

0/5 above the brim, with minimal moulding—do an episiotomy and apply the vacuum extractor, or apply outlet forceps.

1/5 above the brim, with a moulding score of 0 to 1 and fetal distress—do a vacuum extraction or apply outlet forceps.

1/5 above the brim, with a moulding score of 2 or 3 and fetal distress—do a symphysiotomy.

2/5 above the brim, with a moulding score of 0 or 1 or possibly 2 and a live baby—do a trial of vacuum extraction in the theatre, with everything ready for symphysiotomy or section if you fail. Or section her anyway.

2/5 above the brim, with a moulding score of 3 or possibly 2 and fetal distress—do a symphysiotomy, if necessary followed by vacuum extraction.

3/5 above the brim, with a moulding score of 0 or 1—do a trial of vacuum extraction. If necessary and her pelvis is big enough (you can get your finger between the head and her symphysis) do a symphysiotomy.

3/5 above the brim, with a moulding score of 2 or 3—section her, unless you can get a finger between the head and her pelvic wall, indicating that a symphysiotomy might be possible.

If he is dead, the major decision is between craniotomy and Caesarean section.

(1) If his head is firmly impacted in her pelvis, and his head is 2/5 or 3/5 or less above the brim, and her cervix is 7 cm or more dilated, a craniotomy should be fairly easy, provided you can get a finger between his head and her pelvis.

(2) If his head is mobile or more than 3/5 above the brim, a craniotomy will be dangerous. Section, with all its risks, will be safer.

A MENTO-POSTERIOR PRESENTATION. If her cervix is fully dilated and her baby is alive, section her. If he is dead, and her cervix is fully dilated, do a craniotomy.

A CONGENITAL VAGINAL SEPTUM (rare) seldom causes trouble, because it usually quite thin, pushes to one side, and may never even be diagnosed during labour. If it does cause trouble, but is thin, you may be able to divide it. If it is thick, you may have to section her, and excise it later when she is not pregnant.

A VAGINAL STRICTURE (quite common) caused by scar tissue from a previous delivery, or of uncertain cause, feels quite different from a cervix. If it is thin, incise it at 4 o'clock and 8 o'clock, let vaginal delivery proceed, and suture the laceration. If it is wide and fibrous, section her.

AN OVARIAN TUMOUR OR A FIBROID. Section her. If she has an ovarian cyst or tumour, you can remove it at Caesarean section. If she has a fibroid, leave it and remove it subsequently if necessary.

CAUTION ! Never try to remove a fibroid at Caesarean section.

POSTOPERATIVELY AFTER A DIFFICULT VAGINAL DELIVERY

Keep her in hospital for three or four days (14 days for a symphysiotomy). Observe her carefully. Before she goes home, make sure that she understands: (1) what operation she had, and (2) why it was done. This will be important when she becomes pregnant again.

Her baby has a greater chance of brain damage. This may be caused by: (1) The operation itself. (2) Lack of oxygen. (3) Her pelvis being too small for his head. Watch him carefully for signs of twitching, irritability, or fever.

OBSTRUCTION BY TUMOURS

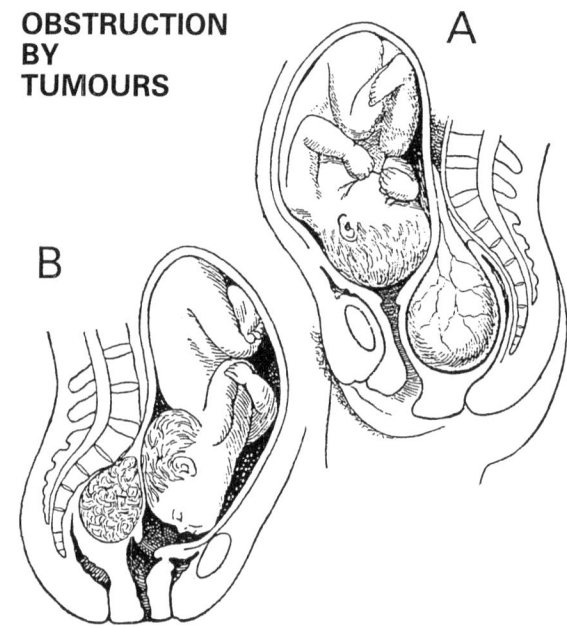

Fig. 18-5 TWO TUMOURS OBSTRUCTING LABOUR. A, an ovarian cyst. B, a cervical fibroid. If a patient has an ovarian cyst or tumour, you can remove it at Caesarean section. If she has a fibroid, leave it and remove it later if necessary. *After Young, James, 'A Textbook of Gynaecology' (5th edn. 1939), Figs. 125 and 168. A and C Black.*

18.4a Oxytocin

Oxytocin is an invaluable drug for making the uterus contract: (1) To *induce* labour. (2) To *accelerate* labour. (3) To stop bleeding after abortion or delivery.

The main dangers are that: (1) If you give too much too fast to a patient of high parity late in labour, her uterus may rupture. The sensitivity of the uterus to oxytocin varies greatly. Early in pregnancy it is comparatively insensitive; it becomes much more sensitive later, especially in multips. So *in a pregnant patient always give it by intravenous infusion,* starting with a small dose. If you do not get the effect you want, give more in an escalating (increasing) oxytocin drip. After delivery, or during an abortion, this rule does not apply, and you can safely give it by bolus intravenous injection, or intramuscularly. (2) In giving oxytocin by infusion, it is possible to give her too much fluid at the same time, especially when you use oxytocin to induce labour early in pregnancy, when you may need high doses. So when you give an escalating oxytocin drip, avoid the danger of water intoxication by giving it in 0.9% saline or Ringer's lactate, not in 5% dextrose, see Section 16.4.

The *primigravid* uterus is sufficiently insensitive for oxytocin to be safe enough for midwives to give routinely to accelerate labour. Using oxytocin to accelerate labour in *multips* can be dangerous, so it should only be given when: (1) The midwifery team is experienced, and able to adjust the 'drops per minute' carefully. And, (2) after the doctor on duty has seen and examined the patient, and has excluded a brow presentation, and CPD (which may not be easy). At least one contributor considers that oxytocin should *never* be used to accelerate labour in multips. In Africa, the head is often high through much of the first stage. Speeding its descent with oxytocin is dangerous for the inexperienced. If a multip's labour is slow, and her previous deliveries were normal, she will probably deliver her present baby eventually, provided he is a cephalic presentation. *So it is likely to be safer to leave her, after examining her carefully to exclude a brow, than to risk rupturing her uterus by giving oxytocin unnecessarily.*

OXYTOCIN

Here are the main methods and indications for the use of ox-

OXYTOCIN

Drops per minute	Units per litre			
	1	5	10	20
	INFUSION RATE IN MILLI-UNITS PER MINUTE			
10	1	3	7	14
20	1	6	14	28
30	2	10	20	40
40	3	14	27	54
50	3	17	34	68
60	4	20	40	80

Fig. 18-5a AN OXYTOCIN TABLE. The dose of oxytocin received by the patient in milliunits per minute depends on the concentration of oxytocin in the bottle and the speed of the drip in drops per minute. The table assumes a standard drip set delivering 15–20 drops per ml. The concentration of oxytocin in the bottle is given in units per litre and *not* in units per 500 ml, as in the text.

ytocin. See also: breech presentation 19.8, and multiple pregnancies 19.11, etc.

ADJUST THE DOSE to the patient— 'titrate it' against the response. Start with a low dose and increase it until you get the response you need. The dose rate ('drops per minute') is critical. Always start with a slow rate, and increase it if necessary every half hour, until she has the contractions she needs (usually 2 or 3 contractions every 10 minutes). Don't give more than 60 drops per minute, or you will give too much fluid. If you need more than 30 drops a minute, double the concentration and halve the drip rate for the next bottle. Note that we give the units of oxytocin to be added to 500 ml of fluid ('one bottle'), and not to one litre.

TO INDUCE LABOUR:

To induce labour between 10 and 28 weeks when the baby is dead (16.4). The uterus is much less sensitive than it is at term, and there is less danger of rupture, so start with 5 units in 500 ml, at 25 drops a minute, and if this does not work, increase the dose the next day, as in Section 16.4. 100 units in 500 ml is the absolute maximum. Read what Section 16.4 has to say about the dangers of water intoxication.

To induce labour at term in primips or in multips <para-4 (19.3). Use 5 units in 500 ml at 10 drops a minute, and increase the speed of the drip to 60 drops/minute as necessary, as in Section 19.3.

If a multip at term is >para-4, use 2.5 units in 500 ml.

If the baby is dead at term, you can use up to 20 units/500 ml, except in multips >para-4.

CAUTION ! (1) Whenever you give oxytocin to induce labour, give it by day rather than by night, when monitoring her reliably will be more difficult. (2) You can increase the drip rate, but don't exceed the concentrations above for particular categories of patients.

TO ACCELERATE LABOUR:

To accelerate labour in primips. Give 2.5 units/500 ml, and *don't increase the concentration*. Start at 10 drops a minute and increase the drip rate by 5 drops each half hour as necessary, to a maximum of 60, until you obtain contractions lasting 45–60 seconds at 2–3 minute intervals.

To accelerate labour in multips. This is controversial, so see above. Give the same dose as in primips, but with *extra special care!* A midwife must monitor the patient all the time. One contributor advises 1 unit in 500 ml. This is also the dose *Primary Mother Care* advises for the acceleration of labour, and then only in primips.

TO MAKE THE UTERUS CONTRACT AND CONTROL BLEEDING after abortion (16.2) or delivery (19.11a). For this purpose you can give oxytocin as an intravenous infusion, or by bolus intravenous injection. You can also give it by intramuscular injection. For this it is best combined with ergometrine as 'Syntometrine' (ergometrine 0.5 mg, oxytocin 5 units in 1 ml).

If you are giving oxytocin in an intravenous drip to control bleeding after abortion or delivery, add 20 or (with a PPH) even 40 units (the maximum) to 500 ml of fluid. Usually quite a modest drip rate is sufficient to control bleeding, but in emergency, you can run the drip in 'fast'.

CAUTION ! (1) Never give a bolus intravenous injection of oxytocin before the baby has been delivered. (2) Intramuscular injections of ergometrine or oxytocin can only be used safely to empty the uterus and expel the placenta and membranes before 16 weeks. After 16 weeks use an oxytocin drip.

BEWARE OF OXYTOCIN IN MULTIPS!

18.5 Vacuum extraction

If you are not an experienced obstetrician, you will find a vacuum extractor invaluable (M 22.3), so if you are not already using one, you must! It has many advantages in the confined space of the reduced pelves so common in many communities. Unlike forceps, the vacuum cup takes up no space in a mother's birth canal, and it is difficult to injure her accidentally. Her baby's head can rotate spontaneously at the optimum level, and if it is deflexed, vacuum extraction will often flex it. Most importantly, a vacuum extractor is less likely to damage his brain than forceps. The indications for its use in a hospital are somewhat broader than those in a health centre (M 22.3).

VACUUM EXTRACTION

INDICATIONS. These indications only apply if the absolute requirements below are met. (1) Delay in the second stage—more than an hour in a primigravida, and 30 minutes in a multigravida, especially delay caused by malrotation of the occiput. (2) To reduce maternal effort if a mother has cardiac failure or gestational hypertension. (3) To minimize the strain on a scarred

WHERE TO PUT THE CUP

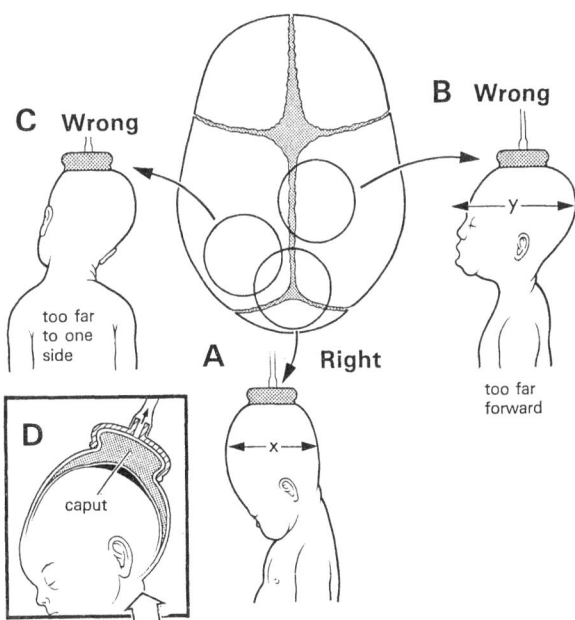

Leave the cup on long enough for caput to be formed inside it before you start pulling

Fig. 18-6 WHERE TO PUT THE CUP OF THE VACUUM EXTRACTOR. You will find a vacuum extractor invaluable. Attach the cup as nearly as you can over his posterior fontanelle.

uterus. (4) *Relative* CPD due to deflexion and malrotation of the head. If there is absolute CPD don't use a vacuum extractor, it will be ineffective and potentially dangerous.

Her cervix should be fully dilated. Some obstetricians apply it at 8 cm, but this can cause tears, and should never be tried if there is any CPD. The rule of 'Three pulls' (M 22.3) still applies, but two 'extra pulls' are allowed to reach full dilatation; then you must deliver her in three pulls. (5) Vacuum extraction is occasionally indicated before full dilatation of the cervix when there is fetal distress in multips without any CPD. (6) Fetal distress in a second twin with a cephalic presentation when the cervix has closed down. The height of the head does not matter in this situation, provided you can get the cup on the occiput. (7) Prolapse of the cord in multips.

CONTRAINDICATIONS. (1) Prematurity, because of the risk of intracerebral haemorrhage. (2) A malpresentation. (3) CPD and a dead baby—outlet forceps or a destructive operation would be safer. (7) An exceptionally uncooperative mother.

CAUTION ! The application of a vacuum extractor before full dilatation is rarely indicated, and is usually dangerous: the only exceptions are (5), (6), and (7) above. Don't apply one for delay late in the first stage. If this does not respond to oxytocin, it is likely to be due to CPD. If (a) she was >3 hrs dilating from 7 to 10 cm on the partogram, or (b) her fundal height is >40 cm (suggesting a large baby), expect difficulty. Do the vacuum extraction in the theatre, and prepare for section.

ABSOLUTE REQUIREMENTS. (1) A proper indication. (2) Good uterine contractions, which means 3 to 4 every 10 minutes lasting over 40 seconds. (3) A cephalic presentation. (4) The baby's head must be 1/5 or less above his mother's pelvic brim. Always determine its station in relation to her pelvic brim, and not to her ischial spines; if her pelvis is shallow and there is much caput, you may be able to feel it below her spines before it is engaged. (5) The head must descend with contractions and bearing-down efforts. (6) You should know where the occiput is, because traction will be more effective if you can put the cup there. Co-operation by a mother who is fully conscious is desirable, but not essential.

18.6 Symphysiotomy

Cutting a patient's symphysis allows the two halves of her pelvis to separate 2 to 2.5 cm. This increases its diameter by 0.6 to 0.8 cm, which is enough to overcome mild or moderate CPD, and so avoid Caesarean section. After delivery, its circumference remains wider by about 1.5 cm, and its diameter by about 0.5 cm, so that her next deliveries may be normal. Symphysiotomy is thus particularly valuable if she wants a large family.

This is one of the most contentious operations in this book. One school of thought considers it a "...barbarous operation done by expatriate doctors on the mothers of the developing world..." Another school, which includes all our contributors who practise obstetrics, considers it an invaluable operation which needs to be reinstated and given its proper place: (1) Unlike Caesarean section, especially with unskilled anaesthesia, it is never fatal, and seldom produces complications, particularly serious ones. (2) It does not leave a mother with a scar in her uterus which may rupture if she does not deliver in hospital when she is pregnant next time. (3) It may save her life if she delivers in a health centre and cannot be referred. Like many other medical procedures it has been evaluated by personal experience rather than by formal trials, and there is a particular lack of good data on how effective it is in the hands of paramedical staff on a community scale. We encourage you to investigate this, since, like the destructive operations, it is one of the few practical procedures which might really alleviate maternal mortality from obstructed labour.

Symphysiotomy has fallen into disrepute because there was a time when it was used to overcome gross CPD, which led to serious complications. It is not used at all in parts of the world where CPD hardly exists, where trends are set—and where most textbooks are written. But, in countries where CPD is common, symphysiotomy is excellent—if it is used for borderline cases only. If CPD is marked, a mother needs a Caesarean section. The skill is to recognize the difference. You will not need to do a symphysiotomy very often, and you will find that deciding when to do one needs more judgement than deciding when to section a mother. If a symphysiotomy fails you can still do a Caesarean section: but you should look upon this as an error of judgement, and try to do better next time.

The indications for symphysiotomy in a hospital and a health centre are different:

In hospital, symphysiotomy is used to its best advantage: (1) At the strategic moment in a well-planned trial of labour, in which there is borderline CPD, and before there are any signs of fetal distress. If the indications are right, it is better than Caesarean section, and it avoids a difficult vaginal delivery. (2) In neglected obstructed labour it avoids a major abdominal operation in a high-risk mother. (3) It is occasionally useful in a breech delivery when the aftercoming head is arrested (9.8). Symphysiotomy is usually done in a primip, but you can do it in a multip. It is especially useful if a mother is isolated and cannot easily attend for antenatal care, if she is infected, and if your anaesthetic facilities are poor.

In a health centre a symphysiotomy is an *emergency* method of delivering a mother, and securing a live baby, when she cannot be referred. It should never be an elective procedure there, because she cannot have a Caesarean section in a hurry if she needs one.

There are two ways of doing a symphysiotomy, either: (1) Open through an incision which is large enough for you to see and feel exactly what you are doing, as described below. Or, (2) closed through an incision which is only just large enough to admit the blade of a scalpel, as described in *Primary Mother Care*. Opinions differ as to which is best. Of those obstetricians who do the operation, the large majority favour the closed method and some think that we should not even have described the open one. One exceptionally able and experienced contributor is however strongly in favour of it. However you do it, you must divide the symphysis through its cartilage, exactly in the midline, because incisions which involve the bone to one side are more likely to lead to chronic pubic osteitis and long-standing pain, both of which are fortunately rare. Local infection in the soft tissue and cartilage is not important and heals without trouble.

Experts can do a closed symphysiotomy through a very small skin incision. If you are not an expert, do it open. Use an ordinary scalpel to cut through the skin and subcutaneous tissue in the midline. Then, when you have found the cartilage, cut through its exact centre with a solid scalpel, or a short ordinary one. *Be sure to support the patient's legs as described below, and don't fail to insert a catheter before you cut!*

SYMPHYSIOTOMY

For closed symphysiotomy, see M 20.7.

INDICATIONS. Mild or moderate CPD associated with any of these problems, most of which are interrelated:

(1) A failed trial of vacuum extraction when failure has occurred by a small margin. It will not work if CPD is gross, and vacuum extraction was done on the wrong indication. This is the most common indication. It is difficult to be sure that vacuum extraction won't work without having a try!

(2) Obstructed labour with a live baby. If his head is deeply jammed into his mother's pelvis, perhaps with caput visible at her vulva, symphysiotomy will be safer for her. If you try to section her, his head will be difficult to deliver, and infection of her deeper tissues is more likely.

(3) A difficult vacuum extraction may succeed, but only after prolonged traction and the risk of damaging the baby. Symphysiotomy will make delivery easier and safer for him.

(4) A prolonged second stage. If the criteria for symphysiotomy are met, and vacuum extraction alone is unlikely to succeed, symphysiotomy is better than trying vacuum extraction first.

(5) Mild or moderate CPD with a live baby, particularly in a primigravida, when his head is 1/5 or 2/5 above the brim, and is too tightly held for vacuum or low forceps alone.

OPEN SYMPHYSIOTOMY

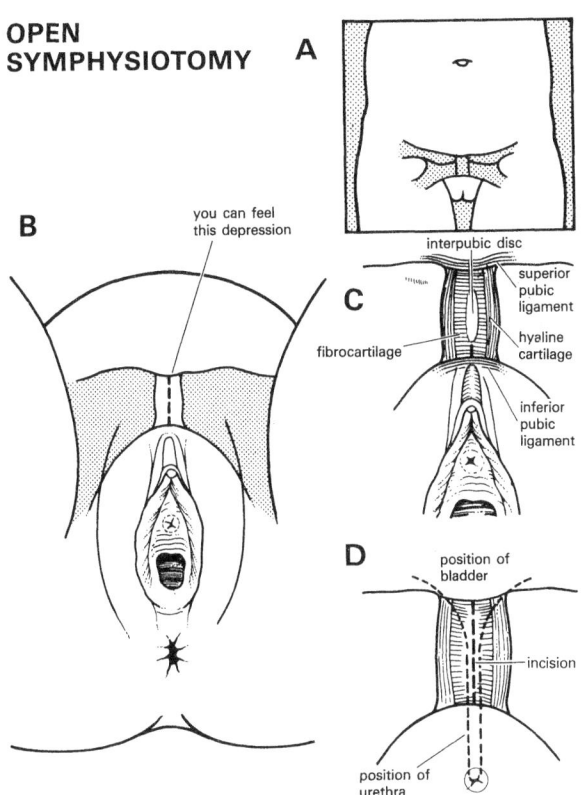

Fig. 18-7 OPEN SYMPHYSIOTOMY. A, the position of the symphysis on the anterior abdominal wall. B, the position of the symphysis in relation to the clitoris. C, the structures to cut. D, the incision in relation to the urethra and the bladder.

(6) To deliver the arrested aftercoming head of a breech— if you are quick!

CAUTION ! Symphysiotomy is normally done at full dilatation, but you can do it when there is still a 1 or 2 cm ring of cervix. Another contributor considers that you should *never* do this!

CONTRAINDICATIONS. (1) Severe CPD. (2) Malpresentations, with the exception of the aftercoming head of a breech (19.8). (3) A dead baby; if there is CPD he should be delivered by craniotomy or section, if there is no CPD a symphysiotomy is unnecessary. (5) A previous Caesarean section. (6) Abnormalities of a mother's legs or spine. (7) Severe obesity is a relative contraindication. (8) A baby more than 4 kg as estimated by the fundal height being >40 cm (who is too big to deliver by symphysiotomy), or less than 2.5 kg (who does not need one). (9) Poor uterine action in spite of an oxytocin drip, especially if dilatation is not complete. (10) A fetal head which remains >3/5 above the brim after rupture of the membranes.

OPEN SYMPHYSIOTOMY

Do a vaginal examination to check the dilation of the mother's cervix, and the descent and position of her baby's head. At this point decide if symphysiotomy is indicated or not.

If his head is 1/5 above the brim a symphysiotomy is unnecessary. If it is 2/5 above symphysiotomy may be indicated. If it is 3/5 above, try to insert a finger vaginally between his head and her pelvis. If your finger passes too easily symphysiotomy is unnecessary. If it passes with difficulty, symphysiotomy is indicated. If it does not pass at all, CPD is too great, so section her. Note that this is somewhat less conservative than the indication for closed symphysiotomy given in *Primary Mother Care*, which advises that midwives should not attempt it, if the head is more than 2/5 above the brim.

Listen to the fetal heart to make sure that he is alive. Put her into the lithotomy position, with her legs outside the lithotomy poles.

CAUTION ! Find two assistants and ask them to support each of her legs, so that her symphysis opens only to a maximum of 3 cm. *This must be their only job;* they must do nothing else. If they allow her legs to flop apart, the fibres of her sacroiliac joint may rupture, and she will have much postoperative pain. You will need these assistants anyway, even if you have lithotomy poles, to prevent too much abduction.

Pass a stiff rubber or plastic catheter. Clean her skin with iodine and spirit. Palpate the bony margins of her symphysis pubis. Infiltrate the skin and subcutaneous tissue over her symphysis with 20 ml of 1% lignocaine with adrenalin (this is a very vascular area). Allow 3 minutes to pass for it to act. Place the index and middle fingers of your left hand in her vagina, to displace the catheter in her urethra to her right side.

CAUTION ! You MUST displace her urethra, or you will cut it. This would be a major disaster!

Incise the skin and subcutaneous tissue over her symphysis pubis in the midline, and find the exact position of the cartilage of the joint. Try locating it with a hypodermic needle first. Then use a standard scalpel to cut down on to it throughout its length. Clamp any superficial bleeding arteries.

When you have exposed the joint throughout its length (it is better felt as a depression rather than seen), divide it using a sharp solid scalpel, or a standard one with a No. 20 or 21 blade. Cut it little by little with your right hand, keeping her urethra to the side with your left hand. Mop up any blood. When the joint is almost divided, it will begin to open. Continue cutting its fibres until it opens fully. Two cm is ideal, *it should never open more than 3 cm*. Its infrapubic fibres may rupture spontaneously, or need cutting. Judge this by how much it opens. If separation is inadequate, cut more joint fibres, usually the superior and posterior ones.

CAUTION ! (1) Always keep her urethra to one side with your left hand. (2) Don't cut above her symphysis pubis, because her uterus or bladder may be protruding there. A small cut in her uterus is not such a tragedy as cutting her urethra. (3) Never do a symphysiotomy without also doing an episiotomy.

If you have operated on the right indications, she will deliver easily—usually after bearing down with 3 or 4 contractions. If she does not deliver spontaneously, apply the vacuum extractor. Give her ergometrine with the birth of the anterior shoulder.

CAUTION ! Don't apply forceps after symphysiotomy, they may stretch her sacroiliac joint too much.

If she bleeds from the incision, apply pressure. Suture her subcutaneous tissue, tie the vessels with 2/0 catgut, and suture her skin with 2/0 or 1/0 monofilament.

Leave a self retaining catheter in place. Leave this in for 48 hours only, provided her urine is not blood-stained (the usual cause of this is obstructed labour), and release it 4-hourly. Keep her in bed for 48 hours—walking will be painful. Allow her to walk on the 3rd to the 5th day. Some patients can do this easily, others, especially the heavier ones, fail to walk until the 5th or 7th day. Remove her sutures on the 7th day. Most patients are walking well, and fit for discharge, on the 10th day. There is no need to bind her pelvis, her symphysis will heal to leave her pelvis larger that it was before.

DIFFICULTIES WITH OPEN SYMPHYSIOTOMY

If she has FEVER postoperatively, suspect urinary infection due to the catheter.

If she DOES NOT PASS URINE when the catheter is removed on the 3rd day, replace it and try on the 5th day.

If she is INCONTINENT OF URINE, especially on standing, it may be partial so that she also passes urine, or it may be total. Insert a catheter and leave it in for 2 weeks. She will probably recover completely or partly. If she still has trouble it is likely to be partial. Advise her to empty her bladder 4-hourly. Incontinence rarely lasts more than 3 months. If necessary (rare), refer her for a sling operation. Loss of the normal angle where the bladder joins the urethra is probably the cause of temporary incontinence. As she heals this angle returns.

If her wound shows signs of LOCAL INFECTION (common), give her ampicillin or chloramphenicol. Insignificant quantities will reach her baby, but avoid tetracycline or sulphonamides, which may harm him. Careful preparation of her skin with iodine and spirit reduces the incidence of infection.

If she BLEEDS from the branches of her epigastric vessels, watch for a haematoma of her wound which may spread up into her abdominal wall. This is said to be more likely when the closed method is used. If necessary, drain it by removing one or two sutures.

If, later, she develops chronic PAIN and DISCHARGE, she has chronic pubic OSTEITIS (rare). Treatment is difficult, treat her pain symptomatically. It probably only occurs when the incision involves bone, so keep strictly to the midline in the fibrocartilage of the joint. This is easier to achieve in the open method than in the closed one.

If you INJURE HER URETHRA, which should never happen, see Section 18.19D.

18.7 Destructive operations

For an obstructed labour with a dead baby a destructive operation is usually, but not always, better than a Caesarean section. You may need to do one for: (1) A cephalic presentation with a normal or hydrocephalic head. (2) A breech delivery when a normal or hydrocephalic aftercoming head has 'stuck'. (3) A transverse lie with a prolapsed arm.

To cope with these situations you can: (1) Open his skull with large scissors, or a special perforator, and remove his brain (craniotomy). (2) Sever his neck from his body (decapitation), and then deliver them separately. (3) Cut his clavicles (cleidotomy). (4) Open his trunk and remove the the organs from his chest and abdomen (evisceration or embryotomy). For a cephalic or breech presentation, craniotomy is usually all you need do. A transverse lie requires decapitation, and often evisceration also, which is more difficult than craniotomy; but even so, it is often wiser than Caesarean section (see Section 18.1), which is particularly dangerous for a neglected infected transverse lie.

These operations are sometimes said to be old fashioned, and to have no place in modern obstetrics. Old-fashioned perhaps, but they have some useful features: (1) They need few instruments and only simple anaesthesia, so that they can be done in the health centre where a mother is first seen. If she cannot be referred, they save her life. If referral is difficult, they avoid the risks and delays of a long journey (they are therefore also described in *Primary Mother Care*). (2) They leave her with an intact uterus, which will be less likely to rupture if she decides to deliver herself at home next time. (3) If she is already infected, they are less likely than Caesarean section to spread the infection to her peritoneum. (4) She stays a shorter time in bed than she does after a Caesarean section.

The case for destructive operations is strongest in unsophisticated communities where people marry as children. A mother may not be fully grown when she first becomes pregnant, so that her pelvis is small and her first labour obstructs. It will continue to grow until she is 25, so, if she can be delivered vaginally with her first pregnancy, her later ones may be normal and without the risks of a scarred uterus.

Besides their distasteful messiness, the main argument against these operations is that, in inexperienced hands, they are liable to be even more dangerous than Caesarean section. This is unlikely to be true—if you follow the instructions carefully! To those who decry them, we reply that, if the obstetric circumstances of disadvantaged communities still existed in advantaged ones, destructive operations would be routine there too.

DESTRUCTIVE OPERATIONS

For destructive operations at Caesarean section, see Section 18.10. For destructive operations at a breech delivery, see Section 19.8.

INDICATIONS FOR CRANIOTOMY. All the following conditions must hold: (1) The baby must be dead. (2) 2/5 or less of his head must be above the brim (if it is higher than this, Caesarean section is usually safer, although if you are expert you may be able to do it at 3/5). (3) His head must be impacted. (4) His mother's cervix must be at least 7 cm dilated, and preferably fully dilated. One contributor gives 5 cm as the minimum. (5) Her uterus must be unruptured, and not in imminent danger of rupturing. If she is multigravid and has been

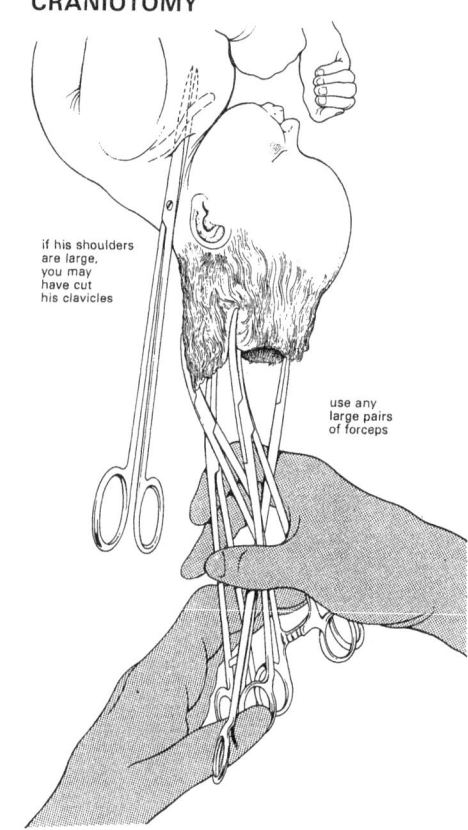

Fig. 18-8 CRANIOTOMY AND CLEIDOTOMY. For an obstructed labour with a dead baby a destructive operation is usually better than a Caesarean section. *Kindly contributed by John Lawson.*

in labour for a long time, her lower segment will be very thin. If it is tender and distended, it is certainly very thin. She can only be saved by Caesarean section; any destructive operation, except pushing a needle into a hydrocephalic head, will rupture it.

PREPARATION. Always do a destructive operation in the theatre with a laparotomy set ready for immediate use; unless you, and your theatre and obstetric team, are very quick and expert indeed (when you can do some destructive operations in the labour ward). You must be able to do an immediate laparotomy, either: (1) immediately instead of a destructive operation, if you find that the indications are unsuitable, or (2) immediately afterwards, if you discover that her uterus has ruptured. You will need an anaesthetist, a scrub nurse, and a 'runner'.

In the labour ward confirm that the baby is dead, set up a drip, take blood for cross-matching, give her pethidine 50 mg and diazepam 10 mg intravenously, and shave her for a vaginal operation and a laparotomy.

PERIOPERATIVE ANTIBIOTICS. Give her chloramphenicol 1 g intravenously. Or, give her penicillin 5 megaunits intravenously with streptomycin 1 g intramuscularly. See also 2.9.

EQUIPMENT. For decapitation use a Blond–Heidler saw (16.1), or large blunt-ended scissors, preferably special embryotomy scissors.

ANAESTHESIA. General anaesthesia *with intubation, especially if she has a transverse lie.* If you cannot intubate her, use subarachnoid anaesthesia or local infiltration anaesthesia.

FOR A CEPHALIC PRESENTATION

CRANIOTOMY. Put her into the lithotomy position, and clean and drape her vulva and perineum.

If you are not using general anaesthesia, give her pethidine 25–50 mg slowly intravenously (check what she was given in the labour ward). And give her diazepam 5–10 mg slowly intravenously until she is just asleep (A 8.8). Infiltrate her perineum with 0.5% or 1% lignocaine (A 5-1).

Catheterize her bladder. Ask your assistant to hold 1 or 2 Sims' specula in her vagina so that you can see the baby's head well.

CAUTION ! Ask another assistant, standing on a footstool if necessary, to steady the baby's head suprapubically, so that it is not pushed upwards whenever you do anything to it.

With a scalpel make an 'X'-shaped incision through the skin of his scalp right down to the bone. Peel the four flaps of scalp off his skull. Put your fingers through her cervix to rest against his skull. Feel for a suture line or fontanelle. Push a closed pair of strong pointed scissors or, better, Simpson's perforator *between the bones*. For a face presentation, choose his hard palate or his orbit. Move the handles back towards her perineum, so as to point the blades at the *centre* of his skull. Open and close them a few times while you turn them round. Brain will flow from the hole. Put your finger into his skull, check that all brain compartments have been opened, and remove any remaining brain. His skull will now collapse.

Try to remove all his frontal and parietal bones. If you don't remove them, they may tear her vagina as he delivers. Remove any loose pieces of bone. Attach 3–4 strong vulsellum forceps, Kocher's or Willet's forceps to his scalp and the remains of his skull. Pull on them and try to bring his posterior fontanelle under his symphysis. If sharp edges of bone stick out, protect her vagina with your finger.

Wait until she has a contraction. Hold the three pairs of forceps together, and pull and twist. His collapsed head should now deliver. His body will follow. If a piece of his skull pulls off, reattach the forceps taking a deeper bite of skull closer to its base. Make a large episiotomy and deliver the remains of his head.

CAUTION ! (1) Don't include folds of her vaginal wall or cervix. (2) Use a good light and a large Sims' speculum, so as to make sure you grasp only his skull.

If delivering his shoulders is difficult, put a hand behind him and try turning him through 90° or 180°. Then try delivering his shoulders again.

If you cannot bring down his shoulders by turning him, bring down his arms one by one. Put a hand behind him in her vagina and feel for his posterior arm. Gently pull it down. Don't worry if it breaks, but don't damage her vagina. Then turn him through 180° and deliver his other arm in the same way. Delivery should now be easy.

Alternatively, cut his clavicles (cleidotomy, see below).

DESTRUCTIVE OPERATIONS FOR A TRANSVERSE LIE

INDICATIONS. Her baby is dead, the lie is transverse, her cervix is 8 cm or more dilated, and her uterus is not ruptured. For a transverse lie, see Section 19.9. For destructive operations at Caesarean section, see Section 18.10.

EXAMINATION UNDER ANAESTHESIA. Prepare her in the labour ward and the theatre as for craniotomy. Good anaesthesia is even more important than it is for craniotomy, because you have to operate higher in her birth canal. Give her a general anaesthetic.

Put her into the lithotomy position, clean and drape her vulva, and catheterize her bladder. Put one hand into her vagina and support her fundus with the other. Observe: (1) The dilatation of her cervix. If it is <8 cm, section is probably safer. (2) The condition of her lower segment; explore it as far as you can without using force. If it is ruptured, section her. (3) The exact position of the baby. Which of his arms have prolapsed? Where exactly, are his head and neck, chest, abdomen, and back?

Choose between these 3 alternatives: (1) If his neck and body are still high in her birth canal, section her (18.10). (2) If you can reach his neck easily, decapitate him. (2) If his neck is difficult to reach, but his body is well down, eviscerate him.

CAUTION ! (1) Don't try an internal version without doing an evisceration first: you will rupture her uterus. (2) Don't attempt decapitation, or evisceration, through her vagina, if he is still high in her birth canal; you will not be able to protect her vaginal wall and cervix adequately. A Caesarean section is her only hope.

DECAPITATION. Pull on his prolapsed arm with one hand, and feel for his neck with your other hand.

If possible, bring an arm down (if it is not already down), and ask an assistant to pull on it. This: (1) prevents him being pushed upwards by your hand in her uterus, (2) prevents her distended lower segment being stretched, and (3) it brings his neck lower and makes it easier to feel.

Feel his neck to find out how large it is, and how easy it is to put a finger round. If he is small and macerated, you can usually cut his neck with strong scissors. If he is larger, you will have to use the saw.

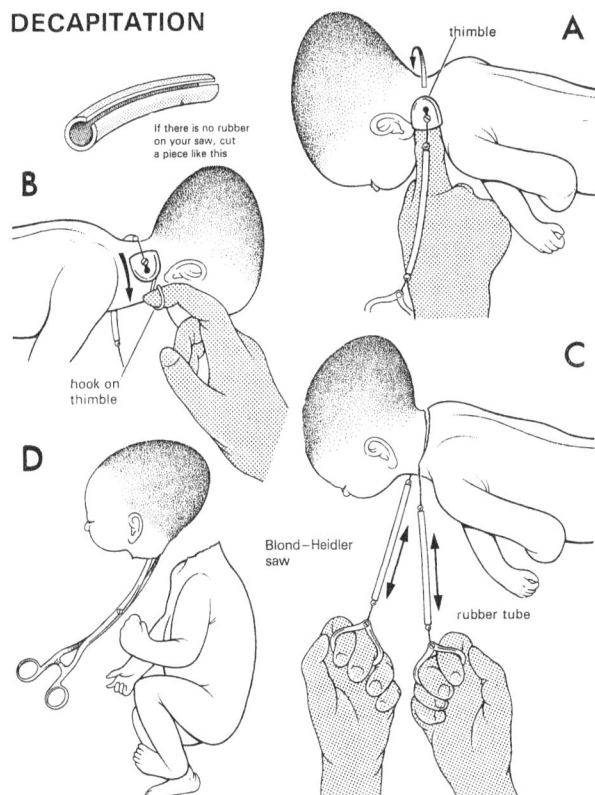

Fig. 18-10 DECAPITATION FOR A DEAD BABY will leave a mother with an intact uterus, which will be less likely to rupture if she decides to deliver herself at home next time. Cut through his neck with a Blond–Heidler saw. A, push the thimble round his neck. B, pull the loop of the thimble down the other side of his neck. C, saw through it. D, remove his head with forceps. Pieces of rubber tube cover the outer third of each end of the saw. *Kindly contributed by John Lawson.*

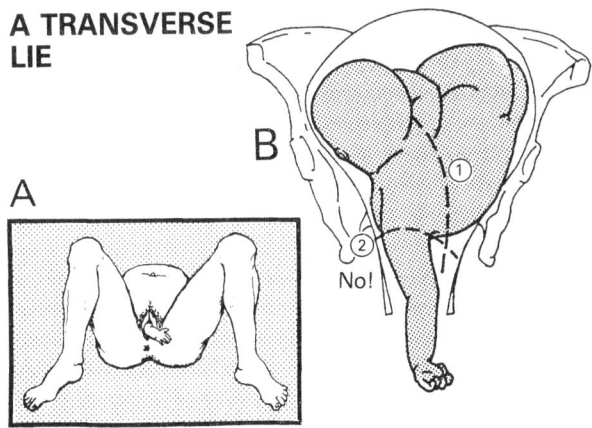

Fig. 18-9 A TRANSVERSE LIE. A, if a community health worker meets this, she is advised to refer the patient to you urgently! B, a shoulder presentation. (1) The incision for decapitation, leaving the head attached to an arm. (2) Caution! Don't try to remove an arm, leave it attached to the head or the body, to help you to bring these down. *A, From David Werner's 'Where there is no Doctor'. B, from Howie, Beryl, 'High Risk Obstetrics', Macmillan, with kind permission.*

If you are using a saw, fix the thimble to it and put this on your right middle finger. Pass the thimble over his neck, and down the other side. If this is difficult, because there is little room between his neck, his head, and his chest, try putting the saw over his neck and under his arm. Or improvise a smaller thimble by fixing something else, such as a piece of wire, to the end of the saw. Remove the thimble, and fix handles to each end of the saw. Insert the rubber sleeves on the saw. Keep the handles close together, so that her vagina is not injured. Protect it with specula. Cut his neck with a few firm strokes.

CAUTION ! Hold the handles close together. If you don't do this, you will cut her tissues.

To deliver his body, pull on his prolapsed arm. As you do so, use your hand to protect her vagina from any jagged pieces of bone in his neck.

To deliver his head, put a hand in her vagina, and turn his head so that his neck points downwards. Grasp the stump of his neck with large forceps, and put a finger in his mouth. Then deliver his head, as if it were the aftercoming head of a breech. This will prevent the stump from injuring her birth canal. If his head is very large, you may need to do a craniotomy. Some operators leave an arm attached to his head to help delivery.

If you delivered his head first, deliver his body by pulling on his other arm. Don't try version, his cut neck might damage her uterus.

If you are using scissors, hook one or two fingers round his neck and pull it down. Ask an assistant to protect her vaginal wall with a speculum. Gently pull his arm. When you do this, you will feel his neck. Try to see what you are cutting with each cut. You can easily cut her uterus or bladder. Cut his neck a little at a time, then deliver him as above.

CAUTION ! (1) Don't cut if you cannot see his neck. After each cut, pull his neck. It will come a little further down with each cut until you have cut right through.

OTHER DESTRUCTIVE OPERATIONS

EVISCERATION for a transverse lie is indicated: (1) when his neck is difficult to reach, but his body is well down, (2) after decapitation. Ask your assistant to pull on his prolapsed arm, and find his axilla. Protect her vaginal wall with one or two specula. With a knife or strong scissors make a large opening in his abdomen or chest. Put one or two fingers into the opening and remove all his internal organs. Make sure you remove his liver, heart, and lungs. If necessary perforate his diaphragm with scissors.

Now reassess the situation, and try whichever of these manoeuvres seems best: (1) Put two fingers behind his pelvis and hook his breech down. (2) Grasp a leg or foot and bring that down. (3) Try to bring his neck down for decapitation by pulling on his arm. (4) If all this fails, don't hesitate to section her.

Alternatively, separate his prolapsed arm at his shoulder. Push the embryotomy scissors through his axilla and divide his internal structures *from inside his skin*, while keeping your other hand between his and her uterus, as a constant guide. Finally, divide his skin and superficial tissues under direct vision, and deliver him in two halves.

CRANIOTOMY FOR A HYDROCEPHALIC HEAD. Push a large needle through her abdominal wall. As the fluid is withdrawn, his head will collapse. Or, guided by your examining finger, you can push a large needle (2 mm × 25 cm) through a suture from her vagina, and drain off as much fluid as you can.

CLEIDOTOMY (division of the clavicles) on one or both sides, will reduce the width of the shoulders of a large dead baby. Use embryotomy scissors to make a small cut in the skin of his neck. Through this, guided by the fingers of your other hand, feel inside his skin, until you can snip a clavicle between the tips of the opened blades. Be sure it is his clavicle and not the spine of his scapula. The ends of his clavicle will then overlap and narrow his shoulders.

DESTRUCTIVE OPERATIONS FOR THE 'STUCK BREECH' see Section 19.8.

POSTOPERATIVELY, AFTER ANY DESTRUCTIVE OPERATION
Remove the placenta manually, and immediately feel for tears of her uterus and lower segment. Give her ergometrine 0.25 mg intravenously as he is delivered. Check her uterus by feeling inside it to make sure it has not ruptured. If it has ruptured, do a laparotomy and repair it (18.17). Check her cervix, vagina, and vulva for tears. If she has a tear of her cervix it will need suturing (18.15).

If her uterus is not well contracted, set up an intravenous oxytocin drip with 5–20 units in 500 ml. Continue the saline drip for 24 hours. Continue the perioperative antibiotics (2.9).

She is at risk from: (1) Postpartum haemorrhage in the first 24 hours. (2) Acute urinary retention in the first 24 hours. (3) Infection of her genital tract after 24 hours. (4) Infection of her urinary tract at 7 to 10 days. (5) A fistula (18.10).

If his head has been impacted in her pelvis for many days, leave a Foley catheter in for 14 days. This will help to prevent a fistula. Obstructed labour with a transverse lie does not cause pressure necrosis of the vagina, so a few days' drainage is enough.

CAUTION ! After any destructive operation, be sure your assistant wraps up the baby immediately he is delivered. His mother must not see him.

AVOID CAESAREAN SECTION FOR OBSTRUCTED LABOUR AND A DEAD BABY, UNLESS YOU THINK VAGINAL DELIVERY WOULD BE TOO DANGEROUS

18.8 Which kind of Caesarean section?

Caesarean section is the commonest emergency procedure in a district hospital. If you are inexperienced it will also be the one which you will be most frightened of doing. In unskilled hands it is often fatal, as the result of: (1) the inhalation of gastric contents, (2) the supine hypotensive syndrome, (3) haemorrhage, or (4) sepsis.

There are several kinds of Caesarean section:

(1) Classical Caesarean section, is done through a vertical incision in the upper segment of the uterus (18.12). It is largely outmoded, but there are some rare occasions when it may be indicated.

(2) A lower segment Caesarean section approaches the uterus through a transverse incision in the peritoneum over the lower segment. It has long been the standard operation because: (a) a scar here ruptures ten times less often than the scar from a classical incision, (b) when it does rupture it does so less dangerously, (c) the incision in the uterus heals better, (d) the danger of spreading infection is reduced, (e) the placenta is less often directly underneath the uterine incision, (f) the gut is less likely to stick to the scar in the uterus, and (g) there are fewer postoperative complications.

But: (a) A lower segment operation needs more skill. (b) It is dangerous if there is intrauterine infection, although less so than a classical one. (c) You may injure the patient's bladder. (d) Bleeding from the ends of the incision is more difficult to control, especially if there are lateral extension tears, as may happen if the lower segment is thin and distended, or the baby is an awkward position, as in a transverse lie. These tears may bleed severely, and in trying to control bleeding you may tie or cut her ureters. (e) You may find it difficult to extract a distorted presenting part through a lower segment incision, and tear it as you do so. A tear will be dangerous, and the only way to avoid one, once you have begun a lower segment operation, is to extend it as an inverted-T incision. Unfortunately, this does not heal well, and is a very bad incision to have to make. So only make the standard transverse incision if it is safe. It is because of these dangers, that we describe the following three alternatives:

(3) The de Lee incision (18.9) is a vertical incision, two-thirds of which are in the lower segment, and one-third in the upper one. It is thus a cross between the classical upper segment operation, and the ordinary lower segment one. Make a de Lee incision if a lateral tear is likely, as can happen if the lower segment is very thin, or the baby is in an abnormal position, as in a transverse lie.

(4) A transverse incision in the upper segment is occasionally needed if there is a transverse lie, or a contraction ring (Bandl's ring).

(5) Extraperitoneal Caesarean section (18.13) is indicated if there is established or potential intrauterine infection. It greatly reduces the incidence of peritonitis, especially if you do not have antibiotics, particularly metronidazole.

(6) Caesarean hysterectomy is occasionally necessary for rupture of the uterus (18.17), when you have to remove the uterus (usually subtotally), and the baby (usually dead). It is also occasionally indicated when the lower segment is severely bruised, or major uterine vessels have been torn, or there is is established or potential uterine infection.

If you enter the abdomen through a lower midline incision, you need not decide whether to do a standard or a de Lee operation, until you get inside. But, if you are going to do an extraperitoneal Caesarean section, you will have to decide to do this before you open the abdomen.

WHICH KIND OF CAESAREAN SECTION?

The indications as to *when* to do Caesarean section are discussed in Sections 18.1, 18.2, and 18.4, and in M 22.12. Here we are concerned with what kind of Caesarean section you do. One indication which is *not* accepted, is the need to tie a mother's Fallopian tubes. There are easier and safer ways of doing this (15.3).

Always do the ordinary lower segment operation unless one of these others is indicated.

CLASSICAL SECTION is indicated if neither a lower segment operation, nor a transverse incision in the upper segment are possible (unusual). This may happen if: (1) The lower half of the patient's upper segment is very vascular, or inaccessible as the result of adhesions from a previous operation joining her lower segment to her abdominal wall. (2) She has had a previous classical incision, which has healed poorly. (3) She has a very vascular lower segment, with many thick veins on it. This may occur with placenta praevia (Type Four, or Types One or Two if the placenta is anterior), or it may sometimes occur with a normally placed placenta. She will bleed much, if you do a lower segment incision in a uterus like this, so a classical one is better. (4) A poorly developed lower segment which does not allow a transverse incision of adequate length. For some special points concerning Caesarean section in placenta praevia, see Section 18.10. (5) You are *very* inexperienced indeed. Alternatively, make a transverse incision half-way up her upper segment, and as you gain experience, transfer the incision to her lower segment. (6) As a preliminary to Caesarean hysterectomy.

CAUTION ! Don't let her wish to have her tubes tied favour the decision to do a classical section.

DE LEE SECTION. Do this if her lower segment is likely to tear, because it is thin and distended, or because there is a transverse lie.

EXTRAPERITONEAL SECTION. Do this if the contents of her uterus are infected and antibiotics are scarce.

18.9 Lower segment Caesarean section

The first steps are to open the mother's abdomen through a lower midline incision, to reflect the peritoneum off her lower segment, and to reflect her bladder downwards at the same time.

If you are not careful, you can easily cut her bladder: (1) When you enter her abdomen. You will be less likely to cut it, if you empty it with a catheter before the operation starts, leave the catheter in, and then carefully reflect her bladder downwards, before you open her uterus. (2) If It is stuck by scar tissue to her abdominal wall or lower segment. (3) Later, if her lower segment tears.

With her bladder well out of the way, you can now open her uterus transversely. The size of the incision is important, and so is the way you make it. It should be about 10 cm long, with its ends curving gently upwards (the 'smile' incision). Both an incision which is too large, and one which is too small can cause serious bleeding from the uterine arteries. These arise from the internal iliac arteries, pass through the paracervical fascia close to the ureters, and then climb up the sides of her uterus.

There are several reasons for severe bleeding: (1) You fail to allow for the fact that her uterus may be rotated—usually to the right. So, before you incise it, check for rotation by looking at her round ligaments. If you don't allow for rotation, you may cut her left uterine artery, because your incision is too far to the left. If you find that the left side of the incision always bleeds excessively, this is probably what you are doing. (2) She will bleed, if you let her uterus tear in an uncontrolled way, by pulling the baby out through an incision which is too small. (3) She will also bleed if you get him partly out, and then try to extend the incision by cutting. Avoid these mistakes by first cutting a small incision, and then extending it as described later. *Never use a scalpel, or scissors, too far laterally towards the sides of the uterus!*

Deliver the baby, then clamp the edges of the incision, especially its outer angles, with Green Armytage forceps, which were designed for this purpose. Most bleeding takes place from the angles of the incision, and these forceps will control it. Wait for her uterus to contract, remove the placenta, and then close her uterus in two layers.

Although you are unlikely to cut her ureters, you can easily obstruct them with misplaced sutures when you close her uterus, especially if there is much bleeding, and you suture wildly with a large curved needle. So: (1) Put a stay suture into her lower segment, just below where you are going to make your incision. This will help you to find it later, when you come to stitch it up. (2) Be sure to suture only her uterus, and not to suture too deeply downwards towards the vault of her vagina. Put a finger behind her broad ligament when you stitch the ends of the wound.

Most operators place abdominal packs on either side of the uterus before they incise it, so as to prevent blood, liquor, and meconium from soiling the peritoneal cavity. Meconium is irritant, and if it becomes infected peritonitis may follow. Others rely on mopping it out afterwards.

Normally, it is best not to bring the uterus out of the abdomen when you repair it: but if there is any problem this may be helpful.

WAMBUE (35 years) had had three previous Caesarean sections, and went into premature labour one evening. The duty doctor took her to the theatre. Her lower segment was very vascular, and there were many adhesions from previous operations. When he incised it, he cut into the placenta (placenta praevia). Section was otherwise uneventful, her uterine incision was repaired, and all bleeding carefully controlled. He noted that her bladder was distended, but assumed that the catheter had come out. When she left the theatre her blood pressure was normal, and she was given a unit of blood. Her urine was however noticed to be bloodstained. Fiften minutes later he was summoned urgently to the ward because she was lying in a pool of blood, with no pulse and a systolic blood pressure of 30 mm Hg. Her uterus was well contracted, she was given ergometrine, and rushed back to the theatre. She was resuscitated and her abdomen was reopened; there was no blood in it. She died on the table. At postmortem she had a large tear in her bladder; the upper edge of her uterine incision had been mistakenly sutured to the upper edge of her bladder, so that the lower edge of her uterus had been able to bleed freely into her bladder. The doctor was overcome by grief and felt very incompetent. LESSONS (1) The anatomy of a patient having her fourth section can be complicated. (2) Always insert a stay suture in the lower segment of the uterus, just below where you plan to make your incision, so that you can recognize it later. This may be difficult after delivery, especially if there are adhesions and the anatomy is complicated (many obstetricians never insert one). (3) If you find an abnormally adherent or vascular lower segment, do a classical operation. (4) As so often, disaster was the result of the combination of risk factors. A lower segment which has been the site of adherence of a placenta praevia, is apt to bleed postoperatively. Had she not also had a placenta praevia, she would probably have escaped with her life, and merely had a vesico-uterine fistula, which could have been repaired. (5) If you have to try to do your best in 20 expert fields simultaneously (see the frontispiece), you will, by the standards of 20 experts, not be as competent as they are, so you will inevitably meet tragedies of this kind, for which you cannot be blamed. One can but do one's best, and what that is will depend on who we are. What is reprehensible is not to care, and not to strive to improve one's standards. (6) A colleague in this condition needs support.

LOWER SEGMENT CAESAREAN SECTION

INDICATIONS. See Section 18.8.

PREOPERATIVE COUNSELLING. Where appropriate, discuss with the patient the advisability of tying her tubes. Her husband, or in some cultures her mother, or preferably both, should consent. The indications are: (1) >2 previous Caesarean sections. (3) Parity >6. (4) Age >35. (5) Medical problems which endanger her life, such as hypertension, diabetes, or heart disease.

PERIOPERATIVE ANTIBIOTICS have been shown to halve the incidence of wound infection after Caesarean section. Most routines are expensive, but here is a cheaper one which is equally effective.

If she is at special risk of infection (membranes ruptured for more than 8 hours, or if you are operating after a failed vacuum or forceps delivery, etc.) give her perioperative chloramphenicol and metronidazole as in Section 2.9. Continue metronidazole for 3 days postoperatively.

If she is a routine case, give her 1 g of metronidazole with the premedication as a rectal suppository or as rectal tablets, and give her another gram 8 hours later.

ASSISTANT. Find yourself a competent assistant. If the head is impacted in her pelvis, ask him to wear two gowns and two pairs of gloves, so that he can disimpact it and then discard the first pair (see below).

A MIDWIFE TO RECEIVE THE BABY. Before you begin make sure that there is a midwife ready to receive the baby, with all the equipment that she needs to resuscitate him (19.12).

EQUIPMENT. Use the Caesar set described in Section 4.12. This includes a large round-ended Doyen's retractor to fit over the bladder and protect it (or use a wide Deaver's or a Morris retractor), and 6 Green Armytage forceps (use sponge-holders if you don't have these). You will need '1' chromic catgut for the uterus, 2/0 catgut for the peritoneum of her vesico-uterine pouch, monofilament for her abdominal wall, and two round-bodied Mayo's needles, a large one for the first layer and a smaller one for the second. A narrow 20 cm steel ruler to measure the true conjugate. The anaesthetist must have a syringe of ergometrine with oxytocin ('Syntometrine') or plain ergometrine ready. You and he will both need suckers.

PACKS. Five or six large abdominal packs with tapes. *NEVER use single swabs,* you can too easily lose them in the peritoneal cavity!

ANAESTHESIA is discussed in detail in Sections 18.2 and in A 6.9 and A 16.6. You have a choice of: (1) Several methods of local anaesthesia (A 6.9). (2) Ketamine (A 8.1). (3) General anaesthesia (A 16.6) for which she *must* be intubated (A 13.3). (4) Subarachnoid (spinal) anaesthesia is satisfactory, provided you know the method and its complications in detail (A 7.1), you put up a drip and give her 1–2 litres of fluid fast, you tilt her to the left, and you observe the contraindications, which are: shock, severe anaemia, hypertension, and heart disease. An augmented saddle block is the safest form of subarachnoid anaesthesia (see below).

If your anaesthetist is an expert, general anaesthesia with cricoid pressure and tracheal intubation will be best (A 16.5), especially if her circulation is unstable due to an APH, or advanced obstructed labour.

If she is shocked, and you are inexpert, and single-handed, local infiltration (A 6.9) will be the safest.

If she is not shocked, an augmented saddle block (A 7.7) is suitable, particularly if you are single-handed. An ordinary saddle block is inadequate, because it does not extend high enough. You need to combine it with local infiltration of the abdominal wall, as in *Primary Anaesthesia* Fig. 7-8.

Explain what is going to happen. Put her on to the operating table before you induce her.

PREVENTING THE ACID ASPIRATION SYNDROME. Don't assume her stomach is empty because she has not taken food for a long time. Labour slows stomach emptying. If she has a general anaesthetic, she is in particular danger from the acid aspiration syndrome (A 16.3). Remove her gastric contents with a stomach tube, give her 30 ml of magnesium trisilicate mixture, or 0.3M sodium citrate within 15 minutes of induction, and then leave a Ryle's tube down. You cannot give her sodium citrate prophylactically throughout labour. If she is given a general anaesthetic, she *must* be intubated using cricoid

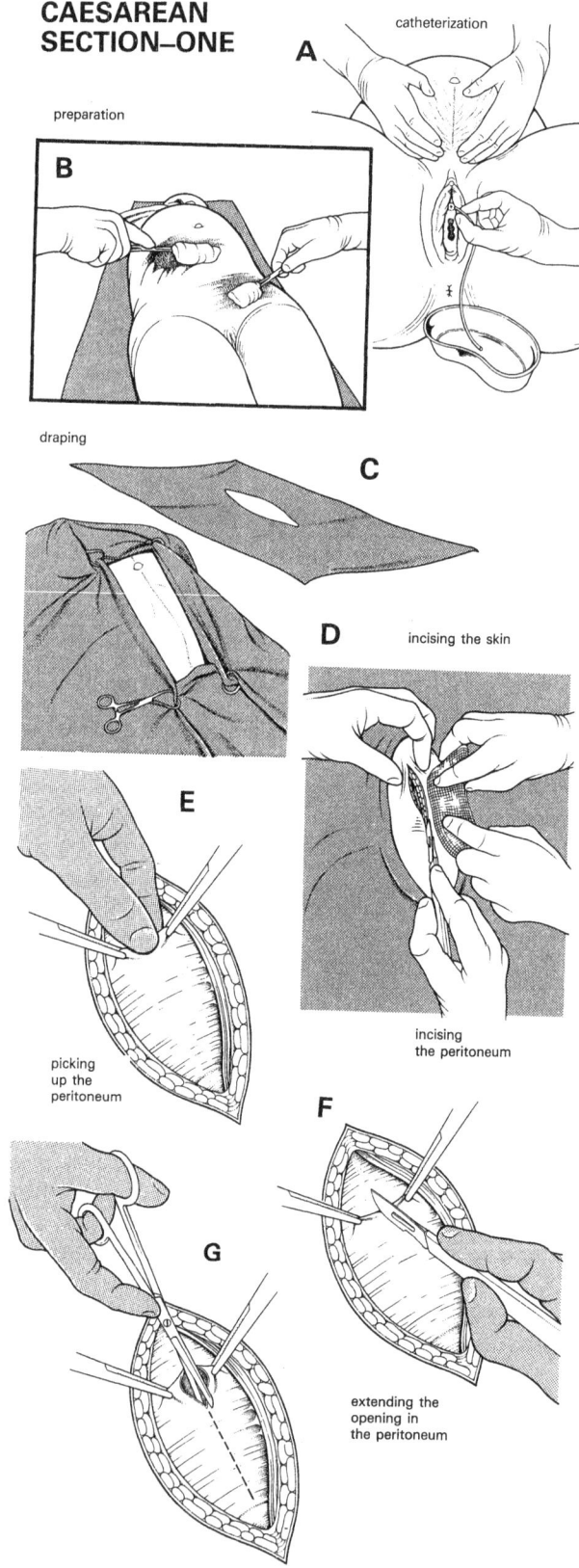

Fig. 18-11 CAESAREAN SECTION—ONE. A, catheterizing the patient's bladder. B, preparing her abdomen. C, draping her and covering her with an abdominal towel. D, incising the skin. E, picking up a fold of peritoneum to feel if there is any gut in it. F, incising her peritoneum. G, enlarging the opening in her peritoneum with scissors.

pressure (A 16.5).

If possible, as prophylaxis against acid aspiration, give her ranitidine 50 mg intramuscularly 1 hour before an elective section, or by slow intravenous injection immediately before an emergency section. Or, if you expect to section her, give her 150 mg by mouth at the onset of labour and then every 6 hours.

POSITION. Stand on her right side. Prevent the supine hypotensive syndrome by tilting her about 5° to the left (A 16.6). Do this, either by tilting the table, or by putting a pillow or sandbag under her right buttock. Find some way of preventing her slipping off the table. A moderate Trendelenburg position will give you better access to her lower segment, and make delivering the baby's head easier, if there is a vertex presentation. It will also be an additional safeguard if she vomits.

PREPARATION. Catheterize her in the theatre while she is still awake, and leave the catheter in (A, in Fig. 18-11). You can also do this in the maternity labour unit. At the same time, do a vaginal examination to make sure you do not miss unexpected progress, and thus the opportunity to do a vaginal delivery if this is indicated.

If you have difficulty catheterizing her bladder before operating, raise the baby's head with your hands. If you fail to pass a rubber catheter on the first occasion, try again after she is anaesthetized, when pushing up his head will be easier. If you have to operate with a full bladder, be very careful as you open her peritoneum. Open it as far cranially as you can, opposite the upper quarter of the incision through her abdominal wall, and empty her bladder with a syringe from her abdomen.

Shave or clip her from her mons pubis to above her umbilicus, and laterally to her iliac crests (optional). Prepare the skin of her lower abdomen (B), drape her with 4 plain towels, and cover these with a towel with a slit in it (C).

LOWER MIDLINE INCISION. Cut through her skin and subcutaneous tissue down to the level of her rectus sheath (D). Extend the incision to within 3 cm of her umbilicus. Try not to carry the incision further down than the upper limit of her pubic hair.

If she has had a previous Caesarean section, see Section 18.10.

Separate her rectus and pyramidalis muscles in the midline as far as her symphysis. If necessary, extend the skin incision further down. A short downwards extension is more effective in improving access than an extension upwards.

Use sharp and blunt dissection to expose her transversalis fascia and her peritoneum. Use two haemostats to pick up peritoneum near the *upper* end of the incision (E). This is especially important if her labour is obstructed, and her bladder is displaced upwards. Feel the fold of peritoneum you have picked up, to make sure there is no bowel or bladder in it. Make a small opening in it with a scalpel (F), and then open the rest of it with scissors (G), longitudinally from above downwards to just above the reflection of her bladder. If you hold her parietal peritoneum with a light shining through it, you will see a constant small vein running transversely across it. If you avoid this, you will avoid her bladder. If her bladder is high deviate to the side of the midline.

CAUTION ! If she has had a previous operation, including a previous Caesarean section, omentum or gut may have stuck to her abdominal wall, so that you can easily cut them. If you cut her gut by mistake, sew it up as in Fig. 9-6. If she has had several previous Caesarean sections, her anatomy will be much distorted by adhesions.

Clamp any active bleeders if they are big, but postpone tying them until later. They usually stop bleeding on their own.

Feel her uterus to find how it is rotated, and identify the presenting part. It is usually rotated to the right, so that her left round ligament is usually more anterior and closer to the midline than the right one. If her uterus is markedly rotated, turn it towards the midline.

Place a large abdominal pack on each side of her uterus, to keep her gut out of the way. Attach artery forceps to the tapes of these packs, to prevent them being lost.

THE CLASSICAL ALTERNATIVE. Consider doing a classical rather than a lower segment section if: (1) her lower segment seems abnormally vascular, or (2) it is abnormally adherent to her anterior abdominal wall. If you decide to do one, see Section 18.12.

THE De LEE ALTERNATIVE. Consider doing a de Lee incision if: (1) Her lower segment is so thin and distended, that it might tear when you extract the baby. (2) She has a transverse lie with a prolapsed arm, and a live baby. (3) A lower segment fails to form, as may happen with a premature delivery in a primip.

To make a de Lee incision, incise her visceral peritoneum transversely, as described below but *high* on her lower segment. Mobilize her peritoneum and her bladder well down. Find the midline of her uterus. Insert a small transverse suture where the bottom end of your incision is going to be, to prevent it extending downwards behind her bladder. Make a longitudinal incision, two-thirds of it in her lower segment, and one-third in her upper segment.

Later, repair a de Lee incision, with two layers of continuous chromic No. 1 or 2 catgut. Make sure you include her uterine fascia in the second layer, or it will continue to bleed. Repair her peritoneum, and pull it up high, so that the top of the incision is covered. If you incised her upper segment over a long distance, tie her tubes on the same indications as in a classical Caesarean section.

THE ALTERNATIVE OF A TRANSVERSE INCISION IN THE UPPER SEGMENT may be necessary if there is a transverse lie or a contraction (Bandl's) ring. Check that her uterus is wide enough. Incise her peritoneum over the lower part of its upper segment with a scalpel. Mobilize it away from the incision with scissors, and incise her uterus transversely in the midline. Enlarge the incision to the right and left, by stretching it with your fingers (it is usually too thick to be cut with scissors), and deliver the baby by breech extraction.

Repair the incision in two layers with continuous chromic No. 1 or 2 catgut. Don't catch the full thickness of her uterine wall in the first layer: it is often too thick. Repair her peritoneum over the incision, preferably with a locking stitch. Tie her tubes.

ORDINARY LOWER SEGMENT CAESAREAN SECTION

If her baby's head is jammed in her pelvis and needs to be disimpacted from below, ask yourself if a symphysiotomy would not have been better, and remember this next time! Ask your assistant to put his hand into her vagina, and to disimpact it to the site where you are going to make your incision. He must do this *before* you incise her uterus. If he waits until after you have incised it, the baby's shoulders may prolapse into the wound, and make delivery difficult. Having done this, ask him to take off his second gown and gloves (see above). Unfortunately, it is difficult to predict that the head needs disimpaction, until after you have opened the uterus.

Pick up the loose peritoneum of her vesico–uterine pouch with dissecting forceps (H). Make a small cut in the peritoneum over her uterus, just below the point where the loose peritoneum becomes firmly attached to the anterior wall of her uterus. This is the abdominal marking of her lower segment. Then put the scissors into the cut, and extend the incision in her peritoneum to left and right, so as to separate it from her uterus underneath (I). As you reach the edges of her uterus, aim the scissors in a more cephalic direction, so that the incision in her peritoneum is curved (J). Aim to leave a bare area about 2 cm wide and 12 cm long. Don't cut into the muscle of her uterus yet.

Use a swab in a holder, or on your finger, to separate the folds of peritoneum on either side of the incision, pressing on her uterus as you do so. This will help to separate her tissues in the right plane, and avoid tearing her peritoneum, or her bladder.

Raise the lower fold, and her bladder with it for about 3 cm (K).

CAUTION ! (1) Take great care to avoid injuring her bladder, especially if this is pulled up high and is oedematous. (2) Don't raise it more than 5 cm. If her cervix is effaced and dilated, you may enter her vagina by mistake.

Put the Doyen's retractor over her bladder, to protect it for the rest of the operation.

Put a stay suture of 2/0 catgut or monofilament into her lower segment (L), and hold the end of it in a haemostat.

Ask your assistant to hold up the stay-suture. A short, full-thickness central incision minimizes the danger of cutting the baby. If you extend it shallowly on either side, the uterus will tear open in the right direction. So, make a 3 cm horizontal incision through the uterine wall in the midline, just above the stay suture (M). Cut only the centre of her lower segment. This should be 2 cm below the peritoneal reflection, and at least 2 cm above her detached bladder. Put a finger either side of the incision and press as you cut (not shown). This will help

CAESAREAN SECTION—TWO

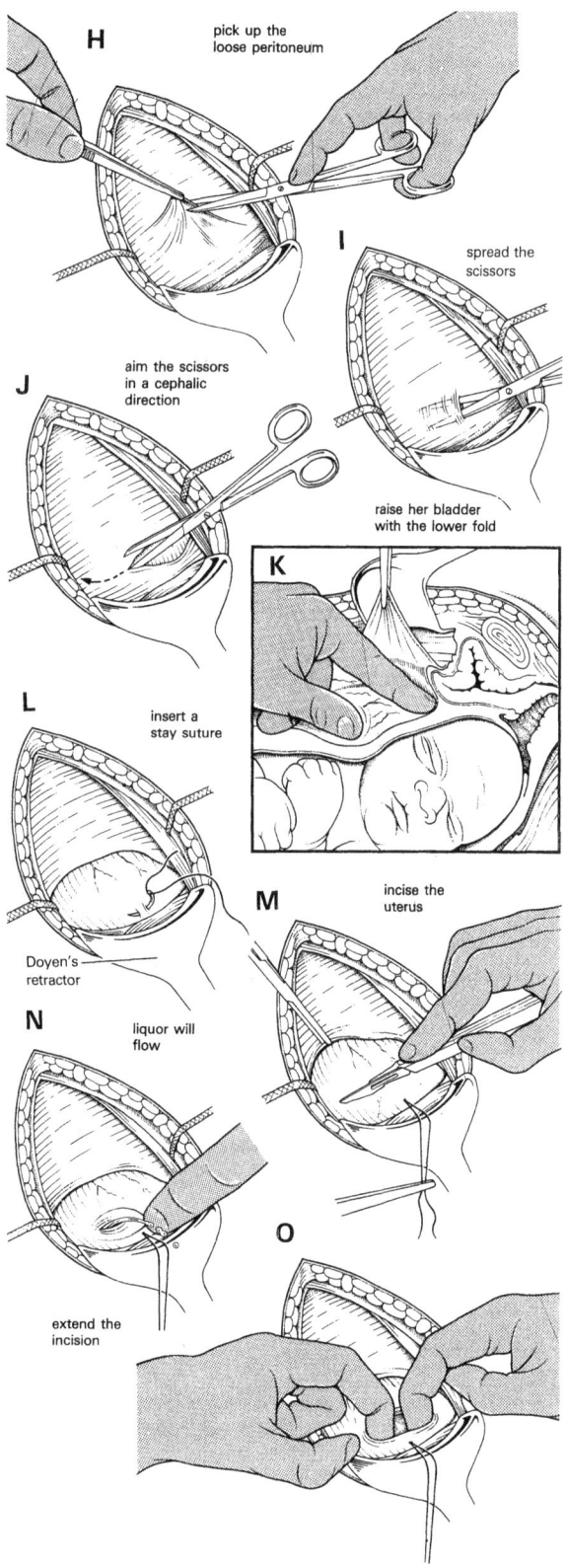

Fig. 18-12 CAESAREAN SECTION—TWO. H, pick up the peritoneum of the patient's vesico-uterine pouch with dissecting forceps and cut it. I, put the scissors into the cut, and open them, so as to separate her peritoneum. J, as you reach the edge of her uterus, cut in a more cephalic direction. K, raise the lower fold of peritoneum with her bladder in it. L, put a strong stay suture in her uterus. M, incise her uterus. N, liquor will spurt out. O, put your fingers into the incision and lengthen it.

you to judge how deeply you are cutting. Deepen it little by little until the membranes bulge into the incision. Cut through them (some operators keep them intact at this stage).

Liquor will spurt out (N). Ask your assistant to suck it away. Insert your closed scissors through the incision, and open them, so as to extend it enough to let you insert both your index fingers. Lengthen the incision by pulling them apart laterally, in the line of the muscle fibres, until it is 10 cm long (O). Her uterus will open naturally, with a curve upwards at each end. If she has had previous Caesarean sections, and her uterus is very fibrotic, you may have to extend the incision with scissors, curving it upwards laterally. Ask your assistant to suck it dry.

Alternatively, and most contributors would say preferably, make a scalpel incision for 2 cm in the midline, without cutting the membranes. Use scissors to cut the uterus, leaving the membranes intact until the incision is complete. Cut in an upward curve from the midline to the left angle of the uterus, and then in a similar curve from the midline to the right angle. If her uterus tears, the tear will then be more likely to run away from the cervix than towards it.

CAUTION ! (1) The lower segment varies considerably in thickness. It is thick before labour and becomes thinner during labour, so be careful not to cut the baby. Protect him with a finger between the membranes and her uterine wall as you cut. (2) Don't make the incision too small, or the uterus will tear as you remove his head. (3) Should you decide to enlarge the incision by cutting, curve it upwards at its ends, so as to avoid the uterine vessels. Also, when you suture it, you will be less likely to suture her ureters.

If she has a scar in her lower segment from a previous Caesarean section, make a shallow cut along it, where you want the rest of it to tear.

If you can feel the baby's vertex through the uterine wall, the placenta is probably lying in the fundus or posteriorly, so you can expect to deliver him without difficulty.

If you cut the placenta as you cut into the uterus, try to detach it, and deliver him round it. Only cut through it if you have to. He can bleed severely from a cut placenta, so clamp his cord quickly. See also Section 18.10.

If the ends of the incision in the lower segment bleed severely, before he has been delivered, quickly deliver him, and then control bleeding as described below.

If there are large veins over her lower segment, incise it precisely and carefully, and deliver him rapidly. The veins will probably stop bleeding as soon as you have delivered him. If necessary, clamp them and insert further haemostatic sutures.

DELIVERING THE BABY AT CAESAREAN SECTION

Remove the Doyen's retractor. Put your finger (only) into the uterus under the baby's head to relieve the vacuum, and make it easier for his head to rise in the incision. Then put your hand *outside* the lower flap of the incision, and lift his head up. If necessary, apply Wrigley's forceps (P). If, when you apply them, the incision is not long enough to deliver him without a lateral tear, extend its ends upwards and laterally with scissors, so as to make a U-shaped flap.

Contributors differ in the way they deliver the head. Some think that you should not put the bulk of your hand into the uterus, because it may cause tears. In practice most do, because it is quicker than forceps.

Now ask your assistant to press on the fundus to assist delivery. He may have to press hard. Do this carefully and gently, without hurrying. Before you deliver the baby's thorax, aspirate his nose and mouth, if convenient. Then deliver his shoulders and trunk.

CAUTION ! Don't try to suck him out with a big Yankauer sucker: it may injure him. Resuscitate him as in Section 19.12.

ERGOMETRINE OR OXYTOCIN. If she has PIH, or eclampsia, or you are operating under local anaesthesia, some operators avoid ergometrine, and give her 5 units of oxytocin intravenously or intramuscularly. Otherwise, give her ergometrine intravenously as soon as you have delivered his head. Ergometrine occasionally makes a conscious patient sick, and may raise her blood pressure.

THE BABY Before you clamp his cord, hold him up by his legs with one finger of your left hand between them, so that the mid-

CAESAREAN SECTION—THREE

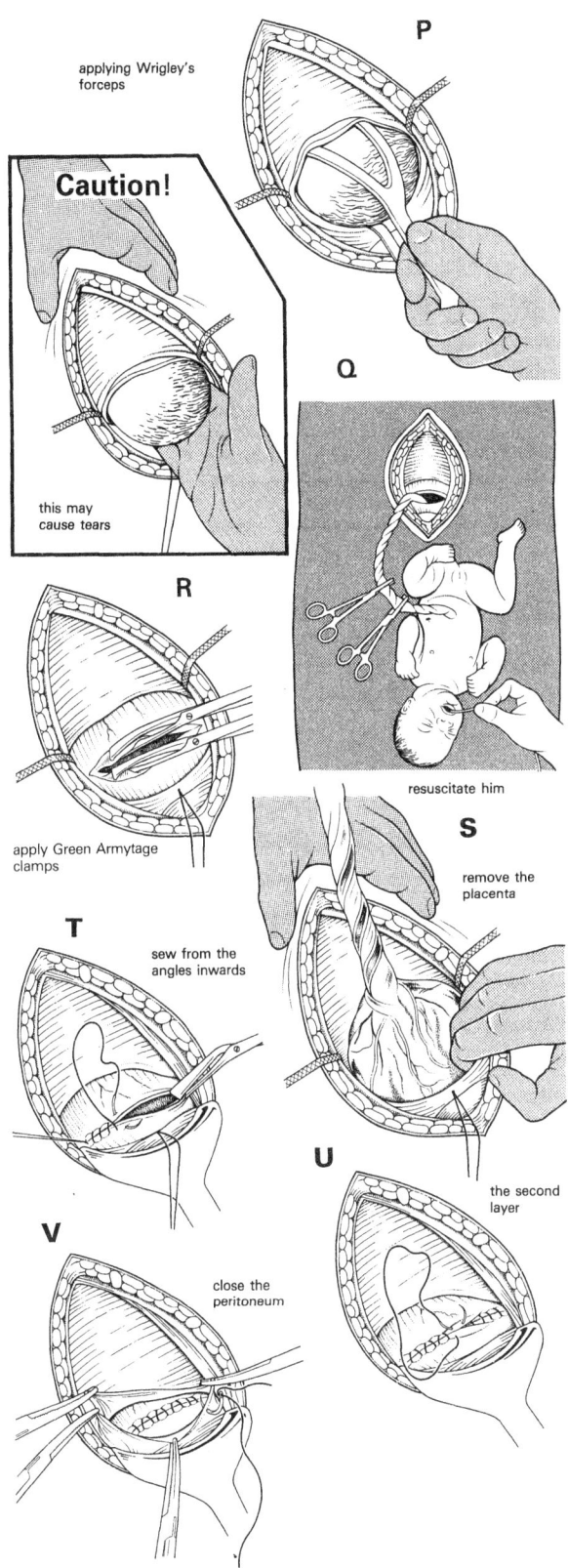

wife who is helping you can suck out his nose and mouth. Lay him head downwards between his mother's thighs (Q). Ask your assistant to put two clamps on his cord and divide it between them, while you care for her wound, especially the angles, which may bleed. In placenta praevia especially, clamp his cord quickly, because he may bleed from the injured sinuses of the placenta. If necessary, resuscitate him (19.12).

CONTROLLING BLEEDING. If you are a quick operator, apply two Green Armytage clamps, one on the upper flap and one on the lower one, just proximal to the angle (R). They will identify the angle for you and allow you to suture it more accurately.

If you are a slow operator apply several Green Armytage clamps (or sponge-holders) all round the cut edges of her uterus, particularly at the angles. Make sure they don't grasp the posterior wall of her empty uterus, as it lies on the promontary of her sacrum; you can easily do this by mistake if bleeding has been brisk. The difficulty in applying many clamps is that they will get in your way.

REMOVING THE PLACENTA AFTER CAESAREAN SECTION

When her uterus is contracting firmly, remove her placenta by a combination of controlled cord traction and fundal pressure (S). If necessary, help it to contract by massaging her fundus from inside her peritoneal cavity. Pull gently on the cord, and press her uterus back with your left hand. This should deliver the placenta easily. If it has stuck, removing it manually from inside her uterus may cause severe bleeding.

When the placenta is delivered: (1) Inspect her uterine cavity *to make sure it is empty.* Wipe it dry with a gauze pack to remove pieces of membrane and clots. (2) Make sure that the placenta is complete. If she has a secondary postpartum haemorrhage, you don't want to have to re-explore her uterus—see 'Stop Press'.

CAUTION ! Don't probe her cervix to improve drainage—keep out of her dirty vagina!

SUTURING THE UTERUS AFTER CAESAREAN SECTION

Do this in two layers using thick chromic catgut and a large round-bodied Mayo's needle. Don't use non-absorbable sutures, particularly not on the inner wall. Ask your assistant to hold the lower edge of her uterus forwards with the stay suture, while you sew from the angles inwards (T). Start the sutures just beyond the right extremity of the incision, work towards the middle, and then start at the left angle. In this way, you secure the angles first.

Alternatively, put a separate stay suture in the right angle, and start a continuous suture from the left angle.

Sew the first layer as a continous running suture. Ask your assistant to hold the free end of the catgut tightly, while you work towards the other end of the incision. Unless the sutures are tight, it will not stop bleeding.

CAUTION ! (1) Start suturing just lateral to the angle. (2) Don't sew the lower edge above the upper one, because this may advance her bladder up her uterus. (3) Don't include her bladder in your sutures. If you find you have included it, you will probably be wise to leave a catheter in for a few days, rather than removing the sutures and starting again, which will cause severe bleeding. (4) If you suture too deeply with a large needle at the angles of incision, you may obstruct her ureters. (5) Don't sew the front and back walls of her uterus together. So, before the first layer of stitches is completed, put two fingers into the uterine cavity, to make sure that its walls are free. If necessary, release the sutures and start again. (6) Don't stitch her gut to the back of her broad ligament. If you are in any doubt, put your fingers down behind it before you start to stitch the lateral extremities of the incision.

COMPLETING THE REPAIR AFTER CAESAREAN SECTION

When the first layer of sutures is completed, make sure again that the ends of the incision are adequately secured. If necessary, put in one or two interrupted sutures, especially if bleeding from the wound continues..

Now start the second layer of continous running sutures (U). Ask your assistant to maintain tension on the stay sutures, so as to show up the edge of her uterus.

Put a large warm pack over her repaired lower segment, and leave it for 2 minutes while you remove the abdominal packs. When you remove it most of the bleeding will have stopped.

Fig. 18-13 CAESAREAN SECTION—THREE. P, if necessary, apply Wrigley's forceps. Don't put your whole hand into the patient's uterus, the extra bulk of your hand may tear it. Q, place the baby on his mother's thighs and resuscitate him as in Section 19.12. R, put clamps on the angles of her uterus, and on any major bleeding points. S, remove her placenta by controlled cord traction and fundal pressure, but wait until her uterus is contracting first. T, start suturing just lateral to the ends of the incision. U, closing the second layer. V, closing the peritoneum.

Look carefully at your completed sutures. If there is still bleeding, put in some more interrupted or mattress 'figure of eight' sutures. Don't close her peritoneum until you have controlled all bleeding.

When her uterus is no longer bleeding, close the peritoneum of her vesico-uterine pouch with continous sutures of 2/0 catgut (V). Again avoid including her bladder with the lower edge of the peritoneum.

If you are going to tie her tubes (15.4), now is the time to do it. Look for ovarian cysts. If you find one which is >5 cm in diameter, consider ovarian cystectomy (20.7).

CLOSING THE ABDOMEN AFTER CAESAREAN SECTION

Clean all blood and debris from her peritoneal cavity, and especially from her paracolic gutters. They will be much cleaner if you previously inserted abdominal packs ('lap pads') beside her uterus. Inspect these by drawing her uterus to the side.

Measure her true conjugate with a steel ruler as in Fig. 18-16. Displace her uterus to the right, and put one end of it on her sacral promontary. Let it rest across her symphysis pubis, and mark the place where it crosses the posterior aspect of her symphysis with your right index finger. Remove the ruler, read off her true conjugate, and record it in her notes and in the summary of labour. It will be invaluable when you come to decide if she should have a trial of scar next time.

Place her greater omentum over her uterus: it will usually reach her bladder. Close her abdomen (9.8). Don't insert a drain.

Bend up her legs, and press on the fundus to express clot from her uterus and vagina. A uterus full of blood will interfere with retraction and encourage infection; you may later mistake blood in her vagina for a postpartum haemorrhage. Clean out her vagina with a sterile swab on sponge forceps.

As soon as she has recovered from her anaesthetic give her baby to her. This close early contact is important in developing the bond between them. If she has had a local or subarachnoid anaesthetic, she can see him before the operation is over.

POSTOPERATIVE CARE AFTER CAESAREAN SECTION

Estimate her blood loss: it will probably be more than you think. The *average* loss is 1 litre. Unless you have expert staff, check her vital signs yourself. Check and chart her pulse, temperature, and respiration half-hourly, until she is awake, and then, when her condition is satisfactory hourly for 12 to 24 hours. Continue the intravenous infusion for 24 hours, or until she can take fluids by mouth and bowel sounds are present. Give her 3 litres of fluid in 24 hours (two bottles of 5% dextrose and one of 0.9% saline). Give her pethidine 100 mg up to 4 doses.

If she bled much, arrange for a fast running drip of saline or Ringer's lactate, and see her yourself in an hour. You will be suprised how often a patient who left the theatre in reasonable condition is now collapsed, because the drip was too slow, or stopped.

CAUTION ! Watch for signs of infection: (1) Fever. (2) A large, soft, tender uterus. (3) Tender thickening in her lateral fornices.

If her membranes had been ruptured for more than 24 hours before the operation, or there are other reasons for suspecting infection, continue perioperative antibiotics (2.9) for up to 5 days.

If she has been in obstructed labour and her urine is bloodstained, leave a catheter in her bladder for 5 to 10 days.

If she vomits, or her abdomen becomes distended, start gastric suction.

CAUTION ! Before she goes home, make sure that she and her relatives know that she must have future deliveries in hospital—*this is ESSENTIAL!* She must come regularly for antenatal care. Give her a card which says why Caesarean section was done, and what she should do about her next delivery. Ask her to show this card at the antenatal clinic, when she becomes pregnant again.

18.10 Difficulties with Caesarean section

Many difficulties attend Caesarean section, and many disasters can follow it, so the list below is long. Torrential bleeding when you cut through a *placenta praevia* can kill a mother. Disasters

CAESAREAN SECTION IN AFRICA, 1879

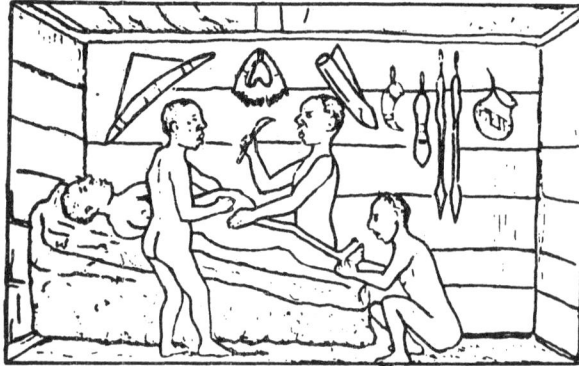

Fig. 18-13a CAESAREAN SECTION IN AFRICA IN 1879, as described by Robert Felkin. The mother was liberally supplied wih banana wine, which was also used to wash the operator's hands and her abdomen. A single rapid lower midline incision opened her abdominal wall and her uterus. Bleeding points were cauterized with a hot iron. After delivery her abdomen was closed with seven thin iron spikes. The baby was put to her breast 2 hours later. Both mother and baby did well. *Felkin RW, 'Notes on Labour in Central Africa'. Edinburgh Medical Journal 1884;29:922. As reported in Medicine Digest 1985;11:17—19.*

with the urinary tract are usually the result of very poor technique. Fortunately, most of the others are rare. Some of these many difficulties are only seen in the developing world, where inexpert operators find themselves working under difficult circumstances.

DIFFICULTIES WITH CAESAREAN SECTION

For difficulties with infection, see section 6.8.

DIFFICULTIES WITH THE INCISION

If a patient has had a PREVIOUS CAESAREAN SECTION, dense adhesions may have formed between her uterus and her abdominal wall. They would have been much less likely to have formed, if her omentum had been placed between her uterus and her abdominal wall, at the last operation. Excise the scar in her abdominal wall with an elliptical incision. If the sides of this might be difficult to join up accurately, make some scratch marks across it and align them later.

Open her parietal peritoneum as far as you can. Lift it between haemostats to stretch the adhesions, and divide them with the points of scissors directed at her uterus. If you find a plane of loose connective tissue, free it with a finger or swab. Cut fibrous bands. If dissecting the adhesions is very difficult (unusual), give up and make an upper segment incision.

CAUTION ! (1) Stay close to her uterus to avoid her bladder. (2) Open her uterus between stay sutures (see the story of Wambue in Section 18.9).

If she has had a PREVIOUS CLASSICAL CAESAREAN SECTION, you would probably be wiser to do a lower segment operation this time.

If after a previous operation, HER BLADDER HAS STUCK TO HER LOWER SEGMENT, so that you cannot mobilize it with a finger or swab, incise the peritoneum on her uterus about 2 cm above her bladder. Lift the lower edge in forceps to stretch the adhesions between her bladder and her uterus. Cut them close to her uterus, keeping the points of the scissors directed at it. If this is difficult, give up and make an incision about 3 cm above where her bladder and her uterus have stuck together.

If the baby's HEAD IS STUCK TIGHTLY UNDER AN OLD SCAR IN HER UTERUS, an incision just above it will probably tear as you deliver him. Instead, make a wide V-shaped transverse incision with the point of the 'V' lying across the middle of the scar. This will divide it and reduce the tension. If her uterus does tear, it will do so near the midline, where you can more easily see and repair it.

If the INCISION IN HER UTERUS TEARS as you remove his head, there will probably be a vertical tear in the corner which will run down behind her bladder, often with heavy bleeding.

If you are alone with the scrub nurse, ask for an extra assistant.

Identify the edges of the incision and the tear. Mobilize her bladder further downwards if necessary.

If you cannot define the extent of the tear, carefully open her broad ligament by cutting her round ligament. This will let you feel her ureter, so that you can avoid it before you apply any clamps. Now apply Green Armytage forceps to the edges of the tear, and draw its angle into view. Apply direct pressure with a dry pack, find the bleeding vessels, and tie them. Use interrupted sutures in the area of the tear. They will be easier to unpick if you catch her bladder or her ureter by mistake.

CAUTION ! After repairing a tear, check that her ureter has not been caught in a stitch by mistake.

If these measures fail, the only way to control bleeding may be to tie her both uterine arteries (See 'Stop Press') or her internal iliac artery on that side (3.5). If you are not able to repair her uterus, do a subtotal hysterectomy (very rarely needed, 20.12).

DIFFICULTIES WITH PARTICULAR PRESENTATIONS

If her labour is OBSTRUCTED WITH A CEPHALIC PRESENTATION, enter her abdomen just below her umbilicus so as to avoid her bladder. If catheterization before the operation was impossible, empty her bladder now with a needle and syringe. Much of the swelling will be oedema, which will not go away. Mobilize her bladder free from her lower segment as usual.

If an assistant is to push the baby's head up from below through her vagina, let him do so now *before* you open her uterus. If he waits until after you have opened it, the baby's shoulder may prolapse into the incision and make delivery more difficult.

Make a transverse incision in the lower segment. Choose its level carefully. If it is too high, delivery will be difficult; if it is too low, you may enter her vagina.

If delivering his head is difficult, don't panic. Everyone finds this a problem, especially when the uterus is tight around him. Take time to push back its wall from around his head, by inserting 2 fingers all round. You will then be able to apply forceps. If you still have difficulty, enlarge the wound upwards and laterally at its ends.

CAUTION ! (1) Don't lever his head out with your whole hand, because this can cause vertical downward tears in the lower segment. (2) If her liquor was purulent or infected, clean her abdomen carefully and wash out her pelvis with warm saline.

If his BREECH is presenting, delivery may be be more difficult than with a cephalic one. Feel for a leg, or better, both legs, and deliver him breech-first as if you were delivering his head. Then deliver his head slowly, or you may damage it. If, by mistake, you take hold of an arm, replace it. Then feel for a leg; recognize it by feeling for his heel. If an arm comes out and will not go back, you are in trouble (unusual). You may have to make an inverted 'T' incision to get him out. When necessary, deliver his arms by a modified Lovset manoeuvre, and his head by a modified Mauriceau–Smellie–Veit manoeuvre (19.8).

If there is a TRANSVERSE LIE, the choice of incision is important. See also 18.9.

If she is in early labour, and her lower segment is poorly developed, with most of the baby in the upper segment, **make a transverse incision in the upper segment and deliver him by breech extraction (19.8).**

If she is in early labour, her lower segment is well developed, and her membranes are still intact, **make a transverse incision in her lower segment, and deliver him by breech extraction.**

If labour is obstructed, and most of him is in the overdistended lower segment, **simple delivery through a transverse incision in the lower segment will cause large tears.** So:

If he is alive make a vertical incision in the lower segment, and extend the incision into the upper one until it is big enough to deliver him.

If he is dead, make a transverse incision in the lower segment, decapitate or eviscerate him, and deliver him in any convenient way. If his hand is outside her vulva, separate his arm at the shoulder joint before Caesarean section starts.

CAUTION ! (1) Don't try to deliver him intact, because this will tear her lower segment severely. (2) Don't make a classical or inverted 'T' incision for a dead baby.

DIFFICULTIES WITH THE PLACENTA

If you anticipate PLACENTA PRAEVIA, expect difficulty, and get help if you can. You can usually use the ordinary transverse lower segment incision. This is contraindicated if: (1) She has a poorly developed lower segment, which would not allow a transverse incision of adequate length. (2) She has a very vascular lower segment with large veins on it. (3) The presenting part is high, and he is lying transversely, indicating that the placenta praevia is probably central. If so, mobilize her uterovesical fold, as for a lower segment operation. Make a low vertical midline (de Lee) incision. Deliver him as for a low classical section. If there is severe bleeding, quickly feel for a foot. His half breech will plug the bleeding area, and you will have the situation under control. Some surgeons make a vertical or transverse incision in the upper segment.

If you find PLACENTA IN THE INCISION: (1) Peel it away from her uterine wall and enter her uterus from above it. (2) If the edge of the placenta is too far away to allow this, cut through it quickly, and deliver him without delay through the hole that you have just made. If you meet his cord, clamp it before you deliver him, but don't waste time looking for it: you can clamp it immediately afterwards. Remember that a baby can easily bleed from an injured placenta. His mother can also bleed, so if you see a large bleeding vessel in the placental bed (unusual), control it with a figure of eight suture.

If she BLEEDS POSTOPERATIVELY (not uncommon with placenta praevia), she is probably bleeding from her lower segment at the site of the attachment of the placenta. Give her oxytocin, and if necessary transfuse her. In desperation, pack her uterus (19.11a).

DIFFICULTIES WITH BLEEDING

See also under 'Difficulties with the incision' and 'Difficulties with placenta praevia' above.

If you have a LOT OF TROUBLE WITH BLEEDING during the operation, it is often helpful to bring the uterus out of the abdomen. You can then reach behind it with your hand and place the sutures at the angle of the incision. It is usually safe to put sutures beyond the end of the incision *provided you suture only into the substance of the uterus.* See 'Stop Press'.

If she has SEVERE VAGINAL BLEEDING 8 to 14 days after delivery (secondary postpartum haemorrhage), the operation site is infected (common after an obstructed labour with sloughing of the tissues). Under perioperative antibiotic cover (2.9) take her to the theatre, and examine her under an anaesthetic. Put a gloved finger into her uterus through her external os and feel: (1) for a piece of retained placenta, and (2) for the inner wall of her uterine scar. If this feels weak, or has broken down, reopen her abdominal incision. You may find a soft necrotic bleeding uterus, with blood and spreading infection in her peritoneal cavity. What was the scar may now be an infected hole in her uterus. Under such circumstances she should have a total or subtotal hysterectomy (20.12). If you don't attempt one, she will die. Expect to find that her parametrium is acutely infected and swollen, so that it feels like cheese.

Alternatively, and less satisfactorily, remove what slough you can and carefully pack the wound. You will probably be unable to find any obviously bleeding vessels. If this fails, you will have to try to remove her uterus or to tie her internal iliac vessels (3.5). Even so, you may fail to save her.

DIFFICULTIES WITH THE URINARY TRACT See also 18.18 and 18.19D

If you OPENED HER BLADDER, identify the hole carefully, hold its edges with Allis forceps, mobilize the surrounding tissues if necessary, and bring its edges together with continuous inverting sutures of fine chromic catgut. Try not to penetrate its mucosa. Drain her bladder continuously with an indwelling catheter for 10 days. On the 10th day spigot it 2-hourly. If she is satisfactory (no leaks, no abdominal discomfort, and a good flow when you release the spigot), remove the catheter on the the 11th day.

If you have INJURED HER URETER at operation, first check that her other ureter is intact. Either, repair it if you can. Or, insert a T-shaped drain into her ureter, bring it out to the surface, and close her abdomen. Later, refer her for expert help. Don't try to do a ureterostomy.

If she has ANURIA: (1) This may be the result of severe hypotension, while she was in obstructed labour (not uncommon). Hydrate her well and give her frusemide 40 mg, intravenously. See Section 53.3. (2) You may have tied both her ureters (fortunately, rare). Refer her. If this is delayed do a temporary nephrostomy on both sides (23.13).

If she complains of a severe dull PAIN IN ONE LOIN postoperatively, you may have tied one of her ureters. Do an IVP to look for a hydronephrosis or a 'nonfunctioning kidney' (actually a poorly functioning one, because insufficient dye is excreted to show the calyces). If you think you have tied a ureter, refer her. If referral is delayed, do a temporary nephrostomy (23.13). Sometimes, when you tie a ureter, neither she nor you are aware of it: her kidney merely stops working.

If URINE DISCHARGES FROM HER VAGINA 2 to 5 days postoperatively, check that: (1) Her bladder is not distended (overflow incontinence). This can happen if it has been bruised. (2) She has not got bladder/urethral incompetence. If you see her urethra leaking, ask her to cough. If urine spurts out, this is what she has. If it is disabling, refer her for a sling operation. (3) She may have a fistula. Treat her with salt perineal baths (Sitz baths). Examine her at 10 days, if necessary under anaesthesia (EUA), when examination will be easier. She may have one of three fistulae:

(A) If urine is COMING FROM HER ANTERIOR VAGINAL WALL: (1) She has a VVF due to pressure from the fetal head during a long and difficult labour. Refer her to have it repaired at 6 weeks, or repair it yourself (see Section 18.18). Or, (2) urine may be leaking from her ureter. To confirm this put cotton wool swabs in her vagina, and instil methylene blue through a catheter into her bladder. If the swabs are stained blue, she has a vesicovaginal fistula. If they are wet, but not blue, she has a ureteric leak (ureterovaginal fistula). The classical test is to insert 3 swabs. If only the lower swab is stained blue, she has stress incontinence. If the middle and upper ones are blue she has a VVF. If the upper one is wet but not blue, she has a ureteric fistula.

CAUTION ! Don't instil gentian violet into the bladder: it causes a chemical cystitis and a contracted bladder.

(B) If she has a URETEROVAGINAL FISTULA (uncommon), it was probably caused by damage to her ureter at Caesarean section by: (1) clamping it in error, not recognizing this, and leaving the clamp on for more than a few minutes, or (b) by including the ureter in a suture closing the uterine wound. An IVP will tell you which side it is on. The kidney on the affected side will show some degree of hydronephrosis. She may or may not have pain in her loin.

A ureterovaginal fistula is more hopeful and less urgent than (a) tied ureter(s), because it means that her kidney(s) will not stop functioning. You will be able to refer her for elective repair. Her ureter may need reimplanting into her bladder, or repair end to end. If she is to retain good kidney function, refer her without delay.

(C) If URINE IS COMING THROUGH HER CERVIX (a vesicouterine fistula), it is the result of cutting her bladder, not immediately recognizing and repairing it, and finally stitching up her uterus so that her bladder communicates with her uterine cavity. Refer her.

If you cannot refer her, wait for 4 to 6 weeks. Open her bladder as for cystotomy for stone (23.15), and repair her uterus and bladder in separate well-defined layers. Drain her bladder as for a VVF; a Foley catheter is an acceptable alternative to the 'button' method (18-23).

OTHER DIFFICULTIES WITH CAESAREAN SECTION

If she has a CONTRACTION RING (Bandl's ring), in her lower segment, or between the lower and the upper segment, deal with it like this: If her baby is entirely above the ring, make a transverse incision entirely above it. If it is round his neck, make a vertical incision across it.

If she has FIBROIDS, leave them unless they are pedunculated and removal is very easy. Otherwise, leave them: they may settle and atrophy. Removing a fibroid, at delivery, from within the wall of the uterus causes severe bleeding.

If she has OVARIAN CYSTS OR TUMOURS, remove them if they are >5 cm. Ovarian cystectomy is possible, but removing the ovary and tube will be quicker and safer. Smaller functional luteal cysts will have usually disappeared spontaneously by the end of pregnancy. See also 20.7.

If she has ADHESIONS, you will have to separate them sufficiently to get good access to her uterus. Don't try to remove them from around her tubes and ovaries; they will ooze and form again.

If you have sewn up her uterus WITHOUT REMOVING HER PLACENTA, it will probably be delivered vaginally in a few hours. The danger is that it might be retained and become infected. Even so, it is probably wise not to reopen her uterus and remove her placenta operatively. If necessary, remove it manually through her vagina.

18.12 Classical Caesarean section

In spite of the long list of rather rare indications in Section 18.8, a classical Caesarean section is seldom done by experienced obstetricians. We describe it mainly because it is slightly easier if you are inexperienced. Because rupture of the uterus is such a danger with subsequent pregnancies, perhaps as early as 28 weeks, sew up the patient's uterus with particular care, and do all you can to persuade her to have her tubes tied. Many steps are the same as for a lower segment operation, so refer to them where necessary.

CLASSICAL CAESAREAN SECTION

See elsewhere for the indications (18.8), the equipment, and anaesthesia (A 16.6).

INCISION. The patient's bladder may be high in her abdomen, so take care not to injure it. Stand on her right side, and make a right paramedian incision, or a midline incision skirting her umbilicus, two-thirds of it below and one-third above her umbilicus. This is best if she has a Bandl's ring or a high bladder.

Look for her round ligaments. Their position will tell you if her uterus is rotated or not. If it is rotated, centre it.

Put large packs each side of her uterus to keep blood and liquor out of her peritoneal cavity (A, Fig. 18-14). If you fail to do this blood will run into her upper abdomen and flanks, and you will have to remove it before you finally close her peritoneal cavity.

Make a 12 cm vertical midline incision in her uterus (B). The uterus is much thicker here than in the lower segment. Make it as low down as possible, extending into her lower segment—*taking care to avoid her bladder.* If necessary, reflect this downwards (as in K, Fig. 18-12). Deepen the centre of the incision steadily, being careful not to wound the baby. As soon as you are in her uterine cavity, put two fingers into the wound and complete it upwards and downwards using scissors to cut between your fingers (C). If the placenta is in the way, try to displace it rapidly, rather than cutting through it.

Search for a leg, and deliver the baby as a breech, guiding his head with your other hand (D). As soon as he is being delivered, ask the anaesthetist to inject ergometrine with oxytocin ('Syntometrine'), or ergometrine 0.5 mg, intravenously. Place two artery forceps on the cord, cut it between them, hand him to the midwife, who should be waiting to receive him, and see that he is resuscitated rapidly. Hold him by his legs with one finger between them as she does so.

As soon as he is delivered, deliver her retracted uterus through the abdominal incision, by hooking your index and middle fingers into its cavity, helped, if necessary, by the fingers of your left hand behind it.

As soon as her uterus has contracted, deliver her placenta and membranes (E). Remove any shreds of membrane that remain by wiping the inside of her uterus with a swab (F). If her membranes were not ruptured before the operation, the appearance of the lower pole of the bag will show you that you have removed them whole.

If her uterus is slow to contract, as may happen if anaesthesia is too deep, wait for the ergometrine to act, and if necessary for lighter anaesthesia. Then, if necessary, remove her placenta manually. Meanwhile wrap her uterus in a hot abdominal towel, and compress it.

Inspect and feel her uterus to make sure that it is not ruptured. Repair it in layers with '1' chromic catgut. For the first layer stitch the decidua and the deep layer of muscle with a continous suture. For the second one, use the sutures shown in G, and H, to invert the peritoneal covering.

CLASSICAL CAESAREAN SECTION

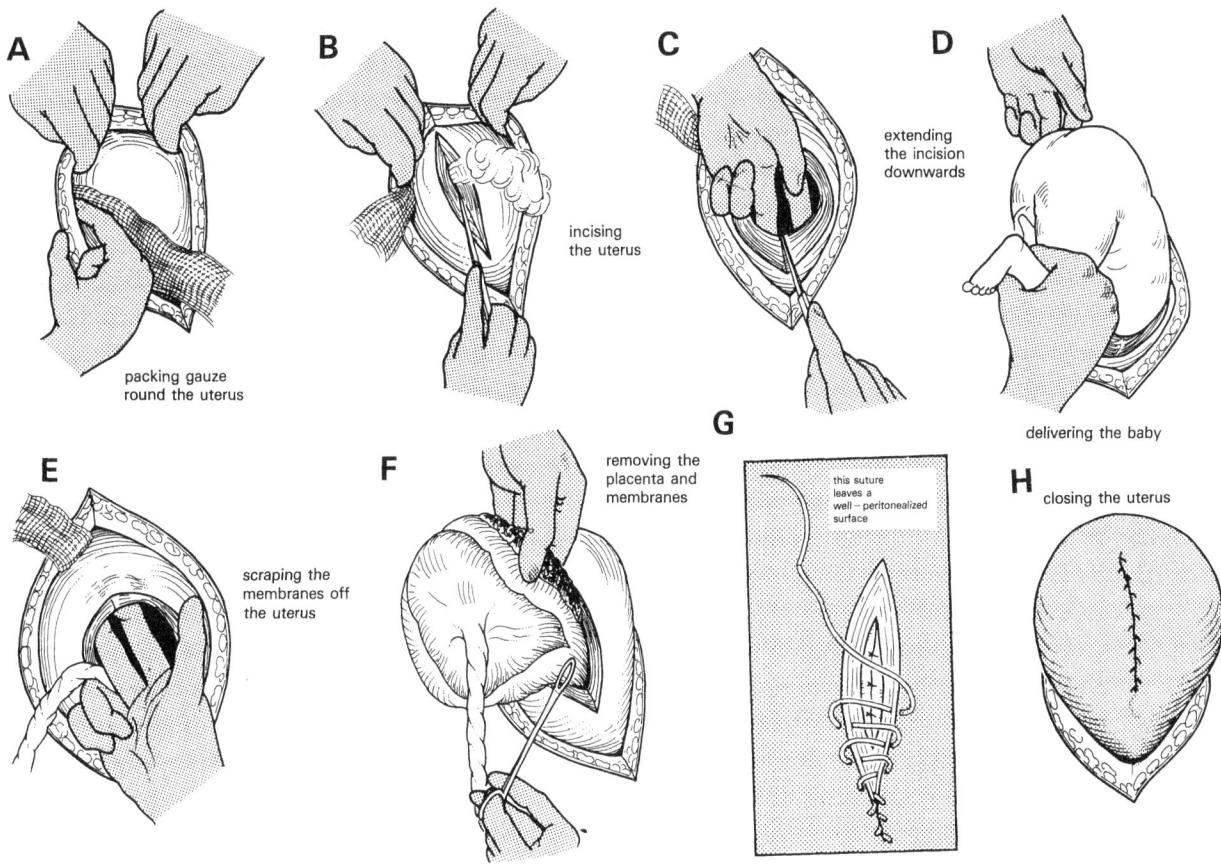

Fig. 18-14 CLASSICAL CAESAREAN SECTION. A, packing gauze round the patient's uterus. B, incising her uterus. C, extending the incision downwards. D, delivering the baby. E, emptying her uterus. F, removing the placenta and membranes. G, an anchor stitch has been inserted, and the wound is being closed by an inverting suture, which pierces each wound edge from within outwards. This buries the peritoneal surface of the wound, and minimizes the formation of adhesions. *After 'Bonney's Gynaecological Surgery', Figs. 331—7. Baillière, with kind permission.*

If a continuous suture is difficult, because her uterine wall is being pulled apart so that each suture cuts out, place several sutures of interrupted silk 1 cm apart. Ask your assistant to pull on all but one of them, so as to approximate the edges of the incision, while you tie the remaining one. The result will be neat and may give a stronger scar than catgut.

If she has agreed to have her tubes tied, now is the time to do it.

Remove and count the abdominal packs. Mop blood and exudate from her peritoneal cavity, and close it (9.8). Alternatively, put tension sutures in her abdominal wall, and leave them in for 10 days. Remove blood clot from her vagina, as in Section 18.9. As soon she has recovered from the anaesthetic, give her baby to her.

POSTOPERATIVELY, follow the same regime as for the lower segment operation (18.9). Explain to her, and to her relatives, that, in her next pregnancy, she must come into hospital, or into a maternity village at 32 weeks. She should have an elective section at the 38th week, or earlier, if there is any suspicion of her uterus rupturing.

18.13 Extraperitoneal Caesarean section

This operation dates from the pre-antibiotic era, and the introduction of metronidazole (2.7) has made it largely unnecessary. But if you don't have metronidazole, and you have to operate in the presence of sepsis, you may find it useful. It is one of the more contentious operations in this book and one contributor doubts its value.

If you section a mother in the presence of intrauterine infection, or after a long labour, she runs the serious risk of multiple peritoneal abscesses or peritonitis. There is quite a chance that she will die. You can reduce the risk of peritonitis by excluding the incision in her uterus from her peritoneal cavity. To do this, reflect her parietal peritoneum from the inside of her abdominal wall, and her visceral peritoneum from the front of her lower segment, and tie them together. This will seal off her peritoneal cavity from the incision that you are about to make into her infected uterus. This takes longer than the standard method, and is not as easy as it looks, but it is worth trying, if she is badly infected.

EXTRAPERITONEAL CAESAREAN SECTION

See also Sections 18.8 and 18.11. Many of the details for the standard lower segment operation apply here also.

INDICATIONS. Any Caesarean section in which the risk of subsequent peritoneal infection is great, when you have no adequate antibiotic cover, and especially no metronidazole. In an obstructed labour the attempt to do an extraperitoneal Caesarean section may be an impractical addition to an already complicated situation.

PERIOPERATIVE ANTIBIOTICS. **Give what antibiotics you can,** as in Section 2.9.

EXTRAPERITONEAL CAESAREAN SECTION

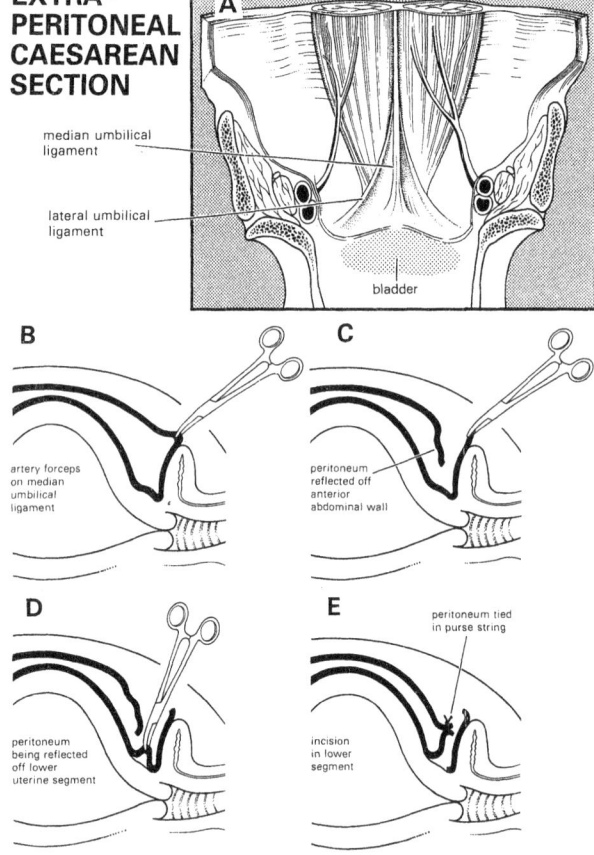

Fig. 18-15 EXTRAPERITONEAL CAESAREAN SECTION. A, a view of the patient's anterior abdominal wall from inside her abdomen, indicating the structures to be cut. B, artery forceps attached to her median umbilical ligament. C, her peritoneum reflected off her anterior abdominal wall. D, her peritoneum is being reflected off her lower segment. E, her peritoneum tied in a purse string. *Kindly contributed by Hugh Philpott.*

INCISION. Enter the patient's abdomen through a vertical incision from her umbilicus to her symphysis pubis. Extend this down to her peritoneum, *but not through it.*

To reflect her peritoneum, attach a haemostat to the root of her median umbilical ligament. Pull on this to allow you to mobilize her parietal peritoneum: (1) laterally towards the walls of her pelvis, and (2) down to the anterolateral aspect of her lower segment.

CAUTION ! Be sure to mobilize her parietal peritoneum superiorly and laterally for several centimetres above the lateral extremity of her uterovesical pouch. If you don't mobilize it extensively the purse string that you are about to make will be too tight, and may leak.

To enter her peritoneum, define and divide her median umbilical ligament. Extend the incision in her peritoneum laterally and downwards on each side towards her lower uterine segment. Cut her lateral umbilical ligaments (obliterated hypogastric arteries) as you do so, and keep close to the point of firm attachment to her bladder. Reflect her bladder downwards.

Attach a curved haemostat to her uterovesical pouch in the midline, where it joins the base of her bladder. Divide her peritoneum between her bladder and her uterus, and extend your incision laterally to join the incision that you have made on entering her peritoneal cavity. Ignore the covering of peritoneum attached to the fundus of her bladder.

Attach artery forceps to the upper incised margin of her uterovesical pouch. Use this to help you mobilize a flap of peritoneum off her lower segment. Mobilize it as far as the point of attachment to the upper segment.

Sew the two layers of peritoneum that you have just mobilized with a continuous suture. Pull it tight to make a bunched-up button of peritoneal tissue. It should look watertight.

Reflect her bladder off her lower uterine segment, and proceed with a lower segment operation in the usual way (18.9).

At the end of the operation, close the incision in her uterus, and control bleeding carefully. If possible, lavage the wound with 2 g of kanamycin or tetracycline dissolved in 200 ml of warm saline. Don't attempt to remove this. If you use water only, remove it.

Insert a 26 Ch fenestrated rubber tube extraperitoneally through her abdominal wall, to lie over the suture line in her lower segment. Introduce a tube drain in her opposite iliac fossa. This will enable you to irrigate her extraperitoneal space postoperatively.

Ignore the peritoneum covering the remainder of her bladder, but stitch the remains of her median umbilical ligament to the back of her rectus abdominis muscle. As you do so, include as much of the overlying transversalis fascia as you can conveniently gather together.

Apply intermittent suction drainage through the rubber tube, and irrigate the antibiotic solution through the tube dressing drain.

If suction drainage is impractical, insert two corrugated drains, one in each iliac fossa, extraperitoneally, leave them in for 48 hours, and then shorten them 3 cm, before you finally remove them.

CAUTION ! Don't try to insert intraperitoneal drains. The aim is to try to keep her peritoneal cavity uninfected.

18.14 Which is it to be? Elective section, 'trial of scar', or section early in labour?

If a mother has had one Caesarean section the alternatives for her next pregnancy are: (1) An elective section, before she goes into labour. (2) Section in early labour. (3) An attempt at vaginal delivery (a 'trial of scar'). How can you choose between these three?

A lower segment Caesarean section is sometimes done for such conditions as fetal distress, placenta praevia, or the prolapse of the cord or an arm, which are unlikely to happen again in a later pregnancy. When a mother like this becomes pregnant again, there is every reason to expect that her labour will be normal, except for the scar that she now has in her uterus. This will almost always give some warning before it ruptures, so you can safely let her have further attempts at delivering her babies vaginally. This is called a 'trial of scar'. She can have as many trials as she likes, provided the previous one was successful, but she must have had only *one* previous Caesarean section. If she has had two sections or more, always section her. Contributors differ greatly in their use of a trial of scar. One only does them in exceptional circumstances.

"TWO CAESARS OR MORE, ALWAYS A CAESAR"

When you do a trial of scar, admit her to hospital and observe her closely. Should her scar show signs of rupturing, section her immediately. These warning signs only last an hour or two, before her uterus ruptures, so you must admit her and observe her with the greatest care.

If CPD was the reason for her Caesarean section, it reduces the chances of a successful trial of scar in this pregnancy, but does not exclude it, because: (1) The pelvis continues to grow up to the age of 25. (2) Uterine action is often poor in the under-16s. An accurate measurement of her true conjugate done at the time of her previous section, as in Fig. 18-16, helps. A trial of scar is unwise if it is <9 cm. It is contraindicated in a breech presentation if the true conjugate is <10 cm. A trial of scar is absolutely contraindicated if her previous Caesarean section was classical.

ONE 'CLASSICAL', ALWAYS A CAESAR

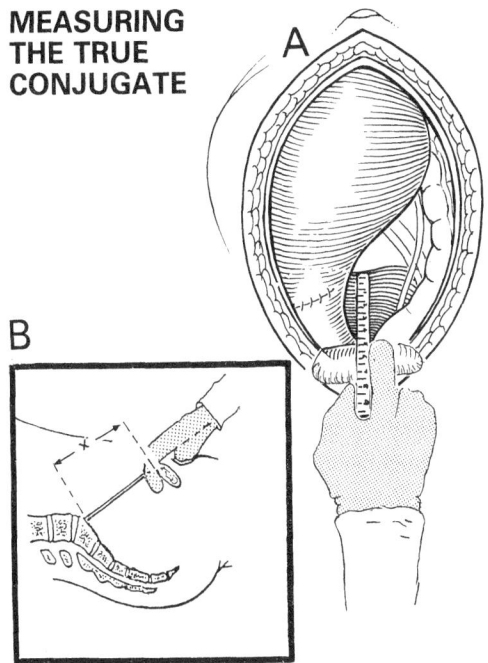

MEASURING THE TRUE CONJUGATE

Fig. 18-16 MEASURING THE TRUE CONJUGATE AT CAESAREAN SECTION. If you pack a steel ruler in the the Caesar set, and measure a patient's true conjugate routinely, it will help you to decide if a trial of scar is indicated next time she goes into labour. If you do it carefully, it will give you an exact measurement, and will enable you to check the vaginal measurement you made of her her diagonal conjugate when you examined her in the antenatal clinic (it is 2 cm less).

A, her uterus has been pushed to the right and the ruler placed across her pelvic cavity. Her bladder has been displaced, partly out of the wound. In reality her symphysis is covered by the lower end of the wound and by her bladder. B, put your finger down behind her symphysis on to its posterior surface, bring your finger and the ruler out together, and see where it comes on the ruler. 'X' is her true conjugate.

Good care during a trial of scar means that her pulse must be taken reliably, and you must be able to section her immediately. If, for example, her uterus shows signs of rupturing at 3 a.m., section must be possible before 4 a.m., not at 10 am the following morning. If the organization and discipline of your hospital are not such that it can provide care of this quality, elective section will give her a better chance of saving her baby, her uterus, and perhaps her life. If it takes several hours to find a driver, to fetch you, and to prepare the theatre, a trial of scar will be dangerous. Ideally, a uterus should never rupture during a trial of scar. If more than the very occasional one ruptures, patients should be referred to wait to go into labour at a larger hospital.

Even when conditions are not ideal, a trial of scar may be justified, because the immediate and future risks of a further section can be considerable. If mothers know that they cannot have a trial of scar in hospital, they may try to have trials themselves at home. A mother will usually understand if you say "We will give you a try, and if you have any difficulty, we will do another Caesarean section".

Ask the clinics to refer all mothers who have had a previous Caesarean section, and who are sure of their dates, at 34 weeks, so that you can assess them as described below. If a trial of scar is not indicated, plan an elective section at 38 weeks, or in early labour, if a mother is not sure of her dates.

The best indication that a uterine scar is going to rupture is a rise in her pulse rate. Take this half-hourly. If it rises above 100, or she has pain between contractions, her scar is probably rupturing, so section her. Other signs are described below.

Elective Caesarean sections are one of the alternatives to a trial of scar, but they are not the complete answer: (1) They may not be popular, so find out what your mothers think about them. If they are unpopular, avoid them, but at the antenatal clinic make the decision to section a mother in early labour. (2) Her dates may be uncertain, but even if they are certain, they need to be confirmed by a corresponding fundal height in mid pregnancy, before 20 weeks. (3) She is easily sectioned too early, so that her baby is at risk from prematurity.

HARBANS KAUR (38, gravida 4 para 3) was admitted at 9 a.m. on a Saturday, for a trial of scar, having had one previous Caesarean section with her first pregnancy. She was 7 cm dilated and had good contractions. At noon she was fully dilated and her baby's head was 3/5 above the brim. During the next half-hour it remained there. The doctor on duty was called for another emergency Caesarean section, so the intern was advised to attempt vacuum extraction. He failed, but in doing so, he included her cervix under the cup, and tore it. At 3 p.m. she developed pain, shock, and abdominal tenderness, and the fetal heartbeat disappeared. She was rushed to the theatre. Her uterus had ruptured, and the tear had extended into her bladder. The superintendent was called. He found that her ureter had been caught in a hastily applied suture. The following day she was found to be leaking urine vaginally. LESSONS. These are many, they include: (1) In multips the second stage should not last longer than 20 minutes. (2) A vacuum extractor was applied when the head was 3/5 above the brim. It should be only 1/5 up or less (except for a trial of vacuum or symphysiotomy). (3) When you apply the cup of a vacuum extractor, you should make sure that you don't include her cervix. (4) When a trial of scar is done, it must be possible to do an immediate Caesarean section if the trial fails.

WARNING SIGNS MAY ONLY LAST AN HOUR OR TWO BEFORE RUPTURE

TRIAL OF SCAR

INDICATIONS. (1) A patient who has had *one* lower segment Caesarean section, and the reason for it is absent in this pregnancy. For example, it might have been done for a malposition or malpresentation, maternal or fetal distress, or CPD due to hydrocephalus, etc. (2) The scar from a myomectomy (provided her uterine cavity was not opened during the operation), hysterotomy, or uterine perforation during a 'D and C'.

CONDITIONS. (1) She must have had not more than one previous Caesarean section. (2) When labour starts, she must either be in hospital, or not more than one hour away from it, with certain access to suitable transport. (3) Caesarean section must be available any time of the day or night, within one hour of the decision to section her. (4) Her pregnancy must have been normal. (5) Her baby must be a vertex presentation in the occipito–anterior position (some obstetricians will do a trial of scar for a breech). (6) There must be no fetal or maternal distress.

CONTRAINDICATIONS. (1) Two or more previous lower segment Caesarean sections. (2) One previous classical Caesarean section. (3) Any degree of CPD, or suspected CPD in this pregnancy, as suggested by a true conjugate of <9 cm or a diagonal conjugate of <11.5 cm. Although this is the ideal figure, it is unrealistic in some countries; in New Guinea, for example, a figure of 10.5 cm is used for the diagonal conjugate. (4) An occipito-posterior presentation. (5) Any other form of malpresentation, or obstetric complication. (6) Sepsis following a previous section is a relative contraindication only. (7) Any need for an oxytocin drip.

A request for tubal ligation favours the decision to do an elective Caesarean section. On its own, it is not a sufficient contraindication to vaginal delivery, because a vaginal delivery followed by tubal ligation will be safer. If a patient arrives in labour, use the same criteria as if she arrived during pregnancy.

ASSESSMENT. See all mothers with a previous section in the antenatal clinic at 36 weeks, and decide whether to do a trial of scar or not. Take a careful history. Assess her pelvis clinically and assess the size of her baby by measuring the height of her fundus; if it is >40 cm, don't do a trial of scar. If you have not previously measured her true conjugate, X-ray pelvimetry is useful but not essential.

METHOD Ask her to avoid heavy work during the last month of pregnancy, or to come in for rest. If she can be sure to reach hospital within an hour of labour starting, let her wait at home until labour starts. Otherwise, admit her at 36 weeks for rest and observation. Allow her fluids only by mouth during labour.

Don't induce labour. Unless your blood bank can be relied upon to have blood available within an hour, have it cross-matched, and ready to give if necessary. Record her pulse and the fetal heart rate carefully.

You may sometimes be able to feel the scar in her lower segment, when you examine her vaginally. This will be easier if you are using epidural anaesthesia. If it bulges or feels weak, section her immediately. The tenderness of a scar is difficult to assess in labour, and is not, on its own, an indication for section. Assist her with outlet forceps, or vacuum extraction, if necessary.

Abandon the trial if: (1) She crosses the alert line on the cervicograph! (2) Her pulse rises to 100. (3) She has pain between contractions. (4) Her pain is generalized. (5) She has unexplained vaginal bleeding. (6) Her uterine contractions cease. (7) She has rectal or vaginal tenesmus.

Stay with her during labour so that you can examine her lower uterine segment vaginally immediately after delivery of the placenta, so as to be sure that it has not ruptured. One contributor considers this impractical, and only recommends it if she has had a PPH; others do it routinely. Examining it is uncomfortable, but does not need anaesthesia. If you find a rupture, repair it at laparotomy (9.2, 18.17).

If she has a postpartum haemorrhage, the scar in her uterus has probably broken open; confirm this by doing a vaginal examination, and repair it abdominally if you find it.

18.15 Injuries of the birth canal

Primary Mother Care describes the repair of episiotomies and first-degree tears; here we describe the repair of more serious injuries. You can nearly always avoid third-degree tears by 'controlled pushing', and by making an episiotomy when this is needed. They follow instrumental deliveries more often than normal ones. Almost all obstetricians meet them sometimes: so recognize this, and don't blame the midwife. She will be upset anyway, and will be tempted to conceal such a tear if you are harsh.

Suture second- and third-degree tears, either within 24 hours of delivery, or after several months, when a tear has epithelialized and is no longer infected. With a recent third-degree tear: (1) Start by stitching the edges of the patient's rectum together. (2) Cover these stitches with a layer of fascia. (3) Suture her anal sphincter with two or three interrupted sutures. (3) Close her vaginal and perineal skin. If a tear is old, you will first have to incise and reflect the skin which has grown over it.

TEARS OF THE BIRTH CANAL

LESSER INJURIES

If a patient has a second-degree tear, and it is less than 24 hours old, suture it (M 24.1). If it is more than 24 hours old, wait, and sit her in salt baths. Use a bowl of water containing enough salt to make it into half-strength saline. Sit her in this twice a day for an hour; after 2 or 3 days she can continue baths at home. Her tear will heal itself in a few weeks, with little deformity of her perineum. Don't try to excise it, or her introitus will stenose later.

If her cervix is torn, it may have a single tear, which is large enough to sew, or numerous small ones. The bleeding from small tears is most easily controlled by packing, see Section 19.11a. Blood is more likely to be coming from a poorly contracted uterus, for which she needs ergometrine and oxytocin.

If she has a haematoma of her vulva (unusual), incise it at its lowest point, and evacuate the clot. Insert a drain, and suture this in position. If it bleeds severely, pack the cavity for 24 hours. If you don't see the bleeding vessel immediately, don't waste time looking for it. These haematomas are usually unilateral, and cause great pain, and occasionally retention of urine and shock.

If her clitoris is torn (rare), undersew it with continuous catgut. It may bleed severely. Enquire what happened; a common mistake is to support the perineum too vigorously, so as to force the head against the pubis, and tear the tissues over it.

A RECENT THIRD-DEGREE TEAR

Repair her tear as soon as possible. Don't wait to let her recover from her labour. If you have to delay >24 hours or there is infection, leave it, and do an elective repair later when it has healed.

CAUTION ! This is *not* a minor operation. The best chance of success is the first attempt. If you fail, she is condemned, at best, to some episodes of faecal incontinence.

EQUIPMENT. One pair of tissue forceps, 6 haemostats, needle-holders, and round-bodied curved needles. Use No.1 chromic catgut for all tissues except her skin.

ANAESTHESIA. (1) Repair her tear in the labour ward, using local infiltration with 1% lignocaine. Often, she has already had a pudendal block prior to vacuum extraction or forceps. Or, (2) take her to the theatre. Give her a general anaesthetic. Make sure you have a competent assistant.

METHOD. Put her into the lithotomy position, with her buttocks hanging well over the edge of the table. Shine a good light on the wound. Clean it and the skin round it thoroughly. Put a large gauze pack with a tape attached to it into her vagina. This will keep the tear free from blood, but be careful that bleeding does not occur above it. Ask your assistant to retract her vaginal wall while you survey the tear.

If the tear goes high up her rectum and vagina (fortunately quite rare), you will find that there is nothing between her rectal mucosa and her vaginal skin. These two must be repaired in separate layers, so first dissect them free from one another. Lower down, her perineal body separates them, so that there is no problem.

Suture her rectal mucosa with interrupted or continuous sutures, starting at the apex of the tear, and tying the knots outside the lumen of her rectum. Use a round-bodied curved needle.

If the tear is very extensive, pick up her prerectal fascia with a second row of sutures. These will reinforce the first layer.

To close her external sphincter ani, look for the torn ends of this muscle. You will find them lying in little pits on each side of her anus. Often, one side is deeply retracted, so that you have to fish for it.

Define the muscle on each side by dipping into the pits with artery forceps. Pull the end of the muscle up, and put artery forceps across it. Do the same the other side. Bring the artery forceps on each side together, and put your little finger into her anus. It should just go in, but be held firmly. If it is not tight, you have not defined the sphincter properly on each side, so fish again. Then insert three catgut sutures through the muscle to exclude the forceps. Don't tie them until you have removed the forceps, as in A, Fig. 18-17. Take a deep bite with the needle laterally, so as to include the fascia surrounding the muscle. Tie the knots without too much tension, or they may tear out. Check that you have not inserted too many sutures, and made her vagina too narrow. You should be able to insert 2 fingers comfortably.

To close her vaginal skin use a single layer of continuous catgut sutures.

To close her levator ani muscles, take deep bites with the needle each side, so as to take a good hold of the muscles and the fascia covering both their surfaces. These thick sheets of muscle and fascia lie deep on each side of her rectum. Begin at the anal end and join them together.

Put in three to five stitches like this. Leave them united until they are all in place. Then tie them with care, so as to avoid excessive tension.

Suture the skin of her anal margin with a few interrupted catgut sutures. Close the skin of her perineum with interrupted monofilament. Put a dry dressing on her wound.

CAUTION ! Don't close her skin and vaginal wall too tight; leave room for drainage, in case she becomes infected or oozes.

POSTOPERATIVELY, keep her on a fluid diet until the third day. If she does not open her bowels by the 4th or 5th day (unusual), give her a small enema. Give her a normal diet from Day 1. Give her liquid paraffin twice daily for two weeks, starting on the third day. Start salt baths from Day 1.

REPAIRING A THIRD-DEGREE TEAR

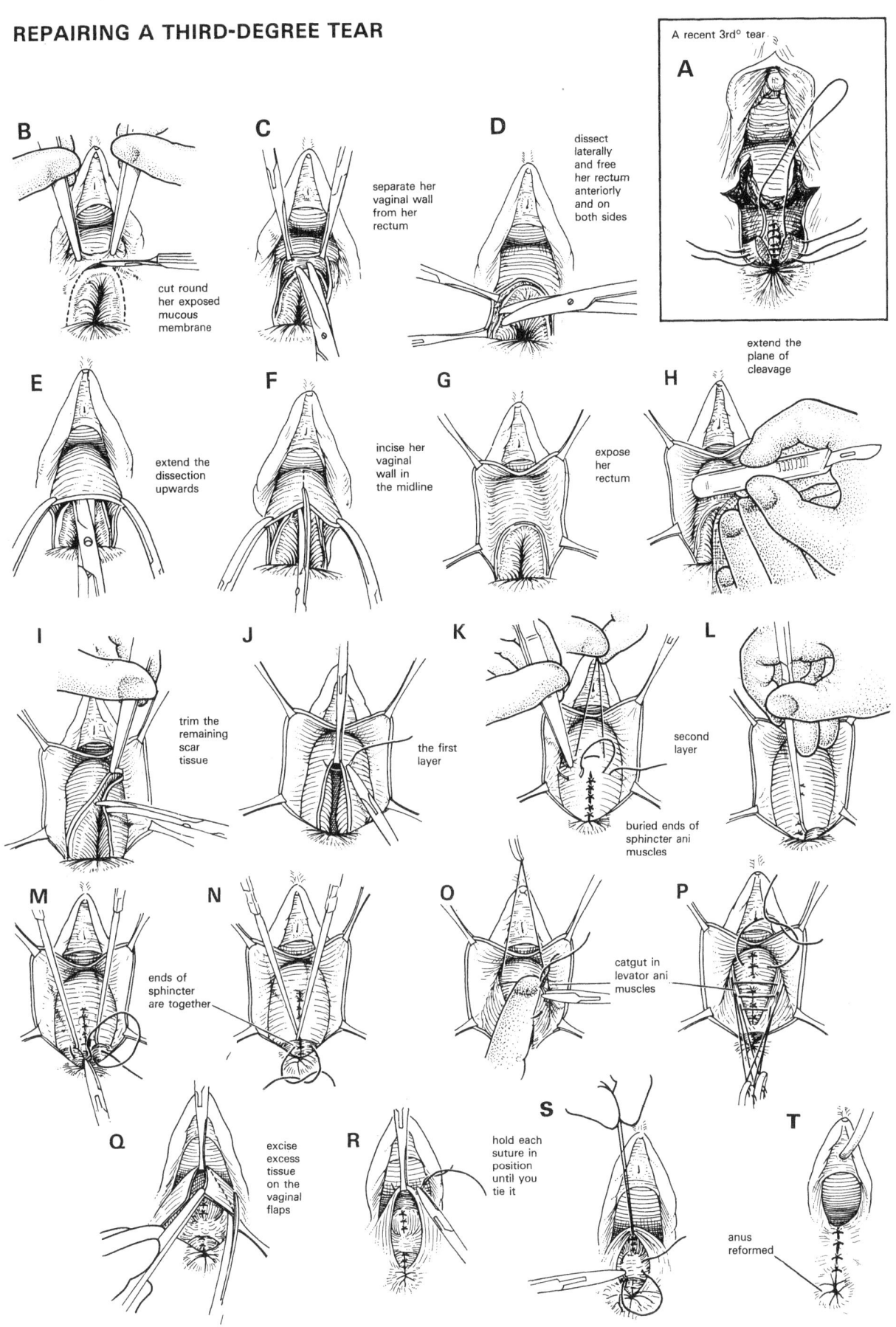

Fig. 18-17 REPAIRING A THIRD-DEGREE TEAR. A, a recent tear, B to T, an old one. *From Parsons and Ulfelder, 'Atlas of Gynaecological Surgery', pp. 259 and 261. W.B. Saunders, with kind permission.*

18.16 Old third-degree tears

If a third-degree tear occurs in hospital, it is usually repaired immediately. If it occurs elsewhere, a patient may present too late for an immediate repair. Or a tear which has been sutured immediately may break down, and need repair later. Sometimes, a tear epithelializes and heals itself. If it is not very extensive, and her levator ani muscles are little damaged, she may not want the operation, and only be incontinent of faeces when her stools are very loose.

AN OLD THIRD-DEGREE TEAR

This is more difficult than the repair of a fresh tear. If possible, refer her. Don't operate for at least three months after delivery, or the last attempt to repair it, because her tissues will still be oedematous and infected.

PREOPERATIVE PREPARATION. Give her a low-roughage diet for 2 days, and then an enema preoperatively.

ANAESTHESIA. Give her a saddle block (A 7.7), or an epidural block (A 7.2), or a general anaesthetic.

INSTRUMENTS. Use those listed in the previous section for a recent tear. A good light, plenty of swabs (she will bleed), an assistant, and a scrub nurse.

METHOD. The patient in B, Fig. 18-17 has torn her perineal body. Cut round her exposed mucous membrane for the full thickness of her vaginal skin. Apply Allis forceps, and use scissors to gently separate her vaginal wall from her rectum (C).

While you exert gentle tension on her vaginal wall, dissect laterally and free her rectum anteriorly and on both sides (D). Apply clamps to the cut edges of her vaginal skin, and hold them downwards. Extend the dissection upwards in the plane of cleavage between her rectum and her vagina, holding your scissors against her posterior vaginal wall (E).

Incise her vaginal wall in the midline (F), to expose her rectum (G). Hold her rectum medially, and use the handle of your scalpel to extend the plane of cleavage between the vaginal flap and her rectal wall (H). If you can mobilize her rectum, you can close it without tension.

Trim the remaining scar tissue from the edge of her rectal mucosa (I). Hold the upper edge of her torn rectum in Allis forceps, and invert its mucosa with a row of fine atraumatic catgut sutures (J). Continue them until you reach the mucocutaneous margin of her anal opening, so as to make her a normal anus.

Reinforce and bury the first layer of sutures with a second layer (K). This will reduce the the size of her rectum, but only temporarily.

Fish for the retracted ends of her sphincter ani muscles, which you will find buried in dimples at either side of her anus. Use hooks (L), or dip in with fairly fine artery forceps. Bring the hooks together to see if you have secured her sphincter (M and N). Bring the ends of her sphincter ani together with at least 3 1/0 catgut sutures.

Place several interrupted sutures in her levator muscles (O and P). When they are all in place, tie and cut them.

Excise any excess tissue on the flaps of her vagina (Q). Bring the raw edges of her vaginal wall together with interrupted catgut sutures (R, and S). Hold each one until the next is in position, and then cut it. When you have closed her vagina, close her perineal skin. The last two or three of these sutures should complete the formation of her anus, so that rugae radiate from it like the spokes of a wheel. If they don't, you have not done the operation as you should.

POSTOPERATIVELY, manage her as for an acute tear (18.15).

18.17 Rupture of the uterus

Uteri can rupture before or during delivery, but in only about two-thirds of cases do you make the diagnosis before you deliver the baby. In the rest you make it afterwards, usually after some difficult obstetric manoeuvre, such as a retained placenta (18.14), or a destructive operation (18.7), or after a trial of scar (18.14).

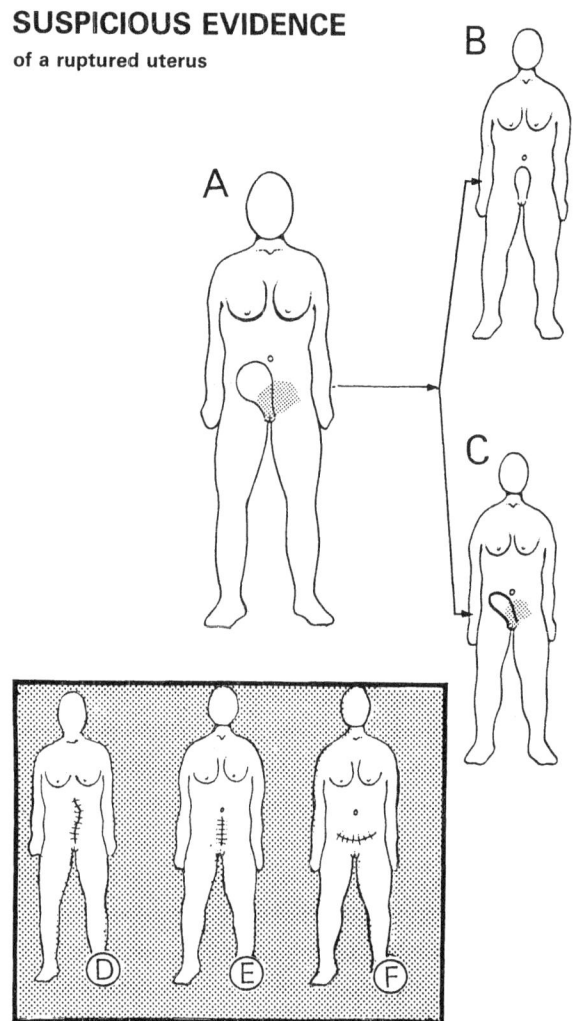

Fig. 18-18 SUSPICIOUS EVIDENCE. If a postpartum patient has a mass contiguous with the uterus (A), which does not disappear on catheterizing the bladder (B), but persists (C), it is probably a haematoma of her broad ligament due to rupture of her uterus. If a previous Caesarean section has left scar D, suspect strongly that it was classical. Scar E, might be either. F, is almost certainly a lower segment scar. *After Nash and Drouin with the kind permission of the Editor of Tropical Doctor*

Here we are mostly concerned with rupture of the uterus before delivery, as a complication of obstructed labour.

Section 18.4 describes the management of obstructed labour. If a mother, particularly a multip, arrives too late, or you do not recognize that she has obstructed, her uterus is likely to rupture. This is a great obstetric disaster. If primary care is really bad in your district, 50% of the mothers referred to you may need an operative delivery, and of these 5% may have ruptured their uteri.

The usual story, which is described in more detail in Sections 18.1 and 18.3, is that a mother is admitted from her village in obstructed labour, having waited a long time in a rural health centre for transport to hospital. She is often sufficiently clear-headed to be able to tell you that she had strong frequent pains which stopped suddenly.

When her uterus ruptures there may be a direct communication between her uterine cavity and her peritoneal cavity (complete rupture), or her peritoneum or her bladder may separate the baby from her peritoneal cavity (incomplete rupture, less common). If her membranes ruptured some time before delivery, the contents of her uterus will be infected, and her uterine muscle bruised and in poor condition for repair.

Never try to deliver a mother with a ruptured uterus vaginally. Aim to: (1) Resuscitate her and operate soon. (2) Remove the baby and the placenta. (3) Control bleeding. (4) Repair or remove her uterus on the indications given below. Unless the rupture is extensive, and her tissues are particularly bruised and oedematous, repairing her uterus is likely to be easier than removing it, because the distortion of her anatomy makes hysterectomy difficult. But even repair is not easy, because the edges of the tear are ragged and not easy to bring together. Hysterectomy takes longer than repair, and causes more bleeding. A subtotal hysterectomy, which leaves her cervix and perhaps part of her lower segment, is easier than a total one; it causes less bleeding, and there is less danger to her ureters. If you have to remove her uterus, try to leave one ovary. The secret of success is to *exert continued traction on her uterus (20.12), and to identify important structures and landmarks before you start to cut or suture them.*

Speed is critical. Most time is lost getting her to the theatre, and in getting it ready, so make sure that it always is ready. *If you are not familiar with the anatomy, study Figures 20-16 and 20-17!*

RUPTURE OF THE UTERUS

DIAGNOSIS. Be aware of impending rupture when labour is obstructed, especially in a multip, and try to prevent it happening by intervening immediately.

Impending rupture: (1) Bandl's ring between the upper and lower segments rises. (2) The lower segment becomes stretched and painful to touch, even between contractions, which increase in strength and duration. (3) The patient becomes anxious and restless, with a rapid pulse and irregular respiration.

Actual rupture: (1) Her uterine contractions stop suddenly and are replaced by no pain (common), or less pain, or severe continuous pain (uncommon). (2) She is shocked and pale before delivery, or she becomes shocked afterwards, and does not repond to transfusion immediately (especially if the placenta is retained). (3) She may bleed from her vagina, sometimes quite severely, sometimes not at all. If the presenting part is jammed in her pelvis no blood can escape from her vagina. In this situation, see if she has a haemoperitoneum by aspirating both her iliac fossae. (4) Her uterus is tender to palpation (it may feel soft, or be permanently tense). Later, her entire abdomen may be tender. (5) The baby may be abnormally difficult to feel (common) or abnormally easy (uncommon). Sometimes, the shape of her uterus changes, and you may be able to feel him outside it (usually his limbs are close under her abdominal wall, a certain sign of rupture). If he is in her broad ligament, you will be unable to feel him. (6) His head may previously have been low in her pelvis, but has now risen higher and may now be no longer palpable vaginally. (7) Bloodstained urine. (8) The absence of a fetal heartbeat, unless the tear is a small one, and he is still in her uterus. (9) The appearance of the placenta at her vulva before he is delivered (uncommon). (10) The prolapse of loops of gut into her vagina (uncommon).

Shock or severe vaginal bleeding may dominate the picture. Her blood pressure is low and her pulse is fast. She is usually lucid, and may even be talkative, which may delude you into thinking she is less ill than she really is.

If she is in obstructed labour, and you are still not sure if she has ruptured her uterus or not, resuscitate her, prepare for laparotomy, give her a general anaesthetic, intubate her, and examine her vaginally in the lithotomy position. The presenting part may have disengaged, so that your hand passes through the rupture into her abdominal cavity, allowing you to feel the inner surface of her abdominal wall. You may find that the presenting part is unexpectedly easy to dislodge, and the attempt to do this is followed by a gush of blood. If it is not easy to dislodge, try to pass a catheter by pushing it up a little vaginally. If this fails, stop for fear of damaging her urethra. Pass your fingers anterior to the presenting part, into her uterus and feel for a rupture. If there is one, you will feel the inner surface of her abdominal wall. If there is no rupture, deliver her vaginally (18.7).

CAUTION ! (1) Dramatic symptoms of rupture are uncommon. (2) If you are about to attempt a vaginal delivery, but have any suspicion that her uterus may have ruptured, take her to the theatre. Be prepared to give her a general anaesthetic and to do a laparotomy, if necessary.

DIFFERENTIAL DIAGNOSIS. Rupture of the uterus is not the only cause of collapse during an obstructed labour, it can also

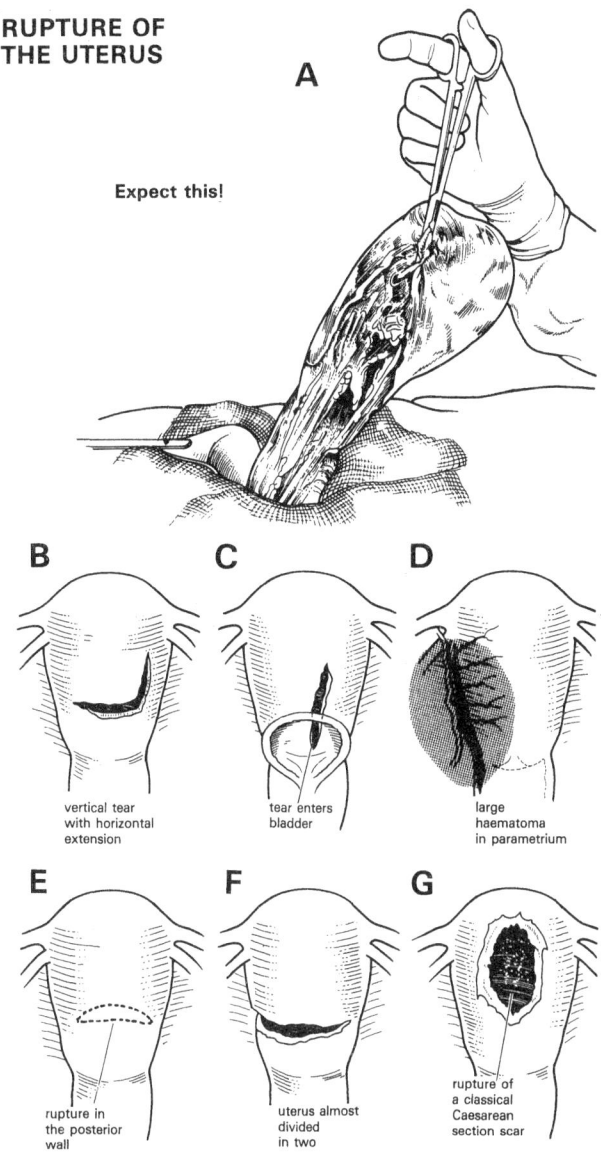

Fig. 18-19 RUPTURE OF THE UTERUS. A, a ruptured uterus may look like this. B, a tear in the anterior wall with a vertical extension at one end. C, a tear involving the bladder. D, a tear in the lateral wall opening into the broad ligament. E, a transverse tear in the posterior wall. F, a tear which almost detaches the uterus. G, the tear from a classical Caesarean section.

be due to septic shock (53.4), electrolyte imbalance, or dehydration (A 15.3) or:

Suggesting abruption with a massive concealed haemorrhage but no rupture—a tense, tender uterus. The important sign of abruption is a closed or nearly closed cervix—it is always open in obstructed labour.

CAUTION ! Beware of diagnosing abruption in a patient with a previous Caesarean section. Rupture is much more likely, even if she has not been in labour long.

RESUSCITATION. Do this vigorously in the theatre or the labour ward. Internal jugular or subclavian puncture (A 15.2) is better than a cut down. Give her at least a litre of 0.9% saline before anaesthesia starts, and 100 mmol of sodium bicarbonate to correct her acidosis. Operate as soon as you can, don't wait too long; adequate resuscitation is impossible if she is still bleeding inside. Continue to resuscitate her while you operate. Put up two drips, one for saline or Ringer's lactate given fast, and the other for blood (53.2, A 16.7).

If she is sufficiently conscious to understand, explain that you would like to tie her tubes. If she is not fit enough to understand, her relatives will. It is seldom necessary to tie tubes without permission. As a general rule, no woman who has had a ruptured uterus should ever become pregnant again (see below). The only exception is an extraperitoneal (partial) rupture through a lower segment scar.

CAUTION ! Don't try to deliver the baby before she is resuscitated, because this will remove his tamponading effect, increase shock, and perhaps extend the tear.

PERIOPERATIVE ANTIBIOTICS. Start these (2.9). Avoid gentamicin before anaesthesia (A 14.3).

EQUIPMENT. A 'Caesar set' and some large curved clamps or artery forceps. You will need a scrubbed second assistant, besides the scrub nurse, the anaesthetist, and a 'runner'.

ANAESTHESIA. Pass a nasogastric tube, aspirate her stomach, and instil 30 ml of magnesium trisilicate. (1) If you give her a general anaesthetic, intubate her under cricoid pressure (A 16.7). (2) If her condition is poor, local infiltration anaesthesia will be safest (A 6.9). (3) A ketamine drip (8.3). Avoid subarachnoid or epidural anaesthesia, because she is already hypotensive.

EXPLORATION FOR RUPTURE OF THE UTERUS

Clip or shave her, wash her abdomen, and pass a catheter. This will prevent you mistakenly opening a high full bladder. Make a low midline or paramedian incision (9.2), and insert a self-retaining retractor.

You will see blood, and a tear in her uterus. Her dead baby (common) and the placenta (sometimes) may be in her peritoneal cavity. If the placenta is still attached to her uterus, he may be alive (rare), even if he is lying free in her peritoneal cavity. If it is detached, he will be dead, wherever he is.

If he is lying free in her peritoneal cavity, the rupture is complete. Remove him.

If he is in her broad ligament, open it. This is most easily done by dividing the round ligament over it.

If he is still in her uterus, as with a posterior rupture, deliver him through a transverse incision in the lower segment, as for Caesarean section.

Suck out blood and liquor. There may be bleeding, or this may have stopped, especially if the tear is transverse across the vessels.

If you have not already given her ergometrine, give it as soon as he is delivered. Lower the head of the table and pack off her gut.

Deliver the empty uterus into the wound and inspect it, especially its posterior wall—there may be a second tear. Find the edges of the tear along its whole length. Divide her round ligament if this makes the tear easier to see.

The tear may: (1) Be in the anterior wall of her uterus, often with a vertical extension at one end, making it L-shaped (B, in Fig. 18-19). (2) Extend into her bladder (C). (3) Extend longitudinally, along the lateral wall of her lower segment, from her fundus to her vagina, opening up her broad ligament and involving a uterine artery (D). Tears of this kind are more common on the left. (4) Extend transversely across the posterior wall of her uterus (E, rare). (5) Detach the uterus almost completely (F, rare). (6) Be in the upper segment through the scar of an old classical Caesarean section (G). Often, one of her uterine pedicles is torn across.

Feel for the placenta and detach it from her uterus with your fingers. Use swabs on a holder to remove as much of the membranes as you can.

Control bleeding from her uterus with No. 2 chromic catgut. Or, clamp the edges of the tear with several pairs of Green Armytage forceps. Control bleeding from her broad ligament temporarily with pressure from a pack. If she has an extensive haematoma tracking up from the torn vessels on one side towards her kidney, evacuate it and tie them.

REPAIR OR HYSTERECTOMY? The indications depend on: (1) The nature and extent of the rupture. (2) Your experience.

If you are inexperienced, only do a hysterectomy if repair seems very difficult.

If you have some hysterectomy experience, factors favouring a repair are: (1) A rupture which is not too large. (2) A rupture with clean edges which are easy to see and are not too oedematous. (3) Little or no infection. Factors favouring a hysterectomy are: (1) Extensive or multiple tears. (2) Edges which are very bruised and oedematous and not easy to define, especially some posterior ruptures, or ruptures extending down into her vagina. (3) Gross infection of her uterus.

THE REPAIR OF A RUPTURED UTERUS

Start by defining the position of her uterine pedicles, her ovarian pedicles, and her round ligaments.

If the tear extends into her cervix or lower segment, reflect her bladder as for a lower segment Caesarean section. *Avoid her ureter.* Ask your assistant to pull her uterus forwards and to the other side. Lift her tube and ovary, so as to make her infundibulopelvic ligament, which carries her ovarian vessels, taut. Put your thumb and index finger on either side of this ligament, and slide them down. Feel for her ureter as a hard round cord near her pelvic brim. From there trace it down to the injured area. See also Fig. 20-16.

Remove all clot. If she bleeds a little, disregard it. If she bleeds much, apply haemostats or transfixion sutures.

CAUTION ! (1) Be sure to keep her bladder well away from the edges of the tear. (2) Don't excise any tissue unless it is obviously dead.

Start at the apex of the tear; if convenient hold it with a stay suture. Suture it as for Caesarean section, using 2 layers of continuous catgut in a large half-circle round-bodied needle (size '2' or '3'). You can suture a vertical tear going down to the cervix from below upwards, but sometimes the other way round is easier. Traction on the suture will help to bring the lower end into view. Don't worry if the inner layer has to be placed inside her uterus. Make the second layer an inverting continuous suture. If necessary, use extra sutures to close off the corners, or repair her vagina (usually anteriorly).

If the rupture is lateral and has extended into her broad ligament, open its peritoneal roof, and tie the bleeding vessels. Control any oozing with under-running stitches. *Avoid her ureter.* With one finger inside her broad ligament and another behind it, feel for her ureter; if necessary, pass a tape under it to keep it out of the way. Start at the apex and work downwards. Exert traction on the running suture to expose the depths of the tear. Stop before you reach the lower edge, so as to leave room for a drain from her broad ligament into her vagina. If there is much oozing, pack her broad ligament with a gauze bandage, bring it out of her vagina, and close the visceral peritoneum over it. Remove the pack 12 hours later.

HYSTERECTOMY FOR A RUPTURED UTERUS

The following description differs from that in Section 20.12, and is modified for rupture of the uterus. Consult the illustrations in that chapter, and particularly the account of the anatomy of the ureters, vessels, and ligaments. Hysterectomy may be surprisingly easy when the tear is extensive and transverse, and the uterus almost completely detached.

INDICATIONS. (1) Complicated rupture of the uterus (also see above). (2) Postpartum haemorrhage, which is not responding to treatment, and when tying the internal iliac arteries (3.5) has failed to control bleeding.

METHOD. Remove the baby and the placenta and clean away most of the blood and liquor. Insert a self-retaining retractor, and lift her uterus from her abdomen. Maintain traction on it with one hand, or insert a traction suture.

Start by identifying: her uterus and round ligaments, her tubes and ovaries on both sides, her infundopelvic ligaments, the avascular area in each of her broad ligaments, her lower segment, her rectum, and especially her ureters. You will find this difficult, because of the size of her uterus, and the disturbance to her normal anatomy caused by bruising and oedema, both near the tear, and far from it.

Deflect her bladder, and trace her ureters over the whole length of the operative field as described above (20-16). Find where they are in relation to the tear, in the distal part of their course.

You will have difficulty deciding where her uterus ends and her vagina begins. Feel for a small ridge of tissue (the remains of her cervix) on the 'inside'—but even this may be absent. If you are still not sure, it will merely mean that you will not know if you have done a total or a subtotal hysterectomy. In view of her present state, this hardly matters.

Find the tear and clamp the obvious bleeding points. Pull her uterus to the left, and divide her right round ligament between clamps about 2 cm from it. This will open the anterior

ANATOMY FOR HYSTERECTOMY

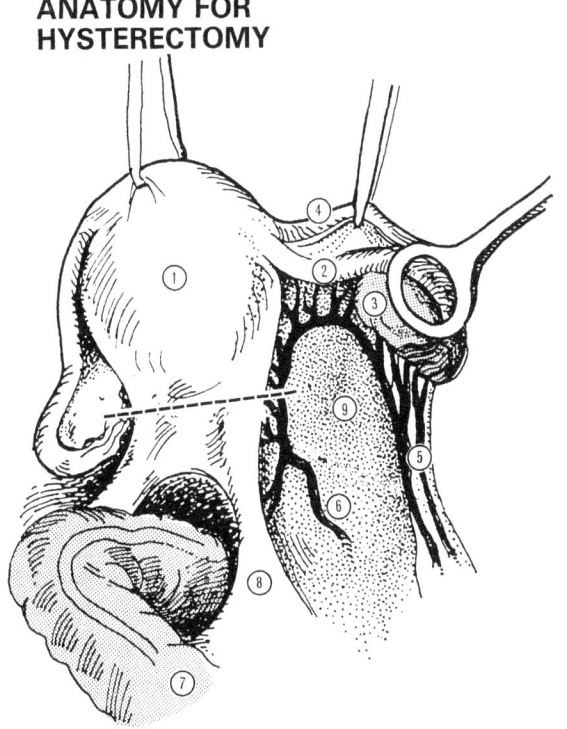

Fig. 18-20 ANATOMY FOR EMERGENCY HYSTERECTOMY. The patient's uterus seen from behind before hysterectomy. It is tilted to the left and her adnexa (ovary and tube) have been lifted up to show them more clearly. For simplicity the tear is not shown.
 1, the body of her uterus. 2, her right Fallopian tube. 3, her ovary. 4, her round ligament. 5, her ovarian vessels running in her infundibulopelvic ligament which is being stretched. 6, her uterine vessels. 7, her rectum. 8, her sacrouterine ligament. 9, the avascular area in her broad ligament. *Kindly contributed by Frits Driessen.*

peritoneal leaf of her broad ligament. Enlarge this opening down towards her bladder. Lift her right tube and ovary with one hand, and push a finger of your other hand from behind through the avascular area in her broad ligament.

CAUTION ! Leave her ovary and tube in place on one or both sides.

On the side on which you will remove her ovary, clamp her infundopelvic ligament between two artery forceps and cut it. On the other side, to retain her tube and ovary, clamp and divide her tube and her ovarian ligament near her uterus. If they are very thick and vascular, you may have to clamp and cut them in two steps.

Transfix the pedicles of her round ligaments and infundibulopelvic ligaments with '2' multifilament or chromic catgut.

Using the clamps that you have already applied, pull her uterus well up in the midline, and cut the peritoneum between her uterus and her bladder. Extend the incision laterally to meet the incisions you have made in the anterior leaves of her broad ligaments.

Push her bladder off her lower segment for 2 or 3 cm with a swab on a holder. Pushing it further down can cause bleeding. If the rupture is anterior, put its edge on the stretch before you separate off her bladder.

Now expose the back of her lower segment by pulling her uterus forwards over her symphysis pubis. Divide the peritoneum over the back of her lower segment at the same level as you did anteriorly. Extend the incisions laterally to join the openings in her broad ligament. Push the lower flap of peritoneum off her lower segment with a swab on a holder; or, if this is difficult, cut it loose with scissors.

On either side of her uterus there will now be a bundle of loose connective tissue containing her uterine vessels. If necessary strip down the peritoneum of her broad ligaments to see them more clearly.

Pull her uterus to the right and clamp her uterine vessels with strong Kocher forceps, just above the level where her bladder is still attached to her lower segment.

CAUTION ! Make sure the points of the forceps are close to her uterus.

Place a second clamp inside the first, and cut her uterine vessels between them. Tie and transfix the pedicle. Use a double transfixion ligature because of its width.

Do the same thing on the other side.

Excise her uterus through its lower segment, just above the level of her cut uterine vessels. Have artery forceps ready to pick up the cut edge of her lower segment, before it disappears in the depth of her pelvis. Clamp any bleeding vessels.

If the tear extends across her lower segment, it will probably serve as the 'line of cutting' to remove her uterus. Examine the edge and remove any very oedematous and bruised tissue, again checking the position of her ureters first.

If there is a downward tear in her cervix, repair this now, after making sure that her bladder and ureters are well out of the way. Alternatively, do a total hysterectomy, and remove her cervix.

Suture the anterior and posterior walls of her lower segment with figure of eight stitches, being sure to include the angles on each side, because these bleed. If there are signs of infection, leave the centre open so that you can insert a drain; otherwise close it.

Her pelvis should now be nearly dry. Tie any remaining bleeders.

If her broad ligaments are oozing, place a drain near them and bring it out through her vagina.

Close her pelvic peritoneum with a continuous suture. Start on the left at the pedicle of her infundopelvic ligament, and suture the anterior edge of her peritoneum to the posterior edge, placing all vascular pedicles under it. Let her remaining ovary and tube hang freely in her pelvis.

CLOSING HER ABDOMEN (after hysterectomy or repair)

Always tie her tubes after a repair, unless you have repaired a lower segment Caesarean scar, and she is likely to return for an elective section at the start of her next labour.

If her condition is unstable, close her abdomen without delay. If it is stable search for additional injuries, especially to her bladder.

Clean and wash her peritoneum with at least two litres of warm saline. Instill 1 g of tetracycline in 1000 ml of warm saline (2.9). Close it with No. 0 or 2/0 catgut. Close her abdominal wall as usual. Monitor her haemoglobin. 'Suck and drip' her (9.9, A 15.5). Keep a catheter in her bladder until her condition is satisfactory, and monitor her urine output carefully: it should be at least 1 ml/kg/hour (A 15.5). If she has a postoperative diuresis, usually at 24 to 48 hours, be sure to give her potassium (A 15.5, 9.9).

Watch for anuria (53.3), respiratory complications (9.11), peritonitis (6.2), and peritoneal abscesses (6.3). Remember her nutrition; if there are no signs of peritonitis, start feeding her orally with a high-energy high-protein mixture as soon as her bowel function allows it, a few days after the operation (58.11). If there are no complications this can usually start on the 3rd postoperative day.

DIFFICULTIES WITH RUPTURE OF THE UTERUS

If her BLADDER IS TORN, its wall near the opening is usually stuck to her lower segment, and needs mobilizing before you can repair it. You may find that her bladder is so torn that it lies flat like a handkerchief.

Use Allis' forceps or Babcock clamps to stretch the wall of her bladder and her lower segment. Suck away the blood. Separate her bladder from her lower segment with a 'swab on a stick', or with scissors. Gently dissect it off the lower segment, taking care not to make the tear any bigger. Free the bladder wall round the opening for 1 or 2 cm.

Close the opening in her bladder with two layers of 2/0 continuous catgut. Put the first layer through the full thickness of her bladder wall, but just submucosal if possible. If this is difficult, include the mucosa. Use the second layer to invert the first one. Insert an indwelling catheter and maintain *open* drainage (an unspigoted catheter) for 10 to 14 days. Unfortunately, complete closure of the bladder is often impossible; its edges are usually thin and necrotic, so that a fistula follows.

If complete CLOSURE OF HER TORN BLADDER IS IMPOSSIBLE, because there is much presure necrosis, or the opening extends far down into her urethra, you may have to close her bladder over a wide-bore suprapubic tube. If she develops a vesico-uterine fistula, repair it later, or refer her to have it repaired.

If you think that you have CAUGHT HER URETER in a suture, unpick it; usually there is no permanent harm. Alternatively, open her bladder and cannulate it. If severe damage is confirmed, the only way to preserve the function of her kidney is to reanastomose it over a splint, or to reimplant it in her bladder. An intravenous injection of methylene blue or indigo carmine may help to show leaks in her ureter (18.10).

If she is ANAEMIC after delivery with a BOGGY PELVIC SWELLING and deviation of her uterus, she probably has a PELVIC HAEMATOMA. This is really a rupture of her uterus which has bled into her broad ligament instead of into her peritoneal cavity. If you see her <24 hours after delivery, do a laparotomy and explore and repair her rupture. If you see her >24 hours after delivery and she is stable, treat her non-operatively in the hope that her haematoma will resolve.

18.18 Vesicovaginal fistulae (VVFs)

Fistulae between the bladder and the vagina are the most exacting gynaecological problem in the developing world. Some hospitals in Northern Nigeria have waiting lists of more than 600 patients, most of whom will never be treated. They were once equally common in Europe.

In the developing world VVFs are usually the result of obstructed labour in a young primigravida (18.3), and less often of a traumatic vaginal delivery (particularly with Kielland's forceps), of unskilled Caesarean section, or of rupture of the uterus into the bladder, especially through the scar of a previous section. They can occur: (1) Near the cervix (juxta-cervical). (2) In the middle of the vagina. (3) Near the urethra (juxta-urethral). (4) As a massive combination of the first three. (5) In the vault of the vagina as the result of vaginal surgery. Wherever the patient's fistula, she usually thinks she is incurable, and, as it does not kill her, she is likely to endure great misery for a long time, especially if she is very young (16 is the average age in Northern Nigeria). She may have lain at home for weeks in a pitiable emaciated state with contractures and bed-sores from lying curled up on her side, expecting to be returned to her parents and divorced by her husband.

Fistulae have the reputation of being almost impossibly difficult to repair. One contributor believes that there is no such thing as an 'easy' VVF, and that only the occasional generalist with 'golden fingers' can do them. Nevertheless, in one district hospital (Chogoria in Kenya) 15 VVFs were successfully repaired without any failures by a succession of general-duty doctors, all working 'from the book', and with no individual doctor doing more than two. So *if you cannot refer VVFs*, you may be justified in attempting to repair the smaller, less difficult ones, which do not involve a patient's urethra. If you succeed, she will be immensely grateful. If you get a reputation for repairing them well, patients will come to you from a long way away. As always, learn from an expert, if you can. *These are very rewarding patients!*

Most VVFs are due to pressure of the child's head during a prolonged labour. The best time to repair them is about 6 to 8 weeks after delivery (one contributor waits 12 weeks), when the slough has separated and the tissues are no longer friable, but before they have had time to become fibrotic. If a patient presents later than this, fibrosis makes the operation much more difficult. As soon as you diagnose a new VVF, keep the patient in hospital and give her salt baths two or three times a day to keep the wound clean.

These fistulae can be repaired abdominally through the bladder, but we only describe the vaginal route. Aim to incise round the edges of the fistula, and free three planes—her vaginal mucosa, her bladder mucosa, and if possible a layer of tissue in between them—if you can define it. If you can sew up these layers separately, you will probably cure her fistula. See also *Primary Mother Care* Section 24.3, and the reference below:

Lawson JB, and Harrison K, 'Obstetrics and Gynaecology in the Tropics'. Edward Arnold. Second edition, expected 1989.

VESICOVAGINAL FISTULAE

ASSESSING THE FISTULA is best done 1 to 3 days before the repair, so that you know what to expect and are not obliged to repair a patient immediately after you have assessed her. Explain that you are only going to examine her. If you find that her tissues are not in an ideal state, examine her again later. If they are suitable for operation, anaesthetize her for examination only, and put her into the lithotomy position. You will be able to see large and medium-sized fistulae with a speculum and a catheter. If you have difficulty finding a smaller one, infuse a coloured fluid, such as dilute methylene blue, into her bladder with a catheter and a funnel. Stress incontinence is the main differential diagnosis.

(1) How big is the fistula? (2) How far it is from her urethral orifice? (3) What is the state of the surrounding tissues? Are they soft and friable, or soft and healthy? Mildly, or severely fibrosed? (4) Is her urethra stenosed or obstructed? (5) Is her vagina narrowed, or almost obliterated by scar tissue? (6) Does she seems to have 'lost her urethra'? See Section 20.14.

INDICATIONS FOR BEGINNERS. If you are a beginner, *and you cannot refer her,* only operate if her fistula is: (1) Less than 1 cm in diameter. (2) More than 2.5 cm from her urethral meatus. (3) Not significantly fibrosed. Otherwise, you are unlikely to succeed until you are much more experienced.

PREPARATION. She may well be malnourished, anaemic, tuberculous, or have some chronic bowel disease. Her urinary leak may have caused an ammoniacal dermatitis which has ulcerated. So be sure to restore her general health and make her as fit as you can before you operate. Build up her morale and enthuse your ward and theatre team. If possible, admit her next to a patient who has just had a successful repair.

POSITION. This is critical and depends on the skill of your anaesthetist, and your personal preferences as to which way you like to operate. (1) If your anaesthetist is skilled, you can lie her on her front, her thighs abducted as far as possible, and her legs supported in double lithotomy stirrups, as in Fig. 18-21.

REPAIRING A VVF

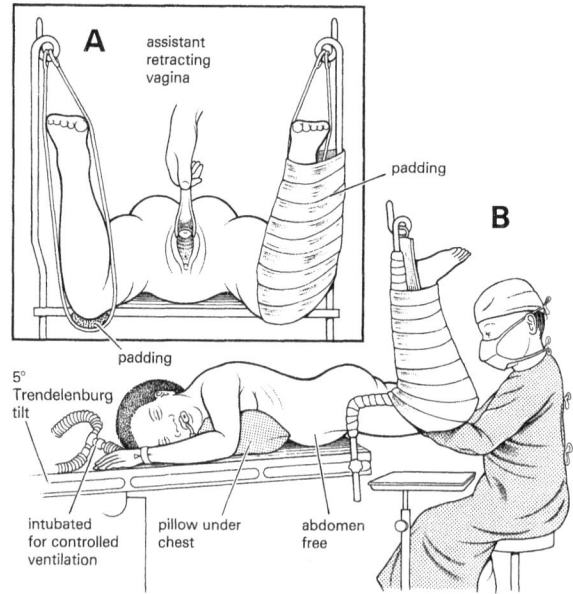

Fig. 18-21 REPAIRING A VVF. Note the way in which the patient's legs are held, and how the supports are padded. There is a pillow under her chest, her abdomen is free, she has been intubated, and the table has a 5° head-down tilt. It can be more steeply tilted (20°) and her legs slightly more flexed than this.

Bandage her legs to the poles, have her buttocks clear of the table, and an overtable just below her. Tilt her 5° head-down, and raise the table to a convenient height to let you see into her vagina. One contributor tilts the table at 20° and slightly flexes her thighs over the end of the table so as to stop her slipping down. This is not an easy position to arrange on many theatre tables. (2) If your anaesthetist is less skilled, operate on her while she is lying on her back in the exaggerated lithotomy position, with a steep (30°) head-down tilt, her buttocks well over the edge of the table, and her shoulders supported by shoulder rests. This is more difficult, and is like working on the sump of a car without a pit. But it is not too difficult—if you get the table high enough with plenty of head-down tilt. Gynaecologists soon get used to it.

ANAESTHESIA. If she is lying prone, use general anaesthesia, intubate her, use relaxants, and control her ventilation. Put a pillow under her chest, and another smaller one under her pubis; make sure that her abdomen is free. Don't rely on spontaneous ventilation, because she will not ventilate adequately.

CAUTION ! No patient should lie prone under general anaesthesia, and be expected to breathe spontaneously. Hypoxia, cardiac arrest, brain damage, and death may follow.

Add a 1 mg ampoule of 1/1000 adrenalin to 100 ml of saline. You will need 10 to 25 ml or more of this solution to infiltrate the tissues round her fistula. It will show up her tissue planes and reduce bleeding.

BLOOD. Cross-match two units.

EQUIPMENT. A knife with a curved No. 12 blade, an ordinary No.10 blade. Sims' specula. Langenbach retractors. Fine 16 cm dissecting forceps, toothed and plain. 12 cm fine curved artery forceps. Two vulsellum forceps. A pair of 20 cm light curved scissors. Two standard needle-holders. A 14 to 16 Ch catheter. A funnel for the catheter. A good sucker, two fine ends for it, and a probe to clear them.

ASSISTANTS. You will need three. (1) An assistant on the right side of the table (viewed from your end), at the level of her abdomen, to hold up her posterior vaginal wall with a Sims' speculum, using both his hands, and resting them against her sacrum if necessary. (2) An assistant immediately on your right. (3) An assistant on your left, with the trolley, to hand you the instruments.

REPAIRING AN EASIER VVF

If her fistula is high in her vagina, near her cervix, it is usually easier to suture the first layer transversely, as in Fig. 18-22 and the description below. If it is low (juxta-urethral) near her vesico-urethral junction, suture it longitudinally, as in Fig. 18-22a. Provided she still has a centimetre or two of good urethra, you can repair quite a low fistula.

Place an ordinary Jacques rubber catheter in her urethra, to make sure that you don't close it by mistake. Distend the layer between her vaginal wall, and her bladder, with adrenalin in saline.

Open the fistula at its margin, as near as possible to the place where her bladder and her vagina meet. If necessary, cut within her vaginal epithelium.

If you cannot see the edges of her fistula, pull downwards with a vulsellum forceps applied to the vaginal wall covering her urethra.

Use a scalpel with a No. 12 blade to open up the layer between her vagina and her bladder, keeping near to her vagina. Extend the separation with scissors, using sharp and blunt dissection, until you have separated a good margin, say 1 cm towards her cervix, and 0.5 cm laterally and towards her urethra. This may be difficult, and you may have to cut with the No. 12 blade.

Try to define and dissect an intermediate layer of tissue (her precervical or pubovesical fascia), by separating it from her bladder wall. This may be difficult, if her fistula is large and fibrotic. One contributor considers the separation of an intermediate layer impractical.

She may bleed. If you can suck the blood away adequately, and it does not obscure your vision, accept it. Bleeding will probably stop. If necessary, use a transfixion suture. Avoid diathermy, especially near the walls of her vagina and bladder, because it destroys tissue, and reduces the blood supply.

Suture her bladder, starting at each end and working towards the middle. Using '0' catgut on a 5/8-circle atraumatic needle,

AN EASIER VVF

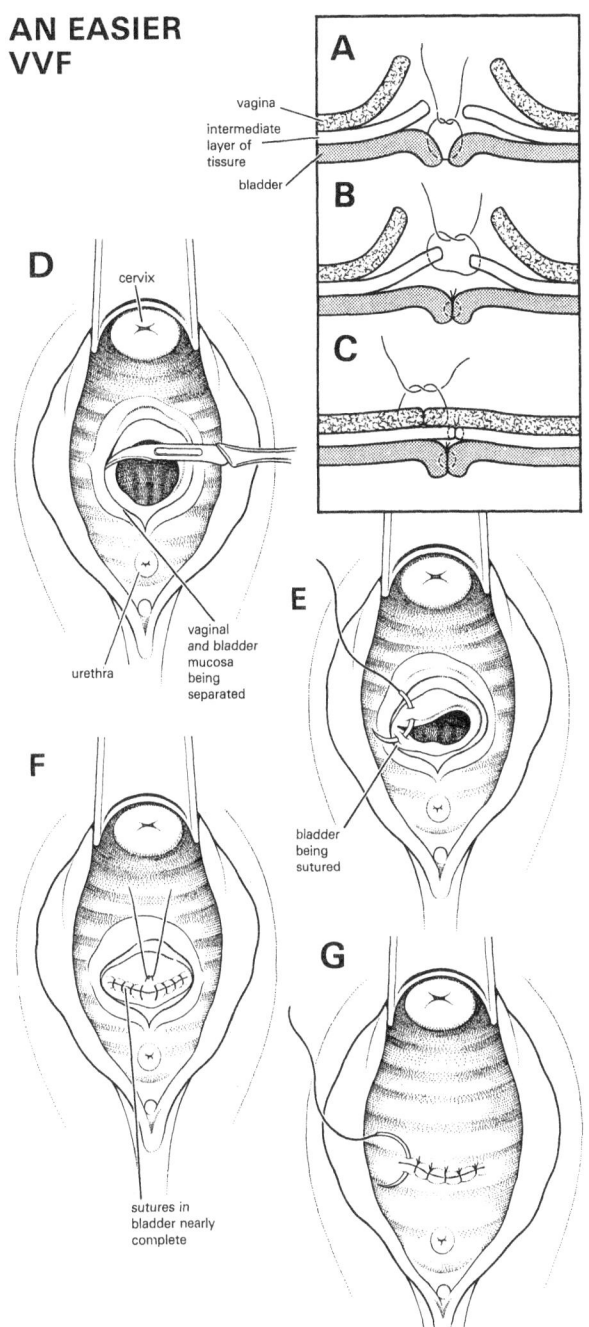

Fig. 18-22 AN EASIER VVF. The patient is lying prone, as in the previous figure. A, the three layers of tissue round her fistula have been separated; the deepest bladder layer is being sutured. B, the intermediate layer is being sutured. C, her vagina is being sutured. Separate the vaginal and bladder layers for at least 0.5 cm. The tissue between them forms an intermediate layer. D, opening the fistula at its margin, as near as possible to the place where her bladder and her vagina meet. E, starting to sew up her bladder. F, her bladder has been sutured, and the sutures from each direction are now about to be tied. G, the intermediate layer has been sutured, and so has the superficial layer. Note that she is prone.

place continuous or interrupted sutures about 3 mm apart. If the fistula is high in her vagina near her cervix (juxta-cervical) it is usually easier to suture the first layer transversely. If it is juxta-urethral, the first layer is best sutured longitudinally.

Check the patency of the repair you have just done by instilling coloured fluid into her bladder. If it leaks, insert more sutures, or take them out and start again.

For the following two layers use reliable '0' slowly absorbed sutures— polyglycolic acid ('Vicryl', best or 'Dexon')—or failing these chromic catgut. Close the intermediate layer (if you have been able to define it) with interrupted sutures, and

A DISTAL VVF

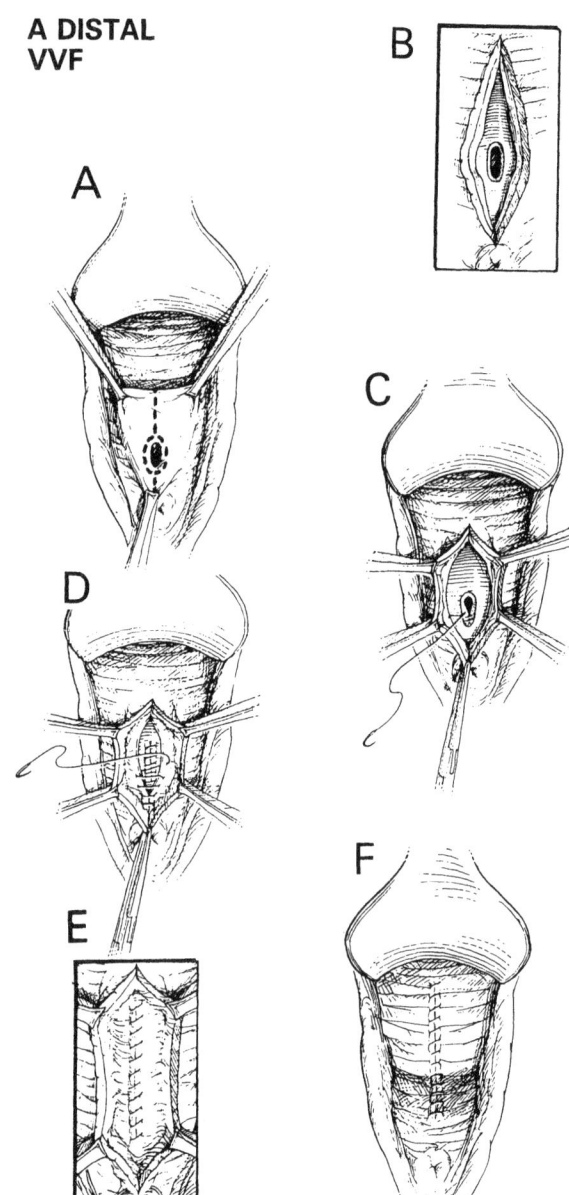

Fig 18-22a REPAIRING A DISTAL (juxta-urethral) VESICOVAGINAL FISTULA at the junction of the bladder and urethra. A, mobilize and excise the fistula track. B, the track excised. C, the fistula is low in the vagina, so it is being closed longitudinally in three layers. D, mobilizing and closing the precervical fascia. E, closure of the precervical fascia is complete. F, the vaginal wall has been closed. *After Poldratz KC, the Mayo Foundation. Permission requested.*

SECURING A CATHETER IN THE BLADDER

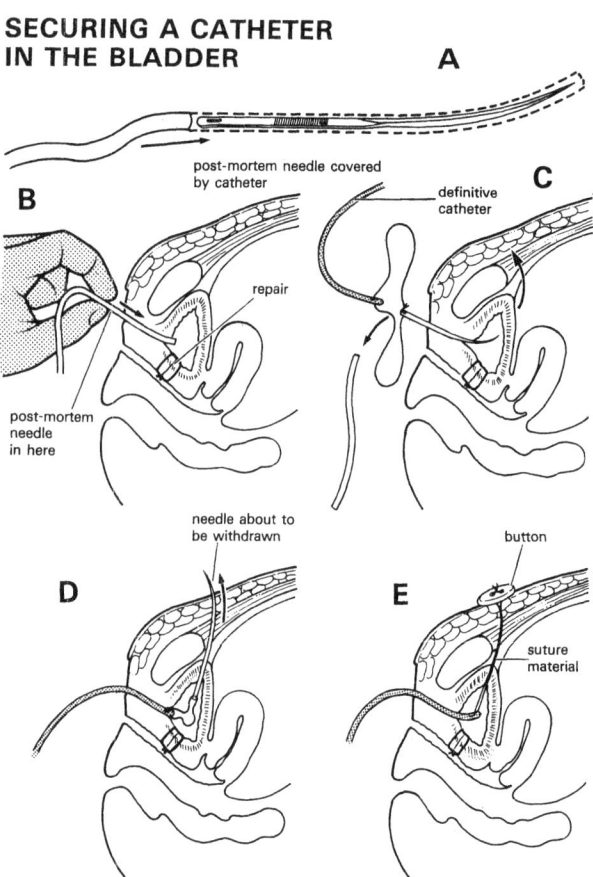

Fig. 18-23 SECURING A CATHETER IN THE BLADDER. The purpose of this procedure is to hold a catheter in the bladder, without its pressing on the site of the repair of a VVF. A, covering a post-mortem needle with a catheter. B, introducing the catheter into the bladder. C, the needle in the urethra, the ensheathing catheter removed, and the definitive catheter being tied to the needle. D, the needle being pushed through the abdominal wall. E, the catheter secured with a suture and button.

Push a piece of plastic tubing, or a catheter with its distal end cut off, over a curved post-mortem needle, so that the point of the needle is protected inside the catheter. Introduce this protected needle through her urethra into her bladder. Remove the catheter, leaving the needle in place. Then, using No. 2 monofilament, tie the catheter which is to be used for drainage to the eye of the needle, leaving a length of 12 cm or more free.

Push the needle through her tissues, so that it emerges through her anterior abdominal wall, just above her symphysis pubis. Pull it through with the suture following, so that the end of the catheter lies in her bladder. Tie the suture emerging from her abdominal wall over a button. The catheter should lie freely in her bladder, and not against its wall, and yet not be so loose that it can be pulled out.

POSTOPERATIVE CARE FOR A VVF

Drain her bladder continuously for 10 (or 12) days. Ideally, use a bag with a non-return valve. Ask the nurses to empty this hourly and sign the chart to make sure that it has been emptied. *If the catheter blocks, the repair is in danger of breaking down.* It is in the greatest danger of doing so between the 5th and the 8th day. On day 11 spigot and release the catheter 2-hourly. On day 12 do it 4-hourly. If this is satisfactory, remove the catheter and for a day or two check that she passes urine normally.

If she leaks, examine her on a couch in the left lateral position, to find out if urine is coming from the fistula, or from her urethra.

If she leaks from her urethra, **this may be because it has been dilated by the catheter.** If so, send her home to return in 6 weeks. This urethral incompetence may settle spontaneously. If she is no better, a urethroplasty may be indicated; refer her.

If she leaks through the fistula, **continue to drain her bladder for 20 days.** It may still close, but this is not very likely. If it does

eliminate all dead space. Close her vaginal wall with interrupted sutures. If possible, place the line of sutures transversely. Otherwise place it whichever way the edges lie easiest. Try to arrange the sutures on the three layers so that they don't immediately overlie one another. Check again that the repair does not leak.

CAUTION ! (1) Don't use non-absorbable sutures. (2) Obliterate all dead space. (3) With larger fistulae take care to avoid her ureters.

Close the intermediate layer (if you have been able to define it) with interrupted sutures, and eliminate all dead space.

Close her vaginal wall with interrupted sutures. If possible, place the line of sutures transversely. Otherwise place it whichever way the edges lie easiest. Check again that the repair does not leak.

INSERTING THE CATHETER. A bladder drain is required, which will not press on the repair, as a Foley catheter might, and will not slip out, as would a simple Jacques catheter. Use a big curved post-mortem needle to insert one in the following way.

not close in 20 days, remove the catheter, start salt baths again, and reassess her in 2 to 4 weeks. If you cannot refer her, and think you might succeed, try to repair her fistula again, about two months after the original operation. In most series of repairs for large VVFs, about 80% succeed the first time; 50% of the remainder heal the second time when the fistula is much smaller. Marion Sims, the pioneer of these repairs, succeeded for the first time on his thirteenth attempt!

If possible, culture her urine just before you remove the catheter, and if it is infected, give her a 5- to 7-day course of the appropriate antibiotic.

Warn her that if she becomes pregnant again she must have a Caesarean section, her repair may break down and a second attempt at repair will be more difficult.

For difficulties with fistulae, see Sections 18.10, and 18.19D.

18.19 Rectovaginal fistulae (RVFs)

Fistulae between the rectum and the vagina (RVFs) are less common than those between the bladder and the vagina (VVFs). When a patient has a large VVF, she often has an RVF too, because both fistulae are caused in the same way—by pressure from the presenting part during a neglected obstructed labour. This causes the adjacent rectal and vaginal walls to necrose; as they heal they unite to form a fistula.

The diagnosis is obvious—faeces start to leak through a patient's vagina 2 to 4 days after an obstructed labour, as necrotic tissue starts to separate. To distinguish an RVF from a third-degree tear, clean away her faeces, and look at her perineum. Closing an RVF can be very difficult, because it is so difficult to get at. If you have not repaired one before, make your decision to do so in her best interests. How difficult will it be to repair her, or to refer her? If you cannot refer her, you may have to try to repair her yourself. Unless someone repairs her fistula, she will have to remain with a permanent colostomy.

RECTOVAGINAL FISTULAE

Keep the patient in hospital, and give her salt baths three times a day. *If possible refer her.* Only if you cannot refer her, consider proceeding as follows.

Make a defunctioning sigmoid colostomy (9.5) as soon as the diagnosis is made, and her condition is satisfactory. Continue with salt baths for about 6 weeks.

ASSESSMENT. Under general anaesthesia explore her vaginally, pass a proctoscope, and, if necessary, a sigmoidoscope to see her RVF. How big is it? Is it clean, with all slough gone? Are its edges oedematous? Decide if it will be easier to close from above or below. If you are going to refer her, do so now, while her tissues are healthy. Delay may lead to the formation of fibrous tissue round the fistula, but less so than with a VVF.

If her fistula is at her pelvic brim (common), plan to repair it from above.

If her fistula is within easy reach vaginally (up to 8 cm from her fourchette, less common), plan to repair it from below.

If she also has a VVF, repair this first. Now that she has a colostomy, faeces no longer leak into her vagina.

REPAIR FROM ABOVE (common)

ANAESTHESIA. (1) General anaesthesia and intubation, with a relaxant if possible. (2) Subarachnoid (spinal) anaesthesia. Blood for transfusion is usually not necessary, but should be available. Pass a nasogastric tube.

POSITION. Lay her supine with a 5 or 10° head-down tilt. Stand on her left.

INCISION. Make a left lower paramedian or subumbilical midline incision. Carefully pack her gut out of the way with a large damp pack, marked by a tape, to which a haemostat is attached.

You will recognize the RVF as the place where her rectum is fixed to her vagina, and often to her bladder also, perhaps with considerable fibrosis. The attachment of her rectum to

FISTULAE

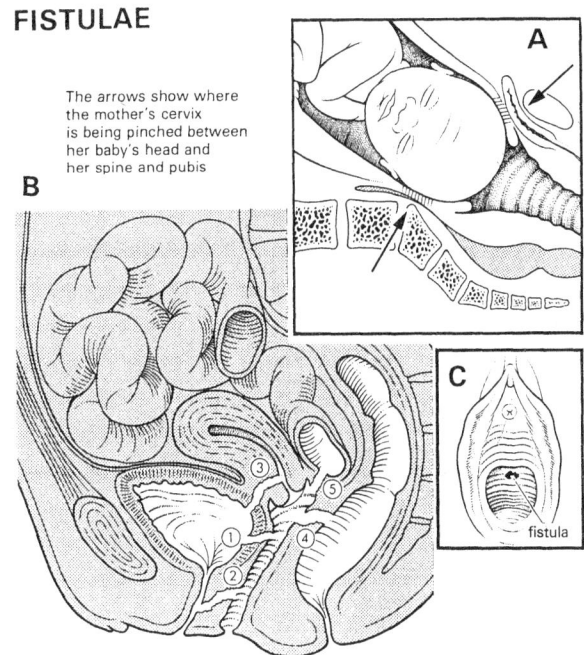

The arrows show where the mother's cervix is being pinched between her baby's head and her spine and pubis

Fig. 18-24 FISTULAE. A, the mechanism of fistula formation. B, various fistulae. C, a vesicovaginal fistula.

1, a vesicovaginal fistula (commonest) is almost always due to pressure from the child's head in a prolonged obstructed labour. 2, a urethrovaginal fistula (not uncommon) is usually an extension from a vesicovaginal fistula, and seldom occurs in isolation, unless it is mistakenly produced surgically. 3, a vesico-uterine fistula (uncommon) is due to damage to the bladder at Caesarean section which is not recognized and repaired (18.10). 4, a rectovaginal fistula (next commonest after a VVF) is usually fairly high in the vagina and is due to pressure necrosis of the child's head against the sacral promontary and upper sacrum. (5) An ileovaginal fistula (very rare). Fistulae between the ureters and and the vagina also occur (rare, 18.10), but are not shown here.

her bladder may obscure her upper vagina. Use fine curved dissecting scissors to separate her rectum from her vagina. As you do this, you will open into the fistula. As you separate her rectum from her bladder and vagina, avoid cutting through any normal tissue—or you may create another fistula! The area is rather inaccessible, because an RVF usually lies at the brim of the pelvis and extends into it.

Freshen the edges of the rectal wound and close it transversely with continuous '0' chromic catgut on a 5/8 atraumatic needle. If it is large, this may be difficult, but avoid closing it longitudinally, because this will narrow her rectum.

If access to her vaginal defect is easy, close it. Otherwise leave it. It will heal spontaneously, now that her rectal defect is closed.

REPAIR FROM BELOW (uncommon)

ANAESTHETIC. Give her a general anaesthetic. Blood is not often necessary, but it should be available.

Lay her supine in the lithotomy position, and work through her vagina. Have an assistant to help you on your right, and a trolley assistant on your left.

Infiltrate the tissues around the fistula with adrenalin solution, as for a VVF. Use a No. 12 blade to dissect the fistula and separate her vagina from her rectal wall. Extend the incision with curved dissecting scissors.

Close her rectum with continuous '0' catgut on an atraumatic 5/8 needle. Use similar, but interrupted, sutures for her vaginal wall. There is no intermediate layer, like the one which you may be able to define between her bladder and her anterior vaginal wall.

POSTOPERATIVELY, (both approaches) care for her as if she had had a large gut repair (9.5). At about 4 weeks, inspect the repair vaginally and with a proctoscope and a sigmoidoscope. Pass a rectal tube (26 to 30 Ch) up to the colostomy. If all is well, close it. If she becomes pregnant again section her.

DIFFICULTIES WITH FISTULAE (VVFs and RVFs)

For vesico-uterine and ureterovaginal fistulae, see Section 18.10.

If she has SEVERE VAGINAL STENOSIS associated with an RVF or VVF, which cannot be reconstituted, she may need a hysterectomy (20.12)—which should be subtotal, if you are inexperienced. She and her relatives may be reluctant to accept this. So you may have to wait until she has pain from a haematometra, before she will accept it. She and her husband or a relative must sign for it, before you do it.

If she has a URETHROVAGINAL FISTULA (not uncommon) it is usually an extension from a vesicovaginal fistula, and seldom occurs in isolation, unless it is mistakenly produced surgically.

If it involves the proximal half of her urethra only, and you are experienced, repair it as part of a VVF repair. If she is still incontinent after this, and her fistula has closed, her bladder/urethral junction is incompetent. Refer her for a sling urethroplasty.

If it is more extensive (rare, unless caused by bad surgery, such as a disastrous symphysiotomy), **refer her.** She is likely to need ureteric diversion.

If you are operating on a JUXTA-URETHRAL VVF or a fistula which involves her urethra, (not advised until you become expert), you will find a Martius graft useful. Repair the first two layers as usual. Leave her vaginal mucosa open for the moment. Make a longitudinal incision in a labium majus and retract the skin edges. Use scissors and dissector to separate a broad-based finger-like pedicle of fibro-fatty tissue from her underlying fascia, taking care to preserve its blood supply. Base it posteriorly and and extend it to about the level of her clitoris: make it long enough to reach her urethra without tension. Before closing her vaginal skin, use scissors to make a tunnel under her labium minor and surrounding skin, through from your present incision to the fistula repair. Stretch the tunnel until it easily accommodates the pedicle. Pass a strong catgut stitch through the tip of the pedicle, draw it into its new bed and suture it over the repair with 2/0 catgut sutures. Finally, cover its tip with her vaginal mucosa. The pedicle will fill dead space, separate her bladder and vaginal mucosa, and improve the repair. If necessary do it on both sides

If she has a 'GISHIRI CUT', it may extend into her bladder or divide her urethra and cause a formidable defect which is almost impossible to close. Traditionally, the Hausas of Nigeria cut the anterior vaginal wall on a variety of indications. Most cuts on non-pregnant women are small and easily repaired.

If SEVERAL ATTEMPTS AT REPAIRING A VVF FAIL, her ureters will have to be diverted into her colon, but only after the most skilled surgeon in the region has done all he can. Diversion of the ureters has an appreciable operative mortality, and urinary infection will shorten her expectation of life.

If she has an unrepaired VVF and succeeds in becoming PREGNANT AGAIN, she is at risk of premature labour. Severe scarring (18.4) may prevent delivery of even a small fetus.

19 Other obstetric problems

19.2 The surfactant test for fetal maturity

The surfactant test is a simple way of estimating the maturity of a baby. It is seldom needed in the developed world, where the length of gestation can usually be obtained from a pelvic examination early in pregnancy, or by an ultrasound scan. Unfortunately, this does not apply in the developing world, where the surfactant test still has a useful place. It is not infallible, so don't rely on it alone—use it in conjunction with an estimate of gestation by dates, and an estimate of the baby's size. It is a test for the surfactant which his alveolar cells secrete, and which is necessary for the expansion of his lungs immediately after birth. If they don't expand, he develops the respiratory distress syndrome, so the test is a measure of the extent to which he is at risk from this.

The test normally becomes positive at 36 weeks, so it is a good sign that he is mature enough to induce. Obtaining amniotic fluid is easy and safe for him and his mother, and is no more painful than an intramuscular injection. Rare complications include rupture of the membranes and injury to his head. Clements (see below) uses varying dilutions; we use only a 1:2 dilution.

Clements et al. The assessment of the respiratory distress syndrome by a rapid test for surfactant in amniotic fluid. The New England Journal of Medicine 1972;286:1077-81.

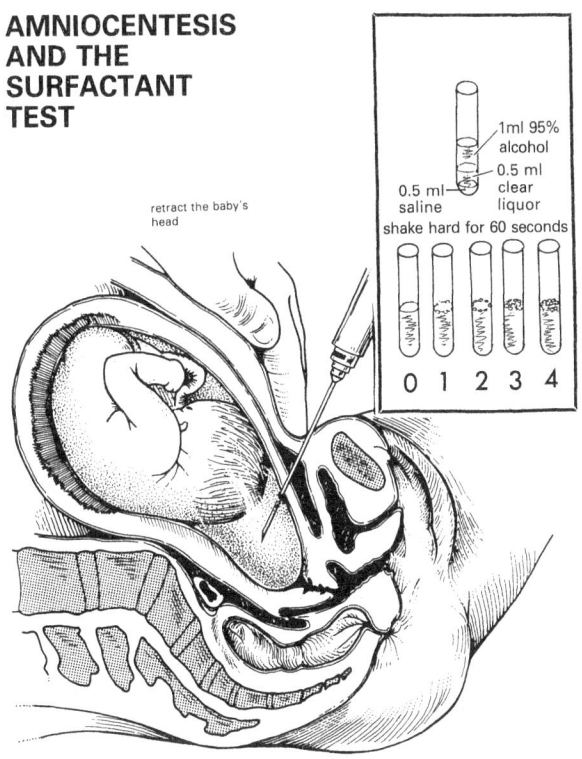

Fig. 19-1 THE SURFACTANT TEST normally becomes positive at 36 weeks, so it is a good sign that a baby is mature enough to induce.

THE SURFACTANT TEST

INDICATIONS. (1) There should be a legitimate reason for induction, but not one which is so strong that you would induce the patient anyway, such as severe gestational hypertension (17.4). Indications include an elective Caesarean section with uncertain dates, suspected growth retardation (19.13), and diabetes (in which the surfactant test is somewhat unreliable, 17.3). (2) If you are able to use ultrasound to localize the placenta, and find that it is in the way of the needle, reassess the need for the test. In practice little harm results from going through it. If however she is Rhesus-negative, putting a needle through the placenta increases the risk of rhesus immunization. (3) She must have a mobile presenting part, showing that she has enough liquor to aspirate. If there is not enough liquor, he is probably mature enough anyway.

ASPIRATION. Take a sterile 10 ml syringe and a long 1 mm needle. If she is very obese, you may need an extra long one. Have a second syringe ready in case the first sample is bloodstained.

Ask her to empty her bladder, so that you don't aspirate her urine. There is no need for local anaesthesia. Prepare the skin over her lower abdomen, preferably with iodine. Lay her supine. The lowest part of the baby is usually his head: feel it, lift it up out of her pelvis as far as you can, and then hold it there with your left hand. This will allow liquor to swirl around it, and fill her lower segment.

While holding his head up, plunge the needle attached to the syringe into her uterus at right angles to the plane of her lower segment, as near to his head as is reasonable, remembering that you don't want to hit it. Remember also that the commonest complication is rupture of her membranes due to inserting the needle too low, too close to her cervix.

Alternatively, aspirate at the level of her umbilicus on the side of his limbs. You need to be able to feel his position clearly. There is usually a good pool of liquor there. Injuring him is very unusual.

Withdraw 5 to 10 ml of fluid. Record it as being clear, or bloodstained (indicating a traumatic tap), and the vernix in it as being absent, scanty, or plentiful. If you fail, try once more and then give up.

EQUIPMENT. You need: (1) 1 ml of clear liquor, uncontaminated by meconium or blood. Only the faintest blood-staining is acceptable—a pale 'rosé' colour at the most. If you cannot avoid blood contamination, centrifuge the liquor hard for 5 minutes and test the supernatant. (2) 95% alcohol. (3) Some completely clean glass test-tubes with an internal diameter 8—14 mm. (4) 'Parafilm' to cover the tubes. If you don't have this, use *new* corks or rubber stoppers. If you don't have these either, a very carefully washed, and even more carefully rinsed, finger is probably better than a used cork or stopper.

METHOD. Take *exactly* 0.5 ml of liquor, 0.5 ml of saline, and 1.0 ml of alcohol (this mixes a 1 in 2 dilution of amniotic fluid with an equal volume of alcohol). Shake the mixture vigorously for *exactly* 15 seconds. Then don't move the tube. Wait 15 minutes before examining it in a good light against a dark background.

No foam, score 0.

An incomplete ring of bubbles peripherally round the meniscus, score 1.

A complete ring of bubbles round the meniscus, score 2.

As above, but foam just covering the whole meniscus, score 3.

Plentiful foam covering the whole meniscus thickly, score 4.

At a dilution of 1:2 as above a score of 1 or more means that his lungs are mature.

CAUTION ! (1) Avoid contamination with anything greasy. (2) Meconium produces a false positive result, so don't do the test if there is meconium in the fluid. (3) Don't shake the tubes a second time.

DIFFICULTIES WITH THE SURFACTANT TEST

If you ASPIRATE NOTHING, have you been brave enough? Push the needle a little deeper and try again.

If you ASPIRATE BLOOD, it may be fetal or maternal blood. Check the fetal heart half-hourly for 4 hours. If it rises steadily, he is bleeding (rare). Section her immediately.

If her UTERUS BECOMES HARD, and there are other signs of placental abruption, she is bleeding behind her placenta (very rare). See Section 16.13.

19.3 Inducing labour at term

If labour does not start when you would like it to, you may be able to start it. If it is going too slowly, you can speed it up. So distinguish between: (1) the *induction* of labour (the subject of this section) when the patient is not in labour, or only in the latent phase, and (2) the *acceleration* of labour, when she is in the active phase with her cervix more than 3 cm dilated. Here we are concerned with induction. For acceleration see M 22.2.

If the continuation of pregnancy would be harmful to a mother or to her baby, and especially if either of them is in danger of death, the logical solution might seem to be to induce labour and deliver them. Unfortunately, induction has its risks for both of them, so there are few indications for doing it in a district hospital. The commonest one is probably *proven* rupture of the membranes (19.5) lasting more than 12–24 hours, when she is near term (>37 weeks). All the other indications below are rare and relative.

Artificial rupture of the membranes (ARM), with an oxytocin drip or oral prostaglandins, is the most powerful way of inducing labour. Don't do it for minor indications, because: (1) You may introduce infection when you rupture her membranes. If labour starts soon, the risk is small, but if it is delayed, the risk is large, especially if the baby is dead. Minimize this by taking the most careful aseptic precautions. (2) If you try to induce her too soon: (a) he will be immature and have less chance of surviving, and (b) her labour is unlikely to start, and if it does start, it may so slow that you have to section her. So only induce labour, when the balance of risks favours it—when the surfactant test shows that he is mature, and Bishop's inducibility test shows that her cervix is ripe, and ready for labour. (3) Inducing labour increases your Caesarean section rate, with all the disadvantages this has (18.1).

There are other risks: (4) Rupturing her membranes may cause the cord to prolapse. (5) Oxytocin may cause her uterus to rupture. And, (6) her placenta may separate. So never induce labour to suit your convenience or hers, but only for the soundest of obstetric reasons.

If her cervix is unfavourable, you can try ripening it with prostaglandins (expensive), or you can insert the balloon of a Foley catheter into her extra-amniotic space (cheap and effective).

INDUCING LABOUR AT TERM

INDICATIONS. (1) Proven rupture of the membranes lasting >12–24 hours when the baby is near term (>37 weeks). (2) Severe pre-eclampsia if the cervix is ripe (17.4). (4) Diabetes (16.3). (5) Abruption (16.3). (6) Postmaturity (19.6) is an uncertain indication, because the diagnosis is rarely made in district hospital practice.

BISHOP'S INDUCIBILITY SCORE. Assess the dilatation of a mother's cervix, its length, its consistency, its position in relation to the axis of her vagina, and the height of her baby's head. Work out the score like this: the higher it is, the more likely it is that induction will succeed. The highest score is 13, and a score of 7 or more is favourable for induction.

Dilatation in cm: 0 cm, score nil. 1 cm to 2 cm, score one. 2 cm to 3 cm, score two. 3 cm to 4, cm score three.

Length in cm: 3 cm, score nil. 2 cm, score one. 1 cm, score two. 0 cm, score three.

Station of the head: 5/5, score nil. 4/5, score one. 3/5, score two. 2/5, score three.

Consistency: Firm, score nil. Medium, score one. Soft, score two.

Position of the cervix. Don't confuse this with the position of the presenting part (OA, OP, etc.): Posterior, score nil. In the middle, score one. Anterior, score two.

RIPENING A CERVIX

INDICATIONS. (1) When the cervix is not sufficiently ripe to enable you to rupture the membranes to induce labour. After ripening, labour will often start without any need to rupture the membranes. See also Section 16.4.

METHODS. Here are three ways of ripening a cervix:

A dinoprostone vaginal tablet in her posterior fornix. Insert one 3 mg PGE_2 dinoprostone ('Prostin E2' Upjohn) tablet in her posterior fornix on the afternoon before you induce labour. Follow this by another 3 mg 6 to 8 hours later if labour is not established, and then, if necessary, a further one, to a maximum of 3.

CAUTION ! (1) The tablet must be close to her cervix in her posterior fornix; merely slipping one into her introitus does not work. (2) Avoid prostaglandins if she is para 5 or above. There may be hyperstimulation. (3) Observe her carefully for at least 2 hours.

A dinoprostone tablet in her cervix. insert a 0.5 mg PGE_2 oral tablet into her cervical canal. Repeat this 6-hourly up to 4 doses.

A Foley catheter in the extra-amniotic space is useful if you have no prostaglandins. 12 to 18 hours before induction, with careful aseptic precautions, and under direct vision, use a Cusco's speculum to insert a 16 to 24 Ch Foley catheter, with a 30 to 45 ml balloon, into her extra-amniotic space. Inflate this with 30 to 45 ml of sterile water, and leave it in place.

CAUTION ! Whenever you induce labour, monitor the baby carefully.

OXYTOCIN TO INDUCE LABOUR AT TERM

INDICATIONS. A high risk-factor, particularly for the baby, such as: (1) Diabetes (17.3). (2) Gestational hypertension (17.4). (3) Placental abruption (16.13). (4) An unstable lie (19.9). (5) A dead baby 3 weeks after fetal movements have stopped (16.4). (6) Postmaturity (19.6).

CAUTION ! (1) For all the above indications her cervix must be favourable, by the score given above. (2) This is oxytocin *to induce labour at term*. It has several other uses, see 16.4 and 18.4a.

CONTRAINDICATIONS. (1) CPD. Never give a multip oxytocin if there is ANY sign of CPD. (2) A previous Caesarean section. (3) Myomectomy. (4) Fetal distress. (5) Malpresentation. (5) Grand multiparity is a relative contraindication, but you can cautiously give a lower dose. (6) Placenta praevia.

METHOD Check the baby's lie and presentation, and try to make sure that one nurse stays with her all the time. Start in the morning with a dose of 5 units to 500 ml of 5% dextrose in water at 10 drops a minute. Vials of oxytocin usually contain 5 units, so this is one vial. *Watch her closely* and increase the drip rate every 30 minutes like this: 10 drops/minute, 20 drops/minute, 40 drops/minute, 60 drops/minute. Increase the infusion until her uterus is contracting 2 or 3 times every 10 minutes. If vaginal examination shows that her cervix is not dilating, increase the infusion to 60 drops/minute regardless of how frequently contractions occur. Don't go above 60 drops/minute.

If you don't get the effect you want and she is a primip, increase the concentration to 10 units in 500 ml and start again at 10 drops/minute.

When her cervix is more than 5 cm, and she is having good

contractions, you may be able to reduce the rate of the drip. Do this gradually. If they go off, increase it again.

If her membranes have not ruptured, and she has not gone into labour by 7 p.m., stop the drip and try again in the morning. If her membranes have ruptured, induction must not stop.

CAUTION ! (1) Higher doses than these increase the uterine tone between contractions, and thus impair the placental circulation. Palpation does not detect this increased tone, unless it is gross. Too much oxytocin will cause prolonged tetanic contractions, and may rupture her uterus (especially if she is a multip). (2) In a multip, reduce the starting dose to 1 unit, and reduce or stop the drip as soon as regular contractions are established. (3) Assess her uterine contractions carefully. If there is no relaxation between contractions, stop the drip. If there is fetal distress, see 'Stop Press'. (4) Oxytocin in high doses (more than 10 units at 30 drops a minute) has an antidiuretic effect. So beware of 'water intoxication', and see Section 16.4. (5) If she is not delivered but is contracting satisfactorily and progressing well, you can use up to 2 l of a solution of 10 units in 500 ml. With more than this volume there is a risk of water intoxication. If she is not nearly delivered, consider Caesarean section. (6) Don't give her >2 l/24 hours without reviewing her carefully.

RUPTURING THE MEMBRANES TO INDUCE LABOUR

CONTRAINDICATIONS. (1) A high mobile head (the cord may prolapse). (2) A dead baby (except in abruption; she will labour fast), because he is much more easily infected (19.5). (3) If she has hydramnios, start by withdrawing some amniotic fluid from her abdomen, so as to reduce her uterus to a normal size. The sudden release of much fluid can precipitate abruption, and make malpresentations, such as a shoulder presentation, more likely.

METHOD. Make sure her bladder is empty. Check the fetal heart, put her into the the lithotomy position, and use careful aseptic precautions.

Flood her vulva with antiseptic solution. Wearing sterile gloves, do a careful vaginal examination and measure Bishop's score (see above).

Spread her labia widely, put two fingers into her vagina and then into her cervix. If necessary, stretch it to admit your 2 fingers. Gently sweep her membranes away from her lower segment without rupturing them. Feel carefully for the placenta, or the cord.

If you can feel her placenta, she has placenta praevia and you have made a horrible mistake. You are unlikely to do this if the head was in contact with the brim. Section her if it is Type Three or Four (16.12).

If you can feel the cord presenting through her membranes, leave them intact, turn her on her side and repeat the examination in about 2 hours. With luck, the cord will have floated away. If it has not and you want a live baby, you will have to section her.

CAUTION ! If she is in labour, rupture her membranes during a contraction, to minimize the risk of prolapse of the cord.

If you cannot feel either the placenta or the cord presenting through her membranes, rupture them with Kocher's forceps. Hold these in your left hand, and guide them through her cervix with your right hand. As you prepare to tear them, ask an assistant to push the presenting part into her pelvis. This will allow the fluid to escape in a controlled way, and will minimize the risk of the cord prolapsing. Grip her membranes and tear them. If fluid flows, or there is fetal hair in your forceps, you have succeeded. Note the amount and colour of her amniotic fluid, make sure the cord has not prolapsed, and check the fetal heart.

Enlarge the opening with your fingers. Keep them in her vagina until the head has descended against her cervix. With your fingers still in her vagina, check the fetal heart again. If she has a sudden persistent bradycardia: (1) She may have the supine hypotensive syndrome (A 16.6), so turn her on her side. (2) The cord may be trapped. Don't raise the baby's head, because the cord will probably prolapse further (19.10). Instead, turn her on her side and listen again; this usually solves the problem.

Alternatively, do a 'membrane sweep' only, and don't rupture her membranes until she is well advanced in labour. This is effective, and there is less risk of infection than when her membranes are ruptured some time before delivery.

19.4 Preterm labour

Strictly speaking, *preterm labour is the onset of regular painful contractions before 37 weeks*. In practice, you can treat labour between 34 and 36 weeks as if it was at term, so that it is only labour before 34 weeks that needs managing differently. It may or may not be associated with rupture of the membranes.

The management of preterm labour is controversial. We think you should avoid tocolytics and steroids. Using them may lead you to think that you are doing something useful when you are not, and divert you away from the treatment of the cause of the premature labour, which may be antepartum haemorrhage, a urinary tract infection, or intrauterine growth retardation (IUGR), etc. In practice, when a mother does go into preterm labour there is little you can do about it. It often stops spontaneously, so that 70% of mothers are not delivered 48 hours later, and go into labour normally nearer term.

PRETERM LABOUR

If a patient goes into labour before 34 completed weeks, find out if her membranes have ruptured, if necessary by the methods in Section 19.5. If they have ruptured, manage her as in that section. If they have not ruptured, manage her like this:

If she is in the active phase of labour (her cervix is >3 cm), don't try to delay delivery.

If she is in the latent phase of labour (her cervix is <3 cm) assess her contractions by palpation.

If she has regular contractions and her membranes are not ruptured, look for a possible cause, although you are unlikely to find one. Put her to bed, sedate her (give her pethidine 100 mg, or phenobarbitone 60 mg). Some obstetricians use tocolytics.

If her contractions are doubtful, consider other common and less common causes of pain. Urinary tract infection (17.6)? Constipation? This is sometimes the result of pica, eating quantities of earth, etc. Abruption (16.13)? Appendicitis (12.1)? Gut obstruction (10.3)? Other abdominal conditions (10.2)? Put her to bed and observe her for 24 hours.

WHEN SHE GOES INTO LABOUR her baby is at high risk, so, if she is a primip, make a liberal episiotomy, and control the delivery of his head with your hands. An episiotomy is usually unnecessary in a multip, because her perineum is no barrier, unless she has had a previous tear or an episiotomy. Handle him gently and keep him warm.

19.5 Premature rupture of the membranes (PROM) and intrauterine infection (IUI)

When labour is normal, regular contractions start and the patient's cervix begins to dilate before her membranes rupture and amniotic fluid escapes. Sometimes, her membranes rupture first, before contractions start, either before 36 weeks (preterm rupture), or at term (prelabour rupture). When her membranes rupture early the risks are: (1) Intrauterine infection or 'IUI', which is much the most important but is usually not common, and (2) premature labour.

Are you going to induce her or not? The *advantages* of expectant treatment (not inducing her) are that: (1) It increases the maturity of the fetus, which is important if she is less than 36 weeks. (2) It avoids the risks of induction, which are: (a) Failure, which means that you will have to section her, because you will have done repeated vaginal examinations. (b) The complications of oxytocin (18.4a). The *disadvantage* of expectant treatment is the risk of infection (chorioamnionitis) which may kill her and her baby. You can minimize this risk by: (1) Totally avoiding vaginal examination with your fingers until contractions are well established. (2) Avoiding speculum examinations as much as possible. (3) Practising reasonable vulval hygiene. (4) Observing her carefully for signs of infection, and inducing her and giving her antibiotics at the very first sign of infection.

Many obstetricians feel that IUI is such a serious risk, after premature rupture of the membranes, that it far outweighs any benefit that might follow from expectant treatment. What are you going to do? If there is little puerperal infection in your hospital, you can manage mothers expectantly. If puerperal infection is common, both mother and child are best delivered within 24 hours. Fortunately, labour usually starts successfully within this time. *If in doubt, induce!*

Midwives often justify vaginal examinations by saying that they are necessary to exclude prolapse of the cord. Tell them that: (1) The risk of prolapse of the cord is small, but the risk of infection is great. (2) Cord prolapse will only harm the baby, but infection will endanger his mother also. (3) If her cervix is sill closed, as it often is, vaginal examination will not rule out cord prolapse. Teach them that *premature rupture of the membranes calls for the suppression of vaginal curiosity!*

Avoid steroids, and give antibiotics only on the indications below.

PREMATURE RUPTURE OF THE MEMBRANES

The patient complains of loss of fluid from her vagina, before the onset of regular painful contractions. If you are not sure of her dates, estimate them from her fundal height using Fig. 19-15. This is not precise, but it may be the best you can do.

EXAMINATION. Start by separating her labia and asking her to cough: Is liquor discharging from her vagina? Is urine coming from her urethra?

If you don't see any fluid, repeat the examination after a few hours, so as not to miss intermittent loss of liquor from a small leak. Do *one* sterile speculum examination, to make sure that her membranes have ruptured, and that she really is draining liquor. Make sure that a senior person does this, so that it need not be repeated. Ask her to cough: you may see it escaping from her cervix. Observe: (1) The dilatation of her cervix. (2) Its degree of effacement. (3) Confirm the presenting part—you may see it if her cervix is open. (4) Exclude prolapse of the cord.

CAUTION ! Don't do a vaginal examination with your fingers: the risk of infection is too high.

Alternatively, avoid this examination, and merely 'wait and see'. If she continues to lose fluid (as shown by checking her pads), she has obviously ruptured her membranes. One contributor does not advise a speculum examination, because he finds that he can manage without it.

If you are not quite sure if the fluid that is draining is liquor or urine: (1) smell it, (2) test its pH (urine and vaginal discharge are acid, amniotic fluid is alkaline), and (3) leave some to dry on a slide. Look at it under a microscope. Liquor, but not urine, or a discharge, will dry as a pattern of ferns. If you have not done this test before, try it with some known liquor.

THE MANAGEMENT OF PRETERM RUPTURE OF THE MEMBRANES

If the diagnosis is confirmed or suspected, admit her, provide her with a clean perineal pad or cloth, make sure she keeps her vulva and perineum clean, check her temperature 4-hourly, and inspect her liquor daily. See also 'Stop Press'.

If no liquor can be seen escaping after 5 days, the diagnosis is not confirmed, so discharge her. 25% of patients stop leaking liquor in 5 days and can be discharged. 75% go into spontaneous labour during this time.

If she is less than 28 weeks, with a live baby, and has no signs of IUI, opinions differ on what you should do. Much depends on how common puerperal sepsis is in your hospital: see above. The chances of her pregnancy continuing long enough for the fetus to survive are small, but not zero. If you are worried about the risk of infection, induce her. If the risk of infection seems small, leave her. She will probably go into labour soon, but she might be lucky, and her pregnancy may continue.

If she is 28–36 weeks and her membranes have been ruptured for less than 48 hours, and she has no IUI, wait 48 hours. If her liquor stops draining, don't intervene. If it continues to drain at 48 hours, induce her, if the risk of infection in your hospital is high. If it is not so high, wait until the fetus is more mature at 36 weeks. Culture her amniotic fluid at delivery. One contributor waits 5 days, by which time nearly all mothers have gone into labour, or stopped draining.

If she is >36 weeks. If labour does not start spontaneously in 24 hours, induce her with oxytocin.

CAUTION ! Be sure to induce her if: (1) Her baby is dead at any stage of pregnancy. (2) She has signs of IUI at any stage of pregnancy. (3) She is more than 36 weeks, and has not gone into labour spontaneously in 24 hours. (3) Infection is common in your hospital.

CAUTION WITH OXYTOCIN ! Remember the precautions for the use of oxytocin (18.4a): (1) Don't give her an oxytocin drip if there are any contraindications to its use (M 22.2). CPD is unlikely to be a problem in preterm babies. (2) If she is a grand multip, avoid oxytocin, and await the spontaneous onset of labour. (3) If she has signs of IUI, use oxytocin with extreme caution, and stop the drip as soon as she is having regular contractions, or you section her. IUI increases the dangers of section, so balance the risks as best you can.

INTRAUTERINE INFECTION, 'IUI'

DIAGNOSIS. IUI causes these signs in this order: (1) Fetal tachycardia. (2) Maternal pyrexia and tachycardia. (3) Uterine tenderness. (4) Offensive, blood-stained liquor.

TREATMENT. She will probably be septicaemic, and may be in septic shock (53.4). If necessary, resuscitate her with intravenous fluids. Give her broad-spectrum intravenous antibiotics; chloramphenicol and metronidazole are suitable (2.9). Empty her uterus as soon as possible, whatever the duration of pregnancy. It will often empty spontaneously. If it does not, give her an oxytocin infusion with caution, and stop the drip as soon as she has regular contractions. Her baby usually dies, if he is not already dead when she becomes infected.

DIFFICULTIES WITH INTRAUTERINE INFECTION

If bubbles of GAS come from her cervix, or you feel crepitus of her cervix or abdominal wall, she has GAS GANGRENE. Her uterus and abdominal wall may be distended with gas. Give her large doses of penicillin, chloramphenicol, and metronidazole, as in Section 54.13, and evacuate her uterus. If the infection has spread to the wall of her uterus, consider hysterectomy.

19.6 The mother who is overdue—postmaturity

Babies who are more than two weeks postmature are at increased risk of stillbirth, so it is the custom in much of the developed world to induce them, although there is no convincing evidence that this reduces the perinatal mortality. You will have to weigh up the risks. Induction may reduce the risk from postmaturity, but an induced labour is longer and more complicated than a spontaneous one, and has its own risks.

In the district hospitals of the developing world the risks of accidental premature induction are much greater than they are elsewhere because: (1) A mother's dates may be wrong, because she conceived while breast-feeding, or soon after stopping, before having had a period since her previous pregnancy. Breast-feeding also results in periods which are less frequent than normal. For example, if periods occur every two months, conception will occur 6 weeks after the last period, instead of 2 weeks. These errors are always such that pregnancy is less advanced than mothers think. (2) Many mothers present so late for their first antenatal visit, that the size of the uterus cannot be reliably used to confirm their dates. The risks of routinely inducing postmature mothers thus outweigh its benefits, so postmaturity is only a relative reason for induction. Ask concerned mothers to keep fetal movement charts (M 28.3).

POSTMATURITY. If a mother is more than 42 weeks, and her dates are certain, admit her and ask her to keep a fetal movements chart (M 28.3). If she has any of these risk factors, induce her with oxytocin and rupture her membranes: (1) She is a nullip over 30. (2) She is a multip over 40. This is unusual, so check her dates, and her baby's 'size for dates'. (3) She has a bad obstetric history. (4) She has gestational hypertension. (5) She has markedly reduced fetal movements. If induction is impossible or fails, section her.

19.7 The hopelessly malformed fetus

With most congenital malformations a baby is not large enough, or misshapen enough, to cause difficulty during labour. The important exceptions are anencephaly and hydrocephaly, for which you should use the methods below. If you have the misfortune to find a double monster, Caesarean section is the method of choice.

Anencephaly is complicated in 90% of cases by polyhydramnios (M 15.4); so when you diagnose this, X-ray a mother to see if her baby has a head. If he has not, he is usually stillborn, and even when he is born alive, he does not survive more than a few hours. When you have explained the diagnosis to her, she will usually insist that her pregnancy is induced.

Hydrocephaly is not always easy to diagnose clinically, and is often missed during pregnancy. A common mistake is to misdiagnose a brow presentation (when the head feels big) for hydrocephaly. If you suspect it, confirm the diagnosis by X-ray. If the diagnosis is then obvious, proceed as described below. If it is doubtful, wait. Even during labour the diagnosis is easily missed, if widely distended sutures and fontanelles cannot be felt.

THE HOPELESSLY MALFORMED FETUS

ANENCEPHALY. **If this is accompanied by polyhydramnios,** drain the mother's amniotic sac slowly by draining her hindwaters with a Drew–Smythe catheter. Alternatively, rupture her forewaters by making a small hole with an amnion hook. Give her an escalating oxytocin drip (19.3), and she will probably deliver promptly.

If anencephaly is not accompanied by polyhydramnios (10% of cases), pregnancy may be prolonged up to a year or more (rare), and make delivery difficult. Try PGE2 pessaries first (the ideal indication for them). Then try surgical induction and an escalating oxytocin drip (19.3). These will probably succeed. If you cannot induce her (19.3), you will have to do a Caesarean section—this is tragic, so avoid it if you can.

HYDROCEPHALY. **If you make the diagnosis during pregnancy,** induce labour, and try to avoid Caesarean section.

If you diagnose hydrocephaly when labour with a cephalic presentation has been in progress for some time, and the baby's head is more than minimally enlarged, you will have to make it smaller before you can deliver him. If he is dead, drain his CSF with a lumbar puncture needle. Some obstetricians would do this even if he is alive (draining his CSF does not kill him), others would wait for his heart to stop. If you are not sure of the diagnosis, or don't feel you can risk sacrificing him, you may be forced to section her.

To perforate his head, wait until dilatation has passed 3 cm, then drain his cerebrospinal fluid with a large needle between his widely separated skull bones, or, less satisfactorily, with Simpson's perforator. His collapsed head will slowly settle into his mother's pelvis, and he will deliver.

CAUTION ! If possible, perforate him before she is 5 cm dilated, because her over-distended lower segment may rupture if you don't.

If you diagnose hydrocephaly during a breech presentation, he will probably deliver spontaneously as far as his umbilicus (19.8). Progress will then be arrested as his hydrocephalic head fails to enter her pelvic brim. Draining his CSF will be less messy than a craniotomy: (1) If, at this stage you see the commonly-associated meningomyelocele, pass a steel or gum elastic male catheter through the spinal defect into his ventricles, to drain off his CSF. If he has no spina bifida, you can easily do a laminectomy with a scalpel, to allow the catheter to enter. Or, (2) pass a needle through his occipital bone into his skull. Or, (3) make sure that her bladder is empty, and then tap his aftercoming head abdominally with a large spinal needle.

19.8 Breech presentation

If a baby presents by his breech, he is about 4 times more likely to die than if he presents by his vertex. This is so, even if you exclude the excess mortality due to the higher rate of prematurity and fetal abnormality that is associated with breech deliveries. This increased mortality is due to: (1) The rapid compression and decompression of his unmoulded head. (2) Asphyxia due to the delayed delivery of his head, if there is any CPD, or if his mother has an incompletely dilated cervix. (3) The aspiration of meconium, if he tries to breathe while his head is still in her pelvis. (4) The increased risk of his cord prolapsing.

External cephalic version (ECV, M 19.1). If you can reduce the number of breeches you deliver, you can reduce the perinatal mortality associated with them. Turning a breech presentation in the third trimester will do this, but it is of little value before 34 weeks in a primip, or 36 weeks in a multip, because many breech presentations spontaneously correct themselves before this. After 36 weeks a baby gradually becomes less mobile, which makes version more difficult. On the other hand, if version does succeed, it is more likely to be permanent.

The knee-chest position (M 19.1) is an alternative to ECV which often works. It is also safer, but has never been objectively evaluated; this is being done as we go to press. Ask a mother to spend 10 minutes three times a day in the knee-chest position. This may allow her baby's breech to disimpact in her pelvis, so that he can turn spontaneously.

If external version or the knee-chest position fail, you can deliver a breech: (1) Vaginally, by assisted breech delivery (M 19.1). (2) Vaginally, by breech extraction. Or, (3) abdominally, by Caesarean section. In breech extraction you, rather than his mother, provide the power for pulling the baby down. You exert traction on his legs, groins and pelvis, so it is potentially more dangerous than an assisted breech delivery, which is the usual way of delivering a breech. Breech extraction is described here, but not in *Primary Mother Care*, and is only indicated on the rather unusual indications given below.

What should your policy be towards Caesarean section in breech deliveries? Liberal use of it will reduce your perinatal mortality, but you will have to weigh this against the increased maternal morbidity and mortality that will follow from it (18.1). In the developed world the risks of breech delivery have fallen so much, that it is hardly more dangerous than delivery by the vertex. This is the result of: (1) Safer Caesarean section. (2) Quicker section if the cord prolapses, or there is unexpected delay in the second stage. (3) Greater emphasis on controlled delivery of the head, often assisted by forceps and epidural anaesthesia. (4) Less CPD owing to better maternal nutrition. (5) An increased readiness to section mothers with borderline pelvises, very small breech babies, and footlings (a breech with one foot down and one up). These factors have combined to make Caesarean section so popular in some centres in the developed world, that their section rate for breeches is now over 50%.

The increased safety of breech delivery in the developed world has made obstetricians there look closely at the small risks of ECV, which include: (1) Knotting of the cord. (2) Placental abruption. And, (3) uterine rupture. In the developed world, the risks of ECV, small though they are, are commonly held to be more than those of breech delivery, so that ECV is increasingly out of favour. However, in the developing world, the risks of breech delivery and section are much greater, and grand multiparity is much commoner, so that ECV still has an important place here. It is therefore described in *Primary Mother Care*. Unfortunately, ECV is not done by doctors as often as it should be, or by experienced midwives (it should not be done by inexperienced ones). If your excess perinatal mortality with breech deliveries is more than 20/1000, after correcting for prematurity and fetal abnormality (see below), the risks of ECV are worth taking. Don't attempt it under general anaesthesia.

If there is any question of CPD before the second stage of labour, section the mother. In communities where contracted pelves are common, the risks of a breech delivery are great, so that if you want these babies to survive, you may have to section 25% of your breeches. A mother with a true conjugate of less than 9 cm should not be allowed to deliver a full term breech baby vaginally.

A baby with IUGR or prematurity presenting by his breech is a problem. Much depends on his age: (1) Under 28 weeks' gestation (< 1000 g) his chances of life are small, the lower segment is poorly formed, and it is questionable if section will be any less traumatic than vaginal delivery. (2) From 28 to 32 weeks (1000–1500 g) he may have a better chance with Caesarean section, especially if he is a footling presentation. However, about 20% of these babies have severe abnormalities, and if you don't have ventilators, even the normal ones have a poor chance of surviving. So, in an area of high parity and high perinatal mortality, you should rarely section a premature baby presenting by his breech.

Symphysiotomy needs skill (see below), and is best kept only for unbooked patients, who are admitted in the second stage of labour, whose pelves you cannot assess, and when there is no time for section. You can do a symphysiotomy to help deliver a baby's shoulders, or you can keep it until unsuspected CPD has delayed the delivery of his head—but you will have to be quick, and have a solid-bladed scalpel and a catheter ready!

Epidural anaesthesia (A 7.2) will prevent a mother bearing down before she is fully dilated, and it will make any manipulations that you have to do in the second stage of a vaginal delivery, much easier. Alas, it is seldom practical under the conditions in which you work.

If the difficulties of vaginal breech delivery worry you, and you are tempted to section all breeches, remember the dangers of Caesarean section from anaesthesia, bleeding, and sepsis. An occasional 'stuck breech', and a dead baby, are more acceptable than a maternal death. As your skill and experience and that of your staff improve, so will your successful vaginal deliveries.

Armon PJ, 'The management of singleton breech presentations'. Tropical Doctor 1984;167-169

Lovset J, 'Shoulder delivery by breech presentation'. Journal of Obstetrics and Gynaecology of the British Empire 1937;44:696.

Thornton JG, 'External cephalic version. Tropical Doctor 1985;173-174.

BREECH PRESENTATION

CORRECTING A BREECH PRESENTATION

THE KNEE-CHEST POSITION. Ask her to spend 10 minutes in the knee-chest position 3 times a day. If this fails try external cephalic version.

EXTERNAL CEPHALIC VERSION can be done at any time after 34 weeks, until labour starts. It is not necessary before 34 weeks. You may not succeed after 36 weeks, but it is still worth trying.

Contraindications. Take a history from her and examine her to exclude: (1) Multiple pregnancy. (2) Antepartum bleeding in this pregnancy. (3) A previous Caesarean section. (4) The need to do a Caesarean section in this pregnancy for some other reason. (5) A diastolic blood pressure greater than 100 mm. (5) A fetal abnormality, if you can detect it. (6) A Rhesus-negative mother and no anti-Rh imunoglobulin to give her.

Method. Explain carefully what you are going to do. Ask her to empty her bladder and lie on her back tilted a little to one side. Make sure your hands are warm and she is comfortable. You may find it helpful to lubricate your hands and her abdomen with glove powder.

Find which side the baby's back is. Count his heart rate. Place one hand below his breech, and your other hand above his head. Flex him between your hands, so that you make him do a forward somersault (turn head over heels). Listen to his heart.

If his heart rate slowed to less than 100, turn her on her side and wait until it is more than 100. If his heart rate has not started to recover within 2 minutes, turn him into his original position. His umbilical cord may be tight round his neck.

If a forward somersault fails, try turning him in a backward somersault.

If you fail, rest her with the foot of her bed raised. If she is anxious give her diazepam 5 mg by month. Try again in an hour. If you fail again, try again at the next visit.

If you succeed, see her again one week later to make sure the presentation is still cephalic.

If you cannot turn her by 37 weeks, manage her as a breech delivery.

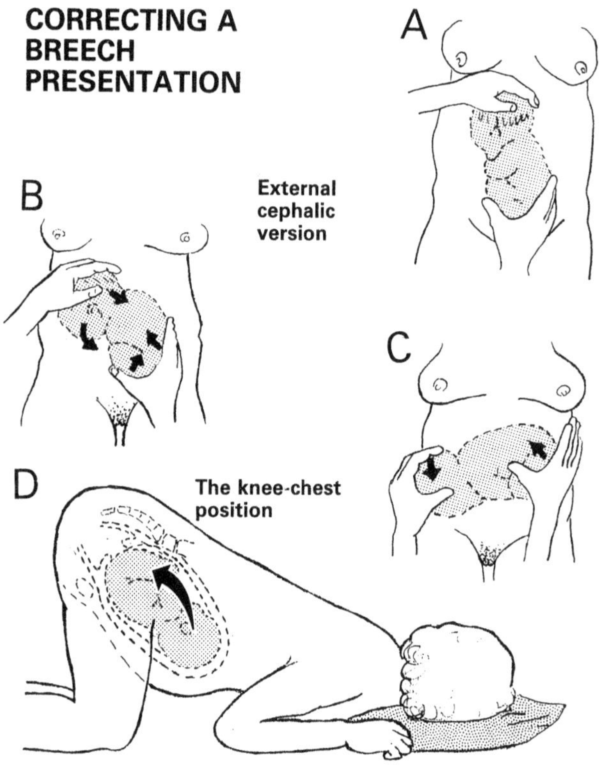

THE INDICATIONS FOR CAESAREAN SECTION IN A BREECH DELIVERY

If she has a normal or or large pelvis, and he is a normal-sized baby, she will probably deliver vaginally. If you cannot touch her sacral promontory easily, and her diagonal conjugate is >11 cm (true conjugate >9cm), she probably has a large enough pelvis. If you can touch her sacral promontory easily, and her diagonal conjugate is less than 11 cm, she has a small pelvis.

Most additional factors, which compromise the wellbeing of a baby, are indications for section. Only a healthy normal-sized mother with a baby less than 3.7 kg (as indicated by a fundal height of <40 cm), who progresses normally in both stages of labour, should be allowed a vaginal delivery. In more detail the indications for section are these:

ANTENATAL INDICATIONS FOR ELECTIVE CAESAREAN SECTION. (1) CPD or suspected CPD. (2) A large baby; feel the size of his head. If he feels as if he is big, that is >3.7 kg (fundal height >40 cm), regardless of the size of her pelvis, section her. (3) The scar from a previous section. (4) Other obstetric hazards, such as placenta praevia, diabetes, gestational hypertension, or APH. (5) An elderly primigravida, or a long history of infertility. (6) A previous stillbirth, especially if it was associated with a breech. (7) Postmaturity >42 weeks. (8) Perhaps a baby with IUGR, or prematurity, weighing 1000-1500 g, especially if he is a footling.

INDICATIONS FOR CAESAREAN SECTION DURING LABOUR. (1) A prolonged active phase. (2) Arrest at the brim, or delay in the descent of the breech during the second stage. (3) A footling presentation. A multip is likely to develop an irresistible desire to push before full dilatation, as her baby's feet enter her vagina. This can result in his head being caught behind her undilated cervix. Other obstetric indications such as: (4) Cord presentation or prolapse. (5) Fetal distress. (6) Prolonged rupture of the membranes.

ASSISTED BREECH DELIVERY

CAUTION ! For breech delivery you need a quiet atmosphere and good communication with the patient. A crowd of supporters crying 'Push, push' is not what you want. Quiet them and explain what is happening. You will need an assistant

THE FIRST STAGE. If her cervix dilates at less than 1 cm per hour in the active phase, or there are any other signs of delay, section her. Until his buttocks are delivered, you can turn back and do a Caesarean section. Only when his buttocks have been delivered have you reached the point of no return. If there is any delay before the delivery of his buttocks, section her.

THE SECOND STAGE. A common fault is to try to deliver a breech through an incompletely dilated cervix, which may extend his arms and make his head difficult to deliver. Full dilatation may not be easy to diagnose in a breech, so don't consider that the second stage has started until his anterior buttock is easily visible. Put her into the lithotomy position (essential if you do the Burns Marshall manoeuvre or apply forceps to his aftercoming head) when his posterior buttock is distending her perineum. As soon as she wants to bear down, do a vaginal examination to make sure that her cervix is fully dilated.

His breech should advance with every contraction. Infiltrate her perineum, and do an episiotomy, when his buttocks are distending it, and you can see a boy's scrotum (or a girl's labia). *Protect his scrotum* (you don't want the episiotomy to castrate him!). His buttocks and legs will then deliver.

Fig. 19-2 CORRECTING A BREECH PRESENTATION. A, to C, external cephalic version. Flex him between his hands so that you make him do a forward somersault. D, the knee-chest position. Ask his mother to spend 10 minutes 3 times a day like this.

THE BURNS–MARSHALL MANOEUVRE

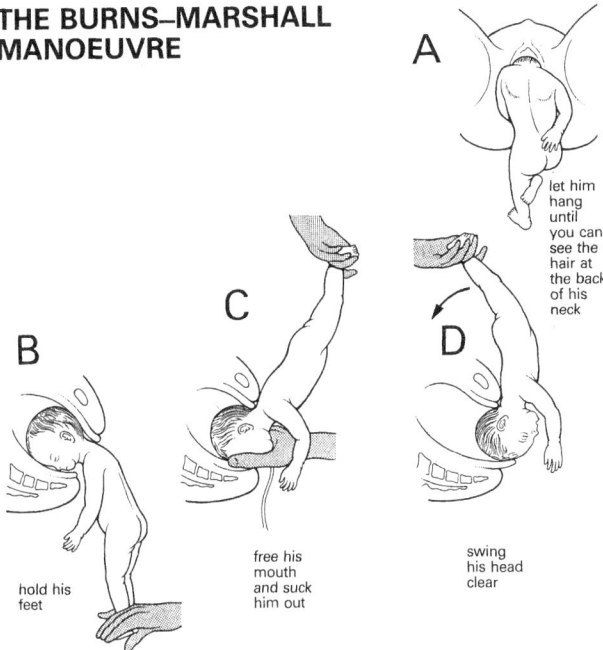

Fig. 19-3 THE BURNS—MARSHALL MANOEUVRE for delivering the head in a breech delivery, if it does not deliver spontaneously. A, allow his body to hang, until you can see the hair at the back of his neck. B, hold his feet. C, swing his feet upwards over his mother's abdomen. Free his mouth and pause while you clean it. D, finish delivery by swinging him over her abdomen.

When his umbilicus delivers there is often a temporary halt in descent. Look at the clock. He should be delivered in 5 minutes.

Wait for progress to resume with the next contraction. His shoulders and arms should deliver with a twisting movement, and his head should follow immediately. *Don't touch him, or try to disentangle his legs, until you see his umbilicus.* Touching him promotes breathing movements and the aspiration of meconium. Put your hand on her fundus, observe each contraction, and keep a steady gentle pressure on his head.

When his umbilicus appears, disengage his extended legs and pull down a loop of his cord, which may be stretched.

CAUTION ! Encourage him to turn so that his back is uppermost. Never allow his ventral surface to face upwards.

When his anterior scapula appears (and not before), search for his arms in front of his chest. If, as is usual, his arms are not extended, they will both be in front of his chest. You should be able to deliver one or both of them. If you have difficulty, feel up to his shoulder and from there feel down his arm, first one then other.

Allow his body to hang, as in A, Fig. 19-3. His own weight will make his head descend through her birth canal. It will have been entering her pelvis, and will be compressing his cord. Assist its descent with gentle suprapubic pressure. He must be able to breathe in the next 5 minutes.

If his head does not immediately deliver spontaneously when his arms are out, try the BURNS–MARSHALL manoeuvre. Wait until you can see the the hairs on the nape of his neck (A, Fig. 19-3). Stand with your back to her left leg, take his legs in your right hand (B), pull him outwards a little and draw him outwards over her pubis. Guard her perineum with your left hand and prevent his head from emerging too quickly. As soon as his mouth and nose appear, pause, and ask your assistant to clear his airways and allow him to breathe (C). Then, carefully deliver the rest of his head (D).

If you cannot get at least his mouth and nose into fresh air with the Burns–Marshall method: (1) use the MAURICEAU - SMELLIE - VEIT manoeuvre, or (2) apply forceps to his aftercoming head (see under 'Difficulties' below). Rest his belly and chest on your right forearm; put your right middle finger in his mouth, and your index and ring fingers on his malar bones. Put your left hand over his back; put your middle finger on his occiput and your index and ring fingers over his shoulders. This will give you some control over the flexion and rotation of his head. Grip his skull and guide it through her birth canal. *Ask her to stop pushing.* Ask your assistant to put his fist on the baby's head, which is still palpable above her pubis, and to press obliquely downwards in the direction of her coccyx. You will feel a 'plop' indicating that his head has gone into her pelvis, and further delivery by the Mauriceau–Smellie–Veit manoeuvre should then be easy.

CAUTION ! This is a method for getting a grip directly on his head. NEVER pull on his shoulders, you can too easily distract his cervical vertebrae and damage his cord.

NOTE: Although Mauriceau–Smellie–Veit is a cumbersome eponym, it is preferred to the alternative which is 'jaw shoulder traction' since this suggests, although it does not intend, traction on the neck, which is very dangerous.

EARLY DIFFICULTIES DELIVERING A BREECH

CAUTION ! (1) Do an episiotomy (except in a grand multip with a very lax outlet) before you do any manipulations, because there is a high risk of a perineal tear. (2) Don't squeeze his abdomen! (3) If his head fails to descend, don't pull on his neck. (4) If his head becomes impacted and he dies, don't sever his neck, or be tempted to open her uterus from above.

If his breech is DELAYED AT THE BRIM, or in midcavity, this is probably a warning sign of CPD; section her. Don't try to deliver her with oxytocin. If section is impossible, consider reaching for his anterior groin with a finger and bringing down his leg. This was once the traditional method, and will probably injure him seriously.

If his breech is DELAYED AT THE OUTLET, make sure that the episiotomy is adequate. There may be CPD. If her pelvis

TWO MORE METHODS FOR DELIVERING THE HEAD

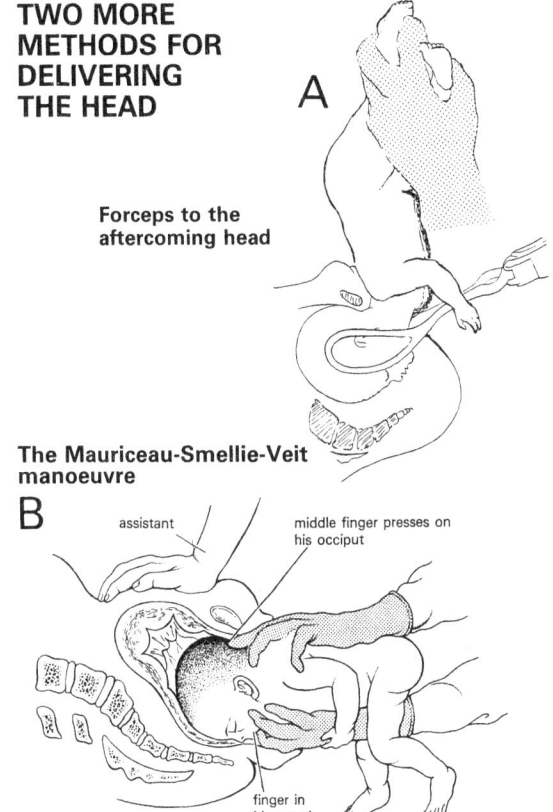

Fig. 19-4 TWO METHODS FOR DELIVERING THE HEAD IN A BREECH PRESENTATION. A, applying forceps to the aftercoming head. B, the Mauriceau–Smellie–Veit manoeuvre is a method for getting a grip directly on a baby's head. Rest his belly and chest on your right forearm; put your right middle finger in his mouth, and your index and ring fingers on his malar bones. Put your left hand over his back; put your middle finger on his occiput and your index and ring fingers over his shoulders. This will give you some control over the flexion and rotation of his head. Guide his head through his mother's birth canal and don't pull on his shoulders. The finger in his mouth is for convenience only.

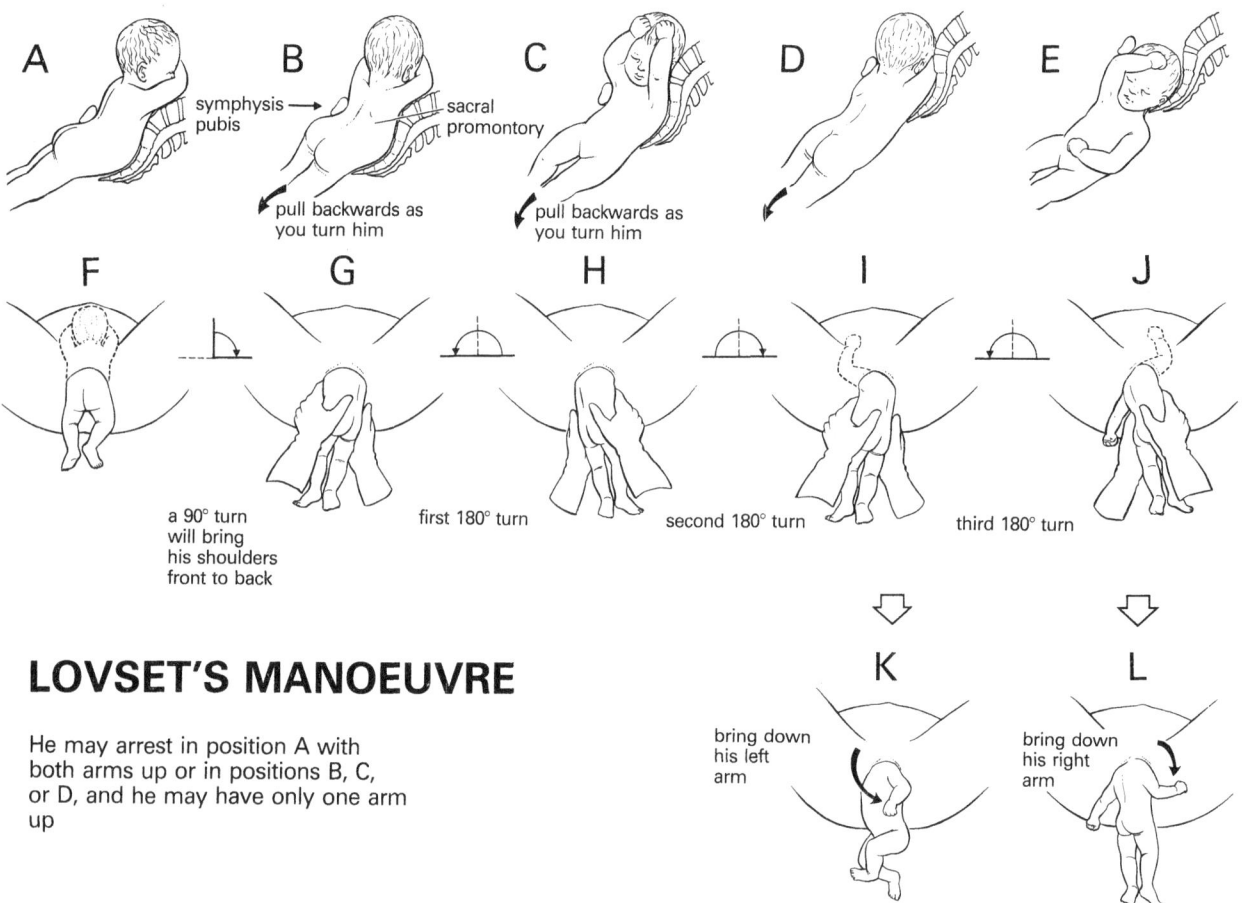

LOVSET'S MANOEUVRE

He may arrest in position A with both arms up or in positions B, C, or D, and he may have only one arm up

Fig. 19-5 LOVSET'S MANOEUVRE for the delivery of the shoulders in a breech presentation. The bottom row of drawings show a view from the patient's perineum. The top row shows the same stage viewed from her left. Remember "If you don't know which way to turn him, keep his back anterior, so that it passes under her clitoris". Many obstetricians merely wiggle him one way then the other, pull, and try to find an arm: but this is the detailed manoeuvre. Practise it on a model.

feels contracted, or he is large, section her. If all is otherwise well, do gentle groin traction, as for breech extraction (see below).

If you have delivered his legs but BOTH HIS SHOULDERS HAVE NOW STUCK above his mother's pelvic brim, his arms are probably extended (A, Fig. 19-5). Normally you can put a finger up her posterior vaginal wall and easily bring them down. If you cannot, they are probably extended. Try LOVSET'S manoeuvre. It is a breech extraction for obstruction late in delivery, and should rarely be necessary. The delivery of his shoulders is prevented by two obstructions at different levels; (1) her sacral promontary is higher than (2) her pubis. The principle of this method is that, by pulling tightly down on to both, and by turning him through 180°, the shoulder which was held up above her pubis will turn to pass into the hollow of her sacrum, and the shoulder which was above her sacrum will now be above her pubis. Two further 'unscrewing' half-turns like this, each bringing his shoulders progressively below these obstructions will deliver him.

Grasp his thighs and pelvis with both hands (if he is slippery use a gauze swab or small towel), your thumbs along his sacrum, your forefingers on his symphysis, and your remaining fingers round his thighs.

If, in the extreme case, he obstructs transversely (A), start by turning him through 90° (A to B), so that his back faces to her left. His left shoulder will then be above her symphysis, and his right shoulder above her sacrum (B). With your first 180° turn (B to C), bring his left shoulder under her sacrum. With your second second turn (C to D) bring his right shoulder under her sacrum. His left arm will now be low enough for you to gently sweep it down. With your third turn turn (D to E) bring his right shoulder under her pubis; it will now be low enough for you to bring his right arm down.

CAUTION ! (1) These three 180° turns are in opposite directions, so that *his back always passes under her clitoris,* and the arm which started posterior always drags across his face. *His belly should never pass under her clitoris.* (2) In the worst case you start in A with both arms extended, so you have to begin with a 90° turn, followed by three 180° turns. If he arrests at a later stage, with only one arm extended, you may only need two turns, or perhaps only one. (3) The first two turns release the shoulder which was arrested above her symphysis when you started it. The third enables you to bring down his right arm. (5) Don't squeeze his belly, or back, or you may rupture his liver, kidneys, spleen, or adrenals (huge in the newborn). If you hold his chest, take care not to compress his abdomen. (6) Remember that the upper part of the birth canal, in which he has stuck, is directed backwards, so start by pulling him backwards.

If LOVSET'S MANOEUVRE FAILS TO DELIVER HIS SHOULDERS (uncommon), it is usually a failure of technique. You may have to be a little firmer, or reach up a little higher to get his arm down. A broken arm will soon heal, so it is no disaster (71.17), and is better than letting him die

DIFFICULTY DELIVERING HIS HEAD

CPD is the most important cause.

IF HIS HEAD IS STUCK ABOVE THE BRIM, you are in trouble. You may be able to draw it into her pelvis with the

Mauriceau–Smellie–Veit manoeuvre. If this fails, he will probably be dead, and the best treatment will be craniotomy (see below).

If HIS HEAD HAS ENTERED THE PELVIS and the MAURICEAU–SMELLIE–VEIT manoeuvre fails to deliver it, rotating his head in her pelvis may help. Stop struggling and think. What is the cause? If it is CPD, and you are an experienced symphysiotomist with an equally experienced obstetric team, a quick symphysiotomy may save him. On the other hand, an unskilful symphysiotomy may cause pelvic trauma and laceration of her urinary tract, so only attempt this if you and your team are expert.

If CPD IS THE CAUSE or SHE IS NOT FULLY DILATED, and you cannot deliver him, let him die and avoid harming her. While she is still in the lithotomy position, sedate her with pethidine 50 mg and let him hang for a while. His head will usually mould, or her cervix will dilate, so that he is delivered in less than an hour.

Alternatively, if his head has stuck in her incompletely dilated cervix (uncommon) either: (1) Apply standard obstetric forceps, such as those of Neville Barnes, inside it. While you apply gentle traction, try to slip her cervix over his head. Or, (2) if this fails, cut her cervix boldly with scissors at 4 and 8 o'clock, and repair your incisions afterwards (M 24.2). Some contributors consider this a relatively safe and successful method, one considers it bloody and dangerous. This complication usually happens to premature breech deliveries, who may not be worth the risk involved.

If the ABOVE MEASURES FAIL and CPD is severe, you may have to do a CRANIOTOMY through his foramen magnum (unpleasant but effective). See Section 18.5 for the general principles of destructive operations. A craniotomy is best done in the theatre under general anaesthesia; but you can do it in the labour ward.

Ask an assistant to pull down his his body. Retract her anterior vaginal wall with a Sims' speculum and expose the back of his neck. Pick up a fold of of the skin over his cervical spine with toothed forceps, and incise it transversely. Use curved Mayo's scissors to cut a tunnel under his skin up to his occipital bone, and push scissors into his head. Open the scissors a few times to break up his brain compartments. Pull gently on his neck while his brain gradually escapes. Or, make a transverse incision over his highest cervical spine and push a straight metal catheter through it on into his his foramen magnum. Or perforate his occiput. He should now deliver quite easily by the Mauriceau–Smellie–Veit manoeuvre.

If he still does not deliver, pass a crotchet up the tunnel and hook it on to the base of his skull.

If he has HYDROCEPHALY, see Section 19.7.

If she is brought in with HIS DEAD BODY PROTRUDING FROM HER VULVA (not uncommon), examine to feel if her cervix is fully dilated or not.

If it is fully dilated, proceed directly to decompress his head with a craniotomy (see above).

If it is not fully dilated, hang a weight of 1 kg on his trunk. His head will usually mould and deliver within an hour. If this fails, do a craniotomy as above.

CAUTION ! Don't try to pull his head forcefully through her undilated cervix. You may cause tears which extend into her lower segment.

If his NECK HAS BEEN SEVERED, and his head has gone back into her uterus, it will be difficult to find and remove. Use craniotomy equipment.

If his CORD PROLAPSES, manage her as you would with a cephalic presentation—section her, unless her cervix is fully dilated, and she is about to deliver. Cord prolapse is more common with breech deliveries, especially with a footling.

OTHER METHODS FOR BREECH DELIVERY

BREECH EXTRACTION uses your pulling forces, rather than her pushing forces. It is a quick way of delivering a small breech baby, usually a second twin. It may be indicated for: (1) Delay with the second twin. (2) Fetal distress with the second twin. (3) Cord prolapse at full dilatation with a breech. (4) A transverse lie in a second twin, following internal version. (5) A dead baby.

Method. She must be in the lithotomy position. Proceed as for an assisted breech delivery. You will need good anaesthesia: a subarachnoid (spinal) anaesthetic, an epidural or a pudendal block. Avoid general anaesthesia. *An episiotomy is vital.*

Hook the index fingers of each hand into his groins and pull, preferably during a contraction.

When his umbilicus appears, hook out his legs by flexing his knees. Do this by applying lateral and dorsal pressure in his popliteal fossae, and by sweeping each leg laterally and downwards. Pull on his pelvis, keeping his back anterior. Pull *posteriorly.* A common error is to pull him towards you, which is not in the axis of her birth canal. When you see his scapulae, hook out his arms. If his arms are not across his chest do Lovset's manoeuvre.

Push his head into his mother's pelvis from above. Then, if necessary, consider applying forceps to his aftercoming head.

The main difficulty is that his arms are more likely to be extended above his head, and his head is more likely to become deflexed. Lovset's manoeuvre and the Mauriceau–Smellie–Veit manoeuvre should solve these problems (see above).

Alternatively, if he is dead: (1) Pull on his leg(s), if you can reach them, or (2) use a combined breech hook and crotchet (Section 15.1a, and Figure 15-2). Pass the blunt hook end of this instrument over an extended leg into his groin, and pull on that. If he is macerated his leg may be pulled off. If it is pulled off, turn the instrument round and hook the sharp crotchet end over his iliac crest.

FORCEPS FOR THE AFTERCOMING HEAD. Standard obstetric forceps, such as those of Neville Barnes: (1) Are not easy to use on the aftercoming head. (2) Are liable to misuse if they are in the labour ward at all. (3) Create the impression for midwifery students that a breech delivery is something that only doctors can do. They must see methods used that they can use themselves at home or in a clinic. Outlet forceps (Wrigley's) are not long enough when you really need them. If they will reach his head they are hardly necessary in a breech delivery.

If you are going to use them, wait until you see his hair line. Ask your asistant to lift him by his ankles, then apply the left blade, followed by the right one. Slowly and gradually deliver his head with them.

THE CORRECTED PERINATAL MORTALITY FOR BREECH DELIVERIES (see above). This should be fairly easy to calculate from your labour ward record books, which should routinely record presentation, birth weight, obvious abnormalities, and live and still births. (1) Work out your perinatal mortality for all babies, excluding breeches, babies <2.5 kg, twins, and babies with obvious malformations. The perinatal period lasts from the 28th week to the end of the first week of life. (2) Do the same for breech deliveries only. Subtract (1) from (2). If the difference is >20/1000, do external version. In many district hospitals it is 50/1000.

19.9 More malpresentations

A transverse lie occurs most frequently in multips, and in mothers with polyhydramnios. When you diagnose it, don't forget the possibility that it may have been caused by twins, a major degree of *placenta praevia,* or CPD. Rarer causes include a congenital uterine abnormality, a grossly abnormal pelvic brim, a fibroid, an ovarian tumour, and an extrauterine pregnancy. When labour is obstructed by a transverse lie, the lower segment is particularly vulnerable, so don't stretch it any more by doing an internal version in advanced labour with a dead baby. Do a destructive operation (18.7).

MORE MALPRESENTATIONS

TRANSVERSE LIE

If a patient is 32 weeks pregnant or more, do an external cephalic version (19.8). This is safe provided there is no antepartum haemorrhage, hypertension with a blood pressure of <100 mm, or twins. If you fail, try again a week later. See also M 19.2. For obstructed labour with a transverse lie, see Sections 18.4

and 18.7 (destructive operations). For a transverse lie with twins see Section 19.11.

If she goes into labour with a transverse lie, when she is less than 30 weeks, or her baby feels as if he is under 1.5 kg, she may deliver spontaneously, although he is unlikely to survive. She also runs an increased risk of prolapse of the cord.

If you see her in the latent phase of labour, when she still has intact membranes and uterine contractions which are not strong, do an external version to produce a cephalic presentation. If this is successful, and she has no signs of CPD, and the position is still unstable, rupture her membranes while an assistant holds her baby's head over her pelvis. If she is of low parity, start an oxytocin drip (M 22.2). Check his lie and fetal heartbeat every 15 minutes, until his head is fixed in her pelvic brim.

If she has a small pelvis with an estimated true conjugate of <9 cm, section her.

If he is alive and she is in the active phase of labour with intact or ruptured membranes, and her cervix is <8 cm, section her. If her membranes are still intact, and you can feel a leg through her lower segment, you can deliver him through a lower segment transverse incision. But if her membranes have ruptured, and especially if his arm has prolapsed, a de Lee incision (18.9) is better, because you can extend this into the upper segment as necessary.

If he is alive and she is fully dilated or nearly so: (1) If she is a primip or a multip with a tight uterus, section her. (2) If she is a multip with intact membranes, and a uterus which is not tight, an internal version and breech extraction is sometimes advised. It is however very dangerous, and at least one contributor considers that the *only* indication for this manoeuvre is the transverse lie of a second twin with intact membranes (19.11).

If he is dead, and her cervix is not yet 8 cm dilated, do a lower segment section, and a transabdominal destructive operation. Use large scissors to decapitate him through the uterine incision (18.9, 18.10).

If he is dead, with an impacted shoulder, and her cervix is >8 cm dilated, and her uterus is not ruptured, do a destructive operation (18.7).

A BROW PRESENTATION

A brow presentation is often missed: (1) During labour. The head is high, but by the time it comes lower, the sutures and fontanelles by which it might have been diagnosed, have become obscured by caput. (2) At Caesarean section a brow presentation is not diagnosed until the typical moulding makes the diagnosis obvious. Unless the baby is premature, or his mother's pelvis is enormous, he will not deliver vaginally.

If you diagnose a brow presentation and she is early in labour, her pelvis is large, and he is of normal size, his head may flex, and he may deliver vaginally. You may be able to assist flexion by putting your hand through her cervix, pushing his head up and trying to flex it. But, if you fail to flex his head, if her membranes rupture, or if she fails to progress, or if there is any sign of obstruction, section her.

A FACE PRESENTATION

If her pelvis is large and there are no signs of CPD, allow her labour to progress. He is most likely to be mento-lateral, and will probably rotate anteriorly and deliver spontaneously. You may be able to help by turning him with your hand. If he remains mento-posterior, you will have to section her.

If she is delayed in the second stage and he is in the mento-anterior position, with less than 2/5 of his head above her pelvic brim, you can do a symphysiotomy if CPD is mild, but section would be wiser. Remember that the head moulds less in a face presentation. If CPD is more than mild, section her.
CAUTION ! (1) Remember the possibility of anencephaly. Anencephalic babies often present by the face, but usually deliver easily. You should be able to distinguish anencephaly, a face, and a breech vaginally, once her cervix is 8 cm dilated; feel for his brow and his mouth. Occasionally, a lateral X-ray is useful. (2) If you are going to use oxytocin, use it with the greatest caution. (3) Never use a vacuum extractor!

19.10 Prolapse and presentation of the cord

If a mother's cervix is not well applied to the presenting part, her baby's cord can *prolapse* when her membranes rupture, especially if his head is high, or she has a transverse lie, a breech, a face presentation, or twins. The cord is said to be *presenting* when it lies below the presenting part, inside her intact membranes. Both prolapse and presentation can obstruct the circulation in it, and so endanger his life. Other presenting parts press less firmly on his cord than does his head, but don't let this delay you.

PROLAPSE AND PRESENTATION OF THE CORD

PROLAPSE. ALWAYS do a vaginal examination immediately a mother's membranes rupture spontaneously, unless: (1) She is <36 weeks and is not having contractions, and you are considering non-operative management. Or, (2) her baby's head is well down (not more than 2/5 above the brim).

If you find a prolapsed cord, DON'T take your hand out of her vagina!

Instead, push his head (or breech) off the cord. While you are holding his head, ask an assistant to insert a Foley catheter and fill her bladder with 500 ml of Ringer's lactate or saline. A full bladder will keep his head away from the cord and inhibit the contractions of her uterus.

Listen to his heart, to find out if he is still alive. It may still be beating, even if his cord is not (cord spasm). Assess his size, and try to exclude gross congenital abnormalities, particularly hydrocephalus.

Remove your fingers, and apply a pad to her perineum, so that the cord remains in her vagina. Turn her on to her side with the foot of her bed raised. Or put her into the knee-elbow position (19-2). Set up an isoprenaline infusion (M 19.6). Put her on a trolley, and take her to the theatre for section as soon as possible. Don't pass a stomach tube; instead give her an antacid. Don't empty her bladder until you are ready to incise her parietal peritoneum.

Always section her unless: (1) She is fully dilated and the head is only 2/5 or less above the brim (unusual). If so, apply forceps (if you are experienced with them because they are quicker), or a vacuum extractor. (2) Prolapse of the cord complicates the delivery of a second twin with a cephalic presentation. If there is no CPD, you can usually apply a vacuum extractor, or do a breech extraction preceded by internal version if necessary.

PRESENTATION OF THE CORD. If you feel the cord vaginally when she has intact membranes, observe carefully for the fetal heart changes which indicate cord compression (M 18.56): (1) Put her into the head-down or knee-chest position. Nurse her with the foot of her bed raised for 24 hours. This will nearly always allow it to rise above his head. Or, (2) before 37 weeks, try external version. Turning him may draw the cord from under the presenting part. Or,(3) section her, unless he is dead or too small to survive.

PROLAPSE OF THE CORD

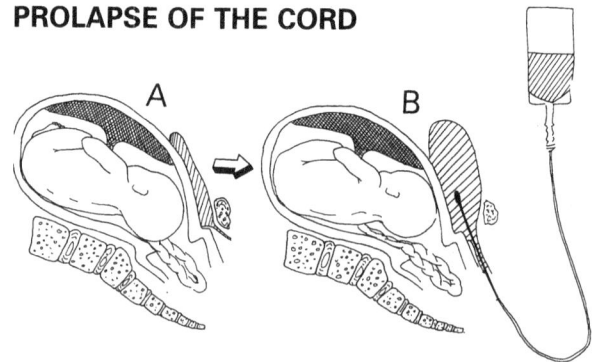

Fig. 19-6 TREATING PROLAPSE OF THE CORD BY FILLING THE BLADDER. A, the head pressing on the cord. B, the patient's bladder has been filled through a catheter, and the cord is now free. A full bladder also inhibits contractions of the uterus.

HOW TWINS PRESENT

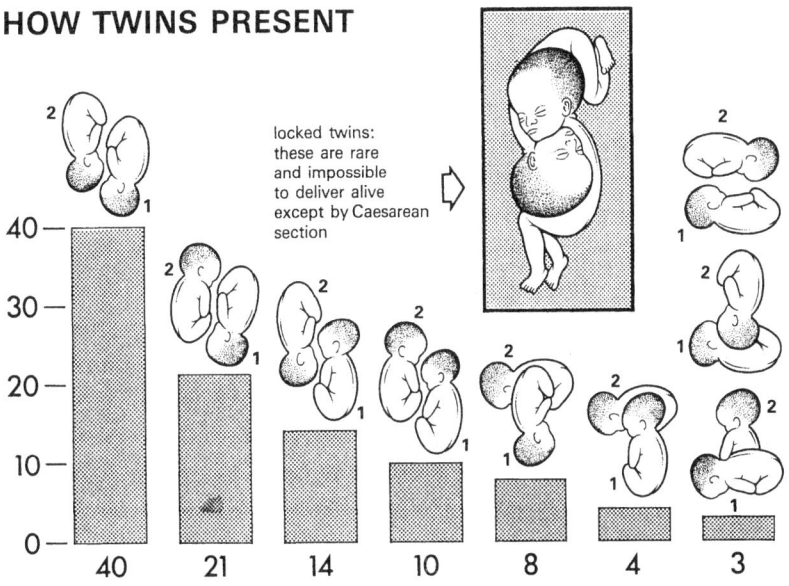

Fig. 19-7 HOW TWINS PRESENT. In 40% of cases both twins are cephalic. In 21% the second twin is a breech. In 14% the first twin is a breech. In 10% of cases both twins are breeches. In all remaining cases one or other twin, or occasionally both, are transverse.

19.11 Multiple pregnancies

You can deliver most twins vaginally, and only section their mother on the same indications as for a singleton pregnancy (18.4). Twins do however have problems: (1) Labour is more often premature, which puts them at risk. (2) Uterine inertia is more common; this delays the first and second stages of labour, and makes postpartum haemorrhage more likely. (3) Malpresentations are more common, especially with the second twin. (4) Prolapse of the cord is also more common. (5) When the first twin has been born, the second may suffer as the uterus retracts and constricts the placental site.

As soon as you diagnose twins plan for: (1) Hospital delivery. (2) Rest from 32 to 37 weeks, at home if possible, or at a hospital or health centre. You will usually have to admit a mother at 34–35 weeks to the mother's waiting area. (3) A clinical pelvic assessment at 36 weeks. She is more likely to become anaemic, so be sure she is on iron and folic acid. Watch for gestational hypertension (17.4). She should not labour for longer with twins than she would with a single pregnancy. If you do decide to use oxytocin, use it with the greatest care. Deliver triplets (or quadruplets) as you would twins. Expect the same problems as with twins, but expect them more often.

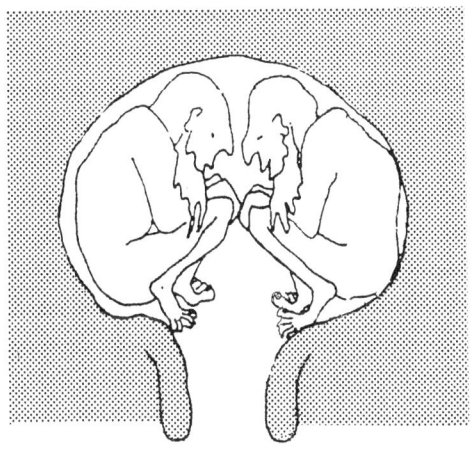

'After you.' 'No, after you'

MULTIPLE PREGNANCIES

FIRST STAGE. As soon as a mother is admitted in labour, determine the lie and presentation of the first twin by abdominal palpation. Confirm this by examining her vaginally, and at the same time assess her pelvis, if this has not already been done at 36 weeks. Manage her as for a singleton pregnancy and use a partogram. If there is delay during the active stage, manage this as for a singleton pregnancy, and apply the same criteria for the use of oxytocin and Caesarean section (see below).

If the first twin is cephalic, or a fully-flexed breech, manage the first stage as an ordinary trial of labour, unless he is very big, or her pelvis is very contracted.

If the first twin has a transverse lie, or is a footling (one leg flexed and one extended), section her, unless he is very small (less than 1.5 kg). He is likely to slip through an undilated cervix, and runs an increased risk of cord prolapse.

SECOND STAGE. Find an assistant who will be ready to look after the first twin, while you deliver the second. Be prepared for an operative delivery of the second twin, and for a postpartum haemorrhage. Have equipment for a drip ready, and ergometrine and oxytocin in easy reach. Preferably, have a drip up routinely.

Deliver the first twin as usual for a cephalic or breech presentation. Immediately he has been born, divide his cord between clamps, and then replace the maternal one by a tie.

CAUTION ! As soon as the first twin is born, look at the clock. Deliver the second twin as soon as possible, but without undue hurry. 20 minutes is a reasonable time.

Feel her abdomen through a sterile towel to find the lie, presentation, and level of the presenting part of the second twin. Then do a vaginal examination to feel how it fits her pelvis. Use 4 fingers or even your whole hand, instead of the usual two; there will always be room for them immediately after delivery of the first twin. The head of the second twin is likely to be high, and you may not be able to reach it with it with two fingers.

If you have a skilled assistant, ask her to do the abdominal palpation and external version of the second twin, and to hold his head steady, while you rupture the patient's membranes.

Listen for the fetal heart, but don't waste too much time doing this; it may be difficult to hear and you will have to deliver him promptly anyway.

CAUTION ! (1) Be sure you know what the presenting part is before you rupture her membranes. (2) The second twin may be larger than the first one. If you are unskilled, a timely section (rarely necessary) is better than the vacuum extraction of a high head, or pulling down the leg of a high-sitting breech. But, if you are expert, a vaginal delivery will always be quicker. Don't be too keen on section: CPD is unusual with twins.

If the second twin is lying longitudinally, rupture his membranes, and deliver him as a vertex or a breech. If he is a vertex, ask your assistant to push his head into her pelvic brim, as you rupture his membranes (to avoid prolapse of the cord).

If the second twin is transverse, correct his lie by manipulating him through a towel on her abdomen, so that his head presents (external cephalic version). The external version of a second twin is usually easy, provided you do it without delay, immediately after the first twin has been delivered, while the membranes remain intact, and before uterine contractions restart. Your assistant can usually do the version, while you check vaginally that he has turned correctly.

If immediate delivery of the second twin in the labour ward by external cephalic version is not possible, try to keep her membranes intact. Rupturing them while he is transverse risks obstructed labour and rupture of her uterus. Arrange for speedy delivery in the theatre by internal podalic version so that you can bring down a leg (see below), or if this fails by Caesarean section.

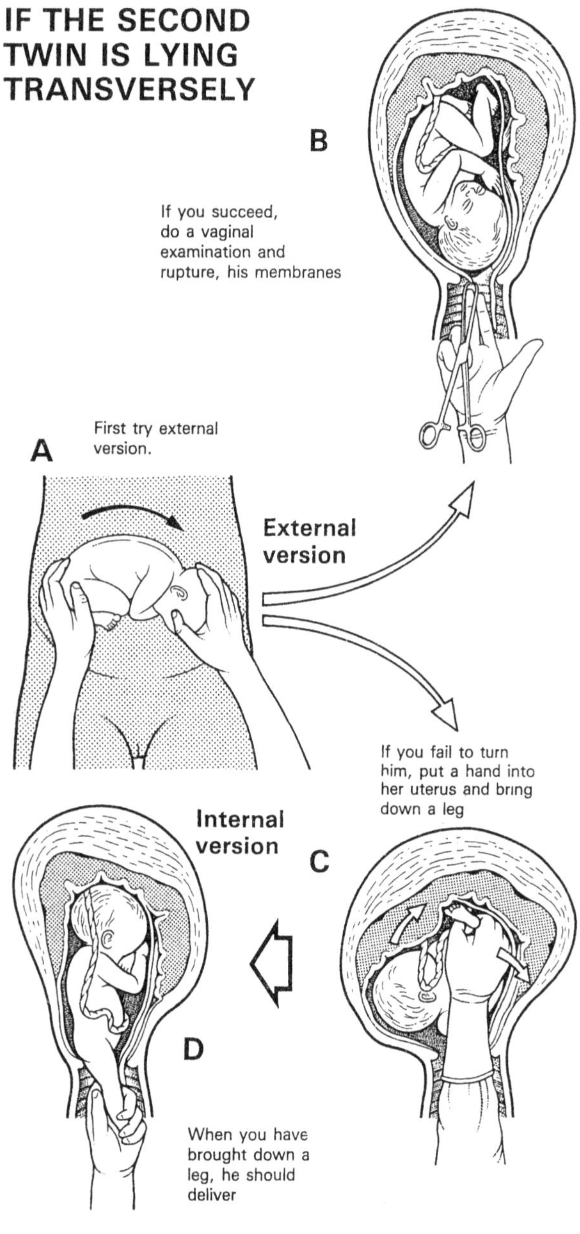

THIRD STAGE. Manage this actively to minimize blood loss. Give her intravenous ergometrine with oxytocin ('Syntometrine') with the birth of the anterior shoulder of the second twin, and then deliver the placentas by controlled cord traction. If bleeding continues or her uterus is lax, also give her 10 units of oxytocin in 500 ml of fluid at 10 drops a minute.

PARTICULAR METHODS FOR MULTIPLE PREGNANCIES

INTERNAL PODALIC ('foot') VERSION can often be done without general anaesthesia. It is kinder however to give her diazepam 10 mg and pethidine 50 mg intravenously.

Put her into the lithotomy position. Make sure her bladder is empty. Prepare her vulva as usual, and preferably her abdominal wall also (sterile sheets are a nuisance, and you want to feel what you are doing).

Wait until she is relaxed between contractions, then put your gloved right hand through her vagina and fully dilated cervix into her uterus, until you can feel her intact membranes. Keep them intact if you can. Often, you have to rupture them before you can get a grip on a foot. Feel her abdomen with your left hand. Grope around for a foot, which you will recognize by its heel. If this is difficult (unusual), work out which way he is lying, and then feel in the direction of his buttocks. Find a leg and follow this down. Use your other hand if this seems easier. When you have found a foot, bring this down. Hold his ankle between your index and middle finger, with your thumb on the dorsum of his foot. Gently pull his foot, so as to bring one of his legs over her pelvic brim, and down her vagina as far as you can, if possible as far as her vulva. His buttocks and other leg will follow. At the same time push his head towards her fundus.

Only now rupture her membranes. Keep pulling on his leg in the direction of the floor. If necessary squat to do this. As more leg appears, hold it higher along its length. When his anterior buttock appears on her perineum, pull horizontally, and then upwards (breech extraction). When his buttocks are out, deliver his shoulders by Lovset's manoeuvre and his head by the Mauriceau-Smellie-Veit manoeuvre (19.8).

Occasionally, it is enough to pull down a leg into her vagina, and let her do the pushing (an assisted breech delivery); but don't rely on this, and be ready to assist her if she is uncooperative or exhausted.

CAUTION ! (1) Internal podalic version is only for the second twin with *intact or recently ruptured membranes*, during a delivery which you have been supervising. It is not suitable if she is admitted with a transverse second twin and ruptured membranes. If so, manage her as a neglected transverse lie: if he is alive section her, if he is dead, do a destructive operation. (2) Make quite sure it is a foot, and not a hand that you are feeling. Don't, in exasperation, bring down any limb—it is sure to be an arm! (3) If you don't know what is presenting, don't waste time waiting for the presenting part to come down. While you wait, her membranes will probably rupture spontaneously, and the presenting part may be an arm!

CAESAREAN SECTION is indicated if she has: (1) A contracted pelvis with a diagonal conjugate of <11 cm, or a true conjugate <9.5 cm. (2) A major malpresentation of the leading baby, such as a transverse lie or an incomplete breech. (3) Lack of progress in labour. (4) A second twin with a transverse lie which you cannot correct. The scar from a previous Caesarean section is a relative contraindication to vaginal delivery.

DIFFICULTIES WITH MULTIPLE PREGNANCIES

If there is DELAY IN THE FIRST STAGE, you can use oxytocin, provided there is no CPD. Rupture the membranes of the first twin.

If CONTRACTIONS STOP after delivery of the first twin, and your are *sure the presentation of the second is cephalic or breech*, rupture her membranes. If contractions don't start immediately, put up an oxytocin drip at 2.5 units to 500 ml, and run this at 60 drops a minute. Try to deliver the second twin within 30 minutes of the first, or preferably less.

If, when you do a vaginal examination after the delivery of the first twin, you feel the head or breech of the second twin,

Fig. 19-8. IF THE SECOND TWIN IS TRANSVERSE, first try external cephalic version. If you succeed, rupture his membranes. If you fail, bring down a leg so as to make him into a breech presentation. This is internal podalic version. Keep the membranes intact if you can, until you have found a foot. In C, and D, they have been broken.

304

but her CERVIX ONLY SEEMS TO BE 7 OR 8 CM DILATED, rupture her membranes and make her push. Her cervix will dilate again, as soon as the presenting part of the second twin comes down. Contraction of her cervix will not delay delivery of the second twin, and is no reason for waiting.

If the SECOND TWIN IS SO HIGH IN HER BIRTH CANAL, that you cannot reach him with your whole hand, and her cervix only admits two fingers, she has a CONTRACTION RING. It may go if you give her pethidine and diazepam, but if it doesn't section her.

If she BLEEDS HEAVILY BEFORE THE DELIVERY OF THE SECOND TWIN, the placenta of the first one has probably separated. Deliver the second twin quickly, and then deliver both placentas together.

If either twin is a BREECH, and she pushes well and the breech descends well, it will be an assisted breech delivery. If there is fetal distress, or delay, or poor pushing, don't hesitate to apply more traction, and turn delivery into a breech extraction (19.8).

19.11a Postpartum haemorrhage—PPH

Perhaps you have just done a vacuum extraction, and are just taking your gloves off, when there is an ominous splashing of blood into the bucket. Or, a midwife calls you in the middle of the night to say that a patient has had a severe postpartum haemorrhage. What are you going to do? A PPH can often be prevented, and can almost always be treated. Here is its management in hospital, which supplements that in *Primary Mother Care*.

PPH is caused by: (1) Bleeding from the placental site because the uterus has failed to contract—much the most important cause. (2) Tears of the genital tract—rupture of the uterus, cervical tears, tears of the upper vagina, and vulval tears, especially near the urethra and clitoris. (3) Occasionally by a clotting defect, especially DIC (disseminated intravascular coagulation), which produces a fibrinogen deficiency.

Aim to resuscitate the patient, to stop the bleeding, and to monitor her carefully. Bleeding most often occurs from the placental site, so your first objective must be an empty well-contracted uterus with the placenta out.

Obstetricians differ in what they do for the few patients who continue to bleed from a contracted uterus with the placenta out, who have no obviously suturable tear or bleeding vessel to tie, and no clotting defect. Some pack the uterus, some stitch quite minor tears (the parturient cervix is normally ragged so they may be stitching the normal), and some do nothing except transfuse. Of those who pack, some explore, inspect, and suture the uterus first, and only pack if they find no tear worth suturing. Others pack, and only explore if packing fails to control bleeding. We side with those who pack when exploring and suturing have failed.

When you pack, do so *on the correct indications, and after all proper steps have been taken*. Packing is messy and time-consuming, and needs large quantities of sterile dressings. If there is a steady ooze, blood is scarce, and HIV common, packing may save a mother's life. In theory, packing is undesirable; in practice it is very useful as a near last resort, before tying her uterine or her iliac arteries, or removing her uterus (see 'Stop Press'). It is much less effective in controlling bleeding from her uterus, than from her cervix. Much the best way to do this is to give her oxytocics to make her uterus contract—if it will.

DIC is probably the commonest cause of a massive PPH, when the uterus is empty, and is satisfactorily contracted. It is the commonest clotting defect, and is an important and preventable cause of maternal death. It is uncommon after a normal delivery, and is more common after abruption (16.13), an obstructed labour (18.3), or an intrauterine death (16.4). Try to keep two bottles of fibrinogen (one gram) in the refrigerator of your maternity unit. This is the only clotting factor which it is practicable for you to stock. If you cannot get it, or any fresh frozen plasma, you will have to give her fresh blood. To do this, you will find it helpful if all your permanent medical and nursing staff know their blood groups, and can be called upon in an emergency.

Bergstrom Steffan. (1) Modrahalsovard I U-Land. (2) Forlossningsvard I U-Land. Reklam and Katalogtryck Uppsala 1988.

IF SHE HAS LOST MORE THAN A LITRE OF BLOOD, OR SHOWS SIGNS OF HYPOVOLAEMIA, REQUEST 2 UNITS OF BLOOD URGENTLY
(decide how much she needs when it comes)

POSTPARTUM HAEMORRHAGE ('PPH')

PREVENTING PPH BEFORE LABOUR

RISK FACTORS FOR PPH IDENTIFIABLE DURING PREGNANCY. If a mother has a history of any of these, she is more likely to have a PPH and should deliver in hospital: (1) Grand multiparity (>5 children). (2) An antepartum haemorrhage in this pregnancy. (3) A postpartum haemorrhage, or a retained placenta, in a previous pregnancy. (4) Multiple pregnancy or other cause of polyhydramnios. (5) Hypotonic uterine action in a previous pregnancy.

RISK FACTORS FOR PPH IDENTIFIABLE DURING LABOUR. (1) Prolonged labour. (2) General anaesthesia, usually with ether or halothane. (3) A full bladder. (4) 'Fiddling with the uterus' during the third stage. (5) Placenta praevia. (6) Placental abruption, mainly because this causes a clotting defect. (7) A clotting defect, especially DIC. (8) Incomplete expulsion of the placenta.

CAUTION ! (1) A postpartum haemorrhage may occur without there being any risk factors. (2) When you 'rub up a uterus', use the flat of your hand on the fundus. 'Fiddling' is all kinds of pushing, pulling, and rubbing, which cause partial separation of the placenta before the uterus has contracted firmly.

PREVENTING PPH DURING LABOUR

Give every mother, especially those with risk factors, an oxytocic drug: (1) Ergometrine with oxytocin ('Syntometrine') 1 ml intramuscularly. Or, (2) 5 units of oxytocin intramuscularly. Or, (3) ergometrine 0.5 mg intramuscularly (usually one ampoule). They will work quicker if you give them intravenously, but there may be nobody around who can do this routinely. Give a mother one of these, as soon as her baby is born—and you are sure there is no twin in her uterus. Then deliver her placenta by controlled cord traction. If supplies are short, you may only be able to give an oxytocic drug to 'at risk' mothers.

If she has a risk factor for PPH, and you have sufficient intravenous fluids and drip sets, set up a drip of dextrose in water before she reaches the second stage. When her baby and her placenta have been delivered, add 20 units of oxytocin to the drip (500 ml), and run this in at about 30 drops a minute for at least 3 hours. Also, give her ergometrine as usual. Unfortunately, this is an expensive routine, and you may have to wait until a mother has already lost 500 ml, before you can afford to put up a drip.

CONTROLLED CORD TRACTION. As soon as her uterus is contracting firmly from the action of oxytocin or ergometrine, put your left hand on her abdomen, above her pubic symphysis, and turn your palm towards her head. Grasp her uterus. As soon as it feels hard from the effect of the oxytocic, push it upwards towards her umbilicus (deliver the placenta more by pushing her uterus up than by pulling on the cord). Wind two or three loops of cord round your index finger and gently pull on the cord, first downwards and backwards, and then more anteriorly as the cord comes out.

As soon as the placenta is delivered check to make sure that: (1) it is complete and that no lobes of it have been left behind (see below) and, (2) that there are no obvious tears in her birth canal. Keep her in the labour ward, and monitor her for at least an hour, before returning her to the ward. Check that her uterus is well contracted and note any bleeding.

Opinions differ about the use of controlled cord traction, without the use of an oxytocic drug. Ideally, you should never apply controlled cord traction before the uterus has hardened under the effect of an oxytocic drug, and if you don't have one,

CONTROLLED CORD TRACTION

Only do this if she has had ergometrine or oxytocin!

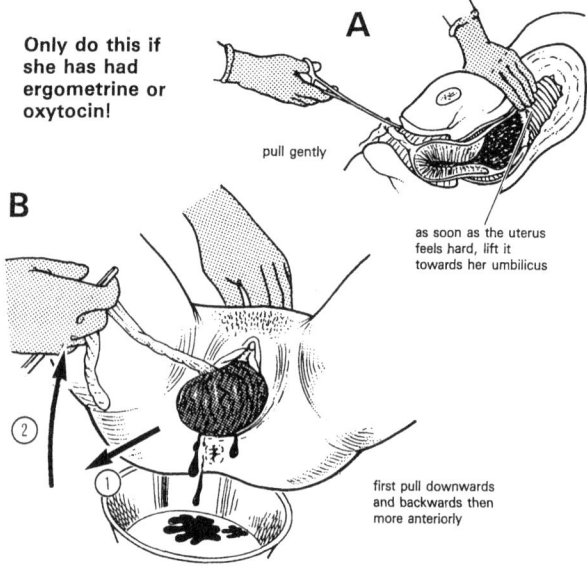

Fig. 19-9 CONTROLLED CORD TRACTION. As soon as her uterus is contracting firmly from the action of oxytocin or ergometrine, grasp her uterus, push it upwards towards her umbilicus and gently pull on the cord, first downwards and backwards, and then more anteriorly as the cord comes out.

you should not use it. In practice, little harm results *provided there are signs of placental separation (lengthening of the cord, hardness and mobility of the uterus)*. Although it is a very valuable procedure, there is a risk, particularly if you do it incorrectly, that you may turn her uterus inside out (inversion of the uterus), see below.

CAUTION ! Don't squeeze her uterus to try to get the placenta out. This is so painful that it may cause shock.

ASSESSMENT AND RESUSCITATION FOR PPH

As soon as you are called to a patient with a PPH, quickly call an assistant: at least 2 people are needed. Assess and, if necessary, resuscitate her vigorously, as you would any other hypovolaemic patient (53.2). What is the state of her peripheral circulation? How much blood has she lost? Is it clotting normally in the receiver used to collect it? It may clot to start with, and then stop clotting later. What has been done so far? Monitor the volume of blood she continues to lose, her pulse and blood pressure, and her urine output.

If she is still bleeding: Is her uterus still contracted? Is the placenta out and complete? Does she have any obvious lacerations of her vulva, vagina or perineum?

If she is not still bleeding, is her uterus well contracted?

CAUTION ! Put someone in charge of her, and make sure that she is that person's sole responsibility, until bleeding has stopped, and her condition is stable. Poor supervision is an important cause of death in PPH.

PPH WITH THE PLACENTA IN

Try to make her uterus contract. (1) If you have not given her ergometrine, or, better, 'Syntometrine', give it now. (2) If this fails to stimulate a contraction, gently massage her uterus ('rub up' a contraction). (3) Remove her placenta by controlled cord traction (see above), as soon as her uterus is contracting firmly. It should deliver immediately.

If controlled cord traction fails to deliver her placenta, remove it manually. Before doing a formal manual removal, you may be wise to do a vaginal examination, and see if it has stuck in her cervix, from which you can remove it quite easily.

While preparing to do a manual removal concentrate on: (1) resuscitating her, and (2) keeping her uterus contracted by putting 20 or perhaps 40 units of oxytocin into the bottle (500 ml) of her intravenous drip (not the tubing, it is needed as a continuous infusion). (3) If the oxytocin does not work, gently rub up a contraction.

MANUAL REMOVAL OF THE PLACENTA can either be fairly easy, or rather difficult. It is usually best done in the the labour ward (which must be equipped for anaesthetic resuscitation, A 3.1) rather than the theatre, which will cause delay and require moving her. You will need stirrups to maintain the lithotomy position and a good light. Before you start, set up a drip of saline or Ringer's lactate, or if she is very collapsed, two drips. If she is already being given an oxytocin drip, stop this just before manual removal to allow her cervix to relax, so that you can get your fingers through it.

Scrub up and gown yourself, then put her into the lithotomy position, and clean her vulva and the protruding cord. Cover her with a lithotomy towel (a towel cut to expose the vulva).

Unless she is very collapsed, she needs analgesia. Give her pethidine 25 to 50 mg and diazepam 10 to 20 mg intravenously. Or, if this is difficult, give her intravenous ketamine (A 8.1). Give them intravenously slowly, into the tubing of the drip, or into a vein. Manual removal without analgesia or an anaesthetic is very uncomfortable, particularly if it turns out to be difficult. Inexpert general anaesthesia, which may be all there is, is unnecessary, and potentially dangerous (18.1a).

POST PARTUM HAEMORRHAGE

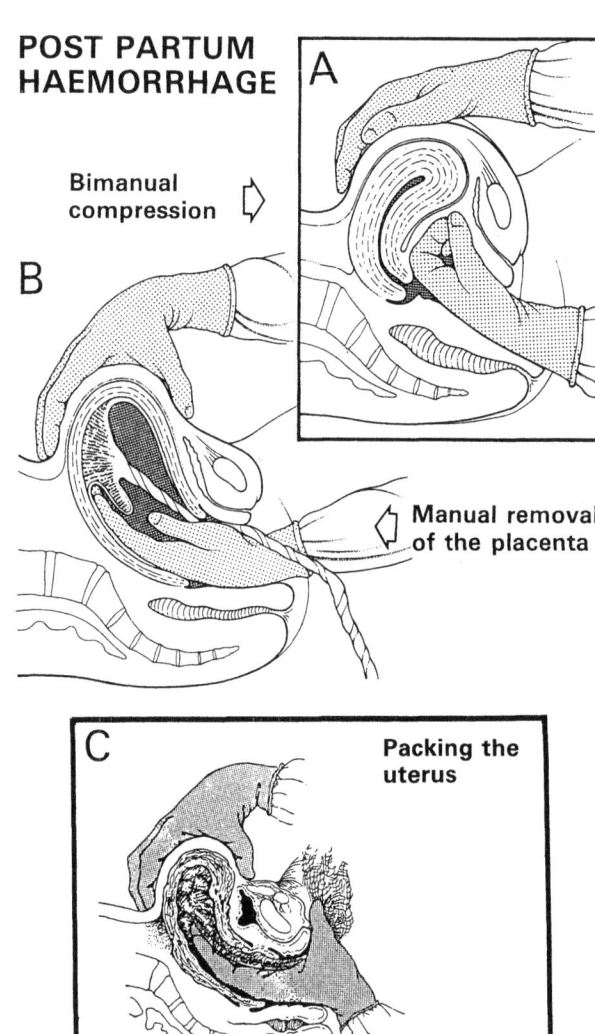

Fig. 19-10. POSTPARTUM HAEMORRHAGE (PPH). A, bimanual compression of a bleeding uterus between a fist in the patient's vagina and a hand on her abdominal wall. B, manual removal of the placenta. Gently separate it from the wall of her uterus with a *slow* sawing movement with the side of your hand. C, packing the uterus is only occasionally necessary. Its main use is to control bleeding from the cervix. It is much less effective in controlling bleeding from the uterus. Much the best best way to do this, is to give drugs to make it contract. C, *kindly contributed by Robert Lange.*

Hold the cord in your left hand. Put the tips of the fingers of your right hand together, and introduce it into the upper part of her vagina. If her placenta has stuck in her cervix, grasp it and slowly remove it. Now let go of the cord, and place your left hand on her fundus (over the towel). Prevent her fundus from being pushed up, as you gradually work your way into her uterus with your right hand. Feel for the part of the placenta which has already separated, and push your fingers between it and the wall of her uterus. Gently separate her placenta from the wall of her uterus with a *slow* sawing movement, with the side of your hand.

CAUTION ! All this time keep your left hand pressing on her fundus, so as to bring her uterus as close to your right hand, as you can. If you don't do this there is a danger you may tear it.

As soon as the placenta has separated, grasp it with your right hand, remove it, and ask your assistant to inspect it. While this is being done, and whether it looks complete or not, explore her uterus for any pieces that may have been left behind, and remove them. Only now remove your right hand from her uterus. Finally, give her a further dose of intravenous 'Syntometrine', or ergometrine (0.5 mg), and wait for her uterus to contract. As it begins to do this, remove your hand. As you do so, check that the lower segment is intact.

Before you finish make sure that there are no other sites of bleeding; so explore her uterus as described below.

Inspect her placenta to see if: (1) a piece of it has been left inside, or (2) a vessel is running off one edge of it. This may lead to an extra lobe which has been left inside. If either of these things have happened, the missing piece of placenta must be removed.

If she continues to bleed, apply BIMANUAL COMPRESSION (A, Fig. 19-10). Put your right hand into her upper vagina. Put your left hand on her abdomen, and use it to push her fundus down onto your right hand. Press for at least 5 minutes, and then review the situation. If she continues to bleed, you are now in the situation of 'PPH with the placenta out', so see below.

Continue the oxytocin drip. Add 20 units of oxytocin to the intravenous fluid (500 ml), and run it in at a rate that will keep her uterus contracted. Continue the drip for at least 12 hours, using more intravenous fluid and oxytocin as necessary. Monitor her carefully. Some obstetricians would also give her an antibiotic. Keep her in hospital for at least 5 days, because of the increased risk of puerperal sepsis, particularly endometritis. A few days later check her haemoglobin.

PPH WITH THE PLACENTA OUT

Failure of the uterus to contract is the most important cause, so aim for an empty, well-contracted uterus.

Feel her fundus. It should be hard and round, and below her umbilicus. If it is soft and difficult to feel, it may be relaxing. Rub it up to make it contract. This may expel some blood and clots. If her bladder is full, catheterize it. Give her ergometrine 0.5 mg, or 'Syntometrine' 1 ml, intravenously or intramuscularly (if she has not already had it).

Resuscitate her. Ideally, put up two drips of saline or Ringer's lactate (in practice you may have to start with a single drip). To the first add 20 units of oxytocin to the intravenous fluid (500 ml). Run it in fast, until her uterus contracts well. Then slow it to 40 drops a minute. Continue this drip for two hours afterwards.

Use the second drip to replace the blood she has lost. Give her a plasma substitute (dextran), or blood. If her blood pressure falls below 80 mm systolic (90 mm is the usual value, but you will probably be worried about HIV), run it in rapidly. As soon as her blood pressure reaches 90 mm systolic, slow it to 40 drops a minute.

Inspect her placenta for missing pieces *with great care,* if you have not already done so. If a piece is retained it will have to be removed. If there are any obvious perineal tears, suture them.

If bleeding stops, continue to monitor her, to resuscitate her if necessary, and to give her intravenous oxytocin.

If she continues to bleed with an empty uterus (5% chance), note the following and take the appropriate action:

(A) Is her uterus still poorly contracted, despite the oxytocin? If so, increase the rate of infusion. If this fails, she may have a piece of placenta remaining inside, or, much less commonly, a ruptured uterus. So explore her uterus (see below), if you have not already done so.

(B) Does the blood coming from her uterus clot normally? If it fails to clot, she probably has a clotting defect (see below).

(C) Does her uterus remain well contracted, but she bleeds in spite of it? If so, explore her genital tract for tears, from her fundus to her clitoris. If you find tears, suture them. If you don't find any tears (and her blood clots), pack her uterus and vagina. If it does not clot, see below.

EXPLORATION FOR PPH

INDICATIONS. (1) As a normal part of any manual removal (see above). (2) A mother who continues to bleed with the placenta out. Also see below on the indications for packing.

METHOD. Scrub up and put on gloves. Towel her, as for manual removal. Catheterize her. Give her intravenous analgesia (see above). Put her into the lithotomy position, get a good light, and find a Sims' speculum, and an assistant to help hold it. Wipe out the blood in her vagina with cotton wool swabs. Look at its walls. Check that her vaginal wall, and her perineal and vulval skin are intact. To inspect her cervix, use two swab-holding forceps. Grasp the front lip of her cervix with one of them. Pull her cervix gently down, and look for lacerations on it. If there are no lacerations in that bit of cervix, use the second forceps to pull down the next bit of cervix, and look at that. Go right round her cervix in this way, looking at every part, as in Fig. 19-11. Then put your hand into her uterus and carefully feel its front, sides, back, and fundus. Feel for a rupture of her uterus (18.17), and for any pieces of adherent placenta.

If she has lacerations of her perineum, vagina, or cervix which are big enough to suture, suture them. Only suture a cervical tear, if it is causing arterial bleeding. A venous ooze is not a sufficient indication for suturing.

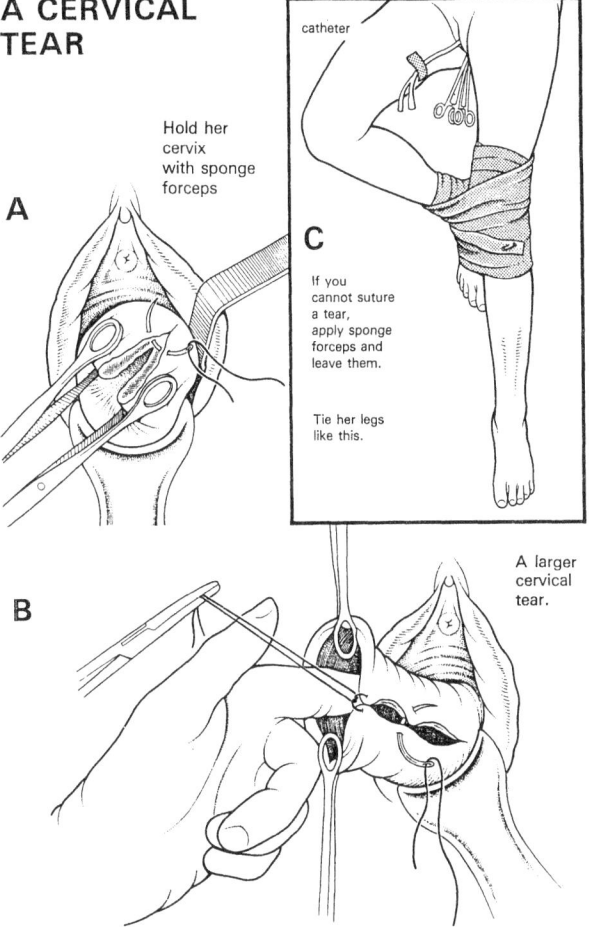

Fig. 19-11 REPAIRING A CERVICAL TEAR. A, search all round the patient's cervix with ring forceps, until you find the tear. B, a longer tear being sutured. C, if midwives cannot control bleeding they are asked to apply ring forceps, tie the patient's legs together, and refer her to you like this.

If she is bleeding from multiple small tears rather than one large one which you can easily stitch, or there is a steady ooze, pack her uterus and vagina as described below.

If a piece of placenta remains inside, scrape it off with your fingers. If you cannot get it all off, she has an abnormally adherent placenta, leave it.

If you find a rupture in her uterus, apply bimanual compression (if the bleeding is severe), until you can get the theatre organized for a laparotomy (18.17).

PACKING THE UTERUS AND VAGINA FOR PPH

INDICATIONS (1) Continued bleeding, when there is no clotting defect, and no tear in the upper vagina, cervix, or uterus, which is large enough to repair surgically, and when *other methods to control bleeding, particularly the adequate use of oxytocic drugs, have failed.* (2) Continued bleeding after a clotting defect has been corrected, or when you are unable to correct it. Note: one contributor packs before exploring and only explores when packing has failed (and the blood clots), see above.

METHOD. Scrub up and glove yourself. Put her into the lithotomy position. Pack her uterus and vagina with a wide roll of sterile gauze, or laparotomy pads, or failing these, maternity pads, which are less satisfactory, because they may get lost inside. Start by packing her fundus and work downwards. Use ring forceps to push lengths of gauze through her vagina into her uterus, until both are firmly packed down to her perineum. Pack tightly to press on her cervix from below. The pack should fill her uterus. However, if both her cervix and her uterus are well contracted, you may not be able to pack her uterus completely. If so, a well packed vagina may press adequately on a bleeding cervix.

CAUTION ! (1) Be sure to pack her *whole* genital tract, from her fundus to her introitus if you possibly can, for which you will need *large* quantities of gauze. (2) Don't only pack her vagina, because she will bleed above the pack and her uterus will fill with blood, the only sign of which may be increasing shock. (3) If you use maternity pads or separate pieces of gauze, you must tie them together, or they will get lost.

When you have packed her uterus, she will have difficulty in passing urine, so pass a Foley's catheter, and connect this to a bag.

If the pack controls bleeding, continue to monitor her and to give her intravenous fluid or blood as necessary. *Remove the pack at 24 to 48 hours, preferably at 24 hours.*

DIFFICULTIES WITH PPH

If a patient is BLEEDING SEVERELY and there is going to be some delay before you can treat her, compress her aorta. Stand on her left and feel for her left femoral pulse with your left hand. Clench your right fist and with your index finger level with her umbilicus and your knuckles in the line of her spine, press firmly through her abdominal wall so as to compress her aorta against her spine. You will feel it pulsating. Press so that you no longer feel any pulsations and obliterate her femoral pulse. If necessary, this method can be kept up for hours, while she is referred or while preparations for surgery are being made, changing hands and workers as required. If her legs become numb, allow a little blood to flow through them. A method described by Staffan Bergström (see above).

If you CANNOT GET YOUR WHOLE HAND THROUGH HER CERVIX TO DO A MANUAL REMOVAL (not uncommon if she has been given a lot of ergometrine shortly before the manual removal is done, or there has been a long delay), you are in difficulty. Avoid this problem, if you can, by using intravenous oxytocin in the drip, rather than ergometrine, and by discontinuing the drip just before manual removal. Try to get one or two fingers through her cervix, and push her fundus well down with your other hand. Usually, her cervix relaxes gradually so that, if you are slow and gentle, you can put your whole hand into her uterus.

If her placenta seems abnormally adherent to her uterus (PLACENTA ACCRETA or increta), remove what you safely can piecemeal, without perforating her uterus, and leave the rest. If her uterus does not contract well, she will not bleed from these areas, but only from the separated ones. The placenta which you have to leave will be slowly absorbed. She is at serious risk from sepsis and secondary postpartum haemorrhage. Continue the oxytocin drip for 48 hours, then stop if she is satisfactory. Give her antibiotics (chloramphenicol and metronidazole, 2.9). Monitor her carefully, and keep her in hospital for 12 to 14 days.

If YOU PUT YOUR FINGERS THROUGH HER UTERINE WALL as you remove the placenta (easily done, but this should be rare if you do the procedure properly), do a laparotomy and inspect the tear. If it is a minor one, you may be able to repair it. If it is a large tear, repair it, and if bleeding is not controlled, tie her internal iliac arteries. If you don't think it is safe for her to labour again, and her relatives agree, tie her tubes. A hysterectomy is seldom necessary.

If her blood FAILS TO CLOT in the receiver as it comes from her vagina, she probably has DIC (DISSEMINATED INTRAVASCULAR COAGULATION). If necessary, you can confirm this with a bedside clotting test (16.13), but don't let this delay you; control is urgent.

Give her 2 g of fibrinogen by rapid intravenous infusion. Give her 2, 4, or 6 units of blood with 10 ml of 10% calcium gluconate after the third bottle. Give her another gram of fibrinogen 15 to 30 minutes later, if necessary. If her problem is DIC causing afibrinogenaemia, this should be enough. If you don't have fibrinogen, give her *fresh* whole blood. Her clotting defect will probably correct itself within 12 hours of delivery of the placenta, so if you can only keep her alive during this period, she will probably live.

If she CONTINUES TO BLEED FROM AN EMPTY UTERUS, DESPITE ALL THE ABOVE MEASURES, try oxytocin 40 units to 500 ml of fluid in a fast running drip and repeated doses of ergometrine 0.5 mg intravenously. Try prostaglandins if you have them. If this fails, tie her uterine (see 'Stop Press') or her internal iliac arteries (3.5), and only if all these measures fail (rare) resort to hysterectomy (20.12). She may have a small rupture of her uterus, which you can only diagnose at laparotomy. Some contributors consider hysterectomy easier than tying the iliac arteries, particularly under inadequate anaesthesia.

If her uterus TURNS INSIDE OUT as her placenta is delivered (rare), she has INVERSION OF HER UTERUS. This may happen spontaneously, or as a complication of controlled cord traction, particularly in elderly multips. Untreated, she can easily die. *Immediately* push it back. If you can return it immediately, it should go back easily. If there is any delay, she

INVERSION OF THE UTERUS

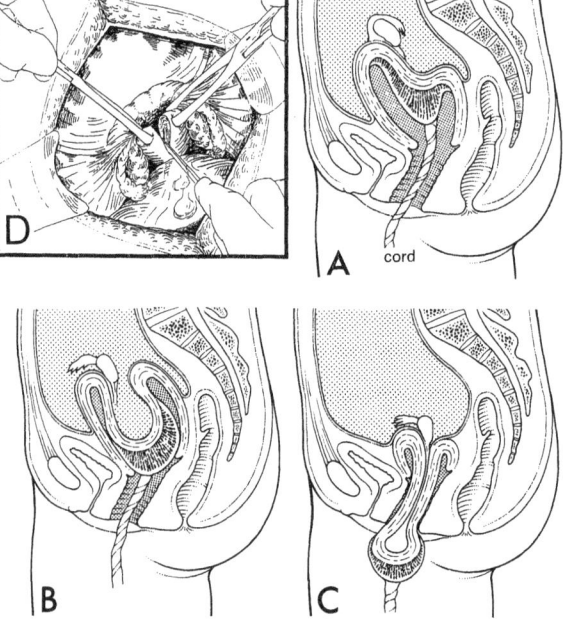

Fig. 19-12 INVERSION OF THE UTERUS. A, B, and C, increasing degrees of inversion. If this happens spontaneously (rare), or as a complication of controlled cord traction, immediately push it back. If there is any delay, replacing it will be much more difficult. D, Haultain's operation for chronic inversion. *After 'Bonney's Gynaecological Surgery', Fig. 431. Baillière Tindall, permission requested.*

may become shocked, and replacing it will be much more difficult. Wash her prolapsed uterus with warm saline, give her an antibiotic, resuscitate her, give her a general anaesthetic, and put her into the lithotomy position. There are two methods. (1) Use an enema nozzle and a douche can of warm saline suspended a metre above her. Wash out her vagina with fluid, insert the nozzle, and close her vagina with you left forearm. The hydrostatic pressure of saline will slowly return her fundus over 15–30 minutes. *Replace it slowly* and manipulate it as little as possible. Check that reduction is adequate. (2) Slowly and gently replace it manually, her fundus last. See also *Primary Mother Care*.

If she presents after several weeks with CHRONIC INVERSION (rare), do a laparotomy. You will probably find that, whereas her uterus is protruding a considerable distance from her vulva, internally it seems to be inverted from her lower segment, which is much congested. Her tubes may enter pits on either side of her evaginated uterus and be attached at their bottoms. Isolate her bladder from the lower part of her uterus and divide its rolled-over rim where it is inverted and constricted. Alternatively, pull it up with a volsellum and incise the posterior rim of the depression in her uterus through both thicknesses of its inverted wall (Haultain's operation, 19-12). This should allow you to withdraw her fundus from inside, aided if necessary by a finger passed through the incision into her vagina. Repair the wound you have made in her uterus in 2 layers.

CAUTION ! (1) Inversion of the uterus is much less common than prolapse of the swollen cervix through the vulva. You can easily push this back and it seldom recurs. (2) See also prolapsed fibroids (20-4).

19.11b Secondary postpartum haemorrhage (puerperal haemorrhage)

This is vaginal bleeding between 48 hours and 6 weeks after delivery, usually between 6 and 14 days, and typically on the 10th day. It is usually due to infection, particularly in association with: (1) Retained pieces of placenta. (2) Obstructed labour, causing necrosis of the cervix and vaginal wall. (3) Caesarean section and breakdown of the the uterine wound (6.8).

PUERPERAL HAEMORRHAGE

If bleeding is mild, observation may be all the patient needs. If she continues to bleed, or has signs of infection, give her antibiotics, such as chloramphenicol and metronidazole (2.9).

If bleeding is severe, she will need antibiotics, resuscitation, and exploration of her uterus for retained pieces of placenta. *Be sure she is well resuscitated before you start exploring her!*

EXPLORING AND EVACUATING A SEPTIC UTERUS is difficult. Sterilize 2 ring forceps (or swab holders), a Sims' speculum, and a *big, blunt* curette. Add them to the vaginal examination tray.

Scrub up, put on gloves and put her into the lithotomy position. Cover her with a lithotomy towel (a towel cut to expose her vulva). Give her ergometrine 0.5 mg, and pethidine 50 mg, and diazepam 10 mg intravenously. Inject the pethidine slowly. Or give her a general anaesthetic.

Clean her vulva with an antiseptic solution. If her cervix is wide open, insert two fingers into her uterus, and try to remove any pieces of placenta that you can feel. They are not easy to find, because her uterine cavity is large and its walls irregular. If you cannot remove pieces of placenta with your fingers, use ring forceps and a large curette, like this:

Put the Sims' speculum into her vagina. Ask a helper to hold it, so that you can see her cervix. Hold the front of her cervix with one ring forceps. Put the other ring forceps into her uterus. Push it in *very gently*, until it is at her fundus. Feel the size of her uterine cavity. Open the handles, turn the forceps and close them again. Pull out any placenta you have grasped. Do this several times in different parts of her uterus, until nothing more comes out.

Curette her uterus. Scrape it down the anterior wall, then the two side walls, and then the posterior wall. Lastly, scrape it across the fundus. Don't scrape too hard, or you may harm its lining. It will still feel irregular when you have finished scraping.

CAUTION ! Emptying a uterus in the puerperium is difficult, and can be dangerous. Its wall is soft, and you can easily perforate it. Never use a small curette, or any small instrument, because they will make a hole very easily. Work gently and carefully, and don't use a sound.

If her uterus is empty and she is still bleeding severely, pack it and her vagina (19.11a).

If packing her uterus fails to control bleeding (very unusual), proceed to laparotomy, and tie her uterine (see 'Stop Press') or internal iliac arteries (3.5). If this also fails (rare) do a hysterectomy (20.12).

If she has a secondary postpartum haemorrhage after Caesarean Section, see 'Stop Press'.

19.12 Resuscitating the neonate

A baby should breathe within a minute of birth, and usually does so. If he does not, he needs resuscitating, which may make all the difference between normality and brain damage. 'Flat' babies, who don't breathe, are often a surprise, but you should be able to predict and prepare for most of them as described below. Most follow difficult deliveries, which are more likely to damage his brain by anoxia during and after delivery, than by trauma during it.

The aim of resuscitation is to make sure that his lungs expand, he is well oxygenated, his circulation and temperature are normal, and he is breathing normally. Mask ventilation and intubation will not help him if he does not need them; so follow the indications below.

Ideally, all your midwives should be able to intubate a baby. They can learn how to do it on a fresh stillbirth. But if normal deliveries are done by a continuously changing succession of midwives in training, you will not be able to train all of them to intubate the occasional baby who needs it. For these babies immediate bag and mask, or mouth to mouth ventilation, will be much better than intubation delayed by the time it takes to call you.

Traditionally, the Apgar score has been used to decide which babies to resuscitate. The instructions given below simplify this, and use only the heart rate and the respirations, on the grounds that if these are unfavourable, the other parts of the score will be unfavourable too. See also *Primary Anaesthesia* Chapter 13.

- *LARYNGOSCOPE, neonatal, straight-bladed, Seward, with two blades sizes O (80 mm) and 1 (110 mm), also ten spare batteries and five spare bulbs, two laryngoscopes only.* You will need a spare laryngoscope—at least one of them must be working *always!*.

- *TUBES, tracheal, neonatal, transparent, plastic or rubber, non-disposable (or disposable but reusable), either Cole pattern with neck and T-piece, or straight pattern with uniform diameter and stylet (optional), sizes 2.5 mm (10 Ch), 3 mm (12 Ch), and 3.5 mm (14 Ch), ten only of each size.* Pack these locally in sets.

- *ADAPTOR, tracheal, neonatal, various sizes, five only.* This fits the tracheal tubes to the Ambu bag.

- *SUCTION CATHETERS, 4, 6, 8, and 10 Ch, ten only of each size.* These fit down the tracheal tubes.

- *AIRWAYS, neonatal, sizes 00 and 000, five only of each size.* One contributor considers these outmoded.

- *MASK, neonatal, soft and clear, sizes 00, 0, and 1, Ambu (AMB) Laerdal, Bennett, or Samson, two only of each size.*

- *BAG, self-inflating, neonatal or infant size 250 or 500 ml, Cardiff, Laerdal, or Ambu (AMB), with reservoir or extension tube, and expiratory pressure release valve, one only.* The pressure release valve will prevent you inflating him at >40 cm of water. The valves must be present and working.

- *SUCTION DEVICE, electric, with overflow bottle and gauge, maximum vacuum 100–120 mm Hg (0.16–0.26 Bar), as 'de Vilbiss 721 Vacu Aide' (deV), one only.* Don't use a standard anaesthetic sucker—it sucks much too powerfully. Alternatively, use a mucus extractor, see below.

- *FOOTPUMP, 'minipump' Ambu (AMB), one only.* You will need this if you don't have electricity, or it fails.

- *MUCUS EXTRACTOR tube and fluid trap, 10 Ch (CHI), five only.* If necessary, you can make these from old drip sets. The danger with a mucus extractor is that you may get secretions in your mouth, which

is not acceptable where HIV is a risk. Unfortunately, there is presently no mouth-operated sucker which avoids this.
• STETHOSCOPE, with small head, one only.

MAKE SURE YOUR MIDWIVES CAN INTUBATE NEONATES

RESUSCITATING THE NEWBORN

'AT RISK' MOTHERS AND BABIES. *Causes arising during labour* (1) Fetal distress. (2) Meconium staining of the liquor. (3) Caesarean section. (4) Vacuum or forceps delivery (except a simple 'lift out'). (5) Abnormal presentation, commonly breech delivery. (6) Prolapsed cord. (7) APH, especially placenta praevia. (8) Prolonged labour. *Maternal conditions.* (1) Diabetes. (2) Fever. (3) Other maternal illnesses. (4) Extremes of maternal age (<16 or >35 years). (5) Heavy sedation. The excessive administration of pethidine (>100 mg 4-hourly during labour). Contrary to popular belief, pethidine in reasonable doses (100 mg 6- to 8-hourly) causes only minimal neonatal depression. (6) Babies whose mothers have severe gestational hypertension (pre-eclampsia) which has required heavy sedation, particularly with diazepam, or phenobarbitone (not advised). *Fetal conditions* (1) Multiple pregnancy. (2) Pregnancy of abnormal length (<37 weeks, or >42 weeks). (3) Prematurity. (4) IUGR (19.13). (5) Isoimmunization. (6) Abnormal babies.

CAUTION ! When you start any operative delivery, make sure that the midwife who is helping you is completely ready to resuscitate the baby.

WARMTH. The first principle in caring for a baby is to keep him warm and keep him fed. Hypothermia is one of the most easily avoidable causes of neonatal death in low birthweight babies, even in 'warm' countries, so keep him warm and dry *during all the procedures which follow!* He can easily lose 3°C in 15 minutes, with dangerous consequences, which include hypoglycaemia, respiratory distress, and acidosis. If you can keep the whole room at 30°C (very uncomfortable for adults), you will not need an additional heater. If you cannot maintain this temperature, keep the room as warm as you can (24–26°C is a good compromise) and provide a radiant heater (a lamp is almost useless) over the resuscitation platform, with sides to prevent drafts. Use *dry* towels and keep them warm near a radiator or in a warm cupboard. Survey the temperatures of babies arriving in your neonatal ward. You may be surprised by how cold some of them are! Later, the best place to keep him warm is between his mother's breasts, which will also assist breast-feeding and bonding.

OXYGEN (with spare cylinders) is desirable, but not essential. It must reach him at a pressure of not more than 30 cm of water (20 cm is the usual working pressure), so there must be a blow-off valve which prevents it exceeding this pressure. Provide one by using a T–tube and a water manometer, as in U, Fig. 19-13, if necessary made from old drip sets. If you don't have oxygen, you will have to ventilate him by mouth (see below).

THE RESUSCITATION PLATFORM can be horizontal, or slightly sloping head-down. It can be the top of a suitably prepared trolley, or a broad shelf attached to the wall at a convenient height.

OTHER EQUIPMENT AND DRUGS should be kept immediately available on a trolley. Besides the special equipment listed above, you will need: Warm towels. Feeding tubes 6 and 8 Ch. Needles 0.5, 0.6 and 0.8 mm. A stopclock indicating seconds and minutes. Scalp vein sets and paediatric infusion sets. 1 cm adhesive tape to secure the tube. 'BMstix' or 'Dextrostix' to measure the blood glucose; note the expiry date, and economize by cutting strips in half lengthwise. Blood sugar bottles.

10 ml ampoules of 8.4% (1 mmol/ml) sodium bicarbonate, 10% calcium gluconate, 5% and 10% dextrose in water, and 0.9% sodium chloride. 10% oral dextrose. Naloxone hydrochloride (expensive but seldom needed): neonatal 20μg/ml for intravenous use, or adult 400 μg/ml. Dilute 1 ml of the adult naloxone with 20 ml of saline for neonatal use. *Don't have both* because you can easily mistake them. 1 mg ampoules of vitamin K_1. 3 ml ampoules of 1:10,000 adrenalin. If you only have 1 ml ampoules of 1:1000 adrenalin, dilute one of these with 10 ml of saline.

CAUTION ! (1) Ask another person to check all drugs before you give them. (2) Don't use nikethamide, caffeine, or aminophylline, or other central stimulants. (3) Older drugs, such as nalorphine and levallorphan, may cause respiratory depression, if you don't give them at exactly the right dose for a particular situation. (4) Keep all drugs in their original boxes and not together as 'mixed ampoules'.

Check the equipment regularly, keep a log book, and sign it. Clean and disinfect the equipment after use (2.5, 28a.2).

INTRAVENOUS INJECTIONS. **Catheterizing the umbilical vein is more likely to cause infection; a scalp vein drip is safer.** If a baby needs intravenous injections, give them into the drip or directly into the umbilical vein with a syringe and needle; be sure you are in the vein and not in the tissues.

IMMEDIATELY AFTER BIRTH

Start the clock. Hold him for a moment with his head lower than his legs, so that fluid drains from his respiratory tract. Place him on the resuscitation platform. Quickly dry him with a warm towel; dry his hair, axillae, and groins. Remove the wet towel and cover him with a dry one.

Leave his cord at least 3 cm long, with the nearest tie at least 2 cm from him, so that it can be used for intravenous injection if necessary. Don't apply alum powder to it for at least 24 hours.

If he is BREATHING NORMALLY AND CRYING VIGOROUSLY, with a good heart rate and normal colour and muscle tone, he usually needs no suction. But if there are copious secretions or blood in his mouth, gently suck out his oropharynx (see below). Briefly clear his nose, and hand him to his mother.

If he has MECONIUM-STAINED LIQUOR, you MUST clear his airway. *If possible, do this as soon as his head is delivered, before he takes his first breath.* When he has been delivered, hold his chest to prevent inspiration, until you have cleared his pharynx and larynx under direct vision with a laryngoscope. This is difficult, and it may be easier to intubate him and suck through the tracheal tube.

If there is only a little meconium, intubate him, and aspirate it with a suction catheter through the tube.

If there is much meconium, aspirate immediately with the largest possible catheter, or quickly connect suction to a tracheal tube. If a catheter or tracheal tube blocks, remove it and quickly replace it with another. Continue until all meconium is cleared, unless there is bradycardia (<60/minute); if so intubate him immediately. If his condition allows it, *avoid ventilation until you have removed as much meconium as you can.*

If his BREATHING IS SHALLOW AND IRREGULAR, estimate his heart rate by listening to it, by feeling his umbilical cord pulsating or his brachial pulse.

If it is >100/min, and he is well perfused, with good tone, apply tactile stimulation and an airway. *Gently* flick the soles of his feet, or rub his back for a few seconds. Be gentle, and if there is no prompt response, stop, suck out his oropharynx and start mask ventilation.

If it is <100/min, insert an airway and start mask ventilation.

If he NEVER BREATHED, or STARTED TO BREATHE AND THEN STOPPED, start bag and mask ventilation. If his heart rate is still <100 after one minute of ventilation (he is usually pale and limp), apply suction briefly and intubate him immediately.

SUCKING HIM OUT

If necessary (see above), first suck out his mouth, then his nose with a sterile, wide, soft rubber or plastic catheter, or use a standard 'disposable but reusable' mouth sucker with a fluid trap. Give one long, strong suck, and don't push the catheter >5 cm from his mouth.

CAUTION ! Before you start to ventilate him by any method, be sure to suck him out. Sucking out his trachea is as important as ventilating him. If you don't suck him out, you may push liquor, mucus, or meconium deeply into his bronchi.

NEONATAL RESUSCITATION

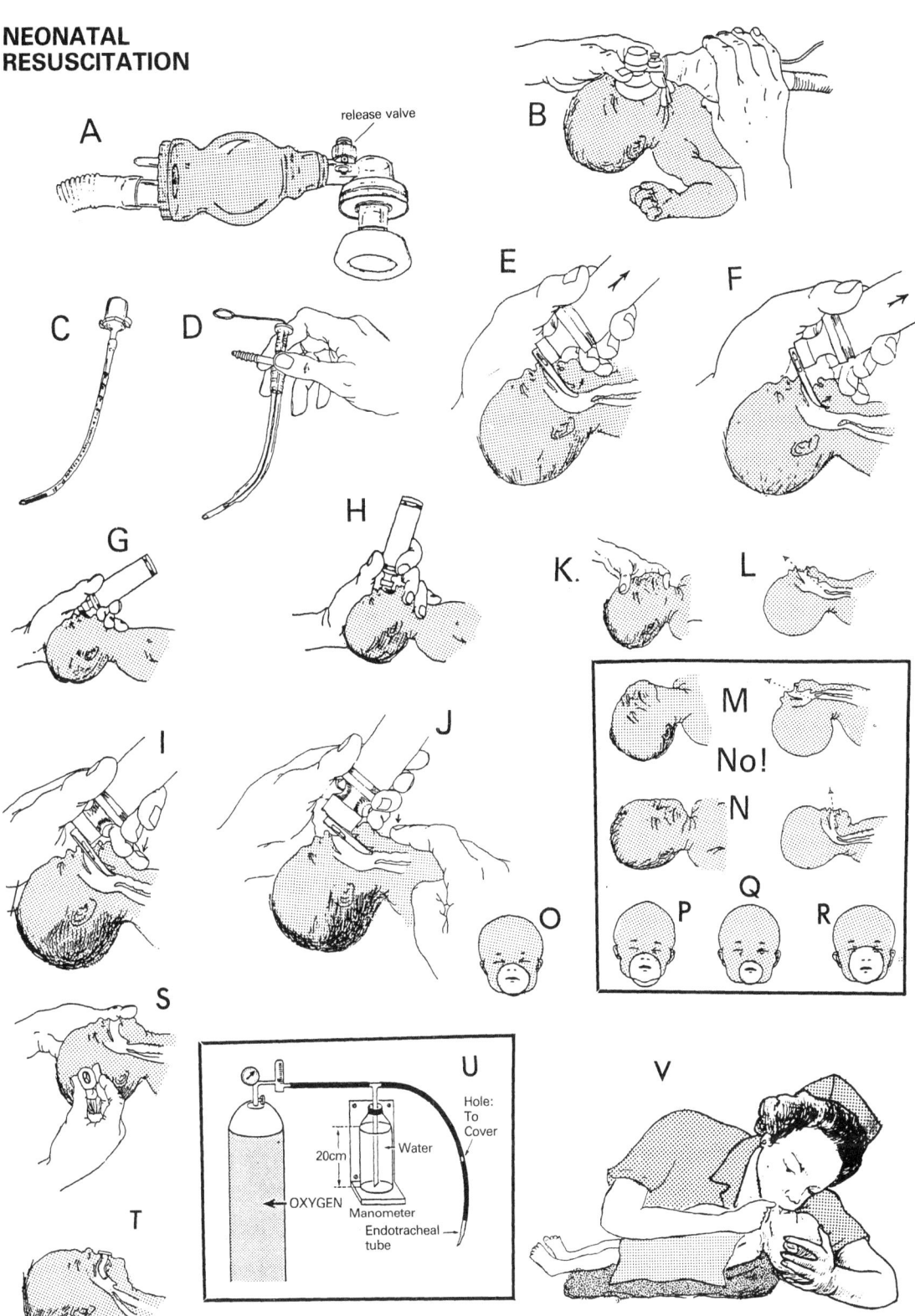

Fig. 19-13 NEONATAL RESUSCITATION. A, a transparent Laerdal self-inflating bag; note the valve. B, compress the bag with your finger tips. C, a straight-sided tube. D, a Cole tube with side arm and stylet (optional). E, lift his epiglottis. Or F, put the blade of the laryngoscope into his vallecula. G, and H, lift his tongue forwards to view his larynx. I, gently press on his trachea with your 5th finger. J, or ask an assistant to do this. K, and L, the correct position for resuscitation. M, his neck is too extended. N, it is too flexed. O, the correct size of mask. P, it overlaps his chin. Q, it is too small. R, it overlaps his eyes. S, and T, inserting infant airway. U, a T-tube and water manometer adjusted so as not to exceed a pressure of 20 cm of water. V, mouth to mouth ventilation. Blow gently from your cheeks only, about 40 times a minute. Lift up his chin, extend his head and keep him warm.

BAG AND MASK VENTILATION

Slightly extend his neck, if necessary with a small pad under his shoulders. Insert an oral airway (optional). Put a finger under his mandible to hold it forwards, without compressing the soft tissues of his neck K, and L, Fig. 19-13. Choose the largest mask which will not overlap his eyes or his chin (O).

Gently compress the bag with your finger tips (B), so as to inflate him 30–60 times a minute with as high a concentration of oxygen as you can, usually at a flow of 2–6 litres/minute. You can increase the oxygen concentration by fitting a reservoir or additional length of hose over the air intake (A). Watch his chest, it should rise with each breath. Don't compress the bag suddenly and forcefully. The object of each inflation with the mask is to expand his lungs and start him breathing.

If his chest does not rise with each breath: (1) Check that the mask makes an adequate seal with his face. (2) If necessary, clear his airway again by sucking out his mouth and nose. (3) Does the bag leak? (4) If necessary, insert an infant airway (S, and T). If this fails, intubate him. If you cannot intubate him, try compressing the bag harder.

If mask ventilation fails, intubate him promptly.

INTUBATION

INDICATIONS. The failure of mask ventilation. Don't intubate him unless his heart rate and general condition deteriorate, and not until after you have sucked out his pharynx and larynx under direct vision. Unskilled attempts at intubation do more harm than good. Most 'floppy' babies can survive without it, provided you ventilate them in some other way.

METHOD. Neonatal intubation resembles adult intubation (A 13.1). Prepare the tracheal tube you think you will need. Cole tubes (C) do not require a stylet. If you use a stylet, curve it to the shape of the tube and don't let it protrude beyond the end.

<1250 g or <28 weeks 2.5 mm tube.

1250 g–2 kg or 29–34 weeks 2.5 or 3 mm tube.

>2 kg or >34 weeks 3 or 3.5 mm tube.

'Big baby' 3.5 mm tube.

Slightly extend his head on his neck (K and L). First try to ventilate him with a mask for a few breaths. Gently insert a laryngoscope with a straight blade (size 0 blade for a small preterm baby and size 1 for a larger one) with your left hand, holding his lips apart with the fingers of your right hand. Guide the blade over the surface of his tongue, pushing it to the left. Continue until you see his leaf-like epiglottis. Either lift his epiglottis gently (E), or insert the blade into his vallecula (F). Lift his tongue forwards, so that you can see his larynx (G and H). If you insert the blade too far into his oesophagus, withdraw it gradually until you can see his larynx.

Clear his vocal cords and posterior pharynx with a sucker. Gently press on his trachea with your 5th finger (I) (or ask an assistant to press it, J) until you can see his cords. Using your right hand pass the tube between his cords from the right, until the shoulder (Cole type) or mark (straight type) is just above his cords.

CAUTION ! (1) Make sure his trachea remains central. (2) Don't force the shoulder of a Cole tube through his cords. (3) If his cords are obscured by secretions, ask your assistant to hand you the suction catheter and gently clear his airway. (4) Don't overextend his neck; the 'sniffing position' (A 13-7) is ideal. (5) If he is seriously in need of ventilation, intubation is best—if you are sure the tube is in his trachea. If you are not sure, mask ventilation is safer.

Rest your hand gently on his face, hold the tube firmly, and gently remove the laryngoscope (and stylet if you are using one). Connect the tube to the oxygen supply, and adjust it to deliver 4 l of oxygen per minute at 20 to 30 cm of water (use a lower pressure for a very small baby).

Inflate his lungs by occluding the outlet of the tube (U), or the T-piece of a Portex tube, and watching the column of air in the manometer. Or squeeze an Ambu bag. If he has never made any inspiratory effort (primary apnoea), his lungs will be more difficult to expand, so apply more pressure (the 'opening pressure') for slightly longer with his first breath. Inflate him for 2–3 seconds initially, and then for about half a second at 30–60 breaths per minute. If he has taken a few breaths and then stopped (secondary apnoea), he will need less pressure to inflate his lungs. Often, you cannot distinguish primary from secondary apnoea.

Observe: (1) His chest moving; and check that the movements are equal both sides. (2) His breath sounds; and check that they are also equal both sides. (3) An increase in his heart rate. (4) An improvement in his colour.

As soon as you are ventilating him effectively, so that his heart rate is >100, dry him and replace the wet towel with a dry one. Continue ventilating him *until he breathes spontaneously himself.* Note the time at which he first breathes.

If he does not start breathing spontaneously in a few minutes, strap the tube in place with tape and continue ventilating.

If you fail to intubate him within 20–30 seconds, withdraw the tube and ventilate him with a mask (to improve his colour and increase his heart rate) before you try to intubate him again.

If his chest movement is poor after intubation, check the flow-meter. Is the oxygen on? Is the oxygen cylinder empty? Is the tube blocked (suck it out) or kinked (straighten it)? If none of these are responsible, it is probably in his oesophagus, so remove it and try again.

If secretions are copious pass a suction catheter down the tube and aspirate them.

If his breath sounds and chest movements are asymmetrical, the tube is probably in his right main bronchus. Slowly withdraw it 0.5 cm at a time, listening for his breath sounds to become equal. If they continue to be inadequate, he may have a pneumothorax, a diaphragmatic hernia, a pleural effusion, or hypoplastic lungs (not described here).

If his heart rate remains <100, check that the tube is not in his right main bronchus (see above). If it is <50 he needs cardiac compression (see below).

ENDING VENTILATION When he is pink and his heart rate is >150, stop ventilation and watch him carefully; if his heart slows, start ventilating him again. Let him try breathing on his own, when his heart rate is >150. He may need an occasional puff before regular breathing restarts. When he is breathing regularly remove the tube.

CARDIAC COMPRESSION

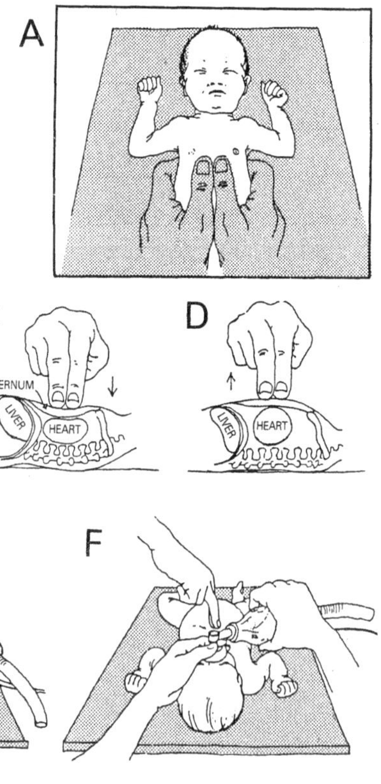

Fig. 19-14 EXTERNAL CARDIAC COMPRESSION. A, grasp the baby's chest with both hands. B, C and D, another method of compressing his chest. E, and F, while you intermittently compress his heart 120 times a minute, ask a colleague to inflate him 30–60 times a minute.

CAUTION ! (1) Don't remove him from the labour ward with the tube in place. (2) Don't leave him on a sloping resuscitation platform: the weight of his liver pressing on his diaphragm will make breathing difficult. (3) If he has been in any way abnormal, watch him carefully for 24 hours.

If he does not start breathing or his heart rate remains <50 for 30–45 minutes, stop. He is unlikely to survive.

EXTERNAL CARDIAC COMPRESSION

INDICATIONS. If his heart beat is <50/minute (bradycardia), compress his heart in the hope of strengthening or restarting it. He is usually pale. If his heart is not beating at birth, external cardiac massage is unlikely to start it.

METHOD. Grasp his chest with both hands and place your thumbs over his sternum at the level of his nipples (A, Figure 19-14). Gently compress his chest 1–1.5 cm. When you relax, keep your fingers on his chest. While you intermittently compress his heart 120 times a minute (B, C, and D), ask a colleague to inflate him 60 times a minute (E and F). Time this by calling out to your assistant "One, two, (compressions)—breathe" (One contributor advises 100 compressions and 30 breaths, in which case it is about three compressions to a breath). Check his heart rate after 30–60 seconds and thereafter periodically. Observe or feel his pulses or listen to his heart.

CAUTION ! (1) Don't press over his liver. (2) He needs cardiac compression *and* ventilation.

DRUGS FOR NEONATAL RESUSCITATION

Prompt ventilation will correct his acidosis and will be safer than giving him a bolus injection of sodium bicarbonate. Difficult intravenous injections have a low priority; ventilation is critical.

If he has persistent bradycardia (<50) in spite of adequate ventilation and cardiac compression, give him 2 mmol/kg of sodium bicarbonate intravenously. Either give 2 ml/kg of 8.4% sodium bicarbonate (1 mmol/ml) or 4 ml/kg of the 4.2% solution (this is a more convenient dilution to give: make it by diluting the 8.4% solution with an equal volume of 5% dextrose or water). One contributor gives sodium bicarbonate to any 'flat' baby. *If you have catheterized his umbilical vein, always flush with 0.9% saline before and after giving sodium bicarbonate.*

If he has persistent bradycardia or no heart beat after bicarbonate, give him 0.1 ml/kg of 1:10,000 adrenalin intravenously, or down the tracheal tube. If necessary, repeat the dose after 10–15 minutes.

If adrenalin fails to improve persistent severe bradycardia or make his heart beat return, give him 1–2 ml (0.1–0.2 g) of 10% calcium gluconate intravenously slowly. *Never give this with sodium bicarbonate.* Flush with saline or 5% dextrose first.

CAUTION ! Continue ventilation and cardiac compression.

If his respiration is depressed and his mother has had a narcotic (pethidine), ventilate him first if necessary, and give him one dose of naloxone. Either 200 μg intramuscularly (60 μg/kg). Or, 40 μg intravenously (10 μg/kg).

HYPOGLYCAEMIA IN NEONATES

DIAGNOSIS. Hypoglycaemia is one of the more preventable causes of death in the first hours or days of a baby's life. He is at risk if: (1) He is underweight, either premature or 'small for dates' (IUGR). (2) He has been hypoxic perinatally. (3) His mother had gestational hypertension ('pre-eclampsia'), uncontrolled diabetes, or severe sepsis.

The symptoms of hypoglycaemia are ill-defined. Think of it in any baby you have resuscitated who is jittery, tremulous, apnoeic, lethargic, hypotonic, or who has an abnormal cry, or who feeds poorly or has convulsions.

MANAGEMENT. Give him 5 ml/kg of 10% dextrose intravenously. If he improves, becomes more alert and stops convulsing, continue giving him dextrose 100 ml/kg/24 hours intravenously and small volumes of expressed breast milk.

If possible, test a heel-prick sample of his blood with 'BMstix', and repeat this 6-hourly, just before feeds, for the first 24 hours or longer if necessary. If 'BMstix' reads <2.5 mmol/l, he is hypoglycaemic. If possible, send a specimen for his blood sugar to be measured in the laboratory. Continue to monitor his blood sugar with 'BMstix' for 48 hours.

Alternatively, if you cannot give him a drip, you may be able to manage him orally. Pass a nasogastric tube, and aspirate his whole gastric contents. This tells you how much of his previous feed, if any, is left in his stomach, and avoids overfilling his stomach, with the risk of regurgitation. Hypoglycaemia reduces the motility of the gut, so this is a danger in 'at risk' babies. If the aspirate contains meconium or blood, lavage his stomach with 10 ml of water or saline. Then give him 10 to 15 ml of 10% dextrose by nasogastric tube, alternating with expressed breast milk 2-hourly, so that he has 100 ml/kg/day of fluid.

LATER IN THE RESUSCITATION OF A NEONATE

Check that he is pink and well perfused, his heart is normal (110–130), his pulses are easily palpable, he has good tone and spontaneous movement, he is warmer than 36°C, his breathing is regular (40—60/min) and is without distress.

Give all 'at risk' babies vitamin K_1 (phytomenadione) 0.5 mg intramuscularly. Avoid synthetic analogues, such as menadiol sodium diphosphate ('Synkavit'), because of the risk of kernicterus.

Give him to his mother. She will have been worried while you were resuscitating him. Even if he needs special care, give her a chance to hold him before you remove him.

In the ward watch his colour and his breathing, and monitor his blood glucose with test strips. Correct his blood glucose as necessary (especially if he has IUGR). An efficient way to keep him warm is in the 'kangaroo pouch' between his mother's breasts, when she is well wrapped up, and he wears a hat (he can lose much heat from his head).

DIFFICULTIES WITH NEONATAL RESUSCITATION

If you DON'T HAVE A BAG AND MASK and CANNOT INTUBATE HIM, what you and *especially your midwives* should do depends on the prevalence of HIV in your area:

IF HIV IS RARE, use MOUTH TO MOUTH VENTILATION. Bend his head gently backwards over a rolled up towel. Put your mouth over his mouth and nose. Blow in gently. Blow with small breaths, about 40 times a minute. Don't blow from your lungs. *Blow from your cheeks only.* You need very little air to blow up the lungs of a small baby—20–50 ml only. If you blow too hard, you will cause a pneumothorax. His chest should move as you blow, as if he was breathing himself. Most babies start breathing with your first two breaths. So stop after two breaths and see if he breathes. After a few inflations he should start breathing and become pink. His heart should beat faster.

IF HIV IS COMMON, use the form of artificial ventilation which is known in some areas (Papua New Guinea) as 'FROG BREATHING'. Gently extend his neck over a rolled up towel, as for intubation. If you have oxygen, pass this through one nostril. Pinch his nose between your finger and thumb. With your other hand pull down his jaw, and then pull it up and close his mouth. This raises his upper ribs and increases the capacity of his chest, so that air is drawn into his lungs. Repeat this rhythmically to imitate breathing. It is surprisingly effective.

If he is VERY PRETERM (<26 weeks) or very small (1000 g), suck him out and do only minimal resuscitation. You will not be able to ventilate him long-term, so don't start. If you keep him warm, he may surprise you and do well. Manage him as in *Primary Child Care* Section 26.22.

If the OXYGEN IS NOT WORKING, *very gently* blow down the tube intermittently using your cheeks. Practise by blowing down the manometer to see what a pressure of 30 cm of water feels like. Don't go above this.

KEEP HIM WARM AND KEEP HIM FED

19.13 Intrauterine growth retardation (IUGR)

It used to be thought that prematurity and IUGR, both of which are difficult to treat, and fetal abnormalities, which are impossible to treat, were the commonest causes of perinatal deaths in the developing world, as they are in the developed world. This does not appear to be so, since most perinatal deaths occur in

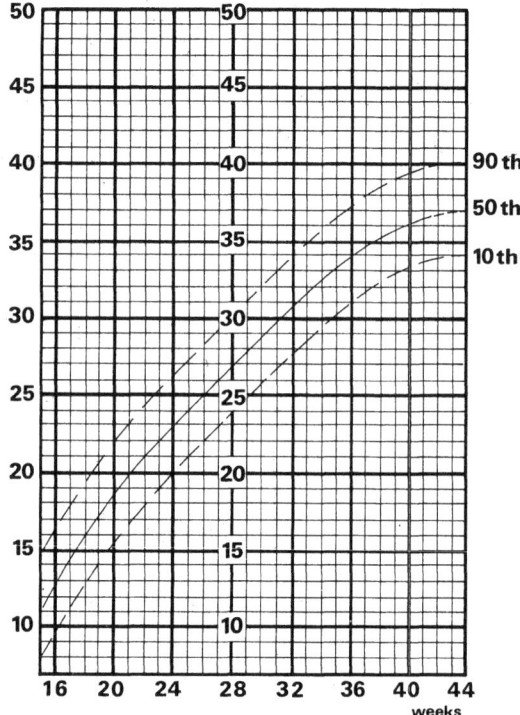

Fig. 19-15 A FUNDAL HEIGHT CHART. If low-birthweight babies are common in your district, you will find many mothers falling below the 10th centile, either because their babies have IUGR or because they are genetically small (the relative importance of these factors is unknown).

normally formed, normally grown babies weighing >2.5 kg, as the result of birth trauma and asphyxia related to CPD, pre-eclampsia, abruption, cord prolapse, and malpresentation. These deaths are much more preventable than those from IUGR.

Babies who are sufficiently small to be classified as being of low birthweight (<2500 g) may: (1) have been born after a pregnancy which was abnormally short, or (2) have grown abnormally slowly during a pregnancy of normal length. These 'small for dates' babies suffer from intrauterine growth retardation or IUGR. In the developing world 25% of babies may be low birthweight, and of these 70% may have IUGR. Its causes in approximate order of frequency include: malnutrition, placental malaria, gestational hypertension, essential hypertension, recurrent antepartum haemorrhage, sickle-cell disease, malformations and chromosome abnormalities, virus infections, smoking, and alcohol. There is also an 'idiopathic' group (30% in the developed world) in whom there is no obvious cause, but who are generally considered to be suffering from uteroplacental vascular insufficiency. A hungry starving baby from any of these causes readily dies, particularly during early labour, when his heart suddenly stops.

Because of the overwhelming importance of malnutrition as a cause, 21 of the 22 million low birthweight babies who are born each year are in the developing world. Their chances of dying are 20 times higher than those of other babies. Malnutrition is also the most potentially preventable cause.

IUGR is not easy to detect clinically. The risk factors for it, some of which are determined by malnutrition, include: (1) IUGR in previous pregnancies. (2) Low weight before pregnancy began. (3) Low weight-gain during pregnancy. (4) Multiple pregnancy. (5) Smoking. Even so, 30% to 50% of cases commonly remain undiagnosed. The only way you have of diagnosing IUGR is to encourage your midwives to measure the fundal height as carefully as they can between 20 and 36 weeks. If the uterus is 5 cm lower than it should be, and there are <10 movements in 12 hours (M 28.3), you can diagnose IUGR. Unfortunately, many mothers are unsure of their dates, and most health workers (including doctors) are unable to record the height of the fundus with sufficient accuracy. Even if we can, it is of little value in multiple pregnancy, polyhydramnios, a transverse lie, or in a very obese mother.

The fundal height chart in Fig. 19-15 is derived from women in Wales (no fundal height charts for the developing world have yet been devised). If low birthweight babies are common in your district, you will find many mothers falling below the 10th centile, either because their babies have IUGR or because they are genetically small (the relative importance of these factors is unknown).

If you diagnose IUGR during pregnancy, and decide to deliver a mother before term (it is not one of the indications for induction in Section 19.3), don't do so before 34 weeks. Do the surfactant test (19.2), in case her dates are wrong. You then have a choice between inducing labour (19.3) and elective Caesarean section (18.9). Babies with IUGR tolerate asphyxia badly.

Babies with IUGR born at term have only a slightly increased risk of a major handicap, such as cerebral palsy or mental retardation. But between 1% and 30% of them have some minimal cerebral dysfunction, such as problems with speech, language, and learning. The babies at greatest risk of some major handicap associated with IUGR, particularly cerebral palsy, are: (1) The badly asphyxiated baby with severe IUGR born at or past term. (2) The baby with IUGR delivered before 34 weeks. Try to diagnose and deliver babies in the 'window' between 34 and 36 weeks—if you can. Delivering a baby whose mother has diabetes (17.3) presents similar problems in judging the best time for delivery, the main difference being that he is too big rather than too small.

Much of the effort of modern obstetrics is devoted to detecting babies with IUGR, monitoring them, and getting them out into the world at just the right moment, when the risks outside the uterus are less than those inside it. If the moment of induction can be judged successfully, it may increase a child's chance of survival. Unfortunately, despite a massive investment in resources, a baby suspected of having IUGR is often found to be normal, and vice versa. It is thus not surprising that IUGR is seldom diagnosed in the district hospitals of the developing world, and even with the sophisticated technology of the industrial world, the diagnosis is often wrong. However, you can treat the more manageable causes of perinatal mortality, some of which express themselves as IUGR—malaria, gestational hypertension, syphilis, obstructed labour, and poorly managed breech and twin deliveries.

20 Gynaecology

20.1 Some of the simpler operations

As with the rest of surgery, the highest incidence of gynaecological disease, and the worst cases are to be found where there are fewest gynaecologists. In a survey of two Indian villages 55% of women had gynaecological complaints, 92% had one or more gynaecological or sexual diseases and the average number of these diseases per woman was 3.6. Only 8% of them had had any gynaecological treatment. This is some indication of how little attention is given to the reproductive health of non-pregnant women, most of whom only encounter the health care system when they are the target of family planning programs.

So there is much gynaecology to do! You can evacuate an incomplete abortion (16.2), drain and marsupialize a Bartholin's abscess (20.4), drain a pelvic abscess (6.5), and tie a patient's tubes (15.3). You may have to do an emergency hysterectomy; but you should, if possible, try to refer a 'cold' one. The standard repertoire of an expert gynaecologist includes an anterior and a posterior colporrhaphy, a Manchester repair, and a vaginal hysterectomy. These are difficult, particularly the latter two, so we have included Le Fort's operation and ventrisuspension.

Bang RA et al., 'High prevalence of gynaecological disease in rural indian women'. Lancet 1989;i:85-87

20.2 Abnormal and 'dysfunctional' uterine bleeding ('DUB')

'Abnormal uterine bleeding' includes any bleeding which is abnormal in its degree and timing. 'Dysfunctional uterine bleeding', or 'DUB', is abnormal bleeding which has no obvious pathology.

In the developing world, abnormal uterine bleeding usually has some obvious pathology. The list of its possible causes is a long one and is given below. Only diagnose DUB after you have excluded obvious pathology. DUB occurs most commonly at the extremes of reproductive life: (1) In young girls for their first few cycles, before these settle into a normal pattern. (2) In older women nearing the menopause, before complete amenorrhoea sets in. DUB should be an uncommon diagnosis in the prime of life; if you make it often, you are probably misdiagnosing abortions or chronic ectopics. In the developing world it seems to be rare, even in older women, perhaps because patients here are more tolerant of minor menstrual irregularities. This is in sharp contrast to the industrial world, where DUB is one of the commonest gynaecological diagnoses.

The commonest cause of DUB is the failure to ovulate. Because ovulation does not occur in the middle of a cycle as it should, the corpus luteum does not develop and produce progesterone normally. The endometrium grows abnormally thick under the influence of unopposed oestrogen, and eventually begins to shed unevenly. Courses of progestogen stop bleeding temporarily, and when these are stopped normal periods usually follow.

The important diseases not to miss are carcinoma of the cervix (very common), and, usually after the menopause, carcinoma of the endometrium (rare in the developing world). The investigation of abnormal bleeding often requires a 'D and C', but you may not have time to do very many of these, so you will probably have to limit yourself to priorities. These are *intermenstrual bleeding*, and especially *postcoital bleeding*, which does not have some more obvious cause. Heavy regular periods are a common complaint, and are usually benign.

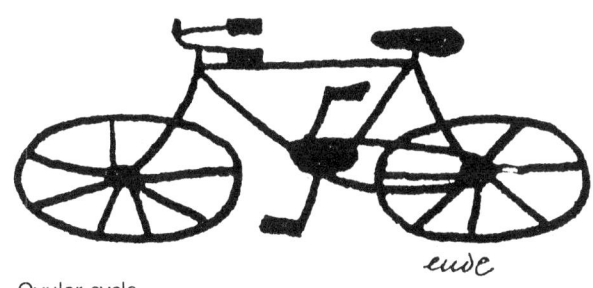

Ovular cycle

ABNORMAL UTERINE BLEEDING

HISTORY. A careful history and examination will nearly always reveal some obvious cause. "*When* did the bleeding start? Last year? At Easter? At the beginning of the cold season? For how many days do you bleed and when?" Ask about the last episode. "Are you bleeding now?" "Were you bleeding last week? Last month?" Describe the bleeding pattern by giving approximate dates and amounts. Make sure the patient distinguishes blood escaping vaginally, from blood in her urine.

CAUTION ! (1) Avoid statements like 'Has periods ×2 a month', 'polymenorrhoea', 'menorrhagia', etc. (2) *Ask about postcoital bleeding*. (3) Bleeding patterns are imperfectly matched to diagnoses, so don't always expect her history to give you the answer.

EXAMINATION. Is she anaemic? Examine her abdomen. Examine her cervix with a speculum. Do a Pap smear (M 29.1).

DIAGNOSIS AND TREATMENT. The treatment of most conditions is described elsewhere. Diagnose 'DUB' by exclusion, and remember that a 'D and C' is not automatic treatment for all forms of uterine bleeding.

Pregnancy-related. Abortion in all its forms (16.2), ectopic pregnancy (16.7).

Contraception-related. 'Depo provera' or a loop (M 3.10).

Hormone treatment elsewhere at a health centre or by a private doctor.

Pathology in the genital tract. Fibroids (20.6), cervical polyp (20.5), chronic pelvic infection (6.6), vaginitis (trichomonas, atrophic menopausal or foreign body), cervical erosion, cervicitis, ovarian cysts and tumours (20.7), carcinoma of the cervix (common, 32.35), endometrial carcinoma (rare, 32.25), choriocarcinoma (uncommon, 32.38).

If she is less than 20, and you have excluded the above pathology, she probably has DUB. Avoid treating her if you can. If treatment seems to be necessary, try cyclical progestogens (see below) first. If they fail and bleeding is severe or persistent, curette her.

If she is between 20 and 40, she can have most of the pathology listed above. Don't miss carcinoma of the cervix. If she has *intermenstrual* or *postcoital* bleeding, be sure to take a wedge or punch biopsy of any hard, friable, or ulcerated area on her cervix. A 'D and C' will not diagnose carcinoma of the cervix (32.35); you can almost always diagnose this by looking at her cervix with a speculum. See also Section 32.35.

If she is over 40, and especially if she has postmenopausal bleeding (bleeding 1 year or more after the menopause), always do a 'D and C' to exclude carcinoma of the endometrium. Other causes include fibroids, especially prolapsed submucosal fibroids (20-4), and senile vaginitis.

If she has a heavy loss and no obvious cause, and emergency treatment is necessary, see below.

CYCLICAL PROGESTOGENS

TO STOP ACUTE BLEEDING NOW, give her norethistrone 5 mg 3 times daily for 5–10 days. Or, give her one 'combined' contraceptive pill twice daily for 10 days. Bleeding will probably stop while she takes these pills. She will get a withdrawal bleed (normal, scanty, or heavy) 2–3 days after stopping them, but this should not last more than a week, after which normal periods should restart. Explain this to her. See her again in a month, to see if treatment has worked, and she has stopped bleeding.

If she has not stopped bleeding: (1) your diagnosis was wrong. Or, (2) she did not take her tablets regularly. Or, (3) her DUB is unsuited to hormonal treatment. So do a 'D and C'.

FOR RECURRENT DUB treat her as for an acute episode, then put her on the 'combined pill', as for contraception without a 'D and C'.

CAUTION ! 'DUB' is only a diagnosis of exclusion, and in many settings an immediate 'D and C' is simpler.

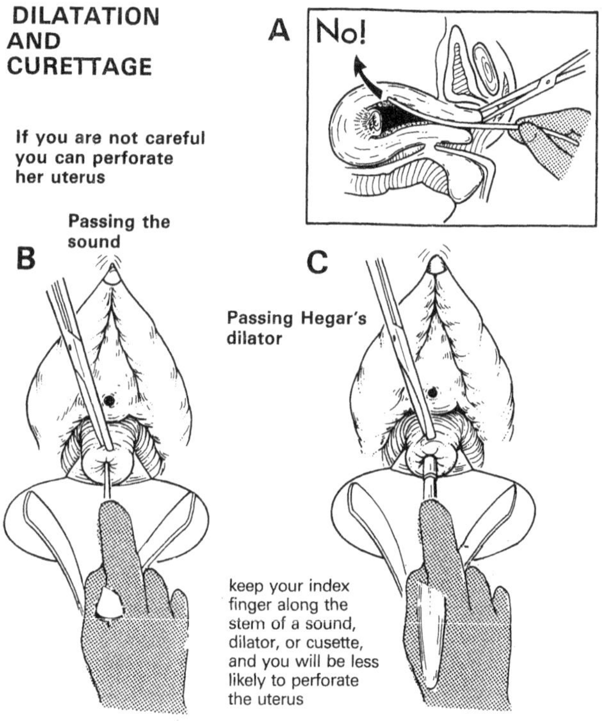

20.3 'D and C'—dilatation and curettage

There are two superficially similar operations: (1) The evacuation of an incomplete, or septic abortion, which does not usually require that the cervix be dilated, and which is descibed in Section 16.2. And, (2) dilatation and curettage of the uterus, which is described here. Although both operations have similar complications, they have different indications.

A 'D and C' is a complement to a carefully taken history and examination, and is not a substitute for them. It is also one of the commonest operations in gynaecology, and one of the the most abused ones, so make sure that you only do it on the proper indications, which are: (1) To diagnose the cause of abnormal bleeding, unless you have already found the cause in a patient's lower genital tract. (2) To exclude carcinoma of the endometrium and tuberculous endometritis. (3) To make sure that a patient is ovulating, when you are investigating her for infertility. (4) To treat DUB (dysfunctional uterine bleeding), when A 'D and C' can occasionally be life-saving.

Ideally, all curettings should be sent for histology. Unfortunately, this is unlikely to be possible, so you will probably have to send only the most urgent ones. If a patient is less than 40, sending her curettings for histology is less urgent, unless they look abnormal macroscopically (profuse, thick, 'cheesy', or infected), or you suspect choriocarcinoma.

Although a 'D and C' is usually simple, the long list of difficulties described below show that it can be dangerous, and even fatal. The main risks are: (1) Perforating the uterus, perhaps followed by haemorrhage or sepsis. (2) Injuring a nulliparous cervix. Most of the complications we list are very rare.

DILATATION AND CURETTAGE—'D and C'

INDICATIONS. **Use dilatation followed by curettage:** (1) To investigate abnormal bleeding. It may reveal: carcinoma of endometrium, endocervical adenocarcinoma (but not squamous

DILATATION AND CURETTAGE

If you are not careful you can perforate her uterus

Fig. 20-1 DILATATION AND CURETTAGE. A, the main danger is perforating the uterus. B, passing a sound. C, inserting Hegar's dilator. Perforation of the uterus is less likely if you use your finger as a guide and steadier like this. *After 'Bonney's Gynaecological Surgery'. Baillière Tindall, with kind permission.*

carcinoma of the cervix, see below), choriocarcinoma, 'chronic endometritis', tuberculous endometritis, chronic anovulation, or submucous fibroids. (2) To treat post-menopausal cervical occlusion causing pyometra, and to exclude carcinoma as its cause.

Use dilatation only, without curettage: (1) To correct cervical stenosis after amputation, or conization (32.35). (2) To permit the insertion of an IUD.

If you are doing and 'D and C' for infertility, its purpose is to decide whether there is histological evidence of ovulation, and to exclude tuberculous endometritis. So always do it in the premenstrual phase. Send the curettings for histology, and make sure you tell the pathologist that this is what you want to know, or he may merely report them as 'normal'. He will usually make the diagnosis of tuberculosis histologically, but consider sending a separate specimen in a sterile bottle, for culture for tuberculosis, if you think that this is the cause, and are working in an area of high incidence. If your pathological services are under pressure, you won't be able to do this very often.

CAUTION ! (1) Don't do a 'D and C' to treat primary dysmenorrhoea, even if other methods have failed. Persevere with analgesics. If necessary give her a 50µg oestrogen combined pill to suppress ovulation. (2) A 'D and C' will not diagnose squamous carcinoma of the cervix, for which she needs a cone or wedge biopsy (32.35). Don't do a 'D and C' if you suspect she has a tubo-ovarian abscess, which you should be able to diagnose clinically. Infection will have fixed her uterus; moving it with dilators may tear it, spread the pus, and cause a fatal peritonitis.

USING A MENSTRUAL REGULATION SYRINGE

If you only want to do a biopsy, consider using a menstrual regulation syringe (M 3.19), which is ideal for assessing whether she is ovulating or not, and for the diagnosis of tuberculous endometritis. You can do it as an outpatient using only a paracervical block (A 6.14).

STANDARD METHOD FOR DOING A 'D AND C'

You can do this as an outpatient. Ask her to empty her bladder. There is no need to catheterize her.

ANAESTHESIA. (1) General anaesthesia. (2) An anaesthetic 'cocktail' (A 8.8). (3) A paracervical block (A 6.14).

EQUIPMENT. A catheter, Sims' and Auvard's vaginal specula, a uterine sound, 2 vulsella, a pair of narrow ovum forceps, sharp curettes of different sizes, and a set of Hegar's uterine dilators. Arrange these in order of size on the trolley.

EXAMINATION. If necessary, empty her bladder. Swab her vulva and vagina. When you dilate her cervix, you will need a mental picture of the shape, length and direction of her uterine cavity. Get this picture by: (1) Examining her bimanually, to feel the size, position, and mobility of her uterus (feel also for disease in her adnexae). Note particularly if her uterus is retroverted, because this increases the chance of perforating it with a misdirected dilator. (2) Measure the depth of her uterus with a sound, except when you suspect an abortion.

DILATATION. Start by making sure that her buttocks are well over the edge of the table. Grasp the anterior lip of her cervix with one, or even two vulsella, and pull it well down. This will bring a sharply anteverted or retroverted uterus towards the axial position, and reduce the risk of perforation. If it is soft, as after labour or an abortion, use sponge forceps.

With the picture of her uterine cavity in your mind, dilate her cervix, starting with the smallest dilator. As you do so, place a finger beside it to act as a 'brake', if you enter her cervix suddenly.

Insert the dilator in the direction which minimizes the resistance to it as far as possible. When it has been in place for at least half a minute, insert the next size without delay, and without waiting for her cervix to contract again. Dilate a large uterus more than a small one. If your purpose is only to do a biopsy, use a fine curette, and don't dilate beyond Hegar size 8—larger sizes may tear her cervix.

CAUTION ! (1) Be gentle. (2) Dilate slowly, leave each dilator in place for at least half a minute. (3) Don't twist the dilators. (4) Be particularly careful not to perforate her uterus, if you suspect a missed or incomplete abortion, or carcinoma of her endometrium. All these make it soft, friable and easily perforated. (5) If you suspect a carcinoma, make sure you dilate her cervix enough to let you explore her uterus adequately. (6) Don't allow a dilator or a probe to become trapped in a false passage. (7) Never use a douche.

CURETTAGE. Do a complete or a partial curettage on these indications.

If all you want is some endometrium to find out if she is ovulating, do a partial curettage. Explore her uterus with long, careful strokes, so that you get long thin strips of endometrium for histology.

If you are curetting for an incomplete abortion, or for the diagnosis of intermenstrual bleeding, or other forms of abnormal bleeding, and are anxious not to miss carcinoma of the corpus, do a full curettage. Start scraping at her fundus, and scrape towards you all round the anterior, posterior, and lateral surfaces of her uterine cavity. Continue until there is a scratching feeling.

EARLY DIFFICULTIES DURING A 'D AND C'

See also Sections 16.2 and 6.6a.

If you CANNOT PASS A SOUND or small dilator, her uterus is probably acutely flexed, either forwards or backwards. Feel it carefully.

If her uterus is anteverted (flexed forwards), pass the sound under direct vision though her external os, remove the speculum, and depress the handle of the sound posteriorly on to her perineum. When it is in the axis of her uterine canal it will probably pass.

If her uterus is retroverted (flexed backwards), it may be held in place by adhesions. If a bimanual examination shows that it is fixed, consider abandoning the operation. But, if she must have a 'D and C', put the volsellum on the posterior lip of her cervix and pull it well down; pass the dilators with their points backwards. If you tear the adhesions that are holding her uterus, she may bleed into her pouch of Douglas, or into her peritoneum. You may then have to open her abdomen (rare), and secure the bleeding vessels.

If her CERVIX IS SO RIGID that the larger dilators will not pass without the risk of tearing it, leave one dilator in place for several minutes, before introducing the next one. If a dilator is tightly gripped as you remove it, reinsert it and leave it in a little longer before inserting the next largest size. Nulliparous and senile cervices are often stiff. Don't use excessive force. You can usually do an adequate curettage with a small, sharp curette, when her cervical canal is only dilated to Hegar 6 (20 Ch).

If LARGER DILATORS DO NOT GO IN as far as smaller ones, you are inserting successive dilators a progressively shorter distance into her uterus. If you fail to realize what you are doing, you may only curette her cervical canal, and not the body of her uterus. Return to the smaller dilators, and start again.

If you find that INSERTING LARGER DILATORS IS UNNATURALLY EASY, stop! You have probably lacerated her cervix, and increased the risk of bleeding and sepsis. The tear may run into her vaginal vault from her external os, or it may start near her internal os, so that the tips of succeeding dilators catch in it, and ultimately enter her broad ligament.

If a DILATOR SUDDENLY SLIPS IN much further than the one before (not uncommon), you have probably perforated her uterus into her peritoneal cavity, or into her broad ligament on either side, or into her bladder. Even experts occasionally do this, especially if a patient is pregnant, postpartum, or postabortion, or if her uterus has been softened by an endometrial carcinoma: (1) Abandon the operation, and don't try to confirm the diagnosis by probing her uterus. (2) Don't irrigate her uterus. What you do now depends on whether she is a clean case, or a septic one.

If she is a 'clean case', take her pulse, blood pressure, and temperature half-hourly. She will probably recover. If her pulse rises and her blood pressure falls, and there are signs of fresh blood in her peritoneal cavity (rare), restore her blood volume and do a laparotomy.

If she is potentially 'septic' as after an abortion, give her antibiotics, and observe her as above.

If you perforate her uterus and a LOOP OF GUT APPEARS AT HER VAGINA (rare), don't: (1) be tempted to resect it and anastomose it at her vagina, or (2) to push it back through the tear and plug her uterus with gauze. Instead, open her abdomen and draw the prolapsed gut back. Clean it, resect it, if it is damaged, and inspect the rest of her gut.

If you SPLIT THE TIGHT VAGINA of a postmenopausal patient with a speculum, suture it if it bleeds.

If the LACERATION which is causing the bleeding runs up from her external os (rare), you may be able to seize the bleeder with a haemostat and secure it with a mattress suture.

LATER DIFFICULTIES WITH A 'D AND C'

If, as she recovers from the anaesthetic, her PULSE RATE IS FASTER than it should be after a simple dilatation, she complains of pain (which she should never do), she is pale, cold, and restless, and has some lower abdominal rigidity: (1) She has probably bled into her peritoneal cavity after a perforation. (2) You may have missed an ectopic pregnancy and ruptured it with your 'D and C'. Immediately explore her pelvis through an abdominal incision. Find and suture the perforation. If it is extensive, and sutures will not control the bleeding (rare), tie her internal iliac arteries. If this fails, remove her uterus. Leave her vagina open to allow free drainage.

If she develops symptoms of low abdominal PAIN AND FEVER, suspect salpingitis, and treat it as usual. This is an unusual complication of a 'D and C'.

If, postoperatively, she has PAIN on one side, and a swelling develops in her broad ligament, a haematoma has formed. Occasionally, it may be so severe as to raise the peritoneum of the side wall of her pelvis, and extend even to her loin. If so, she will have the signs of a mass and of hypovolaemia. You may need to open her abdomen and secure the bleeding vessel.

If she develops symptoms of PERITONITIS (lower abdominal tenderness, and rigidity), her prognosis is worse if they appear early, and you cannot feel a pelvic mass, which shows that the infection is localizing. The difficult decision to make is whether you should explore her abdomen or not.

If her symptoms are not severe or worsening, give her antibiotics (2.7), wait and watch her closely. Her peritonitis or pelvic cellulitis may only be local, and symptoms may subside.

If her symptoms are severe or worsening, or generalized, or you have inadvisedly given her an irritant douche, open her abdomen, repair the tear, and mop out her pelvis. If her peritonitis is generalized, wash out her peritoneal cavity and instil tetracycline (6.2). Don't remove her uterus. Make quite sure that her gut has not also been injured.

20.4 Bartholin's cyst and abscess

If a cyst develops in one of Bartholin's glands, don't try to excise it completely; marsupialize it instead, which means bringing its wall to the surface as a pouch, which will slowly heal. This is easier than trying to excise it, which is more difficult for routine use under the conditions in which we work. Also marsupialize an abscess; this is less easy because its wall is soft and poorly defined. If necessary, merely incise it and marsupialize it later when it is not infected.

BARTHOLIN'S CYST AND ABSCESS

Marsupialization can sometimes be an outpatient operation.

ANAESTHESIA. Give the patient a general anaesthetic, or use ketamine, or subarachnoid or epidural anaesthesia.

MARSUPIALIZING A CYST. Ask your assistant to immobilize the cyst with sponges on forceps. Make a longitudinal incision, with extensions at either end, in the margin between her vulval mucosa and her skin, on the inside of her labium minus. Let the fluid escape. Apply Allis' forceps on the edges of her labium minus, and retract them laterally. If necessary, push the cyst forwards by putting a finger behind it. Use interrupted catgut sutures to tie the edges of the cyst wall to her skin, and to stop bleeding.

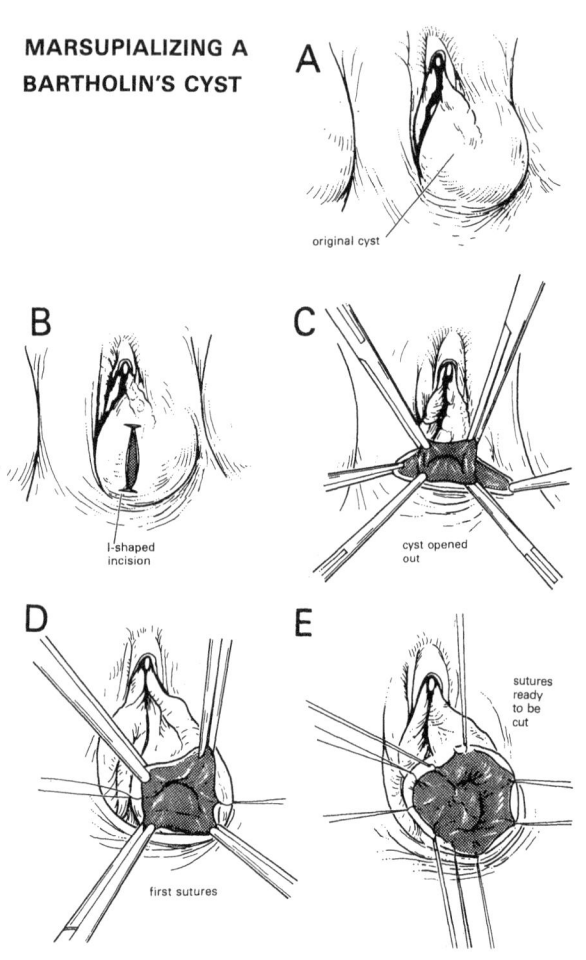

Fig. 20-2 MARSUPIALIZING A BARTHOLIN'S CYST. A, the cyst. B, the incision with its extensions. C, opening out the cyst. D, the first sutures. E, sutures almost complete.

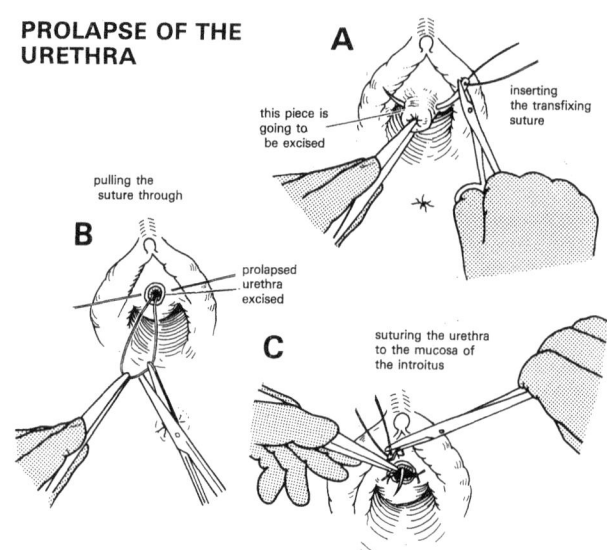

Fig. 20-3 PROLAPSE OF THE URETHRA. A, passing a suture through the prolapsed urethra. B, cutting the suture so as to make two separate sutures at either side. C, inserting further sutures as needed. *After 'Bonney's Gynaecological Surgery', Figs. 92 to 94, Baillière Tindall, with kind permission.*

MARSUPIALIZING AN ABSCESS is a painful minor emergency, which is easier before the abscess ruptures, so operate soon. Excise an ellipse of skin over the abscess, to include the duct, and suture the cyst wall to her skin. Give her antibiotics (ampicillin or tetracycline), advise several salt baths daily, and give her an analgesic.

CAUTION ! Don't try to excise a cyst unless it has recurred after marsupialization. If so, admit her; excision is often complicated by heavy bleeding and haematoma formation.

20.5 Prolapse of the urethra

In some tropical communities prolapse of the mucosa of the urethra is common in young girls between the age 6 months and 8 years. It usually causes no symptoms, but a child may have slight dysuria, or her mother may notice blood on her clothes. While most of her urethra remains in its normal place, its mucosa is gradually extruded at the external orifice to form a deep red or bluish tubular mass, which swells and becomes oedematous, and occasionally even gangrenous. You cannot replace her prolapsed urethral mucosa, so you have to excise it. Be careful to distinguish it from a schistosomal granuloma, or a venereal wart.

PROLAPSE OF THE URETHRA is not as easy to treat as it looks, so refer the patient if you can.

Under ketamine, use a small sound to find her meatus in the prolapsed mass of tissue. Pass a catheter, withdraw it, and then replace this by fine artery forceps. Open the points slightly to distend her urethra. With the forceps as a guide, transfix it from side to side and then from front to back with strands of 3/0 catgut. Use a knife or scissors, or, better, diathermy, to cut off the mucosa distal to the point at which the sutures cross the lumen. Pull the strands of catgut down as two loops, cut them, and then tie each of the four pieces, so as to join the edge of her urethral mucosa to her skin. What little bleeding there is is usually controlled by the sutures.

Insert a Foley catheter for at least 24 hours. As soon as her bladder function is normal, she can go home. Warn her that her vulva will be sore for at least a week.

20.6 Fibroids

Fibroids are uncommon in young women, but common in older ones. In the developing world a patient with fibroids usually presents with: (1) Infertility or subfertility. (2) Recurrent abortion. (3) Abnormal bleeding. (4) An abdominal swelling. (5) Lower abdominal pain. The severity of her symptoms depends less on the size of her fibroids, than where they are; a small submucous fibroid can cause severe bleeding, whereas a huge interstitial one may hardly be noticed. She commonly has PID also, and the pain it causes may be her presenting symptom.

Several operations are possible: (1) Hysterectomy, which should ideally be total, so that her cervix is removed, and with it any risk of cervical carcinoma. (2) Myomectomy, which is usually abdominal, but which can be vaginal. Surgery can be difficult because of associated subacute or chronic PID, her wish not to have a hysterectomy and to continue menstruating, and the technical difficulties of doing a myomectomy.

There is one particular presentation that you should be aware of:

A pedunculated submucous fibroid may prolapse and present as a mass in her vagina, or less commonly at her vulva, as in Fig. 20-4. She may also complain of bleeding, and present as if she had an abortion, with a lump hanging in her vagina. Her cervix dilates to allow it to pass, and remains partly dilated around it. The mass may be large, necrotic, infected, and smelly. Bleeding may have made her very anaemic. The risk in merely tying the pedicle and cutting it off, is that her peritoneal cavity may have come down with it, so that you may open this by mistake. She is also at risk from from infection and bleeding.

FIBROIDS

THE DIFFERENTIAL DIAGNOSIS is that of a pelvic mass: (1) Pregnancy. (2) A full bladder. (3) An ovarian cyst (20.7). (4) A chronic ectopic pregnancy (16.7). (5) PID with an inflammatory mass (6.6).

CAUTION ! (1) A centrally placed fundal fibroid may feel like a pregnant uterus, but is much harder. (2) Pregnancy can occur in a fibroid uterus.

INDICATIONS FOR SURGERY The rate at which a fibroid grows varies greatly. If it causes no symptoms, consider leaving it unless it is the size of a 12-week pregnancy or larger. At this size it will probably cause symptoms, so if she has completed her family, suggest hysterectomy. The indications for removing a fibroid depend more on symptoms (bleeding, anaemia, and premenstrual pain), than on its size. If it is causing symptoms, you may have to remove it when it is quite small. Other reasons for removal include torsion and prolapse. Many patients don't need surgery.

If the patient's uterus and the mass seem fixed and tender, and especially if she has fever, she is more likely to have PID, with or without fibroids. Treat her medically at first. Admit her, give her an antibiotic, and reassess her in 3 or 4 weeks.

If her temperature does not settle after a reasonable time, and her uterus remains tender, examine her under anaesthesia. She may have: (1) A tubo-ovarian abscess which fluctuates and needs draining. If so, leave her fibroids until later. (2) Mobile degenerating fibroids that you can operate on. 'Red degeneration' can occur in a fibroid during pregnancy, and can cause pain and a tender mass, but not the degree of fever that is common with PID or a tubo-ovarian abscess.

If she is younger and wants children, consider doing a myomectomy or referring her for it. Make sure she understands that: (1) If it is found to be impracticable, she may have to have a hysterectomy, or to have her abdomen closed after nothing has been done. (2) She may grow more fibroids later, especially if she does not conceive.

If she is older and does not want children, consider doing a total hysterectomy (20.12).

MYOMECTOMY

INDICATIONS. A patient with fibroids who wants children. Myomectomy is hazardous, and has more complications than hysterectomy. Most patients are better with a hysterectomy, or with no surgery at all. If you are inexperienced, don't attempt it unless she has: (1) A single fibroid <10 cm in diameter. Or,

FIBROIDS

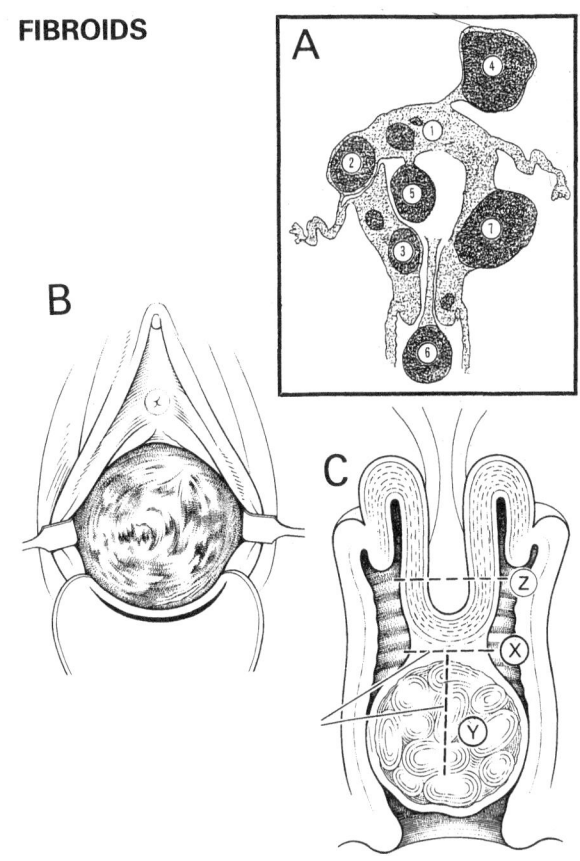

Fig. 20-4 FIBROIDS. A, the surgical pathology of fibroids. B, a submucous fibroid polyp has brought the fundus of the uterus down with it. C, the correct site for incision. First, incise the fibroid longitudinally ('Y') to find the level of its capsule. You can then cut and transfix or twist off the pedicle transversely just above this ('X'), with no danger of entering her peritoneal cavity. Don't incise at level 'Z'!

Fibroids can be: 1, intramural. 2, subserous, distorting the tube. 3, submucous. 4, subserous and pedunculated. They can also project into the uterine cavity (5), through the cervix (6), or into the parametrium (7).

(2) a fibroid which is subserous (pedunculated into her peritoneal cavity), or submucous (pedunculated into her uterine cavity, and usually coming through her cervix into her vagina).

CONTRAINDICATIONS. (1) Multiple fibroids (>3) (2) Active sepsis. (2) Dense adhesions of both tubes which make pregnancy impossible. (3) If she has a large posterior fibroid in her pouch of Douglas, leave it unless you are an expert. Removing this without damaging her bladder or ureters is difficult, and can be bloody.

If you are inexperienced, refer her. If you cannot refer her proceed as follows.

MYOMECTOMY FOR INTRAMURAL FIBROIDS. Bleeding is the great danger. Cross-match 2 units of blood, with due consideration for HIV.

Use tourniquets to prevent bleeding. Make small openings at the base of her broad ligaments. Take three rubber catheters. Pass one round her cervix and the other two round each of her ovarian pedicles. Pull them tight and hold them with clamps to occlude the vessels temporarily. Alternatively, pass a catheter round her cervix and clamp her ovarian vessels with rubber covered bowel clamps. Special vascular clamps are better if you have them. If her anatomy makes applying catheters or clamps difficult, consider abandoning the operation.

Make an incision over the fibroid which exceeds its diameter by 2 or 3 cm. The correct plane to remove it in may not be easy to find. Cut into the fibroid and you should see it. Shell it out. If necessary, remove some of the wall of her uterus to reduce the size of the dead space. Repair her uterus with at least 2 rows of mattress sutures of '1' or '2' chromic catgut.

Remove the catheters. If her uterine incisions bleed, insert more mattress sutures. If bleeding continues, decide whether to do a hysterectomy, or to tie her internal iliac arteries.

Close her abdomen in layers without drainage. Make sure she knows what you have removed, and understands that she must always be delivered in hospital in future.

MYOMECTOMY FOR A SUBMUCOUS FIBROID POLYP. She may have only a single vaginal fibroid. If she has others, they can be removed later by myomectomy or hysterectomy. Bleeding is usually mild, but however you remove a fibroid, it can occasionally bleed so severely that you have to tie her internal iliac arteries (3.5), or to do a hysterectomy (2.12). If necessary, give her an antibiotic and a blood transfusion.

If the pedicle of the polyp is thick and is attached well within the cavity of her uterus, be careful. Incise it longitudinally to find the level of the capsule of the fibroid first, as in Fig. 20-4. You can then cut and tie the pedicle just above this, with no danger of entering her abdomen. Transfix the pedicle as far distally as you can, and divide it distal to the ligature, so that you minimize the risk of opening her peritoneal cavity. If you don't remove it completely, it will recur.

If she has a large submucous polyp presenting at her cervix, but not protruding through it, treatment is difficult. It is sure to be partly necrotic, so that a hysterectomy carries the risk of sepsis. You can: (1) Define it as well as you can with your fingers first and then twist it off vaginally (risky). If she continues to bleed (unusual) see above. (2) Improve her general condition, transfuse her, give her antibiotics, and then do a hysterectomy.

CAUTION ! Don't try to twist off a fibroid polyp, it is usually impossible. The only kind of cervical polyp to twist off is a mucosal one, as in Fig. 20-5.

DIFFICULTIES WITH FIBROIDS

If her FIBROID IS PAINFUL, either spontaneously or on palpation, with perhaps a low fever, this is due to aseptic necrosis (red degeneration), or associated torsion of a pedunculated fibroid.

If you discover a SMALL SUBMUCOUS FIBROID when you are doing a 'D and C' for abnormal vaginal bleeding, you may be able to remove it with the curette.

If she has a MUCOSAL POLYP, it may come from her cervix or endometrium and cause menorrhagia, or intermenstrual bleeding, or both. If it comes through her cervix, you can see it with a speculum and twist it off, as in Fig. 20-5. You will only see an endometrial polyp when you do a 'D and C'.

If she is PREGNANT, don't remove a fibroid, unless it is peduncuated and very easy to remove. See Section 18.7.

REMOVING CERVICAL POLYPI

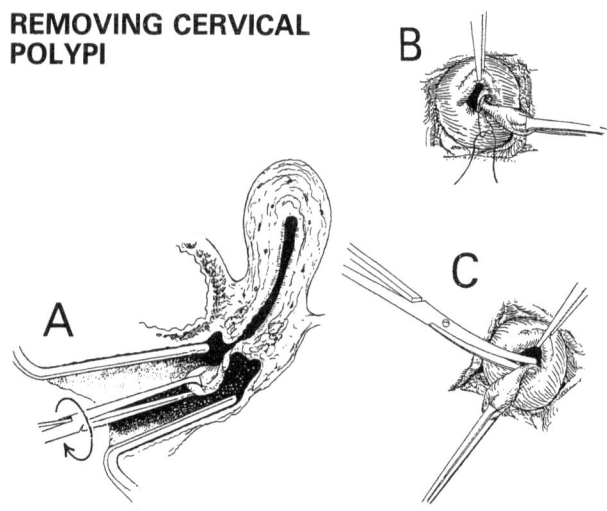

Fig. 20-5 THREE WAYS OF REMOVING MUCOSAL POLYPI. A, by twisting. B, by ligation. C, by section. These mucosal polypi are much more common and are more easily removed than fibroid polyps. Don't try to remove pedunculated fibroids this way. *Kindly contributed by Jack Lange.*

20.7 Ovarian cysts and tumours

Many ovarian tumours are cystic, but some cysts are not tumours and some tumours are not cysts. Their classification is complex, so here is a simplified scheme. First the cysts you may meet. *Benign:* (1) Functional cysts of the follicles and corpus luteum. (2) Benign serous or mucinous cystadenomas. (3) Dermoid cysts (teratomas or hamartomas). (4) Unclassified benign cysts (simple cysts). *Malignant:* (1) Malignant serous or mucinous cystadenocarcinomas. (2) Metastatic carcinomas (from the gut, or breast) (3) Burkitt's lymphoma. (4) Other rarer tumours. 'Pseudocysts' are postinflammatory collections of fluid between adhesions in the pelvis (6.6), and are not true ovarian cysts; but the distinction is not always easy, even at operation.

An ovarian cyst can be of any size, from a pingpong ball to larger than a full-term pregnancy, and may: (1) Present as a mass, or as abdominal distension, which may be massive. If so, the patient may be in poor health, or she may be fairly well. (2) Be found accidentally during a pelvic examination done for some other purpose, such as family planning. (3) Cause abdominal pain due to torsion (see below).

Ask your clinic staff to refer any patient with an ovarian cyst larger than a small orange. If it is not too large, removing it should not be too difficult, provided it has not stuck to surrounding structures. Don't try to biopsy it; instead, remove it entirely, and send a sample for section.

Large cysts are more likely to be malignant than small ones. But huge cysts (larger than a full term pregnancy) are usually benign, or only of low-grade malignancy. They are more common in places where there are few doctors removing small ones, which is why they are relatively common in the developing world. Solid ovarian tumours are more likely to be malignant, and to have spread by the time you see them.

Most large cysts are mucinous or serous cystadenomas; some are cystadenocarcinomas. *Try to remove a cyst without spilling the fluid,* because if you do, you may spread a malignant tumour and harm the patient greatly. If a tumour has not spread through the wall of a cyst, its removal intact without spilling will usually cure her. Aspirating a cyst before you try to remove it: (1) Makes it easier to remove. (2) Requires a smaller incision lower in the abdomen. (3) May make dissection of adhesions easier. (4) Is likely to cause some spillage. Not aspirating a cyst either causes no spillage, or, if it bursts or you cut into it, a much worse spillage than if you had aspirated it first. Should you aspirate or not? Opinions vary; much depends on how skilled you are. As you will see below, we advise you not to aspirate, if you can avoid it. Even large cysts are not too difficult to remove intact—if you make an incision which is large enough (see below).

Most ovarian cysts have few adhesions. If adhesions are dense you may be dealing with: (1) Old PID. (2) A malignant cyst in which the growth is already spreading into the peritoneum. (3) Previous peritonitis that has left adhesions which have stuck the cyst to the peritoneum. (4) A cyst which has previously undergone torsion.

Don't be put off by the difficulties we describe below: some are rare and others only occur with really huge cysts of 20 kg or more. Cysts of the size of a full-term pregnancy or a bit larger commonly cause no trouble. Don't operate unnecessarily, adhesions and infertility may follow. Try to avoid removing both ovaries for bilateral benign tumours (usually dermoids). Remember that operating on a pseudocyst, or a cyst in the broad ligament, is particularly dangerous.

IF YOU ARE INEXPERIENCED, ONLY OPERATE FOR
SUSPECTED ACUTE COMPLICATIONS (torsion)

OVARIAN CYSTS

EXAMINATION bimanually reveals a round solid or cystic mass, which is dull to percussion and separate from the uterus.

OVARIAN TUMOURS

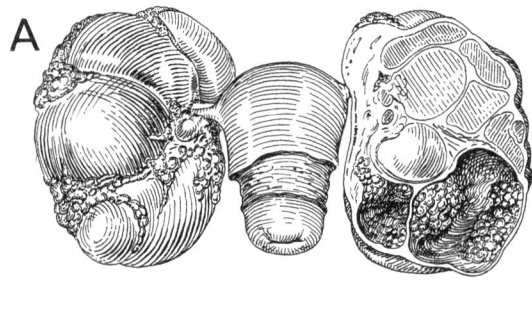
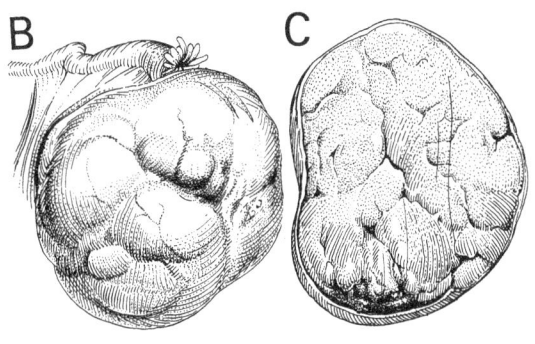

Fig. 20-6 OVARIAN TUMOURS. A, a pseudomucinous cystadeoncarcinoma shown in cross-section on the right. B, a solid primary carcinoma. C, the same carcinoma in cross-section. *Adapted from a drawing by Frank Netter with the kind permission of CIBA-GEIGY Ltd, Basle (Switzerland).*

THE DIFFERENTIAL DIAGNOSIS varies according to the way in which a cyst presents, but there is considerable overlap. Torsion (see below), is more likely to be confused with an inflammatory lesion.

Any presentation of an ovarian cyst may be confused with: (1) Pregnancy. (2) A distended bladder, which may contain up to 5 litres of urine. (3) Pseudocysts. (4) Hydrosalpinx. (5) Fibroids. (6) A chronic ectopic pregnancy (haematocele). (7) A broad ligament cyst arising from the Wolffian ducts. (8) An appendix mass, or a small-gut mass. (9) Mesenteric cysts. (10) An enlarged spleen with a long pedicle. (11) Hydronephros.

Presenting as an acute abdomen (torsion, see below). (1) Appendicitis or an appendix mass (12.1). (2) Acute ectopic pregnancy (16.6). (3) Degeneration, bleeding, or infection in a fibroid (20.6). (4) A mass due to PID (6.6). See also 10.2.

Presenting as an abdominal mass or distension. (1) Ascites (she is dull to percussion in her flanks, rather than in the centre of her abdomen). (2) Obesity (fat is usually generalized). (3) Distension with gas in a false pregnancy.

CAUTION ! (1) Be quite sure she is not pregnant. (2) Always catheterize her before you try to diagnose an intra-abdominal cyst—it may subside dramatically!

THE MANAGEMENT OF AN OVARIAN CYST

If you are inexperienced, refer her. If she is pregnant see below under 'Difficulties'. If you cannot refer her, proceed as follows.

If a cyst is <5–10 cm in diameter, it is usually a functional (follicular or luteal) cyst, and may be associated with fibroids and dysfunctional uterine bleeding (DUB, 20.2). 5 cm is the size of a small orange. Don't include her normal ovary in the measurement. The simple rule is that a cyst like this need not come out. Review her in 6–8 weeks, and only operate if the cyst persists. Most functional cysts will have disappeared. If you find such a cyst at laparotomy for some other condition, leave it. If you must interfere, aspirate it.

If she is <15 (before the menarche), many cysts are benign, but there is an increased risk of malignancy, which is sometimes low-grade. At operation the decision to remove her ovaries is particularly difficult. Only remove large (>10 cm), solid ovarian tumours, and be sure to send them for histology.

If she is 15 to 35 years old, and the cyst is >5 cm, it is probably a dermoid, especially if it is firm. An X-ray may show bone or a tooth. Remove it; to do so you may have to remove the whole ovary. If it is bilateral (15%), try to leave some ovarian tissue.

If she is 30 to 55 and it is large, it is likely to be a cystadenoma, which may be bilateral (20%). The contents may be serous, and there may be papilliferous growths inside its wall (less likely to be malignant), or outside (more likely to be malignant). If it is very large, its contents are likely to be mucinous. Malignant change is unusual. If however the mucin spills into her peritoneum, dense adhesions (myxoma peritonei) may form. Remove these cysts: they may undergo torsion, or occasionally rupture spontaneously.

If she is past her menopause, the risk of malignancy is increased. Be prepared to do a hysterectomy, when you remove the cyst.

If you can remove a serous cystadenoma intact, before there has been any spread, as shown by peritoneal deposits and ascites, her prognosis is very good. If there is peritoneal spread, the cyst will probably be adherent to the surrounding structures, and her prognosis is poor. If you are not an expert, don't try to remove ovarian carcinomas which have spread to the peritoneal surface.

If she presents with a palpable mass, ascites, or oedema of her legs (due to lymphatic obstruction from peritoneal deposits), consider the possibility of a solid adeno- or undifferentiated carcinoma of the ovary, which characteristically presents like this. It is often bilateral, and by the time she reaches laparotomy, it will probably have spread widely. Her prognosis is poor, but rare cases do occasionally regress spontaneously.

If there is peritoneal spread, remove the primary if this is not too difficult; but it will not cure her. There is little to be gained by removing her uterus.

If the tumour is solid, remember the unusual possibility that it may be a fibroma, which is benign, but can cause ascites (Meig's syndrome). Remove it.

If you are in an endemic area and she is between 10 and 25, remember Burkitt's lymphoma (32.3), which is often bilateral.

INDICATIONS FOR SURGERY. The treatment or prevention of complications: torsion, bleeding, or infection. (2) Suspected malignancy. (3) Discomfort due to size.

CAUTION ! Infertility is not an indication.

ANAESTHESIA. (1) General anaesthesia. (2) Subarachnoid anaesthesia.

MORE OVARIAN TUMOURS

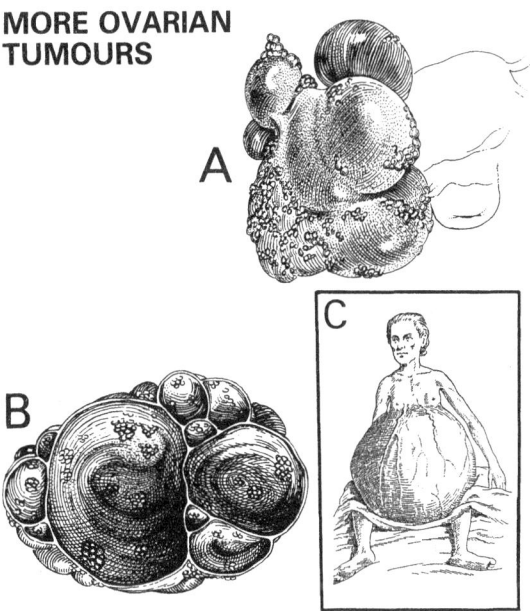

Fig. Fig. 20-7 MORE OVARIAN TUMOURS. A, a papillary serous cystadenoma. B, the same in cross-section. C, a very large ovarian cyst showing dilated veins on the abdominal wall. *A, and B, adapted from drawings by Frank Netter with the kind permission of CIBA-GEIGY Ltd, Basle (Switzerland). C, after James Young.*

REMOVING AN OVARIAN CYST

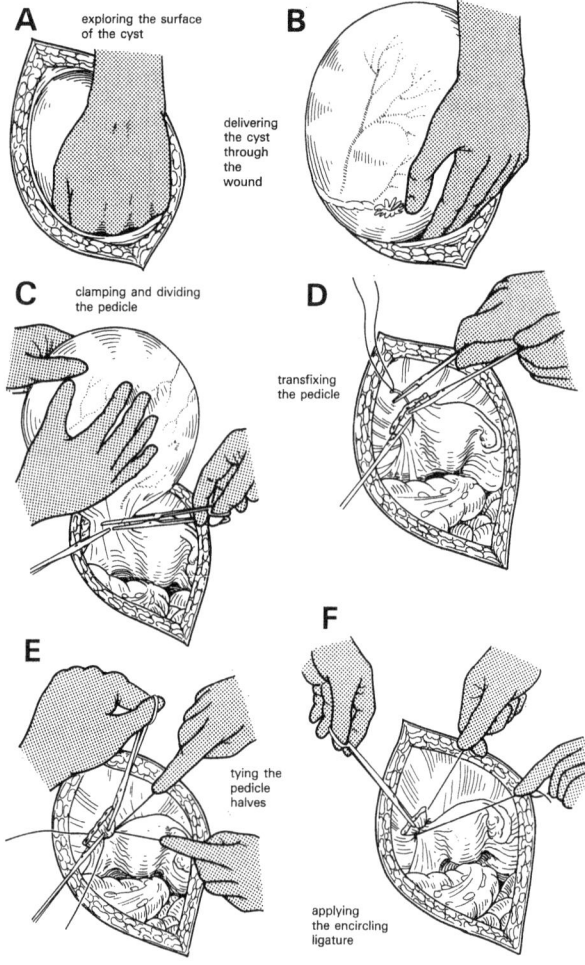

Fig. 20-8 REMOVING AN OVARIAN CYST. A, exploring the surface of the cyst. B, delivering the cyst without rupturing it. C, clamping and dividing the pedicle. D, transfixing the pedicle. E, tying the pedicle in halves. F, applying the encircling ligature. *After 'Bonney's Gynaecological Surgery',* Figs 4.29 to 4.34, Baillière Tindall, with kind permission.

CYSTECTOMY FOR SMALLER OVARIAN CYSTS

INCISION. Make a median or paramedian incision, big enough to allow you insert your hand, and to remove the cyst intact. Feel its whole surface for adhesions—if you find them see below. Search for secondaries in the rest of her peritoneal cavity, over the surface of her liver, and under her right diaphragm. You may need both hands.

When the cyst is free of adhesions, deliver it through the abdominal wound, and hand it to your assistant, taking care not to pull on its pedicle, which may be so thin that it easily tears, causing the proximal end to slip into her pelvis and bleed.

CAUTION ! Before you remove the cyst, examine her other ovary.

If her other ovary is also cystic, and she is relatively young, try to do an ovarian cystectomy (see below), unless there is a suspicion of malignancy. Suspect malignancy on the combination of these factors: (1) she is over 40 years, (2) the tumour is solid or lobulated, (3) there are papillary excrescences on its surface (especially) or inside it, (4) she has ascites, (5) there are secondaries on the surface of her peritoneum, (6) the cyst is fixed and immobile.

If she has a bilateral, papilliferous, or obviously malignant ovarian tumour, what you should do depends on your skills, and how far the tumour has spread: (1) If there is no peritoneal spread, and you can do a total hysterectomy with the removal of both ovaries, do so. Otherwise, do a bilateral oophorectomy (removal of the cyst with the ovary). (2) If there is little or no spread, do a bilateral oophorectomy. It will remove the bulk of the tumour, but it will not cure her, so the benefit will be minimal. (3) If there is wide peritoneal spread, merely biopsy a deposit on her parietal peritoneum.

The pedicle of an ovarian cyst consists of: (1) the infundibulopelvic ligament and ovarian vessels, (2) the ovarian ligament, (3) a portion of the broad ligament, and (4) frequently the Fallopian tube. If it is wide (often it is not), clamp it with several clamps, taking a bite of not more than 2.5 cm in each of them. Cut through the pedicle at some distance from each clamp; it will be less likely to slip off if you do this.

Transfix the pedicle in each clamp with double '1' or '2' catgut sutures, or 'O' or '1' multifilament, taking care to avoid the plexus of veins as you insert the needle. Some surgeons advise that, if a pedicle is very broad, you should apply a chain of 3 to 4 or more ligatures. Finally, ask your assistant to hold the clamps, and pass a further ligature round the entire pedicle. This will tie any veins which may have escaped the other ligatures.

Swab the stump, and, if bleeding has been controlled, cut the ligatures short. Remove the cyst from the operation site, and ask an unscrubbed assistant to open it. If it looks malignant and she is >40, remove her other ovary also, and if you can, her uterus too. If she is younger, wait for histological confirmation of malignancy, and refer for more radical surgery later if necessary.

CYSTECTOMY FOR A VERY LARGE CYST

POSITION. She may develop the supine hypotensive syndrome (A 16.6), if she lies on her back, so lay her with a sandbag under one buttock.

INCISION Make a paramedian or median incision. If you hope to remove the cyst intact, make it at least 5 cm longer than the diameter of the cyst.

If you are not sure if you can remove the cyst intact, make the incision at least 25 cm long and examine the cyst, separating such adhesions as you can see, without too forceful traction on the wound. If you cannot dissect further in safety, enlarge the incision to see the outline of the cyst and any adhesions. Aspirating fluid (see above) may help you do deliver it through the abdominal wall, but seldom helps in dissecting adhesions. A flabby cyst has an edge which is difficult to define, so that vital structures, such as the ureter, are more easily cut. If you do decide to aspirate fluid, use a syringe and needle, don't aspirate more than is necessary, and *don't contaminate the operation site with the fluid you have aspirated!*

NOTE: (1) The size of an incision makes almost no difference to the probability of operative shock. (2) A large one will not affect her adversely, except to increase the incidence of postoperative pain, and slightly increase the risk of wound breakdown. (3) A wound which is too small is dangerous because you cannot dissect safely, and you are obliged to exert excessive traction. This will kill cells in the edges of the incision, and increase the risk of subsequent wound sepsis, and possible breakdown—see Section 9.2.

Remove the cyst by clamping its pedicle as above. Be careful not to pull it so hard that you tear this. Insert tension sutures (9.8), and apply an abdominal binder.

OVARIAN CYSTECTOMY

This removes the cyst but leaves the tissue of her ovary. It is usually not difficult.

INDICATIONS. (1) She is less than 40, especially if her other ovary is also damaged. (2) The cyst is >5 cm. If it is <5 cm, it is probably functional, so leave it. (3) The cyst must be benign, a reasonable amount of normal ovarian tissue should be present. If her cystic ovary is her only remaining one, it is not important if its tube is intact or not. She needs its endocrine function, regardless of possible fertility. You may be able to shell out even quite large cysts, and retain some ovarian tissue.

METHOD. The cyst lies in the substance of her ovary and is covered by the ovarian capsule. Cut around the edge of the cyst, well away from the remaining mass of her normal ovary. Using scissors or fingers, dissect between the cyst and her ovarian tissue. Control bleeding with 2/0 chromic catgut, and close the outer layer of her ovary with continuous locking sutures.

SALPINGO-OOPHORECTOMY

INDICATIONS. Removing a tube and ovary is indicated when cystectomy, or ovarian cystectomy is not desirable, or not possible, because: (1) They have been damaged by torsion, bleeding, or infection. (2) There is a possibility of malignancy. (3) There are extensive adhesions between her tube and ovary. (5) If she is >45-50 a bilateral salpingo-oophorectomy with hysterectomy is likely to be preferable.

METHOD. The tube and ovary receive their blood from two sources which anastomose with one another: (1) The ovarian vessels in the infundibulopelvic ligament (20-17), and (2) the ascending branches of the uterine vessels.

Carefully divide any adhesions between her ovary and broad ligament, approaching them from below and behind. Raise her tube and ovary, find her infundibulopelvic ligament, and identify her ureter, so that you can avoid it. Clamp, divide, and tie her ovarian vessels in her infundibulopelvic ligament. Clamp, divide, and tie her ovarian ligament. Clamp, divide, and tie her tube. Suture her round ligament over the raw area (optional).

CAUTION ! Be sure not to tie her ureter. This is not a problem if the structures are mobile. But if there are adhesions, and especially if her ovary and tube have stuck to the back of her broad ligament, be sure to mobilize them before you resect.

DIFFICULTIES WITH OVARIAN CYSTS

If she has severe, COLICKY LOWER ABDOMINAL PAIN, sometimes with vomiting, suspect TORSION OF AN OVARIAN CYST. Her pain if may come and go, as it twists and untwists. She may not know she has a mass in her abdomen; it may enlarge acutely as the veins in its pedicle become obstructed. For the differential diagnosis see Section 10.2. Rule out retention of urine preoperatively. Do a laparotomy, tie and transfix the pedicle, and excise the cyst.

If she is PREGNANT, you may meet any of these complications.

If the cyst is <5 cm in diameter, it is probably a luteal cyst (very common, and usually disappears after 16-18 weeks). Leave it and follow her up after delivery.

If it is >5 cm, it is probably a cystadenoma, a dermoid, or a cystadenocarcinoma, and delivery may be difficult. Ovarian cystectomy or salpingo-oophorectomy are possible after the first trimester, and before the last few weeks of pregnancy. Don't remove it in early pregnancy, because abortion is more likely. Instead, remove it between the 16th and 24th week, even if you diagnose it earlier. If it is large, operate up to the 30th week.

If it causes pain, this may be due to torsion or haemorrhage. Remove it urgently at any stage of pregnancy.

If you diagnose it after the 30th week, **allow her to deliver vaginally,** unless it is very large (>25-30 cm). The ideal time to remove it is 4 to 6 weeks later.

If she goes into labour with an ovarian cyst and obstructs, see Section 18.4, and especially Fig. 18-5.

If you find an ovarian cyst at Caesarean section, **remove it if it is >5 cm.** See Section 18.10.

If there are EXTENSIVE ADHESIONS, she may have a pseudocyst (postinflammatory cyst), and not a true ovarian one. Don't try to deliver the tumour until you have divided them, or you may lacerate her gut or tear large veins. Separate them using your hands, swabs, or scissors (*not* a scalpel!). Gently pass your hand between the cyst wall and the floor of her pelvis. Don't mistake her parietal peritoneum for the cyst wall. Don't tie off any colon when you tie off adhesions.

CAUTION ! It is safer to leave a little cyst wall on her gut or the bladder, than to remove a little gut or bladder with the cyst wall.

If you meet a collection of PSEUDOCYSTS, there may still be signs of inflammation. Aspirate as many collections of fluid as you can, close her abdomen, give her antibiotics, and hope they will not recur.

If the cyst is NOT FREELY MOBILE, but seems to be embedded in her broad ligament, it may be arising from the remains of her Wolffian duct. Removing it may be difficult. It may be: (1) stuck to her broad ligament, or (2) inside it. The distinction is usually unimportant. If it is inside the ligament: (1) be sure to avoid her ureter, *which may run anywhere over the cyst.* (2) Don't damage the venous plexuses in this region. Study her anatomy carefully before you start.

If the cyst does not shell out easily, and extends down close to her ureter, **you would be wise to remove as much as you can,** and leave the remains open to her peritoneal cavity (marsupialization).

If you can define the cyst clearly by finger dissection, and are able to push her ureter out of the way, **you may be able to remove it completely.** It is covered by peritoneum which you will have to dissect off. Divide her round ligament on the same side, to open up her broad ligament. Then dissect off her peritoneum posteriorly, until you reach her ovarian vessels in her infundibulopelvic ligament. Tie them. Then dissect anteriorly and medially, and divide her tube and ovarian ligament close to her uterus. Finally, slowly and carefully dissect the cyst from the posterior leaf of her broad ligament, so as to avoid her ureter.

If you find BILATERAL BENIGN CYSTS (common with dermoids), try to spare at least some ovarian tissue on one side.

If a cyst looks MALIGNANT, consider her age and her wish to have children.

If she is young and has no children, **remove the tube and ovary** which are involved, and send tissue for histology. If it is found to be malignant, it may be necessary to remove her uterus and other ovary.

If she is older and does have children, **and particularly if you cannot follow her carefully, consider doing a bilateral salpingo-oophorectomy together with a hysterectomy.** This is a difficult operation and a difficult decision, so refer her if you can.

If her INFUNDIBULOPELVIC LIGAMENT IS GROSSLY THICKENED, so that her ovarian vessels are difficult to distinguish from her ureter, open up her peritoneal tissues lateral to them, and extend the incision towards her pelvic brim. Grasp her ovarian vessels and draw them medially. You will then see her ureter attached to her peritoneum, crossing her common iliac artery.

DIFFICULTIES WITH GIANT OVARIAN CYSTS

If she develops CARDIAC FAILURE, which may be delayed for a day or two postoperatively (rare), the reasons for it are not clear. Don't overload her with fluid; if necessary, give her a diuretic.

If she develops RESPIRATORY FAILURE (rare), due to the paradoxical movement of her diaphragm, which is lax and overstretched, now that the the cyst has been removed, give her oxygen and sit her up. If necessary, do a tracheostomy and control her ventilation (A 16.1).

If her ABDOMEN DISTENDS postoperatively (unusual), it is probably due to ileus. Insert a nasogastric tube and give her intravenous fluids (10.13).

If her ABDOMEN IS ABNORMALLY LAX, apply an efficient binder postoperatively.

CAUTION ! Don't be tempted to resect any redundant abdominal wall. This will make the operation much more extensive, and open up more tissue planes. This is a cosmetic procedure; refer her for it later if necessary.

20.9 Prolapse of the uterus

Childbirth may so injure a patient's pelvic organs that her uterus, her bladder, or her rectum may prolapse, either singly, or in combination. If her bladder or urethra prolapse as a cystocele, the standard operation is an anterior colporrhaphy. If her rectum prolapses, it is a posterior colporrhaphy. If her uterus prolapses it is either a Manchester repair, if it is to be left in, or a vaginal hysterectomy if it is to be removed. Prolapse appears to be comparatively uncommon in much of the developing world, despite the much greater multiparity of its mothers, but it is uncertain if this is a real difference; they may merely complain less.

A Manchester repair or a vaginal hysterectomy involve some fairly difficult vaginal surgery, with the risk that, if you are not expert, you may enter her rectum or her bladder and cause a fistula. If her uterus has prolapsed, they are certainly the best operations, so refer her for them if you can. If this is impossible, or she is unwilling to undergo them, Le Fort's operation, or ventrisuspension, are possible alternatives. They are old-fashioned and less effective than the modern operations, so that experts no longer

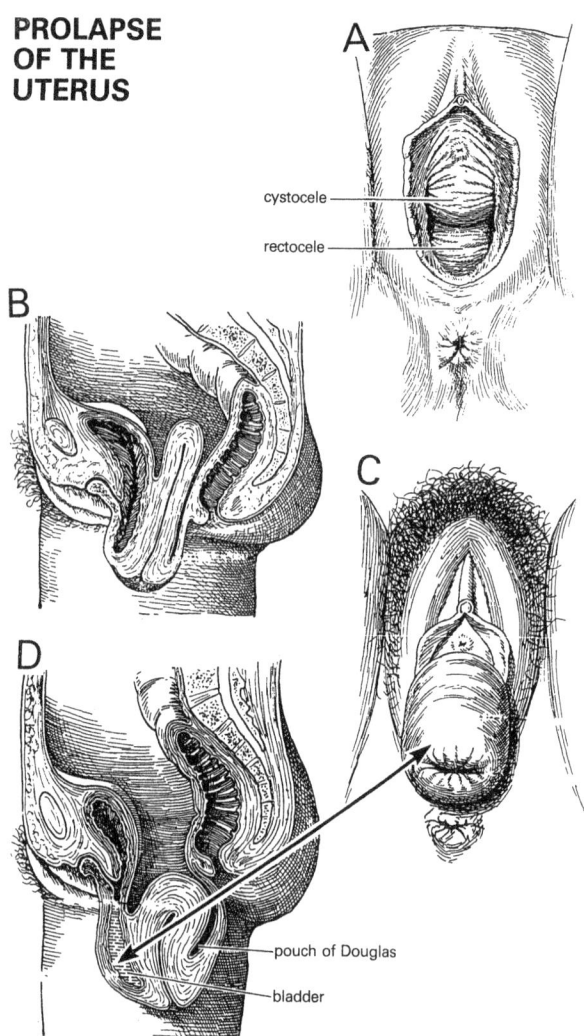

PROLAPSE OF THE UTERUS

Fig. 20-9 PROLAPSE OF THE UTERUS. A, a cystocele and a rectocele. B, a third degree prolapse. C, and D, the same patient with procidentia; her fundus is outside her introitus. Ideally, all these patients need a vaginal hysterectomy and an anterior and posterior colporrhaphy. If you are unable to do this, you could do an anterior and posterior colporrhaphy on A, and a Le Fort's operation on the other two patients. Patient CD is also suitable for ventrisuspension. *After Young James, 'A Textbook of Gynaecology', (5th edn 1939). A and C Black, permission requested.*

do them. But if you are not an expert, you will find that they are your only way of helping an old woman whose genitalia are prolapsing. Contributors differ as to whether we should include ventrisuspension or not. Because it is disputed we have put it in small print; it *may* have a place.

If she has a cystocele or rectocele which are large enough to cause symptoms, *without much uterine prolapse,* you can, if you are sufficiently skilled, do an anterior repair (colporrhaphy), or a posterior one, which is somewhat more difficult or both.

MARY, an old lady of 80, complained that her husband was accusing her of having given him an STD, because he was having pain in pasing his urine. She wanted a letter she could take to the court saying that she was free of any STD. On examination her uterus was grossly prolapsed, ulcerated and stinking, but she had no evidence of any STD. A Manchester repair cured her completely. LESSON A patient's symptoms are not always what they seem.

Pessaries for prolapse. Many old women prefer to avoid surgery, and can be treated with a pessary. Ring pessaries are suitable for most of them. If a patient is comfortable she can leave it in indefinitely, but you should see her from time to time. Menstruation (if she is still menstruating) and sex (if she still wants it) can take place as usual; she may not even be aware that she has one.

• PESSARY, *ring pattern, semi-rigid polythene, 40 to 120 mm, assorted sizes, predominantly the larger ones, 25 pessaries only.*

INSERTING A PESSARY

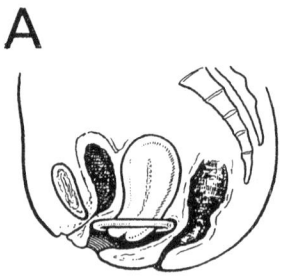 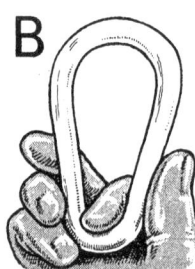

Fig. 20-9a A RING PESSARY IS OFTEN very acceptable to an older patient with moderate prolapse. Choose its size as you would a diaphragm, by measuring the depth of her vagina with your fingers. *After Garry MG, 'Gynaecology Illustrated', Churchill Livingstone, permission requested.*

RING PESSARIES FOR PROLAPSE

INDICATIONS. If surgery is impracticable. Moderate prolapse especially in an older patient; if her perineal muscles are very deficient, they will not hold a pessary. If too big a ring is required, her vaginal wall or cervix may prolapse through it.

METHOD. Choose the size of a ring pessary, as you would a diaphragm, by measuring the depth of her vagina with your fingers. It will usually be about 70 mm. Warm it in hot water to soften it, lubricate it, compress it, and insert it like a diaphragm, with the posterior part behind her cervix, and the anterior part behind her symphysis. It will resume its ring shape and take up a position in the coronal plane. If a 70 mm pessary falls out, try a larger size in 5–10 mm intervals. If it feels very tight and uncomfortable, so that she cannot pass urine, try a smaller size.

See her in 3 months; if all is well then, see her annually and ask her if the pessary is comfortable. Ideally, she needs a new pessary each year. If it is not coated with solid material, you can wash and replace it.

If her pessary keeps falling out, she needs surgery.

If her vagina is ulcerated at her annual checkup, leave her pessary out for a 1–2 months and give her some oestrogen cream to insert nightly. When her ulcers have healed, insert a smaller pessary, and see her in 3 months.

20.10 Ventrisuspension

In this operation a patient's prolapsed uterus is sutured to her anterior abdominal wall. This relieves both her prolapse, and the rectocele or cystocele, which she will probably have also. If it does not, you can do a simple diamond-shaped excision of her anterior or posterior vaginal wall. Ventrisuspension alone does not interfere with her bladder, her urethra, her rectum, or her vagina. It is not difficult, and is a convenient operation if you are inexperienced, because you can do it through a large lower median incision; it does however sometimes fail. The approach is the same as that for a Caesarean section, which you will have to master anyway.

Aim to: (1) Make the anterior wall of her uterus, cervix, and bladder stick to her rectus muscles. (2) Make the peritoneum of her bladder, and the anterior wall of her cervix stick to the back of her pubis, so that there is no chance of an internal hernia occurring between them.

Opinions vary as to whether this operation is advisable in a premenopausal patient who may become pregnant. Pregnancy is possible, but it would seem wise to tie her tubes, if she will let you. You will occasionally find that, when you cut down on an old Caesarean section scar that was infected at the time of the original operation, you will go straight into the amniotic space. Such a patient has, in effect, had an unintentional ventrisuspension.

VENTRISUSPENSION

INDICATIONS. (1) Any patient with a prolapse involving a considerable descent of her uterus. (2) Prolapse in old postmenopausal patients.

METHOD. Open the patient's abdomen through a midline incision, extending well down towards her symphysis pubis. The

VENTRISUSPENSION

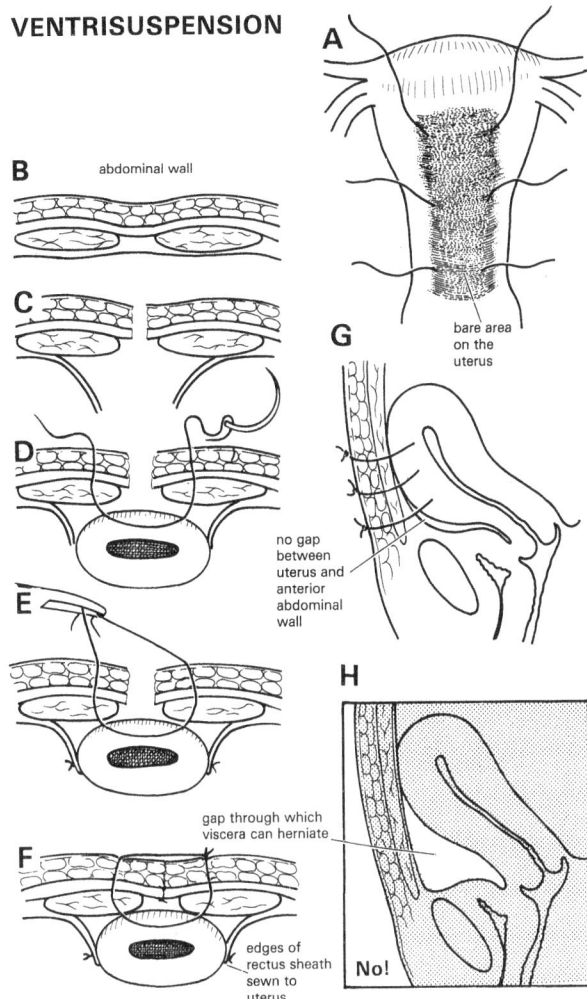

Fig. 20-10 VENTRISUSPENSION. A, the bare area you aim to create on the patient's uterus, with the sutures in place. B, her abdominal wall before starting the operation. C, her abdominal wall opened and her posterior rectus sheath reflected. D, the sutures in place, and the posterior sheath sewn to her uterus. E, and F, closing the sutures. G, a side view of the completed operation, showing her uterus close up against her abdominal wall. H, the space through which gut can herniate that you are trying to avoid. *Kindly contributed by Andrew Boddham-Whetham.*

upper limit of the incision will depend on how far up you can pull up her uterus, when you have examined it.

Separate her uterus and adnexa from any adhesions, bring them into the wound, and examine them.

Identify the peritoneal reflexion of her bladder, so that you can avoid it. Separate her rectus abdominis muscles from their posterior sheath, along their whole length on each side of the wound.

Use a scalpel to vigorously excoriate the anterior surface of the body of her uterus, to within a centimetre of its upper and lateral borders (A, in Fig. 20-10). Don't excoriate her cervix. Instead, elevate and remove a strip of peritoneum about 2 cm wide off her cervix, her bladder, and her anterior abdominal wall, to join up with the skin incision.

Prepare three large curved cutting needles with strong monofilament. Decide how high up her uterus should come behind her abdominal wall.

Pass each needle through the outer surface of her rectus sheath on one side, through her rectus muscle, and then out of its bare posterior surface. Then pass it deeply in and out of the bare area of the anterior wall of her uterus, across into the bare area of her other rectus muscle, and out through her rectus sheath and anterior rectus muscle. As you do this, avoid her posterior rectus sheath, which will fold inwards (B, C, and D). Apply clamps to each suture, and leave them until later (E).

Now comes the tricky part. Using 2/0 monofilament on a round-bodied needle, and starting at the apex of her bladder (but without penetrating it), sew her peritoneum to itself along the line that you have previously excoriated. Leave no gap between her uterus and her anterior abdominal wall. When you have closed this gap, sew her peritoneum and her posterior rectus sheath (which are very thin) to the edges of the excoriated area on her uterus. Use a continuous suture, and make sure that it passes behind the three large sutures that emerge from the body of her uterus.

In this way, close her peritoneal cavity, still leaving most of her uterus and all her adnexae intraperitoneally, but with most of the excoriated area of her anterior uterine wall exposed in the bottom of the wound.

Now bring her rectus muscles lightly together with continuous monofilament sutures. Close her anterior rectus sheath with continuous monofilament, and tie the three large sutures which you previously passed through the anterior wall of her uterus. The main strength of the suspension is the adhesions that are formed, not these sutures.

If a ventrisuspension is not enough, you can do a simple diamond-shaped excision of her anterior or posterior vaginal wall, to tighten up her vagina without doing a full Manchester repair.

20.11 Le Fort's operation

In Le Fort's operation the anterior and posterior walls of a patient's vagina are bared, and sewn together, so that a central longitudinal partition runs down its centre. This gives her a bipartite vagina which cannot prolapse, and which will also prevent her uterus from prolapsing. Prolapse of her bladder and rectum are also almost impossible. She cannot have sex, but there is still sufficient vaginal drainage to allow her to menstruate. This operation is rarely done in premenopausal women, because they usually want to have sex. Unfortunately, prolapse may recur down one side. This operation may not be popular in your community: she must understand what is to be done.

LE FORT'S OPERATION

INDICATIONS. An old postmenopausal woman with procidentia, or advanced prolapse of the second degree, who no longer has sex.

CONTRAINDICATIONS. (1) Premenopausal women. (2) Ulcerations of the vaginal mucosa.

ANAESTHESIA. (1) Saddle block. (2) Ketamine. (3) Local infiltration. (4) Subarachnoid anaesthesia.

METHOD. Put the patient into the lithotomy postion and examine her uterus. If she has any cervical lesions, deal with them—it will be the last opportunity you will have to take a Pap smear.

Using careful aseptic precautions, grasp her cervix and draw it out of her vulva with a vulsellum. Mark out an area on her anterior vaginal wall to be excised (A, in Fig. 20-11). Excise a rectangle of mucosa. Do the same on her posterior vaginal wall. Replace her cervix, and use catgut mattress sutures to unite the bare areas and cover her cervix, except for small channels on either side. If the local circulation is good, and there is no infection, the anterior and posterior walls of her vagina will unite.

20.11a Anterior and posterior colporrhaphy

A patient's anterior vaginal wall, and with it her bladder, may bulge towards her introitus when she coughs or strains (cystocele). The same thing can happen to her rectum (rectocele). If her cervix descends more than a little at the same time, she needs a Manchester repair, or if you cannot do this or refer her for it, Le Fort's operation (20.11), or ventrisuspension (20.10). An anterior and particularly posterior repair are more difficult than these two procedures, but they are much more satisfactory, so learn to do them if you can.

An anterior colporrhaphy mobilizes her bladder, returns

Le FORT'S OPERATION

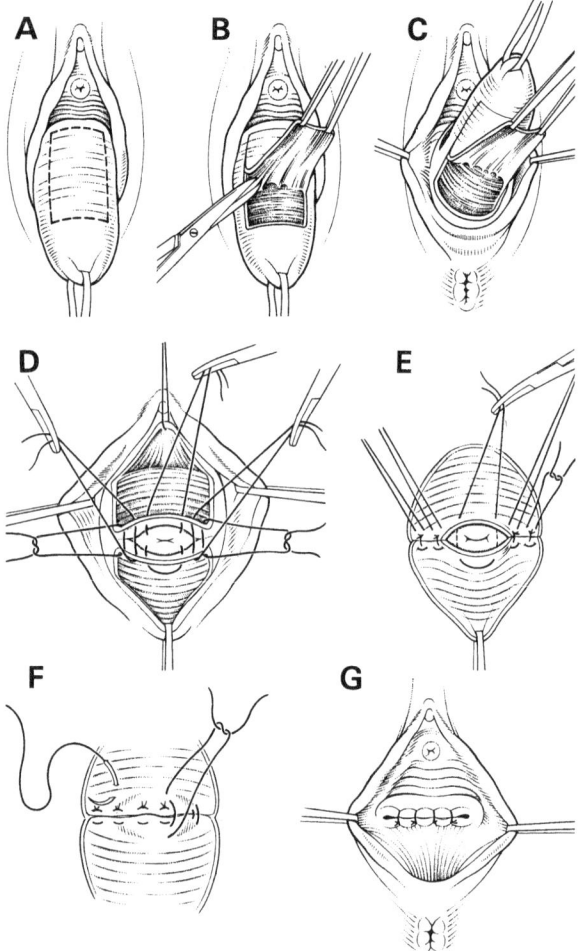

Fig. 20-11 LE FORT'S OPERATION. A, the cervix pulled downwards with vulsella, and the area of vaginal skin mapped out. B, mucosa being dissected off its anterior surface. C, mucosa being dissected off its posterior surface. D, the cervix inverted, and the raw surfaces being united with mattress sutures. E, the raw surfaces being joined together over and around the cervix. F, the cervix has disapppeared. G, the repair, complete with small channels at either side. *Roberts TWD, in Rob C, and Smith R, 'Operative Surgery: Gynaecology and Obstetrics; p. 89. Butterworth, with kind permission.*

it to its normal place, and fixes it there. Cut through the tissues joining her cervix and her bladder, so as to expose the peritoneum of her uterovesical pouch, and then suture the fascia on either side, so as to make a supporting buttress from her urethra to her cervix.

A posterior colporrhaphy, reduces her gaping introitus, reconstitutes her perineal body, reinforces her pelvic diaphragm by approximating her levator ani muscles, corrects her rectocele and eliminates the hernia of her pouch of Douglas. You can feel the levator ani muscles of a normal nullip 5 cm from her introitus. The key sutures in this operation bring her levator ani muscles together in this position.

COLPORRHAPHY

If possible, refer the patient for both these operations, otherwise proceed as follows. If she is postmenopausal, give her a course of oestradiol before starting.

ANTERIOR COLPORRHAPHY (anterior repair)

INDICATIONS. (1) Prolapse of her anterior vaginal wall which troubles her, especially if she has to push it back to micturate, provided there is little or no descent of her uterus. Preferably wait until childbearing is ended, because a prolapse may recur after pregnancy. She can be pre- or postmenopausal.

CONTRAINDICATIONS. (1) Ascites. (2) A severe chronic cough.

EXAMINATION. Lay her on her side in the left lateral position. Insert a Sims' speculum posteriorly and ask her to cough and strain downwards. Her cystocele will then show its full size and the degree of uterine descent. If her cervix comes down to her vulva, she is not suitable for an anterior repair alone. Refer her for a Manchester repair, or if this is impossible, consider doing le Fort's operation, or ventrisuspension. These are mainly for third degree prolapse (when the cervix is at the introitus or lower).

PREPARATION. Her tissues must be clean before you operate. Ask her to bath in a basin of salt solution (10 g/l). If she is already sufficiently clean, do this for 2 days prior to surgery.

ANAESTHESIA. (1) Subarachnoid anaesthesia (A 7.4). (2) Ketamine (A 8.1). (3) General anaesthesia (A 10.1).

METHOD. Put her into the lithotomy position and clean her vulva and vagina. Towel her and suture her labia minora to her skin with catgut about 4 cm from her vulva (optional, shown in I). Infiltrate her tissues, from her anterior urethral orifice to the anterior lip of her cervix, with 1/200 000 adrenalin in saline, or sterile water (A 5.4); you will probably need 20 or 30 ml.

Insert a Jacques (simple rubber) catheter to help identify her urethra. Put vulsellum forceps on her cervix and draw it down.

Incise her vaginal wall covering her cervix about 1.5 cm from her cervical os, and continue this laterally for about 2 cm on each side. Undermine the edge away from her cervix, and continue to within 1 cm of her urethral orifice, using the 'push and spread technique' with scissors (4-8).

CAUTION ! Keep close to her vaginal wall to avoid injuring her bladder. Distending her tissues with adrenalin solution makes this easier. The key to success is to work in the right layer.

Cut the wall of her vagina in the midline (A, Fig. 20-12). Dissect her vaginal wall away from the underlying tissues with a combination of blunt and sharp dissection, until you expose her bulging bladder fully on both sides. Where possible, use a gauze-wrapped finger (B). Take great care to separate her bladder from her vagina in the lateral part of the flap near her cervix. Dissection should be almost bloodless, until you reach the veins which lie well laterally.

Dissect her bladder away from her cervix (C). If necessary, draw up her bladder with dissecting forceps and cut it from her cervix with Mayo's scissors. Separate her bladder from her cervix with a retractor and expose the peritoneum of her uterovesical pouch, but *don't open her peritoneal cavity*. Using gauze dissection, separate the lateral extensions of her bladder from the lateral border of her uterus.

Feel for a stout pillar of fascia on each side of her uterus. The secret of success is wide and courageous dissection, the fascia you want is always there if you go far enough laterally. Use a series of interrupted simple, or, better, mattress sutures of chromic catgut or polyglycolic acid ('Dexon'), to pick up this fascia as far laterally as you can, starting anteriorly (D). If this fascia is difficult to identify, insert the sutures into the fascial envelope of her bladder. When you reach her cervix, take a bite of that. When you have tied the sutures, her bladder will be suspended (E).

Remove redundant vaginal wall (F); this usually needs to have a diamond-shape. If she has a large cystocele, you will have to remove much vaginal wall, but if you remove too much, her vagina will be too narrow. Close it with interrupted sutures. Insert a Foley catheter.

If she has a rectocele, usually accompanied by a deficient perineum, repair this at the same time.

POSTOPERATIVELY, drain her bladder into a bag or bottle. Spigot the catheter and remove it 2-hourly. Remove the catheter on the 5th day. About 6 hours later ask her to pass urine and then recatheterize her.

If her residual urine is <100 ml, let her pass urine normally. Restart salt baths.

If her residual urine is >100 ml, reinsert the catheter for another 2 days and repeat the process.

POSTERIOR COLPORRHAPHY (posterior repair)

INDICATIONS A significant rectocele (bulging of her posterior

COLPORRHAPHY—ONE Anterior colporrhaphy

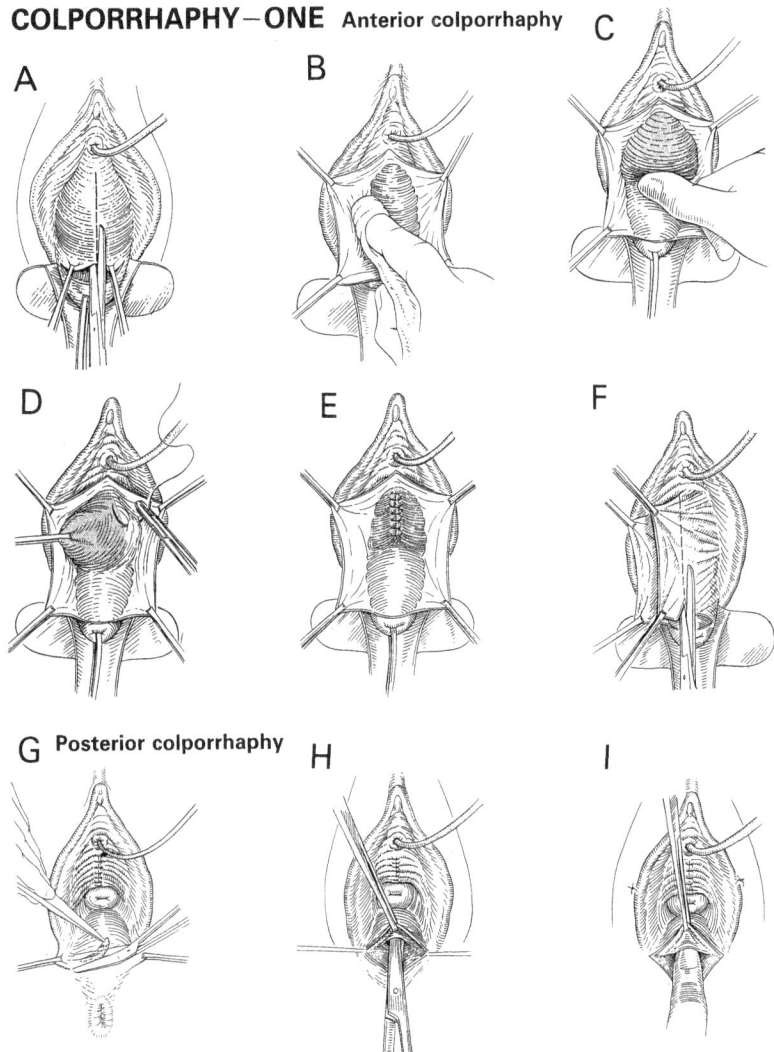

Fig. 20-12 COLPORRHAPHY—ONE. Anterior colporrhaphy: A, incise the patient's anterior vaginal wall. B, mobilize her cystocele. C, mobilize her cystocele from her cervix. D, insert the tightening suture as far laterally as you can. E, the obliteration of her cystocele is complete. F, remove her redundant vaginal wall.

Posterior colporrhaphy: G, excise an ellipse of skin at the junction of her vagina and perineum. H, mobilize her posterior vaginal wall. I, separate her rectocele from her posterior vaginal wall.

vaginal wall), with little or no descent of her cervix. Usually her perineum is deficient also. Do the operation at the same time as an anterior repair (see above).

EXAMINATION. Lay her in the left lateral position, with the speculum placed anteriorly to push her anterior vaginal wall out of the way. Demonstrate her rectocele by asking her to cough and then strain.

PREPARATION. As for an anterior repair. Give her an enema preoperatively.

METHOD. Infiltrate her subepithelial tissues with adrenalin solution as above. On each side place Allis forceps about 2 cm apart over the posterior termination of her labium minus, just inside her fourchette at the level of her carunculae hymenales (the little skin tags remaining from the hymen), and retract them. If you place them lower than this, the repair produces a bridge of skin which, causes dyspareunia. Retract the forceps, and use scissors to remove a little ellipse of skin between them (G).

Hold her posterior vaginal wall with forceps. Use blunt dissection, and the 'push and spread technique' with scissors (H), to dissect to a point where her posterior vaginal wall bulges less. When you have established a plane of cleavage, you can use your index finger (I).

CAUTION ! Keep near her vaginal wall to avoid incising her rectum.

At this point you usually need to excise some posterior vaginal wall (J, and K). How much you remove will decide how tight you leave her vagina. If she does not want sex, remove a generous amount, if she does remove only a little (L, assumes that you have not removed any).

Use 1/0 chromic catgut or polyglycolic acid ('Dexon') sutures on a curved needle to pick up: (1) Her levator ani muscles high in the wound on each side. (2) The fascial layer, which is rather thin, and tie it on each side. This will support her rectal wall (L).

Pick up her transversus perinei muscles on each side to reconstitute her perineal body (M). Finally, close her posterior vaginal wall and skin longitudinally in the sagittal plane (N).

If you have done an anterior and a posterior repair together and she wants to have sex, her vagina should admit 2 fingers easily. If you can only insert one finger, she will have some dyspareunia. Remove the 2 sutures closing her vagina and skin, and reconstitute the margin (fourchette) transversely.

POSTOPERATIVELY, if you have done an anterior repair also, manage her for that. If you have done a posterior repair only, start salt baths on the second day, and give her a full diet on the third day. As soon as her bowels have opened and her

COLPORRHAPHY—TWO

Posterior colporrhaphy—continued

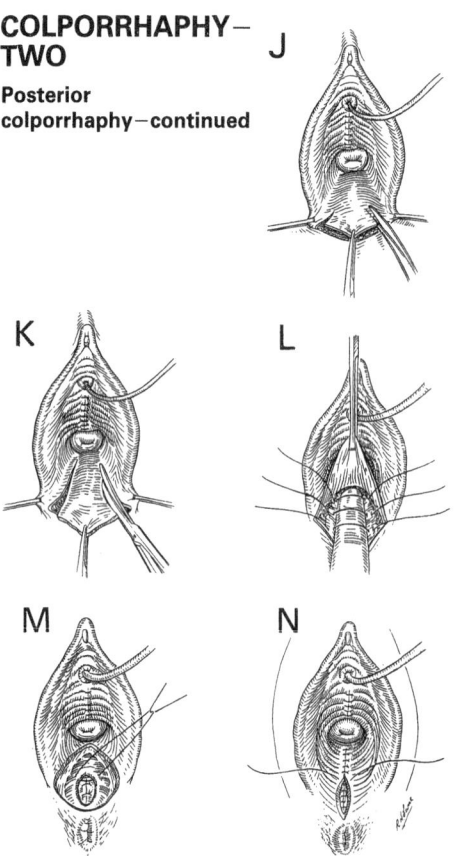

Fig. 20-13 COLPORRHAPHY—TWO. J, removing some skin from the posterior of the vagina. K, carrying the excision up to the apex of the freed vaginal skin. L, obliterate her rectocele by tightening the fascial layer. M, suture her perineal muscles together. N, both operations nearly complete.

wound is satisfactory, allow her home to continue salt baths there.

DIFFICULTIES WITH COLPORRHAPHY

If THERE IS MUCH BLEEDING: (1) If it is venous, inject adrenalin solution and wait 3 minutes or better 5. If necessary, pack her vagina. *Don't try to control venous bleeding with haemostats and ligatures.* (2) Underpin a bleeding artery with a needle and catgut.

If you OPEN HER BLADDER BY MISTAKE, which is unusual if you operate carefully, repair it with a purse string suture and reinforce it with a second layer of Lembert sutures (9-5). Drain her bladder for 10 days.

If you OPENED HER RECTUM BY MISTAKE this is not a disaster. If it is a large wound, close it transversely; if it is a small one, longitudinal closure is adequate.

20.12 Hysterectomy

You may occasionally have to do an emergency hysterectomy if a patient has: (1) A ruptured uterus, and repair is impossible (not uncommon). (2) Uncontrollable postpartum haemorrhage (PPH, uncommon). Hysterectomy for a ruptured uterus differs from the operation described below, and is described in Section 18.17. The only occasion on which you may have to use the method which follows urgently, is for an otherwise uncontrollable PPH; all other indications are nonurgent.

The indications for nonurgent 'cold' hysterectomy include: (1) Severe anaemia, as the result of excessive bleeding, due to fibroids. (2) Carcinoma of the body of the uterus. (3) Severe DUB (dysfunctional uterine bleeding) which you cannot control by other means (rare, 20.2). (4) Removal of the Fallopian tubes with the uterus for chronic pelvic pain due to PID which fails to respond to medical treatment. If possible try to refer all these cases, especially the last. 'Cold hysterectomies' can have disastrous complications, even in the hands of experts, and their patients even die occasionally. So don't do them, unless you are experienced, and cannot refer a patient. Fibroids may cause disability, but they seldom threaten life. If you are going to operate on them, start with nicely mobile uteri, without huge intraligamentary or cervical fibroids.

You can do a total hysterectomy by removing a patient's entire uterus; the advantage of doing this is that you remove her cervix, which is a common site for carcinoma. Or, you can do a subtotal operation, and leave a stump of her cervix behind. Experts almost always remove the whole uterus, so that subtotal hysterectomy is almost obsolete. Subtotal hysterectomy is contraindicated, if there is any suspicion of carcinoma in either the cervix, or the body of her uterus. But it is an easier operation, because you can more easily avoid the ureters. If you are inexperienced, start by doing a subtotal operation, particularly if you are operating for fibroids. But even this can be difficult, if there are adhesions from chronic PID. Don't attempt a radical hysterectomy which also removes her pelvic lymph nodes. It is the only adequate surgical treatment for carcinoma of the cervix, but this really is a task for an expert.

If you start by making a bladder flap, you will see the relations of the patient's ureter, her uterine artery, and her cervix more easily. The great danger is that you may cut, tie or clamp her

AVOIDING THE URETER

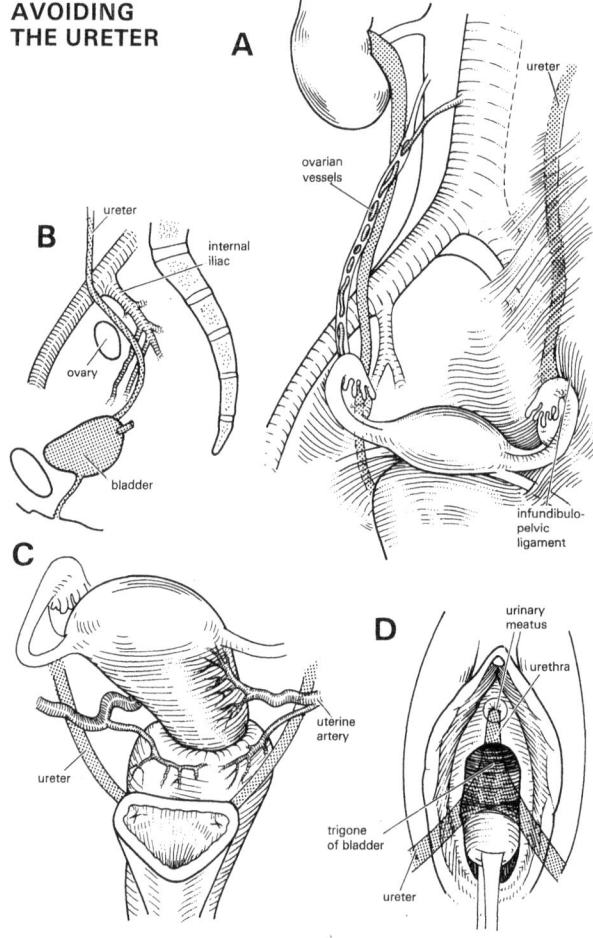

Fig. 20-16 AVOIDING THE URETER. A, notice how the ovarian vessels pass in front of the ureter. B, the ureter passes over the brim of the pelvis, just after the common iliac artery has divided into its internal and external iliac branches. C, the ureter passes close round the vault of the vagina under the uterine artery. D, the relation of the urethra, the trigone of the bladder, and the ureters when you retract the cervix. See also Fig. 3-7 which shows the relation of the ureter to the internal iliac artery when you come to tie it. Garry MG, 'Gynaecology Illustrated', pp. 308 and 309. Churchill Livingstone, with kind permission.

THE LIGAMENTS OF THE PELVIS

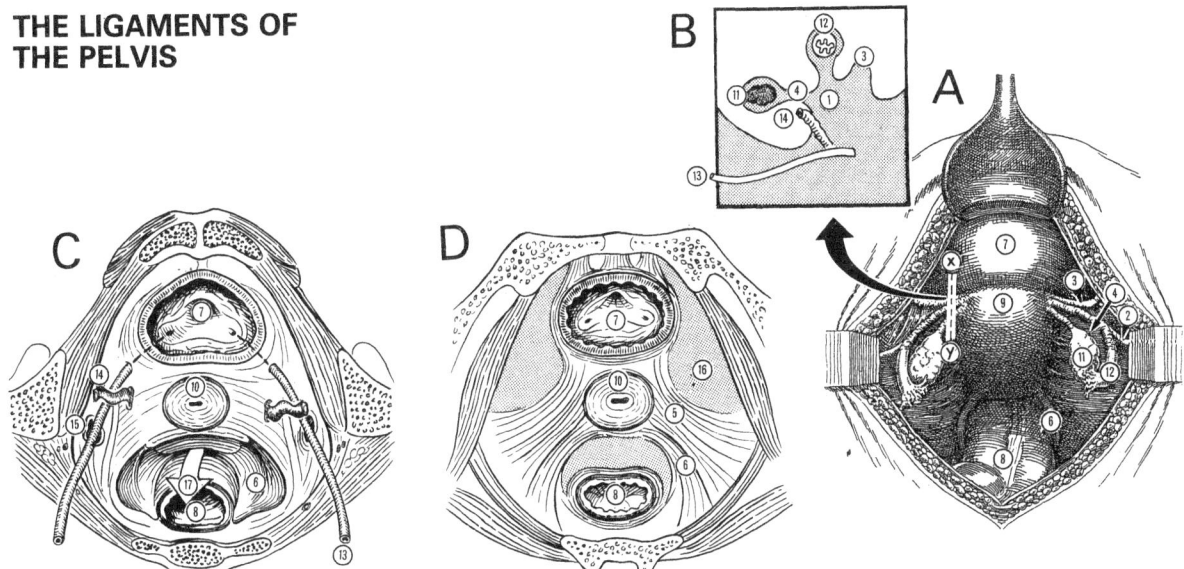

Fig. 20-17 THE LIGAMENTS OF THE PELVIS. A, you are standing on the patient's right and looking down into her pelvis. B, a sagittal section of part of her pelvis along line 'X—Y' in Diagram A. C, a section through a her pelvis, parallel with her pelvic brim. D, the main supporting ligaments of her pelvis viewed from above.

1, her broad ligaments. 2, her infundibulopelvic ligaments. 3, her round ligaments. 4, her ovarian ligaments. 5, her cardinal (transverse cervical) ligaments. 6, her uterosacral ligaments.

7, her bladder. 8, her rectum. 9, the fundus of her uterus. 10, her cervix. 11, her ovaries. 12, her Fallopian tubes. 13, her ureters. 14, her uterine arteries. 15, the veins of her pelvis. 16, fat filling the odd spaces in her pelvic connective tissue. 17, the arrow shows how an opening can be made from her posterior fornix into her pouch of Douglas. *A, after James Young. C, after Last. D, after Jeffcoate.*

ureters. They are at risk at several stages: (1) When you tie her ovarian vessels. So, lift these clear of her ureters before you tie them. (2) In the base of her exposed broad ligament. So before you do anything in this region which might injure her ureters, feel for them carefully. You can roll a ureter between your finger and thumb, and when you pinch one, it slips through your fingers.

Gentle continued traction is the secret of all pelvic surgery: (1) It demonstrates the tissue planes. (2) You are less likely to pick up structures that you do not want to cut. (3) Vessels stand out more clearly. (4) You are less likely to injure her bladder, or her ureter. (5) You can find the relation of her bladder to her cervix and vagina more easily.

Bleeding can be severe, especially from the uterine vessels. Divide these late in the operation, after most of the other structures have been removed from around them. Even when you have divided them, you are still in a bloody triangle at the sides of her vaginal vault.

If you are not careful, you can also cause a vesicovaginal fistula. This will be much less likely if: (1) You develop a bladder flap. (2) You carefully separate her bladder from her cervix. (3) You separate it from her uterine vessels.

All these dangers will be much more likely if you clamp blindly with a large clamp. So: (1) Don't clamp blindly. Only clamp what you can see. (2) Don't include more tissue in a clamp than it can safely hold.

Finally, wound infection is likely to be disturbingly common.

ANATOMY. The most critical items of a patient's pelvic anatomy are her ureters, as shown in Fig. 20-16. 'Ligaments' mean quite different things to gynaecologists and to orthopaedic surgeons. To a gynaecologist a 'ligament' is a fold of peritoneum, or a local thickening of the pelvic connective tissue. Gynaecologists recognize: (1) A patient's broad ligaments which are folds of tissue running from her Fallopian tubes towards the floor of her pelvis. The ureter and the uterine artery lie in the base of the broad ligament; vessels run round its edge, and its middle is avascular (see Fig. 18-20). (2) Her infundibulopelvic ligaments are folds of tissue which run from the lateral ends of her tubes to her pelvic wall. Their importance is that the ovarian vessels run in them. (3) Her round ligaments are folds of tissue which run from her uterus close to its junction with her tubes, anterolaterally towards the brim of her pelvis. They are really anterior folds or leaves in her broad ligaments. (4) Her ovarian ligaments support her ovaries, and hang off the back of her broad ligaments. (5) Her cardinal (transverse cervical) ligaments are thickenings of her pelvic connective tissue which run laterally from her cervix to the sides of her pelvis. (6) Her uterosacral ligaments run from her lower segment to her sacrum on each side of her rectum. They are, in effect, the posterior edges of her cardinal ligaments.

HYSTERECTOMY

INDICATIONS. See above.

CONTRAINDICATIONS TO TOTAL HYSTERECTOMY. (1) An inexperienced operator. (2) Active PID. (3) A uterus, which on clinical examination is 'fixed' in the pelvis. Dense adhesions, such as those due to PID, may pull the ureters out of place and make the operation difficult. (4) Obesity does the same.

ANAESTHESIA. You must be able to keep the gut out of the operative field, so you will need good muscular relaxation, and a moderate head-down tilt. (1) General anaesthesia with a long acting relaxant (A 14.3). (2) Lumbar epidural anaesthesia (A 7.2). (3) Subarachnoid anaesthesia (A 7.6). (4) Ether alone (A 11.3).

Set up a drip, and have blood cross-matched.

EQUIPMENT. A general set, a catheter, a uterine probe and sounds, a suitable self-retaining retractor, preferably Kirschner's, Gosset's, or Balfour's; also a Deaver's retractor and a tenaculum. At least 4 and preferably 6 long curved uterine clamps, either Hunter's or Maingot's. 1% iodine or Bonney's blue or gentian violet, a large damp pack with a tape. '0' or '1' multifilament or '1' or '2' chromic catgut for all pedicles. '1' catgut for the vagina. 2/0 catgut for the peritoneum.

PREPARATION. Make sure that she has signed the consent form and understands that she will have no more children and no periods.

HYSTERECTOMY—ONE

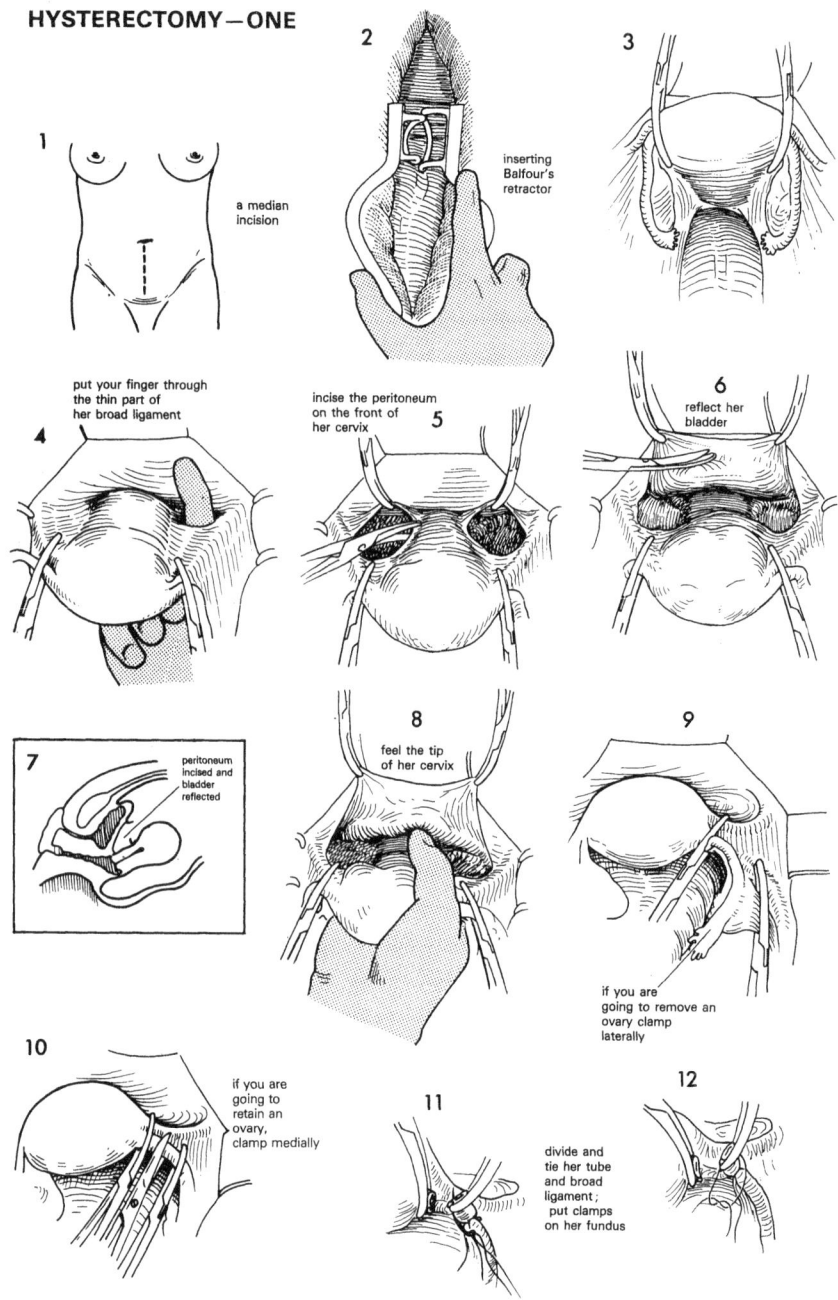

Fig. 20-18 HYSTERECTOMY—ONE. Make the incision (1), open the patient's broad ligament (4), reflect her bladder (6 and 7). Either remove her ovary (9) or retain it (10 and 11). *After Parsons L, and Ulfelder H, 'An Atlas of Pelvic Operations', pp. 21ff. WB Saunders, with kind permission.*

Four hours before the operation give her a gram of metronidazole rectally (tablets or a suppository, 2.9). Find yourself a competent assistant. If he is inexperienced, go through this account with him first.

Catheterize her bladder. Compress it suprapubically to make sure it is empty, and leave the catheter in for continuous drainage.

First put her into the lithotomy position, to paint and drape her perineum. Paint her vagina with 1% iodine, Bonney's blue, or gentian violet. This will make a big difference when you come to open it. Then lay her supine on the table and remove the lithotomy poles. Tip her slightly head-downwards to let her gut fall away from her pelvic cavity. Provided the angle is not too steep, it will not make anaesthesia difficult. Ideally, adjust the break in the table so that her knees are slightly flexed. Abduct her arm on an arm board.

You can choose whether you stand on her left or her right. The illustrations here assume you are standing on her left, which most right-handed surgeons find easier.

INCISION. If you are inexperienced, make a median or a left paramedian incision (9.2), from her symphysis to her umbilicus (1, in Fig. 20-18). If you are skilled, and her uterus is not more than 15 cm high (equivalent to a 14–16 week pregnancy), a transverse (Pfannensteil) incision gives the best cosmetic result. Open her peritoneum in the middle of the incision, and make the first cut upwards, so as to more easily avoid her bladder.

CAUTION ! Make sure your incision is long enough, and that you have divided her rectus sheath and muscles as far as her symphysis pubis (an extra 1 cm at the bottom is worth 5 cm at the top). If necessary extend the incision generously above her umbilicus.

Exploration is the first step. Inspect her pelvic cavity. If you find an inflammatory lesion, don't proceed to explore her upper abdomen, because you may spread the infection.

Otherwise, put your left hand into the wound to feel the organs in her abdominal cavity quickly and thoroughly. Follow a set pattern, for example—right kidney, liver, gall-bladder,

HYSTERECTOMY—TWO

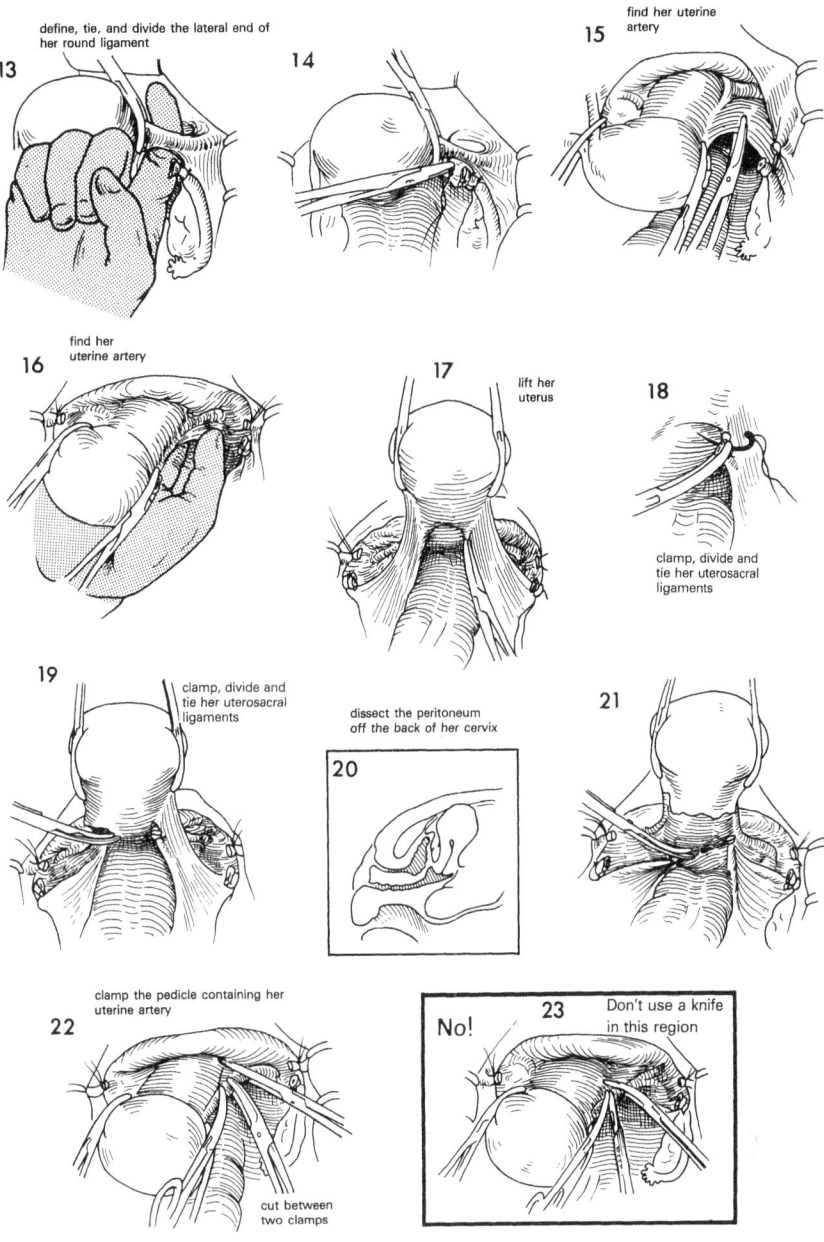

Fig. 20-19 HYSTERECTOMY—TWO. Isolate and tie the patient's round ligaments (13 and 14), find her uterine arteries (15 and 16), tie her uterosacral ligaments (18), reflect the peritoneum off the back of her cervix (21), and clamp her uterine arteries (22). *After Parsons L, and Ulfelder H, 'An Atlas of Pelvic Operations', pages 21ff. WB Saunders Co, with kind permission.*

stomach, duodenum and pancreas, left kidney, spleen, and finally her colon from her caecum to her sigmoid. Look particularly for metastases in her liver.

Clear the operative field. *This is often the most difficult part of the operation.* Don't start removing any organs until you have cleared the site of operation: (a) Clean away any adherent bowel or omentum from her pelvis. (b) Use blunt dissection to free any loose adhesions between her uterus and its surrounding structures—her sigmoid colon, her ovaries, or the walls of her pelvic cavity. Her tubes and ovaries may be stuck down behind her broad ligaments; get your fingers under them and free them from below upwards. Denser adhesions will have to be divided with scissors, or if you think they are likely to contain blood vessels, clamped, divided, and tied. Try stretching them before you divide them. Divide any adhesions between the fundus of her bladder and the fundus of her uterus. (c) Carefully pack her gut out of the way with a large damp pack, marked by a tape, to which a haemostat is attached.

Protect the wound edges with moist gauze, and insert a self retaining retractor (2). You can put the crossbar towards her head or towards her feet, and use the third blade to retract her bladder. Make sure it does not compress her caecum, her sigmoid, her small gut, or her iliac vessels. When necessary, use Deaver's retractor.

Put clamps on either side of her fundus, over her tubes and round ligaments (3). Use them to exert traction, and control back bleeding. Alternatively, if these structures are friable, use a myomectomy screw or traction sutures on the fundus.

Ask your assistant to pull on the clamps, so as to demonstrate the thin part of her broad ligament more clearly. Push your finger through this thin part near her uterus, from behind forwards, to make a hole (4). Do the same on the other side.

Reflect her bladder. Incise the peritoneum on the front of her cervix, near to its vesico-cervical reflexion (5). Dissect her bladder off the front of her cervix, and upper vagina (6 and 7),

HYSTERECTOMY—THREE (SUBTOTAL)

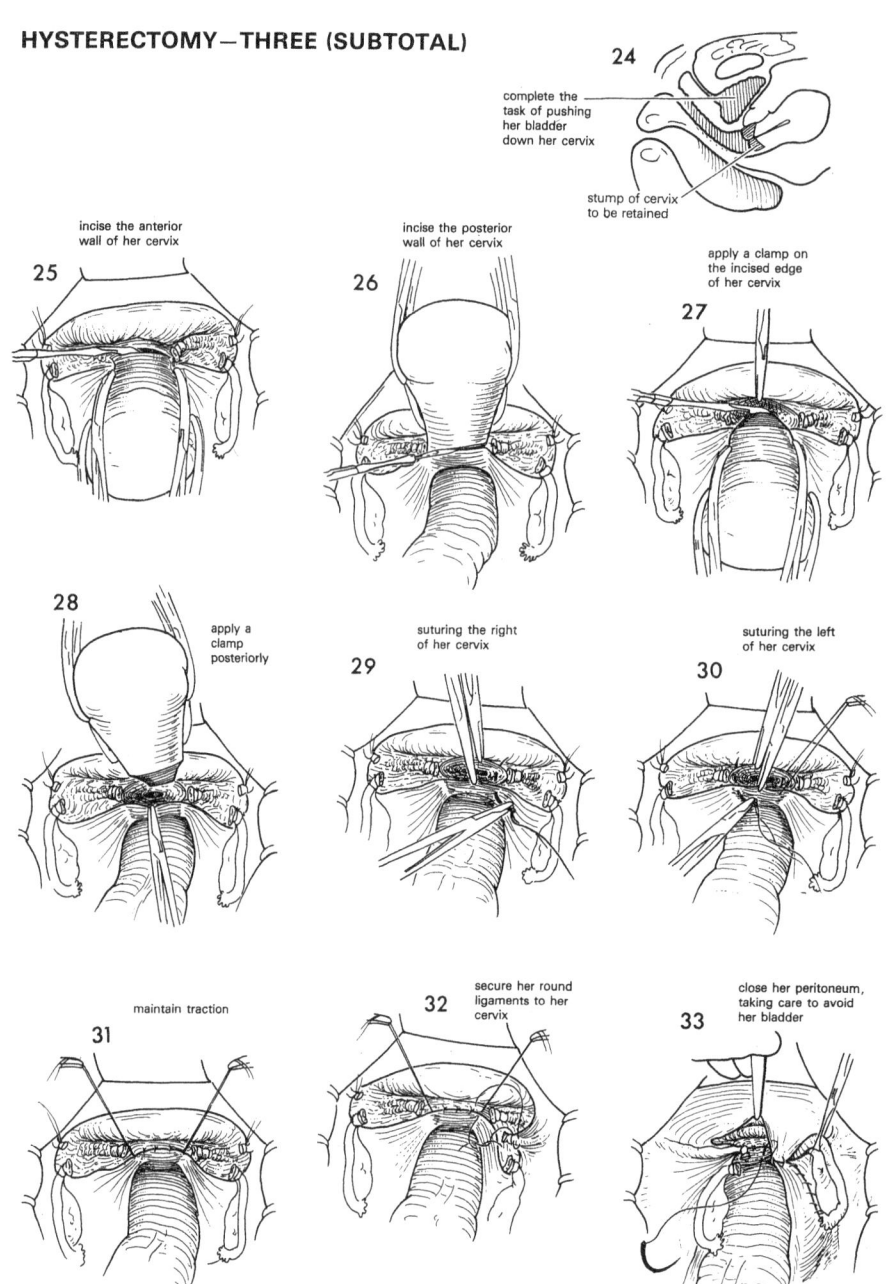

Fig. 20-20 HYSTERECTOMY—THREE, SUBTOTAL HYSTERECTOMY. The part of the uterus to be retained (24). Making a cone-shaped cut to remove the uterus (25 to 28). Suturing the round ligaments to the cervix (32). Closing the peritoneum over the stump (33). *After Parsons L, and Ulfelder H, 'An Atlas of Pelvic Operations', pp. 45 and 47. WB Saunders Co, with kind permission.*

until you can feel the tip of her cervix (8). Feel her cervix from in front and behind. Separate her bladder from the underlying tissues also.

Find her ureters. They enter her pelvis at the bifurcation of her iliac vessels. Trace them distally to beyond the tip of her cervix; recognize them by their feel: they are rather hard, they do not pulsate, and you can roll them between your finger and thumb—see Fig. 20-16.

CAUTION ! Ureters are apt to be easy to find when they are in no danger, and almost impossible to find when you need to find them. If you cannot find them these steps will protect them: (a) Free her adnexa from adhesions before you remove them. (b) Lift her infundibulopelvic ligament and find her ovarian vessels before you clamp them. (c) Carefully dissect her bladder away from her cervix, and the adjoining part of her broad ligament. (d) Cut and mobilize downwards the posterior peritoneal leaf of her broad ligament, and the posterior surface of her cervix.

Deal with her ovaries. You must now decide if you want to retain them or not. If they have multiple cysts, they are better removed, but try to retain at least one if she is premenopausal, or less than 5 years postmenopausal.

If you are going to remove an ovary, **clamp its vessels**, lateral to it, taking care not to clamp her ureter at the same time (9). Divide her ovarian pedicle medial to the clamp, and tie it with a double transfixion suture using No. 1 or No. 2 catgut.

If you are going to retain an ovary, **apply a clamp across the Fallopian tube and its pedicle**, 1 cm lateral to the first clamp that you applied to these structures near her uterus (10). Divide her tube and broad ligament between these clamps (11 and 12). Remove the lateral clamp and tie its pedicle as above.

Do the same thing on the other side, removing or retaining her ovary, as you decide.

Tie her round ligaments. Define, tie, and divide the lateral end of her round ligament. Do this by pushing your finger under it and tying it (13 and 14)

Find her uterine artery. Cut the posterior leaf of her broad ligament with the loose areolar tissue inside it, almost as far as the artery (15 and 16). If your assistant stretches her broad ligament well by pulling on the clamps, you may see the artery through the tissues you are going to cut. Repeat this on the other side.

Ask your assistant to lift up her uterus again (17). This will demonstrate her uterosacral ligaments. Clamp, divide, and tie them (18 and 19). Dissect the peritoneum off the back of her cervix (20 and 21), if it is not too adherent, otherwise leave it. Her uterus will now be much more mobile.

Divide her uterine arteries. Feel for her uterine arteries again. There is no need to dissect them out. Next feel for her ureters on each side of her distal cervix. Again, identify them by their feel—firm cords which you can roll between your finger and thumb.

Clamp the pedicle containing her uterine artery almost horizontally, well away from her ureter, with the tip of the clamp biting the side of her cervix, and leaving 0.5 to 1 cm of tissue on the uterine side (22). Better, use two clamps and divide between them. Use scissors, not a knife, in this region (23).

Complete the task of pushing her bladder down her cervix, if you have not already done so (24). Blunt dissection is usually enough.

You can now decide if you want to do a subtotal or total hysterectomy. If you are inexperienced, do a subtotal one. But, before proceeding, here is an alternative to some of the above steps, as used by one contributor:

An alternative to the above method, and some say a safer one: (a) Divide her round ligaments between clamps, 2–3 cm from her uterus; this opens the anterior peritoneal leaf of her broad ligament. (b) Enlarge the opening. (c) Find the avascular area of her broad ligament and push your finger through it. (d) Clamp and divide her infundibulopelvic ligament (or her tube and ovarian ligament). (e) Do the same on the other side. (f) Divide the peritoneum between her bladder and her cervix. (g) Feel for her cervix. (h) Lift the peritoneum over her bladder while an assistant pulls on her uterus. This will stretch the connective tissue between her bladder and cervix. Cut this with scissors and push her bladder downwards bluntly. Then proceed to deal with her uterine arteries and uterosacral ligaments as above.

SUBTOTAL HYSTERECTOMY

When you are sure you have reflected her bladder adequately (24), pull on the clamps attached to her uterus and incise the anterior wall of her cervix, above the reflexion of her bladder and the stump of her uterine vessels (25). Then draw her uterus sharply forwards towards her symphysis, and incise the posterior wall of her cervix (26). Place a clamp on its anterior incised edge (27). Make a cone-shaped cut, so that you remove the endocervical lining.

Place clamps on the posterior and anterior cut edges of her cervix (28), so that you can maintain traction—making sure that you avoid clamping her bladder!

Bring the two cut edges of her cervix together to control bleeding. Use a cutting Mayo half-circle needle, and place the first stitch in the edge of her cervix, close to the point where you tied her uterine arteries. Control bleeding by placing the sutures through the posterior peritoneal reflection, deep into the muscle of both lips, at the apex of the cone (29, 30 and 31).

Suture her round ligaments to her cervix (32), and close her peritoneum, taking care to avoid her bladder (33).

TOTAL HYSTERECTOMY

Cut through her cardinal ligaments flush with her cervix, until you feel the end on each side (34). Meanwhile, ask your assistant to pull on her cervix to give you good exposure. You should be able to feel her cervix through the wall of her vagina from in front and behind with your finger and thumb (35).

Opening her vagina. Before you do this insert clamps on her vaginal angles immediately below her cervix — these are not shown in (35) and (36) or (37) but they are shown in (38). Ask your assistant to pull up her uterus. Use a broad-bladed or right-angle retractor to pull back her bladder. Plunge the scalpel into her vagina through its anterior wall, just distal to where you feel her cervix is. Hold it at an angle of 45° from the line of her cervix (36). Cut laterally to the left and right, keeping near to her cervix. If you can easily see to complete the cut, cut across her posterior vaginal wall with a scalpel. If not, use curved scissors (37). Complete the incision across her anterior and posterior vaginal walls to remove her uterus (38).

CAUTION ! To avoid damage to her ureters, make sure you find them. Clamp her uterine pedicles away from them, and cut her vaginal wall very close to her cervix.

Use transfixion sutures to tie her uterine pedicles, making sure that you do not include her ureters (not illustrated). Use '1' or '2' catgut, or '0' or '1' multifilament, keeping the ends long as markers.

Closing her vagina. Hold the cut ends of her anterior and posterior vaginal walls with clamps or vulsellum forceps. Close her vagina with '1' continuous chromic catgut (39 and 40). This should stop any bleeding. If it does not, control it with mattress figure of eight sutures—taking care to avoid her ureters!

If you can easily do it, suture her round ligaments to the ends of her vaginal vault (41). This will help to prevent prolapse, but is not essential.

Starting at one end, use '0' chromic catgut to close her peritoneum with one long continuous stitch (42 to 45). Leave her ovaries free in her peritoneal cavity. If you sew them into the extraperitoneal space, or fix them to the side wall of her pelvis, she may have dyspareunia.

CAUTION ! When you close up her peritoneum make sure that you do not pick up her ureters by mistake. They may be very close.

Remove the swab holding her gut, and close her abdomen in the usual way. There is no need for a drain.

CLOSING HER ABDOMEN AFTER A HYSTERECTOMY

Remove and count all packs and sponges. Grasp her sigmoid colon and carefully place it so that it fills the lower part of her pelvis. Place her omentum so that her small intestine is completely covered.

Close her abdomen as usual. Postoperatively, check her vaginal pads to make sure she is not bleeding.

Alternatively, suspend the vault of her vagina by sewing her cardinal ligaments separately from her cervix. Clamp them as far distally as you can from her uterine artery pedicles, before you cut them away from her cervix. Check the position of her ureters before you do this. When you have removed her uterus, use a mattress suture to join her cardinal ligaments to the ends of her vagina, before you close it.

THE SPECIMEN. Open her uterus to see if there is a carcinoma of its body. Do this after the operation, to avoid contaminating the wound with tumour cells if any are present.

DIFFICULTIES WITH HYSTERECTOMY

If ADHESIONS from old PID or endometriosis prevent you starting, begin by dividing her round ligaments. Then put your hand behind her uterus and push a finger through her broad ligament under her tube and out through her divided round ligament. You now have her tube and ovarian vessels and can clamp and divide them safely.

If her UTERUS is so LARGE that it obstructs your access to her pelvis, do a subtotal operation first, and, if necessary, cut across her cervix quite high up. When you have removed the body of her uterus you will have plenty of room to complete the operation.

If you CANNOT FIND HER URETER, but must proceed with the operation, keep close to her uterus. You will nearly always be safe there. Do only a subtotal operation.

If a FIBROID EXTENDS INTO HER BROAD LIGAMENT, this may: (1) Be growing out from her uterus and displace her uterine vessels and ureter downwards and laterally, and her ovarian vessels upwards. (2) Be separate from her uterus and arise *de novo* from the connective tissue in her broad ligament. Both are difficult; if possible refer her.

If you must attempt to deal with (1), **divide both her ovarian vessels and dissect out the upper part of the fibroid.** Then proceed with the operation as usual on the normal side of her uterus only. Clamp and tie her uterine artery and uterosacral ligament. Cut across her vagina. As you reach the affected side of her vagina you will see her uterine artery on that side. Clamp and divide it (it may be large) and shell out the remainder of the fibroid.

HYSTERECTOMY—FOUR (TOTAL)

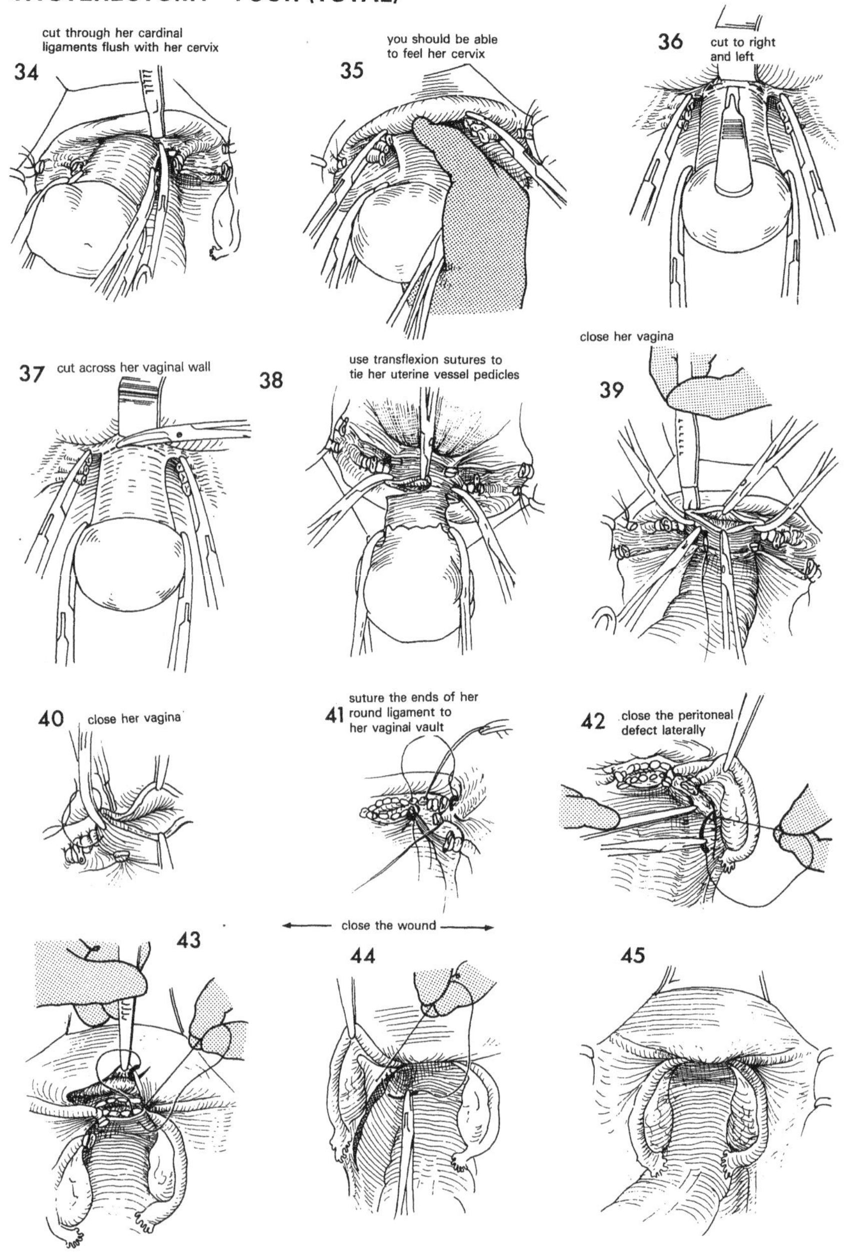

Fig. 20-21 HYSTERECTOMY—FOUR, TOTAL HYSTERECTOMY.
Reflect the patient's bladder (34), feel for her cervix (35), incise the fornices of her vagina (36 and 37), and cut her uterus free (38). Close her vagina (39 and 40). Suture her round ligaments to her cervix (41). Close her peritoneum laterally (42). Close it over her vagina (43 to 45). *After Parsons L, and Ulfelder H, 'An Atlas of Pelvic Operations', pp. 33 and 34. WB Saunders, with kind permission.*

Labels on figures:
- 34: cut through her cardinal ligaments flush with her cervix
- 35: you should be able to feel her cervix
- 36: cut to right and left
- 37: cut across her vaginal wall
- 38: use transflexion sutures to tie her uterine vessel pedicles
- 39: close her vagina
- 40: close her vagina
- 41: suture the ends of her round ligament to her vaginal vault
- 42: close the peritoneal defect laterally
- 43, 44, 45: close the wound

If you must attempt to deal with (2), **open her broad ligament** by dividing her round ligament, as you would for a broad ligament cyst. Her ureter will be attached to the posterior edge of her broad ligament above; lower down it will be displaced downwards and medially by the fibroid.

If there is a FIBROID IN HER CERVIX, removing it can be very difficult. Either do only a subtotal operation. Or, do a subtotal one and then cut down on to the fibroid as for a myomectomy and shell out the fibroid before you remove her cervix.

If you DIVIDE HER URETER and recognize that you have done so, you can: (1) Repair her ureter over a T-tube. (2) Refer her for reimplantation. This is better if the cut end will reach her bladder.

If you OPEN HER BLADDDER, repair it in at least two layers. Leave a catheter in for 10 days. The tear is likely to heal uneventfully.

If you HAVE INJURED HER COLON, repair the tear and do a proximal defunctioning colostomy.

Iif she BLEEDS or there is a PERSISTENT OOZE at the end of the operation, try a warm pack and tie any arterial bleeders. If this fails, don't close her vaginal vault. Instead, insert a purse string suture all round her vaginal vault and pull it tight. This will leave a central hole in her vagina through which any haematoma can escape.

If she suffers from insidious RETENTION OF URINE postoperatively (uncommon), it is likely to be due to detrusor failure, and to be difficult to treat. Try 4 weeks of catheter drainage and urethral dilatation. If this fails, teach her intermittent self-catheterization (64.16), which is effective and safe. Use a clean but not sterile simple plastic catheter, which she can use for at least a week. In a woman a retentive bladder is much better than a leaky one.

20.12 The sequelae of female circumcision

Female circumcision, which includes all deliberate mutilations of a girl's genitalia, is still done in many parts of the world, sometimes as early as 8 days after birth, but usually at puberty, when it is part of a coming of age ritual which is willingly entered into, and endured with stoicism. In some districts all your female patients will be circumcised. The commoner types are:

Circumcision proper (Sunna circumcision) removes only the clitoral prepuce, and is analogous to male circumcision.

Excision removes the prepuce, the glans, and sometimes the clitoris itself, together with part or all of the labia minora.

Infibulation (Pharaonic circumcision) is still almost universal among Muslims of the Sudan. It excises a varying amount of vulval tissue, and partly closes the vaginal orifice. In its most drastic form all or part of the mons veneris, the labia majora and minora, and the clitoris are removed, and the raw areas are left to heal across the lower vagina. A piece of wood (commonly a matchstick) is then inserted, and the girl's legs are strapped together for 40 days while the lesion heals. The final result is a flattened vulva, without labia, made of a membrane of skin which hides her urinary meatus, and is marked by a midline scar extending backwards from her symphysis pubis to her narrowed and scarred vulval orifice, which may only admit one finger, and sometimes not even that.

ZEINAB (6 years) was laid naked across a bed, securely tied by her arms and ankles. With a deep sweep of the razor, the midwife removed the anterior two-thirds of one of her labia, together with her clitoris. The unfortunate girl's shrieks were drowned by "That's nothing to fuss about!"—while the midwife removed her other labium in the same way. As usual, there was a sadistic smile on the face of the operator, and the whole business was thoroughly enjoyed by the priviledged spectators. Haemorrhage is always profuse, and was dealt with as usual. A clamp, made of a bent piece of split cane, was adjusted so as to grip the raw edges together, and its ends tied. For the next three weeks the girl's life was far from being a bed of roses, the clamp remained in place, and her urine had to find its way out as best it could... Derived from Alan Worsley's account of infibulation and female circumcision in the Sudan.

Verzin JA, 'Sequelae of Female Circumcision'. Tropical Doctor 1975;163-69.

Worsley A, 'Circumcision in the Sudan'. Journal of Obstetrics and Gynaecology of the British Empire. 1938;45:686.

THE SEQUELAE OF CIRCUMCISION

COMPLICATIONS. can occur at various times in the patient's life. Their true incidence is not known.

Immediate complications: (1) Haemorrhage (common). (2) Infection. (3) Retention of urine. (4) Trauma to her rectum and anus. (5) Amputation of the urethra, resulting in a vesicovaginal fistula.

Late complications: (1) Implantation dermoids (common) which may be as large as a football, and hang down over her introitus. (2) Coital difficulties due to excessive stenosis. In its extreme form the narrowed introitus will barely admit a fine probe, and may lead to anal intercourse. (3) Infertility; pregnancy can however occur when the introitus is too tight to admit the penis. (4) Keloid formation. (5) Urinary tract infection. (6) Difficulty of micturition may occur after many years. (7) Calculus formation in her vagina. (8) Haematocolpos.

Obstetric complications: (1) The impossibility of making an adequate vaginal examination. (2) Difficulty passing a catheter. (4) Delay in labour due to a tight perineum.

DECIRCUMCISION FOR DYSPAREUNIA. Under local anaesthesia, saddle block (A 7.7), subarachnoid anaesthesia (A 8.1), or ketamine, make a midline incision forwards from her stenosed vulval orifice.

EXCISION OF A DERMOID CYST. Make an elliptical incision round the base of the mass and excise it.

DIFFICULTY IN LABOUR. If pharaonic circumcision is practised the introitus will not be big enough to allow the baby to pass, so it will be the local practice to make an anterior episiotomy ('the cut'). Failure to make one delays or obstructs labour, and may force the baby's head backwards and cause severe perineal lacerations. The anterior episiotomy is usually adequate; but if it is not, make a posterolateral one also.

CAUTION ! Bladder and urethral fistulae have followed carelessly done anterior episiotomies.

REPAIR. After delivery you may be asked to repair her introitus, so that it is narrow once more. If this is a cultural requirement, it may be kind to grant her her wish. On the other hand, she may may be anxious not to be sewn up, and resist your attempts even to sew up her posterolateral episiotomy, which must be repaired.

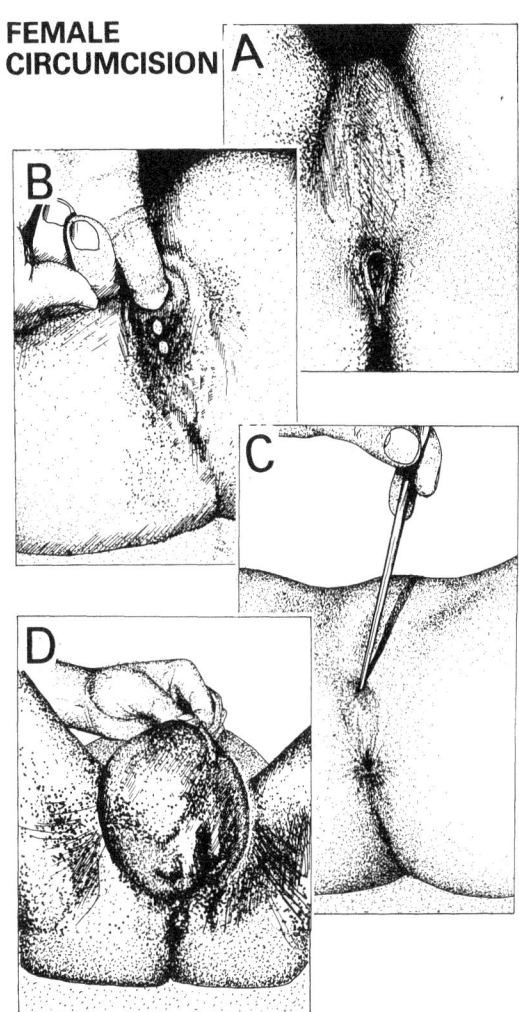

Fig. 20-22 FEMALE CIRCUMCISION. A, the usual appearance of the end result of circumcision. B, a midline circumcision scar healing in patches to give a perforated appearance. C, in its extreme form the narrowed introitus will only admit the point of a fine probe. D, a large implantation dermoid following circumcision. *After JA Verzin, with the kind permission of the editor of Tropical Doctor.*

20.14 Some other gynaecological problems

Here are a few more problems; some, such as congenital abnormalities and injuries, occur anywhere. Others are specifically tropical.

OTHER GYNAECOLOGICAL PROBLEMS

CONGENITAL ABNORMALITIES OF THE GENITAL TRACT

IF A GIRL FROM 14 TO 16 HAS LOW ABDOMINAL PAIN AND AN ABDOMINAL MASS (not uncommon), examine her vagina and vulva. If you find a bulging membrane, her vagina and

HAEMATOCOLPOS

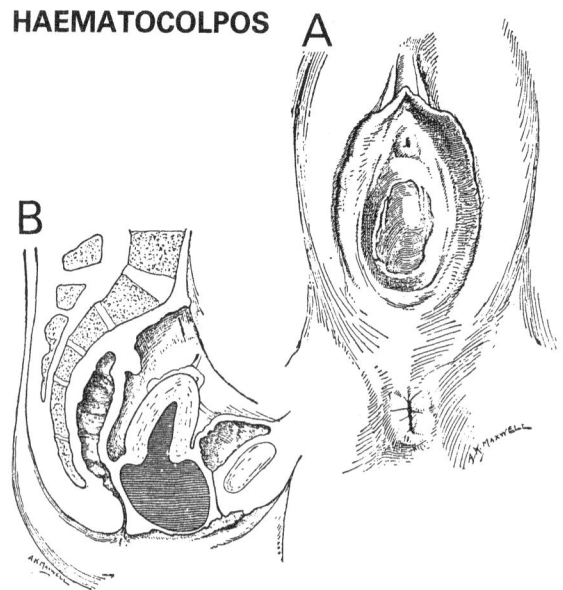

Fig. 20-23 HAEMATOCOLPOS. A, the bulging membrane retaining a girl's first menstrual discharges. B, a cross-section shows that there is also some degree of haematometra. *After Young, James, 'A Textbook of Gynaecology', (5th edn. 1939). A and C Black, permission requested.*

perhaps her uterus are distended with her first menstrual discharges—haematocolpos, perhaps with haematometra, as in Fig. 20-23. Make the diagnosis by inspecting her introitus and by a finger in her rectum. If the membrane feels thin, incise it with a cross-shaped incision. If it is not thin, refer her. Don't do anything more than make a cruciate incision in a thin membrane. *Don't* insert a drain; you risk introducing infection. If the gap between her upper and lower vagina is more than a thin membrane, the operation to establish patency is not easy, and restenosis is common. The problem is not urgent.

If a girl 6 months to 2 years after puberty has a LOWER ABDOMINAL MASS, one of the possibilities is a haematometra in the horn of a *uterus didelphus* (double uterus with two cervices, rare) with one cervix stenosed so that a haematometra develops. You can usually manage her by repeatedly dilating her stenosed cervix.

If she complains of a SWELLING IN HER ANTERIOR VAGINAL WALL behind her urethra, especially before the reproductive years, consider the possibility of a URETHRAL DIVERTICULUM (not uncommon in some tropical communities), and don't confuse it with a cystocele or a urethrocele. If you can squeeze its contents into her urethra, the diagnosis is confirmed. If necessary, do a urethrogram as in Section 34.5. If you cannot refer her, consider excising the diverticulum, which is usually not difficult. Operate with a urethral catheter in place. Repair the small defect in her urethra which was the neck of the diverticulum.

INJURIES OF THE GENITAL TRACT

If an irritant has been placed in her vagina so as to cause a CHEMICAL VAGINITIS, this may be so severe as to involve the whole thickness of her vaginal wall, and be followed by stenosis. Irritants include caustic soda and rock salt and are sometimes used to procure abortions.

If you see her in the acute phase, admit her and remove all traces of the chemical, under anaesthesia if necessary. Douche the lesion with a mild antiseptic, and give her an antibiotic to limit the infection. Continue with salt baths until her wound is clean.

If the whole thickness of her vaginal skin has sloughed, **severe fibrosis and a VAGINAL STRICTURE are likely.** If you cannot refer her, consider inserting a skin graft (57.2) on a large mould, as soon as her vaginal cavity is clean. A dentist may have suitable material for the mould. Make it round a Hegar dilator, and then withdraw this, so as to make a passage for her menstrual fluid to escape. Stick a split skin graft to the outside of the mould with Compound Paint of Mastic BPC, or Compound Tincture of Benzoin BPC. Hold the mould in place with sutures. Remove these 21 days later, and immediately regraft any raw areas.

If PART OF HER URETHRA HAS BEEN DESTROYED, she might have lost the proximal part during labour (18.18) or the distal part from *lymphogranuloma venereum* (see below). Provided the proximal quarter is intact, the loss of the distal three-quarters usually causes no symptoms. An operation for repair of the proximal quarter is difficult, so refer her for this.

CHRONIC INFECTIONS AND PARASITOSES OF THE GENITAL TRACT

If she presents with NODULES OR PAPILLOMAS of her lower genital tract, and you are in an endemic area for S. haematobium or S. mansoni, consider the possibility of SCHISTOSOMAL GRANULOMAS. These take various forms: (1) Frond-like (fern-like) lesions with a narrow base or plaques developing on the vulva, usually before puberty from the age of 6 to 15 years. These are often single, cause no problems, seldom bleed, and can be removed easily. (2) Multiple granulomata of the vagina and cervix in the reproductive years and after them. These also seldom bleed, but they may be so extensive that they distort the bladder/urethral angle and cause incontinence. (3) Ulceration or papillomas of the cervix, closely resembling carcinoma. Look for ova in her urine, stool, vaginal discharge, and tissue scrapings or biopsies. Venereal warts (condyloma acuminatum) are the major differential diagnosis. Give her the appropriate chemotherapy.

CAUTION ! (1) In a schistosomal area don't consider all suspicious vulval or cervical lesions as carcinoma. (2) She may have carcinoma and something else. (3) Don't excise large vulval lesions without doing a biopsy first.

If she presents with CHRONIC ULCERATION OF HER VULVA, the differential diagnosis includes: (1) Small and usually ulcerated granulomata arising in a perineum that is permanently wet from a VVF (salt baths will improve her temporarily). (2) Furunculosis; she may be diabetic, test her urine for glucose. (3) Secondary syphilis; painless, moist, flat-topped swellings. (4) Chancroid; painful shallow ulcers. (5) Tuberculosis (29.1). (6) Amoebiasis (rare); painless ulcers which may mimic carcinoma and usually respond dramatically to metronidazole (31.2). (7) Schistosomiasis (see above). (8) Carcinoma (32.35a). (9) Donovanosis (*granuloma inguinale*); red, angry, destructive lesions with a raised edge. (10) *Lymphogranuloma venereum* (see below, 22.10). Distinguishing between these last two can be difficult, and she may have both. Donovanosis can cause a pseudoepitheliomatous hyperplasia, which may be mistaken histologically for carcinoma. Fortunately, they both respond to tetracycline given for 3 weeks. You can also give chloramphenicol.

If she has LYMPHOEDEMA OF HER VULVA, consider the possibility of tuberculous glands of her groin (29.1), bancroftian or Malayan filariasis, *lymphogranuloma venereum*, secondary or tertiary syphilis, and donovanosis, etc. Massive elephantiasis of the vulva is usually caused by donovanosis or filariasis (31.4). Vulval oedema can sometimes be so gross as to mimic elephantiasis of the scrotum.

Suggesting lymphogranuloma: a fistulated inguinal adenitis with a sour smell, a concealed indolent sore of her vaginal vault, vesicovaginal or rectovaginal sinuses and rectal strictures; painlessness. Histology is often non-specific.

Treat any local sepsis. If elephantiasis has produced a large tumour of her vulva, you may have to excise it, but excision, particularly of enlarged labia majora, is likely to be disappointing. Excise a wide area of skin, so that the incision goes through healthy skin; this will assist healing, and make recurrence less likely. Insert an indwelling catheter to make nursing easier during the first week. Apply a well-padded dressing of vaseline gauze.

CAUTION ! (1) Operate under antibiotic cover. (2) Don't excise her lymph nodes, this will only make the condition worse, since all lymph from the involved areas has to drain through them.

OTHER GYNAECOLOGICAL PROBLEMS

If she complains of a PROFUSE VAGINAL DISCHARGE OR POST-COITAL BLEEDING, one cause is CERVICAL EVERSION (also called a cervical erosion); other more common ones are described elsewhere (M 29.6). The normal columnar endothelium of her cervix bulges out, and you can see it when you do a speculum examination. Cervical eversion usually causes no symptoms. If necessary, cauterize her cervix with a hot cautery or a stick of silver nitrate.

If you use a cautery, make 6–8 radial burns from her external os to the junction of the glandular eversion (the erosion) with her normal squamous epithelium. You will need a cervical block or general anaesthesia.

If you use a stick of silver nitrate, just touch all the glandular epithelium. Warn her that her discharge will get worse for a week before it improves. No anaesthesia is necessary.

If she complains of a small round red LUMP ON THE POSTERIOR MARGIN OF HER URETHRAL ORIFICE, it is probably a URETHRAL CARUNCLE. Usually, it needs no treatment; if it is pedunculated and bleeding, excise it. See also prolapse of the urethra 20.5.

If an OLD WOMAN COMPLAINS OF SUDDEN SEVERE VAGINAL BLEEDING, suspect a vaginal tear (not uncommon), usually in her posterior fornix as the result of sex, especially after a period of abstinence. You will see the tear on speculum examination: (1) If she has stopped bleeding, do nothing. (2) If she continues to bleed, insert one or two mattress sutures. (3) If the tear has gone through her posterior fornix (rare), replace her gut and repair it.

URETHRAL CARUNCLE

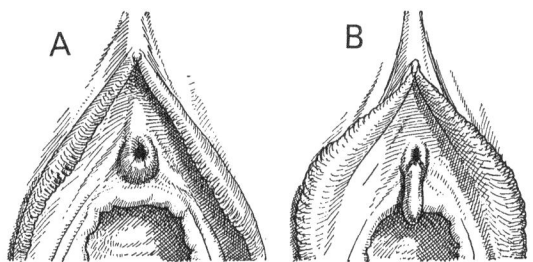

Fig. 20-24 URETHRAL CARUNCLE. **This usually needs no treatment (A); if it is pedunculated (B), excise it.** *After Young, James, 'A Textbook of Gynaecology', A and C Black, permission requested.*

21 The breast and the thyroid

21.1 Introduction

The breast and the thyroid may both be afflicted by a variety of benign and malignant swellings which need surgery. Both may have abscesses which need draining, the breast often, and the thyroid only rarely. We describe a simple and a modified radical mastectomy, but we do not tell you how to remove the thyroid, because this requires a knowledge of anatomy and an expertise that you are unlikely to have.

You will see two kinds of inflammatory lesion in the breast: (1) Acute abscesses, which almost always occur during lactation, but may occasionally occur during pregnancy, and rarely at other times. They are here, rather than with the other abscesses earlier in the book, so that they can be discussed with other 'lumps in the breast'. And, (2) a varied group of subacute or chronic infections, which you will have to distinguish from tumours and tuberculosis of the breast (21.3).

THE BREAST

21.2 Pus in the breast

The importance of a breast abscess is less for a mother than for her child, who may cease to be breast-fed as a result of it, and be subject to all the hazards of being bottle-fed, particularly marasmus. So your main objective must be to see that when you have treated her abscess, she continues to breast-feed.

Acute septic breast infections usually occur during the second week of the puerperium, in a breast which is either engorged, or has a cracked nipple. Antibiotics alone are only effective if you give them *early*, during the phase of acute cellulitis. *As soon as there is a definite lump, incise it.*

Avoid these common mistakes: (1) Don't delay incision, and don't continue with antibiotics alone after an abscess has formed. The mass may fail to resolve, and become so hard (an 'antibioma') that you cannot distinguish it from carcinoma. (2) Don't wait for fluctuation, or for the abscess to point. If you do, she will suffer much unnecessary breast destruction. (3) Provided that she does not present so late that breast-feeding is impossible, don't take her baby away from her breast. He is much the best way of keeping it drained. (4) Don't suppress lactation with stilboestrol, its effects are temporary anyway. Finally, (5) don't forget to insert a drain.

Subacute or chronic recurrent abscesses are unrelated to lactation, and are less painful. They are usually close to the areola, are often associated with inversion of the nipple, and they commonly involve both breasts, either simultaneously, or one after the other. Often, a fistula of a mammary duct is present. If the lesion is localized, you can excise it, as in Fig. 21-1.

BREAST INFECTIONS

For the general method, see Section 5.2.

ANAESTHESIA. Give the patient a general anaesthetic. If you use local anaesthesia, which is not very satisfactory, be sure to premedicate her well with pethidine.

ABSCESSES IN LACTATING BREASTS

INDICATIONS FOR INCISION. (1) An area of tense induration. You will feel this most easily when her breast is empty. (2) Pain which is severe enough to have kept her awake the previous night.

Use the tip of your finger to feel for the point of maximum tenderness. Run your finger firmly across the oedematous swelling: you may feel that its centre is slightly softer than its edges. If you are in doubt aspirate it with a needle (5.1).

CAUTION! Don't wait for fluctuation.

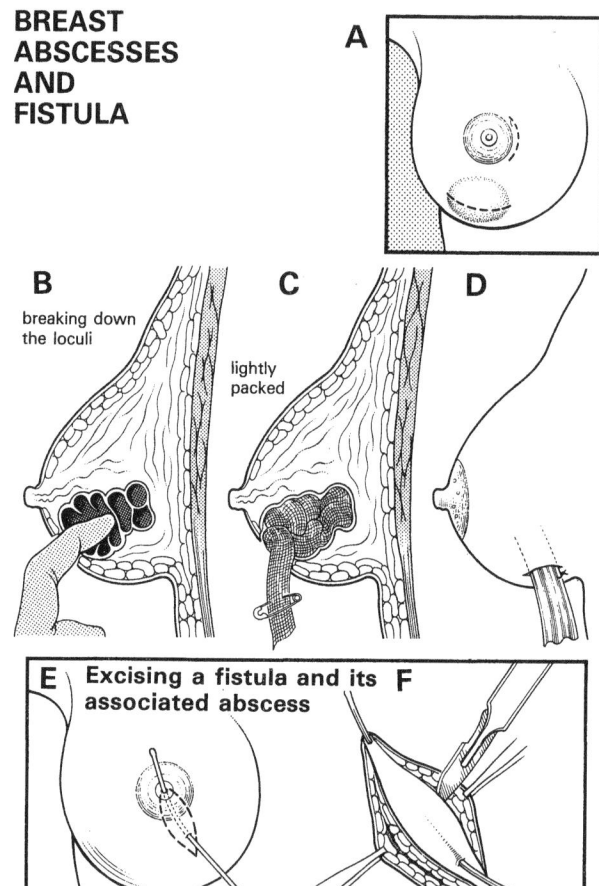

Fig. 21-1 A BREAST ABSCESS AND A FISTULA. A, if an abscess points at the areola, or near it, make a circumferential skin incision at its margin. Elsewhere in the breast, a circumferential incision is preferable to a radial one, which leaves an uglier scar. B, insert your finger and break down all loculi. C, loosely pack the cavity. D, the cavity has extended below the incision, so a dependant drain has been inserted. E, and F, excising a fistula of a mammary duct. Both ends of the fistula are being excised, including 2 cm of skin distal to the distal opening. *After Rob C and Smith R, 'Operative Surgery'; (2nd edn), p. 289. Butterworth, with kind permission.*

INCISING A BREAST ABSCESS

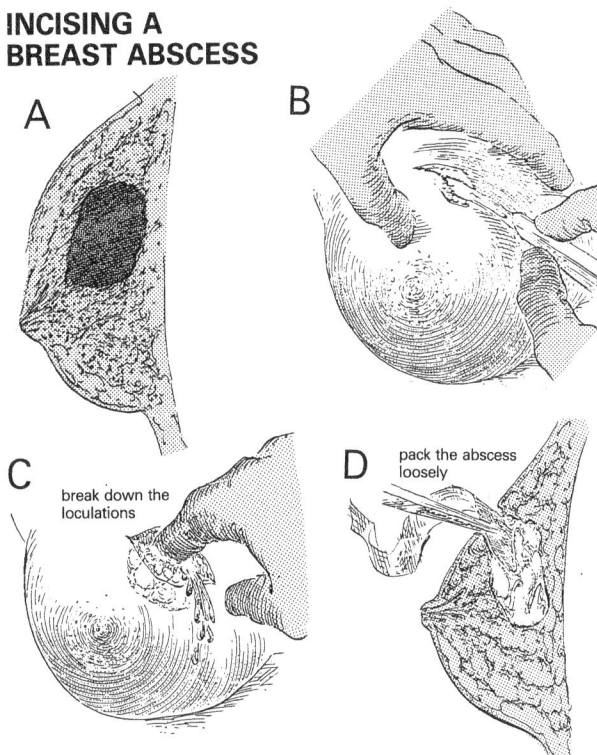

Fig. 21-2 DRAINING A BREAST ABSCESS. This is a less schematic figure than the last one. If the pus could have been reached through a circumareolar incision, it would have left a much better scar! *Adapted from an unknown source.*

INCISION. If an abscess points at the areola, or near it, make a circumferential skin incision at its margin. Elsewhere in the breast, a circumferential incision is preferable to a radial one, which leaves an uglier scar. If you are going to get a finger into an abscess, it will have to be at least 2 cm.

Cut through the skin and subcutaneous tissue. Push a long haemostat into the abscess, and open its jaws. Pus will ooze out. Feel every part of her breast against the haemostat, and try to enter all its loculi. Remove the haemostat, and use your gloved finger to break down any septa between its loculi. If it is in her subcutaneous tissue, feel for a deeper extension.

Insert a drain, and apply a dry dressing. If you wish, you can pack a small cavity; but if you pack a large one, the bulk of the dressings may interfere with breast feeding.

If she has a large abscess in a lower quadrant, make a single incision in the lower part of her breast. There is no need to make a main incision, and then another counter incision inferiorly to provide free drainage.

If you cannot find any pus, the lesion may be an anaplastic carcinoma, so send a biopsy for examination.

If milk flows from the wound, reassure her that it will stop, provided breast-feeding is re-established.

CAUTION ! (1) If she has no fever, or throbbing pain, consider the possibility of a carcinoma. (2) Follow her up carefully. Another abscess may form.

BREAST-FEEDING must *not* stop! Let her baby continue to suck from her normal breast *and, as soon as possible, from her infected breast.* But don't let him suck from the infected breast if: (1) Its nipple is cracked. (2) Pus comes from it. If so, express her milk, by hand or with a breast pump. Discard it if it is obviously mixed with pus, otherwise feed it to him. As soon as he can fix on to the nipple, encourage him to suck from it.

If she presents late, when breast feeding has become impossible, incise and drain her breast, and give her an antibiotic to hasten the resolution of the inflammatory oedema. Start expressing her breast as soon as possible, and don't discharge her until breast-feeding has been re-established.

SUBACUTE AND CHRONIC ABSCESSES. Be sure to take a biopsy for tuberculosis.

If: (1) she has a small opening discharging pus, at or near the areolar margin, or (2) recurrent abscesses continue to reappear at the same site, near her areola, she has a mammary fistula (sinus). Examine her during an quiescent phase. See if you can pass a probe from the site of the abscess, through to her nipple. If you can, a fistula is present and you may be able to excise the whole lesion, as in E, and F, Fig. 21-1. Make the incision round the fistulous track, and continue it 2 cm distal to the fistula. There is no need to remove more than 0.5 cm of skin on either side of the track. Deepen the incision to expose the underlying tissue, and excise the fistula. Be sure to excise the central part of the duct, because if you leave it behind, the lesion is sure to recur.

RE-ESTABLISH BREAST-FEEDING IN AN INFECTED BREAST

21.3 Lumps in the breast

A normal breast is slightly and uniformly nodular; most of its diseases make it lumpy. Sorting out these lumps can be difficult. The important decision is whether or not a patient has carcinoma.

Consider all lumps in the breast as malignant, unless you are sure they are benign. No woman should be left with a lump in her breast, if she can have it removed by aspirating a cyst, or by excision. After the menopause lumps in the breast are more likely to be malignant.

BREAST LUMPS AND OTHER BREAST DISEASES

EXAMINATION

HISTORY. How long has the patient had her symptoms? Has she any pain? Is it associated with her periods? If she has pain, is it in one breast or both? Is there any discharge from her nipple? Is it watery, bloody, or like thin pus?

EXAMINATION. First examine her sitting up undressed to the waist, then lying down. Examine both her breasts, her liver, and her skeleton.

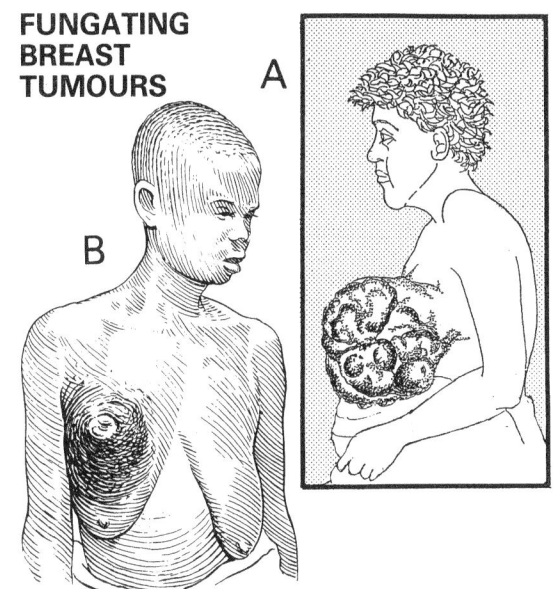

Fig. 21-3 TWO FUNGATING TUMOURS OF THE BREAST. Unfortunately, many patients in the developing world present late when their tumours are already fungating like this. A, a fibroadenoma (uncommon). B, a fungating carcinoma (very common); note the 'peau d'orange' ('orange skin') appearance of the skin over the breast, and the malignant ulcer.

· **Inspect:** (1) Her nipples for position, retraction, and cracking. (2) Her areolae for pigmentation, swelling of Montgomery's tubercles, and a rash. (3) Her skin for prominent veins, sinuses, ulcers, and 'peau d'orange'.

Palpate her breasts: (1) Start with the breast she considers normal, feel each of its 4 quadrants with the flat of your hand, and then its subareolar area. (2) Feel for lumps, note their size and site, and whether they are single or multiple; also their consistency, warmth, tenderness, mobility, and surface. (3) If you find a lump, feel if it is tethered to the skin, or to pectoralis major. Test for the latter by asking her to place her open hand on her waist, and then ask her to press downwards to tense this muscle, while you try to move the lump. (4) Feel with your finger and thumb behind each nipple, and look for any discharge. (4) Feel her axillary nodes—medial (pectoral), lateral, anterior and posterior. Note their number and size, and if they are fixed to her skin, or to deep structures.

A normal breast is slightly and uniformly nodular, especially before the menopause; this nodularity is maximal before the periods. At the menopause the nodularity becomes less, and more fat is deposited.

The classical signs of malignancy are: (1) adherence of the lump to the skin or to pectoralis major, (2) enlarged nodes in the axilla, and (3) 'peau d'orange'. The absence of these signs does NOT exclude carcinoma. Their presence increases the chances of it, but they are not confirmatory, because they can also be caused by tuberculosis, or fat necrosis, etc.

If you are not sure if she has a lump or not, examine her in 2 weeks time, at the opposite phase of her menstrual cycle. Lumpiness of the breast varies with the menstrual cycle.

DIAGNOSING CYSTS IN THE BREAST

If a lump is deep and spherical in all directions, it is probably a cyst; it may or may not be fluctuant, and it can be benign or malignant. Cysts and solid lumps can be difficult to distinguish. You may see any of the following cysts, but only the first two are common.

A mature breast abscess (very common, 21.2) has obvious signs of inflammation, and usually occurs in one breast only, commonly during lactation.

Fibroadenosis (also called fibrocystic disease, common) makes both breasts abnormally granular, usually with premenstrual pain and some tenderness. One or more of these granular areas may be sufficiently obvious to be palpable as a cyst. She is between 25 and 60, there is occasionally an association with malignancy, and there may be a clear discharge from her nipple; rarely, this is blood-stained.

An intracystic papilliferous carcinoma (rare) presents as a cyst. Aspiration yields blood-stained fluid, and does not make the cyst disappear entirely.

Carcinoma of the breast with colloid degeneration (rare), feels cystic. Aspiration yields only a little thick fluid, and does not make the cyst disappear.

Serocystic disease (cystadenoma phylloides, rare) is a rapidly growing benign giant fibroadenoma, which becomes partly necrotic and fluctuant. The skin over it may ulcerate, but is not infiltrated.

A galactocele (uncommon) is a residual milk-containing cyst, the contents of which may solidify.

Hydatid disease (not uncommon in endemic areas, 31.13). Look for cysts elsewhere, especially in the liver.

DIAGNOSING SOLID LUMPS IN THE BREAST

A developing breast abscess (common, see above).

An abscess modified by antibiotics (an 'antibioma', common) is the result of treating an abscess with antibiotics, and not draining it. The lump is usually tender, but not always so. She may have tender axillary nodes and 'peau d'orange'.

A fibroadenoma, (common) is a smooth, well-defined, solitary, and usually painless lump 2 to 5 cm in diameter (but which may be much larger), that moves freely in the breast (a 'breast mouse'). From its hardness such a lump could equally well be a carcinoma; mobility is the important sign, so is lobulation. There are two histological types, a common pericanalicular type, and a less common intracanalicular one. Be careful to distinguish a fibroadenoma, which is an isolated lump, from an area of nodularity due to fibroadenosis, which is a different disease. She is between 15 and 40, and usually between 18 and 25.

Tuberculosis of the breast, (uncommon) is less often seen than tuberculosis of the axillary lymph nodes (31.4), and closely resembles carcinoma. Suspect tuberculosis if a lump is tender or there is a sinus. The mass is painless, and may be attached to her skin or the muscles of her chest wall. Look for signs of tuberculosis elsewhere. Biopsy the mass or her axillary nodes. If you cut across a tuberculous node, you will see areas of caseation. Give the standard tuberculosis treatment. If she has a discharging sinus, you may have to admit her. There is no need for a mastectomy.

CAUTION ! In areas where tuberculosis is common, don't forget the possibility that it it may infect the breast or the axillary nodes.

A giant fibroadenoma (uncommon), presents as a large breast filled with a large, deeply lying, hard, smooth, lumpy, mass (21.5D). It it is untreated it may fungate as in Fig. 21-3. She is usually between 35 and 45.

A neurofibroma (rare) feels hard, like a fibroadenoma, but may be soft, and may be one of many similar tumours elsewhere.

A lipoma (uncommon) feels like breast tissue, but has an indistinct outline separating it from the surrounding normal breast.

An intraduct adenoma (fairly common), or an intraduct carcinoma (less common). A carcinoma is more often palpable than an an adenoma. Both present as a discharge from the nipple, which is usually serous, but may be dark or blood-stained. The prognosis after limited removal is good.

A carcinoma, may be schirrhous or medullary (both common). She has a hard, fixed mass with the criteria of malignancy listed above. *Mastitis carcinomatosa* (rare) is a highly malignant form of carcinoma seen during pregnancy. It is more generalized, and more like inflammation, or Burkitt's lymphoma, than the hard, fixed mass of a typical carcinoma.

Burkitt's tumour (only seen in endemic areas, and uncommon even there) is usually bilateral. She is between the ages of 14 and 25. It may simulate mastitis carcinomatosa, but is not particularly associated with pregnancy. Her skin is stretched, and may ulcerate; she usually has other tumours elsewhere.

Other possibilities include an organizing haematoma (fairly common), and fat necrosis (uncommon).

MANAGING CYSTS IN THE BREAST

If you think a mass is a cyst, proceed as follows. First, exclude hydatid cysts (if yours is an endemic area), by looking for lumps that might be hydatid cysts elsewhere in her body. Aspirate the cyst with a wide bore needle.

If the fluid you aspirate is blood-stained, explore and biopsy the lump.

If the lump remains after you have aspirated it, operate to remove the lump completely, unless it is very large, and send tissue for histology.

If the fluid is clear and the lump disappears, as is usual in fibroadenosis (the commonest cause), no further treatment is necessary. Try to see her regularly. If the cyst appears again, or other cysts appear, aspirate again. If at any time lumps do not disappear, remove them as immediately above.

MANAGING SOLID LUMPS IN THE BREAST

Consider all lumps as malignant, until you are sure they are benign. Biopsy or excise solid lumps and send tissue for histology. The future management of the patient depends on the result.

CAUTION ! Excision of the entire lump for histological examination should be the general rule.

The only occasional exception to this rule, is the lump which is 'almost certain to be benign', for example, it has all the features which suggest a fibroadenoma. If the patient is highly reliable, and does not want her lump removed, you can measure it, and see her every two weeks at first and later monthly, measuring it each time. If it enlarges or changes its character, remove it. Leaving such a lump should be the exception. You can remove most fibroadenomata through a

THE PATHOLOGY OF A FIBROADENOMA

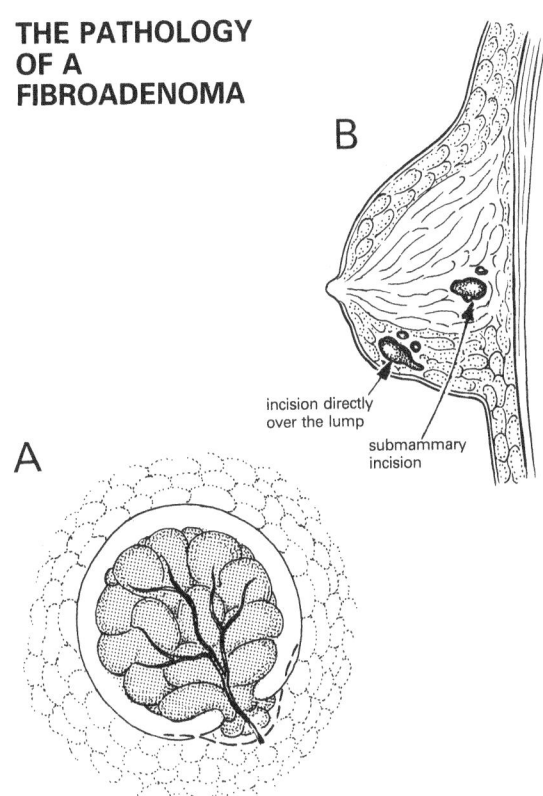

Fig. 21-4 THE PATHOLOGY OF A FIBROADENOMA. A, the tumour is attached to the capsule by a stalk carrying its blood supply. Sometimes the tumour extends into the capsule near the stalk. B, remove a superficial fibroadenoma by incising directly over it. If it is deeper, a submammary incision may be best. *After Rob C and Smith R, 'Operative Surgery', Vol. 1 (2nd edn), (Butterworth), with the kind permission of Hugh Dudley.*

periareolar incision, with a good cosmetic result if the lump is small.

If it is an obvious fibroadenoma by the criteria above, shell it out without removing any normal breast tissue round it, and send part of the specimen for histology.

If she has carcinoma of her breast, see Section 21.4.

If she has a lump and a discharge from her nipple, her prognosis is better, because it is more likely to be a duct adenoma or carcinoma. Excise the duct involved (21.5) and her prognosis will be good.

If you suspect that she has Burkitt's lymphoma of her breast, take a needle biopsy, stain a slide preparation, and interpret it yourself as in Fig. 32-3. Or, less satisfactorily, send a biopsy. If you are not confident that you can interpret a slide preparation, do both; excise the lump, make a slide from it, and send the biopsy for histology. If the tumour is large and ulcerating, excise it, and graft her exposed pectoralis major. If Burkitt's lymphoma is likely and histology slow, start chemotherapy immediately.

MANAGING A DISCHARGE FROM THE NIPPLE

This can be: (1) The normal active breasts of pregnancy (common). Colostrum can be discharged from the 16th week of pregnancy, and even earlier in multigravidae. (2) The normal usually milky discharge after lactation stops (fairly common). This may persist for months and occasionally years, especially if lactation is prolonged. (3) The discharge associated with fibroadenosis (uncommon). (4) The discharge associated with periductal mastitis (plasma cell mastitis, uncommon). (5) The clear, or less often blood-stained discharge, due to an intraduct adenoma (fairly common) or carcinoma (uncommon).

Discharge is more serious if it comes from one duct rather than from many, if it is bloody, or if it is associated with a lump. At the start of the examination, don't palpate the her breast in the normal way, because this may squeeze out any secretion which has accumulated, and you want to see exactly where it is coming from. Instead, ask her to lie back. Gently wipe her nipple clean. Then, press with one finger 3 cm distal to her areola, and move it towards her nipple. Start at 'one o'clock' and move progressively all round her breast to the '12 o'clock' position. If there is any discharge, wipe it away and note its position. Then examine her breast in the usual way.

If she is pregnant, and the fluid is clear and comes from many ducts in both breasts, reassure her.

If both breasts continue to discharge milky fluid from many ducts, even years after lactation has stopped, reassure her.

If she has fibroadenosis, the retention cysts it causes may occasionally cause a disharge from one breast, seldom both. Aspirate the cyst if she has one. If it does not disappear, or if the fluid is blood-stained, do an excision biopsy.

If she has a watery, or bloody, or dark discharge from one duct, usually without a lump, she probably has an intraduct adenoma. If she has a lump, it is more likely to be a carcinoma; even so, her prognosis is good. Excise the lump with the duct (21.5).

If she has a recurrent discharge from several points on her nipple, watery or viscid, green, white, black or occasionally bloody, suspect periductal mastitis (plasma cell mastitis, rare). This can also present as a hard, tender swelling with redness of the overlying skin, which you can confuse with an acute breast abscess, or a rapidly growing carcinoma. It may regress spontaneously.

MANAGING A SINUS OR FISTULA IN THE BREAST

A sinus or fistula may discharge milk, or a non-specific fluid. A milk fistula can follow a breast abscess (fairly common), or village surgery (fairly common in some communities), or tuberculosis of the breast (uncommon). Or it can complicate a carcinomatous ulcer. Other possibilities besides those below are a foreign body, and fungi.

If she has a milk fistula, and is or should be breast-feeding, try to improve or re-establish breast-feeding soon. Her fistula will probably heal. If it does not, it will probably do so when she stops breast-feeding at the normal time.

CAUTION ! A milk fistula is not an indication to stop breast-feeding. Rather, it is an indication to re-establish breast-feeding soon, if it has stopped.

NIPPLE DISEASES

Chronic eczema, (uncommon) is bilateral. Clean her nipples frequently with soap and water. Apply Lassar's paste 1%, or hydrocortisone ointment 1%.

Paget's disease of the nipple, (uncommon) is unilateral, and is a sign that that there is an underlying intraduct carcinoma. 'Peau d'orange' may develop around it. Excise all the area affected, with the underlying lump, including a margin of at least 2 cm of normal tissue horizontally and vertically. Close the wound as for a 'lumpectomy' (21.5).

DIFFICULTIES WITH BREAST DISEASES

If she has evidence of ACUTE INFLAMMATION —a recent history, throbbing pain, and tenderness, don't wait for fluctuation. Treat her for a breast abscess, as in Section 21.2. Acute infection may be difficult to differentiate from mastitis carcinomatosa.

If she is over 70 and has a SOFT FATTY LUMP, which feels as if it might be a lipoma, suspect that it is in fact a carcinoma, which can be as soft as a lipoma at this age.

If BOTH HER BREASTS ARE ENLARGED, with pitting oedema, suspect some generalized disease, such as cirrhosis, the nephrotic syndrome, or heart failure.

If she has ONE SWOLLEN PAINLESS BREAST, with PITTING OEDEMA and NO PALPABLE MASS, she may have:(1) Tuberculosis of her axillary nodes causing lymphoedema of her breast, or (2) non-specific inflammation of them. If she has tuberculosis, her affected breast is larger than the opposite one, is not tender or only slightly so, and almost always shows 'peau d'orange'. Her axillary nodes (usually the lateral pectoral group) are commonly matted together, and may be attached to underlying structures and her skin. She may also have a discharging sinus. Look for signs of tuberculosis elsewhere, especially enlarged nodes in her other axilla, her groins, and her abdomen. X-ray her chest, and do an ESR and a tuberculin test. See also Sections 31.4 and 31.6 and Chapter 29. This manifestation of tuberculosis affecting the breast via the axillary nodes is more common than tuberculosis of the breast itself.

If she has SMALL FIBROTIC NODES IN HER AXILLA, not the typical enlarged matted tuberculous ones, and no signs of tuberculosis elsewhere, she may have chronic non-specific infection following repeated infection of her hand and arm, usually from wounds. Filariasis affecting her axillary nodes is another possibility (31.6).

If a nipple is CHRONICALLY ULCERATED, suspect that this is associated with an underlying duct carcinoma, unless she has a clear history of trauma. Biopsy it: there are also some rare causes such as syphilis and tuberculosis, etc.

If anyone but a female over 10 years has a firm tender discoid SWELLING DEEP TO THE NIPPLE just larger than the areola, and concentric with it, the condition is one of gynaecomastia. This is normal in infants of either sex, in boys near puberty, and in young men. In infants it is nearly always bilateral, and is sometimes complicated by mastitis. In young men it may be uni- or bilateral. Reassure all these patients.

If both an adult MAN'S BREASTS ENLARGE, this is still gynaecomastia. If the clinical findings are not those of physiological gynaecomastia (see above), he probably needs investigation. He may have disease of his liver, testes, adrenals, or pituitary, or he may have leprosy, or have been treated with stilboestrol. Investigate him as best you can. Often, no cause can be found. If you decide to remove such breasts, do so as in Fig. 30-9.

If one of A MAN'S BREASTS ENLARGES, he may have CARCINOMA OF THE MALE BREAST, or gynaecomastia; you can usually distinguish them clinically. If he has carcinoma treat him as if he were female. Excise it, together with some of the skin and the muscle underneath it. Because he has so little fatty tissue, the tumour infiltrates his skin and deeper tissues at an earlier stage, and his prognosis is worse. Orchidectomy usually produces a temporary remission. If he agrees, do the subcapsular operation. This leaves a small palpable 'testis', but even so it is not popular! (23.25).

If ONE BREAST IS VERY MUCH LARGER THAN THE OTHER, but is otherwise normal, the patient may have GIANT HYPERTROPHY (uncommon). This is probably congenital, and may affect both breasts. Such breasts may enlarge more in the third decade, especially following pregnancy.

21.4 Carcinoma of the breast

Carcinoma of the breast is very common in Caucasians, but is less common in Africans. Carcinoma of the African male breast is however not the rarity that it is in Europe. Carcinoma of the breast can occur at any age after 20 years, but is most common between 50 and 70, particularly in non-parous women and in women who started childbearing late; it is also common in the sisters of patients with the disease, and to a lesser extent in their daughters.

Most carcinomas arise from glandular tissue. There are several types: (1) Schirrous carcinomas (75%) contain much connective tissue, and form hard lesions which cut like an unripe pear to produce a greyish cut surface which becomes concave. (2) Medullary (anaplastic) carcinomas (15%) contain less fibrous tissue and are softer. (3) Duct carcinomas (6%) are the least invasive, and present as a watery or blood-stained discharge from the nipple. Clinically, you cannot distinguish them from duct papillomas. (4) 'Inflammatory carcinoma' or 'mastitis carcinomatosa' (uncommon) is the most malignant type, and usually develops during pregnancy.

Breast carcinomas form no capsule; they invade locally through the lymphatics, and spread widely through the bloodstream. A patient's prognosis is related to: (1) the stage at which treatment starts, (2) the number of nodes in her axilla that contain microscopic deposits, and (3), less significantly, the treatment she has. The stage at which the diagnosis is made is critical. Unfortunately, methods of self-examination, which are so effective in educated communities, are seldom applicable in poorly educated ones, in whom carcinoma commonly presents late. There is however one measure you can take—*persuade your staff to examine their patient's breasts on every convenient opportunity.*

Carcinoma of the breast may present as a painless lump in the breast (80%), as enlargement of a breast, as ulceration, or as a discharge from the nipple, which is usually but not always blood-stained.

Treatment is mainly surgical and is controversial—the radical and conservative schools do not agree, but the conservatives are gaining ground. As in any other part of the body, surgery can only cure carcinoma of the breast, if it is local and has not spread elsewhere. If radiotherapy is available (unusual in much of the developing world), it is the preferred treatment for axillary nodes. No known drug is curative, although the regimes below do give short remissions. Many patients present late with foul, stinking ulcers. A mastectomy at this stage, if it is possible (the growth may be fixed to the deep structures and make it impossible) relieves a patient's suffering, and makes her last months more bearable, but only if you can remove the tumour with a margin of normal skin all round it and still close the wound.

CARCINOMA OF THE BREAST

Here we assume that a patient has a lump in her breast, which you think is probably malignant by the criteria in the previous section.

STAGING and PROGNOSIS. Here is the Manchester system of staging. The prognosis of scirrhous and medullary carcinoma is the same. Duct carcinoma has the best prognosis, even after the excision of an entire duct system, and mastitis carcinomatosa the worst.

Stage One The growth is confined to her breast, and is not adherent to her pectoral muscles or to her chest wall. There are no enlarged nodes in her axilla. Adherence to the skin, or ulceration through it, does not affect staging, if it is smaller than the tumour. 68% of all patients survive 5 years, and 54% 10 years.

Stage Two As for stage One, but there are now *mobile* nodes in her axilla. 60% of patients survive 5 years and 40% 10 years.

Stage Three There is skin involvement which is larger than the tumour, but it is still limited to her breast. If any axillary nodes are palpable, they are still mobile. Or the tumour is fixed to her pectoral muscle, but not to her chest wall. Or it is fixed to both. 15% of patients survive 5 years and 4% 10 years.

Stage Four She has distant metastases, either lymphatic, or blood-borne. These include infiltration of the skin beyond her breast, fixed nodes in her axilla, palpable nodes in her supraclavicular fossae, involvement of her other breast; or deposits in her bones, liver, or lungs (unusual). 4% of patients survive 5 years and 4% 10 years.

On microscopic examination the axillary nodes are involved in 10% of patients in Stage One, although they may not be obvious for 20 years. Sadly, most patients in the developing world present in stages Three and Four.

In Stages One and Two, a patient's prognosis depends on the stage of the disease, and where the primary tumour is in her breast. Tumours in the lateral half of the breast have a better prognosis.

If the tumour is in the lateral half of her breast, and her axillary nodes are not involved, there is a 90% chance that she can be cured surgically. If they are involved, she has only a 50% chance of surviving 5 years. There is a 20% chance that it will recur locally.

If it is in the medial half of her breast (less common), her prognosis is worse, because it is more likely to spread to her internal mammary nodes.

THE MANAGEMENT OF CARCINOMA OF THE BREAST

STAGE ONE. Do a 'lumpectomy' (21.5). Excise 2 cm of normal breast round the lump, and send tissue for histology. No further treatment is needed, whether or not the report confirms carcinoma.

INCISIONS FOR LUMPS IN THE BREAST

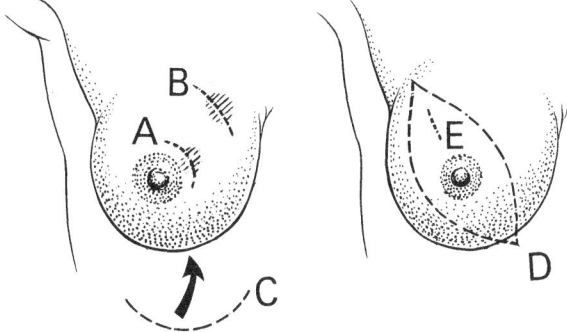

Fig. 21-5 INCISIONS FOR REMOVING LUMPS FROM THE BREAST. A, if the lump is within 5 cm of the the nipple, make a periareolar incision, not larger than half the circumference of the areola. Some scratches across the site of the incision before you make it will help you to align its edges. B, if the lump is further away make a curved circumferential incision over it, parallel to the areola. C, if the lump is deep in the breast, you may be able to use a submammary incision. D, slant a mastectomy incision obliquely towards the axilla. E, if your histology services are good enough to justify taking a biopsy, make a radial incision within the area of a possible later mastectomy, so that you can excise the scar. If either your histological services or the patient are unreliable, don't take a biopsy and then hope to do another operation later.

STAGE TWO. Management depends on whether or not histology is available without undue delay.

If histology is available, first do a biopsy, and then proceed with one of the following operations as soon as the result is available. You have three choices. You can do: (1) A 'lumpectomy' (see below) plus dissection of the axilla preserving pectoralis major. (2) A simple mastectomy plus dissection of the axilla preserving pectoralis major. (3) A 'conservative radical mastectomy' (Patey's operation). (4) Lumpectomy or simple mastectomy combined with radiotherapy to the axilla, if it is available. This is the best because it is least mutilating. If radiotherapy is not available, Patey's operation is recommended.

CAUTION ! For Stage Two, a 'lumpectomy', or simple mastectomy without removing the axillary nodes, is not considered adequate; but it may be all you can do if you are unskilled. We have only described Patey's operation, but operation (2) above is almost the same. See Section 21.5

If histology is not available, or is only available after undue delay, proceed with one of the above definitive operations immediately.

STAGES THREE AND FOUR. Surgery is only palliative, and may not be indicated if the metastases are worse than the primary. Aim to: (1) Prevent the tumour ulcerating through the skin. (2) Remove the primary *in toto* with, if possible, a margin of 2 cm of surrounding breast. Excise as much breast tissue as is necessary to do this. Usually, only a simple mastectomy is required, but you may need to remove part of her pectoralis major muscle. Leave the nodes in her axilla. The only indication for removing them is when they might ulcerate (unusual). This is only possible when they are mobile. Local removal will make life more bearable. Consider combining it with hormone therapy, which is cheaper and much easier than chemotherapy.

MASTITIS CARCINOMATOSA may develop if a patient is pregnant. Try to distinguish it from an inflammatory mass by needle aspiration, and from Burkitt's lymphoma (in endemic areas) by needle cytology (32-3). Do the appropriate operation for the stage of the lesion. Anything you can do will probably only be palliative. Neither abortion nor subsequent pregnancies alter the prognosis.

HORMONAL AND CYTOTOXIC TREATMENT FOR BREAST CANCER

BILATERAL OOPHORECTOMY may help a premenopausal patient with metastases, especially in bone. It produces remission rates (usually partial) of 20% to 40% in premenopausal patients for up to 7 years, but is unpopular in some communities in the developing world. Length of life is not improved.

OESTROGENS. Ethinyl oestradiol in a dose of 1 mg/day is useful for postmenopausal patients, and produces some symptomatic improvement in most patients, especially if they have pain from bony metastases. Or, give her stilboestrol 10 to 20 mg daily in divided doses.

A PROGESTAGEN such as medroxyprogesterone acetate is a possible alternative, if she is postmenopausal.

TAMOXIFEN is a non-steroid oestrogen antagonist which competes with oestrogen for receptor sites on the tumour cells, and has few side effects. Give 10 mg twice daily initially, and continue it indefinitely. Only some tumours are oestrogen-receptor-positive, and only a sophisticated laboratory can identify those that are. Tamoxifen causes partial remissions in postmenopausal patients. The remission rate 0 to 5 years after the menopause is 14%, 5 to 10 years after 30%, and > 10 years after 37%. Tamoxifen has been expensive, but is now (1988) much cheaper from secondary sources.

CYTOTOXIC DRUGS produce remissions of 5 to 12 months in 50% of cases, especially in premenopausal patients with soft tissue lesions rather than bony metastases, but often with considerable toxicity. Single-dose regimes are not very effective. If drugs are short, carcinoma of the breast has a low priority; keep them for Burkitt's lymphoma and nephrobastoma. If you decide to use them, here are two possible regimes—

Use the 'CMF' regime. Give her cyclophosphamide 100 mg/m^2 by mouth daily for 14 days. Give her methotrexate 30 mg/m^2 intravenously on days 1 and 8. Give her 5-fluorouracil 500 mg/m^2 intravenously on days 1 and 8. Repeat the course 28 days after starting for up to a year if she responds. Stop if there is no response.

Alternatively, give her doxorubicin ('Adriamycin') 60 mg/m^2 every 3 weeks or 20 mg/m^2 weekly to a cumulative maximum dose of 600 mg/m^2. This simple regime is effective in a high proportion of cases, but will make her lose her hair.

21.5 Simpler operations for tumours of the breast

If a patient has a carcinoma, or a suspicious lump in her breast, you have a choice of 5 operations: (1) You can 'shell out' a suspected fibroadenoma from the breast tissue around it. (2) You can do an excision biopsy or 'lumpectomy' to remove the mass and 2 cm of normal breast around it. (3) You can do a simple mastectomy. (4) You can do Patey's modified radical mastectomy as described in the next section. (5) You can excise an intraduct carcinoma.

In operations (1) and (2) you do not remove the nipple or any skin, in (3) and (4) you always do. In (5) you remove some skin but leave the nipple. Dissection of the axilla is only described here as part of Patey's operation.

There are two operations to avoid. (1) If either your histological services or the patient are unreliable, don't take a biopsy, and then hope to do another operation later. She may not return, the report may be lost, and there will be too long an interval between the biopsy and the definitive operation. (2) Don't do a full radical mastectomy—it is mutilating and has no advantages over the modified radical operation described here.

SIMPLER BREAST OPERATIONS

'SHELLING OUT' A LUMP

INDICATIONS. This is only indicated if you suspect a fibroadenoma.

METHOD. Proceed exactly as for lumpectomy except that you should shell out the mass without removing 2 cm of normal breast around it.

'SHELLING OUT' AND 'LUMPECTOMY'

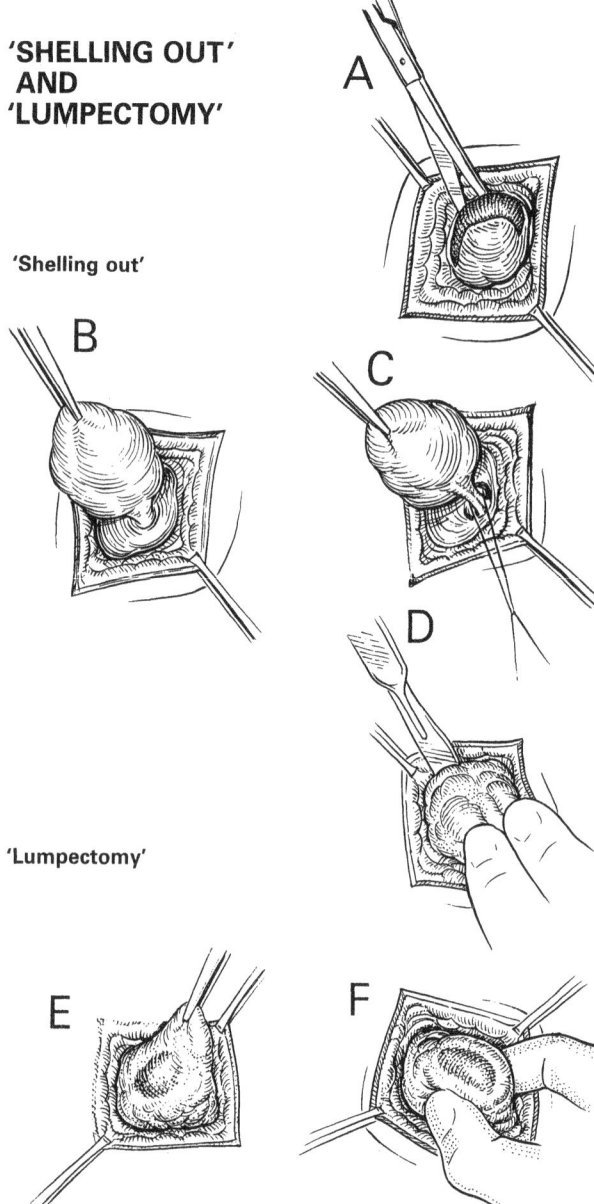

Fig 21-6 'SHELLING OUT' AND 'LUMPECTOMY' for the removal of a fibroadenoma. A, B, and C, you may be able to shell out a fibroadenoma through a small incision with minimal disturbance to the surrounding tissue. D, E, and F, you may have to expose the lesion, and remove it with a small part of the surrounding breast (lumpectomy). *After Rob C and Smith R, 'Operative Surgery' Vol. 1 (2nd edn), (Butterworth) with the kind permission of Hugh Dudley.*

'LUMPECTOMY' FOR A MASS IN THE BREAST

INDICATIONS. (1) Any suspicious lump less than 5 cm in diameter. (2) A lump of unknown nature more than 5 cm in diameter.

ANAESTHESIA. Ketamine (A 8.1) or general anaesthesia.

INCISION. If you are removing a fibroadenoma from a young woman, try not to scar her breast or to compromise future lactation. Use a periareolar, or circumferential (less satisfactory), or submammary incision (21-5). If these are difficult, use any incision which will give good exposure and allow you to remove the lump.

If you make a periareolar incision, you can remove a lump up to 5 cm or even 8 cm from the nipple. Gently dissect radially through the patient's breast from her areola, in line with the ducts.

If you make an inframammary incision and approach the lump from the back, this will be less easy than removing it through a periareolar or circumferential incision. Use it for deep inferiorly placed lumps.

Cut round the infra-lateral quadrant of her breast. In Caucasians and most Asians the crease under it usually forms a pigmented line. Hold her breast up while you make your incision in this line, and free it from her pectoral fascia. Continue to hold it up while you remove the lump from the back. Incise the posterior surface of her breast, until you have exposed the lump. Grasp it with forceps, and then free it from its bed with a scalpel or curved scissors. Remove it with a margin of at least 2 cm of macroscopically normal tissue.

If an inframammary incision is too difficult, make a circumferential one directly over the lump. This may be necessary, but produces an obvious scar. It will however be less obvious than a radial one.

With all incisions, use a sharp knife. If you suspect malignancy, excise the lump *with a margin of at least 2 cm of normal breast*. Otherwise (as in a fibroadenoma) shell it out. If necessary, remove the lump with an elliptical segment of breast tissue, with its long axis placed radially. Bleeding is not usually much of a problem. If it is difficult to control immediately, pack the wound with swabs, apply pressure for 5 to 10 minutes, remove the swabs, and then either transfix and tie the bleeding vessels, or control them with diathermy. Close the cavity with interrupted sutures of plain catgut on a half-circle needle.

If the cavity is too large to be completely obliterated by sutures, consider inserting a drain (some surgeons never insert one). Close her subcutaneous tissue with more interrupted sutures, and her skin with 3/0 or 4/0 monofilament. Postoperatively, apply a tight binder (uncomfortable), or a pressure dressing of adhesive strapping (better).

SIMPLE MASTECTOMY

INDICATIONS. A lump which is known or suspected to be malignant, and which is too large to remove by lumpectomy.

CONTRAINDICATIONS. An uncertain diagnosis—never remove a whole breast when the diagnosis is not proven histologically, and the lump can be removed by lumpectomy (with a 2 cm margin of normal breast). If you don't know the diagnosis, do a lumpectomy.

ANAESTHESIA. Anaesthetize the patient as above. If the mass is ulcerated, suture some gauze squares to it after she is anaesthetized, to minimize contamination.

INCISION. Make an oblique incision from the tail of the her breast superolaterally to its inferomedial margin. Ask your assistant to stretch her skin as you cut. Excise an ellipse of skin to include her nipple. Make it wide enough to let you dissect her breast adequately, and yet not so wide as to make closure difficult. Control bleeding by asking your assistant to press firmly with gauze as you cut.

Dissect back the superomedial and inferolateral flaps, in the plane between her subcutaneous fat (usually 1 to 2 cm thick), and the fat of her breast. Continue the dissection in all directions to the periphery of her breast, where you will meet her pectoralis major muscle. Dissect her breast off this muscle (usually with a knife), clamping bleeding points as you proceed, until you have removed it *in toto* with the ellipse of skin.

CAUTION ! (1) Don't make the skin flaps too thin, or open up tissue planes more than is necessary. The flaps should be at least 1 cm thick. (2) Don't remove her pectoral fascia, or muscle, unless the tumour is sticking to it. (3) Make the flaps of even thickness.

Then enter her axilla, but only far enough to remove the axillary tail of her breast. The tail only extends a short way into the axilla.

If the tumour is fixed to her pectoral muscle, remove part of it with her breast. You can, if necessary, remove most of it. But if you dissect it along her clavicle, be careful not to damage the vessels deep to the muscle. Remember that this is a Stage Three tumour, and you are not expecting a cure, so don't attempt anything too difficult.

Now control bleeding points by diathermy or tie them with 2/0 plain catgut. Irrigate the wound with warm saline before you close it. Remove any redundant skin, so that the edges

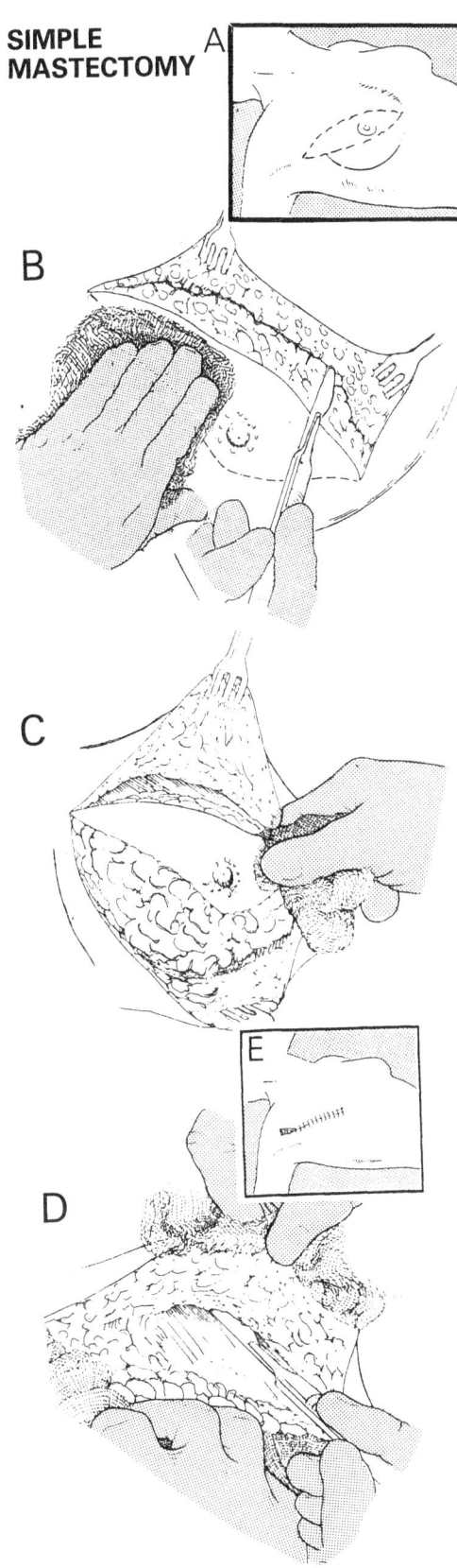

of the incision come together cleanly. If you cannot close the wound completely, cover the bare area with a split skin graft (57.2).

Insert a suction drain inferolateral to the incision. A 'Redivac' tube and reusable suction bottle are best. Or use a catheter with extra holes connected to a suction bottle, or, less satisfactorily, to a drainage bag.

Close her wound with plain catgut for the fatty layer, and 2/0 interrupted monofilament sutures for the skin.

POSTOPERATIVELY, cover her breast with layers of gauze and cotton wool, and hold them firmly in place with adhesive strapping. Apply a pressure dressing for 3 or 4 days. Remove the drain when no more blood or serous fluid comes, usually at 3 to 7 days. Remove the stitches after 7 to 10 days, the alternate ones first. Let her use her arm as much as she wishes. Encourage active movement from the 4th day.

EXCISING A DUCT PAPILLOMA OR CARCINOMA

Aim to excise a single duct system with its surrounding tissue. Try to make sure that neither the patient, nor anyone else, squeezes her breast during the 2 or 3 days before you do so in the theatre.

Under general anaesthesia, find the orifice of the affected duct by squeezing the secretion out of it. You may be able to feel the lesion under her areola (see the method for examining a breast for this condition in Section 21.3). Pass a fine probe or a hypodermic needle with a blunt end along the duct. Ask your assistant to hold this, while you excise an oval of skin and breast tissue with the duct and the lesion. Make sure that you excise the probe with a margin of at least 2 cm of macroscopically normal tissue horizontally and vertically all

AN INTRADUCT PAPILLOMA

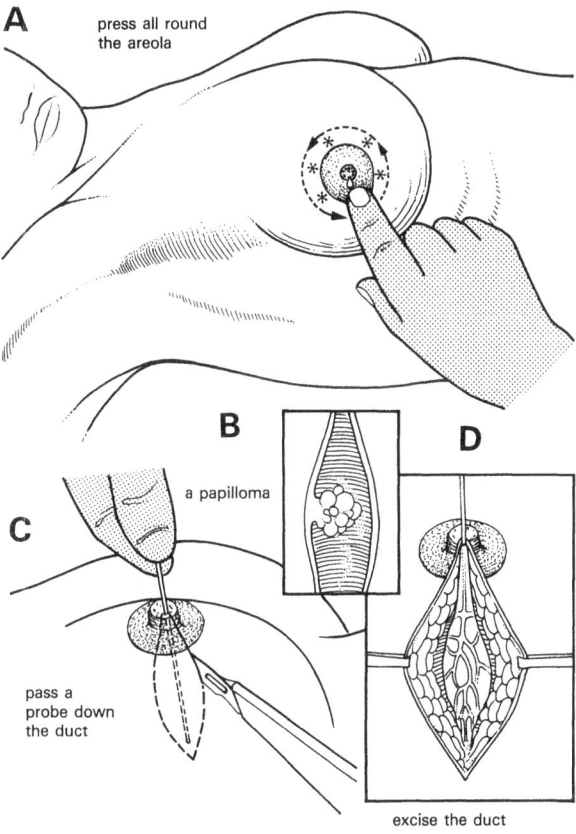

Fig. 21-7 SIMPLE MASTECTOMY. A, make an oblique elliptical incision, centred over the patient's nipple, from its superolateral to its inferomedial margin. B, dissect superolateral and inferomedial flaps. C, continue dissection in all directions to the periphery of her breast. D, dissect it off her pectoralis major. E, close the wound with a drain. A suction drain (preferably 'Redivac') as shown for Patey's mastectomy would be better than the corrugated rubber drain shown here. *After Rob C and Smith R, 'Operative Surgery', Vol. 1 (2nd edn), (Butterworth), with the kind permission of Hugh Dudley.*

Fig. 21-8 EXCISING AN INTRADUCT PAPILLOMA. A, carefully palpate all round the breast to find out which segment the discharge is coming from. B, a lesion in the wall of a duct which might equally well be a duct papilloma or a carcinoma. C, pass a fine probe down the duct, and excise it with some of the surrounding tissue.

EXCISING A GIANT FIBROADENOMA

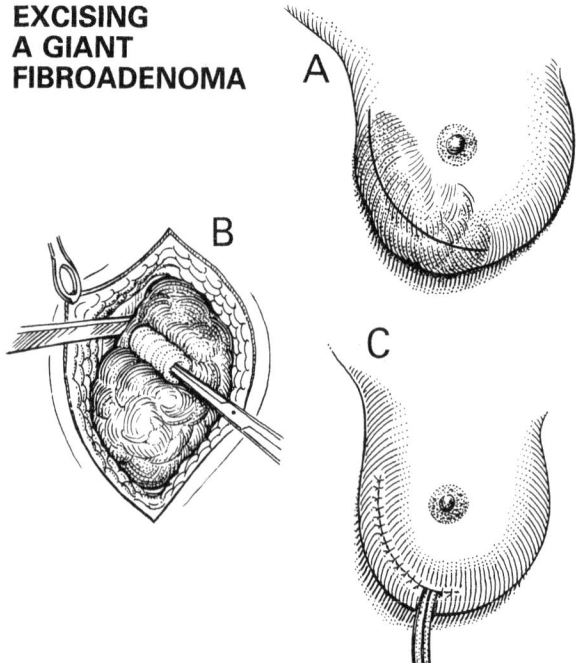

Fig. 21-9 EXCISING A GIANT FIBROADENOMA. If the mass only occupies part of the breast, you may be able to shell it out like this. Otherwise, you may have to do a simple mastectomy. *After Rob C and Smith R, 'Operative Surgery', Vol. 1 (2nd edn), (Butterworth), with the kind permission of Hugh Dudley.*

round the duct, except at the nipple. Suture the deeper layers with plain 2/0 catgut to obliterate the dead space. Close her skin with 2/0 or 3/0 monofilament. There is no need for a drain. If haemostasis is not good (unusual), apply a pressure dressing. Send the specimen for histology. Remove alternate stitches at 7 days.

At the first review, if the pathologist reports a papilloma (75% chance), reassure her. If he reports a carcinoma (15%), follow her up carefully each month for at least 6 months. These carcinomas are low-grade, so the operation itself may be sufficient.

DIFFICULTIES WITH TUMOURS OF THE BREAST

If she presents with a GIANT FIBROADENOMA, simple removal may not be practical, and you may have to do a a simple mastectomy. If it only occupies part of the breast, you may be able to shell it out. If you preserve normal breast tissue where you can, her breast may retain its normal shape afterwards.

If a MASS FORMS IN THE SCAR after you have done a lumpectomy or mastectomy for carcinoma, consider the possibility of a local excision.

21.6 Patey's operation for carcinoma of the breast, modified to remove pectoralis minor

The traditional radical mastectomy (Haagenson, Stiles, and others) removes both pectoralis major and minor. Removing pectoralis major is mutilating, and has not been shown to produce any more survivors than operations which leave it, such as Patey's. In its original form Patey's operation removes pectoralis minor also. This is is easier than preserving it, because it allows you to remove all the tissues containing the lymph nodes in the axilla 'en bloc', up to the axillary vessels and the brachial plexus.

Patey's operation is *for the careful caring operator, who cannot refer his patient.* Its aim is to try to remove her breast, and with it the triangular mass of fibrofatty tissue and lymph nodes in her axilla which is bounded by serratus anterior medially, latissimus dorsi posteriorly and laterally, by coracobrachialis above, and by the axillary apex superomedially. During the operation your assistant will have to retract pectoralis major forwards, so that you

ANATOMY FOR MASTECTOMY

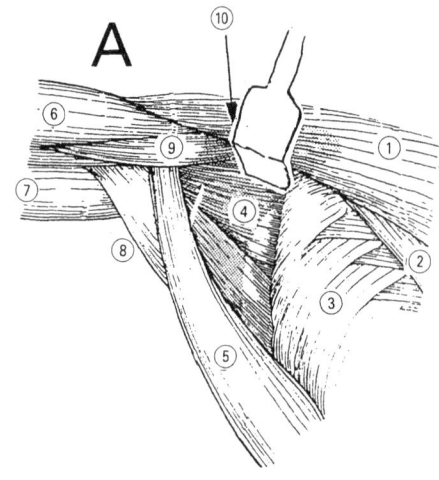

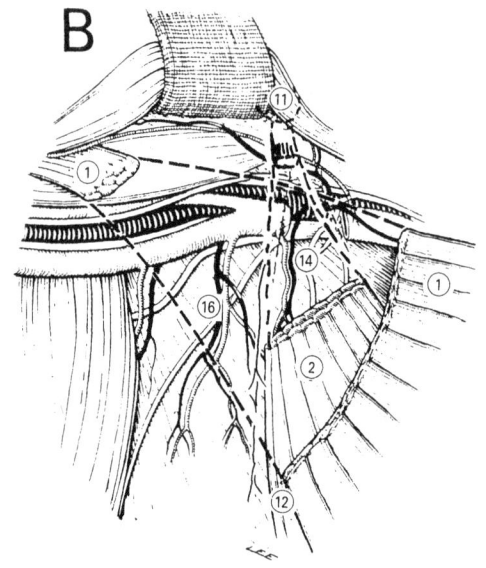

Fig. 21-10 ANATOMY FOR A MODIFICATION OF PATEY'S OPERATION. A, the empty axilla to show its muscles, as if its contents were absent. B, pectoralis major is shown cut away to reveal the structures under it. In reality it is retained.

The key to structures in this and later figures is: 1, pectoralis major (retained in this operation). 2, pectoralis minor (removed in this operation). 3, serratus anterior. 4, subscapularis. 5, latissimus dorsi. 6, biceps. 7, triceps. 8, teres major. 9, coracobrachialis. 10, the axillary space. 11, the coracoid process. 12, the nerve to serratus anterior. 13, the nerve to latissimus dorsi. 14, the lateral pectoral nerve. 15, *After Rob C and Smith R, 'Operative Surgery', Vol. 1 (2nd edn), (Butterworth), with the kind permission of Hugh Dudley.*

can see under it. *The key to dissecting the axilla is to expose the anterior edge of latissimus dorsi, and to find the plane just medial to it, which contains the subscapular vessels and the nerve to this muscle.* Having done this, you will have to remove all pectoralis minor, and the clavipectoral fascia in continuity with it.

The clavipectoral fascia is a sheet of tissue which extends from the apex of the axilla, where it is attached to the clavicle, to the base of the axilla, where it is continuous with the axillary fascia. It encloses pectoralis minor. Aim to remove it completely, together with the fat and lymph nodes that are associated with it.

PATEY'S OPERATION

Refer the patient if you can; if not proceed as follows.

ANAESTHESIA. General anaesthesia. Have two units of blood cross-matched for her.

CAUTION ! For the methods of controlling bleeding, see the previous section.

EQUIPMENT. A general set (4.12). A large right-angled retractor. At least 24 Spencer Wells or similar haemostats. Find two *competent* assistants.

PREPARATION. Sit her up a little, prepare and paint her back and flank on the affected side, and then let her lie back on a plastic sheet covered with a sterile towel, as in A, and B, Fig. 21-11. If you don't do this, the back of her flank will not remain sterile during the operation. Drape her arm so that you can flex and extend it when necessary, without disturbing the drapes.

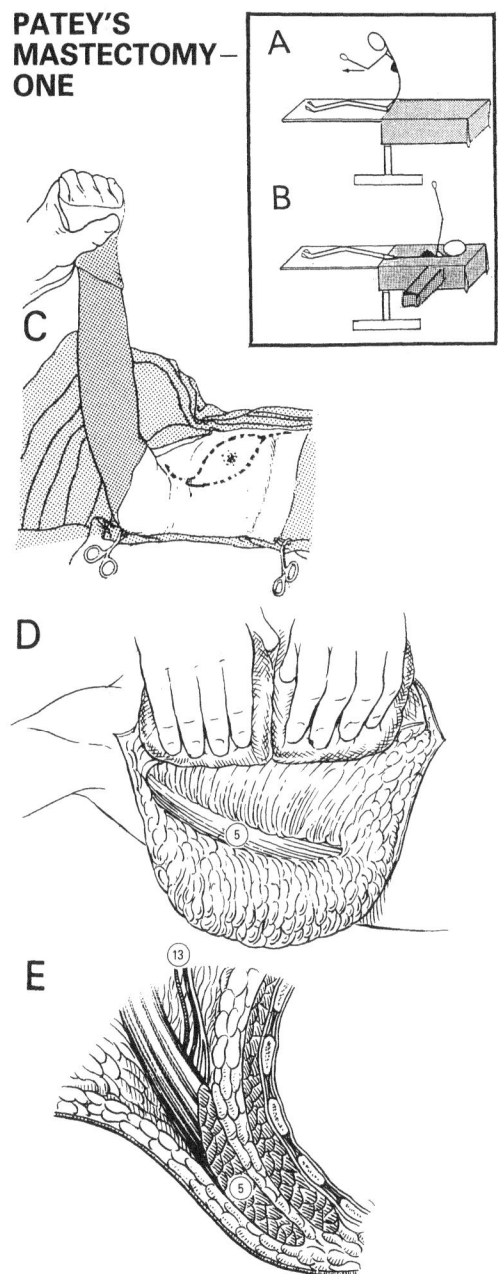

Fig. 21-11 PATEY'S MASTECTOMY—ONE. A, and B, draping the patient. Unless you prepare and drape her like this, the back of her flank will not remain sterile during the operation. C, plan the incision, so that the tumour is in the middle of an island of skin, and at least 4 cm away from any palpable edge of the tumour. D, carry the inferior flap back to just beyond the anterior border of her latissimus dorsi. E, dissect the tissues superficial (not deep) to latissimus dorsi for 5 cm. For a key to numbered structures see caption to Fig. 21-10. *After Rob C and Smith R, 'Operative Surgery', Vol. 1 (2nd edn), (Butterworth), with the kind permission of Hugh Dudley.*

You may need to cover a bare area, so prepare her thigh for skin grafting (57.2). A sandbag behind her lower thigh will make cutting the graft easier (optional).

INCISION. Plan the incision so that the tumour is in the middle of an island of skin, and at least 4 cm away from any palpable edge of the tumour. Make an oblique incision from her coracoid process, which you will be able to feel 2.5 cm inferior to the junction between the middle and outer thirds of her clavicle, to a point about 5 cm superolateral to the xiphoid process of her sternum. Bring the lateral edge of the ellipse well medial to the outer border of her pectoralis major (the anterior axillary fold). Don't extend it down her arm or over the front of her shoulder.

RAISE TWO FLAPS as you would if you were doing a simple mastectomy (21.5). Start with the inferolateral flap, and carry this back to 5 cm beyond the anterior border of her latissimus dorsi. Find the nerve to this muscle, which enters it with her subscapular vessels on its deep surface, near its anterior border. If you have placed your flap correctly, you will encounter latissimus dorsi as in E, Fig. 21-11.

CAUTION ! If you dissect the inferolateral flap too deep you will: (1) make it too thick, (2) leave pieces of breast or lymph nodes in it, (3) endanger the nerve to latissimus dorsi, and (4) find the accompanying subscapular vessels a nuisance.

Now dissect the superomedial flap to reach the edge of her breast. Dissect this from the underlying muscle, as described in Section 21.5 for for simple mastectomy.

TURN HER BREAST LATERALLY starting from the point where the flaps join inferomedially. Begin over her thoracic cage near the root of her xiphisternum. Dissect her breast away from her pectoralis major, clamping the vessels entering its deep surface as you progress. You will now have turned her whole breast over on itself to leave it lying laterally (F).

ENTER HER AXILLA to mobilize the axillary tail of her breast, by dissecting along her chest wall posterior to pectoralis major. Ask your assistant to lift her pectoralis major to make this easier.

You should now see the edge of her pectoralis minor. Dissect towards it. Separate its origin from her chest wall—it arises from ribs 3, 4, and 5 and from the intervening intercostal spaces. Dissect her clavipectoral fascia from her thoracic wall, working superomedially to reach the apex of her axilla, where you will see the fascia carrying her axillary vessels, before they disappear under her clavicle. Your assistant will have to retract her pectoralis major well at this stage.

A cutaneous nerve, the intercostobrachial, crosses through her axillary fat from the chest wall medially (T2), to supply the skin of her axilla and upper arm. You can sacrifice this.

While you are dissecting away pectoralis minor, you will meet some of her lateral pectoral vesels. Clamp these and tie them with 2/0 multifilament, or coagulate them with diathermy.

Now start dissecting her axilla, where you have exposed the edge of her latissimus dorsi. Find the nerve to this muscle, if you have not done so already, and preserve it. Dissect the tissues off the superficial surface of latissimus dorsi for about 3 cm. This will help when you come to close the wound.

Now, start inferolaterally to dissect the contents of her axilla from latissimus dorsi laterally, and from serratus anterior covering her thoracic wall medially.

CAUTION ! Preserve: (1) The nerve to latissimus dorsi as it crosses the posterior wall of her axilla. (2) The nerve to serratus anterior, which lies on the surface of this muscle, on the medial wall of her axilla.

Work superiorly along the anterior edge of latissimus dorsi, towards her axillary vessels (the vein lies inferomedial to the artery) and her associated brachial plexus. You should see the vein first; it is delicate and has several small branches—so be careful!

Dissect the contents of her axilla away from her axillary vein along the line 'X' in G, Fig. 21-12.

As you dissect medially along the vessels and nerves, continuing to expose the inferior and medial aspect of the vein, you will meet from lateral to medial: (1) Her subscapular artery and its two veins. Leave these if you can. (2) Her lateral pectoral artery. (3) Her acromiothoracic artery with four branches, two of which enter the field medially. (4) Her superior pectoral vessels.

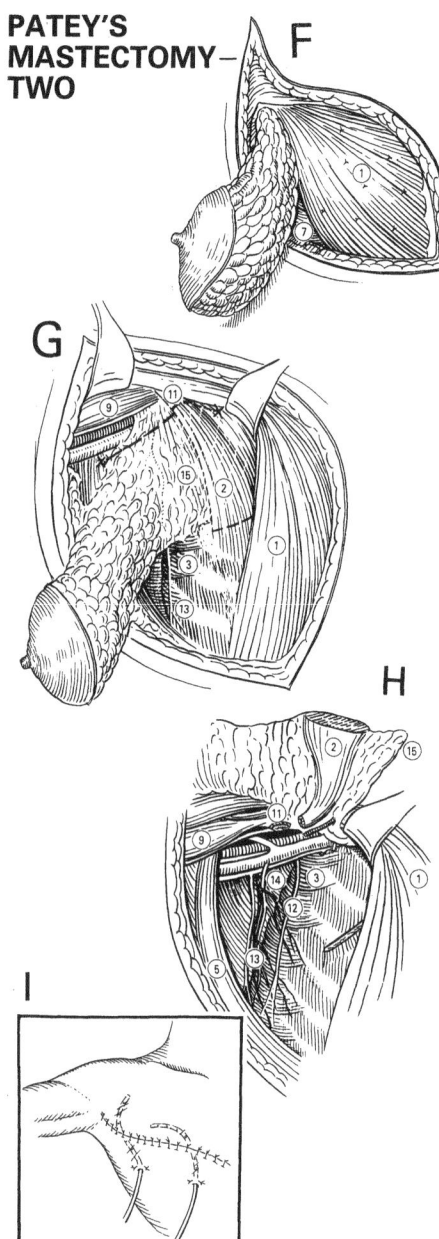

Fig. 21-12 PATEY'S MASTECTOMY—TWO. F, clear the whole of the patient's pectoralis major to its lateral edge. G, the entire contents of her axilla, including her clavipectoral fascia, pectoralis minor, and her breast have been reflected laterally. The insertion of her pectoralis minor into her coracoid process is about to be divided ('X'). H, pectoralis minor has been divided and her clavipectoral fascia is about to be removed. For clarity, the nerve trunks of the brachial plexus are not shown. I, the wound has been closed, and long tubular drains are in place. For a key to numbered structures see caption to Fig.21-10.

Use blunt dissection to separate the fascia anteriorly and posteriorly. While you dissect medially, ask your assistant to lift up her pectoralis major more. Ask another asistant to lift her arm, which has been lying on its arm board.

When you reach the apex of her axilla, you will be able to feel her first rib, and will meet the dissection you have done along her anterior chest wall. Now find the insertion of her pectoralis minor into her coracoid process. To reach it you will need sharp dissection with scissors along her axillary vessels. Divide its insertion near the bone (H). This will enable you to remove the contents of her axilla 'en bloc', including her pectoralis minor and her attached breast.

DRAINING AND CLOSING THE WOUND. If possible insert suction drains (a reusable 'Redivac' bottle and tube is ideal). A two-ended drain is best. Insert two perforated tube drains through separate stab incisions in the inferolateal flap. Corrugated drains can be used, but increase the risk of infection.

Starting at each end, use '0' monofilament to close the wound with simple interrupted sutures, spaced about 1 cm apart and passing through the skin 0.5 cm or less from its edge. Or, use a continuous blanket suture. Avoid mattress sutures, which leave an ugly scar. You should be able to close the wound using skin sutures only, unless she is very fat.

If you cannot close the wound without tension, close its ends first. Then sew the edges of its middle part to pectoralis major, and apply a split skin graft (57.2) to the muscle bed. Place gauze over this graft, and hold it in place with 3 pairs of 'tie over sutures' (57-8) inserted through the skin edges.

Apply a pressure dressing for 3 or 4 days. Remove the drain when no fluid flows, usually at 4 to 7 days. Remove alternate stitches on the 9th day, and the others on the 10th day, or later if necessary. Start arm exercises on the 7th day, especially those for shoulder abduction, internal rotation (ask her to put her hand behind her lower back), and external rotation (ask her to put her hand on the back of her neck).

DIFFICULTIES WITH PATEY'S OPERATION

If you DAMAGE HER AXILLARY VEIN, clamp it above and below with arterial clamps, or with Spencer Wells forceps with rubber tube over their jaws. Sew up the hole with 4/0 or 5/0 multifilament silk or monofilament, not catgut.

If you cannot repair the tear, tie her vein proximally and distally. This will usually only cause temporary ischaemia of her arm, because her cephalic vein is still intact.

If SHE IS UNABLE TO PULL HER SHOULDER DOWN, you have damaged the nerve to her latissimus dorsi. This is not a great disability.

If she has a WINGED SHOULDER, you have damaged the nerve to her serratus anterior. This looks unsightly.

THE THYROID

21.7 The general method for thyroid

The common surgical problem with the thyroid is a painless increase in its size, or the appearance in it of a painless mass. A painful thyroid is either due to haemorrhage (not uncommon in colloid goitre or carcinoma), or an abscess (rare in the developed world, and seen infrequently here, 5.10a). When a goitre or a mass needs surgery, the patient usually needs subtotal or total removal of his thyroid. This is not easy, and we have already given our reasons why you should refer the patients who need this done (21.1). There are however some ways in which you can help patients with surgical diseases of their thyroids.

GENERAL METHOD FOR THE THYROID

DIAGNOSIS. Note the patient's age, his (or more often her) sex, and where he lives. Simple and colloid goitres are common in females in the second and third decades, and in anyone who lives in an iodine-deficient area. How long has it been present? Has there been a sudden increase in the size of the mass in his neck? Is it painful? Does he have difficulty breathing or swallowing?

Inspect his neck from in front, and feel it from in front and from behind. Give him a drink, and confirm that it moves up when he swallows (all thyroid swellings do this). Feel the size of its lobes and its isthmus; feel its surface and consistency, and listen for a bruit.

IS HE HYPERTHYROID? You can diagnose moderate and severe thyrotoxicosis clinically. Minor degrees require measurement of his basal metabolism and/or hormone assays.

Suggesting hyperthyroidism: Loss of weight? Tremor, especially of his outstretched arms and fingers? Sweating? Anxiety? Hyperactivity? Exophthalmos? Lid lag (his upper lid is slow to follow his globe when he looks downwards)? Palpitations? Tachycardia? Cardiac irregularities (flutter, fibrillation)?

SOME THYROID LESIONS

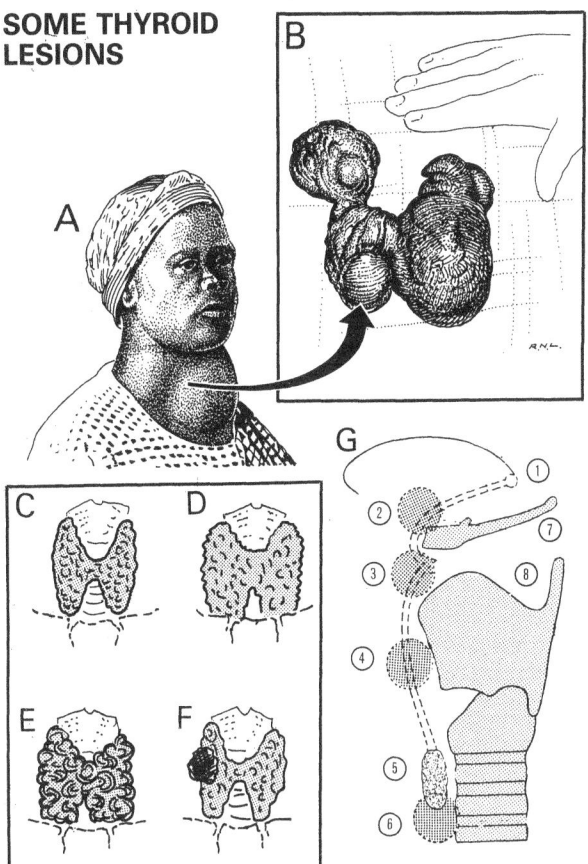

Fig. 21-13 SOME LESIONS OF THE THYROID. A, a patient with a non-toxic adenomatous mass in her thyroid gland. B, the mass removed at thyroidectomy. C, the smooth, soft, symmetrical goitre of puberty or pregnancy. D, the large, smooth firm symmetrical swelling of a colloid goitre, thyrotoxicosis, or Hashimoto's disease. E, a large, nodular, firm, assymetrical goitre. F, the solitary nodule of an adenoma, carcinoma, or cyst. G, congenital abnormalities of thyroid development.

1, the foramen caecum. 2, 3, and 4, positions for thyroglossal cysts. 5, the pyramidal lobe. 6, a mediastinal goitre. 7, the hyoid bone. 8, the thyroid cartilage. *A, and B, after Bowessman, Charles, 'Surgery and Clinical Pathology in the Tropics,' E and S Livingstone, with kind permission.*

Heart failure? His thyroid is usually enlarged, and may or may not be nodular. You can often hear a bruit.

SUDDEN ENLARGEMENT OF THE THYROID GLAND

In order of frequency the causes are: (1) Bleeding into the cyst of a colloid goitre. This will make it painful initially, but the pain may have gone by the time he presents. (2) Increase in the size of the colloid cysts of a goitre (this is not really sudden). (3) Bleeding into a carcinoma. (4) A rapidly growing carcinoma. (5) Acute bacterial infection (5.10a).

Refer him urgently. If dyspnoea is present, aspirate the haematoma or the abscess. If this does not relieve him (unusual) try tracheal intubation (A 13.2) or tracheostomy (52.2, difficult).

A SOLITARY NODULE IN THE THYROID

If he presents with a solitary nodule, first confirm that it is in his thyroid, and then feel carefully for other nodules.

If there are other nodules he probably has a nodular colloid goitre, and he may perhaps be thyrotoxic (unusual).

If it really is a solitary nodule, it is quite likely to be a papillary carcinoma (which has a good prognosis with radical surgery), or a follicular carcinoma (with a worse one). Refer him to an expert, who will explore his neck and do a subtotal, hemi- or total thyroidectomy, as required.

If you have a quick and reliable histology service, consider needle biopsy. Even a good pathologist may have difficulty distinguishing normal thyroid tissue from a low-grade papillary carcinoma. He will however be able to recognize the nodule of a colloid goitre.

CAUTION ! (1) Enucleation is easy, but is not satisfactory because: (a) It does not remove a carcinoma completely. This is particularly important if it is papillary. (b) He may think he is cured, and not report back for radical surgery. (c) It makes a second operation more difficult. (2) Don't explore a solitary nodule unless you can do a thyroidectomy.

If he is unable or unwilling to be referred, follow him up regularly, and measure the nodule. If it enlarges try to persuade him again to be seen by an expert.

DON'T TRY TO EXCISE A SOLITARY THYROID NODULE UNLESS YOU CAN DO A THYROIDECTOMY

21.8 Hyperthyroidism (thyrotoxicosis)

This is much less common in most rural communities of the developing world than it is in the industrial world, but it is becoming more common in towns. Look for the signs listed above (21.7).

HYPERTHYROIDISM

MEDICAL TREATMENT is the first choice for all cases, except where the disease arises in the nodule of a pre-existing nodular goitre (toxic nodule). Unfortunately, the relapse rate after medical treatment is 50%.

Admit the patient and give him:

(1) Tabs propanolol 40 mg three times daily (or some other β-blocker). Within 48 hours there should be a fall in his pulse rate, and a diminution of his tremor, anxiety, restlessness, heat intolerance, and sweating. If there is no response in 48 hours, increase the dose to 80 or even 160 mg four times daily. If necessary continue for 2 or 3 months. Or, use another beta blocker.

CAUTION ! (a) 40 mg of propanolol orally is only effective for about 6 hours. If he presented with severe hyperthyroidism, severe symptoms, or even a crisis may follow the omission of a single dose. Regular doses are especialy important just before and immediately after surgery. (b) Don't use propanolol for long-term treatment.

(2) Tabs carbimazole 10 to 20 mg three times daily. Reduce this dose when his symptoms are controlled. He may experience symptomatic improvement in a week, but you may have to wait 3 to 6 weeks for an objective clinical response. Slowing of the pulse and weight-gain are the most reliable signs of improvement. When you judge him to be euthyroid reduce the dose to between 2.5 to 5 mg three times a day. Continue treatment for 18 months to 2 years if necessary. His hyperthyroidism may remit spontaneously, so that he needs no further treatment. Watch for the side effects of carbimazole (rashes etc.)

If he relapses (>50% chance), advise surgery or a second course of medical treatment. The latter only succeeds in 25% of cases.

SURGICAL TREATMENT. He should be euthyroid before surgery. If possible refer him untreated, so that the expert can assess his clinical state before treatment starts. If this is impractical, treat him with propanolol and carbimazole for 6–8 weeks before the expected date of the operation. Most surgeons give Lugol's iodine 1 ml daily for 10 days preoperatively to reduce vascularity. Beta blockers are continued up to the operation and for 10 days afterwards.

CAUTION ! It is dangerous to operate on thyrotoxic patients who have not had antithyroid drugs for 6–8 weeks preoperatively. Even then, postoperative thyrotoxic crises occur. Thyroidectomy is not an operation for the generalist!

The recurrence of hyperthyroidism after a bilateral subtotal thyroidectomy is very unusual. However, 30% of patients become hypothyroid within 10 years and need l-thyroxine 100 to 200 micrograms daily.

21.9 Thyroglossal cysts

A thyroglossal cyst is a smooth, painless, subcutaneous lump which usually lies on the thyroid cartilage just to one side of the midline (G, Fig. 21-13). These cysts occur in both sexes equally, usually between the ages of 15 and 40, and are formed from the epithelial pouch that gives rise to the thyroid gland. This runs from the junction between the anterior two-thirds and the posterior third of the tongue (the foramen caecum, 21-13), to the pyramidal lobe of the thyroid, just above the isthmus. Cysts sometimes occur within the pyramidal lobe, or in relation to the hyoid bone.

Excision is usually not difficult. Occasionally, however, an extension of the cyst goes up to and through the hyoid bone, which may need to be divided, so refer the patient if you can. If you cannot refer him, proceed as follows.

THYROGLOSSAL CYST

ANAESTHESIA. (1) General anaesthesia with intubation (A 13.1). (2) Intravenous ketamine (A 8.2). (3) Local anaesthesia (A 5.4).

INCISION. Make a 6-8 cm transverse incision in a skin crease over the swelling. Separate the tissues between the patient's strap muscles in the midline longitudinally. If exposure is inadequate, divide these muscles transversely. Also divide the pretracheal fascia covering the cyst. Dissect it out with scissors.

Close the wound in layers. Approximate his strap muscles with 3/0 plain catgut, and his skin with 3/0 or 4/0 monofilament. Remove the sutures on the 5th day.

If an extension of the cyst extends up into his neck through his hyoid bone (uncommon), follow it upwards and divide his hyoid bone if necessary. No vital structures are in the way, and his divided hyoid does not need repair. If a remnant is left behind the cyst may recur.

21.10 Physiological goitre

A physiological goitre presents as a uniform, smooth, painless swelling of the thyroid gland, mainly in girls and women between 15 and 25. It appears to be about equally common everywhere, and does not cause dyspnoea or dysphagia. It often resolves spontaneously as the period of maximal hormonal activity passes.

21.11 Colloid goitre

Colloid goitres are worldwide, but are very common in areas of iodine deficiency (endemic goitre). They can be prevented by the administration of iodine to the entire community, which also prevents the other manifestations of endemic iodine deficiency (iodine embryopathy, etc.).

Colloid goitres occur between the ages of 20 and 50, and affect women more than men. Large ones obstruct breathing by narrowing or displacing the trachea, and they may occasionally obstruct swallowing. Sometimes, they extend into the thorax. They can be 'simple', in which case they are larger and firmer than a normal thyroid and have a regular surface. More often they are nodular. Although the patient may complain of a single nodule, he usually has more than one, with one lobe of his thyroid much larger than the other. There is no bruit over the nodule unless it is a toxic (hyperthyroid) nodule. Treatment, when it is indicated, is surgical. One of the dangers of a colloid goitre is that bleeding into it may cause it to increase in size suddenly.

COLLOID GOITRE

If a colloid goitre is small, and is causing no obvious symptoms, surgery is not really necessary, and the indications for its removal are cosmetic. Discuss this with the patient in the light of the available surgical and anaesthetic skills and priorities.

If he has dyspnoea or dysphagia, or the gland is large, subtotal thyroidectomy is indicated, but is seldom urgent. If there has been a sudden increase due to haemorrhage (unusual) see above.

21.12 Tumours of the thyroid

Adenoma It is doubtful whether a true adenoma of the thyroid exists, because it is difficult to differentiate histologically from a low-grade papillary carcinoma. Adenomas present as solitary nodules. In most communities the commonest nodules are colloid goitres.

Carcinomas are seen occasionally everywhere, and vary from the very slow-growing to the very malignant. In Europe the frequency of the various types is as follows. (In Africa the follicular type is relatively more common.)

Papillary carcinomas (70%), are of low-grade malignancy, and present as a nodule with or without spread to the lymph glands of the neck. The histological appearances of a needle biopsy resemble those of a normal thyroid or an 'adenoma'. Refer the patient for total thyroidectomy and block dissection of his neck on one or both sides, which will probably cure him (5 year survivals 95% and 10 year survivals 90%).

Follicular carcinomas (20%) spread to bone early, so that the first sign may be a bony secondary. He may have a lump or area of thyroid enlargement, or his thyroid may be clinically normal. If the disease is confined to his neck, refer him for a radical thyroidectomy, and a block dissection on one or both sides. If he has metastases to bone or other organs, there is little to be done. Radiotherapy often gives temporary improvement. About 5% of tumours take up radio-iodine, which is very effective. Follicular tumours range from low-grade to high-grade malignancy: (1) If he has a low-grade tumour with no metastases, he has an 86% chance of 10 year survival after radical thyroidectomy. (2) If he has metastases in his neck he has a 44% chance of survival. (3) If he has distant metastases, his prognosis is the same as for an anaplastic carcinoma.

Medullary carcinomas (3-5%) have a familial incidence, and are transmitted as a Mendelian dominant. They have a characteristic histological appearance, a poor prognosis, and may be part of a system of multiple endocrine tumours.

Anaplastic carcinomas (5%) mostly occur in elderly women, and are little helped by radiotherapy; radio-iodine is not taken up. 75% of patients are dead in two years.

21.13 Other problems with the thyroid

You may see the following three non-neoplastic diseases of the thyroid. Apart from lymphocytic thyroiditis they are uncommon, and you may have to do a needle biopsy to distinguish them.

OTHER THYROID PROBLEMS

If a goitre is uniform and feels unusually FIRM and VERY WELL-DEFINED but is not particularly tender, consider the possibility of autoimmune lymphocytic thyroiditis (Hashimoto's disease, not uncommon). The patient is aged 20 to 70, and is usually about 50. Women are more commonly affected than men. Spontaneous resolution is usual but slow. Hypothyroidism often develops, and needs replacement therapy with l-thyroxine 100 to 200 micrograms daily. Prednisolone is of doubtful value.

If a patient's thyroid has become uniformly enlarged, MODERATELY TENDER, and PAINFUL over some weeks or months, he may have subacute thyroiditis (de Quervain's disease, uncommon). This is a non-suppurative inflammation, sometimes with hyperthyroidism. The ESR is raised. It is self-limiting, but you can promote its resolution by giving him prednisolone 30 mg daily, until his pain and swelling subside. He has a 10% chance of becoming hypothyroid.

If his thyroid becomes WOODY-HARD, is fixed to the surrounding tissues, and is either normal-sized or a little enlarged, suspect RIELEL'S THYROIDITIS (woody thyroiditis, rare). Distinguish this from malignant tumours.

22 Proctology

22.1 The general method for the anus and rectum

A patient's rectum and anus can cause him much disability and discomfort. In the tropics he can have most of the diseases which are seen elsewhere, but with a different frequency, and with a few extra ones. You should have little difficulty treating anorectal abscesses (5.13) and fistulae (22.2), piles (22.4), fissures (22.7), pilonidal sinuses (very rare in Africans, 22.8), prolapse of the rectum (22.9), juvenile polyps (22.10), lymphogranuloma venereum (22.10), and some cases of imperforate anus (28.6).

Although the anus is a particularly infected area, so that any surgical wounds near it are sure to become infected, the infection seldom spreads, so that they readily heal—if you let them granulate from the bottom up—make sure your nurses understand this. Don't attempt primary suture, and instead make wide, shallow saucer-like wounds. Don't let his subcutaneous tissues or his skin edges fall together and unite prematurely, before the bottom of his wound has healed. A shallow, open wound with trimmed edges heals better than one with much redundant skin and fat.

PHYSIOLOGY. The purpose of a patient's anus is to keep him continent. Its failure to do this is a social disaster. Continence is mostly maintained by his external sphincters and his levator ani, especially its deep puborectalis part, which forms a sling at his anorectal line, in the angle between his anus and his rectum. The tone in his external sphincters is increased by reflex and voluntary contraction. His internal sphincter, which is under autonomic control, is less important, but helps to keep his anal canal closed and empty. In painful conditions, both his sphincters are in spasm. The lower part of his anal canal is sensitive enough to let him know what is in his rectum—nothing, gas, liquid, or solid. Receptors in the smooth muscle of his upper rectum and the voluntary muscle of his pelvic floor let him know when his rectum is dilated.

Goligher JC, 'Surgery of the anus, rectum and colon'. (4th edn 1980). Ballière Tindall.

- *PROCTOSCOPE, Gabriel, 64×25 mm, one only.* This is the standard instrument for examining the rectum. You will also find an ordinary Sims' speculum useful for examining the anal canal under general anaesthesia.
- *SPECULUM, bivalve, Goligher pattern with detachable third blade, one only.* Use this for doing minor rectal operations, such as division of the internal sphincter.
- *SIGMOIDOSCOPE, Strauss, 330 mm, Luer fitting, in case with bellows, cord and standard endoscope bulb (35.1) complete with biopsy forceps, etc., one only.* Keep sigmoidoscopes and proctoscopes in a case so that their various parts don't get lost.
- *SPONGE HOLDER, for sigmoidoscope, 430 mm, one only.*
- *FORCEPS, for biopsy through sigmoidoscope, Officer pattern, one only.* These are the most expensive part of the outfit. If necessary, you can use them to remove foreign bodies from the oesophagus, or even from the urethra.
- *SUCTION TUBE FOR SIGMOIDOSCOPE, one only.* You can make this from a piece of ordinary copper tube, 15 cm longer than the sigmoidoscope, with a right angle bend at one end.
- *BELLOWS, spare for Strauss sigmoidoscope, Luer fitting, one only.*
- *BULBS, endoscope, standard (35.1), small fitting, ten only.* Endoscope bulbs are very easily blown.
- *BATTERY BOX, for endoscopes, holding D type dry cells, one only.* This must be the same voltage as the standard endoscope bulbs, and have a lead which fits the endoscopes.
- *PROBE, medium-sized, malleable silver, one only.*
- *DIRECTOR, probe-pointed, one only.* This has a groove on it. Pass it through a fistula and then cut down on the groove.

THE PECTINATE LINE AND THE ANORECTAL LINE ARE LANDMARKS

THE GENERAL METHOD FOR THE ANUS AND RECTUM

EQUIPMENT. A rectal tray containing proctoscopes, finger cots or gloves, long cotton-tipped applicators, and testing materials for occult blood. If you are going to pass a sigmoidoscope, you may need a suction tube and a sucker.

PREPARATION. Put a drape over the patient and keep the instruments out of his sight. Tell him what you are going to do, and explain that you will not hurt him. If some pain is necessary, warn him. Be gentle, don't hurry, and use warm instruments.

Lie him on his side with his buttocks extending well over the edge of the table, as in A Fig. 22-2. Flex his hips fully, but keep his knees at 90° so that they are out of your way. It is convenient to have his right upper hip and knee a little more flexed than his left.

DIGITAL EXAMINATION OF THE RECTUM

Draw his buttocks apart and look at his anal region for skin tags, lumps and the openings of fistulae (B). Feel any abnormalities, such as the tracks or openings of fistulae, or tumours (C).

Lubricate the end of your finger well. Insert it so that its larger broad dimension lies in the anteroposterior axis of his anal canal. When you touch the sphincter, it will contract. Wait, give it a few seconds to relax, and then press firmly and gently in the axis of his anal canal. Keep pressing, until you can feel your finger suddenly slip easily into his anus. Note the tone of the sphincter.

As you put your finger into his anus, feel for lesions below and above his anorectal line. Then palpate the entire circumference of his anus between your two fingers (E).

In a man feel each of the two lobes of his prostate separated by a median furrow.

In a woman, look to see if she has a rectocele, feel her cervix and uterus rectally, and feel for swellings in her rectovesical pouch.

Sweep your finger all round the patient's pelvis and examine his coccyx between two fingers (F).

Finally, if you suspect an intraperitoneal mass, a bimanual recto-abdominal examination may be useful in a man (G), and a vagino-abdominal one in a woman.

PROCTOSCOPY. Examine his anus with your finger first. Lubricate the proctoscope and push it firmly in the direction of his umbilicus. Examine the lining of his anal canal as you withdraw it—slowly, and looking for piles as you do so.

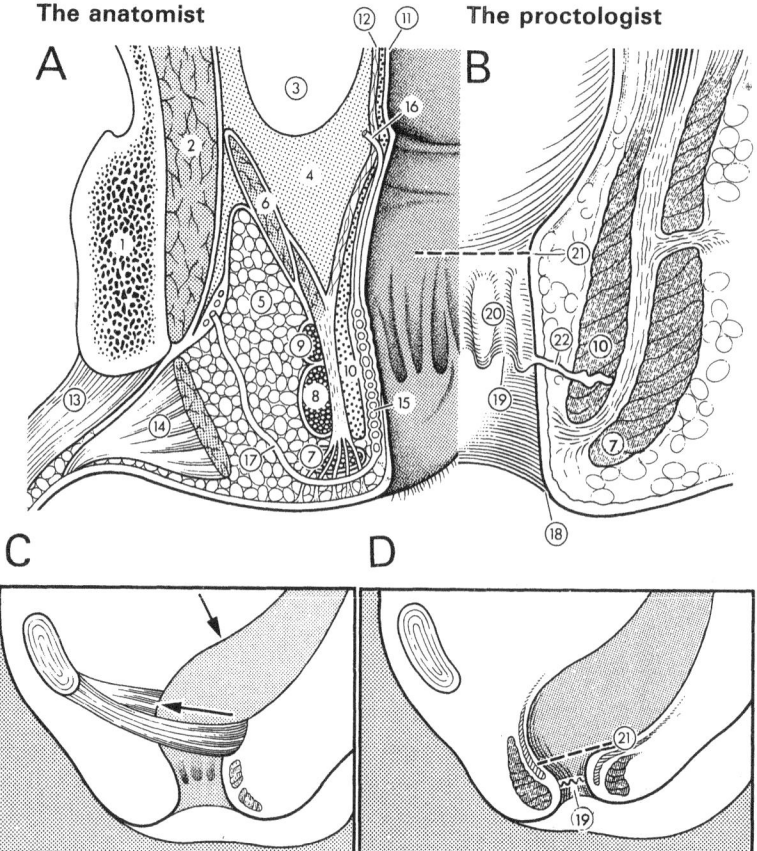

Fig. 22-1 THE ANORECTUM. A, an anatomist's view to show the bony pelvis (1), inside which is obturator internus (2). Below the pararectal fossa (3) lies the pelvirectal space (4). This is separated from the ischiorectal fossa (5) by the levator ani muscle (6). Sphincter ani externus has three parts, a subcutaneous part (7), a superficial part (8), and a deep part (9). Inside the external sphincter lies the internal sphincter (10). This is continuous with the circular muscle of the gut (11), outside which is the longitudinal muscle (12). Two other muscles are also shown, semitendinosus (13), and gluteus maximus (14). The rectal venous plexus (15), is drained by the superior rectal vein (16) and the inferior rectal vein (17).

B, a proctologist sees things more simply and has three reference points. His first is the anal verge (18), where the anal and perianal skin join. His second is the pectinate line (also called the dentate line) (19), where the anal columns (20) and sinuses end. Red, loosely-attached rectal mucosa lies above this line, and pale, tightly-stretched anal lining lies below it. His third reference point is the anorectal line (21), which is the palpable upper border of the complex of anal sphincters. This is something you can easily feel with your examining finger, provided the patient has adequate muscle tone, and has not been anaesthetized and given a relaxant. It is about 2 cm further in than the pectinate line, and the rectum balloons out above it, as shown in D.

Note that the external sphincter (7) comes down a bit lower than the internal one (10).

The anal glands (22), are an important site of infection, and the origin of fistulae and sinuses. They open into the crypts just above the pectinate line.

C, a view of the rectum to show how the puborectalis muscle pulls the anorectal junction upwards and forwards when it contracts. You can easily feel it doing this when you do a rectal examination. During defaecation, it relaxes completely. Increased intra-abdominal pressure pushes the anterior rectal wall down, and so closes the anal canal and prevents incontinence.

D, the relation of the anorectal line to the external sphincter. A, after 'Gray's Anatomy', 8.127 (Churchill Livingstone). B, after MacLeod JH, 'A Method of Proctology', Fig. 1.1. Harper and Row, with kind permission. C, and D, kindly contributed by Brian Hancock.

SIGMOIDOSCOPY

Do a sigmoidoscopy just after he has defaecated normally, or after he has had an enema. There is no need for a general anaesthetic, unless you fail without one and the examination is essential (as for carcinoma). If you are clumsy, you can perforate his gut, so: (1) Always do a digital examination first. (2) Never push a sigmoidoscope further in, if you cannot see the lumen in front of it. Follow the lumen at all times. (3) Never force it. If there is a pocket or a blind area in the way, withdraw it a little, and then advance it again. Your main aim while inserting it is to do so successfully. Do most of the examining as you withdraw it.

Ask him to breathe in and out while you gently insert it, lubricated and warmed with its inserter in place. You will feel the resistance of his anal sphincter suddenly diminish (B, in Fig. 22-3) as it enters his rectal ampulla.

While you look where it is going, turn it 90° posteriorly (C), as you gently manipulate it past the mucosal valves of his rectum. While you insert it, gently pump in enough air to distend the lumen in front of it. Don't blow his sigmoid up too much, or he will feel urgency and cramps.

The first 12 to 15 cm, as far as his rectosigmoid junction is usually easy. You will see his smooth rectal mucosa giving way to the concentric rugae of his sigmoid colon. At this point his gut passes over his sacral promontary, and may turn in any direction. Proceed anteriorly and to the left. You should be able to reach 25 or 30 cm, but don't force it. Be sure you can distend his gut with air, before you push the sigmoidoscope further in.

If you find much stool, send him to the lavatory; if that fails give him an enema, and try again later.

Rotate the sigmoidoscope, as you withdraw it, so that you inspect every part of his mucosa. Be careful to examine the posterior wall of his rectal ampulla. This lies at 90° to his anal canal, and you can easily miss it. Remove some stool, and test it for occult blood.

PREOPERATIVE CARE FOR ANAL OPERATIONS

Do a sigmoidoscopy before all anal operations to exclude coexisting tumours and inflammatory bowel disease. For this to be possible, his bowel must be empty, so give him a small enema or a glycerine suppository preoperatively.

EXAMINING THE RECTUM

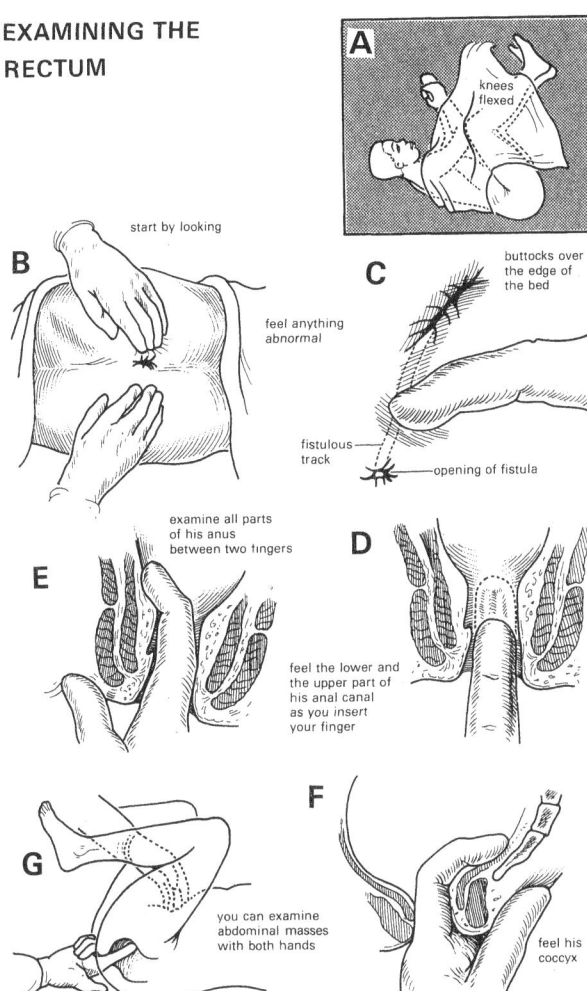

Fig. 22-2 EXAMINING A PATIENT'S RECTUM. A, have his knees well flexed and his buttocks over the edge of the couch. B, start by looking. C, then feel. You may feel the track of a fistula. D, feel his anal canal as you insert your finger. E, feel all round his anus. F, feel his coccyx. G, if necessary, examine his abdomen between your two hands. *After MacLeod JH, 'A Method of Proctology', (179) Figs. 2-1, 2-8, 2-9, Harper and Row, with kind permission.*

POSTOPERATIVE CARE AFTER ANAL OPERATIONS

DRESSINGS are important. Dress an open anal wound with flat pieces of gauze, soaked in hypochlorite ('Eusol' or 'Milton' 15 ml to a litre of water), or some other antiseptic or salt solution. Cover the whole raw surface with a flat piece of gauze. *Tuck an edge of the gauze into any flat crevices.* Insert a corner of the gauze into any extension of the wound towards his anal canal. Use more gauze to fill out the hollow of the wound up to the level of the surrounding skin.

Finally, apply more gauze and wool to the surface, and hold the whole dressing with a T-bandage.

BATHING is more convenient than irrigation. Sit him in a large bowl containing warmed salt solution equivalent to full-strength or half-strength saline.

BOWEL ROUTINE. Give him 15 ml of liquid paraffin twice daily from the day of the operation. If he has not opened his bowels by the evening of the second postoperative day, counting the day of the operation, give him 3.5–5 ml of liquid extract of cascara, or some similar purgative. If his bowels do not act the following morning, do a rectal examination to see what the problem is; his rectum may be empty. If his faeces are impacted give him 850–1000 ml of a soap and water enema, through a tube, a funnel, and a well-lubricated rubber catheter. Ask him to retain the enema as long as possible before using a bedpan. The dressing will probably come away with his bowel action. Give him a bath, and redress his wound.

SIGMOIDOSCOPY

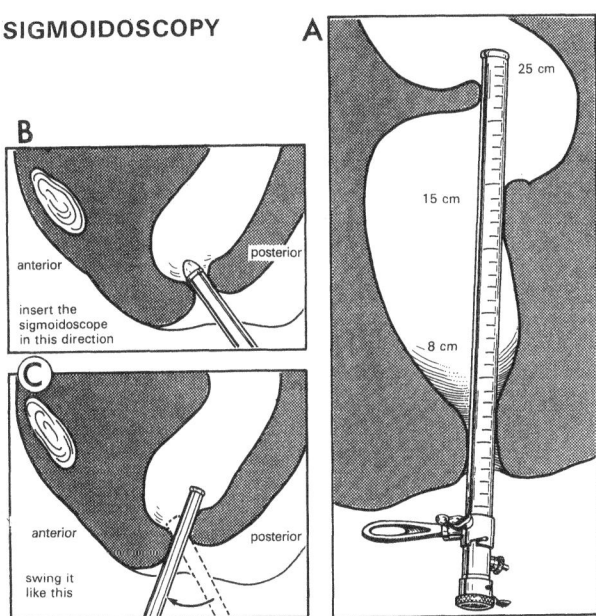

Fig. 22-3 PASSING A SIGMOIDOSCOPE (A) enables you to inspect the last 25 cm of a patient's colon. With your finger you can only feel the last 8 cm. B, introduce the sigmoidoscope, pointing it towards his umbilicus, and when it is through his anal sphincter (C) swing it backwards. *After MacLeod JH, 'A Method of Proctology', (1979), Figs. 2-12 to 2-14. Harper and Row, with kind permission.*

Continue with 15 ml of liquid paraffin each evening, for a week only. If you continue too long, there are numerous side effects, such as the malabsorption of fat-soluble vitamins, and paraffinomas; also his anus may stenose because it is never dilated by a normal stool.

22.2 Anorectal sinuses and fistulae

The anorectal abscesses in Section 5.13, and the sinuses and fistulae described here, are part of the same disease process. An abscess is the acute phase, and a sinus or fistula the chronic one. Both sinuses and fistulae are tracks lined by granulation tissue, which open on to the skin near the anus. The difference between them is that a sinus has no internal opening, whereas a fistula opens into the patient's anal canal, or occasionally into his rectum. Usually, there is only one internal opening, but he may have several external ones. These can either be insignificant little holes, or prominent little nodules of granulation tissue, which heal over temporarily. The treatment of sinuses and fistulae is similar.

Typically, a patient with a fistula starts by having an abscess, which either bursts and fails to heal, or is not drained properly (see Section 5.13), after which he complains of a chronic painless discharge which soils his clothes. His fistula is only painful when it becomes temporarily blocked, so that pus builds up inside it.

Fistulae can take any of the paths shown in Fig. 22-5; they can be subcutaneous (common), low anal, high anal, or intermuscular (rare).

A fistula seldom heals spontaneously, and almost always needs surgery. Cut down on it, deroof it, expose it, and let the wound you have made heal from the bottom by granulation during several weeks. A fistula nearly always goes through the anal sphincters, so that in cutting down on it, you have to cut them. Fortunately, a patient usually has some sphincter capacity to spare, and as his fistula usually goes through his sphincters quite superficially, you can cut the superficial part of them without making him incontinent. *But if his fistula goes deep, and you cut too much of his sphincters, he will become incontinent.* If, on the other hand, you make the opposite mistake of not cutting deeply enough, you may leave part of the track behind, with the result that his fistula recurs.

You have a 50% chance of finding the internal opening quite easily, by passing a probe from the external opening towards his anal canal. One of the worst mistakes is to create an internal opening, where there was none before, in the process of looking for it, by forcing a probe through into his anal canal. This makes a sinus into an iatrogenic fistula, opens up healthy tissue to infection, and makes cure more difficult.

The key landmarks are his pectinate line, and his anorectal ring. If necessary, you can cut both his sphincters below his pectinate line. In doing so, you preserve his anorectal ring (formed by his puborectalis muscle), and he remains continent, although he may have some incontinence of watery stools. Cutting his anorectal ring makes him completely incontinent. Fortunately, fistulae which go deep to the anorectal line are rare. If you find he has one, and cannot refer him, all you can do is to lay open the superficial tracks, curette the deep ones and hope for the best. This is difficult surgery, so examine him carefully and *only operate if he has an easier fistula*—incontinence is worse than the intermittent discharge from a fistula!

Fistulae which have external openings in front of a transverse line across the anus enter directly into it by the shortest path. Fistulae behind this line usually curve round, so that they enter the anus posteriorly at 6 o'clock (Goodsall's rule, Aa, 22-6). In doing so they follow a horseshoe path, and are often bilateral, one side communicating with the other. There are exceptions, and very superficial fistulae behind the line may occasionally track directly into the anus.

You will find that the track of a horseshoe fistula hugs the puborectalis part of the levator ani muscle, as it forms a sling round the sides and back of the anorectal junction, external to the external sphincter. Fortunately, the internal opening of such a horseshoe fistula is usually at the pectinate line, although the fistula itself may go much deeper.

Provided you trim the wound edges well, the common straight superficial fistulae heal with only minimal postoperative care, but this is critical for deep ones. The wound must be laid open widely, and it must granulate from the bottom up. If it heals leaving pockets, it will recur. So try to prevent the opposing granulating walls of the wound, or its skin edges, from touching one another, uniting, and leaving an unhealed pocket underneath them. Your main difficulty in treating these patients is likely to be to persuade them to stay long enough in hospital. If you are short of beds, a relative or the staff of a health centre will have to manage the wound.

PERIANAL ABSCESSES, SINUSES, AND FISTULAE ARE *NOT* HELPED BY ANTIBIOTICS!

ANORECTAL FISTULAE

X-RAY. X-ray the patient's chest: his fistula may be tuberculous (uncommon). If it is tuberculous, surgery is usually unnecessary. He may or may not have an obvious chest lesion.

EXAMINATION IN THE THEATRE. Prepare him for anaesthesia, if necessary. Before you start, warn him that you are going to examine him under anaesthesia to try to find where his fistula runs. Explain that if he has one of the easier fistulae, you are going to operate. Otherwise, you may have to leave it (unusual). Further indications are given below.

If the opening is less than 5 cm from his anus, his fistula is perianal, if it is more than 5 cm away, it is probably high. Multiple openings suggest a horseshoe fistula. Record the position of all external openings carefully on a copy of diagram A, in Fig. 22-4.

Feel for the thickened track which runs from the external opening(s) towards his anus. If a fistula is superficial, you can usually feel its firm, fibrous track quite easily. As you press it pus may exude from the external opening.

Put a finger into his anus and try to feel the internal opening: you may be able to feel an induration at its internal end. Feel the entire circumference of his rectum, as far as your finger

PROCTOLOGY

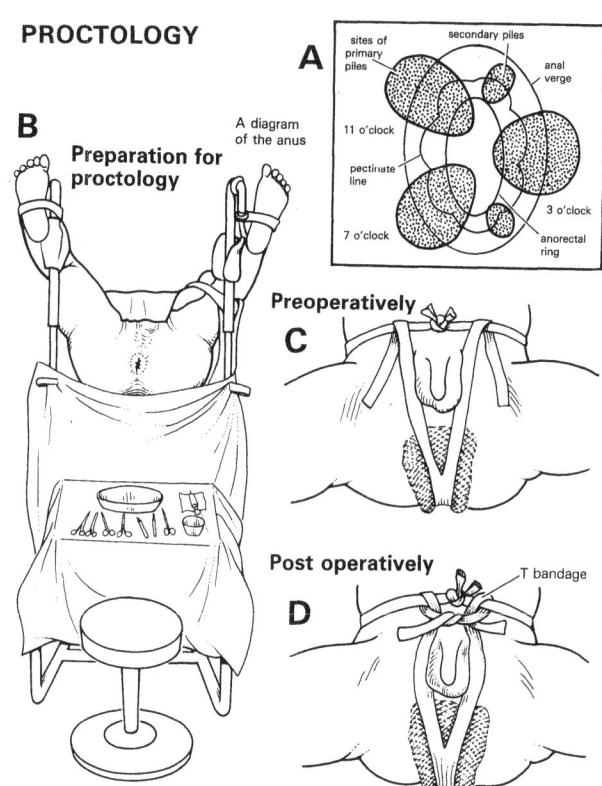

Fig. 22-4 PROCTOLOGY. A, a diagram for recording abnormalities around a patient's anus. This has 3 lines, an inner one for the anorectal line, a middle wavy one for the pectinate line, and an outer one for the anal margin. Record your findings in relation to these 3 lines. Here, the diagram records the sites of the three primary piles, and the common sites of two secondary ones. B, arrangements for operating on a patient's anus. You must also have a light on a stand which will direct its beam horizontally into the wound. C, a T-bandage before the operation, and D, the bandage tied up after it. *After Golighter JC, 'Surgery of the Anus Rectum and Colon', (4th edn. 1980) Figs. 64 and 65, Baillière Tindall, with kind permission.*

can reach. Determine particularly where the fistula might be in relation to his anorectal ring and his pectinate line. Try to feel the track between your two fingers. Does it appear to come to an end low down, or high up in his anus? If you feel induration at the level of his puborectalis or above (rare), he has a complex high fistula.

PROCTOSCOPY. Examine his anal canal with a proctoscope. You may be able to see the internal opening of his fistula, usually at 6 o'clock on his pectineal line. Insert the proctoscope as far as it will go, withdraw the obturator, and then gradually withdraw the instrument itself. As soon as its end becomes obstructed and closed by his anorectal ring, stop. If you can still see the opening of the fistula, it is safely below the critical level of his anorectal ring.

You may be able to feel the track of a horseshoe fistula as a thick horizontal indurated rod, hugging his puborectalis sling.

In 50% of cases you will find the opening easily, in the other 50%, it will be present but tiny. A probe may show it, but if it does not, inject methylene blue (or boiled milk) into the external opening, and look for this flowing into his anus—finding the internal opening is the key to all fistula operations!

PROBING. Don't do this until you have finished your initial inspection. You may need to wait until he is anaesthetized. Decide where a track is probably going to go before you start probing. Pass the probe as far as possible towards his anal canal, and feel for its end in his anus. It may pass through into the lumen, or it may stop before getting there. If his fistula is superficial it will pass horizontally, if it is deep, the probe will pass almost vertically, parallel to his anus.

CAUTION ! (1) If the probe passes vertically, and not towards his mid anal canal (even though there is an opening there), he

ANAL FISTULAE

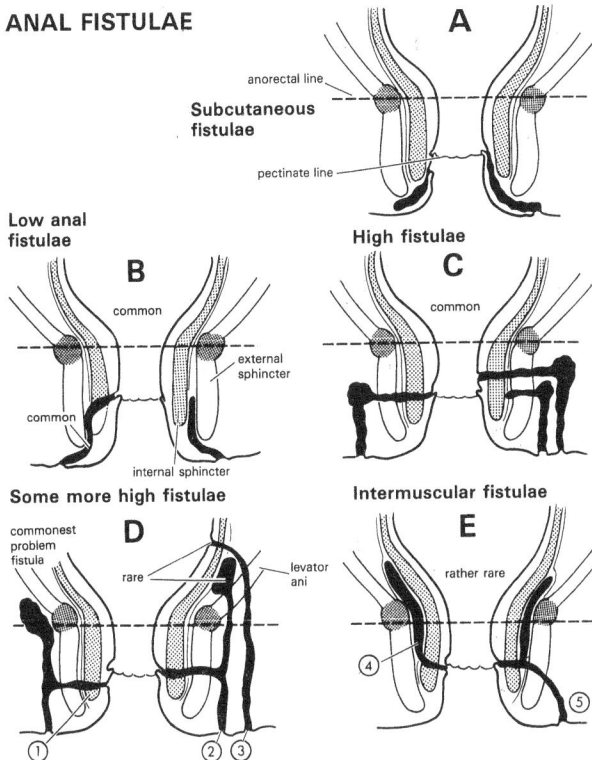

Fig. 22-5. PATTERNS OF FISTULAE. A, two subcutaneous fistulae, one opening at the pectinate line, and one just below it. B, two low anal fistulae. C, several high ones. D, some more high fistulae. Fistula (1) is the commonest high fistula; it goes high towards the levator ani, but does not penetrate it. The high extension is often missed, but it must be explored and laid open. Fistulae (2) and (3) penetrate the levator ani. E, high intermuscular fistulae (rare) may exist alone (4), or be an extension of a low anal fistula (5). *After Goligher JC, 'Surgery of the Anus, Rectum and Colon', (4th edn 1980) Figs. 121 to 126. Baillière Tindall, with kind permission.*

probably has a high complex fistula or a deep sinus. (2) Only pass a probe into the rectum through a fistulous track—don't force it through normal tissues.

DEROOFING AN ANAL FISTULA

INDICATIONS. You should now know where the fistula runs. *Only operate on the easier and more superficial fistulae.* The main risk is incontinence. Refer him if: (1) His fistula has multiple openings, unless you have had some experience with the operation. (2) He has had previous unsuccessful operations. (3) The probe passes vertically upwards. (4) His fistula is palpable in his upper anal canal, or above his anorectal ring (rare).

Other factors which increase the risk of subsequent incontinence are: (1) The liability to attacks of diarrhoea, or a history of soiling, which might indicate reduction of his sphincter capability. (2) A female patient, particularly if she is old.

EQUIPMENT. This includes a medium-sized malleable silver probe, or a probe-pointed director.

ANAESTHESIA. (1) Ketamine. (2) Light general anaesthesia. Avoid relaxants and subarachnoid anaesthesia. You want to be able to feel the anorectal ring, so as not to cut it. Muscular relaxation makes feeling it more difficult, but does provide better exposure.

A SUBCUTANEOUS OR LOW ANAL FISTULA. Carefully confirm the findings you obtained before you anaesthetized him. If you thought that his fistula was blind at the inner end (a sinus), confirm this. Pass a probe or director through the track, from the external opening towards his anal canal, either completely through to its lumen, or as far as it will go. It may enter his anal canal, or it may stop before doing so.

If the probe enters his anus superficial to his pectinate line, cut down on all structures superficial to it, and lay the track open. If you are using a director, cut down to the groove in it.

Look at the velvety track of the opened fistula. If there is no such track, you have probably opened up a false passage. Look carefully for any side openings, and feel among the fatty tissue for nodules of induration, that might be offshoots of the fistula. As a general rule, all fistulous tracks communicate with one another. Using a sharp spoon, curette the tracks, so as to leave only healthy tissue, and trim away any overhanging skin.

Alternatively, make a narrow pear-shaped incision to include both the internal and external openings. Excise both of them, and the track of tissue that still clings to the probe.

If the probe enters his anus deep to his pectinate line, leave the fistula untreated, or refer him. Even experts find these fistulae difficult.

CAUTION ! (1) Don't cut deep to his pectinate line, or you will cut too much sphincter. (2) When you cut down on to a probe or director, do so by the most direct route.

If the probe does not enter his anal canal, he has a sinus. Lay it open in the same way, but without opening into his anus.

A LOW ANAL FISTULA

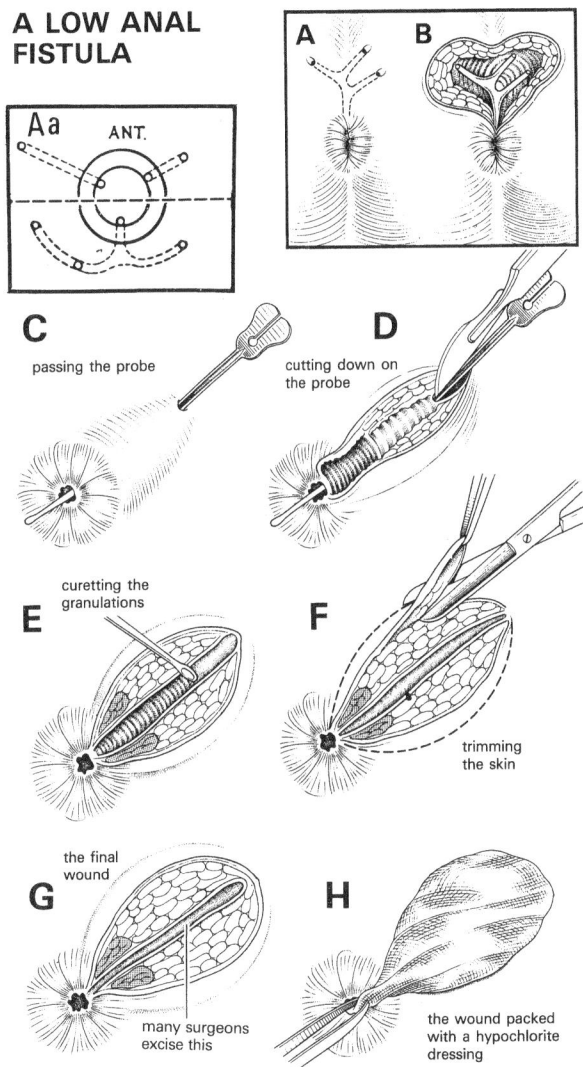

Fig. 22-6 A LOW ANAL FISTULA can have several tracks, as in A, and B, or only one, as in the remainder of these figures. Aa, Goodsall's rule. Fistulae above a horizontal line across the anus usually pass directly into it; fistulae behind the line usually curve round it to enter at 6 o'clock. C, passing a probe-pointed director along the track from the external to the internal opening, and out through the patient's anus. D, cutting down on the director. E, scraping away the granulation tissue with a sharp spoon. F, trimming the edges of the wound. G, the final pear-shaped guttered wound. If there is much fibrous tissue round the track, excise it. H, packing the wound with gauze soaked in hypochlorite. *After Goligher JC, 'Surgery of the Anus, Rectum and Colon', (4th edn 1980) Figs. 139 and 140, Baillière Tindall, with kind permission.*

A HIGH POSTERIOR HORSESHOE ISCHIORECTAL FISTULA

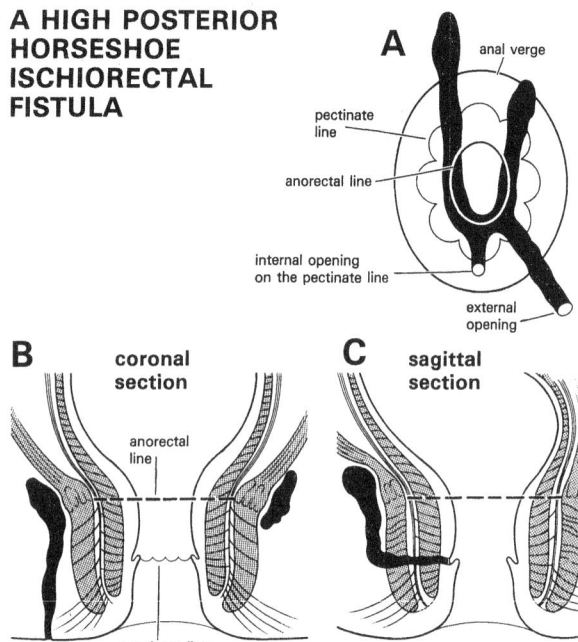

Fig. 22-7 A HIGH POSTERIOR HORSESHOE FISTULA—ONE. A, the fistula shown on a standard diagram of the anus. B, a coronal section. C, a sagittal section. This is the fistula that is being operated on in the next diagram. *After Goligher JC, 'Surgery of the Anus, Rectum and Colon', (4th edn 1980). Fig. 128, Baillière Tindall, with kind permission.*

weeks to heal, and an ischiorectal one 4 weeks. An extensive horseshoe fistula may take 12 weeks. If necessary, trim away any excess granulation tissue.

DIFFICULTIES WITH ANAL FISTULAE

If a FISTULA PASSES FORWARDS from his (or her) anus, it may be an URETHRAL FISTULA (23.8), or originate in Bartholin's glands (23.4).

If a FISTULA IS POSTERIOR, don't confuse it with a PILONIDAL SINUS (22.8). If it is low and immediately behind his anus, it may have arisen in an anal fissure.

If the EXTERNAL OPENING IS SOME DISTANCE FROM HIS ANUS, look out for a long curved fistula, or a high one. Its thickened track will usually show you its course and destination. Probe it, but don't expect it to enter his anus.

If his FISTULA EXTENDS UP THROUGH A HOLE IN HIS LEVATOR ANI, and you cannot refer him, pass a haemostat through the hole and stretch it. Enlarge the opening to provide free drainage. If necessary, cut backwards, laterally or forwards, but not medially. Enlarge the external wound by wide trimming, especially posteriorly, to provide a wide gutter, extending

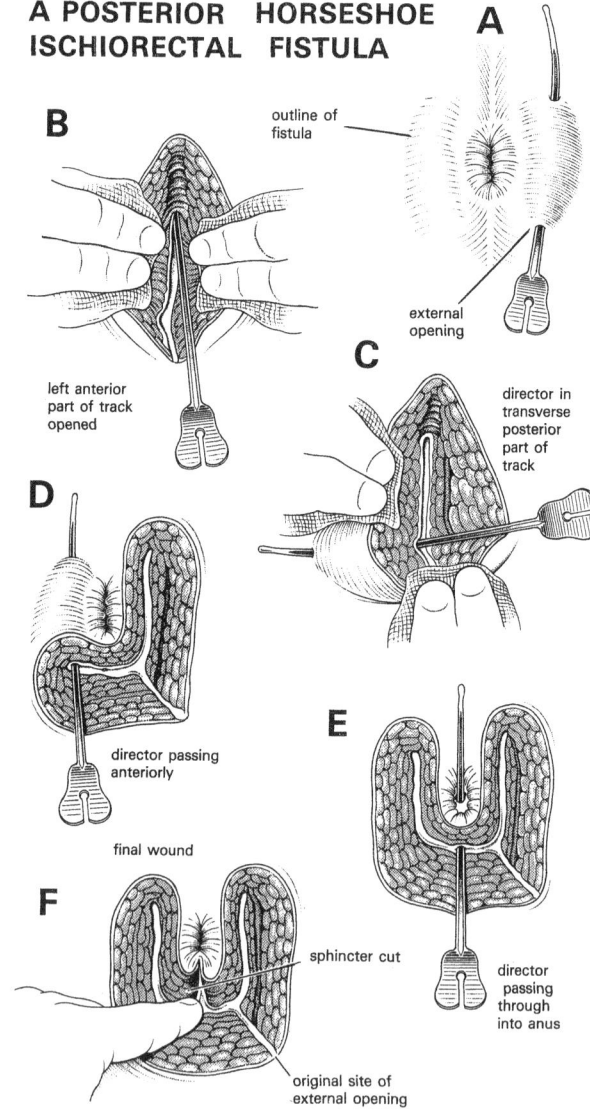

With all sinuses and fistulae, look, feel, and probe for other track openings and areas of induration. If you find any, open them and curette them. Curette the granulation tissue.

Control bleeding with diathermy, or tie off bleeding vessels with 2/0 plain catgut. Excise the skin edges and bevel them, so as to leave a conical or pear-shaped concave raw area. Be sure that there will be no pockets or overhanging edges, when muscle tone returns. If a fistula is complex, you will have to make a deep, wide wound.

Always send tissue for histology to exclude tuberculosis. Apply flat squares of gauze soaked in hypochlorite, or salt solution, pad it with plenty of gauze, and hold it in place with a T-bandage. Avoid vaseline gauze because it may cause a foreign body granuloma ('paraffinoma').

ISCHIORECTAL (horseshoe) FISTULAE usually have two or more external openings. Pass a director into an opening, and lay open one side at a time.

Point the director forwards, make it project against his skin at the side of his anus, and cut down on it. The track will be deeply overhung by fat; trim this. Turn the director posteriorly, and see if you can follow the track across to the other side, and then forwards on that side.

Now see if you can find the opening into his anus posteriorly. If you have seen a definite opening below his anorectal ring, encourage the director to follow it there, and lay the fistula open.

CAUTION ! (1) Most of these fistulae have a posterior opening close to the pectinate line, and if you miss it and don't lay it open, the fistula will recur. If you don't find such an opening, make one. (2) Lay open all side tracks.

If oozing is a problem, apply pressure from adrenalin soaked gauze. Gutter, trim and dress the wound as above. If his fistula is complex and deep, feel it with your gloved finger each day, to keep the edge of the granulating wound smooth, and to make sure that no deep pockets are left, which would lead to recurrent infection. Lay a flat gauze square on it. If you are worried about the way it is healing, take him back to the theatre and further lay the wound open.

POSTOPERATIVE CARE is the same as for any granulating anal wound, with daily, or twice daily, salt baths (sitting in a bowl of saline), regular dressing changes, and measures to ensure soft stools. Warn him that a perianal fistula may take 2

Fig. 22-8 A HIGH POSTERIOR HORSESHOE FISTULA—TWO. This is the fistula in Fig. 22-7. A, passing the director forwards. B, cutting down on the track on the left side. C, passing the director along the posterior part of the track towards the right. D, exposing the track on the right side. E, passing the director forwards through the posterior communication into the patient's anus. G, the final horseshoe-shaped wound, with part of his sphincter divided. *After Goligher JC, 'Surgery of the Anus, Rectum and Colon', (4th end 1980). Fig. 147, Baillière Tindall, with kind permission.*

backwards towards the side of his coccyx. Provided there is no internal opening above his levator ani, or chronic pelvic disease, such as regional ileitis, his prognosis is good.

CAUTION ! Don't look for an opening in his rectum, there almost never is one, unless the cause of the fistula was a penetrating injury.

If you find a HIGH INTERMUSCULAR FISTULA (submucous fistula, unusual), leave it. If it really is submucous, it can be opened into his rectum, but if it happens to be outside his rectal wall, and you cut into it, this will be a disaster.

If he also has PILES, excise them, or they may thrombose and bleed postoperatively. Or, if they are first-degree, do Lord's procedure (22.5), and leave his anus packed.

If he has RECURRENT DISCHARGE FROM THE TRACK, his wound has healed over externally, without healing from below. Operate again. It will not heal with antibiotics. Also consider the possibility of tuberculosis.

If he has ULCERATIVE COLITIS, or CROHN'S DISEASE (both uncommon in the developing world), he is a special case, so refer him.

If there is GREAT NODULAR THICKENING of his subcutaneous tissue, purplish discoloration (in a white skin), numerous sinuses which seldom discharge much pus, and no real cavity or track, suspect SUPPURATIVE HIDRADENITIS (rare).

If he, or more likely she, has MULTIPLE FISTULAE with much scarring and skin bridges between them, suspect LYMPHOGRANULOMA VENEREUM (22.10) or colloid carcinoma of the anus.

22.3 Rectal bleeding

A patient who bleeds severely from his stomach or duodenum, usually vomits the blood, if he bleeds fast. If he bleeds more slowly, it appears as black tarry melaena stools. The higher the source of the blood, the longer it takes to reach his rectum, and the more likely is it to be converted into melaena stools. Although a melaena stool is usually the result of bleeding from his stomach or his duodenum, it can follow bleeding from his small gut. Dark red 'burgundy-coloured' blood mixed with stool can come from the stomach, the duodenum, the small or the large gut, but fresh bright-red blood usually comes from the rectum or anus. Not all dark stools are the result of bleeding, so remember the possibility of iron medication (negative occult blood test), or nose bleeds (often positive for occult blood).

Bleeding from the upper gut is often severe, is usually more serious than it looks, and frequently threatens his life (11.3). Bleeding from the lower gut is often mild, and even a small quantity of bright blood can be alarming. He is usually not as ill as he seems, and you have more time to investigate him.

Rectal bleeding is common everywhere, but its causes differ geographically. In the developing world, where carcinoma is still comparatively unusual, you can treat most patients with rectal bleeding quite easily.

If he continues to bleed from his rectum, and you are not sure why, you will have to decide: (1) if you are going to operate, (2) when, and (3) what you are going to do when you get inside. In most areas, the commonest cause of massive rectal bleeding is a peptic or duodenal ulcer; but in some tropical areas it is bleeding from the terminal ileum, or ascending colon, due to typhoid or amoebiasis.

The major mistakes are: (1) To misjudge the severity of his bleeding. (2) To fail to use your finger, a proctoscope and a sigmoidoscope, to label him as having 'piles' without examining him properly, to fail to investigate him, and so to miss a carcinoma. (3) To miss the more treatable diseases, such as tuberculosis and amoebiasis, as the following case shows.

POUL (53) had passed several bloody stools since the morning, but had no other gastrointestinal symptoms. He was neither anaemic nor hypotensive, but during the next few days he continued to bleed, and his haematocrit fell to 23%. Sigmoidoscopy showed friable, oedematous, reddish-yellow areas in his rectum, but no obvious ulcers. A smear from his rectal mucosa showed amoebae. Metronidazole cured him dramatically. LESSONS (1) Amoebiasis is readily treatable—if you diagnose it. (2) A severe bleed in the absence of previous symptoms of amoebiasis is unusual.

THE GENERAL METHOD FOR RECTAL BLEEDING

See also Section 11.3.

COMMON CAUSES (other than piles 22.4). Peptic ulcer (11.3). Typhoid ulcers of the ileum (bleeding may be severe, 31.8). Amoebiasis (31.10). Schistosomiasis *mansoni.* Bacillary dysentery (diarrhoea with blood and mucus, 31.10). Anal fissures (which may bleed at defaecation, 22.7). Lymphogranuloma (22.10). Polyps, especially juvenile polyps (usually producing a little fresh blood, see below). Intussusception ('red currant jelly stools', 10.8). Also causes of high gastrointestinal bleeding (11.3).

UNCOMMON CAUSES. Carcinomas of the colon, rectum, or anal canal (32.27), tuberculous ulcers of the gut (29.5), non-specific ulcers of the gut (see below), pigbel disease (31.9), Meckel's diverticulum (episodic massive bleeding in the young, 28.5), rectal prolapse (22.9).

RARE CAUSES. Ulcerative colitis, ischaemic colitis, diverticulitis, haemangiomas of the small gut, blood dyscrasias, villous adenomas of the rectum (bright blood with much watery mucus). A foreign body in the rectum.

EXAMINATION. (1) Assess the degree of the patient's hypovolaemia (53.2), and the severity of his anaemia. Does sitting him up in bed make him feel faint, or exercise make him breathless? Examine him for epigastric tenderness, distension, the signs of subacute gut obstruction (10.3), and abdominal masses.

Examine his rectum with your finger and a proctoscope, and don't forget to look at his stool.

CAUTION ! Never forget to do a sigmoidoscopy if an adult presents with rectal bleeding.

DIFFERENTIAL DIAGNOSIS. Bleeding related to defaecation? (an anal or rectal lesion). Blood mixed with stool? (some lesion higher than the rectum). Painful bleeding? (a lesion below the pectinate line; piles arise above this line and are painless, unless they prolapse or strangulate). A feeling of something prolapsing from the rectum? (piles, prolapse, or polyps). Dyspepsia, heartburn, etc.? (peptic ulceration, 11.1). High fever for a week or two? (typhoid fever, 31.8). Loss of weight, anorexia, night sweats, and fatigue? (abdominal tuberculosis; rectal bleeding is unusual 29.5). Vague lower abdominal pain followed by the passage of much dark blood? (non-specific ulceration of the gut, 22.10). Abdominal pain, diarrhoea, fever, prostration? (non-occlusive infarction of the gut, pigbel disease, 31.9).

THE INDICATIONS FOR LAPAROTOMY. (1) Loss of > 1500 ml of blood. If he is *in extremis,* surgery may be life saving. (2) The presence of a mass. The treatment of most causes of rectal bleeding is discussed elsewhere. Most colonic bleeding stops on its own, so don't operate too early.

RESUSCITATION. Replace the blood he has lost, with due regard to the dangers of HIV (28a.2).

ANAESTHESIA. General anaesthesia.

LAPAROTOMY. Enter his abdomen through a long midline incision. Exclude more common causes of bleeding, such as peptic ulceration, then examine his entire gut from his duodeno–jejunal junction down to his rectum. Note the colour of the contents of his gut. What is the highest site in his gut to show bleeding? Look for abnormal vessels going to the bleeding area, and feel for induration or an ulcer. If necessary, do a gastrotomy and enterotomies (open his gut, 9.3) to find the level of the bleeding.

If he is bleeding severely from his right colon, you don't find a lesion, and there is no bleeding more proximally, consider doing a 'blind' right hemicolectomy (66-20). This will not be easy, so don't do it lightly. Afterwards, open the specimen to see where the blood is coming from.

DIFFICULTIES WITH RECTAL BLEEDING

If a CHILD HAS INTERMITTENT CONTINUING RECTAL

BLEEDING, he may have a JUVENILE POLYP. This is a friable, proliferative mass, which lies on his mucosa to begin with, and then develops a stalk. On rectal examination you can usually feel a soft, mobile, pedunculated mass, and see a strawberry-like lesion through a proctoscope or sigmoidoscope. If examination is difficult, you may have to anaesthetize him to examine it.

If a polyp is small, remove it through his anus, tie the stalk, and cut it off. If you cut the stalk without tying it first, it may bleed massively. Or, if tying it is impracticable, leave it to undergo spontaneous strangulation, necrosis, and sloughing.

If the cause of a patient's RECTAL BLEEDING IS NOT IMMEDIATELY OBVIOUS, consider the possibility of NON-SPECIFIC ULCERATION OF THE GUT (uncommon). In the tropics patients sometimes bleed from small punched-out ulcers of unknown cause in the mucosa of their distal ileum and proximal colon. They are usually middle-aged adults of either sex, who present with lower abdominal pain and fever, followed by the passage of a quantity of dark blood rectally. He may be tender in his right iliac fossa; sigmoidoscopy is normal, except for blood coming from above. If bleeding does not stop and you are sufficiently skilled, a right hemicolectomy may save him, because the source of the bleeding is nearly always in his distal ileum, or proximal colon. In good hands he has a 10% chance of death.

His distal ileum and colon are likely to be discoloured by contained blood, and feel slightly oedematous and thickened. The ulcers in his mucosa are rarely palpable.

If you have established the source of the bleeding, and think you could remove it, do an extended right hemicolectomy, and take the last 20 cm of his ileum, his ascending colon, and his entire transverse colon up to his splenic flexure. Do an end to end ileo-transverse anastomosis in two layers.

Open the specimen, and you will find numerous punched-out ulcers in his terminal ileum and right colon, one of which may contain a bleeding artery. Histology shows non-specific changes only, with very little inflammation round the ulcers.

If he has RECTAL BLEEDING ACCOMPANIED BY SEVERE DIARRHOEA, PROSTRATION, vomiting, and fever, consider the possibility of pigbel disease, and see Section 31.9.

22.4 Piles

If the vascular lining of a patient's anal canal becomes swollen and starts to protrude, he has piles. These are common in the industrial world, but are less often seen in patients on high-residue traditional diets. They usually form in the 3, 7, and 11 o'clock positions (when he is in the lithotomy position), and although they usually cause no symptoms, they can bleed and make him severely anaemic; they can prolapse, and they can thrombose and become very painful. Untreated, they eventually shrink to form harmless skin tags.

He may complain of bleeding, of 'something coming down', of a mucus discharge, or of pruritus. If he has diagnosed himself, and says that he has piles, enquire how they affect him. Piles are the commonest cause of rectal bleeding, which is usually painless, bright red, and either streaks the stool, or follows after it. Carcinoma of the colon is the most important differential diagnosis, so exclude this by *always* sigmoidoscoping anyone with rectal bleeding, even in the developing world where carcinoma is uncommon; *even if he has piles*—he may have both!

Piles are reversible in their early stages, and may respond to a high-residue diet, or to dilatation of his anal sphincter. If they are very large and have been present for a long time, you will have to excise them. Never fail to examine him, and remember that ointments are seldom a sufficient treatment.

PILES

EXAMINATION. You can see piles through a proctoscope, but only the patient can tell you if they bleed, or prolapse on defecation, if they retract spontaneously, or if he has to replace them. There are 3 degrees of piles.

First degree piles usually only cause bleeding, and don't prolapse from his anus, so you cannot see them merely by looking at it.

Second degree piles prolapse on defecation, but return spontaneously afterwards. They form distinct swellings at the three main positions. If you pull gently, you may be able to draw them down.

Third degree piles prolapse on defecation, and don't return spontaneously, so that he has to push them back. They form large projecting lumps, their outer parts covered with skin, and their inner parts with purple anal mucosa, separated by a groove.

DIGITAL EXAMINATION is not enough by itself for diagnosing piles, because you cannot usually feel them with your finger. If, however, a pile has been present for some time, you may feel it as a soft longitudinal projection, as you sweep your finger round his anus.

PROCTOSCOPY is the only satisfactory way to diagnose piles. They bulge into a proctoscope like grapes, as you withdraw it and ask him to bear down. Withdraw it just to his anus, and then ask him to continue straining.

If no red mucosa projects beyond his anal verge, his piles are first degree.

If they do project, they are second or third degree.

If they remain prolapsed when he stops straining, and you have to push them back, they are third degree.

SIGMOIDOSCOPY must be done routinely to look for carcinoma, especially if he is over forty and from the industrial world; it is desirable in the developing world. If he presented with bleeding, and you cannot see any piles, it is *essential!!*

INTERNAL PILES

If his symptoms are mild, or merely consist of bleeding, simple measures are usually enough. If he is not already on a high-residue diet, persuade him to eat one. Treat constipation with stool-softeners. If his piles have appeared in association with an attack of diarrhoea, they will probably go as his diarrhoea resolves. If necessary, treat it.

CAUTION ! Don't treat piles, unless they cause symptoms (anaemia for example) that need treating. They often remain asymptomatic for many years. One patient may have classical third degree piles, but no symptoms. Another may collapse from hypovolaemic shock with only first degree piles.

If piles prolapse, the above measures are unlikely to be adequate, so see below for the indications for Lord's anal stretch (22.5), and ligation and excision (22.6).

If he has acutely painful, bluish, fixed swellings at his anus, which make sitting or defecation painful, his piles have probably been squeezed by his internal sphincter, so that they have thrombosed, ulcerated, strangulated, or become gangrenous. Digital examination is painful, and proctoscopy impossible. He may refer to his symptoms as 'an attack of piles'. One differential diagnosis is a 'thrombosed external pile', see below.

If the symptoms from his prolapsed piles are mild, **give him a rubber glove and some analgesic ointment, and ask him to return them to his anus himself.** This, combined with baths, may enable him to overcome his acute attack.

If the symptoms from his prolapsed piles are severe, **bath him and wash the mass.** A warm bath is remarkably soothing. Put him to bed, raise its foot steeply, and give him morphine. Apply a large moist gauze dressing to his anus, and hold it with firm pressure in a T–bandage. Some surgeons apply an ice pack. Don't worry about his bowels for a few days.

Lord's anal stretch under anaesthesia is very good for the early painful stages, and relieves pain, even though his piles remain prolapsed; it may make them resolve more quickly.

The mass will shrink over about a week. Thrombosis leading to fibrosis may cure his symptoms, so that he needs no further treatment. If it does not, excise his piles (22.6) when his oedema has settled.

CAUTION ! Don't: (1) Try to incise thrombosed internal piles, or (2) try to excise them immediately.

If a thrombosed pile fibroses, it may present as a pedunculated fibrous polyp (unusual). Excise it.

If a thrombosed pile becomes infected, treat him with antibiotics, if necessary (rare). Tie and excise his piles as soon as the infection has subsided.

LORD'S ANAL STRETCH — ONE

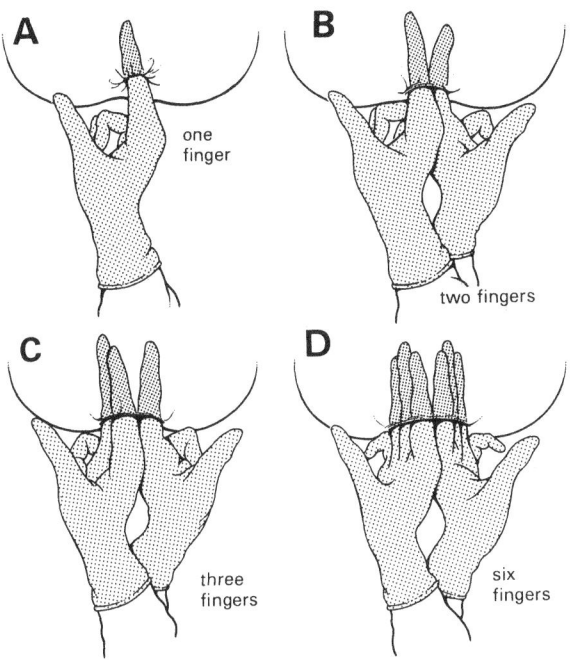

Fig. 22-9 LORD'S ANAL STRETCH—ONE will cure many cases of piles and anal fissures. First, do a digital examination with your right index finger, then introduce two fingers, side by side. Stretch hard, and then put four fingers in. *Dilate the patient's anus gradually over 3 or 4 minutes, so that the sphincters of his anus are stretched, and not torn. Finally, put six or eight of your fingers in.*

If he is admitted because of severely bleeding piles, exclude a bleeding diathesis (measure his bleeding and clotting time) or anticoagulant treatment. Put him to bed, give him morphine, and transfuse him. Many bleeding piles are cured by Lord's anal stretch alone, if they are of first degree, or small second degree. The patients who bleed severely are usually the younger ones with tight anal sphincters.

EXTERNAL PILES

If he presents with a painful anus, and you find a small (0.5 to 1 cm), tense, black, acutely tender swelling just outside his anal verge, it is a thrombosed external pile. First, make sure it is an external pile, and not a thrombosed internal pile, which has prolapsed from higher up. It will probably resolve spontaneously in a week, and eventually become a skin tag.

If you see him within 36 hours, use a fine needle to infiltrate the skin around it with lignocaine, bisect it, squeeze out the clot, and excise it together with 1.25 cm of his adjacent skin. His pain will go immediately. Apply vaseline gauze, and let the pear-shaped wound granulate.

22.5 Lord's anal stretch

If a patient has second degree piles, you have a choice of two procedures: (1) Lord's anal stretch, and (2) excision and ligation. Piles are probably the result of an unduly tight anal sphincter, which may be associated with bands of rigid tissue in his anus. Lord's operation dilates his sphincter and breaks these bands. The indications for it, and for those tying and excising piles are important, and are given below, so follow them with the greatest care. They include the readiness of his piles to prolapse, his age, and the tightness of his anal sphincter. Lord's operation is one of the simplest in surgery. Anaesthetize him, put your fingers into his anus, gradually stretch it, and his piles will be cured. He need only be in hospital for a few hours, so that you can treat him as an outpatient. Tying and excising his piles will keep him in hospital for up to ten days.

LORD'S ANAL STRETCH

INDICATIONS. (1) Piles which prolapse when a patient defecates, after which they either return spontaneously, or he has to push them back. The operation is particularly likely to be successful if he is under 50, and has a tight sphincter, and a history of painful defecation. (2) Acutely prolapsed and strangulated piles. (3) First or second degree piles which are bleeding heavily, especially if he has a tight sphincter. (4) Anal fissure, including an associated anal tag. (5) Constipation caused by a tight anal sphincter. (6) Always dilate his anus after you have have done a colostomy for obstruction, or a resection and anastomosis.

CONTRAINDICATIONS. (1) Piles which prolapse when he walks, sneezes, coughs, exercises vigorously, or passes wind. (2) Piles which are prolapsed most of the time (third degree). (3) A loose sphincter—*never* stretch his sphincter, unless you can feel some tightness in his anal canal—there is no point in doing so otherwise, and it may impair his continence. (4) Chronic diarrhoea.

The operation is less likely to be successful if he is over 50, and he is more likely to suffer from incontinence of wind, or occasionally faeces. Bleeding piles are not a contraindication.

ANAESTHESIA. (1) General anaesthesia, preferably but not necessarily with relaxants is best. (2) Ketamine (A 8.2). (3) Caudal block (A 7.6).

POSITION. If you are using subarachnoid anaesthesia his position immediately after its injection is important—see A 7.6. As soon as the anaesthetic solution has been fixed (about 10 minutes), lay him on his back with his legs up in stirrups, and give the table a slight head-down tilt.

Alternatively, if your anaesthetist is more skilled, lay him on his left side.

SIGMOIDOSCOPY OR PROCTOSCOPY should always follow a careful digital examination. If you don't do this, you may fail to diagnose carcinoma of his rectum.

FEEL FOR THE CONSTRICTING BAND. First, do a digital examination with your right index finger. Insert two fingers of your left hand and pull upwards, and one finger of your right hand and pull downwards, if he is in the lateral position, as in A, Fig. 22-10. Feel for the constricting band, which is usually at the level of his anorectal line (22-1). If his anus feels tight, dilatation is likely to be successful. If it feels loose, proceed to haemorrhoidectomy (22.6).

DILATATION must be gentle and controlled. Start by introducing the index fingers of each hand, then gradually insert more fingers as you overcome the constriction. *Put the strain on the constricting bands in the right and left lateral positions, in the 3 and 9 o'clock positions.* Try to avoid damaging his sphincter at 12 o'clock, and especially at 6 o'clock, where it is weaker. Stretch hard and then

LORD'S ANAL STRETCH—TWO

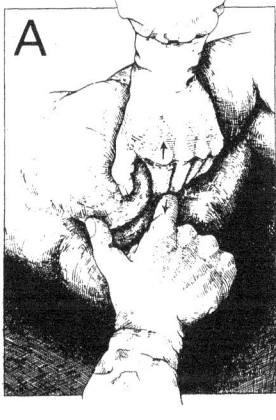

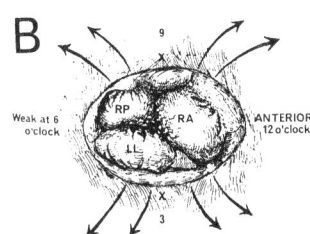

Fig. 22-10 LORD'S ANAL STRETCH—TWO. A, identifying the constriction. B, the direction of dilatation. Pull laterally and avoid the weak 12 and 6 o'clock positions. *After Peter Lord in Rob C and Smith R, 'Operative Surgery: Part 1: Abdomen, Rectum and anus; (2nd edn 1969), (Butterworth) with kind the permission of Hugh Dudley.*

put four fingers in. *Dilate his anus gradually over 3 or 4 minutes, so that the fibres of his sphincter are stretched, and not torn.* Usually, you can insert six or eight of your fingers. The tighter his anus, the more you should stretch it. You may feel constrictions in his lower rectum, as high as your fingers can reach. Make these give way laterally. You should be able to see well up his rectum between your two hands. He may bleed a little, but he will not bleed severely.

CAUTION ! (1) The necessary degree of dilatation varies, and it is better to dilate too little rather than too much. (2) The more severe degrees of dilatation are not indicated for anal fissures (22.7). For a fissure 'four fingers for four minutes' is enough.

Some surgeons put a pack in his anus to minimize haematoma formation, some give him a dilator, others do nothing. If his piles prolapse after the stretch, apply a pad and T-bandage to keep them in place.

Give him 20 ml of liquid paraffin daily for 10 days to soften his stools. There is no need for him to use a dilator. You can usually send him home on the same day.

If you have operated for piles, advise him to eat a high-residue diet.

DIFFICULTIES WITH LORD'S PROCEDURE

If he is INCONTINENT OF FLATUS, reassure him that this will pass off in for a few days to a few weeks.

If he FEELS UNSURE OF HIS SPHINCTER MECHANISM, reassure him. If his outlet was previously very tight, he will need to get used to its new condition. Encourage him, and ask him to do sphincter exercises for a few weeks.

If FAECES STAINED MUCUS escapes from his anus at the 6 o'clock position, causing soiling and soreness (keyhole deformity of the anus, rare), avoid producing it in future by making sure that the strain of dilatation is thrown on the lateral aspects of the anus.

If there is BRUISING, reassure him. It may be extensive.

If his PILES THROMBOSE postoperatively, with much swelling and soreness, reassure him. His symptoms will settle and the result will be excellent.

If his rectal mucosa or a LARGE PILE PROLAPSES postoperatively, and is troublesome, anaesthetize him, clamp the redundant mucosa, and cut it off distal to the clamp. Tape the clamp to his buttocks. Return him to the ward. Remove the clamp an hour later. Or, do nothing, except wait for a few weeks, and then do a haemorrhoidectomy if his piles are still troublesome.

If his PILES RECUR, excise them, do another maximal dilatation of his anus, and excise any skin tags. There is about a 25% chance of recurrence on the first occasion.

22.6 Tying and excising piles

If a patient has piles which prolapse while he walks, or during such activities as digging in his fields, they are too advanced for Lord's operation. Such patients are rare, and form only about 10% of those who present with piles. The alternatives are injection, which is only palliative, and difficult to do well; the application of rubber bands, which needs special equipment, or tying and excision. Tie and excise each of his three piles, together with a triangle of his perianal skin. This is not difficult, but be sure to leave bridges of mucosa between each pile. If you don't, a stricture may form.

MILLIGAN'S HAEMORRHOIDECTOMY

INDICATIONS. Piles which are unsuitable for Lord's procedure on the indications given in Section 22.5. These are: (1) Piles which prolapse while a patient is walking, sneezing, coughing, exercising vigorously, or passing wind. (2) Piles which are prolapsed most of the time, or are permanently prolapsed (third degree). (3) Patients with second degree piles, but with a loose sphincter, which makes them unsuitable for Lord's operation, particularly older patients.

CONTRAINDICATIONS. (1) Septic piles. (2) Acutely thrombosed piles, because it is easy to remove too much mucosa.

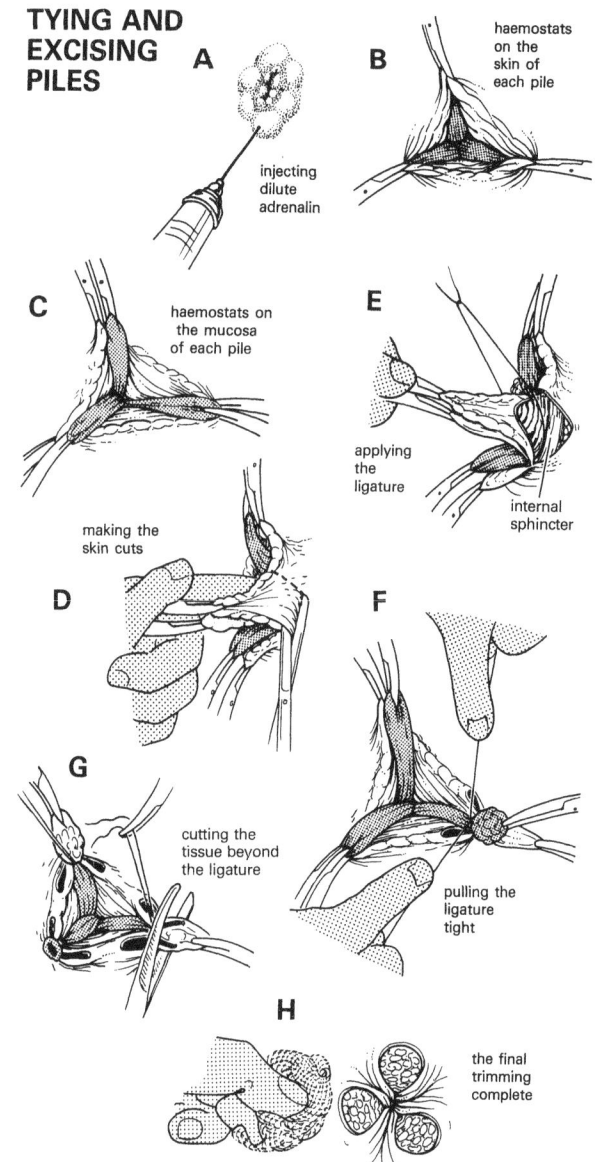

Fig. 22-11 TYING AND EXCISING PILES. A, inject adrenalin in saline to control bleeding. B, apply forceps to the skin of each primary pile. C, apply a second pair of forceps to the mucosa-covered part of each pile. D, make the skin cuts for the 3 o'clock pile. E, nick the mucocutaneous junction at the neck of each pile and tie it. F, pull strongly as you tie a pile, release the forceps as you do so, and allow the ligature to sink into the tissues. G, after you have tied all three piles, excise the 7 o'clock and then the 3 o'clock pile, taking care to leave adequate stumps. H, the final skin wounds have been trimmed. *After Goligher JC, from 'Surgery of the Anus Rectum and Colon', (4th edn 1980) Figs. 80 to 87, Baillière Tindall, with kind permission.*

ANAESTHESIA. (1) General anaesthesia, ether (A 11.3). Relaxation is useful. (2) Caudal block (A 7.6). (3) Ketamine may be adequate (A 8.2).

POSITION AND PREPARATION. Put him into the lithotomy position, with his buttocks well beyond the end of the table. A sandbag under his sacrum helps exposure. Clean his anal region, and arrange the instruments and towels as in Fig. 22-4.

Do a careful digital examination to make sure that he really does have no other pathology. Sigmoidoscope him if you have not already done so.

Some surgeons infiltrate the subcutaneous tissues round his anus with 1:100 000 adrenalin in saline or lignocaine (A, in Fig. 22-11). The adrenalin reduces bleeding, and the lignocaine reduces postoperative pain. Others prefer not to use it, saying that it increases the incidence of reactionary bleeding afterwards. It you decide to use it, insert the needle in the midline, and deposit 15–20 ml in the subcutaneous tissues on either side of his anus.

Push some dry gauze into his rectum, and slowly pull it out. His piles will prolapse with it.

Grasp the skin at the mucocutaneous junction of each pile with haemostats, and pull them outwards (B). This will make their mucosa covered parts protrude.

Take the purple mucosa covered part of each pile in other larger haemostats, and draw them downwards and outwards. This will bring all three piles well out of his anus, so that you see his pink rectal mucosa at their upper ends (C).

Pull on all three piles until you see the rectal mucosa, not only at the upper end of each pile, but also between them. The piles have now been drawn down as far as they will go, which will allow you to tie them at their upper poles, rather than around their middles.

The 3 o'clock or left lateral pile. Grasp the two haemostats attached to this pile in your left hand. Draw them down towards the opposite side, while your index finger rests in his anal canal, and presses downwards and outwards on the pile. Using blunt scissors in your right hand, make a V-shaped cut in his anal and perianal skin opposite this pile (D). The ends of the V should reach the mucocutaneous junction, but not extend into the mucosa beyond it. The point of the V should lie 2.5 to 3 cm from the junction.

If you press your index finger firmly against the end of the scissors as you cut, you will see the lower edge of his internal sphincter laid bare. This is a firm, whitish ring which should be clearly visible. If you hold the pile aside (E), you will see it quite clearly.

Make a slight nick in the mucosa above and below the narrow mucosal pedicle.

Transfix the pedicle of each pile using a 30 cm strand of No. 16 braided silk. Alternatively, use No. 3 chromic catgut, but transfix the pile, because it will be more likely to slip off. As you tie the pile, remove the haemostat grasping its mucosa, and use it to hold the ends of the ligature. Hand both pairs of haemostats to your assistant, and ask him to retract them laterally (F).

CAUTION ! A slipped ligature can cause fearsome bleeding!

The 7 o'clock or right posterior pile. Treat this in the same way. Hold the pile forceps with your right hand and make the scissor cuts with your left hand. When you make your cut, note the position of the cut you made for the 3 o'clock pile, and *make sure you leave a good skin bridge and a bridge of intact mucosa* running into his anal canal.

The 11 o'clock pile. Treat this similarly, being sure to preserve bridges of skin and mucosa between it and his other piles.

Excision. Now excise all three piles, leaving at least 1 cm of tissue beyond the ligatures (G). As you cut the ligatures short, the stumps of the piles will disappear inside his anal canal.

Pass your finger into his anus to assess the tightness of his anal canal. If it is tight, stretch it to four fingers, which may lessen postoperative pain.

Push some dry gauze into his anus, while you examine his skin wounds. Trim any loose edges with scissors, to leave three flat pear-shaped raw areas. The end result should look like a clover leaf ("If it looks like a dahlia it's a failure!")

Pass a lubricated speculum and look at the ligatures. Control all bleeding, either with more ligatures, or with diathermy. Don't allow blood to pool in his rectum. Oozing will stop spontaneously, but all spurting vessels must be picked up and tied, however small.

Apply a hypochlorite or saline dressing, or vaseline gauze, to his anus, and cover this with plenty of dry gauze and cotton wool. Hold it in place with a T-bandage. Start salt baths (22.1) on the first or second day. Let him remove his own dressing in the bath.

If he has passed no stool by the third day, do a rectal examination, and if he has faeces in his rectum, give him a glycerine suppository.

CAUTION ! (1) Always leave mucosal bridges between the excised piles. (2) Do a rectal examination before discharging him to make sure that: (a) His faeces are not impacted, and (b) that he is not developing a stricture. If he is, he must pass a dilator every day. Many surgeons postpone this examination until the second week.

DIFFICULTIES WITH HAEMORRHOIDECTOMY

If he has has ACCESSORY PILES, only excise the main ones, so that that you only make three skin wounds.

CAUTION ! Be careful not to take too much anal mucosa: it is better to leave secondary piles alone.

If he has an associated ANAL FISSURE, treat it by by stretching it with your fingers (Lord's procedure). There is no need to excise it. Large piles and fissures are seldom seen in the same patient.

If he has postoperative PAIN, give him pethidine. If severe pain follows defaecation, a hot bath will soothe it.

If he has DIFFICULTY PASSING URINE postoperatively, try giving him pethidine, or ask him to stand while he passes it. If this fails, give him subcutaneous carbachol 0.5 mg, and ask him to try again in 15 minutes. Only if his fails, catheterize him, and remove the catheter after 48 hours. Or, do a suprapubic aspiration.

If he BLEEDS WITHIN 12 HOURS (reactionary haemorrhage), you may be able to secure the vessel with artery forceps in the ward. If this fails, return him to the theatre, reanaesthetize him, and tie it there.

If he BLEEDS BETWEEN 7 AND 10 DAYS (secondary haemorrhage), he may bleed into his rectum and pass clotted blood with his next stool. Bleeding may stop spontaneously; if it does not, try pushing a lubricated, adrenalin-soaked pack into his anus and lower rectum. If this is inadequate or impractical, insert a large Foley catheter, inflate it, tie a weight to it, and exert traction on the bleeding site. Maintain traction for 3 days. Thereafter, keep his stools soft. Return him to the theatre only as a last resort.

If you FORGOT TO LEAVE BRIDGES OF SKIN AND MUCOSA between his piles, so that his rectal mucosa has retracted up his anus, pull it down and suture it to his perianal skin. He will probably recover uneventfully, but watch for a stricture.

If he develops a STRICTURE (unusual), you probably did not leave adequate bridges of tissue between his excised piles. Provide him with an anal dilator. If you don't have one, he can use a banana, but he must use it with a lubricant.

22.7 Anal fissure

An anal fissure causes suffering out of all proportion to its size. It starts as a crack in the lower part of a patient's anal canal, which makes defaecation, and the half-hour following it, acutely painful. Even the thought of a bowel movement may fill him with such fear that he ignores the urge, so that the hard constipated stools that he eventually passes make his fissure worse, and may occasionally make it bleed.

You will almost always find his fissure posteriorly in the 6 o'clock position, between his anal verge and his pectinate line, directly over the distal end of his internal sphincter. A small oedematous skin tag commonly forms on his anal verge, just posterior to the fissure. This is the 'sentinel skin tag'. Later, his fissure may become indurated and infected, and may lead to a low perianal abscess (5.13), which may discharge through the fissure, and externally, to produce a low anal fistula. His internal sphincter lies directly under his fissure, and after several months of exposure this becomes fibrosed and spastic.

ANAL FISSURE

DIAGNOSIS. A fissure is acutely painful, so don't do a rectal examination, or pass a proctoscope, until the patient is under general anaesthesia. Alternatively, and less satisfactorily, smear his anus with 10% amethocaine ointment for 10 minutes. Can you see a sentinel skin tag? Look for a triangular or pear-shaped slit posteriorly, just inside his anus.

DIFFERENTIAL DIAGNOSIS Other obvious skin changes and cracks? (pruritus ani). Diarrhoea with multiple fistulae away from the midline? (the skin changes following some forms of colitis). More induration than in a fissure, a larger ulcer, and perhaps enlarged inguinal nodes? (carcinoma). Indurated margins, a symmetrical lesion on the opposite margin of his anal canal, and no pain? (primary chancre). The whole region is moist and pruritic, with flat, slightly-raised lesions, which are usually symmetrical on both sides? (secondary syphilis).

TREATMENT depends on how long he has had his fissure. Early presentation is unusual in the developing world.

If it is acute (less than 10 days old), only his epithelium is involved. It may heal, if you keep his stools soft for a week or two with liquid paraffin. When it has healed, warn him that it may return, if he allows himself to become constipated. He may have to continue this treatment indefinitely. Warn him that he must not keep his stools too loose, or they will never dilate his anus, so that it stenoses.

If you give him a local anaesthetic ointment (5% lignocaine), ask him to smear it over the sphincter inside his anus, not outside it.

If, his fissure fails to heal after you have kept his stools soft for 3 weeks, stretch his anus (22.5). Unfortunately the relapse rate with non-operative treatment is high, even if a fissure does heal at first.

If his fissure is chronic (more than 10 days), fibrosed, has a sentinel skin tag, and especially if you can see the exposed fibres of his internal sphincter under it, it will probably not respond to non-operative treatment. First try stretching his anus (22.5). After a day or two, there is a 95% chance that he will be completely free of pain. There is a 15% chance that his fissure will recur later. If it does, don't repeat the stretching, refer him for sphincterotomy.

22.8 Pilonidal infections

The hairs from a patient's back sometimes work their way into the skin of his natal cleft and form a sinus or fistula, just behind his anus. These sinuses are very rare indeed in Indians and Africans.

He is usually a young man who presents with an abscess in his natal cleft. A history of "recurring abscesses at the base of his spine" is almost diagnostic. Incising his abscess may cure him, or he may get others.

Look also for one or more openings, sometimes with hairs coming out of them, exactly in the midline 5 cm behind his anus. Often, he has another sinus, 2–5 cm superiorly, and slightly to one or other side of the midline, with an indurated track joining it to the first one.

Look for hairs coming out of the sinuses. Don't mistake a pilonidal sinus for a subcutaneous or perianal fistula (22.2). If you are in doubt, remember: (1) In a pilonidal sinus there will be no induration between the lowest sinus and his anus. (2) There will be no fistulous opening inside his anus. (3) When you probe the lowest sinus, the probe will pass towards his sacrum, not his anus.

Aim to: (1) excise the sinus with a little surrounding tissue, (2) make sure that the wound heals properly, and (3) prevent hairs growing into it as it heals.

You have two choices: (1) You can do Lord's procedure (which is quite different from Lord's anal stretch). Lay open the main track, and excise the mouth of each sinus, together with a little cylinder of tissue, and then scrape, or preferably brush out, the hairs. If he will reattend regularly for postoperative care, this is probably the best method. (2) You can pass a probe through the sinus, cut down on it, and lay it open, as you would any other fistula. The most important part of the postoperative care, after either method, is to make sure that new hair does not grow into the granulating wound.

PILONIDAL INFECTIONS

ACUTE INFECTION. Incise and drain the patient's abscess through a short incision, taking particular care to remove all hair and granulation tissue with a curette. Insert a drain. If necessary, treat his sinus later.

PILONIDAL SINUS

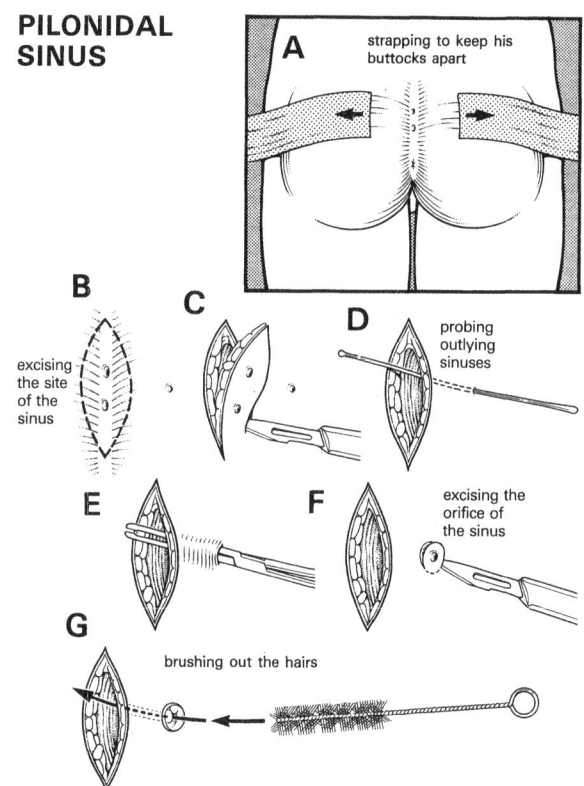

Fig. 22-12 LORD'S OPERATION FOR A PILONIDAL SINUS. Peter Lord developed two operations: (1) his anal dilatation in Figs. 22-9 and 22-10, and (2) his procedure for a pilonidal sinus shown here. A, the openings of the sinuses. B, an ellipse of skin marked out for the removal of the main sinuses. C, the ellipse being excised. D, outlying sinuses being probed. E, a haemostat being passed through the sinus. F, a little nodule of tissue being excised from the opening of the sinus. G, the sinus being brushed out. *After Rob C and Smith R, 'Operative Surgery: Abdomen II', p. 777, Butterworth, with kind permission.*

OPERATIVE TREATMENT FOR PILONIDAL SINUSES

INDICATIONS. Two or more episodes of infection, and a persistent discharge. Be sure to operate at a time when his symptoms are quiescent.

ANAESTHESIA. You can operate on him while he is on his side, with his hips flexed, so there is no need to intubate him (A 16.12). (1) Ketamine (A 8.2). (2) As an outpatient, under local anaesthesia. Don't use subarachnoid or epidural anaesthesia—there is a septic lesion too close to the injection site.

METHOD. Shave the whole of his back thoroughly, especially the area near his buttocks. Put him in the left lateral position, with his buttocks over the edge of the table. Put a piece of gauze soaked in an antiseptic, such as chlorhexidine, over his anus, and towel him. Ask your asistant to stand at the other side of the table, and to retract his right buttock.

Methylene blue injection makes the tracks much more visible, especially to a beginner. Most experts reckon it is unnecessary. Insert a cannula into the sinus, and tie a purse string suture round it. Inject methylene blue while your assistant tightens the purse string.

LORD'S PROCEDURE starts with probing any side-openings to find the direction they run in. Use a No. 11 scalpel to cut round them, and remove a little cylinder of tissue about 5 mm deep, with a 4 mm disc of skin.

Clean the track you have made, if possible with a very small brush (as made for electric razors), or a small curette. Treat all side openings in the same way. When you are sure that there are no more pockets that might contain hairs, apply a gauze dressing, and don't try to pack the cavity.

Postoperatively, regular salt baths (22.1) are important. Inspect the wound from time to time to make sure it is healing from the bottom up, without bridging or fistulae. Keep his back and buttocks shaved free of hairs while his wound heals, or his sinus will recur. Eventually, the scar will become strong enough to withstand them.

LAYING OPEN is done by passing a probe or fistula director into the primary opening, and letting it emerge through any secondary openings. Or, if a track is blind, bring it out to the skin. Incise the skin between the two openings, and lay the track widely open. Remove any hairs and curette the track. If necessary, trim the wound to encourage its edges to remain widely open. Pack it with a hypochlorite, or saline dressing, and treat it as for any other granulating wound in this region (22.1).

CAUTION ! (1) Don't leave any sinuses behind. This is a disaster, and is why some surgeons excise a wedge of involved tissue down to the sacral periosteum.

Hold the raw margins of his wound apart until healing is complete. Let them heal from below, which is difficult, because of the anatomy of the natal cleft. If skin grows too soon, a residual cavity forms, into which hairs can fall or grow. Either pack the wound edges apart with a hypochlorite or saline dressing, or hold them apart by sewing a gauze roll in place. Ask him to run his finger up and down the wound itself each time he changes the dressings. This helps to keep the wound smooth and flat, removes debris, and is not painful. Give him some plastic or rubber surgeons's gloves, and some KY jelly. When he reattends, shave the edges of the wound carefully.

If he is fat, encourage him to lose weight. Ask him to separate the wound at least once a day with lateral traction. Warn him that his sinus might recur.

DIFFICULTIES WITH PILONIDAL SINUSES

If his wound BLEEDS postoperatively, give him some gauze, and ask him to sit on it.

If there is EXCESSIVE GRANULATION TISSUE, curette it. Remove loose hairs.

If his skin forms a BRIDGE ACROSS THE LESION, with a dead space underneath, his sinus will recur. This is the commonest cause of recurrence, and is the result of poor operative technique, or poor postoperative care; so try to get it right next time.

22.9 Rectal prolapse

Occasionally, the rectum prolapses out of the anus. It may prolapse incompletely, so that only a pink fold of mucosa shows, or it may prolapse completely, so that the whole thickness of the rectal wall is turned inside out (procidentia), and may ulcerate. At the same time the patient's anal sphincter may stretch and become patulous, so that he is incontinent. At first his rectum only prolapses with defaecation, later it does so on minimal coughing and straining; finally it is outside all the time.

Although the rectum can prolapse at any age, it commonly does so in children between the ages of 3 and 5 (usually incompletely), and occasionally does so in the aged (usually completely). The reasons are not clear. Prolapse is more common in malnourished children, perhaps because of poor tone and wasting of the anal sphincter mechanism. Prolapse is also associated with diarrhoea. If a child's malnutrition is treated, his prolapse is usually cured also. A chronic cough, especially whooping cough, and worms, particularly *Trichuris*, may also play a part.

A child's rectal prolapse usually presents as his mother noticing that "Something red appears at his anus after defaecation". When she brings him to you, there is usually nothing to see. If there is, you can usually replace his rectum manually, but it is likely to return. If it remains prolapsed too long, it ulcerates. His prolapse will however correct itself as he grow older and his nutrition improves; some surgeons accept this, and don't usually do anything further. You can strap his buttocks as described below. If this does not prevent it recurring, you can usually cure him quite easily with Thiersch's operation. Pass a suture around his anus subcutaneously, tie it just tight enough to prevent his rectum prolapsing, and just loose enough to let him pass his stools.

If you insert a non-absorbable suture, you will have to remove it later. Some surgeons also use gallows traction.

An adult's rectal prolapse is much more difficult to treat. Symptoms are due to the prolapse itself, and to a particular type of incontinence caused by difficulty in regulating bowel action. If you cannot refer him, Thiersch's operation, preferably using wire, quite often succeeds. If it does not, you can hitch his rectum to his sacrum, in an operation which is similar to the ventrisuspension of a prolapsed uterus (20.10), but is more difficult.

RECTAL PROLAPSE

EXAMINATION. If a patient's prolapse is intermittent, he will give a history of "something coming down", but there will be nothing to see. If he is an adult, pass a proctoscope and ask him to strain down. His anal mucosa will prolapse into the hollow of the proctoscope, and extend beyond his anus as you withdraw it. If his prolapse is complete, the whole thickness of his rectum slides out all round, sometimes for several centimetres. When you do a rectal examination, his anal sphincter feels weak.

To find out if his prolapse is partial or complete, put you finger into his rectum, and feel the protruding ring of mucosa between your finger and thumb. If all you can feel is two layers of mucosa, it is incomplete; if you can feel more tissue than merely mucosa, it is complete.

If he is a child, distinguish a prolapse from a rectal polyp, or an intussusception. Examine him immediately after defaecation. Feel the outer aspect of the swelling, up to his anal orifice. In a prolape you cannot enter his anal canal at any point, but you can pass your finger between an intussusception, or a rectal polyp, and his anal wall.

If he is an adult, you will probably find that his prolapse is reduced when you examine him. Ask him to bear down to let you observe it. His anus may be large, and his sphincters abnormally lax. Assess their tone, because this is an important determinant of treatment and prognosis. Put your finger into his anus, and ask him to try to squeeze it. You may feel very little contraction. If it is very lax, he may allow you to put three or four fingers into it without discomfort.

CHILDREN WITH RECTAL PROLAPSE

If a child has diarrhoea, treat it. If his nutrition is poor, treat that first. These are the common causes of prolapse, and *treatng them usually cures him and avoids an operation.*

MANUAL REPLACEMENT AND STRAPPING. Using a glove and KY jelly, replace his prolapse manually. You may have to squeeze it for 15 minutes to do so.

Strap his buttocks securely together with a large gauze pad up against his anus. If this method is to work, the strapping must be adequate, painless, and easily applied. Apply a large square to each buttock. Join these with a 2.5 cm transverse strip, so as to close his buttocks, and leave this strip on during defaecation. Afterwards, remove it, clean his buttocks, and replace it with a fresh strip. Ask his parents to repeat this after each bowel movement, and give them some vaseline gauze, plain gauze, and strapping, with which to do it. After a time, his rectum will stay up where it belongs. Strapping is often all that is necessary.

If, after three or four reductions his prolapse soon recurs after defaecation, leave it out. Try again 3 or 4 days later, when it may stay in. After a week or two it will probably stay in. If it is not controlled after several weeks, and he is fit enough, do a temporary Thiersch's operation using No. 2 chromic catgut. If he is not fit enough, wait longer. Alternatively, consider gallows traction.

CAUTION ! Too much trauma reducing a prolapse causes bleeding, which can be worse than leaving it outside covered by vaseline gauze.

GALLOWS TRACTION is controversial. Some surgeons don't use strapping and proceed immediately to gallows traction. Others consider it ineffective and messy. If you decide to use it, suspend him in the gallows position for a few days to two weeks (78.2). If this fails, consider a temporary Thiersch's operation.

ADULTS WITH RECTAL PROLAPSE

If an adult has an incomplete prolapse and the tone of his sphincter is normal, or only slightly relaxed, you can treat him in much the same was as if he had large third degree piles (22.6). Insert a bivalve proctoscope, and use haemostats to catch catch his redundant mucosa at the 3, 7, and 11 o'clock positions. Use scissors to divide the prolapse into three main portions, like primary piles, with narrow bridges of skin and mucosa between them. Tie and excise the bunches of mucosa, as if they were piles. These 'piles' are broad-based, so apply a transfixion ligature before you excise them. Preserving satisfactory mucocutaneous bridges may be difficult, but if one or even two are cut, the result may still be satisfactory.

If he has an incomplete prolapse and his sphincter is grossly relaxed, treatment is difficult, so refer him. If you cannot refer him, he may possibly benefit from Thiersch's operation (see below).

If he has a complete prolapse, refer him. If you cannot refer him: (1) If his prolapse is <15 cm and his sphincters are not too lax, try Thiersch's operation. (2) Otherwise, and if Thiersch's operation fails, try the operation described below for hitching up his rectum to his sacrum. If you can do a hysterectomy, you can do this, but it is not always successful.

THIERSCH'S OPERATION FOR RECTAL PROLAPSE

INDICATIONS. (1) Children in whom strapping and/or gallows traction have failed. (2) Elderly debilitated adults whose life has been made miserable by rectal prolapse, particularly if you are inexperienced in abdominal surgery.

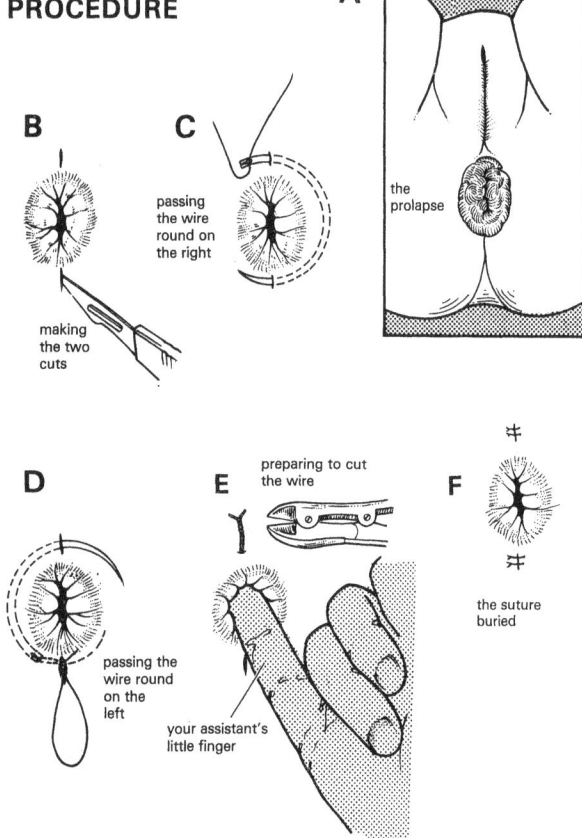

Fig. 22-13 THIERSCH'S PROCEDURE. A, the child's prolapsed anus. B, make two cuts in his skin 2 cm from his anus. C, pass the suture material from 12 to 6 o'clock on the right hand side. D, now pass it round on the other side. E, tighten the suture material with your assistant's little finger in the child's anus. F, finally bury the sutures. *From Goligher JC, 'Surgery of the Anus, Rectum and Colon', (4th edn 1980), Fig. 187 Baillière Tindall, with kind permission.*

ANAESTHESIA. (1) Ketamine for children (A 8.2). (2) General anaesthesia.

SURGERY. Put the patient into the lithotomy position and replace his prolapsed rectum (A, in Fig. 22-13). Put your finger in his anus and feel his sphincter. It may be so loose that you can hardly feel it. Prepare and drape him.

Make short incisions in the 6 o'clock and 12 o'clock positions 2 cm from his anus (B). Then, take a large curved round-bodied needle and thread it. For an adult use fine braided stainless 1 mm steel wire, or '2' braided silk. For a child use '1' or '2' chromic catgut.

Put the needle into his skin in the 12 o'clock position 1 cm from his anus. Pass it subcutaneously round his anus 1 cm from it and out again at the 6 o'clock position (C). Pull the suture material through.

Put the needle back into the 6 o'clock hole from which it has just come. This time pass it round the other side of his anus and out at the 12 o'clock incision (D). Ask your assistant to put his little finger into the child's anus (E) (in an adult he should use his index). Tie the suture round his finger. Secure it with several knots, cut the ends 1 cm long and bury them. Close the two skin wounds with catgut.

CAUTION ! (1) You must be able to get the tip of your little finger into a child's anus and your whole finger into an adult's anus. Getting the tension of the suture material right is difficult. If it is too tight, it will interfere with defaecation, and cause faecal impaction, or the wire may cut out. If it is too loose, it will not cure his prolapse. (2) Don't forget to make sure that he can pass stools normally before discharge.

The major complications are breakage of the suture, and difficulty in passing even a soft stool, if the suture is too tight. Advise an adult to eat his traditional high-fibre diet.

Alternatively pass an ordinary tubular hypodermic needle round his anus from the 12 o'clock to the 6 o'clock positions, and vice versa. Pass the suture material through this, and tie it as above.

POSTOPERATIVELY, an adult is usually old, so leave his non-absorbable suture in.

STITCHING THE RECTUM TO THE SACRUM

Expose the patient's pelvis through a lower midline incision, and pack away his gut. Mobilize his rectum down to his pelvic floor, laterally by incising his peritoneum, and posteriorly by finger dissection, keeping close to his rectal wall. If you don't there will be massive bleeding. Dissection is quite easy, because there is a bloodless plane between the rectum and the sacral fascia. Be careful not to go too far backwards, because there is a plexus of veins just anterior to the sacrum; if you damage this he may bleed severely. Bleeding gets worse with each attempt at ligation.

If you are unlucky and do injure this venous plexus, insert a gauze pack and wait 10 minutes. If bleeding continues, pack the area with ribbon gauze, leave the pack in place, and remove it under general anaesthesia after 48 hours. The prolapse may even be cured.

Divide the lateral ligaments (the sacrouterine ligaments in a woman, 20-17). These contain a few blood vessels, which may need transfixing.

Using non-absorbable '0' or '1' multifilament sutures, pull his rectum firmly upwards towards his sacral promontary, and place about 6 sutures between his pre-sacral fascia and the tissues around the back and sides of his rectum.

If you have an 'Ivalon sponge' or 'Marlex mesh', insert a broad strip of this between his rectum and his sacral periosteum.

CAUTION ! (1) Don't penetrate the wall of his rectum. (2) Be sure to put all the sutures in first and then tie them later. (3) Make sure his rectum is pulled up well out of the hollow of his sacrum.

22.10 Other anorectal problems

Carcinoma of the rectum (32.27) is not uncommon in India, but is still unusual in Africa. Try to diagnose it and refer the patient. Here also are some other problems which you will meet occasionally.

OTHER ANORECTAL PROBLEMS

LESIONS OF THE RECTUM

If a patient has an ULCERATIVE or PROLIFERATIVE LESION OF HIS RECTUM, it might be an amoebic granuloma, which an unusual complication of amoebic colitis (31.10). This can obstruct his colon or his rectum, but is more common in his caecum. An amoebic granuloma of the rectum is softer, and lacks the craggy hardness and friability of a carcinoma. Look for amoebic trophozooites in his stools, and biopsy the lesion. Don't do a colostomy. Metronidazole will usually make the lesion melt away.

CAUTION ! If you think that any granulomatous mass in relation to the large gut might be an amoeboma, try metronidazole.

If he presents with CONSTIPATION, TENESMUS, and the passage of MUCUS, one possibility is a SOLITARY RECTAL ULCER (common in India in adults and older children). Sigmoidoscopy shows a solitary linear ulcer 8-10 cm from his anus. Digital evacuation is an important cause. Instead of asking "Do you put your finger into your rectum?", ask "How often do you put your finger into your rectum to remove the faecal matter?". Treat him with a hydrophilic colloid and the threat: "Although there is as yet no evidence of cancer, persistence with digital evacuation might produce it".

LESIONS AT THE ANUS

If he has a FIRM FUNGATING MASS at his anus, perhaps with enlarged inguinal lymph nodes, it may be a CARCINOMA OF HIS ANAL CANAL. Take a biopsy and refer him.

If you cannot refer him, there is little you can do for advanced lesions, but, if the lesion is small and near his anal margin, infiltrate it with local anaesthetic solution containing adrenalin. Ask your assistant to hold a speculum in position, while you excise the tumour widely.

If he has WARTY CAULIFLOWER-LIKE LESIONS in his perianal area, he probably has CONDYLOMATA ACUMINATA. These are of viral origin, and may extend inwards as far as his pectinate line, and become infected and ulcerated. They move on the underlying tissue (unlike a carcinoma), and the skin between them is normal. If in doubt, take a biopsy.

Infiltrate his perianal skin with dilute lignocaine with adrenalin (A 5.4). Then carefully remove the growths with scissors. Treat the raw areas that are left with hypochlorite or saline dressings, like any other perianal granulating lesion.

If he has a STRICTURE OF HIS RECTUM, which may partly obstruct it and cause alternating constipation and diarrhoea, with faecal incontinence, it is probably due to: (1) Lymphogranuloma venereum (much the most likely cause, see below). (2) Carcinoma. (3) Fibrosis following a corrosive traditional enema (usually a long stricture). (6) Schistosomiasis. (7) Amoebiasis (8) Unskilful haemorrhoidectomy (22.6). A stricture due to lymphogranuloma venereum is usually a localized shelf-like lesion of hard fibrous tissue about 1 cm deep, 5 cm in from the anus, and lined by thin adherent anal skin. Sometimes there is a rectovaginal fistula below the stricture.

If you remove the stricture entirely, he may become more incontinent. Either: (1) Carefully dilate it with Hegar's dilators under general anaesthesia. Try not to tear it, or you will cause further inflammation and fibrosis. Or, (2) put the patient into the lithotomy position, and, preferably using diathermy, make four V-shaped incisions in the 12, 3, 6, and 9 o'clock positions to remove four triangular pieces of fibrous tissue. Or, (3) if obstruction is severe, consider referring him for an abdominoperineal resection and a permanent end colostomy.

If a woman has ULCERATIVE LESIONS ON HER GENITALIA, accompanied by acute inflammation and suppuration of her inguinal nodes, she probably has LYMPHOGRANULOMA VENEREUM. Most chronic cases are seen in women, in whom it causes thickened and oedematous perianal and vulval skin, with anorectal suppuration, fibrosis, fistulae, and a stricture (see above). Meanwhile, her perianal region discharges pus, blood, and mucus. Ultimately, her anus and lower rectum are destroyed, and replaced by a thick fibrotic tube. The demonstration with a probe of 'bridges of skin' virtually confirms the diagnosis. Amoebiasis is the important differential diagnosis. Early, tetracycline and chloramphenicol are effective. Later, they can do nothing, except control sepsis.

23 Urology

23.1 Equipment for urology

Disease of the urinary tract can be very distressing, so much so that some sufferer in the Middle Ages is said to have prayed 'O Lord, take me not through my bladder'. You may not always be able to prevent the Creator taking your patients this way, but you can do much to help them. Urological cases are among the 'smelliest and dirtiest' in the wards. Because it is usually considered sensible to start making rounds at the 'clean' end, you and your staff are likely to arrive tired at the urological patients, and can easily neglect them.

You can treat acute, chronic, and 'acute on chronic' retention (23.5), and urethral strictures, whether they are passable (23.8) or not (23.9). You can remove the prostate, and take stones from the bladder in adults (23.15) and children (23.16) and from the urethra (23.17) and ureter (23.14), but not from the kidneys. You can treat carcinoma of the penis (32.33) and prostate (32.32), but not the bladder (32.31). You cannot do much about the congenital anomalies of the urinary tract, except to remember that the absence of a kidney is the most important one.

The most useful urological investigations are urinalysis, microscopy and culture, and a blood urea, followed, when necessary, by a urogram and cystoscopy. We have included methods for both the latter, although you can usually do without a cystoscope if you have to.

The commonest urological procedure is to pass a catheter to let a patient's urine flow out of his bladder. Catheters are graduated according to the Charrière gauge, which is their circumference in millimetres. If there are two numbers, for example, 18/22 Ch, the smaller one refers to the circumference of the tip, and the larger one to the circumference of the shaft. Think of catheters in three sizes—8 or 10 Ch for simple drainage, 14 or 16 Ch Foley self-retaining catheters for the relief of retention, and large 20 or 24 Ch catheters for postoperative drainage or evacuating blood clots.

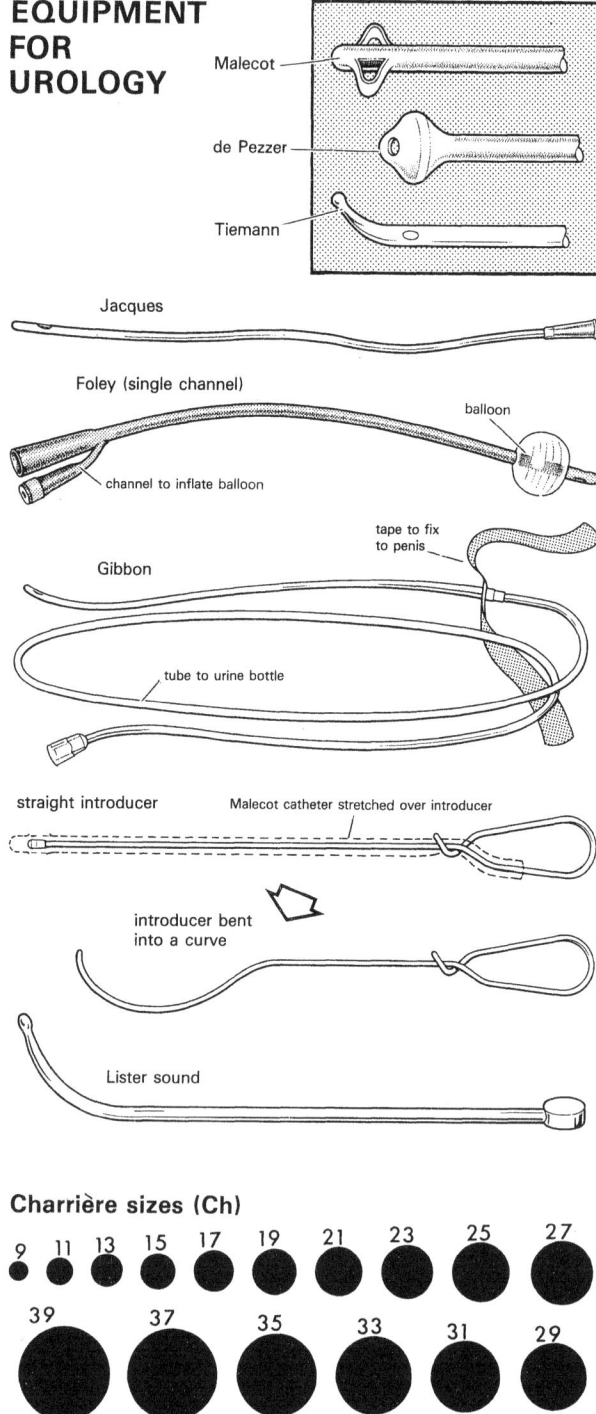

Fig. 23-1 EQUIPMENT FOR UROLOGY. Each catheter has its own special purpose. The Charrière scale shows the actual diameter of each catheter.

• CATHETERS, latex or plastic, Jacques, 380 mm, (a) 8 Ch, ten only. (b) 10 Ch, twenty only. (c) 14 Ch, ten only. (d) 16 Ch, ten only. (e) 20 or 24 Ch, ten only. These are the cheapest, simplest, softest, and safest general purpose catheters. You will be wise to start with them before trying any others.

• CATHETER, Tiemann, rubber or plastic, olive-tipped, (a) 16 Ch, twenty only. (b) 18 Ch, fifty only. (c) 20 Ch, fifty only. These have bent, olive-tipped ends, and you may succeed in passing one round a prominent prostatic middle lobe when you cannot pass a Jacques or a Foley catheter. A 'coudé' catheter is any catheter, like a Tiemann, with a bend near the tip.

• CATHETER, Gibbon, simple polythene, with removable nylon stylet, 10 Ch, twenty only. The nylon stylet of a Gibbon catheter makes it easy to pass, but when it is removed the catheter is soft. It has a tube which you can lead straight into a collecting bottle, and flanges to strap to the penis.

• CATHETERS, Foley, latex rubber, self-retaining, double channel, 30 ml balloon, (a) 14 Ch, twenty only. (b) 16 Ch, forty only. (c) 18 Ch, forty only. (d) 20 Ch, forty only. (e) 22 Ch, forty only. These have a balloon at the end which you can blow up through the second channel, and so keep the catheter in the bladder.

- *CATHETERS, Foley, silicone rubber, self-retaining, double-channel, 30 ml balloon, (a) 14 Ch, five only. (b) 22 Ch, five only.* Keep these expensive silicone Foley catheters for long-term drainage and stricture management.

- *CATHETER, plastic, Foley balloon, three-channel for continuous irrigation, 75 ml balloon, straight tip, 22 Ch, twenty only.* This catheter holds itself in place and allows you to irrigate the bladder. One channel is for the balloon, one is for irrigating fluid going into the bladder, and one for fluid and urine coming out. Use these for Freyer's prostatectomy (23.19).

- *CATHETER, Malecot, self-retaining, rubber or plastic. (a) 20 Ch. (b) 26 Ch. (d) 32 Ch. Twenty of each size.* These are very similar in function to a de Pezzer catheter; which you use is a matter of personal preference. For suprapubic drainage, you can use a Foley as easily as a Malecot or a de Pezzer catheter.

- *Alternatively, CATHETER, de Pezzer, self-retaining, rubber or plastic, 20 Ch, 26 Ch, and 32 Ch. Twenty of each size.* This self-retaining rubber catheter has a circular flange. You can put it on to an introducer, pull it straight to flatten the flange, insert it, and then remove the introducer, whereupon it will regain its original shape, and stay in place in the bladder (or in a caecostomy, 9.5). *Malecot and de Pezzer catheters are only for suprapubic use.*

- *INTRODUCER, catheter, two only.* Keep one of these straight for introducing suprapubic catheters, and bend the other one into a smooth curve for introducing urethral catheters. If you use the same introducer for both purposes and keep on bending and unbending it, it will soon become so kinked that you cannot withdraw it. An introducer can be a dangerous instrument in the urethra, so use it with great care, and only when absolutely necessary.

- *SPIGOTS, plastic, for catheters, (a) small, fifty only. (b) large, fifty only.* If a patient has a spigot in his indwelling catheter, he can walk about with it in, and remove it to drain his bladder. If you don't have plastic spigots, make wooden ones.

- *BOUGIES, neoplex, Porges (POR), filiform, (a) smaller sizes olive-tipped, (b) larger sizes plain, sizes 1 to 20 Ch, two only of each size. (c) Follower to fit, two only.* Use these for dilating strictures, for which they have many advantages over metal bougies—except that they are much less durable. You can control their passage through the anterior urethra more easily, they follow the curve of the posterior urethra, and you will less easily cause false passages, even with small sizes. Cheatle's forceps can crush plastic bougies when they are hot, so tie them into bundles, and handle them only with tapes. Lift them out of the sterilizer and put them into cold boiled water. They will then be the right consistency for use.

- *SOUNDS, metal, large, blunt, straight, plain-end, Powell's, sizes 12 to 20 Ch, one only of each size.* Historically, a 'sound' refers to a metal instrument used to locate stones in the bladder by the sound of the instrument hitting the stone. The terms 'sound' and 'bougie' are now used synonymously. If you are going to use a metal sound, Powell's straight sounds are the safest—a large one is much too large to be led down a false passage.

- *SOUNDS, metal, Otis–Clutton urethral, curved with olive ends, 9/14 Ch, 11/15 Ch, 12/17 Ch, 14/18 Ch, 15/20 Ch, 17/21 Ch, and 18/23 Ch, one only of each size.* Use these for dilating a strictured urethra. The set is deliberately incomplete, because small sounds are dangerous, and can too easily cause a false passage.

- *TROCAR and cannula, gall-bladder, Ochsner, with metal piston and side branch, medium size, one only.* Although this is intended for draining a patient's gall-bladder, it is even more useful for draining his urinary bladder suprapubically.

- *SYRINGE, bladder washout, 50 ml, plastic, boilable, two only.*

- *RETRACTOR, Thomson–Walker, with two pairs of detachable abdominal wall blades, and a long blade for posterior wall, one only.* Use this for a suprapubic prostatectomy. It is designed to reach into the floor of the bladder.

- *URINE BAGS, simple pattern, with drainage outlet at the bottom, plastic, reusable, five hundred only.* Although these bags are intended to be disposable, you can boil them and reuse them many times. Put 20 ml of cetrimide into the bag to help prevent infection, especially in long-standing cases. If you don't have any urine bags, you can wash blood-giving bags and blood-giving sets, cut them, and adapt them.

- *CLAMP, penile with rachet, twenty only.* If a patient is incontinent, he may find a penile clamp useful. You can also use one to retain local anaesthetic before you pass a catheter.

- *BIOPSY NEEDLE, Travenol 'Tru-cut' (TRAV) code 2N2704, one only.* This is for the operative treatment of priapism (23.29). Several punctures with a large ordinary needle or a sharp trocar may be effective.

23.2 Catheters and how to pass them

Before you pass a catheter, think for a moment about what you want to do with it. If you are going to drain urine from a healthy patient, who cannot pass urine after a hernia operation, use a soft rubber Jacques catheter. If it has only to let out urine, its lumen can be narrow. If you expect bleeding, and want to irrigate a bleeding bladder, so as to dilute the blood in it and prevent it clotting, you will need a catheter with an irrigating channel. If you need to suck out clots, choose a large catheter made of stiff material which will not collapse.

If an indwelling catheter has to stay in place for 10 days or more: (1) Avoid red rubber, and use latex, plastic, or ideally silicone, because these will be less irritant. (2) Be sure that it does not fit so tightly that it blocks the mouths of the paraurethral glands. There must be plenty of room beside it for their secretions to ooze out. (3) It must be soft, because a stiff tight-fitting catheter can press on the mucosa of the urethra at the external sphincter or the penoscrotal angle, and cause a pressure sore, and finally perhaps a stricture. So use the narrowest, softest, catheter which will serve your purpose, and remove it as soon as you can. Finally, remember that passing a catheter is a sterile procedure—you can so easily infect a patient and cause him needless misery.

USE THE NARROWEST, SOFTEST CATHETER; AND REMOVE IT SOON

PASSING A CATHETER

EQUIPMENT. 2% lignocaine gel, preferably with chlorhexidine, an antiseptic suitable for the patient's scrotum (1% chlorhexidine), the right selection of catheters, a penile clamp to retain the anaesthetic, receivers, a sterile bottle in which to send urine for culture, a syringe to blow up the Foley balloon, and a sterile connecting tube and bag to receive the urine.

METHOD. Admit him. If he is in severe pain, give him pethidine. This may help him to pass urine. Explain what you are going to do. Make sure you have help. Scrub and put on sterile gloves.

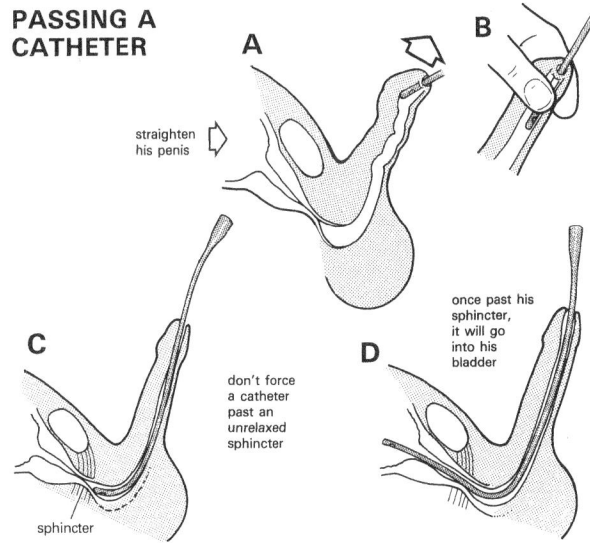

Fig. 23-2 PASSING A CATHETER. A, and B, straighten out the patient's urethra to remove its kinks. C, if the mucosa over his external sphincter is not well anaesthetized, it may go into spasm—never force a catheter past an unrelaxed sphincter. D, when it is past his relaxed sphincter, it will find its way into his bladder, provided it is flexible and well-lubricated.
After Blandy J, 'Operative Urology', Figs. 2.54 to 2.56 Blackwell Scientific Publications, with kind permission.

Sit him comfortably in a good light with his legs apart, and a waterproof sheet under him. Drape him.

Using a syringe without a needle, put 10 ml of lignocaine gel into his urethra, and keep it there for 4 minutes with a penile clamp, or with light pressure from your finger and thumb.

CAUTION ! Allow it to act for at least 4 minutes. Half the trouble in passing a catheter comes from not doing this.

Start with a 14 or 16 Ch Foley catheter (smaller latex ones may be too supple). Hold his penis straight upwards to flatten out its folds. Take the catheter in your other gloved hand. Don't touch either your skin, or his skin. Push it gently into his meatus, and down his urethra, while keeping his penis straight.

If it sticks at the junction of his penis and scrotum, he may have a stricture, because this is the common site.

If it sticks at his external sphincter, wait, be gentle, and get him to relax it. If he tightens it, you will never get the catheter in. Force is dangerous. Be slow, gentle, and crafty. Ask him to "Breathe in and out, and pretend to pass water". If you can catch his sphincter off its guard, the catheter will slip in.

If it sticks in his posterior urethra, his prostate may be enlarged. Put your finger in his rectum, and press on it. You may find that the catheter will now pass onwards.

CAUTION ! Never use force.

If it still does not pass: (1) It may be too large (try a smaller one). (2) His sphincter may not be relaxed because he is frightened (try anaesthesia; see below). (3) His urethra may not be properly anaesthetized (try introducing 5–10 ml more lignocaine, with KY jelly). (4) The catheter may have caught in mucosal pockets in his urethra—you can easily make these into a false passage, if you are not careful. (5) He may have a large prostate, which distorts his urethra, and prevents the catheter following it into his bladder.

You now have two choices:

You can do a suprapubic needle puncture (23.5). This may be your first choice for: (1) Postoperative retention. (2) Longstanding retention with overflow. (3) Retention from any cause in the middle of the night. Often, after aspirating him for 8 or 12 hours, the oedema at his bladder neck may settle, and a catheter may now pass more easily (unless he has a stricture). If a second attempt at catheterization fails, suprapubic drainage ('SPP', 23.6) would probably be wiser. This is safer than persisting with attempts to pass a urethral catheter. *Be prepared to accept failure early* and go straight to suprapubic catheterization, especially in areas where strictures are common. If you leave his urethra alone for two or three days, a further attempt to pass a catheter will often succeed.

Or, you can try other kinds of catheter as follows.

Try a 6, 9, or 12 Ch Gibbon catheter. This has a stiffened removable nylon stylet. Use the two plastic strips incorporated in the catheter to hold it in place in his penis.

If this fails, try a 15 Ch rubber Tiemann catheter. With a little patience, you are almost sure to succeed. If you do, strap it in, and change it for a Foley catheter a few days later. It is stiff, and can damage his urethra by pressure, if you leave it too long.

If the above methods fail on the ward, and as a last resort, and if he has an empty stomach, take him to the theatre. Give him pethidine with diazepam (A 8.8), or a general anaesthetic (seldom necessary). While he is deeply asleep, his sphincter may relax and, with luck, the catheter will slip in. If it does not, try a curved metal introducer to 'lift' a catheter into his bladder—taking great care. When it is in his bladder, remove the introducer.

CAUTION ! (1) Try to avoid using an introducer if you can—this is an instrument for the experienced. If you do use one: (a) lubricate it when you put it into the catheter, and (b) lubricate the catheter when you pass it into his urethra. This will help to prevent it being pulled out with the introducer. (2) Make sure the introducer has a smooth curve. A kinked introducer will be difficult to extract.

CAUTION ! Ask the nurses to change his urine bag at least every 48 hours, aseptically and without getting his organisms on their skin.

DIFFICULTIES WITH CATHETERS

If the BALLOON WILL NOT DEFLATE in a Foley catheter, cut the catheter across, and leave it for 24 hours to empty. It

A CONDOM CATHETER

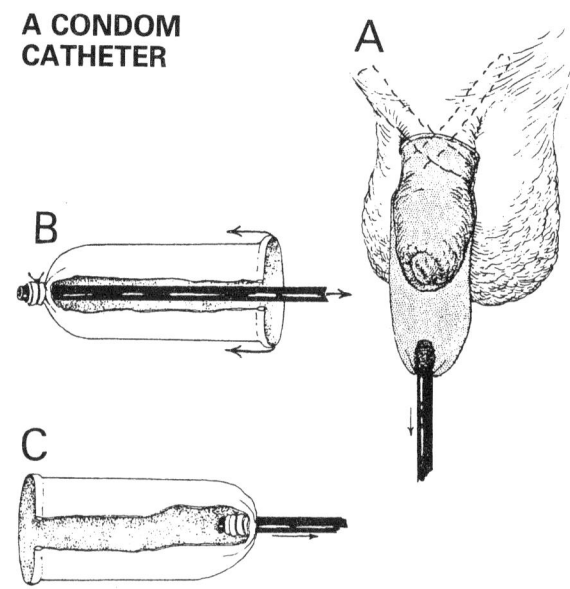

Fig. 23-3 A CONDOM CATHETER. If a patient is incontinent, you will find this very useful. You will not have a proper belt to attach it to, so you will have to use strapping, as in C. *Kindly contributed by Jack Lange.*

will often deflate by itself. If it does not, inject ether up the balloon channel, and you will hear a "pop". Be sure to wash out the ether, and any balloon fragments which may have been left behind.

If you CANNOT REMOVE AN INDWELLING CATHETER, even though you have deflated the balloon, you have probably left it in much too long, so that crusts have anchored it to his mucosa. You will have to pull it out firmly, but in doing so you will damage his mucosa. A latex catheter becomes encrusted in 3 or 4 weeks, and a silastic one in 3 or 4 months. Be safe, and change a silastic one every 6 weeks. Note its state, and if it is good, you can extend the intervals for changing it by 2 weeks to a maximum of 4 months.

23.3 Cystoscopy

Looking at a patient's bladder with a cystoscope is: (1) Often the best way to find out what is going on inside it. (2) Usually more useful than an X-ray. (3) Particularly useful in areas where *S. haematobium* is endemic, because it is the most practical way of diagnosing the cancer of the bladder that commonly complicates this disease, and which also causes haematuria (32.31). For this you only need the simplest instrument, without provision for catheterizing the ureters..

Cystoscopy is an acquired skill, even with modern equipment using a fibre-optic light source and a solid rod lens system.. With the older Ringleb type of cystoscope described here, it is even more difficult—one problem is that bulbs have an infuriating tendency to 'blow', and need frequent replacement. Although we describe the use of such an instrument here, the methods in this manual have been chosen so that you can usually manage without one. If you look after a cystoscope carefully, it will serve you many years. Even so, cystoscopy is on the edge of this system of surgery, and at least one contributor doubts its relevance. The problems are: (1) to get the instrument in (modern practice is always to do this under direct vision, so as to avoid causing damage), (2) to have a good enough instrument to give you a diagnostic view, and (3) to know what the normal looks like.

• *CYSTOSCOPE, simple pattern, Ringleb type, for examination only, 19 Ch, with single irrigating sheath, and 'Autoface' pattern bulb, boilable, with battery box, rheostat, and 25 spare bulbs, one outfit only.* A cystoscope like this can often be obtained free, or secondhand for less than $50. You can examine a patient with it, but you cannot use it to operate on him. It has a thin metal telescope with a side-looking prism

A SIMPLE CYSTOSCOPE

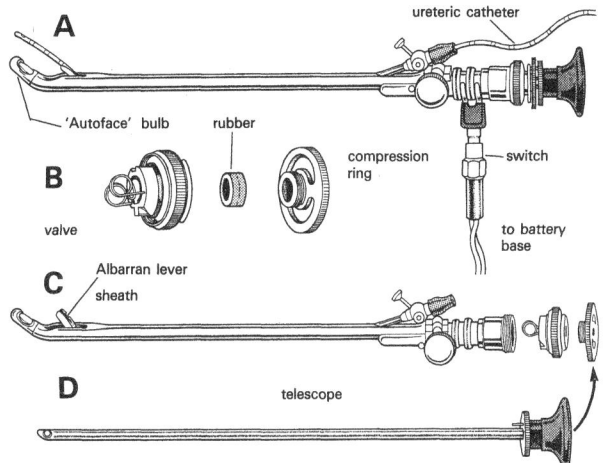

Fig. 23-4 A SIMPLE CYSTOSCOPE, of the Ringleb pattern. A, the assembled cystoscope. B, the parts of the chamber. C, the sheath. D, the telescope. The Albarran lever is for manipulating a ureteric catheter, which is not described here.

at one end, and an eyepiece at the other. Around this is a sheath with an irrigating and lighting system. The 'Autoface bulb' can be twisted to face in any direction, after the thread has been fully engaged. The sheath has a detachable switch which clips on to two rings near its outer end, and is connected through a cord to a battery box.

At the proximal end of the sheath is a chamber, to which a valve is fixed, with a collar and screws. There is a groove on the upper surface of the valve, which fits into a projection on the roof of the valve chamber. At the outer end of the sheath is a washer and a compression ring. When this is tightened, no fluid can leak back along the side of the telescope.

Methods of irrigation differ. Some cystoscopes have a tap with two positions, some have two taps, and in others you have to remove the telescope and fix a tap ('the faucet') in the hole where the telescope was.

- SYRINGE, bladder, Barrington's metal, one only. Use this to wash out the bladder during cystoscopy.

- CAN, douche, metal, 3 litre, with rubber tubing, one only.

CYSTOSCOPY

INDICATIONS. These include: (1) Urinary retention, or difficult micturition, particularly as a prelude to Freyer's prostatectomy. If the patient has an enlarged prostate, cystoscopy may precipitate acute retention, so do it as the first stage of a prostatectomy (23.19). (2) Haematuria over the age of 30 in areas where *Schistosoma haematobium* is highly endemic, see Section 32.31. (3) To diagnose schistosomiasis when it is strongly suspected clinically, but you cannot find ova in the urine. (4) Recurrent urinary infection.

CONTRAINDICATIONS. (1) Acute cystitis, until you have controlled the infection.

TESTING A CYSTOSCOPE. The theatre staff should do this before they sterilize it. Look down the telescope; the image should be clear. If it is misty, there is dirt on the lenses; clean them with spirit-soaked swabs. If it is still misty, water has probably entered the telescope, so return it to the makers or an agent for repair.

If a crescentic part of the visual field is cut off, the telescope has been bent. If this only happens after you have inserted the sheath, this is bent.

To test the bulb, connect up the battery box and set the rheostat to zero. *Place the end of the cystoscope in water to cool the bulb and prevent it burning out.* Gradually turn up the rheostat until the bulb begins to glow. Stop when the loops of the filament appear to coalesce.

If the bulb fails to light, scrape the electrode at the bottom of the bulb socket with a pin. Use a pin to raise the central contact on the bulb. If it still fails to light, replace it. Check that the battery is not exhausted, and that the slide on the battery box is not loose.

STERILIZATION. Even though your cystoscope may be boilable, an antiseptic solution will be safer for it. Keep it in its box until you want to use it. Remove the compression ring and valve, and immerse it in glutaraldehyde solution ('Cidex', Ethicon, 2.5) or 1% chlorhexidine, or 1/1000 mercury oxycyanide, or 1/80 phenol. Ten minutes immersion will kill all bacteria capable of infecting the bladder. Rinse it in sterile water, and place it on a sterile towel. Sterilize a spare bulb at the same time. After use, rinse it in water, and dry it with swabs soaked in spirit.

If it is boilable, and you do decide to boil it, immerse it in its perforated metal box in boiling water for 10 minutes. Then leave it in a sterile towel to cool.

ANAESTHESIA. You can examine a woman as an outpatient without any anaesthesia, unless she has a painful stricture of her external meatus, or a very irritable bladder.

General anaesthesia will be easier if the patient is male and you are inexperienced, or he has carcinoma of his bladder (32.31) or tuberculosis (uncommon).

If you are going to use local anaesthesia, lay him on his back, clean his glans penis with cetrimide, and use the nozzle of a tube of 2% lignocaine jelly to inject 5 g down his urethra. Apply a penile clamp proximal to his glans. Five minutes later inject a further 5 g, and reapply the clamp. Massage his penile urethra, so as to squeeze the jelly into his posterior urethra. After a further 10 minutes he is ready for cystoscopy.

PREPARATION. Put him into the semilithotomy position—flex his hips to only 75° and abduct them 30 to 45°, so as to leave his buttocks further up the table than the poles. Don't use the full lithotomy position. To provide fluid for irrigation, use a douche can a metre above him filled with autoclaved water.

INTRODUCING THE CYSTOSCOPE. Loosen the compression ring, pass the cystoscope into its sheath, and lubricate it with KY or lignocaine jelly.

CAUTION! Because urethral strictures are so common, always start by passing a large (22 Ch) Jacques catheter, before you pass a cystoscope. If you find a stricture bougie him under general anaesthesia (23.8).

If the patient is female, you will have no difficulty, unless her meatus is stenosed. If so, dilate it with sounds.

Clean the glans penis of a man and hold his penis vertically with your left hand. Introduce the cystoscope gently into his urethra, and stretch his penis along it, as it descends under its own weight. When its tip lies against his triangular ligament, swing the eyepiece down between his thighs with a circular motion, and it will slip into his bladder.

If its beak sticks in his external urethra, depress the eyepiece further and it will probably slip in—never try to push it in. If it still will not pass, put your finger in his rectum, or on his perineum and guide it in that way—this is seldom necessary. If the beak is in his bladder, the cystoscope will rotate freely.

WASHING OUT HIS BLADDER. Remove the telescope and plug in the faucet. Collect the urine which comes out. If it is hazy, send it for culture. Crystal clear urine will be sterile.

Fill a bladder syringe with water, and expel any air by holding its nozzle upwards, and depressing the plunger. Then squirt some of the water on to your own hand, to make sure that it is not too hot. Wash out his bladder by injecting 50 ml at a time, until the washings are clear. Alternatively, wash it out with water from the douche can.

INSPECTION. Distend his bladder with 250 ml of water. Put in the telescope and look around. A normal bladder holds 250 to 400 ml. You will see very little, if it holds less than 50 ml. Bladders with advanced carcinoma, severe schistosomiasis, or tuberculosis are often very small, and need very careful handling; they may bleed if you fill them too full.

An object is the correct size when it is 5 cm from the prism: it looks larger if it is nearer, and smaller if it is further away. There is a small knob on the valve chamber in the same line as the prism. If you keep your finger on this as you rotate the cystoscope, you will always know where the prism is pointing.

If you see nothing to begin with: (1) The beak of the cystoscope may still be in his urethra. (2) The light may have gone out. (3) You may have inserted the telescope incorrectly. The small pin in the eyepiece should fit into the expanded end of the valve collar. Try twisting the compression ring a little.

(4) There may be blood or clot on the objective. (5) If you see nothing but a 'red out', you may have failed to run fluid into his bladder.

Examine his bladder systematically, starting with the fenestra (window), looking downwards towards the base of his bladder. Note the size of the median lobe of his prostate as you enter his bladder (it looks like a 'termite hill'). Observe his interureteric bar. This is a ridge of tissue between his two ureteric orifices. It is a useful landmark, but it is sometimes not very conspicuous. Another landmark is the small air bubble which is always present in the top of his bladder. Return to his interureteric bar, and look all round the side walls and roof of his bladder. Turn the cystoscope through 360°, so as to examine a circular strip of bladder wall. Then push it further into the fundus, withdraw it 2 cm and look around 360° again.

Find his ureteric orifices by finding his interureteric bar, and tracing it laterally. When you see an orifice, the cystoscope must be in either the 5 o'clock, or the 7 o'clock position.

Depress the eyepiece to look at the anterior wall of his bladder. This may be impossible to see in a man, unless he is fully relaxed under general anaesthesia.

The mucosa of a normal bladder is a yellow sandy colour, and has fine branching vessels under it. If the fluid in his bladder is bloody, the mucosa may look pink—don't confuse this with cystitis. A normal trigone is pink and vascular.

Finally, partly withdraw it and examine his trigone and his internal urinary meatus. You should be able to see everything except the base when it is obscured by a very large median lobe. When this is very large you may not see his ureteric orifices either.

23.4 Haematuria

Blood in a patient's urine can be the result of almost any pathology at any level, but is much more likely to be coming from his bladder than from his upper urinary tact. He can bleed as the result of injury, bacterial infection, parasitic infestation, stones, or neoplasia.

If schistosomiasis is endemic in your district, a patient with frank haematuria, who is over 30, has a 25% chance of having carcinoma of his bladder, so be sure to cystoscope him. Under the age of 30, frank haematuria is much more likely to be due to schistosoma than carcinoma. The other important cause is prostatic hypertrophy. Other causes are rare (renal tuberculosis, carcinoma of the kidney or pelviureteric junction, and vascular abnormalities). Because cystoscopy is so necessary in the diagnosis of malignancy in areas where *S. haematobium* is endemic, it should be the first investigation after a haemoglobin, a blood urea, a urine microscopy, and (if possible) culture; an intravenous urogram may not be necessary.

Bladder stones seldom cause macroscopic haematuria. Ureteric stones, which are common in much of Asia, but are uncommon in sub-Saharan Africa, usually present with renal colic and microscopic haematuria.

HAEMATURIA

Confirm that there really is blood in the patient's urine by examining it microscopically.

THE TWO GLASS TEST. Ask him to pass his urine into two containers, and watch him do it. You may see: (1) A constant ooze from his urethra, indicating a lesion distal to his external sphincter. (2) Initial or terminal haematuria, indicating a local lesion of his bladder or prostate. Terminal haematuria is typical of schistosomiasis. (3) Total haematuria which is equal in both glasses, and may contain worm-like clots, indicates bleeding from his upper urinary tract or bladder; it is common in schistosomiasis and carcinoma of the bladder.

CYSTOSCOPY is usually best done after he stops bleeding. The exceptions are: (1) A bladder full of clot which needs immediate evacuation. (2) Recurrent haematuria when you cannot find a cause, and you would like to know which kidney blood is coming from (rare).

23.5 Retention of urine

Retention of urine can be acute, chronic, or 'acute on chronic'. Three kinds of patient suffer from it, but the first two are much the most common: (1) The young man with a history of gonorrhoea, followed by a stricture or prostatitis. Sometimes, acute gonorrhoea alone is enough to cause retention, or he may have both. (2) The old man with a large prostate. (3) Less common, the patient with painless retention as the result of an acute neurological lesion, such as injury or tumour of his spine, in which case the signs are obvious, but are often overlooked. Retention is usually a man's problem, but it can happen in women as the result of: detrusor failure complicating pelvic surgery, especially hysterectomy (20.12D), a retroverted gravid uterus, an impacted fibroid in early labour, or a spinal lesion.

Acute retention usually presents in much the same way, whatever its cause. The patient arrives in acute discomfort, often late in the evening, when he has at last realized that he is not going to pass urine before he goes to bed. His bladder is distended to his umbilicus. If you cannot catheterize him easily, you will be wise to drain his urine suprapubically by needle aspiration. This is safer than repeatedly trying to pass a catheter (23.2). No stricture is complete, and the final cause of the obstruction is probably congestion and oedema. This will subside while his bladder drains suprapubically, so that if you try to catheterize him again a week or two later, you will probably succeed. If he has an enlarged prostate, and you can operate on him during the next few days, you can leave his suprapubic catheter in place until you do so. If he has a stricture, you can bougie him as soon as his acute obstruction is over.

SUPRAPUBIC DRAINAGE IS SAFER THAN FORCEFUL CATHETERIZATION

RETENTION OF URINE

First make sure that the patient really has got retention of urine, and is not oliguric or anuric. If you cannot feel or percuss his bladder, the reason for his inability to pass urine must be in his ureters or kidneys. One glance at his face will usually tell you if his retention is acute or chronic—if he is in agony, it is acute. If his bladder is grossly distended, but he is in little pain, his retention is either chronic, or neurological.

Young? (probably a stricture). Old? (more likely a large prostate).

HISTORY. Has he had gonorrhoea, and how was it treated? Does he have to strain to pass urine? (suggests a stricture). Frequency, hesitancy, dysuria, nocturia? (prostatism).

EXAMINATION. Examine his urethra from end to end for a stricture, using your eyes and your fingers. Start at his glans, feel his urethra in his penis, and his perineum, for palpable thickening. Extensive strictures are associated with a large palpable area of scarring in his perineum. You may feel the distended proximal part of his urethra ending in a firm fibrous stricture. Examine his membranous urethra with your finger in his rectum. Exclude phimosis and stenosis of his meatus. Look for scars on his scrotum and perineum. If he has a painful tender area in his perineum, he probably has a periurethral abscess complicating a stricture.

Examine his prostate rectally: (1) The hardness and irregularity of (a) a carcinoma are usually easy to distinguish from the softer, smooth consistency of (b) benign hypertrophy, although the gritty feeling of (c) a calcified prostate may be misleading. (2) A firm mass above his prostate is likely to be carcinoma of his bladder. (3) Tenderness of the prostate is often difficult to assess, but a genuine prostatic abscess or acute prostatitis is usually obvious. (4) An impacted stone in the prostatic urethra (uncommon, the meatus is the common site of impaction).

CAUTION ! (1) The size of a prostate is no indication as to whether it is causing obstruction or not, but it is useful to know its size when planning surgery. (2) If his bladder is distended:

(a) You will have difficulty distinguishing its base from the upper border of his prostate. (b) It may seem enlarged, because it is being pushed downwards by his distended bladder. You may find later, when he comes to operation. that his prostate has disappeared. So if you do think it is enlarged, examine him again, after you have relieved his retention—don't diagnose prostatic enlargement from one examination while he has retention.

Are the nerves to his bladder intact? Can he feel a pin-prick beside his anus? Test his anal reflex during rectal examination, and feel for a patulous anal sphincter. If you suspect any neurological abnormality, examine his spine and legs thoroughly.

Look for heart failure, anaemia, and hypertension, which might be the result of an obstructive uropathy.

SPECIAL TESTS. Later, examine his urine for sugar, protein, and pus. Diabetes can cause retention, and proteinuria may indicate uropathy. Measure his haemoglobin and his blood urea. Take a plain X-ray of his kidney, ureter, and bladder. There is no need for a routine intravenous urogram: reserve it for special indications, such as haematuria when the cause is not found on cystoscopy, or you suspect some abnormality of his kidneys.

RELIEVING OBSTRUCTION OF THE LOWER URINARY TACT
Pass a catheter as in Section 23.2.

RECOVERY DIURESIS AND THE DANGER OF RENAL FAILURE

When you have relieved an obstruction to a patient's urinary tract, his bladder and his kidneys may recover, or they may not. An early sign that his kidneys are recovering, after the relief of chronic obstruction, is a recovery diuresis, which may amount to several litres a day. He needs an adequate fluid intake, whether or not he has a diuresis.

If he has a recovery diuresis, measure his urine output carefully, and give him intravenous fluids, in large quantities if necessary. Don't forget the potassium: he may need say 35–40 mmol for every litre of urine he produces. If possible, measure his serum potassium, and adjust the dose of potassium you give him accordingly. Be guided also by his pulse and blood pressure chart. If you fail to appreciate the danger of this diuresis, he may slip into renal failure again, due to dehydration leading to poor renal perfusion, in spite of an apparently normal fluid intake.

DIFFICULTIES WITH RETENTION

If he has the SYMPTOMS OF PROSTATIC OBSTRUCTION with acute or chronic retention, but no large prostate, there are two possibilities (see also Section 23.20):
DYSKINESIA (formerly called bladder-neck obstruction), is a functional rather than a mechanical obstruction. You cannot diagnose it by the size of his prostate or by looking at his bladder neck. It is not mechanically tight, but fails to open up during a voiding contraction. You can easily insert a catheter, which drains quantities of urine, and cystoscopy shows trabeculation of the bladder.
BLADDER-NECK STENOSIS is a mechanical obstruction due to fibrosis or previous prostatic surgery, or schistosomiasis. As with a urethral stricture, passing a catheter is difficult or impossible. Treatment is by incising the bladder neck, if possible endoscopically, deeply enough to divide all its circular fibres.

23.6 Emergency ('blind') suprapubic cystostomy, suprapubic puncture ('SPP')

If a patient has retention of urine, and you cannot pass a catheter, you will have to drain his bladder from his abdomen. As it distends, it rises up above his pubis and strips the peritoneum off his abdominal wall. This allows you to drain it without going through his peritoneal cavity. Most surgeons have their own favourite ways of doing this. We describe several alternatives: a syringe and needle is best for immediate emergency use; and a thin plastic tube passed through a trocar and cannula is best if drainage has to be continued for more than a few days. The track

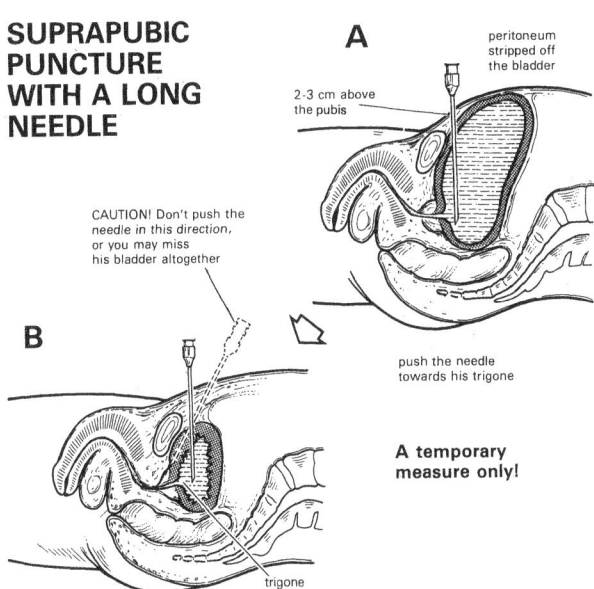

Fig. 23-5 EMERGENCY SUPRAPUBIC PUNCTURE with a long needle is the least satisfactory of the methods described here, and is a temporary method only. *Kindly contributed by Andrew Pearson.*

round a thin tube is less easily infected, although the tube itself is more readily blocked by clots.

EMERGENCY SUPRAPUBIC PUNCTURE ('SPP')

INDICATIONS (1) Acute obstruction with a *full* bladder, such as that from an enlarged prostate, a bladder stone, or a stricture when catheterization has failed. (2) Rupture of the urethra (68.3, 68.5).

CONTRAINDICATIONS (1) An empty bladder. This method is therefore contraindicated, if the patient has extravasation of urine. (2) A carcinoma of the bladder causing retention. A track may form, which is very distressing. So feel for a craggy rectal or suprapubic mass before you do a suprapubic puncture.

CAUTION ! (1) For a blind suprapubic puncture, his bladder must be distended and palpable. If it is not, wait for it to fill, or do a formal cystostomy. (2) The classical site for drainage is half-way between his pubis and the upper limit of bladder dullness. If you are going to remove his prostate later, do the cystostomy (drainage) as high as you can, so that you can open his abdomen below it later, without entering the cystostomy track. If he has a stricture, so that you will not be operating through his abdomen, the site of the cystostomy is less important.

A NEEDLE AND SYRINGE. Scrub and put on sterile gloves. Mount a 0.9 or 1 mm needle on a 20 or 50 ml syringe, preferably with a three-way tap. Check the outline of his bladder. Insert the needle 2–3 cm above his symphysis pubis, and advance it towards his lower sacrum. Aspirate as much urine as you can, and advance the needle a little as you do so.

CAUTION ! Use this method once or twice only, then try catheterization. If this fails proceed to the other methods.

A LUMBAR PUNCTURE NEEDLE *is the least satisfactory of any of the methods here.* It is however an emergency method which a night sister can use.

Find a 0.9 or 1 mm lumbar puncture needle and stillette, or a long exploring needle of the same length. Have these ready in sterile packs or boil them. You will also need an intravenous drip set, and spirit swabs; a container for his urine, such as a measuring jug, or a urine bag; gauze and adhesive strapping.

Lay him down, swab his suprapubic area, and insert the needle 2 or 3 cm above his pubis. Push it downwards. It will enter his bladder for almost its full length. Withdraw the stylet. Urine will escape. If his urine is tinged with blood, withdraw it a little, it may have touched his trigone. Connect it to the bag of a drip set, or a bottle.

CAUTION ! The needle must be a long one. If you use a small one, his bladder will pull itself out of the needle as it contracts down behind the pubis. In emergency you may be able to use the needle of a drip set, but it is too short, and is completely impracticable if he is fat. The danger with any needle, and especially that from a drip set, is that it easily slips out when he turns over in bed, so that his urine extravasates.

USING A POLYTHENE TUBE. The description here applies to retention due to a stricture, but it can also be used for obstruction due to an enlarged prostate.

Use a hydrocoele trocar and cannula, and 1.5 metres of plastic tube of external diameter about 2.5 mm, with lateral drainage holes cut in the first 5 cm. Or, use a Gibbon's catheter. Make an identification mark 15 cm from the tip. A small scalpel blade, a skin needle and suture, local anaesthetic.

Infiltrate the site of puncture with local anaesthetic solution in the midline at the chosen site. Continue to infiltrate down to his bladder; when you get there, confirm it is distended by aspirating a few millilitres of urine into the syringe.

Make a nick in his skin with a scalpel blade. With your left hand on the dome of his bladder to steady it, push the trocar into it with a steady turning movement towards his lower sacrum. If his bladder is lax, compress it with the edge of your hand. You will feel it 'give' as urine gushes out. Push the plastic tube down the cannula to well beyond the 15 cm mark, and withdraw the cannula. Some urine will escape and relieve his distension. Carefully withdraw the tube to the 15 cm mark, and secure it to his skin with a monofilament stitch tied several times round the tube, as in Fig. 23-6. Alternatively, apply pieces of strapping, as in Fig. 65-8.

CAUTION ! (1) Beware of suprapubic scars—if his peritoneum is adherent to his abdominal wall, you may injure his gut. Or, less seriously, the trocar may traverse his peritoneal cavity, and some urine may leak into it, to cause a mild local sterile peritonitis. (2) Puncture his abdominal wall in the direction of his lower sacrum. If you push the trocar too caudally you may enter his retropubic space and fail to enter his bladder. If you push it too cranially, you may enter his abdomen and possibly injure his gut.

Drain the urine into a plastic urine bag, or bottle. Make sure he has a daily fluid intake of at least 3 litres daily—a generous fluid intake is the best way of preventing or clearing infection.

If he has a stricture, drain it for about a week before you attempt to dilate it. After doing so, clip off the tube with artery forceps. You can estimate his residual urine by measuring the volume which drains through the tube, after he has passed urine. If there is no residual urine you have succeeded.

If there are no complications, he may be able to leave hospital in 24 to 48 hours, complete with his drainage system. Don't try bouginage for at least a week, then try it gently at weekly or two-weekly intervals. A few strictures will remain impassable—see Section 23.9.

If instrumentation fails and he is unable to pass urine about the 5th day, **try again at the 10th day. If this fails again, an operation will be necessary.**

48 hours after you have removed the tube the puncture site may be difficult to find.

A MALECOT OR de PEZZER CATHETER, A TROCAR, AND AN INTRODUCER. Under local anaesthesia stab his bladder through his abdominal wall with a sharp scalpel. Make an incision that is wide enough to let the catheter through. Thread a Malecot or de Pezzer catheter over a straight introducer (as in Fig. 23-1), and push it through the stab wound. Withdraw the introducer. Anchor it with monofilament stitched to his skin and tied several times round the tube.

CAUTION ! (1) The catheter must project well into his bladder. If it does not project far enough, it may be pulled out as his bladder contracts. (2) It must not project too far, or it will touch his trigone, and cause discomfort.

DIFFFICULTIES WITH EMERGENCY SUPRAPUBIC CYSTOTOMY

Other difficulties include extravasation of the urine into the suprabpubic space, followed by spreading cellulitis, injury of the prostate, perforation of the bladder wall into the rectum, urinary peritonitis, and perforation of the large or small gut. See also 'Difficulties with retention' Section 23.5.

If there is heavy or prolonged BLEEDING, suspect a bladder tumour, or damage to his bladder neck. Abandon the procedure.

If the TUBE BLOCKS, flush it through with saline from a syringe. It is more likely to block if there is too long a length inside his bladder, hence the importance of the 15 cm mark.

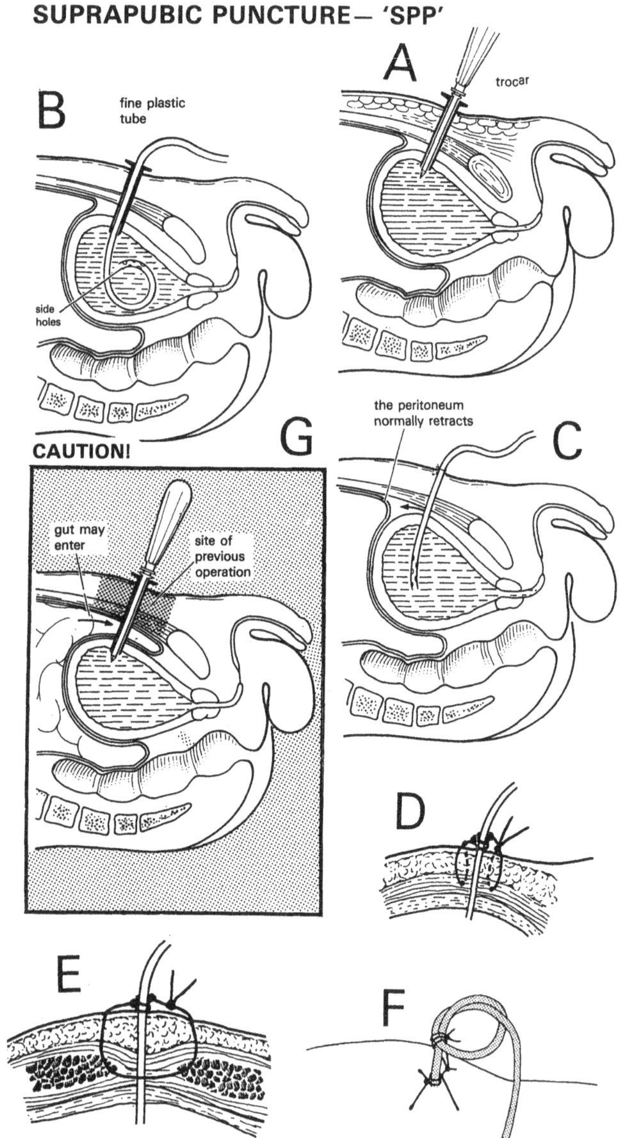

Fig. 23-6 SUPRAPUBIC PUNCTURE WITH A TROCAR and plastic tube—'SPP'. A, inserting the trocar. B, inserting the tube. C, the tube in place. D, and E, anchoring the tube. F, alternatively, make the tube into a loose knot and tie it to the patient. G, if his peritoneum is tethered by the scar of a previous operation, the trocar may traverse his peritoneal cavity, with the risk of damaging his gut. *Kindly contributed by Neville Harrison.*

23.7 Open suprapubic cystostomy

If a patient must have his urine diverted but his bladder is not distended, you cannot do a blind suprapubic puncture, so you have to do an open one. This can happen as the result of extravasation of urine due to trauma or a stricture. A similar operation is needed for the removal of a stone from the bladder (23.15).

SUPRAPUBIC CYSTOSTOMY (Open)

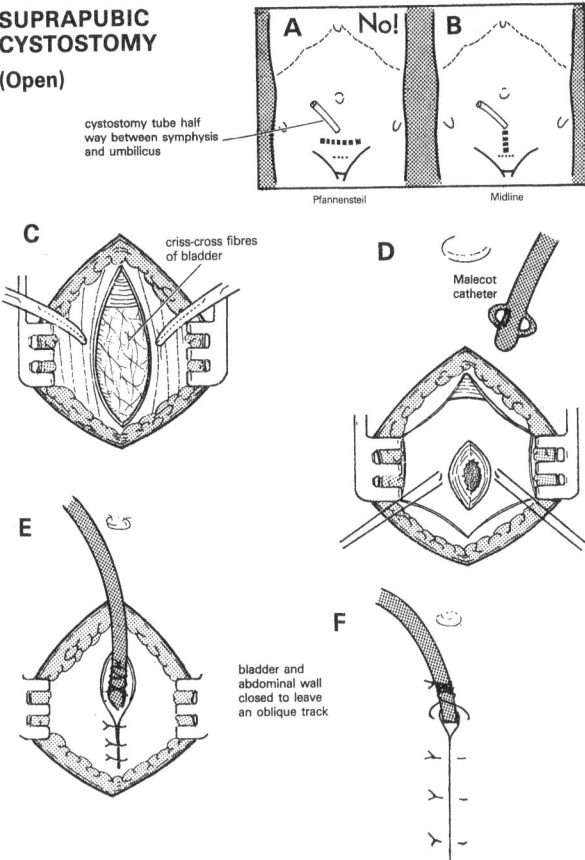

Fig. 23-7 OPEN SUPRAPUBIC CYSTOSTOMY. A, avoid using a Pfannensteil incision. B, a midline incision. The cystostomy tube should emerge half-way between a patient's umbilicus and his symphysis. C, in a midline incision part his rectus muscles to reveal the criss-cross fibres of his bladder. D, open his bladder between stay sutures. E, and F, close his bladder and abdomen, being careful to leave an oblique track, that will be less likely to leak when the catheter is withdrawn. *After Blandy J, 'Operative Urology', Figs. 8.14 to 8.24. Blackwell Scientific Publications, with kind permission.*

OPEN SUPRAPUBIC CYSTOSTOMY

TEMPORARY OPEN CYSTOSTOMY

ANAESTHESIA. (1) Local anaesthesia (A 5.4). (2) Ketamine (A 8.2).

INDICATIONS. (1) The need to divert a patient's urine, when his bladder is not sufficiently distended, or clear in outline, for a blind cystostomy, as with most cases of extravasation of urine. (2) Rupture of the bladder (68.2). (3) The treatment of clot retention. (4) As a necessary step in a urethroplasty. (4) As a permanent measure for an impassable stricture of the urethra, which is so high up (as in the membranous urethra), that a urethrotomy, which would be preferable, is impossible.

CONTRAINDICATIONS. Avoid doing a suprapubic cystotomy if a patient has carcinoma of his bladder (common in areas where *Schistosoma haematobium* is endemic), or is suspected of having it, because it may lead to a permanent and distressing urinary fistula.

METHOD. Make a midline vertical suprapubic incision. A 5 cm incision is adequate unless he is fat. Divide his linea alba, and retract his rectus muscles. Use your forefinger, covered with a gauze swab, to push the cellular tissue and peritoneum upwards, away from the anterior surface of his bladder. Dissect the loose fatty tissue away from in front of it.

Recognize his bladder by its characteristic pale appearance with some tortuous blood vessels. Aspirate it first, unless it is impalpable (as with trauma causing extravasation). Insert stay sutures, superiorly and inferiorly, at the proposed ends of your vertical bladder incision. They will make useful retractors when it sinks into his pelvis. Take urine for culture, open his bladder with a longitudinal 5 cm incision, and explore it.

If you are going to leave a suprapubic catheter in place, pass a Malecot, de Pezzer, or Foley catheter into his bladder through a separate stab incision above or to the side of the main one. Make it a snug fit and hold it in place with a purse string suture (many surgeons pass it through the main wound).

Close the main bladder incision with 2 layers of 2/0 or 1/0 chromic catgut sutures. Close the wound with the catheter emerging through a long, oblique, mid-line track. Extend the wound proximally if necessary. If it is likely to be infected by contaminated urine, as it may be if you are operating for extravasation, insert a retropubic drain.

See also Section 23.10 on extravasation of urine, especially if you have to continue suprapubic drainage more than a month.

CAUTION ! Make sure the suprapubic catheter emerges high, so that the track closes easily, and will not interfere with an approach to the bladder later.

PERMANENT OPEN CYSTOSTOMY

INDICATIONS. Some impassable urinary obstruction: a very tight stricture, or prostatic hypertrophy where catheterization has failed, and he is too ill for surgery. Where surgery is even reasonably good, a permanent cystotomy should rarely be necessary.

METHOD. Pass a Foley, a Malecot, or a de Pezzer catheter suprapubically by the method just above, or that in Section 23.6, using a trocar and cannula. If necessary, he can go home with the catheter leading into a bag, or closed with a spigot, which will need to be released 4-hourly. The bag will need cleaning and replacing after 2 weeks.

Change his catheter monthly. If you use an introducer, you should have no difficulty replacing his catheter, once a track has been established after the first 10 or 14 days. Replacing it earlier may be almost impossible. If you leave it in for longer, phosphatic encrustation, both inside and out, will make it difficult and painful to remove. A high fluid intake and acidifying his urine will minimize encrustation. The leak round the tube should not be too inconvenient. To leave him with a 'hole' is distressing, because he will be wet all the time.

He faces the certainty of infection, and the probability of an early death.

23.8 Postgonococcal urethral strictures

Gonorrhoea is common everywhere, but for quite unknown reasons, strictures are much more common in some communities than in others. In Uganda in 1963, for example, the attack rate for young adult males was estimated to be about 15% per year, with one patient in 50 getting a stricture. If yours is a 'high stricture area', like Uganda, treating them will be your most common urological task, so that you will need to hold a regular 'bougie clinic'. You will also see a few strictures which are the late results of schistosomiasis, trauma (68.7), prostatectomy (unusual), tuberculosis (rare), or of an operation on the urinary tract. Whatever its cause, you should, if possible, refer a patient with a stricture for a urethrogram, urethroscopy, and the release of his stricture with an optical urethrotome. If this is impossible, you will have to bougie him yourself, and if this fails, to treat him as in Section 23.9.

Strictures can be of any length from 5 mm to 10 cm. The commonest sites for gonococcal ones are: (1) the bulbous urethra, (2) at the junction of the penis and scrotum, and (3) in the glans penis—in this order. Gonococcal strictures are the result of fibrosis in the corpus spongiosum. Meatal strictures are described in Section 23.28.

A urethral stricture increases the resistance to micturition, which causes the detrusor muscle of the bladder to hypertrophy. This may produce an adequate flow for a time, but as time passes, sacculations and diverticula form in the bladder, it no longer empties completely, and the high residual urine it contains leads to frequency of micturition, and infection. Sensation from it is diminished, as its wall is increasingly replaced by fibrous tissue. Finally, the patient develops 'retention with overflow', and becomes incontinent. Bilateral hydronephroses form, and his blood urea rises; this completes the picture of secondary renal failure (obstructive uropathy).

Besides: (1) acute painful retention, and (2) chronic painless retention with overflow incontinence, the many other complications of a stricture include: (3) False passages. (4) Periurethral abscesses causing: (a) extravasation of urine, with gross distension of his penis and scrotum (sometimes leading to gangrene), and (b) external fistulae. (5) Infection of his urinary tract. (6) Infection of his seminal vesicles, epididymes, and testes. (7) Chronic non-specific infection ending in elephantiasis. (8) Obstructive uropathy ending in renal failure. (9) Bladder neck stenosis, and detrusor failure. These are common and may explain why bouginage and external urethroplasty often fail. (11) The results of straining, such as hernias or prolapse of his rectum. (12) Stones in his urethra and bladder. (13) Carcinoma of his urethra or bladder. (14) Infertility and impotence.

Acute and 'acute on chronic' retention are the common presentations, but a stricture may present as any of the many complications listed above. Prostatic obstruction is the main differential diagnosis (23.18). Chronic retention distends the bladder greatly, but is painless, so that decompression is not needed so urgently as it is in acute retention.

If he has a stricture and you cannot refer him, you will first have to calibrate it (find out how big it is), and then you will have to dilate it gently with bougies. There are two phases: (1) Initial bouginage, preferably with plastic bougies, to stretch it. (2) Maintenance bouginage with metal sounds to keep it stretched. Strictures are never cured, so maintenance bouginage must continue for the rest of his life. Bougie him every week or so to begin with, and then at gradually increasing intervals, until you are dilating him only once every 6 or 12 months. Even if the stenosis of his urethra is relieved, his bladder may fail to empty because its detrusor muscle has failed as the result of long-standing obstruction.

The key to success is to start bouginage early, *before* passing urine becomes really difficult. The more difficult it is, the more difficult will it be for you to pass a bougie. Passing one may be so unpleasant that he will not return again until he is desperate, by which time bouginage may be almost impossible. The only way to prevent this vicious circle is to start early, when his urine flow is only starting to fall off. He will probably find that the calibre of his stream deteriorates, before its pressure falls. Encourage him with the thought that strictures can be controlled, even by dilatation, especially if they are well treated and complications are avoided. Persuade him that, unless he returns regularly, his problems will be much greater.

Watch his kidneys and measure his blood urea. If you are in doubt as to how to manage the complications of a stricture, the rule to remember is "If in doubt divert" the urine stream with suprapubic drainage.

**START BOUGINAGE EARLY
DILATE THE PATIENT FOR LIFE**

STRICTURES

This is the patient in Section 23.5 with retention of urine, in whom you have been unable to pass a catheter, and who you think has a stricture.

DIAGNOSTIC BOUGINAGE. If he has been on suprapubic drainage and you last attempted to pass a catheter some days ago, try again now. The oedema round his obstruction may have subsided, and you may succeed. Using careful aseptic precautions, try to pass a 14 Ch soft rubber blunt-nosed Jacques catheter.

If this passes easily into his bladder, he has not got a stricture.

If it is held up, note exactly where it is held up, and start with smaller bougies.

INITIAL AND MAINTENANCE BOUGINAGE FOR THERAPY

CONTRAINDICATIONS. Don't drain an acutely inflamed stricture. The causes of inflammation include acute retention, periurethral or prostatic abscesses, and extravasation of urine. If he has any of these, drain him suprapubically until the inflammation has settled down in about 4 weeks, then dilate him. Some surgeons do this as early as 10 to 14 days.

EQUIPMENT. Soft plastic 'Neoplex' bougies sizes 1 Ch to 20 Ch. Powell's straight metal sounds 13/17 to 18/22 Ch. Lister's curved metal sounds 9/14 to 18/23 Ch. KY jelly. Ideally lignocaine jelly 2% in tubes. A penile clamp. A ureteric catheter is sometimes useful in a passable stricture. Sterilize all instruments except plastic ones by boiling. Keep plastic ones in a large tray of antiseptic solution (2.5).

ANAESTHESIA. Minimizing the pain of his first bouginage is important, because if it is too painful, he may not reattend. (1) General anaesthesia (best). (2) Lignocaine gel supplemented with intravenous thiopentone while taking the proper precautions (A 12.1). Clean his meatus with an antiseptic, not spirit. Use a syringe without a needle, to inject some 2% lignocaine jelly into his anterior urethra. Massage it well back into his perineum. With old attenders anaesthesia may unnecessary.

ANTIBIOTICS. Fever and rigors are common after dilatation, so give him give him a broad spectrum antibiotic at bouginage or, better, just before it such as: (1) gentamicin 120 mg. Or, (2) trimethoprim 200 mg. Or, (3) amoxycillin 250 mg with clavulanic acid 125 mg ('Augmentin', expensive). Also, instil 5 ml of chlorhexidine 0.05% in glycerine into his urethra 10 minutes before you dilate his stricture. These measures will not prevent all bougie reactions, but they should prevent septicaemia.

TO PASS A PLASTIC BOUGIE lay him down and hold his penis straight up. This will convert its natural 'S' shape into a 'J'.

To calibrate his stricture, ask him to breathe deeply (to relax his external sphincter). Then pass a well-lubricated 15 Ch plastic bougie down his urethra. If you cannot pass it, try a smaller one. If this does not pass, try a still smaller one.

Dilation. Now you know how wide his stricture is, you can start to dilate it.

CAUTION ! (1) If possible start with a medium-sized bougie (15 Ch) first, because it is less likely to make a false passage than a small one. (2) Don't overstretch his urethra. If a bougie is gripped—stop! (3) Pass each bougie only just beyond the stricture. When a stricture grips a bougie there is a loss of touch, which makes passing it safely through his prostatic urethra difficult, so that you can easily damage his prostate, and cause severe bleeding.

The first time you try, you may only be able to dilate his stricture a little. Try to dilate him 2 Ch at each visit, for example from 4 Ch to 6 Ch. Next week you may be able to dilate him to 8 Ch. But if you have not hurt him, he will find that his stream improves. *Don't dilate his stricture more than 2 Ch, or at the very most 6 Ch, at any one time,* because you may tear it and cause more fibrosis.

See him again each week until he reaches 20 to 22 Ch. Some surgeons are content with 15 Ch, which is adequate for normal voiding. Then lengthen the intervals at which you see him, until he is attending only once in 3 to 6 months.

PASSING METAL SOUNDS. Use plastic bougies until his stricture is stable, preferably at 20 to 22 Ch, then use metal sounds. Don't use them before his stricture is 12 Ch, because you can easily damage his urethra with smaller sounds, and make a false passage. *Straight sounds are safer than curved ones,* because they give you a safer 'feel' and lack leverage. You can use them for nearly all strictures, except those in the bladder neck. Usually, you only need to pass a curved sound to make a final check of his whole urethra. Pass them in the same way as bougies, but remember they are much more dangerous.

Look carefully at his notes to see what size of sound was used before. Use a straight one for the anterior urethra, and

PASSING A METAL BOUGIE

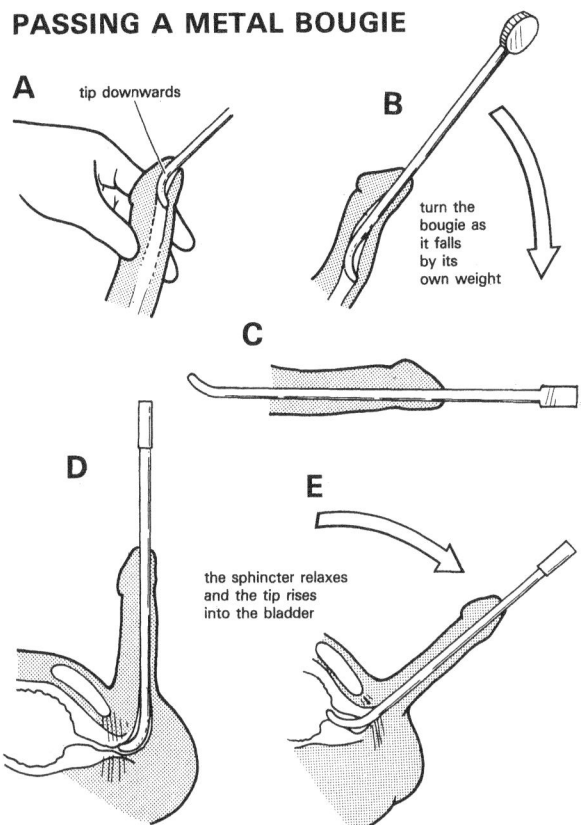

Fig. 23-8 PASSING A METAL SOUND. A, put the tip of the sound into the patient's urethra, point downwards. B, and C, as the sound drops gently down his urethra, rotate its handle. D, there is always a little resistance as the tip of the sound meets his external sphincter: wait for the sphincter to relax. E, the sphincter relaxes as the handle falls, and the tip of the sound rises up into his bladder. *After Blandy J, 'Operative Urology', Figs. 14.21 to 14.23. Blackwell Scientific Publications, with kind permission.*

a curved one elsewhere. Hold his penis upright, and *let the sound fall into his urethra by its own weight, as in Fig. 23-8.* Don't push! If it meets with resistance, guide it *very gently* on its way. When you feel the resistance of his perineal membrane, depress it between his thighs, and it will slip into his bladder (the 'tour de maitre', or 'touch of the master').

You will know when a sound is in his bladder by: (1) The ease with which it passes through his perineal membrane into his bladder. (2) The fact that it is exactly in the midline. (3) The ease with which you can rotate the handle of a curved sound. This test does not apply to a straight one.

Eventually, try not to dilate him at intervals of less than 3 weeks, because it takes this time for any local reaction to subside. If his stricture needs dilating more often than this, it is unstable, so consider surgery.

CAUTION ! The signs of a false passage are: (1) Pain. (2) The sound deviates from the midline. (3) You cannot turn the handle of a curved sound freely. (4) He bleeds as you withdraw it. (5) Later, a perineal haematoma develops.

When you have successfuly dilated his stricture, pass a catheter and check his residual urine by passing a catheter after micturition and seeing how much urine remains in his bladder. You will find that the residual urine will be persistently high in about a third of patients; if so, see below.

NYLON FILIFORM BOUGIES are useful if you have failed to pass a sound. You will need several of these, as in Fig. 23-9. Pass the first one, until it is held up by the stricture, either in a fold or a false passage. Continue with more filiform bougies, until with luck, one gets through. Then remove the bougies that have failed to get through, and screw on flexible 'followers' of increasing size. The filiform bougie will curl up in his bladder as you advance it. This is a useful method, even if you have no followers.

MAINTENANCE BOUGINAGE. Make sure that he knows that he may need dilatation once a fortnight for 3 months, then once a month for 6 months, then every 3 months for a year, then every year ever afterwards. Remind him to come a week after his birthday! If possible, teach him self-dilatation with the bougie in C, Fig. 23-9.

CAUTION ! Adjust maintenance bouginage to his needs. Progressive extension of the interval is not always possible, and you may have to stabilize him with more frequent dilatations.

INDICATIONS FOR SURGERY. (1) His stricture is persistently impassable. (2) He needs bouginage at frequent intervals, with many failures. (3) He has an established false passage. When this happens, a curved metal sound passes easily through his false passage, but he still has chronic retention, and urethrography shows the false passage. (4) He has bladder-neck stenosis. (5) He cannot attend regularly, for example, he may not be able to afford transport.

23.9 Difficulties with strictures

Here are the difficulties you may meet in dealing with a stricture. Most of them are characteristically a problem of gonococcal strictures. Extravasation of urine is described in the next section, and impassable strictures in Section 23.11.

EARLY DIFFICULTIES WITH STRICTURES

If BOUGINAGE FAILS but the patient CAN PASS URINE, it is not a disaster. Let him go home and wait a week or two. When he returns, bouginage may be easier. If you again fail to dilate him, and cannot refer him, see Section 23.11.

If BOUGINAGE FAILS and he CANNOT PASS URINE, admit him for some method of suprapubic cystotomy, preferably small-bore suprapubic puncture (23.6). As soon as the acute episode has resolved, he can leave hospital with his suprapubic tube, and reattend the bougie clinic a week or so later. You will probably be able to pass a bougie, if not at the first visit, then at a later one when his stricture has settled down. If necessary,

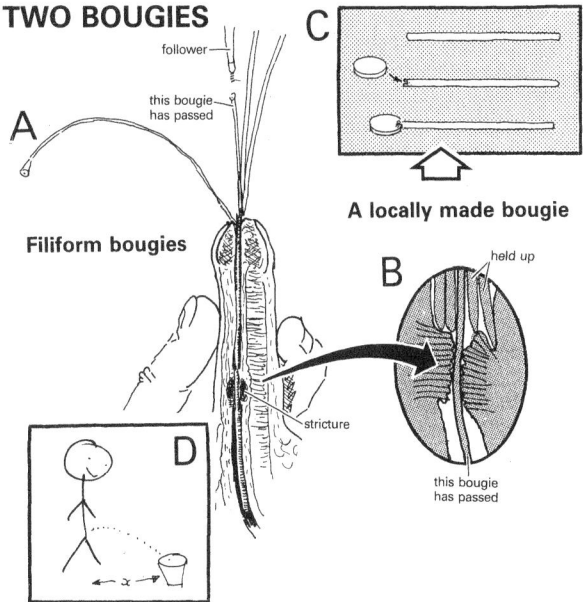

Fig. 23-9 TWO BOUGIES. A, several long thin filiform bougies have been inserted into this patient's urethra looking for a passage through his stricture. Most have been held up at the stricture, or in false passages. In doing so, they have made it easier for the successful bougie to pass through the tiny hole, which is all that remains of his urethra. This bougie is now going to be screwed on to its follower. B, a close up of the stricture. C, a locally made straight metal bougie that you can give to a patient with a stricture in his penile urethra, so that he can dilate himself. A brass disc has been brazed to a metal rod with a smooth round end. D, a simple way to measure patency of his stricture. How far can he urinate? 'X' is a measure of its patency.

try again at weekly or 2-weekly intervals. With patience and perseverance most strictures will yield. Once you have passed a 7 or 8 Ch bougie, his urine flow will be adequate, and you can remove his suprapubic tube. Or, you can spigot it, and make sure he can void adequately, before you remove it. If his urethra is of adequate calibre, his suprapubic puncture track will rapidly close. His stricture is now manageable—but is not cured!

If on the above regime, his stricture remains impassable, see Section 23.11.

If his STRICTURE BLEEDS stop dilating—immediately! You have damaged his mucosa. If you continue, you may create a false passage, and make further treatment more difficult. Try again two weeks later. The corpora cavernosa can bleed briskly, and, to the patient, alarmingly. Bleeding usually stops, but he may return in a few hours with retention of urine. You are much more likely to damage his urethra, if you try to dilate it under general anaesthesia.

If he has PAINFUL RETENTION WITH HAEMATURIA and urethral bleeding, he has CLOT RETENTION. The combination of a painfully distended bladder and blood loss may cause shock, so he may need intravenous fluids or blood. Open his bladder suprapubically (23.7) and remove the clot.

If he develops a FALSE PASSAGE it is the result of: (1) failure in the art of bouginage, (2) doing it when his urethra is acutely inflamed, or (3) under anaesthesia. The bougie goes through the false passage, whereas urine will not, so the his symptoms are not improved, and bleeding, extravasation, and abscess formation may follow. Ideally, a bougie should be passed through the correct route, under the direct vision of an endoscope.

If there is no extravasation, merely drain him suprapubically.
If there is extravasation, see Section 23.10.

If the bougie goes into his RECTUM, which it should never do, drain his bladder suprapubically, give him prophylactic antibiotics, consider doing a temporary colostomy (which is unikely to be necessary), and refer him.

If he has RIGORS, after instrumentation, these are likely to be transient and self-limiting.

If he develops COLLAPSE AND SHOCK after bouginage, suspect Gram-negative septicaemia, which is uncommon, but very dangerous, and may kill him. Take a blood culture, and start parenteral broad-spectrum antibiotics (gentamicin and metronidazole).

Other early complications include transient incontinence (uncommon).

LATE DIFFICULTIES WITH STRICTURES

If he has CHRONIC RETENTION with a HIGH BLOOD UREA, divert his urine suprabubically by blind (23.6) or open (23.7) cystostomy. But be careful, the relief of chronic obstruction is often followed by an obligatory polyuria, which may amount to several litres a day. See Section 23.5.

If his BLADDER CONTINUES TO EMPTY INADEQUATELY, or not at all, after you have dilated his stricture, try a period of continuous bladder drainage for up to 6 weeks to keep it empty. This may be followed by successful voiding.

If he develops a TENDER PAINFUL SWELLING in his perineum, he probably has a PERIURETHRAL ABSCESS, which may or may not be associated with retention of urine. The diagnosis is not difficult, but you can easily overlook it in the presence of retention of urine—see also Section 5.14.

If he develops a FISTULA, it is the consequence of an inadequately treated periurethral abscess, or he may give no history of an acute episode, and his fistula may appear spontaneously. Multiple fistulae may involve his perineum, scrotum, and penis, his perianal region and the inner aspects of his thighs (the 'watering can perineum' in Fig. 23-10). You may be able to demonstrate these fistulae radiologically. Sometimes, a fistula forms between his urethra and his rectum.

If his fistula is recent, give him a course of antibiotics, dilate his stricture, and divert his urine by suprapubic drainage. You will probably have to do this by open cystostomy (23.7), because his bladder will not be distended.

If his fistula is an old one, with epithelialized tracks, treatment is difficult. In theory, excising all the tracks and diverting his urine should allow slow healing. In practice, teatment is prolonged and disappointing.

A 'WATERING CAN' PERINEUM

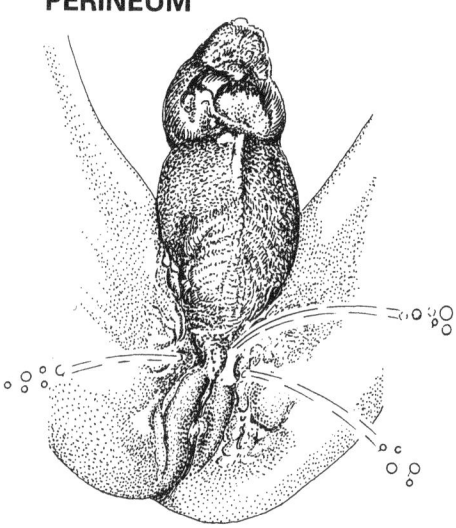

Fig. 23-10 A 'WATERING CAN PERINEUM' is the late result of a complex gonococcal stricture, or rarely a tuberculous one. Multiple chronically infected and epithelialized fistulae have involved this patient's penis, scrotum, perineum and thighs. A sullen ooze of purulent discharge is more usual than the shower of urine shown here. *Kindly contributed by Neville Harrison*

If his fistula fails to close, suspect tuberculosis or carcinoma, and exclude these histologically.

If chronic fistulae and periurethral sepsis lead to gross ELEPHANTIASIS (uncommon), consider excising his chronically oedematous tissue, and retaining his skin by raising flaps at least 1 cm thick. If necessary, excise his oedematous tissues totally and graft the bare area with split skin.

If his TESTES AND EPIDIDYMES SWELL, he has developed acute epididymo-orchitis. Treat him non-operatively with antibiotics (ampicillin or trimethoprim).

If his PERINEUM, LOWER ABDOMEN, OR PENIS SWELL, he has EXTRAVASATION of urine (23.10).

If HIS BLADDER REMAINS DISTENDED AFTER HE HAS PASSED URINE (he has a high residual urine), this is either due to detrusor failure, or bladder-neck stenosis, or both. Or, he may have a stricture and benign (or malignant) prostatic hypertrophy. Bladder-neck stenosis is probably caused by chronic infection. You may feel it as a prominent lip when you pass a straight metal bougie, or you may see it radiologically (34.5). You can: (1) Refer him for a transurethral resection, if his urethra is wide enough to pass the instrument. Or, (2) open his bladder and either incise his bladder neck, or remove his prostate.

CAUTION ! A prominent bladder neck, felt or seen, does not always indicate stenosis. Only a tight bladder neck can be diagnosed in this way.

If he develops STONES, they are the result of infected stagnant urine, and may form in his dilated urethra proximal to the stricture. They will remain until you remove them by cystotomy or urethrotomy. Then treat his stricture and his infection.

If he BLEEDS FROM HIS URETHRA, and this is not associated with instrumentation, consider the possibility of a BLADDER TUMOUR (32.31), and don't necessarily attribute the bleeding to the stricture, or its treatment. By the time the diagnosis is made, the tumour may have extended beyond his bladder, and may have appeared through a cystostomy track, or a urethral fistula. You will not be able to see the lesion until you have dilated his stricture to at least 18 Ch to take a cystoscope. You may also see it as a filling defect in a cystogram. If it has already extended beyond his bladder, it is inoperable, and palliation merely prolongs his misery.

A FORCED PASSAGE IS A FALSE PASSAGE

23.10 Extravasation of urine complicating a stricture

The effects of extravasated urine are dramatic. The combination of urine and infection produces severe oedema of a patient's scrotum and abdominal wall. If this is not treated, the skin over his scrotum, penis, and anterior abdominal wall may slough. He may be very ill, toxic, febrile, dehydrated, anaemic, or uraemic, or all of these things. If his renal function is impaired, as it often is after a long standing stricture, extravasation may kill him.

Urine can extravasate from a stricture spontaneously, through a periurethral abscess, or as the result of bouginage. The other important cause is trauma (68.7). The attachments of Camper's (Buck's) and Colle's fascia limit its spread so that: (1) From a hole in his bulbous urethra it can track into his scrotum, up over his pubis and into his lower abdominal wall. (2) From a hole in his penile urethra the swelling is limited to his penis.

EXTRAVASATION OF URINE

Exclude cardiac, renal, and hepatic causes of oedema.

Assess the patient's fluid and electrolyte state before surgery. He will probably benefit from intravenous fluid replacement, which may be life-saving.

Control infection with antibiotics. Chloramphenicol will probably be suitable.

DIVERT HIS URINE FLOW so that it no longer leaks into his tissues. His bladder will probably not be palpable because: (1) his urine has 'passed' into his tissues, and (2) oedema may obscure his swollen bladder, even if it is distended. You will probably have to do an open cystostomy (23.7), because: (a) his bladder is unlikely to be dilated enough for a blind one, and (b) you are unlikely to be able to negotiate his stricture with a urethral catheter. Make a formal suprapubic cystostomy, and divert his urine through a high, oblique, midline track.

Later, treat his stricture (23.8). Remove his suprapubic catheter, as soon as regular progressive dilatation has opened up his urethra enough to provide an adequate flow (7 or 8 Ch). If his urine flow is adequate, the high, oblique, midline, suprapubic track that you have made should close satisfactorily.

If you have to continue suprapubic drainage for more than a month, change the suprapubic catheter at 4- to 6-week intervals—see Section 23.7.

DRAIN THE URINE OUT OF HIS TISSUES. Lay him supine, give him a general anaesthetic and perioperative antibiotics (ampicillin, trimethoprim, or gentamicin). Clean his abdomen, penis, and scrotum, and the upper half of his thighs with 1% cetrimide, followed by 1% alcoholic iodine.

(1) Make 5 cm incisions on each side of the base of his penis. Insert your index finger, and open up the tissue planes widely towards his abdomen, and down the shaft of his penis. (2) Make 5 cm incisions on the inferolateral aspects of his scrotum, and use your finger to open up the tissue planes as far as possible. Place two long corrugated rubber drains into the depth of each wound in each direction, and suture them in place. Dress the wounds with gauze and cotton wool. Bath him in a bowl of salt water each day. The swelling will usually settle in about 5 days. Shorten the drains 5 cm a day. Areas of necrotic skin and subcutaneous tissue will form. These will take a long time to separate spontaneously, so excise them. When infection has subsided, close the skin incisions by secondary suture, and graft the bare areas (57.2). Don't attempt bouginage again until he is much improved, say at 4 to 6 weeks.

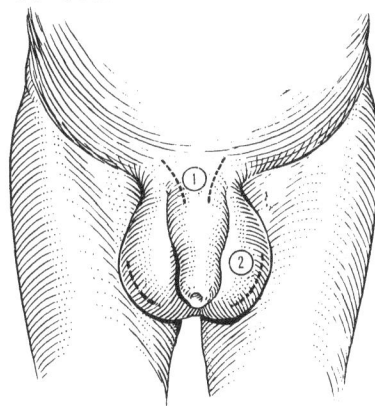

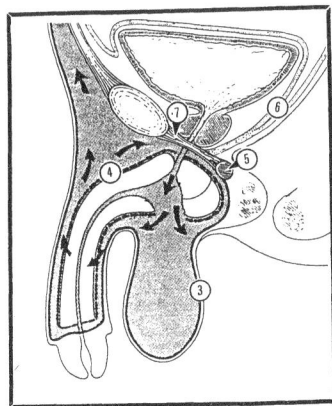

Fig. 23-11 EXTRAVASATION OF URINE. A, the fascial planes concerned with the superficial extravasation of urine. B, incisions for drainage. C, a dissected drawing (not an operation!) showing the directions in which urine can track (C, Fig. 68-6 shows another way to drain extravasated urine).

1, and 2, incisions for drainage. 3, Colles' fascia. 4, Camper's fascia. 5, the transversus perinei muscle. 6, Denonvillier's fascia. 7, the triangular ligament. A, from 'Hamilton Bailey's Emergency Surgery', edited by HAF Dudley, Fig. 50.11 (John wright). With the kind permission of Hugh Dudley.

23.11 Impassable strictures

A stricture which you cannot bougie is a difficult problem. A short traumatic one can be excised, and the ends of the patient's urethra anastomosed end to end. If however it is the result of inflammation, it is likely to be longer, and to need a formal urethroplasty in at least two stages, in which a new urethra is made with scrotal skin. This is a lengthy and difficult procedure, which many patients will not submit to. Unless a stricture is very short, a urethroplasty is work for an expert urologist, so refer all patients with impassable strictures if you can.

If you cannot refer a patient, you may be able to:

(1) Assist bouginage by putting a finger into his bladder through a cystostomy.

(2) Leave him with a permanent opening between his bladder and the outside (a suprapubic drain or cystostomy). His drain will need to be changed every few weeks (23.7).

(3) Leave him with a permanent artificial opening between his urethra and the outside by doing the first stage only of a Blandy's posterior urethroplasty. This will leave him with a permanent urethrostomy orifice in his perineum, through which he will pass urine 'like a woman'. It will not effect his potency, but he may not like his semen coming out of 'the wrong place'. The first stage is not easy, but is much easier than the second, for which you may be able to refer him. Even the first stage may do him much good, and is much better than a permanent suprapubic drain, which may be the only alternative. It is not easy to get a good channel which will not restenose, and bleeding can be a nuisance. This is one of the operations for a 'careful caring operator' (1.8). You can do it for an impassable stricture anywhere in the urethra, even as high as the verumontanum.

(4) Do a simple urethroplasty if a stricture is short enough. Unfortunately, few strictures are short enough, and relief is likely be temporary only, especially in Africa, because African patients have a particular tendency to make scar tissue.

(5) Do an external urethrotomy with closure, if his stricture is fairly short, and is anterior enough in his membranous urethra for there to be some normal urethra above it. Fortunately, although gonococcal strictures may be long, there is almost always some normal urethra above them. Strictures without normal urethra above them are likely to be the less common traumatic ones of the posterior urethra (see below under 'Difficulties'). An external urethrotomy is: (a) not nearly as good as an expert internal urethrotomy or a urethroplasty, (b) not an easy operation, so try to avoid doing one if you can.

To do an external urethrotomy you will need to find both ends of the stricture, cut down on it, pass a plastic (not rubber) tube through it, and let his urethra heal round this. He will need dilating for life, but he will at least be able to pass his urine through his penis.

You can easily find the distal end of a stricture, by passing a sound down his urethra. Finding its proximal end is more difficult. There are two ways of doing this: (a) You can open the dilated part of his urethra and pass a bougie forwards. If you do this, you cannot go astray in a false passage, and you can find the lumen of the stricture more easily. (b) You can open his bladder and pass a curved C-shaped sound forwards through a cystostomy incision into his urethra.

Stom J H, 'Management of urethral strictures in a rural hospital in Ghana', Tropical Doctor 1982;12:32-34.

IMPASSABLE STRICTURES

BOUGINAGE ASSISTED BY A FINGER IN THE BLADDER

This may avoid external urethrotomy, so try it first. Do an open suprapubic cystotomy, and introduce a large urethral sound through the patient's external meatus. With a finger in his bladder, guide the tip of the sound through the stricture. Fix a plastic catheter to the tip of the sound, remove the sound, and draw the catheter into his urethra in a retrograde manner from above.

PERINEAL URETHROSTOMY, the first stage only of Blandy's posterior urethroplasty.

INDICATIONS. Impassable strictures. You can do a urethrostomy, suitably modified, anywhere in the urethra, even if the stricture reaches as high as the verumontanum.

ANAESTHESIA. General anaesthesia; an erection will increase bleeding.

PREPARATION. Put him into the cystoscopy position to allow access to his suprapubic region. Shave his perineum, and prepare his skin with care.

METHOD. Make an inverted 'U'-shaped scrotal flap with rather a flat apex to end just in front of his ischial tuberosities (A, Fig. 23-12). The key to the operation is access, so the flap must go far back. Cut through his skin and dartos, tying and coagulating vessels as you go, and allow the flap to hang down.

CAUTION ! (1) Allow a generous lining of fat on the flap. (2) Try not to disturb the vessels in its base. (3) Don't use diathermy on the flap, or you may coagulate them.

Pass a 24 Ch bougie down to the face of the stricture, and ask your assistant to hold it in the midline. Feel for it, and dissect down to it, until you see his bulbospongious muscle (B). Dissect the muscle from the bulb and reflect it on either side (C). Cut down on to the bougie (D), and immediately insert a 4/0 continuous catgut suture on either side, to close his spongy tissue and prevent bleeding. Incise until you reach healthy tissue; in a bulbar stricture you may have to cut to within a few millimetres of his 'veru', and you have completely divided the stricture. Cut 1 cm at a time, and control bleeding by continuing your haemostatic stitch down each side of his split corpus spongiosum (E).

CAUTION ! Be sure to carry the incision past his stricture. The only way to be sure about this is to pass your finger past the stricture, to make sure there are no strands of fibrous tissue remaining.

Inspect his stricture and his 'veru' with a nasal speculum (F). Divide all fibrous bands until you see his 'veru'.

Partly straighten a 3/0 chromic catgut atraumatic needle (H). Hold it in a needle-holder, so that it almost points straight ahead, and pass it under the edge of his urethra, until it emerges into the lumen (G). Grasp it with a long needle holder or haemostat and advance it up towards his bladder, until the catgut emerges; then withdraw it backwards. Pass it through the apex of the flap and hold it in a haemostat. Pass 5 sutures like this. Clip each haemostat to the drapes, so that they cannot be muddled up (I). Push the flap towards his bladder. Tie one throw on each knot until it is tight. Reinsert the speculum, and check that the edge of the flap is neatly up against the defect in his urethra, before completing the series of knots. If not, readjust and replace the suture which was at fault. When you are sure the flap is in the right position, put several more throws on each knot, and cut their free ends. Withdraw the speculum and complete the work of sewing in the flap, trimming away surplus skin where necessary (J). Use fine monofilament to bring the edges of his scrotum to the edges of his urethra (K). Leave the catheter in.

POSTOPERATIVELY, give him frequent salt baths (22.1), remove the catheter at 5 days, and the sutures, after premedication, at 14 days. Make sure that there are no cross-adhesions between the suture lines. If a bridge has formed, part it, and ask him to keep the passage open by inserting his finger daily in the bath. If possible, refer him for the second stage at 3 months.

DIFFICULTIES with a Blandy's posterior urethroplasty. Curiously, incontinence is uncommon.

If the TIP OF THE SCROTAL FLAP of a posterior urethroplasty necroses, take it down, trim it and resuture it; there is usually plenty of skin.

If a HAEMATOMA forms, take him back to the theatre, take down the wound, evacuate it, and secure haemostasis.

A SIMPLE URETHROPLASTY

INDICATIONS. A stricture <2 cm long.

CONTRAINDICATIONS. A stricture more than >2 cm. One contributor considers even a shorter one is contraindicated, if there is intense fibrosis in an African patient.

METHOD. Do an open suprapubic cystotomy (23.7). Pass a straight metal sound through his external urinary meatus, up to the distal face of the stricture, as above. Open his skin, subcutaneous tissue, bulbocavernosus muscle, and corpus spongiosum at the tip of the sound, over the area of the stricture. A 2.5 cm incision is usually enough.

Pass a curved metal sound through the cystostomy wound, into his urethra, and down to the proximal face of the stricture. Incise his urethra longitudinally between the two sounds.

If the stricture is long, you will have to do an external urethrotomy, as below.

If the stricture is short, sew it up transversely, using 2/0 chromic catgut on a cutting needle, or better 'Vicryl'. Slight trac-

---

Fig. 23-12 PERINEAL URETHROSTOMY. This is the first stage of Blandy's urethroplasty. A, the outline of the flap. B, the flap allowed to fall down. C, reflect the patient's bulbospongiosus from his bulbar urethra. D, open his urethra on to a bougie just distal to his stricture. E, oversew his corpus spongiosum to control bleeding. F, inspect his urethra with a nasal speculum and continue to incise it, until you emerge into healthy mucosa, and can see his verumontanum (his 'veru'). This is normally a cystoscopic landmark, and is a posterior midline swelling in his urethral mucosa. It is just proximal to his external sphincter and his ejaculatory ducts open onto it. G, use a modified atraumatic needle to insert sutures at the edge of his divided urethra. H, how to bend the needle. I, lead 5 sutures through the apex of the flap. J, the top 5 sutures tied, bringing the flap into his opened-out urethra. K, his scrotal skin approximated to his urethra all round.

1, the scrotal flap. 2, his ischial tuberosities. 3, the flap reflected. 4, his bulbospongiosus. 5, his urethra. 6, his bulbospongiosus being incised. 7, the bougie. 8, the sutured edge of his corpus spongiosum. 9, his 'veru'. From Blandy J, 'Operative Urology', Figs. 14.43 et seq. Blackwell Scientific Publications, with kind permission.

PERINEAL URETHROSTOMY

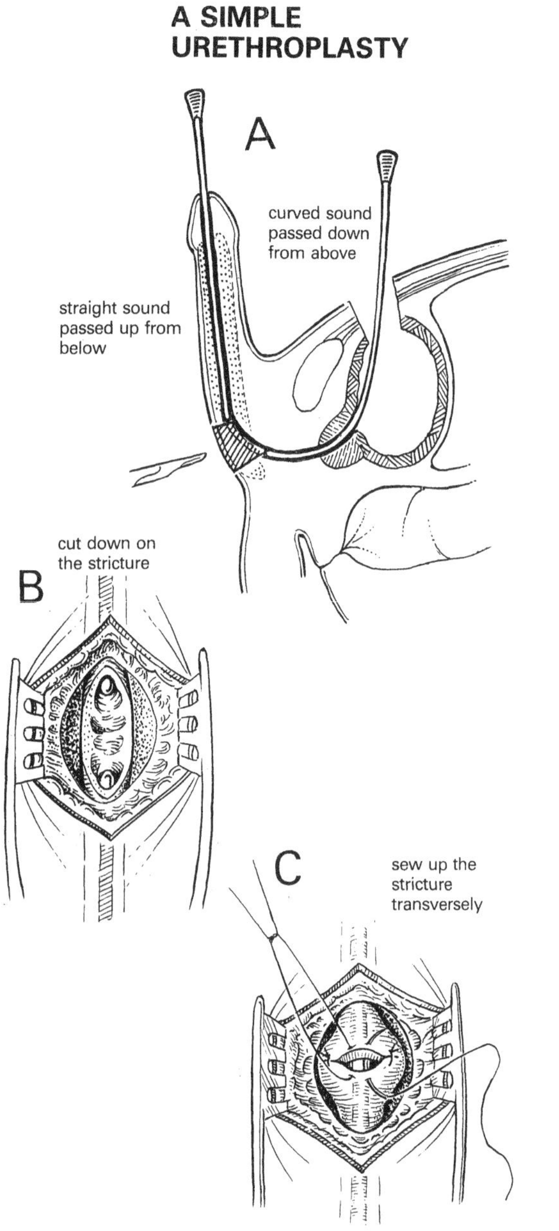

A SIMPLE URETHROPLASTY

EXTERNAL URETHROTOMY

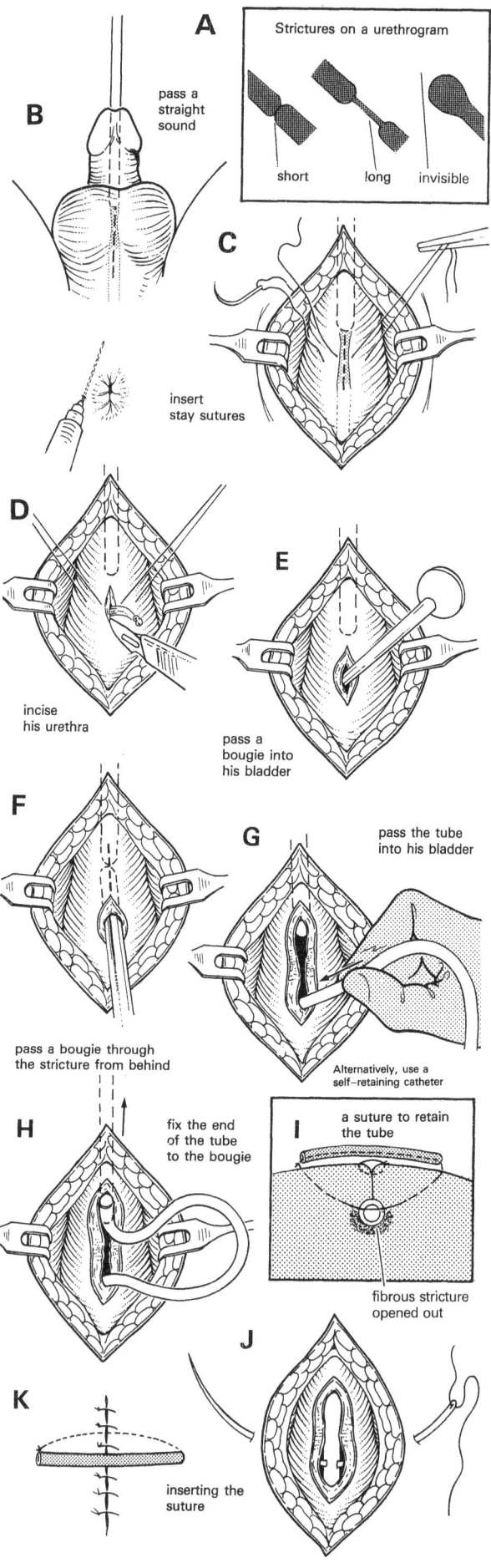

Fig. 23-13 A SIMPLE URETHROPLASTY. A, pass a straight metal sound up to the distal face of the stricture, and a curved one down to its proximal face through the cystostomy wound. B, cut down on the stricture. C, if it is short, sew it up transversely. *Kindly contributed by JH Stom.*

tion on the sutures will not jeopardize the end result. Insert a small-bore catheter, and leave it in place for 14 days.

Close the wound in layers. If much pus discharges from the external ostium of his urethra, remove the catheter on the 7th day.

EXTERNAL URETHROTOMY

INDICATIONS. An impassable stricture.

EQUIPMENT. Make a solution containing lignocaine 2% 20

Fig. 23-14 EXTERNAL URETHROTOMY. A, different kinds of strictures as seen on a urethrogram. B, pass Powell's sound in the urethra to find the distal end of the stricture. C, place stay sutures. D, open the bulb of his urethra, by cutting between the stay sutures. E, pass a straight bougie into his bladder. F, pass a bougie forwards to find the proximal end of the stricture. G, pass the tube into his bladder. H, pass the tube down his distal penile urethra by first fixing it to the end of the sound. I, J, and K, if you are not using a self-retaining catheter, anchor the tube like this. *After Davey, 'Companion to Surgery in Africa', (1st edn), p. 334. Churchill Livingstone, with kind permission.*

380

ml, hyaluronidase ('Hyalase') 1 ml, adrenalin 1/1000 1 ml, and 0.9% saline 80 ml. Even if you operate under general anaesthesia, use this fluid; it is essential for controlling bleeding. If you don't use it, alarming bleeding will obscure the anatomy. Apart from the hyaluronidase, which is not strictly necessary, it is the 'jungle juice' recommended in Primary Anaesthesia (A 5.4). A straight Powell's sound. About 45 cm of 7 mm tube; ideally, silastic, or, less satisfactorily some other plastic. Don't use red rubber—it is too irritant. The tube should not be too big—about 18, or at the most 20 Ch, so that there is enough space between it and the urethra for secretions to drain. Some surgeons cut small side holes to promote drainage. Alternatively, use a self retaining catheter, and don't sew it in place.

ANAESTHESIA. Use general or local anaesthesia, with the patient well premedicated with pethidine or morphine.

METHOD. Put him into the lithotomy position and pass a Powell's sound, until it meets the anterior end of the stricture (B, in Fig. 23-14).

Start to infiltrate his perineum 3 cm in front of his anus and carry the infiltration well forwards, past the tip of the Powell's sound.

Start to incise 2.5 cm in front of the place where you can feel the tip of the sound, back to a point 5 cm in front of his anus. Cut his deep fascia. Use blunt dissection with scissors in the midline to display the muscles round the bulb of his penis.

The thick spongy tissue of the bulbus spongiosum through which the urethra passes easily slips away from your scalpel, which may stray from the midline. So, before you cut it, anchor it with *deep* stay sutures, and use them to pull the bulb of his penis forwards on to the knife, which can now cut boldly, exactly in the midline through the median raphe of his bulbospongiosus muscle (C).

As you open his urethra, urine will spurt out (D). If it does not, assist it with a hand on his abdomen. To make sure you have found the lumen, pass a straight bougie into his bladder (E). Withdraw it, and push it gently forwards from the urethral opening, to find and pass through the stricture from behind (F). Divide the stricture by cutting down on this bougie, until there is a clear passage into his urethra anteriorly.

Take the 45 cm length of 7 mm tube, pass one end back into his bladder, and the other end forwards out through his external meatus (G). The easiest way to do this is to thread it on to the end of the Powell's sound (H).

This tube must remain in his urethra for 3 weeks. So fix it with a Colt's needle through all the layers of his perineum, and let the needle take a bite of the tube on the way (I, J, and K).

Close his muscle and fascia loosely with interrupted catgut, and his skin with monofilament. Finally, anchor the stitch that you passed through the tube, and prevent it cutting into his skin, by passing it through a short length of plastic tube (K).

Apply a pad and a firm T-bandage for 24 hours to prevent a haematoma forming. Raise his scrotum with strips of broad strapping, and fix it to his thighs to to minimize the swelling that may follow.

Give him a sulphonamide for 7 to 10 days, and make sure that he has a daily fluid intake of at least 3 litres.

At 10 to 14 days, remove all sutures except the one which anchors the tube. Get him up with the tube spigotted for 2 or 3 hours at a time. If he is able to reattend easily, you can now discharge him.

At 3 weeks, cut the anchoring stitch and remove the polythene tube. Pass a large (22 Ch) bougie, and ask him to return for regular dilatation.

CAUTION ! Make sure that he understands that he is not cured, and that he must continue to attend for regular dilatations for the rest of his life.

DIFFICULTIES WITH EXTERNAL URETHROTOMY

If there is a STEADY OOZE from the cut surfaces of his cavernous tissue, after he has returned to the ward from a urethrotomy, you may need to take him back to the theatre, reopen his wound and search for the bleeding point. Pack it with dry or haemostatic gauze.

If his STRICTURE IS SO HIGH in his urethra that you can find no normal urethra above it (rare), it is probably a TRAUMATIC STRICTURE. If you cannot refer him, he will have to live with a permanent suprapubic cystostomy (23.7).

23.12 Stones in the urinary tract

Stones in the urinary tract vary greatly in their prevalence. For example, they are common in North India and the Sudan, but are rare in East and Central Africa. In the 'stone belts' of South East Asia and South America, they are very common, even in children. You should be able to: (1) Relieve the excruciating pain of renal colic. (2) Do a nephrostomy for calculous anuria—this can be life-saving, but is rarely needed (23.13). (3) Remove a ureteric stone (23.14). (4) Remove an adult's (23.15) or a child's (23.16) bladder stone. (5) Remove a stone impacted in a child's urethra (23.17). Removing a stone from anyone's kidney, or his renal pelvis, is too difficult to be described here.

Stones are of two kinds: (1) Primary or metabolic stones. (2) Secondary stones resulting from obstruction, or repeated infection. Primary stones are most common in men between 30 and 50, and usually form in the renal pelvis; the lower calyx is the next most common site.

The size and position of a stone determines what it does. If it is small, and remains in the periphery of the kidney, or in a calyx, it may cause few symptoms; if it enlarges it may obstruct part of the kidney. A small stone may pass down the ureter, cause acute renal or ureteric colic as it does so, and later be voided in his urine. If it is too big to do this, it may obstruct the upper end of the ureter, and cause a hydronephrosis which will ultimately destroy the kidney.

Stones in the bladder don't usually return when you remove them, but those in the upper urinary tract often do. "A gram of prevention is worth a kilo of pills, or a megatonne of surgery", so warn a patient with a stone in his upper urinary tract that he has about a 50% chance of getting another one during the next 10 years. Advise him according to the instructions below. The most useful preventive measure is a high fluid intake.

Most stones are radio-opaque, so learn where to look for them; an occasional exception is a urate stone in a child's bladder, but even these usually contain enough calcium to let you see them on an X-ray film.

URINARY STONES

SPECIAL TESTS. The presence of microscopic haematuria is the most useful test. If there are pus cells, or a patient's urine is alkaline, it is infected.

X-RAYS. Take a plain film of his kidneys, ureters and bladder (a 'KUB'). You can easily miss a stone if: (1) the film is poor, (2) it is only moderately radio-opaque, or (3) it is obscured by bone. Look for kidney stones opposite his second lumbar vertebra. For ureteric stones, see Section 23.14. Don't mistake a gallstone, or a calcified lymph node, for a urinary stone. They are easily distinguished. In a lateral X-ray of his abdomen gallstones are anterior and renal and ureteric stones overlie his lumbar spine.

An intravenous urogram: (1) Will tell you if his kidney has stopped functioning or not. If no contrast medium is excreted, it has stopped functioning, or is excreting so little dye that this is invisible. (2) May help you to find the site of an obstructing stone that is not be visible on a plain film. Take films at 1, 3, 12 and even 24 hours. Enough contrast medium may have accumulated to show up his urinary tract, down to the site of the obstruction.

If contrast medium is concentrated in his kidney (a 'nephrogram'), but does not show up in his renal pelvis, a stone may have blocked its pelviureteric junction, and caused the contrast medium to be retained in his kidney tissue. This is a hopeful sign, because it shows that he still has good renal function.

DIFFERENTIAL DIAGNOSIS. The simplest situation is the patient with colic and a stone in his ureter, described in Section 23.14. Here are some other possibilities:

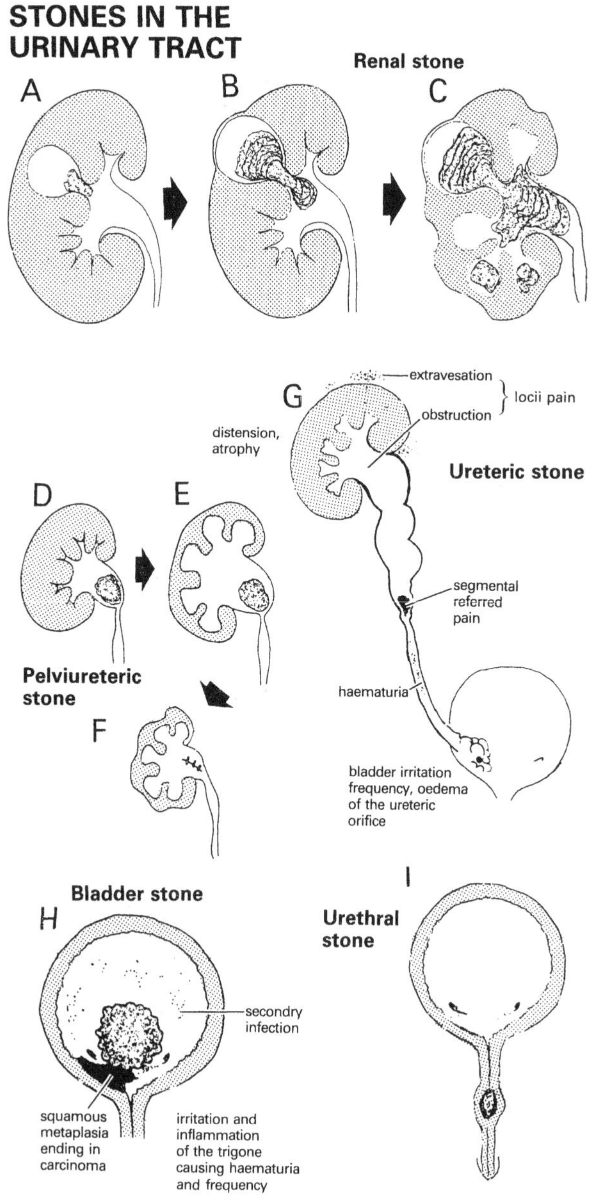

STONES IN THE URINARY TRACT

Fig. 23-15 STONES IN THE URINARY TRACT. A, a stone jammed in a calyx causing hydrocalyx. B, the parenchyma over the dilated calyx has atrophied. C, a staghorn calculus has formed, and there are several stones elsewhere in the kidney. D, a stone has impacted at the pelviureteric junction. E, the calyces have dilated. F, the stone has been removed, but not before the patient's kidney has been severely damaged by obstruction and infection. G, a stone in the ureter causing loin pain, segmental referred pain, haematuria, and frequency. H, a bladder stone with squamous metaplasia ending in carcinoma (rare in Africa). I, a stone in the urethra. *After Blandy J, 'Operative Urology'. Blackwell Scientific Publications, with kind permission.*

If he has moderate pain in his costovertebal angle, a high fever, chills, an obviously infected urine, and an intravenous urogram shows that his renal pelvis and calyces are normal, he has acute pyelonephritis.

If he has a palpable tender renal mass, he probably has a hydronephros. If in addition he has fever, toxaemia, and leucocytosis, it is probably a pyonephros.

If he has a dull ache, with occasional fever and pyuria, suspect that he has a stone which is not obstructing his urinary tract.

If he has anuria and renal failure, this can be due to stones on both sides, but it is more likely to be due to chronic interstitial nephritis or pyelonephritis.

CAUTION ! Some stones cause no symptoms, even when they are large.

TREATMENT FOR URINARY STONES

If he has a stone in his ureter, see Section 23.14.

If he has a small kidney stone (<0.5 cm), which is peripheral in his kidney, and is causing no symptoms and no infection, leave it, but watch it carefully, to see if it moves into his renal pelvis and obstructs this.

If it is obstructing his renal pelvis, it should be removed. The risk of hydro- or pyonephros is too high to leave it. If he has stones on both sides, the side with the better function should be operated on first.

If he has renal colic for few days, after which he gradually becomes oliguric, and then anuric, he probably has calculous anuria (23.13). This can arise from bilateral obstruction, or, more commonly, from the obstruction of a single kidney. Catheterization of his bladder produces no urine. A plain film confirms the diagnosis. His blood urea rises. The episode may relieve itself spontaneously as the result of the oedema in his ureter settling, and the infection being brought under control. Watch him for 24 to 48 hours.

If you have a cystoscope and can pass a ureteric catheter, it may slide past the stone; you can then leave it in place for 2 or 3 days, which will relieve the acute situation, perhaps for long enough for you to refer him. Or the catheter may dislodge the stone back into his renal pelvis.

If he does not rapidly improve, you will have to do an urgent nephrostomy (23.13), and refer him.

TO PREVENT RECURRENT STONES ask him to take plenty of fluids. If he has an associated infection, treat it.

If he has a uric acid stone try to raise the pH of his urine. Make it alkaline with sodium bicarbonate tablets three times a day, or potassium citrate mixture 20 ml three times a day. If possible, measure his serum uric acid. Only give him allopurinol if he has recurrent uric acid stones.

If his serum calcium is consistently high, it suggests a parathyroid adenoma, or some other generalized disease. A raised urinary calcium is more common; advise him to restrict his intake of dairy products.

23.13 Nephrostomy for calculous anuria or hydronephrosis

Other sections in this chapter deal with obstruction to the outflow of urine down the urethra by strictures or enlargement of the prostate. Here we are concerned with the obstruction of his upper urinary tract: his ureters or the pelves of his kidneys. Because these are bilateral, his life is only in danger if both sides are obstructed simultaneously, or he has obstruction in a solitary kidney. When this happens he passes no urine and soon dies of uraemia, unless something is done quickly. Obstruction can be the result of: (1) *Schistosoma haematobium* causing strictures at the junctions of his ureters and his bladder, so producing hydronephroses. (2) Stones obstructing his renal pelves (or a staghorn calculus on one side, and no function on the other). (3) Mistakenly tying both a woman's ureters, while removing her uterus (22.12) or doing a Caesarean section (18.10).

A chronically obstructed kidney is usually large, *so whenever you diagnose renal failure, always feel for enlarged kidneys.* Permanent relief of the obstruction requires expert surgery, so you will have to refer the patient for this. Meanwhile, with luck, you may be able to keep a patient alive long enough to refer him (or her) to an expert, if you put a tube into one of the patient's obstructed kidneys to decompress it, and remove the risk of uraemia. Chronic obstruction of this kind is not uncommon in areas where stones or *S. haematobium* are endemic.

Nephrostomy is not an easy operation, because the kidney is deep and difficult to get at. It is easier for schistosomal hydronephrosis of slow onset, than it is for stones, because the kidney is always large. Having exposed his kidney, you can either push a catheter through a dilated calyx, if you can find one, or you can open his renal pelvis and pull a catheter through his kidney into it. If a stone is the cause, and you can easily remove it, and his condition is good, consider doing so.

NEPHROSTOMY

If a patient has stones on both sides, decompress the side on which he has had recent pain or discomfort, because this is the side which is most likely to regain its function.

ANAESTHESIA. Give him a general anaesthetic, intubate him, and give him a relaxant (A 14.3).

POSITION. Place him on his side with the kidney to be operated on uppermost, as in B, Fig. 23-16. If your table has a kidney bridge, place his 12th rib on the underside over it. Then raise it, so as to open up the space between his rib cage and his pelvis. If you don't have a kidney bridge, place him on 3 or 4 sandbags or folded pillows. If you have a table that can be broken (the head or foot end can be lowered separately), use it to give you more room.

Flex his lower knee, straighten his upper knee, and put a pillow between them. Support his upper arm on a cushioned Mayo table, to prevent his trunk rotating. Take a wide strap, or a long piece of wide adhesive strapping, and wrap this round his pelvis and trochanters, so that his pelvis will not rotate. Have him leaning forwards a little, rather than strictly on his side.

NEPHROSTOMY —ONE

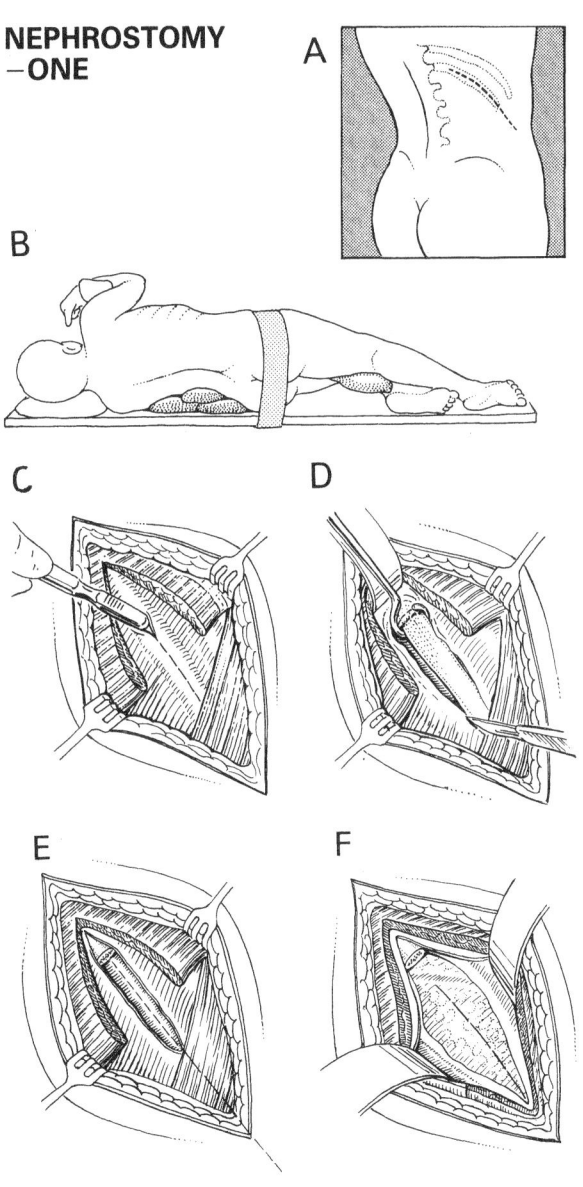

Fig. 23-16 NEPHROSTOMY, ONE—EXPOSING THE KIDNEY. A, the incision over the patient's 12th rib. B, he is ready for surgery, with sandbags under his loin and his arm supported. C, latissimus dorsi has been cut and the periosteum is being stripped over his 12th rib. D, and E, removing his rib. F, his rib removed, and his perirenal fat exposed. Alternatively, make an incision just below his 12th rib and don't remove it.

INCISION. Here we assume that you are going to remove his 12th rib. You can, if you wish, approach his kidney just below and parallel to it, without excising it, especially when his kidney is large, as with a hydronephros. If necessary, make a short incision forwards from his 12th rib.

Mark his 12th rib with a felt pen, A, in Fig. 23-16. Then prepare and drape him, so as to leave an area about 20 cm wide over his 12th rib, from the midline of his back to his umbilicus.

Stand at his back, and make a skin incision starting at the lateral margin of his sacrospinalis. Cut along the line you have drawn over his 12th rib. Proceed anteriorly, and stop 5 cm short of his umbilicus, at the lateral margin of his rectus sheath. A shorter incision will do if he has a marked hydronephros.

You will have to cut much muscle. If possible, use a cutting diathermy, turned down low enough to cut through muscle and coagulate the vessels in it at the same time. Or, use a scalpel, and carefully control the bleeding points as you meet them.

Start by cutting his latissimus dorsi over his 12th rib, until you can see it (C). Then remove his 12th rib subperiosteally with a scalpel, or cutting diathermy. Cut the periosteum down the middle of his rib as far as its tip. Using a periosteal elevator, push the periosteum off its raw surface down its entire length. Reflect the flaps of periosteum. Take a curved periosteal stripper, and gently insert it under the distal part of the rib. Slide it up and down, until the rib is completely clear of periosteum (D, and E,). Cut the narrow strand of external oblique muscle attached to the tip of the rib. Use rib shears, or bone cutters, to cut off the rib as close to its neck as is convenient. Don't punch towards the neck of the rib, *it is too close to his pleura!* Smooth its stump so that it will not tear your gloves.

Cut the three muscles of his anterior abdominal wall in line with the skin incision. The first two, his external oblique and internal oblique, can be cut boldly. When you get down to his transversus, stop temporarily. His peritoneum is under it, and you don't want to risk opening it and flooding it with urine.

Return to the bed of his rib, and use the tip of a scalpel to cut its lowermost half. Carry the incision down on to the remaining fibres of his transversus muscle. Split this in the direction of its fibres.

You will now see his peritoneum, with his liver and part of his colon under it (F). Using a sponge on a holder, gently push the peritoneum down and away from you forwards and upwards. Use a self retaining retractor to separate his rib cage above, from the crest of his ilium below, and so open up the whole area.

Feel for his kidney up against his posterior abdominal wall. If you are not sure if it is his kidney, try moving it up and down. Use a scalpel to make a short incision in the fascia over it. Insert your fingers, separate his perirenal fat, which may be extensive if he is obese; and feel the shape, size, and consistency of his kidney. The tissues around it will probably be engorged and oedematous.

If his kidney is enlarged and soft and feels cystic, it is probably hydronephrotic, but it may be polycystic, in which case nephrostomy does not help. If it is hydronephrotic, it is probably safe to drain it through a dilated calyx, without exposing his renal pelvis (nephrostomy through the cortex).

If his kidney looks and feels fairly normal, expose its pelvis, and drain that (nephrostomy through the renal pelvis).

CAUTION ! (1) Be careful not to damage his fragile and often flattened renal vein, which enters his renal hilum anteriorly, and may cover part of his renal pelvis—which is why you should approach it from behind. (2) The end of the catheter must go into the drainage system, and not into the kidney itself.

NEPHROSTOMY THROUGH THE CORTEX is easier, but does not provide such good drainage. Choose an area on the convex surface of his kidney, where his renal parenchyma is thinly stretched over a tense fluctuant area, and which feels as if there is probably urine under pressure close below it. To confirm that you have found a dilated calyx or pelvis, aspirate it with a fine needle and syringe. Be sure that you are not dealing with an isolated renal cyst.

Take a fine haemostat and plunge this into the fluctuant area. If urine pours out, you are in the right place. Suck it out. Take a small Malecot catheter, flatten out its tip with a haemostat, and push this far enough into his kidney to get a good flow of urine (G, in Fig. 23-17). Remove the haemostat and leave the catheter in. If blood oozes around it, insert a haemostatic suture of fine plain catgut. Bring the nephrostomy tube to the surface.

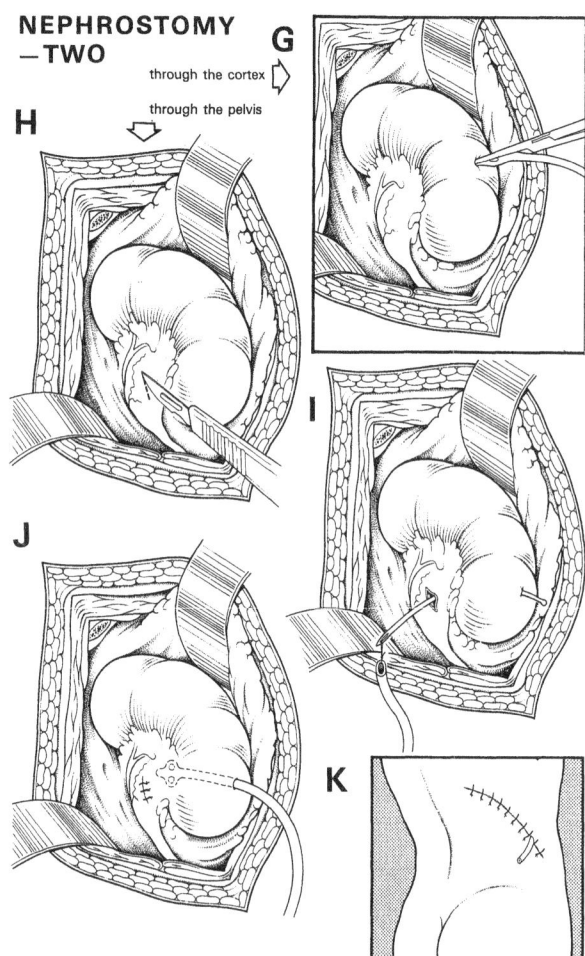

Fig. 23-17 NEPHROSTOMY TWO—DRAINING THE KIDNEY. G, to drain a kidney through its cortex, push a Malecot catheter into a tense fluctuant area. H, to drain a kidney through its pelvis, make a short incision in the posterior of the patient's renal pelvis, well away from its junction with his ureter. I, pass a probe through this incision out through the cortex of his kidney, and tie a Malecot catheter to it. J, the catheter in place. K, the wound closed with the nephrostomy tube in place.

NEPHROSTOMY THROUGH THE RENAL PELVIS drains a kidney better, but is more difficult, because you have to mobilize it. His renal pelvis lies posteriorly, so to get at it you have to turn his kidney forwards and medially, using finger dissection. When his perirenal tissues are oedematous and thickened, separating his kidney from the fat around it is not difficult. You will see his tense distended renal pelvis, which is the most posterior of the structures at the hilum.

Holding his kidney so as to expose his renal pelvis, confirm that urine is present by aspirating with a syringe and fine needle. Make a short incision in his renal pelvis, well away from its junction with his ureter. Urine should gush out (H).

Pass a curved probe through this incision. With your other hand, feel for an area on the convex surface of his kidney, where its cortex feels thin. Carefully (to minimize bleeding) push the tip of the probe out through this point (I). Tie the probe to a Malecot catheter, and draw it back and out through his kidney (J). Close the pyelostomy opening with two fine catgut sutures. If his kidney bleeds where the catheter emerges, apply a purse string catgut suture. Bring the catheter straight to the surface in a position in which he will not occlude it when he lies down (K).

If there is no area of thinned cortex, as may happen with a stone, consider removing the stone through an incision in his renal pelvis, and let the nephrostomy catheter drain from there.

Irrigate the tisses round his kidney, and close all the muscles over it together in one layer. Close his skin, and suture the nephrostomy tube to it. Finally, as an extra precaution, tape the nephrostomy tube to his skin. Connect it to a bedside collecting bottle.

If at any time you open his pleura, see Section 9.2D.

POSTOPERATIVELY, if urine drains freely, you have succeeded, and his uraemia should improve. Watch for the nephrostomy tube kinking or blocking. If it blocks, try irrigating it. He may develop a massive recovery diuresis, so make sure that he gets enough oral or parenteral fluid. See Section 23.5.

Refer him for definitive surgery, when his general condition permits.

23.14 Ureteric stones

The stone that obstructs a patient's ureter originates in his kidney. Once it is free in his renal pelvis, it may pass into his ureter, and it can stick anywhere, but it is most likely to stick: (1) at his pelviureteric junction, (2) in the upper or (3) in the lower third of his ureter, or (4) at the entry of his ureter into his bladder. A stone is usually rough, so that some urine can usually leak past it to begin with. Later, obstruction becomes complete, so that after some weeks or months, he develops a hydronephros or a hydroureter, which may become infected.

As the stone passes down his ureter, it causes severe ureteric colic—even a tiny one causes agony. He has a sudden severe pain in his loin, radiating to his groin, perineum, and testis (or to a woman's labia). He vomits, sweats, and rolls about to get relief. If, at the same time, his urine is infected, he has fever and rigors. His urine may be 'smoky', but is seldom grossly blood-stained. He may be slightly tender in the area of the referred pain, and he may have had attacks like this before. If his stone impacts, the severe pain of ureteric colic gradually subsides.

There is an 85% chance that his ureteric stone will be passed into his bladder, and then out through his urethra. So give him plenty of fluids, and treat his pain.

Don't try to remove a stone from the renal pelvis. This has to be done through a lumbar incision, as for a nephrostomy (23.13); the undilated pelvis is difficult to isolate, and you can easily injure important blood vessels. You can however remove a stone from the middle third of the ureter extraperitoneally, as described below. Ideally, a stone at the lower end of the ureter should be removed with a cystoscope and a Dormia basket, which is difficult and expensive, and needs a modern cystoscope. If you cannot do this, or have tried and failed, you can remove the stone extraperitoneally at open operation, as described below.

URETERIC STONES

SPECIAL TESTS. There are red cells in the patient's urine. A plain ('KUB') film may show the stone. Often, it does not, because he has an associated ileus, and his distended gut obscures it. Look for it along the course of his ureter, as this crosses the tips of the transverse processes of his lumbar vertebrae, runs over his sacroiliac joint, and descends in a gentle arch to a point just medial to his ischial spine, whence it turns medially to enter his bladder. Here, you can easily mistake a stone for a phlebolith. Most ureteric stones are slightly elongated.

If the diagnosis is in doubt, and you want to exclude some disease, such as appendicitis, which requires an urgent operation, take an intravenous urogram at the time of the pain. Otherwise it is unnecessary. Take a film soon after injecting the contrast medium, another at one hour, and a further one at 1½ hours, after he has emptied his bladder, so that contrast medium does not obscure the lower end of his ureter. The delayed excretion of contrast medium into his renal pelvis and dilatation suggest a stone. If they are not present at this stage, take further films at 3, 12, and possibly 24 hours. A totally normal urogram *during the presence of pain* excludes a diagnosis of ureteric colic.

THE DIFFERENTIAL DIAGNOSES include: (1) Appendicitis (for which an intravenous urogram is often necessary). (2) Ovarian

REMOVING A STONE FROM THE MIDDLE AND LOWER THIRDS OF THE URETER

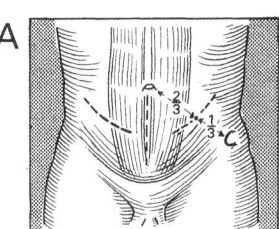

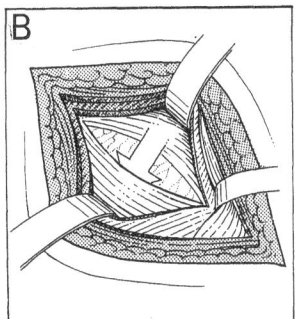
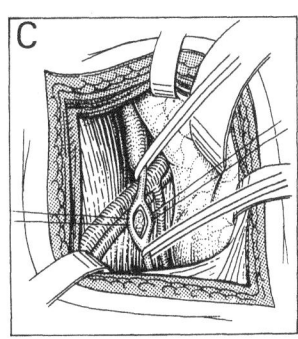
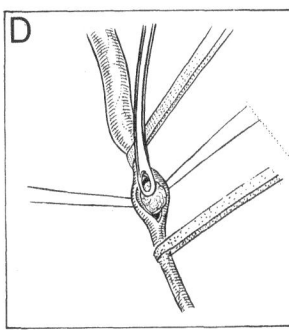
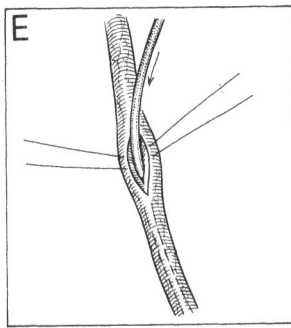

Fig. 23-18 REMOVING A STONE FROM THE LOWER TWO-THIRDS OF THE URETER. A, centre the incision on McBurney's point; for the middle third carry it laterally in the line of the inguinal ligament, for the lower third carry it medially in the line of this ligament. Alternatively, for the lower third use a midline incision. B, divide the external oblique in the direction of its fibres. Cut the internal oblique muscle to expose the transversalis fascia. C, sweep the peritoneum medially to the bifurcation of the common iliac artery. Find the ureter and the stone. Pass catheters, or tapes, round the ureter above and below the stone. Cut on to it with a small knife. D, carefully remove it with Desjardin's forceps. E, pass a thin rubber catheter upwards and downwards to ensure patency. *Kindly contributed by Samiran Nundy.*

causes. (3) Salpingitis. (4) Colic due to the passage of blood clot in the ureters, resulting from trauma, or a neoplasm.

MANAGEMENT. Leave a stone of <5 mm to pass spontaneously, unless there is some complication. A stone of >5 mm is less likely to pass.

An impacted stone may remain in the ureter for weeks or even years, with contrast medium flowing past it and no upper urinary tract dilatation. There is no immediate need to remove a stone which is causing neither symptoms nor harm.

NON-OPERATIVE TREATMENT. Relieve his pain with pethidine (not morphine, because it causes spasm of the smooth muscle of the ureter), intravenously if necessary. Also give him atropine. Repeat these as required. Give him plenty of fluid, a tablet of frusemide 40 mg, and encourage him to walk about. Strain his urine to look for the stone. Repeat the plain X-rays on alternate days.

INDICATIONS FOR SURGERY. (1) Symptoms persist, and serial X-rays taken at 6 to 8 week intervals show that a stone of 5 mm or more is impacted (if it is not causing symptoms or obstruction, it does not necessarily have to be removed, but it is desirable to do so, and there is more time for referral). (2) Pain comes and goes over days or weeks without any further descent of the stone. (3) An intravenous urogram shows a hydronephrosis or a hydroureter, or no excretion of contrast medium. (4) Infection supervenes with fever, chills, rigors, pyuria, and toxaemia.

If possible, refer him; removing a stone from his ureter is not an immediately life-saving procedure, and it can be difficult. If you cannot refer him, proceed as follows.

X-RAYS. Take a plain X-ray of his abdomen just before you operate to make sure that the stone has not moved.

ANAESTHESIA. (1) General anaesthesia using intubation and a relaxant. (2) Subarachnoid (spinal) anaesthesia.

THE RENAL PELVIS OR UPPER THIRD OF THE URETER

This is difficult surgery. Refer him. If you cannot refer him quickly, do a nephrostomy.

FROM THE MIDDLE THIRD OF HIS URETER

Lay him supine. Start your incision at McBurney's point (A, 23-18), and carry it *laterally* for 7 cm parallel to his inguinal ligament. Divide his subcutaneous tissues, and his external oblique aponeurosis in the direction of its fibres; divide his internal oblique in the same direction. Divide his transversalis fascia, and sweep his peritoneum medially, until you reach the inner margin of his quadratus lumborum muscle, and the bifurcation of his common iliac artery into its internal and external iliac branches (3-7, 20-16). You will see his ureter lifted up by his peritoneum. Don't injure his spermatic vessels, which lie lateral to his ureter.

Feel for the stone in his ureter. Carefully pass a long Lahey forceps round his ureter, and pass two fine rubber catheters, or tapes, above and below the stone. This will prevent it slipping upwards or downwards. Cut longitudinally on to the stone with a No. 15 blade. Remove it carefully with Desjardin's forceps. Wash the area free of grit with warm saline. Pass a small rubber catheter up into his kidney, and down into his bladder, to make sure that no other stones are left behind.

Leave the ureteric incision open. Place a No. 12 Malecot catheter near this site, and bring it out through a separate stab incision. Close the abdominal incision in layers, using interrupted chromic catgut for the muscle, and monofilament for his skin. Connect the catheter to a closed drainage system.

CAUTION ! Make sure you find the stone and encircle his ureter above the catheter. If it slips upwards into his kidney, don't try to remove it by extending the incision, or using a traumatic instrument. Close the incision and refer him.

POSTOPERATIVELY, the catheter will drain up to 1000 ml of urine daily, but the volume will gradually diminish. By the 7th day his ureteric incision should have closed, and drainage ceased. If the volume draining remains undiminished, there is an obstruction in his ureter distal to the site of the incision, or it is diseased locally. Wait another week, and refer him.

FROM THE LOWER THIRD OF HIS URETER

X-ray and anaesthetize him as above. Empty his bladder by passing a urethral catheter. Lay him supine, with a slight Trendelenberg position. There are two possible approaches. Remaining outside his peritoneum, which should be your aim, is easier in the first one.

Start your incision at McBurney's point and carry it *medially* parallel to the inguinal ligament. Incise his external and internal oblique, and open his transversalis fascia.

Or, (2) make a lower midline, or paramedian incision, starting at his pubis, and ending at his umbilicus. Incise his transversalis fascia (a transverse incision can also be used).

Carefully strip his peritoneum upwards with a gauze swab. Look for his ureter at the bifurcation of his common iliac vessels (Figs. 3-7 and 20-16) and follow it downwards to his bladder. It is crossed anteriorly by his vas deferens. You may have to divide his superior vesical artery so as to let you mobilize his bladder sufficiently to allow you see his ureterovesical junction easily.

Find the stone, and pass a rubber catheter under his ureter to prevent the stone slipping upwards. Make a longitudinal incision over it, and remove it carefully. Close the wound, leaving behind a rubber Malecot catheter connected to a closed drainage system as above. Care for him postoperatively as above.

DIFFICULTIES WITH URETERIC STONES

If his ureteric colic goes, but THERE IS NO EVIDENCE THAT HE HAS PASSED A STONE, don't be surprised, this is not uncommon. It has probably passed without him being aware of it, especially if it is small.

If a stone becomes impacted at his pelviureteric junction, and HE ONLY HAS ONE KIDNEY, do a nephrostomy and refer him quickly.

If a stone is FIRMLY IMPACTED AT HIS URETEROVESICAL JUNCTION deep in his pelvis, try to squeeze it into his bladder or upwards into a more accessible part of his ureter where it will be easier to remove. Alternatively, make an incision 3 cm above the site of impaction, and try to remove the stone carefully with Desjardin's forceps.

23.15 Bladder stones in adults

Bladder stones can be primary, when there is no obstruction, or secondary, when there is. In the industrial world, primary bladder stones were once common in adults and children, but have now almost disappeared. A few secondary stones are seen in adults with urinary obstruction. Primary stones are however still common at all ages in a 'stone belt' which includes North Africa, the Near and Middle East, Pakistan, India, Burma, Thailand, Vietnam, Laos, Kampuchea, southern China, and Indonesia; mostly, but not only, in the poor.

If you are not in the stone belt, and you do find a bladder stone in an adult, be sure to exclude distal obstruction. If you remove a stone from his bladder, and there is obstruction, a fistula may form and refuse to heal.

Most bladder stones in adults cause no pain, or slight pain in the perineum, or, if a stone is big, a 'bumping feeling' as the stone moves about.

The operation to remove a bladder stone in an adult is similar to that for the first stage of a Freyer's prostatectomy, and the open suprapubic cystostomy described in Section 23.7. The exact way in which you close the bladder is not important, you can use continuous, or interrupted, sutures, of plain or chromic catgut. There is no need to oppose the mucosa precisely, nor is it now considered important to avoid penetrating the mucosa with stitches. But be sure to: (1) Keep the bladder empty with an indwelling suprapubic or urethral catheter. (2) Drain the retropubic space, so that blood and urine cannot accumulate.

When you have removed a bladder stone it does not usually recur, so the strict measures for preventing the recurrence of stones in the upper urinary tract are less necessary in the bladder.

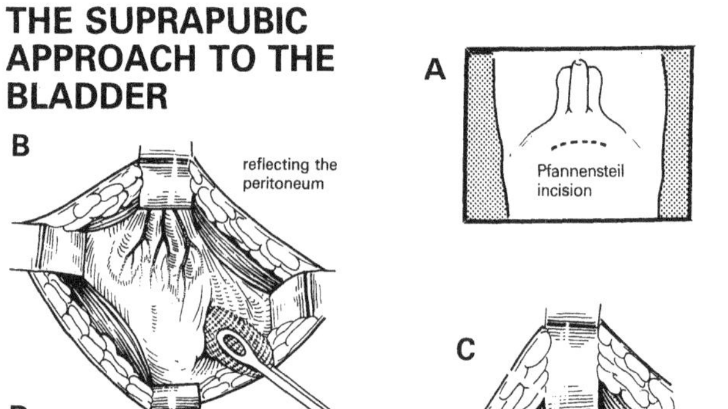

THE SUPRAPUBIC APPROACH TO THE BLADDER

A, Pfannensteil incision
B, reflecting the peritoneum
C, if you want to displace his bladder upwards, you may need to divide his puboprostatic ligaments.
D, opening his bladder between Allis forceps
E, the first layer of sutures
F, sutures complete; the stone removed

Fig. 23-19 THE SUPRAPUBIC APPROACH TO THE BLADDER FOR THE REMOVAL OF A STONE. In this view you are standing on the patient's left side, so that his bladder appears upside down. A, the site of a Pfannensteil incision. B, displace the reflection of his peritoneum upwards. C, if you need to reflect his bladder upwards, you can divide his puboprostatic ligaments; most surgeons don't do this. D, hold his bladder in Allis' forceps and open it. E, the first step in closure. F, complete the second layer of sutures. Figure 23-21 shows the method of closure in more detail. *After Flocks RH and Culp DA, 'Surgical Urology', (4th edn 1975), Plates 69 and 70. Yearbook Medical, with kind permission.*

BLADDER STONES IN ADULTS

X-RAYS confirm the diagnosis, because bladder stones in an adult are usually radio-opaque. Other retropubic calcifications include: (1) Calcification of the bladder wall due to bilharzia (very common in endemic areas and gives no trouble). If necessary, confirm this by showing that the shadow is a different size when the bladdder is full and empty. (2) Calcification in a uterine fibroid. (3) A calcified mesenteric lymph node.

DIAGNOSIS. If this is in doubt, pass a sound, and feel it grating against the stone (the classical way of diagnosing one).

ANAESTHESIA. (1) Local infiltration of the skin, subcutaneous tissues, and muscle layers of the abdominal wall will produce enough anesthesia for short operations. If he is debilitated, this is the method of choice. (2) If the operation is a long one, or you need muscle relaxation, use general anaesthesia, or a low subarachnoid (A 7.6).

PREPARATION. If his bladder is going to be difficult to find, consider inserting a urethral catheter and filling it with fluid; you can use the same catheter for postoperative drainage. A steep Trendelenburg position will make exposure easier.

A PFANNENSTEIL INCISION (23-20) makes it easier to keep low, and avoid opening his peritoneum, as it passes from his abdominal wall to his bladder.

Incise his skin and subcutaneous tissue transversely. Either: (1) part his rectus muscles to expose his peritoneum in the midline. Or, (2) cut his rectus muscles transversely in line with the skin incision, little by little, until you see the inferior epigastric vessels in the deep surface laterally. This will give you better exposure, and you will be less likely to incise the peritoneal reflection over his bladder in error, which may spread infection into his peritoneum.

Alternatively, make a paramedian incision.

Find the reflection of his peritoneum and displace this upwards. Grasp his bladder with stay sutures on either side of the midline, or with two Allis' forceps, holding the entire thickness of its wall. Make a vertical incision in his bladder, unless you want to remove a large stone—then make a transverse one. You can suture a transverse incision more easily, but it will bleed more than a vertical one. Suck away his urine as it gushes out.

Put your finger into his bladder to feel if the stone is lying free, or is impacted in a diverticulum. Feel for a tumour or other pathology. Remove any free stones with your fingers, a scoop, or lithotomy forceps.

THE PFANNENSTEIL INCISION

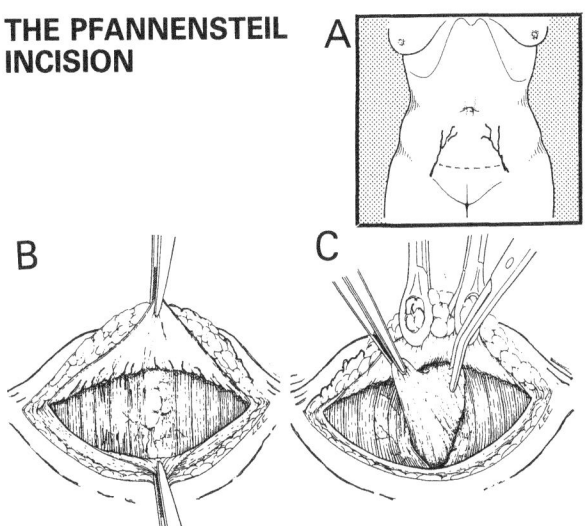

Fig. 23-20 DETAILS OF THE PFANNENSTEIL INCISION. A, the incision. The inferior epigastric arteries lie at the ends of the incision on the deep surface of the rectus muscles. B, reflecting the anterior layer of the rectus sheath. C, the rectus muscles have been parted and you are preparing to enter the abdomen. Alternatively, you can cut them transversely little by little, until you reach the epigastric vessels on the deep surface. *From 'Hamilton Bailey's Emergency Surgery', edited by HAF Dudley, (John Wright). With the kind permission of Hugh Dudley.*

CAUTION ! Repeatedly wash out his bladder before you close it. If you leave any stony fragments, they will act as the nuclei for the formation of more stones.

Close his bladder in two layers with continuous or interrupted 2/0 catgut or 'Dexon'.

Most surgeons rely on a urethral Foley catheter to provide drainage, and don't feel that a suprapubic one is necessary; it does however allow the patient to have a trial of voiding. Be sure to drain his retropubic space; bring the drain out through a stab wound.

POSTOPERATIVELY, remove his retropubic drain after 48 hours. Leave the Foley catheter in place for 8–10 days, to keep his bladder collapsed while it heals. Take a specimen of urine for culture a day or two before you take it out.

DIFFICULTIES WITH BLADDER STONES IN ADULTS

If he develops a FISTULA, which is not uncommon, it will probably be the result of some obstruction to his urethra. Leave his urethral catheter in long enough for his fistula to heal.

23.16 Bladder stones in children

In some parts of Asia, smooth stones, up to 5 cm in diameter, form in the bladders of underprivileged children (mainly boys). Even an infant may suffer from them. In India a third of all urinary problems in childhood are caused by bladder stones. Why they form is far from clear, because the kidneys of these children show no special tendency to form them. When you have removed a bladder stone, it is unlikely to recur.

A child's mother will say that he cries every time he passes urine, and pulls at his penis as he tries to relieve his pain. Frequency and strangury make his life unbearable; sometimes he passes blood. Other symptoms include: interruption of the stream, frequency, dysuria, and suprapubic pain.

There are few physical signs. His bladder may be distended, and his foreskin red and swollen from being pulled on. You may be able to feel the stone when you examine him rectally. It is likely to be made of urates, but it will probably contain enough calcium for you to see it on an X-ray.

Removing a stone from the bladder of a child is not too difficult. When you have done so, there is no need to drain his bladder with a catheter, either suprapubically or through his urethra—if you have sutured it securely.

ASHVIN (3 years) had repeated urinary infections which had been treated with antibiotics on many occasions, but his symptoms always returned. He then saw another doctor, who remembered that repeated urinary infections in children should always be investigated, so he X-rayed Ashvin's bladder and was surprised to see a large stone. At operation, the stone was difficult to remove, and appeared to be lying in a diverticulum. Afterwards he had no more urinary infections. LESSON Don't forget the possibility of stones in children, especially if you are in a high-stone area.

CHILDREN'S BLADDER STONES

ANAESTHESIA. Give the child a general anaesthetic (A 18.3). A relaxant is helpful. Ketamine, tracheal intubation, and relaxants (A 8.5).

PREPARATION. As soon as he is asleep, prepare his lower abdominal wall, thighs and genitalia, and drape him. If you are new to this kind of surgery, distend his bladder with water before you start, so that you can find it more easily. Pass a small plain catheter; then, using a 20 or 50 ml syringe, inject 100 to 200 ml of water into his bladder, depending on his size.

INCISION. Make a midline skin incision, starting at his symphysis pubis and extending up to a point 5 cm below his umbilicus. Reflect the skin flaps 1 cm on either side.

Divide his linea alba strictly in the midline, without entering his peritoneal cavity. Keeping his umbilicus in view to help you stay in the midline, make a vertical incision through the whitish aponeurotic fibres of his linea alba. Continue the incision down to his symphysis pubis, where you will meet his pyramidalis muscle on each side. With a sponge on a holder, gently push his rectus muscles laterally, so that you can see his posterior rectus sheath. Insert a small self-retaining retractor to keep his rectus muscles apart.

Feel for his distended bladder: it should be easily palpable as it rises out of his pelvis. Using a sponge, or your index finger, gently break down the thin layer of his posterior rectus sheath, and open his retropubic space. At the same time displace his peritoneum, so that you don't enter his peritoneal cavity. You should now be able to feel and see his distended bladder.

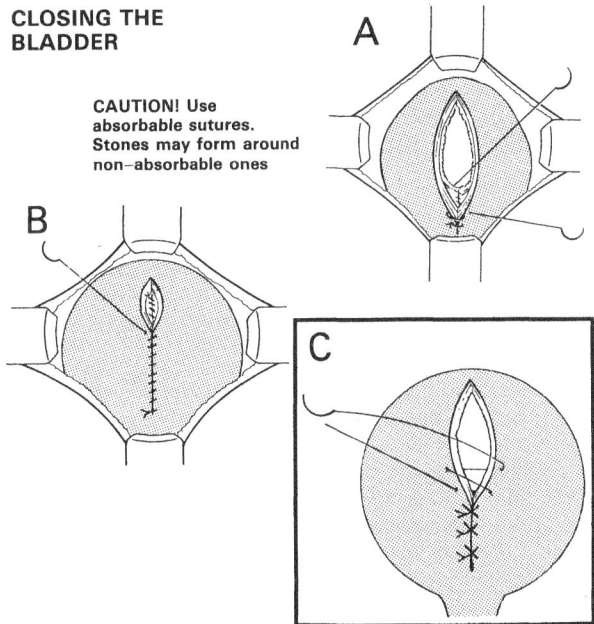

Fig. 23-21 CLOSING THE BLADDER IN TWO LAYERS. This is the standard way of closing the bladder in adults. In a child you can usually use a single layer. A, and B, use continuous or interrupted plain or chromic 2/0 or 3/0 catgut sutures on an atraumatic round-bodied needle. Don't use non-absorbable sutures because they may be the focus of stone formation. C, if his bladder is very thin and weak, close it with figure of eight sutures like this. *After Blandy J, 'Operative Urology', Figs. 8.10 and 8.11. Blackwell Scientific Publications, with kind permission.*

Insert stay sutures, and apply a haemostat on each side of the midline at the most easily accessible part of his bladder. This will prevent it slipping away. Get the sucker ready. Then with a scalpel, or cutting diathermy, make a 2 cm incision in the bladder wall, between the two stay sutures. Water will squirt out.

With your index finger, feel through the hole in his bladder for the stone. Remove it with stone forceps or a sponge-holder. If the hole is not big enough, enlarge it. Having removed one stone, feel again to make sure that he has not got another one.

Close his bladder carefully with continuous 3/0 chromic catgut or 'Dexon' on an atraumatic needle. Include all layers, and make the bites not more than 5 mm apart. The longer the incision, the more care you need in closing it.

CAUTION ! Make a small stab incision just beside the wound and insert a small soft rubber drain down to the suture line. Don't forget to do this. Even if you think you have closed his bladder securely, it may still leak. If urine extravasates, it may cause a serious cellulitis.

Sew up his linea alba with 2/0 catgut. Make sure that you have controlled all bleeding, and then close his skin. If you think that his bladder may leak, or if you have had to make a large incision, insert a Foley catheter and connect this to a bedside drainage bottle for 4 to 5 days. Otherwise, don't insert one. Some surgeons always insert a small suprapubic catheter and use it for a trial of voiding.

POSTOPERATIVELY, he will probably pass urine without difficulty later that day. If urine leaks through the suprapubic drain, insert a urethral catheter, and leave it there for a few days. Otherwise, remove his suprapubic drain after 3 to 4 days. He is unlikely to get another stone, but his siblings may.

23.17 Urethral stones in children

Most stones in the bladder are passed spontaneously in the urine. Occasionally, one impacts in the urethra, especially in boys in areas where bladder stones are common. The patient is usually able to pass urine around it, but pain, strangury, and dribbling are severe. Suspect that he has a urethral stone, if he has severe pain and dribbling, a distended bladder, and you can feel a hard mass somewhere along the course of his urethra.

URETHRAL STONES IN CHILDREN

Feel along the child's urethra for a calculus. He may be able to show you where it has stuck.

Removal by manipulation under general anaesthesia may succeed.

If an X-ray suggests that it might be wedged in the neck of his bladder, try to feel it rectally. You may be able to push it back up into his bladder. If you fail, insert a well-lubricated Lister's sound into his urethra, until it strikes the stone. You may be able to push it back into his bladder.

If this fails, ask your assistant to exert upward pressure on the stone, with his finger in the child's rectum, while you manipulate it with the sound. If you can move the stone back into his bladder, proceed to remove it suprapubically, as above.

If it impacts between his bulbous urethra, and his fossa navicularis, remove it by external urethrolithotomy.

If it impacts at his external meatus or his fossa navicularis, you may be able to 'milk' it free.

If it has developed in a diverticulum (rare), you may have to cut down on this.

URETHROLITHOTOMY. Give him a general anaesthetic (A 18.3), or ketamine (A 8.5), and place him in the lithotomy position.

Clean and prepare his genitalia, the medial surface of his thighs, and his perineum. Feel for the stone in his urethra, and steady it between the thumb and index finger of your left hand.

Make a 3 cm midline incision over the stone, on the ventral surface of his penis. Cauterize or tie off the bleeding points. This is a very vascular area. If you don't control bleeding, everything will be obscured. Ask an assistant to retract the skin flaps with rake retractors.

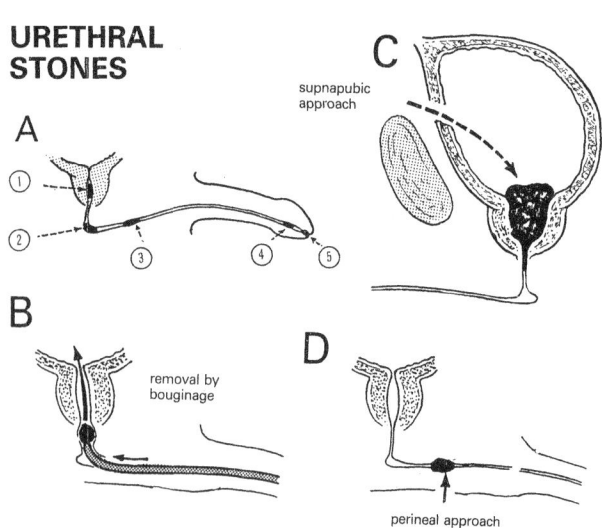

Fig. 23-22 URETHRAL STONES. A, the sites where stones can impact in the urethra. B, removing a stone by bouginage. C, the suprapubic approach. D, the perineal approach.
1, the prostatic urethra. 2, the bulb of the urethra. 3, the perineal urethra. 4, the fossa navicularis. 5, the external meatus.

Incise the part of his urethra containing the stone. Make the incision just big enough to deliver it. Lift it out with stone forceps or a haemostat. Try not to break it.

Insert a small (10 or 12 Ch) Foley catheter into his urethral meatus, and up past the incision into his bladder. Inflate the balloon. Don't try to close his urethra, its edges will fall together and heal naturally. Close his skin.

Connect the Foley catheter to a bedside drainage bottle, and remove it after a week.

23.18 Prostatic obstruction

If urine can no longer pass through a patient's prostate, as the result of benign enlargement, carcinoma, fibrosis (bladder-neck stenosis), or bladder-neck dysfunction, you will have to relieve his obstruction. He can present with:

(1) Prostatic symptoms before his urinary flow is completely obstructed. He may have: (a) Frequency of micturition which interferes seriously with his sleep, (b) difficult voiding, or (c) a poor stream. Unfortunately, this is an unusual method of presentation in the developing world.

(2) Acute retention of urine (23.5), perhaps precipitated by a recent drinking bout. If you catheterize him, he will usually start to pass urine again, but his retention will probably recur, so he should have his prostate removed after his first attack.

(3) Chronic retention. His bladder remains distended when micturition is over, and he may dribble urine continuously and painlessly (retention with overflow).

(4) 'Acute on chronic' retention. He has had a poor flow for some time, and his bladder is large and has recently become *painful*. He may progress to retention with overflow.

If he presents with retention, he may be not be well enough for you to remove his prostate immediately, because: (1) His acute retention may be the final episode in a long period of obstructive uropathy; his blood urea may be high and his urine infected. (2) He may have been precipitated into retention by a serious illness, such as pneumonia, or fracture of the neck of his femur. If you try to remove his prostate while he is like this, he will probably not survive the operation. He is more likely to live if you wait, drain his bladder for a week or two, and investigate him meanwhile.

If he presents with retention, and you expect to remove his prostate within 2 weeks, pass a urethral catheter and drain his urine into a closed sterile system. If you have to delay beyond

2 weeks, do a suprapubic cystostomy (23.6). Some surgeons try to avoid doing a suprapubic cystostomy, if they possibly can, and are prepared to leave a plastic urethral catheter, or a polythene tube, in place for several weeks if necessary, changing it every week, or even every 2 or 3 weeks.

If you are in an area where *Schistosoma haematobium* is endemic, and commonly causes carcinoma of the bladder, try to avoid doing a suprapubic cystostomy. In some areas this is responsible for up to 10% of cases of urinary obstruction. If a patient does have carcinoma of his bladder, and you do a suprapubic cystostomy, it will never close.

If possible, examine him under anaesthesia (do an EUA) and cystoscope him some days before you remove his prostate. This will confirm the diagnosis, distinguish carcinoma of his prostate from carcinoma of the base of his bladder infiltrating his prostate, and enable you to diagnose associated bladder diverticula and stones. An EUA and cystoscopy will also make it easier to plan your theatre lists, because they are are quickly done, whereas a prostatectomy takes time.

URINARY OBSTRUCTION

PLAN OF INVESTIGATION. Here is an ideal scheme: do as much of it as you can. Assess the patient's general condition, feel for palpable kidneys, feel the size of his bladder, feel his urethra for strictures and do a rectal examination, having first measured his acid phosphatase, as evidence of carcinoma of his prostate with local or bony secondaries (32.22). If he is in retention, catheterize him. A day or two later, or when his blood urea is down if it was previously raised, examine him under anaesthesia and cystoscope him. Operate at your convenience.

CAUTION ! Measure his acid phosphatase *before* you do a rectal examination, or more than 48 hours afterwards (32.32).

RENAL FUNCTION. Measure his blood urea. Chronic retention with a blood urea of up to 12 mmol/l is common in the elderly, but provided underlying causes, such as heart failure, are corrected, it is no great risk in itself.

If he has retention of urine with a blood urea of over 15 mmol/l, pass a plastic urethral catheter, or a piece of polythene tubing. Only pass a suprapubic catheter if you fail to pass a urethral one. Drain his bladder for a week to improve his renal function. If his blood urea remains high, say at 15 mmol/l, you can operate, but at only at greater risk. There is no need to try to decompress an obstructed bladder slowly, this is almost impossible, and it does not reduce the incidence of bleeding.

X-RAYS. A straight X-ray of his pelvis is important. Look for: (1) Stones (they are almost always radio-opaque). If you find one, remove it at the same time as his prostate. (2) Secondary deposits from carcinoma of his prostate, which may be osteolytic or osteosclerotic.

An intravenous urogram is unnecessary in acute retention: it gives only incidental information and is expensive. Most of what you need to know can be found from other tests. If you do one, look for: (1) Dilated kidneys or ureters. (2) Signs that he has enough renal function to excrete the contrast medium. (3) Stones or diverticula.

ANAEMIA. Measure his haemoglobin; it should be above 10 g/dl. Don't operate unless you can transfuse him.

ANTIBIOTICS. If his urine is infected, give him an antibiotic. If necessary, catheterize him to make sure it drains adequately.

CYSTOSCOPY. Do this, as in Section 23.3, while he is anaesthetized and in the lithotomy position. If you have difficulty getting the beak of the cystoscope past his prostatic urethra, be gentle. Any force will make it bleed. If it sticks at a urethral stricture, dilate this, or do a suprapubic cystostomy and send him back to the ward.

Allow his urine to flow out. Note the volume of his bladder, and if it looks infected or not. Start by inspecting his internal urinary meatus, with the fenestra of the cystoscope placed so that the edge of the meatus bisects the field of view. Normally, the posterior part of the urinary meatus is flat, and the rest is part of a circle. Look for: (1) carcinoma of his bladder, (2) bladder stones, (3) benign enlargement, (4) fibrosis of the bladder neck (uncommon), (5) diverticula.

Enlargement of the prostate: (1) Enlargement of its lateral lobes will make his prostatic urethra appear as a cleft before you enter his bladder. (2) His median lobe will project from the posterior aspect of his bladder like 'a termite hill', and may make it difficult to see the ureteric orifices (B, 23-23). (3) His bladder may be trabeculated, showing that its outflow is obstructed.

Diverticula. You will see thick muscle bundles intersecting one another, perhaps with small saccules between them. Diverticula are merely extra large saccules, and are usually above and lateral to the ureteric orifices, with radiating folds around their openings. You may be able to get the beak of your cystoscope inside one. Diverticula rarely matter, once outflow obstruction has been relieved, and diverticulectomy is seldom necessary.

Bladder-neck dysfunction causes retention of urine but cannot be diagnosed cystoscopically.

Bladder-neck fibrosis can be diagnosed cystoscopically, but needs experience. Suspect it if: (1) His bladder is obviously obstructed, as shown by muscle hypertrophy, residual urine, and perhaps diverticula. And, (2) his prostate is small, he has no urethral stricture and no CNS disease. And, (3) the neck of his bladder is tight as you pass the cystoscope.

CAUTION ! There is very little relationship between the appearance of the prostate and the presence or degree of outflow obstruction.

EXAMINATION UNDER ANAESTHESIA. Let the urine out of his bladder, remove the cystoscope, and examine his prostate bimanually with one finger in his rectum. Note its size, and any suspicion of malignancy as shown by its hardness, nodularity, and spread outside the prostatic bed. If it feels malignant, biopsy it with a Vim Silvermannn needle (32.26, 32.22) through his rectum. Or, you may find that he has not got an enlarged prostate, but that it merely felt enlarged, because it was pressed on by a full bladder.

IS PROSTATECTOMY INDICATED?

The indications and contraindications are the same for Freyer's transvesical (23.19), and for Ghadvi's perineal method (23.21).

INDICATIONS. (1) Significant symptoms due to outflow obstruction. (2) The harmful effects of outflow obstruction, which are: (a) Difficult voiding and deterioration of his urinary stream. (b) Frequency of micturition (due to outflow obstruction) which interferes seriously with his sleep. (c) Acute retention of urine. (d) Chronic retention with overflow.

Conditions which do not by themselves indicate prostatectomy include: (1) Frequency and nocturia. (2) Haematuria (which is quite common in prostatic hypertrophy). (3) An increased residual urine (difficult to assess).

CONTRAINDICATIONS. (1) A patient whose general condition is very poor. (2) Very poor renal function, which does not improve after catheterization. (3) Severe sepsis. (4) Limited mobility and senility (rather than age alone). A very senile old man is likely to be permanently incontinent anyway, and will be better with permanent urethral drainage through a small Foley catheter, or, if you cannot pass one, with a permanent suprapubic cystostomy. (5) A malignant prostate is a contraindication to Freyer's and especially to Ghadvi's prostatectomy, but is very suitable for transurethral resection, which you will not be able to do. Manage a malignant prostate with oestrogens and catheter drainage, as in Section 32.32.

If he is too sick for prostatectomy, he may be suitable for treatment by the injection method (23.22).

23.19 Freyer's transvesical prostatectomy

If a patient needs his prostatic obstruction relieved, there are three ways you can do it. You can use: (1) A modification of Freyer's method in which prostatic adenomas are removed through the bladder. (2) Ghadvi's method (23.21) in which they are removed laterally through the perineum. (3) The injection method in Section 23.22 which scleroses them with a mixture of glycerine and phenol.

Of the possible alternatives, Millin's retropubic operation is nicer for the patient, but it is more dependent on preliminary

PROSTATECTOMY

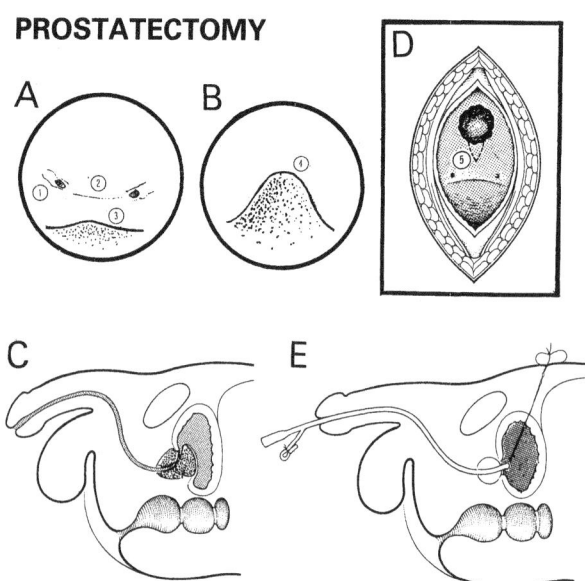

Fig. 23-23 PROSTATECTOMY. A, the normal cystoscopic appearances of the base of the bladder, with the ureteric openings (1), the interureteric bar (2), and the middle lobe as a hardly visible swelling (3). B, in benign prostatic hypertrophy the middle lobe (4) projects into the bladder to obscure the interureteric bar and the ureteric openings. C, enlargement of the middle lobe. D, the position of the wedge to cut out of the neck of the bladder (5). E, the prostate has been removed and a Foley catheter left in the bladder, and secured with a stitch round a roll of gauze on the abdominal wall.

cystoscopy and is more difficult. It also needs good lighting, more help, and better postoperative care. Transurethral resection needs much skill and an expensive resectoscope. The advantages of Freyer's method are: (1) If you cannot cystoscope a patient, you can look into his bladder to exclude diverticula, carcinoma, and stones. (2) You can control bleeding more easily. (3) When well done, mortality is low. One of its disadvantages is that it normally requires large quantities of irrigating fluid, although we describe ways of doing without this.

When a prostate enlarges benignly, it does so because adenomas form in its lateral lobes. These are joined anteriorly by a narrow anterior commissure, which is the most anterior part of the prostate. As the adenomas form: (1) They compress the normal tissues of the prostate around them to form a false capsule. (2) They compress the prostatic urethra from side to side. Posteriorly the median lobe of the bladder enlarges superiorly and extends upwards into the bladder. With Freyer's method you open a patient's bladder through his abdomen, insert your finger in the plane between the adenomas and the false capsule, and shell them out. Doing this without injuring his membranous urethra needs skill.

One of the difficulties of any prostatectomy is that the raw bed of the prostate bleeds after you have removed its adenomas. There are several ways to reduce this bleeding: (1) You can use diathermy (if you have it) during the operation. (2) You can put a suture or two into his prostatic bed. (3) You can compress the walls of his prostatic bed with the balloon of a Foley catheter (the standard method). (4) As a last resort you can pack his prostatic bed, and leave the pack in place.

If he bleeds, the clot may obstruct his urethra and distend his bladder (clot retention). This opens up the vessels in his prostatic bed, makes the bleeding worse, and is the great hazard of prostatectomy. Prevent it by washing away the blood, as it collects, in any of the following ways. Base your choice on the availability of catheters and irrigation fluid: (1) You can leave a three-way irrigating Foley catheter (preferably plastic rather than rubber) in his urethra, and wash away the blood in his bladder with a stream of irrigating fluid. One channel is for the fluid to go in; one is for fluid, blood, and urine to come out; and one is to blow up the balloon. (2) You can insert a two-way Foley catheter through his urethra, and introduce fluid into his bladder through a suprapubic catheter. This can be either a rubber tube, as in C, and D, Fig. 23-26, or another Foley catheter. (3) You can put a two-channel Foley catheter in his bladder, give him quantities of intravenous fluid and frusemide, and let his urine wash the blood out of his bladder this way. (4) You can use suprapubic suction and no irrigation. (5) You can leave a large suprapubic tube in his bladder and remove clots with forceps. This is what Freyer did, but the suprapubic fistula you make takes a long time to close. It can use huge quantities of gauze, and urine may overflow from the suprapubic tube into the patient's bed. Not surprisingly, nurses hate this method! We describe two versions of it; one using bladder washouts which is highly recommended under difficult circumstances. (6) You can leave a catheter in his urethra, pass a de Pezzer catheter suprapubically, and pack his prostatic bed as in Fig. 23-27.

If you are going to irrigate his bladder, you will need about ten litres of fluid. This can be: (1) Intravenous saline—which is expensive and is likely to be scarce. (2) Sterile saline made from tap water. The disadvantage of this is that it may enter his circulation through his prostatic sinuses, and if it is not pyrogen free, it may give him rigors. (3) Sterile 3.8% sodium citrate (which is no better than saline).

If you have not been able to cystoscope him, you can inspect his bladder through his operation wound to exclude diverticula and tumours, and pass a sound to exclude a stricture. Unfortunately, you cannot always exclude bladder-neck fibrosis until you have felt inside his bladder. If you find this condition, you will have to cut a wedge out of his prostate as in D, Fig. 23-23, D, Fig 23-24, and J, Fig. 23-25.

MODIFIED FREYER'S PROSTATECTOMY

INDICATIONS. Benign enlargement of the prostate—see Section 23.18. Carcinoma is better treated with oestrogens as in Section 32.32. If however, you happen to find a carcinoma incidentally, you can open up a sufficient channel to relieve the obstruction, as described below.

EQUIPMENT. An abdominal set (4.12), Langenbeck or bent copper retractors, a self-retaining retractor, such as Walton's, a vulsellum or Littlewood's forceps, suction, diathermy (if available), preferably a three-way irrigating Foley balloon catheter with a 75 ml balloon, or the alternatives described below.

ANAESTHESIA. (1) Ketamine with a relaxant (A 8.4). (2) Subarachnoid or epidural anaesthesia. (3) General anaesthesia. You can manage without a relaxant, but anaesthesia has to be deeper. Preferably, have at least two units of blood crossmatched (with due care as to HIV, Chapter 28a), and a drip running.

POSITION. Lay the patient on his back and give the table a mild head-down tilt. Stand on his left side, so that your right hand is in the most convenient position to enucleate his prostate, and so that you can, if necessary, put your left index finger into his rectum.

SOUNDING. If he does not already have a catheter in, and you have not done a cystoscopy, pass a sound to make sure he has not got a urethral stricture. If all is well, pass a catheter, and leave about 300 ml of saline in his bladder to make it easier to find when you operate

THE INCISION depends on whether he has already had a suprapubic cystostomy.

If he has had no suprapubic cystotomy, make a Pfannensteil (Fig. 23-20), or less satisfactorily, a 7 cm midline incision immediately above his pubis longitudinally between his recti.

If he has had a suprapubic cystostomy, dissection will be easier if you start in an unscarred part of the wound. Make an elliptical incision round the wound, excise the skin edges and the suprapubic track, and split his rectus muscles. Dissecting the peritoneum off his bladder will be difficult, so cover your

FREYER'S PROSTATECTOMY – ONE

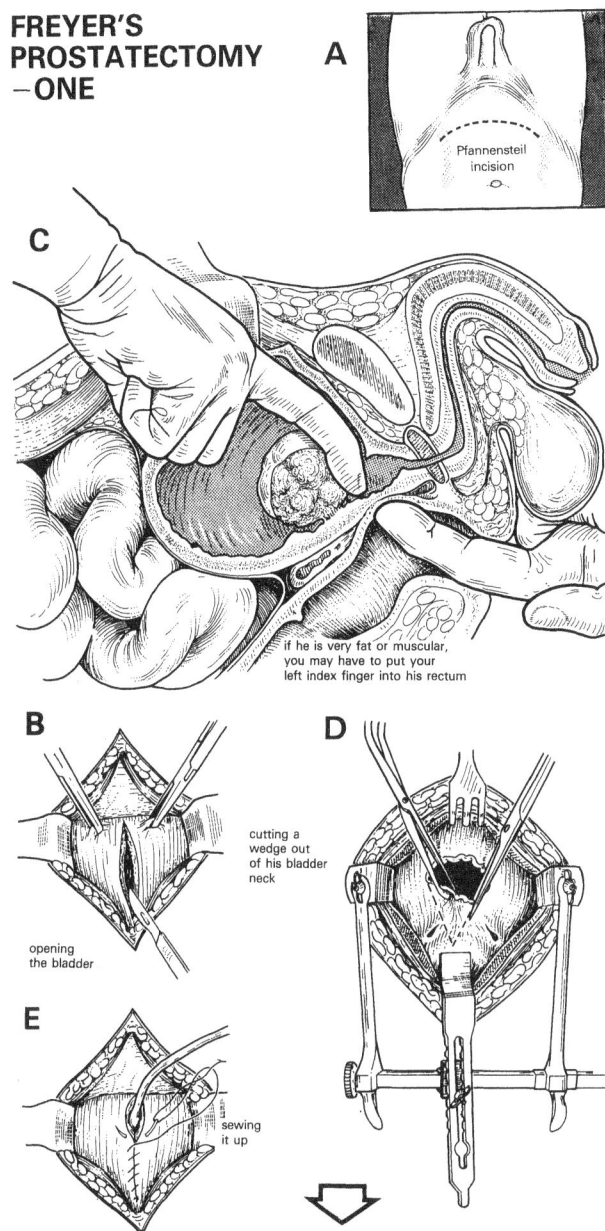

Fig. 23-24 FREYER'S PROSTATECTOMY–ONE. A, the incision. B, open the patient's bladder. C, put your finger into his internal meatus and remove his enlarged prostate. A finger in his rectum is only sometimes necessary. D, cut a wedge out of his bladder neck, E, close his bladder. *Adapted from a drawing by Frank Netter, with the kind permission of CIBA-GEIGY Ltd, Basle (Switzerland).*

right index with gauze. Keeping the pulp of your finger in contact with his pubic symphysis, push your finger into his retropubic space. When you reach his prostate, rotate your finger through 180° and peel the peritoneum off the anterior surface of his bladder.

Insert stay sutures into the anterior wall of his bladder (A, Fig. 23-25), and then incise it in the sagittal plane.

CAUTION ! Don't enter his peritoneal cavity. If by mistake you do so, immediately suture it.

Put two fingers of your right hand into his bladder. Feel inside to exclude neoplasms and the orifices of diverticula. You can easily miss these. Feel his prostate and his internal urinary meatus.

If his prostate is enlarged, and you can easily get your fingers into his internal urinary meatus, enucleate the prostate as described below.

If his prostate is not enlarged, and he has a tight internal meatus which you cannot put your finger into, he has bladder-neck fibrosis, so see Section 23.20.

TO ENUCLEATE HIS PROSTATE, remove the self-retaining retractor. Put your index finger into his prostatic urethra. Use your left index finger to split into the recess between the anterior commisure (which should remain *in situ*) and the left lateral lobe of his prostate at about 10 o'clock. Open up the plane between the gland and the false capsule as far distally as you can. Separate it through at least 90°, and preferably 150°. Use your right index finger to repeat the procedure on the right side starting at about 2 o'clock, so as to free his prostate from within its bed (false capsule). There is usually a residual attachment distally. Pull his prostate up into his bladder to make this taut. Divide it near his prostate, either blindly with curved dissecting scissors or with your finger.

CAUTION ! (1) Divide the attachment close to his prostate, or you may damage his internal sphincter which surrounds his membranous urethra, deep and superficial to his perineal membrane. (2) Preserve his anterior commisure. Damage to either may lead to incontinence of urine or a stricture.

Remove his entire prostate, including its median lobe, by bringing it into his bladder with your index finger. If it is still lightly attached proximally to the mucosa of his bladder, separate it with scissors. Removing each lateral lobe separately may be easier. One will bring the median lobe with it.

If he is very fat, or muscular, you may be unable to reach the lower border of his prostate. So you will have to push it upwards with your left index in his rectum while you enucleate the adenomas from above. To do this, cover your left hand with two gloves, and protect your forearm with a sterile towel under the drapes.

When you have turned the lateral lobes into his bladder, feel the inside of his prostatic cavity, to make sure that no adenomatous masses have been left behind.

CAUTION ! You can easily leave a large mass of adenoma behind, so compare one side with the other. Use your fingers, sponge holders, or vulsellum forceps to grasp and twist off any remaining pieces of adenoma.

TO ENLARGE HIS BLADDER NECK, first check the position of his ureteric orifices. Cut a wedge out of his bladder neck in the 6 o'clock position level with his ureteric orifices and between them (J, in Fig. 23-25). The mucosa of the bladder overhangs the prostatic cavity, and if you don't do this he may get retention of urine later ('bladder-neck obstruction').

TO CONTROL BLEEDING insert two figure of eight sutures in the 4 and 8 o'clock positions (I, 23-25), *taking care to avoid his ureters*. Then put a tight gauze pack in his prostatic cavity. After 3 minutes, take it out and assess the amount of bleeding.

Put a purse string of catgut in the floor of his bladder, around what was his internal meatus. Blow up the balloon of a 50 or 75 ml Foley catheter, until it fits snugly in his prostatic bed (usually 30–50 ml is required). This will help to stop bleeding. Then tighten up the purse string round it to hold it in place (L, 23-25). It will usually remain in his prostatic bed. Some surgeons put a *large* balloon in the prostatic bed directly without an initial purse string suture. It must be large: if you don't have one, insert a purse string suture first.

Alternatively, if bleeding is still brisk (unusual), tightly repack his prostatic cavity, and leave the pack in place for 15 minutes. Remove it. If his prostatic cavity is still bleeding, you may need to suture substantial bleeding vessels on either side of the bladder neck (if you have not already done so). Pack his prostatic cavity a third time, but this time pass a Foley catheter into his bladder. Either don't inflate the balloon, or inflate it when it is well up in his bladder. Use a long length of sterile 10 cm gauze, pack it round the Foley catheter, and bring the end out through the abdominal incision as in Fig. 23-27. Some surgeons have never had to do this.

Insert a '2' monofilament suture through his abdominal wall and his bladder, and then through the holes in the catheter to hold it in place. Knot it over a button (L, 23-25). If he is confused postoperatively, this will prevent him from pulling out his catheter, even if the balloon bursts.

IRRIGATION OR DRAINAGE FOR FREYER'S PROSTATECTOMY

The purpose of irrigation is to remove blood clots, which encourage infection and block the drainage tube. Some surgeons don't irrigate routinely, and only do so if bleeding has been

FREYER'S PROSTATECTOMY —TWO

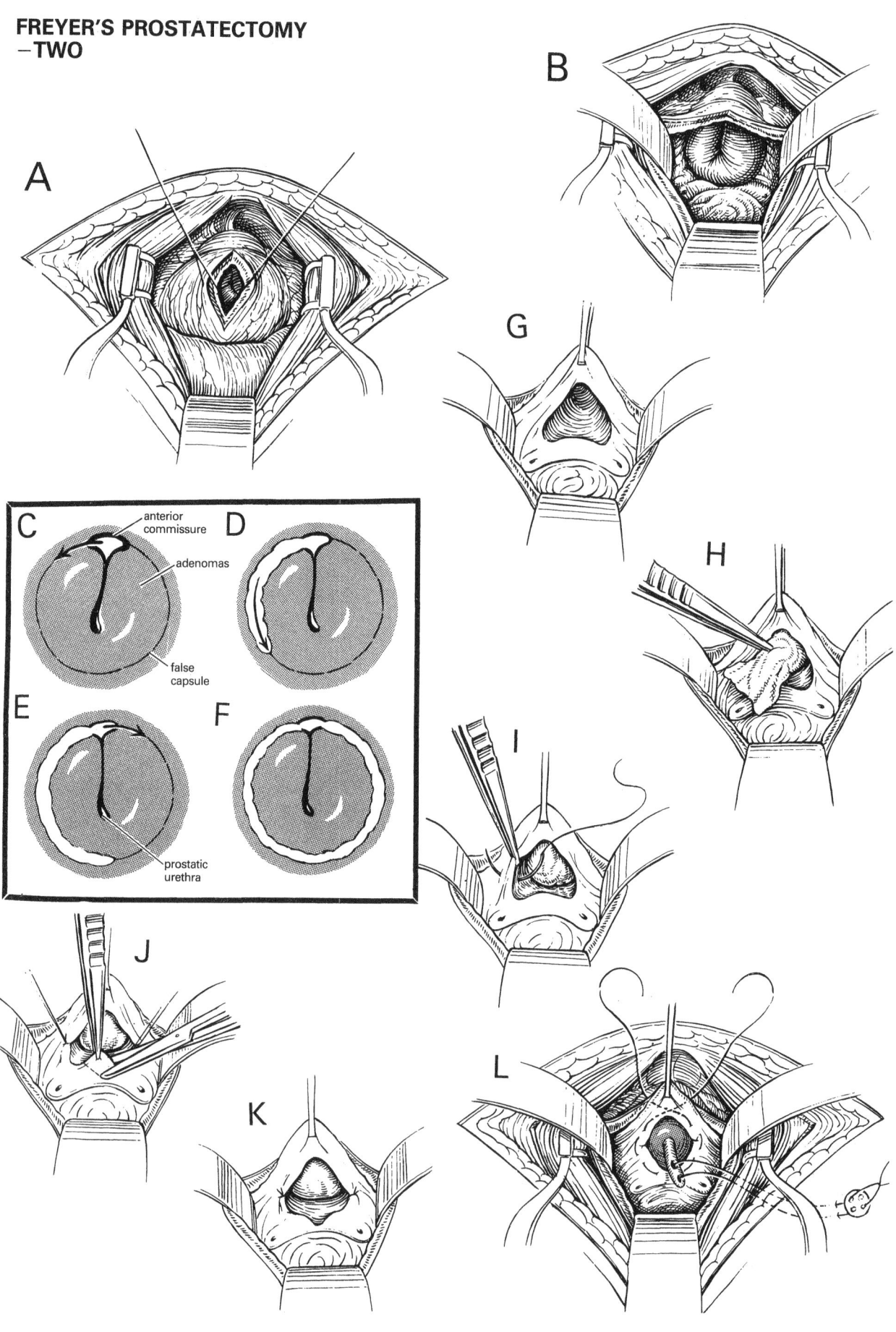

392

IRRIGATION FOR PROSTATECTOMY

A three-channel Foley catheter

A two-channel Foley with suprapubic drainage

Dislodging clots

you can use another Foley

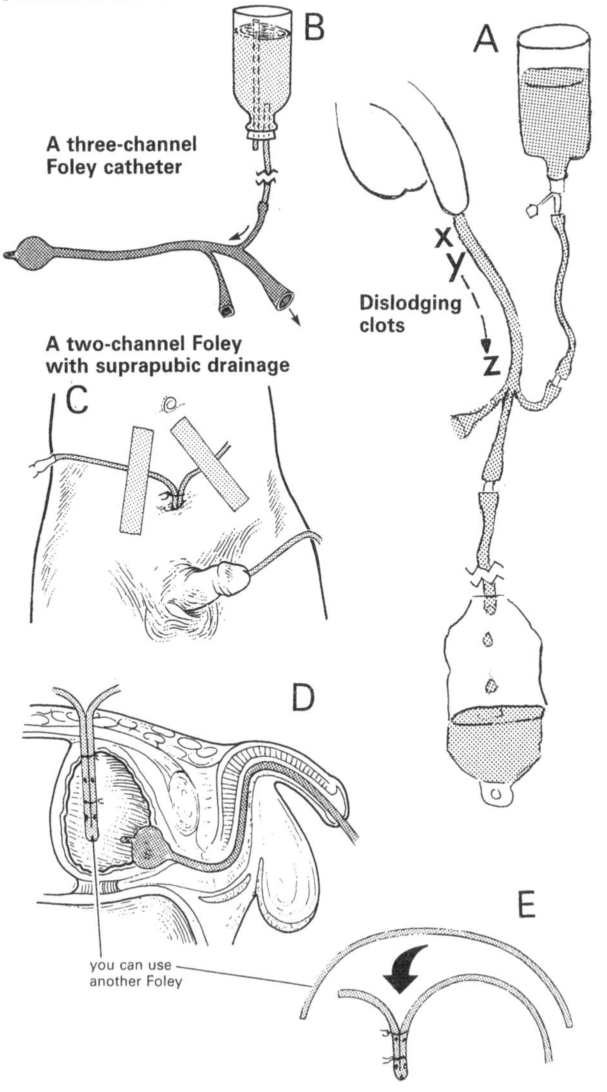

Fig. 23-26 IRRIGATION FOR PROSTATECTOMY. A, a three-channel Foley catheter. B, how to 'milk' a catheter to dislodge clots. Pinch it at 'x' between the finger and thumb of your left hand. Pinch it just distally with your right hand ('y'). Move the fingers of your right hand down the catheter ('z') keeping its lumen closed. Then suddenly stop pinching with your left hand. There will be suction along the catheter into the bag. C, a two-channel Foley catheter with suprapubic drainage through a rubber tube. D, how the tube enters the bladder. E, how it is folded.

A second two-channel Foley catheter is an alternative.

brisk. If you have had to pack his prostatic cavity to control immediate bleeding, he will probably need irrigating.

Choose one of these six methods. (1) is the best because there is no abdominal wound to leak. (5) and (6) are the least satisfactory, but are useful if there is severe bleeding which you cannot control, or you lack irrigation fluid. Where you can, tie the catheter in place with a suture to his abdominal wall (L, 23-25).

Fig. 23-25 FREYER'S PROSTATECTOMY—TWO. A, insert stay sutures and open the patient's bladder by making a stab incision between two Allis' forceps. B, inspect his bladder. C, to F, use your right and then your left index finger to open up the plane between the gland and the false capsule. G, his empty prostatic cavity. H, mopping out his prostatic cavity. I, sutures being placed at 4 and 8 o'clock to control bleeding. J, cutting a wedge out of the neck of his bladder. K, the wedge complete. L, suturing a Foley catheter in place. *After Maxwell Malament, from a publication by Ethicon Ltd, with kind permission.*

(1) A THREE-CHANNEL IRRIGATING FOLEY CATHETER. Introduce saline down one channel, and let it drain through another. Remove the catheter on day 8 to 12. There is no need to use a three-channel catheter if he also has a suprapubic catheter.

(2) A PAIR OF TWO-CHANNEL FOLEY CATHETERS one through his urethra and the other suprapubically. Pass a large 20 to 24 Ch two-channel Foley catheter through his urethra into his prostatic bed. Pass another (8 to 10 Ch) into his bladder through an oblique high suprapubic track. An oblique track will close more easily than a straight one. Introduce fluid through the abdominal catheter, and drain it through the urethral one. This is the best method for a beginner. If you don't have a second Foley, you can use a Malecot or a de Pezzer catheter suprapubically.

Remove the suprapubic catheter when the fluid is no longer bloody, usually on day 3 or 4. If you leave it longer it tends to leave a track which leaks. Remove the urethral one on day 8 to 12.

(3) A TWO-CHANNEL FOLEY CATHETER AND FRUSEMIDE. Give him a bottle of 5% dextrose alternating with one of 0.9% saline every 6 hours, with frusemide 40 mg twice daily for two days. In this way he will irrigate himself. Remove the catheter on day 8 to 12. This is expensive in intravenous fluids.

(4) CONTINUOUS SUPRAPUBIC SUCTION. Cut multiple side holes in a rubber tube, as in E, Fig. 23-26, bend it double, insert it into his bladder, and apply continuous suction with a pump or with jerricans (10-8). You can use this method with a pack, or a Foley catheter, in his urethra. If your pump exerts more suction than 10 cm of water, fit it with a bypass, as in Fig. 19-13.

(5) SUPRAPUBIC TUBE. Put a large (2 cm) rubber tube with two side holes into his bladder, so that it does not quite reach his trigone. Stitch it to his skin. Allow it to drain into dressings. Don't connect it to a bottle, because its purpose is to allow clots to be extruded. If clots block it, remove them with spongeholders. Nurse him on a plastic sheet. Insert a urethral catheter.

On the 3rd or 4th day, when there are no more clots, withdraw the large suprapubic tube, and put in a small one. Cut two eyes in this, transfix it with a safety pin, and fix it to his abdominal wall with strapping.

On the 10th day remove the suprapubic tube, and allow the fistula to heal. To make sure that the torn end of his urethra is not obstructed by adhesions, pass a sound through it, or tie in an 18 Ch plastic catheter. This will keep him dry until his fistula has closed. Wash out his bladder daily with mercury oxycyanide 1/6000, or plain water.

Alternatively, here is a method which is highly recommended under difficult circumstances. Insert a large suprapubic drain into his bladder, and a urethral catheter. Wash out his bladder with water through his urethra, and let it wash the clots in his bladder up and out through the suprapubic tube. Continue washouts until clots have stopped, and the fluid which comes out is only a pale pink. When this happens, let him pass his urine through his urethral catheter, and leave the suprapubic tube in a little longer as a safety measure. With this method you can see the clots coming out, and make sure that his urethral catheter never blocks.

(6) PACKING THE PROSTATIC CAVITY. After you have enucleated his prostate, pull the urethral catheter further into his bladder, and pack his prostatic cavity firmly with a roll of gauze. Bring the end of the gauze out through the abdominal incision, as in Fig. 23-27. Place a de Pezzer catheter in the upper end of the incision. Start irrigating as soon as you have closed his bladder. Remove the pack at 24 hours if bleeding is controlled, and at 72 hours if it is not. Remove his urethral catheter at 10 days.

CLOSING THE ABDOMINAL WALL AFTER FREYER'S PROSTATECTOMY

This is the same with all methods. Close his bladder with two layers of continuous '0' or 2/0 chromic catgut, preferably on an atraumatic needle. Preferably insert the first one through the mucosa only, and use the second one to invert the muscle coat.

Insert a 2 cm wide corrugated rubber drain in his retropubic

PACKING THE PROSTATIC CAVITY

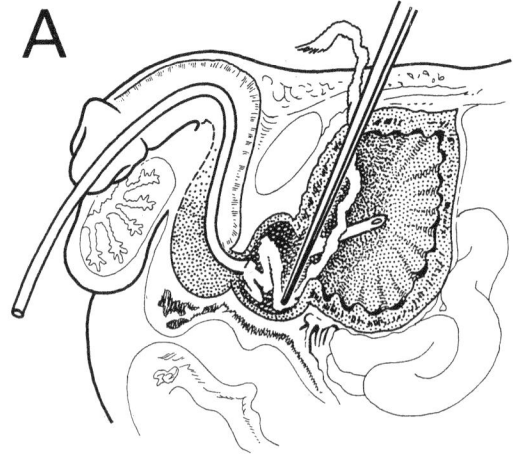

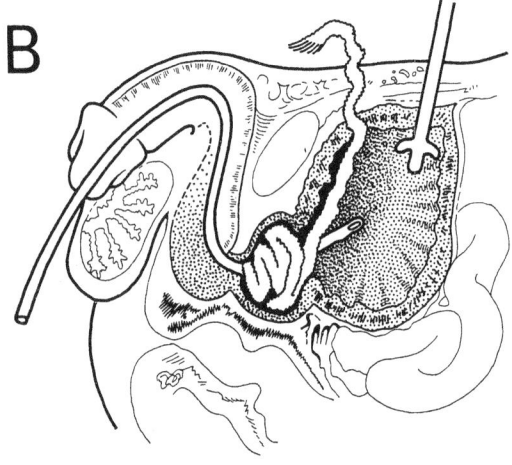

Fig. 23-27 PACKING THE PROSTATIC CAVITY. Where technology and facilities are limited, this method may still have a place in controlling bleeding at operation and afterwards. A, inserting the pack. B, the prostatic cavity packed, with one end of the pack coming out of the wound, for removal after 24 hours.

space, through a new incision, below the original Pfannensteil one. If you made a midline incision, put the drain to one side. Stitch it in place. Bring his rectus muscles together with a few catgut sutures, and close his anterior rectus sheath with continuous chromic catgut. Close his skin. There is no need to tie his vasa, because this does not influence the incidence of postoperative epididymo-orchitis.

POSTOPERATIVE CARE AFTER FREYER'S PROSTATECTOMY

He must pass plenty of urine. So each 24 hours give him 2 or 3 litres of 0.9% intravenous saline, alternating with 5% dextrose, until he can take fluids by mouth (A, 15.5).

IRRIGATION METHODS. Teach the nurses to milk the catheter hourly (B, 23-26), until all the clots have gone, usually in 2 to 4 days. In methods (1), (2), and (3) continue irrigation with saline, just fast enough for his urine to be pale pink. It is usually necessary for 24 to 48 hours. You will need about 4 bottles of fluid in the first 24 hours, and less the next day. You may need to continue irrigation until the 4th day.

CAUTION ! Don't raise the irrigation bottle too high. If it is more than 60 cm above his bladder, and haemostasis has been poor, the fluid in his bladder may enter his circulation, especially if the outflow catheter is obstructed. Keep the drainage bottle on or near the floor, to make use of gravity.

Let down the balloon on the third day, unless there is much bleeding; if so, wait until bleeding stops. His prostatic cavity will then become smaller naturally, and there will be less danger of secondary haemorrhage.

Most patients are fit for discharge about the 10th day, unless they have been left with a fistula which has not yet healed, as in methods (5) and (6).

DIFFICULTIES WITH FREYER'S PROSTATECTOMY

Besides the normal anaesthetic risks, and those listed below, the postoperative difficulties you will meet include epididymitis, septicaemia, deep vein thrombosis (unusual in the developing world), ileus (10.13), uraemia and oliguria (53.3), postoperative shock (53.1), and bladder tamponade.

If you find that he has CARCINOMA of his prostate, you will not be able to shell it out, because this causes *much bleeding,* and is difficult. So remove enough tissue with scissors (or diathermy) to leave an adequate channel for his urine. You should have reduced the chances of finding carcinoma of the prostate inadvertently by measuring his acid phosphatase, by X-raying his pelvis for secondaries, and by cystoscopy.

If when you open his bladder you find that THERE ARE NO ADENOMAS, he probably has BLADDER-NECK DYSFUNCTION. Relieve this by incising the neck of his bladder, as in the next section.

If you find DIVERTICULA in his bladder, leave them: they will become smaller now that you have relieved his obstruction, unless they were very large. Removing them is difficult, so try to refer him for this later.

If he BLEEDS from his prostate after his return to the ward, within 48 hours of the operation (reactionary haemorrhage, not uncommon), all that is usually necessary is to keep the catheter clear by milking it hourly. If his urine is a deep red-wine colour, speed up the irrigation, and consider washing out his bladder. Raise the foot of his bed if his blood pressure is low. Give him morphine. If necessary transfuse him. Occasionally, you may have to take him back to the theatre, reopen his wound, and control bleeding from his prostatic bed.

If he has a DISTENDED PAINFUL BLADDER and no urine drains, he has CLOT RETENTION. This is one of the most feared complications of prostatic surgery, and occurs within the first 72 hours. He has bled severely, and the blood in his bladder has clotted and obstructed the catheter. Transfuse him as necessary. Take a metal ear syringe and inject 50 ml of sterile saline into his bladder and immediately aspirate it.

CAUTION ! Don't inject more than 50 ml, or you may burst his bladder, and don't try this method more than once. If you are lucky, you will dislodge the clot.

If you fail to dislodge the clot, take him to the theatre, remove the catheter under general anaesthesia, insert a 24 Ch *metal* catheter, wash out his bladder through this, and replace the Foley catheters. If this fails, open his bladder, remove the clots, and pack his prostatic cavity, as in Fig. 23-27.

If he BLEEDS 8—12 DAYS AFTER THE OPERATION (secondary haemorrhage, quite common), it usually settles. Many cases are not severe, and will stop on their own. If he does not stop bleeding (rare), dilate his suprapubic fistula (if he has one) with Hegar's dilators, and remove the clots from his bladder with sponge forceps. Reinsert a urethral catheter, and wash his bladder through this until the fluid is nearly free of blood. Then put in a large suprapubic drain, and send him back to the ward. You may occasionally need to pack his prostatic cavity with gauze (23-27); but avoid doing this if you can, because it requires formal re-opening of the wound. If it is necessary, take him back to the theatre, reopen his prostatic bed, and control bleeding. If he does not have a suprapubic fistula, this is what you will have to do.

If he is INCONTINENT OF URINE, you can reassure him that this is almost certain to improve during the next 3 months. It is more likely if you damaged his external sphincter at operation, and it can be permanent. The symptoms of urge incontinence are common in patients who had these symptoms preoperatively; they usually resolve spontaneously.

If he develops a SUPRAPUBIC FISTULA, it will probably close spontaneously before he leaves hospital. If it is slow to heal, his lower urinary tract is probably still obstructed. So drain his bladder with a urethral catheter for up to 10 more days.

If he has a FURTHER ATTACK of retention of urine some months or years later, dilate him with bougies (23.8). If this fails, you may have to do a wedge resection of the neck of his bladder. This is very unlikely to happen, if you routinely excise a wedge of tissue from the back of the neck of the bladder when you remove the prostate.

23.20 Other causes of urinary obstruction— dyskinesia and bladder-neck fibrosis

There are two causes of urinary obstruction in which a patient's prostate feels normal rectally, with no sign that it is enlarged, but in spite of this his urine cannot pass. Between 5 and 10% of cases of prostatic obstruction are like this. He is usually younger than most patients with benign prostatic hypertrophy. You can pass a sound (or a cystoscope), and so exclude a stricture.

If you are able to examine such a patient through a cystoscope, you will find that his bladder is obviously obstructed, as shown by trabeculation, a hypertrophied interureteric bar, and perhaps diverticula. But you cannot see any sign of an enlarged prostate. Instead, the posterior lip of his urinary meatus is unduly prominent (difficult to see with an ordinary cystoscope).

These cases were formerly grouped together as the 'small fibrous prostate', a term which is no longer used. Instead, urologists now recognize: (1) Dyskinesia or bladder-neck dysfunction. This is a disorder of function, and cannot be diagnosed by feeling the internal meatus. (2) Bladder-neck stenosis, which is a true fibrosis of the bladder neck. One cause of this is a schistosomal fibrosis of the submucosa of the trigone.

You can treat bladder-neck dysfunction medically, with alpha blockers, or surgically, by cutting the fibres of the neck of the bladder.

BLADDER NECK DYSFUNCTION

If you suspect the diagnosis before you operate, try phenoxybenzamine hydrochloride ('Dibenylene'), an alpha blocker, 10 mg daily or twice daily. This is symptomatic only, so treatment has to continue indefinitely. Orthostatic hypotension can be a problem.

If you set out to do a modified Freyer's operation, you may find, when you open the patient's bladder, that his prostate is not enlarged. Instead, he has a tight internal meatus, which you cannot put your finger into.

METHOD. Get adequate exposure—you cannot expose his internal urinary meatus through a short incision. Approach the inside of his bladder as for Freyer's prostatectomy (23.19).

Put a self-retaining retractor into his bladder, open it, and tilt the head of the table downwards slightly. Use a Langenbeck retractor, or a bent copper retractor, to draw the anterior wall of his bladder against his pubis, so that you can see his internal urinary meatus.

Identify the orifices of his ureters. Make deep cuts in his bladder neck in the 5 and 7 o'clock positions, sloping towards one another so as to excise a wedge of his bladder neck, as in J, Fig. 23-25. They must go deep enough to divide the circular fibres of the neck of his bladder. When you have cut them the neck of his bladder will spring open, and his obstruction will be relieved.

If *Schistosoma haematobium* **is the cause,** there will be more fibrosis, and you will be cutting fibrous tissue rather than muscle.

CAUTION ! (1) Take great care not to injure his ureters, as they enter his bladder. A wise precaution is to pass a 7 Ch catheter (or a feeding tube) into each of them. (2) If you find diverticula, leave them.

POSTOPERATIVELY, use any of the methods of irrigation or drainage in Section 23.19. Remove the urethral catheter on the 5th or 6th day. If his bladder was large and atonic at operation, insert a 16 or 18 Ch Foley catheter, and drain his bladder for 3 or 4 weeks into a bottle.

23.21 Ghadvi's lateral perineal prostatectomy

The place of his operation in the hospitals for which we write is not clear, which is why it is in small print. Earlier descriptions of it were incomplete, so that some operators appear to have neglected the critically important step of incising the prostatic capsule, and entering the prostatic urethra inside it, rather than outside it. How common incontinence and stricture are with less skilled operators remains to be determined, and to be compared with the complication rate of Freyer's operation, in the same hands and under the same circumstances. More extensive trials are in progress. Meanwhile, the place of this operation is uncertain, but it may turn out to be a very useful method. At least one contributor has advised its deletion: others disagree.

About 1500 BC Sushruta removed bladder stones through a lateral incision in the perineum. More recently, Ghadvi has adapted this approach to remove the prostate, and it is now used by a number of surgeons in East Africa. It has several advantages: (1) Most importantly, there is no need for postoperative irrigation, and the 15 or 20 bottles of fluid that Freyer's method may need. This makes it very popular with the nurses. (2) There is less bleeding, so that few patients need a blood transfusion. (3) There is very much less risk of clot retention, than with other methods. This is because the balloon of a Foley catheter can be used to compresses a pack in the prostatic cavity most effectively, and with much less tendency for it to slip up into the bladder than with Freyer's method. (4) The operation is quick—about 30 minutes. (5) The incision is small and the scar hidden. (6) You seldom need an assistant. (7) You need only the minimum of equipment. (8) It is painless. (9) It has a low mortality rate. (10) Recovery is rapid. (11) There is little danger of injuring the rectum. Preliminary cystoscopy is desirable, but not absolutely necessary. (13) It is well adapted to adversity—to overcrowded wards, and the very minimum of equipment and facilities.

Like all operations, it has some disadvantages: (1) Enucleating a prostatic adenoma through the perineum needs more experience than removing one through the bladder—you will find it more difficult to be sure what you are feeling at the end of your finger, and preferably you need a very long finger. You should therefore be familiar with Freyer's method before you start. (2) The prostatic capsule cannot be sutured in the depth of the wound, so you have to let it granulate. This means that a postoperative catheter is required for 10 to 14 days, which is the same time as with Freyer's method, but is longer than with Millin's retropubic prostatectomy (5 days), which allows you to suture the prostatic capsule. (3) In the original series of 400 patients temporary incontinence was seen in 10% of cases. About 1% of the series needed a penile clamp 6 months after the operation. The complication rate is thus much the same as with other methods of prostatectomy. The reasons for incontinence with this method, as with the others, is not altogether clear. It may be due to fibrosis in the membranous urethra, or because the hypertrophied lower part of the lateral lobes protrudes through the dilated fibres of the sphincter urethrae. When this happens these overstretched fibres may not regain their tone and their power to compress the urethra. Postoperative incontinence is said to be more common in patients who already have preoperative incontinence with overflow.

Ghadvi NP, 'Sushruta's lateral perineal approach for prostatectomy', Proceedings of the Association of Surgeons of East Africa 1978;1:28-32

Loefler IJP, 'Ghadvi's prostatectomy', Proceedings of the Association of Surgeons of East Africa 1983;6:51-52.

GHADVI'S PROSTATECTOMY

INDICATIONS. (1) As for Freyer's method. (2) Many patients requiring prostatectomy under difficult circumstances. (3) It is an excellent way of taking a biopsy of the prostate.

CONTRAINDICATIONS. (1) An inexperienced operator doing his first prostatectomy. You will be wise to have done a few operations by Freyer's method first. (2) Carcinoma of the prostate. (3) Dyskinesia and bladder-neck fibrosis ('small fibrous prostate', 23.20). (4) Obesity; if a patient is very obese, you can examine his prostate through his rectum without difficulty, but obese buttocks make it difficult to remove his prostate through his perineum; your finger is not long enough. If you try and have difficulty, you may damage his urethra, and a stricture may follow.

EQUIPMENT. Two haemostats, ovum forceps, a guarded knife as in Fig. 5-6, or pointed scissors; a straight urethral sound. A bladder irrigation syringe, or an ear syringe, or a bottle of saline hanging from a drip stand. 2 Foley catheters, a catheter introducer, a roll of sterile gauze or a uterine pack.

ANAESTHESIA. (1) Ketamine drip (A 8.4). (2) Caudal epidural anaesthesia (A 7.3). (3) Saddle block (A 7.6). (4) General anaesthesia—relaxants are not essential (A 11.3). (5) You can premedicate a very old man with pethidine, and then use local infiltration only.

GHADVI'S PROSTATECTOMY

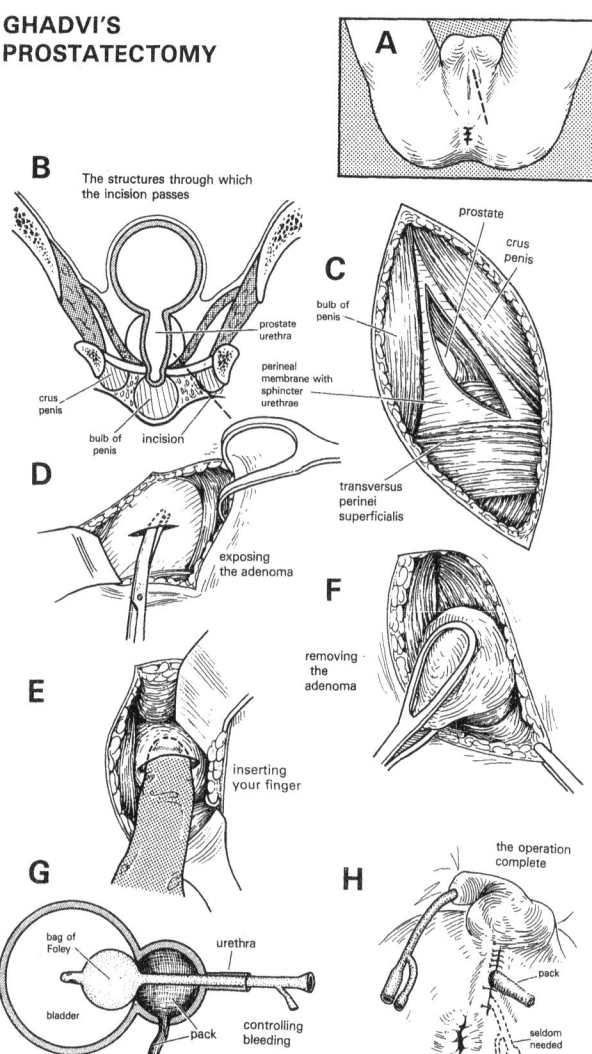

Fig. 23-28 GHADVI'S LATERAL PERINEAL PROSTATECTOMY. A, the incision. B, a cross sectional view of the structures through which the incision passes. C, a schematic view of the structures through which it passes. D, the capsule of the patient's prostate being incised with scissors. E, insert your finger through the incision. Reach for the top of his prostate and avoid his external sphincter. F, remove the adenoma. G, a diagram of the way bleeding is controlled with a pack in the prostatic cavity. H, the finished operation, showing the urethral catheter, the pack in the wound, and an additional catheter (dotted), should one be needed. *Kindly contributed by NP Ghadvi.*

INCISION. Prepare him, put him into an exaggerated lithotomy position. Pass a metal urethral sound up into his bladder, to make sure he has not also got a stricture, and to identify the position of his urethra.

Make a left sided oblique 6 cm incision, as in A, Fig. 23-28, extending from his subpubic angle to his ischial tuberosity. Anteriorly the incision should be about 1 cm lateral to the median raphe, and extend further from it posteriorly. Incise his subcutaneous tissue and undermine flaps on each side, as far as the bulb of his urethra, and the crura of his penis.

Split Camper's fascia vertically, as it stretches over his ischiocavernosus and bulbocavernosus muscles. Open the groove between these two muscles between the bulb and the crura of his penis. Deep to them, use a pair of scissors to split his perineal membrane. Extend the gap vertically with your index finger. The upper limit of the gap is his subpubic angle, and its lower limit the resistance his deep transversus perinei offers to your finger.

Incise his prostatic capsule with pointed scissors, and push your finger through the incision. Feel for the tip of the sound, and let this guide you to his urethra. Feel for the top of his prostate, split the commissure anteriorly, and try to get your finger underneath it so as to enucleate it (some surgeons don't use scissors or a guarded knife, and push their fingers straight through the prostatic capsule).

Put your right index finger into his prostatic urethra, through the torn capsule of his prostate, and withdraw the sound.

CAUTION ! (1) Don't try to enter his urethra outside his prostatic capsule below his perineal membrane, because this is where his external sphincter is, and you must not tear it. Leaving it intact is the critical step in preserving continence. (2) You must have a sound in place, because this tells you where his urethra is.

With your right hand in his suprapubic region, push his prostate downwards.

Split the anterior commissure of his prostate with a hooking movement of your right index finger, and separate the lobes from the capsule by encircling them, as with Freyer's method.

The incision is small, so you cannot remove his prostate in one piece. Instead, remove it lobe by lobe with ovum forceps.

Your finger will not be long enough to reach far enough into his bladder, to let you remove the intravesical protrusion of his middle lobe. So use a pair of ovum forceps to twist all the remaining portions of his middle lobe from the capsule.

CAUTION ! In all cases put your finger into his bladder to dilate its internal sphincter.

Insert a Foley catheter. Pack his prostatic cavity with a roll of sterile gauze to control bleeding. Wash out his bladder with saline. Suture only his skin. Apply mild traction to the catheter by strapping it to his thigh.

POSTOPERATIVE CARE. Antibiotics are not necessary routinely. As soon as his urine is clear, and not mixed with frank blood, give him intravenous diazepam and remove the pack, usually at 24–48 hours; removing it is not difficult and bleeding is rare. Remove the skin stitches and the urethral catheter between 10 and 14 days.

DIFFICULTIES WITH GHADVI'S PROSTATECTOMY

If a piece of **ADENOMA ESCAPES INTO HIS BLADDER,** remove it with ovum forceps; if this fails, you will have to do a small suprapubic cystotomy and remove it that way.

If he has **BLADDER-NECK FIBROSIS (a 'small fibrous prostate'),** you will not be able to get into his prostatic urethra with your finger, so you will have to use a guarded knife, as above. This, if you diagnose it preoperatively, is normally considered a contraindication to this method.

If he has a **MALIGNANT PROSTATE,** you may be able to enucleate the adenomatous zone, before it has been infiltrated from the peripheral carcinomatous zone. Send a biopsy for histological examination. A preoperative diagnosis of carcinoma is a contraindication to this method. It is likely to bleed much.

If the operation is **DIFFICULT,** protect his rectum from injury by putting your left index into it, while your assistant stabilizes his prostate by downward and forward suprapubic pressure.

If **YOUR FINGER GOES INTO HIS RECTUM** insert 2 or 3 stitches of '0' or '1' catgut on a curved atraumatic needle through his rectal wall and his prostatic bed. Keep him on a liquid diet for a week. Some surgeons insert no sutures when this happens.

If **URINE IS NOT DRAINING into the bag, and his bladder is distending,** he has clot retention. Take him to the theatre, remove his skin stitches, and the perineal pack, and evacuate the clot in his bladder through his perineal wound. Remove the clot with ovum forceps. Leave a large three-channel Foley catheter in the wound, repack his prostatic cavity, and irrigate his bladder, as with Freyer's method.

If **URINE LEAKS from his wound,** it will probably start do so between the 7th and 10th day, after which his fistula will heal spontaneously in 2 weeks. Leave his urethral catheter in place, and cauterize the fistulous track with diathermy. No permanent perineal fistulae have been recorded.

If he is **INCONTINENT OF URINE after removing the catheter,** reassure him that this is likely to be only temporary, and that he will probably gradually gain control of micturition. If he is unlucky enough to be permanently incontinent, fit him with a penile clamp.

If he starts to develop a STRICTURE, dilate him regularly (23.8).

23.22 The injection method for benign prostatic hypertrophy

If you are not able to do Freyer's prostatectomy, or a patient is too old or too sick for it, try injecting his prostate with phenol, which will make it slowly necrose and fibrose. The method is an old one from India, and dates from the days before prostatectomy was as safe as it now is in skilled hands and with good facilities. The following account is that of Gray and Visser, who consider that it is a reasonable alternative to a transurethral or suprapubic prostatectomy, in a primary care hospital, where there is no trained urologist. It should not replace prostatectomy entirely, even when there is no urologist, but if you do introduce it, you will find that it will dramatically reduce the number of prostatectomies that you need do.

Injection is straightforward and at least 90% successful. Like most surgeons, Gray and Visser report an occasional death from prostatectomy, but none from injection. In 42 cases it did however cause epididymitis twice, and a perineal fistula once; only two patients needed their prostates removed surgically, and all were discharged without a catheter. The procedure is not difficult, and could probably be learnt by a technician.

Success depends on placing the needle *close to, but not actually in,* the patient's urethra. The response seems to depend on the size of his prostate, the extent to which its subcervical lobe is involved, and how close your injection is to his urethra. You will find that the needle is easier to place when his prostate is small, and if so, it will probably respond after only four injections. Large prostates need more injections, and the method is most likely to fail if a prostate is huge. Injection does not take long, and you will probably find that the most efficient way to manage a series of cases, is to do them together on the same days of the week, in a minor theatre.

This method enjoyed a brief period of popularity in Europe in the 1970's, and also for very poor risk patients. Perineal pain was found to be a problem, and contrast studies showed that the injection often went far outside the prostate.

Herman Gray and Hendrik Visser, Mkar Christian Hospital, PO Gboko, Benue State, Nigeria. Personal communication.

THE INJECTION METHOD FOR PROSTATIC HYPERTROPHY

INDICATIONS. (1) Lack of the facilities or the skill to do Freyer's suprapubic prostatectomy. (2) The patient with moderate enlargement, who is in poor medical condition, as the result of uraemia or malnutrition.

CONTRAINDICATIONS. If his prostate is huge, and his medical condition is good, he should have a prostatectomy.

THE SOLUTION. Take 0.6 ml of phenol, 0.6 ml of glycerine, and 0.6 ml of glacial acetic acid. Add 28 ml of water. Put the mixture into 'water for injection' bottles and autoclave it.

ADMISSION AND CATHETERIZATION. You will probably already have had to catheterize him, to relieve his retention of urine. If he merely has symptoms of prostatic obstruction, without actual retention, you may be able to treat him as an outpatient without catheterizing him.

INJECTION Put him into the lithotomy position, and leave his catheter in place. Infiltrate his perineum with lignocaine.

Put your finger into his rectum. Push a 0.9 or 1 mm spinal needle from his perineum into one of the lateral lobes of his prostate. You will feel a woody resistance as you enter it. Inject 1.5 ml of the solution. Inject another 1.5 ml on the other side.

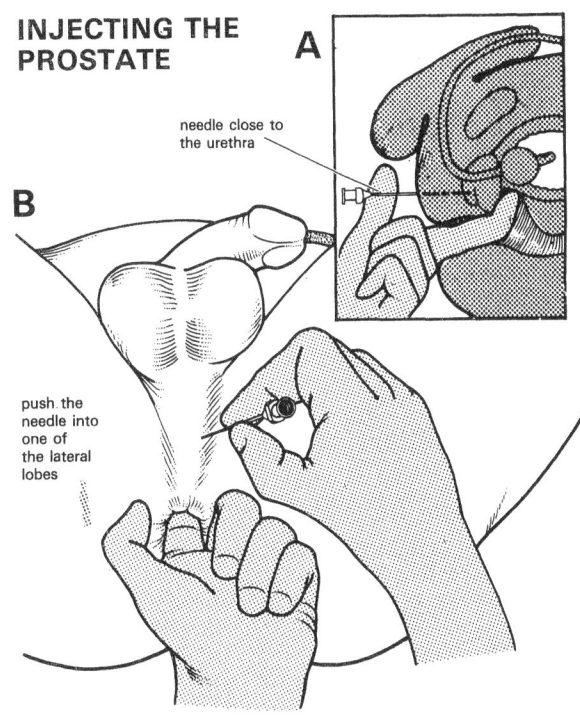

INJECTING THE PROSTATE

Fig. 23-29 INJECTING THE PROSTATE WITH PHENOL for benign prostatic hypertrophy. A, success depends on placing the needle close to, but not actually in, the patient's urethra. B, put your finger into his rectum, and push a spinal needle into one of the lateral lobes of his prostate; you will feel a woody resistance as you enter it. *Kindly contributed by Hendrik Visser, of Mkar Christian Hospital.*

CAUTION ! If he complains of a burning sensation during injection, stop. The needle is not in his prostate. If he has a burning pain in his penis, the needle is in his urethra. Wait until next week and try again, leaving the catheter in meanwhile.

Give him a series of 5 injections 4 days apart, while leaving the catheter in. After 5 injections, remove the catheter.

If he can urinate, good. Discharge him and ask him to reattend if his symptoms recur.

If he cannot urinate, reinsert the catheter and give him 4 more injections at 4 day intervals.

If he still cannot urinate after the second course of 4 injections, you will have to decide whether to give him a third course of 4 injections, or to remove his prostate surgically. If prostatectomy is impractical, or he is unfit for it, and the third course of injections fails, he will have to put up with a catheter indefinitely.

If you do remove his prostate surgically when injections have failed, it will be more fibrotic, it will shell out easily, and there will be less bleeding than there would have been if you had not injected it. It may be like putty.

23.22a Epididymo-orchitis and associated conditions

A patient with acute epididymo-orchitis presents with an acute painful swelling of one testis and epididymis. A few cases are viral: the important viral cause is mumps. Chronic epididymo-orchitis is common in the developing world after the age of 25. It is the result of: (1) Previous untreated or imperfectly treated attacks of acute epididymo-orchitis, which is usually gonococcal. (2) Non-specific urinary infection (usually due to *Esch. coli*). (3) In endemic areas, schistosomal epididymitis. This is usually confined to the tail of the epididymis, causes little pain, less swelling, and no signs of inflammation except mild tenderness. (4) Tuberculosis (uncommon).

EPIDIDYMO-ORCHITIS AND ASSOCIATED CONDITIONS

ACUTE EPIDIDYMO-ORCHITIS

DIFFERENTIAL DIAGNOSIS AND TREATMENT. In gonoccocal and non-specific urethritis, either only a patient's epididymis is affected, or his epididymis is affected more than his testis, usually unilaterally.

Suggesting acute gonococcal epididymo-orchitis—a urethral discharge or a history of it. If possible isolate the causative organism, and give him the appropriate antibiotic. Tetracycline 500 mg 8-hourly for 7 days will usually be appropriate.

Suggesting acute nonspecific epididymo-orchitis—a previous urinary infection. There is no discharge but pain on micturition is common. If possible, culture his urine and give him the appropriate antibiotic. If not give him ampicillin 250 mg 6- to 8-hourly for 5 days, or trimethoprim 200 mg 12-hourly for 5 days.

Suggesting mumps orchitis—his testis is affected and his epididymis may appear normal. Usually unilateral but occasionally bilateral, not necessarily simultaneously. He will settle without treatment, but if both his testes are affected he may become infertile, especially if he is an adult.

Suggesting schistosomiasis haematobium—small 3 to 5 mm nodules in his epididymis, nearly always in the tail.

CHRONIC EPIDIDYMO-ORCHITIS

DIFFERENTIAL DIAGNOSIS. For the differential diagnosis of chronic epididymo-orchitis from tumours, see Sections 23.25 and 32.34a.

MANAGEMENT depends on the cause.

If the cause of his chronic epididymo-orchitis is chronic infection, give him an antibiotic such as ampicillin or trimethoprim, guided by his urine culture. His infection will probably settle. If it does not, look elsewhere for tuberculosis, and consider biopsy.

If he has schistosomal epididymitis don't treat him unless it causes symptoms: if so, give him antischistosomal drugs.

If he has severe recurrent attacks of pain which do not settle, consider excising his testis and epididymis (rarely necessary). You will have to remove both, because you cannot remove his epididymis without his testis: there will be too much bleeding. See Section 23.25.

23.23 Hydroceles in adults

In Europe the cause of hydroceles is unknown. In the tropics they are one of the commonest manifestations of Bancroftian filariasis. You will see all the anatomical varieties, but you will find the common infantile and vaginal ones difficult to differentiate, because most vaginal ones come up close to the patient's deep inguinal ring—see Fig. 14-15.

If a hydrocele is small, leave it, but if it is so large that it makes sex difficult, or is an unwelcome weight, operate. If it is only a modest size, turn it inside out, so that the fluid which it secretes drains into the lymphatics; if it is larger, excise its secreting surface. Aspirating smaller hydroceles every 3–6 months is popular with many patients, but it is not a cure.

The scrotum is famous for its tendency to bleed postoperatively, develop a haematoma, and swell. Complete haemostasis is important: (1) Sharp dissection causes less bleeding than blunt or gauze dissection. (2) If necessary, sew over the cut edge of the tunica postoperatively with continuous or simple haemostatic sutures of chromic catgut, as in G, Fig. 4-7.

Mlay SM and Philip PJ. 'Combined scrotoplasty and radical excision of the sac in the treatment of large vaginal hydroceles'. Proceedings of the Association of Surgeons of East Africa. 1980;3:149-153.

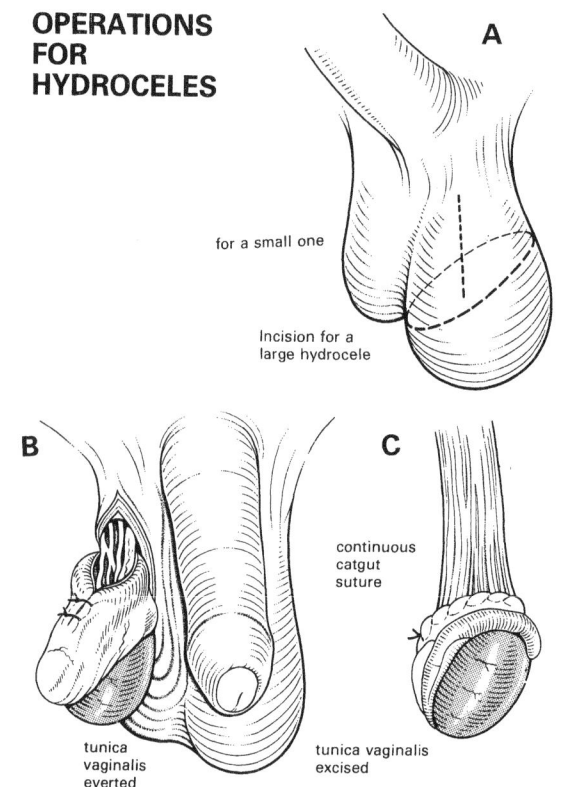

Fig. 23-30 OPERATIONS FOR HYDROCELES IN ADULTS. A, if the patient's hydrocele is a small one, make a vertical incision just lateral to the median raphe. If it is large, make an elliptical incision, and excise the skin within the ellipse, after which you can turn his processus vaginalis inside out (B), or you can excise it (C).

HYDROCELES IN ADULTS

For congenital hydroceles in children, see Section 14.5. If the patient also has epididymitis, or prostatitis, control this first.

ANAESTHESIA. (1) Low subarachnoid anaesthesia. (2) General anaesthesia.

INCISIONS. If his hydrocele is a small one, make a vertical incision just lateral to the median raphe. If it is large, make an elliptical incision, and excise the skin within the ellipse. Adjust the size of the ellipse to the size of his hydrocele.

EVERSION OF THE TUNICA

INDICATIONS. Fairly small, thin-walled hydroceles. This is a simple, quick operation, with little risk of a postoperative haematoma.

METHOD. Hold his scrotum in such a way as to stretch the skin over his hydrocele. Make a vertical incision, as in A, Fig. 23-30. Carefully deepen the incision, until his hydrocele extrudes out, and you see his tunica vaginalis. Control bleeding.

Make a small incision in the avascular upper and anterior aspect of his tunica vaginalis. This should be only just big enough to allow you to deliver his testis through the opening. When you have done this, evert his tunica vaginalis, and suture it behind his testis. If you have made the incision in the sac small enough, his testis cannot return through it. If it might be in danger of doing so, put a few sutures through it (B).

CAUTION! (1) Make sure you evert the whole sac. If it has an upward prolongation and you fail to evert this, it may recur. To evert it put a haemostat into it, pull it inside out completely, and pass a mattress suture though it.

Close his skin with monofilament, and leave a corrugated rubber drain in the wound.

EXCISION OF THE SAC OF A HYDROCELE

INDICATIONS. A large hydrocele with a greatly thickened wall, perhaps covered with a layer of cholesterol crystals.

METHOD. If his hydrocele is large, resect a large piece of his scrotal skin. Excise the entire sac of his hydrocele, except for a cuff about 1 cm deep around his testis and epididymis, as in C, Fig. 23-30. The cut edges will bleed profusely. If you don't have a cautery, pass a simple continuous or haemostatic chromic catgut suture along the whole cut edge.

CAUTION ! (1) The cleft between his testis and his epididymis may be greatly enlarged by the extension of his hydrocele, so take care not to injure or remove his epididymis with his tunica vaginalis. (2) In the hope of minimizing swelling and the formation of a haematoma in his scrotum afterwards, operate gently, and control bleeding with the greatest care, before you close his skin.

If there is no ooze at all, don't insert a drain. If an ooze persists, insert one. Warn him that oedema may temporarily make his scrotum even bigger than it was before.

SCROTOPLASTY AND RADICAL EXCISION

INDICATIONS. As above, very large bilateral hydroceles. This operation removes most of the loose scrotal tissue, minimizes the cavities into which oozing can take place, and gives good cosmetic results.

METHOD. Stretch the skin over the hydrocele and make two crescentic incisions, meeting anteriorly and posteriorly near the median raphe, and outlining just over half the skin area. Make the upper part of the incision first, and tie the bleeding vessels to make the lower incision relatively bloodless. Stretch his scrotal skin to control bleeding, and cut down to his internal spermatic fascia. Separate this by sharp dissection from his tunica vaginalis, and remove redundant scrotal tissue.

Dissect his tunica vaginalis from the rest of his scrotal wall by finger dissection, and open the sac. Excise the redundant sac close to his testis, and oversew the free edge with haemostatic continuous chromic catgut sutures, as in C, Fig. 23-30. For the insertion of drains and the closure of the wound see above.

DIFFICULTIES WITH HYDROCELES

If he is a NEONATE or a CHILD, see Section 14.5.

If he has a really ENORMOUS HYDROCELE, it may extend upwards through his inguinal canal, as an inguinoscrotal hydrocele. Its upward prolongation may lie anterior or posterior to his peritoneum, and may contain several litres of fluid. Don't mistake it for a distended bladder combined with an infantile hydrocele. Excise the abdominal sac, and if possible his tunica vaginalis also. If he also has an indirect inguinal hernia, excise the sac of that too. Such a hernia may accompany or follow a hydrocele.

23.24 Torsion of the testis

Torsion of the testis is a surgical emergency which needs operation without delay. The consequences of not operating are so serious, that it is never wrong to operate to exclude torsion.

Occasionally, a patient's tunica vaginalis ends abnormally high up his spermatic cord, so that his cord can twist and obstruct the blood supply to his testis and epididymis. When this abnormality (the 'bell-clapper' testis) is present, his testis usually hangs transversely, and does so on both sides. Unless you can untwist his cord, his testis will necrose, become a purple-black, and fill his tunica vaginalis with a blood-tinged fluid. If you don't relieve the torsion before this happens, his testis will atrophy. If you are going to save it, you must operate within 4 to 6 hours of the start of symptoms.

Torsion can occur at any age, but is more common in the first year of life and in adolescence (12–20 years). Typically, a teenage boy wakes with sudden severe *pain in his groin or lower abdomen* (due to the surface representation of his testis), rather than in his scrotum. Sometimes, he has severe nausea and vomiting, and mild fever. His testis becomes tender and swollen, and the skin of his scrotum may become red.

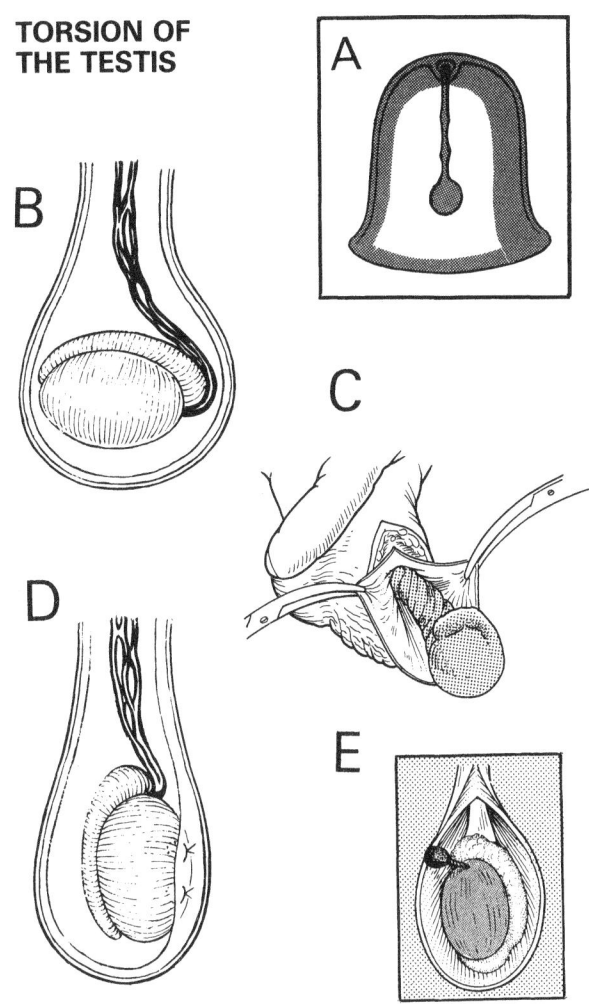

Fig. 23-31 TORSION OF THE TESTIS. Occasionally, a patient's tunica vaginalis ends abnormally high up his spermatic cord, so that his cord can twist and obstruct the blood supply to his testis and epididymis. This abnormality is the 'bell-clapper' testis. A, is a bell with its clapper. B, is such a testis, with its long intravaginal spermatic cord hanging horizontally. C, torsion of the spermatic cord. D, the cord untwisted and anchored to prevent torsion recurring. E, torsion of the epididymis of the testis.

TORSION OF THE TESTIS

THE MAIN DIFFERENTIAL DIAGNOSIS is acute epididymo-orchitis.

Suggesting torsion —the sudden onset of pain in an adult or a teenager, with a non-tender prostate, typically with no urinary symptoms, no signs of urethritis, and a sterile urine. No fever, or mild fever if he presents late. His testis lies higher on the involved side than it does on the normal one. Examine him standing. You may see his *normal* testis lying horizontally. His spermatic cord is enlarged and painful. You cannot feel the normal plane of cleavage between his epididymis and his testis. The slow onset of pain does not exclude torsion.

Suggesting epididymo-orchitis —the slower onset of pain in an adult with a tender prostate, urinary symptoms, signs of past or present urethritis, and an infected urine. Usually mild fever. In the standing position his normal testis is in its usual oblique attitude.

CAUTION ! (1) Don't diagnose anyone under the age of 18 as suffering from epididymo-orchitis, unless the physical signs make this certain. If there is any doubt, operate. You will not harm orchitis by exploring it, but antibiotics will not relieve torsion. Except for the orchitis of mumps, orchitis is very rare in young boys. (2) Treat painful testicular enlargement in an infant or neonate as torsion.

MANIPULATIVE REDUCTION is temporary and is never adequate or definitive treatment. It is only appropriate in the first hour or two, so the opportunity for it seldom arises. Even if it is successful, torsion may recur, so proceed to operation and orchidopexy early.

ORCHIDOPEXY FOR TORSION OF THE TESTIS

ANAESTHESIA. (1) Ketamine. (2) General anaesthesia. (3) Low subarachnoid anaesthesia if he is over 15 years old.

INCISION. Make a vertical incision in his scrotum, over the area of tenderness. Cut through his subcutaneous tissue and fascial layers down to his tunica vaginalis. Open it. You will find it filled with blood-tinged fluid, and you will see his twisted spermatic cord. Untwist it.

If there seems no chance that his testis will survive, transfix his spermatic cord, and excise it.

If you are not sure if his testis is viable or not, wrap it in a warm, moist swab and inspect it again in 5 minutes. Bright bleeding when you incise his tunica albuginea is a promising sign. If you are in doubt, preserve it, especially if his symptoms have lasted less than 10 hours, and it has twisted less than one and a half times.

If untwisting relieves the vascular congestion, suture his testis to his tunica vaginalis to prevent the torsion recurring, as in D, Fig. 23-31. Align his testis with its head placed superiorly. Anchor it to his tunica vaginalis laterally with two non-absorbable sutures.

CAUTION ! Always anchor his other testis in the same way, the condition is usually bilateral.

If the twisted testis is viable, operate on the normal one at the same time.

If the twisted testis is not viable, infection is a possibility, so operate on his normal one soon after the wound has healed.

Control bleeding. Close the skin incision.

DIFFICULTIES WITH TORSION OF THE TESTIS

If you find that his TESTIS ITSELF IS NOT TWISTED, but instead there is a small, twisted structure attached to it (more likely in an infant), he has TORSION OF AN APPENDIX OF HIS TESTIS OR EPIDIDYMIS. These are the remains of the pronephros. Tie off the twisted structure, and excise it.

If he is an INFANT, AND ESPECIALLY A NEONATE, you may find that his whole tunica vaginalis with its contained testis and spermatic cord is twisted (supravaginal torsion). Deal with it in the same way.

If an UNDESCENDED OR MALDESCENDED TESTICLE STRANGULATES, you can mistake it for a strangulated hernia (14.6).

If he has ALREADY LOST ONE TESTIS because of torsion and atrophy, be sure you anchor the other side, if this has not already been done.

If his TORSION REDUCES ITSELF SPONTANEOUSLY, warn his parents that it can recur, and advise them that both his testes should be anchored.

23.25 Orchidectomy

You may occasionally need to remove a patient's testes. If he has a seminoma or a teratoma, remove one of them (32.34a). This is much safer than biopsying it, which may spread his tumour. If he has a carcinoma of his prostate, and you decide not to treat him with oestrogens, you can remove both of them, either by doing a total orchidectomy or a subcapsular one. If you do the latter, you can tell him that you are only removing 'the part of the testicle which produces the hormones', which may be more acceptable to him. The remnant is small but is easily palpable. Even so, you will probably find that subcapsular orchidectomy is more unpopular than stilboestrol (32.32).

ORCHIDECTOMY

Don't mistake mumps orchitis for a tumour. This causes rapid

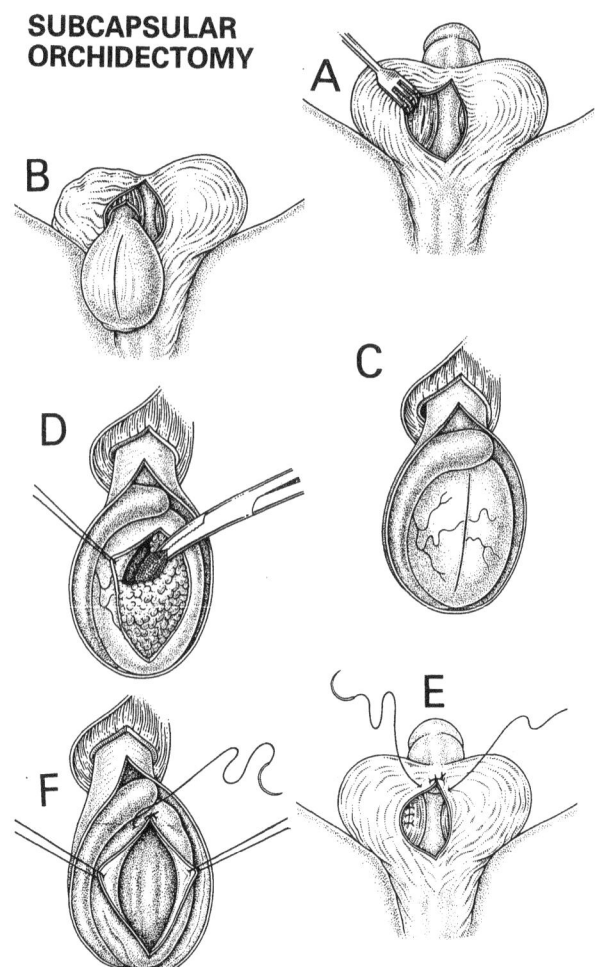

Fig. 23-32 SUBCAPSULAR ORCHIDECTOMY FOR CARCINOMA OF THE PROSTATE. A, make a longitudinal incision in the patient's scrotum. B, evaginate his testis. C, incise his tunica albuginea. D, separate the substance of his testis from the inner surface of his tunica albuginea. D, close his tunica, E, close his skin. *After Rob C and Smith R 'Operative Surgery': Urology', pp. 667 and 668 (Butterworth). With the kind permission of Hugh Dudley.*

enlargement, and some pain (minimal in the case of a tumour). Mumps orchitis may cause little pain, so if you are in doubt, wait for a few days rather than remove his testis.

You will have to exert some traction on the cord, but beware of its upper end slipping out of the clamp and retracting out of sight. Take great care to secure haemostasis, before you close the wound. If possible, apply diathermy to the smaller bleeding vessels, and tie off the larger ones. Close the patient's skin with continuous horizontal mattress sutures of catgut.

SUBCAPSULAR ORCHIDECTOMY FOR CARCINOMA OF THE PROSTATE

Raise his scrotum, and incise his stretched skin and dartos muscle, to expose both his testes (A, Fig. 23-32). Evaginate each testis with its coverings, and incise its tunica vaginalis vertically to expose his testis and epididymis (B). Incise his visceral tunica vertically over the globe of his testis. Use sharp and blunt dissection, to separate the substance of his testis from the inner surface of his tunica albuginea (C). Control bleeding carefully at the upper pole. Remove all testicular tissue, and close his tunica with continuous 3/0 plain catgut sutures (D). Close his scrotum in 2 layers with continuous 3/0 chromic catgut, without inserting a drain. After a few weeks, blood clot in his tunica will become organized to form a small palpable nodule, like a small testis.

ORCHIDECTOMY FOR A TESTICULAR TUMOUR

You will need to remove his cord with his testis, so open up his inguinal canal as for a hernia with an inguino-scrotal incision (14-4). Pick up his cord within its covering of cremaster.

TOTAL ORCHIDECTOMY

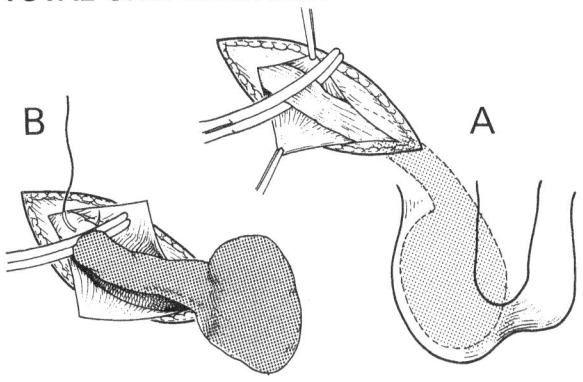

Fig. 23-33 TOTAL ORCHIDECTOMY FOR A TUMOUR. A, apply a soft bowel clamp to the patient's cord before you do anything else. B, make an inguino-scrotal incision and remove his cord with his testis. *After Blandy J, 'Operative Urology', (1978), Figs. 15.37 and 15.40. Blackwell Scientific Publications, with kind permission.*

Apply a soft bowel clamp to it, before you do anything else. Deliver his testis from his scrotum by pushing it up from below. If his tumour is large, you will have to extend the incision further into his scrotum.

If you feel a hard irregular mass, which is not chronic epididymo-orchitis, doubly transfix and tie his cord proximal to the clamp as near his internal ring as you can, and excise his testis. If he has a seminoma, he should have radiotherapy to his retroperitoneal nodes.

ORCHIDECTOMY FOR CHRONIC INFECTION (rare)

If you do not suspect malignancy, and there is an overlying skin lesion on his scrotum, arange your incision so as to excise this, and remove it attached to the structures under it. Enter his scrotum away from any diseased area. Deliver his testis and any skin which is attached to it. Pull *gently* on his testis, to free about 6 cm of his cord; divide it between two clamps, and tie it twice with strong catgut. Divide it between them. If it is very thick, separate its structures and tie them separately. Leave the wound in his scrotum unsutured to drain freely, dress it loosely, and close it by delayed primary suture.

23.25a Undescended or maldescended testes

About 3% of newborns and 0.5% of older boys have a testis missing from their scrotums, and in 20% of them it is missing on both sides. An *incompletely descended* testis lies along the track of descent of the testis, the common sites for it are in a child's inguinal canal, or inside his abdomen. A *maldescended* testis may lie in his suprainguinal pouch, just superior to his external ring deep to the membranous part of his superficial fascia, in his perineum, or on the medial aspect of his thigh. The distinction between incomplete descent and maldescent may be difficult. A testis which is absent from the scrotum will make hormones but not sperms. So if neither of his testes are in his scrotum, he will have his normal secondary sex characteristics, including potency, but he will be infertile. The less complete the descent, the greater his chance of infertility. If a testis is absent on one side only, he will probably be fertile, but his misplaced testis is more easily injured, and is about 30 times more likely to become malignant. Even so, because malignant testicular tumours are so rare anyway, this is a small risk.

Spermatogenesis is normal in an incompletely descended testis and in a maldescended one, until the age of 6. This is also the age at which nearly all 'retractile testes' (see below) will have settled normally into the scrotum. So wait until the age of six before you advise orchidopexy. If neither of his testes are in his scrotum by this time, orchidopexy may make him fertile. If one of them is, he will probably be fertile anyway, and it is uncertain if the small risk of malignancy will be altered, so orchidopexy has little point. Its main effect is psychological. Maldescended testes are usually good ones, which can be brought down more readily. Unfortunately, the evidence for orchidopexy improving fertility is still inconclusive.

UNDESCENDED TESTES

If neither testis is present in a newborn's scrotum, the possibilities are: (1) Retractile testes (very common). (2) A genuine undescended or maldescended testis. (3) An intersex (rare). He may look male, but really be a female with the adrenogenital syndrome.

If the testes of a boy under 2 years retract into his groin to lie at his external ring or even a little within it, especially when he is cold, but can be manipulated downwards (retractile testes), consider him normal. By puberty they will probably be permanently in his scrotum. Follow him at least to the age of 16. If at any stage his testes cannot be manipulated into the correct position in his scrotum (unusual), see below.

If neither of his testes can be manipulated into his scrotum, refer him for orchidopexy at the age of 6 or as soon after as possible.

If only one of them is missing, orchidopexy is much less important.

If he has a hernia and an undescended testis on the same side, orchidopexy should be done at the same time as herniorrhaphy; it will be much more difficult later.

ORCHIDOPEXY FOR UNDESCENDED TESTIS

INDICATIONS. Testes which are not in place in the scrotum by the age of 6, and cannot be brought down to their normal position. If possible refer him. If you really cannot refer him and are experienced, consider proceeding as follows. The important part of the operation is getting enough cord length, the method of fixation is less important.

ANAESTHESIA. (1) General anaesthesia (10.1). (2) Ketamine (8.1).

METHOD. Aim to mobilize his spermatic cord to obtain more length, and then to fix his testes in their normal places. Deal with incomplete descent and maldescent in the same way.

To mobilize his spermatic cord, make a 5 cm incision from just lateral to his mid inguinal point to the root of his scrotum. Open his inguinal canal from his external to his internal ring. Find his spermatic cord containing his spermatic vessels and vas. Use sharp dissection to mobilize his cord and testis from all surrounding structures, including his dartos muscle. If he has a hernia remove the sac. Avoid any trauma which may cause bleeding.

If you now have enough length of cord to bring his testis down into his scrotum, stop here.

If not, incise his external oblique and transversus muscles lateral to his inguinal ring and open his peritoneal cavity. Dissect his cord from the peritoneum covering it for about 5 cm. This is not easy, so don't attempt it unless you have had some experience.

To fix his testis in his scrotum, insert your finger into his scrotal sac to open it up. Then place his testis in his scrotum. Insert a non-absorbable suture from his skin into his testis, and then out again, as a mattress suture. Tie this over small pieces of gauze. Or open the midline septum of his scrotum, and push his testis to the other side. Narrow the hole in the septum round his cord, with multifilament. Close his skin wound with monofilament.

If you fail to bring down his testis fully, a two-stage procedure will be necessary. Fix his testis as far as you have been able to bring it with a mattress suture as described above. If he has bilateral incompletely descended testes do nothing on the other side. Refer him for a second operation on this side, or for an operation on the other side.

If his testes are maldescended, manage them as for incomplete descent.

CAUTION ! (1) Be sure to discuss with his parents what you can achieve by operation on an incompletely descended testis. (2) Take great care not to damage the blood supply of his testis. (3) At the end explain the outcome of the operation.

23.26 Circumcision

Don't circumcise a child, unless his parents have very strong religious reasons for wanting it, or because there is some surgical indication for doing so. Remind them that the normal adhesions between the glans and the foreskin disappear as a child grows older. In areas where the incidence of carcinoma of the penis is high, circumcision can be considered good preventive medicine, but improving standards of hygiene would be better. A further argument against circumcision is that the prepuce is useful raw material for plastic surgery.

Aim to leave a 2 or 3 mm fringe of the inner layer of his prepuce. One of the purposes of the foreskin is to provide enough skin to allow the penis to erect, so when you do circumcise him, be careful not to take off too much skin, or his pubic hair will later be drawn up the root of his erected penis. On the other hand don't leave too much, or he runs the risk of recurrent phimosis. The method is the same in adults and children, except that an adult foreskin needs more dissection, and is more likely to need a dorsal slit.

A STORY FROM MULAGO HOSPITAL. Horrible shrieks used to be heard from the theatre whenever circumcisions were being done. A caring surgeon put Fig. 23-34 on the wall whereupon they stopped completely, to the gratitude of the staff—and the patients! Ten years later this event was still remembered.

CIRCUMCISION

INDICATIONS FOR INFANTS. (1) Phimosis. (2) Extreme desire by the parents. Dissuade them if you can.

INDICATIONS FOR ADULTS. (1) Phimosis; recent balanitis, such as that due to diabetes. (2) The relief of paraphimosis following the dorsal slit operation. (3) A suspected malignant lesion confined to a small area of the foreskin.

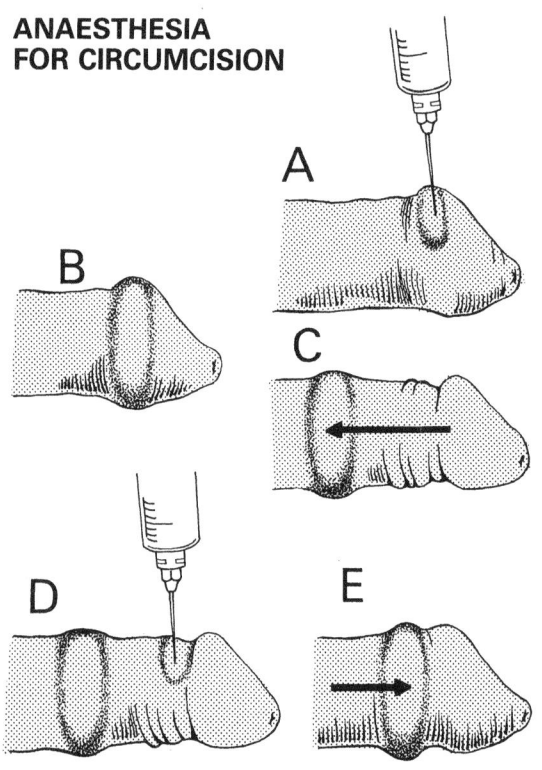

Fig. 23-34 ANAESTHESIA FOR CIRCUMCISION for patients over 15. Under 15 use ketamine (A 8.1). A, and B, with the patient's prepuce forward, infiltrate a ring of anaesthetic solution *without* adrenalin at site of section. C, pull back his prepuce. To do this you may have to infiltrate a little more solution and make a dorsal slit in it. D, and E, infiltrate another ring of solution, at the site of section, just behind his glans. Pull his prepuce forwards again, and all is ready for circumcision to start.

CIRCUMCISION

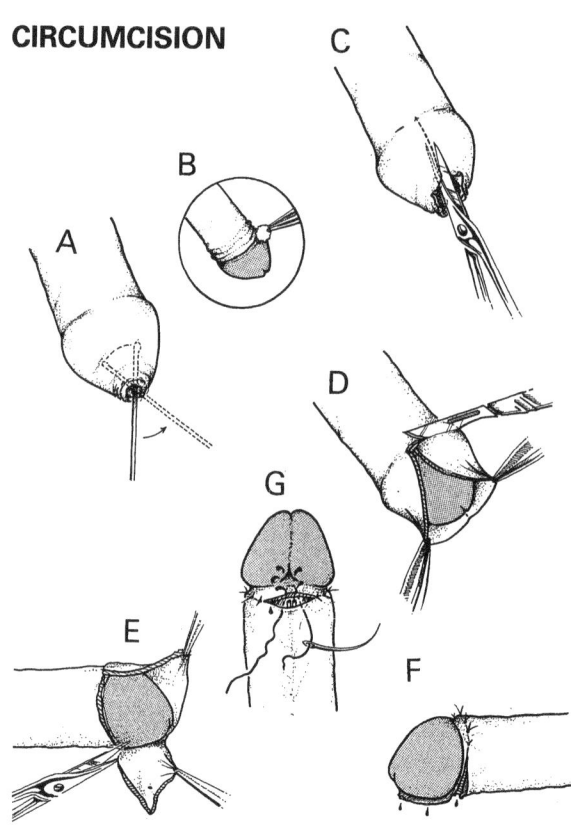

Fig. 23-35 CIRCUMCISION. A, free up the patient's prepuce. B, retract his foreskin and clean his glans. C, make a dorsal slit. D, cut the outer skin only with a scalpel. E, cut the inner layer with scissors leaving a 2 mm fringe at the corona. F, stitch the fringe of prepuce to the skin of the shaft. This will control most of the bleeding. G, control frenal bleeding with this special stitch.

ANAESTHESIA. Admit an older child or adult, and starve him. (1) If he is <15 give him ketamine. (2) If he is >15 use local anaesthesia, as in Fig. 23-34. You will have to cut the inner and outer skin of his prepuce, so you will have to infiltrate them both. A, and B, with the prepuce forward, infiltrate a ring of anaesthetic solution *without* adrenalin at site of section. C, pull back the prepuce. To do this you may have to infiltrate a little more solution and make a dorsal slit in it. D, infiltrate another ring of solution at the site of section just behind his glans. E, pull his prepuce forwards and do the circumcision. Or, (3) do a ring block round the base of his penis with 7–10 ml of 0.75% bupivacaine or 2% lignocaine. Or, (4) give him a general anaesthetic.

METHOD. Paint and drape him for surgery. If adhesions or a tight phimosis prevent you pulling his prepuce back, paint up and drape as best you can. Use a probe to free up the prepuce from adhesions to the glans (A, in Fig. 23-35). Retract his foreskin if you can (B), clean up thoroughly and then pull it forwards again. With his penis in its normal relaxed position, feel for the bulge of the corona of his glans. Use scissors to cut a dorsal slit in his prepuce up to the level of the bulge in his corona (C).

CAUTION! Make sure that the point of the scissors is not in his meatus.

Now cut the outer skin only round his corona (D). Cut the inner layer with scissors, leaving a 2 mm fringe at his corona (E). Use 2/0 or 3/0 plain catgut to control bleeding, by stitching the fringe of his prepuce to the skin of the shaft of his penis (F). Finally, control bleeding from his frenal vessels with a special encircling stitch (G). Dress the wound with vaseline gauze. No dressing is needed after 24 hours. The sutures will fall out on their own.

CAUTION! (1) Don't cut his glans. (2) Don't use diathermy on the penis, it can cause gangrene of the whole organ. (3) Never use adrenalin in a local anaesthetic for the penis, this too can cause gangrene.

DIFFICULTIES WITH CIRCUMCISION

If you CANNOT SEPARATE HIS PREPUCE AND HIS GLANS, because the cleft between them is obliterated, you may find yourself dissecting his glans from his thick adherent prepuce. If necesary, work slowly and carefully with a sharp scalpel. This will leave a raw area. Allow this to granulate on its own, and don't try to graft it with split skin.

If an adult has postoperative PRIAPISM, sedate him. Do this as a routine, if it is a problem in your area.

If he BLEEDS, insert one or two more interrupted sutures.

23.27 Phimosis and paraphimosis

Distinguish three conditions: (1) Phimosis, in which the orifice of a patient's prepuce (foreskin) is too small for his foreskin to be retracted over his penis. (2) Paraphimosis, where his foreskin has retracted, and stuck behind his glans, so that it cannot be brought forward again. (3) A meatal stricture (32.28), in which the external opening of his urethra (his external meatus) is abnormally constricted.

Paraphimosis is the result of forcible retraction of the foreskin. It is common in adolescence, and is fairly common between 8 and 14. Part of his foreskin is tight, so that it becomes oedematous distally. The oedema may be severe. If it has been present for more than a few hours, the base of his penis may be oedematous also. Try to get his foreskin into its normal place over his glans.

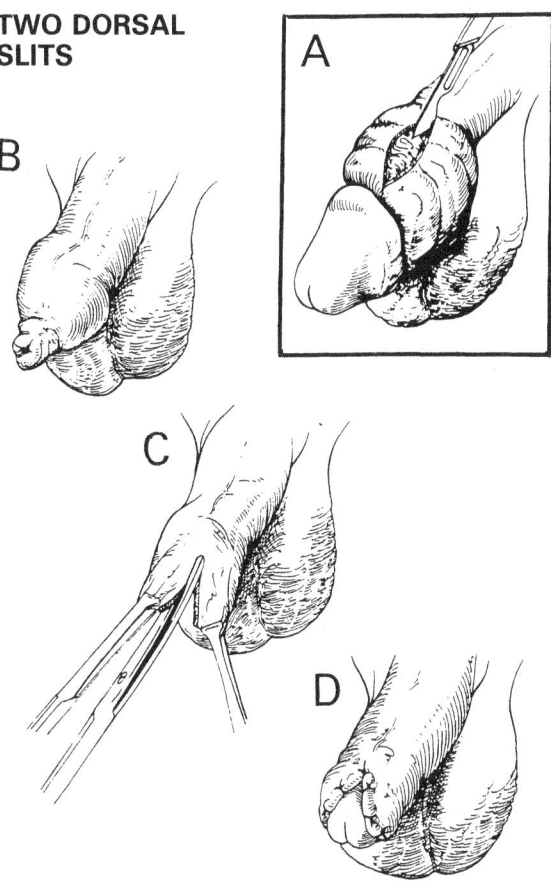

Fig. 23-37 TWO DORSAL SLITS. A, a dorsal slit for paraphimosis. The slit is in the tight circumferential ring, which causes oedema of the foreskin and glans beyond it, and which has been forced back over the shaft of the penis. B, C, and D, a dorsal slit for phimosis, to enlarge the orifice of the foreskin. *Kindly contributed by Jack Lange.*

PHIMOSIS AND PARAPHIMOSIS

PHIMOSIS.

Under local or general anaesthesia make a dorsal slit (A 6.15) as in Fig. 23-37.

PARAPHIMOSIS

ANAESTHESIA. (1) Ketamine. (2) General anaesthesia.

METHOD. Squeeze the patient's swollen foreskin between the thumbs and index fingers of both your hands, so that the fluid which is making it swell, goes up into the tissues of the shaft. If the swelling is severe, wrap layers of gauze over it and squeeze them. When his foreskin is in its normal place, any residual swelling will usually subside in 24–48 hours.

Alternatively, inject hyaluronidase ('Hyalase'), and local anaesthetic solution, into his oedematous foreskin. This will help manual reduction. If you can bring his foreskin forwards intact, circumcision or a dorsal slit will be easier.

After several minutes of firm squeezing, when the swelling is much reduced, push his glans proximally with your thumbs, and draw his foreskin over it with your fingers.

DIFFICULTIES WITH PARAPHIMOSIS

If you FAIL TO REDUCE HIS PARAPHIMOSIS, the constricting band is too tight. Incise it dorsally and try again.

If HIS PARAPHIMOSIS RECURS, wind a strip of zinc oxide strapping round the end of his penis, leaving the tip of his foreskin free, so that he can micturate. Remove it in 24–48 hours. He may need circumcision later (unusual).

If he PRESENTS LATE, when his foreskin has become infected as the result of a spontaneous split, give him an antibiotic and salt baths three times daily. Sloughing is unusual.

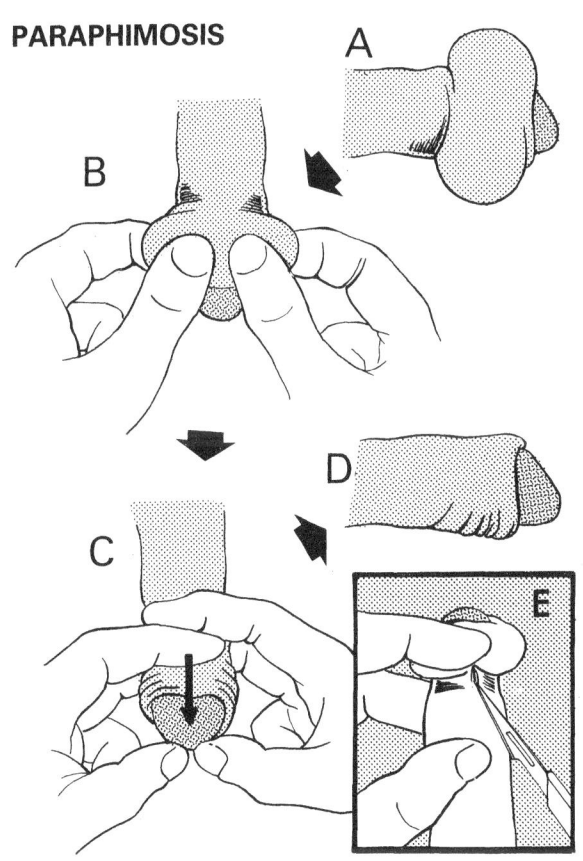

Fig. 23-36 PARAPHIMOSIS. A, paraphimosis as the patient presents. B, use the thumbs and forefingers of both your hands to squeeze his swollen foreskin. C, slide the roll of foreskin forwards over his now thinner glans. At the same time push his glans back. D, successful reduction. E, if manual reduction fails make a small dorsal slit and then try again. This is a dorsal view.

MEATOTOMY

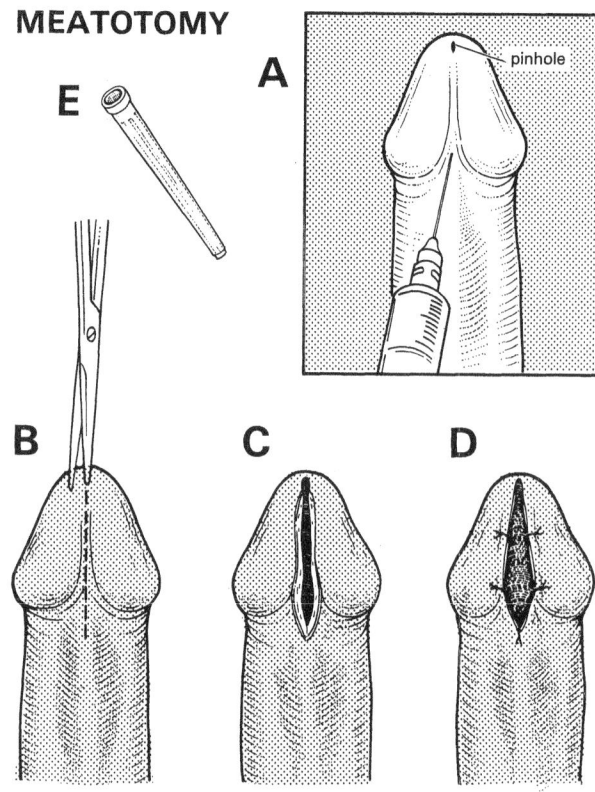

Fig. 23-38 MEATOTOMY. A, although general anaesthesia is preferable, you can infiltrate a patient's fraenum and glans with anaesthetic solution. B, introduce one blade of a pair of fine scissors into his urethra. C, cut 1.5 cm beyond the stenosis. D, suture his mucosa to his skin. E, the plastic cover of a disposable needle makes a good dilator. *Kindly contributed by Neville Harrison.*

23.28 Meatal strictures

Strictures of the meatus have quite a different cause and prognosis from the gonococcal ones in Section 23.8. You may see them in children, or adults, and they may be congenital, or acquired. The most important acquired cause is infection associated with instrumentation and catheterization. In adults a meatal stricture may be due to the skin disease called balanitis xerotica obliterans ('BXO', also called lichen sclerosis atropica). This also involves the foreskin, so there is usually an associated phimosis also.

MEATAL STRICTURES

Dilatation should nearly always preceed meatotomy.

If a meatal stricture develops in a child, give his mother a plastic rod to keep it dilated. The rounded plastic containers used for disposable needles are very suitable. Ask her to lubricate it with vegetable oil. If necessary do a meatotomy as described below.

If a meatal stricture develops in an adult, first try dilatation as above. Although general anaesthesia is preferable, you can, if necessary, infiltrate his fraenum and his glans immediately under it with anaesthetic solution. Alternatively, do a ring block of the base of his penis as in Section 23.26. Put one blade of a pair of fine-pointed scissors into his meatus, and cut its ventral aspect in the midline. To stop his stenosis recurring, cut 1.5 cm beyond his meatus, and suture his mucosa to his skin. Use the first two stitches on either side as retractors to open the wound, and expose the mucosa of his urethra. Insert a suture at the apex of this incision to control bleeding from his frenal artery. His meatus may restenose, so give him a dilator.

If there are signs of BXO (see above), hydrocortisone cream will help to prevent recurrence. Let him apply it into his meatus from the nozzle of a small tube, which will then act as a dilator.

23.29 Priapism

If a patient has a persistent painful erection, either rigid, or merely turgid, he has priapism, which is a urological emergency. If this is secondary to sickle-cell disease (in which it is common), leukaemia, or some neurogenic cause, such as paraplegia, it usually settles with sedation and without impairing subsequent erections. The danger is that if priapism from any cause persists too long, his corpora cavernosa may become ischaemic and fibrotic, so that he becomes permanently impotent. So treat him early.

You can: (1) Sedate him; always try this first. (2) Inject an adrenergic drug. *Don't persist too long with sedation and anaesthetics.* Use an adrenergic drug sooner rather than later. (3) Drain his distended corpora cavernosa by making two small fistulae on each side which allow them to drain into his glans penis.

Winter CC, 'Priapism cured by creating fistulae between the glans penis and the corpora cavernosa'. Journal of Urology 1978;119:227-8.

PRIAPISM

SEDATION. First try heavy sedation with pethidine and chlorpromazine. This will usually cure a patient, especially if his priapism is due to sickle-cell disease.

If he does not respond to heavy sedation in an hour or two, give him a general anaesthetic, or intravenous pethidine and diazepam, and/or try an adrenergic drug.

ADRENERGIC DRUGS. Aspirate his corpora cavernosa with a 1 mm needle; this alone may cure him. If it does not rapidly do so, inject: (1) Metaraminol ('Aramine') 1 mg in 5 ml of saline. Or, (2) a dilute (0.001 mg/ml) solution of adrenalin. Make this by diluting the contents of a 1 mg ampoule to 100 ml in saline. Massage his penis to distribute the drug through both corpora. The venous spaces of his corpora connect, so you only need inject one of them. Repeat the procedure after 10 minutes if detumesence fails to occur.

CAUTION ! (1) Monitor his blood pressure, at 5 minute intervals. Both metaraminol and adrenalin raise it. Deaths from ruptured aneurysms have been reported with metaraminol. (2) Adrenaline is dangerous in a local anaesthetic solution when used subcutaneously as a ring block on the penis or finger (A 5.3), where it may cause gangrene, but not in the corpora cavernosa.

If this is not rapidly effective (unusual), proceed to make a fistula while he is still under general anaesthesia.

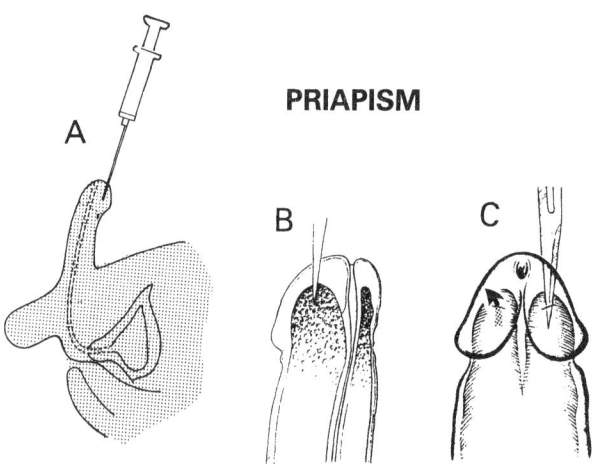

Fig. 23-39 PRIAPISM. If sedation and adrenergic drugs fail (unusual), you will have to resort to surgery. Aim to create fistulae, which will allow a patient's corpora cavernosa to drain into his glans penis. In priapism his turgid corpora cavernosa project up under, and into, his glans penis. A, aspirating his corpora cavernosa through his glans. B, and C, use a sharp knife to make an incision on each side between his glans and his corpora. Alternatively, use a needle and syringe, or a special biopsy needle. *After Rob C and Smith R, 'Operative Surgery: Urology'. p. 584, (Butterworth). With the kind permission of Hugh Dudley.*

MAKE A FISTULA BETWEEN THE CORPORA AND THE GLANS. Under general anaesthesia, aspirate his corpora cavernosa through the tip of his glans penis (A, 23-39). Then, using the same needle, irrigate his corpora cavernosa with saline (preferably with some heparin). This initial aspiration and irrigation can be omitted.

Introduce a 'Travenol' biopsy needle (23.1) in the closed position through the same skin wound, and push it through his glans to the coronal septum (between his glans and his corpora cavernosa), taking care to avoid his urethra. Note that the ends of his erected corpora cavernosa project well into and under his glans. You may need considerable force. Open the biopsy needle by extending its obturator blade through the septum, and close it by pushing the sheath over the fenestrated tip, twist it, and remove it. You should withdraw tissue consisting of fibrous septum, and the contents of his corpus cavernosum. Repeat the manoeuvre in another site close by and then do the same thing with his other corpus cavernosum. By doing this you will create two fistulae on each side

His penis should now become flaccid rapidly, and remain so. Control brisk bleeding from the puncture site by pressure or with a figure of eight absorbable suture. There is no need for a pressure dressing, or an indwelling catheter.

If you don't have a 'Travenol' needle, make 2 or 3 cuts (B and C) each side with a No. 11 blade, or use a large sharp needle.

23.30 Other urological problems

The injuries to a patient's penis and scrotum are discussed in Section 68.8. Here we describe the foreign bodies that can enter his lower urinary tract, and some urological problems.

OTHER UROLOGICAL PROBLEMS

For a periurethral abscess, see Section 5.14.

If a patient says that a FOREIGN BODY body has entered his urethra, try to remove it with as little damage as possible. Give him a general anaesthetic. Ideally, identify it with a cystoscope with a 0° telescope to look down his urethra. Failing this, locate it in his penis by palpation and with X-rays. Try to disimpact its distal end from the wall of his urethra. Use alligator forceps and, perhaps, a large bore cannula. If necessary, do a urethrotomy, and cut down on his urethra through the ventral surface of his penis.

If the foreign body is far back in his urethra, try to dislodge it into his bladder, and if you cannot remove it endoscopically, do so through a small suprapubic cystotomy.

If it is a pin, you will have to remove it head first, so put its point through the wall of his urethra, and turn it round.

If the opposing SURFACES OF HIS GLANS AND PREPUCE ARE ACUTELY INFLAMED, he has acute BALANITIS. Test his urine for sugar to exclude diabetes. The primary treatment of balanitis is better hygiene, and the application of an antiseptic. Show him how to retract his foreskin. Ask him to do this at least 3 times daily, to wash with soap and water and to apply a mild antiseptic, such as chlorhexidine or 'Savlon' (cetrimide and hexachlorophene). Systemic antibiotics should not be needed. If he has associated phimosis, circumcise him or make a dorsal slit when the infection has subsided.

If PAIN AND SWELLING DEVELOP WITH EXPLOSIVE RAPIDITY in his penis or scrotum, and he becomes very ill, suspect that they are about to slough as the result of FOURNIER'S GANGRENE (more appropriately called acute necrotising subcutaneous infection). This is more common in diabetics, and may follow surgery to his scrotum or penis, or extravasation of urine. It resembles cancrum oris, and may follow measles. It is caused by a synergistic combination of organisms, including anaerobes. *Cl. Welchii* is sometimes responsible, and may form gas in his scrotum. It may spread rapidly, eat away much of his scrotum, penis or abdominal wall, and end in Gram-negative septicaemia and death.

Control the infection with gentamicin, or a cephalosporin *and metronidazole*. Apply wet dressings of saline or povidone iodine. Alcoholic iodine is effective, but very painful. The sloughs will probably separate rapidly to expose his testes. Excise all dead tissue as soon as possible, sacrificing some living tissue if necessary. If necessary expose his testes and the shaft of his penis. When the infection has settled, attempt secondary suture (54.6) or split skin grafting as appropriate. You may have to bury his testes in his abdominal wall.

If he passes MILKY URINE, he has CHYLURIA due to a fistula between his lymphatics and his urinary tract. Sometimes he passes chyle and blood (haematochyluria). The endemic form of chyluria is due to *W. bancrofti* (but not *W. malayi*) blocking his lymphatics and promoting fistulae between his lymphatic system and his urinary tract. Where *W. bancrofti* is endemic chyluria is not uncommon, elsewhere it is rare. Chyluria debilitates, through a persistent loss of fat in the urine, but does not kill. Treatment is medical, with diethyl carbamazine 2 mg/kg ('Heterazan') three times a day for 14 days, repeated at intervals. Don't ask him to restrict his diet. He has a 50% chance of remitting spontaneously. No surgical method is effective, or simple enough, to be described here.

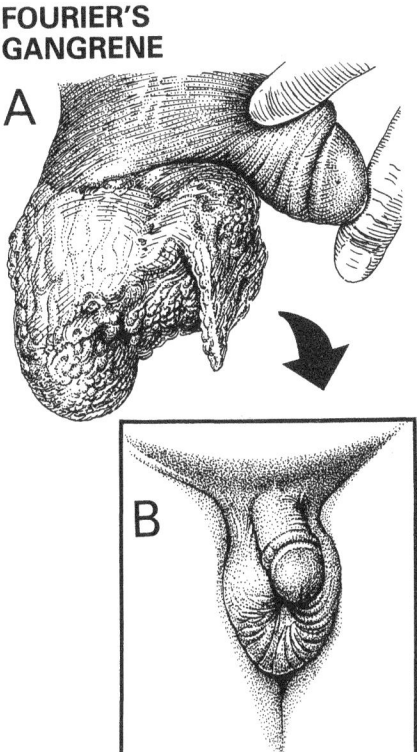

FOURIER'S GANGRENE

Fig. 23-40 FOURNIER'S GANGRENE OF THE SCROTUM. A, as the patient presented. He is usually much worse even than this. B, as he healed without skin grafting. *After Charles Bowesman, 'Surgery and Clinical Pathology in the Tropics'. E and S Livingstone, with kind permission.*

24 The eye

24.1 The general method for the eye

There are 30 million blind people in the world. Half of them are blind from cataracts, and a quarter from trachoma. The other major causes of blindness are glaucoma, vitamin A deficiency, corneal infections, and onchocerciasis. In the industrial world two people in a thousand are blind, but in the developing world blindness is ten times more common—one or two in every hundred. Cataract can be treated, and glaucoma can be arrested; trachoma and vitamin A deficiency can be prevented. It is unfortunate therefore that ophthalmology scares most doctors, who imagine that the eye must be impossibly difficult. This is not true: you can diagnose 90% of eye diseases with a torch and an ophthalmoscope.

Someone in the district must be able to do cataracts and trabeculectomies. Surgery inside the eye is difficult, so learn these operations by apprenticeship from an expert; they are not described here. They can also be done by a medical assistant.

Here is the basic eye equipment—it does not include equipment for operating inside the eye. Look after it with the greatest care.

• CHARTS, visual acuity, (a) Snellen and (b) illiterate E charts, both for use at 6 metres; one chart only of each. These are essential, and can usually be produced locally. They have patterns of 'Es' of different sizes in different positions, and can be used by patients who cannot read.

• TEST TYPE, reading pattern, one set only. Optional. Use this for examining older patients with presbyopia who need glasses. If necessary, you can also use a book or newspaper.

• TORCH, for focal illumination, local pattern, preferably pencil type, with 'lens bulb', one only. A locally available torch is adequate: it can be easily replaced, as can its bulb and batteries.

• LOUPE (magnifying spectacles), binocular, surgical, Bishop Harman headband type, ×2–×8, one only. Some simple form of magnification is useful for examining the front of the eye, for removing superficial foreign bodies, and for other kinds of fine work, such as suturing nerves.

• TONOMETER, Schiötz, one only. You must be able to measure the intraocular pressure (IOP) if you are going to diagnose glaucoma. Digital measurement is simple but unreliable, unless the pressure is very high (>40 mmHg), by which time there may be advanced loss of vision.

• OPHTHALMOSCOPE, simple pattern, Keeler type, battery handle, one only. An ophthalmoscope is very useful, but you can do much good eye work without one.

• SLIT LAMP MICROSCOPE, on stand, simple pattern, as Inami 911SX or equivalent, one only, optional. You will find a slit lamp useful, although you can diagnose uveitis without one. Read the pamphlet with the instrument, and spend some time with an experienced operator.

• NEEDLES, retrobulbar, 7 cm, blunt tip, very fine, one box only. These are the best needles for retrobulbar blocks, but you can use any long thin needle.

• SPECULUM, ophthalmic, lid, solid blades, hinged with screw adjustment, one only. You can only insert a lid speculum after a patient has been anaesthetized with drops of a local anaesthetic.

• SCISSORS, ophthalmic, lid, blunt points, one only. If necessary, you can use any fine scissors.

• FORCEPS (clamp), tarsal cyst (chalazion), 8 mm ring, Lambert pattern, one only. This has two blades, one with a ring and the other with a plate. Use it to hold an eyelid while you incise a tarsal cyst.

• CURETTE, chalazion (tarsal cyst), one only.

SOME EYE ANATOMY
The flow of aqueous

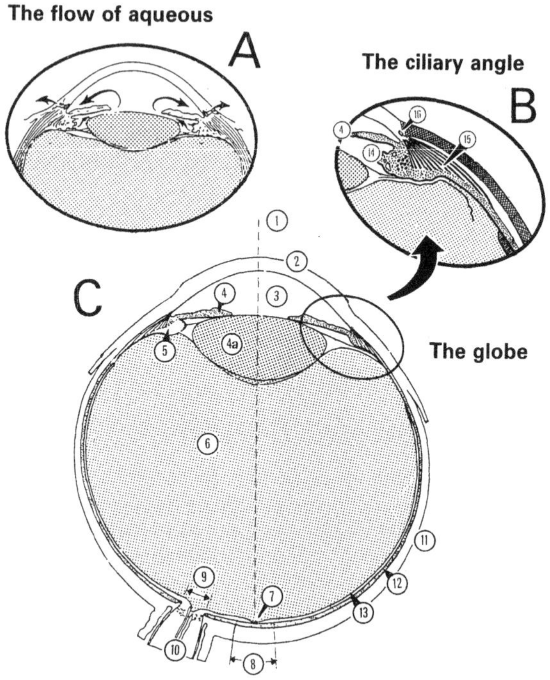

Fig. 24-1 SOME EYE ANATOMY. A, the flow of aqueous from the ciliary body into the posterior chamber, through the pupil into the anterior chamber, then through the trabecular apparatus into the scleral sinus (canal of Schlemm). B, the ciliary angle. C, the globe.

1, the visual axis. 2, the cornea. 3, the anterior chamber. 4, the iris. 4a, the lens. 5, the ciliary body (the section on the left passes through a ciliary process, on the right it passes between them). 6, the vitreous. 7, the fovea. 8, the macula. 9, the optic disc. 10, the optic nerve. 11, the sclera. 12, the choroid. 13, the retina. 14, the ciliary process. 15, the ciliary muscle. 16, the scleral sinus.

• CAUTERY, simple type, ball pattern, two only. Heat this on a spirit lamp.

• CLAMP, eyelid, entropion, Desmarre's or Snellen's, (a) medium and (b) large, one only of each. Use this to hold a patient's eyelid when you operate for entropion.

• SCISSORS, ophthalmic, spring pattern, Westcott's or Castroviejo's, two only. These are particularly delicate instruments which need treating with special care.

• FORCEPS, fine, toothed, St Martin's, two only.

• RETRACTOR, eye, Desmarre's, one only. Use this for examining children.

• NEEDLE HOLDER, ophthalmic, curved with lock, Castroviejo pattern, (a) light, (b) heavy, one only of each type. Use the light pair for suturing a corneal laceration, and the heavier pair for lid surgery.

• TRIAL LENSES, basic set with trial frame, spherical lenses only, cylindrical lenses not required, one outfit only. These are for prescribing glasses to correct refractive errors, and are a luxury unless spectacles are easily available.

• GLASSES, simple frames, second-hand if necessary, spherical lenses +1 to +3.50—the most commonly needed glasses are +2 and +2.50, several hundred assorted. If you can stock glasses you can deal simply and effectively with the reading difficulties of most patients.

• BASIC DRUGS. *Antibiotics*. Topical antibiotic: enriched tetracycline (or chloramphenicol) eye ointment 1%. Subconjunctival antibiotic: Gentamicin injection 40 mg/ml. *Drugs acting on the pupil*. For diagnosis: cyclopentolate 1% or phenylephrine 10%. For treatment: atropine 1% as ointment. Pilocarpine 4% for glaucoma. *Local anaesthetics*. Lignocaine hydrochloride 4% or amethocaine hydrochloride 0.5%. *Steroids*. Hydrocortisone 1% (a weak formulation). *Vitamins*. Vitamin A capsules 200,000 iu. *Diagnostic materials*. Fluorescein papers.

Sandford Smith J, 'Eye Diseases in Hot Climates', John Wright.

Schwab L, 'Primary Eye Care in Developing Nations', Oxford University Press.

Galbraith JEK, 'Basic Eye Surgery, a Manual for Surgeons in Developing Countries'. Churchill Livingstone, 1979.

Parr J. 'Introduction to Ophthalmology', Oxford University Press, (2nd edn 1982).

THE GENERAL METHOD FOR AN EYE

HISTORY

Always take the patient's history carefully, it may be critically important. Occasionally it is misleading. He is likely to have: (1) An acute red painful eye(s), which has occurred spontaneously (24.3), or is the result of trauma (Chapter 60). (2) Gradual or sudden impairment of vision in one or both of his eyes (24.5). (3) Gradual difficulty reading, usually in patients over 40 (presbyopia, 24.8). (4) Other less common but often important eye symptoms, such as squints (24.9), protrusion of the eye (proptosis, 24.11), or difficulty opening his eye (ptosis, 24.15) or closing it (lagophthalmos, 30.3).

If he has pain, try to distinguish: (1) The deep pain caused by an abrupt increase in intraocular pressure. (2) Foreign-body pain from irritation of his conjunctiva. (3) Superficial pain in an eyelid. (4) Photophobia, which is eye pain on exposure to light. (5) Minor discomforts which may result from inadequately corrected refractive errors. (6) Headaches.

EXAMINING AN EYE

The standard examination of an eye is time-consuming to do well, so train a nurse or medical assistant to test a patient's visual acuity and examine his eyes. At first he will refer many patients to you. Later, he will be able to see 90% of the patients himself. Your consulting room must be at least 6 metres long and you should be able to darken it. You *must* have a good light. Most examinations can be done while a patient sits in front of you.

MEASURING HIS VISUAL ACUITY.

ALWAYS test his visual acuity. Explain to him that you want to test his eyes. Begin by testing them separately (with distance glasses if he wears them); test them again each time you see him; and record your results, so that you will know if his vision is deteriorating or not. If he can read, test each eye separately with Snellen's type.

Stand him 6 metres from the well-lit chart, and close his left eye with a piece of paper or your left hand. Ask him to start at the top and tell you whether the "three legs go up, down, right, or left", until he cannot read any more. The top figure is the distance in metres to the test chart, the bottom one is the distance at which a person with normal vision can read that line. The usual sequence of tests getting progressively worse is: 6/6, 6/9, 6/18, 6/60, 3/60. CF 3 m (count fingers at 3 metres) is equivalent to 3/60. If he cannot CF at 1 m, try hand movements (HM), and then test for the perception of light (PL). If you shine a torch into each of the 4 quadrants of his visual field, can he tell you where it is coming from?

Visual acuity can be usefully divided into four groups: (1) Good vision 6/6-6/18; (2) poor vision 6/24-6/60; (3) blind CF 5 m-PL (he can count fingers at 5 metres to perceive light); (4) blind to light NPL (he cannot perceive light). Blindness is 'a loss of vision which results in the patient being unable to con-

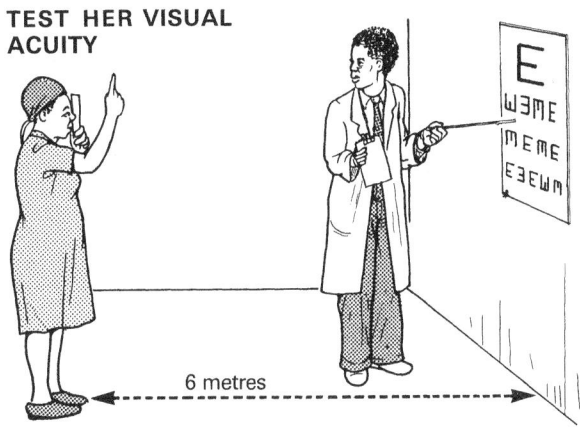

TEST HER VISUAL ACUITY

Fig. 24-2 TEST THE PATIENT'S VISUAL ACUITY before you do anything else. Stand him 6 metres from the test chart and ask him to tell you if the "three legs go up, down, right, or left". *From a TALC slide set.*

tinue with his normal life, and to walk unassisted'. It is usually equivalent to binocular vision of <3/60, which is the same as <CF 3 m. Before you decide that he is completely blind, test him with a very strong light. If an eye cannot see any light, and its pupil does not react to light, it is sure to be beyond help, so there is no point in referring him. If his vision is normal and remains normal and his eye is white, referral is rarely necessary.

EXAMINING THE OUTER EYE WITH A TORCH

Start by looking at his face. Note any abnormalities of his lids, lacrimal apparatus, puncta and canaliculi, his lacrimal glands and sacs, and also any epiphora (tearing). If he is in much pain, and his eyelids are in spasm, one drop of a sterile local anaesthetic will make examination easier.

Do his eyelids open and close normally? You can see this best when he blinks. Check his lids for swellings, and check that his lashes are in their normal position.

Are his conjunctivae white? Note particularly the distribution of any redness. If it is maximal near his corneoscleral junction, it is ciliary hyperaemia (this occurs in iritis and corneal ulcer). If it is maximal at the periphery but often extending all over, it is likely to be conjunctivitis. To examine the conjunctiva of his upper lid, evert it as in H to K, Fig. 24-5.

Look for pus or mucopus in his inferior fornix. This is present in all cases of bacterial conjunctivitis, and in some cases of viral conjunctivitis. Look also for signs of vitamin A deficiency: dry-looking conjunctivae, or Bitot's spots (white patches on the temporal side of his conjunctiva).

Are his corneae bright, shining and clear? Surface irregular? (corneal ulcer). Pannus superiorly? (trachoma, 24.13). Haziness? (oedema from trauma, keratitis, or glaucoma).

Is the surface of his cornea normal? Ulcerated? Instil one drop of 2% fluorescein, or dip the end of a fluorescein impregnated filter paper inside his lower lid for a few seconds. Mop out the excess fluorescein with tissue paper. Shine a light on his eye at an angle. Gaps in the corneal epithelium stain green (foreign bodies, ulcers, abrasions).

Is his anterior chamber normal? Note its depth. Is there any blood (hyphaema, 60-7), or pus (hypopyon, Fig. 24-7) on the bottom of his anterior chamber?

Are his pupils black? Do they react to light? Pupils grey or white? (opacities in the lens, cataract). Note their size and shape. Is their outline irregular? (adhesions of his iris to his lens, called synechiae, due to iritis). A pupil which is large and does not react to light in an eye that cannot see? (most likely optic nerve damage, commonly caused by glaucoma).

SPECIAL EXAMINATION METHODS FOR THE EYE

THE PIN-HOLE TEST is a useful way of screening for refractive errors. If he has poor vision, place a card with a 1 mm hole (punched with a pencil) in front of his eye. If he has an uncorrected refractive error, his vision will be improved. If he has a lesion of his retina or optic nerve, it will be worse.

DIGITAL TONOMETRY to measure the intraocular pressure (IOP). Ask him to look down and keep looking down, but not to actively close his eyes. Put the tips of both your index fingers on one of his globes, so as to feel his sclera through his upper lid above the upper border of his tarsal plate. Gently press with alternate finger tips towards the centre of his globe: (1) Gently fluctuate it from one finger to another. (2) Indent it with one finger and estimate the sense of fluctuation imparted to your stationary finger. (3) Estimate the indentation of his sclera as you relax your indenting finger. You can judge his eye to be 'soft' (<10 mmHg), 'normal (10–35 mmHg), or 'hard' (>35 mmHg). This is a crude test, and he must have a significant rise of pressure (>30 mm Hg) before you can detect it.

SCHIOTZ TONOMETRY Clean the instrument with a pipe cleaner and ether. Using the standard 5.5 gram weight and the metal footpad, make sure the instrument is calibrated to zero. Explain what you are going to do, lie him flat and instil a local anaesthetic into his conjunctiva. Ask him to open both his eyes, and look straight up at a target placed on the ceiling.

With the 5.5 g weight in place, put the tonometer plunger gently on the centre of his cornea with his eye open, and read the scale. If in doubt, repeat the reading 3 times. Use the tables provided with the instrument to calculate his IOP from the scale reading.

The normal IOP is 7 to 25 mm Hg. In practice, using the 5.5 g weight, a scale reading of 2 or less (>28 mmHg) indicates a raised IOP. A reading of 3 or above (<25 mmHg) is 'normal'. If his IOP is >40 mmHg, his cornea is likely to become oedematous (the characteristic 'hazy cornea' of glaucoma), and you can see this with a torch. This is usually a late sign of glaucoma.

OPHTHALMOSCOPY to examine the fundus and media of a patient's eye. You *must*, either, dilate his pupils with a short-acting mydriatic such as cyclopentolate 1%, or examine him in a dark room.

(1) Ask him to keep both eyes open and look straight ahead. (2) Start with the '0' lens in the ophthalmoscope (unless you have a refractive error and are not wearing glasses; if so select the appropriate correcting lens and use this as '0'). (3) Use your right hand for his right eye and your left hand for his left eye. (4) Hold the sight hole of the ophthalmoscope close to your eye, resting it against your nose and orbit, and move it with you as if it was attached to your head. To find this position, look through the sight hole at some distant object. (5) With your thumb on his forehead gently raise his upper lid clear of his pupil. (6) Start with the ophthalmoscope 20 cm from his eye, and shine the light into his pupil; it should glow uniformly red (the red reflex). (7) Move closer and watch for any opacities in his media silhouetted against his red reflex. If you see a shadow, use the + lenses (+5 to +12) to see it more clearly. (8) Ask him to look straight ahead, and move as close as you can to his eye without touching his eyelashes or cornea. (9) Find and look at his optic disc: it is 15° to the nasal side of the optical axis of his eye. (10) Turn the wheel with your forefinger to get the best view of his disc. Examine: (a) The vertical cup/disc ratio (a ratio of >½ suggests glaucoma, 24.6). (b) His disc margins; if these are blurred all round (360°) it suggests papilloedema (refer him). (c) His blood vessels, looking for haemorrhages and exudates suggestive of diabetic retinopathy. (d) His macula, for black and white pigmentation which may suggest choroiditis involving his macula (maculopathy).

SLIT LAMP MICROSCOPY. Position his head by placing his forehead and chin on the rest. Vary the angle of the light as convenient. Examine his eye layer by layer: conjunctiva→cornea→anterior chamber→lens.

Conjunctiva: Foreign body? *Cornea:* Foreign body embedded in his cornea? Ulcer? Note its size and shape after instilling fluorescein and using the blue light. On the back of the cornea look for keratic precipitates (KP, these are clumps of white cells, and indicate uveitis). *Anterior chamber:* look for cells and flare, pus and blood; estimate its depth. *Lens:* Posterior synechiae from his iris? Opacities? *Vitreous:* Particles from a recent posterior uveitis, or bleeding?

SCHIOTZ TONOMETRY

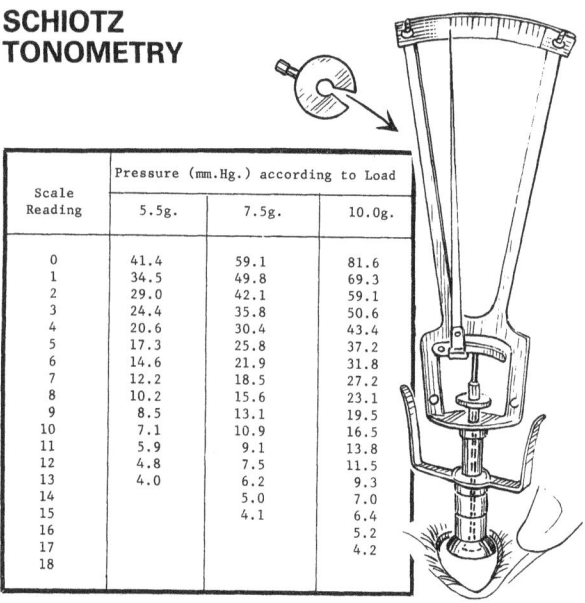

Scale Reading	Pressure (mm.Hg.) according to Load		
	5.5g.	7.5g.	10.0g.
0	41.4	59.1	81.6
1	34.5	49.8	69.3
2	29.0	42.1	59.1
3	24.4	35.8	50.6
4	20.6	30.4	43.4
5	17.3	25.8	37.2
6	14.6	21.9	31.8
7	12.2	18.5	27.2
8	10.2	15.6	23.1
9	8.5	13.1	19.5
10	7.1	10.9	16.5
11	5.9	9.1	13.8
12	4.8	7.5	11.5
13	4.0	6.2	9.3
14		5.0	7.0
15		4.1	6.4
16			5.2
17			4.2
18			

Fig. 24-3. SCHIOTZ TONOMETRY. The scale is merely an example; use the scale which is supplied with your instrument. Three weights are usually supplied with each instrument.

SLIT LAMP MICROSCOPY

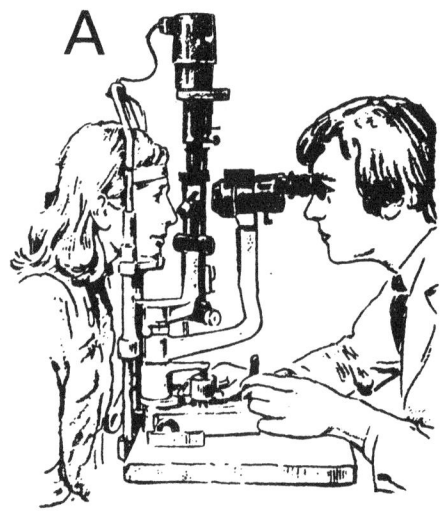

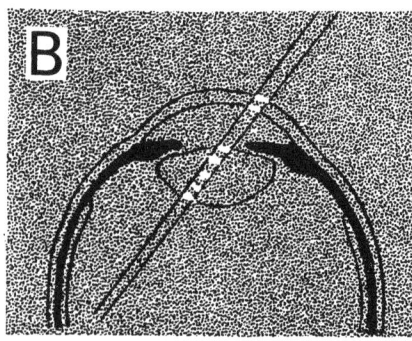

Fig. 24-4 SLIT LAMP MICROSCOPY. A, a narrow pencil of light illuminates the patient's eye from an angle while it is examined with a low-power microscope. B, the layers of his cornea and lens are demonstrated. Particles (not shown) in his aqueous and vitreous reflect light, like dust particles illuminated by a sunbeam in a darkened room.
After Parr, John, 'Introduction to Ophthalmology', (2nd edn 1982). OUP, with kind permission.

MOVEMENTS. Test the movements of both his eyes together, and then test each eye separately, in all directions, including convergence. Note any squint (24.9).

DIAGNOSIS. You have now examined his eyes and should be able to make a provisional diagnosis.

BASIC METHODS FOR THE EYE

BASIC DRUGS. Here is a list:

Antibiotics: Tetracycline or chloramphenicol eye ointment, and eye drops. Ask your pharmacy to make up eye drops in used injection bottles and autoclave them. A little gentamicin for subconjunctival injections will go a long way. Don't use penicillin locally on the eye, either as drops or as subconjunctival injections; it does not keep well and may cause hypersensitivity, especially in light-skinned people. You can get high concentrations of an antibiotic inside his eye by: (1) Injecting it subconjunctivally (see below). (2) Applying it frequently (not less than 4-hourly) as drops into his conjunctiva. If an eye infection is severe, give him systemic antibiotics also. Systemic chloramphenicol will enter his eye.

Drugs acting on the pupil: You will need mydriatics to dilate it. Atropine 1% as ointment or drops will dilate his pupil for a week, so only use this for treating iridocyclitis. Cyclopentolate 1%, or phenylephrine 10%, will dilate it for some hours only, so use these when you want to examine him with an ophthalmoscope.

Steroids may be indicated in iridocyclitis. They quieten the inflammation, reduce photophobia and lachrymation, and make the eye white. Use hydrocortisone or prednisolone as a 1% suspension. The frequency of administration depends on the degree of inflammation; you may have to administer them every 3 hours night and day.

CAUTION ! (1) Steroids can cause viral and fungal corneal ulceration, glaucoma, and cataracts. They are dangerous in the hands of the nonexpert, so prescribe them with the greatest care. (2) Don't use any steroid unless you are certain about the diagnosis, and then use the weakest commonly available one, which is hydrocortisone 1%. (3) Avoid more powerful steroids, such as dexamethasone, because they are more likely to induce glaucoma in a susceptible eye. See also Section 24.5.

Local anaesthetics: Lignocaine hydrochloride 4% or amethocaine hydrochloride 1% (A 5.8).

CAUTION ! The great danger of an anaesthetized eye is that a foreign body may get into it, of which he is unaware, or that he may abrade it, so shield it.

Diagnostic materials: Fluorescein papers are better than fluorescein drops, because you can more easily keep them sterile.

Placebo: If he wants something for his eyes and you need a placebo, give him saline eye drops 0.5%.

EYE DROPS. Pull his lower lid down so that you can see his conjunctiva. Ask him to look up. Put drops or ointment into the outer third of his conjunctiva. Close his eye *for two minutes* to allow the drug to enter his eye. Don't let the dropper touch his eye, or it may become contaminated. If possible, each patient should have his own drops, because of the danger of cross-infection.

TO MAKE CHLORAMPHENICOL EYE DROPS dissolve two 250 mg capsules in 100 ml of water. Filter the solution into sterile 10 ml dropper bottles. Screw the caps on loosely, and sterilize them in a hot water bath at 100°C for 30 minutes, without letting the water splash over the necks of the bottles. Refrigerate them; their shelf-life is 2 months at 2-8°C. The shelf-life of commercial drops is only 4 months, so this is a useful method.

SUBCONJUNCTIVAL ANTIBIOTICS are indicated if he has a severe corneal infection or ulceration, especially with hypopyon. You can inject a volume of 0.5 ml (max 1.0 ml) under his conjunctiva. If this contains 0.2 ml of a local anaesthetic, such as 2% lignocaine, the injection will be almost painless. Use a sharp 0.4 mm needle on a 2 ml syringe, as in E, Fig. 24-5.

CAUTION ! Be careful which antibiotics you mix in the same syringe. Don't mix crystalline penicillin and lignocaine. Gentamicin alone is not too painful.

Anaesthetize his eye with a few drops of local anaesthetic solution. Ask him to look up. Pull down his lower lid, with your finger on his cheek. Rest the needle flat on the conjunctival surface of his globe, with the bevel facing away from it. Push the needle under his conjunctiva, parallel to the surface of his globe, rotating it gently as you do so. If it is in the right layer, you will see its point under his conjunctiva. Then inject.

Inject gentamicin 40 mg (the standard antibiotic for this purpose), or chloramphenicol 100 mg, or soframycin 50 mg, or methicillin 100 mg, or ampicillin 100 mg. Make these up in a volume of 1 ml. Don't use penicillin, because of the danger of hypersensitivity. Systemic chloramphenicol enters the eye; so if his eye is severely infected, give him 500 mg 4 times a day for 10 days.

If his infection is getting worse, repeat the injection, daily, for 2 or 3 days (3 is the maximum) until you are quite sure that there is going to be no endophthalmitis. A severely infected eye is likely to improve, or be lost, in a few hours, so subconjunctival injection is usually only done once, or occasionally twice, on successive days.

WARM SOAKS are an old method, but are an effective one for soothing a painful eye. Ask him to wrap a cloth round a spoon, to dip this into very hot water, and to hold it as close to his eye as he can bear. Soaks are useful for a stye (infected eyelash follicle).

PAD HIS EYE if he has had a minor injury with no suspicion of perforation (60.4). An eye pad, with gentle firm pressure, will reduce his discomfort, and promote healing by preventing his lids moving over the injured area.

Shut his eye, put a pad of gauze over it; place two pieces of adhesive strapping diagonally across the pad, from his forehead to his cheek, to hold the pad in place. Change the pad daily, and look for signs of ulceration or infection.

CAUTION ! The great danger of an eye pad is that it may rub against an anaesthetized eye, and cause an abrasion. So his eye must be shut when you apply the pad. A layer of vaseline gauze on the pad will help to ensure this. Opinions vary as to

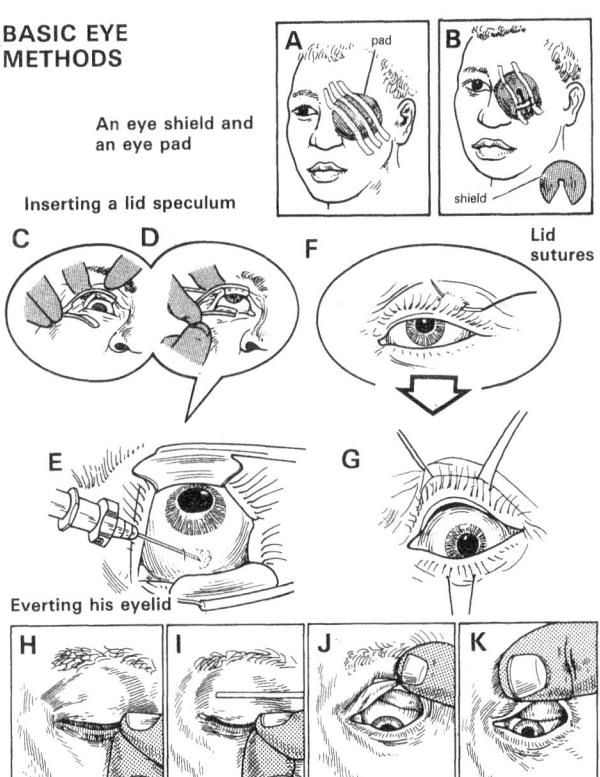

Fig. 24-5 SOME BASIC EYE METHODS. A, an eye pad. B, an eye shield. C, inserting the upper blade of a lid speculum while the patient is looking down. D, inserting the lower blade while he is looking up. E, subconjunctival injection is an effective way of getting a high concentration of an antibiotic inside his eye. F, inserting the first lid suture. G, lid sutures in place; two for the upper lid and one for the lower lid. H, to K, steps in everting the upper lid.

whether you should ever pad an anaesthetized eye. If you do pad it, there is a risk of the pad pressing against the eye. If you don't pad it, dust may get into it of which he is unaware!

SHIELD HIS EYE: (1) After any severe injury, especially if there is a perforation. (2) After any operation. Shielding it allows it to open and close, without anything extraneous touching his cornea, and perhaps scratching it. A shield is the safest way to protect an anaesthetized eye, and is very helpful for a painful inflamed eye with photophobia.

Put a piece of sterile gauze across his orbit without touching his eye. Hold this in place with a strip of adhesive strapping diagonally across his orbit. Cut an 8 cm diameter circle from cardboard, or an old X-ray film. Cut a radius in this, fold it into a cone, and maintain the cone with a piece of strapping. Hold the cone in place with two pieces of adhesive strapping, or plastic tape from his forehead to his cheek.

CAUTION ! Never occlude the eye of a child under 7 years for several days, because this may cause amblyopia (24.9).

24.2 Operating on an eye

Unless you have received special training, limit your surgery to operations on a patient's lids: entropion (24.13), tarsal cysts (chalazion, 24.12), tarsorrhaphy (30.3), and evisceration, enucleation, and perhaps exenteration of his eye (24.14).

Trauma is described in Chapter 60. Although Section 60.4 describes the repair of a perforating injury, this needs good magnification, 8/0 or 9/0 sutures, and skill. So you would probably be wise to treat him non-operatively, and to give him subconjunctival gentamicin and atropine eye ointment.

EYE OPERATIONS

EQUIPMENT. Don't operate with the large instruments of a basic set. Use the fine eye ones in Section 24.1. For operations on a patient's globe, an operating loupe and a bright focal beam are almost essential, preferably a 12 volt spotlight from a battery, or a transformer from the mains. A spirit lamp.

5/0 and 8/0 polyglycolic acid, silk, or monofilament sutures, all on 7.5 mm curved atraumatic needles. Monofilament sutures are better than silk on the cornea. 8/0 sutures are the finest ones that you can use without a microscope. Use virgin silk or nylon for the cornea, and catgut or polyglycolic acid for the conjunctiva. Nylon irritates if it is exposed.

PREPARATION. Prepare his face from his hairline to his chin and from ear to ear, using povidine-iodine 10%, or a non-alcoholic lotion which will not harm his eyes, if it enters them accidentally. Other surgeons use iodine and spirit, and take care to keep them out of his eyes.

Make a special drape with a slit from the middle of one end to the centre. Place this under his chin, and up each side of his face. Fold it over his head and keep it there with a towel clip. Place another drape across his forehead over his eyebrows, and clip this to the first one. If he is intubated, place a third drape over his nose and the catheter mount. If he is having a local anaesthetic, don't cover his nose or mouth.

ANAESTHESIA. You can usually use local (A 6.5) or general anaesthesia (A 16.9). Use general anaesthesia for a perforation (if local anaesthesia is complicated by retrobulbar haemorrhage, it may aggravate loss of eye contents).

POSITION the table so that you can sit comfortably, with your knees under it. If necessary, put his head at the foot end, or rest it on a plank, or sheet of wood, pushed under the mattress, and projecting beyond the table.

Sit your assistant on your right for a right eye, and on your left for a left eye. Keep your own eyes on the wound; ask him to place the instruments in your outstretched hand, and to hold them by their proximal ends, without touchng their tips.

You can use a speculum, or lid sutures, to hold an eye open while you operate on it.

TO INSERT A SPECULUM, on a conscious patient instil two drops of local anaesthetic. Ask him to look down, grasp his top lid with your finger, and slip the top blade of the speculum under it. Then ask him to look up, grasp his bottom lid, and slip the lower blade of the speculum under that. Adjust the arm of the speculum until his eye is exposed, and then tighten the locking nut.

LID SUTURES are not for suturing wounds, but to hold the lids away from an eye while you operate on it. They avoid the risk of a speculum, which may press on his eye, and perhaps scratch his cornea.

In his upper lid insert two 3/0 silk or monofilament sutures, just above his lash line and down to his tarsal plate. In his lower lid insert one suture just below his lash line. Don't penetrate the conjunctiva of either lid. Hold these sutures with haemostats.

BLEEDING. The cornea is avascular and cannot bleed. If his conjunctiva or sclera bleed, apply a pad and very gentle pressure. Or flood the wound with saline from a syringe and an irrigating needle, or an undine attached to a tube and silver cannula. The blood will stream in the clear saline, so that you can see the exact point where it is coming from, and control it with a cautery. Heat a squint hook or a small cautery in the flame of a spirit lamp, until it is hot, but not red hot. Touch the bleeding point with this, through the stream of saline. This will cool its tip enough to prevent burning, but will leave it hot enough to seal the bleeding vessel. Don't use diathermy.

EXAMINING A BABY'S EYES

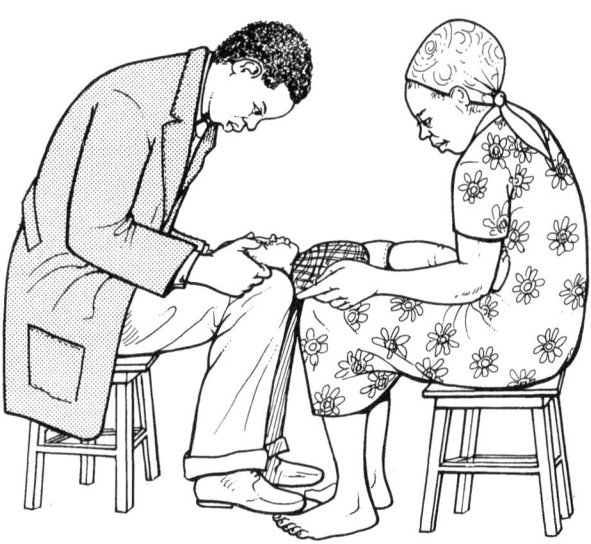

Fig. 24-6 EXAMINING A BABY'S EYES. Sit him on his mother's lap and hold his head between your knees.

24.3 The red painful eye

Acute red painful eyes are due to: (1) conjunctivitis (much the most common cause at any age). There are two particularly important forms of conjunctivitis in different age groups. (1a) Ophthalmia neonatorum in newborn babies. (1b) The conjunctivitis associated with recent measles in children between the ages of 6 months and 6 years. There are also some important, but less common causes of an acute red eye: (2) A corneal ulcer. (3) Acute iritis. (4) Acute glaucoma. (5) Trauma is another cause, but the diagnosis is usually obvious from the history (Chapter 60).

The problem in a busy clinic is that conjunctivitis is so much more common than the rarer causes of a red eye, that these are easily missed. So your *first task* in managing red eyes is to make sure that these rarer causes are recognized. Twenty patients may have conjunctivitis, and the twenty-first a corneal ulcer, or acute glaucoma. A patient's history, his visual acuity, and the examination of his eye with a torch should enable you to decide which he has.

Conjunctivitis can be bacterial, viral, allergic, or chemical. Bacterial conjunctivitis is common in the developing world, and may be mild, or so severe that a patient's conjunctiva pours out pus, and his lids swell so much that he cannot open his eyes. Neglected bacterial conjunctivitis may be followed by a corneal ulcer and a corneal scar, or by perforation and endophthalmitis. Bacterial conjunctivitis needs an antibiotic. Viral conjunctivitis usually resolves spontaneously without one, if the cornea is not involved.

Besides infecting a patient's conjunctiva, bacteria can infect his lids (blepharitis), or his cornea, where they can cause: (1) Changes in the stroma (keratitis and sometimes a corneal abscess). (2) A corneal ulcer, which is a loss of surface epithelium. The danger of a corneal ulcer is that infection may spread inside his eye as an endophthalmitis, which may blind him.

A corneal ulcer may be due to: (1) Bacteria. (2) Herpes simplex virus. (3) Fungi. (4) Other conditions such as leprosy, causing lagophthalmos and exposing his cornea (30.3). Bacterial corneal ulceration can follow even a minor injury which damages the epithelium, or it can be spontaneous. Corneal ulcers are most easily seen when they are stained with fluorescein, which is why this is so useful.

When bacteria enter an eye through a corneal ulcer the first place they get to is the anterior chamber. If pus gathers here, and the patient stands upright, it falls to the bottom, with a straight upper fluid level called a hypopyon, as shown in C, Fig. 24-7.

Endophthalmitis may be the result of: (1) A corneal ulcer, especially a bacterial one. (2) A perforating injury of his cornea or sclera, especially if a foreign body has been left inside his eye (60.9), or if a wound is neglected (60.4). Once bacteria have entered his eye, the chance of total blindness is high. If you see him early, when the infection is fairly localized, he may retain some useful vision; but if you see him late, the best you can do is to control infection, because his eye will be blind. If you cannot control it, you will have to eviscerate his eye (24.14).

RED PAINFUL EYES AND OTHER EYE INFECTIONS

For the general method see Section 24.1. Acute iritis (24.5) and acute glaucoma (24.6) are described here as part of the differential diagnosis of a red eye, but are dealt with more fully later. Make sure you examine the patient in a good light.

THE DIAGNOSIS. If he has conjunctivitis, his discomfort or pain varies from mild to severe: (1) Both his eyes are usually involved. (2) His visual acuity is normally good. (3) He usually has a purulent discharge. (4) His conjunctivae are red, especially in his fornices. (4) His cornea is clear and does not stain with fluorescein (unless his conjunctivitis has caused a corneal ulcer). (5) His pupils are normal. (6) The tension in his globe is normal.

THE DIFFERENTIAL DIAGNOSIS OF CONJUNCTIVITIS. Distinguish particularly between the redness of conjunctivitis, which is typically maximal at the periphery, but is often uniform everywhere (very common), and redness which is most marked at his corneoscleral junction (ciliary injection, less common).

CAUTION ! Look for mucopus in his inferior fornix—it is always present in bacterial conjunctivitis; hesitate to diagnose conjunctivitis if you don't find any.

Conjunctivitis is usually bilateral: its important differential diagnoses are usually unilateral:

Suggesting acute iritis—one (sometimes two) moderately painful red eye(s) with no discharge. His pain is often only mild, and he may complain of headache. Reduction in visual acuity, which may be only mild. Ciliary hyperaemia. A clear cornea. A small constricted pupil, which becomes irregular when you dilate it, due to posterior synechiae (adhesions). Look for an inflammatory exudate in his anterior chamber, preferably with a slit lamp: his aqueous is not as clear as it should be. The beam from the lamp shows a flare, like a beam of light shining across a dusty room. You may also see little lumps of cells (keratic precipitates or KP) sticking to the back of his cornea, and posterior synechiae between his iris and the front of his lens. The inflammatory cells in his anterior chamber may form a sterile hypopyon. His IOP (intraocular pressure) may be increased due to secondary glaucoma (24.6).

Suggesting acute angle closure glaucoma—one (seldom two) very painful red eye(s) with severe unilateral headache, and slight watering. Severely impaired visual acuity, often down to hand movements or perception of light only, with haloes, and sometimes even blindness. Ciliary hyperaemia (mild in the early stages). A hazy cornea (due to raised IOP) without its normal lustre. A shallow anterior chamber; this is best seen by shining a torch from the side. A vertically oval *dilated* pupil which does not react to light. A raised IOP (24.1).

Suggesting a corneal ulcer—one severely painful red eye with reduced visual acuity (if the ulcer is central), redness most marked round the limbus, photophobia, swollen eyelids, and watering. Look for a grey-white spot (the ulcer) on his cornea, which stains with fluorescein. If it is not obvious, look for a defect in the smooth surface of his cornea in the reflection from a focused light. If his ulcer is central, hyperaemia is equal all round his limbus. If it is near the edge, hyperaemia is more marked there. If his infection is severe, pus cells sediment at the bottom of his anterior chamber, with a fluid level (hypopyon). His pupil is usually regular. For treatment see below.

Suggesting a foreign body. The signs of an abrasion (60.4), and a foreign body (60.9), are similar to those of a corneal ulcer—unilateral pain, photophobia, a watery discharge, sometimes impaired vision, and ciliary hyperaemia, which may be localized to the region near the lesion. See also Section 60.4.

ACUTE INFECTIVE CONJUNCTIVITIS

TREATMENT. Clean his eyes with a cotton swab and saline. Instil chloramphenicol eye drops or ointment hourly in severe infections, and 3 hourly in less severe ones. Or use tetracycline ointment, with or without polymyxin and bacitracin. An eye ointment at night will prevent his lids sticking together. Continue treatment for two days after symptoms have resolved. Allow the exudate to escape, clean his eyes with a clean cloth and water, and don't pad them.

CAUTION! If his conjunctivitis is severe, watch carefully for a corneal ulcer, and if necessary examine his cornea with fluorescein.

If his corneae are not clear and his visual acuity is poor, he has a corneal ulcer (see below) and his sight is in danger.

CORNEAL ULCER

TREATMENT is an *emergency*. Start aggressive treatment with antibiotics urgently. Admit him. He may be more comfortable with a pad or shield (24.1).

If his ulcer is severe, and particularly if he has hypopyon, give him a subconjunctival injection (24.1) of gentamicin 40 mg, or chloramphenicol 100 mg. Also, apply chloramphenicol drops, or tetracycline eye ointment *hourly*. Also give him systemic chloramphenicol (24.1, 2.9).

If his ulcer is not so severe, and he has no hypopyon, *hourly* conjunctival antibiotics and atropine ointment 3 times daily may be adequate.

Also, with any corneal ulcer, provided it has not already perforated, give him atropine eye ointment 2 or 3 times a day to keep his pupil dilated. This will prevent adhesions forming between his iris and his lens (posterior synechiae). Advise warm soaks (24.1). If there is any suspicion that he may be short of vitamin A, give it (see below). Complications include: (1) Diffuse scarring of his cornea (24.4). (2) A dense white scar (leucoma, 24.4). (3) Perforation of his cornea, with adherence of his iris, and perhaps staphyloma (an opaque protrusion of his cornea). (4) Endophthalmitis.

If his corneal ulcer is very severe, so that his whole anterior chamber fills with pus, he has endopthalmitis.

If his corneal ulcer has proceeded to the point where it has weakened, softened, and distorted his globe (pthisis bulbi) you will have to eviscerate it (24.14).

ENDOPHTHALMITIS (panophthalmitis)

His anterior chamber is full of pus. Subconjunctival and parenteral antibiotics (24.1) are essential, but it usually too late

THE IRIS AND THE CORNEA

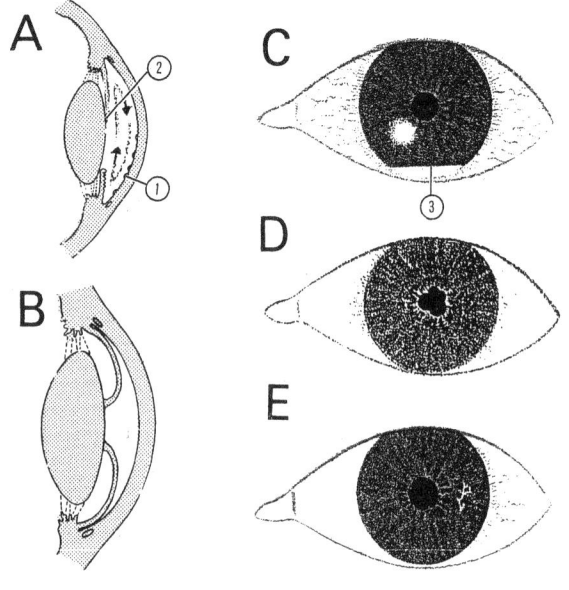

Fig. 24-7 THE IRIS AND THE CORNEA. A, a vertical section of the eye to show the flow pattern of the aqueous. B, iris bombé—the iris is adherent to the lens all round and is bulging forwards. C, an acute bacterial corneal ulcer with a hypopyon. D, acute iridocyclitis. The pupil is small and irregular, because posterior synechiae have formed. E, a dendritic ulcer of the cornea, the result of herpes simplex infection.

1, some KP on the back of the cornea. 2, a posterior synechia (adhesion between the lens and the cornea). 3, a hypopyon. *After Parr, John, 'Introduction to Ophthalmology', (2nd edn 1982). OUP. with kind permission.*

for them to be successful, because the inside of his eye has become an abscess.

If his endophthalmitis is early, with some hope of vision, refer him *urgently* if you can. If not, try to control infection and minimize pain. Give him subconjunctival and parenteral chloramphenicol for 5 to 7 days. His infection may settle.

If his endophthalmitis is due to a foreign body in his eye, remove it. It is usually superficial, so that you can remove it through the wound by which it entered, which is usually in his cornea, even if this has to be enlarged (60.9). Remove any prolapsing iris, and suture his cornea (60-6). Continue subconjunctival and parenteral antibiotics. Remove the sutures at 7 days.

If he presents late, with no hope of vision and an anterior chamber full of pus, and shows no improvement in 48 hours, eviscerate his eye (24.14). The chances of sympathetic ophthalmia are negligible, so this is not a determining factor in deciding to remove it (60.10).

DIFFICULTIES WITH RED PAINFUL EYES

If a NEONATE has RED SWOLLEN CONJUNCTIVAE with a PURULENT DISCHARGE, a few days after birth, he has OPHTHALMIA NEONATORUM, which may be gonococcal or chlamydial. His cornea is usually clear, but may have an ulcer. This is an acute emergency, which may blind him. Clean away the pus with a swab and water, put tetracycline ointment into his eyes *every hour*. Give him penicillin, for example crystalline penicillin 30 mg/kg/day in 4 divided doses intramuscularly. Or, less satisfactorily, give him procaine penicillin forte 0.5 ml (30 mg) daily. Continue penicillin for 5 days.

If his conjunctivitis is very severe, and especially if he has a corneal ulcer, **instil chloramphenicol eye drops every minute for one hour, every hour for one day, and then 3-hourly until he is better,** and give him penicillin as above.

If he has an ACUTE RED EYE BETWEEN THE AGES OF 6 MONTHS AND 6 YEARS, the important condition is the combination of malnutrition, vitamin A deficiency, and recent measles. Look for: (1) Night blindness (inability to see in dim light). (2) Bitot's spots (white foamy spots on his lateral conjunctiva). (3) Xerosis (dryness of his conjunctiva with inability to produce tears, or a dry hazy cornea). (4) Keratomalacia (corneal ulceration, softening of his cornea). Give any child with any of these signs vitamin A 200,000 iu by mouth immediately, again after 24 hours, and again after 1 week. Also, give him a topical antibiotic such as tetracycline 1% 3 times daily. If his cornea is ulcerated, give him atropine eye ointment 1% once daily, and an eye pad. Improve his nutrition, and encourage his mother to give him plenty of dark green leafy vegetables.

If he has a CHRONIC LOW-GRADE CONJUNCTIVITIS with yellow-grey dots (follicles) under his upper eyelid, and he comes from an endemic area, he almost certainly has TRACHOMA caused by *Chlamydia trachomatis*. This goes through three stages described in Section 24.13; the important one to recognize is the second. During the acute stage, make sure he puts tetracycline eye ointment 1% or 3% into his eyes twice a day for six weeks. If his trachoma is severe, also give him a 14-day course of a sulphonamide or tetracycline.

Teach him to wash his face and hands well several times daily, and to avoid rubbing his eyes. Explain that his disease is due to the entry of dirt, often from flies. *Apply tetracycline eye ointment to any case of acute red eyes, particularly when these occur as epidemics of conjunctivitis.*

If LARGE GELATINOUS VEGETATIONS have formed on his upper tarsal conjunctiva, and look like cobblestones, or on the bulbar conjunctiva surrounding his limbus, suspect ALLERGIC CONJUNCTIVITIS. This is common in children and young adults. Their eyes are very itchy and water much. Suppress the inflammation with antihistamine drops or a very weak steroid. Beware of steroid glaucoma (24.5, 24.6D), because steroids, once started, may be needed for many years.

If he complains of PAIN AND WATERING WITHOUT ANY HISTORY OF A FOREIGN BODY, consider the possibility of a DENDRITIC ULCER. Stain his cornea with fluorescein and look for a branching irregular ulcer, which may also resemble the outline of an amoeba, or a country on a map. This is due to infection with the herpes simplex virus. He may think (wrongly) that "something has got into his eye". Dendritic ulcers occur all over the world, especially after fevers, particularly measles, malaria, and meningitis. In the industrial world they are now the most common and most damaging form of corneal ulcer; they commonly recur, and treatment is difficult. Refer him.

If you cannot refer him, if possible give him an antiviral agent: idoxuridine ointment (×5 daily), trifluorothymidine drops (hourly), or acylovir ointment (×5 daily). If his lesion is severe, combine this with mechanical removal of the epithelium containing the virus. Apply a topical anaesthetic, and stain his cornea with fluorescein. Using a loupe, a good light, and a ball of cotton wool on the end of an applicator, *gently* scrub the surface of his cornea in the region of the ulcer to remove its epithelium. A chronic stromal keratitis with corneal scarring and blindness can complicate herpetic eye diease.

CAUTION ! Never apply steroids, because these may spread the infection to the stroma of his cornea, and make his condition worse.

If a CHEMICAL has got into his eye, his conjunctiva is intensely red (more so than in infective conjunctivitis), his cornea may be opaque (from keratitis or an ulcer), and his vision impaired. Unlike infective conjunctivitis, mucopus is absent. He may admit to having used traditional medicine for a painful eye, which has made it worse. If the chemical is still present, wash it out with much water. Give him an analgesic, and shield his eye. Instil an antibiotic ointment; its vaselene base will be soothing, and the antibiotic may prevent secondary infection.

If he has an acutely inflamed and oedematous lid or face, with a BLACK SLOUGH, and surrounding brawny oedema, and hides are used in the district, consider the possibility of ANTHRAX. His eyelid may be completely destroyed, but his eye is normal. Give him high doses of penicillin and sulphonamides. Anthrax responds rapidly to penicillin. Later, if necessary, toilet the slough and graft the raw area. If you leave raw lids ungrafted, severe scarring and a scar-induced ectropion may follow.

24.4 Loss of vision in a white eye

This is one of the common presentations of eye disease. Loss of vision in a white eye can be slow or fast. If a patient loses his vision slowly over months or years, he may have: (1) A corneal scar. (2) Cataracts. (3) Glaucoma. (4) A refractive error. Or, (5) disease of his retina due to: (a) Senile macular degeneration. (b) Retinitis pigmentosa. (c) Chloroquine maculopathy. (d) Old macular scars. Or, (6) optic atrophy. If he loses his vision suddenly over minutes or days, the cause is usually inflammatory or vascular (see below). If he complains that he cannot read, he usually has has presbyopia (24.8).

Corneal scars cause 70% of blindness in children and 25% in adults in the developing world. A corneal scar can be: (1) Diffuse. (2) A circumscribed white patch (leucoma). (3) A staphyloma, which is a bulging of the cornea forwards between the lids, due to the thinning, caused by previous ulceration. (4) Pthisis bulbi, which is disorganization of his entire eye, leaving it small and shrunken. Bilateral scarring follows ophthalmia neonatorum, vitamin A deficiency, traditional eye medicine, and trachoma. Unilateral scars are more likely to be caused by corneal ulceration due to bacteria, the herpes simplex virus, fungi, or trauma.

Cataracts cause about one half the blindness in the developing world, where they blind about one person in 200. 85% of cataracts are 'senile', and the rest are either congenital or familial, or due to trauma, iritis, or diabetes. A patient with a cataract presents with gradual loss of vision, in one or both his eyes. His corneae are clear, and there is an opacity in his pupil(s). A cataract can be immature (making his pupil grey), or mature, or hypermature (making it white). Sometimes a cataract swells, pushes the iris forwards, occludes the angle of his eye, and causes secondary glaucoma.

Removing cataracts is a standardized and repetitive task; it is also a skilled one and is never urgent, so it is not described here. If you want to remove them, apprentice yourself to an expert for several months, and try to remove at least 50 under supervision. Or, send an assistant to learn this skill. Cataracts can also be removed on a mass scale, particularly in Asia, in special 'eye camps'.

In good hands the chance of success is over 90%. If a patient is operated on for the right indications, even moderate success in one eye only will enable him to be independent again. He is usually happy if he can see well enough to find his way about his home area. You will have to weigh up the benefits, and the risks, because vision without a lens is not normal vision.

There are two methods: (1) Removing the whole of his lens, within the capsule of the cataract (intracapsular extraction), which is the preferred method in the developing world. (2) Opening the anterior capsule, removing the cortex and lens, and leaving the posterior capsule (extracapsular extraction). This is safer in younger people (<30 years).

LOSS OF VISION IN A WHITE EYE

One or both eyes? Gradual or sudden? Family history? Any external factors such as trauma?

COMMON CAUSES OF GRADUAL LOSS OF VISION

This is the patient who cannot see normally, and whose eyes are not reddened by conjunctivitis or ciliary injection. Examine him as in Section 24.1.

CORNEAL SCARS

If the cause of the scar is still present, and it is getting worse, arrest it. Causes include scratching of the cornea by the inturned eyelashes of trachoma (trichiasis, 24.13; vitamin A deficiency causes an acute ulcer in young children, and does not cause progressive scarring). When you are sure that you have done all you can to prevent his scar progressing, manage him like this:

If he still has adequate vision in his other eye, he will not be severely disabled, and no treatment is indicated.

If he cannot see light at all, explain that nothing can be done.

If he is blind, and has a central leucoma which obscures his pupil, with an area of clear peripheral cornea, refer him for a optical iridectomy. This will give him an artificial pupil peripherally, behind his area of clear cornea, and should give him enough vision to make him mobile. It is contraindicated if he already has enough vision for mobility, or if he has no clear peripheral cornea.

If he is blind due to diffuse corneal scarring which has not made his eye perforate, consider referring him for corneal grafting. This is difficult and is usually impractical, because grafts and experts are scarce. Preferably, his cornea should have few vessels in it or none.

If his eye is blind and painful, consider eviscerating or enucleating it (24.14).

If he has any other kind of corneal scar, for example a unilateral corneal scar or pthisis bulbi, there is no point in referring him.

CATARACTS

(1) Measure his visual acuity accurately in both eyes. His pupils should react briskly to light. If they don't, suspect that he also has some other condition, such as optic nerve disease. (2) Measure his IOP to make sure his loss of vision is not due to glaucoma (24.6). (3) Dilate his pupil and examine his red reflex with an ophthalmoscope to assess how dense his cataract is, especially if it is immature. If you can easily see his optic discs, his cataract is not yet dense enough to be worth extracting.

INDICATIONS FOR EXTRACTION. (1) To improve his sight. (2) To treat complications, especially secondary glaucoma.

If he has bilateral cataracts, operate when his acuity in both eyes has fallen to <6/60 (CF at 6 m).

If he has a unilateral cataract, surgery is only indicated to treat or prevent secondary glaucoma, or uveitis. It will not improve his sight.

If he has already lost the sight in his other eye for any reason, and he now has a cataract in his remaining eye (cataract in an only eye), delay surgery until he has difficulty getting around by himself and is nearly blind (<CF 3 m), because any complication will make him totally blind.

If he has already had one cataract removed and is happy with his aphakic spectacles, his second cataract can be operated on at any time. But, because he can now see, he will be a low priority.

If his cataract is not ready for extraction, or if extraction is impossible, atropine ointment weekly, or minus (concave) glasses may improve his sight.

CONTRAINDICATIONS. (1) Unilateral cataracts with adequate sight in the other eye. (2) Bilateral small immature cataracts with acuity >6/60 in both eyes together—review his progress in 3-6 months.

If a cataract extraction is indicated, refer him.

POSTOPERATIVELY, if you have to care for him after he has been operated on by someone else, watch for a leaking wound (with or without iris prolapse), infection, bleeding, and a raised IOP. Gently open his lids, and examine his eye with a torch. If there is any iris prolapse, he must go back to the theatre, and have the iris excised and the wound resutured.

If his cornea is hazy with a striate pattern (striate keratitis), it will probably settle.

If his anterior chamber is shallow, the wound may be leaking. A firm double pad and bandage applied to his eye for 24-48 hours may stop the leak.

If there is blood in his anterior chamber (hyphaema), pad his eye and keep him in bed.

If there is pus in his anterior chamber (hypopyon), it may indicate postoperative infection (endophthalmitis). His eye is likely to be painful and his visual acuity very low. Give him subconjunctival gentamicin (24.1), topical antibiotics hourly and chloramphenicol by mouth.

If his red reflex is absent, there is some opacity in his media.

If he complains of much pain and his cornea is hazy, his IOP is probably raised (aphakic glaucoma); measure it. (1) His vitreous jelly may be blocking his pupil. Immediately dilate his pupil with cyclopentolate and phenylephrine drops, followed by atropine ointment for several weeks.

If his wound is tight, his cornea clear, his anterior chamber deep and clear, and his pupil black, all is well. Give him +10 aphakic spectacles and discharge him between the 3rd and 10th postoperative day.

RARER CAUSES OF GRADUAL LOSS OF VISION IN A WHITE EYE

Examine his macula and his optic cup with particular care.

If an old person has gradual loss of central vision, atrophy, and irregular pigment at his maculae, suspect senile macular degeneration. There is no treatment.

If he has pale, white, flat optic discs (distinguish these from the pale cupped discs of glaucoma), and normal maculae, he has optic atrophy. Try to find the cause (there are many, including a space-occupying lesion around the optic chiasma). There is no treatment.

If he has gradual loss of vision at any age, often starting with night blindness, a family history, and dark pigmentation which follows his retinal vessels and takes the form of 'bone spicules', suspect retinitis pigmentosa. There is no treatment.

If he has gradual loss of central vision and has taken excessive doses of chloroquine (>10 tablets weekly for >1 year), suspect chloroquin maculopathy. His macula has a typical 'bull's eye' pattern with a dark centre and a paler surrounding ring. Stop chloroquin. There is no treatment.

If he has old macular scars (large white areas with black edges, often around his optic disc and his macula), they may be due to previous toxoplasmosis or toxocariasis. There is no treatment.

SUDDEN LOSS OF VISION IN A WHITE EYE(S)

He has lost his vision over minutes or days, in one or both eyes, which are white.

If at any age he has steadily lost his vision over 24 hours, in one eye or occasionally both his eyes, suspect posterior choroiditis due to toxoplasmosis or other causes. The important sign is inability to see his retinal vessels due to hazy media caused by inflammatory cells in his vitreous. He may respond to systemic steroids, and he may resolve spontaneously. Give him atropine until the inflammation has resolved.

If symptoms started with a flash of light followed by black objects floating in his field of vision, and then a curtain or cobweb across it, suspect retinal detachment. Part of his retina may look grey-green. Dilate his pupil and examine his fundus. You will see an abnormal red reflex in one part of his fundus, with elevation of part of his retina, and tortuosity of its vessels, which are difficult to focus on. Expert surgery may save his sight.

If he has instantaneous loss of vison, suspect occlusion of his central retinal vein (a swollen disc with many haemorrhages all over his retina), or artery (a swollen disc, oedema of his retina, and often a cherry-red spot at his macula). There is no immediate treatment. If he has central retinal vein thrombosis, follow him for at least 3 months, because he may develop secondary glaucoma, which needs treatment.

If he has loss of central vision with an abnormal pupil response to light, suspect optic neuritis (any age, usually in the 3rd and 4th decades, and usually unilateral). His media and optic disc are usually normal. He will usually improve over about 8 weeks. Bilateral optic neuritis following methyl alcohol or drugs (quinine) is permanent. There is no specific treatment.

24.5 Uveitis; iritis and iridocyclitis (anterior uveitis), and choroiditis (posterior uveitis)

Any part of the uveal tract can become inflamed—the iris (iritis), the ciliary body (cyclitis), or the choroid (choroiditis). More than one part may be involved at the same time (iridocyclitis). The terms 'iritis' and 'uveitis' are often used loosely and interchangeably, and we will do the same here. Although iridocyclitis may be caused by bacteria invading the eye through a corneal ulcer (24.3), it and other forms of uveitis are more often due to a sterile inflammation, usually from an unknown cause. Uveitis of several kinds is common in the developing world.

Iritis (more strictly iridocyclitis) has several consequences: (1) A patient's inflamed iris may stick to his lens by posterior synechiae (adhesions, common) or less often to the back of his cornea by anterior synechiae. (2) If the entire margin of his pupil sticks to his lens, his iris balloons forwards (iris bombé, B, 24.7), and he has secondary glaucoma (24.6). (3) Small separated pieces of iris may stick to his lens, or less often to his cornea. (4) Abnormal proteins enter his aqueous, and cause an aqueous flare, which you can see with a slit lamp. You can also see leucocytes as tiny particles floating in his aqueous. (5) These particles may stick to the back of his cornea as keratic precipitates (KP), and they may be numerous enough to gather at the bottom of his anterior chamber as a hypopyon. Unlike the hypopyon that results from the entry of bacteria through a corneal ulcer, the hypopyon of iridocyclitis is usually sterile. Untreated iridocyclitis eventually subsides spontaneously, typically in about 6 weeks, leaving his eye severely damaged. It may relapse, or it may be insidious and chronic, with few symptoms except progressive loss of vision.

Uveitis presents in two ways (or in both of them together, panuveitis, see below): (1) Anterior uveitis (iritis) presents as an 'acute red eye'; it is thus one of the important differential diagnoses of of this condition, and particularly of conjunctivitis (24.3). He has pain in and around his eye varying from mild to severe, photophobia, watering, and often blurred vision. He has ciliary hyperaemia, and often general hyperaemia also. His pupil is constricted. (2) Posterior uveitis (choroiditis) presents as progressive loss of vision, without other obvious symptoms, in a white eye (24.4).

Iritis is usually a sterile reaction to one of the infections listed below. If onchocerciasis (24.7) is endemic in your district, it will certainly be the most common cause. Usually, no cause is found, and iritis is presumed to be an autoimmune disease.

Atropine will keep his pupils well dilated, and break down synechiae.

Steroids are controversial. Opinions differ as to their long-term benefit, and whether they are safe in non-expert hands. They probably hasten resolution, and justify the risks associated with their use, but only provided that you *don't use them if there is any sign of infection, especially a corneal ulcer.* Remember also that: (1) Steroids will make a red eye white, regardless of the cause, without necessarily curing it. (2) They will suppress the normal inflammatory response, without killing the causative agent. (3) They may raise his intraocular pressure, and may cause a secondary glaucoma that could blind him (unusual). (4) If you give steroids long term, they may cause a cataract, but they will not do this during the few weeks that are necessary to treat acute iritis.

UVEITIS, iritis, iridocyclitis, choroiditis

DIAGNOSIS. Uveitis may be unilateral, or bilateral, and presents in various ways.

Acute anterior uveitis (iritis, iridocyclitis) presents as a red, painful eye, with photophobia and tearing; for the differential diagnosis see Section 24.3.

Posterior uveitis involves mainly a patient's choroid, and presents as fairly sudden loss of vision over 24–48 hours in a white and usually painless eye, due to damage to his retina and an exudate of cells and pigment into his vitreous. After dilatation, you can see these as a vitreous haze with an indistinct retina. At a later stage, when the haze has cleared, you may see foci of white depigmentation, surrounded by heaped up black pigment which results in impaired vision, especially if it involves his macula.

Panuveitis (quite common) is a combination of anterior and posterior uveitis, and causes loss of vision in a red, painful eye.

SPECIAL TEST. Dilate his pupil and look for posterior synechiae which will confirm the diagnosis of iritis.

CAUSES. You will probably find no cause, but if he has any of these, it may be responsible: syphilis, leprosy, herpes, tox-

SOME LEFT OPTIC DISCS

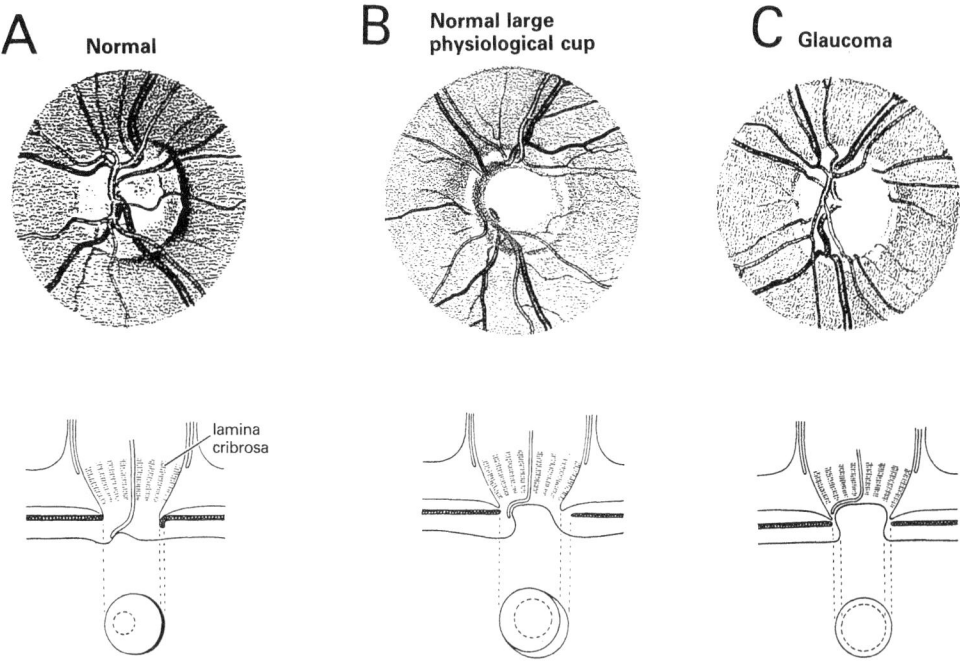

Fig. 24-8 SOME LEFT OPTIC DISCS. A, a normal optic disc with a moderately sized cup and the lamina cribrosa shown stippled. B, another normal optic disc. This has a large physiological cup and a temporal scleral crescent. C, the optic disc of a patient with gross 'chronic' open-angle glaucomatous cupping. *After Parr, Jon, 'Introduction to Ophthalmology', (2nd edn 1982). OUP, with kind permission.*

oplasmosis, toxocariasis, onchocerciasis (24.7), tuberculosis (29.1), trauma, or the leakage of the lens protein from a hypermature cataract.

TREATMENT. Dilate his pupil with short acting mydriatics (cyclopentolate and phenylephrine). When his pupil is dilated, maintain him on atropine ointment 1% three times a day, until his uveitis is no longer active, as shown by the absence of KP bodies and redness. This will prevent posterior synechiae, which would lead to the blinding complication of secondary glaucoma and cataract. So, *keep his pupil dilated until all the inflammation has subsided.*

If his disease is unilateral, cover his eye with a shield (24.1) if it is severe, and a shade if it is not. If it is bilateral, give him eye shades made from exposed X-ray film.

STEROIDS. His iritis will subside spontaneously, but topical steroids will hasten its departure.

CAUTION ! NEVER give steroids if: (1) There are signs of infection. (2) He has a corneal ulcer.

If he has anterior uveitis (iridocyclitis), instil hydrocortisone drops 1% into his conjunctival sac 3 hourly.

If he has posterior uveitis, give him tablets of prednisolone 20–30 mg/day for 3 to 6 weeks. Don't continue beyond 6 weeks. Tail these off for a week at the end of the course.

If his IOP is raised, also give him acetazolamide 250 mg 6-hourly, until the inflammation is under control. Double the dose if it remains raised. If possible monitor his IOP weekly by tonometry.

DIFFICULTIES WITH UVEITIS

If POSTERIOR SYNECHIAE develop, they may be followed by a cataract. Or they may occlude his pupil and cause pupil block glaucoma (iris bombé), with an increased IOP. Be sure to dilate his iris vigorously with atropine, so that it does not stick to his lens.

If he gets SECONDARY GLAUCOMA, his pupil will not dilate. You can refer him for an iridectomy, but it is usually too late.

24.6 Glaucoma

Glaucoma is a group of blinding diseases in which a patient's intraocular pressure (IOP) is usually raised, causing damage to his optic nerve, and resulting in loss of vision. There are four kinds: (1) Primary (chronic) open-angle glaucoma (POAG). (2) Primary angle closure glaucoma (ACG). (3) Secondary glaucoma as a complication of trauma, swollen cataract, iritis, etc. (4) Congenital glaucoma (buphthalmos).

POAG occurs in eyes in which the angle between the iris and the cornea is normal, and is probably due to a block in the drainage of intraocular fluid at the trabeculum. POAG causes 10–20% of blindness in developing world, 90% of glaucoma in Caucasians, and most cases of glaucomatous blindness in Africans. Up to 1% of the over-40s may have it. POAG is bilateral, but is often asymmetrical; it is insidious and progressive, and causes no symptoms until a patient has lost much of his sight. Glaucoma cannot be prevented, and even early treatment cannot restore lost vision. The best that can be done is to recognize it *early,* and to prevent his vision getting worse. For this to be possible, *all health workers must be aware of the possibility of glaucoma in any patient who complains of loss of vision.* The key to early diagnosis is to pick up early changes in the optic discs and a raised IOP, both of which can be recognized by eye assistants. The aim of medical and surgical treatment is to lower the IOP to a level which will stop further damage to his optic nerve, and therefore preserve his vision at its present level. Trabeculectomy (not described here) is a relatively simple operation, with a reasonable chance of preserving what vision he still has. It should be available at a referral hospital, or at another district hospital, where there is a surgeon interested in doing it. Learn it from an expert at the same time that you learn cataract extraction.

The symptoms of POAG are non-specific. The patient complains of slow loss of vision in one or both his eyes over months or years ('loss of vision in a white eye', 24.4). Sometimes, he has marked loss of vision in one eye, while his other eye is normal, or nearly so. Occasionally, he has pain and headache, but this is late. Glaucoma is often familial, so inquire about blindness in his relatives.

Angle closure glaucoma (ACG, acute glaucoma) usually occurs over the age of 35, in women more often than men, with an abnormally narrow angle between the iris and the cornea. If this angle should happen to close a little more than usual, it causes a sudden abrupt rise in a patient's IOP, so that he presents with unilateral episodic attacks of pain, misty vision, and rainbow-coloured haloes round lights. Between attacks his eye is normal. Sooner or later, an episode of raised IOP does not resolve, and he presents with classical acute congestive glaucoma ('loss of vision with a red eye', 24.3). Acute glaucoma is relatively uncommon, and is rare in Africa. Its incidence is highest in Inuits and Mongolian peoples, in Burma, and in South East Asia.

The dangers of atropine in glaucoma result from its effect in dilating the pupil: (1) This keeps the iris away from the lens, and prevents adhesions (synechiae) forming between them, which is valuable in iritis when you want to prevent this happening. (2) Dilatation of the pupil crowds the iris into the angle of the anterior chamber, where it impedes the drainage of aqueous. This is never a desirable effect, but it does not matter in a normal eye or in iritis; *it can however blind an eye if drainage is already impaired by glaucoma!* So, do give atropine in iritis, but *don't* give it in glaucoma!

IF AN OLDER PERSON COMPLAINS OF POOR VISION, CHECK FOR GLAUCOMA.

GLAUCOMA

PRIMARY OPEN-ANGLE GLAUCOMA, 'POAG', 'chronic glaucoma'

DIAGNOSIS. Measure the visual acuity of any patient who presents with loss of vision. A hazy cornea or a pupil which does not respond normally to light should make you suspect glaucoma. If his IOP is >28, or his cup/disc ratio is >0.5, he may have glaucoma. The end stage of glaucoma is a patient with a blind, or nearly blind eye, with a large pupil that does not react to light. Aim to diagnose it long before this with the following three tests. Loss of visual field is an early sign, but is not easy to test for with simple equipment.

CAUTION ! (1) The IOP is useful in confirming glaucoma, but is not absolute. (2) Glaucoma can occur with a normal IOP (30% of patients with glaucoma have an IOP of <22 mmHg). (3) A raised IOP is not always associated with optic nerve loss. (4) The IOP fluctuates, so if you are in doubt, repeat the measurements over a few days.

(1) LOSS OF VISUAL ACUITY is not an early sign in POAG, but it is a quick one. Always measure a patient's visual acuity, whenever he presents with an eye complaint (24.1).

(2) CUPPING OF THE OPTIC DISCS is the important sign. Chonic glaucoma causes the discs to become deeper and wider, and the remaining rims of disc tissue to atrophy. One eye is commonly affected more than the other, so that a definite difference between a patient's two eyes is probably abnormal. Enlargement starts at the upper or lower margins, so that a vertically ovoid cup with a cup/disc ratio of >0.5 is probably abnormal. Eventually, the margin of the cup approaches the margin of the disc, so that only a narrow rim of tissue remains. Its wall becomes steep, so that vessels bend abruptly as they reach the level of the surrounding disc. If the edge of the disc overhangs the cup, you may lose sight of them until they appear over the edge of the cup. A large physiological cup can be difficult to distinguish from an early glaucomatous one.

With practice, eye assistants can distinguish 'normal discs', 'suspicious discs' and 'advanced glaucomatous cupping'. If you can only do one test, changes in the discs are the most useful one. If necessary dilate his pupils.

Normal discs: (1) The discs are the same in both eyes. (2) The ratio of the optic cup to the optic disc is 0.5 or less. (3) The cup is circular and the periphery of the disc (the optic nerve rim) is pink. (4) The appearance of the disc remains constant over time.

Signs suggestive of glaucoma: **(1) A cup/disc ratio of greater than 0.5. (2) A vertically oval cup, perhaps with notching at the upper or lower poles. (3) An area of pallor >30% of the disc area. (4) Asymmetry of the cup/disc ratio between the two eyes.**

(3) ABNORMAL PUPIL RESPONSES are a useful way of testing for glaucoma, and only need a torch. Initially, one pupil does not react as briskly as the other. Finally, there is no response at all.

If you shine a light into a normal eye in a semidark room, its pupil will constrict (direct response), and so will the other pupil (consensual response).

GLAUCOMA

The visual field

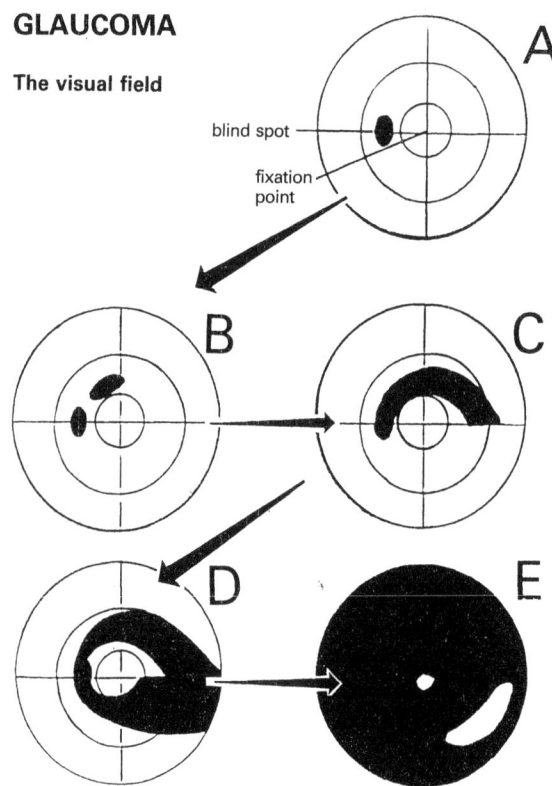

The optic discs

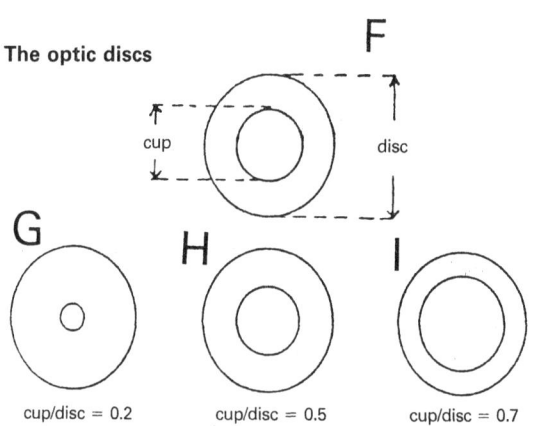

Fig. 24-9 GLAUCOMA. A, a normal visual field with its normal blind spot. B, a paracentral scotoma (blind area) in early glaucoma. C, an arcuate scotoma in early glaucoma. D, a ring scotoma in early glaucoma. E, complete loss of visual field apart from a small central island, and a larger temporal island, in advanced glaucoma. Unfortunately, there is no easy way of monitoring the visual field in glaucoma.

F, a schematic representation of the cup/disc ratio. G, a normal optic disc with its physiological cup. H, a cup/disc ratio of 0.5, the borderline of normality. I, pathological cupping of the optic disc due to glaucoma with a cup/disc ratio of 0.7. *Kindly contributed by Allen Foster.*

If his optic nerve is completely destroyed, there will be no direct or consensual response (total afferent pupil defect).

If his optic nerve is partly destroyed (for example 90%), his pupil will constrict slowly when the light shines in it (partial afferent pupil defect), showing that only a little optic nerve is functioning.

The swinging torch test, is a useful test for early asymmetrical optic nerve damage, and does not need an ophthalmoscope. It is theoretically difficult, but is easy in practice. In a semidark room shine a light into his good eye, and then swing it across into his bad eye (the eye with reduced vision).

As the light shines in his good eye, the pupil of his bad eye will constrict. As you swing the light quickly across to his bad eye, its pupil, which was previously constricted, will now dilate. This indicates a relative afferent pupil defect, early optic nerve damage, and a difference in function between his two optic nerves.

The practical test is to swing the torch from one pupil to the other and back again in a semidark room. *If one pupil consistently dilates as light shines on it,* that eye has a reduced pupil response, relative to the better eye, and should be investigated for optic nerve disease, perhaps POAG.

THE RISK FACTORS FOR POAG are: (1) Age >40. (2) A positive family history in first-degree relatives. (3) Race, POAG is more common in Africans than in Caucasians. (4) A vertical cup/disc ratio of >0.5. (5) An IOP of >28 mmHg (<2 with a 5.5 g weight).

MANAGEMENT will preserve what sight he has, but will not improve it.

If he is already blind in both eyes and unable to walk about by himself, it is too late to help him.

If he has any sight left (he can walk about by himself with either eye), refer him immediately for trabeculectomy. Even when his sight is as poor as CF 1 m (24.1), he may still derive some benefit from treatment. If you cannot refer him, or do a trabeculectomy yourself, you will have to try medical treatment:

Medical treatment can lower his IOP, but it has to be constant, consistent and *continue for life,* which is usually impracticable, so that immediate surgery is better. The drugs are: (1) Pilocarpine 4% 4 times daily. (2) Timolol 0.5% twice daily (expensive). This is a β-blocker which reduces the secretion of aqueous. (3) Acetazolamide tablets 250 mg 4 times a day. Start him on pilocarpine or timolol, and if this fails to maintain his IOP <20 mmHg, also give the other drug. If both drops fail to lower his IOP below 20 mmHg, give acetazolamide 250 mg 1 to 3 times daily for short periods (side-effects may occur with continued use). To treat him effectively, you will have to measure his intraocular pressure, and monitor his visual fields regularly. This has to be done in a specialist clinic.

Surgical treatment is a trabeculectomy which removes a piece of the filter (the trabecular meshwork), and so allows his intraocular fluid to drain under his conjunctiva; this increases drainage and reduces his IOP. The operation has an immediate success rate of >80%, and is the recommended treatment for most patients with POAG in the developing world.

'ACUTE GLAUCOMA'

This is is usually due to 'ACG' (angle closure glaucoma), but secondary glaucoma (see below) may occasionally present acutely.

DIAGNOSIS. He presents with an 'acute red eye' at any age (one of its rarer causes, 24.3), severe unilateral headache in and around his eye, and sudden profound loss of vision. When you examine him, his vision is reduced, his eye is red, his cornea is hazy from oedema, his anterior chamber is shallow, his pupil is usually dilated, and his intraocular pressure is usually over 40 mmHg.

CAUTION ! He will go blind unless you treat him quickly.

TREATMENT. Admit him as an emergency. Refer him to an ophthalmologist as soon as possible, who will decide whether to do a trabeculectomy or peripheral iridectomy, or whether to treat him medically. If referral is delayed, start treatment before he goes. If you cannot refer him, you will have to treat him medically yourself. Give him an analgesic to ease his pain, and treat both his eyes. Aim to:

(1) Lower his IOP by increasing the drainage of aqueous. Give him acetazolamide 500 mg orally followed by 250 mg 6-hourly, as soon as his nausea has subsided.

(2) Keep his pupils constricted. This will keep the periphery of his iris away from the angle of his eye, where the aqueous flows out, and so help it to drain. Treat both his eyes with drops of pilocarpine 1–4% every 15 minutes, for 2 hours. If this makes his pupil constrict, the angle will be opened.

(3) If necessary, you can also lower his IOP by increasing the tonicity of his blood. Give him 50 ml of flavoured glycerine by mouth. If he is nauseated, he may not tolerate this. Or, give him 200 ml of 20% mannitol intravenously during 20 minutes.

When medical treatment has reduced his IOP to normal, he needs a peripheral iridectomy soon, to prevent a future attack, and probably a prophylactic one on the other side also.

CAUTION ! (1) He can become totally blind in 12 hours, so treatment is urgent. (2) Rainbow-coloured haloes round lights, and misty vision, are important prodromal signs, and need urgent investigation and treatment. (3) Atropine can precipitate an attack in a patient with a shallow angle, so avoid it in such people.

SECONDARY GLAUCOMA

This complicates: (1) Trauma, including hyphaema (blood in the anterior chamber, 60.8). (2) Swollen cataract (see below). (3) Some cases of iritis. Treat the primary condition, and refer him. If you cannot refer him, treat him with acetazolamide, mannitol, or glycerol as above.

DIFFICULTIES WITH GLAUCOMA

If he has an acute RED PAINFUL EYE, a shallow anterior chamber with a hazy cornea, and a FIXED, DILATED WHITE PUPIL, he has a SWOLLEN CATARACT, causing secondary glaucoma. Give him acetazolamide 500 mg immediately followed by 250 mg 4 times daily, and refer him for removal of his cataract.

If he has LOSS OF VISION and has been using steroid drops for several months, suspect STEROID GLAUCOMA. Topical steroids cause a genetically determined rise in IOP in a third of people. This is sometimes severe enough to cause glaucoma, exactly like POAG. Stop steroids.

If a child has BIG EYES, which may be associated with photophobia, blepharospasm, and tearing ("...such beautiful big eyes"), suspect CONGENITAL GLAUCOMA (buphthalmos, ox-eye, rare), due to maldevelopment of the angle of his anterior chamber. The sclera of a child are soft, so that his eyes enlarge when his IOP rises. Other signs are: an increased IOP, a corneal haze (variable), sluggish reaction of his pupils to light, and enlargement of his cornea (>12 mm), or of his whole globe. If necessary, treat him medically and refer him immediately.

24.7 Onchocerciasis

Onchocerciasis is a parasitic infection of the skin and eyes caused by *Onchocerca volvulus,* which is endemic in parts of West and Central Africa, with foci in East Africa and Latin America. In hyperendemic areas 60% of the population are infected: in such areas blindness rates may vary widely, but may be as high as 15%. Microfilariae invade all parts of the eye: the cornea (keratitis), the anterior chamber (iritis), the retina (chorioretinitis), and the optic nerve (optic neuritis). Blindness and irreversible eye lesions are most often found in men of 30 and older. Try to identify the patients at high risk from the blinding complications, and to arrest their disease.

ONCHOCERCIASIS

A patient from an endemic area complains of itching, with or without a rash. He may have skin nodules, night blindness (enquire about this), gradual loss of vision in both his eyes, and sometimes tearing and photophobia. Look for microfilariae in snips from his skin.

CORNEA. He has a sclerosing keratitis with opacification of the lower third of his cornea. Tongues of opacification invade his cornea from the 3 and 9 o'clock positions, or from anywhere in the lower half, where they may form an apron across his cornea. If he is not treated, opacification slowly advances upwards over his pupil, until all that may be left is a clear area at 12 o'clock.

Slit lamp microscopy shows 0.5 mm linear and fluffy opacities at all levels in the stroma, and minute wriggling microfilariae in his anterior chamber.

IRIS. The final stage is a small, non-reactive, down drawn, pear-shaped pupil. Earlier stages are a loss of pigment in the margin of his pupil, exudation in front of, across, or behind it, posterior adhesions which turn it inwards, and small keratic precipitates (KP). A gelatinous exudate sometimes drags the lower margin of his pupil down and everts it.

Posterior synechiae and peripheral anterior synechiae lead to secondary glaucoma.

RETINA AND OPTIC DISCS. Look for: (1) Diffuse white areas and black pigmented ones most marked temporal to his macula (the Ridley fundus). (2) Optic atrophy, with sheathing of the vessels close to the nerve.

TREATMENT. Ivermectin ('Mectizan') is the drug of choice. Ongoing (1988) community trials are using an annual dose of 150 µg/kg with encouraging results. The traditional drugs diethylcarbamazine (DEC) and suramin cause so many complications, including visual deterioration, that they are not recommended. Nodulectomy is usually only recommended for children with head nodules.

If he has an onchocercal iritis, dilate his pupil with atropine and give him topical steroids (24.5). If he develops secondary glaucoma (24.6), treat his onchocerciasis and then refer him for surgery.

24.8 Refractive errors, difficulty reading, and presbyopia

In terms of comfort, increased efficiency and the number of people who benefit, the prescription of glasses is among the most valuable procedures in medicine. So do what you can to supply them. The refractive errors are: (1) Myopia (short sight). (2) Hypermetropia (long sight). (3) Astigmatism (the refractive mechanism is aspherical). (4) Presbyopia (the common long-sightedness of old age) (5) Aphakia ('no lens') after cataract extraction.

Presbyopia is part of the normal process of ageing: it appears earlier in the tropics than in higher latitudes, and is easily diagnosed and treated. It is responsible for 85% of the need for glasses.

Whereas a myopic child has to be specially fitted, because his eyes may not be the same, a presbyope can, if necessary, be left to choose the glasses which best suit him from a pile of second-hand ones. Astigmatism is more difficult to correct, but it is usually so mild that it needs no correction. In the developed world, its correction is often overemphasized.

The visual acuity of all patients with refractive errors improves when they look through a pin-hole, which uses only their central vision. This is the basis of the pin-hole test (24.1).

REFRACTIVE ERRORS

If a patient has astigmatism or hypermetropia, he needs retinoscopy, which you will not have been trained to do, so refer him.

If he cannot see at a distance but can read, he is myopic. Test each eye alone with minus spherical glasses starting with −0.5 dioptres, and increasing in 0.5 dioptre steps. The smallest minus number that gives him the best acuity is the prescription he needs.

If he is a child with reduced visual acuity due to refractive errors or squint, refer him.

If he is aphakic after a cataract extraction, try him with +10, 11 or 12 lenses for distance, and +13, 14 or 15 lenses for reading.

DIFFICULTY READING PRESBYOPIA

If a patient complains of difficulty reading books or newspapers, (1) Ask him his age. If he is under 40 he does not need reading glasses for presbyopia, so explain this to him. (2) Measure his visual acuity. If it is not good, see Section 24.4, otherwise proceed. (3) Examine his eyes to make sure they are white, and that he has no serious problems. If they are otherwise normal, you can give him glasses.

TO PRESCRIBE READING GLASSSES give him those with the lowest number (the weakest pair) which will let him read easily. A useful guide is: age 45 +1.00, 50 +1.50, 55 +2.00, 60 +2.50, 65 +3.00. If he is choosing from a pile, he needs the weakest satisfactory pair (usually +2.00). Explain that they are only to be worn for reading and other close work, not for seeing in the distance.

24.9 Disease of the neuromuscular system of the eye (squints, amblyopia, and diplopia)

If a patient's eyes do not look in the same direction, he has a squint. Squints are common in the developing world, and are usually accepted with resignation. Although treating a squint needs relatively simple technology, it is time-consuming and needs skill, so squints will probably be low in your list of priorities.

If his eyes do not look in the same direction, he will see two images. This causes confusion, and to avoid it he tends to suppress the sight in one of them. If this suppression continues for long enough, he may lose vision in that eye. This is called amblyopia, which is a reduction in vision, due to lack of use of an apparently normal eye. If amblyopia is not corrected by the age of 7, it becomes permanent. So try to diagnose and refer squints before this age.

SQUINTS AND AMBLYOPIA

SQUINTS

DIAGNOSIS. The corneal light reflex and the cover test will demonstrate a manifest squint.

The corneal light reflex. Shine a pen torch directly in front of you, and ask the patient to look at it. If each of his eyes is properly fixing the torch, its reflection from his corneal mirrors will be the same, and more or less central on each cornea. Are the reflections from your torch equally centred on his pupils?

The cover test. Ask him to look straight ahead at some target in the distance. Cover his left eye with a piece of paper. If his right eye moves, in or out, to fix on the distant target, it was previously squinting. If it does not move, it was looking straight at the target.

Now put the paper in front of his right eye. If his left eye moves as you remove the paper, it was previously squinting in or out. If it does not move, he does not have a manifest squint, and both eyes look straight.

MANAGEMENT is limited.

If an adult has a squint and no double vision it may be the cause of reduced vision in the squinting eye (amblyopia). There is no treatment at this age.

If an adult has a squint and double vision, this suggests a serious recent disease of his extraocular muscles or their nerves, such as diabetic neuropathy, myasthenia gravis, or raised intracranial pressure. He needs a full medical and neurological examination.

If a child under the age of 7 years presents with a squint:
(1) Dilate both his pupils, and use an ophthalmoscope to make sure that his squint is not due to a retinoblastoma in one of his eyes (an uncommon cause of squint, 32.7). Look for a yellowish mass on his retina.

(2) If his retinae are normal, try to assess his visual acuity in both eyes. This may be possible if he is >3 years, but rarely if he is younger.

If he has reduced vision in either eye, or a definite squint, and he is under 7, refer him. He may need glasses, occlusion therapy to treat amblyopia, and perhaps surgery on his extraocular muscles.

CAUTION ! Never occlude the eye of a child under 7 years for several days, because this may cause amblyopia.

If you cannot refer him, correct any refractive error and occlude the eye that he normally uses. Occlude it for 1/2 to 2 hours a day while he is doing close work, reading, or drawing. The duration of treatment depends on the duration of his ambylopia. If treatment is prompt, a 6–8 weeks of occlusion may be enough. If it is delayed he may need it for a year, or it may fail.

AFTER THE AGE OF 6 MONTHS NO SQUINT SHOULD BE IGNORED

24.10 Diseases of the lids and nasolachrymal apparatus

Diseases of the eyelids and nasolachrymal system include tumours, deformities of the lids, and watering (epiphora). Globally, the most important disease of the lids is trachoma, which scars them, and causes them to turn inwards (entropion, 24.13). The commonest and usually the most harmless disease of the lid is a stye.

THE LIDS

If a patient has a red swelling on his lid margin, with an eyelash coming out of it, he has a stye (hordeolum). This is a staphylococcal infection of the follicle of an eyelash. Pull the eyelash out of the swelling, and give him an analgesic. Antibiotics are only necessary in recurrent styes, or if there are signs that infection is spreading beyond his lid (carotid sinus thrombosis is a rare complication, 5.5). Suggest that he tries hot spoon bathing (24.1).

If he has a swelling in either lid, some distance from its margin, pointing towards its conjunctival surface, he probably has a tarsal cyst, (chalazion, Meibomian cyst). Avoid an external scar by incising his conjunctiva wherever the cyst points.

If a few lashes turn in on the eye (trichiasis), remove them with a pair of forceps (epilation). They regrow, and need removing at regular intervals.

If most of his lashes or the margin of his lid is turned in (entropion), he needs surgery (24.13).

If the margin of either lid is everted (ectropion), usually as the result of scarring, seventh nerve palsy, or leprosy, surgery may be necessary (unusual).

THE NASOLACHRYMAL APPARATUS

If a mother brings you her young child saying that he has had a watering eye since birth, he has congenital atresia of his nasolachrymal duct. It will probably resolve spontaneously by the age of 18 months. Reassure her, and give her a topical antibiotic to apply if he gets conjunctivitis. If his eye is still watering at the age of 2 years, his nasolachrymal duct needs probing and syringing. Refer him.

If something interferes with the drainage of an adult's tears, his eye waters (epiphora) even if there is no local irritation. He can usually learn to live with it, but epiphora can occasionally be so severe that it needs surgery (dacryocystorhinostomy). Refer him.

If he has a tender swelling between his eye and the side of his nose, he probably has acute dacryocystitis (an abscess in his tear sac). Give him a systemic antibiotic, an analgesic, and warm soaks (5.5).

24.11 Proptosis

If there is a space occupying lesion in a patient's orbit, it pushes his eye forwards. Proptosis is always serious, and it can be difficult to diagnose; so it is fortunate that it not common. Some of its causes (orbital cellulitis and Burkitt's lymphoma) need chemotherapy. Most of the patients who need surgery are either going to die from malignant tumours anyway, no matter what is done, or they have slow-growing benign tumours, which you have time to refer. So your ability to help a patient with proptosis is limited; but you should try to make a diagnosis.

Proptosis can occur slowly over years, or rapidly over days. Its causes vary geographically, and with the age of the patient. Here they are, the more common ones first; the later ones are mostly very rare:

An adult may have: (1) A retrobulbar haematoma following an injury (common, 60.8). This is only an incident in a head injury, and the diagnosis is obvious. (2) A mucocele of his frontal sinus (the commonest cause), due to an infection followed by an obstruction, which prevents his sinus draining into his nose. (3) Orbital cellulitis, or an orbital abscess, usually following frontal or ethmoid sinusitis (5.5), or occasionally trauma. (4) A pseudotumour of his orbit due to a granuloma of unknown cause. (5) An epidermoid or dermoid cyst, which may be of the 'dumbbell' type, and extend into his anterior cranial fossa. Don't operate on these, unless you are skilled enough to dissect widely, and have made an accurate diagnosis. (6) A mixed lachrymal tumour (lachrymal adenoma). (7) A haemangioma or hamartoma; you may be able to empty a haemangioma temporarily by pressing it back into his orbit. (8) A hydatid cyst, if he comes from an area where these occur (31.13). (9) Cavernous sinus thrombosis (5.5). (10) A secondary tumour. (11) A malignant melanoma (32.20). (12) Carcinoma of his maxillary or ethmoidal sinuses (32.39) invading his orbit. (13) The hyperophthalmopathic form of thyrotoxicosis (dysthyroid eye disease, Graves's disease). (14) A meningioma of his sphenoid.

A child may have: (1) A retinoblastoma in the first 5 years of his life (32.7). (2) Acute ethmoiditis, commonly when he is about 2. (3) Burkitt's lymphoma, if he comes from the 'Burkitt zone' (32.3). He will probably have a jaw tumour also. (4) A rhabdomyosarcoma (32.9). (5) Some other kind of lymphoma (32.4, 32.5). (6) A neuroblastoma. (7) A secondary tumour.

You can treat orbital cellulitis, abscesses, and cavernous sinus thrombosis (5.5) with systemic antibiotics. If you diagnose a retinoblastoma (32.7) early enough, you can enucleate the globe. Burkitt's lymphoma usually responds dramatically to chemotherapy.

PROPTOSIS

HISTORY. Long history? (benign lesion). Short history? (malignant lesion or acute infection). Acute onset with pain? (infection).

EXAMINATION. Sit the patient down, stand behind him, look down on his eyes from above, and observe the relative positions his globes. This will help to distinguish pseudoproptosis, due to the relative widening of one palpebral fissure.

Hold a ruler horizontally, and measure the position of each cornea from the midline. If he has two proptosed globes, and they are both equidistant from the midline, he probably has thyrotoxicosis (the most likely cause of bilateral proptosis). If they are not equidistant, one globe has probably been pushed out of place by an orbital mass.

Examine his fundi for papilloedema and optic atrophy. Search him for signs of a primary malignant tumour.

CAUTION ! Don't confuse proptosis with a staphyloma due to a neglected corneal ulcer (24.3). His normal intraocular pressure has caused his previously weakened cornea to bulge, in a manner which you can mistake for a tumour. His globe is however in its normal position.

X-RAYS may demonstrate: (1) Erosion of the bones of his orbit. (2) Sclerosis (typical of a meningioma). (3) Calcification (sometimes in a retinoblastoma).

BIOPSY may be practical.

If a tumour is palpable externally, explore over it and take

PROPTOSIS

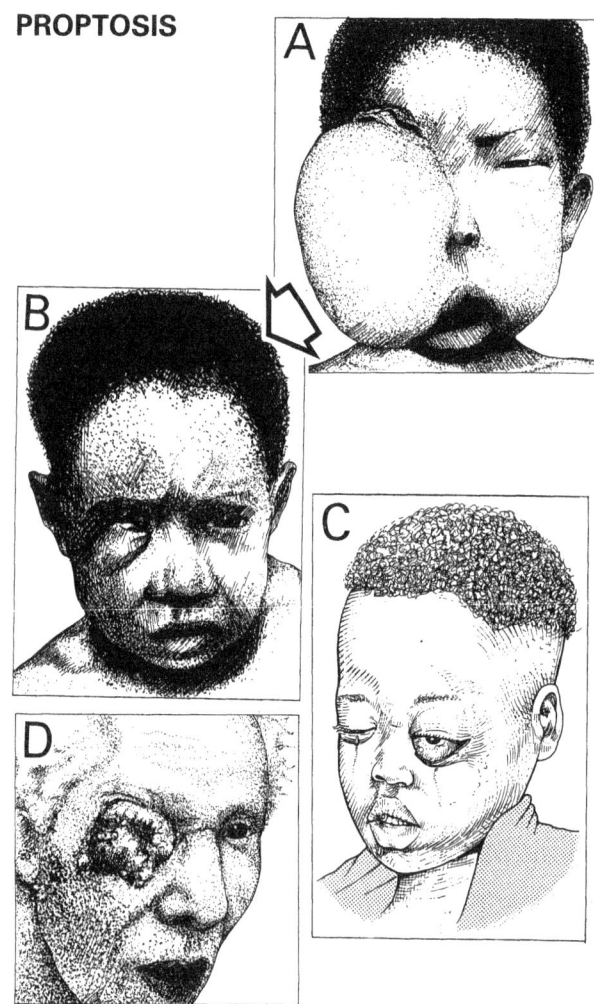

Fig. 24-10 PROPTOSIS. A, and B, Burkitt's lymphoma, before and after treatment. C, proptosis, cause not yet established. D, carcinoma of the maxillary antrum extending into the orbit. *A, B, and D, after Parsons GA, and Berg D, 'Proptosis and orbitotomy in Papua New Guinea', Tropical Doctor 1977;7:129-33. C, kindly contributed by Edward Kasili.*

a biopsy, except for lachrymal adenomas, which should never be biopsied.

If it is not palpable externally, a lateral orbitotomy which splits his temporal bone may be indicated. Refer him.

DIAGNOSIS AND MANAGEMENT. See elsewhere for the management of orbital infections (5.5), especially draining pus (drainage through the lower or upper fornix is usually best), retinoblastoma (32.7), and Burkitt's lymphoma (32.3).

Acute (<3 months) in an adult: orbital cellulitis, trauma, pseudotumour.

Acute (<3 months) in a child: acute ethmoiditis, retinoblastoma (0–5 years), Burkitt's lymphoma (5–15 years).

Chronic (>3 months) in an adult: frontal mucocele, thyrotoxicosis, lachrymal tumour, meningioma.

If his proptosis arose acutely, and his lids are red and swollen, perhaps with a fever and tachycardia he has orbital cellulitis, or an orbital abscess. Give him systemic antibiotics. If he has an abscess drain it.

If a child of about 2 years has sudden unilateral proptosis, with swollen lids and conjunctiva, fever and tachycardia, suspect acute ethmoiditis. Give him systemic antibiotics.

If he is very sick and with an acute pulsating proptosis, which may be unilateral initially, but soon becomes bilateral, with engorgement of the veins, and total inability to move his eye, perhaps with an associated meningitis, suspect cavernous sinus thrombosis (5.5).

If he has a swelling which has enlarged slowly (weeks or months) in the superior nasal quadrant of his orbit, pushing his eye downwards and outwards, he probably has a mucocele of his frontal sinus (common). Drain it through an approach between his periosteum and his frontal bone, keeping outside his orbit. Enter his sinus and drain the mucopus. Place a drain from his sinus into his nose. Suture his skin in layers. Remove the drain at 6 weeks.

If he is between 15 and 35, and his proptosis occurred over several weeks or months, suspect a pseudotumour. The diagnosis is largely by excluding other causes. It will respond well to prednisolone 80 mg daily for 1 week, falling slowly to 5 mg daily by the 4th week. Maintain him on 5 mg a day for several months, or it will recur.

If he has a swelling of the upper lateral quadrant of his orbit, pushing his eye downwards and inwards, which has grown slowly over many months or years, he probably has a lachrymal adenoma. Don't be deceived by the small mass of tumour palpable externally: most of it will be inside his orbit behind his eye. It needs removing through a lateral orbitotomy. Refer him.

If the proptosis of thyrotoxicosis does not respond to medical or surgical treatment (21.8), try high dose systemic steroids. If this fails, refer him for the surgical decompression of his orbits.

SYMPTOMATIC TREATMENT FOR HIS EXPOSED CORNEA. Examine his cornea to make sure that it is not ulcerated. Apply antibiotic eye ointment 3 or 4 times daily, and especially at night. If necessary, protect it by tarsorrhaphy (58.28). *Padding can be dangerous, because the pad may abrade and ulcerate his cornea.*

24.12 Tarsal cysts (chalazions or Meibomian cysts) and granulomas

Cysts sometimes form in the Meibomian glands on the conjunctival side of a patient's tarsus. They present as a swelling in either lid, which may become chronically or acutely infected. Small asymptomatic ones need no treatment, and may resolve spontaneously. Incise an acute infection and curette a chronic one. These cysts are common everywhere, so that treating them is a common outpatient eye operation. Sometimes, they present as granulomas.

TARSAL CYSTS

EQUIPMENT. Chalazion clamp, No. 11 scalpel blade and curette.

ANAESTHESIA. Anaesthetize the patient's conjunctiva with drops of lignocaine 4%, or amethocaine hydrochloride 1%. Infiltrate his lid with lignocaine and adrenalin around the chalazion. Insert the needle at the upper margin of his upper tarsus,

A TARSAL CYST

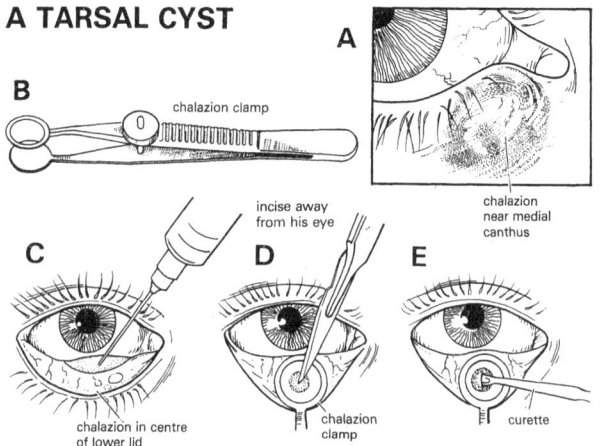

Fig. 24-11 CURETTING A TARSAL CYST. A, a chalazion close to a patient's medial canthus. B, chalazion forceps. C, local anaesthesia. D, the chalazion clamp in place ready to incise a chalazion in the centre of his lower lid. E, curetting it.

and the lower margin of his lower tarsus. Carry it forwards to his lid margin, on either side of the chalazion.

CURETTAGE. Evert his lid slightly. Put the chalazion clamp over the cyst, so that the solid blade lies on the skin of his eyelid, and the ring lies on his conjunctiva over the cyst. Close it so that it holds the lid and the cyst. Insert the tip of a No. 11 blade, *so that it cuts away from his eye.* Alternatively, make a cruciate incision. Swab its contents clean.

CAUTION ! Take care to curette away any pockets of granulation tissue, which may be hidden by a flap of conjunctiva, or have herniated themselves through his tarsal plate into his orbicularis muscle. If you don't do this, it may recur.

Remove the clamp and pinch his lid until it stops bleeding. If this is troublesome, wash it with warm saline. Place antibiotic ointment in his conjunctival sac 3 times a day for a week.

If the MATERIAL YOU INCISE IS HARD, and not gelatinous, suspect a carcinoma. Send it for histological examination, and refer him.

24.13 Entropion

Trachoma is the commonest eye infection in the tropics, and in its blinding hyperendemic form is the second commonest single cause of blindness and impaired vision (cataract is the first one). It is a chlamydial infection, which spreads from the eyes of one person to another, especially among children, in the poorest and most disadvantaged communities, particularly those in the Middle East and Africa. Trachoma is a chronic follicular conjunctivitis; it scars the conjunctiva of the eyelids and the cornea, and goes through four stages (see also Section 24.3):

1. The patient has a mildly red watery, eye due to bilateral conjunctivitis, especially of his upper lids, but without any distinguishing features.

2. Under his upper lid he has dilated blood vessels and hyperaemic, oedematous epithelial tissue (*papillae*). He also has yellow-grey swellings (*follicles*). Look at his corneoscleral junction with a loupe. If the edge of his cornea looks mildly grey, due to an arcuate (crescent-shaped) grey infiltration, and blood vessels go beyond the grey area into his cornea, he has *pannus* (meaning a curtain). This starts at the 12 o'clock position, and extends to 9 and 3 o'clock. Follicles and pannus indicate second stage trachoma. Follicles are not diagnostic, but pannus is.

3. The follicles in his lids become coarser and pannus spreads, sometimes across the pupillary area of his cornea. Scarring makes the margin of his upper lid irregular, and turns his upper tarsus inwards (entropion), taking his lashes with it, so that they scratch his cornea each time he blinks (trichiasis). This causes recurrent attacks of keratitis, which eventually end in a corneal opacity that blinds him.

4. Fibrous tissue replaces the follicles in his lids. This is the stage of cicatrized, or healed trachoma. His cornea is grey and scarred, his vision severely impaired, and his lids are deformed.

If you work in an endemic area, you are likely to have so many patients with entropion that you cannot refer them, so learn how to correct their eyelids yourself, and if necessary train an assistant to do this. The operation is always worth doing, even if his lids are severely scarred–his sight may recover suprisingly. Even if you fail, you are not likely to make his sight worse.

Several operations are possible:

A tarsal plate rotation with a mucosal graft from his mouth, is best. Unfortunately, this is more difficult and takes more time, which is important when you have many patients to treat. Instead, we describe two others. Opinions differ as to which is best. The difficulty is that if you do them and fail, you have crippled his lid, so that it is difficult for anyone else to do anything more.

Radical eyelash excision (Malcolm Phillips) removes the lashes that scratch the cornea. This is simple; one contributor considers it the best operation and another the worst. If you can remove his lash follicles completely, his lashes cannot regrow, and so cannot scratch his cornea. Removing them is little cosmetic disability if he has a dark skin, and the relief that follows is dramatic.

Tarsal eversion is possible if his tarsal plate is firm enough to hold sutures. Cut a strip from its free margin, by incising from his conjunctiva outwards. This will free the edge of his upper lid, so that you can turn it through 180° and sew it in place over the rest of his lid. This will give his upper lid a new edge, and make it about 3 mm shallower; but it will still meet the lower one when it shuts.

ENTROPION

If only a few lashes are turning in, try pulling these out with forceps (epilation) without local anaesthesia. They may grow back so you may have to repeat this several times.

INDICATIONS. Trachoma which has distorted a patient's upper tarsus, so that it has curled inwards and made his lashes scratch his globe. Operate as soon as possible after entropion occurs.

You can operate on both his eyes at the same time, but if you do, you will have to admit him for 3 days, to allow the oedema of his eyelids to subside. Catgut sutures allow him to be discharged without needing to reattend.

EQUIPMENT. An eye set, a scalpel with No. 15 blade, 4/0 silk or chromic catgut.

ANAESTHESIA. Anaesthetize his upper lids through his skin with 1 ml of 2% lignocaine with adrenalin. Anaesthetize his conjunctiva with 2 drops of amethocaine, or lignocaine, or 4% cocaine.

RADICAL EYELASH EXCISION FOR ENTROPION (Malcolm Phillips)

Start with his right eye. Use a scalpel to incise the margin of his upper lid, at the lateral end of his lashes, to a depth of 3 mm as in Fig. 24-12.

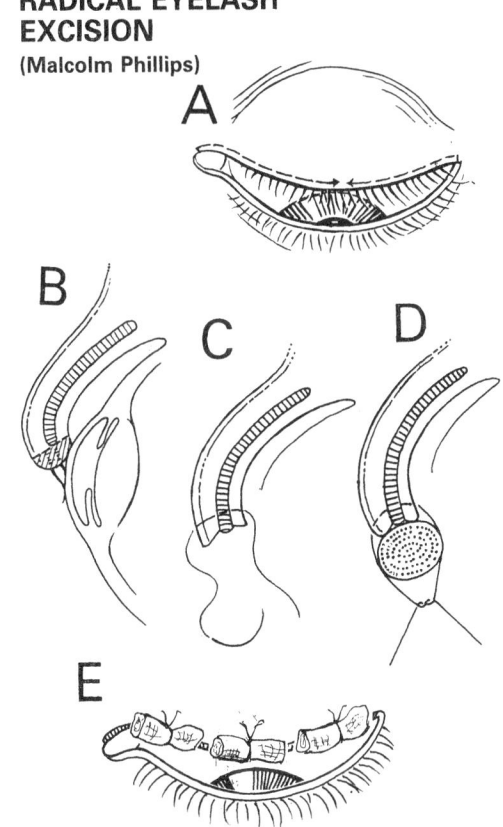

Fig 24-12 RADICAL EYELASH EXCISION (Malcolm Phillips). A, the direction of the incision. B, the part of the inverted eyelash to be excised. C, a suture passed through the lid. D, a small gauze pad tied to the eyelid. E, the operation complete.

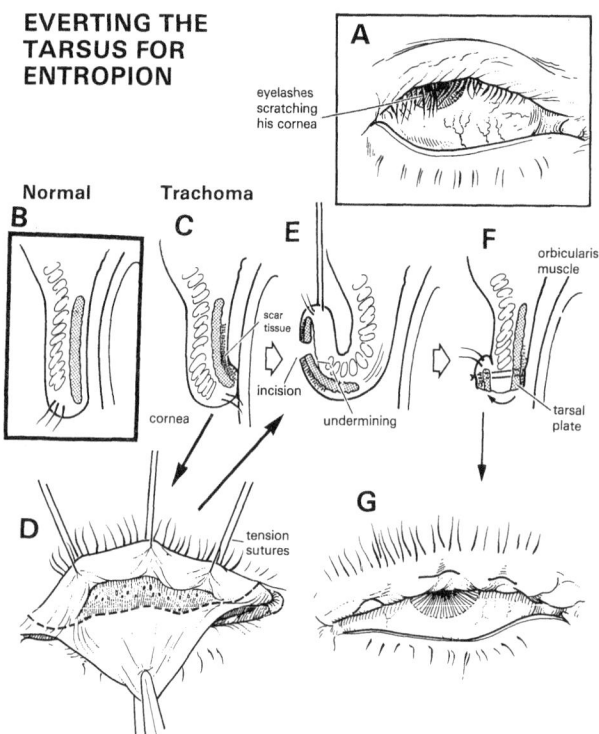

Fig. 24-13 EVERTING THE TARSUS for late trachoma. A, the patient, showing his inturned upper lid, with his lashes scratching his cornea. B, a normal eyelid. C, a lid scarred with trachoma, with its lashes rubbing against his cornea. D, making the incision. E, his lid everted with tension sutures. The incision has been made, and the superficial surface of the tarsus gently undermined in both directions. F, the margin of the lid has been rotated and sutured in place. G, the completed lid. *Kindly contributed by Roy Pfaltzgraff.*

Starting from either end, and using small sharp scissors, remove the margin of his lid bearing the roots of his lashes. Cut towards the medial end and preserve his punctum. Evert his lid as you do this, by pressing it with a swab. On his left eye, start at the medial end (if you are a right-handed operator).

Control the considerable bleeding that will result by suturing his conjunctiva to the skin of his eyelid with 3/0 catgut sutures on a cutting needle. Insert about 5 sutures, 5 mm apart, and use them to hold little rolls of gauze. Apply an eyepad for 24 hours. Remove the sutures in 7 days.

TARSAL EVERSION FOR ENTROPION

For this method, his tarsal plate must be stiff enough to take sutures. Using the anaesthetic method described above, place traction sutures of black braided silk in the centre of his upper lid, and at the junctions of its medial and lateral thirds with the middle third. Evert it over a roll of gauze, and clamp the sutures to a drape.

Using a No. 15 scalpel, make an incision about 3 mm from the inner margin of his lid, and parallel to it. Cut through his conjunctiva and the full length of his tarsal plate, at 90° to its surface, so as to free a strip from its edge. Curve each end of the incision towards the free edge of his lid, so that you can evert the strip of lid that bears his lashes.

Use skin hooks to retract the free edge of his lid. Use the tip of your scalpel to free the tissues from the anterior surface of the strip of tarsal plate for about 2 mm, until you see the follicles of his lashes in the base of the wound. Now undermine the anterior surface of the main part of the plate to a depth of about 4 mm. A *little* undermining like this will help you to mobilize the free edge of his tarsus. Do this in the plane between his orbicularis muscle and the insertion of his levator palpebrae superioris tendon.

CAUTION! Take care not to buttonhole his skin.

You can now rotate the distal fragment through 180° as in F, Fig. 24-13. Insert 3 small mattress sutures of 4/0 chromic catgut, and knot them tightly so that they bury themselves and need not be removed. Or use cotton sutures, and remove them later. Put tetracycline eye drops into his conjunctiva 3 times a day for a week.

24.14 Destructive methods for the eye

If a patient has a blind painful eye, he *may* be better without it. This is one of the occasions on which the indications are more critical than the operation. If you cannot refer him, you will have to treat him yourself.

Evisceration is the least radical procedure; scrape out the contents of his globe and leave his sclera intact. This is is the only safe procedure if his eye is infected, because a sleeve of dura containing CSF surrounds his optic nerve. Other operations require that you cut it, and so open up a potential path of infection to his meninges. You may need to eviscerate his eye: (1) When antibiotic therapy fails to control a severe infection causing suppurative endophthalmitis, leading to orbital cellulitis, and oedema of his lids. If you don't eviscerate his eye and drain the pus from it, the infection may spread and cause cavernous sinus thrombosis and meningitis. (2) When he has a chronic less urgent infection in a blind painfull useless eye.

Enucleation (excision) removes his globe by dividing his conjunctiva, the extrinsic muscles of his eye, and his optic nerve. This can be done where there is no active infection; it is contraindicated when there is.

Exenteration is a bloody, mutilating operation. It removes the entire contents of his orbit, together with its periosteum, his globe, and all its extrinsic muscles. Consider doing this when he has a fungating malignant tumour of his eye or orbit. It will not prolong his life, but his last days will at least be more comfortable. He will be left with an empty orbital cavity, which you can line with split skin, or allow it to granulate. One contributor considers that exenteration has no place in this manual.

Removing an eye is not an operation to be done lightly: (1) The main indication for enucleation is persistent severe pain in a blind eye (see below). (2) If it has been injured, always try to repair it first, no matter how hopelessly injured it is (60.1). (3) He is unlikely to get a prosthesis, and the best one is his natural eye, even if it is blind.

DESTRUCTIVE METHODS FOR THE EYE

Before you start any destructive operation: (1) Get *signed* permission from a child's parent or guardian. (2) Make sure you operate on the correct eye!

CAUTION ! (1) Unless you are operating for malignancy or acute infection to save a patient's life, his eye must be totally blind. Test this with a strong light. (2) When pain is the main indication, it must be considerable. Pain is subjective, so make sure, if you can, that he really does have severe pain. See him on several occasions. If he has *any* sensation of light, leave it. It may become quite useful six months later. Don't take it out unless he implores you to.

EQUIPMENT. A basic eye set (4.12), a curette.

EVISCERATING AN EYE

INDICATIONS. (1) The failure of antibiotic therapy to control a suppurative endophthalmitis. (2) A blind, persistently painful eye, especially if it is infected.

ANAESTHESIA. (1) General anaesthesia. (2) If there is no significant infection, you can use the combination of a facial and a retrobulbar block (6.5).

METHOD. Incise his conjunctiva at its junction with his cornea, using fine-toothed forceps and fine scissors. Cut through the margin of his cornea with scissors. Excise his entire cornea. Scoop out all the contents of his eye with a curette or a periosteal elevator.

Pack his sclera for a few minutes to control bleeding. Then

EVISCERATION OF THE EYE

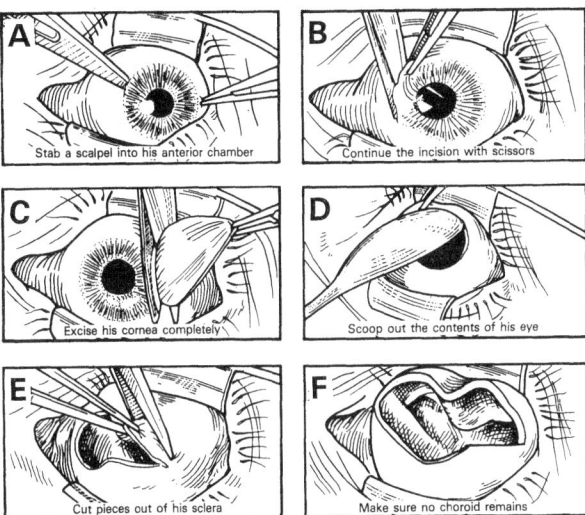

Fig. 24-14 EVISCERATING AN EYE. A, the patient's conjunctiva has already been incised and undermined. Stab a No. 11 scalpel blade through his cornea into his anterior chamber. B, continue the corneal incision with scissors. C, excise his cornea completely. D, scoop out the contents of his eye with a curette. E, cut a triangular section out of each side of the hole in his sclera. F, inspect the inside of his eye to make sure that no choroid remains. *After Galbraith JEK, 'Basic Eye Surgery' (1979), Figs. 9-17 to 9-24. Churchill Livingstone, with kind permission.*

look inside to make sure that no black choroid remains. If necessary, wipe it away with gauze. If any does remain, he runs the remote risk of sympathetic ophthalmitis (60.10).

If you are operating for acute infection, leave it open to drain.

If you are operating for chronic infection. excise a 5 mm triangle of sclera from each side, to help make his globe collapse. If you wish, fill the remains of his globe with antibiotic drops. Suture the edges of his sclera together with 5/0 plain catgut, or leave them open.

If he can get an artificial eye, insert a plastic conformer shell.

POSTOPERATIVELY, control bleeding by bandaging two eye pads firmly over the socket. Leave the dressing on for two days. Clean his lids and lashes twice daily, and put two drops of chloramphenicol 0.5% into the socket. Discharge him. He will be ready for an artificial eye in a month.

ENUCLEATING (EXCISING) AN EYE

INDICATIONS. (1) A malignant intraocular tumour (retinoblastoma or melanoma) is an absolute indication. (2) A blind, persistently painful eye, which is *not* infected (evisceration is an alternative). (3) A penetrating wound, especially in the ciliary region, complicated by plastic iridocyclitis, and entanglement of the iris, lens capsule, and vitreous. If you leave an eye like this, sympathetic ophthalmitis may follow. Steroids are so effective that enucleation is very rarely necessary for sympathetic ophthalmitis (60.10). It is useless, if the second eye is already involved.

ANAESTHESIA. (1) General anaesthesia. (2) A retrobulbar block using not less than 6 ml of lignocaine, combined with a 7th nerve block (A 6.5).

EQUIPMENT. A minor surgical set.

METHOD. Incise his conjunctiva at its junction with his cornea, using fine-toothed forceps and fine scissors. 'Circumcise' it, and undermine it back to the insertion of his extraocular muscles, about 8 mm from the edge of his cornea. Push closed scissors through his conjunctiva to open up the plane between his conjunctiva and his globe. Open them to expose his sclera, anterior to the insertion of his rectus muscles. Snip Tenon's capsule between the insertions of these muscles. Pass scissors through the incision, until you have defined the muscle insertions.

ENUCLEATING AN EYE

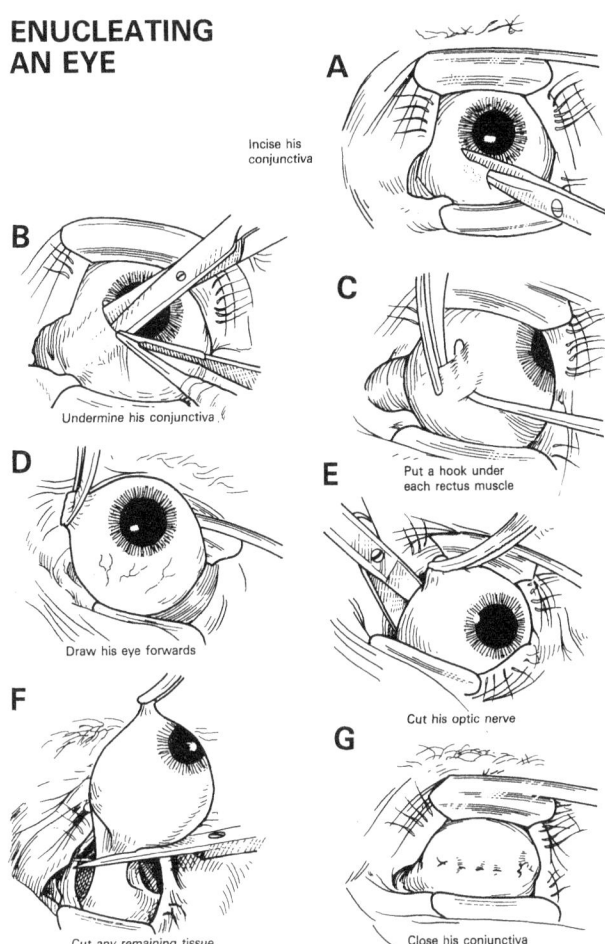

Fig. 24-15 ENUCLEATING A PATIENT'S EYE. A, incise his conjunctiva. B, undermine his conjunctiva for about 8 mm. C, slip a muscle hook under each rectus muscle, bring it forwards into the wound, and cut it. D, draw his eye forwards by pulling on the insertion of his medial rectus muscle. E, cut his optic nerve from the medial side. F, cut any remaining adherent tissue. G, suture his conjunctiva with catgut. *After Galbraith JEK, 'Basic Eye Surgery' (1979), Figs. 9-9 to 9-15. Churchill Livingstone, with kind permission.*

Slip a squint hook under his medial rectus muscle, and pull it into view. If he is to have an implant, lift the muscle and insert a mattress suture of chromic catgut through its belly, about 3 mm from its insertion. Clamp its insertion, remove the squint hook, and cut the muscle with scissors.

Separate each rectus muscle in the same way. Leave the stump of his medial rectus tendon a little longer, so that you have something to hold his globe with.

Make his globe prolapse forwards out of his orbit by closing the arms of the speculum behind it, and pushing them backwards. If his eye is so enlarged, that it will not fit between the blades of the speculum, pull it forwards by holding the stump of his medial rectus muscle with a haemostat.

Pass a pair of curved scissors, with their blades closed, down the medial side of his orbit, feel for his optic nerve behind his eye, open the scissors, and cut it. If you are excising it for a malignant tumour, cut it as far posteriorly as you can, because it may have been infiltrated by tumour.

Pull his eye forwards, and cut any tissue that remains attached to it. Put a hot wet pack into his orbit, and press on it until bleeding stops.

If he is to have an implant, it will probably be a simple glass globe. Place it in the muscle cone, and Tenon's capsule, and suture his conjunctiva over it.

If he is unable to have an implant, close his conjunctiva and Tenon's capsule separately with 5/0 catgut. Irrigate his socket with 0.5% chloramphenicol.

EXENTERATING AN EYE

INDICATIONS. A malignant tumour of his orbit, usually a

retinoblastoma, which has penetrated his globe and caused proptosis.

ANAESTHESIA. You must use general anaesthesia. Have blood for transfusion available.

EQUIPMENT. A general set, periosteal elevators.

METHOD. If his lids have been involved by the tumour, suture their margins together with 3/0 silk. Use a No. 15 scalpel blade to cut round the margins of his orbit. If his lids are not involved, incise closer to his scleral margins, so as to save all, or some, of the skin from his lids to line his empty orbit.

If he bleeds profusely from the upper inner margin of his orbit, control it with diathermy. If you don't have diathermy, operate swiftly, and apply a pack. Incise the periosteum round the margin of his orbit, and reflect it as far posteriorly as you can. It is firmly adherent at the suture lines.

CAUTION ! (1) The bone on the medial wall of the orbit is very thin, so elevate the periosteum here with special care. (2) The tumour may have eaten through the wall of his orbit, into his brain. If so, you may find it difficult to know where you are.

The periosteum should strip easily until you reach his orbital fissures, and his nasolacrimal duct. Cut this. Separate his palpebral ligaments, his trochlea, and his inferior oblique muscles from the bone with his periosteum.

Use curved scissors to cut the structures entering through his orbital fissures. Pull the contents of his orbit forwards, and cut the tissues at its apex with strong scissors as far back as you can.

He will bleed profusely. Remove the contents of his orbit, and then control bleeding.

Turn the skin at the edges of his orbit back into it. Graft its raw surfaces with split skin, either now or as a secondary procedure in 10–14 days. Gently pack his orbit. If you are not grafting it, dress it with acriflavine wool, and apply a firm bandage.

DIFFICULTIES WITH DESTRUCTIVE METHODS FOR THE EYE

If he REFUSES TO HAVE A PAINFUL EYE enucleated or eviscerated, consider injecting absolute alcohol behind it to destroy its sensory nerves. You can use any strength of alcohol, provided it is more than 50%, but you may need to repeat the injection if pain returns. Permanent relief is uncertain.

Retrobulbar alcohol is very painful for about 30 seconds, so give him a retrobulbar block of lignocaine 1 ml (A 6.5). Remove the syringe and needle. When the block is effective, put another syringe on the needle and inject 2 ml of alcohol. His orbit will become severely oedematous for 10 days. Give him chloramphenicol eye drops 4 times daily for a week.

24.15 Other eye problems

Here are some of the other eye problems you may meet.

OTHER EYE PROBLEMS

If he has a BLIND, PAINFUL EYE, it may be better removed. See Section 24.14.

If CANNOT OPEN HIS EYE he has PTOSIS. This may be congenital (refer him), traumatic (refer him), acute as the result of an oculomotor palsy (refer him), or the result of myasthenia gravis (treat him).

If he has A SMALL YELLOWISH-WHITE LUMP adjacent to his cornea in the region exposed by his palpebral opening, he has a PINGECULA. It is harmless, reassure him.

If he has a wing-shaped vascular THICKENING OF HIS CONJUNCTIVA which grows on to his cornea, usually from the medial side (common), this is seldom serious. If his vision is good, leave it. If it is advancing over the centre of his cornea and impairing his vision, refer him. If you cannot refer him, under local anaesthesia excise the pterygium off his conjunctiva, and dissect it off his cornea. Leave his sclera bare, and gently diathermy it. Up to 50% recur.

If an old person has a complete or incomplete WHITE RING ENCIRCLING HIS CORNEA about 1 mm within the limbus, he has ARCUS SENILIS. It is harmless, reassure him.

If A PATIENT IS WORRIED ABOUT HIS EYES, they are both white, they have good visual acuity, and he is under 40 years old (that is, he is not presbyopic), and there is nothing obviously abnormal, you can reassure him that his eyes are normal.

25 The ear, nose, and throat

25.1 Introduction

The ear, nose, and throat have been particularly neglected in primary care, both by community health workers and in health centres. Most of the workers who provide it don't even possess an otoscope, let alone any batteries for one, and very few can even see the ear-drum. So do what you can to improve their standards. Here we are concerned with the patients they refer to you. A third of these may need a foreign body removed. You can also treat otitis media (25.3), and open the mastoid cortex to allow pus to drain, or perhaps do a cortical mastoidectomy (25.4). Unfortunately, a radical mastoidectomy for the many serious complications of acute-on-chronic mastoiditis is an expert's task.

You can treat a patient's bleeding nose (25.6), remove foreign bodies from it (25.5), treat frontal and maxillary sinusitis (25.7), and remove nasal polypi (25.10). About the only surgery you can do on the throat is to remove foreign bodies and drain pus (5.6, 5.7). Don't try to remove tonsils and adenoids; this is seldom justified, unless you are able to give plenty of blood if necessary. If you are skilled, and have a bronchoscope, you may be able to remove foreign bodies from his bronchi (25.13) and oesophagus (25.14).

Here are some of the common mistakes to avoid: (1) Don't use penicillin powder or drops in the ear: they cause sensitivity too easily. (2) Be very careful in using streptomycin or gentamicin parenterally; both are ototoxic, and may cause deafness and giddiness.

This is the equipment you will need:

- *HEADLIGHT, with forehead band and cords, 6 volt 3 watt bulb, and pin terminals to use with battery, one only. ALSO, 25 spare bulbs.* This is less effective than the ENT surgeon's traditional type of head mirror, but is easier to use.
- *HEAD MIRROR, with webbing or fibre headband, one only.*
- *EXAMINATION LAMP, Chiron, on base with castors, with Bedford Russell extending arm, one only (optional).* Ideally, you need this special spotlight with a head mirror, but you can use an ordinary 100 watt light bulb.
- *ANGLEPOISE LAMP, preferably with internally reflecting bulb giving a parallel beam, one only.*
- *OTOSCOPE, Keeler, new standard halogen type, with rechargeable handle, with: (a) 5 nylon specula, (b) mini-charger, state voltage (normally 240 volts), (c) adaptor for disposable specula, (d) box of disposable (but reusable) 3 mm specula, one outfit only.* This is the new Keeler standard otoscope with a rechargeable handle, a charger, and some disposable specula which you can reuse.
- *TUNING FORK, Hartmann's, with foot, 512 Hz, one only.*
- *PROBE, Jobson Horne, 178 mm, with one serrated and one ring end, one only.* Remove wax with the ring end, and wrap cotton wool round the serrated one.
- *HOOK, wax, St. Bartholomew's pattern, one only.* Remove wax and foreign bodies with this.
- *HOOK, Quire's, one only.* This marvellous instrument is sadly neglected, because it is so little known. You can use it in the nose, and sometimes in the ear, where it works better than an ordinary hook, because it does not have to be rotated to be inserted.
- *SYRINGE, aural, Bacon's, for one-hand use, one only.* This has a rubber bulb, a tube, and a valve. It delivers a steadier stream of fluid than a metal syringe, and can be used with one hand. If you don't have an ear syringe, use an ordinary 20 ml syringe with an eccentric nozzle. If you wish, you can fix a small plastic cannula to its tip, and cut it short to prevent it being pushed in too far.
- *FORCEPS, aural, alligator, Hartmann's, one pair only.*
- *FORCEPS, aural, Wilde, one only.* These are standard ear dressing forceps.
- *FORCEPS, aural, Omerod, elongated cup, crocodile action jaws, one only.*
- *FORCEPS, nasal, dressing, Tilley, one only.* You will need long narrow forceps to reach into the ear.
- *SPECULUM, nasal Thudichum, Mark Hovell modification, size 7, five only* Use these for examining the nose. Dangle one on the distal IP joint of your index finger, and control it between the sides of your middle and ring fingers.
- *SUCTION TUBE, Lempert, one only.*
- *TROCAR, antral, stainless steel with metal handle, Luer fitting, size 7, Tilley Lichwitz, one only. ALSO, rubber syringe with male mount for use with the antral trochar, one only.* Use this for washing out a patient's antrum. If the rubber bulb perishes, use a 20 ml syringe and attach this to the trocar with a piece of catheter.
- *MIRROR, laryngeal, with metal stem, boilable, 24 mm, one only.* You will need these to look at the larynx.
- *MIRROR, rhinoscopic, with metal stem, St Clair Thompson boilable, 14 mm, one only.* Use this for examining the nasopharynx.
- *LAMP, spirit, one only.* This is to warm a laryngeal mirror.
- *SNARE, polypectomy, nasal, Glegg's, (a) one snare only. (b) Five spare wires for the snare.* Using topical anaesthesia, pass the wire loop of this snare round the base of a polyp, gently pull it out and cut it off. If you don't have one, you can use Luc's forceps (see below).
- *FORCEPS, nasal turbinate, Luc's, one only.* If you fail to remove a polyp with a snare (unusual), you may need these.
- *TONGUE DEPRESSOR, Lack, adult, one only.*
- *DRESSINGS AND DRUGS.* (1) 5 mm selvage ribbon gauze, 50 metres only. (2) Magnesium Sulphate Paste BPC (magnesium sulphate 38% in phenol 0.5% in anhydrous glycerol), 1 kg only. The gauze is for packing the ear, impregnated with magnesium sulphate for boils.

For nausea and vertigo: (1) Tab prochlorperazine ('Stemetil') 5 mg. Give 5 to 10 mg three times daily. Ampoules 12.5 mg in 2 ml. Give 12.5 mg intramuscularly 6-hourly. (2) Tab. Cinnarizine ('Sturgeron') 15 mg, one or two tablets three times daily.

Silver nitrate applicator stick, for epistaxis (AVO), packet of 50 applicators, one packet only.

Drugs acting on the nose: (1) Ephedrine nasal drops BPC (ephedrine hydrochloride 1%). Put a half-full dropper into each nostril. (2) Beclomethasone dipropionate (a steroid) in metered 50 µg dose aerosol; 200 dose applicator. Three puffs into each nostril three times daily.

Bull TR, 'A Colour Atlas of ENT Diagnosis', Wolfe Medical.

Ludman H, 'ABC of ENT', British Medical Association 1971.

Bull PD, 'Lecture notes on Diseases of the Ear, Nose and Throat', (6th edn), Blackwell Scientific Publications.

25.2 Deafness

Severe deafness cripples a patient's mind by preventing him communicating with other people. It is thus a serious handicap, and, alas, a neglected one. About 5 million people in the world are profoundly deaf and a further 200 million partly so; as usual, most of them are in the developing world. Try to find out the incidence of deafness in your district, and the common causes for it. The most common one will probably be chronic suppurative otitis media of the tubotympanic, mucosal, or 'safe' type.

Deafness can be: (1) Conductive, due to disease in the external canal and middle ear cavity, up to the oval window. (2) Sensorineural, due to disease of the cochlea, eighth nerve or brain.

Much conductive deafness in the rural tropics is the result of chronic suppurative otitis media, which persists because of a patient's poor general health and nutrition. His middle ear becomes acutely infected, and his drum perforates. He fails to get the prompt, short (2 day), high doses of antibiotic (preferably ampicillin) that would cure him. Instead, his acute otitis media fails to resolve, his drum does not heal, his ear continues to discharge, and its ossicles are damaged. This is less likely to happen with the common tubotympanic 'safe' type of chronic otitis media, than it is with less common attic, bony, or 'unsafe' type (25.3). Unfortunately, chronic middle ear disease is not suited to the 'eye camp' approach, which is so successful in treating blindness due to cataracts.

Sensorineural deafness is usually high-tone and incurable, but a properly fitted hearing aid helps. You are unlikely to have an audiometer, so make good use of a tuning fork.

Prevent deafness by making sure that: (1) Middle ear disease is diagnosed and treated in primary care. (2) Anyone working in a very noisy environment wears ear plugs, or muffs. (3) In areas where genetic, early, progressive sensorineural deafness is common, as it is in parts of India, do what you can to discourage cousins from marrying one another.

Very many deaf people, of any age from infancy onwards, can be helped by a modern hearing aid, which usually helps conductive deafness, if there is not too much high frequency loss and no discharge. Unfortunately, hearing aids are expensive, and need to be fitted carefully; heat and moisture rapidly inactivate them, and batteries are difficult to get. One health worker advertised for second-hand ones in Europe, and received a hundred, mostly working. This source, and methods of finding, selecting, and importing the most suitable second-hand ones for particular patients, needs following up.

A useful source of information, and of hearing aids, is: The Commonwealth Society for the Deaf, 105 Gower Street, London WE1E 6AH.

DEAFNESS

EXAMINATION (adults)

Always do the next two tests as a pair; separately they will not give you the information you need. Unlike an audiometer, a tuning fork is robust.

RINNE'S TEST. Strike a tuning fork (512 Hz) gently against your knee or elbow (not against a hard surface, or unwanted overtones will be produced). Place the foot of the vibrating fork firmly on the patient's head, just above and behind the ear to be tested; press with sufficient pressure to need your other hand to support the other side of his head. Then place the fork, still vibrating, with the flat side of its tines towards his ear canal. Ask him "Which sound is loudest?" If air conduction is better than bone conduction, sound is being conducted normally to his cochlea, but he may still have a sensorineural loss. If bone conduction is better than air conduction, he has a problem with sound conduction (middle ear disease).

CAUTION ! Beware of the false negative Rinne test. If he has severe sensorineural deafness in one ear, bone conduction may be better than air conduction (wrongly indicating conduction deafness or middle ear disease), because the sound is conducted through his head, so that he hears it in his other ear. Weber's test will distinguish this.

WEBER'S TEST. Strike the tuning fork against your knee, place its foot on the top of his head, and ask him to say which ear

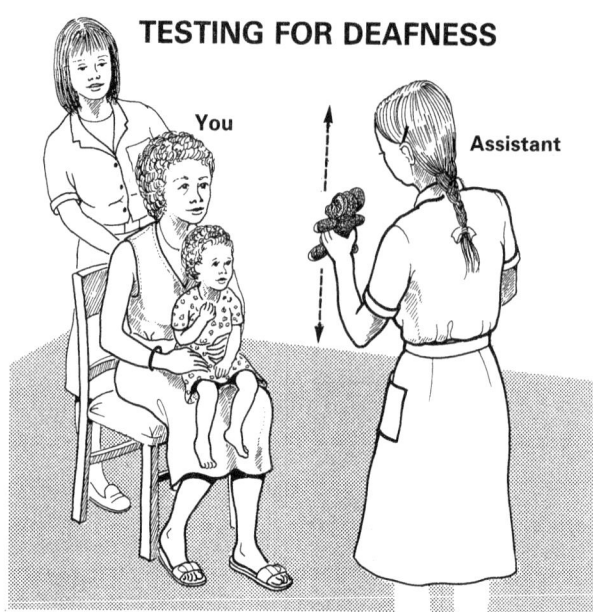

25-1 TESTING FOR DEAFNESS. Sit the child on his mother's knee facing your assistant. Meanwhile remain out of sight behind his mother.

hears the sound loudest. If he has conductive deafness in one ear (a negative Rinne's test, bone conduction heard better than air conduction), he will hear the tuning fork better in that ear. If he has sensorineural deafness, the sound will be loudest in his better functioning cochlea.

EXAMINATION (children)

In a child under 3 years neither a tuning fork nor an audiometer are useful. Unless you have special equipment you have to use: (1) His parents' account of an abnormal behaviour response, or his failure to make proper speech sounds. Or, (2) the distraction test, which is effective in most young children.

THE DISTRACTION TEST is a valid screening method. Find a sensitive and understanding assistant, and practise making the test noises, which are the syllables of the word "shoe", spoken separately as two tests, a high-pitched "Shsh..." and a low, sung "Ooo...". Make them softly, just loud enough for your assistant to hear.

Sit the child on his mother's knee facing your assistant. Meanwhile, remain out of sight behind his mother. Ask your assistant to gain the child's attention a little, by moving a toy up and down in a vertical line, while making the test sound. Then, ask him to hide the toy and break eye contact. At this exact moment, make a "Sh..." sound about 60 cm from the child's ear, and level with it, while you remain out of his sight. A normal child immediately turns towards the source of the sound. Reward him with some encouragement. Now test his other ear with an "Ooo" sound, before returning to the first ear with an "Ooo" sound, and then the second ear with a "Sh..." sound. To avoid false results, be sure to test his ears alternately.

If there is no response, try louder sounds. Then try a visual or tactile stimulus. If he still does not respond, suspect mental retardation, or some non-audiological problem. If he does respond, repeat the sound stimuli at 2 or 3 metres, first in a louder voice and then in a normal one.

CAUTION ! (1) This is a very reliable test—if you do it carefully. Otherwise, you can easily get false positives, and false negatives. (2) Before the test itself, practise both the manner of attracting the child's attention, and the sound to be made. (3) Timing is critical. (4) Make sure his mother does not give him any clues, consciously or unconsciously. (5) You will get a false positive if you show yourself, or let him see the test object either directly, or reflected in a window, or some reflective object, or give him some tactile clue. You will get a false negative if he is bored, tired, or distracted by other things. If this happens, don't persist; try again later.

THE MANAGEMENT OF DEAFNESS

The above tests should tell you where the lesion is. Here is a guide as to what it is.

IN THE EXTERNAL EAR conductive deafness can be caused by wax, and foreign bodies (25.5), or external otitis. Rarely, a tumour is responsible, or a child is born with a closed external canal.

IN THE MIDDLE EAR conductive deafness is caused by fluid in the middle ear (often associated with a cold), and acute or chronic otitis media. Otitis media is indicated by a discharging ear.

If he has conductive loss and his drum is normal, suspect otosclerosis, especially if he has a family history. This is not found in pure West Africans (or Japanese), and is rare in other Africans, but is not uncommon in Indians. A hearing aid is safer than stapedectomy by anyone but a real expert. 'Dead ears' are not uncommon, even after the 'best' surgery.

IN THE COCHLEA AND BEYOND sensorineural deafness is often congenital, but may be due to mumps, measles (not uncommon), rubella, other viruses, bacterial meningitis, and excessive noise ('boilermaker's deafness', 'disco deafness'; all Trinidad steel band players are profoundly deaf over 2 kHz). Commonly, it is due to old age (presbyacusis), sometimes Menière's syndrome (deafness, vertigo, and tinnitus), and very rarely to an acoustic neuroma. This probably never occurs in Africans—look for signs of involvement of his fifth and seventh nerves, and for imbalance due to involvement of his cerebellum.

In children, the severest acquired deafness follows meningitis. The deafness that follows mumps is usually unilateral, so it is not much of a handicap.

DIFFICULTIES WITH DEAFNESS

If a BABY IS BORN DEAF, this will usually be suspected by his family. A mother who says that her baby is deaf is usually right. Don't ignore her. His intelligence will probably be normal, and an 'island' of residual hearing may remain. His parents and older siblings must make the most of this. Instruct them like this: "Let him watch you speaking. Use speech and signs together, because you will not know which he will later find easiest. Speak slowly and clearly, and indicate familiar objects as you name them. If necessary, repeat the word close to his ear. Show you are pleased, whenever he tries to use a word, however indistinctly. Include him in as much play, and as many activities, as you can. As always, success builds on success".

CAUTION ! Children who are born deaf cannot learn to speak unless they heave special teaching, from their parents, or someone else, from as early in life as possible.

25.3 Otitis media and externa

Otitis externa exists in two types. A patient may have: (1) An infected hair follicle near the entrance of his meatus (a staphylococcal boil), which is very painful, because the skin here is tightly bound down to the perichondrium of the elastic cartilage of his ear. His boil is always near the entrance to his meatus, because there are no hair follicles to become infected in the deeper bony part. (2) A diffuse inflammation of his whole ear canal resembling eczema. The common causes are: (a) excessive self-cleaning of the ear, (b) 'stress' and (c) excessive humidity.

Acute otitis media is typically a disease of children. A child presents with acute earache, and fever; if he is very young, he may vomit, or have fits. At first, the margin of his drum and the handle of his malleus are red; later, his entire drum is red and bulges, so that it obscures his malleus. A few hours later his drum may burst, and give him instant relief. Otitis media is most common in children under one, and is often recurrent. *Haemophilus influenzae* or *Streptococcus pneumoniae* are usually responsible. Antibiotics are effective, if you give them in good doses promptly. There is no need to continue them beyond 48 hours.

Chronic otitis media is usually the result of failure to treat the acute stage. It too exists in two types.

The tubotympanic type is much more common, and is also known as the mucosal or 'safe' type, because it rarely leads to serious complications. The patient has a profuse mucopurulent discharge from his ear, without a very bad smell; he has a central perforation of his drum (a hole surrounded on all sides by drum), and moderate deafness. This type is the result of a low resistance to infection, due to poor health and nutrition.

The attic, bony type is also known as the 'unsafe' type, because it is more likely to lead to complications if the disease becomes advanced. A cyst lined with epidermis develops in the upper part of the patient's middle ear, and fills with scales to form a 'cholesteatoma'. This is surrounded by inflammatory tissue, and may erode through the bony walls of his middle ear and create a pathway for infection. He has a perforation on the edge of his drum, in its pars flaccida, or in its posterosuperior region. He has a small volume of very smelly discharge, and is usually severely, but variably, deaf. This type is common in India and South East Asia, but is less common elsewhere. Erosion and infection may spread: (1) Into his labyrinth, causing giddiness. (2) Through the roof of his middle ear, causing an extradural or subdural abscess in his temporal lobe, or in his posterior fossa. (3) To his lateral sinus, which may thrombose, and make him very ill with a high fever. (4) To his meninges; this is uncommon because infection is usually well localized. (5) To involve his facial nerve. Refer all these complications; he needs expert surgery, including a mastoidectomy, perhaps with tympanoplasty to preserve his hearing, and perhaps his life.

OTITIS

THE DIFFERENTIAL DIAGNOSIS of acute otitis media is mainly otitis externa (particularly a boil in the ear), and in young children, 'teething'.

Suggesting otitis externa—the patient is an adult with *normal hearing* (unlike otitis media), no fever or only a low fever, less malaise and prostration than with otitis media. He has *pain when his pinna and canal are moved*. He may also have a swollen, tender node just behind his ear. Don't confuse this with the tender bone of mastoiditis.

OTITIS EXTERNA

If he has a boil in his ear, give him a strong analgesic, and a high dose of an intravenous or intramuscular antibiotic, effective against penicillin-resistant staphylococci. Apply an ear wick of magnesium sulphate or glycerine and ichthammol.

CAUTION ! (1) Don't incise a boil *unless it is clearly fluctuant,* because there is a danger of perichondritis and collapse of his pinna. (2) A boil in the ear is very painful, so don't forget the analgesics.

If he has the diffuse form of otitis externa, keep his ear clean. Syringe it, and be sure to mop it dry afterwards. Give him antiseptic steroid ear drops. If he is a 'self-cleaner', treat the condition that is causing him to touch his ear, and persuade him to leave it alone.

If it is subacute or chronic, clean his ear with boracic or 50% spirit drops. If he also has a low-grade skin infection, give him a broad spectrum antibiotic systemically.

ACUTE OTITIS MEDIA

TREATMENT. Give antibiotics early. Give him a high dose of ampicillin or amoxycillin for 2 days. Or, less satisfactorily, give him penicillin. Aim for good compliance over this short period. If he is very unwell, give the antibiotic intramuscularly. Avoid chloramphenicol as a first choice, and use erythromycin only if he is allergic to penicillin. Relieve his pain, and apply local heat to his ear (the mother of one contributor, who had otitis media as a child, used to wrap a hot baked potato in a woolly sock and apply this to his ear—marvellous!). As soon as he is well, and his drum is no longer bulging, stop the antibiotics.

If his pain and fever continue, and his drum is still bulging after 24 hours of treatment, the organism is probably insensitive to the antibiotic you are giving him, or you are not giving him enough. Change the antibiotic or increase the dose.

If acute otitis media fails to resolve after 5 days of antibiotic treatment, change to another one. If this fails, stop: don't persist with antibiotics indefinitely. Some surgeons incise the drum (see below) when pain has not improved after 3 days of antibiotic treatment.

If you see a child after his drum has already perforated, and is discharging, culture the discharge and give him penicillin for a week. If necessary, change the antibiotic when the result becomes available. Teach his parents, or a nurse, to dry-mop the discharge with cotton wool ('Primary Child Care' Section 17.5). If this is not done often enough, otitis externa and a persistent discharge may follow. Monitor his hearing. If it does not return to normal, refer him. In the developed world, where otitis media is normally treated early, a persistent discharge after acute otitis media already suggests mastoiditis. It may not do so elsewhere.

If his mother has difficulty getting cotton wool to swab his ear, ask her to put a toilet paper wick (assuming she has any) into it for a minute, three times, and to repeat this three times a day.

CAUTION ! Don't attempt myringotomy (incising the drum)—it is not for the occasional operator, because you can easily dislocate the incudo-stapedial joint. The only absolute indication for it is acute otitis media, with a facial palsy (see below).

CHRONIC OTITIS MEDIA

DIAGNOSIS. This is the patient with a perforated ear-drum which discharges continuously or intermittently, and who may or may not give a history of a previous acute attack. Smell the discharge. An offensive, thick, pasty discharge is characteristic of a cholesteatoma, and thus of serious disease. His prognosis, and the urgency of referral, depend on where the perforation is in his drum, rather than on how big it is.

If the perforation does not extend to the edge of his drum, and does not involve its pars flaccida (the superior part of his drum), it is central and is not dangerous, because a cholesteatoma is rare. He complains of increasing deafness, recurrent discharge, and occasionally earache, but pain is rare. Referral is less urgent. Teach him the importance of a careful aural toilet.

If the perforation extends to the edge of his drum, and particularly if it involves the pars flaccida, it is marginal and is dangerous, because it implies bone destruction. A cholesteatoma is common. Try to refer him.

TREATMENT FOR CHRONIC OTITIS MEDIA. Mop out his ear canal, and try to see the peforation. If there is much discharge, rinse out his ear with warm sterile water or saline; mop his ear dry, and you will then be able to examine it. You can syringe a discharging ear, but it is probably wise not to syringe one with a cholesteatoma. Try to keep his ear mopped dry with cotton wool, in the hope that the perforation in his drum will heal. Spirit drops may dry it out.

He may develop any of the many complications listed under 'Difficulties with chronic otitis media' below.

DIFFICULTIES WITH ACUTE OTITIS MEDIA

If he has SEVERE EARACHE, WITH A NORMAL DRUM, suspect referred pain from dental caries, or an impacted wisdom tooth. If these are not responsible, suspect referred pain from his pharynx, or his temporomandibular joints. If an adult has earache, a normal drum, and an enlarged node in his neck, suspect that he has carcinoma of his pharynx (32.28), or larynx.

If you see a FLUID LEVEL or BUBBLES in a child's ear, with an indrawn drum, he has SEROUS OTITIS MEDIA (secretory otitis media). This may be the result of obstruction of his Eustachian tube by enlarged adenoids, and is common in children recovering from otitis media, or it may occur spontaneously. He usually has no pain, and little hearing loss. If there are bubbles or a fluid level, enough air remains to maintain his hearing; with all the air gone, deafness is more marked. Middle ear effusions usually resolve spontaneously, so wait several weeks if necessary. If his effusion persists, it may it may alter his behaviour, and impair his speech, even if it does not cause marked hearing impairment. If his school behaviour or progress is poor, or the acquisition of speech is affected, consider referring him for myringotomy, perhaps with the insertion of a grommet for ventilation.

If he has acute otitis media, and develops a FACIAL PALSY, myringotomy is essential. Refer him. Distinguish this from herpes zoster of the geniculate ganglion, which is excruciatingly painful, and is accompanied by vesicles in his meatus and on his drum.

If he has TENDERNESS, redness, and swelling over his mastoid process, he has ACUTE MASTOIDITIS. This is usually accompanied by persistent fever, and a red, bulging drum, with pus discharging through a perforation. Tenderness is acute *high* on the mastoid proces. Note that a meatal boil (furuncle) may also produce postauricular swelling, due to the infection of an adjacent lymph node. If he is an infant, acute mastoiditis causes a swelling above and behind his ear, displacing it outwards and *downwards*. If he has a boil in his meatus, the swelling is evenly distributed up and down his postauricular groove, displacing his ear outwards, but *not downwards*.

If AN ADULT DEVELOPS SEROUS OTITIS MEDIA for the first time, consider the possibility of obstruction of his Eustachian tube by a nasopharyngeal tumour.

If your workers delivering primary care are NOT ALLOWED TO USE ANTIBIOTICS, and so cannot use them to treat otitis media, instruct them like this. Clean the ear, syringe it with a rubber rat-tailed syringe, using water or, better, 30% spirit in saline. Then insert drops of 50% spirit. With the ear held uppermost for 2 minutes, insert 2 or 3 drops twice daily after cleaning. Although attic disease and a cholesteatoma should not be syringed, the risks in the routine use of this treatment are small.

DIFFICULTIES WITH CHRONIC OTITIS MEDIA

If he has a TENDER SWELLING OVER HIS MASTOID, he has ACUTE-ON-CHRONIC MASTOIDITIS, and needs a radical mastoidectomy. If you cannot refer him for this, do a cortical one (25.4). Temporary drainage may be lifesaving, and allow you more time to refer him.

If he has earache and fever with bilateral chronic discharge, the side with the ache is the side on which he has acute-on-chronic mastoiditis.

If he has chronic otitis media, and has earache, this is ominous. Pus is gathering under pressure somewhere, and, unless it is released, it may track internally, with serious results. If he also has fever, he needs referral for a radical mastoidectomy soon, *even if he has no signs of other complications.* Antibiotics *alone* will cure none of the complications; but always start them before you refer him.

If PERMANENT DEAFNESS develops as the result of bilateral chronic otitis media, he will need a hearing aid.

If he has chronic otitis media and develops a FACIAL PALSY, a cholesteatoma is invading his facial nerve. Refer him for radical mastoidectomy.

If he has a chronically discharging ear and suffers from SEVERE VERTIGO, perhaps with VOMITING, he has LABYRINTHITIS. These symptoms are worse when he moves his head. He usually also has fever and is unwell. Look for a fine horizontal nystagmus, and see if this is made worse when you close his ear canal with your finger, and gently press it (the fistula sign). Admit him, and give him penicillin in high doses, as described below, with chloramphenicol and metronidazole. He needs a radical mastoidectomy, as soon as his labyrinthitis has settled.

If he has a chronically discharging ear which suddenly becomes PAINFUL, and he has HEADACHES, VERTIGO, NECK STIFFNESS, or LOSS OF CONSCIOUSNESS, his condition is serious, because the infection has spread from his middle ear to his dura, meninges, or brain. Admit him, give him penicillin with chloramphenicol and metronidazole, and refer him rapidly.

If he becomes VERY ILL with severe headache, vomiting, and fever, he has MENINGITIS. Neck stiffness, photophobia, and a positive Kernig's sign will soon follow. Confirm the diagnosis by lumbar puncture. Examine his CSF by Gram's method, and culture it.

Either give him 600 mg penicilllin G intramuscularly every 4 hours for 3 days, then 6-hourly. And inject 10 000 units intrathecally every day. And give him chloramphenicol and metronidazole, as in Section 2.9.

Or, if you have no chloramphenicol, combine the penicillin with metronidazole and sulphadiazine 2 g 4-hourly.

Continue these drugs for 2 weeks, but stop the intrathecal penicillin after 3 days. Make sure he has an adequate fluid intake. When his meningitis has settled, he needs a radical, or failing that, a cortical mastoidectomy.

If, in addition to the signs of meningitis (above), he develops

NOMINAL APHASIA (difficulty in naming familiar objects), or PYRAMIDAL SIGNS, suspect a BRAIN ABSCESS. Refer him: he is best treated by drainage through a burr hole (a hazardous operation because of the nearness of the sigmoid sinus) and antibiotics, followed by a radical mastoidectomy.

If he has RIGORS, and is comparatively well in between, suspect LATERAL SINUS THROMBOSIS. Do a lumbar puncture, and when the manometer is in place compress his jugular vein, first on one side, and then on the other. If his CSF pressure rises on the normal side, but not on the side on which he has ear symptoms, his lateral sinus is thrombosed on that side (Queckenstedt's test). Give him high doses of penicillin, and refer him.

25.4 Acute mastoiditis

Acute mastoiditis is typically a disease of children, and may complicate neglected acute or chronic otitis media. It is rare where primary care is good. In babies, it occasionally presents as a swelling over the mastoid process.

If acute mastoiditis complicates acute otitis media (uncommon), the child continues to have fever, and his ear continues to discharge pus in increasing quantity through a perforation in his drum.

If acute mastoiditis complicates chronic otitis media, the patient has: (1) A dull nagging pain; this may either be a new pain, or an increase in an old pain. (2) Increasing discharge; he is so used to a discharge anyway, that he does not usually complain about this. (3) Increasing deafness. Chronic otitis media will already have made him deaf, and he may not notice that his deafness has been getting worse. (4) Tenderness over his mastoid process. (5) Sometimes, oedema of the skin over his mastoid process, due to underlying infection, giving it a 'velvety feel'. (6) A swelling in the posterosuperior wall of his meatus. (7) Anterior rotation of his pinna, so that his ear sticks out more on the affected side than on the normal one. This is a very characteristic sign, and should make you suspect the diagnosis, as you see him walking through the outpatient department; it can however also be caused by a swollen postauricular lymph node, by a meatal boil, or by cellulitis of his scalp.

Four operations are possible: (1) If pus has gathered under his periosteum you can simply open this and drain the pus. (2) You can open his mastoid cortex to allow pus to drain. (3) You can remove all the cortex overlying his mastoid antrum, and saucerize the opening, by removing some or all of the air cells of his mastoid (cortical mastoidectomy). Depending on how many air cells you open, this is potentially much more dangerous than simply opening his mastoid cortex—his dura, his sigmoid sinus, and his 7th nerve are all at risk. (4) If he has chronic mastoiditis, an expert can do a radical mastoidectomy.

ACUTE MASTOIDITIS

X-RAYS are seldom necessary. Normal mastoids differ greatly in the number of air cells they contain, so compare both sides for differences in density and structure. The early sign is diffuse haziness of the cells. After about 2 weeks the bony septa between them break down.

If a mastoid is sclerotic and its air cells poorly developed, suspect that the mastoiditis is acute-on-chronic. This makes mastoidectomy less urgent, which is fortunate, because it is more difficult.

THE DIFFERENTIAL DIAGNOSIS includes inflammation of the postauricular node, a boil in the patient's external auditory canal, and inspissated wax in his ear.

Suggesting mastoiditis, no pain on pulling his ear. Pain on deep pressure over the *upper* part of his mastoid at 11 o'clock in relation to his right external auditory meatus. Don't test for tenderness over the tip of his mastoid. A profuse mucopurulent discharge, a swelling on the *inner* bony part of his meatus at 11 or 12 o'clock, marked middle ear (conductive) deafness, and cloudy mastoid air cells on the X-ray.

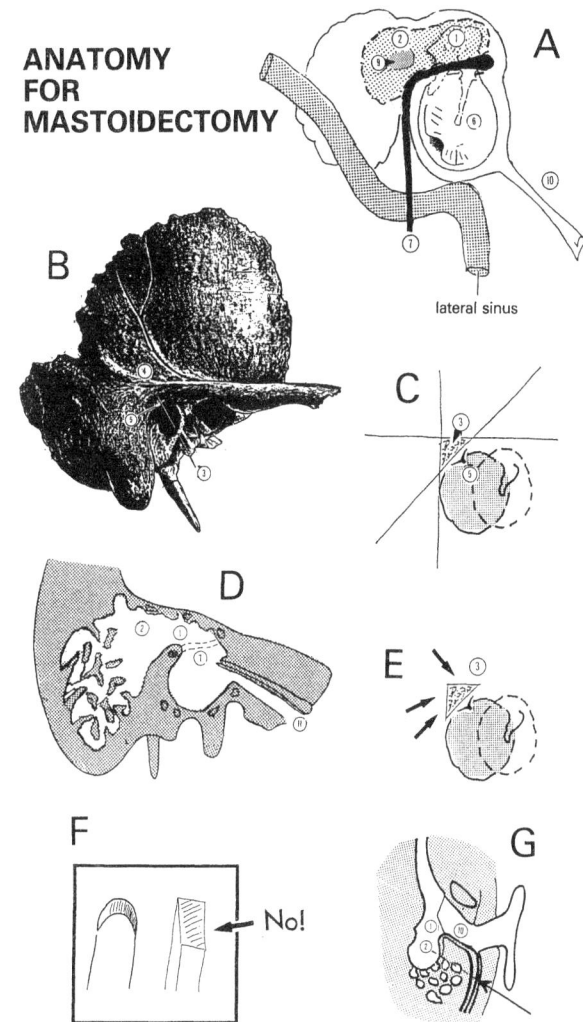

Fig. 25-2 ANATOMY FOR MASTOIDECTOMY. A, a schematic view of the tympanic antrum with the horizontal semicircular canal in its medial wall. B, the squamous temporal bone, showing the position of the suprameatal (MacEwen's) triangle. C, a diagrammatic view of this triangle bordered by the three tangents, showing the drum lying anteriorly. D, the cavity of the middle ear and its connecting air spaces. E, gouge into the triangle from these directions. F, use a gouge not a chisel. G, a horizontal section through the external auditory meatus, showing the approach to the mastoid. Note that the meatus runs anteromedially.

1, the attic. 2, the antrum. 3, the suprameatal triangle. 4, the posterior extension of the zygomatic process (the suprameatal ridge). 5, the spine of Henle. 6, the handle of the malleus. 7, the facial nerve. 8, the lateral sinus. 9, the lateral semicircular canal. 10, the external auditory canal. 11, the eustachian tube. *Kindly contributed by Christopher Holborrow, Ian Kennedy and Patrick Beasley.*

CAUTION ! The mastoid is always tender during the first few days of an attack of otitis media, before the drum has burst. Only diagnose acute mastoiditis, when tenderness and fever appear in a patient who has had a discharge for several weeks (mastoiditis is uncommon in acute otitis media).

Suggesting postauricular lymphadenitis and swelling of the tissues round it—some septic lesion on his scalp or neck, particularly infected ringworm or impetigo, or following lice in his scalp; his pinna may be pushed forwards; no discharge or deafness, a normal drum. Swollen lymph nodes are usually at 8 or 9 o'clock in relation to his right ear, whereas the swelling of mastoiditis is at maximal at about 11 o'clock.

Suggesting a boil (furuncle) in his external auditory meatus (25.3, rare in a child)—swelling in the *outer* cartilaginous part of his meatus, and his mastoid is not tender. His hearing is diminished if his meatus is blocked, but becomes normal if you are able to open it by pulling his pinna upwards and backwards. Pain on pulling his ear and on chewing, a history of other boils, thick scanty discharge. If you can see his drum, it is normal. If the boil is on the posterior wall of his meatus, his pinna may be pushed forwards. X-rays show a normal mastoid.

DRAINING THE PERIOSTEUM FOR ACUTE MASTOIDITIS

If pus has already found its way to the surface of his mastoid, and is lying under his periosteum, there is no need to do a cortical mastoidectomy. Incise the skin and periosteum close behind his ear as in A, Fig. 25-3, but stop there. Insert a drain for a few days. If his infection does not resolve, deeper drainage or cortical mastoidectomy will be necessary.

DRAINING THE MASTOID CORTEX FOR ACUTE MASTOIDITIS

If you cannot refer him and do not feel able to do a cortical mastoidectomy, be content with draining his mastoid cavity. *This could be life-saving!* Incise behind his ear, as described below, and open his periosteum—there may be pus under it. Then use a gouge to open the cortex of the bone for about 1 cm, and expose some of his mastoid air cells, which will be full of pus. Dress the wound as described below.

CORTICAL MASTOIDECTOMY FOR ACUTE MASTOIDITIS

INDICATIONS. Acute mastoiditis. Draining the mastoid is not quite the urgent operation that it was in the days before antibiotics, so give them and try to refer him. If you cannot refer him, give him antibiotics for 2 to 4 days, and operate when his infection has settled a little. His mastoid must be drained soon, to reduce the risk of infection spreading to cause thrombophlebitis of his lateral sinus, or a brain abscess.

ANTIBIOTICS are necessary. The most suitable ones are likely to be chloramphenicol with metronidazole.

THE EQUIPMENT includes bone gouges and a mallet, a periosteal elevator, a self retaining retractor, a headlight and suction (both essential), curettes (preferably Collier and Morris), and bone wax (3.1) to control bleeding.

CAUTION ! Use a gouge; the angle of a chisel is more likely to enter his dura or his lateral sinus.

ANAESTHESIA. (1) Ketamine (A 8.1). (2) General anaesthesia (A 10.1).

INCISION. Shave the hair behind his ear. Lay him on his back, with his head on a sandbag, turned towards the other side. Put two towels under his head, and fold the upper one round it. Feel for the site of his suprameatal triangle, just inferior to the posterior end of his zygomatic process. Make a curved incision about 0.5 cm behind his pinna, and following the same curve. Start it just beyond his zygomatic process superiorly, and extend it just beyond the tip of his mastoid inferiorly.

CAUTION ! (1) Don't extend the incision beyond the tip of an infant's mastoid, because his facial nerve is very superficial just there, and you may cut it. There is no real mastoid tip in a baby; the incision must be high. (2) Don't include his temporalis muscle in the upper part of the incision, because it will bleed unnecessarily.

Deepen the incision down to the bone. You will see his temporalis muscle at the upper end of the wound, and his sternomastoid at the lower end. Use a periosteal elevator to raise them both, with his periosteum. Elevate his periosteum forwards, as far as the lateral end of his posterior bony meatal wall, backwards for a few millimetres, and upwards with his temporalis muscle, to the level of the upper attachment of his pinna. Expose a wide enough area of bone to identify the following three landmarks:

(1) Henle's spine, at the junction of the superior and posterior bony walls of the meatus. Define the edge of the canal carefully, and you will find this spine. It overlies the entrance to the mastoid antrum, which lies about 12 mm below the surface in an adult: follow the posterior meatal wall inwards to find it.

(2) The suprameatal ridge, which is a posterior prolongation of the zygomatic process, and marks the lower limit of the dura of his middle fossa.

(3) His antrum lies under a well-defined pitted triangle, the suprameatal (MacEwen's) triangle (C, Fig. 25-2) formed: (a) Superiorly by his suprameatal ridge (and the superior tangent of his external auditory meatus); (b) Anteriorly by an oblique tangential line across his posterior meatal wall at the spine of Henle; and (c) Posteriorly, by a vertical tangent to the posterior wall of his meatus.

Insert a self-retaining retractor to keep the flaps away from the field of operation, and to help control bleeding.

Remove the cortex of his mastoid with a gouge and hammer in the directions shown in E, Fig. 25-2. Remove chips of bone little by little. Chip forwards towards his external auditory meatus, away from the place where his lateral sinus is nearest the surface. If you chip too far backwards, you will enter it. Start working widely and shallowly with the largest gouge, and gradually deepen the cavity with smaller ones, until you reach his antrum. The bone usually changes colour as you reach it. You may have to chip away quite a lot of bone. If pus is working its way to the surface, his antrum will be easier to find.

CAUTION ! (1) As long as you keep below the superior tangent of his external auditory meatus, you will be safe. There is not always a very clear depression in the suprameatal triangle, but if you work into its centre behind Henle's spine, you will reach the antrum. (2) Remember that the antrum lies about 12 mm deep in a adult, but is only a few millimetres deep in an infant. (3) If you reach his dura, STOP! Don't remove any more bone, or you may damage it. If you do, you may cause meningitis, or uncontrollable bleeding from his lateral sinus. (4) Take special care not to damage the medial, or the anteromedial, wall of his antrum, because you may damage his lateral semicircular canal, or his facial nerve. (5) Remember that the tip of the long process of his incus is in the floor of the entrance to his antrum–don't disturb it. (6) Preserve his posterior meatal wall, and don't dissect the skin from it.

As soon as you remove the cortex of his temporal bone, pus may flow from his mastoid air cells. Use swabs and a curette to carefully remove all pus, granulation tissue, and loose pieces of necrotic bone from his antrum and mastoid air cells. Chip

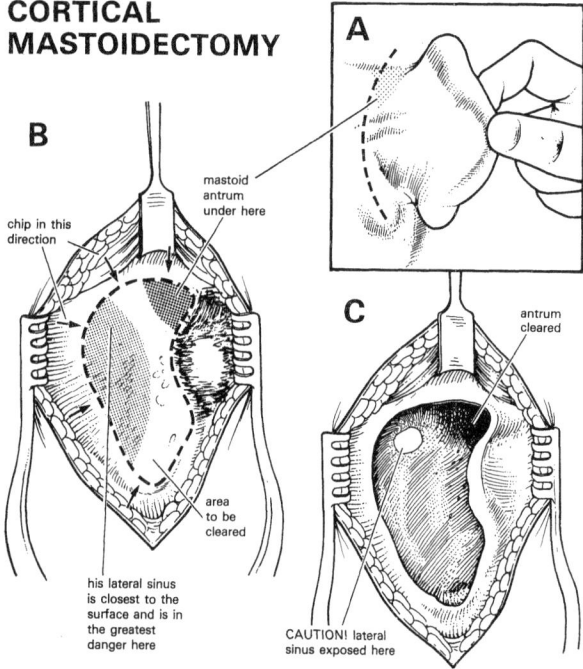

Fig. 25-3 CORTICAL MASTOIDECTOMY. A, the incision behind a child's pinna, showing the approximate position of his antrum. B, the surface of his bone has been cleared. This diagram also shows the surface markings of his mastoid antrum, the area to be cleared, and the danger area where his lateral sinus is closest to the surface, and thus in the greatest danger of being injured. Gouge away from it towards his external auditory meatus. C, the surface of his temporal bone has been chipped away and the more superficial air cells cleared. Note that his cleaned out antrum is the deepest part of the wound. His lateral sinus is more at risk lower down.

and scrape away bone containing air cells, including his antrum, which is the deepest area to be cleaned.

Make the bony cavity saucer-shaped, so that the flaps will fall into it and obliterate it. Syringe it with warm saline, insert a corrugated drain, and start to shorten this after 48 hours.

25.5 Foreign bodies in the ear

Foreign bodies in the ear are more difficult and dangerous to remove than those in the nose—the dangers include a perforated drum, total deafness, and a facial palsy, or all three. So refer the patient if you can. The middle (isthmus) of the auditory canal is narrower than either its outer, or its inner end. If a foreign body is impacted outside the isthmus, removing it should not be difficult. Try syringing first. If this fails and you cannot refer him, and you have to use instruments, be sure to anaesthetize him first, especially if he is a child. The foreign body may be a seed, a live cockroach, a piece of paper or a broken matchstick. Two-thirds of patients are usually under five years.

MOHAMMED ASLAM (10 years), the son of a local VIP was admitted with a ball-bearing in his ear. The consultant ENT surgeon was on leave, and so a junior took the case over. It seemed a pity to give the child a general anaesthetic, and as he seemed co-operative, it was decided to remove the ball-bearing with a wax hook. Unfortunately, after two unsuccessful attempts, during which the ball-bearing was driven deeper in, some bleeding began, which other obscured the view, but the ball-bearing was eventually removed. However, in the blood clot were found the remains of his malleus, his incus, and his stapes. LESSONS (1) If you are inexperienced, simpler methods may be safer, even if they are less dramatic. Syringing is not clever, but it is 'brilliant' compared with inadvertent stapedectomy. (2) The less experienced you are, the more necessary is it to remove a foreign body under general anaesthesia. A struggling child is no subject for delicate surgery.

FOREIGN BODIES IN THE EAR

First try to syringe the patient's ear, if necessary under ketamine, as if you were removing wax. Use a 20 ml syringe, or an ear syringe containing water at body temperature. Pull his ear upwards and backwards, and direct the stream of water up along the roof of his ear canal, so that it gets behind the foreign body and pushes it out. Syringing will remove most foreign bodies.

If syringing fails (rare), try gentle suction with a piece of catheter on the end of the sucker. If this too fails, refer him.

If you cannot refer him, admit him and *always* anaesthetize him. Ketamine is ideal. A foreign body is seldom urgent, so you have time to starve him.

Lay him down, and use a forehead mirror, and a good source of light. Or use an auriscope with a large speculum and an open lens. Rest your hand on his head. Use an aural hook, a cerumen hook, or a paper clip bent exactly as shown in Fig. 25-4, smoothed with a file or on a stone, and held in mosquito forceps. Put the hook into his auditory canal, so that it lies against the wall. Then, when it is past the foreign body, twist it, so that it lies behind it, and allows you to pull it out.

CAUTION ! Be very gentle so as: (1) Not to push the foreign body beyond the isthmus of his auditory canal, and (2) not to damage his tympanic membrane. (3) Don't try to use dissecting forceps.

If it has gone beyond the isthmus, so that you cannot remove it with a hook, make a small vertical incision from the back of his pinna at its attachment to his mastoid, through into his ear canal; hold his pinna forwards, and remove the foreign body under direct vision. An incision like this does not get you a long way in, but it may help. Inspect his drum and close the incision with 2 monofilament sutures. Then pack his canal with ribbon gauze to prevent oedema and granulations. If possible impregnate the gauze with 'BIPP' (Bismuth and Iodoform Paste). Remove the pack in 5 days.

DIFFICULTIES WITH FOREIGN BODIES IN THE EAR

If there is an INSECT IN HIS EAR, put a few drops of oil into his ear to kill it, then try syringing it out. If this fails, which is seldom, anaesthetize him.

If a VEGETABLE FOREIGN BODY SWELLS, and jams in the

REMOVING A FOREIGN BODY FROM THE EAR

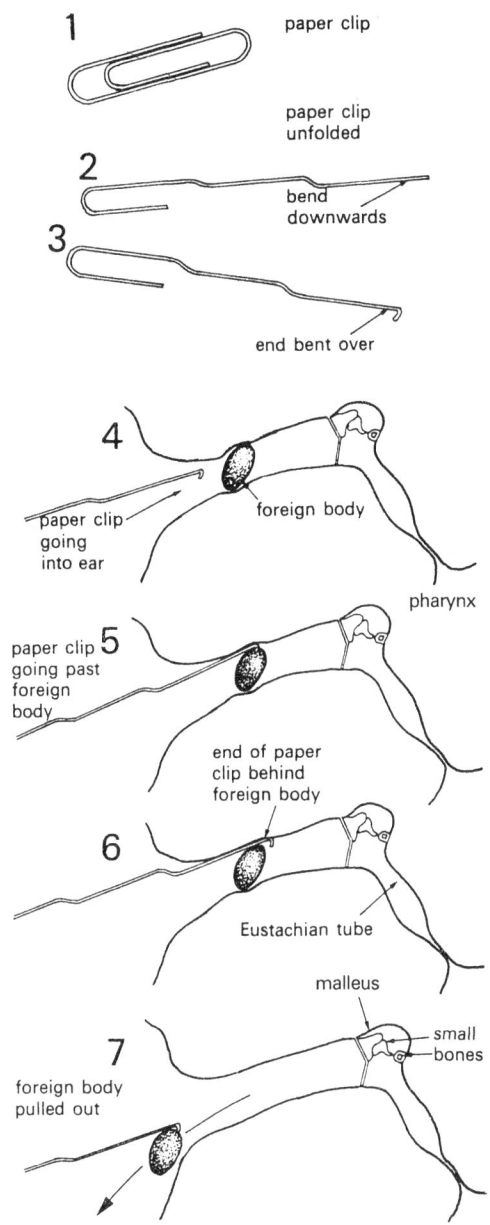

Fig. 25-4 REMOVING A FOREIGN BODY FROM THE EAR. Start by trying to syringe it out. If this fails, and if you don't have the proper hook, you can use a bent paper clip. Bend it exactly as shown and hold it in mosquito forceps. Be sure you anaesthetize the patient first.

canal, leave it and try again later.

If his TYMPANIC MEMBRANE IS RUPTURED, try to prevent infection, and let it heal spontaneously. Keep it completely dry for 6 weeks. Don't dust it with antibiotics, or pack the canal. Mopping is unnecessary, unless his middle ear discharges; if so treat him as for otitis media. A drum may rupture during unskilled attempts to remove a foreign body, or as the result of an explosion, or a blow, or by penetration with a sharp object.

CAUTION ! Don't syringe a ruptured drum, and do as few manipulations as possible.

25.6 Epistaxis

A bleeding nose can be a very unnerving emergency; if you don't treat a patient correctly, it can be fatal. The measures described here will control the severest bleeding, but it commonly recurs.

Nose bleeds are rare in infancy, common in childhood, uncommon in young adults, and more common again in the elderly. Most bleeding is easily controlled, and has no obvious cause. Blood usually comes from the anterior septal vessels in the front of the nasal septum (Little's area, F, in Fig. 25-5). You can see these with a nasal speculum and a good light (try the sun) behind you; you will see them better with a head mirror. When bleeding comes from anywhere else, it usually comes from far back in the patient's nose. This is difficult to get at, and he is usually both elderly and hypertensive.

Try the simpler methods first. If you teach them to your nurses and auxiliaries, they will be able to treat most patients. You will need suction, and if possible a headlight and BIPP (4.11).

NOSE BLEEDING

EXAMINATION. Sit the patient upright looking straight ahead. Ask an assistant to stand behind him, and hold his head. If he is bleeding from the anterior half of his nasal cavity, most of the blood will come from his nostrils. If he is bleeding from the posterior half, much of it will be trickling down his pharynx.

A child is almost certainly bleeding from his anterior septal vessels; so are most adults. In the remaining cases, the bleeding is posterior, and is occasionally caused by a systemic disease.

DIFFERENTIAL DIAGNOSIS. Did the blood come first from his nostrils, or his nasopharynx? This will be some help in deciding where he is bleeding. Apart from obvious hypertension, there is usually no time to speculate on the cause. Other causes include trauma, a foreign body, tumours, onyalai, leukaemia, scurvy, purpura, and the prodromal stages of diphtheria, measles, varicella, and scarlet fever.

IMMEDIATE TREATMENT. Sit him forwards a little, drape him in a mackintosh, and hold his nose over a receiver. Tell him not to swallow the blood, but to spit it out. *Avoid a stomach full of blood!* If he cannot sit up lay him on his side.

Squeeze his nose, so that you press its soft mobile parts against his septum, while he breathes with his mouth wide open. Do this yourself, or delegate a nurse to do it. If bleeding is more than minimal, keep pressing for 5 minutes by the clock. If it is minimal, ask him to do it himself. If necessary, sedate him. If squeezing fails, try it again. If you wait long enough the bleeding will usually stop, and you will have done nothing to damage his mucosa.

If you decide that bleeding is not going to stop, put up a drip, take blood for cross-matching, and give him pethidine 50 or 100 mg intramuscularly, or slowly intravenously. He will now tolerate your manipulations more easily. Proceed with anterior packing.

ANTERIOR BLEEDING FROM THE NOSE

ANAESTHESIA. All packing, intranasal manipulation or cauterization needs local anaesthesia, either by spray (A 5.8), or on a gauze or wool swab wet with 4% lignocaine.

ANTERIOR PACKING aims to provide a focus for the development of a firm clot close to the bleeding point. You will need a head mirror, with a good light shining on to it from behind his shoulder, a nasal speculum, and dressing forceps, preferably Tilley's. If you don't have a head mirror, a good light behind you will do. For each side of the nose you will need about a metre of 13 mm gauze packing, or a 13 mm roller bandage. To make this easier to remove later, smear it with vaseline, or 'BIPP' (4.11). If you lack BIPP, soak it in 1/100,000 adrenalin solution.

Pack the nostril which is bleeding most. Sit him upright, and ask an assistant to stand behind him and hold his head. Warn him that he will find the procedure very uncomfortable. Clear his nasal cavities by asking him to blow his nose, or clear his bleeding nasal cavity with a sucker and cannula. Your previously applied lignocaine pack should have produced some anaesthesia.

Focus your light on the speculum, and put it into his bleeding nostril. Grasp the end of the gauze with forceps and place it

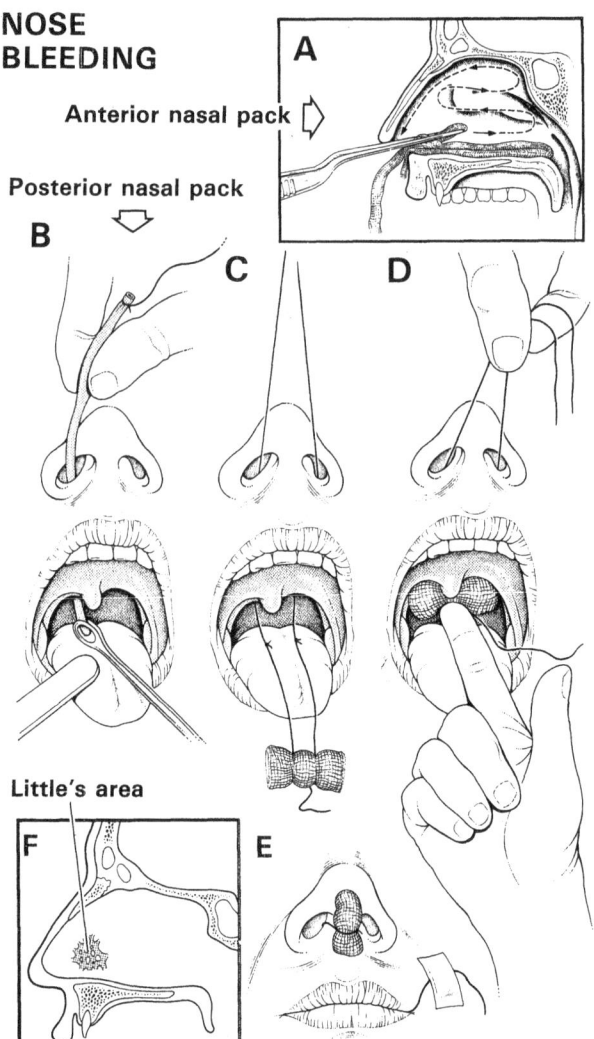

Fig. 25-5 EPISTAXIS. A, inserting an anterior nasal pack. B, to E, inserting a posterior nasal pack. B, passing a catheter. C, a gauze roll ready to be pulled into place. D, pushing the gauze roll into place. E, the gauze roll tied in place. F, a patient's anterior septal vessels (Little's area) have about a 50% chance of being the source of the bleeding. *After Loré JM, 'An Atlas of Head and Neck Surgery', Plate 51 WB Saunders, with kind permission.*

as high and as far back as you can. Try to pack his nasal cavity in an orderly way in horizontal layers, starting on its floor and working towards its roof. This is difficult, and you will probably find yourself putting gauze wherever it will go, until his nose is full. Leave both ends of the gauze protruding from his nostrils. If necessary, pack both sides of his nose, and secure all the four ends of the gauze with a safety pin. Strap a pad of folded gauze across the front of his nose, and wait a few minutes.

If an anterior pack controls bleeding, leave it in place for 48 hours. Then gently remove it, preferably early in the day, so that you can more easily repack his nose if necessary. Observe him carefully for 24 hours before you discharge him.

If an anterior pack does not control bleeding, remove it, insert a posterior one, and then repack his anterior nasal cavity as above.

CAUTERIZATION (optional). Soak a small piece of ribbon gauze in 4% lignocaine and adrenalin solution, squeeze out the excess, and apply this to the bleeding area for 10 minutes, or use a local anaesthetic spray. Use a nasal speculum, or a wide-bore aural speculum, and a good light, to find the bleeding vessels in Little's area. Touch them along their course with an applicator that has had a bead of silver nitrate fused to its tip. His mucosa will turn white.

If you fail to control bleeding, reinsert the lignocaine and adrenalin pack. If this too fails, hold a silver nitrate stick over the bleeding area for a few moments, and then roll it away to one side before you remove it (if you pull it off, bleeding may restart).

If you fail again, try a galvanocautery with a hot wire loop. If necessary, use any thin wire heated in a spirit lamp. Gently touch the bleeding area. You can also use diathermy, preferably under general anaesthesia. Leave the scab, and dress it with vaseline.

CAUTION ! (1) Don't cauterize both sides of his nasal septum at one time with silver nitrate or heat, because it may perforate.

POSTERIOR BLEEDING FROM THE NOSE

POSTERIOR PACKING may be necessary if: (1) An anterior pack fails to control anterior bleeding. (2) There is severe posterior bleeding.

Take him to the theatre. Spray his pharynx and palate with 4% lignocaine.

Use a Foley catheter (often very effective). Start with this. Pass a Foley, with a reasonably sized balloon, gently through his anaesthetized nostril, until you see its tip just behind his soft palate. Inflate the balloon with air, and gently withdraw the catheter, so that the balloon impacts in his posterior nasal opening. Tape it to his cheek, then pack his nose from in front as described above.

CAUTION ! (1) Don't inflate the balloon in his nasal cavity, because this can quickly cause pressure necrosis of his mucosa, which may make bleeding worse. (2) The tube of the catheter can ulcerate the rim of his nasal entrance, so spread out the pressure by putting a little gauze pad under it.

Use a pack of folded or rolled gauze sponges of sufficient bulk to plug his posterior nares. If possible give him a general anaesthetic, and intubate him. You will need two packs, of at least 5 cm square for an adult. Tie 50 cm of soft string, or umbilical tape, to a small (18 Ch) rubber catheter, as in B, Fig. 25-5. Put this into one nostril, and pull it out of his mouth, leaving the string in place. Do the same thing on the other side.

Tie the oral ends of the strings to the pack, and tie a third piece of string to it. Pull the pack up into the back of his nose, and press it into place with your finger in his throat. Make sure that it has gone behind his soft palate, and that this has not folded upwards.

Then pack his anterior nasal cavity, as above.

Tie the nasal ends of the string over some gauze. Let the third string protrude from the corner of his mouth, and tape it to his cheek. Or keep it in place with a plastic umbilical cord clamp.

CAUTION ! (1) Insert packs with great gentleness: you can easily cause more bleeding as you insert them. (2) Withdraw the packs, or the Foley catheter, slowly after 48 hours. Don't leave any pack or catheter, either anterior or posterior, in his nose for longer than this, or you will increase the risk of suppuration, especially in his sinuses. The only possible exception is a pack impregnated with 'BIPP' (4.11), which you can leave for a week. If you are using a Foley, deflate it a little first to see if bleeding is controlled. (3) Remove a pack slowly, bit by bit.

When you remove a posterior pack, do so in the theatre, with a light and the necessary equipment ready, so that you can if necessary repack without delay.

Because epistaxis may recur when you allow him home, make sure he knows how to hold his nose, to breathe through his mouth, and to sit forwards in the correct position.

GENERAL MEASURES FOR EPISTAXIS

Try to estimate how much blood he has lost. If he has been bleeding severely, watch for signs of shock. Keep him propped up in bed. Give him aspirin or paracetamol, if necessary. Pethidine or morphine can be helpful. Monitor his blood pressure, his respiration, and his haemoglobin. Most severe epistaxes are precipitated by infection, so give him a broad-spectrum antibiotic (ampicillin or chloramphenicol and metronidazole, 2.9) for at least 5 days. If you have to transfuse him, use *fresh* blood.

DIFFICULTIES WITH EPISTAXIS

If anterior and/or posterior PACKING FAILS, make sure that the packs have not become loose. If so, replace them. Use not less than a metre of ribbon in each nostril. It is not possible to bleed through proper packing.

If he has been properly packed and CONTINUES TO BLEED whenever the packs are removed, anaesthetize and intubate him (you should be removing them in the theatre anyway). Failure of packs to control bleeding on one occasion is common, but they usually work eventually. The ultimate measure is to tie the arteries supplying his nose: (1) Start with his anterior ethmoidal, which is the easiest. (2) Alternatively, tie his external carotid (3.3). There is such an extensive collateral circulation that this often fails to help. (3) His internal maxillary artery can also be clipped, behind the posterior wall of his antrum, but this is an expert's task.

To tie his anterior ethmoidal artery, make a small incision 1 cm medial to his inner canthus. Cut down to bone, raise his periosteum, particularly posteriorly, so as to make a passage along the medial wall of his orbit. As you raise his periosteum, you will find it tethered at the point where his anterior ethmoidal artery crosses from his orbit to enter bone. Carefully dissect it. Diathermy it, clip it, or tie it with a small suture.

If he BLEEDS PERSISTENTLY, check for signs of a bleeding disorder. Look for petechiae, ecchymoses, and a large spleen. If possible, measure his clotting (16.13) and bleeding times, his prothrombin index, and his blood urea. If you find any abnormality, investigate him further. He may have leukaemia or thrombocytopenia, etc. Don't pack his nose. Instead, control the ooze by soaking oxidized cellulose sponges in topical thrombin solution (if you have it), and place these in his nose. If this fails or you cannot do it, you will have to pack his nose. He may die.

If HE IS ELDERLY, suspect that his bleeding nose may be serious. Enquire carefully for a history of illness, trauma, medication, or a bleeding disorder. If he is hypertensive, bleeding may be difficult to stop. He too may die.

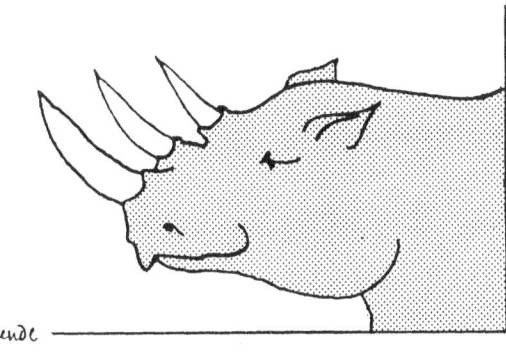

Augmentation rhinoplasty?

25.7 Blocked nose and the general method for sinusitis

The sinuses lead off the nose, so that disease in them usually follows disease in the nose. Sinusitis has some common features, regardless of which particular sinus is infected, so we will discuss these first, and deal with frontal (25.8) and maxillary (25.9) sinusitis later.

The common presenting symptoms in a patient's nose are: (1) discharge, (2) obstruction of his nasal airway, and (3) facial discomfort or pain.

Nasal obstruction is usually due to engorgement of the erectile vascular tissue in the mucosa over his inferior turbinates due to: (1) Labile control of his mucosal vessels, as the result of a wide variety of 'constitutional' and environmental factors. His mucosa swells and obstructs his airway, often with a watery nasal discharge, and bouts of sneezing. Psychosomatic factors may also affect the nose ('honeymoon rhinitis'). (2) An inherited atopic state. (3) Reaction to a specific allergen. (4) A foreign body can also obstruct his nose (25.11), as can (5) infection and (6) nasal polypi (25.10).

Facial pain or discomfort may be due to sinus disorders. Engorgement of his nasal mucosa may obstruct the natural ventilation of his sinuses, and cause a feeling of pressure in his cheeks, or forehead.

Acute sinusitis often follows a viral upper respiratory infection, and usually involves one of a patient's sinuses only. He presents with fever, a copious purulent discharge, and: (1) Pain, or a sense of pressure in his cheek (sometimes wrongly thought to be 'toothache'). (2) Obstruction of his nasal airway, often without the discharge of mucus or pus. (3) Swelling of his face (this is much more likely to be due to a dental abscess, 5.8). Tenderness over an infected sinus is not a useful sign.

Chronic sinusitis may follow acute sinusitis, if his resistance is low, or if he has nasal polypi, which prevent his sinuses draining. Pain is not a major feature, but he may have a dull ache in his face, usually later in the day. Bending his head forward can be uncomfortable.

BLOCKED NOSE AND SINUSITIS

BLOCKED NOSE

See also frontal (25.8) and maxillary sinusitis (25.9).

DIAGNOSIS. Exclude polypi (25.10) and foreign bodies (25.11).

MANAGEMENT. Enquire for psychosomatic factors and do your best to allay them.

If there is no more treatable cause, try a nasal steroid spray (beclomethazone, 'Beconase', or budesonide, 'Rhinocort') puffed into each nostril 3 or 4 times twice daily. Continue for 2 weeks before assessing its benefit. Try this for 3 or 4 weeks, and only continue it if there is improvement.

ACUTE SINUSITIS

TREATMENT. Give him a broad-spectrum antibiotic (ampicillin or amoxycillin), and an analgesic (sinusitis is painful). Nasal decongestant drops are not helpful, and are uncomfortable to instil in the head-down position.

CHRONIC SINUSITIS

EXAMINATION. Look for: (1) Obstruction (usually on one side only). (2) A discharge from the front of his nose, and a bead of yellow pus high above his inferior turbinate. (3) Pus on the dorsum of his soft palate. (4) Also, look at his handkerchief (if he has one), which may be stiff from dried pus (this does not happen with a watery discharge).

TREATMENT. Give him a broad-spectrum antibiotic, and encourage him to blow through his nose without pinching it to restrict his airway. The Venturi effect of doing this will draw pus out of his infected sinus. If he does not improve, wash out his antrum under local anaesthesia (25.9).

DIFFICULTIES WITH THE NOSE

If he presents with dull red mucous membranes, and his nose contains many dried crusts, suspect CHRONIC ATROPHIC RHINITIS. There is little you can do for him, except not to mistreat him. This mostly means not giving him vasoconstrictor sprays and drops (including ephedrine), and persuading him not to buy them himself. They will only give him temporary relief, after which his symptoms will get worse. He will get some relief from a saline solution, sniffed as many times a day as is practical.

25.8 Frontal sinusitis

Frontal sinusitis starts with localized pain above a patient's eye. If he presents late, he may have gross orbital swelling, proptosis, and diplopia. If large doses of penicillin, chloramphenicol, and metronidazole do not control his symptoms rapidly, you may have to drain his frontal sinus. Frontal sinusitis is always secondary to maxillary sinusitis and obstruction of his frontonasal duct, so be sure to wash out his antrum.

FRONTAL SINUSITIS

See also Sections 5.5 (infections in the orbit), 7.14 (osteomyelitis of the cranium), and 24.11 (proptosis).

EXAMINATION. Examine the patient's nasal cavity for pus, a deflected nasal septum, and signs of past surgery. Look for associated abnormalities in his maxillary antrum by transillumination (25.9). Antral puncture may reveal pus in it.

X-RAYS. Take an erect film, and look for increased density of the shadow of his frontal sinus on the abnormal side, and a fluid level. A bilateral opacity suggests mucosal thickening, a unilateral one is more likely to be pus.

NON-OPERATIVE TREATMENT. Give him large doses of penicillin and 0.5% ephedrine nose drops instilled in the Moffat position (25-8). Inhalations of tincture of benzoin, or menthol and eucalyptus, will give him useful symptomatic relief.

TO DRAIN HIS FRONTAL SINUS, if you cannot refer him, give him a general anaesthetic, incise under his eyebrow from a point above his pupil to beside his medial canthus. Tie his angular vein. Use a small gouge, or dental drill, to cut a hole in the floor of his frontal sinus, to expose its lumen. Insert a small drain. Also, wash out his maxillary antrum through a cannula inserted through his inferior meatus (25.9). If necessary, refer him for definitive surgery.

TO REMOVE FRONTAL SEQUESTRA see Section 7.14.

CAUTION ! Wash out the maxillary antra of all patients with frontal sinus infections, because this is often the primary source of infection.

25.9 Maxillary sinusitis

If the ostium of a patient's maxillary sinus is blocked, he has pain in his cheek. If it is full of pus he has fever, and perhaps signs of inflammation on his cheek. Ephedrine nose drops may open his blocked ostium, but if his sinus is chronically full of pus, it needs puncturing and washing out, which is not difficult. Opinions differ as to whether a Caldwell-Luc operation should be in the repertoire of the generalist, so try to refer a patient who needs one. Fortunately, it is rarely necessary. Its main indication is chronic infection of the antrum which fails to respond to non-operative treatment.

MAXILLARY SINUSITIS

TRANSILLUMINATION needs to be interpreted with care, because antra are often asymmetrical. Take the patient into a darkened room, shine a small torch with a bright beam on to his hard palate, and close his lips around it. If his maxillary antrum is normal, his cheek on that side glows red. If one antrum transilluminates less well than the other, it may contain thickened mucosa, pus, blood, a tumour, a polyp, or a foreign body.

X-RAYS tell you more than transillumination. Take an AP film with his head tilted backwards. If you take an erect film, you may be able to see a fluid level.

BLOCKED OSTIUM. Give him 0.5% ephedrine nose drops in the head-down position, so that they run into the higher part of his nose. Lay him on his back with his head over the end of the couch, as in Fig. 25-8, and let him sniff them up during 10 minutes.

ANTRAL WASHOUTS FOR SINUSITIS

INDICATION. Pus in the maxillary antrum.

METHOD. Ask an assistant to stand behind him to steady his head. Obtain good local anaesthesia, *especially under his inferior turbinate where the trocar will penetrate:* (1) Anaesthetize the anterior

THE MAXILLARY ANTRUM

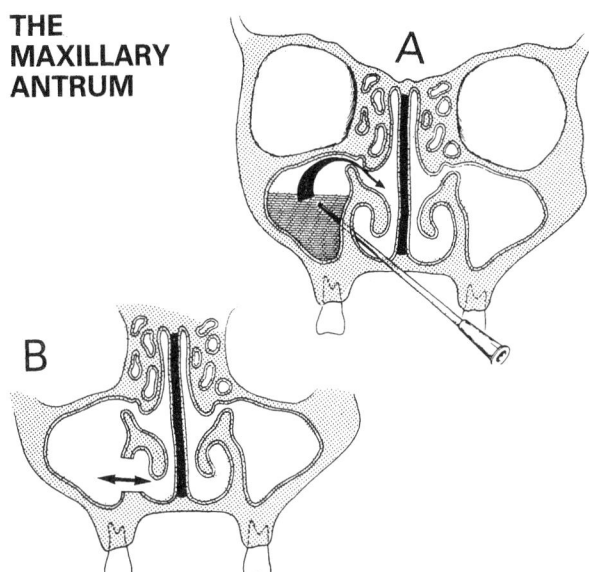

CALDWELL–LUC ANTROTOMY

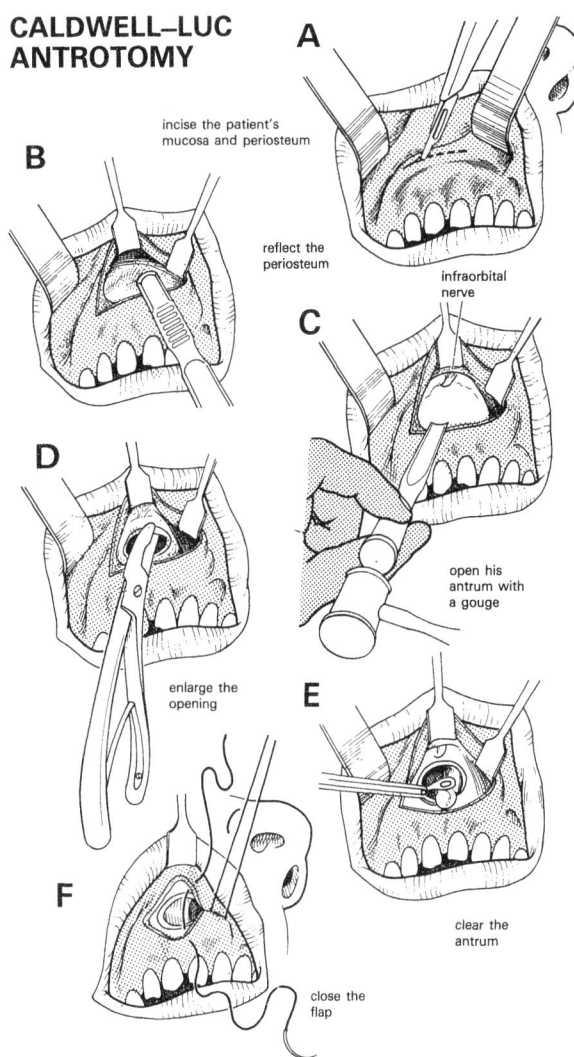

Fig. 25-6 THE MAXILLARY ANTRUM. A, an antral washout. Push a cannula into a patient's antrum through the lateral wall of his nose in his inferior meatus. Wash the contents of his antrum out through the ostium. B, an intranasal antrostomy. *After Bull PB, 'Lecture Notes on Diseases of the Ear, Nose and Throat', (6th edn). Blackwell Scientific Publications, permission requested.*

end of his inferior turbinate with lignocaine 4%, applied on gauze, or as a spray. (2) Twist cotton wool on to the serrated end of a Jobson Horne probe. Load this with cocaine paste, or soak it in 4% lignocaine. Gently paint under his inferior turbinate. Or, (3) use a long thin needle to inject lignocaine into it. Give the local anaesthetic a few minutes to act.

Take an antral trocar. Grasp the side of his head with your fingers behind it and your thumb over his zygoma. With your finger along the trocar to prevent it going in too far, push it along the floor of his nose, under his inferior turbinate. Slide it along the wall, then push it laterally towards the outer canthus of his eye, until it will not go any further. About 5 cm should go inside.

Aspirate the contents. In most diseased antra aspiration is impossible, because the ostium is blocked. If you aspirate air, it suggests that his antrum is normal. Ask him to lean forwards over a bowl, and to breathe through his mouth. Pump saline through the needle with a 20 ml syringe, or a Higginson's syringe, and let it run out through the ostium into the bowl.

If his ostium is sufficiently blocked to prevent the saline draining (rare), insert a second needle to let it drain.

CAUTION ! (1) Don't go right through his antrum into his cheek. You should be able to waggle the tip of the trocar slightly when it is inside his antrum. (2) Keep the Higginson's syringe full of saline. If you blow air in, and his ostium is blocked, he may possibly die of air embolism (very rare).

CALDWELL–LUC OPERATION

INDICATIONS. (1) Chronic infection of the antrum which fails to respond to non-operative treatment. (2) Exploration. (3) To obtain a biopsy, and reduce the bulk of the tumour, in suspected carcinoma of the maxillary antrum. Refer him if you can.

ANAESTHESIA. (1) General anaesthesia with tracheal intubation and a pack in his throat. (2) Intravenous ketamine.

METHOD. Using a dental syringe and cartridge, infiltrate his mucosa with an adrenalin containing local anaesthetic to reduce bleeding. Starting over his canine tooth, make a 5 cm incision through his mucous membrane and his periosteum, in the sulcus between his gum and his lip, well above the sockets of his teeth. Raise the periosteum and reflect flaps upwards and downwards. Reflect the upper flap to just below the floor of his orbit. As you do so, find and preserve his infraorbital nerve. If you damage it, he will have numbness of his lip and cheek. Reflect the insertions of his facial muscles with his periosteum.

Use an osteotome to open the anterior wall of his antrum—well above his tooth sockets, and the floor of his antrum. Start by making a small hole, and enlarge it with nibblers, a punch, or bone forceps. Use a small dissector to remove all damaged mucous membrane. Remove benign tumours and cysts with forceps and scissors.

CAUTION ! (1) Take care when you approach the the roof of his antrum, because the bony covering of his infraorbital nerve is thin and easily damaged. It supplies sensation to an area of his cheek and upper teeth. Remove all bony fragments. (2) Don't try to clear the sinus blind, try to see into it. Don't damage the roots of his teeth, which often project into it.

If the cavity is severely infected, with very diseased muscosa, make an opening from the medial wall of his antrum through into his nasal cavity, under his inferior turbinate (intranasal antrostomy, B, 25-6). The medial wall of his antrum bulges inwards, so you can do this easily. Use a small gouge to lift away the bone and reveal the mucosa of the inferior meatus of his nose. Incise this anteriorly, superiorly, and posteriorly, to allow an inferiorly hinged flap to fall into his antrum.

Fig. 25-7 CALDWELL–LUC OPERATION. A, incise the patient's mucosa and periosteum well above his tooth sockets in his canine fossa. B, elevate his periosteum. C, open the anterior wall of his antrum with an osteotome. D, enlarge the opening with bone cutters. E, clear his antrum. F, close the opening with a mucosal flap. *After Lorê JM, 'An Atlas of Head and Neck Surgery', p. 73. WB Saunders, with kind permission.*

If you have difficulty controlling bleeding, pack his antrum (seldom necessary) with the tail of the pack coming through his antrostomy into his nose. Impregnate the pack with 'BIPP' (4.11), or, less satisfactorily, gauze soaked in saline. 48 hours later remove the pack through his nose

CLOSE THE WOUND in his oral mucosa with several small absorbable sutures. If you don't close it securely, he may develop an oro-antral fistula.

25.10 Nasal polypi

A patient with nasal polypi is usually an adult, who presents with long standing nasal obstruction, which becomes complete from time to time, with or without a nasal discharge. He has grey fleshy masses in both his nasal cavities. When you remove them, they look like skinned grapes. Polypi are common and treatable. Try non-operative treatment first, and if this fails, remove as many as you can surgically. Some polypi of the maxillary antrum are so large that they project through the ostium into his nasopharynx, and have to be removed through his mouth. If a polyp is on one side only, it may be malignant (or, very rarely a meningocele), so treat it as such, until you have proved it is benign.

NASAL POLYPI

NON-OPERATIVE TREATMENT. Ask the patient to place 2 drops of betamethasone (50 µg) into each nostril twice daily for 4 weeks, while he is in the Moffat position in Fig. 25-8, and ask him to remain in this position for three minutes afterwards.

REMOVING POLYPI UNDER LOCAL ANAESTHESIA. Premedicate him thoroughly. Sit opposite him, and ask a nurse to stand behind his head. Spray or douche his nose with lignocaine 2% with adrenalin 1/100,000. Be careful not to exceed the maximum dose (A 5-1). Wait for 5 minutes.

With a good light coming over your right shoulder, open his nostrils with a nasal speculum. Pass a Glegg's polypectomy snare, manoeuvre the loop to catch a polyp round its base, and remove it. If polypi do not come out with the snare, pull them out piecemeal with angled forceps.

Repeat the process, until you have removed as many polypi as you can. If he feels pain, spray more anaesthetic and wait another 5 minutes. If he bleeds excessively at the end of the operation, pack his nose as for epistaxis (25.6).

THE MOFFAT POSITION

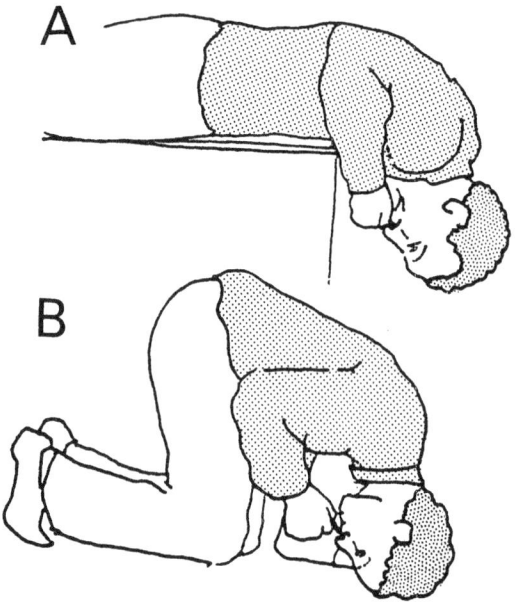

Fig. 25-8 THE MOFFAT POSITION FOR PUTTING DROPS IN THE NOSE. A, over a table. B, on the floor. If a patient inserts drops in either of these positions, and remains in them for 3 minutes afterwards, the drugs they contain are more likely to remain in contact with his mucosa for long enough to be effective.

REMOVING POLYPI UNDER GENERAL ANAESTHESIA enables you to remove them more completely than under local anaesthesia, but there will be more bleeding. Avoid ketamine, because the laryngeal and pharyngeal reflexes are partly preserved, and cause trouble. Give him a general anaesthetic, intubate him, and pack his throat with a large pack. Be sure the throat pack is visible all through the operation, or has a stout thread fixed to it. Have good suction available. Large clots can form in his pharynx, and be aspirated when you remove the tube. *So clear his throat first, and remove the pack with care.*

When you have removed all the polypi you can, pack his nose with an anterior pack each side (25.6). Send him back to the ward lying on his side.

25.11 Foreign bodies in the nose

If a child puts something, such as a maize seed or a bean, into his nose, it will have to be removed, or it will cause chronic suppuration and obstruction. Removing it is seldom an emergency, and is easier and much less dangerous than removing a foreign body from the ear. Commonly, the child or his parents know that there is a foreign body inside, and know where it is. Suspect one when: (1) One side of a child's nose only (usually the right) is blocked or discharges (common). A unilateral *foul-smelling* bloody nasal discharge, with obstruction is a foreign body unless it is a tumour (rare in most communities). (2) He has a perforation of his palate (rare).

FOREIGN BODIES IN THE NOSE

Clear his nose and try to see the foreign body. If you cannot see it (rare), take a lateral X-ray. Try to get the child to blow or sneeze the foreign body out. Close his other nostril and tickle his nose to make him sneeze.

CAUTION ! (1) If you suspect a foreign body, assume it is there, until you are absolutely certain it is not. (2) Don't believe a negative X-ray.

ANAESTHESIA. (1) Local anaesthesia is suitable, if you can see it, it is not too far back, and he is reasonably co-operative. It will minimize the risks of inhalation, if your anaesthetist is not skilled. (2) Intravenous ketamine, if local anaesthesia is unsuitable. (3) Give him a general anaesthetic. Pass a tracheal tube, and pack his pharynx to prevent him inhaling the foreign body.

EQUIPMENT. You will need a good light, suction, angled forceps, and some kind of hook, such as a Eustachian catheter, a bent probe, or a bent paper clip held in a haemostat. Put a large speculum on an auriscope, and remove its back lens.

THE METHOD varies, depending on the anaesthesia you use.

If you are using local anaesthesia, spray his nose well with local anaesthetic solution (without exceeding the dose, see A 5-1), and wait for 5 minutes. Ask his mother to sit him on her lap, hold his legs between hers, and to put her arms round him. Ask a nurse to hold his head. Put your chair close to his mother's, with your legs outside hers. Either use a head mirror, or have a good light behind you.

If you are using general anaesthezia, lay him on his side, so that if you push the foreign body into his pharynx, it will not go into his airway.

Try to bring the foreign body out anteriorly—if you push it posteriorly, he may inhale it (this should not happen if his throat has been adequately packed).

If the object is firm, pass your chosen hook beyond it, usually above it, turn the hook behind it and deliver it. Don't try to grab it with forceps, or you will push it further in. Try to draw it towards the floor of his nose, and away from its roof. Then use angled forceps to remove it. A foreign body is most likely to impact in the roof of his nose. Here it is dangerously close to the floor of his anterior cranial fossa and the medial wall of his orbit.

If the foreign body is soft, use forceps. You may be able to suck small foreign bodies away. Otherwise, use small alligator forceps, or any forceps with blunt angulated tips.

If he bleeds, use gentle suction. Packing (25.6) is seldom necessary.

CAUTION ! Make sure there are no more foreign bodies present.

25.11a Laryngoscopy

A laryngoscope, which enables you to look directly at the larynx, and push a tube through it, is one of the most useful of all instruments, but don't forget the advantages of indirect laryngoscopy, with an angled mirror. Its great advantages are that you can do it on an outpatient, it needs only simple equipment, and it can be very informative. But it is not easy, and you will have to do it fairly often, if you are going to become competent with it. The main indication for indirect laryngoscopy is to examine the vocal cords in order to: (1) Distinguish chronic laryngitis from a polyp or carcinoma. (2) Check the movement of the cords, when one of them is suspected of being injured, as after thyroidectomy, or by a carcinoma of the bronchus on the left side.

LARYNGOSCOPY

DIRECT LARYNGOSCOPY. Do this as for tracheal intubation, see A 13.2. You can more easily get a good view; take a biopsy with Magill's forceps or straight alligator forceps, but be careful not to damage the patient's cords.

INDIRECT LARYNGOSCOPY

INDICATIONS. Hoarseness lasting more than 4 weeks. He is more likely to have laryngitis, but he may have a polyp, or carcinoma.

EQUIPMENT. A good light coming from behind him and slightly to one side. A head mirror with a band, laryngeal mirrors and a spirit lamp, 4% lignocaine in a laryngeal spray.

INDIRECT LARYNGOSCOPY

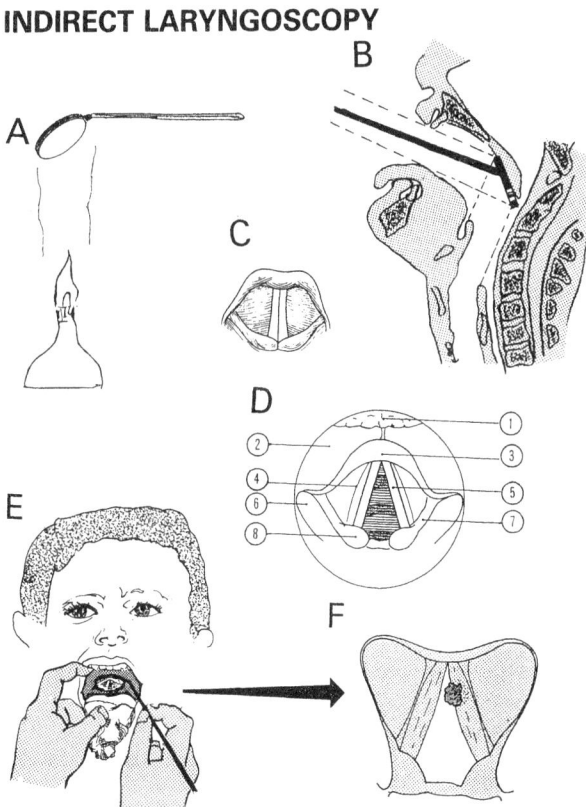

Fig. 25-8a INDIRECT LARYNGOSCOPY. A, warming the mirror. B, the light path to a patient's larynx. C, his cords opposed. D, his cords separated. E, a view of his larynx. F, a carcinoma of his glottis—see Section 32.39.

1, the dorsum of his tongue. 2, his vallecula. 3, his epiglottis. 4, his vestibular folds. 5, his vocal cords. 6, his pyriform fossae. 7, his aryepiglottic folds. 8, his arytenoid cartilages.

METHOD. Sit opposite him, and arrange the light so that it comes from over his shoulder.

Wrap gauze round his protruding tongue, and pull it forwards with your left hand. Spray his fauces, soft palate and pharynx with lignocaine.

Warm an angled mirror in the flame of a spirit lamp, and test its temperature on the back of your left hand; it should feel just warm, but not hot. Place the back of the mirror against his soft palate, push a little and look down at his larynx. Identify his cords.

Normal cords are white. Laryngitis makes them red, and chronic laryngitis also makes them swell. If you see a lump, it is probably a polyp. A ragged ulcer is likely to be a carcinoma.

Ask him to say "Eee..." and note the movement of both his cords.

To examine his nasopharynx, depress his tongue with some soft instrument, and place a smaller (14 mm) rhinoscopic mirror in his pharynx, so that your line of sight passes up behind his soft palate.

25.12 Bronchoscopy: inhaled foreign bodies in the larynx and tracheobronchial tree

If a patient flexes his neck, and extends his head sufficiently, he can align his mouth with his trachea or oesophagus, so that a rigid tube can be passed down them. This is the 'sword-swallowing position', and is the basis of rigid bronchoscopy and oesophagoscopy. In theory, these are simple procedures—the traditional type of bronchoscope is merely a long tube with a light at one end. In practice, however, removing a foreign body with one requires such skill, that it is one of the most difficult procedures we describe, and is at the very limits of *Primary Surgery*. Anaesthesia is difficult, and the skill of your anaesthetist is the main determinant of success. You need a range of intruments to cover all sizes of patient, and also a variety of forceps. There are many opportunities for disaster, particularly tearing the patient's lower trachea and bronchi if he struggles, so causing mediastinal emphysema and mediastinitis. Many hospitals don't have bronchoscopes; this is for those that do. If you have other instruments with fibre-optic illumination, make sure that your bronchoscope is compatible with that system. You will need good suction.

You will find bronchoscopy useful for: (1) Sucking out a patient's stomach contents from his trachea, if he has been unfortunate enough to aspirate them during a general anaesthetic (A 16.3). Make this your first priority, especially if you are new to bronchoscopy. (2) Sucking out the secretions which have gathered in the bronchi of a desperately sick patient postoperatively (9.11). (3) Removing foreign bodies, especially peanuts inhaled by children. This is more difficult than the other two indications, so don't start with it, if you can avoid doing so. (4) Diagnosing carcinoma, and other diseases of the larger airways.

Inhaled foreign bodies in the larynx and tracheobronchial tree, particularly peanuts or watermelon pips, are common. If a child is lucky, his first immediate bout of coughing expels the nut. If he is not so lucky, wheezing and coughing stop without expelling it. This may be followed by a latent interval, during which there are no signs, especially if the nut has gone far down his bronchial tree. This latent interval is then followed by fever, a cough, and the symptoms of chest infection. Antibiotics may relieve his symptoms temporarily, but they always return when treatment stops. He is often misdiagnosed as having tuberculosis.

If coughing, or the 'upside down thump' described below, fail to remove a foreign body, it has to be removed through a bronchoscope. Even if you can successfully pass one, removing a foreign body is difficult, and sometimes impossible. Yet if you cannot refer him, and leave it inside him, suppuration and chronic disability, or death, are certain.

• BRONCHOSCOPE, rigid, Negus, conventional lighting, distal illumination, complete with cords, Wappler fitting, battery box, two lamp carriers and 2.5 v lamps with 10 BA thread, (a) infant lumen 5.4×4.1 mm,

(b) child 7×5.7 mm, (c) adolescent small 8×6.7 mm, one only of each size, (optional). ALSO, 25 spare bulbs. If you are going to remove foreign bodies from the lower respiratory tract, you will need these. This is not the complete range, which includes the adolescent large, the small adult, the adult, and several for the lower bronchus. Darken the theatre so that you do not have to use the bulbs at voltages which shorten their lives.

• FORCEPS, for bronchoscope, (a) Chevalier Jackson, 2/2 teeth on 50 cm shaft, one only, (b) Haslinger tubular shaft or sliding shaft type for small bronchoscopes (both optional). If you have bronchoscopes, you will need forceps for them. Mark the shaft of the forceps with tape, so that you know when the tip is beyond the bronchoscope.

BRONCHOSCOPY

INDICATIONS. See above.

CAUTION ! This is not an easy procedure, so refer the patient to an expert, or call one in, if you can. Usually, this is impossible, so that, if you don't bronchoscope a patient, nobody else will. You will need a good anaesthetist and a good nurse.

BRONCHOSCOPY UNDER LOCAL ANAESTHESIA. Premedicate him. Give an adult chlorpromazine 50 mg, and atropine 0.6 mg. Sit him up and inject 5 ml of 4% lignocaine into his trachea with a short stiff fine-bore needle; aim to produce a fine spray. Go through his cricothyroid membrane (A 13.5). Check that you are in his trachea, by aspirating before you inject. Before you pass the instrument, spray his cords with more lignocaine and wait 2 minutes.

CAUTION ! Don't exceed the dose of lignocaine, particularly in a small child (A 5-1). 10 ml of 4% lignocaine is the absolute maximum for an adult.

BRONCHOSCOPY UNDER GENERAL ANAESTHESIA. Give him a general anaesthetic and a short-acting relaxant.

BRONCHOSCOPY FOR THE ASPIRATION OF STOMACH CONTENTS

He will probably be in the theatre, and be partly or completely anaesthetized already, so there is no need for anaesthesia. He will not resist for long. Insert the bronchoscope, as rapidly as you can, and aspirate with a long sterile catheter.

BRONCHOSCOPY FOR THE RETENTION OF SECRETIONS

INDICATIONS. He is likely to be a very sick adult, who has been unable to cough his airway clear of secretions postoperatively (see Section 9.11). His breathing is bubbly, and parts of his lungs may have collapsed. He is so ill that he will die, unless his lower respiratory tract is cleared.

METHOD. If you cannot call in anyone who is more expert, take him into a side ward, or better, the theatre. Have an anaesthetist and a competent nurse to help you. Sit him up in bed with pillows behind his back. Use local anaesthesia as above. Blindfold him, and wear spectacles to protect yourself from showers of sputum. Stand behind him on a firm chair, with the bronchoscope and sucker ready. Ask him to look upwards.

Now pass the bronchoscope gently behind his tongue. Look for his uvula and his epiglottis. This will lead you in the midline to his vocal cords, as when intubating. As soon as you see them, aim the bronchoscope in the same direction as his trachea. Slip its beak between his cords and advance it downwards, sucking out the secretions as you do so. Clear his airway and remove the instrument. This will produce a paroxysm of coughing—which will benefit him greatly.

CAUTION ! (1) Make sure you are not going down his oesophagus (you must recognize his cords on entry). (2) Very little movement should be possible between the bronchoscope and the patient. So hold its handle in your right hand. Hold its shaft between the index and middle fingers of your left hand. Rest your left thumb on his upper front teeth, and keep his lower lip out of the way with a gauze swab, held in your ring finger. If you hold the bronchoscope against his teeth like this, it and his head will turn as one and less damage is likely.

Alternatively, demonstrate his cords with a laryngoscope, before you pass the bronchoscope.

FOREIGN BODIES IN THE BRONCHI

IMMEDIATE TREATMENT—THE 'UPSIDE DOWN THUMP'. If

BRONCHOSCOPY

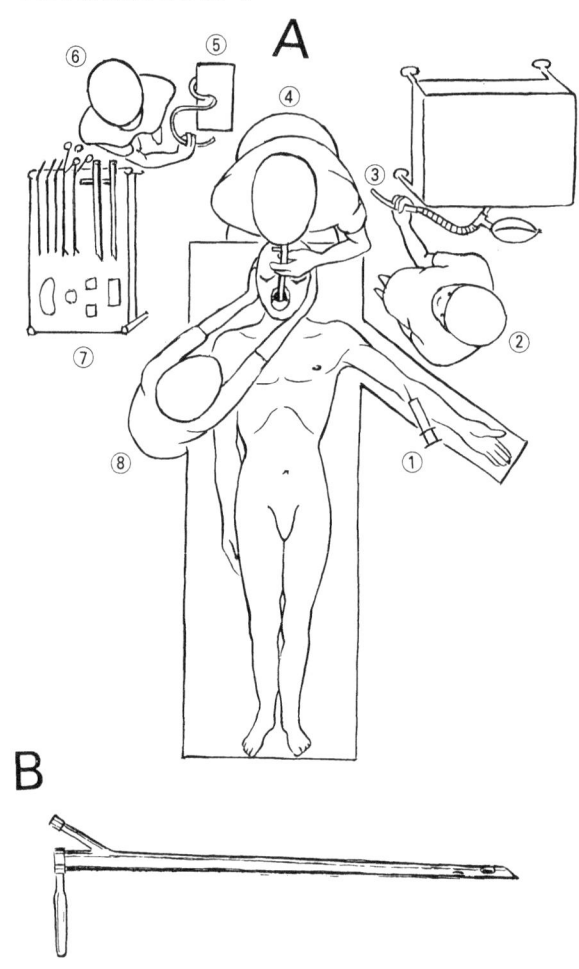

Fig. 25-9 ARRANGEMENTS FOR BRONCHOSCOSCOPY. After induction the anaesthetist moves to the patient's left.
1, a syringe in a vein. 2, the anaesthetist. 3, the oxygen line. 4, the surgeon. 5, the sucker. 6, the trolley nurse. 7, the trolley with sucker tubes. 8, the nurse who controls the patient's head.

you are present when a child inhales a foreign body, turn him upside down and bang the back of his chest—he may cough it out. This is a very valuable procedure (and once saved the editor's life!).

HISTORY AND EXAMINATION. If he presents later, take a careful history, look for impaired movement on one side of his chest, and listen for localized wheezing.

X-RAYS. Look for a radio-opaque object, localized collapse, pneumonitis, consolidation of a segment or an entire lobe; and mediastinal shift. There will be obstructive emphysema if a foreign body allows air into a bronchus, but not out of it.

CAUTION ! (1) If a mother comes to you saying that her child has inhaled a peanut, believe her, she is almost certainly right. (2) Most plastics are radiolucent, so you will not see them on an X-ray film. (3) Negative X-rays never exclude a foreign body, unless everyone is sure it is radio-opaque.

BRONCHOSCOPY FOR THE REMOVAL OF A FOREIGN BODY

EQUIPMENT. A suitable size of bronchoscope. A long piece of bent wire with a hook on it (see below). Switch on the light, insert the grasping forceps, and practise picking up peanuts from an assistant's hand before you start.

ANAESTHESIA must abolish the child's cough reflex; local anaesthesia *alone* will not do this adequately: (1) Ketamine or thiopentone followed by intermittent suxamethonium (A 14.2), with oxygen intermittently introduced into the bronchoscope through an uncuffed tube. Be sure you have a drip up. (2) Suxamethonium followed by a long-acting relaxant, if the anaesthetist is skilled.

CAUTION ! Be sure to spray the child's larynx with lignocaine, because this will prevent laryngeal spasm as you pass the bronchoscope, and minimize difficult airway problems as he recovers.

You will need two tracheal tubes, one for 'normal' intubation between attempts at bronchoscopy, and a larger one which fits snugly into the end of the bronchoscope, so that you can ventilate him while the bronchoscope is in place, if his pulse rate falls, or if he becomes cyanosed. There is usually some leakage, so you will need a good flow of oxygen. Blow oxygen into him intermittently, watching his pulse rate meanwhile. A *falling* pulse is a sign of anoxia. Only proceed to remove the foreign body, if his pulse is satisfactory. Oxygen through the side tube will not by itself ventilate him adequately, if he is paralysed. The anaesthetist and the surgeon share the patient. The anaesthetist is in charge, and decides when he must give oxygen.

CAUTION ! (1) His chest must expand during ventilation. If it does not, remove the bronchoscope, intubate him, and then try to bronchoscope him again.

METHOD. Lay him flat on his back, with his head raised on the flap of the table (if it will raise), or on a cushion. Ask a nurse to stand on his right, to hold his head with the palms of her hands over his ears, and to move his head from left to right as required.

Spray his larynx (see above), anaesthetize him, and intubate him. When he is intubated, ask the anaesthetist to show you his cords with the laryngoscope. Holding the bronchoscope as described above, put your left thumb on his upper incisor teeth, guide it forwards over the dorsum of his tongue, obliquely across his mouth from the right. His palate is a useful guide to the midline. Lift it so as to draw his lower pharynx forwards, as if you were passing a laryngoscope, taking care not to injure his teeth.

Slowly flex his neck into the 'sword-swallowing position' as you pass the bronchoscope (the position is the same as for oesophagoscopy in B, and C, Fig. 25-10). As the bronchoscope goes down, you will need more extension of his head, then flexion of his neck. You should see his uvula first, then his epiglottis, and then his larynx with its cords. Pass the bronchoscope through them (they will remain open under general anaesthesia). Turn it through 90° as you do this, so that its bevel is in the long axis of his glottis. When you are through his glottis, turn it back again. Aim it in the line of his trachea.

Look for the foreign body in his bronchi: the common site is just distal to his carina in his right main bronchus. The right main bronchus is shorter, more vertical and wider than the left. Most foreign bodies enter the right one.

If his carina is normal, pass the bronchoscope down one or other bronchus, preferably the normal one first. When you withdraw from the right main bronchus and enter the left one, you will have to move his head to the right as you do so.

With luck you will see the foreign body, and perhaps the bronchi to particular lobes. If it is up a side bronchus (unusual) there is no way you can get it out. Try to bring it out on the end of the sucker. If this fails, grasp it with the forceps. If it will come up the bronchoscope, good. If it will not, gently withdraw the bronchoscope and the foreign body together. If there is much pus, suck that out too.

CAUTION ! (1) Hold the bronchoscope lightly in your fingers, so that if he moves, it will move with him, instead of injuring his respiratory tract. (2) Take care not to damage his teeth. (3) Remove it promptly if he struggles. (4) If you fail, and the anaesthetist says "That's enough", obey him, he is master of the team!

If you want to identify his bronchi, on the right, look for his right upper lobe bronchus in the 2 or 3 o'clock position, his apical lower lobe bronchus at 6 o'clock, and his right middle lobe bronchus at 12 o'clock. Then look into the bronchi of his lateral, anterior, posterior, and medial basal lobes.

On the left, look for his left upper lobe bronchus in the 10 o'clock position, his apical lower lobe bronchus at 6 o'clock, and then into the bronchi for his lateral, anterior, and posterior basal lobes.

DIFFICULTIES WITH BRONCHOSCOPY

If he is SUFFOCATING AND BLUE from the procedure, wait and try again next day. If he is suffocating because of the foreign body, you will have to persist.

If a FOREIGN BODY BREAKS INTO PIECES, bring it up bit by bit. If it slips off while you are withdrawing it through his cords, try again. If necessary, squirt a little saline down the bronchoscope with a syringe.

If you are looking for a CARCINOMA, look for abnormalities of the wall, and biopsy any growth. It will be easier to remove a piece from the carina.

If the FOREIGN BODY ROLLS UP AND DOWN HIS TRACHEA, but you cannot get it past his cords, tip the table steeply head down, and manipulate it past them with the piece of hooked wire that you have prepared for this eventuality.

25.13 Foreign bodies in 'the throat'

A patient with a foreign body in his pharynx, or oesophagus, usually knows what has happened and is usually right. It can stick in his tonsils, his vallecula, his pyriform fossa, or in his postcricoid region.

Most fish bones stick in accessible regions, usually the back of the tongue or tonsils. Foreign bodies seldom stick in the larynx itself, except when an affluent, elderly, and often intoxicated diner gets a piece of steak caught in his larynx, as a result of which he gasps and collapses. Treat him immediately, as described below.

FOREIGN BODIES IN 'THE THROAT'

EMERGENCY TREATMENT. If a patient is obviously choking, and you are present at the time, sit him up, grasp his tongue with gauze, pull it forward, and ask him resist retching. Hook it out with your finger.

If there is a piece of food in his larynx, try Heimlich's manoeuvre—immediately, like this: Stand behind him, put your fist under his xiphoid and give a short sharp upward push, at the same time that you compress his chest with your arms. This will rapidly compress his lungs, and may push out the food.

If he is asphyxiating, put your finger into his larynx, and try to hook the foreign body out. If you fail, insert a wide-bore needle (or a blade) through the cricothyroid membrane of his larynx (52.2) to create an airway (not to remove the foreign body!).

EARLY PRESENTATION. This is the patient 'with something in his throat' who presents within 2 or 3 hours without severe dyspnoea. Take a careful history. Where and how severe is his pain? Feel his neck. Surgical emphysema? Take X-rays, especially a lateral view. Look for air in his tissues. If a large fish bone has stuck, you should see it, but you will not see a small one.

If there is no convincing evidence that it has lodged in his pharynx, and pain is mild, it probably only scratched him and passed on. Treat him expectantly. Persuade him to eat dry bread. A small sharp object may enter his oesophagus and pass on through him.

If you can see it, or there is air in his tissues, or if for any other reason you suspect it has lodged in his pharynx, examine his pharynx under general anaesthesia with tracheal intubation. Or, less satisfactorily, use intravenous ketamine and intermittent suxamethonium and oxygen (A 14.2). Have good suction available. Use a laryngoscope to carefully search his tonsils, his valleculae, and the back of his pharynx. Take the opportunity to have a look at his larynx, even though a foreign body here does cause different symptoms (25.12). Grasp it with Magill forceps.

CAUTION ! (1) Relaxants are dangerous unless you can inflate his lungs (A 13.1). (2) Keep his head well down all the time.

If you don't find it, proceed to oesophagoscopy.

If there is a perforation of the wall of his pharynx, spreading aerobic and anaerobic infection may be dangerous. If there is a large wound, try to suck it out (difficult). If necessary, consider opening up the tissues of his neck (also difficult). Refer him, or get more experienced help if you can. Give him chloramphenicol and metronidazole.

If there is a piece of food in his larynx, try Heimlich's urgent tracheostomy (52.2). It may save his life until you can refer him. The smaller he is the more difficult this will be, especially in an emergency. Try inserting a wide (1.8 mm) needle first to establish an airway. Follow this by laryngoscopy, and bronchoscopy, as soon as possible. Avoid passing the bronchoscope through the tracheostomy, which is difficult and dangerous. Only attempt it if the bronchoscope will not pass his cords.

If possible, refer him. Only attempt to remove a foreign body yourself, if his respiration is so distressed that referral is impossible.

LATE PRESENTATION (3 hours to several days later). If the foreign body has not caused a wound, his symptoms should have settled. If there is a wound, there will be signs of air in his tissues and/or infection, especially after 24 hours. Refer him if you can. Give him antibiotics and metronidazole. If you cannot refer him, proceed as above.

25.14 Oesophagoscopy

Passing an oesophagoscope, even more so than passing a bronchoscope, might be considered to be outside the range of *Primary Surgery*. It is however the easier of these two procedures. An oesophagoscope looks like a bronchoscope except that it has no side tube for oxygen, and no ventilation holes at its distal end, because the patient does not need to breathe through it.

Fortunately, most ingested foreign bodies pass through the gut, but if they stick, they have to be removed. 90% stick in its upper 5 cm, just below the cricopharyngeus muscle before the oesophagus enters the thorax. This is fortunate, because this is the easiest place from which to remove them. They are commonly coins, buttons, safety pins, or bones. The patient may have almost no symptoms, or he may be distressed, refuse food, drool saliva, choke, gag, or cough (typically in paroxysms). If he is a child he may merely 'fail to thrive'. If he is older, he may complain of pain, or the sensation of a foreign body behind his sternum. If it is large enough to compress his trachea, he may have stridor, or episodes of cyanosis and recurrent pneumonitis (unusual). If he is very young, or mentally incompetent, there may be no history that he has swallowed anything. Symptoms may have lasted hours or years. The diagnosis is usually obvious, but a foreign body which is missed, can cause persistent dysphagia and loss of weight, so that you may suspect a carcinoma.

A TRUE STORY. The examining surgeon at a nurse's training school (St Francis Hospital, Katete, in its early days): "What instrument would you use for oesophagoscopy?" Enrolled nurse: "A sigmoidoscope". When it was explained that this was wrong, she repeated (correctly) that this was indeed the instrument that she had seen used at her rural hospital! LESSON If necessary improvise.

• OESOPHAGOSCOPE, (a) infant, (b) child, (c) adult, *with forceps and suckers that are long enough to go through them. One only of each.* If you don't have an oesophagoscope, you may be able to use a bronchoscope to remove coins from the oesophagus, or bougie a carcinoma, before passing a Celestin tube. The more protruding beak of a bronchoscope is, however, more likely to perforate the oesophagus.

• BOUGIES, oesophageal, neoprene, *standard set, alternate sizes only, one set only.* The old fashioned gum elastic ones are satisfactory.

THE SECRET IS TO FLEX HIS NECK AND EXTEND HIS HEAD

OESOPHAGOSCOPY

INDICATIONS. (1) The removal of foreign bodies. (2) To check the nature of a stricture, whether fibrous or malignant after a barium swallow, and to take a biopsy. (3) Bouginage for carcinoma of the oesophagus. (4) Bouginage for a stricture.

OESOPHAGOSCOPY

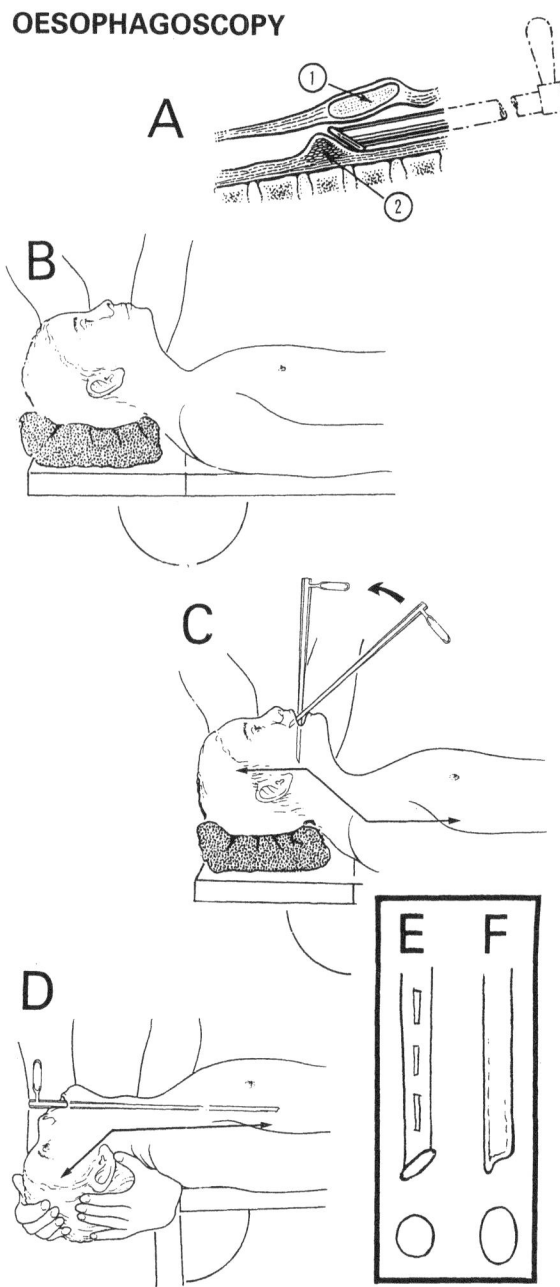

Fig. 25-10 POSITIONING THE HEAD FOR OESOPHAGOSCOPY. A, the difficult part is passing the patient's cricopharyngeus. This will be easier if you keep the handle of the instrument up, so that it slides over this muscle. B, keep his head on a pillow with his neck flexed and his head extended in the 'sniffing position'. This position will allow you to oesophagoscope him as far as the deepest part of his thoracic kyphosis. C, introduce the oesophagoscope obliquely and move it vertically, as it reaches his pharynx. D, if you need to examine the lowest part of his oesophagus (less often necessary), straighten or slightly extend his neck, until he is in the sword-swallowing position. E, a bronchoscope is circular, and has air holes. F, an oesophagoscope is oval, and has none. *Adapted from 'Hamilton Bailey's Emergency Surgery', edited by HAF Dudley, Figs. 22.1 and 22.3. John Wright, with kind permission.*

ANAESTHESIA. (1) General anaesthesia with a short-acting relaxant and tracheal intubation. (2) Ketamine is a poor second.

POSITION. *Keep the patient's head on a pillow throughout.* This will flex his neck. Then extend his head on his neck to bring him into the 'sniffing position' shown in A 13-7. This position will allow you to pass the oesophagoscope into the deepest part of his thoracic kyphosis. The most common reason for failure is insufficient flexion of his neck, and extension of his head.

If you need to view the very lowest part of his oesophagus

(unusual), straighten, or slightly extend, his neck, so that his pharynx and his oesophagus are in a straight line to let the oesophagoscope pass (the 'sword-swallowing position'). *Otherwise, keep it flexed.* If your table does not have a headpiece that drops down, ask an assistant to hold his head over the end of the table, to control its movement—this is not easy, and is dangerous!

INSERTION. Aim the oesophagoscope vertically downwards at his uvula. Angle it so as to pass the base of his tongue (aim at the foot of the pedestal of the table). When his larynx comes into view, avoid the midline, and pass it laterally, through one or other pyriform fossa, to reach his oesophagus, which is again in the midline.

Going through his cricopharyngeus is the difficult part. It should look like the the anus: aim for the centre of the pit. If you have difficulty, pass a tube or bougie first, and use this to guide the oesophagoscope through.

CAUTION ! (1) Never advance the oesophagoscope blind, or you may perforate his oesophagus. (2) Keep the lumen of his oesophagus in the centre of your field of view, as you slide the instrument down.

OESOPHAGOSCOPY FOR REMOVING A FOREIGN BODY

THE X-RAY DIAGNOSIS may be straightforward, if the foreign body is opaque. In the oesophagus coins lie in the coronal plane, so that you see their full diameter in a PA film. In the respiratory tract they lie sagittally, so that you see them end-on. A barium swallow may be useful, but it makes oesophagoscopy soon afterwards more difficult; diatrizioate meglumine ('Gastrografin') is better.

CAUTION ! (1) A normal X-ray does not exclude a radiolucent foreign body. (2) If he has swallowed a foreign body that may cause trouble, X-ray his whole abdomen and his pelvis also.

METHOD. First try laryngoscopy. You may be able to feel the foreign body with a probe, and remove it with a long clamp.

If laryngoscopy and simpler methods fail, pass the oesophagoscope, as above. As soon as you can see the foreign body clearly (usually a coin), pass the biopsy forceps and grasp it firmly. If it moves distally, withdraw the forceps, pass the oesophagoscope a little further, and try to grasp it again. When you have grasped it, bring it and the oesophagoscope out together.

CAUTION ! (1) The great danger is perforating his oesophagus: (a) usually at the level of his cricopharyngeus, which keeps the entry closed, or (b) at a lower level where the foreign body impacts—beware of his aorta! (2) Safety pins, bones, and lumps of food, such as meat, should, if possible, be removed by an expert—they are particularly difficult, and dangerous. (3) Don't advance the oesophagoscope, if you cannot see the lumen of his oesophagus beyond it.

DIFFICULTIES WITH OESOPHAGOSCOPY FOR REMOVING A FOREIGN BODY

If you DON'T HAVE AN OESOPHAGOSCOPE, you may be able to use a sigmoidoscope (as the nurse saw done in the story above). After you have identified his cricopharyngeus, use the obturator to negotiate it. If the foreign body is blunt, you may be able to pass a Foley catheter beyond it, inflate the balloon and pull it out with that (difficult).

If a FOREIGN BODY IS TOO LARGE TO REMOVE WHOLE, as with an impacted denture, you may be able to break it and remove the pieces.

If you FAIL TO REMOVE A FOREIGN BODY, refer him, probably for its open removal through the side of his neck.

If, soon after he is back in the ward, he develops PAIN in his neck, behind his sternum, or in his back, with dyspnoea, suspect PERFORATION OF HIS OESOPHAGUS. Look for air in his neck, pleural cavity or mediastinum (the earliest sign is a translucent crescent overlying the aortic knuckle). Consider giving him some contrast medium ('Gastrografin' *not* barium) and taking another film. Refer him for an immediate pharyngotomy (if the tear is in his cervical oesophagus) or thoracotomy. Delay is likely to be fatal.

If the above symptoms are delayed, he has FEVER and his chest X-ray is normal, suspect MEDIASTINITIS. Antibiotic treatment is more likely to succeed. Do a temporary gastrostomy to rest the abrasion in his oesophagus.

If an EMPYEMA develops, evacuate all fluid and air, insert intercostal drains (65-2), give him nothing by mouth, and consider a feeding jejunostomy (9.7, a gastrostomy is less effective because feed can reflux into his oesophagus).

If he develops a RETROPHARYNGEAL ABSCESS, treat him as in Section 5.7.

If he develops a STRICTURE, treat him as in Section 25.15.

OESOPHAGOSCOPY FOR INVESTIGATING A STRICTURE

Pass the instrument with care, using one of small diameter first. Suck out and advance the instrument under direct vision. If entry is easy, and vision is poor, with a small instrument, withdraw it, and try a larger one. Continue distally under direct vision, until you see the lesion, sucking out any fluid you find.

OESOPHAGOSCOPY FOR CARCINOMA OF THE OESOPHAGUS

Give him a general anaesthetic and a short-acting relaxant, intubate him, and control his ventilation. Pass the oesophagoscope, suck out the debris, then pass it further distally. Try to dilate him with graduated bougies. Take two biopsies for histology.

25.15 Corrosive oesophagitis, and oesophageal strictures

Corrosive oesophagitis is not uncommon in some communities, as the result of a patient swallowing caustic soda (for making soap), sulphuric acid, or some other corrosive chemical. You will have to treat him in the acute stage, and if necessary in the other stages also. It is useful to be able to oesophagoscope him, but you may be able to manage without doing so. If you don't have the correct bougies, try to improvise them. For malignant strictures, see Section 32.24. *Bouginage is always dangerous!* Do it with *infinite* care, if you want to avoid perforating his oesophagus, and killing him.

Martinson FD, 'Corrosive oesophagitis in Nigeria', Tropical Doctor 1978;8:123-126

CORROSIVE OESOPHAGEAL STRICTURES

THE ACUTE PHASE

After swallowing a corrosive substance, a patient has immediate retrosternal or abdominal pain, he drools, and he may vomit food or blood. He may also have stridor, or symptoms due to the poisonous nature of the substance he has ingested. You may see patches of burnt mucosa on his lips, mouth, or pharynx.

Find out what he took and when. Give him an analgesic. If you see him *within 6 hours,* when the corrosive agent is still present, lavage his stomach *urgently!* If there is delay, avoid lavage. Add the antidote to the lavaging fluid. For a corrosive acid, use magnesia, chalk, or washing soda. For an alkali, use vinegar, or the juice of 5 lemons.

If he is unconscious (unlikely in corrosive poisoning), intubate him first.

To lavage his stomach, lay him prone with his head over the end of the bed, remove any false teeth, and preferably insert mouth gags on each side of his mouth. Pass a safety pin through the wall (not the lumen) of a large rubber stomach tube (10 mm for an adult, 8 mm for a child under 2 years), to mark the distance it should pass (adult 50 cm from the tip, 25 cm in a child under 2 years). Pass tepid water into his stomach, never more than 500 ml at time in an adult, and 250 ml in a child. Send the first washouts for analysis. Continue washing out with 500 ml at at time, until you have used 5 litres.

CAUTION ! Check the volume of fluid you have used. A marked discrepancy suggests that his stomach has perforated.

After you have lavaged his stomach, pass a small nasogastric tube (14 to 19 Ch). This will maintain a lumen, reduce adhesions, and let you to feed him.

Set up a drip, and give him an antibiotic. *Don't oesophagoscope*

GASTRIC LAVAGE

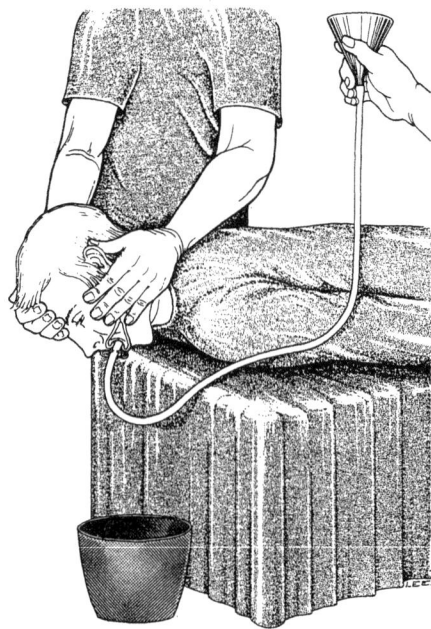

Fig. 25-11. GASTRIC LAVAGE is urgent if a patient has swallowed a corrosive substance. *After 'Hamilton Bailey's Emergency Surgery', edited by HAF Dudley, John Wright, with kind permission.*

him now! In a few days, he will be able to swallow round the tube, as the latent stage is approached.

You may be able to persuade a child to swallow a piece of string coated whith honey, one end remaining outside, while the other goes into his stomach. This will maintain a lumen, however small, and may be a useful way of performing retrograde bouginage later.

If possible refer him, if not proceed as follows.

THE LATENT STAGE

If he has no severe complications immediately, his pain and dysphagia improve, and he may think himself cured. However, during the next 6 weeks (or much longer), the granulation tissue in his oesophagus steadily contracts, and become densely fibrous.

You may be able to oesophagoscope him at 14 days. Don't try to inspect the whole length of his oesophagus with a rigid instrument.

If you cannot refer him, bougie him after 2 weeks and repeat this with care. How often you should bougie him, whether or not you should replace the nasogastric tube, and the time you should leave it in, will depend on how he progresses. Do a barium or 'Gastrografin' swallow, and X-ray his chest.

THE CHRONIC STAGE

If he has not been bougied in the latent stage, he will notice a reversal of the improvement he previously enjoyed. His dysphagia gets worse, but because he has no pain, he does not seek treatment, until he finds he cannot swallow fluids. He is hungry and thirsty, he loses weight, and may vomit due to the obstruction in his oesophagus or stomach. The overspill of his oesophageal contents, held up above the stricture, may cause pulmonary symptoms.

Continue to bougie him as often as is necessary, until you can pass a large bougie (preferably 40 Ch), at 4-monthly intervals, over the period of a year. Most patients will not bougie themselves, and permanent gastrostomies are not accepted, except by patients with malignant strictures, who hardly ever return for follow-up.

DIFFICULTIES WITH CORROSIVE OESOPHAGEAL STRICTURES

If you CANNOT PASS A BOUGIE through his mouth, and you cannot refer him, do a gastrostomy (11.8), and pass a fine Jackson or filiform bougie, with a strong silk thread attached to it, up through his oesophagus, and out through his mouth. Or, use the piece of string he swallowed previously, to pull graded Gabriel-Tucker bougies up his oesophagus to dilate the stricture. After reasonable dilatation, pull a nasogastric tube of appropriate size, as well as a fresh piece of string, up and out of his nose. Use the string for further retrograde bouginage later.

Insert a large de Pezzer or Foley catheter (28 or 30 Ch) through the gastrostomy to keep it open for the same purpose, until you can restart bouginage orally. After a few weeks the acid from his stomach will eat through the balloon, so you will have to replace it.

If all this fails, or if he has a long tight stricture, or multiple ones, he will have to be referred for a stomach, jejunum or colon bypass operation.

REMEMBER, BOUGINAGE IS *EXQUISITELY* DANGEROUS!

25.16 Other problems in the ear, nose, and throat

Here are some other ENT problems which you might meet; most of them are rare. Respiratory obstruction will cause you much anxiety. Dysphagia and hoarseness come second. Some laryngeal emergencies are part of a general illness.

OTHER ENT PROBLEMS

For carcinoma of the maxillary antrum, see Section 32.39.

THE EAR

If a patient develops SLOWLY PROGRESSIVE DEAFNESS IN ONE EAR, becomes unsteady on his feet, and has rare attacks of severe vertigo, suspect an ACOUSTIC NEUROMA (rare). Look for a loss of corneal sensation, slight facial paralysis, and an increased protein in his CSF. Refer him.

THE NOSE AND PARANASAL SINUSES

If a patient has a SWELLING ON HIS NASAL SEPTUM it may be a HAEMATOMA or an ABSCESS. The same incision is suitable for both. Move the tip of his nose from side to side; you will see that swelling is continuous with the columella on both sides, and is fluctuant. Soak a length of 1 cm ribbon gauze in 4% lignocaine, mixed with a few drops of adrenalin, and place it over the red mucosal part of his septum. Wait a few minutes, and then make a vertical incision over the swelling. Remove a small piece of mucosa to enlarge the hole, and insert a drain. Or try aspirating it.

THE LARYNX—STRIDOR

Here are some causes of stridor with the most important causes first. The later ones are all rare. Stridor is always worse on inspiration, unless otherwise stated. Remember also retropharyngeal (5.7) and peritonsillar abscesses (5.6).

If a patient of any age has the RAPID ONSET OF HOARSENESS AND STRIDOR, worse on inspiration, suspect ACUTE LARYNGITIS (not uncommon). Steam and antibiotics will usually cure him. Tracheostomy may occasionally be necessary, but avoid it if possible, especially in a young child. If there is a membrane in his throat, he is likely to have a streptococcal infection (common), or DIPHTHERIA (uncommon).

If a child, particularly, has PROGRESSIVE DYSPHAGIA, continual drooling from his mouth, STRIDOR, COUGH, a red swollen epiglottis, and is ill and febrile, suspect ACUTE EPIGLOTTITIS (not uncommon), which is much more serious than acute laryngitis. If he is old enough to speak, he may have the characteristic 'hot potato' speech, which is different from the hoarseness of laryngitis. Give him chloramphenicol or ampicillin intravenously. Be prepared to intubate him, followed if necessary by tracheostomy. If he is not rapidly and correctly treated, his chances of death are considerable.

If a patient of any age has SLOW PROGRESSIVE HOARSENESS, leading to STRIDOR which is worse on expiration, suspect a papilloma of his larynx, or a carcinoma in older smokers (both not uncommon, 32.39). Tracheostomy and endoscopic removal may be necessary. Biopsy an adult's lesion, and look for malignant change. Recurrence is more common in children, and deaths have occurred.

If a patient of any age has SUDDEN STRIDOR, particularly on inspiration, AFTER INGESTING FOOD, suspect a foreign body (not uncommon). Remove it (25.12).

If a child (usually) has HOARSENESS and variable progressive STRIDOR of RAPID ONSET AFTER FEVER, with severe dysphagia and a bleeding mouth and nose (rare), suspect GANGRENOUS PHARYNGITIS. Give him antibiotics and oxygen. Feed him through a small nasogastric tube, and aspirate his pharynx periodically to remove blood and slough. Mortality is high.

If a baby has STRIDOR SOON AFTER BIRTH, worse on any exertion or crying, but he looks well and his cry is normal, suspect LARYNGOMALACIA (rare). Endoscopy shows a markedly folded epiglottis, with its aryepiglottic folds sucked in towards the larynx during inspiration to cause stridor. Reassure his parents that he will probably recover spontaneously between 3 and 5 years.

If an INFANT OR YOUNG CHILD has sudden, spasmodic STRIDOR, usually at night, which ends spontaneously with another deep inspiratory effort and collapse, suspect LARYNGISMUS AND TETANY (rare). He is normal between attacks. Give him parathyroid hormone and calcium between attacks, and his prognosis will be good.

If a child has had STRIDOR and DYSPNOEA ON EXERTION SINCE BIRTH, perhaps with hoarseness which is progressive with his growth, suspect a LARYNGEAL WEB (rare). Symptoms depend on the degree of stenosis. Tracheostomy may be necessary. Expert surgery can give good results.

If a patient of any age has SUDDEN STRIDOR, worse on expiration, following food, medicine or a sting, suspect ANGIONEUROTIC OEDEMA (rare). Give him an antihistamine or intravenous hydrocortisone. Tracheostomy may be necessary. His prognosis with treatment is good.

If a patient of any age has SUDDEN SEVERE STRIDOR, usually without much hoarseness (rare), suspect LARYNGEAL PARALYSIS due to infection, trauma, poliomyelitis, or nutritional deficiencies. Give him vitamin B complex. Occasionally, a permanent tracheostomy is necessary.

THE OESOPHAGUS

If, after a heavy meal, a patient, who is usually between 20 and 40, VOMITS, AND HAS AN INTENSE PAIN IN HIS LEFT (rarely his right) CHEST radiating to his neck, suspect that he

A DISTAL OESOPHAGEAL TEAR

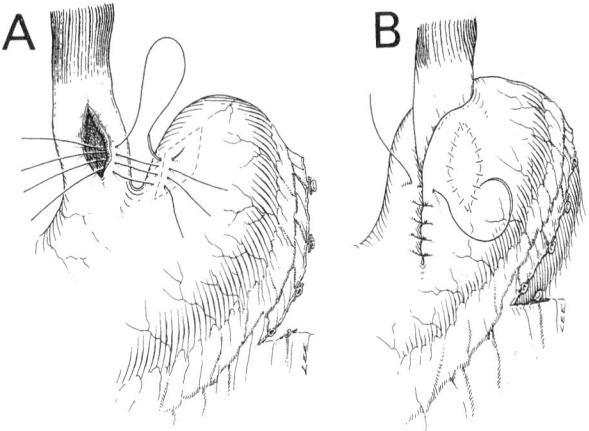

Fig. 25-12. A DISTAL TEAR IN THE OESOPHAGUS is being patched with the stomach, which is wrapped round it. *After 'Hamilton Bailey's Emergency Surgery', edited by HAF Dudley, Fig. 22.4. John Wright, with kind permission.*

has RUPTURED HIS OESOPHAGUS during the act of vomiting. Feel and listen with a stethoscope for surgical emphysema (a fine crackling) in his neck or chest. He is intensely thirsty, but sips of water make the pain worse. If one lung is hyperresonant with no breath sounds, his pleura has perforated, and he has a hydropneumothorax. One differential diagnosis is a perforated peptic ulcer, but here the pain comes *before* the vomiting. When he ruptures his oesophagus the pain comes *as he vomits*. Other differential diagnoses include a spontaneous pneumothorax, acute pancreatitis, and coronary thrombosis. Take a chest X-ray; it may show a pneumothorax, perhaps with a fluid level; if so aspirate this. Confirm a rupture by asking him to swallow 10 or 20 ml of 'Gastrographin', *avoid barium*. This may show a leak. Many of these patients are mistakenly operated on for a perforated peptic ulcer.

CAUTION ! (1) His upper abdomen is usually rigid. (2) Early, he has no clinical or X-ray signs in his chest; these come later when treatment may be too late.

Before you refer him, resuscitate him and pass a nasogastric tube (check radiologically that it is not in his mediastinum). Insert a chest drain with an underwater seal (65.2).

If you cannot refer him, a feeding gastrostomy (11.8) will keep him alive, and a wide bore intercostal tube will evacuate his pleura, and hopefully allow it to seal on to his oesophageal tear.

If you ever find a DISTAL TEAR in the oesophagus, consider mobilizing the stomach, suturing it over the tear as a diamond-shaped patch, and then wrapping the stomach round the oesophagus and suturing them as in Fig. 25-12.

26 Dental and oral surgery

26.1 Introduction

In this chapter we consider those parts of the expertise of the dentist, periodontologist, and oral surgeon that are within your scope. Dental abscesses are described elsewhere (5.8), and so is your role as a maxillofacial surgeon (62.1). Don't forget that a hospital can play a key role in dental health education—improved oral hygiene is one of the main ways to combat caries, and periodontal disease, and to keep the community's teeth in its mouth. When treatment is needed, dental auxiliaries are the main way of giving the community the care it needs at a cost it can afford.

Anaesthesia for operations round the mouth. As so often, much of what you can do will be limited by your anaesthetic skills, or those of your assistant. You can however do much with local infiltration, and with maxillary or pterygopalatine blocks (A 6.3 and 6.4). You can also do many procedures under ketamine (A 8.1), and although this is not usually recommended for work in the mouth, it is likely to be safer than an inexpert general anaesthetic, especially for babies and children under 2 years, as an alternative to intubation. If a patient as small as this is to be intubated, the tiny tracheal tube that he needs is easily blocked. When you use ketamine, you must share with the anaesthetist the critical task of clearing blood from his airwway whenever necessary, and have a swab on dissecting forceps, and a sucker, with a catheter at its tip, instantly ready (see also A 8.1).

Here is the basic equipment you will need:

• CHAIR, operating dental, one only. A dental chair is expensive. If you don't have one you may be able to adapt a strong chair, and fit it with a rest to support the patient's head, when it is pushed firmly backwards, especially when you extract upper teeth.

• DENTAL MIRROR, serrated handle, with No. 4 size plane head, as A, Fig. 26-1, one only.

• DENTAL PROBE, single-ended, as Ash No. 14 (B, 26-1), one only.

• DENTAL DRESSING TWEEZERS, Guttman, as Ash No. 13 (C, 26-1), one only.

• 'PLASTIC INSTRUMENT' Ash No. 6 (D, 26-1), one only. This is for inserting filling material into a cavity.

• SPATULA, metal, for mixing filling material (E, 26-1), one only.

• SCALER, dental, Cumine, as Ash No. 152 (F, 26-1), one only.

• DENTAL MATERIALS, clove oil for dental use, 100 ml only. Zinc oxide powder, 1 kg only. When mixed together on a glass slab with the spatula listed above, these make an effective analgesic and a mildly antiseptic dressing for a dental cavity.

Halestrap DJ, 'Simple dental care for rural hospitals, (4th edn 1981). The Medical Missionary Association, 6 Cannonbury Place, London N1 2HJ.

26.2 Gum disease

The gums of healthy teeth are close up round their necks, and extend up between them, as in G, Fig. 26-2. If gums are diseased by periodontitis, they recede down the necks of the teeth (H, and I, 26-2), which ultimately become loose and are lost. Besides causing sore, bleeding gums, periodontal disease causes more lost teeth in many communities even than caries.

Periodontal disease is the result of a vicious circle. Food particles and plaque accumulate between a tooth and its gum, and cause the gum to slowly recede. This makes the pocket larger, so that food accumulates even more easily. In more severe cases the diseased gums swell, bleed easily (gingivitis), and discharge pus (pyorrhoea), often with severe fetor.

The prevention, and most of the treatment, is improved oral hygiene—better tooth-brushing, as in Fig. 26-2, and, when necessary, scaling to remove calculus (hardened plaque) that has accumulated in the crevices (J, 26-2).

You will not find yourself scaling many teeth yourself, but there must be someone in your hospital who does this, and you should be able to teach him how to do it.

PREVENTIVE DENTISTRY

CLEANING TEETH

Explain to the patient that he should always start with his toothbrush (or toothstick) on his gums, and move it up over his lower teeth, and down over his upper ones, at least 10 times, during at least 2 minutes. This is not easy behind the lower front teeth, and needs much practice. After this, he should rinse out his mouth. If he does not have toothpaste, he can use common salt, or nothing—brushing is more important than paste.

SCALING TEETH

INDICATIONS. One of the causes of bleeding gums is plaque (tartar) round the teeth. Measure the depth of his gum pockets.

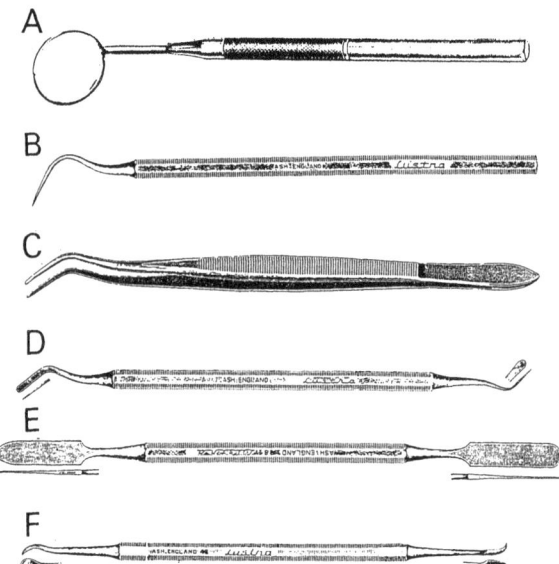

Fig. 26-1 SOME DENTAL INSTRUMENTS. A, a mirror. B, a probe. C, forceps. D, a 'plastic instrument' for putting filling into a tooth. E, a spatula. F, a Cumine scaler. *From the Ash instrument catalogue.*

DENTAL HYGIENE

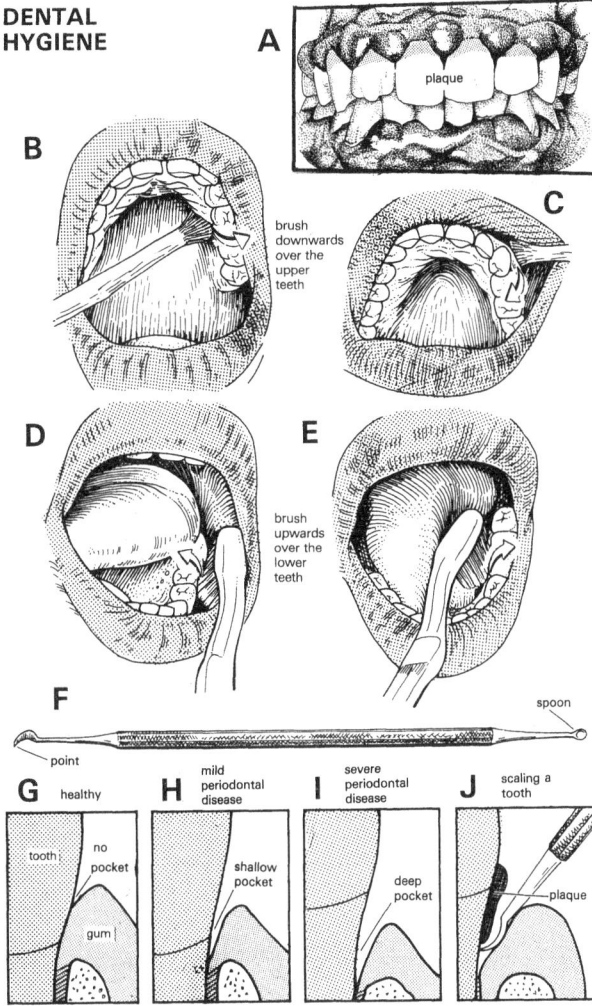

Fig. 26-2 PREVENTIVE DENTISTRY. A, calculus around the lower front teeth. B, and C, using a toothstick on the upper teeth. D, and E, using a toothbrush on the lower teeth. Explain to the patient that he should move the brush vertically from his gums up and over his teeth, and not horizontally along them. F, a dental scaler. G, to J, sections of a tooth and gum. G, healthy gum. H, early periodontal disease. I, severe periodontal disease. J, removing calculus with a scaler. *Halestrap DJ, 'Simple Dental Care for Rural Hospitals' (4th edn 1981), pp.7 and 11. The Medical Missionary Association, with kind permission.*

If these are less than about 5 mm, scaling may be all he needs, but if they are deeper than this, refer him for gingivectomy. If this is impractical, consider extraction.

Use the spoon end of a scaler (F, in Fig. 26-2) to remove deep calculus (hardened plaque, J, in this figure). This starts just below the gum. Removal may be difficult, because the calculus may stick so firmly to his teeth that scraping it off can cause mild pain and bleeding. Use the point of the scaler to remove plaque from between his teeth. Ask him to rinse his mouth out thoroughly, and then show him how to clean his teeth.

CAUTION ! The most important part of the treatment is to show him how to clean his teeth effectively.

26.3 Extracting teeth

You should be able to extract a patient's teeth, either for severe toothache due to irritation of his dental pulp, or abscess formation, or less often, for periodontal disease. This makes teeth so loose that they almost fall out.

Try to remove his tooth with all its roots, and without damaging anything else in his mouth. The secret of success is to force the beaks of the forceps over the visible crown of his tooth, and under his gums, between the periodontal membrane and the alveolar bone, so as to grip its roots firmly. Then, while still grasping his tooth firmly, gently rock it or rotate it depending on the kind of tooth you are removing (as in D, or E, Fig. 26-5). This will break down the periodontal membrane, and widen its socket. The common idea of 'pulling teeth' is false—the important movement is the early one of *pushing* the beaks of the forceps into his jaw around the root of his tooth.

Each forceps has handles, a hinge and a pair of blades. Forceps for the upper jaw are straight, or slightly curved; those for the lower jaw have blades at right angles to their handles.

Ideally, forceps should avoid the crown, and fit the whole surface of the neck and root of a tooth. The blades must be sharp, so that they can easily slide between a tooth and its gum. If necessary, sharpen them on the outside of their tips.

If a tooth has one root, you can loosen it by twisting it (D, 26-5). The teeth which have one root are: the upper incisors and canines, and the lower incisors, canines, and premolars. All other teeth have more than one root, so you cannot twist them. Instead, you have to rock them (E, 26-5). You will need two forceps for upper molars—one for the right and another for the left. Upper molar forceps are curved, so as to avoid the lower lip. The buccal blade with a beak on it is designed to grip the two outer roots, and the palatal blade is designed to grip the one inner root. One pair of lower molar forceps is enough.

* *FORCEPS, dental, set of six with the following Ash numbers: (a) Upper anteriors (Nos. 1 or 2). (b) Upper right molars (Nos. 17 or 94). (c) Upper left molars (Nos. 18 or 95). (d) Upper premolars and roots (No.7). (e) Lower molars (Nos. 73 or 22). (f) Lower anteriors and roots (No. 74N). One only of each.*
* *Alternatively, FORCEPS, dental, universal, set of two, upper universal (No. 36), and lower universal (No.74), one only of each. Dental forceps are expensive, so you may have to manage with these two universal forceps, but they are not so easy to use.*
* *ELEVATORS, dental, (a) upper jaw, straight inclined plane, Coupland, (b) and (c) set of two lower jaw, Cryer's, mesial and distal. One only of each. Coupland's elevator is a small gouge on a metal handle. You will need it to remove roots; if you don't have one you may be able to use the narrow blades of anterior forceps.*
* *PROP, dental, one only. You may find this useful to keep a patient's mouth open while you extract his teeth.*

EXTRACTING TEETH

INDICATIONS. A patient with: (1) A painful, severely carious tooth. (2) A periapical abscess. (3) A periodontal abscess. (4) Severe periodontal disease.

If he has severe periodontal disease and his teeth are firm, but have swollen gums round them, leave them until other remedies have failed—you may be able to save them. But if one or more of his teeth are loose in their sockets, and his gums are red and swollen, and bleed easily on light pressure, remove them.

CONTRAINDICATIONS. Don't try to extract: (1) Buried or impacted teeth. Refer him. If you cannot refer him, see Section 26.4. (2) Displaced teeth. (3) Teeth which have no visible crown. (4) Teeth in very dense bone. Some of these will give you and most dentists much difficulty. (5) Teeth from a patient with a personal or family history of excessive bleeding, particularly bleeding after a previous tooth extraction—refer him. (6) A tooth with an apical abscess, from a patient with heart disease. Refer him; if impossible, proceed as below.

If a small hole in the tooth seems to be responsible for the pain, consider non-operative treatment, and refer him. Clean out the cavity. Use a mixing spatula on a glass surface to make a paste of zinc oxide powder, clove oil and cotton wool fibres. Dry the hole and pack it off with cotton wool to keep it dry. Pack the mixture into the cavity with a plastic hand instrument (D, 26-1), or some substitute for it.

CHILDREN'S TEETH. If he is aged 6 to 12, be very careful when you remove a deciduous tooth, lest you remove or damage the permanent tooth under it.

EXTRACTING TEETH

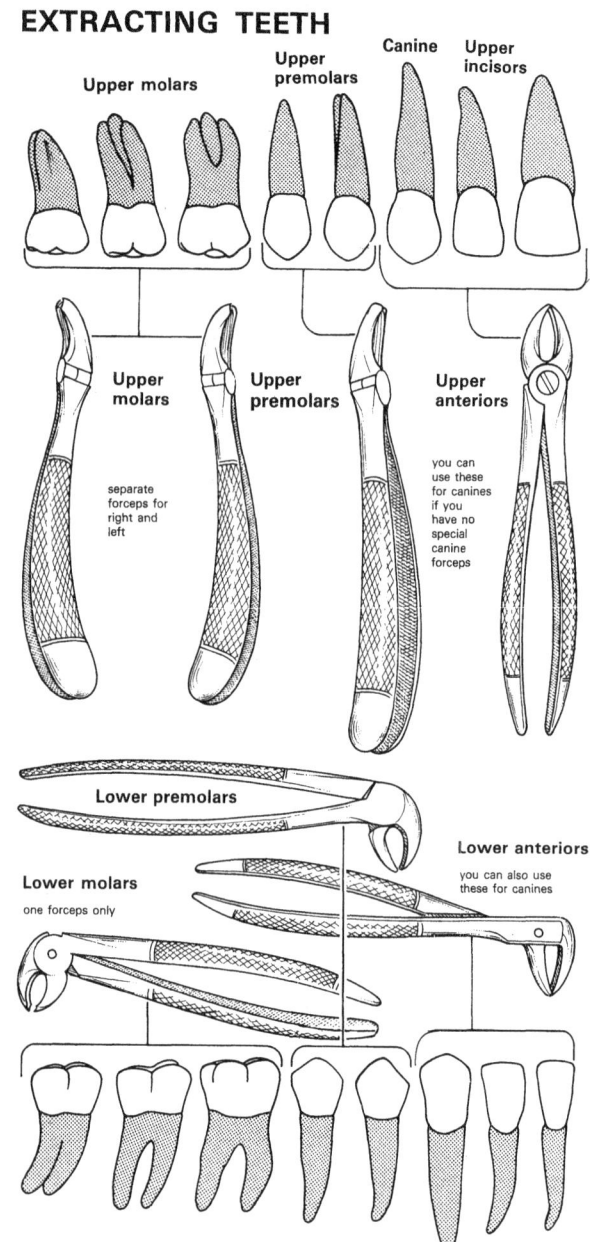

Fig. 26-3 TEETH AND FORCEPS FOR THEM. Forceps for the upper teeth are straight, and those for the lower teeth are cranked. There are separate forceps for the upper molars, right and left; all other forceps can be used on either side. The beak of a pair of molar forceps is always on the outside, where it fits between the two buccal roots. *Kindly contributed by Hanif Butt.*

MEDICAL HISTORY. Don't forget this. If he has any form of heart disease, extract his teeth under antibiotic cover.

WHICH TOOTH? If he has toothache, he usually knows which tooth is causing it. Occasionally, when the pain is referred, he is wrong even about which jaw it is in. So don't necessarily remove the tooth which he thinks is at fault. The offending tooth may: (1) Have a large hole in it. If you cannot immediately see any carious areas, use a dental mirror to look for them on the adjacent surfaces of his teeth. (2) Be broken, black, or brown. (3) Look grey under its enamel. (4) Be loose, and surrounded by severe periodontal disease. (4) Be tender on gentle tapping. Tap each tooth in turn with the handle of a dental mirror. The most sensitive one is likely to be the cause of his toothache.

X-RAYS. If a tooth is displaced or impacted, X-ray it.

ANTIBIOTICS. If he has an apical abscess (5.8), give him an antibiotic for 24 hours beforehand, and continue it for three days afterwards.

EXTRACTING TEETH

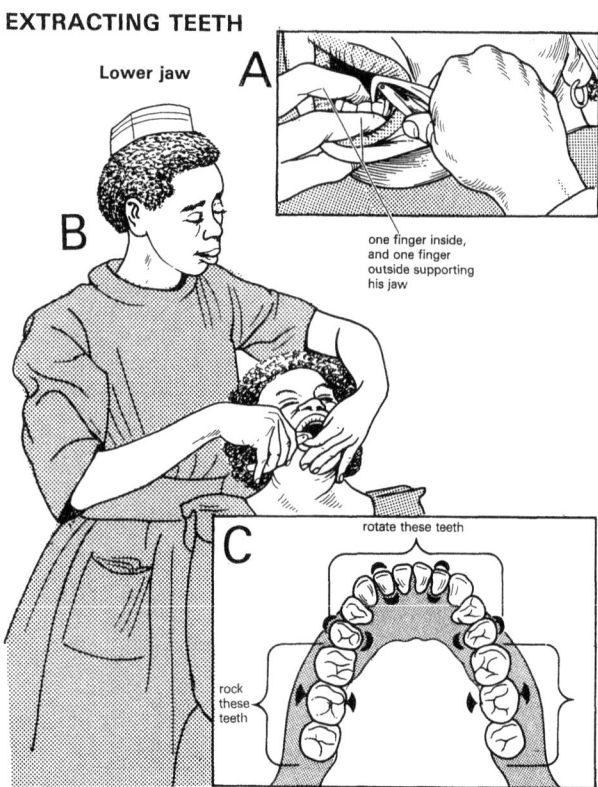

Fig. 26-4 EXTRACTING A LOWER RIGHT TOOTH. Stand behind the patient. If you cannot get low enough, stand on a box or something stable. Support his jaw with one finger inside it and one outside it. *From 'Common oral diseases', Fig. 2.9.3. WHO, with the kind permission of Martin Hobdell.*

ANAESTHESIA. Use local anaesthesia (A 6.3). Make sure that a tooth is properly anaesthetized, by pushing a blunt probe into the gingival crevice on its buccal and lingual surfaces. If he feels pressure but not pain, anaesthesia is adequate. If he feels pain, inject more anaesthetic.

POSITION. Sit him down so that his head is level with your chest as you stand. Position yourself and him correctly. The stance of the operator in B, Fig. 26-5 is ideal.

IF YOU ARE EXTRACTING A LOWER TOOTH, use right-angled forceps and press downwards. First, where to stand and how to position him:

If you are extracting a lower front tooth or a lower left molar or premolar, sit him upright in the chair, and low enough for his mouth to be level with your elbow. If he is too high stand on something. Grip his alveolus between the first and second fingers of your left hand, and put your thumb under his mandible.

If you are extracting a lower right premolar or molar tooth, **stand behind him (B, Fig. 26-4).**

If you are left handed, **stand behind him** for extracting all lower left premolar and molar teeth. For all others, stand in front of him, but to the left of his legs.

Lower teeth. The beaks of lower molar forceps are both pointed to fit between the two flattened roots. Use small rotating movements combined with a sideways movement between his tongue and his cheek. Use constant downward pressure, and support his jaw in your other hand.

To extract a lower incisor tooth, stand in front of him, push the beaks of the forceps down round the root, and apply a gently backwards and forwards movement.

To extract a lower canine, which has a more rounded root, use gentle rotating movements (D, 26-5).

To extract lower left premolars, turn his head towards you and use gentle rotating movements.

To extract lower right premolars, move to his right, or even stand behind his right shoulder.

EXTRACTING TEETH

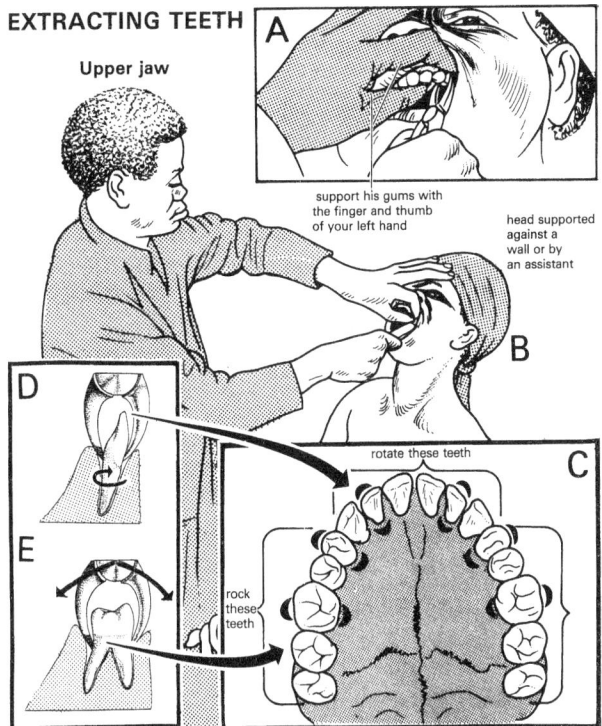

Fig. 26-5 EXTRACTING TEETH FROM THE UPPER JAW. A, support the patient's gums between the finger and thumb of your left hand. B, tilt his head backwards and support it against a wall, or ask an assistant to support it. Note the excellent stance of the operator in this figure. C, the teeth to rotate (those with single roots), and the teeth to rock (those with more than one root). D, rotating a tooth with a single root. E, rocking a tooth. *From 'Common oral diseases', Fig. 2.9.2, WHO, with the kind permission of Martin Hobdell.*

To extract a lower right molar, stand behind his right shoulder, and use a side-to-side rocking action (E, 26-5).

If you have difficulty extracting his lower third molar, this may be because its roots are deformed, and need to be dissected out with bone chisels—see Section 26.4.

IF YOU ARE EXTRACTING AN UPPER TOOTH, tilt his head backwards. If your chair does not have a head rest, support his head against a wall, or ask your assistant to support it. Stand in front and to the right of the patient's legs. For all upper teeth, put the finger and thumb of your left hand on either side of his gums.

CAUTION ! (1) Make sure that the long axis of the blades is in the long axis of the tooth. (2) Don't grasp his tooth and his gum together. (3) Carious teeth are brittle and will break, if you put too much sideways pressure on them—don't use the forceps as a 'nut cracker'. (4) Don't start extracting movements when you have only grasped the crown of his tooth. (5) When you rock a tooth, feel if it is responding to reasonable pressure; if it does not respond and seems very firmly fixed, refer him.

An upper incisor, or an upper canine has a single conical root, so rotate the tooth at the same time as you press it firmly in the direction of its tip (D, 26-5). Finally, tilt it outwards.

An upper premolar has delicate roots (the first premolar often has two), so be as gentle as you can. So make *small* side to side and rotating movements while you push upwards with considerable force. When the tooth is loose, pull it downwards.

An upper molar has three roots, two on the buccal side, and a single large one on the inside next to the palate. The roots of the third molar are sometimes fused together. Choose the correct molar forceps (right or left), so that the pointed blade slips down outside the crown between the roots on the buccal side. Press upwards *firmly* until the beaks are beside the roots, while you make *slight* side-to-side rocking movements to loosen it (E, 26-5). Finally, increase these movements, and exert pressure in an outward direction, until you can draw the tooth out of its socket into his cheek.

CAUTION ! Make sure you support his alveolus firmly between your finger and thumb, because you can easily break off part of it, especially when you extract a third molar, and break his maxillary tuberosity.

AFTER ANY EXTRACTION, examine the tips of the roots you have removed. If they are not complete, see below.

POSTOPERATIVELY AFTER TOOTH EXTRACTION

Allow him to rinse out his mouth *once only.* Remove loose bits of bone and tissue. Push the lingual and labial sides of his empty socket together. Place a tight ball of gauze over his socket, and tell him to bite on this for 15 or 30 minutes—make sure it presses *on to* the socket. When you remove it 15 minutes later, bleeding should have stopped. If it has not, see below.

Ask him not to spit, or wash to out his mouth again for 24 hours—it may wash away the blood, which should be clotting in his empty socket. The following morning, he can start rinsing out his mouth with saline, using a small spoonful of salt to a cup of water. If his empty socket does not bleed after you have removed his tooth, use a dental probe to scratch around inside it until it does bleed. A socket which does not bleed is more likely to become infected (see below under 'dry socket'). Tell him not to meddle with the socket.

CAUTION ! If you have extracted his tooth for an abscess, make sure he returns for antibiotic treatment if his swelling does not rapidly improve.

DIFFICULTIES DURING TOOTH EXTRACTION

If there is a constant OOZING during the operation, swab, suck, and apply packs. If necessary, press a dry pack over the wound for 2 minutes *timed by the clock.*

If his tooth is IMMOVABLE, and fails to yield when you apply reasonable force with forceps, or an elevator, it probably needs dissection. So stop and refer him: it may have curved roots or be ankylosed.

If the crown or a ROOT BREAKS as you extract a tooth, examine it carefully to see how much you have left behind. What you should do depends on how much is left.

If it is only a root apex, less than 5 mm in its greatest dimension, removing it is going to need much dissection. Leave it. If he is healthy, the retained apex of a vital tooth is unlikely to cause trouble.

If the root is larger than 5 mm, try to extract the fragment of the broken root with a Coupland's inclined plane elevator as in Fig. 26-7. Wiggle the elevator between the root and its socket.

CAUTION ! (1) Hold the elevator with your index finger near its tip in case it slips. (2) The roots of the upper premolar and molars are very close to the antrum, so that you can easily push a root into it.

If his ALVEOLUS BREAKS as you remove his tooth, examine the socket. Remove any bony fragment which has lost over half its periosteal attachment. Grip it with haemostatic forceps, and dissect off the soft tissues.

If you DISPLACE A TOOTH INTO HIS ANTRUM, refer him. If you cannot refer him, see below.

If, while you are extracting an upper molar, you feel SUPPORTING BONE MOVE WITH HIS TOOTH, you have FRACTURED HIS MAXILLARY TUBEROSITY, and are in danger of opening his antrum. If only a small piece of tuberosity has broken off, remove it. If a larger piece has broken, refer him. Removing the tooth and the detached fragment will open his antrum. He will need to have a mucoperiosteal flap made to cover the gap. Warn him that if he has the same teeth extracted on the other side, the same thing may happen again.

If, when you remove his upper molar, YOU SUSPECT YOU HAVE MADE A FISTULA, ask him to grip his nose and to try to blow air through it. This will raise the pressure in his antrum, make blood in his socket bubble, and deflect a wisp of gauze if you hold it over the socket. Refer him to have the fistula closed with a flap. If you cannot refer him, see below. Meanwhile, don't allow him to rinse out his mouth until the defect has been repaired, and don't put any instrument through the fistula— you may infect his antrum.

If extraction of a tooth has CAUSED A FISTULA, you see him within 24 hours, and cannot refer him, close it immediately, by incising the periosteum, and advancing a buccal mucoperiosteal flap over the defect, as in E, Fig. 26-7, and sew it in place. Postoperatively, give him an antibiotic and inhalations of tincture of benzoin.

If you see him after 24 hours, the edges of the wound will probably be infected, so that if you close it now, the suture line will probably break down. Allow the area to heal, excise the fistulous tract, and close the fistula with a buccal flap.

You can remove most teeth or roots from the antrum through the original defect enlarged if necessary. Failing this, the Caldwell–Luc approach will give you better access (25-7).

If you LOSE A TOOTH while you are extracting it, immediately bring his head forwards, and hope he will cough it out. X-ray the socket and his chest. If he has inhaled it, refer him to have it removed by bronchoscopy during the next few days, before a lung abscess develops. If you cannot refer him, you may have to bronchoscope him yourself (25.12).

If you BREAK HIS MANDIBLE (62.7) or dislocate it (62.6), treat these injuries as described elsewhere.

If you INJURE HIS TONGUE, and the wound is small, it needs no treatment except mouth washes. If it is larger, pull it forwards and suture it.

If he has an EXTRA TOOTH, it is usually conical, and may present almost anywhere on his jaw, and even in a nostril. Removing it may call for skill and ingenuity. If necessary use a dental elevator to clear away the soft tissues of his gum before you apply forceps.

BLEEDING AFTER TOOTH EXTRACTION

His socket may bleed too much or, more rarely, not enough. If it fails to bleed adequately, it is more likely to become infected (see below). Bleeding during the first few hours is likely to be reactionary haemorrhage. Later bleeding is the result of infection.

After any tooth extraction, squeeze his gums between your finger and thumb for a few minutes. Then allow him to rinse gently with clean water. If he continues to bleed, follow these steps in order. If one fails, try the next.

(1) Ask him to bite on a pad of damp cottonwool, or gauze, for 15 minutes.

(2) Ask him to bite on it for a further 30 minutes. Make sure the pad really does press on to the socket this time.

(3) Soak a small ball of cotton wool in the contents of a 1 mg ampoule of adrenalin. Press this into his bleeding socket for 30 minutes.

(4) Stitch his gums. Use a half-circle cutting needle in a needle-holder and 3/0 black waxed silk, or any suitable suture material, to hold a plug of haemostatic gauze over his bleeding socket, as in A, Fig. 26-6. If you don't have haemostatic gauze, use cotton wool; but be sure to remove it in 48 hours.

Alternatively, bring the edges of his gum together. If they will not come together, chip away the bone from the crests of the socket until they do. This will put his gum under tension, and make it less likely to bleed. Send him home biting on the pack.

CAUTION ! Don't be content with inadequate suturing, it will only cause more problems later.

INFECTION AFTER TOOTH EXTRACTION

He may return some days after a tooth extraction complaining of:

(1) PAIN AND BLEEDING. His empty socket is probably infected. Irrigate it, remove clot and food debris, pack it with haemostatic gauze, and suture it. Place a firm gauze pack on it and ask him to bite on this. Give him an antibiotic. Don't let him rinse out his mouth, which may restart the bleeding; instead, clean it with wet gauze. If you don't have any haemostatic gauze, suturing it without gauze is probably better than suturing it over ordinary gauze.

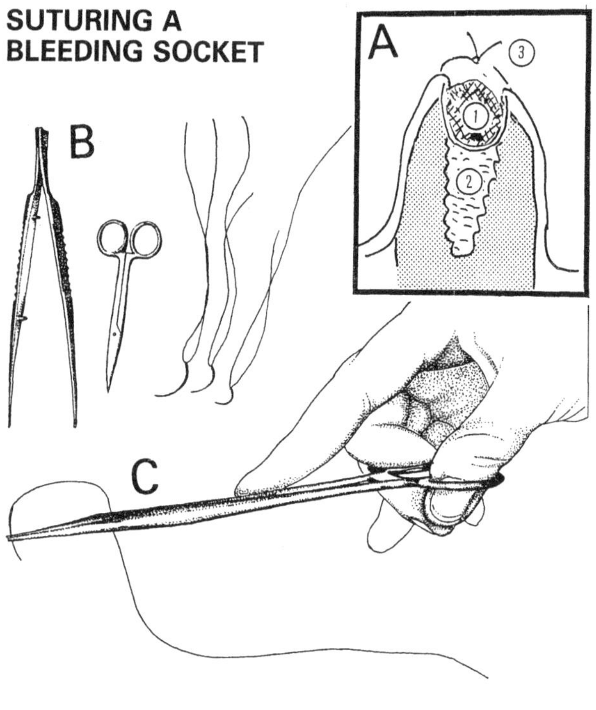

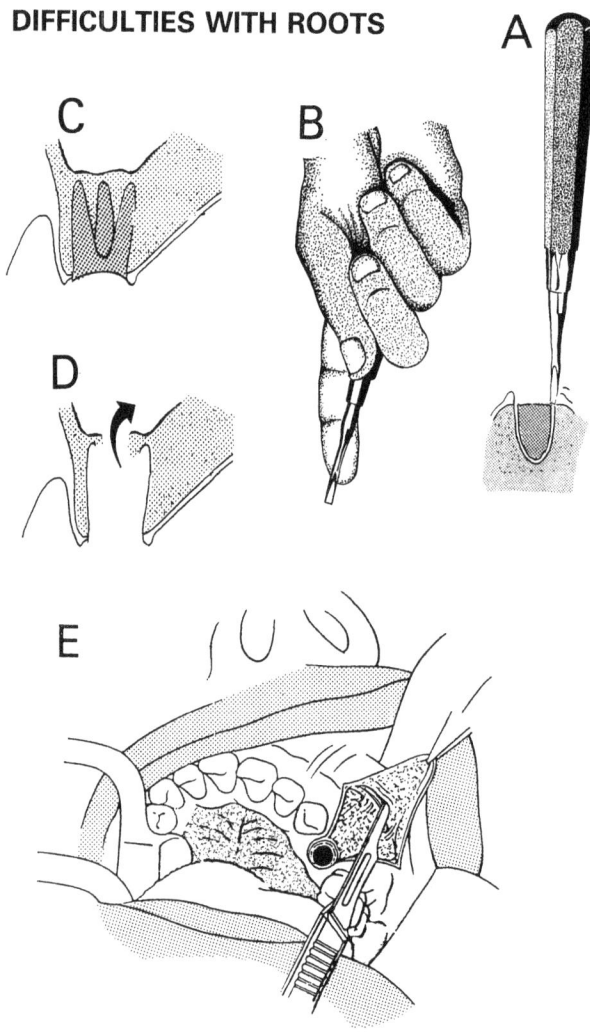

SUTURING A BLEEDING SOCKET

Fig. 26-6 SUTURING A BLEEDING SOCKET. A, a ball of haemostatic gauze (1), soaked in adrenalin and plugging a clot filled socket (2), which is closed by stitches (3). B, the equipment. C, how to hold the needle. *B, and C, from 'Common oral diseases', WHO, with the kind permission of Martin Hobdell.*

DIFFICULTIES WITH ROOTS

Fig. 26-7 DIFFICULTIES WITH ROOTS. A, Coupland's inclined plane dental elevator (not to scale with the tooth socket). B, how to hold this with your finger close to the end, to act as a guard. C, the roots of a patient's upper teeth are close to his maxillary antrum. D, be careful not to cause an oro-antral fistula. E, a relieving incision being made through the periosteum (only) on the under surface of a mucoperiosteal flap, which will be moved across to close an oro-antral fistula. *A, to D, kindly contributed by DJ Halestrap. E, after 'Hamilton Bailey's Emergency Surgery' edited by HAF Dudley, Fig. 16.45 (John Wright), with the kind permission of Hugh Dudley.*

(2) An acutely PAINFUL EMPTY SOCKET, without any clot in it. He has a DRY SOCKET. This is a local osteitis of the condensed bone that lines it. The danger is that osteomyelitis may follow. If you cannot refer him, irrigate it with warm saline and remove any food and degenerating blood clot. Under local anaesthesia, scratch around inside it to make it bleed. Try to excise any sharp bone spurs. When it has bled, and a clot has formed, it will probably heal. A dry socket is very painful, so make sure you give him adequate analgesics.

(3) FEVER and a very painful socket, a mandible which is exquisitely tender, and perhaps numbness of his lips (due to involvement of his mental nerve). He has acute OSTEOMYELITIS. Admit him and treat him as in Section 7.14a.

BROKEN ROOTS AFTER TOOTH EXTRACTION

If a ROOT BREAKS OFF as you remove a tooth, leave a small piece (less than a third of a root) in place. Remove a larger piece. You may be able to do this with the narrow blades of a pair of anterior forceps, or by passing Coupland's inclined plane elevator between the root and its socket, as in A, Fig. 26-7. Try to push the elevator towards the bottom of the socket, while you press it firmly and rotate it a little each way. As you do so, hold it with your thumb near its tip, to prevent it doing any unnecessary damage (B). It should act like a wedge and move the root out of the socket. You can also use this elevator for loosening very firm teeth.

If you FAIL TO REMOVE A ROOT, destroy its pulp by pushing a dental probe down it, cover it with a zinc oxide and oil of cloves dressing, and explain that you have left a root behind. Ask him to return in a few weeks time. Then try again; removing it this time may be easier.

CAUTION ! Don't try to remove a fractured maxillary root by passing instruments up the socket. You may enter his antrum and cause a fistula (D, 26-7). This is much more likely to occur with molars and premolars, than with incisors and canines.

OTHER DIFFICULTIES WITH CARIOUS TEETH

If he presents with a SMALL GRANULOMA with a discharge and underlying thickening, on his lower face, jaw, or chin, or inside his mouth on the surfaces of his alveoli, it is probably a DENTAL SINUS. An abscess around an infected residual root has caused an abscess in the bone under it, which has tracked through his soft tissues, to discharge on his gums or on the surface of his face. X-rays show a carious tooth, or a residual root, opposite the sinus. Give him a general anaesthetic, or ketamine, and remove the root with a dental elevator and forceps. Curette away the granulation tissue on his face. The discharge will stop in 48 hours, and the granuloma will not recur. If X-rays show signs of osteomyelitis, give him an antibiotic.

26.4 Impacted third molars ('wisdom teeth')

A lower third molar sometimes fails to erupt because it faces forwards, or lies horizontally impacted against the second molar. A pocket or flap of gum (operculum) may overhang it, so that food is trapped and inflammation results. The patient, who is usually a young adult, but who may be an old one, complains of pain, which may be referred to his ear, and sometimes trismus. Secondary infection may follow.

IMPACTED THIRD MOLARS

Gently syringe the space between the crown of the patient's unerupted tooth, and the flap of gum over it, with warm saline. Then insert a pledget of cotton wool soaked in oil of cloves under the flap. Give him an antibiotic, and ask him to use hot saline mouth washes. His infection may settle down.

AN IMPACTED WISDOM TOOTH

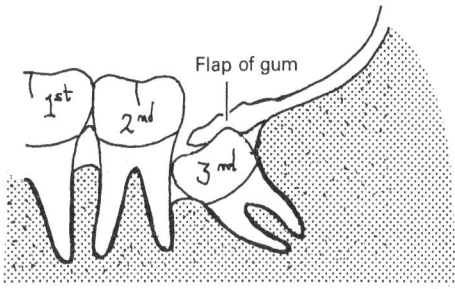

Fig. 26-9 AN IMPACTED WISDOM TOOTH. This patient's third molar is lying obliquely in his jaw and is covered by a flap of gum. Food may be trapped and inflammation result. *Kindly contributed by James Gardiner.*

If his infection does not settle, and you cannot refer him, you may be able to incise the gum round the edge of the apex of his tooth, so that food no longer packs around it.

If a third molar is pressing on the gum flap, and making his condition worse, refer him to have it removed, when the acute infection has subsided. If necessary, control infection and trismus with mouth washes, syringing, and antibiotics. If this fails, refer him. If you cannot refer him, give him an inferior alveolar and lingual nerve block (A 6.3).

If his second molar is carious, remove it to leave space for his third.

If his second molar is normal, and his impacted third molar is at a nearly normal angle, use bone forceps or dental forceps to nibble away his jaw behind it.

If his third molar is completely horizontal, split it with a chisel, and then extract it in two parts, with any convenient forceps.

26.6 Cancrum oris

Cancrum oris is now rarely seen in the industrial world, but in many developing countries it is not uncommon. It is a gangrenous process of the mouth, which starts suddenly, rapidly involves the adjacent tissues of the face, quickly becomes well demarcated, and then spreads no further. It most often affects one or both sides of the jaw, and occasionally the front of the face (mouth,

DENTAL SINUSES

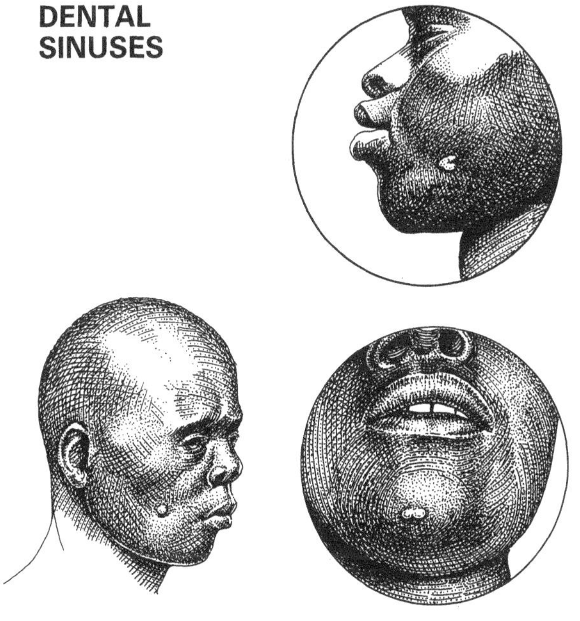

Fig. 26-8 THREE DENTAL SINUSES. A dental sinus is caused by a chronically infected residual dental root which has caused an abscess in the bone around it. This erupts on the gums, or, less often, on the surface of the cheek. *After Charles Bowesman. 'Surgery and Clinical Pathology in the Tropics'. E and S Livingstone, permission requested.*

lips, nose, and chin). *Fusiformis* and *Borrelia* are largely responsible, but it is not contagious. It resembles Fournier's gangrene of the scrotum (23.30), and may be associated with simultaneous extraoral gangrenous lesions of the limbs, perineum, neck, chest, scalp, or ear, etc.

Although cancrum oris can occur at any age, you will see it most commonly in a malnourished child between 1 and 5, whose general health has been further weakened by some infectious disease, usually measles, but also malaria, gastroenteritis, typhoid, whooping cough, tuberculosis or leukaemia, etc. Sometimes, there is no antecedent infection.

The lesion starts inside a child's mouth, in association with acute ulcerative gingivitis, and then spreads to his lips and cheeks. The earliest stage, which is seldom seen, is a painful red or purplish-red spot, or indurated papule, on his alveolar margin, most often in his premolar or molar region. This lesion rapidly forms an ulcer, which exposes his underlying alveolar bone. If you see him at this stage, he has a sore mouth, a swollen, tender, painful lip or cheek, profuse salivation, and an extremely foul smell, with purulent discharge from his mouth or nose. Within the next 2 or 3 days, a bluish-black area of discoloration appears externally on his lips, or cheek. The gangrenous area is cone-shaped, so that much more tissue is destroyed inside his mouth, than his external wound might indicate. After separation of the slough, his exposed bone and teeth rapidly sequestrate.

Quite extensive superficial lesions can heal suprisingly well. But destruction of his deeper tissues, teeth and skeleton can produce such appalling disfigurement that you have to refer him for expert plastic surgery—if he is lucky. This may include: the correction of gross mutilation, 'dental anarchy', trismus (particularly difficult) and a salivary leak. You can however treat him during the acute stage, as described below. Untreated cancrum oris is almost always quickly fatal, due to the associated illness (measles, typhoid, diarrhoea etc.) or a complication, such as septicaemia or aspiration pneumonia. Secondary haemorrhage is most unusual. and cavernous sinus thrombosis (5.5) has never been reported.

Tempest MN, 'Cancrum oris'. British Journal of Surgery, 1966;53:11, 949-69.

Tempest MN, 'Cancrum Oris'. Tropical Doctor 1971;4:164-169

THE ACUTE STAGE OF CANCRUM ORIS
Start emergency treatment immediately, and aim to build up the child's general resistance. If possible admit him. There is no need to isolate him. If admission is impractical, outpatient treatment is possible.

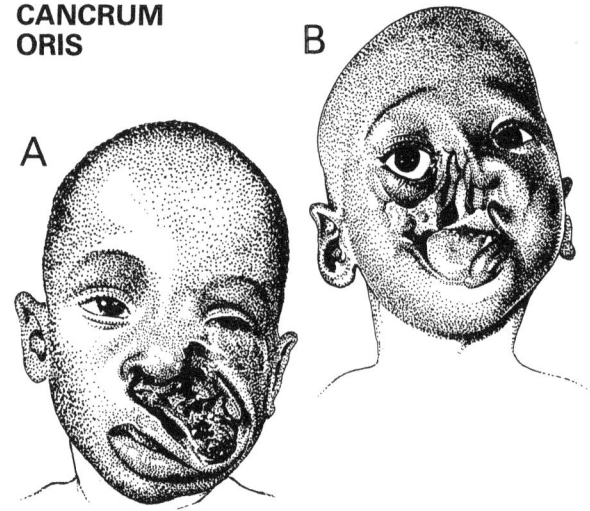

Fig. 26-10 CANCRUM ORIS. **A, cancrum oris in the acute stage, showing well-demarcated gangrene of the upper lip and adjacent cheek. B, a typical example of the gross facial mutilation that follows.** *After Michael Tempest with the kind permission of the editor of Tropical Doctor.*

FEEDING AND ELECTROLYTES. You can usually correct his protein energy malnutrition, by feeding him by mouth. If his mouth is too sore, feed him through a nasogastric tube.

CORRECT HIS ANAEMIA; give him folic acid, iron, ascorbic acid, and the vitamin B complex, particularly nicotinic acid.

ANTIBIOTICS. Give him penicillin in large doses and metronidazole.

CARE FOR THE LESION by repeatedly irrigating it with saline. Chewing raw pineapple, or slices of orange, will help to clean his mouth. Pack cavities with gauze pads soaked in hypochlorite ('Eusol'), saline, or BIPP. Change these dressings often, and keep them moist by adding more solution to the outer layers. Avoid vaseline gauze (which acts like a foreign body), especially when it has been impregnated with antibiotics.

If he is fit enough for surgery, cut away any separating sloughs, and remove any loose teeth or sequestra. When quite large sequestra are ready to separate, you may be able to remove them under ketamine.

If he is too ill for surgery, allow the dead tissues to separate spontaneously. Sequestra occasionally drop out. More often, they have to be removed after 3 or 4 weeks, when his condition has improved enough for surgery to be safe.

CAUTION ! There is no place for radical surgery at this stage, except to control bleeding (rare).

REFER HIM FOR REPAIR at 3 to 6 months, before marked trismus develops. This will allow his scars to mature, his local tissues to become soft and pliable, and his health to improve. Meanwile, do your best for his nutrition, and for his oral hygiene.

26.7 Jaw swellings

Lesions which make the jaws swell are comparatively more common in the developing world than they are elsewhere. Apart from trauma (62.1), the jaws can swell as the result of conditions which include: (1) Infection: an alveolar abscess (5.8), a dental sinus which is sometimes misdiagnosed as an early jaw tumour (26-8), and osteomyelitis (7.14a). (2) Any of the cysts described below. (3) Tumours: Burkitt's lymphoma (32.3), ameloblastoma (see below), carcinoma, salivary tumours (32.23), and giant cell tumours (D, 26-12, A, 32-1). (4) A complex group of fibro-osseous lesions which will not be discussed further here.

In managing tumours, and particularly cysts of the jaw, be aware of the possibility of: (1) A giant cell tumour which is only locally invasive, but may grow very large if it is not treated, as in Figure 32-1. (2) An ameloblastoma (adamantinoma). This arises inside the jaw from the enamel organ of a tooth, and slowly destroys the surrounding bone. It may be solid or cystic, it is locally invasive like a basal cell carcinoma, and does not metastasize. You are unlikely to miss an ameloblastoma if you remember that: (a) The radiolucent lesions it produces are commonly multilocular (the cysts below are mostly unilocular). (b) The solid tissue from around any 'cyst' should be sent for histology, which is the only certain way of making the diagnosis (the cysts below are filled with liquid). If you think that a patient might have an ameloblastoma, refer him for its radical removal.

The following cysts originate from the teeth, and present as smooth, slowly enlarging, painless swellings, usually on the buccal surface of the lower jaw, or on either surface of the upper one. They may be hard, tense, or fluctuant. If the bone over a cyst is thin it may crackle like an eggshell when you press it. Tenderness and pain are signs that a cyst has become infected. These cysts are benign, they can be treated without too much difficulty, and with the exception of an odontogenic keratocyst, they seldom recur.

A dental cyst forms round the apex of a chronically infected, and usually non-vital, tooth, commonly in an older patient. Chronic infection causes the epithelial remnants in the periodontal membrane to grow, and become cystic. Dental cysts are usually quite small, and are commonly symptomless. Occasionally, they grow large enough to expand the alveolus in which they arise. In the maxilla they may encroach on the antra, or the nasal fossae.

The fluid they contain is usually clear, but may contain cholesterol crystals. X-rays show a clearly defined, well corticated, unilocular radiolucency, unless the cyst is infected, which causes it to lose its cortex.

A dentigerous cyst usually arises in a young adult from the follicle of a normal unerupted, or erupting, permanent tooth. It expands the outer table of his jaw while the stronger inner one prevents a pathological fracture. The tooth which forms the cyst usually fails to erupt, and you can see that it is missing from its normal place in his mouth. X-rays show a well corticated unilocular radiolucency *containing the unerupted tooth*. If this tooth is normally placed, opening the cyst may allow it to erupt. Often, it is so misplaced that it cannot erupt, and you will have to enucleate it.

An odontogenic keratocyst (rare) is filled with keratinized epithelial squames. These make the contents creamy, so that it looks like pus, and can only be distinguished from pus microscopically. Don't confuse this cyst with an abscess; there are no signs of infection. X-rays show a well corticated uni- or multi-loculated radiolucency. These cysts are particularly likely to recur after they have been removed (20–60%), so refer him.

Developmental cysts (rare) are not associated with teeth. The commonest one is a nasopalatine cyst, which develops from epithelial remnants in the incisive (nasopalatine) canal, immediately behind the upper front teeth. If it is causing problems it should be enucleated. If this is impractical you may have to marsupialize it, taking care not to injure his incisor teeth and the vessels to them.

Although dental cysts are more common, they are usually small and symptomless, so that dentigerous cysts are more likely to present to you for treatment. There are several ways of treating cysts, and each type of cyst has its preferred method: (1) You can marsupialize a cyst, by removing the mucosa over it, together with the immediately underlying bony wall and lining, washing it out, and then suturing the lining of its floor to the surrounding mucoperiosteum. This relieves tension, stops further expansion, allows drainage, and lets the space the cyst occupied slowly fill up from the bottom. (2) You can pack a cyst open. (3) You can decompress a dentigerous cyst, by opening it, and allowing the tooth in it to erupt. (4) An expert can enucleate a cyst by reflecting a periosteal flap, opening it, removing all its lining, and then replacing the flap. This is more difficult than the preceding methods, and is not described here. (5) An expert can also excise a piece of jaw with the lesion. This is the treatment of choice for an ameloblastoma, a giant cell tumour, an odontogenic keratocyst, an ossifying fibroma, a carcinoma, and also for fibrosarcoma. Although resected jaw can be replaced with bone or metal, this is not absolutely necessary, because life without a mandible is still worth living, because a patient's tongue is strong enough to crush his food against his palate.

SWELLINGS OF THE JAWS PARTICULARLY
CYSTS

EXAMINATION. Stand exactly in front of the patient and inspect his face carefully for asymmetry, especially of his mouth, nostril, and the level of his inner canthi. Feel the mass carefully. Most dental cysts which arise from an apical infection are small (<1 cm), most dentigerous cysts are quite large (3–8 cm). Examine and count his teeth.

If a tooth is missing (and has not fallen out), it may be hidden in a dentigerous cyst.

If one tooth in a line of permanent teeth is much smaller than the others, it might be a persistent milk tooth, with the missing permanent one hidden in a dentigerous cyst.

Aspirate and examine the fluid from the swelling with a wide-bore needle. If you withdraw clear yellow fluid it is a cyst. If you withdraw a substance that looks like pus, it is either true pus from an infection, or a mixture of keratinous squames from an odontogenic keratocyst. Microscopy will tell you which of these it is. Look for dental sinuses (26-8) on his gums or face.

X-RAYS. Take films in two planes. Compare the density of the sinus shadows on either side. A cyst is an area of radiolucency surrounded by a radio-opaque line. If there is a tooth in the cyst it is dentigerous, otherwise it is probably dental.

CAUTION ! (1) Be careful to distinguish a cyst in the maxilla from a normal part of his antrum—this can be difficult. (2) The signs that indicate that the lesion is not a simple dental cyst, but a more aggressive lesion are: (a) A multilocular ('honeycomb') radiolucency, indicating an ameloblastoma, an odontogenic keratocyst, or a giant cell tumour. (b) A loss of cortex, indicating an aggressive lesion, particularly a carcinoma. If a benign cyst is infected, it may also lose its cortex.

MANAGEMENT depends on the type of cyst.

If a dental cyst is small and symptomless, leave it.

If it is small but is causing symptoms, remove the tooth and curette the cyst.

If a dental cyst is large, and especially if it is in his upper jaw (unusual), refer him if you can. The danger is that you may create a fistula between his mouth and his nose or his antrum. He may need to have the fistula closed surgically.

If he has a dentigerous cyst which is smaller than about the end of your thumb, you may be able to operate on it, especially if it is in his lower jaw.

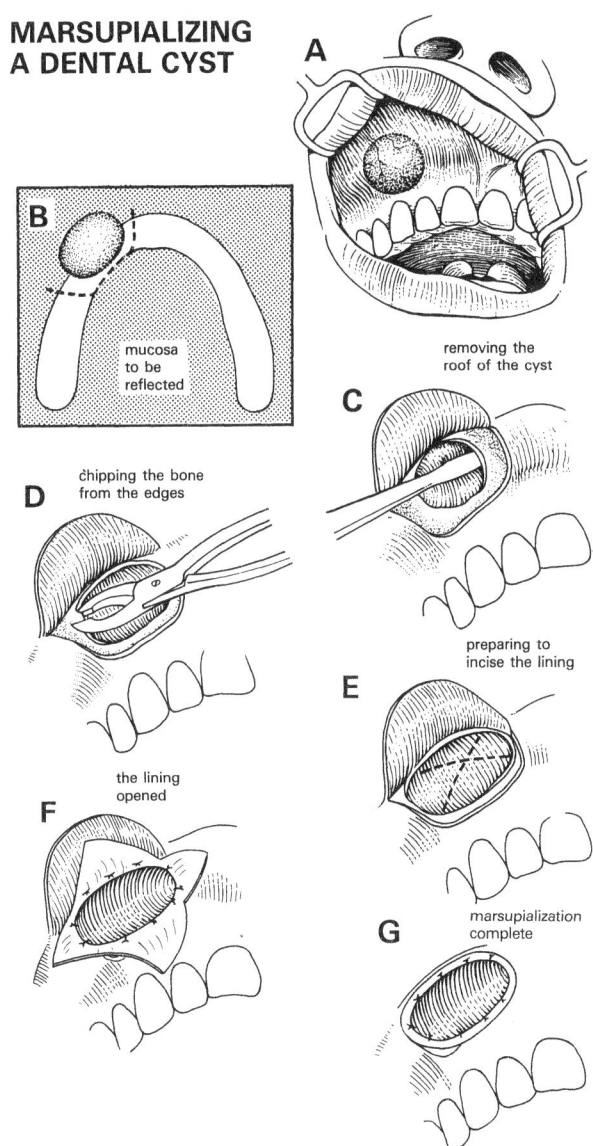

Fig. 26-11 MARSUPIALIZING A CYST. A, a cyst on the gum. B, the area of the mucoperiosteal flap to be reflected. C, removing the bony roof of the cyst. D, trimming the bone from the edges of the cyst. E, preparing to incise the lining of the cyst. F, the cyst opened. G, marsupialization complete. *Adapted from Howe and Zamet, 'Minor Oral Surgery', Fig. 194. John Wright with kind permission.*

MARSUPIALIZING A CYST

INDICATIONS. (1) An easier alternative to enucleation for a larger dental cyst. (2) A dentigerous cyst. (3) An elderly patient, in whom there is a risk of pathological fracture.

ANAESTHESIA. Use a combination of local infiltration and pterygopalatine (A 6.4), and mandibular blocks (A 6.3). Thoroughly clean his mouth first.

INCISION. You can approach all cysts from inside his mouth, unless his jaw is to be resected (not described here).

Approach the cyst from the side of the jaw on which the swelling is greatest. If it is equal both sides, approach it from the buccal side. Reflect a large mucoperiosteal flap. Remove bone over the same site. Remove the superficial part of the lining, so as to expose the cavity widely, and render the deeper part of its lining continuous with his oral mucosa. Wash out the cyst, and examine its lining for signs of neoplastic changes. If there is more than a little tissue in it, suspect that it might be an ameloblastoma. Send any material you remove for histology.

If you are marsupializing a dentigerous cyst, be sure to remove all the epithelium, or it may grow again. To do this, remove all the soft tissues on the outside of the bony cyst wall. Remove the tooth at the same time. Leave it open to granulate.

If a dental cyst is related to a permanent tooth, it is likely to be non-vital. It might be saved by root canal treatment, but you will probably have to remove it. If it is related to a deciduous tooth (unusual), remove the tooth.

If the bone is much expanded and the bony wall of the cyst is thin, consider compressing it to reduce its size.

Pack the cavity, and remove the pack at 48 hours or earlier. Continue with thorough mouth washes until it has healed. Ask him to wash out his mouth after meals.

CAUTION ! (1) Be sure to make a wide opening. If it is too small, it will close, and the cyst will recur. Ideally, it may need an acrylic obturator to stop it closing over; failing this pack it.

PACKING OPEN A CYST

INDICATIONS. An infected or 'messy' cyst, with a lining which you cannot completely remove, or a flap which has to be sacrificed.

METHOD. Remove the tooth associated with a dental cyst, unless it can be root-treated. Open the cyst, remove as much of its lining as you can, and then pack it with BIPP impregnated gauze, or plain gauze. Reduce the bulk of this over several weeks, to allow the cavity to granulate slowly from its base.

THE DECOMPRESSION OF A CYST

INDICATIONS. A dentigerous cyst which is small enough for this to be practical (unusual).

METHOD. Remove the surface of the cyst and allow the tooth to erupt.

ENUCLEATING A CYST

If possible, refer the patient. General anaesthesia with tracheal intubation is essential. Approach a cyst in his upper jaw through the labial aspect of his alveolus. Approach a cyst in his lower jaw through an incision 1 cm below the lower border of his mandible, or inside his mouth, through the labial side of his alveolus. Infiltrate the tissues with adrenalin in saline (3.1). Clear the bony covering of the cyst, fracture its eggshell surface, and remove a piece of bone from its most prominent part. Nibble away more bone, and push the cyst off the bony wall of the cavity in which it lies. If it is a dentigerous cyst, its lining will be held round the tooth it contains.

26.8 Cleft lip and palate

If milk comes from a baby's nose as he sucks, suspect that he has a cleft palate. You will not be able to repair either a cleft lip or a cleft palate, but you should know how to manage a child who has one, and when to refer him.

Cleft lips are not too difficult to repair well. They may be: (1) incomplete, (2) complete, (3) premaxillary, (4) complete with a cleft palate. (1) and (2) cause no problem with breast feeding, and (3) seldom does, but (4) makes breast-feeding very difficult. If a baby cannot suck, get him on to breast milk with a cup and spoon. Refer him for repair when he is 5 kg.

Cleft palates are much more difficult to repair. This should be done at 12 to 18 months, before he tries to speak, and when he should be fit enough for a major operation, if he has been adequately fed. Breast-feeding is a major problem, except for minor clefts of the soft palate only, which need no treatment. Try a cup and spoon. If this fails, he will have to be fed through a nasogastric tube, until he is stronger, when cup and spoon feeding may be possible. Some contributors are against all feeding bottles at any time anywhere!

A special plate, supported by two wire arms on his cheek, can be constructed in the first few days of life, to bridge the gap in his cleft palate.

26.9 Other dental and oral problems

The range of possible oral pathology is large, so that we can only describe a few of the conditions you might might see. Some of the more important ones are tumours. Cysts of the jaw have been described in a previous section. An epulis is a mass arising from the gum. If you take a biopsy, be sure to take samples from different parts of the lesion.

OTHER DENTAL AND ORAL PROBLEMS

ULCERS OF THE MOUTH

If a patient has a recent, shallow, painful ULCER in his mouth, it is likely to be an APTHOUS ULCER, or a recurrent HERPETIC ULCER (both very common). The distinction between them is not important, since there is little you can do about either of them, and they will resolve spontaneously. Advise mouth washes, and try folic acid 5 mg weekly, both as prevention and treatment. These ulcers are more common in people taking proguanil ('Paludrine')

If he has a RAGGED ULCER of his gums, cheek or the floor of his mouth, suspect that he has a CARCINOMA (uncommon), especially if it has a raised edge. Send tissue for histology and refer him for deep radiotherapy, or radical surgery. See also Section 32.22.

LUMPS ARISING FROM THE ALVEOLUS

Consider also carcinoma of the mouth (32.22).

If he has a FIRM LUMP ON HIS GUM, it is probably a FIBROUS EPULIS (common). Some of these lesions are fast-growing, and if a lump is soft, bluish, and grows rapidly it may be a sarcoma (very unusual). Excise it, or treat it by diathermy (if small, unusual), and send tissue for histology. If it is very extensive, try to refer him to an expert periodontologist (if you can find one!) or a maxillofacial surgeon. It may be one of a wide range of obscure, rare, fibro-osseous lesions.

If a patient has a SOFT SWELLING ON HIS (or her) GUM, between two teeth, or on the palate, and associated with chronic infection, it is probably a PYOGENIC GRANULOMA (granulomatous epulis, 34.2, common) and is particularly likely to occur during pregnancy (B, 26-12, pregnancy epulis), when it is often very vascular, and may simulate a malignancy. Pyogenic granulomas are common inside the mouth, and can also occur on the tongue. If a patient is pregnant, leave the lesion and don't try to excise it. Otherwise, excise it, and provided the infection is eradicated, it will not return. Send any material you obtain for histology. Make sure there is no underlying osteomyelitis (7.14a); if there is, treat it.

If a CHILD IN THE 'BURKITT ZONE' has a LOOSE TOOTH, with a swollen jaw, or SWELLINGS OF HIS JAW, suspect that he has BURKITT'S LYMPHOMA (32.3). Typically, his teeth are displaced.

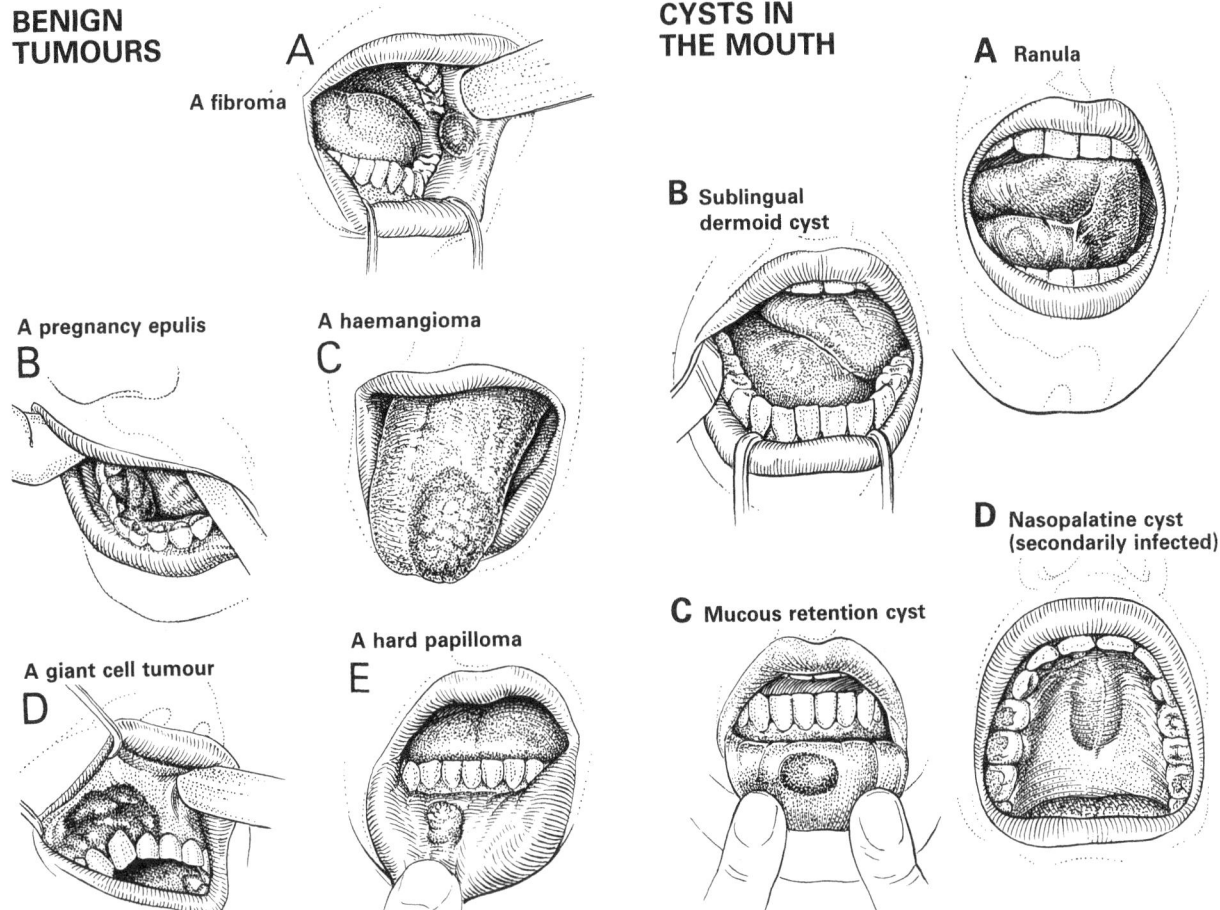

Fig. 26-12 BENIGN TUMOURS OF THE ORAL CAVITY. A, a fibroma. B, a pregnancy epulis. C, a haemangioma of the tongue. D, a giant cell tumour. E, a hard papilloma. *Adapted from drawings by Frank Netter, with the kind permission of CIBA-GEIGY Ltd, Basle (Switzerland).*

Fig. 26-13 CYSTS IN THE MOUTH. A, a ranula. B, a sublingual dermoid cyst. C, a mucocele of the lip. D, a secondarily infected nasopalatine cyst. *Adapted from drawings by Frank Netter, with the kind permission of CIBA-GEIGY Ltd, Basle (Switzerland).*

LUMPS ARISING ELSEWHERE IN THE MOUTH

If he has a PEDUNCULATED SWELLING on his cheek (or tongue), it is probably a FIBROEPITHELIAL POLYP or a fibroma (A, 26-12). This is commonly associated with irritative trauma, particularly that from an ill-fitting denture. Excise it and it will not recur, provided the trauma is removed.

If he has a PAPILLOMA (wart) inside his mouth, it may be viral (verruca vulgaris), and he may have similar lesions on his hands. If necessary, excise his oral lesion.

If he has an EXPANDING TUMOUR OF HIS MANDIBLE, with an X-ray showing large loculi and a honeycomb appearance, suspect that he has an AMELOBLASTOMA (rare). See Section 26.7.

CYSTS OF THE MOUTH

If he has a bluish, translucent, RAISED VESICLE several millimetres to a centimetre or more in diameter, it is probably a MUCOUS RETENTION CYST (C, 26-13, common). These cysts may arise from the mucous glands anywhere inside his mouth, including his tongue, but are most common inside his lower lips. They may arise in a few days, persist for months, periodically discharge their contents, and then recur. Try to excise the lesion; if you merely incise it, it is likely to recur.

If a CHILD has a circumscribed, fluctuant, often BLUISH SWELLING of his alveolar ridge, over the site of an erupting tooth (common), it is probably an eruption cyst. This is usually symptomless, and bursts spontaneously to allow the tooth under it to erupt. If it does not, give him ketamine, grasp it with toothed forceps, and excise it. A little dark blood will escape, and the underlying tooth will erupt during the next few months.

If he has a slowly enlarging painless MASS on one side of the FLOOR OF HIS MOUTH, with normal mucosa over it, it is probably a RANULA (A, 26-13, uncommon). This is a particular form of retention cyst, arising from the inferior aspect of the tongue, and caused by blockage of the submandibular duct. If you remove it entirely by careful dissection, it will not recur. If this is difficult, deroof it; it will probably not recur.

It may also be a SUBLINGUAL DERMOID CYST (B, 26-13, rare), which is a developmental cyst in the line of fusion of the first branchial arches. The epithelium lining it is thicker than that of a ranula. Although it arises in the midline, it usually displaces the tongue to one side. Dissect it out cleanly, and take care not to injure his submandibular duct.

If he has a midline swelling in the roof of his mouth, it is probably a NASOPALATINE CYST (D, 26-13, 26.7, rare), which may have become secondarily infected. More likely, it is a pleomorphic adenoma (mixed salivary tumour) in an ectopic site.

27 Primary orthopaedics

27.1 The scope of primary othopaedics

Most of your orthopaedic problems will be the fractures that are described in detail from Chapter 69 onwards. Many of the non-traumatic conditions you will see are also described in other chapters: they include osteomyelitis (Chapter 7), septic arthritis (7.16), and tuberculous bone and joint disease (Chapter 29). The orthopaedics which remains to be considered here consists of the important subject of contractures in general (27.2), polio (27.3 to 27.7), talipes (27.15), and a few minor orthopaedic probems that you can treat without difficulty, such as epicondylitis ('tennis elbow', 27.9), stenosing tenosynovitis (27.10), ingrowing toenail (27.16), and a few others (27.17).

Try to obtain the following superb manual, which describes the management of all kinds of disability in the community:

David Werner, 'Disabled Village Children, A Guide for Community Health Workers, Rehabilitation Workers and Families'. Hesperian Foundation Box 1692 Palo Alto California CA 94302 USA.

27.2 The general method for contractures

A contracture is a deformity which prevents the movement of a joint through its normal range. Structurally, contractures are the result of shortening of the soft tissues of a limb, and/or tightening of the ligaments of a joint. This can happen as the result of: (1) Disuse (see below). (2) Soft tissue or bony injuries, especially burns (58.24 to 58.26) and fractures. (3) Muscle imbalance, due to weakness of the nerves supplying a group of muscles. This can be temporary, when you expect the nerve to recover, or permanent, when you expect it not to. (4) Poliomyelitis, and other lower motor neurone lesions, which weaken one muscle group more than another. (5) The spastic paralysis of an upper motor neurone lesion, such as that following a cerebrovascular accident, the cerebral diplegia or paraplegia of a birth injury, encephalitis, or a head injury. (6) Sepsis in bones (osteomyelitis, 7.2), joints (septic arthritis, 7.16), or lymph nodes with periadenitis (iliac abscesses, 5.12).

That 'prevention is better than cure' is never more true than with contractures. *If a joint is to remain useful, it must move regularly through its full range.* Anything which prevents it from doing this eventually causes a contracture. The soft tissues surrounding a disused joint become shorter, and less elastic, and its muscles waste and will not extend normally. Ultimately, its bones change their shape, and become deformed; it lacks a full range of movement, or becomes fixed near one end of its range, usually flexion.

The two important principles in prevention are: (1) Most importantly, *to keep all joints moving whenever you possibly can.* The need to do this is well shown by the the patient with the severe buttock injury in Figure 54-10. When she was admitted, both her elbows were normal, but as she lay on her front for several weeks, she kept them flexed, and never moved them. The result was that when she was discharged, she had severe contractures in both her elbows, which had been perfectly normal on admission. The burnt child in Fig. 58-1 developed contractures in his unburnt joints because he did not move them. Contractures like this can happen quite unnoticed, and when you do notice them, it may be too late. (2) When movements are temporarily difficult, or inadequate for any reason, prevent deformity by splinting or skin traction (70.10), as with the burnt child in Fig. 58-17.

Treatment starts with a careful assessment, so begin by deciding:

(1) Which tissues are causing the patient's contracture? If his joint is merely stiff, releasing it should not be too difficult. If only his skin, subcutaneous tissues, and muscles are involved, you should also be able to release them. But contractures of his tendons, or nerves (as in his popliteal fossa), are more difficult. Involvement of a joint can be due to: (a) Mild or dense adhesions. (b) Shortening of its capsule or ligaments. (c) Destructive changes, as the result of past infection. (d) A fibrous ankylosis. (e) A bony ankylosis. If his bones are not deformed, you should be able to release his contracted soft tissues. If they are deformed, you will have to refer him for an osteotomy.

(2) What range of movement is there in the joint? Record the movement he still has.

(3) How much power is there in his muscles? This is important if he has a lower motor neurone lesion, such as that following polio, or an upper motor neurone lesion as the result of paraplegia. Muscle power is graded from 0 to 5. The important grade is 3, because this is the grade at which a muscle is just able do its work against gravity. It varies with the muscle; the quadriceps, for example, has to lift a heavy leg against gravity, whereas the extensor of the little finger has only a finger to lift. Any muscle which can lift its part of a limb against gravity, must have a power of at least 3. Charting is difficult to do accurately, especially in young children. In an older patient trick movements can easily deceive you.

Try non-operative methods first. You have several choices: (1) You can use active and passive movements. These might seem the simplest, but they need a determined physiotherapist, or someone, such as a nurse, with some physiotherapy training. (2) You can apply skin or skeletal traction (70.10, 70.11). (3) You can manipulate a joint. (4) You can apply serial corrective casts. Manipulation and casts can often be usefully combined. For example, you can manipulate a joint, and then apply a cast almost at the limit of its range of movement. Later, you can manipulate his joint again, and replace the cast with another one, in which his joint is nearer to the limit of its normal range of movement. If manipulation is to be thorough, you will have to anaesthetize him. The danger is that, during manipulation, a joint may bleed, and the blood in it may organize and cause more adhesions. You can easily break a bone when you manipulate it, so follow the instructions we give, which are designed to prevent this happening. You can also wedge a cast, as in Figs. 70-8 and 70-9. This is economical in plaster, but it has the disadvantage that you cannot combine it with manipulation. (5) You can release soft tissues surgically. Polio contractures are easier to release than the contractures which follow burns, because there is less scar tissue, and no skin loss.

PREVENTING CONTRACTURES IS EASIER THAN TREATING THEM

GENERAL METHOD FOR CONTRACTURES

PREVENTION. Most contractures can be prevented by: (1) Putting a patient's joints through their full range of active and passive movement, several times a day, as with paraplegia (64.13). This is such a simple measure, yet it is so often forgotten. You probably won't have physiotherapists, but this is something that all nurses can do—so show them how. (2) Appropriate splinting, as for burns (58.24), tuberculosis of the knee (29.3), or a radial nerve palsy, as in Fig. 69-2. (3) Skin traction for burns, as in Fig. 58-17. (4) Early movements in bone and joint injuries, as with Perkins traction for a fractured femur (78.4), or fractures of the femoral condyles (79.15). (5) The early drainage of pus, as with septic arthritis of the hip, which readily causes a flexion contracture (7.18). (6) The early grafting of wounds and burns over joints (58.32). (7) Early manipulation and immobilization, as for neonatal talipes equinovarus (27.15).

Often, you will need to do *several of these preventive measures at the same time.* For example, you may need to combine splinting and active and passive movements.

ASSESSING A PATIENT WITH A CONTRACTURE

Where relevant, assess him lying, sitting, standing, and walking. Remember that abduction is movement away from the midline, and adduction is movement towards it. 'Varus' is a deformity towards the midline from the line of a long bone, and 'valgus' is a deformity away from it. In an equinus deformity of the ankle the foot points downwards, like that of a horse (*equus*, a horse), in a calcaneus deformity his foot points upwards so that his calcaneus is downwards.

RANGE OF MOVEMENT. In the anatomical position all joints are at 0°, so record the movement he has from this position (69-1), and state whether they are active or passive.

For example, the range of movement for a normal hip could be: flexion 0°/120°, that is from 0° to 120°. Its other movements might be extension 0°/10°, abduction 0°/40°, adduction 0°/30°, external rotation 0°/60°, internal rotation 0°/30°. 'Normal' people vary somewhat.

A patient with a flexion contracture might have: flexion 30°/110°, extension −30°/−30° (this means that there is no extension in his hip, movement starts at −30° of extension and ends there), abduction 0°/20°, adduction 0°/20°, internal rotation 0°/10°, external rotation 0°/40°. This means that his hip is flexed, but will not extend at all; it will flex a bit more, but not as much as normal. In other directions its movements are slightly limited.

MUSCLE POWER and movements are usually assessed by a physiotherapist, but if you don't have one, you will have to assess them yourself.

Grade 0—no power, not even a flicker.
Grade 1—a flicker of movement, but no more.
Grade 2—movement with gravity eliminated.
Grade 3—movement is just possible against gravity.
Grade 4—movement is possible against gravity and some resistance.
Grade 5—full normal power.

PARTICULAR JOINTS. A contracture of one joint can affect movement in another, so assess him like this.

Hip. If you are assessing a flexion contracture of his hip, flex his other hip as far as it will go. This will correct any lumbar lordosis, which may disguise as much as 60° of fixed hip flexion. Extend and adduct his hip, because a tight abduction contracture may be responsible for most of his deformity.

Knee. If you are assessing a flexion deformity of his knee, do so with his hip in both the neutral and the flexed positions. Assess a varus or valgus deformity from the line of the shaft of his femur. Assess backward, or lateral subluxation of his tibia on his femur as mild, moderate, or severe. Assess external rotation of his tibia on his femur with his knee extended as much as possible.

Ankle. If you are assessing an equinus deformity of his ankle, do so with his knee flexed and extended, because this will help in deciding management. If the deformity is in his ankle joint, it will be the same whether his knee is flexed or extended. But if the deformity is in his gastrocnemius muscle, the range of movement in his ankle will vary with the position of his knee. This is because the gastrocnemius muscle spans both the knee and the ankle. So, if this is short an equinus deformity of his ankle will be less if his knee is flexed, than if it is extended, because his gastrocnemius is not being stretched by an extended knee.

X-RAYS. If necessary, X-ray the bones and joints involved in his contracture. Look for: deformity of the joint surfaces, evidence of active disease, and the degree of osteoporosis.

TREATMENT FOR CONTRACTURES

The need for treatment usually means that prevention has failed. See elsewhere for burns (58.25, 58.26), for polio contractures (27.3 to 27.7), and for paraplegia (64.13). Here are some general methods which you can apply to most contractures. The first two are the safest.

ACTIVE AND PASSIVE MOVEMENTS FOR CONTRACTURES

These may gradually stretch a patient's shortened soft tissues

MUSCLE CHARTING

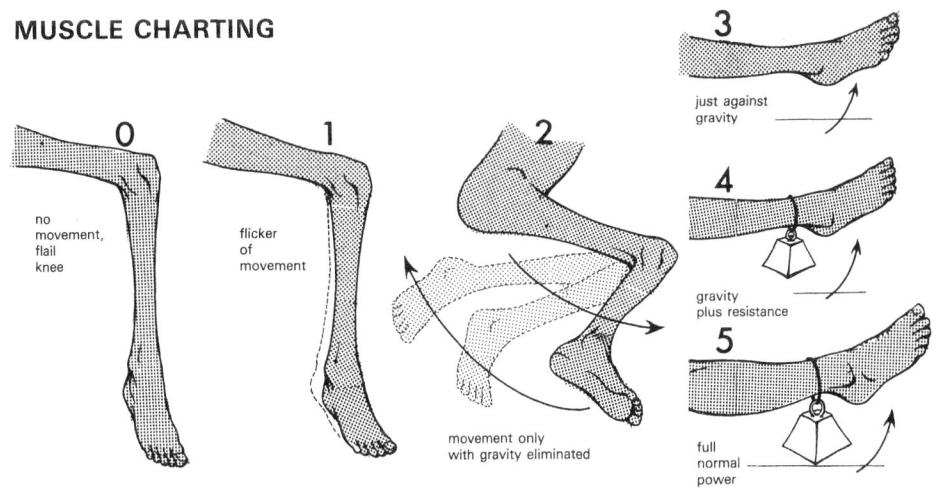

Fig. 27-1 MUSCLE CHARTING. Grade three is the critical one, because this is the grade which allows a patient to lift his limb against gravity. You can test all other muscle groups in the same way. *Kindly contributed by Ronald Huckstep.*

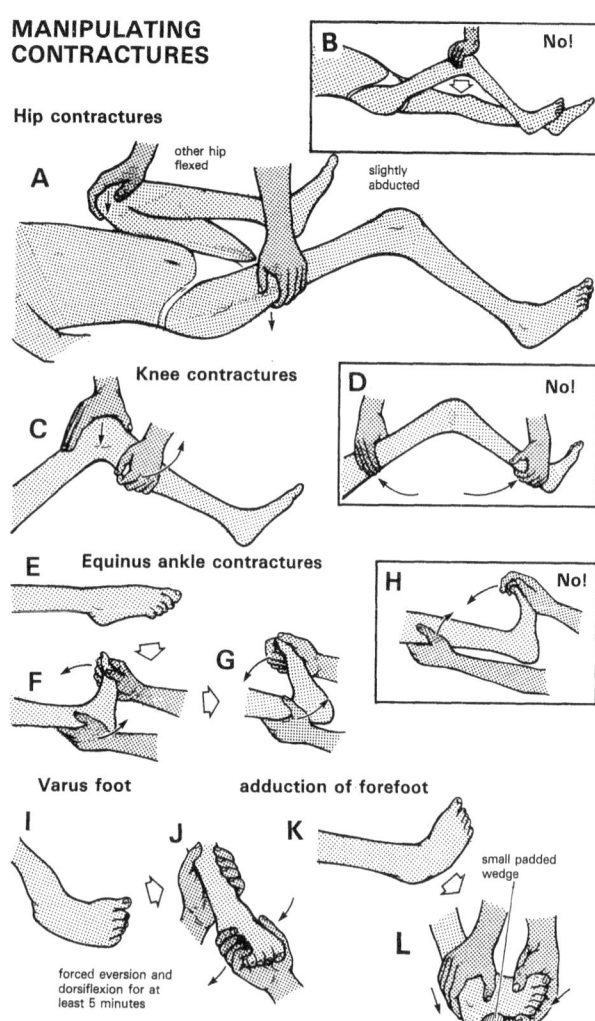

Fig. 27-2 MANIPULATING POLIO CONTRACTURES. When you manipulate a patient's joint under anaesthesia, always exert pressure close to a joint, or you may break a bone or displace his epiphyses. A, when you manipulate his hip, flex his opposite hip, and grasp his thigh. Push it down in extension and slight abduction. B, don't push down on his knee! C, exert pressure near his knee, and not as in D! For an equinus deformity of his ankle (E), grasp him near his ankle, and dorsiflex it (F, and G), not as in H! For a varus deformity of his foot (I), evert it and dorsiflex it for at least five minutes (J). Manipulate an adduction deformity of his forefoot firmly and gently over a wedge (K and L). *Kindly contributed by Ronald Huckstep.*

and correct his deformity. If possible, encourage him to do them himself (active movements). Or, they can be done by a physiotherapist, or nurse (passive movements). Most useful are 'assisted active movements': (1) Support his limb while he gently moves it himself. This eliminates gravity and gives him a greater feeling of security. (2) At the extremes of movement use a little passive movement, as he moves his limb himself assisted by you. Chart the range of its movement at least every week.

TRACTION FOR CONTRACTURES

If satisfactory correction is not possible by exercises alone, consider skin traction (70.10), or skeletal traction (70.11).

MANIPULATION FOR CONTRACTURES

This is often combined with casting.

INDICATIONS. (1) Joints in which active and passive movements or traction have failed, or are not possible because the deformity is too great. (2) Hip contractures of less than 45°. (3) Knee contractures of less than 30°. (4) Ankle contractures of less than 20°.

ANAESTHESIA. If you decide to anaesthetize him, ketamine will be adequate.

METHOD. Press firmly *for at least five minutes* in a direction opposite to that of the contracture. If necessary, repeat the manipulations fortnightly.

CAUTION ! Before you begin, remember that a bone which has not been moving is soft and breaks easily. To prevent this, reduce the leverage that you can exert, by holding a patient's bones close to his contracted joint, as in Fig. 27-2.

HIP. Flex his opposite hip to eliminate a lumbar lordosis. Press the upper third of his thigh backwards, to bring his leg down on the table in slight abduction. This will also stretch his adductors, which will probably be tight.

'Laying the patient prone' is a very useful nursing procedure for preventing and treating flexion contractures of the hip. If he will tolerate it, lay him face down with a pillow under his lower thigh. He is more likely to accept this uncomfortable position if his head faces towards the middle of the ward, rather than the wall.

KNEE. Hold his knee close to the joint. If you don't, you may break his tibia or his femur, displace his epiphyses, or sublux his tibia on his femur.

CAUTION ! Don't try to release contractures of his knee too forcibly, or you may injure his popliteal nerve, or damage the joint.

ANKLE. If he has an equinus deformity, support his ankle, and firmly dorsiflex his foot. If he has a varus deformity, or an adduction deformity of his forefoot, be especially firm and gentle. Don't push up his forefoot only; this may merely extend his mid tarsal and tarsometatarsal joints, without extending his ankle.

CASTING FOR CONTRACTURES

Apply a well-padded plaster cast, close to but *not* at the extreme range of movement of the joint. If you do, pressure on its cartilage may cause necrosis and osteoarthritis later. So let it relax a little, before you apply the cast. A few weeks later, if necessary, manipulate his joint again, and replace the cast with another one, in which his joint is nearer to the limit of its normal range of movement.

CAUTION ! (1) Never put a joint, especially a knee, into a cast under tension. (2) Don't wedge a cast to correct a knee contracture. Both these mistakes may cause an early painful osteoarthritis, in what was previously a painless mobile joint. These are both *very important* rules. Fortunately, osteoarthritis and painful joints are rare in polio; it is tragic to create them unnecessarily.

OPERATIVE METHODS FOR CONTRACTURES

You can release his soft tissues if he has a burns contracture (58.25 and 26). If he has polio, you can release the tendons of his ankle (27.7), his knee, or his hip (27.6). If his contracture is severe and long-standing, you may be able to refer him for a release combined with a myocutaneous flap, or by an osteotomy.

27.3 Preventing contractures in the acute and subacute stages of poliomyelitis

If a child has paralytic polio, teach his parents how to prevent contractures as soon as his pain allows—they can start only a few days after the acute illness. Preferably four times a day, his joints must be stretched in the direction opposite to that in which a contracture might form—for example, stretch an equinus ankle contracture dorsally. Teach them the methods in Fig. 27-2. Fit him with a caliper, as soon as his tender muscles will allow. In the acute stage, leave this on for most of the day and the night. Or, use a plaster gutter splint.

Start to assess the power of his muscles (27-1) as soon as the tenderness allows, usually about three weeks after the start of paralysis. If you assess the degree of recovery each time you see him, you will be able to judge how far he will recover finally. Three months from the onset of paralysis, you will know whether he needs calipers or not.

CONTRACTURES CAN FORM IN A FEW DAYS

27.4 Managing chronic polio

The children of the developing world pay a high price for acquiring their natural immunity. A survey from Ghana showed seven in every thousand to be lame, and although nearly 90% of these children could walk without mechanical aid, many of them had scoliosis and needed calipers.

Poliomyelitis destroys the anterior horn cells of a patient's spinal cord. This causes a flaccid lower motor paralysis, without impairing sensation. The flexor and extensor muscles of a normal limb are arranged so that they oppose one another's action. Polio can weaken both groups mildly or severely, equally or unequally. When, as is usual, the muscle groups are involved unequally, it is commonly his extensors which are most affected. When this happens, his stronger flexors pull his limb into a flexion contracture. If all the muscles of his limb are weak, he has a flail limb. If he is a child, growth will cause further deformity. All this can happen in varying degrees to his hips, his knees, or his ankles, on one or both sides, to cause many patterns of paralysis. His arms are less commonly affected, and are usually less of a disability, so we say nothing about them here, nor do we discuss the effects of polio on the spine.

These are your opportunities: (1) Do all that you can to promote the immunization campaigns that should now be taking place in your district in response to WHO's expanded programme of immunization (EPI). (2) Try to prevent contractures developing immediately after the acute phase of the illness. (3) If they do develop, use serial plasterings, traction, or tenotomies to release some of the milder ones. More complex operations, such as osteotomies, arthrodeses, and tendon transfers, are tasks for an expert, so are all operations on the arms and spine, on the rare occasions when these are necessary. (4) Provide patients with the necessary calipers, crutches, and plaster splints. (5) Follow them up for many years, if necessary, and help them to find places in schools, and to find jobs. As always in medicine, but particularly in polio, consider a patient's total needs. Never treat a single joint without considering the other joints in his limb, his other limb, and the adaptations that he has already made to his disability.

Your results should be good if: (1) you operate carefully on the right indications, (2) you give him simple calipers, and (3) you are able to provide the necessary physiotherapy and follow-up. These last two are likely to be your main constraints. The methods we describe are adapted from those of Huckstep. In some countries they are mostly done by orthopaedic assistants.

Huckstep RL. 'Poliomyelitis: A Guide for Developing Countries, including appliances and rehabilitation' ELBS version. Churchill Livingstone, 1975.

Nicholas D, et al. 'Is poliomyelitis a serious problem in the developing countries?—The Danfa Experience'. British Medical Journal 1977;1:1009-12.

A GENERAL METHOD FOR CHRONIC POLIO

A patient with chronic polio can have any of the following patterns of paralysis:

THE HIP IN CHRONIC POLIO

A MILDLY WEAK HIP (common) needs no treatment, especially if he also has a mild equinus deformity of his ankle, which helps to compensate for the shortening caused by his hip.

A FLEXION AND ABDUCTION CONTRACTURE OF THE HIP (common) due to weakness of its extensors and adductors.

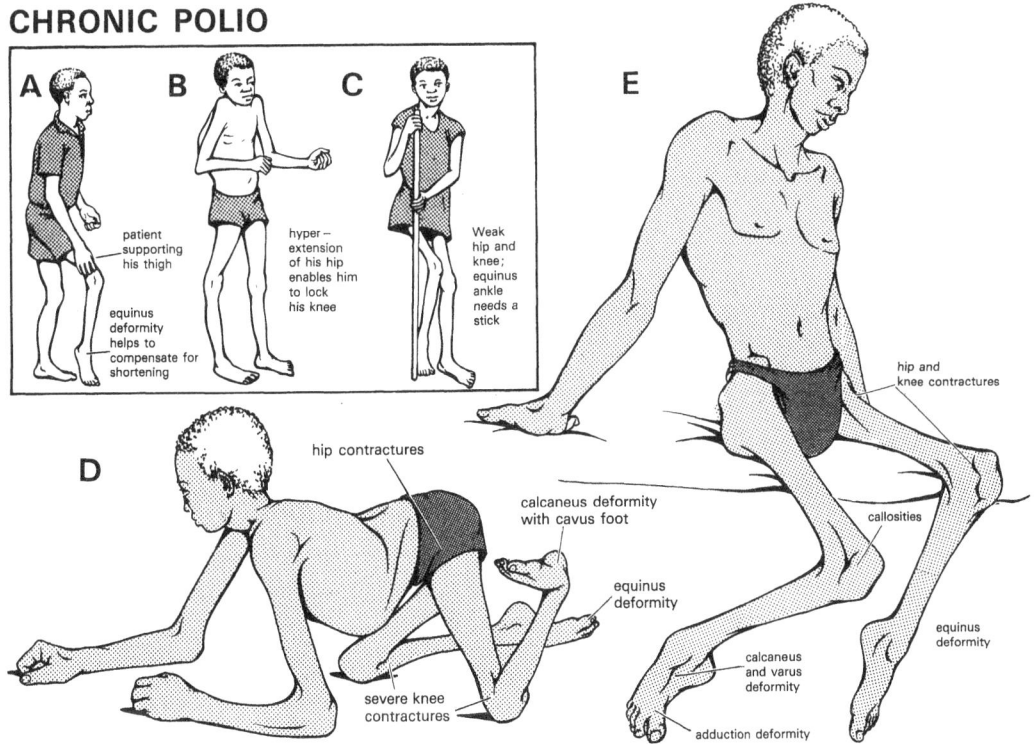

Fig. 27-3 CHRONIC POLIO. A, a patient with a weak hip or knee may be able to walk by putting his hand on his thigh, or by locking it in hyperextension, using the extensors of his hip (B). C, if his whole leg is weak, he will have to use a stick. D, if he has severe contractures of both knees, he may crawl on the ground. E, an adult 'crawler' seated. Note the large callosities on his knees. *Kindly contributed by Ronald Huckstep.*

If an adult or child has an isolated flexion contracture of his hip of <30°, he is probably walking adequately, and needs no treatment, provided he has no other serious contractures. The stability of his hip may even be improved, and shortening compensated for, by a small adduction and flexion contracture.

If an adult or child has an isolated flexion contracture of >30°, consider releasing it.

A FLAIL HIP (fairly common) due to paralysis of all its muscles. Give him a pair of crutches.

DISLOCATION OR SUBLUXATION OF THE HIP (rare) may occur in a flail hip. Reduce his dislocation, and put him into an abduction spica (77.3). Give him crutches. Occasionally, he may need an osteotomy, an arthrodesis, or a psoas transfer. Reducing a dislocated hip can be difficult. Some surgeons would leave a flail hip because it so easily redislocates.

If his dislocation is recurrent, it may be best left untreated. Unfortunately, most dislocations are recurrent, because there are no functioning muscles left around the hip to hold it in place.

THE KNEE IN CHRONIC POLIO

Not all weak knees need a complete caliper. Some patients may be able to manage with a knee splint.

A FLEXION CONTRACTURE OF THE KNEE (common) due to weakness of its extensors.

If a patient has an isolated flexion contracture of his knee of <30°, apply serial casts for a child (27.2), and skin traction for an adult.

CAUTION ! Never put a cast on a knee (or any other joint) while it is held under tension, or osteoarthritis will follow (27.2).

If a patient has an isolated flexion deformity of his knee of >30° but <90°, consider releasing it surgically (27.6). The operation described in Fig. 27-8 is a very limited open tenotomy suitable for a patient: (1) who needs a bit more extension, so that he can be put into skin traction, and (2) whose biceps femoris tendon is tight, but not his semitendinosus and semimembranosus tendons, which are attached medially. Feel his tendons when his knee is extended to its limit. If all his tendons are tight and need surgical release, refer him.

If an adult has a flexion deformity of >90°, correction is going to be difficult, and he may subsequently have a stiff painful knee. If he has *one* contracted knee, either leave him alone, or consider referring him for an osteotomy or an arthrodesis. Don't ever consider straightening two contracted knees in an adult.

A VALGUS DEFORMITY OF THE KNEE (common) is usually associated with a flexion contracture, for which he needs a

MORE POLIO DEFORMITIES

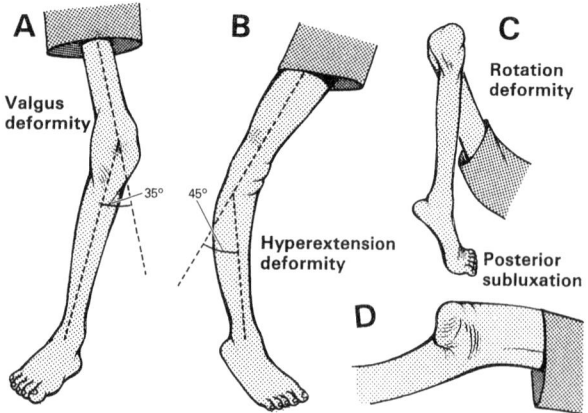

Fig. 27-4 MORE POLIO DEFORMITIES OF THE KNEE. The common and most treatable ones are the flexion contractures shown by patients D, and E, in the previous figure. A patient can also have a valgus deformity (A, in the present figure), a hyperextension deformity (genu recurvatum) (B), a rotation deformity (C), or posterior subluxation (D). All these are much less easily treated. *Kindly contributed by Ronald Huckstep.*

surgical release and a caliper. If necessary, bend his caliper, or fit it with a valgus knee strap, to prevent it rubbing against his knee.

If a small child has a severe valgus deformity of his knee, refer him for an osteotomy, or stapling of his medial epiphysis by an expert.

LATERAL ROTATION OF THE TIBIA ON THE FEMUR, or LATERAL SUBLUXATION OF THE KNEE (common). He usually also has a flexion contracture of his knee. You may be able to correct rotation and subluxation at the same time that you correct his flexion contracture. More often, the deformity is structural by the time you see him, and cannot be corrected by simple tenotomies. If rotation and subluxation are his only deformities, they are usually asymptomatic, and do not require specific treatment.

A HYPEREXTENSION DEFORMITY OF THE KNEE (genu recurvatum, fairly common) is due to early weight-bearing on a weak knee.

If a child's knee has less than 10° of hyperextension, leave it untreated.

If a child has >10° of hyperextension, fit him with an above knee caliper with a posterior strap.

If an adult has a hyperextended knee, leave him untreated, provided it is not getting worse, or causing complications. Otherwise, he may need an osteotomy.

COMBINED HIP AND KNEE CONTRACTURES. If these are less than 30° and he is walking, leave them. If they are > 30°, consider releasing them, provided there are no contraindications.

FLAIL KNEE. He may be able to walk adequately without a caliper, if he has good hip extensors, and if his foot is in a good position.

THE ANKLE IN CHRONIC POLIO

AN EQUINUS DEFORMITY OF THE ANKLE (very common) due to paralysis of its extensors.

If he is a child and flexion of his knee allows you to bring his ankle up into neutral, correct his deformity by serial casting (27.2). If he has a greater degree of deformity than this, do a tenotomy.

If he is an adult, the decision as to whether an operation would improve him is difficult, and depends on: (1) the degree of equinus of his ankle, (2) the power in his knee and hip, (3) the condition of his other leg, (4) whether he can or cannot use crutches, and (5) whether he will need calipers after surgery and can get them.

A CALCANEUS DEFORMITY OF THE ANKLE (rare) due to weakness of his calf muscles.

If his calcaneus deformity is mild, a lace-up boot may be all he needs.

If his calcaneus deformity is more severe, fit him with a below-knee caliper with a front stop.

A VALGUS DEFORMITY OF THE ANKLE (common) is usually associated with some degree of equinus.

If his valgus deformity is mild, correcting his equinus deformity and fitting him with a caliper will probably be enough.

If his valgus deformity is severe, consider referring him for transfer of his peroneal tendons, and perhaps a triple arthrodesis.

A VARUS DEFORMITY OF THE ANKLE (rare) is due to weakness of the evertors of his foot. His foot is inverted and his forefoot may be adducted.

If his varus deformity is mild, fit him with a below-knee caliper.

If his deformity is severe, you will probably have to refer him for soft tissue correction, or a subtaloid triple arthrodesis.

AN ADDUCTION DEFORMITY OF THE FOREFOOT. Try several manipulations as in L, Fig. 27-2. You will probably have to refer him for surgical correction.

A CAVUS FOOT. You may need to refer him for tenotomy, tendon transfer, or arthrodesis of his toes. Surgery is complex, so that scarce orthopaedic skills are probably be best reserved for other patients.

COMBINED DEFORMITIES IN CHRONIC POLIO

A common pattern is a flexion deformity of his hip and knee, and an equinus deformity of his ankle. Provided there are no contraindications (27.6, 27.7), treat these as if they were isolated deformities. If they are all severe enough to need release, consider releasing his hip and knee first, and then his ankle. Refer him if you can.

SHORTENING IN CHRONIC POLIO

Apparent shortening is due to tilting of his pelvis, as the result of an adduction or abduction deformity of his hip. True shortening is a real shortening of his leg, and in polio is due to the failure of a paralysed leg to grow.

If necessary, correct an abduction contracture of the hip, a flexion contracture of the knee, or an equinus contracture of the ankle.

If his shortening makes walking difficult (usually > 4 cm), raise his short leg with a clog or with boots. If necessary, fit calipers.

DIFFICULTIES WITH CHRONIC POLIO

If he BREAKS HIS FEMUR OR HIS TIBIA, fit him with a cast, use the opportunity to correct any deformity, and keep him walking. His knee and ankle are unlikely to be functional, so stiffness will not be a problem. Perkins traction (78.4) may be useful for a short period initially.

27.5 Appliances for polio

When you have released a patient's contracture, the muscles of his leg will still be weak, so you will probably have to provide him with a brace, or a crutch, or both. A weak hip needs crutches, a weak knee needs a long caliper, and a weak ankle needs a short one. *If you cannot provide him with calipers, don't try to release his contractures!*

There are four types of orthopaedic appliances of increasing sophistication:

(1) Appliances of the traditional type, such as the pads, kneelers, sticks, peg legs and crutches, that are used in traditional societies everywhere. Unfortunately, there are no traditional calipers.

(2) Appliances of the Huckstep type, shown in Fig. 27-6. These can be made in a hospital workshop using locallly available iron, galvanized wire, wood, and leather, and can be repaired by a bicycle mechanic, a cobbler, or a blacksmith. If they are properly made with hardwood, a child will usually outgrow them, and need a larger size before they wear out. If they are made of soft wood they wear out quickly.

(3) Appliances of an intermediate type are more durable than Huckstep's. They are cheaper than appliances of type (4), and are less dependent on imported materials. An example is a modified Bata shoe with a metal tube to support the end of the iron bar. If these shoes have an open toe, they will fit feet of various sizes, but are less durable in wet weather. The leprosy shoes in Section 30.5 are of this kind.

(4) The expensive high-technology appliances that are standard in the industrial world. These need imported materials, particularly duralumin and special plastics, and can only be made and repaired by a skilled prosthetist. Unfortunately, many prosthetists consider it a matter professional pride to make only the most sophisticated appliances of this type, which patients cannot afford. Resist their efforts, and encourage them to make appropriate appliances in sufficient quantity.

If you cannot get ready-made appliances from an orthopaedic service, ask your hospital workshop to make those of Types (2) or (3). All large or medium-sized hospitals, doing much surgery, need a workshop making a wide range of appliances of level (3). You will need above- and below-knee calipers, fitted when necessary with backstops or frontstops. These differ only in length, in the diameter of the ring, and in the presence of a knee piece in an above-knee caliper. Calipers of Types (2) and (3) have irons each side of the leg. Although the single outside or inside irons of the calipers of Type (4) look more elegant, they are weaker, they are more difficult to make and adjust, and they are usually less effective than double ones.

Use calipers to prevent deformities in a weak limb, and to straighten and support a child's leg *after you have corrected his contracture.* There are few indications for fitting calipers on an uncorrected contracture. Fit them as soon as he starts to walk, and replace them with a larger size as he grows. Encourage *all* children, who have muscle weaknesses which might lead to deformities, to wear calipers until they have stopped growing, even if they can walk without them.

The indications for fitting an adult with a crutch, or a caliper, are the same as in a child, except that an adult has usually had polio many years ago in childhood, so that his deformities are now stable, in that he is unlikely to get new ones.

ORTHOPAEDIC APPLIANCES FOR POLIO

ABOVE-KNEE CALIPER

If you are uncertain if a knee or ankle caliper is going to be useful or not, consider applying a suitable plaster cast of the same function for 4 to 6 weeks. If it is helpful, make a caliper. In this way you will avoid making calipers that do not help.

PARALLEL BARS FOR POLIO

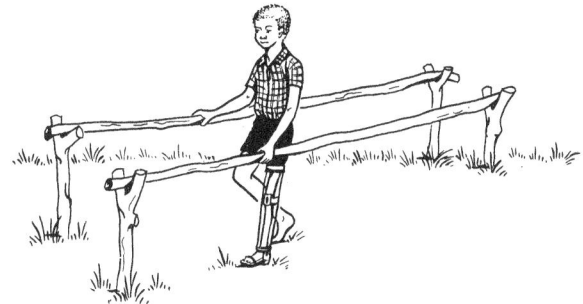

Fig. 27-5 PARALLEL BARS FOR POLIO are helpful when a child is learning to walk. *Kindly contributed by Ronald Huckstep.*

INDICATIONS. Fit a child with an above-knee caliper if: (1) His knee is so weak that he is unable to lift his leg against gravity (the power in his quadriceps is <3). If he can lift it against gravity, a caliper will not help him. (2) He is likely to develop a contracture as the result of muscle imbalance. (3) He has a *mild* knee contracture of less than 30° that a caliper could correct, if he wore one during the day or at night. (4) He is developing a hyperextended knee, as the result of trying to lock and stand on it. (5) He has weak quadriceps, and at the same time too much equinus to let him swing his leg, and lock his knee.

CONTRAINDICATIONS. Don't fit him with an above- or a below-knee caliper, or crutches, if: (1) He is able to walk reasonably well with a flail ankle—walking may be easier without them. (2) He is able to walk reasonably well with a weak knee. He may have learnt to use his hamstrings to extend his thigh, and lock his knee. (3) He needs crutches (because of weak hips), but does not have enough power in his triceps, shoulders, or trunk to use them. (4) You have not corrected his deformity (unless it is a very mild one, and the caliper is designed to correct it).

FITTING. Choose a caliper which reaches about 2 cm below his ischial tuberosity when he is standing, make the straps fairly tight, and make sure that the knee piece gives his knee adequate support anteriorly. Make the posterior strap slightly loose, unless his knee is abnormally hyperextended.

If he has a mild flexion deformity of his knee, fit him with an ordinary caliper with a loose posterior strap, and a tight knee piece, which may need to be padded.

If his knee is hyperextended (genu recurvatum), you can correct this easily, so apply only slight tension to the posterior strap.

If he has a valgus knee, bend the caliper to avoid his bony points, and fit him with an inner knee pad tied to the outer side of his calipers, to prevent his knee from rubbing against the inside iron, especially when he is bearing weight. Fit it so that it presses on the medial side of his knee, and corrects the deformity as he walks.

CAUTION ! A long caliper keeps a knee straight, and lets him walk. But, because his knee does not bend, it may become fixed in extension, and be a nuisance when he sits. So make quite sure that when he takes his caliper off, he puts his knee through a full range of passive flexion. This should not be a problem, if he takes off his caliper each night.

BELOW-KNEE CALIPERS FOR CHRONIC POLIO

INDICATIONS. Provided there are no complications (see above), fit him with a below-knee caliper if his foot is flail or drooping, or is tending to go into varus or valgus, *provided the power in his quadriceps is* >3. If it is <3, he needs an above-knee caliper.

FITTING. Choose a caliper that will allow his knee to flex fully, with a socket which will fit firmly, and not allow too much movement. Always fit a supporting ankle strap.

If his calf muscles are so weak that his foot dorsiflexes excessively, fit him with a front stop.

If he has little power in his dorsiflexors, so that his foot goes into equinus, fit a backstop.

If his ankle is inverted or everted, fit the appropriate inner or outer T-strap.

FOLLOW-UP. Try to see him at least every 6 months. Replace his caliper with a larger one as he grows. A long caliper is no use if it ends just above his knee! Make sure that his family understands that he will need a caliper for life. Do all you can to help him with his education.

OTHER APPLIANCES FOR CHRONIC POLIO

CRUTCHES. You will need a variety of sizes. If possible, make them to measure. If necessary, you can use any straight stick with a handle and a bar for the axilla. He will find a crutch useful if polio has weakened his hips. Let him try one and see how he manages with it. His grip must be strong enough to hold it, his triceps must be strong enough to propel him forwards, and his spine must be strong enough to allow him to sit without help.

A crutch is likely to help him if: (1) Both his legs are in calipers. (2) One leg is in calipers, and his opposite leg or his spine are weak. (3) One leg is in a caliper and is very weak, and his hip on the same side is weak.

Fit crutches as in Section 77.1. The length and the position of the hand grip must be right. Many patients who are given crutches could manage equally well with a stick. It you try him with a stick, teach him to hold it on the *opposite* side to his weak or weakest leg. If his hands are too weak to hold ordinary crutches, he may be able to use forearm crutches.

CAUTION ! Make sure that he does not lean on his crutches, while they are in his axilla. He may paralyse his radial nerve, or even all the nerves to his forearm and hand, and they may take 6 months to recover.

A TOE SPRING may be of great help if he has foot drop. Fix a suitable spring, or a piece of bicycle tubing to the toe of his shoe and to a strap below his knee (30-5). Alternatively, fit a back stop, which is easier to fit.

AN ANKLE SPLINT will be useful if he is in danger of foot drop while he is in bed. Make a suitable splint from plaster, or padded boards, to keep his foot at 90° to his leg.

A RAISED SHOE will help him if one leg is >4 cm shorter than the other. Any cobbler will raise it for him. If he has <4 cm of shortening, do nothing (78.1).

27.6 Contractures of the hip and knee

Before you decide on any operative treatment, assess the function of the patient's limbs in detail, and what he needs to do with them. He may have already achieved remarkable mobility, and although a straight leg may look better, it may not work better, especially if it needs calipers. If a child's legs are so weak and contracted that he crawls along the ground, you must get him walking, because the psychological effect of doing this will be tremendous—his parents will now think that he is worth educating. But if he is an adult, consider his whole future carefully first. He may be able to crawl fast and cultivate his fields on his hands and knees, but if he can only walk slowly and stiffly in calipers, he may die of starvation. So a cultivator may be better crawling, especially if his arms are too weak to use crutches, whereas a clerk, for example, may benefit from calipers. *Sometimes an operation is an obvious disservice,* for example lengthening a patient's Achilles tendon, when he walks on the ball of an equinus foot, and this is compensating for a short leg.

A severe polio contracture can: (1) cause the skin over a patients's joint to shrink, (2) shorten his muscles, intermuscular septa, nerves, and vessels, (3) contract his joint capsule, (4) deform his epiphyses. Undoing all this is difficult, and may be impossible, *so only try to relieve milder contractures,* and follow the indications we give carefully, or you may damage important structures, or cause infection or skin loss. A child's contractures are easier to correct than an adult's—he probably only needs a tenotomy, whereas an adult may need an osteotomy, or an arthrodesis.

The contractures of a patient's hip and knee, are often associated. You may have to release: (1) His iliotibial band, in several places down his thigh. In a young child, one or two incisions may be enough, and you may not need the complete set of four incisions described below. When you have divided it in his thigh, there may be no need to divide it at his knee. (2) The tight structures on the front of his hip, particularly, his iliopsoas. (3) The tendon of his biceps femoris in his popliteal fossa. (4) His medial hamstrings (occasionally).

You can cut tight bands and tendons in two ways: (1) You can push a long thin tenotomy knife through a small skin incision, and cut the bands by feel. This is satisfactory *for the less severe contractures,* provided you do it correctly, and as extensively as

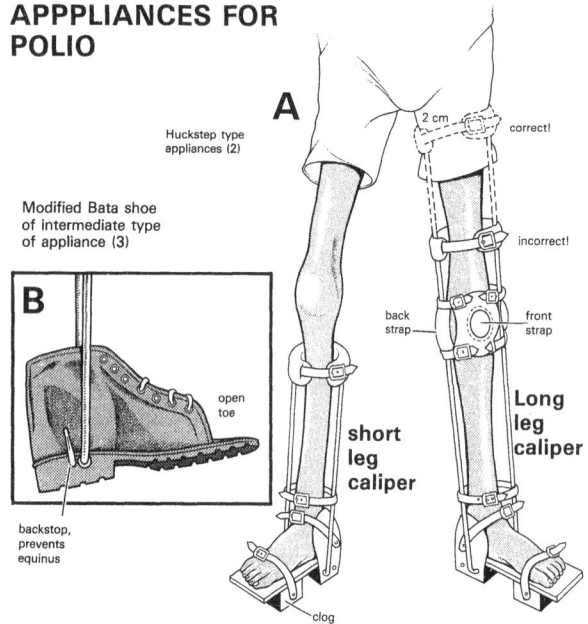

Fig. 27-6 APPLIANCES FOR POLIO. A, calipers of the Huckstep type. Note that long leg calipers should reach to 2 cm below the groin. They will be useless if they only reach to just above the knee. B, a modified shoe, as an example of an appliance of Type 3. *Kindly contributed by Ronald Huckstep.*

necessary. (2) You can cut tight structures under direct vision. *In the thigh,* this is the best method, especially for severe contractures, but it needs more skill and the wound may break down, so use the closed method. *Behind the knee,* the common peroneal nerve is very superficial, so the only safe way to divide the tendons there is by open operation.

Don't try to treat a contracted hip by manipulation and serial casting in a spica—surgery is better.

The knee is the most difficult of the three joints on which you may have to operate, especially in an adult, whose tibia can be rotated backwards and laterally, as well as being flexed. *Be safe, and don't try to release a contracture of > 90°.* If you try, his tight popliteal vessels and nerves may be stretched; and pain, paralysis, and even gangrene may follow. Even a contracture of <90° may be difficult. After you have released it as much as you can by tenotomy, you can obtain the final correction by one of these three methods. You can:

(1) Manipulate his knee and apply a cast.

(2) Apply a cast and wedge it; this may be useful if plaster is scarce, but manipulation and a fresh cast will give better results. A cast by either of these methods will mobilize him earlier, and is economical in the use of beds; but it will not be effective, if the operation has left him with a contracture of 45°, or more. It also increases the risk of a stiff, painful knee, and of osteoarthritis later.

(3) Put him into Hamilton Russell traction. This will keep him in bed for 2 or 3 months, but it does have these advantages; (a) it is better if he is an adult, and his contracture is severe, (b) it reduces the risk of pain and osteoarthritis, (c) it is the only way of treating a contracture which remains >45° after the operation, (d) it helps to control an associated contracture of his hip, (e) it is less likely to cause backward subluxation of his tibia on his femur than extension traction (78.3). Hamilton Russell traction is commonly used for treating fractures of the upper femur and hip, but Perkins traction (78.4) is better and simpler.

(4) Use reversed slings on a Thomas splint.

(5) Use skeletal traction with a pin through the lower tibia, a simple and very useful method (70.11).

ANATOMY. The common peroneal (lateral popliteal nerve) descends obliquely along the lateral side of the popliteal fossa to the head of the fibula, close to the medial margin of biceps femoris. It lies between the tendon of biceps femoris and the lateral head of gastrocnemius, and winds round the lateral surface of the neck of the fibula deep to peroneus longus.

HIP AND KNEE CONTRACTURES TREATED OPERATIVELY

INDICATIONS. (1) An isolated hip contracture of >30° at any age. (2) A child with an isolated flexion contracture of his knee of >30°. (3) An adult with an isolated flexion contracture of his knee of <90°. (4) Combined hip and knee contractures of >30°, provided there are no contraindications. If you have many patients, start by operating on the younger ones with lesser deformities first.

THE CONTRAINDICATIONS to any release operation are: (1) Weak arms. The patient will need crutches, so he must have two strong arms, especially if both his legs and his trunk are weak. There are exceptions to this rule, and a really determined adult, or child, sometimes manages surprisingly well with limited weakness in one or both his arms, provided his trunk is strong. (2) A patient with mild contractures, who is walking reasonably well, is probably best left as he is. This includes a patient with: (a) a contracture of his hip alone of 30° or less, especially if it also has a mild abduction deformity, which may increase its stability and compensate for shortening. (b) An isolated knee contracture in a child—treat him with fortnightly manipulations under anaesthesia. (3) An adult who is earning his living as a 'crawler', and is happy to go on doing so; leave him. (4) Don't operate on any patient unless you can provide him with calipers.

CAUTION ! Scar tissue is not stable for at least 6 months, so when you correct contractures, you must find some way of maintaining the position of his limb for at least 6 months, or longer, if there is still muscle imbalance, or much scar tissue.

CUTTING THE ILIOTIBIAL BAND

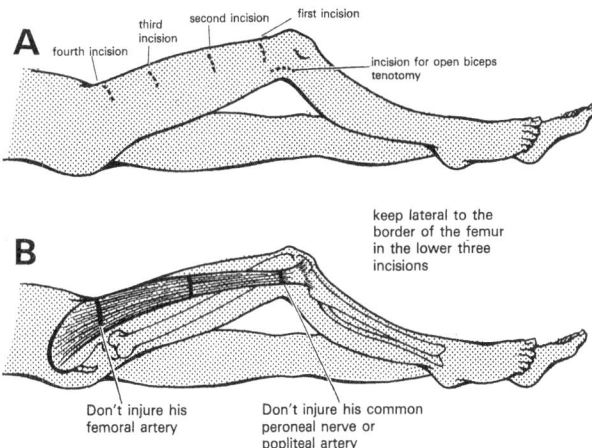

Fig. 27-7 CUTTING THE ILIOTIBIAL BAND. A, the position of the incisions. B, the structures to be cut. *Kindly contributed by Ronald Huckstep.*

TENOTOMY FOR THE HIP AND KNEE

DIVIDING THE ILIOTIBIAL BAND. Use a narrow tenotomy knife, or an old cataract knife, or a No 11 scalpel blade altered as in Fig. 27-10, so that only its tip is sharp. Operate under full sterile precautions, and prepare both his legs, even if you are only going to operate on one of them. Squeeze all blood out of the incisions periodically during the operation, and at the end. His hip incision may bleed considerably.

Release his hip and knee before you release his ankle. The structures you are going to divide must be tense, as you divide them, so keep his hip in as much extension and adduction as you can, while you cut. Feel the tight structures through his skin, to make sure that you have left no tight bands undivided.

First incision. Make this on the outer side of his thigh, about 2 cm above his knee. You can usually feel his tensor fascia lata as a tight band. Push the knife horizontally into the outer side of his thigh, just behind the tight band, until it just touches the lateral side of his femur. Rotate its blade, so that its cutting edge is upwards; then cut all the subcutaneous structures anterior to the blade, and lateral to his femur. Provided you make the incision in the right place, and only cut anteriorly, you will not cut anything important. Don't cut posteriorly, or you may cut his popliteal artery, or his lateral popliteal nerve.

Second and third incisions. Make these one third and two-thirds of the way down the outer side of his thigh. Some surgeons only make one incision in the middle of the thigh. Feel for his tensor fasciae latae, and push the knife in along its posterior border down to the bone, exactly as for the first incision. Then rotate it through 90° and cut anteriorly and laterally to the outer side of the shaft of his femur.

If you cannot feel his tensor fasciae latae, insert the knife where you think it should be and cut exactly the same way. There are other tight structures to be cut, including his vastus lateralis.

The fourth incision is the one which releases his hip. Make it one finger's breadth below his anterior superior iliac spine.

CAUTION ! (1) Don't damage his femoral vessels and nerve. *Don't push the knife further medially than a point 2 cm lateral to his mid-inguinal point* (where you can feel the artery). (2) Feel for his inguinal ligament, and take care not to divide that.

Push the knife in subcutaneously, below his anterior superior iliac spine, from a lateral to a medial direction, so that its flat surface is in the plane of the skin just caudal to his anterior superior iliac spine. Stop 2 cm lateral to his mid-inguinal point (see above). Then rotate it 90°, so that its edge faces *backwards,* and cut all the tight subcutaneous structures.

If his contracture is severe, cut all tight structures lateral to the branches of his femoral nerve. Cut right down to the front of the trochanter of his femur.

When you have cut the tight structures anteriorly, twist the knife so that it cuts laterally, and cut all the tight structures on the antero-lateral side of his hip.

OPEN BICEPS TENOTOMY

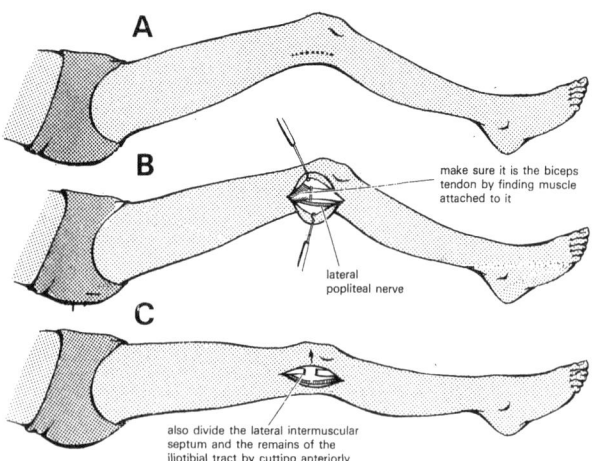

Fig. 27-8 OPEN BICEPS TENOTOMY to release a contracture of the knee. A, the site of the incision. B, be quite sure you find the patient's lateral popliteal nerve, before you cut anything. C, his biceps femoris tendon divided. *Kindly contributed by Ronald Huckstep.*

CAUTION ! (1) When the tip of the knife is deep, angle it caudally, so that its blade is parallel with his inguinal ligament, and will not cut it. (2) Don't cut further back than the coronal plane of the anterior part of his hip joint. Leave the abductors posterior to this, to give lateral stability to his hip. (3) Keep his hip in as much adduction and extension as you can, while you divide the tight structures. Feel them through his skin during the operation, and don't leave any tight deforming bands behind.

OPEN BICEPS FEMORIS TENOTOMY FOR A POLIO CONTRACTURE

INDICATIONS. This is only indicated if his knee contracture is >30° but <90°. The method which follows is a very limited open tenotomy suitable for a patient: (1) who needs a bit more extension, so that he can be put into skin traction, and (2) whose biceps femoris tendon is tight, but not his semitendinosus and semimembranosus tendons, which are attached medially. Feel his tendons when his knee is extended to its limit. If all his tendons are tight and need surgical release, refer him.

METHOD. Make an incision on the lateral side of his knee, as shown in Fig. 27-8. Feel for, and find his biceps tendon under direct vision, hook it out of the wound, and cut it.

CAUTION ! Be sure that it is his biceps tendon, and only his biceps tendon. Be careful you have not got his lateral popliteal nerve with it. They both look very similar. Look for muscle fibres being inserted into the tendon before you cut it. Be sure the nerve has not stuck to the back of the tendon.

Put your finger into the wound, and feel for any other tight structures which need cutting. You may need to cut the posterior part of his iliotibial band, and his lateral intermuscular septum. Sometimes, the anterior part of the deep fascia lata also needs cutting.

Put him into skin traction, or into a well-padded cast.

CASTING AND MANIPULATION. If the contracture of his knee is <45°, apply a cast. If it is >45°, Russell traction is better, but you can apply a cast, if necessary.

Apply a well-padded cast with his knee *just short of the full extension to which it is capable.* It must not be under any tension, or it will be painful and .

CAUTION ! NEVER put a knee into a cast under tension, or wedge a cast to correct a knee contracture, or its articular cartilage may necrose, and early painful osteoarthritis may follow, in what was previously a painless mobile joint.

Check the hip incision again (if you have released his hip at the same time), as soon as you have applied the cast, and squeeze out any clot which has formed, under full sterile precautions. Pad the incision and apply light adhesive strapping.

Every two weeks, remove the cast, and manipulate his hip and knee, until his knee is in at least 5° of hyperextension, and there is <10° of flexion deformity ('fixed flexion') in his hip. Manipulate him as in Section 27.2, and spend 5 to 10 minutes on each joint. Be sure to flex his knee fully, and to rotate his tibia medially and laterally, to maintain these very important movements. Correct or avoid backward subluxation of his knee. If necessary, correct the lateral rotation of his tibia on his femur.

After each manipulation apply a *well-padded* above-knee cast, with his ankle firmly dorsiflexed. *As always, don't put his knee under tension!.*

As soon as the flexion deformity in his knee is less than about 40°, fix a walking piece on the bottom of his cast, and encourage him to walk with crutches.

Leave the final cast on for 2 weeks, and then replace it by an above knee caliper, with its posterior strap loose. Tell him to wear it day and night for 2 or 3 weeks, until the risk of recurrence of a flexion contracture of his knee is less. Later, he can wear it by day only, for up to 6 months, when the tendency for the contracture to recur will have passed, or indefinitely if he needs it to stabilize his knee.

If possible, provide him with physiotherapy, or assisted exercises, after the cast has been removed. If the postoperative care is not properly done, he may end up with a stiff, painful knee, in which his tibia is subluxed posteriorly on his femur.

HAMILTON RUSSELL TRACTION. If he is an adult, and his contracture is >45° after the operation, Russell traction for 2 or 3 months, as in C, Fig. 27-9, is better than casting and manipulation.

Every day, stretch his knee and hip passively. As his contracture improves, make the traction more longitudinal, so that it

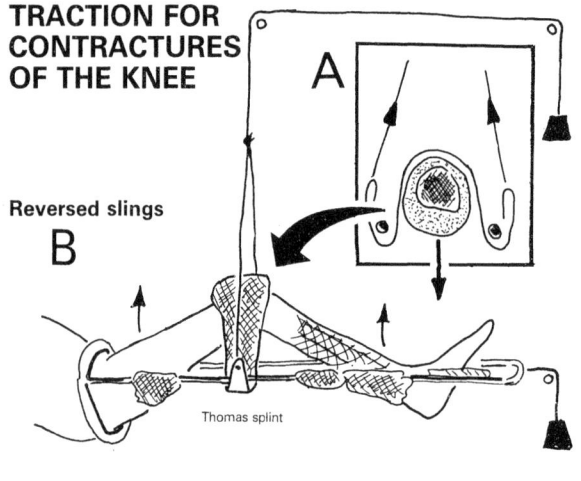

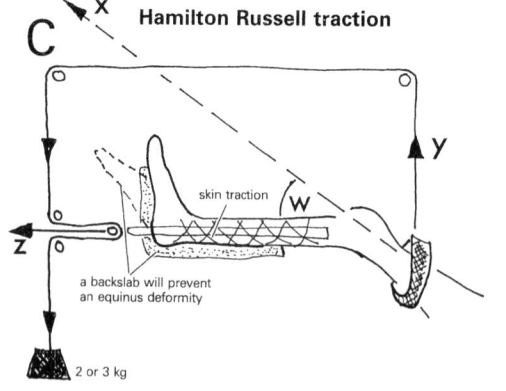

Fig. 27-9 'REVERSED SLINGS' AND HAMILTON RUSSELL TRACTION for contractures of the knee. A, a cross-section of the knee, showing how a reversed sling is passed round it. B, the principle of reversed slings. C, Hamilton Russell traction. Force 'x' is the resultant of forces 'y' and 'z'. Angle 'w' is normally about 45° when Russell traction is set up. As a knee contracture improves, it slowly becomes less. Prevent an equinus deformity with a backslab. This method of traction can also be used to treat fractures of the hip and femur. *Kindly contributed by Hugh Roberts.*

becomes more like extension, or straight leg traction (78.3). You will probably not need to manipulate him under anaesthesia, except for the last 15° of a flexion contracture, which may be difficult to correct, and require a cast in addition. Apply a plaster backslab to his ankle, to prevent an equinus deformity recurring during prolonged Russell traction. Also, stretch his ankle passively each day to correct any deformity, or prevent it.

REVERSED SLINGS are an alternative to Russell traction. Put him into a Thomas splint. Put slings under his calf and his thigh. Pass a sling round the splint, and his knee as shown in A, Fig. 27-9. Lead the cords from this to pulleys. Apply light skin traction of about 2 kg to stabilize his leg.

GET HIM MOBILE out of bed and into a chair as soon as possible. If he is a child, you can usually do this in a few days. If he is an adult, full mobilization may take a month or two. Prop him up gradually in bed or a chair, before he tries to get up. He may need crutches or a caliper; crutches must fit properly, as shown in Fig. 77-1.

DIFFICULTIES RELEASING POLIO CONTRACTURES OF THE KNEE

If his KNEE IS PAINFUL and stiff, (which, so it is said, should never happen if he has been properly treated), reassure him that this is (alas!) a common complication, and that his knee will slowly recover some, or all, its movement in a few weeks or months. His pain will probably go, even if his knee does not regain its full movement. If pain and stiffness persist, try intensive physiotherapy or Hamilton Russell traction. An arthrodesis is necessary occasionally.

27.7 Equinus deformity of the ankle

This is the most common polio deformity in a child, and is fortunately the easiest one to correct. Provided he has no severe valgus or varus deformity, you can correct a *milder* equinus deformity with serial casts, each of which will release his deformity a little more. Specialized polio services caring for large numbers of children tend to neglect casts in favour of tenotomy, which is less trouble. But if you are inexperienced, you will find serial casts very useful.

If a child has a more *severe* deformity, he needs his Achilles tendon lengthened. You can do this: (1) open or (2) closed. The closed operation is simpler, and there is less risk of infection, or keloid formation. The advantage of the open method is that it is possible to divide the posterior capsule of his ankle joint, if this is necessary, as it may be in polio. The risk in both these methods is that you may cut his posterior tibial nerve and vessels, and cause gangrene of his toes, but this should never happen, if you follow the instructions carefully. Contributors differ on the place of the open method. Ronald Huckstep feels that it now has no place in the management of polio. James Cairns uses the open method for more severe deformities, because he can do a posterior release of the ankle at the same time.

Closed tenotomy is done by making two cuts through a patient's Achilles tendon at different levels and dorsiflexing his contracted foot strongly. This stretches his Achilles tendon, so that its fibres slide over one another. They rotate about 90° as they go down his leg, so you will have to make the two cuts in different directions, to allow for this.

LENGTHENING THE ACHILLES TENDON

SERIAL CASTING

INDICATIONS. Mild degrees of equinus deformity (see also Section 27.4). Flex the patient's knee *as far as it will go.* If this relaxes his calf muscles enough to let you bring his ankle into neutral (90°), you will be able to correct his deformity with casts. If both his legs are involved, correct them one at a time, or he will be confined to bed.

METHOD. Don't anaesthetize him. Apply a below-knee cast (81.5), *while his knee is flexed to 90°,* to allow you to achieve more

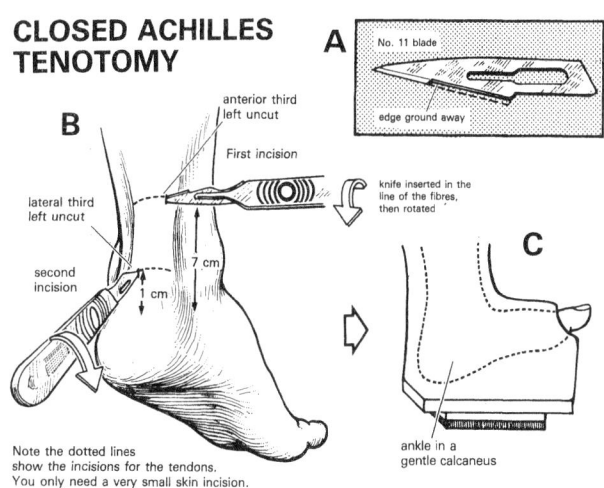

Fig. 27-10 CLOSED ACHILLES TENOTOMY. A, if you don't have a tenotomy knife, make one by grinding away a No 11 blade. B, the two incisions. Make only tiny incisions in the skin. Insert the knife with its blade in the plane of the fibres, and then twist it before you cut. This shows the patient's left foot. The upper scalpel is being inserted from the medial side. C, put the patient's foot into a cast in gentle calcaneus.
Kindly contributed by John Stewart.

dorsiflexion of his ankle. You may not be able to get his foot into neutral on the first occasion.

When the cast is dry, apply a walking heel, and get him walking. Encourage him to progressively extend his knee as he walks. As soon as he is walking normally in his cast with his knee fully extended, repeat the procedure and apply a further cast, until his foot will reach the neutral position with his leg extended.

SUBCUTANEOUS ACHILLES TENOTOMY FOR POLIO

INDICATIONS. See above and also Section 27.4. You can do the operation, if he also has a minor varus or valgus deformity, provided it is not so severe that it will prevent you fitting calipers. If necessary, you can release his ankle on the same occasion as his knee and his hip.

CONTRAINDICATIONS. If he is a child, tenotomy is contraindicated if: (1) His equinus ankle is helping to compensate for a short leg, or to stabilize an unstable knee, and so enabling him to walk satisfactorily. (2) He will never walk because his arms are weak. (3) His deformity is minimal, and he is managing well with a shoe or boot, with or without a caliper. (4) His feet are infected; if so, delay the operation. (5) He has a severe valgus or varus deformity which will make fitting a caliper impossible.

ANAESTHESIA. General anaesthesia, subarachnoid anaesthesia or ketamine.

METHOD. Use a small tenotomy knife, or the improvised one shown in Fig. 27-10. Use full sterile precautions, scrub up, gown yourself, use gloves, and apply a tourniquet (3.9).

To make the first incision, cut through the posterior two-thirds of his Achilles tendon, about 7 cm above its insertion. Do this by pushing the knife into the tendon from the medial side, in the line of its fibres, at the junction of the anterior third and the posterior two-thirds. Rotate the knife 90°, and then cut posteriorly, until you feel the knife cutting very easily, which shows that you have now cut the posterior part of the tendon.

To make the second incision, push the knife into his tendon in the line of its fibres, at the junction of its lateral third and medial two-thirds, about 1 cm above the insertion of his Achilles tendon. Then, rotate the knife through 90°, and cut medially, until you can feel the blade under his skin (these incisions cut all the fibres, at one level or the other, because of the way they rotate).

CAUTION ! (1) Use full sterile precautions, and drape him with sterile towels. (2) Use a gentle sawing motion, and don't break the blade. (3) Don't cut his posterior tibial vessels and nerves, which lie anteromedial to his Achilles tendon, as in Fig. 27-11. (4) Don't try to divide the tight posterior capsule of his ankle joint in this method. This is not tightened in poliomyelitis, unless there is an associated varus deformity, which must be corrected at open operation.

To manipulate his ankle, flex it dorsally. Apply force as close to the joint as possible. If you apply it at the end of his tibia, you can easily break it. In a young child with polio, you should be able to get 20° of dorsiflexion (calcaneus); in an adult or older child you may get less. If necessary, manipulate him again two weeks later.

If his ankle does not reach the neutral position (90°), check that his tendon has been divided properly, by reinserting the tenotomy knife in the same two tenotomy sites. If his ankle is still not fully corrected to 90°—wait, and plan to increase correction by applying serial casts every 2 or 3 weeks.

POSTOPERATIVELY, squeeze out all subcutaneous clot. Bleeding is usually slight. Apply a small dressing.

If his knee is stable, apply a well-padded below-knee walking cast, with his foot near the maximum correction, *but not at the extreme limit of extension.* Elevate his leg, and send him home in a day or two. See a young child in 3 weeks, and an older child or adult in 6 weeks. Remove his cast and apply a below-knee caliper with a backstop.

If his knee is unstable and has no contracture, apply an above-knee cast. Treat him exactly as above, except fit an above-knee caliper instead of a below-knee one.

DIFFICULTIES WITH CLOSED TENOTOMY. **If you have CUT HIS WHOLE ACHILLES TENDON by mistake,** don't be alarmed. It will almost always heal satisfactorily in the lengthened position. Don't try to repair it.

If his DEFORMITY RECURS, it probably did so because he did not wear a caliper, or wore one without a backstop. If he does not wear one initially, his deformity is sure to recur. Six or 12 months later he may be able to do without a caliper. Follow him up carefully, so that you can decide about this.

If you FRACTURE HIS LOWER TIBIA because you have manipulated him too vigorously, fit him with a cast.

OPEN ACHILLES TENOTOMY FOR POLIO

INDICATIONS. Equinus contractures of the ankle, in which there is a contracture of the posterior capsule of the ankle joint that requires release. This is an alternative to the closed method.

METHOD. Give him a general anaesthetic, squeeze the blood out of his leg, and apply a tourniquet to his thigh (3.9). Place him on his side, with the leg to be operated on uppermost. Prepare his skin as usual.

Make a longitudinal incision over the lower third of his leg, extending proximally from the attachment of his Achilles tendon to his calcaneus.

Dissect out his Achilles tendon. You may see the small tendon of his plantaris on its anteromedial side. Make two incisions half way across his Achilles tendon: (1) The lower one 1 cm above its insertion, either from the medial to the lateral side, or vice versa. If there is any varus deformity of his foot leave the lateral side intact. If there is any valgus deformity, leave the medial side intact. The aim of doing this is to help the distal attachment of the tendon to correct the deformity. (2) At a suitable level, about 4 to 10 cm proximally (depending on his size and the degree of plantar flexion to be corrected), make a small incision opposite the first one, as in Fig. 27-11.

Then push up his foot. The fibres of his Achilles tendon will pull out. You should be able to put his foot into normal dorsi-plantar flexion, without too much force.

If you fail to put his foot into a satisfactory position, make a longitudinal incision down the middle of the tendon joining the two cuts. If this still does not correct the position of his foot, dissect down to the posterior aspect of his ankle joint, under direct vision. Divide the posterior capsule of his ankle joint transversely, from lateral to medial, and open up his ankle, by dorsiflexing the posterior part of his foot.

CAUTION ! Be careful not to cut: (1) his flexor hallucis longus tendon, or (2) his posterior tibial nerve and vessels, which lie on the medial side of the posterior aspect of his ankle joint.

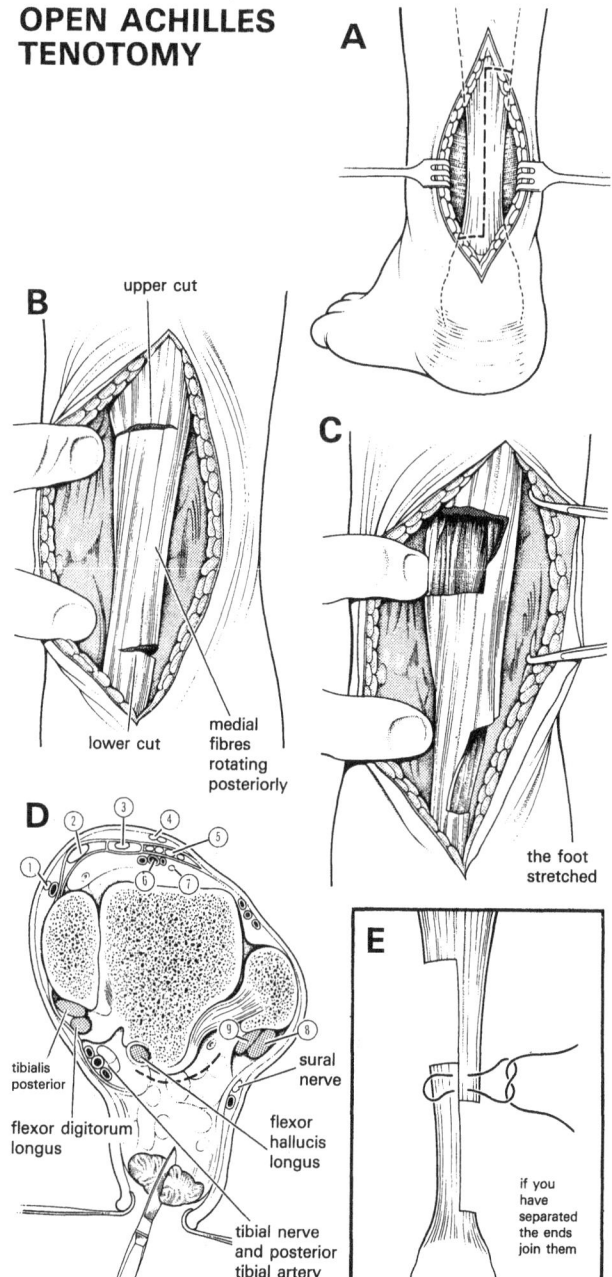

Fig. 27-11 OPEN ACHILLES TENOTOMY. A, the patient's left Achilles tendon exposed. B, the cuts in his tendon. C, his tendon lengthened. D, the anatomy of his ankle joint. E, if you have had to separate his tendon, bring its two halves together with mattress sutures. Note how the fibres of his tendon twist so that the medial ones come to lie posteriorly.

1, the saphenous nerve and vein. 2, tibialis anterior. 3, extensor hallucis longus. 4, the superficial peroneal nerve. 5, extensor digitorum longus and peroneus tertius in the inferior extensor retinaculum. 6, the dorsalis pedis vessels. 7, the deep peroneal nerve. 8, peroneus longus. 9, peroneus brevis.

These structures are only in danger if you divide the posterior capsule.

If you have divided his tendo Achilles completely, bring its ends together with a mattress suture. Close his skin with 2/0 monofilament. Pad his leg, apply a below-knee cast with his knee flexed to 90°, and release the tourniquet.

POSTOPERATIVELY, raise the foot of his bed, expose his leg on a pillow, and check the circulation in his toes hourly. Next day, add a 'shoe' to his cast. Discharge him on crutches, and check his cast in 3 weeks. Remove it or change it at 6 weeks.

REHABILITATION

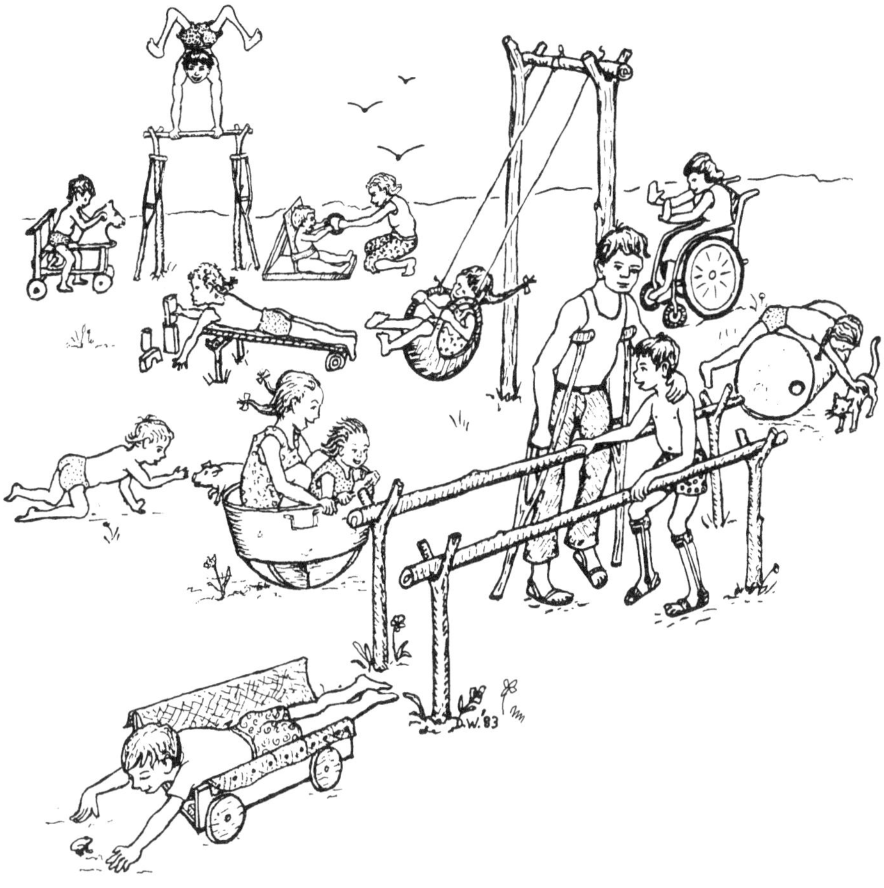

Fig. 27-12 REHABILITATING CRIPPLED CHILDREN. *With the kind permission of David Werner.*

27.8 Back pain, lumbar disc lesions

'Backache' is a common symptom. Your task, as often, is to sort out those patients who need specific and sometimes urgent treatment, from those whom you can only help symptomatically. 'Discs', together with osteoarthritis and senile osteoporosis in the very old, make up most 'backaches'. The important backaches not to miss are the much less common infective ones, particularly in children: pyomyositis (7.1), osteomyelitis (7.15), septic arthritis (7.16) and tuberculosis (29.4). Other causes of back pain include malignant deposits in the spine, back injuries including ligamentous sprains (Chapter 64), spondylosis, spondylolysthesis and ankylosing spondylitis.

Lumbar disc lesions are due to the protrusion of the nucleus pulposus of an intervertebral disc through a weakened area in its annulus fibrosus. This is the ring of firm fibrous tissue that holds the softer nucleus pulposus in place. Prolapsed tissue from the nucleus pulposus presses on a nerve root, and causes pain down the leg. Almost all lumbar disc lesions occur in the spaces $L_4/_5$ or L_5/S_1. Pressure on the S_1 root causes pain down the back of the thigh, calf, and outer side of the foot. Pressure on the L_5 root causes pain on the lateral aspect of the thigh and leg, and the dorsum of the foot. A protrusion from the L_5/S_1 disc usually presses on the S_1 root (not on L_5), but a protrusion from the L_4/L_5 disc may press on the S_1, or on the L_5 root. Occasionally, when the protrusion is central, other roots are involved, and these may cause urinary problems. Disc protrusions are more likely to occur in a back which has been weakened by a sedentary occupation, and may follow sudden flexion of the spine, or bumping in a sedentary position, as with lorry drivers on bad roads.

The patient is usually a middle aged adult, or occasionally a younger one, who presents with sudden severe pain in the front of his thigh, the back of his thigh (sciatic pain, which is present in most patients), his calf, or his foot. Movement, coughing, or sneezing all make pain worse. The dorsum of his foot may be numb, and its dorsiflexors weak, occasionally on both sides. You can usually diagnose a disc lesion clinically without the use of X-rays; atypical cases are more difficult. Most disc lesions are benign and self-limiting, and can be managed non-operatively, although they often recur. Refer him for possible surgery on the indications given below—he probably has a central disc protrusion. At operation, the protruding disc material is removed, and his is disc scraped out.

BACK PAIN

EXAMINATION. Examine the patient's back as in Fig. 27-13. Examine a man's prostate rectally, and a woman's breasts.

LUMBAR DISC LESIONS

EXAMINATION. His lumbar spine is flattened, with loss of its normal lumbar lordosis, and slight scoliosis. He may be tender over his interspinous ligaments, at the site of the lesion, or on gently tapping his spinous processes. Movement of his lumbar spine is usually severely restricted. Forward flexion is always restricted, and is accompanied by spasm. Lateral flexion may be free, in one or both directions.

Lay him flat and raise his leg by his ankle. Straight leg raising is limited and flexing his ankle makes it worse. His ankle jerk (S_1) may be diminished or absent.

BACK PAIN

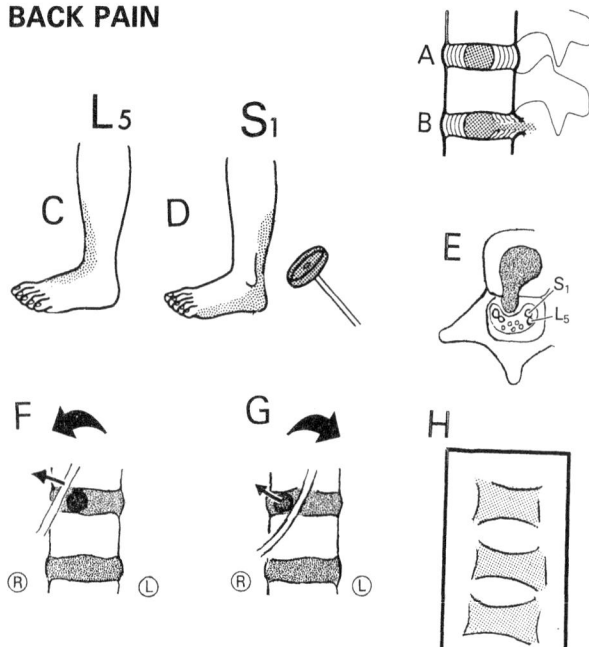

Fig. 27-12a BACK PAIN. A, a normal disc. B, a ruptured annular ligament, with the nucleus protruding. C, an L_5 lesion causes loss of sensation on the dorsomedial aspect of the foot, and weakness of the dorsiflexors of the ankle, with sparing of the ankle jerk. D, an S_1 lesion causes loss of sensation on the lateral border of the foot, weakness of plantar flexors, a tender calf, and a diminished ankle jerk. E, a prolapsed disc pressing on the large L_5 and S_1 nerve roots; S_2, S_3, S_4 and S_5 are all small, control bladder function and are less often involved. F, a medial protrusion causes flexion of the lumbar spine, which tends to lift the root away from it. In this case the spine is convex to the left. G, a lateral protrusion causes flexion of the spine, which tends to lift the protrusion away from the disc. Here the spine is convex to the right. H, in severe osteoporosis X-rays show bulging of the discs into the demineralized vertebral bodies.

He may also have lost sensation in the relevant dermatomes, as shown in Figures 64-2, and A 6-8.

X-RAYS may or may not show confirmatory signs. Look for mild scoliosis, loss of his normal lumbar lordosis and narrowing of the disc space. The X-rays must be well centred to show this. If the film is taken obliquely, any disc space will look narrow.

THE DIFFERENTIAL DIAGNOSES include the following, and those listed below under 'Difficulties':

Suggesting bony secondaries—an older patient with persistent spinal pain, both when active and at rest. The X-rays of his spine may be normal initially. Typically, he has a patchy osteoporosis of the bodies, and/or the arches, of his vertebrae (some secondaries are sclerotic, especially those from the prostate). He may have a pathological fracture, especially of a vertebral body. His discs are spared. Look for the primary in the prostate (32.32), the breast (21.4), the bronchus (32.29), the thyroid (21.12), and the kidney (32.30) and for signs of myelomatosis (32.17).

Suggesting an acute infective cause, pyomyositis (7.1), or osteomyelitis of the spine (7.2, 7.16)—an acute onset with fever in a child or young adult, who is obviously very ill.

Suggesting tuberculosis—a slow onset with loss of weight, malaise, mild fever, and a gibbus.

CAUTION ! (1) Young children don't have disc lesions, so assume that all back pain in a young child is serious, until you have proved it is not. (2) Back pain and fever are a serious combination. (3) Don't forget the possibility of tuberculosis (29.4).

TREATMENT. Put him to bed in his most comfortable position, which is usually with his hips and knees flexed. Don't put pillows under his knees; they will immobilize his legs and promote deep vein thrombosis. Put fracture boards under the mattress. Give him an analgesic (if necessary pethidine or morphine for the first few days), and don't let him get up, even to go to the toilet.

Many patients improve without traction (70.9). If you apply it, tie a band round his pelvis, and apply a total of 7 to 10 kg to both sides of it for a maximum of 3 to 5 days. Raise the foot of his bed to apply counter traction. Alternatively, apply 4 or 5 kg of traction to each leg with adhesive strapping.

Start active and passive movements of his legs, as soon as his acute pain is over. When his pain is sufficiently improved, start back extension exercises.

If his symptoms improve, keep him in bed for 3 weeks. Then allow him up to go to the toilet, keeping his back straight. If he wants to stoop, he must do this with his hips and knees, and keep his back straight.

INDICATIONS FOR REFERRAL. (1) If he has perineal numbness or incontinence of urine or faeces, referral for probable surgery is urgent. If you fail to do this, incontinence may become permanent. (2) More than mild weakness of his dorsiflexors (L_5) or plantarflexors (S_1). (3) Failure of his pain to improve, despite 3 or 4 weeks in bed.

DIFFICULTIES WITH BACK PAIN

If an OLDER PATIENT complains of PAIN WHEN SITTING OR STANDING, or following manual activities, he is probably suffering from OSTEOARTHRITIS. X-ray him to exclude other diseases. If necessary, give him analgesics and keep his spine

EXAMINING THE SPINE

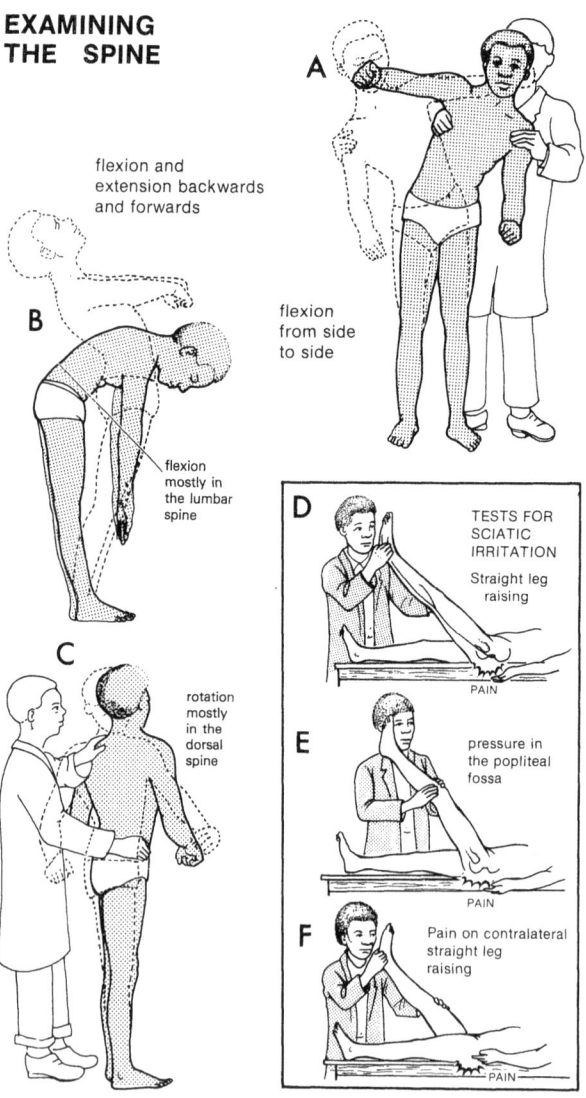

Fig. 27-13 EXAMINING THE SPINE. A, flexion from side to side. B, flexion and extension forwards and backwards. C, rotation. D, straight leg raising to test for sciatic irritation. E, if a patient has a disc lesion, and you raise his leg straight, and then press in his popliteal fossa, it may cause sciatic pain. F, if you raise his other leg, it may also cause pain if he has a disc lesion.

as mobile as possible with exercises. If he is obese, reduce his weight.

If an old patient, especially an OLD WOMAN, has a MARKED KYPHOSIS, think of SENILE OSTEOPOROSIS, with a generalized loss of matrix and calcium, especially from the bodies of her vertebrae. Her discs expand and compress her weak vertebral bodies. Painful pathological fractures are common, and she may have root pain.

Treat her symptomatically with analgesics, and encourage her to keep moving, if necessary with the aid of a stick. Oestrogens are useful, if they are started soon after the menopause before the condition is established. This requires the identification of risk factors, such as her family history. Give her stilboestrol 1 mg daily. The effect of this on a possible increased incidence of carcinoma of the breast is not known.

If an adult or older child complains of BACK PAIN, WORSE ON STANDING, and often episodic, consider the possibility of SPONDYLOLITHESIS. In this condition the body of a vertebra (commonly L_5) slips forwards on the vertebra below it. It is often asymptomatic, and even if you find it, it may not be the cause of his pain, so exclude other causes. If you find it by chance, when there is no pain, do nothing. If he has pain, refer him.

If a YOUNG MAN complains of BACK PAIN and later STIFFNESS, perhaps with inflammatory involvement of his other joints, consider the possibility of ANKYLOSING SPONDYLITIS (common in in India, rare in Africa). Typically, the pain wakens him from his sleep in the early hours of the morning, is relieved by getting up and walking, and, unlike most other pains, is made worse by rest. His upper legs may ache, but radiating pain is unusual. He may be ill. Test for bilateral sacroiliac tenderness, and pain over his sarioiliac joints on springing his pelvis (both early signs). All movements of his lumbar spine are restricted, sometimes with muscle spasm. His chest expansion is also restricted (an objective early sign). Look for uveitis (24.4). His ESR is raised. The earliest X-ray sign is bony erosion of the lower third of both his sacroiliac joints (invariable), followed later by secondary ossification and ankylosis of the whole joint. Early, his lumbar X-rays are normal; later he has a calcification of his intervertebral ligaments ('bamboo spine').

Teach him exercises to help prevent severe curvature of his spine, and retain mobility. In the early painful stages anti-inflammatory drugs may help, especially indomethacin 25 mg three times daily. Keep his major joints mobile, and if they do become fixed, try to ensure that this happens in the position of function (7-16).

27.9 Epicondylitis (tennis elbow)

This is a common condition in people who use the extensor muscles of their forearms vigorously, and not only in tennis players. It is caused by minute tears in the origin of the forearm extensor muscles. The patient complains of pain just distal to the lateral epicondyle of his humerus, without any history of trauma. The pain is worse when you press over his radio-humeral joint during pronation and supination. It lasts for months, or years, and may eventually disappear spontaneously. You can hasten its departure like this.

EPICONDYLITIS. Inject hydrocortisone suspension 2.5 ml with an equal volume of 2% lignocaine into the tender area. One injection has an 80% chance of success, and a second one 2 or 3 weeks later another 10%. *Take very careful aseptic precautions,* and don't give him more than three injections. If his disability is severe, refer him for a muscle slide on the extensor origin.

27.10 Stenosing tenosynovitis

This is a chronic benign condition, in which a patient's tendons no longer run smoothly in their sheaths. His symptoms depend upon which tendon is involved. This disease appears to be less common in the developing world than it is elsewhere.

If he complains of pain (and sometimes an abnormal prominence) over his radial styloid, which may be worse on extending and/or abducting his thumb, its abductor and short extensor tendons are constricted in their sheaths, as they pass over the groove in the end of his radius (de Quervain's disease). They are tender, and you can usually feel a thickening in the tendon sheath. Flexion and adduction of his thumb causes pain over his radial styloid.

If he complains that, when he flexes one of his digits it locks, ('trigger finger' or thumb), so that he cannot extend it again, until he does so passively and forcefully, his flexor tendons are involved. His powerful flexors are able to pull the swollen part of the tendon proximal to the constriction, but his weaker extensors are unable to extend his finger again unaided.

STENOSING TENOSYNOVITIS

If the abductor and short extensor tendons of a patient's thumb are involved and the disease is early, inject the lesion with 0.5 ml of lignocaine mixed with 0.5 ml of a suspension of hydrocortisone *using the most careful sterile precautions.* Place the point of a very fine needle into the palpable swelling, just distal to his radial styloid, and inject between the tendon sheath, and the bone of the groove of his styloid. If you are successful, you will see a wheal appearing on the proximal side of the tendon sheath.

If injection is not successful (50% of cases), make a small transverse skin incision over his radial styloid. Use a fine tenotomy knife to make a longitudinal incision in the sheath to release the tendon. Leave the sheath open, suture his skin only, and start active movements immediately. The result will be good.

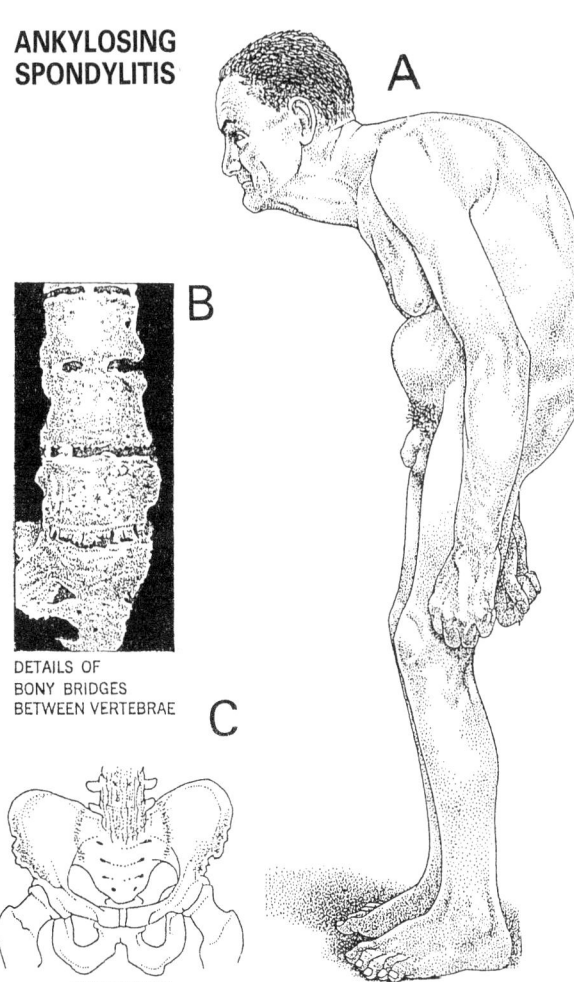

Fig. 27-13a ANKYLOSING SPONDILITIS. A, the characteristic 'question-mark' posture of ankylosing spondylitis. B, bony bridges forming between the patient's vertebrae. C, his sacroiliac joints have fused and only the ghost of the old joint line is visible. *J Robins in 'The Independent', permission requested.*

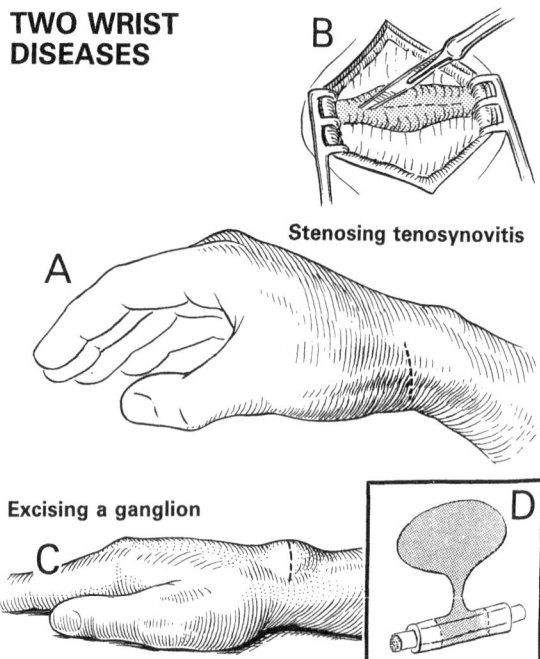

Fig. 27-14 TWO WRIST DISEASES. A, when a patient has stenosing tenosynovitis of the extensor tendons of his thumb, make a transverse incision in the skin of his wrist. B, divide the constriction in his tendon sheath longitudinally with a No. 15 scalpel blade. C, avoid operating on a ganglion if you can. D, if you have to operate, remove the ganglion, and a little of the adjacent tendon sheath, which will reduce the probability of its recurring.

CAUTION ! (1) Avoid the cutaneous branch of his radial nerve, so look for it immediately you incise the skin. (2) Don't try to pare down the tendon. (3) There may be several slips to the tendon, and thus several compartments in the sheath; make sure each is free.

If the flexor tendon of his thumb is inolved at his MP joint ('trigger thumb'), first try steroid injection, as above. If this is not successful, and you cannot refer him, operate. Give him an intravenous forearm block (A 6.19), or a median and ulnar nerve block (A 6.20). Apply a tourniquet; you will need skin hooks and very small retractors. Make a 1 cm incision in the midline of his thumb, on its volar aspect, in the crease of his MP joint, and release the stenosis as above.

CAUTION ! The danger with this operation is that you may cut his digital nerves, so you must know where they are. Review the anatomy before you operate.

If the flexor tendons of his fingers are involved (commonly his ring or middle finger, occasionally his little finger), refer him. If this is impossible, make a 1 cm transverse incision on the palmar surface of his hand, half way between his distal palmar crease and the flexion crease of his finger. Insert retractors and carefully deepen the incision. Take care to find his digital nerves, so that you don't cut them.

When you find the narrowed tendon sheath cut it longitudinally with a No. 15 blade. Insert a small pair of pointed scissors, and run them distally to cut the stenosed sheath. As soon as you have done this, you can flex his finger.

27.11 Ganglions

A ganglion is a round cystic swelling that develops on the back of a patient's wrist, or less commonly on the dorsum of his foot, usually in connection with a tendon sheath, or a joint capsule. Flex his wrist over your knee; this will usually make the fluid in the cyst tense. Bang the tense cyst with a large object, such as a heavy book. It will usually disperse the fluid. If it fails, repeat it under general anaesthesia using a rubber mallet, or a similar object. The chances of it recurring are not much higher than those following surgery. Avoid operating if you can, and only do so on the indications below. If you fail to remove a ganglion completely, it is more likely to recur, and if you dissect too energetically, you may damage a tendon.

REMOVING A GANGLION

INDICATIONS. A ganglion which causes pain, or is large and unsightly, and which has recurred twice after rupture, or could not be ruptured.

ANAESTHESIA. An axillary block, an intravenous forearm block, or general anaesthesia.

METHOD. Apply a tourniquet (3.9). Incise transversely in the line of the skin crease over the ganglion. Dissect out the cyst without damaging tendons, nerves, or vessels. Try not to rupture it, because this will make removing all its extensions more difficult. Excise it, and a short length of the tendon sheath from which it arises (leaving the tendon naked is unimportant). If you fail to do this, it is more likely to recur, which it may do anyway.

Let down the tourniquet, control bleeding, sew up the skin with 2/0 or 3/0 monofilament, and apply a pressure dressing for 24 hours.

27.11a The carpal tunnel syndrome

This occurs more often in women than in men, and is often worse during pregnancy, and before menstruation. It is the result of pressure on a patient's median nerve, as it passes through her carpal tunnel, on the front of her wrist. It causes: (1) Pain, pins and needles and reduced sensation in the distribution of her median nerve (her thumb, her index and her middle finger, and the radial side of her ring finger). (2) Weakness and wasting of the muscles of her thenar eminence; her hypothenar muscles are spared. (3) Pain in her wrist, usually referred pain to her lower forearm, and sometimes even pain referred to her elbow and upper arm. Her pain is worse at night, and she may get some relief by hanging it out of bed. Tapping over her flexor retinaculum (Tinel's sign) may bring on her symptoms.

CARPAL TUNNEL SYNDROME

NON-OPERATIVE TREATMENT. (1) Reduce the patient's oedema with a thiazide, such as hydrochlorthiazide 25 to 50 mg twice daily during pregnancy. Don't operate while she is pregnant, unless her symptoms are severe. (2) Encourage her to lose weight. (3) Inject her carpal tunnel with hydrocortisone suspension 2.5 ml and lignocaine 2.5 ml.

INDICATIONS FOR SURGERY. (1) Wasting of the muscles of her thenar eminence. (2) Failure of non-operative treatment.

ANAESTHESIA. Axillary block (A 6.18), intravenous forearm block (6.19) or general anaesthesia (A 11.3).

METHOD. If you cannot refer her, apply a tourniquet to produce a bloodless field (3.9). Make an L-shaped incision over the creases on the front of her wrist, as in Fig. 27-14a. Incise longitudinally for 4 cm in her thenar crease, and then transversely for 2 cm in her wrist crease. Divide her flexor retinaculum in the line of her arm. Look for her median nerve, but *don't injure it.* Opposite the proximal edge of her retinaculum you should see an incomplete annular depression, most marked anteriorly, which is the site of pressure. Don't sew her deep tissues. Sew up her skin only with 2/0 or 3/0 monofilament. Apply a pressure dressing for 48 hours. Raise her arm in a roller towel (B, 75-1).

POSTOPERATIVELY, watch the circulation in her hand hourly; if there is any problem with this, remove all dressings. She will probably find that her pain is relieved immediately.

27.12 Congenital dislocation of the hip (CDH)

Congenital dislocation of the hip causes no symptoms at birth,

THE CARPAL TUNNEL SYNDROME

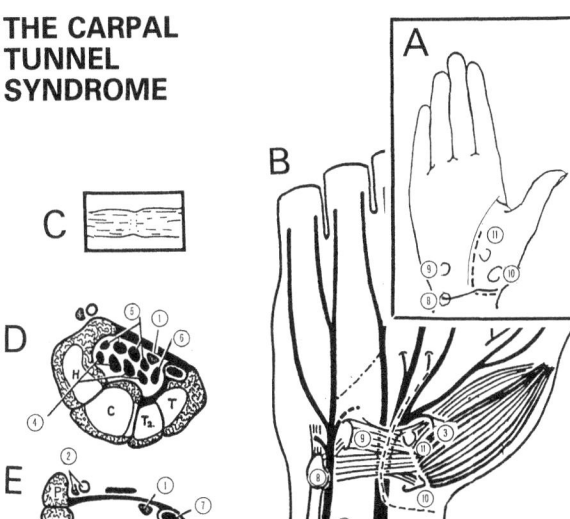

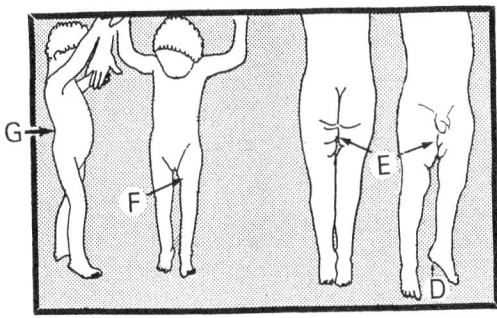

Fig. 27-14a THE CARPAL TUNNEL SYNDROME. A, and B, landmarks for the incision. C, the median nerve with an annular constricting ring round it, caused by pressure from the edge of the flexor retinaculum. D, the distal and E, the proximal row of carpal bones and the carpal tunnel.

H, the hamate. C, the capitate. T, the trapezium. T_2, the trapezoid. L, the lunate. S, the scaphoid. Tq, the triquetrum. P, the pisiform.

1, the median nerve. 2, the ulnar nerve and artery. 3, the muscular branch of the median nerve. 4, the profundus tendons. 5, the superficialis tendons. 6, flexor pollicis longus. 7, flexor carpi radialis. 8, the pisiform bone. 9, the hook of the hamate. 10, the tuberosity of the scaphoid. 11, the tuberosity of the trapezium. *After 'Grant's Method of Anatomy', (9th edn 1975), edited by JV Basmajian), Figs. 32.17 and 32.20. Williams and Wilkins, permission requested.*

so it has to be diagnosed by screening all newborn babies. The danger is that it may cause premature osteoarthritis in later life. If however you can recognize a baby's dislocated hip at birth, reduce it, and hold it in place with a simple splint, you can usually cure him and prevent later complications. In many communities (Africa) it is rare, but in those where it is not, it is worth screening for.

If he is not diagnosed at birth, he may present with a limp (often very mild) when he starts to walk. His leg may then be shortened and his hip unstable. If however his dislocation is bilateral, you will not be able to diagnose shortening, and he may appear to walk normally, although careful observation should show a slight waddle. Baby girls are more likely to dislocate their hips than baby boys.

CONGENITAL DISLOCATION OF THE HIP

DIAGNOSIS. In communities where CDH is sufficiently common to make routine screening worthwhile, examine all children soon after birth. CDH can be confirmed radiologically, but the methods of doing so are not described here.

In a baby do Ortolani's test. Fig. 27-15 shows the test being done in a girl. She *must* be relaxed, preferably after she has been fed. Flex her knees and hold so them so that your thumbs are along the medial sides of her thighs, and your fingers are over her trochanters (A). Flex her hips to 90°. Starting from a position in which your thumbs are touching, abduct her hips smoothly and gently (B).

If a hip is dislocated or subluxed, you will feel the head of her femur slipping into her acetabulum as you approach full abduction (C). You may hear a 'clunk', but this is not essential for the test to be positive. Restriction of abduction may indicate an irreducible dislocation. If the test is positive she must be treated.

If a patient is older, one leg may be slightly shorter, and the hip externally rotated (D). The skin folds of the thigh may be asymmetrical (E), but this sign is not very reliable. If both hips are involved the perineum is usually widened due to their

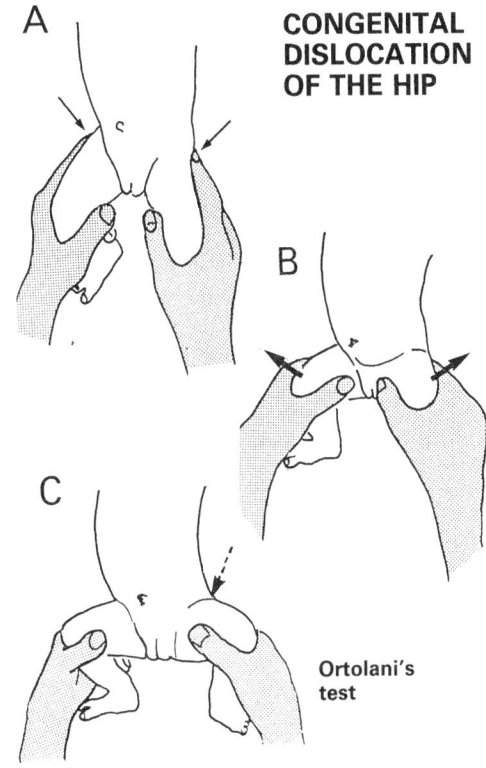

Fig. 27-15 CONGENITAL DISLOCATION OF THE HIP. A, B, and C, Ortolani's test. D, if a patient is older, his leg may be slightly shorter, and his hip externally rotated. The skin folds of his thigh may be asymmetrical (E), but this sign is not very reliable. If both hips are involved the perineum is usually widened owing to their displacement (F). If a patient has been walking his lumbar lordosis may be increased (G). *After Ronald McRae, permission requested.*

displacement (F). If walking has started, the lumbar lordosis may be increased (G).

THE TREATMENT OF CDH

If she is a neonate, treat her in double nappies which will hold her hips in flexion and abduction. Examine her again at one week. If her displaced hip has become stable, apply double nappies for a further 3 weeks, and examine her again. If it is still stable, one nappy only is necessary.

If instability persists, he needs a more substantial splint. Ideally use the von Rosen splint (B, 27-15a). Alternatively, the simplest splint is a sheet of stiff polythene, padded round its edges, which passes between her abducted legs over her nappy. The edges of the sheet are held together at either side by two pieces of 'Velcro' strapping. If you cannot obtain such a splint, you may be able to improvise one.

Apply the splint for 3 months. Then examine her hip again and X-ray it. If there is any doubt that it is not in place, refer her.

SPLINTS FOR CDH

A paddled plastic splint

A von Rosen splint

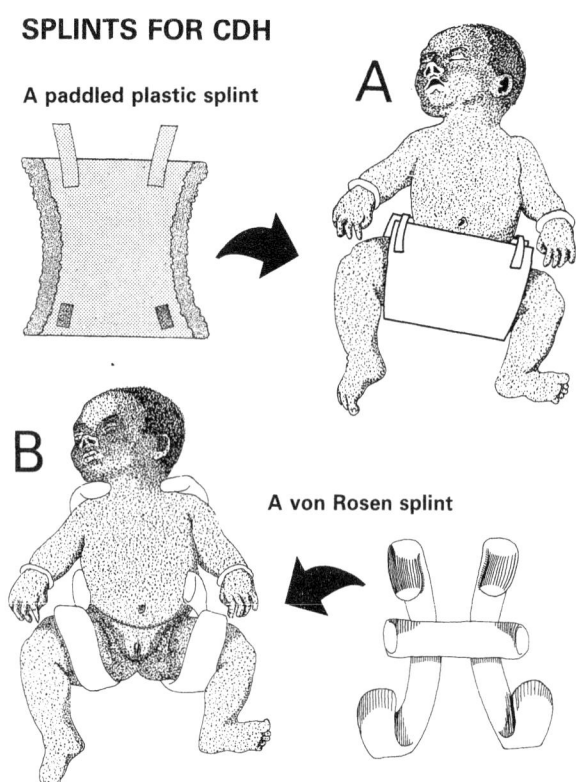

Fig. 27-15a A SPLINT FOR CONGENITAL DISLOCATION OF THE HIP. A, the simplest splint is a sheet of stiff polythene, padded round its edges, which passes between the child's legs over her nappy. B, ideally use the von Rosen splint made of washable malleable padded metal.

DIFFICULTIES WITH CDH

If you DIAGNOSE CDH LATE (over the age of 3 months), she needs skilled surgery, so consider referring her. If she is over 8 years this will be difficult. If a good range of movement is particularly important, as in societies where people squat, an unstable mobile hip may be preferable to a stiff one, whatever the risk of later arthritis.

If REDUCTION IS DIFFICULT or impossible, consider other causes for the dislocation: (1) Partly treated septic arthritis or tuberculous arthritis. (2) A congenital abnormality, and particularly ARTHROGRYPOSIS (rare), as shown by: (a) the absence of skin creases, (b) generalized rigidity of the muscles often of both legs, and sometimes of all four limbs. If you recognize this condition, don't attempt reduction, which may be impossible—refer her. X-rays should distinguish between (1) and (2).

27.13 The child with a painful hip or a limp

Hip disease in a child can present as: (1) A painful hip. (2) A painful hip and a painful, but otherwise normal, knee, due to the referral of pain along the obturator nerve. (3) A painful knee with no pain in the hip. (4) A painless limp. Some hip disease is potentially so serious, that everyone delivering primary care should be on the look out for these four signs, which may be due to several diseases. The most important ones not to miss are the infective ones, especially tuberculosis and septic arthritis, because they need *early* treatment—septic arthritis needs it in the first few hours! The least serious condition is a poorly understood one known as known as 'transient synovitis', which may recover spontaneously, or proceed to Perthes' disease. In the early stages some causes of an irritable hip may be indistinguishable from one another, so observe the child carefully.

A PAINFUL HIP PARTICULARLY IN CHILDREN

DIFFERENTIAL DIAGNOSIS. Don't forget that abdominal and spinal conditions can also cause pain in the hip. Remember also the possibility of disease near the hip (periadenitis, pyomyositis, etc.—see Sections 5.12, 7.1). In Zambia the causes of a painful hip in a child are approximately as follows, in decreasing order of frequency

Suggesting transient synovitis—no X-ray changes, spontaneous resolution in a few weeks without further episodes. Some cases are viral, notably those due to the parovirus, and several joints may be involved. There may be a history of mild trauma.

Suggesting septic arthritis/osteomyelitis (7.18, 7.10)—an acute onset, often in a few hours. His hip is acutely painful, and he cannot move it in any direction. The general symptoms of an acute infection. There are no bony changes for about 2 weeks. If the film is a good one you may see displacement of the fat shadow, or a widened joint space, indicating fluid in his hip joint. Partially treated cases are more difficult to distinguish clinically and by X-ray.

Suggesting sickle-cell disease—pain in other parts of the body also. A positive sickle-cell test.

Suggesting rheumatic fever—age 5 to 20 years. Transient symptoms and the involvement of other joints.

Suggesting tuberculosis (29.3)—any age, but common in childhood and adolescence. Generalized rarefaction of the bone round the joint, localized areas of erosion, a joint space which is either narrowed or widened.

Suggesting Perthes' disease (27.14)—age 4 to 9 years (occasionally 2 to 18 years). His hip is slightly painful when you move it, and all movements are slightly to moderately diminished. No general symptoms. X-rays as in Fig. 27-16.

Suggesting rheumatoid arthritis—from childhood to 40 years (at the onset). The involvement of several joints is usual, although monarticular disease does occur.

Suggesting gonococcal disease or Reiter's syndrome—a urethral discharge, conjunctivitis and/or anterior uveitis. A gonococcal arthritis is usually acute. Reiter's syndrome often follows a chlamydial infection, for which tetracycline may be beneficial.

Suggesting a slipped epiphysis (77.10)—age 12 to 18. Usually a history of an acute onset, sometimes with a fall. X-rays show slipping of the upper femoral epiphysis as in Fig. 77-9. A fixed external rotation deformity.

CAUTION ! (1) If you diagnose transient synovitis, follow up the child carefully—some of these children develop Perthes' disease later. (2) Pain in the knee is often due to hip disease.

A PAINFUL HIP IN A YOUNG CHILD IS
INFLAMMATORY, UNTIL PROVED OTHERWISE

27.14 Perthes' disease (osteochondritis)

Like congenital dislocation of the hip (CDH) and slipped epiphyses (77.10), Perthes' disease causes only minor symptoms in childhood, but may cause severe osteoarthritis in later life. It is a very controversial disease: nobody knows how to treat it, or how to classify it.

A child with Perthes' disease is between 4 and 9 (occasionally between 2 and 18), and is three times more likely to be a boy. *If he presents early,* he does so with intermittent episodes of pain in the front of his thigh, knee or groin, and a limp; in the early stages he is normal between these episodes. Sometimes he has no limp, but only some minimal abnormality of his gait, such as a tendency to walk with his leg turned inwards. Usually (but not always) all the movements of his hip are mildly limited, by discomfort rather than by pain, especially abduction and internal rotation. He may also have some fixed flexion. If his movements are limited, he usually also has spasm, particularly in his adductor and psoas muscles. His thigh and buttock may be wasted.

He may be vaguely tender around his hip, but he is otherwise perfectly well. *If he presents late,* after the disease has run its course, his only signs may be a slight loss of the normal range of abduction, extension, and medial rotation of his hip, or he may have no symptoms or signs. In Africa, most patients don't present until they have permanent deformity.

Perthes' disease is an avascular necrosis of all or part of the epiphysis of the head of the femur. Essentially, the disease passes through five stages during 2 to 4 years: (1) To begin with the child's X-rays are normal. (2) All or part of the head of his femur looks abnormally dense on the X-ray, which indicates reduced vascularity. The cartilage surrounding it does not die; instead, it continues to enlarge, and makes the joint space appear larger. (3) The epiphysis may fragment. (4) New blood vessels gradually grow in, and the epiphysis looks less dense. The epiphysis and metaphysis may soften, so that his metaphysis bends and causes a mild coxa vara (the head and the neck of his femur are angled more medially from the shaft). (5) Eventually, the head returns to its normal density, but it remains flatter, and the neck remains wider than normal.

Catterall classifies Perthes' into four groups, which are complex, disputed, and difficult for the inexpert. Hips in Group One and in Group Two (without risk factors) will do well without any treatment. Most Group Four hips do badly, even if they are treated. A child is more likely to to get osteoarthritis later in life, if the head of his femur flattens. The older he is, and the more misshapen the head, the worse his prognosis. But, even if it is seriously flattened, he will probably not get symptoms until he is middle aged. Unlike slipping of the heads of the femoral epiphyses, the involvement of both hips is unusual in Perthes' disease (15% of cases, mostly in younger children).

The hope of treatment is to prevent deformity, as long as the epiphysis and underlying metaphysis are soft, which is during the avascular phase and during revascularization. There are various possibilities, either alone or combined: (1) Prolonged traction (1–2 years) produces little benefit, and is quite impractical. (2) Any attempt to avoid weight-bearing by restricting a child's activity is also impractical in the developing world. (3) Some contributors consider that weight-bearing calipers don't work and should be avoided. (4) Salter's Toronto splint is expensive and impractical. (5) Surgery has never been proved to be better than non-operative management. What are you to do? We give you two very different regimes. The second is the more practical one.

PERTHES' DISEASE

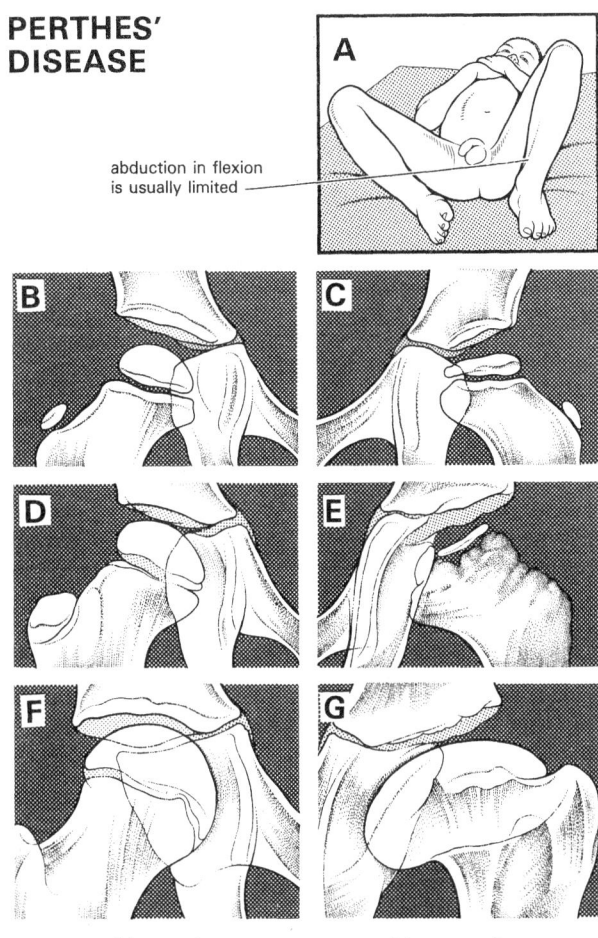

abduction in flexion is usually limited

Normal   Abnormal

Fig. 27-16 PERTHES' DISEASE. This shows the progression of a patient in Catterall's Group Four. A, in Perthes' disease there is always limitation of abduction. B, and C, on the abnormal side the head of the femur is smaller and denser, and the joint space looks increased. E, patchy fragmentation follows. G, the head becomes wide and flattened. Meanwhile, the opposite hip, (B, D, and F) has been growing normally. *After Apley AG, 'System of Orthopaedics and Fractures', Fig. 26-12 18.20, with kind permission.*

THE AIM OF MANAGEMENT IS TO PREVENT LATE OSTEOARTHRITIS

PERTHES' DISEASE

TESTING FOR SPASM

SPASM IN EXTENSION. Lay the child on his back, place your hands on his affected thigh, and roll it backwards and forwards, as in Fig 7-17. Compare both sides. If there is no spasm in extension, test it in flexion.

SPASM IN FLEXION. Flex his hip and knee to 90°. Rotate his leg inwards and outwards. Rotation is usually more limited than abduction or adduction.

ABDUCTION IN FLEXION is usually limited (A, 27-16).

X-RAYS. Take an AP and a lateral view. Abduct his hips, rotate his femurs inwards, and take an AP view to include both hips, so that you can compare them.

GROUPING (Catterall, modified) determines prognosis and treatment. Group him when he presents.

Group One. There is an increase in radiodensity in the head of his femur, but no loss of height and no sequestration. An AP view may show lytic areas in the epiphysis. The metaphysis is normal.

Group Two. In a lateral view the area of sequestration and fragmentation is less than two-thirds of the width of the epiphysis. Loss of height is mild. There is radiolucency in the metaphysis under the affected epiphysis.

Group Three. There is markedly increased density, indicating sequestration of most of the epiphysis, but with a margin of normal bone. There is obvious loss of height. Metaphyseal changes are usually generalized.

Group Four. The whole epiphysis is involved and collapses, so that it has almost no height. The epiphysis extrudes and becomes mushroom-shaped. Metaphyseal changes are marked.

Risk factors. (a) Lateral subluxation of the head leaving it partly uncovered. (b) A translucent area in the lateral third of the epiphysis. (c) Specks of calcium lateral to the epiphysis. (d) Severe radiolucency of the metaphysis. A fragmented upper femoral epiphysis which appears to be extruding from the acetabulum is a poor prognostic sign.

DIFFERENTIAL DIAGNOSIS. See Section 27.13 on the child with the painful hip.

FIRST REGIME. The younger he is, and the less of the head that is involved, the better his prognosis. This is also influenced by the stage of the disease and the presence of risk factors, so weigh them up carefully.

Group One cases usually resolve spontaneously without treatment. Let him walk, but not run, or do violent exercise. X-ray him monthly for 3 months, then 3-monthly for a year, then stop unless he progresses to a worse grade.

Group Two without risk factors. Treat him as Group One.

Group Two cases with risk factors and cases from Group Three. He is likely to progress unless he is treated. Treatment will improve his prognosis, but there is still a chance that he will get osteoarthritis later. Keep him in bed in extension traction (78.3) for about a month, until the spasm in his hip joint has gone. 2 kg will probably be enough. Traction is the best way of making sure that a small child stays in bed.

Then, either: (1) Refer him to an orthopaedic surgeon, who may do an operation to contain the head of his femur in the socket of his acetabulum. Or, (2) continue to apply traction in bed for 1–4 years! A long period of rest in bed is unlikely to be practical, so try to give him as much rest as you can. Then start him walking, but not weight bearing. A weight-relieving caliper is best. This is longer than his leg, and prevents his foot from reaching the ground. Place the ring so that his weight is transmitted from his pelvis to the caliper. If both his hips are involved, the only way you can prevent him bearing weight is to keep him in bed, if necessary for months. Review him regularly: one stage can progress to another, although this is unusual.

Group Four. Deformity of the head is inevitable. Untreated, all patients progress to osteoarthritis. If treated as for Group Three 25% have a good outcome.

SECOND REGIME. Admit him for for a short (3–4 weeks) period of bed rest on traction. *Make sure that he he has got Perthes' disease and has not been misdiagnosed;* avoid supposedly 'weight-relieving' calipers and long periods in bed. In a hard-pressed orthopaedic unit surgery for Perthes' disease has little if any place.

27.15 Neonatal talipes equinovarus

A child is sometimes born with shortening of the soft tissues of the flexor aspect of his leg, and the medial side of his foot, which causes his talus to point downwards (equinus), and inwards (varus). At the same time, his forefoot is adducted at its tarso-metatarsal joints. This may happen to one or both of his feet. If his deformity is very severe, his navicular bone may be pulled medially, and sometimes even away from the front of his talus. If his foot remains like this, its bones may break in the middle to form a 'rocker bottom foot'. Occasionally, he is born with his feet pointing in other directions. Some cases of talipes are due to paralyses, for example those associated with meningomyelocele (28.9).

You should be able to treat 75% of children with talipes using only non-operative methods—if you see them early enough and follow them up thoroughly. The remaining 25% will need expert surgery at some stage. Even if these children are not operated on, they can walk adequately and painlessly, although their feet are ugly, and will not fit into ordinary shoes.

When you treat a child with talipes try to: (1) Correct the position of his foot, as soon as possible after birth. (2) Hold it in a corrected position, until its bones have had a chance to grow in their new position. As soon as he starts walking, his foot is probably safe. Treatment must begin soon—it has been said that if a club foot is diagnosed at the beginning of a breech delivery, manipulation should start then! If treatment is delayed until a child is 6 months old, correction will take longer, but non-operative treatment is still worth trying, even as late as this. Any foot which is not fully corrected at 6 months needs surgery. Where skills and facilities are good, it is often done at 3 months, and sometimes as young as 6 weeks.

You have a choice of: (1) Zinc oxide strapping or, (2) plaster casts. Strapping has to be applied in such a way that each time a child kicks it pulls his leg straight. It can be applied by primary care workers, or by his mother—if she is sufficiently intelligent, and reliable, and you teach her carefully. Talipes and the strapping method have been described in 'Primary Child Care' (26.52), so that all primary health workers should know about it, and how important it is to start treatment early. Some of them may be able to apply it. The strapping method needs a certain skill to do well, and careful supervision.

Plaster casts are more reliable, but they have to be applied in a hospital outpatient department, preferably by yourself, or a carefully trained and supervised orthopaedic assistant, or other paramedical. The disadvantage of strapping is that a less educated village mother may remove it, or not realize that it needs replacing as soon as it becomes loose, so her child may be better with a cast; but she must bring him every two weeks to have it changed.

There are two types of talipes equinovarus: (1) False talipes which is positional only, and does not need treatment, and (2) true talipes which does. There are two varieties of true talipes, (2a) an easy type which responds readily to treatment, and (2b) a resistant type, which does not. You will not know which type a child has, until you have treated him for a few weeks. Rarely, the condition of his muscles which causes his talipes also involves his other muscles, and makes them rigid. This is arthrogryposis.

TALIPES

TRUE OR FALSE TALIPES? Can you bend a newborn baby's ankle, so that the outer side of his foot touches the outer side of his leg? If you can, he has false talipes and he needs no treatment. If you cannot do this, he has true talipes.

MANAGING TRUE TALIPES. **If there is no cleft on the inside of his foot or his heel,** his talipes is sufficiently mild for non-operative treatment to have a good chance of success—*especially if it starts in the first day or two after birth.*

If there is a cleft on the inside of his foot or his heel, his talipes is too severe for non-operative treatment, so refer him to an expert early. Operative treatment can start as early as 3 weeks under ideal conditions, and should be done by 6 months. 3 months is a good compromise. Meanwhile treat him non-operatively.

If he is a true arthrogrypotic, with multiple other deformities, refer him, but it is doubtful if any treatment is worthwhile.

CAUTION ! (1) Start non-operative treatment as soon after birth as possible. (2) Look for other congenital abnormalities, especially spina bifida. Make sure he can move his legs. If he also has a meningomyelocele, he will also be incontinent of urine, and treating his feet will not be worthwhile.

ZINC OXIDE STRAPPING FOR TALIPES

Use zinc oxide strapping. Elastic strapping will not work. If possible, put tincture of benzoin on his leg before you apply

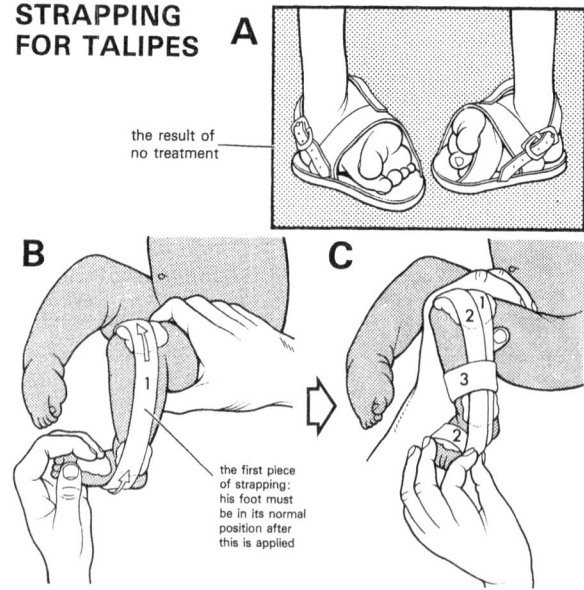

Fig. 27-17 STRAPPING FOR TALIPES. A, the consequences of neglect. Fortunately, this child's deformed feet are not likely to be painful. B, the first piece of strapping. When this is on the child's foot must be in its normal shape. C, the second and third pieces of strapping. *Kindly contributed by John Biddulph.*

the strapping. This will stick it to his leg, and help to prevent sores.

Put pieces of cotton wool over his knee, behind his toes, and on his lateral malleolus. Put the first long piece of strapping (1, in Fig. 27-17) from under his heel up over the cotton wool outside his ankle. Bring it up outside his leg, and over the cotton wool on the top of his knee. Bend his ankle straight, as you put on this strapping. When this piece of strapping is on, his foot must be in its normal shape.

Put on a second piece of strapping (2) round his foot near his toes, up the outside of his leg and his knee.

Put a third piece (3) round his leg. This will keep the two long pieces in place.

Count all his toes and make sure they are pink and warm. If they are blue and cold, you have stopped the blood flowing. This is dangerous. Take the strapping off, and put it on looser. When his feet have been successfully strapped, raise his feet on a pillow as much as possible, especially for the first 5 days. Change the strapping twice a week for a month, then once a week until he is four months old. Follow him up as for a cast (see below).

PLASTER CASTS FOR TALIPES

Let him suck quietly at his mother's breast. There is no need for anaesthesia. Practise manipulating his foot before you apply the cast.

Apply a thin sheet of cotton wool padding from his upper thigh to his toes, with his knee bent to 90°. Apply the cast in two stages. Immobilize his bent knee in plaster first. With his knee immobile, you can then plaster his foot in the correct position more easily.

Use a narrow (2.5 cm) plaster bandage, to immobilize his bent knee. When this has set, extend it by applying a cast from his toes, leaving them visible. As this sets, push his foot into as much dorsiflexion, and eversion of his ankle, as he will tolerate.

As you do this, press behind his metatarsal heads rather than over them, or you will give him a rocker-bottom foot.

When the cast has set, add extra plaster as required, and smooth and trim its edges. Raise his feet on a pillow as much as possible, especially for the first 5 days.

Ask his mother to bring him back to have his cast changed, at first every week, and then every two weeks. If they live far away, every 4 weeks is acceptable. In the wet season, casts don't last long, so if necessary she should come more often. Before you see him, arrange to have his cast removed, under sedation if necessary, for example with chlorpromazine or promethazine elixir 2.5 mg/kg.

CAUTION ! (1) His toes must be visible. (2) Don't leave a deep thumb mark over his anterior tendons, or they will slough. (3) This is a circular cast, but it is not practicable to split it (70.3). Gangrene of the foot can occur, so warn his mother that if his foot becomes cold or blue, or he cries excessively, she must come back immediately. If she lives far away, she must soak off the plaster immediately.

FOLLOW UP. As soon as his deformity is fully corrected, hold it like that for at least a further 6 more months. If it is fully corrected, take off his cast when he starts walking—not before.

Follow him carefully until he is walking normally, and you are sure that his foot is normal and not relapsing. See him regularly until he is at least 5.

Refer him for surgery if: (1) his Achilles tendon is still too short at 3 months. (2) He shows any tendency to relapse. (3) His deformity is not fully corrected when he starts walking.

DIFFICULTIES WITH TALIPES

If at 3 months a child is NOT RESPONDING TO TREATMENT, he probably has the resistant type of talipes, so refer him for surgery as soon as you can. When he has been operated on, continue to apply casts or strapping until he is ready to start walking.

If his FOOT IS DORSIFLEXED (rare), it will usually be in valgus also (talipes calcaneovalgus). Make sure his hip is not dislocated at the same time. This deformity usually disappears spontaneously. If it is severe and persistent, manipulate and splint it.

If his FOREFOOT IS ADDUCTED only, you will probably be able to correct it by manipulation and splinting.

27.16 Ingrowing toe-nail

Ingrowing toe-nails are unusual in barefooted people. One of the hazards of a shoe is that it may press on the sides of a patient's big toe over a long period, and make the side of his nail grow into his soft tissues and cause pain, inflammation, and the discharge of pus from his nailfold. Carefully cutting away his nail may relieve his symptoms, but if this fails, more radical surgery is indicated. If his toe-nail is not deformed, you can excise a wedge of soft tissue (A, in Fig. 27-19); but if it is deformed, he will have a more comfortable toe if you remove his whole toe-nail, including its bed. Use a hexagonal incision, excise the distal part of his terminal phalanx, and reflect the plantar flap dorsally. The V-shaped parts of the hexagon at the sides of his toe will make the incision easier to close, make his nail bed easier to remove, and give his toe a better shape. A slightly short big toe is no disability.

INGROWING TOE-NAIL

INDICATIONS Non-operative measures have failed.

ANAESTHESIA Digital block (A 6.21).

A PLASTIC OPERATION ON THE SKIN FOLD **If the patient's nail is not deformed,** excise an elliptical piece of his skin fold and nail bed, as in A, Fig. 27-19. Suture the edges of the incision so as to draw the remains of the fold away from his nail.

RADICAL EXCISION OF THE NAIL BED **If his nail is deformed,** make a hexagonal incision round it, as in D, Fig. 27-19. When you cut the distal part, insert your scalpel obliquely in order to prevent the skin flap curling when you close the wound.

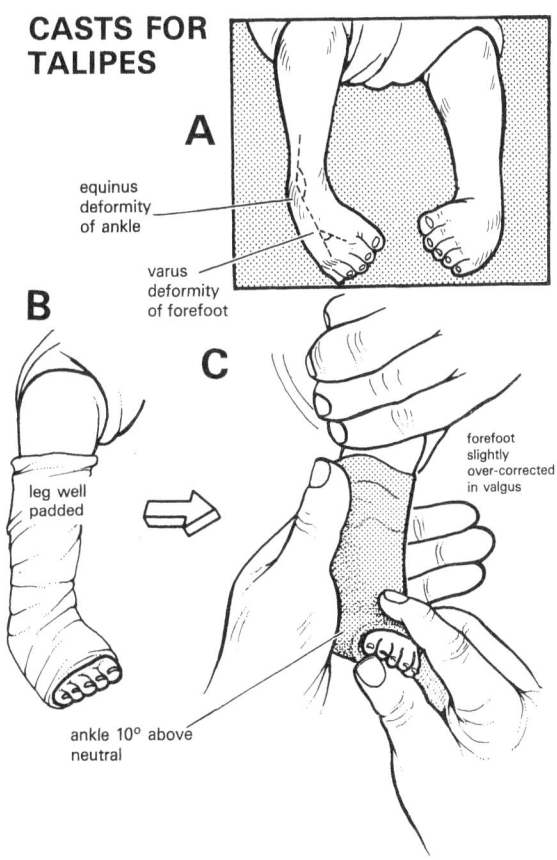

Fig. 27-18 CASTS FOR TALIPES. A, a child with the common type of talipes has an equinus and varus deformity of his ankle, and an adduction deformity of his forefoot. B, first pad his leg well. C, apply the cast. While it is still wet, hold his foot 10° above the neutral position, with his forefoot abducted. Overcorrect it a little, so that his foot is in slight valgus and is slightly everted. *Kindly contributed by John Stewart.*

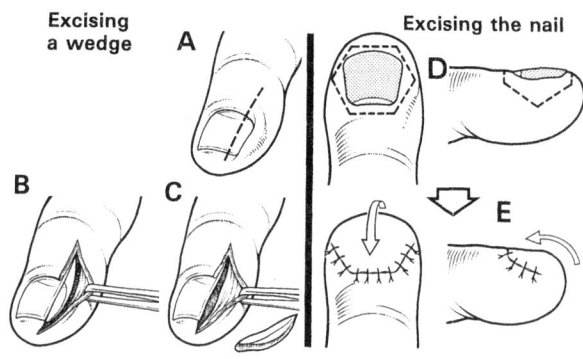

Fig. 27-19 INGROWING TOE-NAIL. If non-operative measures have failed, you can excise a wedge from the side of the patient's nail bed (A, B, and C), or you can excise his whole nail bed, shorten his distal phalanx, and turn the end of his toe over as a flap (D, and E).

Insert a periosteal elevator, or a narrow osteotome into the distal part of the incision, under his nail bed, so as to raise it from his terminal phalanx. Remove the entire contents of the hexagon, including the lateral roots of his nail bed, so as to leave the bone bare and clean. Dissect out and excise the terminal half of the phalanx. Raise the plantar flap of skin and subcutaneous tissue, so as to close the wound.

CAUTION ! The lateral roots of his nail bed may extend round the base of his phalanx, as far as its plantar surface. Be sure to excise them completely.

27.17 Other orthopaedic problems

There are many of these. Here are some of those you can help.

OTHER ORTHOPAEDIC PROBLEMS

PROBLEMS IN NEONATES

If a child is born with an EXTRA DIGIT (common and often bilateral), it usually consists of skin and subcutaneous tissue only. If so, tie cotton tightly round its base; it will soon necrose and fall off. If it is larger and contains bone, leave it for six months, when anaesthesia will be safer, and do a formal amputation (75.24).

If his FINGERS ARE FUSED TOGETHER, (syndactyly, fairly common), this is serious, especially if several of them are involved. Don't try to separate them with straight cuts through the webs, because a severe flexion contracture will follow. When he is 2 or 3 years old he needs multiple Z-plasties, an inverted 'V' procedure for the web, and skin grafts for the defects, so refer him. The importance of doing this depends on: (1) how many fingers are involved, and (2) which fingers are involved. A web between his index and middle finger is more serious than one between his ring and little finger.

If his TOES ARE FUSED TOGETHER, leave them.

If he is born with CONSTRICTIONS OF A LIMB OR LIMBS (rare), they are probably due to compression by bands in the wall of the amnion—AMNIOTIC BANDS. A scar is formed which leads to amputation *in utero* (as in E, Fig. 27-20), or to circumferential constriction. If nothing is done, his limb may become ischaemic, because the constricting tissue does not

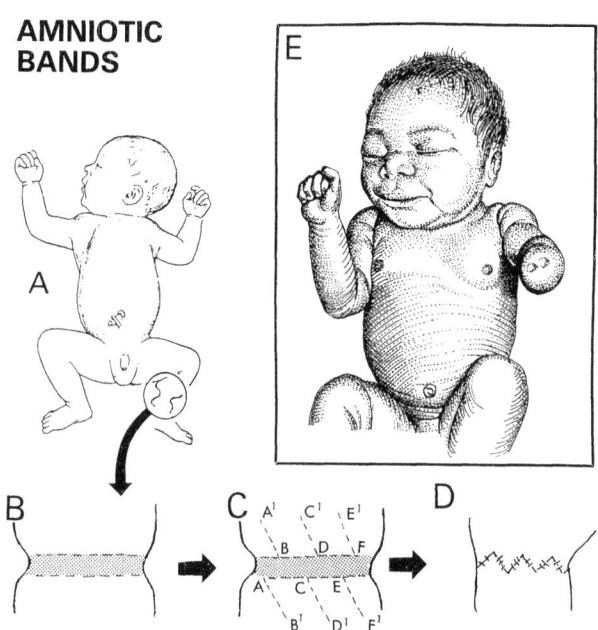

Fig. 27-20 AMNIOTIC BANDS sometimes amputate a limb in utero, as in the neonate E. If they merely cause a constriction (A), excise the constricted area (B), plan multiple small flaps (C) and do a Z-plasty (D).
Kindly contributed by Jim Thornton.

grow. If possible refer him; surgery is not urgent.

If you cannot refer him, operate under ketamine or general anaesthesia. Apply a tourniquet; but not above 150 mm or for <30 minutes.

Excise the lesion down to normal tissue (usually, only his skin and subcutaneous tissue are involved) as in B, Fig. 27-20. Sew up the defect with multiple Z-plasties. Bring A to A^1 and B to B^1, etc. See also G, I, or K, Fig. 58-20. If you join the skin edges side to side, the constriction is more likely to recur.

If he is born with his LEGS FOLDED IN 50° OF HYPEREXTENSION (genu recurvatum), flex them to 45° and hold them there with plaster backslabs for 3 weeks. He will probably grow normally without any disability. Occasionally, this is due to a true congenital contracture of his quadriceps which needs surgery.

PROBLEMS IN OLDER PATIENTS

If a patient, usually a child, develops a LESION WHICH LOOKS CYSTIC ON X-RAY, usually in the shaft of his humerus or femur, the possibilities include a benign bone cyst, fibrous dysplasia, benign osteoblastoma, non-osteogenic fibroma, enchondroma, Brodie's abscess, and tuberculosis. If it is benign, it is probably a BENIGN BONE CYST, or an area of fibrous dysplasia. Aim to avoid a pathological fracture. Refer him to have the cyst opened, scraped out, and filled with a cancellous bone graft. If his bone fractures across a small cyst, it will probably heal spontaneously.

If a patient has a BONY OUTGROWTH on a metaphysis, complete with a marrow cavity and a normal bony structure, he has an EXOSTOSIS (diaphyseal achalasia). He may have one or many. If possible, leave it until he has stopped growing, unless it is in an an awkward place, and is causing disability. Then chip it off with an osteotome. If you have to remove a prominence before growth has stopped, take care not to damage the epiphyseal line. If you damage it, a severe growth deformity may result.

28 Paediatric surgery

28.1 Surgery in children

There are two periods in paediatric surgery: (1) The surgery of the neonatal period, which is mostly concerned with those congenital malformations which need urgent treatment at birth. The few you can treat are described here, but you may feel that most of them are too difficult, and unrewarding, to come high in your list of priorities. (2) The surgery of the rest of childhood, most of which is more conveniently described in other chapters, particularly in those in Volume Two on trauma, which describes children's fractures (69.6) and burns (Chapter 58). Other important aspects of paediatric surgery are most kinds of sepsis, particularly abscesses (5.2), pyomyositis (7.1), and osteomyelitis (7.2); intestinal obstruction by Ascariasis (10.6) and intussusception (10.8); inguinal hernias (14.5), the urological problems of childhood (Chapter 23), poliomyelitis (Chapter 27), talipes (27.15), Burkitt's lymphoma (32.3) and other childhood tumours. Such surgical paediatric problems as do not more conveniently fit anywhere else are here. Many of them will probably have a low priority. If possible refer them.

The fluid requirements of children are described in Chapter 15 of *Primary Anaesthesia* and their anaesthetic requirements in Chapter 18. Very young children tolerate fluid and electrolyte loss badly: they don't have the normal postoperative sodium and water retention of adults, they cannot pass a concentrated urine, and they easily become dehydrated and hypoglycaemic.

PAEDIATRIC SURGERY

ANAESTHESIA. See A 18.1.

If you want to use local anaesthesia on a neonate, sedate him with 1 mg of diazepam: (1) You can dilute 1 ml of 2% lignocaine to 20 ml, and use this as the maximum dose. (2) You can infiltrate the line of the incision with 0.5% procaine, or 0.25% lignocaine. The maximum dose is about 5 ml—see Fig. A 5-1. Avoid adrenalin in the neonate.

General anaesthesia is better if your anaesthetist is good. Use Ayer's T-piece, awake intubation (A 13.6), followed by general anaesthesia and intramuscular suxamethonium, as in A 18.2.

If a neonate requires an urgent operation, operate at 24 hours, or as soon afterwards as possible. Lung function is poor if you

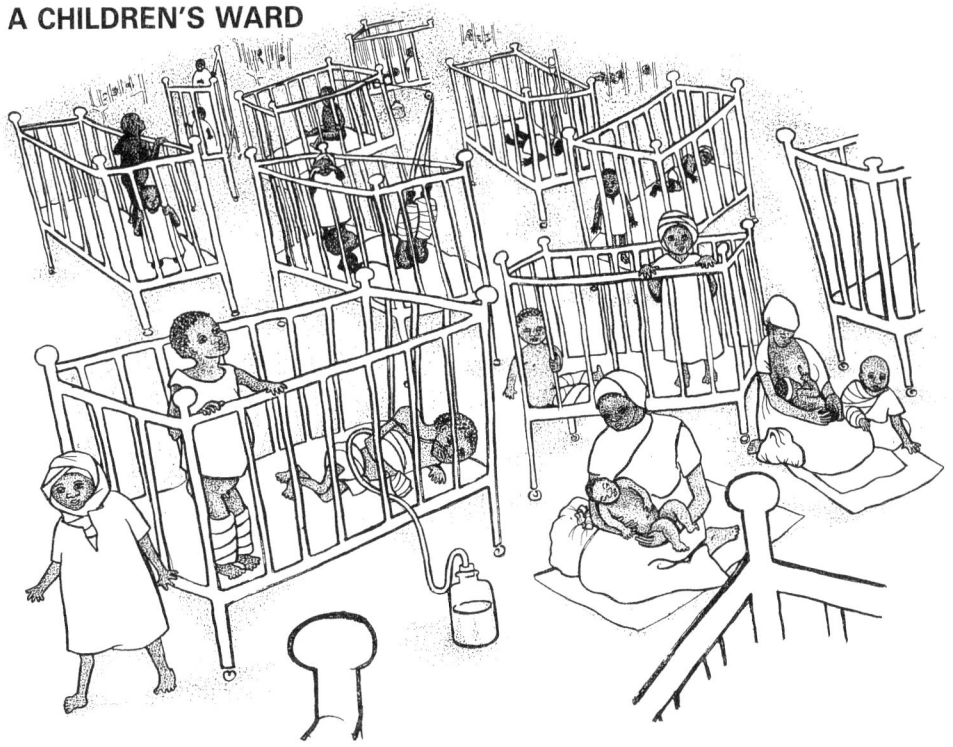

Fig. 28-1 A CHILDREN'S SURGICAL WARD as sketched by a student during her elective term in Africa. There are so many sick children that cots have to be shared. Mothers have been admitted so that they can breast-feed and comfort their children. *Kindly contributed by Celly Bacon.*

operate before 24 hours, when his lungs are not yet fully expanded. Weigh him and put up a drip. Give him vitamin K(,1) 1 mg, and start him on ampicillin 100 mg/kg/24 hours in 3 divided doses.

Make sure the theatre is warm. Place him on a well-padded cross made of two splints, and bandage his arms and legs to it. Cover the rest of his body except for his abdomen with cotton wool. Monitor and replace his blood loss with the greatest care (3-1). If HIV is common in your area, try to use blood from his father or mother. Weigh all blood-soaked swabs accurately, on a scale borrowed from the pharmacy if necessary. Replace blood ml for ml if more than 5 ml are lost. During the operation he will probably need 5 to 10 ml/kg/hour of 5% dextrose in Ringer's lactate.

INTRAVENOUS LINES. An infant requiring general anaesthesia should have a scalp vein drip, a cut-down (A 15.2), or a central venous line (A 19.2).

FLUIDS AND ELECTROLYTES. Replace *all a child's initial fluid deficit* (A 15.3) during the 3 to 6 hours that you are starving him, *before you start to operate*. Prescribe his postoperative fluids yourself, as in Figure A 15-4. Don't leave this to the nurses, and don't exceed 100 ml/kg in 24 hours.

For major surgery, where possible, pass an indwelling catheter. This is not appropriate under the age of 3 years; so, for a boy, use about 50 cm of plastic Paul's tube of suitable size; strap a plastic bag around the perineum of a girl. A child should pass 1 ml/kg/hour, or:
 0 to 1 year, 10 to 20 ml an hour.
 1 to 4 years, 20 to 24 ml an hour.
 4 to 7 years, 24 to 28 ml an hour.
 7 to 10 years, 28 to 30 ml an hour.
 10 to 12 years, 30 to 35 ml an hour.
 More than 12 years, 50 ml an hour.

POTASSIUM. If a child is not taking oral fluids by 24 hours, he needs a potassium supplement. Add 10 mmol to 500 ml of intravenous fluid (20 mmol/litre). Don't give him more than 10 mmol/hour or 3 mmol/kg/day. Or, use half-strength Darrow's solution, which contains 18 mmol/litre. Potassium replacement can be very dangerous in children, if it is handled incorrectly.

If he becomes drowsy postoperatively, and his gut becomes silent, suspect ileus, and give him potassium.

NUTRITION. Interrupt feeding as little as you can. Don't starve a child for more than 4 hours before the operation, and *get him feeding again as soon afterwards as you can*. Listen every 6 hours for the return of bowel sounds, and note whether he has passed faeces or flatus; these signs show that feeding can start. Bowel sounds alone are not so reliable in children, so some surgeons adjust the time of feeding to the nature of the operation, and decide if it is safe to feed a child by aspirating his stomach hourly, before each intake of feed.

Where possible, give him the fluid he needs as half-strength Darrow's solution in 5% dextrose (A 15-6). If he was not starved for more than 4 hours, and feeds are restarted soon, he is not going to be short of energy.

If you are able to give him 50% glucose through a central venous line (unlikely), use it to replace his energy deficit resulting from starvation. Reckon that, if he cannot feed orally for more than 3 days, he needs 1 to 2 g/kg/day. Test his urine and watch for glycosuria and an osmotic diuresis.

Alternatively, dilute 25 ml of 50% dextrose in 500 ml of half-strength Darrow's solution and increase the concentration gradually.

In working out the energy content of various fluids, use Figure 15-6 in *Primary Anaesthesia*, or remember that a litre of 10% dextrose contains 1700 kJ (400 cal). A child's daily postoperative energy needs are—
 A newborn child needs 190 to 210 kJ/kg (45 to 50 cal/kg).
 From 3 to 10 kg he needs 250 to 335 kJ/kg (60 to 80 cal/kg).
 From 10 to 15 kg he needs 190 to 270 kJ/kg (45 to 65 cal/kg).
 From 25 to 35 kg he needs 145 to 190 kJ/kg (35 to 45 cal/kg).
 From 35 to 60 kg he needs 125 to 145 kJ/kg (30 to 35 cal/kg).
CAUTION ! If he becomes drowsy, or unconscious or behaves strangely, suspect hypoglycaemia, or less commonly, water intoxication from lack of electrolytes relative to water.

If you are operating proximal to the upper jejunum, a jejunostomy at the time of the operation is a good way to feed him. See also 28.3.

28.2 Intestinal obstruction in the first few days of life

When a newborn baby vomits repeatedly he may have: (1) Some severe infection, such as septicaemia, originating in an infection of his umbilicus. (2) Intestinal obstruction, due to the conditions described in this chapter. (3) Meningitis. (4) Intracranial haemorrhage. The first three of these are often readily treatable—if you diagnose them early.

Most babies vomit a few times during the first few days of life, but bile-stained vomiting soon after birth almost always indicates gut obstruction. A childs's gut can be obstructed at the level of his oesophagus, his duodenum, his small gut, or, rarely, in his colon; but it is most often often obstructed at his anus. Anorectal malformations form a separate group, and present as the failure to pass meconium, combined with abdominal distension, rather than vomiting; so they are described separately in Section 28.4. Here we are concerned with obstruction higher up a child's gut.

Congenital obstruction of a child's small gut presents as bilious vomiting shortly after birth, and often (but not always) the failure to pass meconium. If the obstruction is proximal to the middle of his small gut, his abdomen does not distend, but if the obstruction is below this point, it does. The distension may be localized or generalized.

An obstructed gut is an emergency. Electrolyte loss and energy lack affect a baby sooner than an adult, so he needs urgent treatment, usually a laparotomy, within a few hours. If you are a careful, nimble operator, you *may* be able to save a few of these children with some of the most technically demanding methods described in this manual.

Hypertrophic pyloric stenosis presents later, as a previously healthy baby 2 to 3 weeks old who starts to vomit, and does not have diarrhoea. This form of obstruction is readily treatable and is described in Section 28.4. In Africa it is about as common as duodenal atresia.

NEONATAL GUT OBSTRUCTION

EXAMINATION. Assess the distension of the child's abdomen, look for visible peristalsis. Feel for the mass of a hypertrophic pylorus. Examine for visible and palpable coils of terminal ileum, that feel as if they might be filled with inspissated meconium (meconium ileus, not described here).

CAUTION ! Neither the passage of meconium during the first 3 days, nor the absence of distension, excludes obstruction.

X-RAYS. After 12 hours he will have swallowed enough air to assist diagnosis. If possible, take erect straight films before you start aspirating his stomach.

Don't use contrast media introduced from *above*, except as described in oesophageal atresia. It is particularly dangerous in obstructions lower than the midgut, and may make them worse.

CAUTION ! (1) The neonatal jejunum, ileum, and colon all have the same smooth outline, and normally contain a few fluid levels. (2) Don't use contrast media.

THE DIFFERENTIAL DIAGNOSIS OF NEONATAL GUT OBSTRUCTION

Suggesting septicaemia—a site of origin for the infection, such as an infected umbilicus; he is more ill than you would expect from obstruction alone; a positive blood culture.

Suggesting raised intracranial pressure —signs of cerebral irritation, a swollen fontanelle (enlargement of the head and papilloedema are late signs).

Suggesting some other cause of abdominal distension —a part of the abdomen which is dull to percussion. Causes include distension of the bladder in urethral obstruction, tumours, ascites, and congenital cystic kidneys, etc.

GENERAL MANAGEMENT. As soon as you suspect the diagnosis, pass a nasogastric tube, strap it to his face, see that it is aspirated at least every 30 minutes, and let it decompress into a bag—aspiration is a common cause of death. Put up

ATRESIA OF THE SMALL GUT

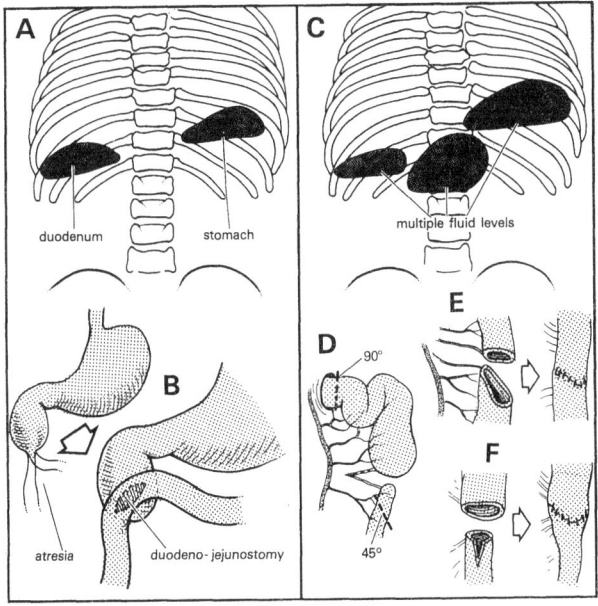

Fig. 28-2 TWO CAUSES OF NEONATAL GUT OBSTRUCTION. A, an X-ray showing the 'double bubble' of duodenal atresia. B, duodenal atresia relieved by a duodeno-jejunostomy. C, an X-ray showing the multiple fluid levels of jejuno-ileal atresia. D, jejuno-ileal atresia showing how the proximal dilated loop is resected at 90°, and the narrower distal one at 45°. E, a single layer end to end anastomosis. F, if, despite the 90°–45° manoeuvre, it is still difficult to anastomose the ends, you can make a nick in the antemesenteric border of the distal end. *Partly after Ravitch et al., 'Textbook of Paediatric Surgery'. Yearbook Medical, with kind permission.*

a drip. Keep him warm. If possible refer him—urgently. If not, consider operating as soon as possible (28.3).

SPECIFIC CONDITIONS OBSTRUCTING THE NEONATAL GUT

OESOPHAGEAL ATRESIA is often associated with a tracheo-oesophageal fistula. The proximal oesophageal pouch fills with saliva, so that he dribbles excessively. If he is given milk or water, he is likely to aspirate it into his trachea. He froths, coughs, and becomes cyanotic. If oesophageal atresia is common in your area, pass a nasogastric tube on all neonates. It has a higher incidence in underweight babies.

Confirm the diagnosis by passing a small (8 Ch in a full term baby and 5 Ch preterm one) firm (you don't want it to curl up) nasogastric tube with a radio-opaque line in it as far as it will go, and then taking AP and lateral chest X-rays. This will show his oesophagus ending in a blind pouch. Suck out the contrast medium immediately afterwards.

Refer him immediately with the tube reaching the blind end of his proximal oesophagus. Frequent aspiration is particularly important to prevent him aspirating saliva. Also, give him a small dose of atropine (A 2-4) to minimize secretion. Make sure that the staff who accompany him understand that they must continue to aspirate the tube, and suck out his pharynx during transport, to prevent fluid entering his lungs. If you cannot refer him, there is little you can do.

DUODENAL ATRESIA AND STENOSIS present as vomiting on the first day of life. His vomit is usually bile-stained, because the obstruction is usually below the ampulla of Vater. His upper abdomen is distended. If the obstruction is above the ampulla of Vater, there will be no bile in his vomit. The absence of dribbling saliva and cyanosis after feeding distinguishes duodenal from oesophageal atresia.

Erect AP and lateral films show a characteristic 'double bubble', with no air (or very little) in his small gut beyond. The bubble on the right is in his distended duodenal cap, and that on the left is in his stomach. He may also have Down's syndrome.

If you cannot refer him, you may possibly be able to do a duodeno-jejunostomy or a duodeno-duodenostomy (28.3).

JEJUNO-ILEAL ATRESIA OR STENOSIS may occur at any point in the small gut. Typically, it presents as bilious vomiting within 24 hours of birth—slightly later than with duodenal atresia, perhaps an hour after the first breast-feed; but it may be delayed for 2 or 3 days. If he has jejunal stenosis rather than atresia, it may be delayed for as long as 2 weeks. Obstruction in the upper jejunum is more common. If the obstruction is low, it presents more slowly, with distension more evident than vomiting. About half these children pass some meconium. Hydramnios is common in the mother.

Erect AP and lateral films show considerable gaseous distension, ending at the site of obstruction, usually with several fluid levels—one or two are normal. Unfortunately, by the time that several fluid levels are present obstruction is advanced.

If you cannot refer him you may be able to resect and anastomose his gut (28.3).

VOLVULUS OF THE SMALL GUT may present in older children, as in Section 10.9, with sudden abdominal pain, distension and shock, or it may present in the first week of life, usually very soon after birth, as an acute abdomen with bile-stained vomiting and abdominal distension. Volvulus usually involves the distal small gut and proximal colon, and is due to a congenital malrotation. If Ladd's bands (see below) are responsible, surgery is simple, because there no need to anastomose gut. Strangulation obstruction develops rapidly.

28.3 Operating for a neonatal acute abdomen

Anastomosing neonatal gut is no easy task, but if you are surgically nimble, are well-experienced with adult gut, and have the right sutures and devoted nurses, you may succeed. You have one advantage—the contents of a neonate's gut are sterile, so that contamination of his abdominal cavity is less of a hazard than it is later on. Anaesthesia is a major problem, but you can use local anaesthesia, although the absence of relaxation does make the operation more difficult. Whatever the difficulties, you may be sure that if you cannot refer him, and don't operate, he will surely die.

An abdominal wound easily breaks down in an infant. It is least likely to do so if you make a transverse muscle-cutting incision. A muscle splitting paramedian incision is next best for healing, and gives good exposure. A child grows, so suture his gut and his wound with interrupted sutures to allow him to do so. Suture his fascia meticulously, with good bites on each side.

You will find that that distal end of an obstructed neonatal gut is so collapsed, and small, that an end-to-end anastomosis is difficult. So make an end-to-side or a side-to-side one. The disadvantage of doing this is that, later, the cul-de-sac that you make may become a refuge for bacteria, and cause the malabsorption syndrome, especially in the small gut. These anastomoses can however be revised later, if necessary.

NEONATAL ACUTE ABDOMENS

ANAESTHESIA AND PREPARATION. See Section 28.1. If you cannot refer a child, operate at 24 hours, or as soon afterwards as possible.

INCISION. Make a right muscle-splitting paramedian, or supraumbilical transverse incision. Examine his whole gut, because there may be more than one obstruction.

DUODENAL ATRESIA takes various forms, including one in which the pancreas is all round the duodenum (annular pancreas, very rare). Anastomose the first part of his duodenum to the first loop of his jejunum behind his colon. If this is difficult, make the anastomosis in front of his colon. Do a side-to-side anastomosis in one 'all coats' layer, or in two layers with interrupted sutures. One of the difficulties is that you cannot see his pancreatic or bile ducts, and if you injure them he will certainly die. Bring up a loop of his proximal jejunum through his gastrocolic omentum, and anastomose it to his distended duodenum. Anastomosing collapsed jejunum is difficult.

JEJUNAL ATRESIA. You may find a variety of lesions, perhaps combined with malrotation, volvulus, meconium ileus, and meconium peritonitis (uncommon). Most often, there is a short segment, or segments, of atresia, or marked stenosis.

Anastomose his dilated jejunum above the stenosed segment to his collapsed jejunum below it. They will be very different in size, so do a side-to-side anastomosis. Unfortunately, a cul-de-sac will form, which will tend to grow.

Alternatively, if there is enough gut, resect the proximal loop to a point where it is about 1 to 1.5 cm in diameter. Cut it off at at 90°, and the distal one at 45°. If there is still a difference in size, make a short incision in the antemesenteric border of the distal segment, as in F, Fig. 28-2.

VOLVULUS OF THE MIDGUT. When you open his abdomen, you see distended coils of small gut, which may be cyanotic and congested, and obscure his right colon. Deliver his small gut to the surface, and protect it with warm moist packs. Examine the base of his mesentery to see which way it has twisted (usually anticlockwise). Untwist it, and hope that its normal colour will return. If it is viable, lay it back in place. If it is not viable, resect the gangrenous part, and anastomose viable gut. If you have to resect much gut, his outlook is poor. Before you close his abdomen make sure that: (1) there is no band of tissue obstructing his duodenum (band of Ladd, see below), and (2) his duodenum is patent. Do this by manipulating his stomach contents through into his small gut.

OBSTRUCTION BY BANDS (arrested rotation). If you find that his duodenum is obstructed by a band of tissue (band of Ladd) running from his caecum or ascending colon towards the right of his abdomen, this is the result of arrested rotation of his gut. These bands are often present but cause no problem.

If a band does appear to be causing obstruction, divide it. Divide the attachment of the band to his parietal peritoneum on the right side of the second part of his duodenum. Displace the right half of his colon to the left. If you see a second band extending from the midline to the start of his jejunum, divide that also. There may be a third band running from his ileum to his ascending colon. His caecum will now be free; leave it on the left side of his abdomen, and don't try to put it back it in its normal place.

OBSTRUCTION BY A REMNANT OF MECKEL'S DIVERTICULUM. Sometimes a cord of tissue runs from his ileum to his umbilicus, causing his gut to strangulate round it (28-4). If so, check its viability, resect it if it is strangulated, and remove the 'cord'.

ANASTOMOSING AN INFANT'S GUT see also Section 9.3

Use the finest haemostats, and handle his gut with the greatest care. Hold it with stay sutures, and don't use clamps—its contents are sterile, so contamination is unimportant. Tailor its ends so that their sizes are a little more equal (see above). If you cannot do this, make a side to side anastomosis. Use a catheter to suck the proximal end clear of any inspissated meconium that would otherwise block the anastomosis. Make a single layer of instrument-tied interrupted sutures, using atraumatic 3/0 chromic catgut, or, better, 4/0 polyglycolic acid ('Dexon'), or 5/0 silk. If you have none of these sutures, don't operate. In most situations there is no room for a second layer.

Gently invert the posterior wall of his gut, as you insert the first sutures. If you can do this satisfactorily, inverting the anterior wall should not be difficult. As you go round the corner from the posterior wall of the anastomosis, to the anterior one, continue to invert the sutures.

POSTOPERATIVELY, see also Section 28.1. Give him 80 to 100 ml/kg/day of fluid. Either give him 0.18% saline in 5% dextrose to which you have added 2 mmol/kg/day of potassium (A 15.1). Or, give him half-strength Darrow's solution in 2.5% dextrose, which will contain the necessary potassium. Replace clear gastric losses with 0.45% saline in 5% dextrose. Replace greenish gastric aspirate with 5% dextrose in Ringer's lactate.

Start oral feeding as soon as possible—when signs of bowel function return. Start with 5 ml of expressed breast milk 2-hourly, and increase this gradually as he tolerates it. This should be possible on the 2nd or 3rd day. Either give it by nasogastric tube, or better, through a tube passed down his gut beyond the anastomosis (making an enterostomy beyond the anastomosis is difficult, because his gut is so small).

DIFFICULTIES WITH NEONATAL GUT OBSTRUCTION

If you find part of his TERMINAL ILEUM IS FILLED WITH THICK FLUID, and that distal to this is some putty-like material, and distal to that again, some meconium pellets just above his caecum, he has meconium ileus (rare). Emptying his gut operatively is difficult, and is not sufficiently rewarding to be described here.

If you find that his SMALL GUT IS DUPLICATED, anastomose the parallel parts to one another at either end.

If you find extensive GANGRENOUS GUT, he has: (1) a volvulus, or (2) twisting round a band or cord (see above), or (3) neonatal necrotizing enterocolitis (rare). Exteriorize the gangrenous part, and close his abdomen. His chances are poor.

28.4 Hypertrophic pyloric stenosis

Hypertrophic pyloric stenosis presents as forceful bile-free vomiting, with constipation rather than diarrhoea, in a baby about three weeks old—the range is 5 days to 5 months. It is more common in boys than in girls, and in the eldest child. To begin with he vomits one or two of his feeds each day, but as the obstruction gets worse, his vomiting becomes more constant and more projectile. Occasionally, he vomits brownish 'coffee grounds'. If he is not treated, he becomes dehydrated, alkalotic, hypochloraemic, hypokalaemic, *and constipated;* he loses weight, and becomes malnourished. Pyloric stenosis is not diagnosed as it should be, and is too often thought to be yet another case of 'gastroenteritis'. But he does *not have diarrhoea!* Misdiagnosis is a tragedy, because surgery is not too difficult and is very effective.

You should be able to feel a child's hypertrophied pylorus as a smooth olive-shaped swelling to the right of the midline in his upper abdomen. If he cries you certainly won't be able to feel it, so sit him on his mother's lap, and feel for it while she feeds him from the breast. If you have difficulty, return a few minutes later, while she is still feeding him. Sit opposite her, look for waves of gastric peristalsis passing from his left upper quadrant towards the right. As they do so, his pyloric swelling will harden under your finger. Feel for the lump again. If you are persistent, you should be able to feel it in all cases—it establishes the diagnosis.

RAMSTEDT'S OPERATION

RESUSCITATION. You can correct minor degrees of dehydration with oral fluids, but if a child becomes severely dehydrated and needs intravenous fluids, give him 20 ml/hour of half-strength Darrow's solution, and reduce this to 10 ml/hour when he is passing urine. Don't give him >150-180 ml/kg/24 hours. Provided he is not severely dehydrated, he should be ready for operation in 4 to 6 hours. Most children need intravenous fluids for about 4 hours preoperatively. He will usually stop vomiting as soon as his stomach is empty. If not, aspirate it through a nasogastric tube.

Alternatively, depending on what fluids you have, you may find this regime useful:

If he is only minimally dehydrated, with no significant electrolyte disturbance, give him 60 ml of Ringer's lactate orally. When his renal function is satisfactory, add 3 mmol of potassium chloride to each feed.

If he is moderately dehydrated, Fgive him the first half of the calculated replacement intravenously as 5% dextrose in 0.45% saline, followed by 5% dextrose in 0.3% saline. As soon as he has passed urine, add 20 to 40 mmol/l of potassium to his intravenous fluid, depending on how ill he is.

If he is severely dehydrated, give him part of his initial replacement intravenously as 5% dextrose in 0.45% saline, partly as 0.9% saline, and partly as 5% dextrose in 0.3% saline. Add potassium as above.

ANAESTHESIA. (1) Ketamine (A 8.5). (2) Local anaesthesia. (3) Awake intubation and general anaesthesia. Sedate him preoperatively with chloral hydrate 300 mg, and place him on a Dennis Browne crucifix, with his limbs bandaged to prevent excessive movement. He will not be able to clear his throat,

RAMSTEDT'S OPERATION

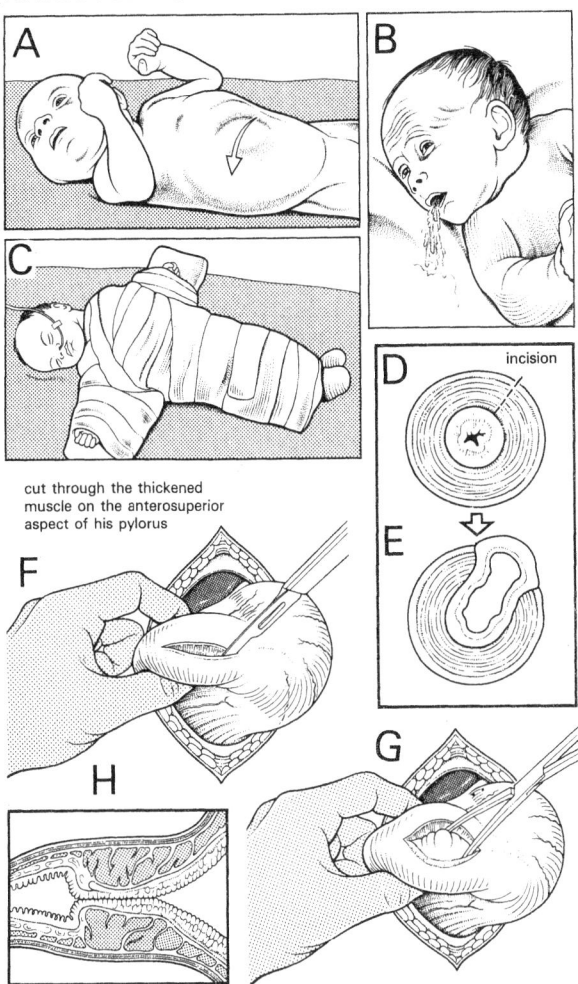

Fig. 28-3 RAMSTEDT'S OPERATION for hypertrophic pyloric stenosis. A, waves of visible peristalsis passing across the abdomen. B, the wrinkled forehead and pitiable expression of a child with pyloric stenosis. C, the child anaesthetized in a Dennis Browne crucifix; use this for all neonatal operations. Note the nasogastric tube. Cover his chest loosely and expose his abdomen (not as shown). D, the thickened muscle of the pylorus, showing the site of the incision. E, intact mucosa pouting out of the incision. F, incising the pylorus. G, opening the incision in the muscle to reveal the mucosa. H, a longitudinal section of the pylorus. *Partly after Harlow W, 'An Atlas of Surgery', (1958) Figs. 50 and 51, Heinemann Medical, with Kind permission.*

so suck out his pharynx frequently. Aspirate his stomach just before you anaesthetize him, and leave the tube down.

The maximum dose of 2% lignocaine you can use is 1 ml, so dilute this in 20 ml of saline and use it to infiltrate his skin and rectus sheath.

INCISION. Open his abdomen through a transverse incision, centered over the swelling to the right of the midline; it is usually half way between his xiphisternum and his umbilicus. Divide all his tissues in the line of the incision. Open his peritoneum.

Make the incision long enough (about 2.5 cm) to deliver the swelling into the wound. It may be quite difficult to find at first, because it may lie deep, partly covered by his transverse colon. Feel it with your finger. A small retractor may help to deliver it into the wound—it is always mobile. Hold the swelling between the thumb and index finger of your left hand. Keep your left middle finger against the distal extremity of his swollen pyloric muscle. Turn this so as to expose its antero-superior border.

Cut through the circular muscle along the length of his pylorus. *Start just proximal to the white line* (the junction of his pylorus and duodenum); at this point (the distal end of the swelling) the wall of his gut becomes thin suddenly. Extend the incision along the whole length of his thickened pylorus (the proximal end is less clear, because his stomach wall is also thickened). Spread its circular muscle, without harming the submucosa, which should bulge out of the incision. You are less likely to harm this, if you use the tip of a haemostat to separate the deeper muscle fibres.

Still using the tip of the haemostat, separate the fibres distally on the duodenal side, under the white line, so as to divide all circular fibres without perforating his duodenal mucosa. As you do this, continue to mark and protect his duodenum with the middle finger of your left hand.

CAUTION ! (1) Don't cut the white line at the site of the pyloric vein, or you may open his duodenum. (2) Don't sew up the muscle incision.

If, by mistake, you open his duodenal mucosa, close it with a few 4/0 atraumatic sutures, and suture omentum over the hole to fill the defect made by incising the muscle layer.

If a vessel bleeds, press with gauze for a few minutes; if this fails transfix it with 4/0 multifilament.

Return his stomach to his abdomen, and place omentum over the operation site. Close his peritoneum and posterior rectus sheath with continuous 3/0 chromic catgut. Close his anterior rectus sheath with interrupted 4/0 monofilament. Bring the skin edges together with fine monofilament.

POSTOPERATIVELY, if you succeeded in not perforating his duodenal mucosa, remove the nasogastric tube as he recovers from the anaesthetic. If you perforated it, leave the tube down for 24 to 48 hours, before you remove it and start feeding him. If he is alert and sucks well, start breast-feeding at 6 hours.

If he vomits frequently during the first 24 hours, wash out his stomach to remove the excess mucus.

If he is taking insufficient fluid by mouth to maintain an intake of 100 ml/kg/day, give him half-strength Darrow's solution.

If he continues to vomit after 24 hours, you may not have divided his pylorus adequately. If necessary, operate again. Wait until 14 days, if you can; but it is better to operate earlier than to let him get worse.

28.5 Disorders of the omphalo-mesenteric duct (Meckel's diverticulum)

In fetal life the intestinal tract and the yolk sac are joined by the omphalo-mesenteric or vitelline duct. Remnants of this may persist and present as: (1) A persistent discharge from the umbilicus which is occasionally faecal. (2) Gastro-intestinal bleeding from ectopic gastric mucosa in Meckel's diverticulum. (3) Gut obstruction caused by gut twisting around a persistent vitelline duct, as described in Section 28.3. You may occasionally have to resect and anastomose gut in connection with any of these three, or, rarely, with the other abnormalities in Fig. 28-4.

28.6 Anorectal malformations

Anorectal malformations are not uncommon. A child who has the misfortune to be born with one presents soon after birth with abdominal distension and the failure to pass meconium. Some lesions are incomplete, and present later with difficulty passing faeces, small faeces, or distension.

There are many kinds of lesion, but what matters most is whether a child's rectum ends above or below his puborectalis sling. If his rectum extends below it (infralevator lesions), you can make him an anus, or dilate a stenosed one without difficulty. But if his rectum ends above this sling (supralevator lesions), you will have to make a temporary colostomy, and refer him later for his sigmoid colon to be pulled through to his perineum. This is difficult, but continence can be achieved in most cases.

A child's anus or rectum may fail to develop entirely (agenesis), they may partly fail to develop (atresia), or his rectum or anus may be narrowed (stenosis). Agenesis (but not the other lesions)

ABNORMALITIES OF THE OMPHALO-MESENTRIC DUCT

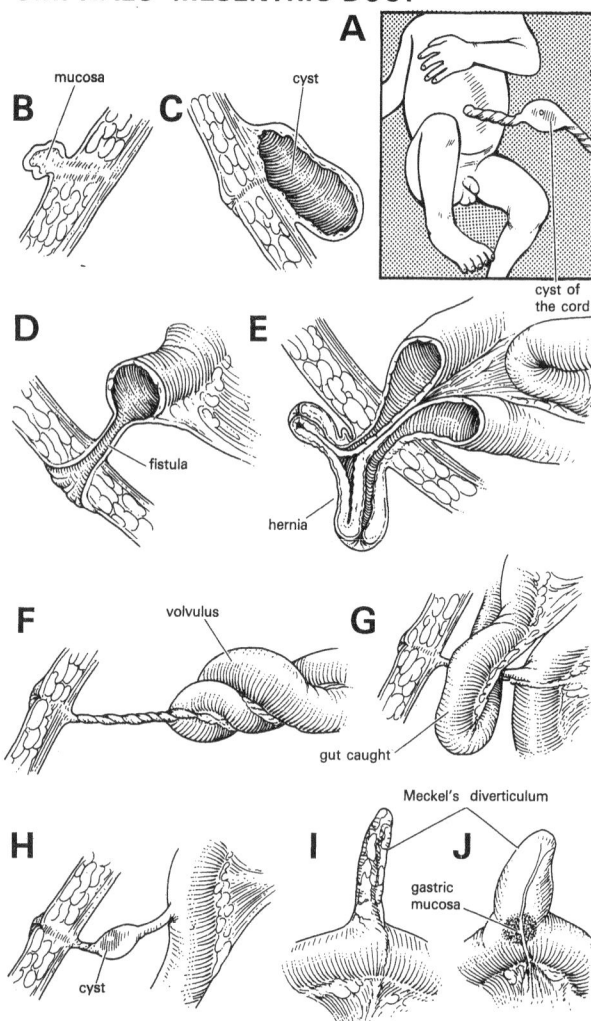

ANORECTAL MALFORMATIONS

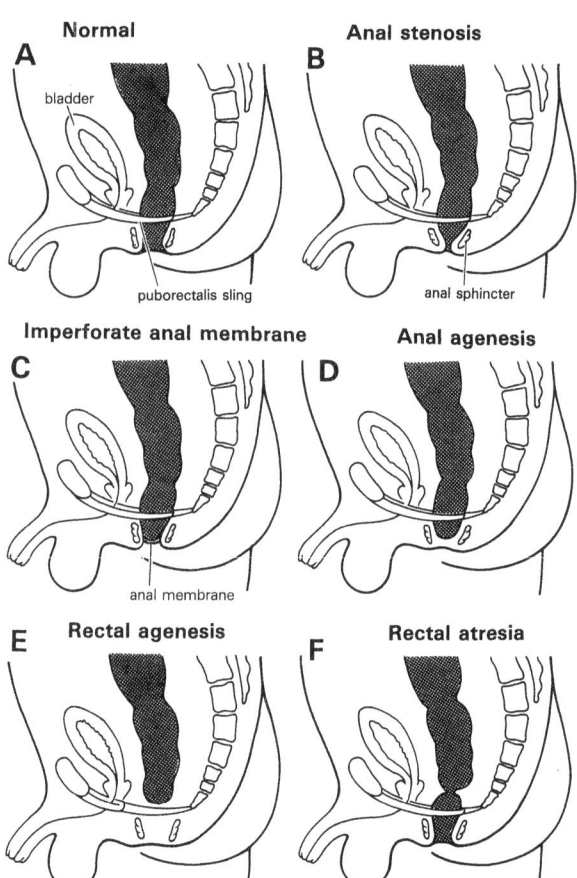

Fig 28-5 ANORECTAL MALFORMATIONS. Low lesions go below the puborectalis sling, high ones remain above it. You should be able to treat the low ones without too much difficulty. You will have to do a colostomy and refer the high ones. *Adapted from Ravitch et al., 'Paediatric Surgery', Fig. 98-2. Yearbook Medical, with kind permission.*

Fig. 28-4 ABNORMALITIES OF THE OMPHALO-MESENTERIC DUCT, are mostly rare. A, a harmless cyst in the cord. B, an umbilicus covered with red intestinal mucosa, which may dip down into the abdominal wall. Don't confuse this with an umbilical granuloma, which is much more common. C, a mucosa-lined cyst communicating with the skin. D, a communication between the ileum and the umbilicus. E, gut may herniate through this communication. F, the duct may persist as a cord around which a volvulus may form (28.3). G, a loop of gut may be caught across this cord. H, the duct may form a cyst. I, the remains of the duct may persist as Meckel's diverticulum, and become inflamed. J, some gastric mucosa in the duct may ulcerate and bleed. *Adapted from Ravitch et. al., 'Paediatric Surgery'. Fig. 88-17, Yearbook Medical, with kind permission.*

may be combined with fistulae between the rectum, and the urinary, or genital tracts, of either sex. These variables combine to produce a complex series of lesions. Some fistulae are useful, because you may be able to dilate them to make an anus. About 75% of cases are low lesions with fistulae.

LOW ANORECTAL LESIONS

Anal stenosis in boys or girls (rare).
Imperforate anal membrane (3%) in boys and girls.
Low rectal (anal) agenesis without a fistula. If there is a fistula (75%), it is rectoperineal or rectourethral in a boy. In a girl it is rectoperineal, rectovaginal, or rectovulvar.

HIGH ANORECTAL LESIONS

High rectal agenesis in boys or girls without a fistula (7%). If there is a fistula (15%), it is rectourethral or rectovesical in a boy. In a girl it is rectovaginal or rectocloacal.
Rectal atresia in boys and girls (rare and not discussed further). There is a normal looking anus in the normal place, low

gut obstruction (no meconium, abdominal distension and vomiting late). A contrast enema is safter than probing.

You should be able to diagnose which kind of lesion a child has from the clinical signs and a simple X-ray (28-6). The risk in trying to repair an anorectal lesion is that, if the lesion is higher than you expect, you may so damage his rectal anatomy that even an expert cannot repair it later. If you find you are operating below skin level, *stop*, do a colostomy, and refer the child for repair later. *Don't divide any muscle.* If you are in any doubt, a colostomy would be wiser, even though you may occasionally do one unnecessarily. *The penalty for failure is incontinence.* Make a transverse colostomy rather than a sigmoid one, because it will make the secondary procedure easier, although it will cause more fluid loss.

ANORECTAL MALFORMATIONS

If possible, refer these children, unless they need dilatation only.

EXAMINATION. Ask your midwives to examine the anuses of all children. Ask them to refer: (1) any child with an abnormal anus, (2) any child who passes no faeces for 12 hours, and whose abdomen distends. Examine him, and if necessary, pass a rectal thermometer or a stiff catheter. If he has no anus, an opening must be provided before he distends. Look for other congenital abnormalities.

If there is a mass of irregular epithelium where the anus should be, the diagnosis is almost certainly anal stenosis. Probe it and look for even a trace of meconium to confirm the presence of an anus.

If the anal skin is smooth, there must be some other kind of lesion, other than stenosis.

If there is a thin veil of epithelium overlying the anal orifice,

surrounded by normal puckering and rugae, there is an imperforate anal membrane (only 3%).

If the anus looks normal, until you put a probe into it, when you find that the rectum is almost or completely blocked, the diagnosis is rectal atresia. You may find a very small hole which you can dilate.

LOOK FOR FISTULAE IN ANORECTAL MALFORMATIONS

If a boy has low rectal (anal) agenesis, look for: (1) meconium in his urine. If you don't find it, he has probably not got a fistula. (2) Examine his perineum, and his perineal raphe along his scrotum. If you see any sign of a black head of meconium, he probably has a fistula leading to a low lesion.

If a girl has low rectal (anal) agenesis, examine her perineum and vulva for fistulae. If you find a suspicious opening, probe it gently—it may extend downwards and backwards under the skin of her perineal body, and confirm that she has a low lesion.

If a boy has high rectal agenesis, examine his urine for meconium.

If a girl has high rectal agenesis, look for a fistula on the posterior wall of her vagina, below her introitus. It may connect with a cloaca where her urinary tract, vagina, and rectum come together into a common channel.

X-RAYS FOR ANORECTAL MALFORMATIONS

Wait until 12 to 16 hours after birth, when the gas the child has swallowed has reached the blind lower end of his gut.

Turn him upside down so that his anus is uppermost. Flex his knees. Strap a *small* piece of metal such as the metal adaptor of a needle flat on the skin where his anus should be.

Take a lateral film. The bubble of gas in his gut will be uppermost. The distance between it and the metal will show you how much tissue there is between the bottom of his gut and his skin.

Interpret the film in two ways: (1) If the gas bubble is less than 2 cm from his anus, he has a low lesion. If it is more than 2 cm from his skin, he probably has a high one. (2) Draw a line between the posterior part of his pubis, and the lowest segment of his sacrum. If any blind dilated bowel has gone beyond this line, he has a low lesion. If it remains above this line, his lesion is high.

CAUTION! (1) X-rays are useful but not completely reliable. There may not have been enough gas in his gut, or he may have a fistula higher up. (2) He may have a vesicorectal fistula and a fluid level in his bladder (uncommon). Exclude this by taking a supine lateral film.

OPENING A LOW LESION

If a child has a low lesion, operate early, especially in a boy. His obstructed gut is going to distend, so, as soon as he has swallowed enough air to help make the X-ray diagnosis, pass a nasogastric tube. Keep him hydrated and give him vitamin K.

ANAESTHESIA. (1) Ketamine (A 8.5). (2) Chloral hydrate and local infiltration anaesthesia. (3) Awake tracheal intubation and general anaesthesia.

ASPIRATION. Immediately before you operate, aspirate his perineum with a syringe and large-bore needle. This will tell you the exact level of his anal pouch, while he is relaxed and anaesthetized.

CAUTION ! If you are in doubt, do a colostomy.

ANAL STENOSIS (boys and girls). If the opening is very small, use a filiform urethral catheter with a metal follower or the smallest Hegar dilator. Continue to dilate the child about every 2 weeks with your little finger. Later, this can be done by a nurse or the child's mother.

IMPERFORATE ANAL MEMBRANE (boys and girls). Incise the epithelial covering of the anus, and dilate it with a Hegar dilator. Continue to dilate it as above.

LOW RECTAL (anal) AGENESIS WITHOUT A FISTULA. **Make a cross-shaped incision so as to mobilize four separate flaps, as in A, Fig. 28-7.** Contributors then differ. One says: *don't divide any muscle;* if you don't immediately find the rectum under the skin, stop, make a colostomy and refer.

Another says: as soon as you have found the external sphincter, divide it at 12 o'clock, and dissect towards the blind end of the gut, up to 2 cm from the skin. Mobilize the blind gut for a few more centimetres, so that you can relax it, and bring it down to the skin within the cut external sphincter. Cut four triangular flaps, so that they interdigitate with the skin flaps. Join them with interrupted stitches of fine catgut (B, and C). *Don't make the anastomosis under tension, if it is tight, you have not mobilized gut enough.*

LOW RECTAL (anal) AGENESIS WITH A FISTULA IN A GIRL. This is the commonest anorectal lesion in a girl. Her sphincter muscles pass round the fistula. You can do two things: (1) is much the best; only do (2) if you cannot do (1).

(1) You can dilate her fistula until it makes an adequate anus. Start by using a rectal thermometer, and later a uterine sound.

IMPERFORATE ANUS

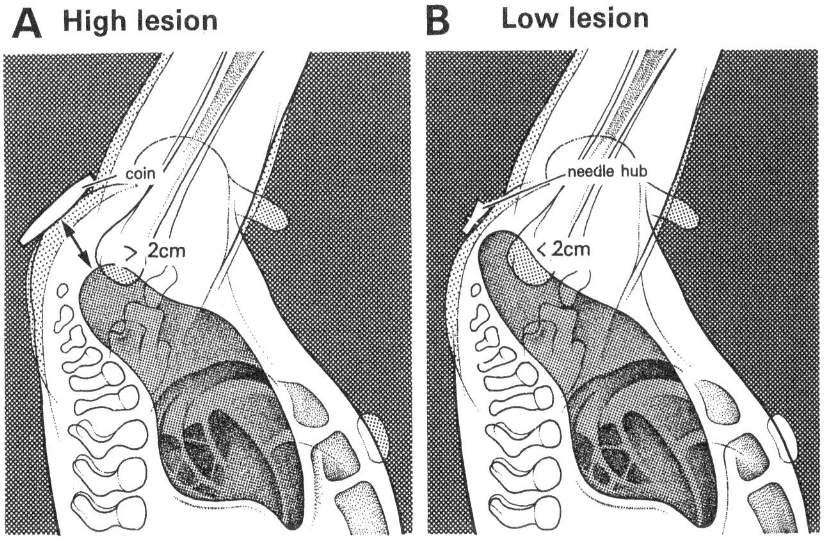

A High lesion   **B** Low lesion

Fig. 28-6 AN 'IMPERFORATE ANUS' showing high and low rectal lesions. The child has been turned upside down and a piece of metal has been placed over his anus. A, shows a high lesion with the gas bubble in his rectum, more than 2 cm from a coin which has been placed over his anus. B, is a low lesion in which the metal hub of a needle has been used, and is less than 2 cm from the gas bubble. The hub of a needle is better than a coin because it fits into the anal cleft.

LOW RECTAL AGENESIS WITHOUT A FISTULA

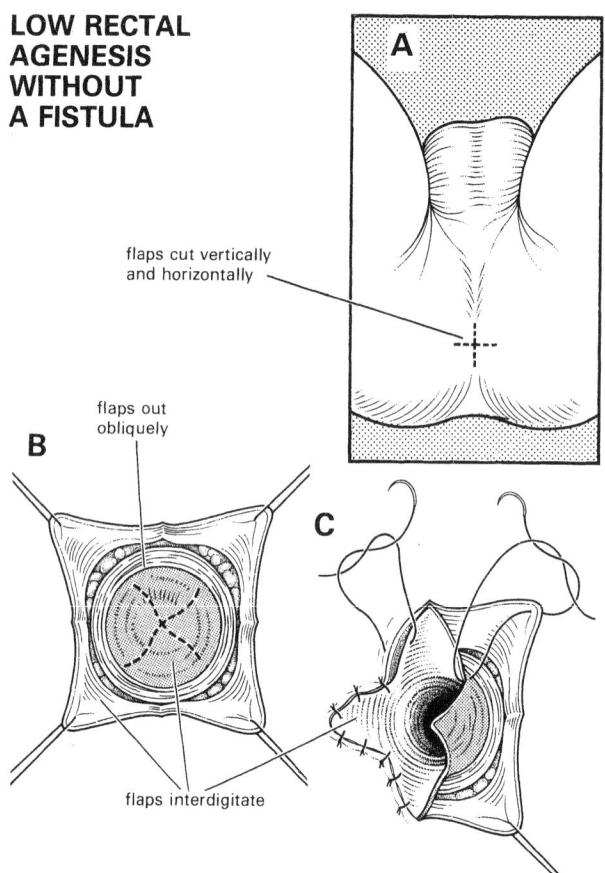

Fig. 28-7 LOW RECTAL AGENESIS WITHOUT A FISTULA. A, make a cross-shaped incision over the child's external sphincter. B, reflect 4 skin flaps, and then cut interdigitating flaps from his anal membrane. C, close these so that they interdigitate with one another. *Adapted from Ravitch et al., 'Paediatric Surgery', Fig 98-3. Yearbook Medical, with kind permission.*

ANAL AGENESIS WITH A FISTULA

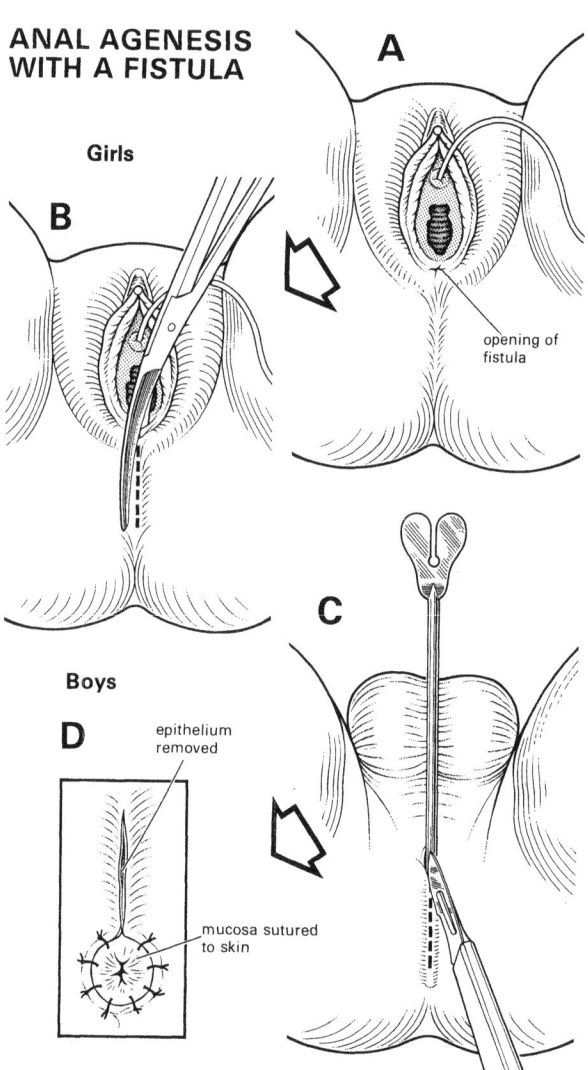

Fig. 28-8 ANAL AGENESIS WITH A FISTULA. A, a girl, showing the fistula opening close to her introitus. B, the cutback operation; note that the scissors point directly backwards, and are superficial. C, a fistula in a boy is being incised on a grooved director. D, the epithelium of the track has been removed, and his anal mucosa has been stitched to his skin. *Adapted from Ravitch et al., 'Paediatric Surgery', Fig. 98-4. Yearbook Medical, with kind permission.*

Then at 6 months, refer her to have her anus brought back to its proper place in her perineum. If this is impractical, it is not a disaster, but it will mean that she will always defecate from her fourchette. This is much less of a disability than it might seem, because it is compatible with a normal sex life, and her husband may be quite unaware of it!

(2) You can do a cutback operation, as in B, Fig. 28-8, but only if, before you cut, your scissors point *directly backwards and are superficial.* If they point in any other direction, and especially if they point deeply, she probably has a high lesion, not a low one, and she may subsequently become incontinent.

After you have cut, mobilize the posterior 180° of the cut, so as to bring the apex of the incision comfortably down to her skin. Join her gut and her skin with interrupted sutures.

LOW RECTAL (anal) AGENESIS WITH A FISTULA IN A BOY. His fistula is usually perineal, and his lesion is low. Unroof the fistulous track, as in C, Fig. 28-8. This will lead back to a normal anorectum, which you can open and dilate (D). Stitch his rectal mucosa to his skin. Finally, remove the mucous membrane lining the fistula.

POSTOPERATIVE CARE (all low lesions). Follow the child up carefully. The anus will probably need dilating at least once a week for a month or more. Warn the child's mother that toilet training will be delayed.

TRANSVERSE COLOSTOMY FOR HIGH ANORECTAL MALFORMATIONS

PREPARATION. Pass a nasogastric tube and suck out the child's stomach frequently. Check his temperature, and put him in a warm bath if it is low. Put him on an electric blanket on the operating table, and bandage his arms and legs in cotton wool to conserve heat.

ANAESTHESIA. (1) Ketamine (A 8.5). (2) Give him a general anaesthetic, as in section 28.3. (3) Local anaesthesia as for the other operations described here.

INCISION. Make a short transverse incision in his right hypochondrium (see Section 9.5). Identify his transverse colon, from its connection by a short omentum to the greater curvature of his stomach.

CAUTION! Don't deliver his sigmoid colon.

Deliver his transverse colon through the wound, and pass a plastic rod under it through a hole in its mesentery, to make sure it remains outside his abdomen. Connect its ends with a rubber tube. Place some catgut sutures between the muscle of his gut and his abdominal wall.

Open the exteriorized loop immediately with a longitudinal incision. Suck out the contents of the proximal loop to decompress his abdomen. Refer him early if fluid loss from his colon is serious; otherwise refer him for definitive repair at 6 months.

DIFFICULTIES WITH ANORECTAL MALFORMATIONS

If you are NOT SURE WHAT TO DO, remember that a fistula is a favourable lesion because there is already an opening between the gut and the outside. If it is narrow, dilate it. If it is wide, there is no need for an urgent colostomy unless: (1) he has signs of intestinal obstruction, or (2) his urinary tract is involved. If so, a colostomy is urgent.

If his ANAL MUCOSA EVERTS after you have operated on his imperforate anus, there is little you can do about it. This is not uncommon during the first three months.

If his ANUS BECOMES STENOSED, it will probably do so because it is fibrosed. Unfortunately, regular dilatation perpetuates the cause of the fibrosis. There may come a time when you will have to balance the softening that will follow dilating less often, with the widening that will follow dilating more often.

If he LOSES FLUID EXCESSIVELY FROM HIS COLOSTOMY, wait for 14 days, while giving him extra fluid to maintain a satisfactory fluid balance. His stools will usually become formed; if they don't, refer him.

If his PROXIMAL TRANSVERSE COLON PROLAPSES, this is a nuisance, but is not serious. You may be able to reduce it by pushing it back with vaseline gauze, or KY jelly, on a glove. If necessary, teach his mother to do this.

28.6a Hirschsprung's disease

In this not uncommon disease, the parasympathetic plexi of a child's rectum and distal colon do not develop normally, so that his faeces are not propelled onwards as they should be. The length of the aganglionic segment varies, and may stretch from his upper rectum, to half-way along his transverse colon. He becomes constipated, and his abdomen distends; and in acute cases his gut may obstruct. He may present at any time during childhood in any of the following ways:

HIRSCHSPRUNG'S DISEASE

If a child presents soon after birth with subacute obstruction, its onset is more gradual than with complete mechanical obstruction, but it is still fairly acute. Rectal examination is normal. X-rays show fluid levels and an upside-down X-ray shows air as far as his anus. His distal large gut may look narrow. Do a transverse colostomy, as for a high rectal malformation (28.6), and refer him.

If he presents later, during the first three years, with abdominal distension, and his condition is not acute (usual), refer him for resection of the diseased segment. If it is acute (very unusual), and if it is essential for his health, do a transverse colostomy before referring him.

If he presents up to the age of 10 years as 'a child whose abdomen is large and who does not open his bowels easily', refer him. The surgeon will have to distinguish Hirschsprung's disease from 'chronic constipation', by doing a biopsy which includes the submucosa, and with it the faulty plexi. At operation, he will have to decide where the faulty plexi end, excise the diseased segment, and anastomose the colon to the distal rectum.

28.7 Congenital abnormalities of the female genital tract

The female genital tract occasionally fails to develop normally. The more common abnormalities are fortunately quite easy to treat. If the vagina fails to communicate with the vulva, a patient may present at birth with hydrocolpos (rare, described below), or at puberty with haematocolpos (uncommon), as described in Section 20.14.

FEMALE GENITAL ABNORMALITIES

If you are shown a baby girl with an ABSENT VAGINA, examine her carefully and consider the possibility of labial fusion. This is common, whereas an absent vagina is rare. If her labia minora are not obviously present and normal, and you can see even the faintest line of adhesions, this is what she has. Gently separate them with a probe. Ask her mother to clean her vulva with tepid boiled water daily for a week, and to bring her to a nurse at one week and two weeks.

If you feel a LOW ABDOMINAL MASS IN A GIRL BABY (rare), examine her vulva and vagina. If you find a bulging membrane just above her vagina, her uterus and vagina are full of watery fluid—hydrocolpos.

If the membrane feels thin, incise it with a cross-shaped incision. *Do nothing else, or you will increase the risk of infection.* She will settle down.

If there is no thin membrane, her vagina is absent through all or part of its length. You have a difficult problem. Refer her.

28.8 Omphalocele (exomphalos)

Not uncommonly, a child is born with a defect in his abdominal wall which involves his umbilicus, and leaves his viscera covered only by a translucent layer of peritoneum and amnion. In *omphalocele minor* there are only a few loops of gut in the sac, but in *omphalocele major*, it may contain most of his abdominal organs,

OMPHALOCELE (major)

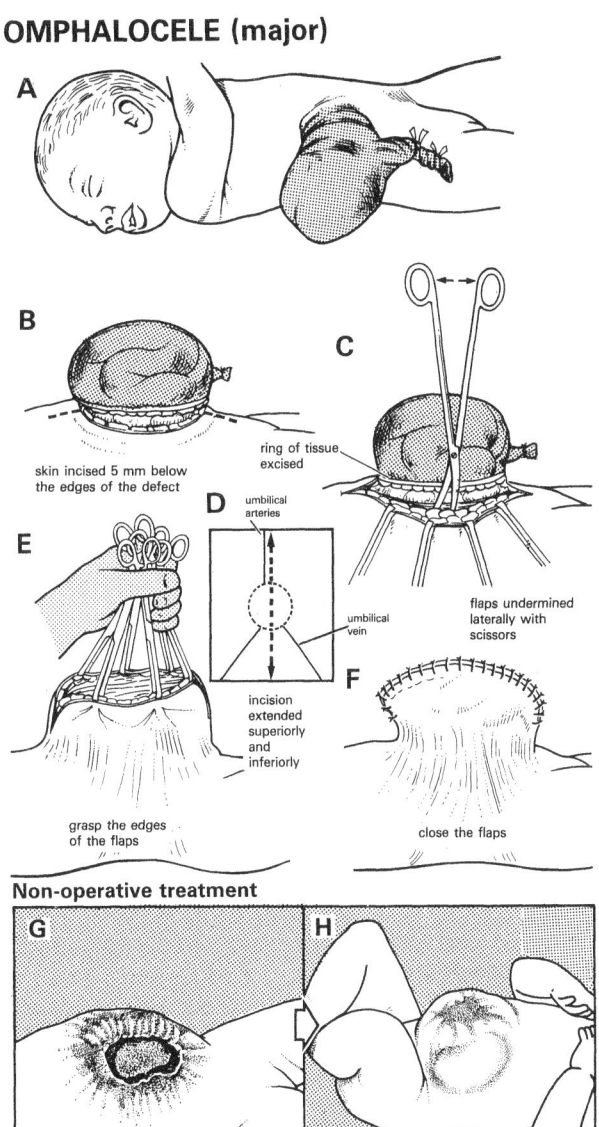

Fig. 28-9 OMPHALOCELE. A, this hernia is too large to reduce in a single stage (omphalocele major); its sac is intact. B, incise the skin 5 mm below the edge of the defect. C, separate skin flaps with scissors. D, extend the incision superiorly and inferiorly. E, hold up the skin flaps with haemostats applied to the subcutaneous tissue to reduce the viscera. F, close the flaps. G, and H, early and late stages in the non-operative treatment with spirit dressings. *Partly after Ravitch et al., 'Paediatric Surgery'. Yearbook Medical, permission requested.*

including even his liver. Often he has no other defects, so he is well worth saving.

The sac of an omphalocele is weak, and easily ruptures or becomes infected, causing peritonitis. If it ruptures during delivery, surgery is urgent. If it survives delivery intact, you have the choice between operative and non-operative treatment. Surgery is the usual method; non-operative treatment needs particularly good nursing care.

If you can reduce the contents of the sac, he has omphalocele minor, which you can treat without difficulty. If you cannot reduce them, he has omphalocele major, which has to be managed surgically in two stages: (1) Undermine skin flaps to make an artificial hernia, and bring them together over his herniated viscera, which will then lie subcutaneously. (2) At nine months to a year, his abdominal cavity should have grown enough to allow you, or an expert, to reduce the hernia into it.

OMPHALOCELE (exomphalos)

As soon as the child is born, apply warm saline soaks to the omphalocele, to keep it moist and to prevent him getting cold. Wrap him up well.

If his omphalocele has ruptured, or is threatening to do so, operate betwen 6 and 24 hours. If its covering appears stable, you can wait a few days. If possible refer him, especially if his omphalocele is large.

NON-OPERATIVE TREATMENT FOR OMPHALOCELES

If the sac is intact and its coverings are fairly strong (common with small omphaloceles, but not with large ones), you can, if necessary, treat omphaloceles of any degree this way. It is however second best, so repair them if you can.

Clean the sac with an antiseptic, and dress it with spirit. Don't use mercurochrome. Apply spirit to the sac hourly for the first 48 hours, and then less often as an eschar forms. This will separate from the periphery, as epithelialisation takes place, but it may take several weeks. He will then be left with a large skin-covered ventral hernia (H, Fig. 28-9) which will need repair later.

THE SURGICAL REPAIR OF OMPHALOCELES

ANTIBIOTICS. Always give these if the sac ruptures before or during the operation. Give him ampicilllin 10 mg/kg 6-hourly, and metronidazole 7.5 mg/kg 8-hourly.

ANAESTHESIA. Set up a scalp vein drip or do a cut-down. Give him a general anaesthetic (A 18.1) or ketamine, tracheal intubation, and suxamethonium (18.2). You can use local anaesthesia for a small omphalocele (not easy), but not for a large one because you need muscular relaxation. If he has an omphalocele major, have blood available, and replace any blood he loses meticulously (3-1).

REPAIRING AN OMPHALOCELE MINOR

INDICATIONS. His omphalocele is small enough for you to be able to: (1) reduce it while he is anaesthetized and breathing spontaneously, and (2) bring the edges of the sac together, without embarrassing his respiration. If it is embarrassed, do a two-stage repair.

REDUCTION. Prepare his skin, including the hernial sac and drape him. Tie and divide his cord, as it emerges from the sac, with '0' chromic catgut (monofilament cuts through too easily).

Try to reduce the contents of the sac into his abdominal cavity. If you fail, manage him as an omphalocele major. If you succeed, incise the skin 0.5 cm, or less, from the edge of the defect (B, in Fig. 28-9). Find and tie his umbilical arteries in the 5 and 7 o'clock positions; tie his umbilical vein superiorly in the 12 o'clock position. Expose the edge of his fascia and peritoneum, and remove a ring of tissue. Excise any tissue of doubtful viability from the sac wall.

Reduce his hernia, and close the defect in three layers. If necessary, hold up the edges of the defect with haemostats (E). Close his peritoneum with 3/0 catgut. Close his fascia with 2/0 monofilament mattress sutures. Close his skin with simple sutures of 2/0 monofilament.

Postoperatively, feed him with expressed breast milk by nasogastric tube, until he is sucking well, usually in 2 or 3 days.

REPAIRING AN OMPHALOCELE MAJOR

This is an omphalocele which you cannot reduce in a single stage (A, in Fig 28-9).

FIRST STAGE. Incise his skin and subcutaneous tissue 0.5 cm or less from the edge of the sac (B). Find and tie the vessels as above. Excise any tissue of doubtful viability from the wall of the sac, including the stumps of the vessels. Extend the incision in the midline superiorly and inferiorly (D). Use scissors to extensively undermine a superficial layer of skin and subcutaneous tissue, and separate this from the muscles of his abdominal wall and the aponeurotic layer. Reduce dissection over his thorax to the absolute minimum that will provide enough skin cover. The flaps must cover the hernia without undue tension.

Hold the edges of the wound up in haemostats applied to the subcutaneous tissue, and reduce the contents of the sac so that they lie subcutaneously. Close the wound in two layers. Use 2/0 chromic catgut for the subcutaneous tissue and 2/0 monofilament for the skin.

Postoperatively, care for him as for omphalocele minor, but continue tube feeding for longer.

SECOND STAGE. Do this at nine months or a year, and refer him for it if you can.

If you cannot refer him, give him a general anaesthetic, and try to reduce the contents of the sac into his abdominal cavity. If you cannot reduce most of them, delay the operation and try again six months later.

If you can reduce all the contents, excise the sac, as for the first operation. Disssect out skin flaps down to the edge of the defect in his abdominal wall. Divide any adhesions between the subcutaneous tissue of the flaps and the sac, or his abdominal organs. Define the peritoneum and fascia at the edge of the defect. Then close the peritoneum and fascia longitudinally if you can (unusual).

If you cannot reduce all the contents into his abdominal cavity, reduce what you can. This will help his abdominal cavity to enlarge. Make his hernia smaller by suturing his subcutaneous tissue to the muscles of his abdominal wall with catgut. Then close his subcutaneous tissue and his skin as before. Operate again about a year later. The greater volume of his abdominal contents will help his abdominal cavity to enlarge.

28.8a The surgery of neonatal jaundice

Most neonatal jaundice is 'medical', and only occasionally is it 'surgical'. Surgically, a child's biliary tract can be blocked by epithelial debris or biliary sand (less common), in which case it may be temporary and clear spontaneously, or by atresia of his biliary tree (more common), for which his only hope is surgery. If much of his bile-duct is not canalized (25%), nothing can be done. If however his bile duct is sufficiently canalized for his gallbladder to be distended, and in connection with his proximal duct system (75%), it can be anastomosed to his proximal jejunum. If he has an extra-hepatic stump, this too can be anastomosed. Without surgery, he will die. Even in experienced hands his outlook is only fair. If a neonate passes clay-coloured stools, try to refer him before 8 weeks.

NEONATAL JAUNDICE

The time of onset is of great diagnostic value.

If a child starts to become jaundiced in the first 6 to 24 hours, his jaundice is likely to be haemolytic as the result of: (1) Septicaemia from an umbilical infection. Look for signs of infection of his cord and the surrounding tissues (septicaemia from cord infection can also occur later). (2) Haemolytic disease of the newborn (uncommon in Africa). Usually, he is D+ve, his mother is D−ve and has anti-D antibodies as the result of having had a previous D+ve child or abortion, or of having been given D+ve blood. Other blood group incompatibilities may have the same effect (for example ABO). (3) Congenital syphilis (severe infection).

BILE-DUCT ATRESIA

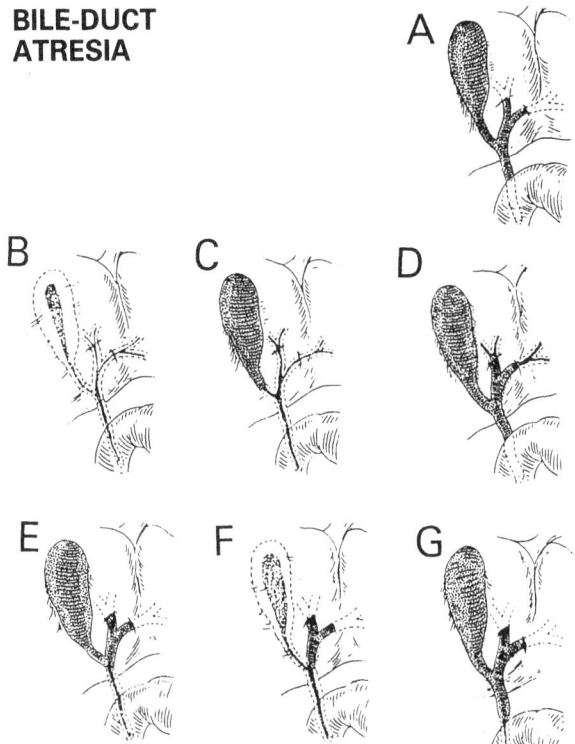

Fig. 28-9a BILE-DUCT ATRESIA. A, normal. B, total atresia of all ducts. C, atresia of all ducts except the gall-bladder. D, intrahepatic atresia. E, atresia of the common ducts. F, atresia of the common bile-duct and gall-bladder. G, segmental atresia of the distal common bile-duct. *After Seymour I. Schwartz, 'Surgical Disease of the Liver', (1964). McGraw-Hill, permission requested.*

If he starts to become mildly jaundiced at 24–72 hours, he is likely to have 'physiological jaundice' due to a deficiency of glycuronidase (common, especially in 'small for dates' babies). This usually clears spontaneously, but can be helped by sunlight and phenobarbitone 1–2 mg/kg 12-hourly.

If he starts to become jaundiced at 24–72 hours, and is severely jaundiced by the 3rd to the 5th day, he may have G6PD (glucose-6-phosphate dehydrogenase) deficiency. This is common, especially in SE Asia and the Mediterranean littoral; a less severe form occurs in parts of sub-Saharan Africa.

If he has little or no jaundice for 3 to 6 weeks, by which time his liver is enlarged, and his stools are clay-coloured, he probably has some 'surgical' reason for his jaundice. Sometimes he is slightly jaundiced at birth, or becomes so a few days later; his urine is dark brown early.

CHOLECYSTOJEJUNOSTOMY

Surgery and anaesthesia are difficult, so refer him if you can; he is very small, and tends to bleed. If you cannot refer him and decide to operate, give him vitamin K₁ (water-soluble) 2 mg intramuscularly, and operate next day.

ANAESTHESIA. (1) General anaesthesia. (2) Intramuscular ketamine, followed by small intravenous doses.

INCISION. Make a subcostal transverse or right upper paramedian incision. If he has a distended gall-bladder, proceed. If he has some inoperable anomaly, close his abdomen.

Anastomose the fundus of his gall-bladder to his jejunum using interrupted sutures of 3/0 catgut or 4/0 multifilament (e.g. silk). See Fig. 13-5.

Postoperatively, manage him as in Section 28.3.

28.9 Spina bifida, meningocele, and myelomeningocele

Congenital abnormalities of the spinal cord and vertebral column are not uncommon. You may see:

Spina bifida alone, in which the arches of a child's vertebrae remain open, usually in his lumbar region. He often has a Mongolian spot over the defect (this is less easily seen in a dark skin, but it is there if you look for it), and/or some extra hair and fatty tissue. Uncomplicated spina bifida is usually symptomless, but watch him carefully. If his legs become weak, refer him: he may have a bifid spinal cord separated by a bony spur (diastematomyelia, rare).

A meningocele is a CSF-filled extension of his spinal canal, without any spinal cord or spinal nerves in it; commonly in his lumbar region, and usually associated with spina bifida. His cord is normal and he has no neurological abnormality. It is a relatively simple procedure to obliterate the sac, close his spinal membranes at the level of his laminae, and then to close his skin. This is a closed lesion, so there is no hurry.

A myelomeningocele is more common than a simple meningocele, and takes two forms: (1) He may have a closed swelling containing spinal cord and/or spinal nerves. (2) More often, his spinal canal is open and leaks CSF, with his flattened cord forming a plaque on its surface. Both varieties may occur in the cervical (rare), thoracolumbar, lumbar, or lumbosacral regions, and other abnormalities are frequent, particularly hydrocephalus. Most children have irreversible paralysis of their legs, and loss of sphincter control, so that surgery merely prolongs their misery, and that of their parents. You may however be justified in operating on sacral myelomeningoceles, as described below.

MENINGOCELE

DIAGNOSIS. If the swelling on the child's back is covered by skin, his legs are not weak, his anus is not lax, and he micturates normally, he probably has a simple meningocele. Otherwise, you cannot tell a meningocele from a myelomeningocele from its site, or its covering. Transilluminate it; you may occasionally see nerves outlined inside it.

If he has any neurological signs, he certainly has a myelomeningocele. These signs are: (1) No movement in his legs. (2) An absent or meagre response to tickling or pin-prick. (3) A lax anal sphincter which does not contract on digital examination. (4) Observe the way he passes urine; he may pass it as a jet at specific times (normal), or it may leak out from time to time (abnormal).

Look for other anomalies, particularly talipes (27.15). Measure the circumference of his head, now and later; he may develop hydrocephalus.

MENINGOCELES

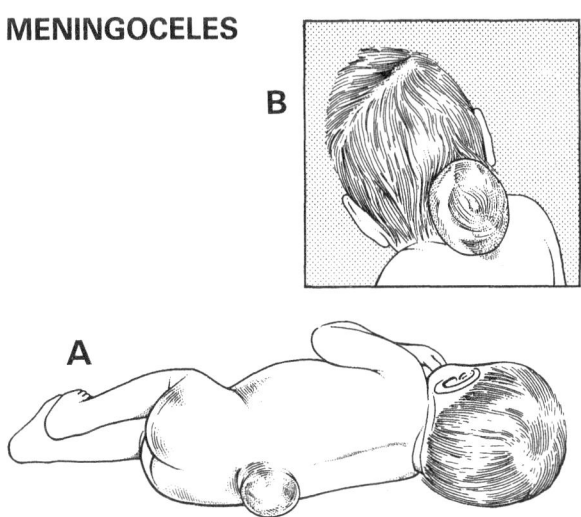

Fig. 28-10 MENINGOCELES. A, a skin-covered sacrolumbar meningocele. If you cannot refer a child like this, you may be justified in operating on him. B, a cervical meningocele. Don't operate on this child.

MANAGEMENT OF MENINGOCELES

If his meningocele is covered with normal skin (usual), surgery is not urgent. Operate when convenient, normally at about 6 months.

If his meningocele is not covered by skin (unusual), surgery is urgent, because it is easily damaged, and may become infected. If he is fortunate and well cared for, it may epithelialize.

If the mass is in his cervical or thoracic regions, it is more likely to be a simple meningocele, so try to refer him. Don't try to operate on lesions in these sites yourself.

If: (1) the central canal of his spinal canal is open to the surface, or (2) he has a myelomeningocele with neurological signs (commonly in the thoracolumbar or lumbar regions), there is nothing to be done, except compassionate palliation.

If he has a sacral myelomeningocele, with normal power in his legs (normal sphincter control is unusual), urgent operation may be justified—see below.

CLOSING A MENINGOCELE

If you cannot refer him, proceed as follows. Take the strictest aseptic precautions and be careful not to damage his cord.

INDICATIONS. A fairly small sacral or lumbar meningocele, with no neurological signs, no hydrocephalus, and no other congenital abnormalities.

CONTRAINDICATIONS. (1) Complete or virtually complete denervation below the level of the lesion. (2) Progressive hydrocephalus. (3) A very large lesion, in which you will have difficulty closing the skin and subcutaneous tissues without tension. (4) Lesions in sites other than the lumbar or sacral region.

ANAESTHESIA. (1) General anaesthesia, with precautions, particularly tracheal intubation, for the prone position (A 16.12). (2) Ketamine (A 8.5). If you use ketamine without intubating him, lie him semiprone (which will make surgery more difficult), when his breathing should be satisfactory.

PREPARATION. Lay him prone with the head of the table depressed at least 30°, to minimize the loss of CSF when you incise the sac. Prepare and drape a wide operative field.

Clean the sac meticulously and aspirate it *slowly* with a 0.8 mm needle until it collapses.

If the swelling is covered by skin, make a longitudinal elliptical incision, through normal skin at the base of the swelling. Cut through the subcutaneous tissue to the deep fascia, and define the neck of the sac by blunt dissection. The defect in the fascia will usually be quite small, and easy to expose. Free all surfaces of the sac, and open it over its dome.

If there are no nerve filaments, amputate the sac at its base, and close it with continuous 4/0 or 5/0 catgut.

If you find nerve filaments, he is not a case of simple meningocele, and his prognosis is poor. Preserve the nerve filaments with the greatest care, try to free them from the sac, close it, and try to cover every filament.

Complete the repair by overlapping his deep fascia and closing his skin.

If you have difficulty closing his skin: (1) Raise flaps by undermining extensively, and making lateral relaxing incisions if necessary. Or, (2) use double pedicle advancement flaps (57-19), with split skin grafts to cover the raw areas. Seal the wound meticulously, and nurse him in the prone position.

SACRAL MYELOMENINGOCELE

This is the child with a sacral myelomeningocele and normal power in his legs, as described above.

Dissect the sac from his cauda equina, being careful not to damage it. Close his dura with continuous 4/0 catgut. Raise flaps of skin and subcutaneous tissue by undercutting with scissors, making lateral relaxing incisions if necessary. Close his skin with 4/0 monofilament, apply a dressing, and nurse him as above.

28.10 Congenital vascular lesions

Congenital vascular lesions are not uncommon, and may worry

CONGENITAL VASCULAR ANOMALIES

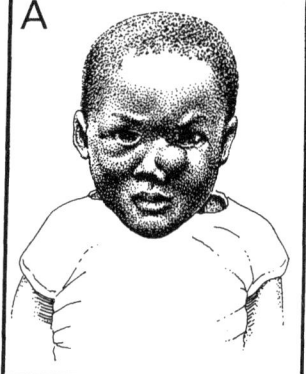
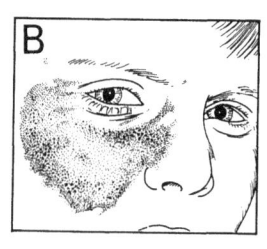
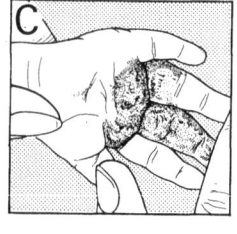
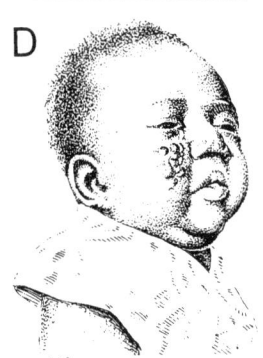
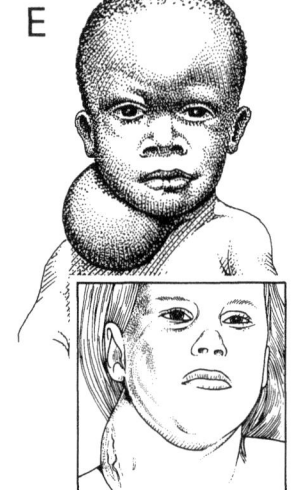

Fig. 28-11 CONGENITAL VASCULAR ANOMALIES. A, a cavernous haemangioma. B, a port-wine stain. C, a capillary cavernous haemangioma of the hand. D, a capillary haemangioma of the face. E, and F, cystic hygromas. *A, D, and E, after Charles Bowesman, 'Surgery and Clinical Pathology in the Tropics'. E and S Livingstone, permission requested.*

a mother, so you should know how to advise her. There is little you can do for most of them except, to watch a child carefully, and refer him when necessary.

A capillary haemangioma, or 'strawberry naevus' (D, in Fig. 28-11) is a skin lesion, and is commonest on the face. It is bright red, and a little raised, sometimes quite markedly. It may occur on the mucous membranes and may bleed severely. A baby is usually normal at birth; the lesions appear one to four weeks later, and enlarge for a few months. Rapid growth is unusual after six months, but slow growth is common up to a year. If you leave them alone, 95% will resolve spontaneously. The first sign that this is happening is the appearance of a lighter, flatter area. Resolution may be precipitated by trauma, but this usually causes only minor scarring. Advise his mother that his lesion will probably disappear slowly. Warn her not to allow traditional healers to scarify the lesion, which may cause bleeding, infection, and worse scarring. If resolution is slow, or she presses you, refer him.

A port-wine stain (B, in Fig. 28-11) consists of cavernous channels, and usually occurs on the face or neck, but is not uncommon on the trunk. It is usually present at birth and does not progress, but it may be quite extensive. The texture of his skin is normal, and is not usually thickened; occasionally there is some hypertrophy and irregularity.

If a lesion is particularly ugly, as in a light skin, cosmetic creams may help. Otherwise, there is no treatment. Reassure his mother that his lesion will not enlarge.

Lesions on the face, in the area of distribution of the ophthalmic and maxillary branches of the fifth nerve, may be associated with vascular abnormalities of the cerebral cortex (Sturge–Weber syndrome), and present with seizures. Glaucoma of the ipsilateral eye sometimes occurs, and is treatable (24.6). Refer him to a neurosurgeon.

A **capillary cavernous haemangioma** consists of abnormal capillaries, arteries, and veins, and is partly compressible. It is usually present at birth, and commonly occurs on a child's face, axillae, or neck, where it may extend into his mediastinum. It may occasionally resolve spontaneously over several years (unusual), or it may enlarge rapidly.

Watch him carefully, and at each visit use a measuring tape to record the exact size of his lesion in two dimensions at right angles. If it does enlarge, refer him—surgery is likely to be difficult, and bleeding severe.

A **lymphangioma** is a congenital capillary cavernous lesion, which is usually present at birth, in the same sites, commonly the neck, as a haemangioma. Some are well circumscribed, but others merge with the surrounding tissues. Some become slowly smaller, others enlarge, sometimes quite quickly, and cause pressure effects in the chest. Most eventually need surgery, which can be difficult and may not be complete.

Watch him and measure his lesion regularly. Refer him if it enlarges, especially if it enlarges rapidly.

A **cystic hygroma** (E, and F, in Fig. 28-11) is a fluctuant, lobulated, translucent mass of abnormal lymphatic vessels, which presents as a soft, diffuse swelling in the posterior triangle of the neck, or occasionally the axilla. It appears early, and may be present at birth. The mass is not attached to the skin, and does not move on the deep tissues. A cystic hygroma usually causes no serious problems, and usually enlarges slowly. Occasionally, it advances rapidly and causes pressure symptoms at the root of the neck, or, rarely, it may regress spontaneously. The main differential diagnoses are: (1) A lymphangioma. (2) A branchial cyst; this is unilocular and low in the neck, along the anterior border of the sternomastoid; aspiration yields a thicker opalescent fluid, instead of the thin, clear, watery fluid from a hygroma. (3) A capillary cavernous haemangioma.

Surgery can be difficult, because a hygroma may penetrate deeply, or have lymphangiomatous extensions. Watch him carefully, and unless it is clearly regressing, refer him. If it is very large, it should be operated on earlier. If it is not so large, removal will be easier when he is more than a year old.

28.11 Other paediatric problems

Here are some of the other problems you may meet, and which do not require complete sections to themselves. Intussusception (10.8), and *Ascaris* obstruction (10.6) are described elsewhere.

OTHER PROBLEMS

PROBLEMS IN NEONATES

If a neonate or an infant has RETENTION OF URINE with overflow, the neck of his bladder is probably obstructed, by the contraction of his internal meatus, or more commonly by URETHRAL VALVES. These usually present in the first six months of life, but they can occur at any age, and even into adult life. They can present as retention, urinary tract infection, dribbling incontinence or renal failure. You may feel that an infant's bladder is distended, and you may be able to feel his kidneys. His distended bladder may simulate a rhabdomyosarcoma of the bladder, but will disappear on catheterization. Pass a urethral catheter (a 6–8 Ch feeding tube is suitable) under ketamine or general anaesthesia. Alternatively insert a suprapubic catheter. Treat any infection and refer him. A urethral catheter is unsatisfactory, because its bore is so narrow that it soon blocks. A suprapubic tube is better, but even this does not drain his ureters or kidneys well.

If a neonate is born with a LARGE SOLID MASS BELOW HIS SACRUM, it is probably a coccygeal teratoma or hamartoma (benign or malignant). Refer him for surgery soon.

PROBLEMS IN OLDER CHILDREN

If a child DISCHARGES URINE FROM HIS UMBILICUS and his urethra, he has a persistent urachus (rare). Sometimes urine discharges in a small spurt during micturition. He may not present until he is a year old or later. Excising the track is not difficult. See Section 28.5.

If he has a dirty UMBILICUS WHICH DISCHARGES, smells, and occasionally bleeds, he has a GRANULOMA OF THE UMBILICUS (very common), caused by an infected remnant of his cord (28.5). Clean it with spirit daily, apply alum powder (Paediatric Alum and Zinc Dusting-powder BPC), and keep it dry. Alum powder is also preventive, because it quickly dries the stump of the cord.

If a boy's URETHRA OPENS ON THE VENTRAL SURFACE OF HIS PENIS, he has hypospadias. Refer him at 3 years, so that the necessary plastic surgery can be completed by the age of 6.

If a child has RECURRENT ATTACKS OF CHOLANGITIS which may lead to JAUNDICE, suspect cystic dilatation, usually of his common bile-duct (CHOLEDOCAL CYST). An expert should be able to anastomose the fundus of his gall-bladder to his jejunum, and excise the cyst. If this is impossible, anastomosis alone is of some value.

28a Surgery, AIDS, and hepatitis B

"One night after I had been doing some blood tests in a rural area with some local medical colleagues, they went off with some girls from the town. They slept with them, and only one of them used a condom. In the morning I asked them how they could possibly have taken such a risk, since we all knew that the prevalence of HIV was quite high in the region. They laughed, saying that you couldn't give up living just because you might get a disease".

A research worker in Central Africa reported in the March 1987 PANOS Dossier.

28a.1 Introduction

While this system of surgery was being written, a disease appeared which seems likely to change the face of the developing world, and perhaps the entire world—AIDS, the acquired immunodeficiency syndrome, caused by the human immunodeficiency virus (HIV). Not the least of its consequences are those for surgery. Some of these are shared by HBV, the virus of hepatitis B, which provides some illuminating parallels and contrasts in what promises to be a pivotal chapter in these manuals.

Although AIDS overshadows hepatitis B, it is significant that during the production of this book, two of its contributors became infected with HBV, and one of them died of fulminant viral hepatitis. Both almost certainly acquired their infections in the theatre. This chapter is based on the experience of Central Africa, particularly Zambia, and applies less to more fortunate countries.

28a.2 AIDS

Where HIV came from is a mystery. It is a retrovirus (RNA virus), and it is also a lentivirus (slow virus), which progressively destroys the immune system and infects the brain. It is one of the most genetically variable of all human viruses, and is spreading as a virgin-soil pandemic. In some studies, up to 50% of seropositive subjects have developed AIDS, but it is possible that some infected people may remain symptom-free for the whole of their natural lives. WHO considers that AIDS is likely to become a pandemic of such severity that it may cause more deaths than any previous pandemic in recorded history.

Although HIV has been isolated from blood, semen, saliva, vaginal secretions, tears, breast milk, and urine, only blood and blood products, semen, and vaginal secretions seem to be important sources for transmission.

The simple rule is that HIV is spread by: (1) Heterosexual intercourse—the dominant method in sub-Saharan Africa. (2) Homosexual intercourse—the dominant method in some communities in the developed world. (3) Blood transfusion and blood and tissue products. (4) Vertical transmission from a mother to her baby. (5) The shared needles and syringes of drug abusers, in which the blood that is drawn into a needle by one addict infects another. (6) Inadequately sterilized needles and equipment in hospitals and health centres, and by traditional practices, such as scarification, which pierce the skin.

The simple rule also is that HIV is *not* spread by: (1) Social and family contact, including sharing the same eating utensils or toilet facilities. (2) Nursing patients with AIDS. (3) The medical treatment of patients with AIDS. (4) Mosquitoes or bed bugs.

These simple rules require qualification, because the routes by which HIV spreads vary greatly in their efficiency. Worldwide, the vast majority of cases of AIDS (probably more than 90%) are the result of penetrative vaginal or anal intercourse. The only other routes of public health importance are the transmission of HIV from a mother to her child, and by the administration of blood and blood products.

THE SPREAD OF AIDS

Evidence for the efficiency of some routes is still incomplete.

VERY EFFICIENT ROUTES. Although blood transfusion is the most efficient route, it is not the most common one.

Blood transfusion is at least 90% efficient.

Needles shared by drug abusers especially if there is much blood in the shared needle or syringe.

Penetrative sexual intercourse. The efficiency of particular methods varies. The male is a more efficient transmitter than the female; the rectum is more vulnerable than the vagina. The transmission rate per single contact is estimated to vary from 1/100 to 1/1000. The presence of GUD (genital ulcer disease) caused by another STD (syphilis, chancroid, or donovanosis) strongly promotes the heterosexual transmission of HIV, and so does traumatic bleeding, classically caused by the first intercourse (defloration). GUD is one reason why vaginal intercourse seems to be a more efficient route in sub-Saharan Africa than it is elsewhere. Another appears to be the greater frequen-

THE AIDS VIRUS

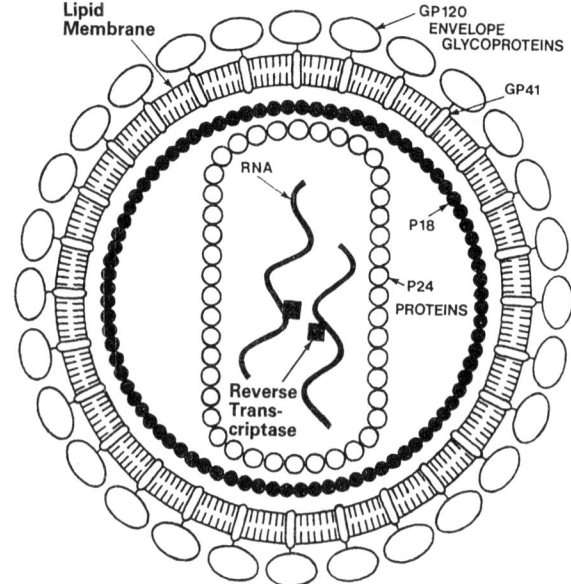

Fig. 28a-1 HIV, THE AIDS VIRUS. The outer lipid membrane is pierced by a glycoprotein (gp41) to which another larger glycoprotein (gp120) is attached. Inside are the core proteins (p18 and p24). When the virus enters a host cell, the enzyme reverse transcriptase makes a DNA copy of the viral RNA, which is permanently integrated into the host's DNA.

cy of intercourse with multiple partners. Risk is graded here from high to less high:
Receptive anal intercourse.
Receptive vaginal intercourse.
Insertive vaginal intercourse.
Insertive anal intercourse.
Oral intercourse (penile, vaginal, or anal).

From mother to child *in utero* or perinatally. 25–50% of the children of HIV positive mothers become infected.

THE FAIRLY EFFICIENT ROUTES. Evidence is incomplete.

Improperly sterilized surgical equipment, needles and cannulae, etc., may also be fairly efficient vehicles of infection, so also may some traditional methods of scarification.

Breast-feeding during, but probably *only* during the post-infection peak of infectivity where HIV was acquired after delivery, especially if it was acquired by blood transfusion (see below).

Sex of any kind with a condom. A condom reduces the risk of HIV transmission, but does not eliminate it (some contributors would put this among the inefficient routes).

THE INEFFICIENT ROUTES. It is fortunate for health workers that the needlestick route is as inefficient as it is.

Needlestick injuries to health workers. About 0.5% per episode (the corresponding rate for hepatitis B is 20%).

Breast-feeding when a mother was infected before or during pregnancy. The added risk of breast feeding is likely to be small (see below).

ROUTES WHICH HAVE NEVER BEEN IMPLICATED IN TRANSMITTING HIV, BUT ARE PROBABLY NOT ENTIRELY SAFE. 'Wet kissing'; deep or vigorous tongue-kissing probably carries some risk.

RISK EXTREMELY LOW OR NON-EXISTENT. Shared bedding, toothbrushes, or eating utensils, etc. 'Ordinary family contact', and 'ordinary nursing care'. 'Dry kissing'.

NO RISK. Ordinary contact at school, in the community, and at work. Shaking hands, hugging. Swimming pools, toilets, telephones, door handles, food and cups. Insects or insect bites, including mosquito bites. Water. Droplet infection by coughing and sneezing (so far). Routine immunizations in childhood, or at any other time, with *effectively sterilized needles and syringes*.

CAUTION ! Beware of false positives and false negatives in diagnosing AIDS in babies. (1) HIV antibodies are transmitted passively from mother to child *in utero,* so beware of diagnosing infection in a seropositive child. Maternal antibody may persist for at least 6 months. (2) An infected child may not seroconvert for 18 months or more (rare). As a result a neonate may be positive, and then become negative as his mother's antibodies wane, only to become positive again as he makes his own antibodies.

Fortunately, in transmitting HIV, each of the above methods is orders of magnitude less efficient than it is in transmitting HBV.

'Ordinary family contact' and 'ordinary nursing care' are general terms which include a wide variety of possible routes of infection, some of which are not absolutely safe, despite the simple rule above. The risk is merely very small, rather than zero. A mother has been infected by her infant son, a woman has been infected while providing home nursing care for a sick neighbour, a nurse has been infected by contaminated blood on her hands and face. *But these cases are exceptional and very rare.* For those who are unaccustomed to weighing up risks (which is most people anywhere in the world), you are probably justified in using the 'simple rule'.

Fortunately for health workers, and especially for surgeons, the routes through which we are exposed in our work are very inefficient. The difficulty is that, although these routes are inefficient, we are exposed to them repeatedly over a long period. Needlestick injuries and infected body fluids, especially blood on our skin, are our main risks. They are not easy to avoid because surgeons commonly injure themselves as well as their patients; they puncture their gloves in up to 30% of operations and injure themselves with needles or knives in 15–20%. So take care where you put the point of your needle, and keep infected body fluids away from your skin. Gloves will keep body fluids away from your hands, but they are little protection against needlestick injuries. They can also put up a psychological barrier between a health worker and his patient, so don't use them unnecessarily.

HIV attacks helper T cells. This reduces the body's ability to resist both the recognized pathogens and the normally harmless commensal organisms, which are thus able to cause opportunistic infections. The result is that a patient with AIDS may suffer, either simultaneously or in sequence, from a wide variety of infections which vary geographically. In Africa, he presents with: (1) Continuing severe loss of weight (hence the Ugandan name 'slim disease'). (2) Intractable diarrhoea due to *Cryptosporidium, Microsporidium,* and *Isospora belli.* (3) Oral and oesophageal candidiasis (thrush)—which is almost invariable. (4) Generalized mild enlargement of his lymph nodes, which are firm enough to be seen under his skin, particularly in his occipital and lateral cervical regions. (5) Mild pyrexia. (6) Anaemia. (7) Recurrent multidermatomal attacks of herpes zoster. (8) Tuberculosis, which is often extrapulmonary, and may fail to respond to treatment (very common). (9) Neurological problems, such as encephalitis and bizarre forms of peripheral neuritis. (10) Septic infections: recurrent boils and abscesses (common), perianal sepsis (5.13) and PID (both of which are made worse by HIV, 6.6), and periostitis (rare, 7.6D). (11) Increased sensitivity to drugs. (12) Bleeding due to thrombocytopenia. (13) 'AAKS', or atypical African Kaposi's sarcoma (fairly common, 32.21). (14) Cryptococcal meningitis (common in Zaire, but not elsewhere). (15) *Pneumocystis carinii* pneumonia (rare in East and Central Africa, but occurring in Zimbabwe). (16) Toxoplasmosis. (17) Cytomegalovirus (probably). (18) Children present with multiple septic infections and failure to thrive (common).

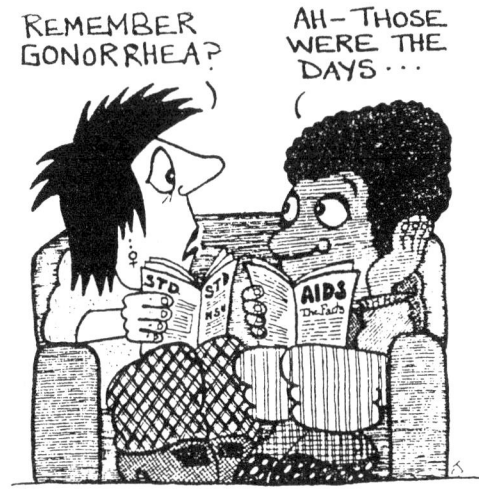

Drawn by Cath Jackson, with the kind permission of the Terence Higgins Trust.

A few weeks after infection with HIV, seroconversion is occasionally accompanied by a self-limiting mononucleosis-like illness (and rarely by encephalitis). A patient then remains relatively well, although he may have fluctuating minimally painful lymph node enlargement, tiredness, malaise, and a little fever and weight loss. After several months he recovers symptomatically (although his enlarged nodes may persist), often for years, before he develops further symptoms.

Although AIDS can usually be diagnosed clinically, all hospitals should be able to test for HIV antibodies. Unfortunately, both the equipment and the reagents are expensive; but there are aid agencies which are prepared to assist with their purchase. The standard method is an ELISA technique, which is not completely reliable, because the virus can be present for up to 3 months (sometimes 6 months) before the ELISA test becomes positive, and even after this it may *occasionally* give false negatives (depending on the assay method; it also gives a significant number of false positives). The competitive immunoassay ('Welcozyme') test gives almost no false positives, but may give some false negatives. A few AIDS cases also give false negatives, either because no antibody is present at the time of presentation, or because the antibody is to a virus which is not detected by the test being used (there are two types of virus, HIV_1, common in East and Central Africa, and HIV_2, common in West Africa).

There is presently no vaccine, and the prospects that there will ever be one are uncertain. So the only methods of control are: (1) No sex before marriage. (2) No sex outside marriage. In default of this a single partner, or a reduction in the number of partners, reduces the risk. Multiple partners greatly increase it. Unfortunately, no sex outside marriage does not help if your partner is already positive. (3) Condoms, which reduce the risk, but do not eliminate it; they are frequently used improperly, and do not completely prevent infected body fluids coming into contact with skin. The message that sex with a condom is therefore 'safe sex' is thus dangerously misleading: it is only 'safer' sex. Sex with a condom is less risky, but it is still risky. (4) Restricting the use of blood and blood products, and where possible testing the blood you give. (5) The effective sterilization of needles and syringes, and anything which may be used on another patient, such as any instrument, cannula, or intravenous fluid set. If the sterilization practices of a hospital are imperfect, and HIV is common, the infection of one patient by another is a major potential risk. This is *iatrogenic* infection (infection as the result of the activities of health workers) and *must* be prevented. (6) Care in preventing needlestick injuries.

IATROGENIC INFECTION *MUST* BE PREVENTED

The fact that HIV enters the human genome makes the prospect of a radical cure even less likely than that of a vaccine. Azidothymidine (AZT) can produce remissions for up to a year at a cost of about $5000 and numerous blood transfusions. Unlike a patient dying of cancer, an AIDS patient is usually young, and may sometimes live for several years, so he may need more than merely 'terminal' care. You can do much to help him and his relatives: (1) Prevent and treat all infections early and efficiently. Warn him that STDs are dangerous, and treat AAKS. It has been said that, in Africa, the effective and early treatment of tuberculosis would do more good than AZT. (2) Encourage good nutrition. (3) Advise a woman that pregnancy may accelerate the disease, and will probably produce an infected child; provide her with contraception. (4) Discourage potentially harmful traditional practices, such as scarification, emesis, and purgation, but be neutral towards harmless ones. (5) Provide a patient with good nursing care. Understand and counsel him sympathetically, and encourage your staff and the hospital chaplain to do so too; shake hands with him. (6) Support his relatives and advise them how to care for him. (7) Set up outreach services to help him and them. Emphasize the simple rule that spread does *not* occur by social contact, or through nursing care.

HIV is potentially present, in greater or lesser concentration, in all a patient's body fluids. Outside the body, it may survive for a variable period if it is wet. It is however an enveloped virus and is highly sensitive to drying, detergents, heat, alcohol, formalin, and hypochlorite (bleach). The ordinary methods of disinfection in Section 2.5 will kill HIV on instruments and dressings. The most practical disinfectant to use on clothes, bed linen, and blood spills, etc. is hypochlorite, either as common bleach, or as tablets of sodium dichloroisocyanurate (NaDCC); or you can use Virkon (see below).

Breast-feeding. The vertical transmission of HIV is responsible for most paediatric AIDS. 25–50% of the children of HIV positive mothers become infected *in utero* or during birth; but how much infection occurs *in utero* and how much during birth is not known. Only the remaining children are at potential risk of HIV in breast milk, but the added risk of breast-feeding is likely to be small. If however a mother is infected after delivery as the result of an infected post-partum blood transfusion, the risk may be greater. It may also be greater if she acquired her infection while she was breast-feeding (usually from her husband). There is a period of viraemia soon after infection, and it has been suggested that breast-feeding during this phase may be more dangerous than at other times.

You will have to balance the benefits and risks of breast and artificial feeding, and follow the guidelines below. Advice suitable for the industrial world where laboratory services are good, and a safe artificial feed is practical, differs from that for the developing world, where neither of these things obtain. *The critical priority is that the potential risk of HIV infection should not halt the present global drive for the return of breast-feeding, and the avoidance of artificial feeding.*

Melbye M, Njelesani EK, Bayley Anne, Mukelebai K, et al., 'Evidence for heterosexual transmission and clinical manifestations of human immunodeficiency virus infection and related conditions in Lusaka, Zambia. Lancet. 1986;ii:1113-1115.

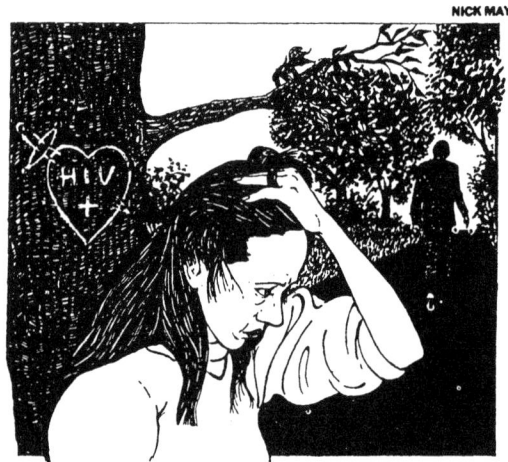

Drawn by Nick May, with the kind permission of The Independent.

AIDS

PREVENTING SPREAD BY BLOOD TRANSFUSION

INDICATIONS FOR TRANSFUSION. In areas where HIV is highly endemic there is *only one indication for blood transfusion*—when the patient's life is in danger. Any transfusion which is not indicated is contraindicated!

METHOD. Try to establish HIV testing in your hospital. Minimize the risk of infection by: (1) Screening all donor blood. Unfortunately, this is not completely effective (see above). (2) Question all donors, and don't take blood from anyone who has had an STD in the previous 5 years (not easy to verify). (3) Don't take blood from high-risk groups, such as prisoners, drivers, or the army. (4) Try to establish a tested donor panel from social groups at low risk (and prepare for its rapid shrinkage). In an 'anti-AIDS club', or church group, the desire to remain publicly a 'safe donor' may encourage saying 'No' to extramarital or premarital sex. (5) Reduce the need for transfusion by treating anaemia medically, particularly the anaemia of pregnancy, and by the efficient care of patients with sickle cell anaemia.

Instead of using blood to treat hypovolaemia use: (1) Saline, which stays in the circulation for about 2 hours. (2) Gelatin ('Haemaccel'), which is expensive but does not interfere with cross-matching. (3) Dextran ('Dextraven'); which is cheaper, but makes cross-matching more difficult. (3) The patient's own blood by autotransfusion (16.10), as with an ectopic pregnancy (16.6), or rupture of his spleen (66.6) or liver (66.7). Avoid blood transfusion, unless it is life-saving. Major paediatric surgery is an exception, because a child has such a small blood volume. Where possible, take blood from a close relative, a spouse, or a parent, who is likely to have the same HIV status as he has. In one African country the only relative who can be almost guaranteed to be HIV negative is the patient's grandmother.

If you need blood for elective surgery, take a unit from him 1 week and 2 weeks preoperatively, store them and give him iron. If necessary, 3 or 4 units can be obtained this way.

CAUTION ! Never give a single unit of blood to an *adult* patient who can do without one, unless it was his own, donated previously. If it happens to contain HIV, it may be fatal. He is likely to need at least 2 units or none.

MIDWIFERY. If a mother is HIV positive, her blood will contain HIV, so will the placenta. Wear gloves and an apron, and don't let her blood get into an open cut or wound. If possible, don't let it get on your skin. So, wash your hands and cover open cuts. Make sure that your staff also follow these rules!

BREAST-FEEDING. Advise people like this:

If a woman is HIV-positive, persuade her strongly not to become pregnant because this encourages the progression of the disease. Unfortunately, her husband may want more children and she may have little choice.

If a mother is HIV-positive before birth, the added risk from breast-feeding, if any, is small:

If a safe artificial feed is impractical (most likely), **she must breast-feed her baby.** The immuological, nutritional, psychological and child-spacing benefits of breast-feeding outweigh the small added risks of infection.

If a safe artificial feed is practical (unlikely under the conditions for which we write), **opinions are divided.** Some would advise breast-feeding and others not.

If a mother becomes infected during or after delivery, the problem is largely theoretical, because you are unlikely to diagnose infection, until it is too late to alter her management. The manner in which she became infected may however determine the risk of transmission:

If she was infected by a blood transfusion during delivery, **her infectivity may be greater, and an artificial feed is advisable.**

If she was infected in some other way while breast feeding (usually by her husband), **she may be infective during the early viraemic phase of her infection.** The risk of infection may however be less than if she is infected by blood transfusion.

If a mother is at high risk of HIV, but you don't know if she is HIV-positive or not, advise her to breast-feed.

If she and her baby are both infected, advise her to breast-feed.

If you run a milk-bank in an area of HIV prevalence, be on the safe side and pasteurize the milk intended for another baby at 60°C for half an hour, or boil it. This will impair some of its immunological activity, but it will still be better than formula.

BLOOD PRODUCTS include plasma and human immune globulin, and factors for the treatment of clotting defects. If they are derived from the pooled plasma of many donors, they are particularly likely to be contaminated by HIV. Unless these products are certified as being HIV-free, avoid them.

IN THE LABORATORY treat all blood as potentially contaminated, and kill HIV in serum by heat-treating it (56°C for 30 minutes) before you test it, making sure that this will not upset the test first. Improve laboratory hygiene, and especially avoid pipetting by mouth.

DISINFECTION FOR HIV AND HBV

CAUTION ! Clean all instruments thoroughly before you disinfect them. If HIV prevalence is high, try to give them a preliminary soaking in a chemical disinfectant first, before they are cleaned, so as to reduce the risk to the staff who clean them.

HIV and HBV are both destroyed by: (1) The standard methods of autoclaving at 121°C (1 kg cm^2) for 20 minutes. This is the method of choice for reusable instruments. There is a special WHO/UNICEF portable steam sterilizer for this purpose. (2) A hot-air oven (including a domestic oven) at 170°C for 2 hours. This temperature will destroy reusable plastic syringes. (3) Boiling for 20 minutes; HBV is destroyed by a few minutes' boil-

Recommended dilutions of chlorine-releasing compounds

	Clean condition (e.g., cleaned medical equipment)	Dirty condition (e.g., blood spills, soiled equipment)
Available chlorine required	0.1% (1 g/litre, 1000 ppm)	0.5% (5 g/litre, 5000 ppm)
Dilution		
Sodium hypochlorite solution (5% available chlorine)	20 ml/litre	100 ml/litre
Calcium hypochlorite (70% available chlorine)	1.4 g/litre	7.0 g/litre
NaDCC (60% available chlorine)	1.7 g/litre	8.5 g/litre
NaDCC-based tablets (1.5 g of available chlorine per tablet)	1 tablet/litre	4 tablets/litre
Chloramine (25% available chlorine)	20 g/litre	20 g/litre

Indicative prices of disinfectants for high-level disinfection

Disinfectant	Price in Europe (US$)	Price for 1 litre of ready-to-use solution (US$)	Price for 1 litre of ready-to-use solution when air-freighted (US$)
calcium hypochlorite (70% available chlorine)	6.00/kg	0.04 (7 g/litre)	0.13
sodium dichloroisocy-anurate (1.5 g of chlorine/tablet)	0.07/tablet	0.28 (4 tablets/litre)	0.32
chloramine (1 g/tablet)	0.02/tablet	0.4 (20 tablets/litre)	0.52
sodium hypochlorite (5% available chlorine)	0.50/litre	0.05 (1:10 dilution)	1.15
formaldehyde (35–40%)	1.70/litre	0.17 (1:10 dilution)	1.30
polyvidone iodine (10%)	5.00/litre	1.25 (1:4 dilution)	2.10
hydrogen peroxide (30%)	3.20/litre	0.65 (1:5 dilution)	4.60
glutaral (glutaraldehyde) (2%)	3.20/litre	3.20 (undiluted)	6.50
2-propanol (100%)	4.20/litre	3.00 (7:10 dilution)	10.70
ethanol (90%)	3.10/litre	2.50 (8:10 dilution)	11.30

As examples, the prices in the right-hand column have been estimated on the basis of the average purchase price in Europe in 1987 plus approximate air-freight costs for a distance equivalent to that from Europe to Africa and special packaging costs for inflammable and corrosive substances.

Fig. 28a-1a DISINFECTANTS FOR HIV. *WHO AIDS Series (2), 'Guidelines on Sterilization and High-Level Disinfection Methods Effective Against the Human Immunodeficiency Virus (HIV). Geneva 1988.*

ing, and HIV probably is too. WHO recommends 20 minutes to be sure.

CAUTION ! In practice, chemical disinfectants are not reliable, because: (1) They may be inactivated by blood or other organic matter. (2) They must be prepared carefully. (3) Some of them rapidly lose their strength when stored in a warm place. *Chemical disinfection must not be used for needles and syringes,* and should only be used for skin-cutting and invasive instruments as a last resort, and then only after the instruments have been properly cleaned, and disinfected in solutions that are correctly used.

Both viruses are also destroyed by the following solutions applied for *not less than 10 minutes* and preferably for longer: (1) Chlorine-releasing solutions, see below. (2) Ethanol 70% (higher and lower concentrations are less effective). (3) 2-propanol (isopropyl alcohol) 70%. (4) Povidone iodine 2.5% for 15 minutes. (5) Formaldehyde 4% (40% solution diluted 1:10) for 30 minutes); this is corrosive, so rinse equipment thoroughly. (6) Glutaraldehyde 2% activated (made alkaline) with a powder supplied with the solution. (7) Hydrogen peroxide 6% (30% solution diluted 1:4). See also Sections 2.4 and 2.5, and make sure that all instruments are *thoroughly washed* before being immersed in disinfectant.

CAUTION ! The following methods are NOT recommended: (1) Solutions of spirit less than 70%, and especially less than 50%. (2) Cetrimide ('Cetavlon') and chlorhexidine ('Hibitane') are not effective, although the 70% spirit in which they are usually made up is effective. (3) 0.1% formalin (stronger concentrations are effective). (4) 'Dettol', 'Roxenol', flavine, etc.

SPECIAL CAUTION ! Washing instruments and then immersing them in 1% cetrimide for 3 minutes between cases is NOT safe!

CHLORINE releasing compounds are excellent disinfectants. Their power is expressed as 'available chlorine': % for solid compounds, and % or parts per million (ppm) for solutions. 0.0001% = 1 mg/litre = 1 ppm. 1% = 10 g/litre = 10,000 ppm. Chlorometric degrees (° chlorom) are sometimes used, 1°chlorom = 0.3% available chlorine.

Chlorine corrodes iron and stainless steel, so don't store these disinfectants in stainless steel containers, or use them repeatedly for disinfecting good quality stainless steel equipment. Immerse such equipment for less than 30 minutes and rinse it well.

Sodium hypochlorite solutions (liquid bleach, 'eau de Javel' etc.) are unstable. Neat disinfectant solutions ('Domestos', 'Chloros', 'Sterite') contain about 100,000 ppm. Strong hypochlorite solution BP contains not less than 80,000 ppm. Most supermarket brands contain about 50,000 ppm; 'Milton' contains about 10,000 ppm. Hypochlorite is readily inactivated by blood and organic matter, which need increased concentrations to disinfect them.

5000 ppm will inactivate HIV in 1 minute, 50 ppm take 10 minutes. Hypochlorite is very unstable at this dilution, so make up the solution freshly and then discard it.

Calcium hypochlorite (70% available chlorine) and bleaching powder (35% available chlorine) are sold as granules, tablets, or powder, and decompose gradually if they are not protected from heat and light.

Sodium dichlorisocyanurate (NaDCC, 60% available chlorine) is comparatively stable.

Chloramine T, tosylchloramide sodium (25% available chlorine) as powder or tablets is also comparatively stable.

Use chlorine solutions like this:

For general disinfection for wards, theatres, and laboratory benches, **use solutions of 1000 ppm.**

For disinfecting blood, body fluids, excreta, etc., on surfaces flood the area to be disinfected with a solution of hypochlorite diluted to not less than 5000 ppm, and leave it on for half an hour before rinsing. Finally, wipe the area with more hypochlorite.

CAUTION ! (1) When cleaning spills wear gloves. (2) Dilution of the virus by washing is simple and important. (2) If you use alcohol, wipe the surface several times, because alcohol evaporates. (3) Establish the rule "You spill it, you clean it". (4) Make sure your hospital disposes of its contaminated materials safely, and does not put them on a rubbish tip where they may be 'reclaimed' by scavengers.

VIRKON (ANT, also from ECHO), a proprietary antiseptic, is a balanced stable blend of peroxygen compounds (mainly inorganic salts), surfactant, and organic acids in an inorganic buffer system at pH 2.6. It is a stable pink/grey powder in sachets of 50 g or in buckets, and is non-corrosive, non-bleaching, and non-toxic, and is not a transport hazard. For disinfecting needles and syringes, use it as a *fresh* 1% solution for at least 10 minutes; 30 minutes is better.

PREVENTING AIDS AND HEPATITIS B DURING SURGERY

Wear gloves whenever you deal with body fluids, and an apron, and a gown when you operate. Double gloves are little extra protection. Avoid getting blood on your skin, and especially into cuts or wounds. Full glasses will protect your eyes, if an artery spurts blood into them; aerosol and splash injury to the conjunctiva has not been recorded as transmitting either virus. If you do get blood or body fluids on yourself, wash immediately.

SYRINGES, NEEDLES, AND NEEDLESTICK INJURIES. Shortage of needles is going to compel you to reuse them.

In practice, make sure that anyone who cleans and washes needles and syringes uses gloves, so that any HIV in them does not get into any cuts he may have on his skin. The best method of sterilization is heat, by boiling or autoclaving, or where practical in a hot-air oven (provided they have been well cleaned first). If you use a disinfectant such as 'Virkon' or hypochlorite, the criteria for killing HIV and HBV must be fulfilled (see above). Ask staff on the wards to squirt syringes and needles through with water, to immerse them in 'Virkon' or hypochlorite, and to send them for sterilizing.

Ideally, use a new needle for each patient and discard the old syringe, needle, and protective sheath into a safe puncture- and leak-proof container (a 'sharps bin': if necessary an old beer can, as the small hole makes a 'non-return' valve), *without resheathing the needle*. This is the occasion when you are most likely to puncture yourself accidentally.

BED LINEN, etc. It is impractical to destroy contaminated linen, or to ask AIDS patients to wash their own linen. You are unlikely to have enough disinfectant (hypochlorite or lysol) to disinfect it, or to be able to boil it. The only practical steps you may be able to take are to sluice it using gloves (the usual practice anyway), to launder it (preferably hot) as best you can with a detergent, and to hang it out in the sun; and to require that the laundry staff should wear gloves for general hygiene, and avoid frank blood and faeces. In practice, ordinary domestic or institutional laundery using heat and detergent in a washing machine is effective. If facilities are stretched, laundry from AIDS patients should have priority.

HEALTH EDUCATION. (1) Emphasize that healthy carriers, not AIDS patients are the main means of transmission. (2) Make sure that you and your staff do all you can to tell the community how HIV is spread, and how it is not spread. Organize lectures, seminars, and group discussions for community leaders, government leaders, church leaders, hospital and health centre staff, and student nurses and paramedicals. Secondary *and primary schoolchildren* are important target groups. Include AIDS in the health education talks you give to all inpatients and outpatients, and especially to all antenatal mothers. Make the most of drama groups. Place posters in public places. Discuss methods of spread with the relatives and contacts of AIDS patients, who should be screened.

SYMPTOMATIC TREATMENT FOR AIDS

An AIDS patient has usually to be cared for at home. As with a terminal cancer patient (33.1), admit him to establish the diagnosis, and start what treatment is possible for his main problems. Base your decision to admit him subsequently on: (1) How ill he is at a given time, (2) how far away he lives from a hospital or health centre, and (3) his home circumstances.

Here are a few of the many conditions you may have to treat:

Diarrhoea. Rehydrate him with oral rehydration salts (ORS). *Isospora belli* responds to co-trimoxazole. Most AIDS-related diarrhoea (*Cryptosporidium*, etc) is incurable, but symptoms fluctuate, and loperamide ('Imodium') usually improves them.

Tuberculosis. Treat this. Suspect HIV if a patient with tuberculosis does not improve on treatment, or if he develops some new manifestation of it while he is being treated, or has an adverse drug reaction. Watch out for tuberculous lymph nodes (29.2).

Oral candidiasis. Nystatin is ineffective and ketoconazole may not be absorbed if he has achlorhydria (common).

Atypical African Kaposi's sarcoma (AAKS, 32.21) is well worth treating by chemotherapy.

Pneumocystis pneumonia. Suspect this if you see widespread fluffy opacities in his chest X-ray (in Zambia these are more likely to be due to AAKS); you will be unable to confirm it. Give him trimethoprim for 6 weeks, but expect only temporary improvement.

If an HIV-positive person in Africa develops pulmonary symptoms suspect: (1) bacterial or viral pneumonia (the former normally responding to antibiotics). (2) Tuberculosis, which may be radiologically atypical (29.1). (3) Pulmonary Kaposi's sarcoma (look for purple patches on his palate or gums). (3) Other infections, not yet identified.

If he has malaise and fever without clear symptoms or signs suggesting a cause (common), try erythromycin or trimethoprim empirically for 7–10 days.

If he is paralysed and immobile, treat any bed sores he develops as in Section 33.2.

SUMMARY

AIDS is a serious threat to mankind. Health workers in the developing world have a particular responsibility: (1) *To really care* for AIDS patients. Get close to them, examine inpatients frequently; greet them, and be seen to shake hands with them. (2) Control the spread of HIV through blood and blood products. (3) Establish a means of testing for HIV. (4) Make sure that syringes, needles, and instruments don't spread it. (5) When you operate, try not to prick yourself or your assistants.

DIFFICULTIES WITH AIDS

If you want to SCREEN a patient preoperatively for HIV, and have no means of testing him, the following signs will be some help: the multidermatome deep scars of herpes zoster (90% HIV-positive in Central Africa), symmetrical lymphadenopathy, oral thrush (patchy erythema on his palate, or small deposits in his gingivobuccal sulcus), and unexplained weight loss.

If you want a set of CLINICAL CRITERIA for the diagnosis of AIDS, use the BANGUI CRITERIA. The presence of *at least two major symptoms and at least one minor symptom* is sufficient to make a clinical diagnosis of AIDS:

Major symptoms. (1) Unexplained fever for longer than a month. (2) Unexplained diarrhoea for longer than a month. (3) More than 10% weight loss.

Minor symptoms. (1) A maculopapular rash. (2) Oral candidiasis. (3) Herpes zoster. (4) Aggressive or uncontrollable herpes simplex. (5) Unexplained cough for more than a month. (6) Large nodes in more than one extrainguinal site.

If DIAGNOSIS IS DIFFICULT, consider BIOPSY. Symmetrical nodes of modest size (<2.0 cm) don't need it. For nodes which make you suspect Kaposi's sarcoma, see Section 32.21.

If a group of nodes is asymmetric (a group of nodes in one axilla or on one side of the neck), **biopsy one.** You may find tuberculosis or lymphoma, both treatable. Solitary enlarged nodes are rare.

HEALTH EDUCATION IS THE WAY TO PREVENT AIDS

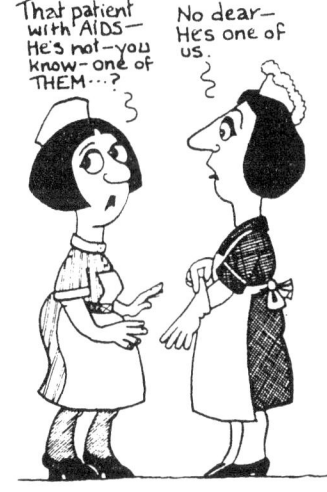

Drawn by Cath Jackson, with the kind permission of the Terence Higgins Trust.

28a.3 AIDS and surgery

Although the complete surgical pathology of HIV is unknown, it is likely to alter the practice of surgery in several ways:

(1) HIV influences the surgical diseases that a patient presents with, because it alters his response to infections. If he is HIV-positive, infections which would normally be only a minor nuisance, may become serious abscesses (5.1). A minor genital infection may become PID (6.6). There is also a peculiar and unusual type of osteitis described in Section 7.6D. Surgical tuberculosis (29.1) is also more common.

(2) HIV may alter his response to surgery, and therefore the indications for major surgery, in a way which varies geographically. In London, HIV-positive patients and patients with frank AIDS disorders, such as pneumocystis or serious gastrointestinal infections, can heal their wounds and deal with bacterial sepsis much as a normal person would. In Central Africa, an HIV-positive patient is surgically normal and heals well unless: (a) He has chronic sepsis *at the operation site,* as with a perianal, or ischiorectal abscess, or a fistula, which is unlikely to heal normally when it is excised or laid open. If however the operation wound does not go through an area of chronic sepsis (as with an amputation), you can expect him to heal normally. (b) He is very ill with AIDS. If so, a surgical wound through normal tissue (as with an amputation), will heal badly; just as it would do if he was cachectic from a terminal cancer.

There appears to be an increased rate of infection in orthopaedic implants, and of the breakdown of reconstructive procedures (VVFs, 18.18, etc).

HIV-positivity is not necessarily therefore a contraindication to surgery. However, in Africa: (a) If he has chronic sepsis at the operation site, you will have to weigh up the effects of not operating, with those of a poor response if you do operate. (b) If he is seriously 'ill' with frank AIDS, you can expect that healing will be impaired. In general, if you expect him to live for years, months, or even some weeks, operate. If not, as with a terminal cancer patient, don't.

(3) HIV is a potential risk to the surgical team. Fortunately, this risk appears to be low, and to be much less than that of acquiring HBV. The most serious, but least likely event, is a needlestick injury that results in the actual injection of contaminated blood, or some other body fluid. This has only been recorded as having happened with certainty on four occasions, whereas several hundred health workers have pricked themselves without converting serologically, or developing AIDS.

Nevertheless, AIDS in a highly endemic area has added to the risks of surgery. When only an occasional patient is HIV-positive, the risk is negligible. Nobody knows how high it is when 20% of the ordinary surgical patients are HIV-positive, say one in every list, during a surgical career of 30 years. As we write, one and probably two doctors in sub-Saharan Africa are known to have contracted AIDS in the course of duty. Of the health workers presently suffering from AIDS worldwide, 95% have been found to have non-occupational exposures that have put them at high risk of acquiring it.

An infected person is thought to shed HIV for life, but he is probably most infectious soon after exposure, before antibodies have developed, and later about the time when the p24 antibodies decline, and clinical illness ('preAIDS') starts. Clinical disease, or markers of progression (falling T4 counts), do however increase the chance of infecting sexual partners or children, and the same may be true in the theatre.

Should you operate? You cannot screen all surgical patients before you do, although you can suspect HIV infection (28a.2D). We argue most strongly that, on the correct indications, you should operate. In addition to the general indications as to when and when not to operate, which are given in Section 1.8, you will need to consider a patient's response to surgery, as described above.

Several contributors work under conditions where the HIV rate is 5 to 30%, and believe that the risk to a careful surgeon is low. We advise you how to reduce this risk, although you cannot, alas, abolish it. Wear goggles, use two pairs of gloves, use scissor dissection where possible, and don't operate on an HIV-positive patient when you are tired at the end of a list and therefore less likely to be careful.

In common with many other callings, the care of the sick has often involved risk, and probably always will. Before the discovery of penicillin, streptococcal septicaemia from a finger prick not uncommonly killed surgeons (see the story of Hamilton Bailey, 2.10). For a period of about 40 years (1945 to 1985) antibiotics changed all that, and left only hepatitis B as an appreciable risk. With AIDS, we are back were we were. Surgery has risks and, whether we like it or not, is nobler by having them.

Life is dangerous, and is 100% fatal, in that we are all going to die some time. Much of the skill of living it depends on taking a proper view of the risks that might end it. The risks of dying from AIDS contracted in the theatre are likely to be much less than at least two others: (1) Dying on the roads, which continues to kill many doctors in the developing world. One contributor to this manual died in this way while it was being written, and the senior editor has himself had two very narrow escapes. So fasten your seat belt, and see Section 50.2. (2) Contracting AIDS promiscuously. The safety precaution here is clear.

Sim AJW and Dudley HAF, 'AIDS and the surgeon'. Br Med J 1988;296:80

28a.4 Hepatitis B

Although hepatitis in its various forms is an important cause of disease all over the developing world, its importance in district hospital surgery is mainly restricted to: (1) The need to distinguish hepatitis from surgical obstruction to the bile ducts (32.26). (2) The danger of hepatitis virus B (HBV) to you and your staff.

HBV invades the cells of the liver and releases a complex series of antigens. These and the antibodies to them can be detected in the blood. You will not be able to detect them, so no more will be said about them here, except that, in an acute attack which is successfully recovered from, the surface antigen (HBsAg) appears in the blood and is then replaced by the antibody (anti-HBs). In chronic hepatitis, when the patient becomes a carrier, HBsAg persists, and no anti-HBs appears. Highly infectious carriers ('super carriers') are also HBeAg-positive.

Hepatitis B has a low prevalence in the industrial world, but is highly endemic in China, South-East Asia, sub-Saharan Africa and in the Amazon basin. In these areas most people are infected at birth, or in early childhood; 5–30% of the population become chronically infected with the virus or carriers of it, and most adults show serological evidence of having had it.

The virus persists in the liver of carriers (see below), and is present in the blood, semen, milk and other body fluids. Transmission is the result of the accidental inoculation of minute amounts of blood, or body fluids, which enables HBV to spread: (1) Vertically from a carrier mother to her infant; this usually occurs during delivery, and infection during pregnancy (i.e in utero) is rare. This is the common route of infection in China, South-East Asia, and Africa. (2) Horizontally among children through scratches and small sores. This is another common route in Africa. By the age of 25 years 75% of people in some endemic areas in the developing world have been infected by one or other of these routes. (3) Through blood transfusions and imperfectly sterilized needles. (5) By vaginal or anal intercourse. (6) Among the inmates of institutions, such as those for the mentally handicapped.

If an infant is infected, there is a greater than 90% chance that he will have a subclinical infection; and a small chance that he will have a clinical attack, which is usually mild. There is also a a significant chance that he will progress to chronic active hepatitis (CAH), or to chronic progressive hepatitis (CPH), as the result of becoming a carrier. Many cases of CAH progress to cirrhosis, and some of these to hepatoma, which is the commonest malignant tumour in the developing world (32.26).

If an adult is infected, there is a 90% chance that he will have an acute clinical attack of hepatitis, with or without jaundice (fulminating and commonly fatal in about 1%), and a 5% chance that he will become an asymptomatic carrier. If he becomes a carrier, he has a 4% chance of developing CPH or CAH, perhaps leading to cirrhosis and hepatoma.

If the surface antigen (HBsAg) persists for more than 6 months after an attack, the patient is a carrier. The earlier he is infected,

HEPATITIS B

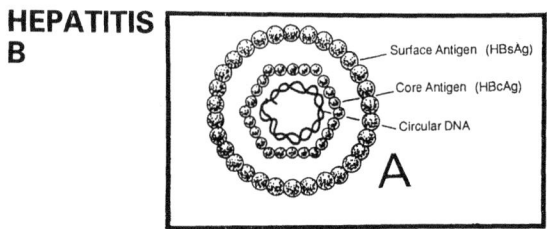

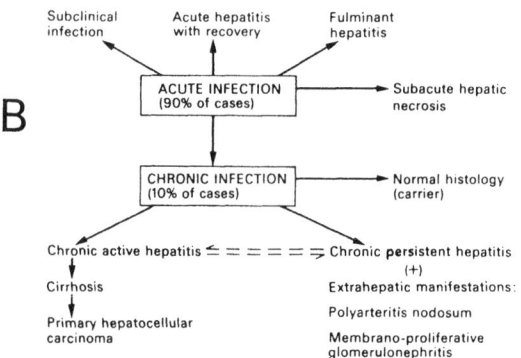

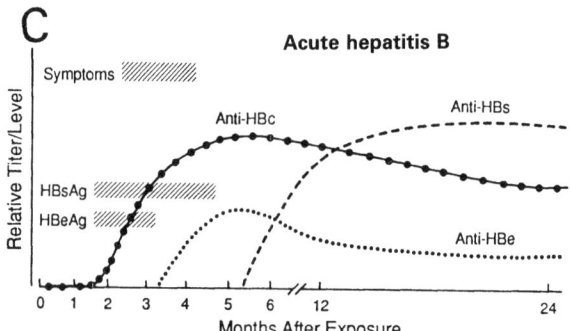

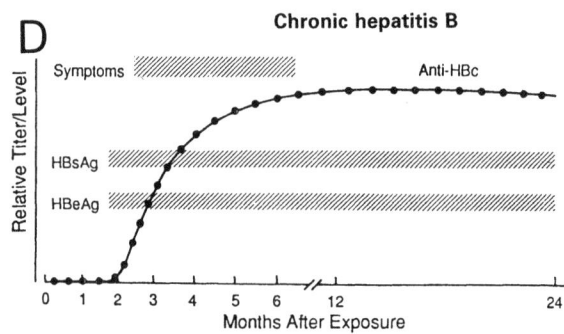

Fig. 28a-2. HEPATITIS B. A, the structure of the virus. B, the clinical syndromes associated with acute and chronic HBV infection. C, antigen and antibody levels in acute hepatitis. D, antigen and antibody levels in chronic hepatitis. *A, C, and D, Program of Appropriate Technology in Health (PATH), Vol 6, No. 3, Figs 1 and 2. B, from the Oxford Textbook of Medicine. Both with kind permission.*

the more likely he is to become one. At birth, the risk is 80 to 90% if a child's mother is a carrier (HBsAg and HBeAg positive, a 'super carrier'). The risk is about 50% during the first 5 years of life, and only about 5% if the infection occurs in adult life. The carrier state usually lasts for life.

Chronic hepatitis is hepatic inflammation which lasts longer than 6 months. It takes two forms, which may be associated with hepatitis B, or with other conditions: (1) Chronic persistent hepatitis (CPH), in which inflammatory cells are confined to the portal tracts; the patient is asymptomatic, with no physical signs of liver disease, and only minor biochemical abnormalities. His prognosis is good, and he seldom gets cirrhosis. (2) Chronic active hepatitis (CAH), in which inflammatory cells extend beyond his portal tracts, and he is unwell and jaundiced, with abnormal liver function tests; he is likely to become cirrhotic, and is at increased risk of hepatoma.

The risks of hospital-acquired infection differ in the industrial and the developing world. In the industrial world carriers are uncommon, but when they occur health workers are at risk, because they are unlikely to have met the virus before. In the developing world many chronic carriers come to surgery, but as most indigenous health workers will already have been infected, usually subclinically in infancy or childhood, subsequent reinfection in the theatre is unimportant. The risk is that, in caring for a carrier patient, a small quantity of blood or body fluid will enter the circulation of a non-immune health worker, and infect him with HBV, the commonest cause of infection being a needlestick injury. Unlike HIV, a very small quantity of blood may be infectious. The risk varies according to state of the infected patient, and the circumstance. High risks are: (1) Patients with acute hepatitis B. (2) HBsAg and HBeAg positive 'super carriers'. (3) HBsAg positive carriers, who do not at the same time have antiHBe.

HEPATITIS B

For sterilization and prevention during surgery see Sections 2.5 and 28a.2.

If you grew up in the developing world, you are probably immune from reinfection. If however you come from the urban elite, and so may not have met the virus before, you may still acquire it.

If you grew up in the industrial world and work in the developing world, you are at particular risk, because you will probably not have met the virus before, and will treat many chronic carriers. If you become infected, your chances are those of any other adult, as described above— a 1% chance of fulminant hepatitis, a 4% chance of CAH, and a 5% chance of becoming a carrier. You would be wise to be immunized.

PASSIVE IMMUNIZATION. Hepatitis B immunoglobulin (HBIG, expensive) gives immediate protection which lasts about 6 months. A dose given early in the incubation period will either be protective, or modify the attack considerably.

ACTIVE IMMUNIZATION. Vaccine is expensive, but advances in genetic engineering promise to make it cheaper. It can withstand being out of the cold chain for 30 days. Give three doses at months 0, 1 and 6. Give infants and children under 12 5—10 μg, give adults 10—20 μg. It is 95% effective.

If a baby has a 'super carrier' mother (HBsAg and HBeAg positive), he is at risk of becoming a carrier. Unfortunately, you are unlikely to be able to test for the carrier state. Give him vaccine within the first 3 days of birth, preferably on the first day, accompanied by HBIG 0.5 ml into the other thigh. Repeat the vaccine only at 1 month and 6 months. It is 95% effective, if HBIG is also given, and only 80–90% effective without it.

HAVING 'Dr' IN FRONT OF YOUR NAME DOES NOT MAKE YOU IMMUNE!

---

29 The surgery of tuberculosis

29.1 Chemotherapy for tuberculosis

In addition to treating pulmonary tuberculosis, you may have to treat 'surgical' tuberculosis in a patient's lymph nodes (29.2), his bones and joints (29.3), his abdomen (29.5), his urinogenital tract (29.6), and in a woman's breasts, where it can present as a lump (21.3), or as an oedematous swelling, due to the involvement of her axillary nodes (31.6). Diagnosing tuberculosis can be difficult. In the developing world, and particularly if BCG has been given, a positive tuberculin test strengthens the diagnosis, *only if it is strongly positive* (for example Mantoux test > 30 mm at 72 hours). A persistently negative one makes the diagnosis of tuberculosis unlikely, unless the patient is severely ill (as with miliary tuberculosis), is HIV-positive (see below), or is very malnourished, or has some other severe illness.

If you can send tissue for histology, especially a lymph node, the diagnosis of tuberculosis is easily confirmed. If this is impossible, or will take too long, you can usually tell if tissue is tuberculous, by cutting it across and looking for caseous areas. Finally, "If you can't think of a diagnosis, always remember the possibility of tuberculosis".

The same drugs that are used for pulmonary tuberculosis are highly successful in surgical tuberculosis—if a patient takes them regularly, and completes the course. The great danger is that he will stop taking them as soon as he feels a little better. The regime that you choose to use will have to depend on: (1) how much money there is for drugs, (2) how easy it will be for him to attend a clinic for injections of streptomycin, (3) if (based on (1) and (2)) you decide to admit him, and (4) if drug resistance is likely. It is unlikely, except in patients who have been partly treated before. We give several alternative regimes below, and there will probably be a standard one in your area. Most regimes have an initial intensive phase, followed by a continuation phase. Never treat tuberculosis with a single drug, because of the risk of acquired resistance.

Isoniazid is the main drug, and if rifampicin were not so expensive, it would be the best companion drug to go with it. Because it is so expensive, you will probably have to use thiacetazone with isoniazid in a compound tablet. Thiacetazone is widely used in Africa, but some communities elsewhere show an unacceptably high frequency of adverse reactions to it. Fortunately, the prices of rifampicin and ethambutol are falling. In India, streptomycin, INAH, and thiacetazone are provided free at tuberculosis centres; the difficulty is getting patients to go to them. Unfortunately, there are times when even these drugs are not available.

Supervise a patient carefully. If he does not complete his course of treatment, the organisms infecting him may become resistant, his disease may progress, and he may need extensive surgery—if he can get it. If he fails to attend for outpatient treatment, see that somebody visits him at home.

Treat surgical tuberculosis with drugs, and try not to drain tuberculous abscesses, unless you have to. If they have to be drained, close the wound without inserting a drain. For a tuberculous spine, or a large joint, use a suction drain. The danger is that they may become secondarily infected. Before the introduction of chemotherapy, draining a tuberculous abscess often led to a persistent sinus, and was sometimes fatal.

HE MUST CONTINUE TO TAKE HIS DRUGS

HIV and tuberculosis. Highly pathogenic organisms, such as *Myc. tuberculosis* may infect HIV-positive patients early, before immune deficiency has fully developed. Less virulent ones, such as *Myc. avium-intracellulare*, strike later, when immune deficiency is complete. Tuberculosis may thus precede AIDS by several months. The risk of an HIV-positive patient acquiring tuberculosis depends on the prevalence of the disease in the local population. In Zambia, where both diseases are common, about 50% of new tuberculous patients are HIV-positive, commonly with multibacillary forms of the disease.

Fever, fatigue, and weight loss are common in both diseases. In an HIV-positive patient, tuberculosis affects the lungs less often than other parts of the body, and may become widely disseminated to involve: the lymph nodes (these cannot be distinguished from those enlarged by HIV alone), the joints, the spine, the blood (miliary tuberculosis), the genitourinary tract, the liver, the peritoneum, and the central nervous system (tuberculomas, cerebral abscesses, and meningitis). There may be little or no granuloma formation, and few lymphocytes in the lesions ('areactive' tuberculosis).

The X-ray appearances of pulmonary tuberculosis are often atypical in an HIV-positive patient. His hilar and mediastinal lymph nodes are commonly enlarged, as are his middle or lower lobes, while his upper ones are spared; cavitation is rare. There is only a 40% chance that he is tuberculin-positive, and when he is, the reaction is weak and often becomes negative later.

Give him a standard course of treatment. Bacilli will probably disappear from his sputum in one to three months. Treat him for 9 months, and consider giving him daily isoniazid after that to prevent relapse. HIV increases the incidence of adverse drug reactions, particularly, it is said, to thiacetazone, so suspect HIV when these occur.

IF YOU CAN'T THINK OF A DIAGNOSIS, THINK OF TUBERCULOSIS

CHEMOTHERAPY FOR TUBERCULOSIS

ISONIAZID (INAH). Daily dose 300 mg, children 10 mg/kg. Intermittent adult dose 15 mg/kg, with pyridoxine 10 mg per dose to prevent neurotoxicity.

THIACETAZONE. Daily dose 150 mg, children 4 mg/kg.

STREPTOMYCIN. Daily dose: if a patient is less than 50 kg give him 750 mg daily, if he is more than 50 kg give him 1 g daily if he is under 40, and 750 mg daily if he is over 40; children 20 mg/kg. The disadvantage of streptomycin is that it has to be injected, but in some communities injections are best.

RIFAMPICIN. Daily dose: less than 50 kg give the patient 450 mg, more than 50 kg give him 600 mg; children 10 to 20 mg/kg. Intermittent adult dose 600 to 900 mg.

PYRAZINAMIDE. Daily dose, less than 50 kg give him 1.5 g, more than 50 kg give him 2.0 g; children 30 mg/kg. Intermittent dose 3 times a week: give him 2.0 g if he is less than 50 kg, and 2.5 g if he is more than 50 kg. Intermittent dose twice a week: give him 3.0 g if he is less than 50 kg, and 3.5 g if he is more than 50 kg.

ETHAMBUTOL. Daily dose 25 mg/kg for 2 months, then 15 mg/kg; children as for adults if aged 12 years or more. Intermittent dose three times a week 30 mg; twice a week 45 mg.

REGIMES

(1) Daily throughout. The common regime in India and in East and Central Africa is daily streptomycin for 60 days at 20 mg/kg. Starting at the same time, give thiacetazone and INAH as a compound tablet ('Thiazina' or 'Isozone Forte') for 12 or 18 months. For an adult this contains thiacetazone 150 mg (3 mg/kg) and INAH 300 mg (6 mg/kg). It has a 92% success rate in previously untreated cases—if he completes the course. The drugs for the entire course cost $30. You may occasionally have to admit him to give him his streptomycin, which will add to the cost, but the cost of 2 months' admission is low compared with the cost of rifampicin.

(2) Daily throughout. Two months of daily streptomycin, isoniazid, rifampicin, and pyrazinamide, followed by 6 months of daily isoniazid and thiacetazone. Total duration 8 months, success rate 98%.

(3) Partly intermittent. Streptomycin, isoniazid, rifampicin, and pyrazinamide daily for 2 months. Then streptomycin, isoniazid, and pyrazinamide twice a week for 6 months. Total duration 8 months.

(4) Intermittent throughout. Streptomycin, isoniazid, rifampicin, and pyrazinamide 3 times a week for 4 months, then isoniazid, rifampicin, and pyrazinamide 3 times a week for 2 months. Total duration 6 months.

CAUTION ! Always aim to give antituberculous treatment as a complete regime. Shorter courses are likely to be ineffective, and promote drug-resistance.

ADMISSION. If he does not live near a clinic, where he can get injections, admit him to give him his streptomycin.

NO ADMISSION. If you are not going to admit him, and can afford rifampicin, use one of the intermittent regimes. They all contain isoniazid, rifampicin, and pyrazinamide. If giving him an injection is likely to encourage his compliance, then the regime should contain streptomycin. A completely oral intermittent regime of ethambutol, isoniazid, rifampicin, and pyrazinamide is equally effective, but more expensive.

If cost is critical, give him regime (1). But if he lives near a clinic, a fully supervised regime like regime (3) is likely to prove more successful and less toxic.

If cost is less critical, use regime (4).

If, in the local community, there is a high prevalence of strains of bacilli which are resistant to streptomycin and isoniazid, you will have to use a four-drug regime. This is only likely to be the case when there are many people who do not complete their treatment. If so, your follow-up programme needs improvement.

TOXICITY

Be aware, and make your staff aware, of the the toxic reactions of antituberculous drugs, *especially those outlined below like this*.

ISONIAZID (INAH). (1) Peripheral neuritis, ±30%. Painful 'hot' soles of the feet, especially in patients whose livers metabolize the drug slowly. You can usually continue treatment, if you notice the condition early. Give him pyridoxine 20 or 25 mg/day. If pain forces you to stop INAH, give another drug. (2) *Psychoses*, ±0.5%, reversible, stop INAH immediately. (3) *Jaundice* <0.5%, reversible if you stop INAH fairly soon.

THIACETAZONE. (1) *Dermatosis*. 30% of light-skinned persons (Caucasians and mongoloids), ±5% of Africans. Typically itchy, black, 2 to 4 cm patches with a centre that may peel. Also, diffuse darkening of the skin with itching (less common). If noticed immediately, partially reversible.

STREPTOMYCIN. (1) *Rash*, ±5%, typically small widespread maculopapules usually accompanied by fever. Stop the drug.

(2) Drug fever, ±5%. Stop the drug. (3) Dysfunction of the vestibular branch of the 8th nerve (vertigo, giddiness). If mild, continue. If moderate to severe, stop the drug. (4) Dysfunction of the cochlear function of the 8th nerve (*deafness*). Stop immediately: irreversible unless the drug is immediately discontinued.

RIFAMPICIN. (1) Transient jaundice usually 2 or 3 weeks after starting treatment. Unless jaundice is progressive, continue the drug. Liver function tests nearly always show some abnormality. (2) If his urine becomes orange-red, this is not a sign of toxicity, it always happens. (3) Gastrointestinal symptoms, usually minor. (4) Drug fever (uncommon). (5) An MOI (monoamine oxidase inhibitor)-like action (uncommon), with intolerance to cheese, fish and meat extracts, and sensitivity to alcohol.

PYRAZINAMIDE. Arthralgia, hepatotoxicity, and urticaria are all unusual.

ETHAMBUTOL. (1) *Visual impairment*, ±1%, reversible if recognized quickly and the drug is stopped. *Test the visual acuity (24.1) of all patients on this drug* every 2 weeks, and make them aware that they must report any slight deterioration in acuity.

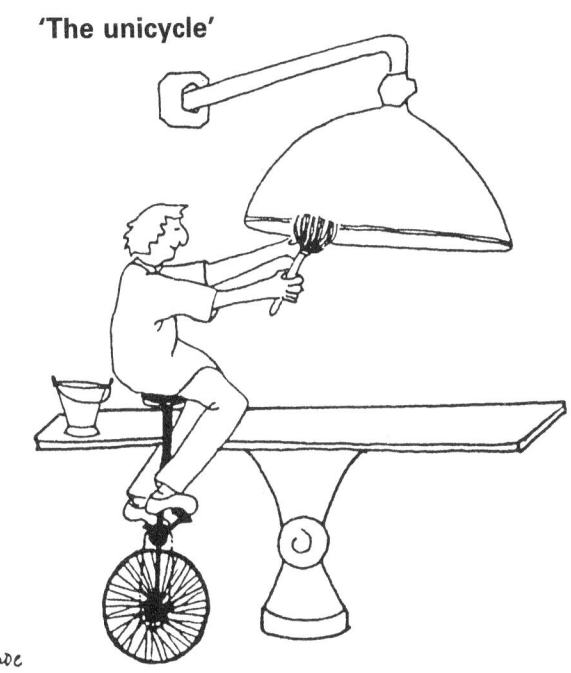

'The unicycle'

29.2 Tuberculous lymphadenitis

Widespread tuberculosis of the lymph nodes is not uncommon in many areas. It usually involves the nodes of the neck, or less often those of the axilla, iliac region, or groin, mainly in children and young adults, although no age is exempt. All four triangles of neck may contain matted masses of glands. If these are not treated, abscesses may form and discharge through the skin, to leave sinuses which may become secondarily infected. After many months, these abscesses may heal spontaneously, to cause severe fibrosis and lymphatic obstruction in the leg (31.4), arm, breast (31.4), or vulva (20.14).

TUBERCULOUS LYMPHADENITIS. Biopsy a lymph node to confirm the diagnosis. You may find that tuberculous lymphadenitis is so common that you cannot biopsy every suspect node. But remember that biopsy is simple, and needs only local anaesthesia.

Give chemotherapy (29.1). Don't excise the enlarged nodes. Don't be alarmed if they enlarge temporarily during chemotherapy, or, rarely, after it, without microbiological relapse. This is due to hypersensitivity to tuberculoprotein. All nodes become smaller in time

29.3 Tuberculous bones and joints

When tuberculosis involves a patient's skeleton, it is the involvement of his joints that matters most—his spine, hips, knees, feet, elbows, wrists, and shoulders, in this order of frequency, and occasionally his other joints also. Bacilli reach his joints from some focus elsewhere. So look for lesions in his lungs, and for signs of surgical tuberculosis in other parts of his body. Look particularly for enlargement of his lymph nodes.

He is usually a young adult, or a child over 6 years, although children as young as a year and older people can also be infected. He complains that one or more of his joints has become progressively painful and stiff during the previous few weeks. If his leg is involved, his first complaint is a limp. His infected joint fills with fluid, and the muscles round it waste. He usually has only mild to moderate pain, except on forced movement. Tuberculous arthritis is 'cold', which means that the skin over his infected joint is the same temperature as his normal skin. His joint is not 'hot', as it is in septic arthritis. Sometimes he has systemic symptoms, such as mild fever, night sweats, or loss of weight or appetite. Pain and fever may be quite marked. He may also have signs of tuberculosis in his chest, or a family history of it.

In a synovial joint, the disease starts in the synovium and grows slowly over the cartilage; it then extends through the cartilage into the underlying bone, which decalcifies. In the spine, disease starts in a disc. If you can treat him before his cartilage is destroyed, his joint will recover fully, or nearly so. If you start later, his articular cartilage will be destroyed, so that even if his disease is arrested, his joint will develop a fibrous ankylosis (except in the spine, when ankylosis is always bony). Sometimes, cold abscesses and sinuses form, become secondarily infected, and may track for a considerable distance.

If a tuberculous joint is secondarily infected, the ankylosis that results is always bony.

His diseased limb develops a flexion contracture, and its joints may subluxate or dislocate, especially his hip, knee, shoulder, or elbow.

You can treat tuberculous joints successfully and cheaply—if you diagnose them early enough, and can make sure that a patient takes his drugs. 'Early', here means the first few weeks. But even if treatment starts late, when his joint surfaces have already been destroyed, he can expect a fairly good result—if you can prevent deformities and contractures.

There are no certain diagnostic signs, so the secret is always to be suspicious. Whenever you see *any* chronic bone or joint disease, ask yourself: "Might this be tuberculous?" If it is, you can treat it. Biopsying a node or the synovium will confirm the diagnosis in about half the cases (see below). If you cannot send tissue for biopsy, you will probably have to rely on the characteristic X-ray changes. Even so, your error rate should be small.

Try to: (1) Give him the drugs he needs in adequate doses for an adequate period—much the most important. (2) Rest his joint; if his arm is involved, you can usually treat it in a sling, but if he has tuberculosis of his leg, you will probably have to admit him. (3) If he has disease of his hip or knee, apply traction. This will overcome spasm, prevent his softened bone from collapsing, and keep his inflamed joint surfaces apart. Experts can do major operations to remove or drain a tuberculous lesion, or promote ankylosis. For these, you will have to refer him.

TUBERCULOUS ARTHRITIS

X-RAYS. Look for: (1) Generalized rarefaction—the patient's whole joint is less dense than it should be. The earliest stage is a lack of definition—his joint is not as sharp as it should be. (2) Localized areas of erosion or decreased density, caused by caseous lesions in the bone. (3) The joint space may be abnormally narrow or wide. (4) In late cases it is irregular.
CAUTION ! Joint destruction in tuberculosis is always more severe than the X-ray appearances suggest. (2) Remember to X-ray his lungs.

SPECIAL TESTS. (1) A positive tuberculin test is only of limited value (29.1).

(2) If a joint is swollen, aspirate it by the methods in Section 7.17, and examine the fluid as in Section 79.3. Great patience may occasionally find AAFB in a stained film of the exudate. Most laboratories reckon that this is not worth doing. If possible, send the fluid for culture, and guinea-pig inoculation (even then it is not always positive). You will not know the answer for several weeks.

(3) If he has any enlarged lymph nodes that might be tuberculous, biopsy one. The biopsy of synovial tissue is indicated in special cases only. Taking a biopsy from his spine is difficult, but you may be able to take one from his hip. Use the anterolateral approach, as for septic arthritis (7.18). Biopsy his knee by the methods in Section 7.17. When you take a biopsy, use the opportunity to examine his articular cartilage. A biopsy is useful for distinguishing tuberculosis from late, imperfectly-treated staphylococcal arthritis.

CAUTION ! Biopsies are fallible, so accept a negative biopsy with caution. About 50% of cases of tuberculous synovitis are reported as 'non-specific chronic inflammation'.

DIFFERENTIAL DIAGNOSIS. Septic arthritis is the main one.

Suggesting septic arthritis —a history of onset over hours or days, rather than weeks; a 'hot' joint, which is acutely painful to move in any direction. He is 'ill', with a high fever and a leucocytosis. Aspiration produces frank pus, rather than slightly cloudy fluid. Bacteria (usually staphylococci) are visible in a Gram stained film. If septic arthritis has been partly treated, diagnosing it may be difficult.

If his hip is involved, flex his knee to 90° and then flex his hip. If his leg goes into external rotation, as you do this, as in Fig. 7-17, it is a sign that his upper femoral epiphysis is slipping. This is much more likely to happen in septic arthritis (or spontaneous slipping of the epiphysis, 77.10) than it is in tuberculosis.

Both tuberculosis and septic arthritis eventually involve the bone of the pelvis. If it is already involved when you first see him, this suggests tuberculosis.

Suggesting trauma —a history of injury, or a haemarthrosis: the X-ray may be normal, or show widening of the joint.

Suggesting other forms of arthritis —a history of dysentery, brucellosis, or gonorrhoea.

If a joint looks like tuberculosis, but tests are negative, he may have rheumatoid arthritis presenting in a single joint. Other joints may flare up later. If possible, take a biospy, do a Rose–Waaler test, and/or a latex test. Remember that tuberculosis is commoner than monarticular rheumatism in most of the developing world.

If he is a child and his hip is involved, consider Perthes' disease (27.14), or a slipped epiphysis (77.10).

If he is old, or had an injury previously, consider the possibility of osteoarthritis and look for lipping, areas of increased density (eburnation), and sometimes associated cysts (especially in his hip).

TREATMENT FOR SURGICAL TUBERCULOSIS

Start by admitting him in order to: (1) Confirm the diagnosis. (2) Give him the confidence that he can be cured. (3) Convince him that he needs long-term treatment. (4) Apply traction to his lower limb, if this is needed. (5) Give him his initial course of streptomycin, if he lives far from a clinic.

CHEMOTHERAPY. Treat him as in Section 29.1. Do all you can to persuade him to continue treatment to the end. Review him regularly. When his course of treatment is completed, warn him that his joint may flare up again at any time. If so, he must return for further treatment.

POSITION OF FUNCTION. The range of movement of his joint may be limited or absent, so make sure that it is kept in the position of function in Fig. 7-16.

ANKYLOSIS. A fibrous ankylosis may be acceptable, even in his leg, especially if he is a child. It is also acceptable in his arm, provided it is near the optimum position of function—see Fig. 7-16.

PARTICULAR JOINTS INFECTED BY TUBERCULOSIS

SHOULDER. Aim for a loose fibrous ankylosis. Rest his arm in a sling, and then gradually encourage him to do without it. If it is painful at the end of treatment, refer him for an arthrodesis. This will not be a significant disability, because of his scapulo-humeral movement.

ELBOW. An elbow fixed in the position of function as in Fig. 7-16, is likely to be better than a stiff painful one. If non-operative treatment fails to give him a pain-free elbow, refer him for an excision/arthroplasty. This will give him a considerable range of movement, but little stability. Fusion is rarely necessary.

UNTREATED TB OF BOTH HIPS

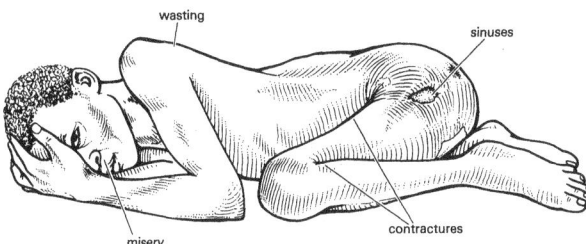

Fig. 29-1 NEGLECTED TUBERCULOSIS OF BOTH HIPS for 29 years. This patient could not even crawl. He dragged himself along in a sitting position, with both his hips and knees fully flexed. *Kindly contributed by Ronald Huckstep.*

HIP. He is usually a child who presents with a painful hip or a limp. For the differential diagnosis, see Section 27.13. Symptoms may start slowly, but he ultimately becomes ill, and fretful, with painful restriction of the movements of his hip. To begin with it is flexed and abducted; later it is flexed and adducted, his leg is shortened, his thigh is wasted, and he may have abscesses in his buttock or groin, as in Fig. 29-1. There is loss of joint space, and a characteristically severe rarefaction of the bone round his hip. If possible, aspirate or explore it, so as to confirm the diagnosis bacteriologically.

Give him chemotherapy and rest his hip, at first in bed only, and then, when pain is a little less, apply skin traction (70.10). If there is abscess formation, and the whole of the head of his femur is necrotic (uncommon in tuberculosis), refer him for the removal of necrotic tissue.

If his hip is in spasm (as diagnosed by rolling it), or his hip or knee show any flexion deformity, apply extension traction (78.3) for several weeks. This will control pain and prevent a flexion contracture.

If there is only narrowing of the joint space, and no bony destruction, allow him up, usually after about 2 months, and let him use his leg cautiously, starting with partial weight bearing, using crutches and a patten (raised shoe) on his normal leg to keep his diseased one off the ground. Skin traction should have corrected any flexion contracture (if present) by this time.

If there is considerable bony destruction, especially of the head of his femur, he still has some hope of a reasonably functioning joint. Don't worry about whether his ankylosis is fibrous or bony. Apply skin traction for 3 months and then get him up on crutches.

Alternatively, and less satisfactorily, put him into a hip spica, in the position of function (7-16). Start him on full weight-bearing. After 3 months, remove his spica and fit him with a removable splint of plaster, leather, or metal, which he can take off for bath or bed. He may need some kind of splint permanently, or until his hip has fixed.

If, after 4 to 6 months, he still has a painful joint with very limited movement or no movement, except under anaesthesia (unusual), consider referring him for operative arthrodesis of his knee, or of his hip. Both these operations should be done during the first two years, while he is still on chemotherapy.

KNEE. He presents with a limp, mild pain, a swollen knee, marked wasting of his quadriceps, limitation of movement (especially extension), and a flexion deformity.

Put him into a Thomas splint, or extension skin traction (78.3), for at least 3 months, and then get him up on crutches. Gradually increase the weight his leg bears, until he is walking as well as he can. If his disease is advanced, or if his pain continues, you may have to fit him with a long leg plaster cylinder; otherwise avoid one.

If a child requires an arthrodesis of his knee, try to delay this until growth has stopped.

ANKLE. Give him chemotherapy, and apply a short leg walking cast (81.5).

TENDON SHEATHS. If he develops a chronic swelling of the tendon sheaths of his hand, or the bursae round his shoulder, don't forget that tuberculosis can involve any of the synovial membranes.

DIFFICULTIES WITH A TUBERCULOUS JOINT

If his symptoms are mild so that DIAGNOSIS is DIFFICULT, you can: (1) Wait 4 to 6 weeks, before committing him to long-term treatment—provided you are sure you are not missing acute untreated septic arthritis. During this time some diseases (transient synovitis and rheumatic fever) will settle, and others may reveal themselves (partly-treated septic arthritis). Tuberculosis will not advance much during this time. (2) Explore the joint, biopsy the synovial membrane, and remove a lymph node for biopsy. An ESR may also be useful.

Alternatively, and less satisfactorily, you can start a trial of treatment with streptomycin and isoniazid for a month. If your diagnosis was correct, the spasm in the muscles round his tuberculous joint will become less, and his general symptoms will improve.

If you are not sure if he has septic arthritis, or tuberculosis, even after opening the joint, treat him for both, and review him later when the histological report is available.

If DEFORMITY PREVENTS SATISFACTORY WALKING, corrective surgery is essential. If an arthrodesis is needed (more likely in the knee than the hip), it is usually best done 6 to 8 weeks after chemotherapy starts.

If an OLD TUBERCULOUS JOINT IS INJURED, observe him closely. A fibrous ankylosis is always unsafe, and can flare up at any time. If pain, etc. continue, and he has no bony injury and no ligament rupture, give him another full course of chemotherapy.

If a COLD ABSCESS develops, leave it, unless it is very big and is causing pain and discomfort. All but the big ones settle on chemotherapy in 12 months. If you have to aspirate a cold abscess (unusual), do so repeatedly with a wide-bore needle. If you can introduce the needle through a long oblique track, a sinus is less likely to form. If it is very large, explore it, clear out its contents, and close it to prevent the entry of secondary infection.

CAUTION ! Don't leave a drain in a cold abscess, or it will become secondarily infected.

If a SINUS develops, it is the result of an abscess opening on to his skin, and is a sign of low resistance. Sinuses are rare

TUBERCULOUS OSTEITIS

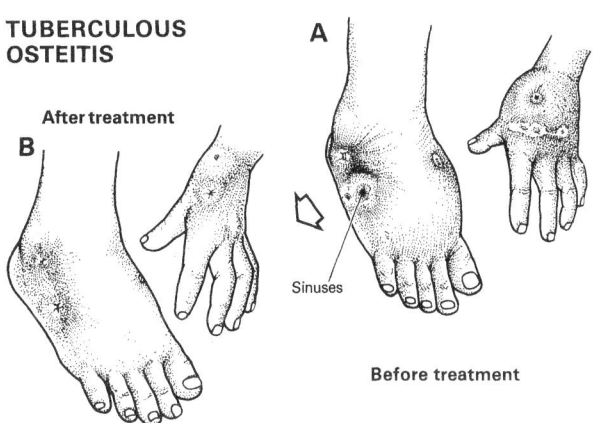

Fig. 29-2 TUBERCULOUS OSTEITIS in this patient improved rapidly on chemotherapy, and his sinuses healed. *Kindly contributed by Gerald Hankins.*

once chemotherapy has started, although an old one may open up temporarily. Chemotherapy will usually close it. A sinus may become secondarily infected, but does not require specific treatment. A biopsy from the track is unlikely to confirm tuberculosis, because non-specific granulation tissue lines it.

If A JOINT BECOMES WARM AND TENDER, with deteriorating X-ray signs, and he has general symptoms, he is experiencing a flare-up. This is unlikely to happen if he has completed his course of treatment, and is a sign that chemotherapy has failed. Consider some other disease, such as septic arthritis, gonococcal arthritis, monarticular rheumatism, or gout. Give him a further course of treatment.

If his LEG ends up SHORT, raise his shoe.

ANY PERPLEXING JOINT IS TUBERCULOUS UNTIL PROVED OTHERWISE

29.4 Tuberculosis of the spine (and idiopathic scoliosis)

The spine is the most common and the most dangerous site for skeletal tuberculosis. It takes two forms: (1) In the first, the patient's general symptoms are mild. The infection usually starts in the anterior part of a disc, and spreads to the adjacent surface of the body of a vertebra, or to two adjacent ones. It seldom involves his neural arches. The result is that, as the bodies of his vertebrae collapse, his spine angles forwards to produce a kyphus (an increase in the normal convex curve of the spine: a scoliosis is a lateral curvature). The shape of his spinal deformity depends on how many of his vertebrae are diseased. Commonly, as his deformity gets worse, a sharp angle (the gibbus) appears. Uncommonly, the destruction is not symmetrical, so that his spine rotates. (2) In the second form his general symptoms are more severe, several of his vertebrae are involved widely in his spine (including perhaps some in his neck), and his disc spaces may not be narrowed.

His first symptom is pain in his back, and his first sign is increasing kyphosis. Later, pus from his diseased vertebrae may track along tissue planes to present as a cold abscess in unexpected places, particularly in his groin (psoas abscess). He may become paraplegic (29.4a).

In a child spinal tuberculosis is an important cause of back pain. He will probably be unwell and have lost weight, but not always so. He may resent examination, be tender over his low thoracic or upper lumbar spine, and show any of the signs seen in adults.

Give him chemotherapy as an outpatient, without applying a plaster jacket. The former practice of giving all patients with spinal tuberculosis a plaster jacket is now outmoded. You will find that his spine will heal quicker if you let his vertebrae collapse down and fuse. As it does so, his pain will go and his vertebrae will recalcify. His deformity will probably increase by about 5° to 25° during treatment. Only extensive surgery, in the most expert centres, gets better results than this. Its main advantage is that it establishes bony fusion in 2 years, instead of in 4 years.

Idiopathic kyphoscoliosis is one of the differential diagnoses of a tuberculous spine. It is a disease of unknown cause, in which a child's spine slowly develops a curve. It may start as early as 3 years, but it more often starts at 7 or 8; it progresses most rapidly between the ages of 12 and 14, and gets worse until he stops growing. If possible, refer him to a special centre, which can fit him with a Milwaukee or similar brace, and if necessary fuse his spine at the appropriate time. If you cannot refer him, reassure his parents that, although he will always be a hunchback, he will be normal in most other ways. Spinal compression is rare, but a moderate or severe lesion will affect the function of his lungs by reducing the size of his thoracic cage.

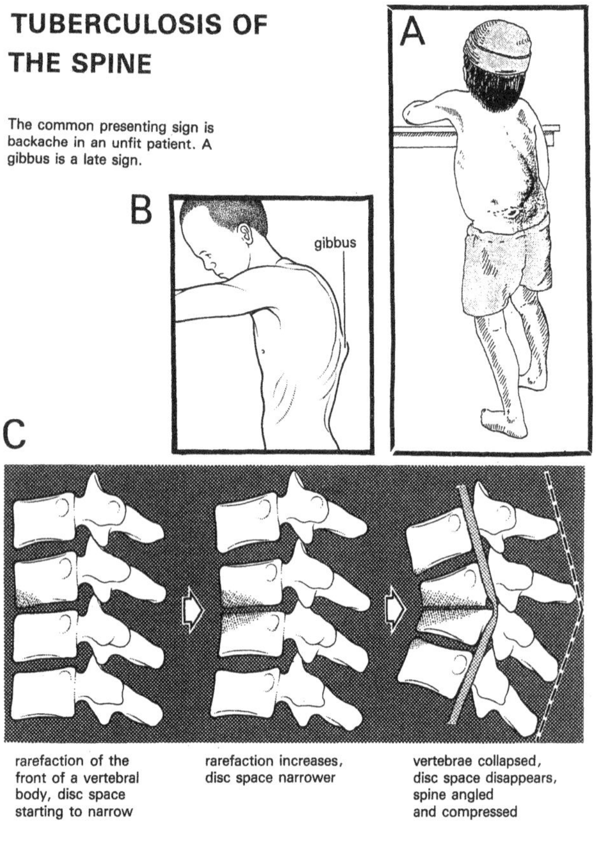

SPINAL TUBERCULOSIS

EXAMINATION. Examine a patient as in Section 27.8. Examine him from the side; look and feel for: (1) a kyphus, (2) reduced movement of his lumbar spine, (3) cold abscesses in his paraspinal area, loin, and groin, (4) sinuses. Test the reflexes in his legs, and their tone, power, and sensation.

X-RAYS are critical, see Fig. 29-3. X-ray his chest also.

Look for: (1) Narrowing or obliteration of a joint space, involving at least two vertebral bodies and the disc between them (this is the typical late picture). Sometimes several vertebrae disappear into the space normally occupied by one or two. So count his vertebral spines, because these may be all that is left when his vertebral bodies have been destroyed. (2) Look for forward collapse of his spine. (3) You may also see: (a) the shadow produced by a paravertebral abscess in his thoracic region (this strongly suggests tuberculosis, but it can be produced by staphylococcal and other forms of bacterial osteitis), and (b) calcification in his psoas sheath, showing that a psoas abscess is forming. Evidence of a paravertebral abscess increases the probability of tuberculosis being the cause, but is not necessary for diagnosing it. (4) Osteophytes and bridging (rare). If you do see bridging, it is more likely to be due to late staphylococcal infection.

SPECIAL TESTS. The ESR is useful and may be very high. A falling ESR is an indication of response to treatment, but is less important than an improvement in his clinical condition, as indicated by decreasing pain and tenderness.

THE DIFFERENTIAL DIAGNOSIS OF A TUBERCULOUS SPINE

Suggesting pyogenic osteitis—a more rapid onset, less bone destruction, and a higher temperature. Confirming the diagnosis may have to depend on the aspiration and examination of pus from his spine, or on costotransversectomy, see Section 29.4a.

Suggesting poliomyelitis—weak, wasted, flaccid legs. If

TUBERCULOSIS OF THE SPINE

The common presenting sign is backache in an unfit patient. A gibbus is a late sign.

Fig. 29-3 TUBERCULOSIS OF THE SPINE. A, a boy from Nepal. B, another patient with a gibbus. Note that in both these patients the lower thoracic region is involved (the common site). C, the X-ray signs (see text). A, *kindly contributed by David Nabarro.*

C, rarefaction of the front of a vertebral body, disc space starting to narrow → rarefaction increases, disc space narrower → vertebrae collapsed, disc space disappears, spine angled and compressed polio involves his spine, it is almost sure to involve his legs too. Scoliosis rather than kyphosis.

Suggesting idiopathic scoliosis—the curve is smooth, with no gibbus, or muscle-wasting. Apart from the curved shape of his spine, there are no other signs; his X-rays are normal, and no vertebrae are destroyed. The disease starts in childhood.

Suggesting a congenital hemivertebra causing scoliosis (usually mild)—half of one of his vertebrae is missing. The half which remains forms the apex of the curve. On an X-ray this is almost triangular, its edges are smooth and well formed, and there are no signs of disc destruction in the vertebra above or below. This kind of scoliosis does not progress with age, and needs no treatment.

Suggesting kyphoscoliosis due to lung disease—a previous history of empyema. By making his lung collapse, an empyema may collapse his thoracic cage. Other causes of fibrosis of a lung, or pneumonectomy. His spine itself needs no treatment.

Suggesting secondary deposits—involvement of the bodies of his vertebrae without involvement of their discs. His serum alkaline phosphatase is raised. If the primary is in his prostate, his acid phosphatase will be raised also.

Suggesting a senile kyphosis—an old woman with osteoporosis of all, or most, of her spine, and normal discs, which bulge into her softened vertebrae. Her kyphus is gradual. Treatment is difficult (27.8).

Suggesting Burkitt's lymphoma—the patient is a child. In the endemic areas this is the commonest cause of paraplegia in children (32.3).

TREATMENT.

Give him chemotherapy, as in Section 29.1. If his back is painful at first, admit him for bed rest, but allow him up if he wishes. If he can walk, encourage him to do so.

Warn him that he *must* continue with his drugs, and that they will take some months to have much effect. During this time, he may find his kyphoscoliosis getting worse, before it stabilizes. If he thinks your treatment is not working, he may default, and go to a traditional practitioner. If he does default, do all you can to trace him.

DIFFICULTIES WITH A TUBERCULOUS SPINE

See also Section 29.3.

If his CERVICAL SPINE is involved, treat him with an orthopaedic collar, or failing this, a plaster cuirasse (64-10) and chemotherapy. His spinal canal is larger in his neck than in his thoracic region, so his spinal cord is less likely to be compressed.

If he complains of CLUMSINESS, WEAKNESS, OR INCOORDINATION, he is becoming paraplegic, so see below.

29.4a Tuberculous paraplegia, costotransversectomy

If a patient with spinal tuberculosis complains of clumsiness, weakness, or incoordination of his legs, he is becoming paraplegic. Later, the voluntary power of his legs is reduced, their muscle tone is increased, and his plantar responses become extensor. Later still, he has flexor spasms, and finally contractures.

Paraplegia is the major complication of spinal tuberculosis. In early cases it is due to an inflammatory oedema round a paraspinal abscess, and later to compression. Paraplegia may be his presenting symptom, and is usually treatable. In most cases it is motor only (unless it comes on very rapidly), because the abscess presses on the anterior columns of his cord rather than on the posterior ones. Although tuberculous *osteitis* affects the various regions of the spine in the following order of decreasing frequency: low thoracic, lumbar, upper thoracic, and cervical, you will see tuberculous *paraplegia* most commonly in the thoracic region, sometimes in the cervical region, and seldom in the lumbar region. This is because the spinal canal is wide there, and the cauda equina running through it is less easily affected than the cord.

There are two types of tuberculous paraplegia: (A) The common early type is due to inflammatory oedema which responds well to chemotherapy, and surgery, if this is necessary. (B) A less common later type, due to pressure and stretching from a bony deformity, when bony union has not occurred. It is the result of no treatment, incomplete treatment, or late treatment. Its prognosis is poor with chemotherapy alone, and even with specialized surgery (not described here), it is not good.

TUBERCULOUS PARAPLEGIA

THE PROGNOSIS AND MANAGEMENT are different in the two forms of the disese in Section 29.4. The patient's bowels and bladder are sometimes involved in Stage (3) below and always in Stage (4); their improvement mirrors that of his his limb muscles. If his prognosis is good he should be operated on:

(A) If his paralysis is fairly recent (<3 months) and his deformity is <60° (common) inflammatory oedema is the likely cause, and if the indications for surgery are followed, his prognosis is good. Even if he has >60° of deformity, he is worth managing as if oedema was the cause, but his prognosis will not be so good.

(1) If his weakness is mild (<grade 3, see 27.2), he is almost sure to recover fully.

(2) If his weakness is severe (grade 0–3) without muscle spasms, he will probably recover.

(3) If his weakness is severe with extensor spasms, he has >50% chance of a full recovery, and if not, he will probably have a partial recovery.

(4) If weakness is severe with flexor spasms, he can expect little or no recovery, and he has little chance of walking without special aids.

(B) If his paraplegia is due tp pressure or stretching from a bony deformity of his neural canal (uncommon in most areas and usually of late onset), the clinical picture is the same, except that the onset of paraplegia is late when kyphosis is marked. However, even if he has marked bony deformity with no paraspinal abscess visible on X-ray, his paraplegia may possibly still be due to inflammatory oedema, so refer him for surgery if you can. If you cannot, try chemotherapy alone: but don't operate yourself, the surgery of this kind of paraplegia is too difficult.

TREATMENT FOR TUBERCULOUS PARAPLEGIA

NON-OPERATIVE TREATMENT. Admit him, and put him to bed. There is a very good chance that he will recover. If chemotherapy and bed rest don't cause neurological improvement in 6 weeks (unusual), review him. Your diagnosis is likely to be wrong, but if you are sure that he is tuberculous, consider costotransversectomy.

CHEMOTHERAPY. Give this as in Section 29.1.

NURSING CARE is the same as for traumatic paraplegia, so manage his morale, his skin, his urine, and his bowels as in Section 64.13.

COSTOTRANSVERSECTOMY

INDICATIONS. Costotransversectomy is also indicated for osteomyelitis of the spine, as described in Section 7.15. (1) Paraplegia due to osteitis (usually tuberculous), provided a paraspinal abscess (tuberculous or pyogenic) can be demonstrated on X-ray. (2) A large paraspinal abscess (tuberculous or pyogenic) when there is no paraplegia. (3) To obtain tissue for histology, when the cause of an osteitis is still in doubt, after considering the clinical condition and the X-rays.

If possible, refer him, if not proceed as follows.

ANAESTHESIA. (1) General anaesthesia (A 9.1). (2) Ketamine (A 8.1). You must intubate him (A 13.2) and give him a relaxant (A 14.1), because you will have to lay him prone (A 16.12) with his chest supported on pillows, and control his ventilation. A prone patient cannot breathe spontaneously unassisted.

PREPARATION. Have 2 units of blood for him in reserve. Diathermy is useful.

Find the vertebra or vertebrae most markedly involved, by noting the site of any gibbus, and examining his X-rays. Clean

COSTO-TRANSVERSECTOMY

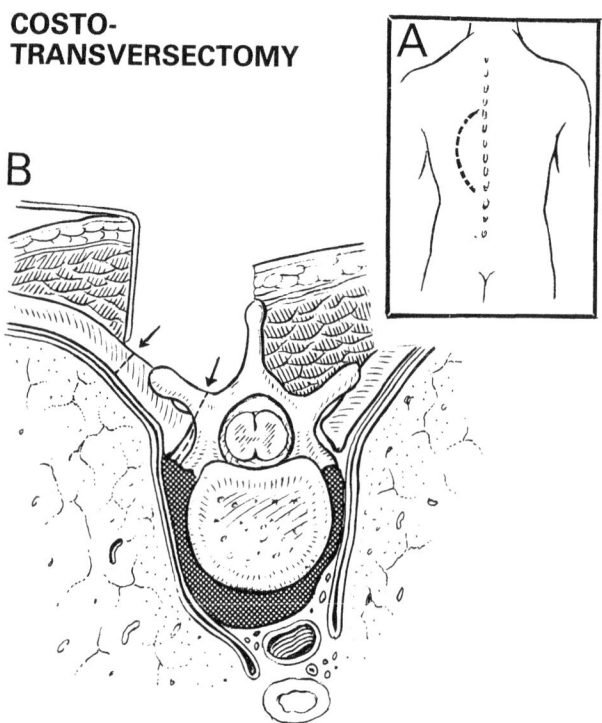

Fig. 29-3a COSTOTRANSVERSECTOMY for a tuberculous or a pyogenic paraspinal abscess. A, the incision. B, the approach to the ribs and transverse processes. *After Campbell's Orthopaedics, Fig. 13-10, with kind permission.*

his back, and cover it with a laparotomy towel with a central hole, or with 4 surrounding towels.

INCISION. Stand on his left and make a 20 cm incision centred on the affected vertebrae, curved to the left, and reaching his spinous processes at each end. Raise a flap of skin and subcutaneous tissues, and turn this medially, to expose his supraspinous ligament.

CAUTION ! (1) Approach the abscess from the left, so as to avoid his azygous vein (at some levels) and his vena cava. You are unlikely to damage his aorta. (2) Later, gentle dissection near his vertebral bodies will help you to avoid damaging his pleura and entering his pleural cavity.

Use a knife to divide his left trapezius near its origin from his spinous processes, and his latissimus dorsi, as this arises from his lower six thoracic vertebrae. Open the plane between his spinous processes, and his sacrospinalis muscle, by cutting at first, and then by dissecting off the muscle from the bone with a stout periosteal elevator. If he bleeds much, pack the wound tightly with a laparotomy pad, and wait up to five minutes.

Expose the transverse processes and the related ribs of his maximally involved vertebrae, together with one vertebra above and below these. Expose the whole of each transverse process and 5 cm of rib distal to its tip.

Cut the periosteum of a rib longitudinally, and elevate it with a periosteal elevator all round. This will help to separate it from the tissue covering his underlying pleura, and protect his intercostal vessels and nerve.

Cut the rib with rib cutters (or carefully with bone cutters), 3 cm from the tip of its related transverse process. *Try to avoid damaging his pleura.* Then resect the medial part of the rib and the transverse process at its base. Repeat this for at least one other rib.

Now look for his paraspinal abscess. Insert your index finger along the side of his vertebral bodies, and separate the tissues gently. You may need some sharp dissection with scissors—if so keep *very* close to the bone. This will lead you to the abscess, and not to his pleura!

Tuberculous pus is watery, with debris in it. Pus from osteomyelitis is yellow and creamy. Drain and culture what you find. Pass your finger round the anterior surface of each vertebra, up and down to ensure thorough drainage.

If you find no pus, check the X-ray, you may have chosen the wrong level. If so, remove a further transverse process and its related rib and feel again.

If you still find no abscess, take some tissue from the disc space for histology. The best place to biopsy is felt more easily than seen. Use forceps designed to biopsy the cervix, or use dissecting forceps and a No. 15 blade mounted on a long handle.

CLOSURE. Preferably use suction drainage ('Redivac', 4.10). There is no need for an intercostal drain, unless you damage his pleura. Approximate his muscles to his spine by sewing his trapezius and latissimus dorsi to his supraspinous ligament with 1/0 multifilament, or chromic catgut. Close his skin with continuous 1/0 or 2/0 monofilament. Apply a dressing. Nurse him on his back and sides, changing his position 2-hourly. He should be able to turn the upper part of his body by 48 hours, but he will still need 2-hourly assistance with turning. He may show no improvement for *up to 6 weeks*. If he has not improved by this time, his outlook is poor. If improvement starts by 6 weeks expect it to continue for 6 months. It will be hastened and improved by the drainage of a significant abscess.

If his paraplegia continues as before, see Section 64.13.
CAUTION ! Avoid an indwelling catheter. If he needs help, use intermittent sterile catheterization—see Section 64.16!

If you DAMAGE HIS PLEURA, see Section 9.2D.

29.5 Abdominal tuberculosis

Abdominal tuberculosis is now rare in the industrial world, but is common in developing countries. In India and Nepal it is responsible for about 10% of gut obstructions. You are most likely to see it when you are expecting something else.

There are three main types, and several less common ones. In Africa the order of their frequency in adults is: (1) The type which presents as ascites. (2) The plastic type, which causes intestinal obstruction. (3) The glandular type, which involves the mesenteric nodes. In India the order of frequency of these types in adults is (2), (3), (1). In children in Africa their order of frequency is (3), (1), (2).

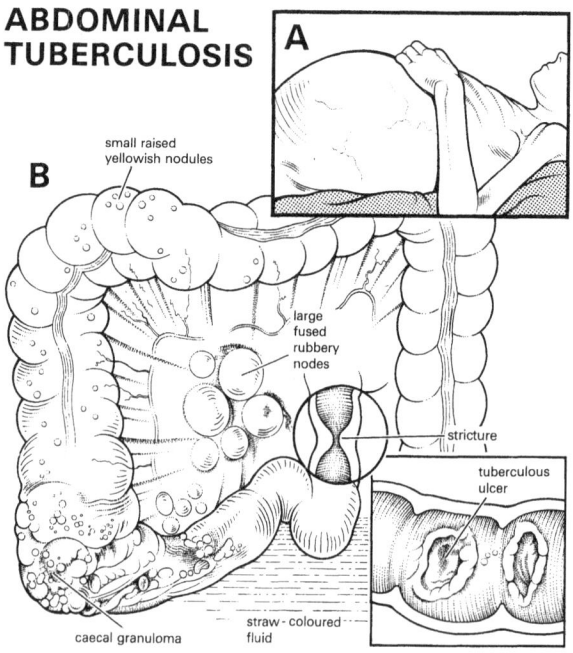

Fig. 29-4 ABDOMINAL TUBERCULOSIS can present in many ways. Patient A's abdomen is distended with ascitic fluid. You may not diagnose some of the other forms of tuberculous peritonitis until you do a laparotomy. *Kindly contributed by Gerald Hankins.*

MORE ABDOMINAL TUBERCULOSIS

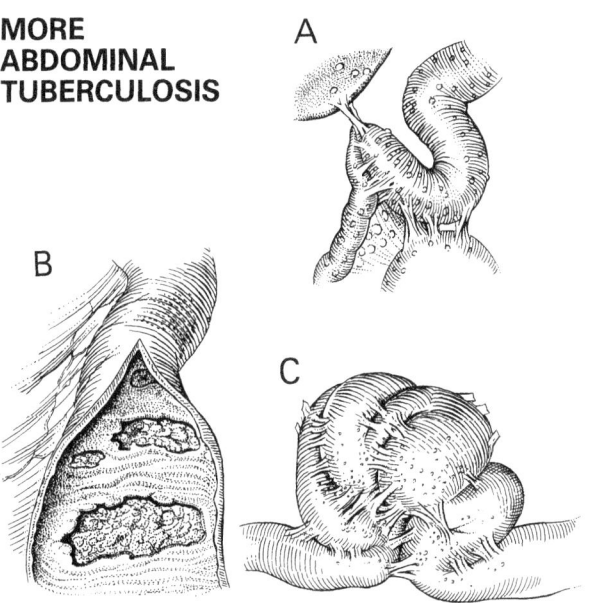

Fig. 29-5 MORE ABDOMINAL TUBERCULOSIS. A, an adhesion causing obstruction. B, tuberculous ulcers. C, coils of gut matted together. *Adapted from a drawing by Frank Netter, with the kind permission of CIBA-GEIGY Ltd, Basle (Switzerland).*

These three types are described in detail in later sections. Less commonly, you may also see:

(4) Tuberculous strictures anywhere in a patient's gut, but usually in his caecum and distal small gut, where they are caused by the shrinkage of a tuberculous ileocaecal mass to form a fibrous constriction.

(5) Tuberculous ulcers (unusual) can occur anywhere in his gut, but are most often seen in his ileum, caecum, rectum, or sigmoid colon. In his small gut, a tuberculous ulcer can cause diarrhoea. On the rare occasions when the ulcer is in his stomach or duodenum, it can closely mimic a peptic ulcer, or a carcinoma. Caseating lymph nodes will lead you to the correct diagnosis. A tuberculous ulcer may perforate his gut, or bleed; because it usually occurs distally, he usually bleeds from his rectum.

(6) Tuberculous fistulae form occasionally.

All this pathology can present in so many ways, and with so few distinguishing signs, that diagnosis is difficult. With all forms of tuberculosis he loses his appetite, he loses weight, and he feels ill, just as he does with tuberculosis elsewhere. He has vague abdominal pain and tenderness, and may vomit. Depending on the type of tuberculosis he has, he may have the symptoms of abdominal swelling (the ascitic type), obstruction (the plastic type), abdominal masses (the glandular type), or bleeding or perforation (tuberculous ulcers).

If he is not obstructed, or bleeding, you can treat him medically. But you will have to operate if his gut obstructs completely (the plastic type) or, rarely, if he bleeds (tuberculous ulcers).

29.6 The ascitic type of abdominal tuberculosis

In Africa, about 70% of patients with abdominal tuberculosis present with ascites; in India only about 10% of them do. In Zambia tuberculosis is responsible for 20% of all cases of ascites. The patient presents with a swollen abdomen containing many litres of straw-coloured fluid. A child with advanced abdominal tuberculosis typically has 'a ballooned abdomen and matchstick legs', but in many children the diagnosis is far from obvious. The fluid accumulates as the result of large numbers of miliary tubercles on his peritoneum. The only certain way to make the diagnosis is to do a minilaparotomy ('minilap'), which will also enable you to diagnose cirrhosis, periportal fibrosis (due to Schistosomiasis mansoni), carcinomatosis of the peritoneum and hepatoma (usually with cirrhosis). Experts can usually diagnose miliary tuberculosis with their naked eyes; but even they can be wrong, so take a biopsy of his parietal peritoneum and/or his liver.

ASCITIC ABDOMINAL TUBERCULOSIS

SPECIAL TESTS. X-ray the patient's chest, and examine his ascitic fluid. If the cell count is over 50 µl, with at least 70% lymphocytes, he is fairly likely to have tuberculous peritonitis. Your lab will be unlikely to find AAFB in it, because they are very sparse. If the fluid has fewer lymphocytes than this, his ascites is more likely to be caused by cirrhosis, or periportal fibrosis.

Measure the protein in his peritoneal fluid. In tuberculous peritonitis it is usually 3 to 10 g/l, but it may be up to 20 g/l, or higher. Most patients with >20 g/l, or more, have carcinomatosis.

If it contains more than 4 g/l of protein, it is likely to be an exudate. If it contains less than 4 g/l, it is likely to be a transudate. Cirrhosis usually produces a transudate; so does periportal fibrosis, if it produces any fluid at all (uncommon).

Blood in the fluid suggests carcinomatosis or a hepatoma.

THE DIFFERENTIAL DIAGNOSIS of ascitic tuberculous peritonitis (for the plastic type see later):

Suggesting ascitic tuberculosis—miliary nodules on the peritoneum, each about 1 to 2 mm in size, slightly raised and whitish. The nodules of carcinomatosis, which is the main differential diagnosis, are larger—usually more than 3 mm—more vascular, and more irregular. You will soon learn to distinguish them. He is not as ill as he would be with a malignant effusion of the same size.

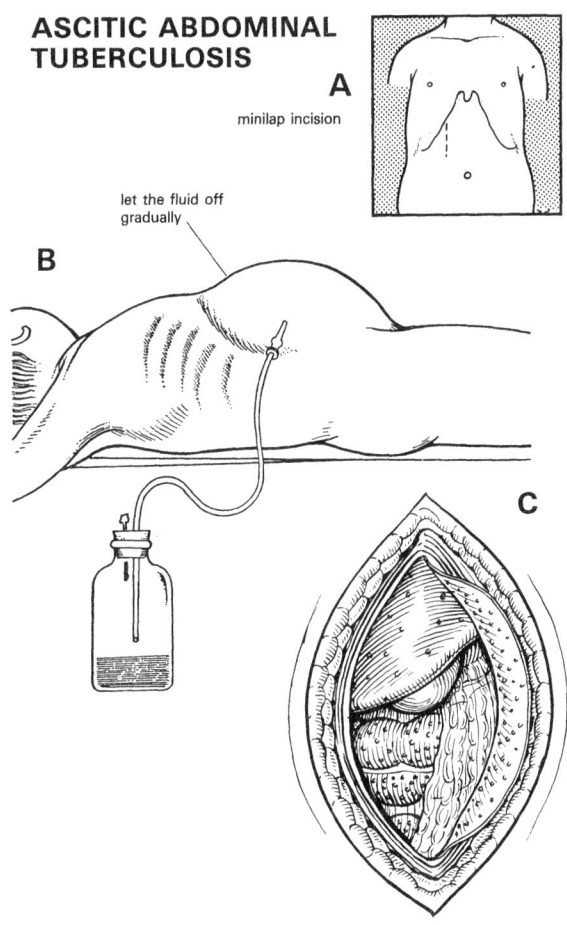

Fig. 29-6 ASCITIC ABDOMINAL TUBERCULOSIS. A, the minilap incision. B, draw off the fluid slowly before you start. C, miliary tubercles of the parietal peritoneum, liver, and gut.

Suggesting ascites secondary to liver disease—his liver may be enlarged, hard, and irregular, or small and hard to feel; his spleen is usually large; there are usually <4 g/l of protein in his peritoneal fluid.

Suggesting the nephrotic syndrome—his ascites is less marked than his generalized oedema. If he has ascites, he usually also has marked ascites of his abdominal wall. There are usually <4 g/l of protein in his peritoneal fluid.

Suggesting nutritional oedema (hypoproteinaemia)—other signs of protein deficiency, but these may also be present in tuberculosis. There are usually <4 g/l of protein in his peritoneal fluid.

Suggesting heart failure leading to cirrhosis and ascites—a raised jugular venous pressure, and other signs of heart failure; <4 g/l of protein in his peritoneal fluid.

Suggesting carcinomatosis of the peritoneum—hard deposits in the pouch of Douglas or rectovesical pouch; usually >20 g/l of protein in his peritoneal fluid.

A MINILAP TO DIAGNOSE THE CAUSE OF ASCITES

INDICATIONS. Ascites of uncertain cause. In the developing world, especially, a patient can have more than one diagnosis, for example, cirrhosis and tuberculosis peritonitis. Ascites predominating over other signs usually requires a minilap. It is seldom indicated when the ascites is not predominant, as in the generalized oedema of heart failure, or renal disease. Check his blood urea before you proceed.

CAUTION! ! (1) A minilap is NOT suitable for exploring the abdomen. (2) You can diagnose tuberculous abdominal glands this way, but they are better biopsied elsewhere, for example in his axilla.

DRAINING THE ASCITES. If he has more than a mild ascites, draw off most of the ascitic fluid slowly before you begin. If it all escapes suddenly, as you open his abdomen, his circulation may collapse. So draw off one litre every 2 hours, starting 48 hours preoperatively, to a maximum of 6 litres. If there is still significant ascites, after you have withdrawn 6 litres, wait until next day before you draw off more. Use a wide-bore intravenous cannula, a drip set, and a sterile bottle.

CAUTION ! To avoid possible injury to a large spleen, which may be difficult to feel because of the ascites, drain the fluid from his right lower abdomen.

ANAESTHESIA. Use local anaesthesia in an adult or ketamine in a child. Avoid general anaesthesia, because he may have cirrhosis.

INCISION. Make a 5 to 6 cm right upper muscle-splitting paramedian incision 4 or 5 cm from the midline. This will allow you to see and examine his liver, and will be less likely than a midline incision to leak ascitic fluid postoperatively.

Look for miliary tubercles and secondary deposits on his peritoneum. Tubercles are remarkably uniform in size, and fairly uniform in appearance (like salt grains). Take a biopsy from his parietal peritoneum. Take a needle biopsy of his liver under direct vision, if this is indicated (32.26), or take a wedge biopsy. Close the incision in the usual way, but don't insert a drain, or it will leak continuously.

TO BIOPSY HIS PERITONEUM remove an elliptical piece of his parietal peritoneum 2×0.5 cm, from the edge of the abdominal incision. This is only necessary if it is abnormal macroscopically.

WEDGE BIOPSY OF THE LIVER

INDICATIONS. The histological examination of any suspicious lesion in the liver.

METHOD. Insert 2 '0' chromic catgut atraumatic sutures near the anteroinferior border of his liver, as in Fig. 29-7. Tie these so as to 'squeeze' his liver, adjacent to the segment you are going to incise, to stop it bleeding. Remove a wedge of his liver 0.5×1.5 cm. Bring the cut edges of his liver together with two more mattress sutures, placed transverse to, and outside, the first two.

TREATMENT FOR ASCITIC TUBERCULOSIS

Give him chemotherapy. Don't expect miracles, if he has acute

WEDGE BIOPSY OF THE LIVER

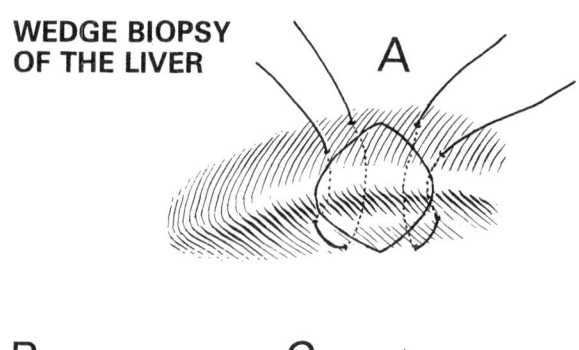
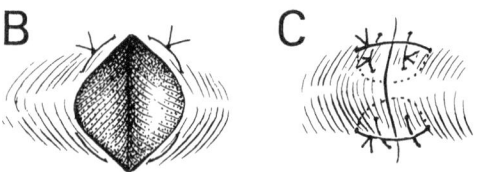

Fig. 29-7 WEDGE BIOPSY OF THE LIVER. A, insert sutures to control bleeding before you cut the liver. B, the wedge excised. C, the wedge closed.

disease and ascites. Before 2 months, the failure of the fluid to reaccumulate will show that he is improving.

29.7 The plastic peritonitis type of abdominal tuberculosis

This is the result of a tuberculous granuloma, which causes a patient's omentum, and the other structures in his abdomen, particularly loops of his distal small gut, his caecum, and his ascending colon, to mat together with many adhesions. The affected coils of his gut are thick and rubbery, with characteristic transverse lesions on his small gut. Loops of his small gut may obstruct, and be difficult to separate. Carcinoma, amoeboma, and Crohn's disease can all cause a plastic peritonitis; but in the developing world tuberculosis is more common than all these others combined. Amoebiasis makes loops of small gut stick to the descending colon, without causing a true plastic peritonitis.

The obstruction in his gut is commonly incomplete, so that his symptoms are subacute or chronic, and may have lasted months or years. The adhesions which mat the loops of his gut together are extensive and difficult to separate, so *manage him non-operatively if you can*. Give him chemotherapy, a light diet, or fluids only, if necessary intravenously, for a few days. A tuberculous granuloma of the small gut usually resolves without a stricture; but in the ileocaecal area fibrosis and stenosis often follow.

Occasionally, you may have to operate for persisting complete obstruction. Even then, if you know tuberculosis is the cause, you will be wise to try non-operative treatment for a few days first—if there is no strangulation. When you do operate, you may find that there is no stricture in the wall of his gut, and that you can relieve the obstruction by dividing adhesions only. This is much preferable, if it is possible, because, if you open his gut, there is always a danger that a fistula may follow. If you have to open his gut, you have a choice between: (1) A 'stricturoplasty', if there is a narrow stricture in his his small gut, as in A, Fig. 29-8. (2) A local small-gut bypass (D, 29-8). (3) A bypass (ileotransversostomy) between his ileum and his transverse colon (9.6). This will relieve his obstruction, and you can refer him for definitive surgery later. (4) A right hemicolectomy (66-20). If you are skilled enough to do it, this will remove the focus of infection, and is better than an ileotransversostomy.

Avoid these common mistakes: (1) Don't try to make a diagnosis without understanding the nature of the disease. Make it by weighing up the signs and symptoms carefully. (2) Don't be too eager to start a therapeutic trial without confirming the diagnosis: he may have some other disease. He will almost certainly be well enough for a 'minilap' under local anaesthesia (29-6).

OBSTRUCTIVE ABDOMINAL TUBERCULOSIS

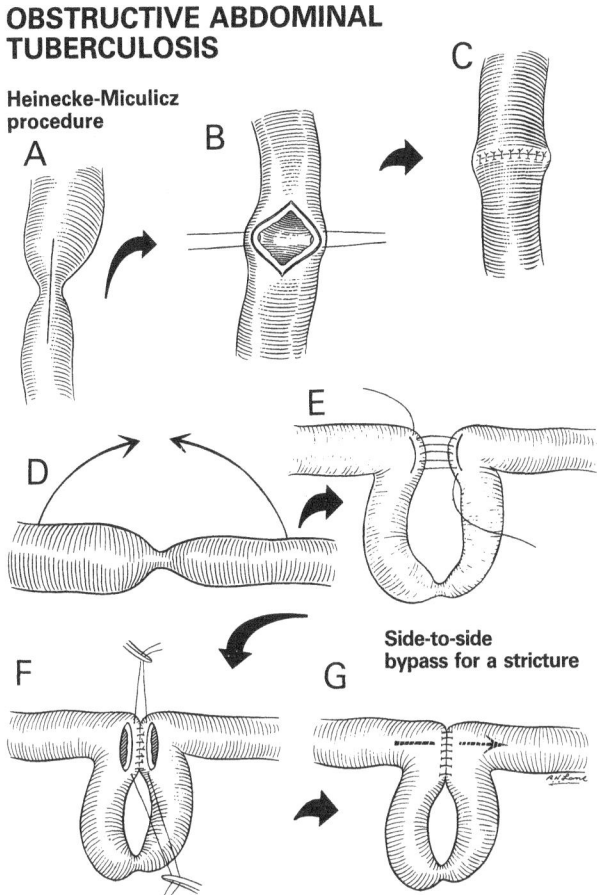

Fig. 29-8 OBSTRUCTIVE ABDOMINAL TUBERCULOSIS. A, to C, the Heinecke–Miculicz procedure for a stricture of the small gut. A, incise the gut longitudinally. B, insert stay sutures beside the middle of the incision, pull them out, and sew up the gut transversely. C, the completed procedure. D, to G, side to side anastomosis to bypass a stricture. D, the stricture with the loops of gut either side of it about to be apposed. E, place a layer of continuous seromuscular sutures between the loops, before you open them. F, the next step is a layer of continuous over and over sutures between the two loops. G, the completed anastomosis. See Fig. 9-12 for further details. *Kindly contributed by Samiran Nundy.*

(3) If you cannot make a diagnosis, don't wait too long before exploring his abdomen. (4) If he has subacute obstruction, which does not respond to non-operative treatment, you will have to relieve it surgically. (5) If he is desperately ill, don't make meddlesome and dangerous attempts to resect grossly scarred gut, or to free difficult adhesions.

PLASTIC ABDOMINAL TUBERCULOSIS

SYMPTOMS. The pattern of signs and sypmtoms described here applies to abdominal tuberculosis as it presents in India and Nepal, where the plastic type of the disease predominates. The different presentation of the ascitic type is described elsewhere (29.6).

Weight loss (all cases), the patient may have lost much weight.

Weakness, malaise, fatigue, and anorexia (75%) are common. He may also have nausea and vomiting, fever and night sweats (60%).

Abdominal pain (90%) is usually constant, central, and not severe. If it is in his right lower quadrant, it suggests ileocaecal tuberculosis. In the ascitic type pain is often mild, and may be absent.

Symptoms of obstruction (30%) include alternating constipation and diarrhoea, cramps, and gurglings. Typically, he describes a 'ball of wind' moving in his abdomen.

Rectal bleeding is rare, but may be severe.

Steatorrhoea with pale, bulky, and offensive stools is sometimes seen.

A chronic cough and blood-stained sputum are rarer than you might expect.

SIGNS OF ABDOMINAL TUBERCULOSIS

Abdominal tenderness (60%) is ill-defined, and is usually maximal in the middle of his abdomen. It is absent in about half the cases. Experts say that they can recognize a peculiar 'doughy' feeling in a tuberculous abdomen.

An abdominal mass (40%) may be present. He may have one or two well-defined tender rubbery masses, either in his ileocaecal region, or at the base of his mesentery. A mass is unusual in the ascitic type.

Signs of obstruction to his lower small gut may be acute or subacute.

He is usually moderately anaemic, and he may have dependent oedema as the result of hypoproteinaemia.

X-RAYS. If you suspect acute or subacute bowel obstruction, take films in the erect and supine positions (10-6, 10-7). Avoid a barium follow through in the acute stage: it may make an incomplete obstruction complete.

SPECIAL TESTS. Measure his haemoglobin and his ESR, and examine his stools. X-ray his chest, and examine his sputum. Do a tuberculin test (29.1). If he has palpable ascites, examine it as described earlier.

Examine him carefully for enlarged axillary or cervical lymph nodes; if you find one, biopsy it. An inguinal node is less likely to be diagnostic, unless it is very large.

THE DIFFERENTIAL DIAGNOSIS OF PLASTIC ABDOMINAL TUBERCULOSIS

Suggesting ascaris infection—he is a child with vague abdominal pain, and subacute obstruction but no weight loss or fever. Tenderness is not constant, and palpable masses of worms are unusual. See Section 10.6.

Suggesting an appendix abscess—a short history, and an acute onset.

Suggesting amoebiasis—a history of passing blood and mucus rectally, and trophozoites in his stools.

Suggesting carcinoma of the colon—a Western life style. It does occur in villagers but is unusual.

Suggesting cirrhosis or a liver tumour—an iregular firm or hard liver, prominent ascites, and a large spleen, a previous attack of hepatitis, alcoholism. A bruit is often present (32.26).

Suggesting Crohn's disease (rare)—loss of weight and diarrhoea are the main symptoms. The differential diagnosis may be impossible until tissues are examined histologically.

NON-OPERATIVE TREATMENT FOR ABDOMINAL TUBERCULOSIS

INDICATIONS. (1) You are reasonably certain of the diagnosis. He is either not obstructed, or his obstruction is subacute. (2) There are no signs of strangulation.

REGIME. Give him chemotherapy (29.1). If he is an adult, his abdominal symptoms and masses are unlikely to respond for about 2 months, although a child may respond sooner. Don't expect chemotherapy to work miracles, if he has acute disease and ascites. If he fails to respond to tuberculosis treatment, consider the possibility of: (1) AIDS in addition to tuberculosis. (2) Carcinoma, or an abdominal lymphoma.

If he is subacutely obstructed, pass a nasogastric tube, give him intravenous fluids, and resuscitate him as in Section 10.5. If he improves and his obstruction passes off, good. If it does not, you may have to operate to divide adhesions, but there is no guarantee that they will not form again.

A DIAGNOSTIC LAPAROTOMY FOR PLASTIC ABDOMINAL TUBERCULOSIS

A minilap for ascitic tuberculosis is described above. A standard laparotomy through an ordinary incision is a more extensive procedure, which may involve you in further surgery. Do one if he has a persistent vague abdominal pain, perhaps some intestinal symptoms, weight loss, and a raised ESR. Open his peritoneal cavity through a right paramedian incision, mostly below his umbilicus, and look for the findings listed above.

If you cannot find peritoneal tubercles or rubbery lymph nodes easily, take a biopsy from his parietal peritoneum. Incise his peritoneum and biopsy a lymph node. If the site of the biopsy bleeds, control it with packs or with a 3/0 figure of eight suture which underlies the bleeding point on both sides.

If you find a firm mass at his ileocaecal junction, perhaps with adhesions to adjacent structures and a normal peritoneum, the diagnosis is more difficult. Cut across an enlarged node. If you see caseous areas, you have confirmed the diagnosis. Even so, take a specimen for histology. Avoid taking a biopsy from the wall of his gut—this may lead to a fistula.

If the nature of an ileocaecal mass is uncertain, and it might be neoplastic, biopsy an enlarged node nearby and proceed as immediately below. Start chemotherapy postoperatively, and await the histological report.

If his ileocaecal mass is probably tuberculous, leave it if it is not is causing obstruction. If it is causing obstruction, do an ileotransversostomy, or if you are experienced, do a right hemicolectomy. If he is debilitated, an ileotransversostomy would be wiser, however skilled you are. Some surgeons would do one or the other of these operations whether or not the mass is causing obstruction.

If he is bleeding rectally, or has a tuberculous ulcer, treat him non-operatively if you can. Only do a hemicolectomy if bleeding is severe and continuous.

If you find a thick fibrotic segment of small gut and his ileocaecal region is normal, you can resect it and anastomose the ends if it is not too long, and there is not too much scarring or too many thick adhesions. If it is very short, do a stricturoplasty as in A, Fig. 29-8.

If a tuberculous ulcer has perforated his terminal ileum, oversew and patch it, as you would with a typhoid perforation (31.8). Or, treat it by resection and end to end anastomosis (9-9).

If loops of his gut are stuck down by plastic peritonitis, don't do too much dissection—the risks are too high. Instead, if he really is obstructed, do a simple side to side enteroenterostomy. Use the same technique as an ileotransversostomy. This will bypass the diseased segment, and avoid much stressful surgery.

ILEOTRANSVERSOSTOMY FOR OBSTRUCTION DUE TO PLASTIC TUBERCULOSIS

See also Section 9.3. Do it side to side, as in Fig. 9-12, but without dividing the gut and closing the ends, because there is no gut to be resected.

PREPARATION. If he is obstructed, make sure you correct his electrolytes first, as in Section 10.5. If you have time, prepare his gut. Give him a fluid diet, cleansing enemas for two days before, and a suitable course of a bowel-sterilizing agent, such as neomycin with sulphaphthalazole.

INCISION. Make a right paramedian muscle-splitting incision. Choose a point on his ileum which is at least 3 cm proximal to any stenosed or diseased gut, and apply a Babcock clamp to the antemesenteric border, lifting the gut out of the wound as you do so. Apply a second Babcock clamp about 3 cm proximal to the first one.

Reach up and draw his transverse colon into the wound. If necessary, extend the incision upwards.

Lift up the omentum which hangs below his transverse colon. It is attached to the anterior surface of his colon by a relatively bloodless fold. Divide this fold with scissors. Displace the freed omentum upwards, and so expose 6 cm of the anterior surface of his transverse colon. Place two Babcock clamps on the taenia of his colon 4 cm apart. Bring the clamps on his ileum up towards those on his colon, so the two parts of his gut lie side by side.

To minimize spillage and contamination, milk the central segment of his transverse colon empty. Then apply non-crushing clamps to each end of the denuded area. Squeeze away the contents of his ileum, and apply light occluding clamps to it in the same way.

Make a two-layer side to side anastomosis with a 3 cm stoma as in Fig. 9-12, but without resecting gut and closing the ends.

Make it 2 mm from the edge of the taenia to give extra strength. Use interrupted or continuous Lembert sutures. Open his colon over a distance of about 3 cm.

Draw his omentum down and tack it lightly to the site of the anastomosis with a few interrupted sutures through the serosa only. Replace his gut in his abdomen.

29.8 The glandular type of abdominal tuberculosis

This presents as irregular lumps in a child's abdomen, sometimes with ascites, and with little tendency to obstruct. His mesenteric nodes are large, and not very mobile. They may be so large that you can feel them through his abdominal wall. They are matted together, and firm to hard, with characteristic pale yellow areas of caseation on their cut surfaces.

Often you can be fairly certain of the diagnosis. If many lymph nodes are involved, biopsy one from his neck, axilla, or groin. Non-specific adenitis is common in the groin, so only biopsy an unusually large one. You may see enlarged nodes in a chest X-ray. If you cannot establish the diagnosis in any other way, you may have to do a laparotomy and take a node for section. Lymphoma is the important differential diagnosis (32.3 and 32.4).

29.9 Urogenital tuberculosis

Suspect that a patient has tuberculosis of his urinary tract, if he has a persistent cystitis, which fails to respond to antibiotics, and has pus cells and red cells in his urine, but no bacteria are cultured from it by routine methods. He is usually a young adult without signs of tuberculosis elsewhere. Urinogenital tuberculosis is common in Asia, but is very uncommon in sub-Saharan Africa. Treatment is usually easy, cheap, and effective—if the disease is not too far advanced, and he takes his drugs conscientiously. He may improve dramatically, especially if you treat him early, and even strictures of the ureter have been known to heal. So watch for urogenital tuberculosis, and be prepared to treat him on the suspicion that he might have it. The surgery that he may need if he presents late is beyond you. Unfortunately, his disease starts so insidiously that he may not complain of it until late.

Bacilli reach one of his kidneys (usually only one, but sometimes both) in his blood, after which caseation slowly destroys it. Only when the disease has eroded into its calyces do bacilli spread in his urine down to his ureter and bladder, infect them, and cause frequency and pyuria. Eventually, most of his kidney is destroyed, after which the disease may spread outside it, to form a palpable mass in his loin, perhaps with a discharging sinus.

Tuberculosis inflames the mucosa of the bladder and forms tubercles which may ulcerate, coalesce, and form shallow ulcers, especially round the orifices of the ureters and on the trigone. Ultimately, much of the wall of the bladder is destroyed, so that it ends up scarred, red, and contracted. A ureter which drains a tuberculosis kidney is flooded with bacilli, and becomes thick, fibrosed and strictured, usually in its lower third. Above this, his urinary tract dilates to form a hydro- or pyonephrosis.

He may present with: (1) The symptoms of chronic cystitis—frequency and dysuria. This later progresses to the burning nocturia and strangury of a small shrunken bladder, which may become secondarily infected. These symptoms make his bladder appear to be the cause of his disease, rather than his kidney. (2) A painless intermittent microscopic haematuria, or sometimes obvious bleeding (a renal carcinoma usually causes obvious bleeding). (3) A dull discomfort in his loin, which gets steadily worse, especially when tuberculosis is complicated by a pyogenic infection (20% of cases). His kidneys are not enlarged or tender, until late. (4) Malaise and the usual general symptoms of tuberculosis. (5) A painless, non-tender, craggy, and occasionally fluctuant tuberculous mass on one side of his scrotum. Otherwise, any genital tuberculosis he may have usually causes no symptoms.

TUBERCULOSIS OF THE URINARY TRACT

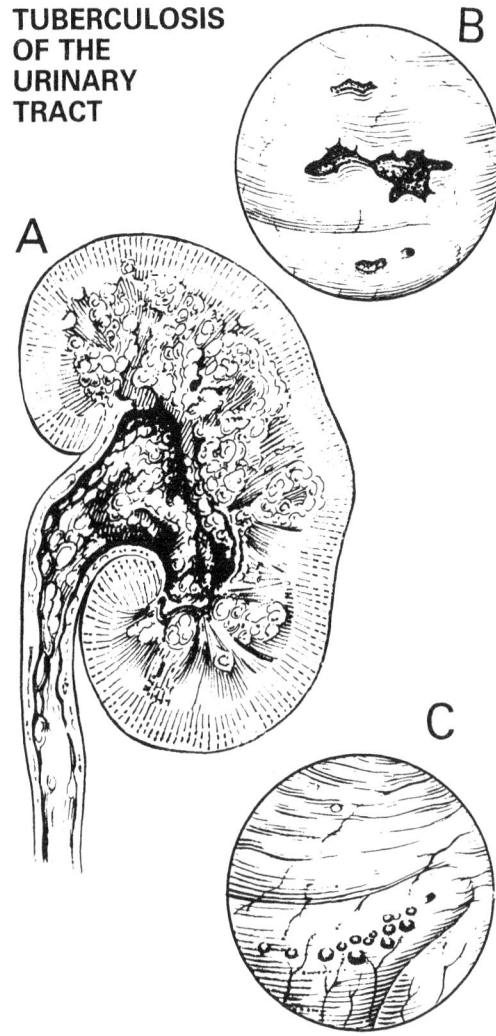

Fig. 29-9 TUBERCULOSIS OF THE URINARY TRACT. A, tuberculosis of the kidney involving the pelvis and the ureter. B, tuberculous ulcers of the bladder. C, tubercles near the orifice of the ureter. *Adapted from a drawing by Frank Netter, with the kind permission of CIBA-GEIGY Ltd, Basle (Switzerland).*

RENAL TUBERCULOSIS

EXAMINATION. Examine the patient's kidneys. Several parts of his urinary tract may be involved at the same time, so also feel his testes, his cords, and his prostate for painless nontender enlargement. A tuberculous prostate feels irregular and boggy; tuberculous vesicles thick and boggy. A tuberculous epididymis feels thick, woody, and craggy. It may caseate, and form sinuses, or it may involve his testis, and cause a secondary hydrocele. His distal spermatic cord is thick and oedematous.

SPECIAL TESTS. Urine with pus cells and red cells, but no bacteria on standard culture (unless there is secondary infection), is strongly suggestive.

A 24-hour urine, or an early morning urine specimen (after a period of dehydration), may show AAFB in a stained film. Repeat the examination 3 times. This needs little equipment, but it does require considerable skill, and much time. So you will probably have to rely on finding pus cells and red cells only. If possible, culture his urine for AAFB.

If you are in an endemic area and routine examination shows no ova of *Schistosoma haematobium*, examine the deposit from a specimen passed at midday (the time when most ova are passed) on 3 consecutive days.

He is usually anaemic, and his sedimentation rate is raised.

CYSTOSCOPY (23.3), will confirm the diagnosis, show the degree of involvement of his bladder, and exclude schistosomiasis.

X-RAYS. Look for the outline of an enlarged kidney, calcification, and obliteration of his psoas shadow.

An IVU will only be positive if disease is advanced. Look for 'moth-eaten calyces', and dilatation of his renal pelvis, and ureter. If it is very advanced, his kidney will not be functioning.

DIFFERENTIAL DIAGNOSIS. In endemic areas schistosomiasis haematobium is the main one, and is much the most common cause of pain on micturition with pus cells and red cells in the urine, compared with urinary tuberculosis, which is uncommon or rare.

Suggesting schistosomiasis—(1) small 3 to 5 mm nodules in his epididymis, nearly always in the tail. (2) Calcification of his bladder wall, as shown by a line in the shape of his bladder, which collapses after micturition. (3) Do a cystoscopy before an IVU, which is much more expensive. (4) The special test above.

TREATMENT OF RENAL TUBERCULOSIS

Treat him as an outpatient, with the standard tuberculosis chemotherapy (29.1). If his renal function is impaired, avoid streptomycin, or ethambutol, or give them intermittently. Rifampicin, INAH, and pyrazinamide are safe. Ask him to return every 2 months for regular assessment, including the examination of his urine, and a further supply of drugs.

If he relapses, and you think that he has not taken his drugs faithfully, consider changing to a regime using second-line drugs.

INDICATIONS FOR SURGERY. Operations for renal tuberculosis are beyond the scope of this manual. Refer him.

If his IVU shows no function, or has a moth-eaten appearance, with flecks of calcium, refer him for nephrectomy. Hypertension is an additional reason. If he is toxic and febrile, suggesting that he has a pyonephrosis, or a perinephric abscess, this is urgent. Otherwise, give him 6 weeks of chemotherapy first, to improve his condition for surgery.

If he has a ureteric stricture, refer him for urological investigation before starting chemotherapy. If you cannot refer him, all you can do is to give him chemotherapy. In endemic areas, schistosomiasis is a commoner cause of a stricture.

If he still has extreme frequency and dysuria, after 3 to 6 months of chemotherapy, suspect that he has a small contracted bladder. Confirm this by cystoscopy and a cystogram. Surgery may be possible.

30 The surgery of leprosy

30.1 Introduction

The best way to deal with leprosy is to recognize it early, and treat it adequately. If this fails, a patient needs surgery, because leprosy affects his nerves. Destruction of their sensory fibres makes the surface of his body anaesthetic, and thus liable to the injuries that result in open wounds and ulcers. Destruction of their motor fibres causes paralysis, wasting, and sometimes contractures of his muscles. Most nerves are mixed, so that both these things happen at the same time, with the result that his arms and legs become paralysed and anaesthetic. Because he has little sensation of pain, he does not know when he is injuring himself. This makes him neglect his painless surface injuries, so that they become steadily progressive ulcers. *The contractures, ulcers, and deformities that result are not an inevitable part of leprosy.* In a well-conducted leprosy program, there should be few of them when patients first present, and none later. They are the purpose of this chapter, and you should not see them very often.

Leprosy most commonly involves a patient's legs, but it can also involve his hands (30.4) and his eyes (30.2, 30.3). Pyogenic organisms readily enter through the lesions that leprosy causes in his skin, so that you may need to drain abscesses (5.2), treat bone, joint, and tendon sheath infections (Chapter 8), and enucleate his eye when its globe has become infected (24.14). Admit him to the general ward. If the staff behave naturally towards him, the other patients will too.

Here we assume you know about the medical treatment of leprosy. Surgically, your task is to: (1) Care for his primary and secondary impairments. (2) Set and record measurable objectives for preventing and limiting his disabilities, and plan how you are going to reach them. (3) Provide him with protective footware and aids. (5) Teach him self care to prevent further disability. (6) Teach the rest of the health care team how to do these things. Most leprosy work should be done by paramedical workers, and the present trend is for vertical programmes, with a specialized cadre of leprosy assistants, to be replaced by horizontal ones which manage many diseases. Much of what is described here can be done by paramedicals—if you teach and encourage them.

There are many practical details which we have little space for, so if you see many leprosy patients, try to get the TALC slide set by Grace Warren, and the manuals listed below.

Fritschi EP, 'Surgical Reconstruction and Rehabilitation in Leprosy'. Available by purchase from: The Leprosy Mission, 80 Windmill Road, Brentford, Middlesex, TW8 0QH.

Neville Jane, Ed. 'A Footwear Manual for Leprosy Control Programmes, Parts I and II'. The German Leprosy Relief Association (DAHW) Postfach 348, D-8700 Würzburg 11 West Germany. Also available free from The Leprosy Mission, see above.

Watson Jean, 'Preventing Disability in Leprosy Patients'. Available from the Leprosy Mission, see above.

Brand P, 'Insensitive Feet, A Practical Handbook on Foot Problems in Leprosy'. Available free from The Leprosy Mission, see above

Warren Grace, 'The Care of the Nerve Damaged Limb' TALC slide set. Teaching Aids at Low Cost, The Institute of Child Health, 30 Guilford Street, London WC1N IEH

DISABILITY IN LEPROSY

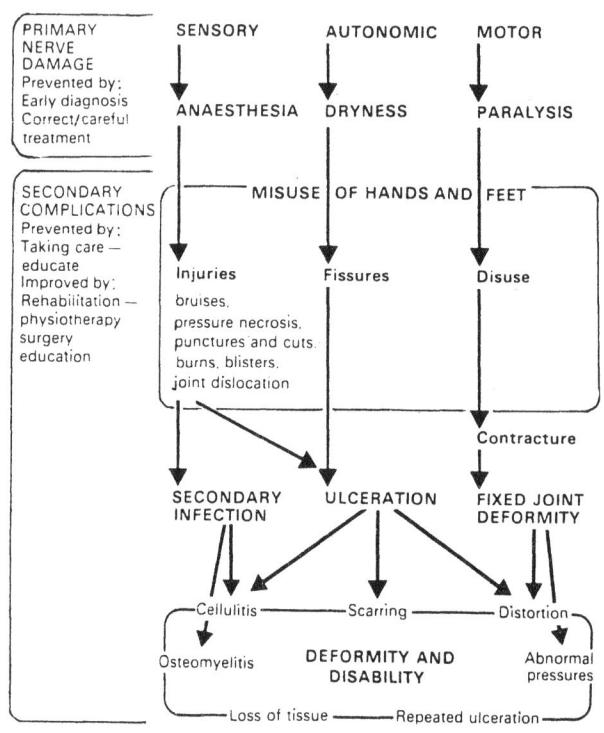

Fig. 30-0 THE CAUSES OF DISABILITY IN LEPROSY. Damage to the sensory, autonomic and motor components of nerves is folowed by anaesthesia, dryness of the skin and paralysis. A further cause of damage is direct invasion of the tissues by *Myc. leprae*. From Bryceson A, and Pfaltzgraff RE, 'Leprosy', (2nd edn 1979), Fig. 9.1. Churchill Livingstone, with kind permission.

30.1a Managing paralysis, especially during lepra reactions

A patient's nerves are involved early in tuberculoid and borderline leprosy, and later and less severely in lepromatous leprosy. This involvement can be slow, progressive, and irreversible. Or it can can occur suddenly during a Type One (see below).

Paralysis, whether slow or sudden, involves his nerves selectively: (1) His facial nerve, so that he cannot close his eye (lagophthalmos, 30.3). (2) His ulnar nerve at his elbow or wrist, so that his hand becomes clawed. (3) His median nerve at his wrist, so that he cannot oppose his thumb. (4) His radial nerve, so that his wrist drops (in the arm the ulnar nerve is most often affected, then the median, then the radial). (5) His lateral popliteal nerve at the neck of his fibula, so that he cannot dorsiflex his foot ('foot drop'). (5) His posterior tibial nerve behind his ankle, so that the intrinsic muscles of his foot become paralysed, his toes clawed, and his sole anaesthetic.

Both kinds of lepra reaction can cause paralysis, but need different management:

Type One reactions (also called non-lepromatous, reversal, or upgrading reactions) often cause sudden reversible paralysis in treated BT, BB, BL and rarely in LL leprosy. They make all the leprosy lesions in his skin and nerves swell acutely. His nerves become suddenly paralysed, and feel large and soft. They may be painless, or tender. His skin lesions may ulcerate, and the fibrosis that results may lead to a contracture. Recovery may take months, *so don't let a contracture develop meanwhile!* The sustained physiotherapy described below will prevent it. *If he has an acute paralysis* (but not otherwise), give him steroids for 6 to 12 weeks, as described below.

Type Two reactions are also called 'erythema nodosum leprosum' (ENL) reactions and occur in 50% of treated LL patients and occasionally in untreated LL or treated BL patients. During a few hours a crop of painful erythematous papules develop, typically on the extensor surfaces of his limbs, but in severe attacks over much of his body except his scalp. His skin may be thickened, especially over the backs of his hands and on his legs, where contractures may form. Meanwhile, his nerves are painful, and become steadily paralysed. Unfortunately, they are less likely to recover than after a Type One reaction. Give him clofazimine in high doses, and aspirin. *If he has a severe acute episode,* you can, if necessary, give him a *short* (10 to 21 days) course of steroids. If you prolong it, he is liable to all the long-term consequences of steroid therapy.

LEPROSY

LEPRA REACTIONS

SUPPRESSION is indicated if a lepra reaction has caused paralysis, or uveitis (30.2). Continue the patient's antileprotic drugs in both types of reaction.

Suppress his Type One reactions with steroids for 6 to 12 weeks, or as long as there is activity. Start with a maximum of 30 mg of prednisolone daily in the mornings. As soon as the acute stage of reaction (swelling, redness, and pain) has subsided, gradually reduce his steroids, even if there is no sign of nerve-function returning. Reduce the dose by 5 mg daily each successive week (30 mg of prednisolone daily for a week, then 25 mg daily for a week..., until you are giving none).

His nerves may start to recover within 3 weeks, or they may not improve for 3 months, or a year, or longer. Meanwhile, manage them as described below.

Suppress Type Two reactions with clofazimine and aspirin or thalidomide (provided there is no possibility of pregnancy), as long as there continues to be any sign of them, however slowly improvement takes place. If you are going to use steroids, give him (or her) a short course only. Some contributors consider that the risks of steroids outweigh their benefits.

PHYSIOTHERAPY IN LEPROSY

A limb which is paralysed by leprosy needs physiotherapy to strengthen its muscles and prevent contractures, especially if paralysis is recent, actively progressing, or possibly only temporary, as in either type of leprosy reaction. Particular physiotherapy for his eyes (30.2), hands (30.4), and feet (30.5) is described elsewhere.

As long as there are signs of weakness, someone, preferably the patient himself, must put all his paralysed joints through their full range of movement each day, even if they cannot be actively maintained in their positions of function.

Protect his paralysed muscles by splinting his joints in their positions of function during sleep, and never allow a muscle to be overstretched. Make sure he does active physiotherapy to retain the mobility of all his joints. Even if all the intrinsic muscles of his hand are paralysed, it will be more useful to him if its joints are kept mobile with the daily exercises in Fig. 30-3. Start this protection the first day you diagnose a reaction.

When he shows signs of recovery, as shown by his pain decreasing, his nerves becoming softer, and his sensation and motor function returning, he must: (1) increase his range of active movement and strengthen his muscles with carefully graded active exercises. And, (2) practise any skilled coordinated movements that he will need later when he returns to his normal life. Tell him to start his exercises as soon as the acute symptoms of neuritis have subsided. Begin by doing each exercise 5 times, increasing to a maximum of 30 times, repeated 3 to 5 times daily. Teach him to do his exercises himself at home: but if he is to have reconstructive surgery, he may need more intensive preparation.

30.2 The eyes in leprosy, iritis (uveitis)

You will need a system of priorities when you approach a leprosy patient. The most important function you need to preserve is his sight. If he has also lost the feeling in his fingertips, blindness will separate him from his environment almost completely.

Leprosy causes: (1) Paralysis of his facial nerve, so that he cannot close his eye (lagophthalmos, 30.3). (2) Loss of sensation in the ophthalmic division of his fifth cranial nerve, which makes his cornea anaesthetic. (3) An acute iritis (uncommon), which is usually associated with a Type Two reaction. (4) A chronic iritis (common) causing atrophy of his dilator pupillae and a small unreactive pupil (see also Section 24.5).

Iritis is common in lepromatous leprosy. It usually comes on so slowly that he may not notice that there is anything wrong with his eyes, until they are severely damaged, and he starts to lose his sight from synechiae, cataracts, or secondary glaucoma (rare). An acute uveitis occurs mainly in patients who have a Type Two lepra reaction, and is less common if they are on clofazimine.

To detect uveitis, use a corneal loupe, and preferably a slit lamp microscope. Grossly, you may see mild ciliary hyperaemia on his conjunctiva next to the limbus. This is a good indication of activity, and you can always see it with a good light; but be careful to distinguish it from conjunctivitis. If you press his globe he may complain of pain. With a slit lamp, the earliest signs are keratic precipitates (KP) on the back of his cornea, a flare, and cells floating in his anterior chamber; these are also the last signs to disappear. If you are in any doubt, and you don't have a slit lamp, dilate his pupils. Any irregularity due to synechiae will then be diagnostic, but it will not tell you if his iridocyclitis is active. If dilatation relieves his pain it probably is active.

THE EYES IN LEPROSY

ROUTINE EXAMINATION. Examine the eyes of all leprosy patients regularly to detect. (1) Lagophthalmos and corneal exposure. (2) Chronic iritis, which may cause secondary glaucoma and blindness. See also Sections 24.1 and 24.5.

(1) Measure the patient's visual acuity. (2) Assess his normal eyelid closure as in sleep (not his forced eyelid closure). If his lids don't touch he has lagophthalmos. (4) Dilate his pupil with a short-acting dilator to see if it is irregular (a sign of iritis). (5) Stain his corneae with fluorescein to look for ulcers due either to lagophthalmos or an ananaesthetic cornea.

IRITIS IN LEPROSY

TREATMENT. Dilate his eyes with 1% atropine eye ointment, or atropine drops, hourly for three hours, or until they are dilated, and then once daily. Give him hydrocortisone or cortisone eye drops or ointment 3 or 4 times daily. If synechiae persist, continue atropine twice daily. If redness or pain persist, or if his corneae are cloudy, he may need steroids by subconjunctival injection, or rarely by mouth. If you give them, he must be taking his leprosy drugs at the same time. He should respond well, if you treat him early. If he has a chronic Type Two reaction (ENL), he may need atropine once weekly and steroid ointment daily for many months.

If his intraocular tension is raised (secondary glaucoma, 24.5), also give him acetazolamide 250 mg 6-hourly, until the inflamation is under control. Use phenylephrine eye drops 10%

3 times daily to lower his intraocular pressure, instead of atropine. Refer him if you can.

CAUTION ! (1) If his eyes are not much better, and he still has pain after 7 days, refer him—urgent treatment may be necessary to save his sight. (2) Make sure that his eyes are examined every week and his pupils are regularly dilated.

If the disease has progressed far enough for 'ring synechiae' to be present, and his intraocular pressure is raised, refer him for a broad iridectomy to save his sight. Ideally, this should not be done until his eye is quiet and white, but this is usually impossible, because he will be blind before it happens.

If he develops a secondary cataract, this will need surgery, but it should not be done at the same time as the iridectomy. Always delay cataract extraction until you are absolutely sure an eye is quiet. This may take years! If his cataract is extracted too soon, while his uveitis is still active, he may become blind.

30.3 Lagophthalmos in leprosy

When leprosy involves the ophthalmic division of a patient's fifth nerve, his cornea becomes anaesthetic. When it involves the zygomatic branch of his seventh nerve, his orbicularis muscle is paralysed, so that he cannot shut his eyes properly (lagophthalmos). The combination of these two lesions can have a devastating effect on his sight.

An anaesthetic cornea prevents him from noticing that he has something in his eye, or that it is dry. He loses his blink reflex, so that, even if he still has enough power in his seventh nerve to blink, he does not wash and wet his conjunctiva automatically. As a result, his cornea may be unprotected, especially while he sleeps, so that it may develop exposure keratitis, and ulcerate. If the centre of his cornea becomes opaque, his sight is spoilt. So warn him of the danger of an anaesthetic cornea, and examine his eyes regularly.

To decide if his cornea has been damaged, look for superficial scars, and use fluorescein drops, or papers, to search for central staining. If his cornea is anaesthetic, his eye is at great risk. If he has lagophthalmos, but his cornea is not anaesthetic, he may have enough sensation to complain of discomfort or burning.

To find out if he has significant lagophthalmos, ask him to close his eyes. If his cornea is *completely* covered, all is well. But if *any* part of it remains exposed, something *must* be done to protect his sight. Several operations are possible, but we only describe two methods of tarsorraphy. Both aim to reduce the gap between his lids when he tries to shut them. Tarsorrhaphy has cosmetic disadvantages, but it does save sight, and it is not difficult, so you should be able to do it if you care for leprosy patients. One of the most effective procedures, transfer of the temporalis muscle, is too difficult to be described here.

LAGOPHTHALMOS IN LEPROSY

If a patient has any weakness in his eyelid muscles, teach him exercises for them, such as screwing up his eyes as strongly as he can.

INVESTIGATION. Test the sensation in his cornea with a wisp of cotton wool. Examine his lachrymal apparatus. If patency is in doubt, dilate the punctum and irrigate the sac with saline. You may be able to flush out the system. If it remains blocked, but there is no sign of infection and no regurgitation of mucus, you can operate, but he will need an antibiotic postoperatively.

NON-OPERATIVE TREATMENT. **If his paralysis is recent,** treat him medically for a few weeks to see if it will recover. Warmth protects nerves in leprosy, so in cold weather ask him to keep his face warm with a woollen Balaclava helmet or a scarf.

If he has anaesthesia but not lagophthalmos, the stimulus to blink will be missing, but not the power to do so. So teach him to blink regularly.

(1) Artificial tears or even paraffin drops twice daily will help to protect his cornea. If you don't have medicinal paraffin, use the domestic kind. (2) Apply antibiotic eye ointment 3 times daily, especially at night. (3) Strap his upper lid to his cheek to prevent exposure of his cornea.

If he has a Type One reaction, give him steroids, as in Section 30.1a.

If his cornea is already ulcerated, give him antibiotics and atropine (24.3) until his cornea heals.

If he has iritis, dilate his pupil with atropine, and consider giving him topical steroids (24.5).

INDICATIONS FOR TARSORRAPHY. Any part of his cornea remaining exposed when he tries to shut his eyes. (1) Leprosy; if his cornea is already damaged, or he has reduced or absent corneal sensation and lagophthalmos, tarsorraphy is urgent. (2) Burns (58.28). (3) Facial paresis or paralysis; Bell's palsy. (4) Degloving injuries.

CONTRAINDICATIONS. (1) A cornea which is already damaged. (2) Lagophthalmos which is only temporary and will recover when the neuritis of a leprosy reaction recovers.

TARSORRAPHY (Margaret Brand)

CHOICE OF SITE. You can do a medial, or a lateral tarsorraphy. Close the medial or lateral half of his palpebral fissure with a pair of forceps, to determine which site is likely to be best, and how long the tarsorrhaphy should be. A medial one keeps the punctae in touch with the globe, and helps to relieve excessive tearing, which is common when the lower lid sags, as in A, Fig. 30-1. It is better cosmetically, but is more difficult,

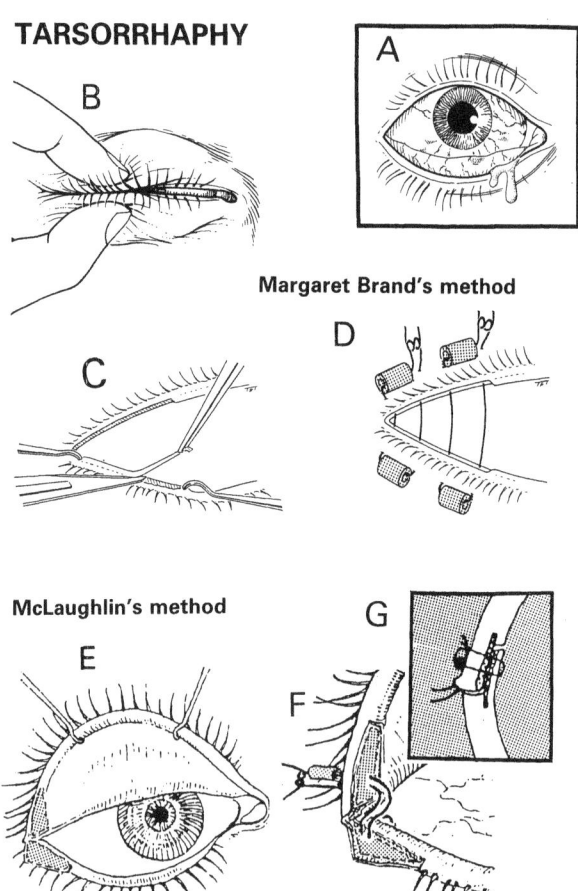

Fig. 30-1 TWO METHODS OF TARSORRAPHY FOR LAGOPHTHALMOS. This is a condition in which a patient's eye will not shut and waters excessively (A). B, pinch his lids together and tell him to open them. This will tell you how long a tarsorraphy needs to be to protect his eyes and still allow him to see. C, the incisions for Margaret Brand's tarsorraphy. D, two mattress sutures inserted. E, the incisions for McLaughlin's method. F, the suture about to be tied. G, the lid sutured. *A, B, C, and D, from 'Watch Those Eyes' by Margaret Brand, with kind permission. E, F, and G, after McLaughlin from McDowell F and Enna CD, 'Surgical Rehabilitation in Leprosy', (1973). Williams and Wilkins, with kind permission.*

because the punctae and canaliculi are close to the operation site, and must not be damaged.

CAUTION ! The tarsorraphy must be large enough to enable him to cover his whole cornea, when he tries to close his eyes. A common mistake is to make it too small, so that it is ineffective. You may have to do medial and lateral tarsorrhaphies at the same time, leaving a small opening through which he can just see.

A temporary central tarshorraphy may be indicated, if ulceration threatens his cornea, or has already occurred, particularly if sensation is poor.

METHOD (lateral tarsorraphy). You can operate on both eyes at the same session. Pinch his lids together to decide how much lid to suture. Mark the appropriate length of lid with a little gentian violet. Instil a few drops of amethocaine 2%. Inject 1 ml of local anaesthetic solution with adrenalin (optional) into each lid near the margin (A 5.3).

Hold his lids apart and make an incision along the grey line (just behind the lash follicles), between the marks you have made with gentian violet. Make another incision parallel to the first one and 1 or 2 mm from it. Dissect away a strip of tissue between these two incisions. Repeat the procedure on the second lid to leave two opposed, raw, bleeding areas. Join these areas with monofilament mattress sutures every 5 mm. Swab away all blood clot, and tie them over lengths of fine rubber or plastic tube, to prevent them cutting into his skin.

CAUTION ! Make sure that no lashes project back between the sutures.

Preferably, cover his eye with a light dressing for 24 hours, and remove the sutures on the 14th day. If you have operated on both his eyes at the same time, leave them uncovered, and insert antibiotic drops 3 times daily until his lids have healed.

LATERAL TARSORRAPHY (McLaughlin)

Incise his lower lid margin along its intermarginal line (the line where his lids touch anteriorly) medially from his outer canthus for 5 or 6 mm. Remove a piece of the anterior lamella of the lower lid. Split the intermarginal line of his upper lid for the same distance, and remove a similar sector of tarsus and conjunctiva.

Evert his upper lid, and insert a 4/0 mattress suture from the skin to the bare area. Insert it through the bare area of his lower lid towards his conjunctiva. Then return, making a mattress suture about 3 mm long tied over a piece of fine rubber or plastic tube. When you tie it, his palpebral fissure will be shortened, and his lids will overlap.

30.4 Leprosy of the hands

A patient with leprosy can lose the feeling in his hands suddenly during a lepra reaction, so that he complains of an immediate numbness, or so slowly that he hardly notices it. When this happens, neglected bruises, blisters, and cuts cause scars that progressively destroy the pulps of his fingers. Painless cigarette burns are a common presentation. To prevent this happening he must learn how not to injure himself. *Persuade him that it is the injury to his hands which leads to wounds, and not the disease itself.* If he fails to care for his fingers, and presents you with a severely disabled hand, there is little you can do, except to maintain such mobility as he has with physiotherapy. Patients are usually able to use their deformed hands quite well, and don't like having their fingers amputated.

Tendon transfers and arthrodeses are sometmes helpful, and a Z-plasty can be done to widen the web of the thumb, but these are all expert tasks.

Severe hand infections are common in leprosy patients, and usually present late. You will see abscesses (8.1), osteomyelitis (8.16), tenosynovitis (8.12), and gangrenous fingers.

HANDS IN LEPROSY

Protect a patient's hands during hard work, either by making sure he wears protective gloves, or by adapting the handles of the tools he uses. He is more likely to consent to wear gloves,

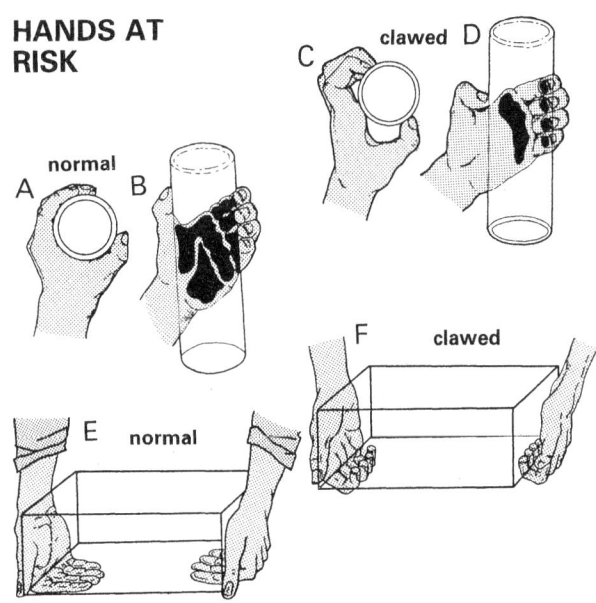

Fig. 30-2 HANDS AT RISK. The area of skin in contact with the cylinder is black. A, and B, when a normal hand bears the weight of a block or a cylinder, most of its surface bears its weight. C, and D, when a clawed hand does the same too much of its weight is borne by the finger tips. E, and F, the same phenomenon when a patient lifts a box. This misuse of the finger tips is an important cause of finger absorption. *From Brand Paul W, 'Clinical Mechanics of the Hand', (1985) Mosby, with kind permission.*

than to use modified tools. If he smokes (persuade him not to) he must use a cigarette holder. Make sure that his insensitive hands are soaked and oiled in the same way as his feet (30.5).

If the flexor surface of his finger cracks, don't let it heal with a short scar which will be likely to reopen when it is stretched—splint it straight while it heals. Use plaster strengthened with a stiff longitudinal wire, or a short length of stiff plastic hose pipe, cut with a tongue which projects into his palm. Observe his finger carefully for blueness. Initially, remove splints at night, until you are sure they are not occluding his circulation.

If the dorsum of his hand is scarred, so that his MP joints become hyperextended, severe disability will result. This can happen as the result of a lepra reaction, when a thick sheet of inflammatory tissue scars and perhaps ulcerates. Put his hand through a full range of movement daily during the reaction to keep it mobile. Later, a skilled surgical release may be possible.

If he has severely deformed finger(s), such as a terminal phalanx bent to 90°, consider amputation or, better, an arthrodesis with shortening of the bones to allow for the contracted tissue on the front of the joint. If his fifth finger is badly deformed, remove it with half its metacarpal (75-28). Its absence will hardly be noticed.

If paralysis is acute (within 3 months, and perhaps up to 6 months, but certainly no more), he has probably had a lepra reaction, and so has some hope of recovery. Give him full antileprosy treatment and steroids for 6 to 12 weeks. Splint his hand in the position of function (75.3) at night, and be sure he moves it by day. Ensure that all the joints of his hand are put through their full range daily, using the exercises D, and E, in Fig. 30-3.

If his ulnar nerve is acutely involved, rest his arm in a sling with his elbow at 90°, and put his whole arm through its full range of motion at least once a day.

If his lumbricals are involved, he is in danger of developing a claw hand, so teach him the exercises in F, and G, Fig. 30-3.

If his median nerve is involved, his thumb web may need stretching. Ask him to grasp the distal end of its metacarpal (not its phalanges), and pull it away from his fingers (not shown).

If paralysis is chronic and slowly progressive, recovery is unlikely, so ask him to do the exercises in Fig. 30-3. A paralysed hand is more useful if it is mobile rather than stiff, and is less likely to be damaged at work.

INFECTIONS IN LEPROUS HANDS (common)

Watch for heat and swelling. Tenderness is often absent and fluctuation is too late to be useful. His first complaint may be painful glands in his axilla. The same principles apply as in normal hands (Chapter 8), with one great difference—the pain which prevents a normal person from using his infected hand cannot protect an anaesthetic one. So make sure that a leprosy patient *rests* his infected hand, and apply a splint to make sure he does. Apply it in the position of safety (75.3) with his MP joints flexed, his IP joints almost fully extended, and his thumb abducted, as if he were holding a tennis ball.

CAUTION ! Antibiotics without rest are a waste of time, money and his fingers!

If infection starts as a macerated skin crease in a paralysed finger, splint it with a posterior splint in just sufficient extension to open out the finger and expose it to the air. If a posterior splint is difficult, use a palmar one. If there is any discharge, give him an antibiotic also.

If you feel rough bone at the base of an ulcer or sinus in his hand, and pus oozes from a joint he has osteomyelitis or septic arthritis (8.15).

If you feel rough bone at the bottom of a sinus over the tip of his finger, he has osteomyelitis of his terminal phalanx. If only part of a phalanx is dead, allow dead bone to separate spontaneously. Otherwise, you are likely to open the joint, and he will lose more finger length. If most of a phalanx is dead, disarticulate the joint and remove the base.

If he has septic arthritis, aim for a fibrous arthrodesis, or a bony ankylosis. Splint his hand and fingers as nearly as possible in the position of function (7.16), and give him an antibiotic. Immobilize his infected joint for at least 4 to 6 weeks after the infection is controlled, and the ulcer healed, while putting all his other joints through their full range of movement daily. If splinting one finger is difficult, you may be justified in splinting it with one of its neighbours (75-14), depending on their condition. Curette dead bone and granulations, and pack the cavity with hypochlorite ('Eusol') or sugar (57.3) to encourage sequestra to discharge and granulations to fill the cavity. An ankylosis usually takes 12 weeks and a fibrous arthrodesis 6 to 8 weeks.

If his septic arthritis does not heal, excise the joint. Make a dorsal incision, remove the joint surfaces, and any dead tissues, and splint the joint in a position of function (75.3). Pack the cavity that remains, and allow it to heal by granulation. Keep the joint splinted in the position of function, and wait 12 weeks for an ankylosis.

If he has septic tenosynovitis, it is likely to be the result of spread from a pulp infection. Splint his hand in the position of function. If drainage is not free make a further opening in his middle palmar crease.

If he has a grossly swollen hand, with pitting oedema of the dorsum, and obliteration of the concavity of his palm, he has a midpalmar space infection—see Section 8.9.

30.5 The care of anaesthetic feet

A patient's feet are even more important than his hands. He may be able to work with a paralysed hand, but if he cannot walk, he will probably be unable to undertake the essential activities of daily life. All over the world, leprosy patients who are being adequately treated medically, are being allowed to walk about on ulcerated feet. The dressings that cover their ulcers *do not prevent them from deepening, and widening, and involving the bones underneath*. The quiet progressive destruction of these feet is not inevitable—and can be minimized. It may be a losing game, so play it as cleverly as you can, and try to retain the usefulness of a patient's foot as long as possible.

Ulcers can be caused by: (1) Constant mild pressure, which causes necrosis by impairing the blood supply to the tissues, as in paraplegic ulcers (64.13). In a normal person ischaemia soon causes pain, so that the ischaemic part is moved, and its blood

HANDS AND FEET IN LEPROSY

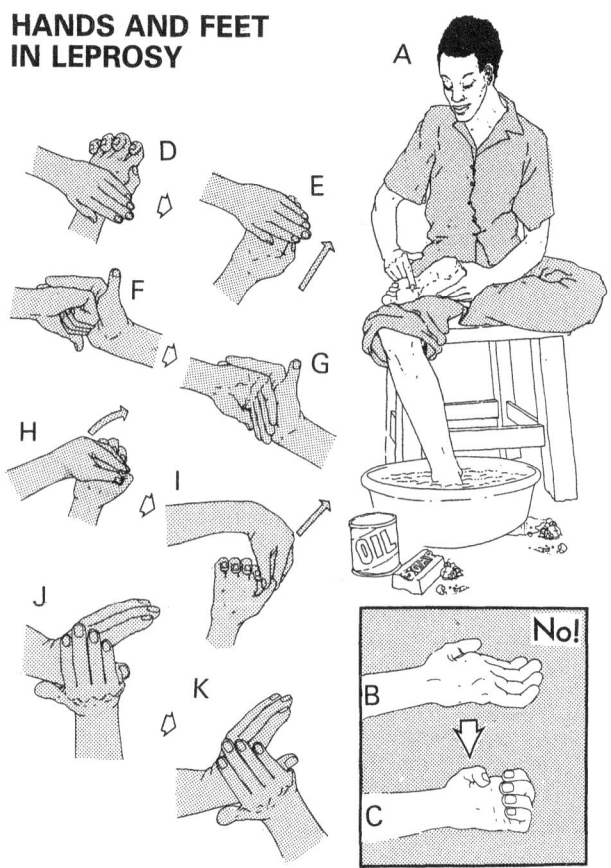

Fig. 30-3 HANDS AND FEET IN LEPROSY. A, a patient inspecting his anaesthetic feet to find early wounds and 'hot spots'. He is soaking them, and is about to rub them with oil. The exercises shown here are for acute and chronic paralysis, and will prevent a hand like (B) from becoming a stiff claw hand (C) which physiotherapy cannot cure. Instruct him like this: D, ''...rest the back of your hand on your thigh, or on a table padded by a cloth. E, use your other hand to rub your fingers as straight as they will go, taking care not to crack any weak skin. F, cup your knuckle joints in your other palm and keep them firmly bent. G, then straighten the end two joints of your fingers, as firmly as you can. H, and I, use your other hand to straighten the end joint of your thumb, as straight as it will go. Pull gently and firmly, as if you were trying to lengthen your thumb, but don't pull it backwards. J, and K, rest the little finger side of your hand on your thigh. Use your other hand to support the back of your thumb firmly (to keep its MP joint flexed), then straighten the end joint of your thumb as firmly as you can...' *After Watson Jean M, 'Preventing Disability in Leprosy', The Leprosy Mission International, with kind permission.*

supply restored. In an anaesthetic limb there is no pain, so that the ischaemic tissue is allowed to become necrotic and ulcerates. (2) A strong force which cuts, shears or tears the tissues. In the foot, the strength of the force is less important than the small area over which it is applied. (3) The frequent repetition of moderate forces, which cause inflammation that weakens the tissues. This is an important cause of ulcers, so try to keep the pressure on a foot low. (4) Forces which spread infection to soft tissues and bone. An infected foot is so painful to a normal person, that he has to rest it—a leprosy patient does not do this spontaneously. (5) A previous ulcer. This is the commonest cause. If a patient has never had an ulcer, he may escape without one— if he is careful. If however he has already had nine ulcers, he will probably get a tenth.

The key to preventing ulcers is: (1) To teach a patient how not to injure himself in the first place, and (2) to teach him 'self care' for any injuries he does receive, in their *earliest* stages. *All* primary care workers should be able to teach this. When his tissues have been damaged, they will usually heal, if he *rests them completely*. Surgery is much less important than rest, at the right time, and for the right length of time. Antibiotics without rest will not heal ulcers.

Ulcers commonly start in the deeper tissues, and develop slowly over several days, so teach him to recognize an ulcer as a 'hot spot' *in its 'pre-ulcer' stage*, before the skin over it has been broken. A hot spot is a warm area of skin, usually with swelling, that occurs after activity, and persists during at least 2 hours of rest. In an anaesthetic foot, a hot spot may be the only indication of some underlying pathology, such as a fracture, disintegrating bone, a strain, or an abscess. Any of these may break through to the surface, and form an ulcer. The patient, or a friend, must learn to look for hot spots, because they mean "Stop!" He must take them seriously, and rest his foot until all signs of inflammation have gone. Rest at the hot spot stage is the only way to avoid the serious damage that starts the downhill road to amputation.

The risk of an anaesthetic foot developing an ulcer depends partly on his shoe (if he has one), and partly on how much he walks. The less he walks the better. Perhaps he can ride a donkey, or a bicycle? The kind of shoe he needs depends on the state of his foot, as defined by the 'degree of risk' below. Many patients with moderate, or even high risk feet, can remain free from ulcers without moulded shoes if: (1) they practise self care, (2) they have microcellular rubber insoles in their sandals or shoes, (3) they limit their walking, and (4) they take small steps. Moulded shoes are more difficult to make, and many hospitals manage without them. With a little instruction a local cobbler should be able to make a suitable unmoulded shoe in the local style, with the necessary insoles and straps, and using only the local materials. If you want him to make a moulded shoe, he will need these special materials:

• *MICROCELLULAR RUBBER, 5 m² × 10 mm only.* This has a closed bubble structure, and is much more resilient than ordinary 'foam rubber'. Some shoe factories can provide it. It is not the same as the foam plastic used for cheap sandals, which is less resilient. Car tyres make good soles, and inner tubes can make uppers.

• *FOAMED POLYETHYLENE, 1 cm thick, as 'Plastazote' (Smith and Nephew) 5 m² only.* This is a light thermoplastic which a skillful cobbler can use to make a moulded shoe, for a moderate- or severe-risk foot. It resists wetting and is easily cleaned, but it does need an oven. Its main disadvantage is that it wears away in less than 6 months. Heat a piece of sheet to exactly 140°C in an oven and hold it at that temperature for five minutes: place it on a 10 cm polyurethane foam pillow; and then ask the patient to stand still on it until it is cool, or let him sit while you force his foot down on it, as in C, Fig. 30-5. It will not burn him, and will set in the shape of his sole, as in illustrations D, and E, in this figure. Be sure to support moulded 'Plastazote' with microcellular rubber, or cork and latex, built up to produce a flat sole; it is not resilient enough to make an insole by itself.

• *FOOTPRINT MAT, also called a Harris mat, rubber, (DOW Canada), two only of each thickness (optional).* This is a mat with little rubber ridges which you ink. Place a piece of paper on the inked mat and ask the patient to walk on it. The greater the pressure, the blacker the ink impression. If you are really interested in the care of leprosy feet, get a footprint mat: its use is described in Paul Brand's book on insensitive feet (30.1).

**LOOK FOR SWELLING AND REDNESS
FEEL FOR 'HOT SPOTS'**

FEET IN LEPROSY

'SELF CARE'. Teach a leprosy patient to: (1) Recognize that his anaesthesia is abnormal. (2) Care for his anaesthetic limbs, so that they are not injured. (3) Inspect his limbs daily, so that he can remove any thorns, and recognize and care for any wound, either open or closed, while it is still small, and before it gets worse. (4) Rest his limbs when they are injured. (5) Recognize and understand the seriousness of 'hot spots'. (6) Treat his first ulcer as the calamity that it really is.

CAUTION ! (1) Persuade him that it is injury to his anaesthetic feet and not the disease itself which leads to ulceration and loss of tissue. (2) He *must* limit his walking, if he has a hot spot,

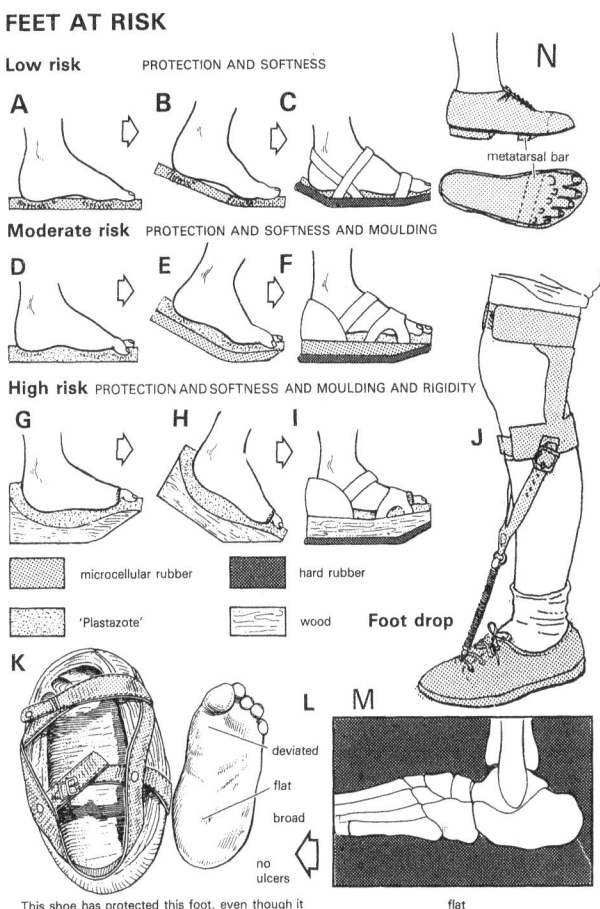

Fig. 30-4 FOOTWARE FOR FEET AT RISK can be made by any cobbler if you are prepared to teach him.
LOW RISK FEET. A, microcellular rubber distributes the pressure. B, hatching indicates the areas of increased pressure on walking. C, a car tyre sole applied.
MODERATE RISK FEET. D, the first layer of 'Plastazote'. E, a layer of microcellular rubber. F, a layer of car tyre.
HIGH RISK FEET. G, a layer of 'Plastazote' in a carved wooden clog distributes the weight evenly. H, when the patient walks, his foot does not flex, and weight continues to be spread evenly. I, the completed sandal.
J, a toe-raising strap for a dropped foot. *This is a very helpful device for any dropped foot, so don't fail to fit one when it is needed.* If necessary, use canvas or plastic straps and make the 'spring' from a car inner tube. K, a properly made shoe can protect a badly damaged foot. Note that it has no ulcers, even though it has lost its arches, and its toes are clawed and deviated. It has remained free from ulcers because the patient limited his activity, and because the shoe has a layer of microcellular rubber built up under a moulded 'Plastazote' insole. M, the foot belonging to the owner of the shoe; its arches have flattened, so has his calcaneus; even so, his shoe has managed to protect him. N, the simplest modification for an ulcerated foot is a metatarsal bar, stuck or stitched to the outside of the sole, just behind the metatarsal heads, proximal to the ulcerated area.
From Bryceson A, and Pfaltzgraff RE, 'Leprosy' (2nd edn 1979), Figs 11.1 to 11.3. Churchill Livingstone, with kind permission.

or an area of deep tenderness.

EXAMINING AN INSENSITIVE FOOT. Look for swellings, injuries and callositis. Are any of his toes pushed apart (with oedema from an injury)? Examine the arches of his feet as he stands, and look for flattening. Feel his whole foot. Warmth or swelling suggest active pathology, and the need for extra care. Press deeply over the common sites of ulceration in A, and B, Fig. 30-6. He may still feel deep pain, when he has lost all ordinary sensation.

Watch him walking barefoot. You can easily miss a dropped foot, if it is also short. Ask him to walk on his heels. He cannot do this if his anterior tibial or peroneal muscles are weak. Finally, don't forget to look at his shoes!

SKIN CARE. Denervation of the skin reduces its natural secretions and makes it dry, so that it more easily cracks, fissures, and becomes infected. Softening dry skin reduces these dangers, and may allow any fissures that have formed to heal. So ask him to get plain water, without detergents, into his dry feet (or hands) by soaking them for 15 to 20 minutes at least twice a day. Then ask him to cover his skin with petroleum jelly ('Vaseline'), or any kind of grease or oil (including car oil). It is the water that is important, not the grease which keeps it in.

If fissures are already well established, pare away the thick callus with a knife, or ask him to rub it away with a pumice or other stone. Remove rough callus regularly, because it may split and crack, or cause ulcers by pressure.

OTHER WAYS TO PREVENT ULCERS. When necessary remember to: (1) Correct deformities. If he has a dropped foot, fit a toe raising strap (J, 30-4). (2) Ask him to take short steps, which will reduce the pressure on the front of his foot and his heel. (3) Ask him to avoid any hard edges or knots in his shoes or socks. (5) Beware of newly healed ulcers. The scar will not have had time to become supple, and is in danger from any shearing force applied to it.

'PRE-ULCERS'. Try to recognize a 'pre-ulcer foot', because 3 days to 3 weeks of immediate bed rest at this stage may prevent a serious ulcer forming. Look for: (1) swelling of his sole, (2) separation of his toes, (3) necrosis blisters at the side of his foot, caused by fluid which has tracked from the necrotic area above his plantar fascia, as in G, Fig. 30-6, (4) 'hot spots', (5) redness, (6) pain (if he still has any sensation), especially pain on deep pressure.

FEET AT RISK FROM LEPROSY

A LOW RISK FOOT is anaesthetic, but has little or no scarring. It needs protection and a resilient sole. The possibilities include: (1) A resilient insole in a well-fitting shoe, which is one size larger than one he usually wears. This may be enough. Don't make the insole too thick, and make sure his shoe is well fastened, so that it does not slip and produce blisters. (2) A car-tyre sandal with an insole of microcellular rubber.

A MODERATE RISK FOOT is anaesthetic, has multiple scars, and has lost some of the subcutaneous fat pad on its sole. A shoe for a foot like this needs to be moulded, to take the weight off the metatarsal heads, and spread it evenly over the entire sole. Such a foot will however do fairly well in a simple car-tyre and microcellular rubber sandal—*if* he keeps the callus well pared down. Or, make a piece of moulded 'Plastazote' as described above. When it has set firm, build microcellular rubber up underneath it, and then fit this to a car-tyre sole. If it is made as a sandal, it will need a retainer for the heel moulded into it. A shoe with a moulded sole is better than a sandal at preventing the foot slipping out, but it *must* have a well-fitting upper with buckles, laces, or straps, so that it remains in its correct relationship to the foot.

A HIGH RISK FOOT has, in addition, a mild deformity, such as flattening of the arches, and shortening, or loss, of toes. It needs a shoe which is moulded to conform to it completely, and has a rigid sole. Build microcellular rubber up under a sole of moulded 'Plastazote', and carve a wooden rocker clog to fit it; then fit this with a hard rubber sole. A clog is rigid, so its front end must be boat-shaped as in G, Fig. 30-4. Some of these feet do well in microcellular rubber sandals—if their owner looks after them carefully.

A DISINTEGRATED FOOT has a major bony deformity such as fragmentation of its tarsal bones, or is 'boat-shaped', or has a dislocated ankle. Rehabilitation is difficult; he may need reconstructive surgery and a proper orthopaedic boot. See also Section 30.6D.

PROTECTIVE FOOTWARE FOR LEPROSY

Instruct a cobbler to make the footwear described above, and to follow the local styles where he can. Make the straps broad, and adjustable with buckles or laces, so as to allow for swelling or bandages. The simplest protection for an ulcerated foot is a metatarsal bar, stuck or stitched to the outside of the sole, just behind the metatarsal heads, as in N, Fig. 30-4.

CAUTION ! (1) *Never* use nails or wire to make or repair shoes for leprosy patients—glue and sew them. (2) If his foot is significantly inverted or everted, only major surgery will allow him to walk satisfactorily. (3) New shoes need special care. Warn him to walk short distances only until the leather has become adjusted to his foot—meanwhile he should use his old ones most of the time.

PARALYSIS OF THE FEET IN LEPROSY

If paralysis developed quickly and is acute (and is still within 3 months, and perhaps up to 6 months, but certainly no more), he has probably been in reaction (Type One) and has some hope of recovery. Give him full antileprosy treatment and steroids for 6 to 12 weeks (30.1a). Treat him as described below.

If he has a posterior tibial nerve palsy, either: (1) Apply a firm bandage to limit friction at the back of his ankle. Combine this with a heel retainer, to minimize the use of the small muscles of his foot, and trauma to his anaesthetic sole. Or, (2) apply a padded plaster boot.

If he has an acute common peroneal nerve palsy, or a palsy of its branches, so that he has a flapping gait and foot drop,

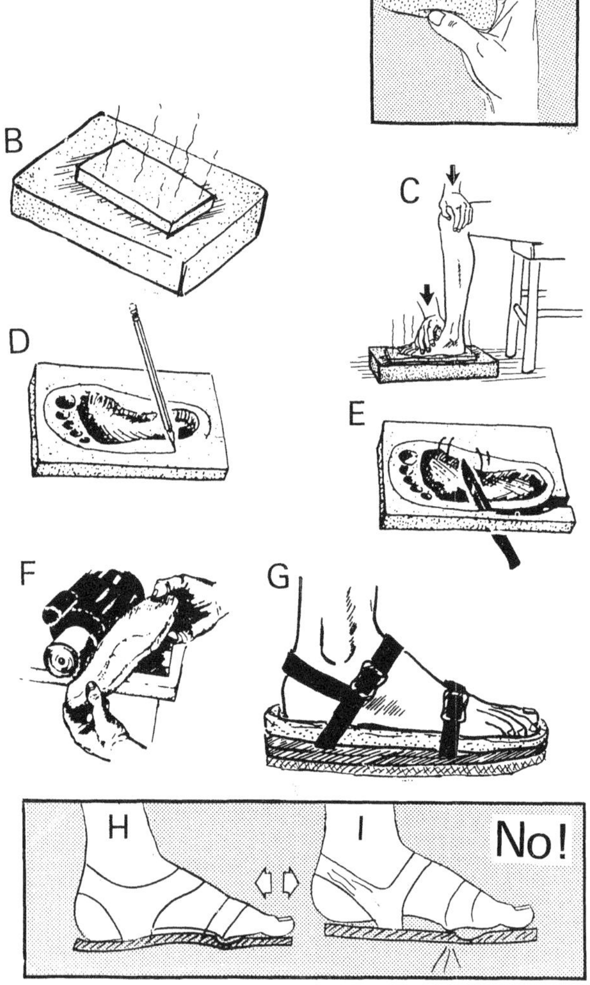

Fig. 30-5 PROTECTIVE FOOTWARE FOR LEPROSY. A, the right kind of microcellular rubber can be squeezed to half its thickness; if it is flatter than this it is too soft, if it is thicker it is too hard. B, a sheet of hot 'Plastazote' laid on soft foam. C, take the mould by applying even pressure and holding it for 3 minutes. Mark it out (D), and cut it (E), so as to project 0.5 to 1 cm in front of the patient's toes and behind his heel. Shape it (F), smooth it on an electric buff, and support it with a layer of microcellular rubber and stick it to a hard rubber sole. G, the completed shoe made from moulded 'Plastazote' supported by layers of microcellular rubber, and soled with car tyre. H, and I, a moulded shoe must be anchored to his foot and must not be allowed to move about. *After Brand Paul,'Insensitive Feet: A Practical Handbook on Foot Problems in Leprosy'. The Leprosy Mission International, with kind permission.*

passive exercises will help to stretch his Achilles tendon and prevent a contracture: (1) Ask him to squat with his heels flat on the ground. (2) Ask him to stand erect about 70 cm from a wall, to keep his feet flat on the ground, and with the palms of his hands flat on the wall to do 'press ups' in the vertical position.

He also needs some protective device. Either: (1) By day, fit him with a toe-raising spring as in J, Fig. 30-4. If he is co-operative, this will be easier and cheaper, and will allow him to do some work. By night, apply a posterior plaster slab to hold his ankle in neutral. Or, (2) apply a complete plaster cast, including his foot and leg up to the middle of his thigh, with 15° of flexion of his knee, and with his ankle in neutral, taking care that the cast does not press on the nerve. Leave it on for 6 weeks.

If his common peroneal nerve paralysis has persisted 6 months in spite of medical measures and physiotherapy, it is probably permanent. He may be helped by the lengthening of his Achilles tendon, and the transfer of his tibialis posterior tendon to the front of his foot to make it into a dorsiflexor (30.8). If this is impossible, or while waiting for surgery, fit him with a toe-raising strap.

If he also has plantar ulceration with his foot drop, be sure to use a posterior slab or a cast. If his ankle is not supported, his tendo Achilles is likely to contract on bed rest. Give him crutches while his ulcer heals, so that he does not even take one step on it.

If he has clawed toes, transfer his flexor longus tendon to the extensor expansion on each toe (N, and O, 30-9).

FIND A CAPABLE COBBLER AND HELP HIM TO HELP YOUR PATIENTS

30.6 When feet have ulcerated

An *uncomplicated* ulcer is only skin deep, does not involve bone or deeper structures, and usually heals easily if the patient rests his leg. A *complicated* ulcer has involved the bone underneath it. It has a deep sinus, or marked infection, and is much more difficult to heal.

When a leprosy patient has his *first* ulcer: (1) Help him to find the cause of his injury. Never let him accept that the cause was leprosy. Was it caused by repeated stress, or by a blow, a puncture, or a burn? (2) Concentrate all your educational energies on him. You can do much more for a patient with his first ulcer, than for one whose foot is already mostly destroyed.

If you can find some way of *resting* an ulcer it will usually heal. This means that he must 'not take one step' on it, until it has finally closed over, and all the scabs are off. If it is uncomplicated, this takes 4 to 6 weeks. You can: (1) Rest it in bed. Unfortunately, this is rarely achieved because: (a) staff do not understand the need for it and explain it to him, and (b) he has no pain, and thus has little incentive to stay in bed. (2) Get him to use a splint and crutches, *continuously* until his ulcer has healed. He won't do this unless you educate and supervise him carefully. (3) Make him a special curative shoe, with a rigid rocker bottom, and a specially moulded upper surface. Making shoes of this kind needs much skill, and is not described here. (4) Put his foot in a cast.

A plaster cast is one of the most practical ways of resting an ulcerated foot. It immobilizes the foot, it spreads the strain of weight-bearing, it is quick to apply, and it is easy and effective. You can apply one in a remote clinic and send the patient home—provided you tell him that he must provide himself with door-to-door transport. If you apply a cast on the indications listed below, it will usually allow an ulcer to heal in 6 weeks.

Unfortunately, although resting a patient's foot in a cast may heal an ulcer, it weakens his bones and ligaments, even if he walks in it. Bones only retain their normal strength if they are regularly used. Rest causes them to lose their minerals, and ligaments to lose their strength. The result is that when his cast is finally removed, he may be delighted to find that his ulcer is healed, but he may not realize: (1) that anaesthesia is preventing him from experiencing the stiffness and pain that protects a normal foot after a cast is removed, and (2) that he needs to practise self care to keep his ulcer healed. Consequently, he may be tempted to use his anaesthetic foot too vigorously, with the result that it dislocates, or its tarsal bones fracture, and he ends up with a neuropathic foot. So: (1) Use casts cautiously, and remember their risks. (2) When you remove one: (a) warn him of the sad consequences of energetic early exercise, (b) start a programme of 'walking training', which will return him slowly to full activity during 7 to 10 days, (c) be sure that he learns 'self care', (d) be sure also that both you and he watch carefully for 'hot spots', and (e) most important, *admit him for at least a week at the time the plaster is removed, so that you can supervise him carefully while all this is done.*

Bone damage is common, and serious, and may be the result of: (1) Sepsis spreading from an ulcer, particularly if he walks on it. (2) Mechanical strain, which is particularly likely to occur when the protective mechanism of pain is absent. (3) Disuse atrophy in bed, or in a plaster cast. (4) Invasion of the bone by leprosy bacilli (leprosy osteitis), which is common in lepromatous and borderline leprosy, but is seldom severe enough to cause collapse. (5) Steroid osteoporosis, which may predispose to fractures.

The best way to minimize bone damage is to treat ulcers carefully, so that bone is not damaged in the first place. There are however also some additional principles: (1) Keep the weight-bearing surface of his sole as large as you can. (2) When you remove bone surgically, don't do so unnecessarily. Make sure it really is dead or infected. Dead bone is usually grey or black; it has no periosteum, and so feels rough to a probe. When you nibble it with forceps its fresh surface is pale, and not pink. Ideally, you should allow a sequestrum to separate before you remove it, but this takes several weeks, during which time the ulcer will not heal. You can shorten this time by removing dead bone as described below.

When bone has been damaged, clean up the mess it has caused. For example, if there is a deep sinus under an ulcer, with bone involvement, rest the leg for a few days to localize the infection. Then remove the dead soft tissue and bone—perhaps one or more metatarsal heads, leaving his toes if you can.

The short equinus foot of leprosy is one of its end results, and is due to the absorption of bone, which may be due to: (1) Neglected ulcers and infections. (2) Paralysis of his extensor muscles. (3) Unduly radical surgery. Muscle imbalance may pull his heel up too much, or push his forefoot down too much, so that it increases the pressure on his metatarsal heads, and so causes worse ulceration and more shortening.

A boat-shaped foot is another of the late effects of neglected leprosy. His arch is destroyed, and instead of being concave, it becomes convex, often with ulcers and bony spurs on the convexity.

FOOT ULCERS IN LEPROSY

ACUTE ULCERS

Put the patient to bed. Splint his foot and raise it to encourage drainage and prevent oedema. *This is much the best treatment.* Ambulant treatment seldom works. Either admit him, or make sure he does not walk *one single step* at home. Let him use bed pans, or crutches to reach the toilet. If necessary, fix a piece of wood to the dressings, as in B, Fig. 30-8, to make sure that he does not walk. If bed rest is impossible, see below under 'Difficulties'.

Local applications to an ulcer make little difference, so there is no need to change the dressings on it at short intervals. Dress it 2 or 3 times a week with hypochlorite ('Eusol'), hypertonic magnesium sulphate, sugar (which is best used daily, 57.3), or some mild antiseptic. Or, soak it, scrape it regularly to remove excess callus, oil it, and dress it daily. When discharge stops, you can apply a cast, leave the dressing unchanged for 6 weeks, and send him home. Or, you can continue daily care as a means of teaching him self care.

If he has fever and other signs of generalized infection, give him an antibiotic. Splint his leg to rest it and stop him walking.

PLANTAR ULCERS in leprosy

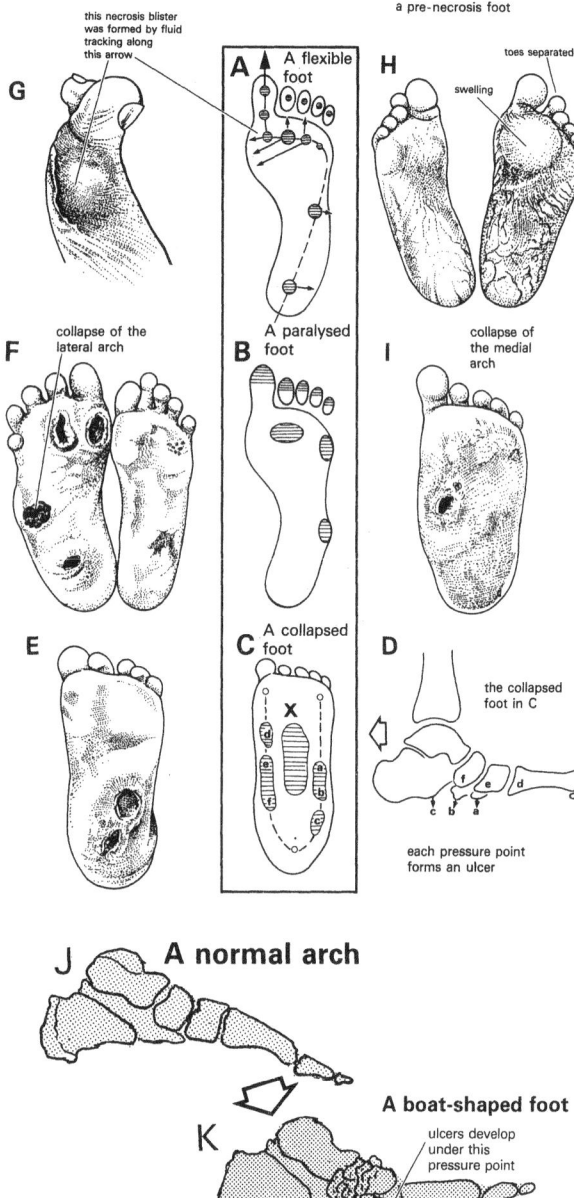

When the acute stage is subsiding, and there is no sign of spreading infection, explore the ulcer with a sterile blunt probe to find out if there is exposed bone in its base.

If bone is exposed, feel if there are any loose pieces or sequestra, and remove them. Pack the ulcer with hypochlorite until it is healing well, and continue to rest his leg.

If bone is not exposed and infection is controlled, either apply a cast and let him walk about, or continue bed rest with a splint and crutches.

A SHORT LEG WALKING CAST FOR LEPROSY

INDICATIONS. A chronic *non-inflamed* ulcer, whose base is visible without any necrotic bone, tendon, or other necrotic tissue. If there is necrotic tissue, remove it before applying the cast.

CONTRAINDICATIONS. (1) Signs of inflammation or infection: heat or oedema of the dorsum opposite the ulcer, excessive discharge, or regional adenitis. (2) Involvement of a joint or synovial sheath (synovial discharge). (3) Dead bone or tendon or capsular sloughs in the base of the ulcer. (4) A long deep sinus with small openings whose base you cannot see.

METHOD. Here is the basic method, which assumes that the patient's toes will be open. Some surgeons cover them to keep out stones and sand. See also Section 70.6 on plastercraft.

Measure his feet for shoes before he goes into his cast—when he comes out of it he must not take a single step without them. Shape the Böhler stirrup (walking iron, 81.3) to his leg before you apply the plaster.

Dress his ulcer with dry gauze or a simple ointment. Cover,

Fig. 30-6 PLANTAR ULCERS IN LEPROSY. A, where ulcers form in a flexible anaesthetic foot with intact muscles; the arrows show where 'pre-ulcer blisters' may track to. B, where ulcers form in a paralysed foot. If the patient has a peroneal palsy, he has ulcers at the lateral side of his foot; if he has complete foot drop his ulcers are anterior on the ball of his foot, under his metatarsal heads, or on his toes. C, and D, shows the same foot with a collapsed arch. Each of its bony prominences (a) to (f) has produced an ulcer. E, two ulcers in just such a foot. F, plantar ulcers and a lateral ulcer caused by collapse of the patient's longitudinal arch. G, a necrosis blister caused by fluid from a necrotic area tracking to the side of the foot. H, a 'pre-ulcer foot', with a swollen metatarsal pad, and separation of the first and second toes, due to fluid in the foot forcing the metatarsals apart. Try to recognize a foot at this stage before ulcers form. I, collapse of the medial arch. J, a normal arch. K, a boat shaped foot. The arch is reversed; ulcers form under the 'keel' of the boat. *After McDowell F, and Enna CD, 'Surgical Rehabilitation in Leprosy', (1973) Figs. 40-1, 40-2, and 40-9, The Williams and Wilkins Company, with kind permission. J, and K, kindly contributed by Grace Warren.*

CAUTION ! Antibiotics have *no* place in treating uncomplicated ulcers—what they need most is rest!

If he has a profuse discharge, or tender groin glands, raise his leg, and give him an antibiotic. Don't let him get out of bed, and don't give him a walking cast.

A PLASTER CAST FOR LEPROSY ULCERS

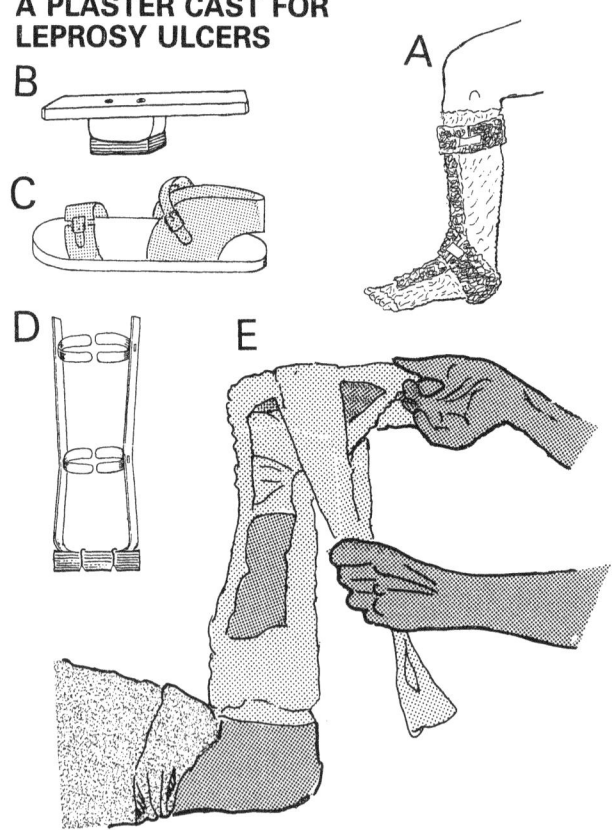

Fig. 30-7 A PLASTER CAST FOR LEPROSY ULCERS. A, sites for extra padding under a plaster cast. B, a wooden rocker shod with car tyre. This has a single bar. If a patient has casts on both legs, double bars on the rockers will enable him to walk more easily. C, a rubber-soled sandal with plastic straps to wear over a plaster cast. D, a locally made Böhler walking iron shod with car tyre. E, apply the cast while he lies face downwards. Ask your assistant to hold his toes up and to pull downwards on a loop of bandage placed as shown. This will flex his ankle, and help to form a better arch if one is needed. Apply the plaster over the bandage. *Kindly contributed by Grace Warren.*

but *do not pack* the wound; discharge must be able to escape easily.

Apply stockinette, a nylon stocking, or an *evenly applied* gauze bandage. Apply the minimum of padding to bony prominences only. Use strips of adhesive tape to fix 3 strips of padding as A, Fig. 30-7, but don't apply the tape directly to his skin. If you don't have padding, use many layers of bandage instead.

Lay him on his abdomen with his knee at 90° and his leg vertical. Apply a thick layer of plaster to his leg without pressure. End the cast 5 cm below the head of his fibula, to avoid pressure on his common peroneal nerve, and leave his toes open. Apply a back slab and circular reinforcing layers. Then fit a Böhler iron or a walking board (wood with a piece of car tyre, F, 81-3). Let it dry for 48 hours. The cast must be *dry* before he walks on it.

Alternatively, a thin well-moulded layer of plaster, covered by a layer of fibre glass, will make a more long-lasting cast. Preferably, use fibreglass tape rather than sheet, because it lasts longer.

CAUTION ! (1) Don't mould the cast under pressure to obtain the required position, or you may cause ulcers and gangrene. (2) Ask an assistant to hold his ankle at exactly 90° or slightly dorsiflexed, as in E, Fig. 30-7, until the plaster has set; it must not be plantar-flexed or inverted or everted. (3) Don't press into the plaster with your fingers, or you may produce pressure points where more ulcers will develop (F, 70-5). (3) Remember that he cannot complain of pain. *A wrongly applied cast may cause ulcers!* So don't apply excessive pressure over a tight bandage.

If he has an ulcer on both feet, he may need a wheel-chair. If he has to move about on the floor, give him 'hand sandals' to protect his hands. Make these with a piece of microcellular rubber, and give them a single strap. If he has casts on both feet, double bars on the walking boards will allow him to walk. Or make flat casts and sandals to go over them as in B, Fig 30-7.

Leave the cast on for 6 weeks. When you remove it, the shoe that you measured him for earlier should be ready. Make sure that he has a period of 'walking training' before he resumes full activity (see above). Apply a firm bandage, and start him walking in a carefully graduated way. Check his foot for swelling or an increase of temperature. Rest it again if signs of inflammation return. Tell him to walk as little as possible, to take short steps, and to avoid uneven ground, sudden strains, and long walks.

If his ulcer has not completely healed in one cast, apply another.

BONE INVOLVEMENT IN LEPROSY

THE INDICATIONS FOR REMOVING BONE. **Consider** removing bone if: (1) There is osteitis. (2) It is loose. (3) It is projecting into a septic cavity with no obvious blood supply around it. (4) It is projecting after an ulcer has healed, so that it forms a pressure point; if so cut it horizontally (see Section 30.7 on calcaneal spurs). (5) One metatarsal is obviously longer than the others, and the skin over it is ulcerating. Apart from the first metatarsal, which may usefully be longer, they should all be on the same line across his foot, so that he can walk without one of them sticking out prominently and taking extra stress.

Admit him. If this is impossible, give him a splint and crutches. Give him antibiotics pre- and postoperatively.

TO REMOVE DEAD BONE apply a tourniquet (3.9), try to loosen the bone, and cut it off at the line of separation. If this line has not yet formed, nibble it at the point where you see the periosteum is adherent again.

CAUTION ! (1) Don't remove bone from the base of an ulcer unnecessarily, especially in the heel. (2) Probing an ulcer will tell you if bone is exposed, but not if it is dead. Exposed bone may be healthy, but the soft tissues will take time to grow over it. (3) Never strip the periosteum unnecessarily, because this may kill the bone under it.

DIFFICULTIES WITH LEPROSY FEET

IF BED REST IS IMPRACTICAL: (1) Give him a splint and crutches, and ask him not to bear weight on the foot with the ulcer. The splint can be plaster (expensive and short-lasting), wood, plastic, wire (mesh fencing wire), or even a roll of paper or cardboard. Or, (2) apply a below-knee cast, as described above, for 6 weeks. Or, (3) attach a projecting bar to his foot as in B, Fig. 30-8, and give him crutches.

If a PLASTER CAST FOR AN ULCER IS IMPRACTICAL, you can: (1) Fit the kneeling leg prosthesis in D, Fig. 30-8, which is suitable for limited activity only. (2) Fit a 'healing shoe' which is less cumbersome than a cast, but also less effective. It must have: (a) a rigid sole with a central rocker, (b) an insole (ideally 'Plastazote') moulded exactly to the shape of his foot, (c) an upper strapped round his foot and ankle, so that they cannot move in relation to his shoe.

If his ULCER RECURS, check the way he cares for his feet. Does he inspect them and soak them *daily* and remove rough callus? Look at his shoes: (1) Is there increased pressure in some area which has caused necrosis? (2) Are the straps so

MORE METHODS FOR LEPROSY

A patient's first ulcer is a critical time for health education

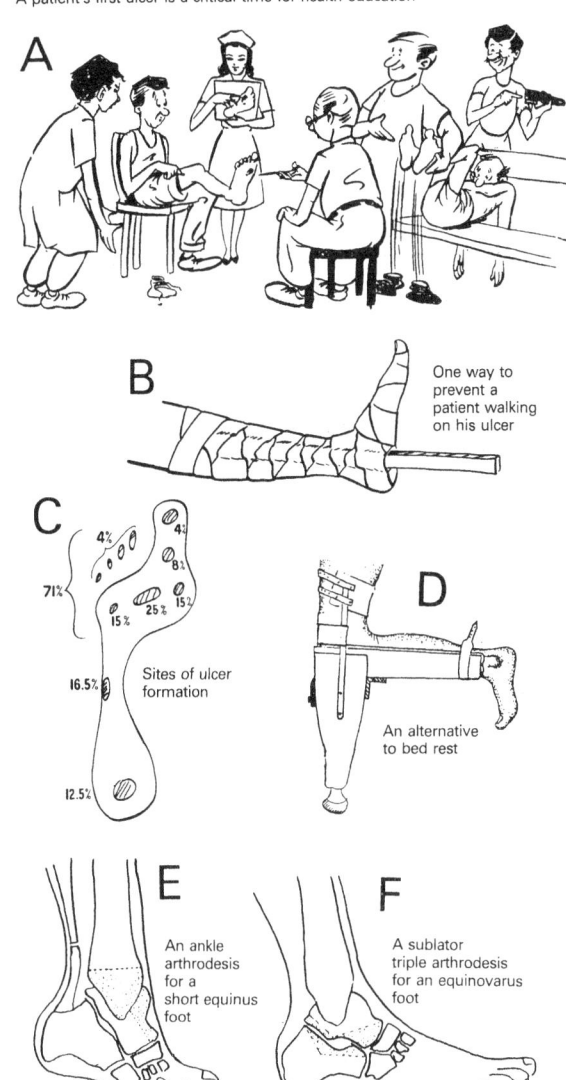

Fig. 30-8 MORE METHODS FOR LEPROSY. A, a patient's first ulcer is a critical time for health education. B, one way to prevent him walking on his ulcer while it heals, is to bandage a wooden bar to his leg. C, the sites of ulcer formation. Feel for warmth and deep tenderness in these sites when you examine his foot. D, if you cannot rest his ulcers by putting him to bed, you may be able to treat him in a walking prosthesis like this. E, an arthrodesis of the ankle joint, or F, a subtalar triple arthrodesis may be necessary if he has a severely equinus or equinovarus foot. A, to D, after Paul Brand, 'Insensitive Feet, A Practical Handbook on Foot Problems in Leprosy'. With the kind permission of the Leprosy Mission International. E, and F, after Ernest Fritschii.

loose that they allow movement of his foot in relation to the shoe, or so tight that they cut into him? (3) Can the contour or fit of his shoes be improved? (4) Does he always wear them?

Also, check how he walks. How far does he walk without resting? Can he walk less, or walk with less pressure on the ulcer, or more slowly or with shorter steps? Ask him to practise walking with his ankles tied with string, to limit his steps to 30 cm.

There are two possibilities: (1) You may be able to excise the ulcer, and all the scar tissue under it, and then graft it with split skin. This may provide a more suitable bed for the regrowth of subcutaneous tissue than the original scar tissue. Some surgeons think that split skin grafts break down too easily, and consider that better quality skin results from the next alternative. (2) You may be able to excise the scarred area, and close the gap you have made with monofilament sutures. This often requires the use of a relieving incision on the dorsum or side of his foot, and packing the cavity with hypochlorite ('Eusol') to encourage healing from the *base or bottom of the wound*. See Section 30.7 on the excision of metatarsal heads.

If he looks after his feet carefully and wears the right shoes, his ulcer should not break down again. If it does, *and he is caring for his feet properly*, there is some underlying abnormality, such as: (1) Sequestration of the bone under the ulcer. Remove sequestra surgically. (2) A bone spur which may need excising as described below. (3) A thick scar which splits under tension as he walks. (5) Inadequate subcutaneous tissue over his metatarsal heads. (5) Malignant change in the ulcer. (6) Claw toes which repeatedly ulcerate. Treat him as described below or refer him.

CAUTION ! When you treat ulcers avoid cutting into living bleeding tissue unless it is to: (1) Open an abscess. (2) Improve drainage from a deep sinus. (3) Remove necrotic tendon, muscle, or bone. (4) Remove a free lying sequestrum. (5) Remove bone that is so placed that healing and normal function are mechanically impossible.

If there is an ULCER ON THE LATERAL BORDER OF HIS FOOT (F, 30-6), it is likely to be associated with peroneal paralysis. Treat it by bed rest and splints or casts. When it has healed a toe-raising strap attached to the area of his fifth metatarsal head may help to prevent recurrence.

Alternatively, if the ulcer is in the middle of the lateral border, you can try to promote healing by surgically paring his cuboid or the base of his fifth metatarsal, and removing any infected tissue. Do this through a dorsolateral incision, which leaves a sufficient bridge of tissue between the incision and the ulcer. Turn back the infected tissues by subperiosteal dissection, trim the bone, remove necrotic tissue, excise the ulcer with an elliptical incision on the sole, and close this with monofilament to achieve primary healing of the plantar wound. Pack the dorsolateral wound, and allow it to close by granulation. Keep the mouth of the wound wide open until the depth of the cavity is clean and closing. A toe raising spring may help to prevent recurrence.

BONY DIFFICULTIES IN LEPROSY OTHER THAN NEUROPATHIC BONE DISINTEGRATION

If a TERMINAL PHALANX PRESENTS in an ulcer at the tip of a toe (or finger), nibble it away with a bone nibbler. If it is badly infected, disarticulate it. If necessary, use a fish mouth incision over the top and down the sides, which will leave the pulp intact.

If you need to REMOVE PART OR ALL OF THE MIDDLE OR PROXIMAL PHALANGES, approach them through incisions at the sides of a toe (or finger).

If BONE IS EXPOSED UNDER A HEEL ULCER, be very careful about removing it from his calcaneus—you can easily remove too much, and a foot without a heel can be a problem. Patients can however walk on very little calcaneus or even none, if you provide them with a rubber heel-pad. Look for a calcaneal spur (see below).

If he has a SHORT FOOT, examine him carefully to see if his heel is taking its proper share of his weight. You can easily miss foot drop in a short foot. Ask him to walk on his heels; if he cannot do so, some of his muscles are weak. Lengthening his Achilles tendon may help, even to the point of making his calf muscles useless, because this will make him walk mainly on his heel, and less on the front of his foot. If he has definite paralysis of his dorsiflexors, he will be better with a tendon transfer (30.8). If this is not practical, fit him with a toe-raising spring.

NEUROPATHIC BONE DISINTEGRATION IN LEPROSY

If his foot is HOT AND SWOLLEN, there are several possibilities.

If he has signs of an acute infection with lymphadenitis, **treat him** with rest, an antibiotic, and if necessary, drainage. His bones may not be neuropathic, and his foot may merely have a soft tissue infection.

If he has no lymphadenitis or signs of general infection, **his hot foot may be the result of neuropathic bone disintegration.** This can also follow a fracture. Admit him. Splint, bandage and rest his foot in bed. The heat and swelling should subside within a week. Then apply a firm supportive bandage and start 'walking training' (see above).

If heat and swelling do not return, he had a sprain or minor injury.

If they rapidly return and persist, there is active pathology, so apply a cast for 6 weeks, check again, X-ray him again and plan treatment accordingly. After this interval stress fractures and other bony lesions will have caused enough osteoporosis to be seen. If you are in doubt, or have no X-rays, have another trial of walking. If heat and swelling return a second time, he has definite neuropathic bone disintegration, so reapply a well fitting walking cast for 6 to 12 months, depending on its site and severity.

If his TARSAL BONES DISINTEGRATE, you may see him in any of these three stages.

In the first stage, his foot is hot, it may be swollen, but its shape is unchanged. **Raise it** to allow swelling to subside. Apply a cast moulded to the shape of his foot, but without trying to change it, usually for 3 to 6 months.

In the second stage, his foot is still hot with active disintegration; its shape is abnormal, and it may be hypermobile. **Raise it** in a splint for 3 days to reduce swelling. Then lay him on his face as in E, Fig. 30-7, mould his foot into as functional a position as you can, accentuate its arch as much as possible, and apply a cast. Leave this on for for 6 to 12 months, and then mobilize him with care. If necessary, treat him for the complications of the third stage (see immediately below).

In the third stage, his foot is no longer hot, showing that his bone lesions are no longer active. If there are rough bones, which will be likely to cause ulcers, trim them. A high-risk shoe may keep him ulcer-free. You may be able to refer him for an arthrodesis, after which he may need a walking cast for 6 to 9 months. If he is lucky his foot will revert to the 'moderate risk' class; if it does not, he may continue to need a special prosthetic shoe or brace. Many of these patients can manage to live well in a simple sandal, with daily skin care.

If there is NO PRACTICAL WAY TO ESTABLISH A GOOD ARCH, at least try to get its bones healed and sclerosed. If the arch of his foot becomes completely flat, he should remain ulcer-free, but if the bottom of his foot becomes convex and boat-shaped, it will be more likely to ulcerate. If his talus and calcaneus are totally destroyed, consider amputation (see below).

If he has an old fixed deformity which cannot be altered, **refer him** for reconstructive surgery or supply him with a special moulded high-risk shoe.

If he has a residal BONY SPUR on the under surface of his calcaneus or elsewhere under an ulcer or scar, try conservative management with special footwear and daily skin care. If ulceration continues, excise it (30.7). Spurs may form under any prominent bone in a boat-shaped foot.

CLAWED TOES IN LEPROSY

Ulcers are often associated with clawed toes.

If he has GRADE 1 CLAWED TOES, (weakness of the intrinsic muscles only, and mobile toes without contractures), his metatarsal heads will have to take excessive pressure, which may cause ulcers. Transferring his flexor tendons gives good results in this stage of clawing (30.7).

If he has GRADE 2 CLAWED TOES, (moderate contractures), you may be able to treat him with a tendon transfer only, or you may need to remove the metatarsal heads at the same time.

If he has GRADE 3 CLAWED TOES, (severe contractures

with or without dorsal subluxation of his MP joints), he will probably have ulcers over his metatarsal heads. To straighten them, you may have to remove at least one phalanx, or the metatarsal head, or both. If the remains of his toes will not bear weight, because they are so badly scarred, do a transmetatarsal amputation (see below).

ANKLE DIFFICULTIES IN LEPROSY

If his ANKLE BECOMES SWOLLEN AND WARM, three things may have happened: (1) He may have sprained his ankle. This is particularly likely to happen if he has a shoe with a rocker sole (the benefit from which may however outweigh the increased probability of a sprained ankle). His ankle needs immobilization. If the sprain is less severe, a firm bandage may be enough. If it is more severe, immobilize his ankle for 3 months in a plaster cast. (2) He may have neuropathic bone disintegration (see above). (3) His ankle joint may be infected (see below).

If he has a DISLOCATED ANKLE that you cannot reduce, or a fixed deformity of it, refer him for surgical correction.

If he has an EQUINUS or EQUINOVARUS FOOT, he may be able to walk quite well, but he will need elaborate footware to keep him ulcer-free. If walking is difficult, and particularly if he has fixed plantar flexion or inversion, refer him for an ankle arthrodesis (E, or F, in Fig. 30-8). When this has been done, an ordinary high moulded shoe, or a sandal of microcellular rubber, may be adequate to keep him free from ulcers.

If his FOOT IS INVERTED, a simple canvas shoe like a tennis shoe may be enough. If not, refer him to have it corrected surgically. When this has been done an ordinary high moulded shoe or a sandal of microcellular rubber may be enough to keep him free from ulcers.

SEPTIC DIFFICULTIES WITH LEPROSY FEET

If SEPTIC ARTHRITIS involves the IP joint of a TOE, excise it through a dorsal incision, remove the remains of its ligaments and cartilage, pack the cavity, and keep his toe *straight* at its IP and MP joints, while it heals by granulation.

If SEPTIC TENOSYNOVITIS complicates an ulcer, draining the tendon sheath may assist healing. Drain it through an incision along the arch of his foot. Clean out all the infection, as far back as is necessary, to find and remove the infected tendon stump. Close his skin with monofilament, so as to leave the smallest possible scar on the weight bearing area. But leave both ends open, so that you can irrigate the lesion until it is clean. Allow it to heal by granulation.

If a SEPTIC TOE REQUIRES AMPUTATION, use a racquet incision on the dorsum (as in Fig. 75-28), leave the metatarsal head, and only resect the surface cartilage if there is septic arthritis of an MP joint. Drain or pack the wound dorsally.

If plantar ulceration is complicated by OSTEITIS of a METATARSAL HEAD, you may need to excise it. This will move the weight-bearing area proximally, so that more ulceration is likely. If you can save a toe in good position, it will help to protect the area of the new 'metatarsal head'. If you can save the distal part of his first toe, it will help to protect his second metatarsal head, which may otherwise soon ulcerate. Sometimes, you may have to remove several metatarsal heads. Do this through dorsal longitudinal incisions between them. If there are plantar ulcers over his metatarsal heads, excise them, and close the incisions in his sole with monofilament. Leave drains or packs in dorsally.

MALIGNANT DIFFICULTIES IN LEPROSY

If a SQUAMOUS CELL CARCINOMA complicates a long-standing ulcer, the alternatives are local excision and amputation. You may be able to excise smaller lesions that don't involve bone, and are distal to his mid foot.

30.7 Operations on the feet in leprosy

Most leprosy ulcers don't need an operation, but there are some simple operations which you should be able to do. Try to correct clawed toes, because they predispose to ulcers at the tip of a toe, on the knuckle, and under the metatarsal head. Apart from the correction of clawed toes, most other tendon transfers are work for an expert. The only other possible exception is a posterior tibialis transfer for foot drop (30.8).

FOOT OPERATIONS FOR LEPROSY

ANAESTHESIA. If a patient's hand or foot are sufficiently anaesthetic, you may be able to operate under sedation alone, especially if he is co-operative. He may even be sufficiently

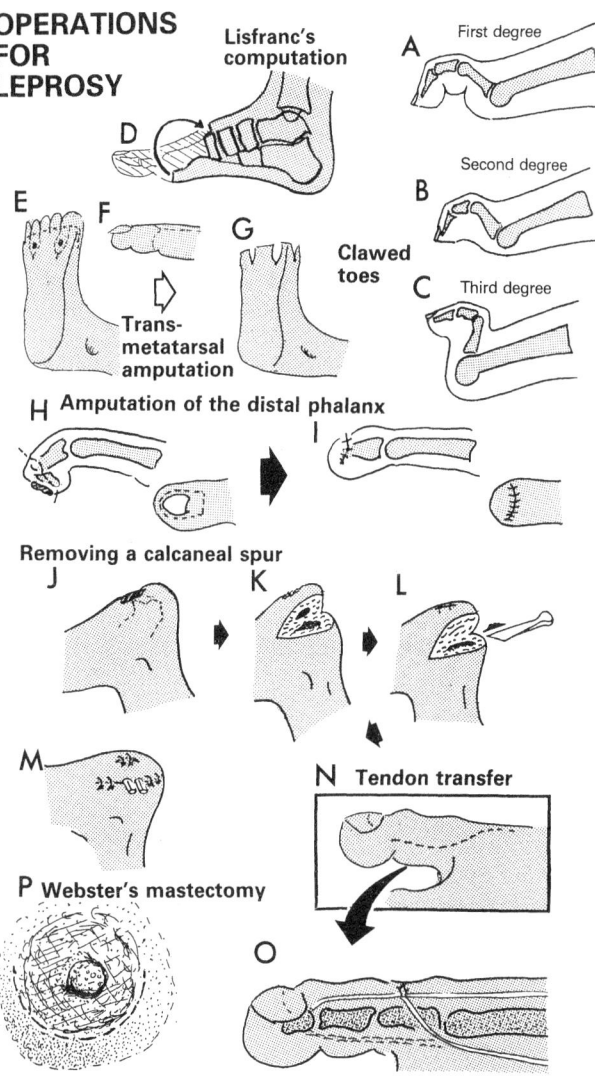

Fig. 30-9 SOME OF THE SIMPLER LEPROSY OPERATIONS. A, clawed toes due to weakness of the intrinsic muscles, but without skin or joint contractures (Grade One). B, clawed toes with contractures (Grade Two). C, clawed toes with severe contractures, and dorsal subluxation of the MP joints (Grade Three). D, Lisfranc's transmetatarsal amputation, in which most of the metatarsals are removed, and the tissues of the sole turned dorsally. E, F, and G, a transmetatarsal amputation for an ulcerated foot, including the excision of the ulcers on its sole. This amputation may be possible when there is not enough tissue to make the long sole flap needed by Lisfranc's amputation, or when there are open ulcers, and thus potential sepsis. F, the longitudinal incision on the side of the big toe, nearer the dorsum than the sole. G, the stump ready for the longitudinal incisions to be closed by suture, and the end of the foot allowed to heal by granulation. H, amputating the distal phalanx. I, the completed operation. J, a heel ulcer over a bony spur. K, expose the bone from the back and side. L, remove the spur with an osteotome. M, close the wound over a rubber drain. N, the incision to transfer the long flexor tendon of a toe to the dorsum. O, the transfer completed. P, Webster's incision for excising the breast. *Mostly after Paul Brand 'Insensitive Feet, A Practical Handbook on Foot Problems in Leprosy'. E, F, G, N, and O, kindly contributed by Grace Warren.*

anaesthetic to tolerate a tourniquet if you sedate him well. If necessary use axillary (A 6.18), wrist (A 6.20), hand (A 6.21), or ankle (A 6.24) blocks, or subarachnoid (spinal) anaesthesia (A 7.4), or ketamine (A 8.1).

ULCERS

If you are excising an ulcer or scar on his sole, you may be able to close the gap you have made by primary suture. This will allow healing by first intention, and will improve the quality of his plantar skin. To do this, excise the ulcer with an elliptical incision, and close the wound with deep mattress sutures (4-7) of '0' monofilament to eliminate dead spaces. Keep the wound dry, and leave the sutures in for 3 weeks. If you can only close an ulcer under excessive tension, consider using a lateral or dorsal relieving incision, right down to the bone. Loosely pack the dorsal incision, and leave it to granulate as described below. Make sure the bridge of skin, between the ulcer and the relieving incision, is adequate to maintain the circulation.

CAUTION ! Only close clean surgical incisions by primary suture. Even some of these need drains to minimize haematoma formation. Remove the drains after 48 hours.

If you are excising a deep ulcer with a sinus track leading from it, put gentian violet into the track. If you cut away all the violet tissue, you should have removed the base of his ulcer, tracks and all.

If you are excising a heel ulcer, make a 'fish mouth' relieving incision around the back or lateral margin of the sole of his heel, as in K, Fig. 30-9. Excise and suture the plantar defect, as described above. Consider packing the 'fish mouth' wound as described below, and allowing it to heal by granulation.

If you are doing some other operation on a foot and it happens to have an open, and potentially infected, ulcer pack it as described below.

PACKING A WOUND OR ULCER. *Loosely* pack it with gauze strips or bandages and allow it to heal by granulation. If you use gauze squares, be sure to leave part of each piece outside the wound, so that it will not be forgotten inside. Soak the packs in hypochlorite, sugar solution, acriflavine emulsion, magnesium sulphate and glycerine, or normal saline. Remove the dressings at 5 days. Provided there is no deep infection, lightly repack the depth of the wound, but keep its mouth widely open. Repeat this every 2 or 3 days, until it has healed by granulation.

TO EXCISE A CALCANEAL SPUR (OR OTHER BONY PROJECTION)

A normal calcaneus has a spur which projects forwards along the line of the plantar ligaments parallel to the ground; this is harmless. If an abnormal spur, associated with an ulcer, projects vertically downwards, remove it. Also remove any irregular bone that has developed because of a fracture or an infection, and which threatens to cause ulcers by pressure from within. *Don't remove these bony projections through the ulcer, because this will make the plantar scar bigger.*

Instead, paint the ulcer with gentian violet. Then make an incision round the back or lateral side of the patient's heel, as in J, to M, in Fig. 30-9, so as to avoid his medial calcaneal vessels. Deepen the incision to the bone, and lift his heel pad off the bone by clean sharp dissection. Continue the incision, so as to raise a flap of heel and plantar fascia, and mobilize the ulcer. Then excise and suture it as described above. Trim his calcaneus with an osteotome to leave a flattened surface. Don't remove bone unnecessarily, or leave new sharp edges or corners to form new ulcers.

If his ulcer had already healed before the operation, insert a drain and stitch the flap back, provided there is no tension.

If his ulcer is open, excise its edges, and sew it up with deep stitches, leaving a pack in place under it, and coming out of the relieving incision as described above. The skin wound from his ulcer should heal by first intent, leaving a gap round the edge of his heel flap to heal by granulation.

If he has osteitis, excise or curette the sinus tracks and insert a pack.

If osteitis is already draining through the centre of his heel, curette and pack the lesion, without trying to excise the ulcer. Stop all weight-bearing until his ulcer is healed; give him a splint. When the infection is controlled, trim any rough bone. Alternatively, as soon as his osteitis is controlled, you may be able to excise the ulcer scar, pack the lesion laterally, and allow it to heal by granulation.

Don't let him walk on trimmed bone for 6 weeks, or until his wound is fully healed, and its scabs are off—unless he is in a plaster cast.

AMPUTATIONS IN LEPROSY

INDICATIONS. Conserve as much bone and soft tissue as you can. The only absolute indications for a below knee amputation are: (1) malignancy, which cannot be removed in any other way. (2) Gangrene. (3) Grossly infected ulcers with inadequate bone, so that they are no longer weight-bearing.

METHOD. Ideally the stump should have sensation. If not, he will need a good prosthetist and careful training. Use one of the methods below, and only do a below-knee amputation as a last resort: it may however be the operation of choice if the tibial area is sensitive. The method of Anderssen and Perssen was specially devised for leprosy. Use a tourniquet (3.9), and see Sections 56.1 and 56.8. The longer his tibial stump, the easier it will be for him to learn to walk with a prosthesis. If he is a healthy young adult, you may be able to take skin flaps almost to his malleoli. If his circulation is poor make a shorter stump. If you amputate through his foot, try to leave as large a weight-bearing surface as you can.

If his foot has become shortened, his toes may remain projecting, and make it difficult to fit a shoe, or they may be subject to excessive pressure. If so amputate them.

If the soft tissue under his metatarsal heads has become so scarred that it constantly reulcerates, remove the distal ends of his metatarsals through dorsal incisions. Keep his toes in line with his sole by bandaging them to a flat board while they heal.

If his foot is chronically scarred and ulcerated, and he has lost part of all his toes, but has good sole tissue proximally, do a transmetatarsal amputation, as in D, Fig. 30-9. Make a dorsal incision and divide the bones along a line proximal to the scar. Without removing tissue from the sole, turn a long sole flap, including the scar up, and around the ends of the bones, bringing the suture line dorsally. The most proximal line for this amputation is through his tarsometatarsal joints (Lisfranc amputation). At this level, you will have to saw through the neck of his 2nd metatarsal, the base of which is more proximal.

CAUTION ! Foot operations leaving shorter stumps are prone to develop complications. So avoid them, unless arthrodeses or stabilization of the ankle are possible.

If he has severe ulceration, poor toes, and not enough sole tissue for a long sole flap, make an incision right round the dorsal and plantar surfaces of his forefoot, at the base of his toes. If possible try to keep some of the skin of his toes on the foot flap (E, in Fig. 30-9). The dorsal skin flap does not need to be as wide as the plantar one, so when you incise his foot laterally to make them, do so as far dorsally as you can (F).

Starting at the base of his toes, strip the soft tissues off the bones, and remove all rough infected pieces of bone, far enough back for the most distal part of the remaining healthy bone to lie over a fairly healthy area of skin. Trim all his metatarsals to a suitable length, so that one does not stick out in front of the others. Smooth the rough bone ends. The dorsal and plantar flaps should meet in front of his foot. Excise any ulcers on the sole of his foot, and suture the gaps you have made with monofilament longitudinally as described above.

CAUTION ! Don't suture the end of his foot. Instead, pack it and allow it to heal by granulation. This will increase the tissue over the ends of his metatarsals, and allow you to operate while he is still infected and ulcerated.

Try to stop him walking for at least 6 weeks. If absolutely necessary, put him into a walking cast, with his ankle in good dorsiflexion, and with sufficient plantar protection to stop him bumping the healing area. Leave the end of his granulating foot protruding for dressings.

If his heel pad has some sensation and a good prosthetist is available, consider doing a Symes amputation (56.9). A Symes stump is too short and too small to be used for weight-bearing unless he has a good elephant boot.

TENDON TRANSFERS FOR CLAW TOES (Girdlestone type)

INDICATIONS. Mobile clawed toes in Grades One or Two (30.6). This operation allows his toes to take more part in weight-bearing, and so protects his metatarsal heads.

ANAESTHESIA. (1) Toe or ankle blocks (A 6.21). (2) Ketamine (A 8.1). (3) Subarachnoid anaesthesia (A 7.4).

METHOD. Under a tourniquet, incise along the midline of the medial side of the middle and proximal phalanges of the toe whose tendon you want to transfer. Proximally, curve the incision dorsally to reach the dorsum of his foot at the distal end of the web. Find his long flexor at his DIP joint. Hold it in forceps, and cut it distally. Cut his flexor sheath back to the middle of his proximal phalanx. Lift the skin and soft tissue off the dorsum of his proximal phalanx and interphalangeal joint, and transfer his long flexor tendon so that it runs diagonally across his proximal phalanx, and reaches the long extensor tendon of that toe. Suture it to his long extensor tendon, proximal to his PIP joint. If his flexor digitorum longus is transferred at this level it will remain a flexor of his MP joint, but will now extend his PIP and DIP joints. Close his skin with monofilament. Splint his foot on a flat board for 3 weeks, and don't allow him to walk. There is no need for physiotherapy.

REMOVING TOE TIPS FOR LEPROSY

INDICATIONS. (1) Fixed flexion of his toes, so that he is walking on the tips of his toes, or on his nails. (2) Repeated ulcers on the tips of his toes.

METHOD. Cut round his nail and across the skin over his DIP joint. Dissect out his distal phalanx, leaving all pulp possible (H, Fig. 30-9). Close the incision with a few mattress sutures (I), and don't worry about dog ears: they will soon atrophy.

EXCISING METATARSAL HEADS FOR STIFF, CLAWED LEPROSY TOES

INDICATIONS. More than one stiff, clawed toe of Grades Two or Three, or ulcers under his metatarsal heads. Sepsis is not a contraindication, because you leave the dorsal wound open and pack it.

Aim to reduce the scarred area, by shortening the metatarsals of one or all of his toes, so bringing his toes down to take some weight. Keep all incisions dorsal where you can, and aim for a mobile pseudarthrosis, not an ankylosis.

METHOD. Over his stiff toe make a dorsal incision which is long enough for you to see his MP joint, and 2 cm of his metatarsal. Elevate his periosteum, and remove his metatarsal head with bone nibblers or cutters. Base the site of bone section on the thickness and quality of his plantar skin. Save as much plantar surface as you can, provided it is of reasonable quality. Smooth the remaining shaft with a small bone file or nibbler. You should now be able to straighten his toe; if it is still dorsiflexed, remove a little more metatarsal. If there is much scarring under his metatarsal heads, consider removing all of them. Don't leave one metatarsal obviously longer than the others. Excise any ulcers on the sole, as above, and close the gaps with monofilament.

Try to avoid damaging his proximal phalanges. If you can find any flexor digitorum longus tendons, release them distally and anchor them over his proximal phalanges, as in the claw toe method above.

For each toe, cut the branches of extensor digitorum longus and brevis to prevent extension. Tack the proximal cut end of the tendon to the remains of his metatarsal to prevent it reattaching itself to the distal end.

Leave the dorsal incision open, pack the wound, and allow it to heal by granulation. Splint his toes straight on a board for three weeks or longer, while his foot heals. When excessive discharge has stopped, consider applying a cast with a window and letting him walk. Ideally, he should not walk, unless he is in a walking cast, for a minimum of 6 weeks, or until his foot is fully healed and the scabs are off.

If you are operating on the head of his 1st or 5th metatarsal, do it in the same way. Make an incision on the medial or lateral side of his foot, but make sure there is enough width in the skin bridge to prevent it necrosing. The width of the flap of skin between the excised ulcer and the relieving incision must be at least half its length (as in making flaps and pedicles).

If all his toes are affected, you can remove all his metatarsal heads through 3 or 4 longitudinal incisions.

If he has marked osteoporosis, apply a walking cast for 2 to 5 months to allow his damaged bones to recalcify, as they will do when infection is controlled. His bone will still look osteoporotic on X-ray; but, provided he returns to walking gradually, it should recalcify without breaking.

30.8 Tibialis transfer for foot drop, from leprosy and other causes

A dropped foot, which a patient is constantly tripping over, is a great disability, *but it is also a treatable one, whatever its cause:* (1) If he has a strong tibialis posterior and gastrocnemius, and a mobile ankle, you may be able to transfer his tibialis posterior tendon. (2) If surgery is impractical, you can fit him with: (a) A toe-raising spring, as in Fig. 30-4, if necessary made with canvas or plastic straps, and using the rubber from an inner tube as the 'spring'. Or, (b) calipers, which will need careful fitting on an anaesthetic limb, if they are not to cause friction burns.

When leprosy has paralysed his lateral popliteal nerve, he cannot dorsiflex his ankle, so that as he walks he is liable to injure the lateral side of his foot, his toes, and the ball of his foot. Severe ulcers and marked deformity may follow. Transferring his tibialis posterior tendon to the dorsum of his foot will restore the dorsiflexion of his ankle, and reduce the risk of ulcers. Refer him if you can, but if you cannot, learn how to do the operation yourself under expert instruction. If this too is impossible, *and you are a careful caring operator,* follow the method below. It is the most complex method described here, and it right at the edge of *'Primary Surgery'.* If leprosy is common in your district, it will be a procedure which is well worth learning, but only provided that there is someone who can prepare him for surgery, and re-educate him afterwards. Reconstructive surgery without physiotherapy is useless; but you can do the physiotherapy yourself, if you take enough time. Tibialis posterior and gastrocnemius are normally used together in walking. An important part of physiotherapy is getting him to separate these actions.

Detach his tibialis posterior from its insertion into his navicular, and divide its distal end into two slips. Thread these under the skin of the front of his leg and foot. Weave the medial slip into the distal end of his tibialis anterior tendon. Weave the lateral slip into: (1) the distal end of his peroneus tertius tendon (only 75% of people have one; it is really the fifth tendon of extensor digitorum longus, and is inserted into the medial part of the dorsal surface of the fifth metatarsal). This is the First Method, D, in Fig 30-11. Or, (2) if he lacks a peroneus tertius, and his peroneal muscles are weak enough to be sacrificed, weave the lateral slip into the distal end of his peroneus brevis tendon (E, the Second Method). Or, (3) if his peroneal muscles are not weak enough to sacrifice, or if the lateral slip of his tibialis posterior is too short to reach the lateral side of his foot, take a piece of tendon and use this as a free graft (not illustrated).

Make four incisions: Incision One, above and behind his medial malleolus, to let you free the muscle belly of his tibialis posterior. Incision Two, over his navicular, to free the insertion of its tendon. Incision Three, on the medial side of the dorsum of his foot, to let you weave the medial slip of his tibialis posterior tendon into the tendon of his tibialis anterior. Incision Four on the lateral side of the dorsum of his foot, to let you weave the lateral slip into his peroneus tertius or brevis. With the Second Method, you may have to make three more incisions, Five, Six, and Seven.

(1) Be sure to join his various tendons at just the correct length and tension, to get the right degree of dorsiflexion and *eversion* of his foot (this is the position in which the lateral side of his foot is higher than the medial side). His foot must be tightly dorsiflexed when you put it into plaster. To help you we tell you how to make a special foot-drop-positioning splint. This is critical.

(2) If your tendon weave gives way, your work is wasted, so be sure to keep his foot dorsiflexed until it has united firmly. (3) Avoid subsequent toe drop by suturing his transferred tibialis posterior to the extensor tendons of his toes. (4) Don't be tempted to anchor his tibialis posterior to a hole drilled in his foot. This may work with other diseases, but in leprosy it will promote the disintegration of his tarsal bones.

TIBIALIS POSTERIOR TRANSFER—'TPT'

Grace Warren's method

EXAMINATION. Check the power of: (1) The patient's tibialis posterior. Ask him to invert his foot against resistance (move it medially). The only other inverter is tibialis anterior, which is usually powerless or very weak in patients needing this transfer. (2) His peroneal muscles. Ask him to evert his foot, and feel his peroneal tendons contracting behind his lateral malleolus (if they are strong, you don't want to sacrifice them).

INDICATIONS. (1) Foot drop from any cause, provided he has a strong tibialis posterior and gastrocnemius (see below), and a mobile ankle. (2) If he has leprosy all these conditions must apply: (a) His leprosy must have been controlled, and he must have been free of reaction for at least 6 months. (b) His lateral popliteal nerve should have shown no sign of improving after 6 months of chemotherapy and the use of a toe-raising spring. (c) His tibialis posterior must be at least 'Power 4', and preferably '4+ or 5' (27.2). (d) He must have no ulcers or infections. (e) Preferably, he should be skin-smear negative. (f) His ankle must be suitably mobile, so test it like this:

Flex his knee to 90°. If you cannot passively dorsiflex his ankle beyond 0°, tendon transfer alone is contraindicated.

Straighten his knee. If you can passively dorsiflex his ankle to 15° (unusual), a tendon transfer alone is enough. If you cannot do this (usual), you will have to combine tendon transfer with lengthening his Achilles tendon at the same time. *Not lengthening his Achilles tendon is a common cause of failure.*

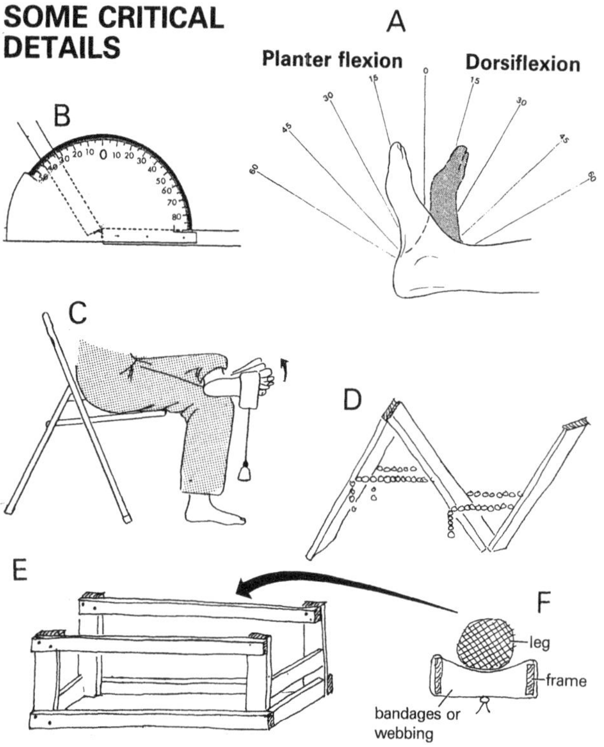

If his ankle is too stiff to dorsiflex without inverting, he will not get a good gait. So refer him for a wedge osteotomy, perhaps with a tendon transfer later.

TENDON TRANSFERS FOR HIS TOES. If a foot is not being dorsiflexed normally, its toe flexors shorten. If you correct his foot drop, his toes will remain abnormally flexed, unless you do something to correct them. So his clawed toes also need tendon transfers (see 30.7), either at the same time that you transfer his tibialis posterior, or later. If you don't do this, he may walk with his toe-nails turned under his toes, which will ulcerate.

RECORD THE PROGRESS OF HIS FOOT. Do this as a baseline preoperatively. Do it again when he comes out of plaster, and at regular intervals afterwards. Record the angles of rest, active dorsiflexion, and active plantar flexion with his knee straight, and passive dorsiflexion with his knee at 90°.

PREOPERATIVE PHYSIOTHERAPY is necessary to strengthen his tibialis posterior. Ask him to sit with his affected foot resting on his other knee and to invert it *without* using his Achilles tendon as in C, Fig. 30-10. Hang a weight (starting with 500 g and increasing to 4 kg, as the muscle strengthens) on the front of his foot, and ask him to lift this by inverting it. This exercise will help him to localize the action of the muscle that is to be transferred, so that it is easier for him to use afterwards.

ANAESTHESIA. (1) Subarachnoid anaesthesia (A 7.1). (2) Ketamine (A 8.1). (3) General anaesthesia (A 10.1). (4) Pethidine and diazepam (A 8.8); his foot will be partly anaesthetic anyway.

PERIOPERATIVE ANTIBIOTICS. An infected tendon transfer is a real disaster, so give him him chloramphenicol and metronidazole (2.9).

EQUIPMENT AND TECHNIQUE. Make a foot-drop-positioning splint, as in D, 30-10, from hardwood, hooks, hinges, screws, and two short chains. Boil or autoclave it. Ideally, you should use a 22 or 30 cm curved Anderssen tunneller, but you can use long Kocher's forceps. You will also need a leg rest, or cradle, to hold his leg about 20 cm above his bed after surgery. Ask your carpenter to make a tubular metal or wooden frame with webbing across it (E, 30-10).

For tendons use 2/0–4/0 braided multifilament (nylon, prolene, polyglycolic acid ['Dexon'], 'Vicryl,' or silk [less satisfactory]) or stainless steel (*not* catgut), on round-bodied, preferably trocar-pointed needles, or use Mayo cervix needles. For skin use nylon monofilament or steel.

For a tendon use several small stitches rather than one large one, and make sure that no single stitch bites more than half its thickness (which makes it liable to break later). Rough tendon ends are harmless on the dorsum of the foot, but if a tendon needs to glide, as when you weave peroneus brevis to tibialis posterior above the ankle, use fine (6/0) nylon monofilament to close over and bury the ends of both the tendon and the larger sutures, so as to prevent them sticking to surrounding structures.

CAUTION ! (1) Clamp a tendon as close to its cut end as you can, and excise the crushed area, which should be as short as possible. (2) Watch for and avoid the main vessels. There is no need to tie off all small ones.

PREPARATION. Lay him on his back, apply a tourniquet to his thigh (3.9), and sterilize his whole leg and foot below his knee. Clip a sterile towel round his thigh, so that you can lift his sterile leg without breaking sterility. A sandbag under the drapes will steady his leg, until you place it on the footboard.

INCISION ONE. Make a gently curved incision on the medial aspect of his leg, starting 2 cm above his calcaneus and 1 cm in front of his Achilles tendon, running parallel to the tendon for 5 cm, and then curving up to reach his tibia about 14 cm above his medial malleolus. Cut his fat and deep fascia, and find his Achilles tendon. Open its sheath, and lengthen it by one of the procedures in Fig. 27-11. Suture it so that his ankle will dorsiflex to 15–25° with his knee straight.

Lift the tissues proximal to his medial malleolus, until you see the tendons, under his deep fascia. Slit this to find his tibialis posterior tendon which lies deeper than his flexor digitorum longus, F, 30-11, also D, Fig. 27-11. Make sure you have

SOME CRITICAL DETAILS

Fig. 30-10 SOME CRITICAL DETAILS. A, measure the movement of his ankle like this (see also Fig. 69-1). B, a locally made goniometer. Hinge two boards together and nail a protractor, partly covered by a piece of card, to one edge. Mark the angles of dorsi- and plantarflexion on it. C, exercises for tibialis posterior. D, a locally made foot-drop-positioning splint made in three parts, hinged together, and adjusted by chains. E, the frame for a leg rest (24×24×36 cm). F, how the leg rests on webbing, cloth, or bandage stretched across the frame. *Kindly contributed by Grace Warren.*

TIBIALIS POSTERIOR TRANSFER

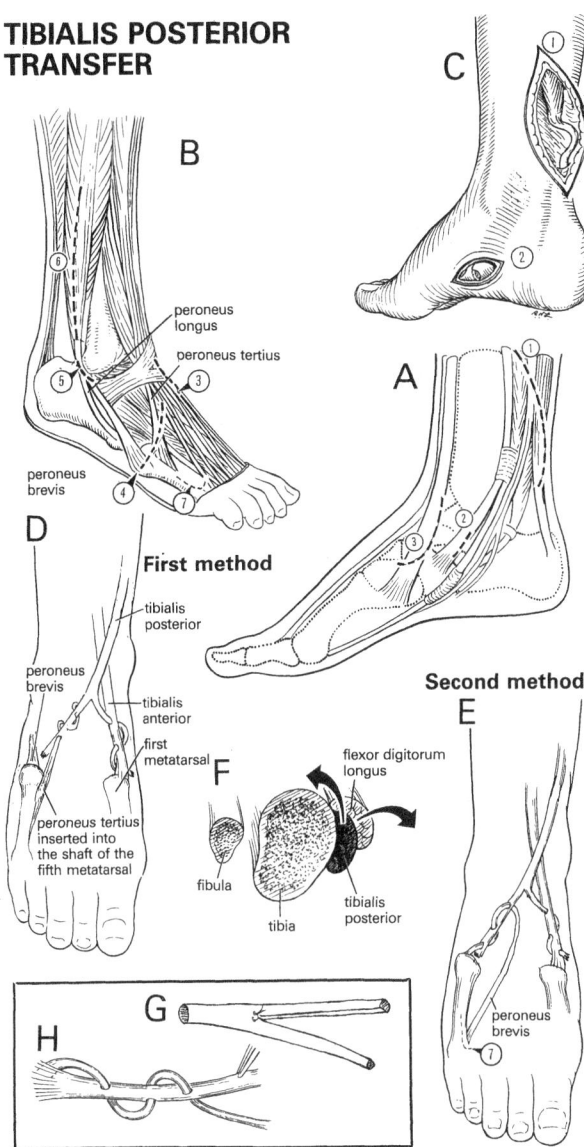

Fig. 30-11 TRANSFER OF THE TIBIALIS POSTERIOR TENDON for foot drop in leprosy and other diseases. A, the medial side of the foot with the first three incisions. B, the incisions on the lateral side of the foot. C, tibialis posterior is being pulled up into Incision One. D, the First Method, using peroneus tertius. E, the Second Method, using the full length of peroneus brevis. F, the relationship between tibialis posterior and flexor digitorum longus. G, split and suture the tendon of tibialis posterior. H, weaving the tendons. *Kindly contributed by Grace Warren.*

INCISION THREE. Find his tibialis anterior on the dorsomedial aspect of his navicular. It is the most medial of the tendons on the front of his ankle. Twist his foot into dorsiflexion and abduction to see it more clearly.

Make a 'J'-shaped incision, with its long arm along the medial side of his tibialis anterior tendon, from the lower end of his tibia to his naviculo-cuneiform joint, and its short arm crossing the tendon laterally for 1 cm. Reflect the flap at the level of his deep fascia, and try not to cut his dorsalis pedis artery. Find his tibialis anterior tendon (check that you are not pulling on his extensor hallucis longus), and open its sheath.

INCISION FOUR is a quarter-circle curved incision, with its convexity towards his toes, extending from 2.5 cm lateral to the distal end of Incision Three, and passing across the dorsum of his foot, to reach the base of his fifth metatarsal, but not extending over the bone itself. Use big scissors and the 'push and spread technique' (4-8) to raise all his superficial tissues off the deep fascia over the dorsum of his foot, so that you can see his toe extensors, his peroneus brevis, and his peroneus tertius (if he has one) inserting into the shaft of his fifth metatarsal. Define and dissect out his peroneus tertius as far from its insertion as you can, above his extensor retinaculum. Cut its tendon free proximally, separate it from its muscle fibres, and leave it free, attached distally to its insertion.

Keeping above his extensor retinaculum, raise his skin and superficial fascia to join Incisions Three and Four, and make a skin bridge.

CAUTION ! His superficial fascia is thin here. Be careful not to cut his extensor retinaculum, which is his deep fascia at this point.

Use finger dissection, and blunt Kocher's, to tunnel up under his skin above his extensor retinaculum, keeping in the midline initially, and then turning medially towards the proximal end of Incision One.

Return to the proximal end of Incision One. Starting about 7 cm above his ankle, raise his skin from the deep structures. Complete the tunnel joining incisions One, Three, and Four. Tunnel under his skin and preserve his long saphenous vein. Make a pocket into which the muscle belly of his tibialis posterior will fit. If necessary, cut the deep fascia over the crest of his tibia, but avoid cutting his tibial periosteum (if you do it will promote adhesions later).

Above his medial malleolus put a finger under his tibialis posterior tendon, remove Kocher's forceps from its distal end in Incision Two, and pull the tendon up into Incision One (C, in Fig. 30-11). Reclamp its distal end, and use the clamp to give you a good grip for traction, while your finger frees its muscle belly from the surrounding tissue at the back of his tibia.

CAUTION ! (1) Be careful to retract flexor digitorum longus posteriorly, so that tibialis posterior comes to lie anteriorly (F, 30-11 shows the anatomy of these tendons), between his flexor digitorum longus and his tibia (you don't want tibialis posterior to twist round digitorum longus). (2) Be careful not to damage his main vessels, the muscle fibres of his tibialis posterior, or his periosteum.

Using finger dissection, a Langenbach retractor, and if necessary scissors, free his tibialis posterior, until it will lift up and roll easily round the edge of his tibia in an oblique direction towards the base of his fifth metatarsal (which it will usually reach), crossing the centre of his leg about 4 cm above his ankle joint. Enlarge the tunnel if necessary.

When you have freed the tendon sufficiently to reach the dorsum of his foot, clamp its distal end with two Kocher,s, and divide it between them. Pull the two slips apart into a 'Y' with 6 cm arms. To prevent them separating any further, put a stitch where they meet, so that it will lie inside them when they lie together (G).

If his tibialis posterior will not reach the dorsum of his foot, check that you have freed its belly sufficiently.

Pass long Kocher's proximally, in the midline of his leg, from Incision Four for about 10 cm, and then deviate towards the proximal end of Incision One. Pick up both slips of his tibialis posterior, and pull them through on to the dorsum of his foot.

Pass the Kocher's from Incision Three to Incision Four. Pull one slip of tendon into Incision Three and leave the other one in Incision Four. Keep a Kocher's on each slip.

Pass your finger along his tibialis posterior tendon to make sure it lies easily in its new bed, that it runs smoothly round his tibia, and that no fascia obstructs its direct pull.

got the right tendon by pulling on it and seeing what it does—tibialis posterior inverts his foot, and does not flex his toes.

CAUTION ! Keep his exposed tendons moist by covering them with saline-soaked gauze.

INCISION TWO. Pull his tibialis posterior above his medial malleolus to find where it is inserted into his navicular. Make a 2-3 cm incision along the plantar side of the tendon, from his navicular proximally. Incise into the tendon sheath and raise the tendon with a blunt hook or curved forceps.

CAUTION ! Make sure you have got the right tendon. It is the only one which is inserted into his navicular, and is usually thick and strong and the size of your little finger.

Clamp his tibialis posterior tendon with Kocher's forceps, as far distally as you can easily reach it, on the medial aspect of his foot, and cut it distal to this (don't follow or try to cut it where it inserts distally, among the arches of his foot). Pull it up into Incision Two, and free it from any adhesions, which would make it difficult to pull out of its sheath later. If there is a large sesamoid bone in it, remove this and reattach the Kocher's. *Don't pull it out of its sheath yet.*

Use everting monofilament sutures (4-7) to close Incisions One and Two, without closing his deep fascia.

Put his foot on the positioning splint, to hold his knee at 80–90° of flexion, and his ankle at 20–25° of dorsiflexion, with his foot everted. While you adjust the tension in his tendons, ask an assistant to hold his foot in this position; or tie it to the foot splint with sterile bandages.

CAUTION ! (1) Don't let his foot invert. (2) Get his heel into the angle of the board.

Through Incision Three, place a Kocher's across about a quarter of his tibialis anterior tendon 2 cm from its insertion. While your assistant holds the distal part of this tendon tense, use a No. 15 blade to make a small *longitudinal* incision in it (Stab One), just distal to the Kocher's. Push a haemostat into Stab One, enlarge it a little and pull the slip of tibialis posterior tendon through it. Make Stab Two at 90° to Stab One 0.5 cm distal to it, and then pull the tendon slip through that. Make Stab Three 0.5 cm further distally again, and pass the tendon through that, as in H, Fig. 30-11 (if the tendon is not long enough, two stabs will do). Don't suture this 'weave' yet.

Turn to Incision Four.

THE FIRST METHOD is indicated if he has a peroneus tertius of suitable size. Holding the distal end of his tibialis posterior tight in Kocher's, weave the distal end of his peroneus tertius through it, in the same way that you wove his tibialis posterior through his tibialis anterior. Make Stab One in his tibialis posterior about level with the proximal end of his fifth metatarsal, just distal to his extensor retinaculum; make Stabs Two and Three more proximally. When the two tendons are woven together, work them along one another, until there is no slack tendon. Then, holding both firm so that they are just in tension, with his foot on the positioning board and his ankle everted, join them with 6 small sutures, passing through a little of each tendon, as in D, Fig. 30-11.

CAUTION ! As you suture the tendons, make sure they lie in the line of the pull of tibialis posterior, and are not raised away from his foot. If they are not in this line, they will be loose subsequently.

If there is spare tibialis posterior tendon left over, suture it to his peroneus brevis, or his extensor retinaculum, and tuck in any loose ends, so that they grow into the periosteum. If there is any spare peroneus tertius left over, stitch it so that it cannot attach itself above his ankle and limit movement.

Return to Incision Three. Move the woven tendons along one another until they lie snugly, and the tension in the medial slip is the same as that in the lateral one *with his foot in the correct position on the splint.* Suture the medial 'weave' in the same way.

CAUTION ! Don't make the medial slip too tight, or his foot will invert.

Check the position of his toes. While your assistant holds them as straight as he can, use a few small stitches to join the slips of his tibialis posterior to his extensor digitorum and extensor hallucis, as they cross.

THE SECOND METHOD is indicated if he has no peroneus tertius tendon, or it is too small:

If his peroneus brevis is paralysed (most patients), use it. Proceed as above until you have woven his tibialis posterior and his anterior together. Peroneus brevis is inserted into the base of his fifth metatarsal. Slip a blunt hook under it, and pull it, so that you can feel it under his lateral malleolus.

Make Incision Five over his peroneus brevis tendon as it passes *under* his lateral malleolus. Peroneus brevis lies deep to peroneus longus under his lateral malleolus, so you will have to hook out the deeper of the two tendons you find there. Pull it distally, and cut it off as far proximally as you can. This will leave the distal tendon as long as possible, without the need to make Incision Six. Return to Incision Four, you should be able to pull 8 cm of peroneus brevis into it. Weave peroneus brevis into the lateral slip of tibialis posterior and suture them as above. Close Incision Five.

If his peroneal muscles are still functioning (unusual), so that they had better not be sacrificed, take a free tendon graft from either: (1) his plantaris tendon from beside his Achilles tendon, or (2) a toe extensor. Weave and suture this free graft into his peroneus brevis as far distally as possible (to provide the best toe lift and eversion), and then into the lateral slip of his tibialis posterior, as described above. If you use plantaris and it is long enough, use it double for added strength (this method is not illustrated).

WITH BOTH METHODS check that the position of his ankle is satisfactory by lifting his leg off the splint, keeping his knee well flexed, and checking the angle of his foot and ankle—it should be in 15–20° of dorsiflexion and show no inversion. If it drops to 10° or inverts, undo some stitches and tighten them. Don't worry if it is high (20–25°): it will stretch later.

If sure you have cut no major arteries (usual), leave the tourniquet on until you have applied the cast. Otherwise, let it down, control bleeding by applying pressure for 5 minutes, carefully keeping his foot in position on the splint, and then close Incisions Three and Four.

CAUTION ! Don't plantarflex his foot while you do this.

THE CAST must keep his foot dorsiflexed and everted, and leave the dorsum of his ankle free. For this it needs a backslab and two side struts or braces.

Ask your assistant to stand beside the patient, facing the foot of the table, to flex his knee, and to flex and externally rotate his hip. His knee should rest on your assistant's abdomen. Your assistant's hand which is furthest from the patient should be flat on the sole of his foot (to avoid pressure areas), with its little finger over the head of his fifth metatarsal, its fingers straight, and with the patient's ankle 20–25° dorsiflexed and everted. His hand must stay in this position until the cast has set. Ask him to support the patient's calf with the flat of his other hand, moving it as the cast is applied.

CAUTION ! The patient cannot complain of pain because his foot is anaesthetic, so pad his heel well, or he may get pressure ulcers.

With his foot in this position, firmly but not too tightly bandage on wool, with extra layers over his heel. Apply an 8-layer 15 cm backslab from the tips of his toes to his mid upper calf (your assistant's hand will be between the backslab and his sole). Secure the slab with a 10 cm bandage. Start at his big toe (A, 30-12), go across his sole medial to lateral, and pass three turns round his forefoot, just proximal to his toes. Then pass two turns round his lower leg (this will leave a strut of bandage at the lateral side of his ankle, and enable you to give

A VERY SPECIAL CAST

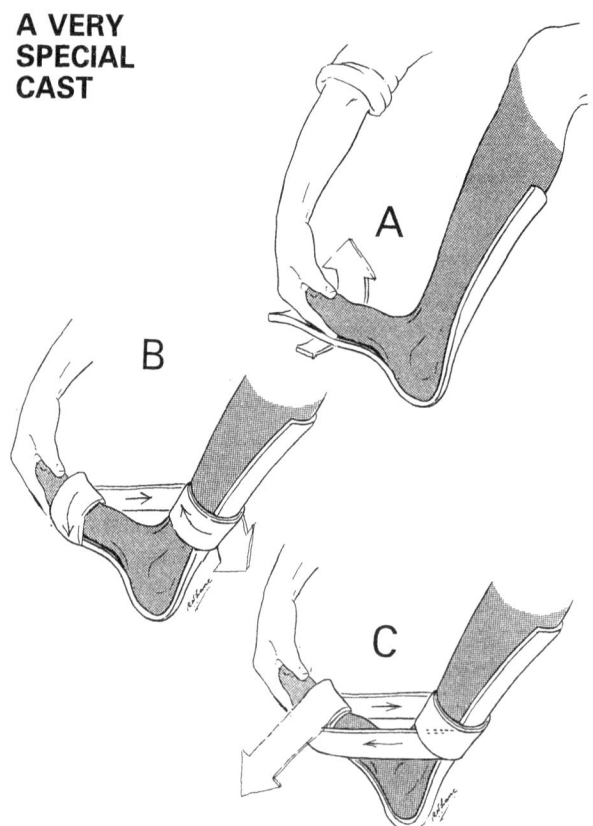

Fig. Fig. 30-12 A VERY SPECIAL CAST for a patient who has had his tibialis posterior transferred. A, the backslab applied with his foot dorsiflexed and everted. B, the lateral strut of plaster. C, the medial strut applied and the plaster being passed round his toes. *Kindly contributed by Grace Warren.*

his foot a good everting tilt as you do so). Then bring the bandage down the medial side of his ankle (to provide a medial strut) and run a turn or two round his forefoot. Continue until the bandage is finished. Apply another 10 cm bandage at the upper end of the backslab. Only now should your assistant remove his hand. Strengthen the side struts and the foot, *but leave the front of his ankle and his toes open.*

CAUTION ! (1) Make sure his toes are not dorsiflexed. (2) Don't leave finger depressions in the cast (F, 70-5). (3) Don't pull the bandages tight.

POSTOPERATIVELY, raise his foot on 2 pillows or in a special splint (E, Fig. 30-10), so that his tibia is parallel to his bed, but about 20 cm above it, and his knee is bent. If necessary (unusual in leprosy), give him morphine. Check the colour of his toes and his pulse hourly for 24 hours.

There will be blood marks on the cast. If the circulation to the toes is impaired, bivalve the cast, open it at least 1 cm, rebandage it, but don't remove it.

On Day 4 get him up on crutches, without weight-bearing.

Fourth week. (fifth week if physiotherapy supervision is limited). Readmit him, and bivalve his cast down the two sides, so that the struts are left attached to the posterior half of the cast (reinforced if necessary), which he can use as a protective resting splint while he is being rehabilitated.

CAUTION ! (1) Keep his foot dorsiflexed when you remove his sutures. If you don't, his flexors, aided by gravity, may pull away his healing tendons. Start exercises the day you remove the cast.

Fifth week. (first week after removal of the cast) Teach him to use his transfer in its new position. Lie him on his back (with his hips flexed and externally rotated, and his knees flexed), with both his feet in the frog position, so that the soles of his feet are almost touching each other. Ask him to do the inverting movement he did before surgery, his *unoperated* foot first. When he does that satisfactorily ask him to do it with both his feet together, and with his eyes closed (the movement produced by the transfer is not what he is used to seeing). Hold his operated foot with your palm flat on his sole, so that it cannot plantarflex. When he can do this without looking, let him look; the first movement may be very slight. Then let him graduate to doing it with only one leg.

Concentrate on getting him to dorsiflex his foot *without* using his gastrocnemius muscle, while trying to get a long, slow pull on his foot. Slowly increase the range and strength of the exercises with his leg horizontal in bed. Once he can do them, let him sit and watch them. After about 5 days, when he can move his transferred muscle easily and on command, sit him on the edge of his bed, and let him dangle his legs over it. Once he sits, he is lifting his foot against gravity, so he must not start doing this until he can isolate his transferred muscle and use it without gastrocnemius.

CAUTION ! (1) These exercises are fatiguing. During the first week, encourage him to do them many times a day for 5 minutes only, with 10 minutes rest periods with his foot back in its cast. (2) He must not plantarflex his foot: his strong gastrocnemius can easily pull the sutures out of his tendon transfer.

Sixth week. If he can isolate his transfer, and has good movement, let him stand with crutches or in parallel bars. Instruct him like this: "Put your operated foot on the ground behind your other foot. Lift up your toes (by contracting your transferred muscle), lift up your foot as if you are walking, and put it down heel first in front of your other foot. Lift it up and put it back again behind the other one". Progress to walking carefully with crutches. Make sure that every step uses the transferred tendon, and that contraction is held until his foot reaches the ground again. Let him walk for periods of 10 minutes and rest for 10 minutes.

Seventh week. While he walks with crutches, check that he uses his transfer with each step. Practise on steps, slopes and stairs. When he is confident, graduate to walking without crutches.

When he is not doing physiotherapy, bandage on the posterior half of the cast, until he learns to control his foot without trying to plantarflex it. He should be walking reasonably well at the end of the seventh week, and be able to discard his cast by day. Continue the protective splint at night until the end of the third month.

When he is off crutches, he can start rising on tiptoe while supporting himself with his hands on a table. His tendon join will gradually stretch, and his muscles will adapt to the range of movement required of them—provided you did not damage his periosteum, and so promote the formation of adhesions above his ankle.

CAUTION ! (1) Don't try to force his foot into plantar flexion: it will gradually come down as he walks. (2) He must not start plantar flexion too early, or he will lose the power of dorsiflexion. (3) Unless he learns to walk using the transfer with each step, he will not get a good gait; but even if he doesn't use it properly he should be much improved.

DIFFICULTIES WITH THIS TENDON TRANSFER

The main difficulty is to persuade him to care for his feet for years to come.

If his TIBIALIS POSTERIOR TENDON IS SHORT, or is badly scarred, so that its whole length cannot be used, transfer what tendon is available, and insert it into his tibialis anterior tendon more proximally. Then attach his peroneus brevis as in Method Two, taking it long so that it bypasses the scarred region.

If the lateral slip of his TIBIALIS POSTERIOR WILL NOT REACH the lateral side of his foot without causing excessive eversion, and his peroneal muscles are not functioning, use a longer piece of peroneus brevis than that described in the second method. If necessary, there is 25 cm of free tendon. Don't make Incision Five but instead make Incision Six 10 cm long, starting 1 cm behind his lateral malleolus and running up his leg in line with his fibula. Cut down until you see his deep fascia, cut this in the line of the tendon, and find peroneus brevis (usually deep to peroneus longus). Cut it out of the muscle (which will not be used), pull it back into his foot at Incision Four, weave it into the lateral slip of his tibialis posterior, and repair Incision Six.

CAUTION ! Check his peroneal tendons behind his lateral malleolus, because peroneus longus and brevis are often attached together there. If necessary cut his peroneal retinaculum, behind but not below his lateral malleolus, so that you can pull his peroneus brevis down and out at the base of his fifth metatarsal without harming the tendon.

Weave, adjust, and suture his peroneus brevis to his tibialis posterior as in the Second Method. Then tunnel its free end back under his skin and, through a small J-shaped Incision Seven, suture it to the periosteum on the neck of his fifth metatarsal, as in E, Fig. 30-11. This will give him a better anterior lift if he has a very mobile foot.

If PRESSURE OF THE DRESSING causes sloughing and infection, dress and graft the bare area.

If his wound becomes INFECTED, his tibialis posterior tendon may adhere to other structures, or break. Splint his leg and apply a hypochlorite ('Eusol') dressing. Rest it until you have controlled infection, then slowly resume exercises.

If he DOES NOT USE HIS TRANSFER, he was not taught adequately. Good physiotherapy is essential.

If his TOES CURL UNDER HIS FOOT, ulcers may form and he may lose them. Keep exercising them to prevent stiffness, and correct them surgically if necessary.

If his FOOT IS SLACK ON THE LATERAL SIDE, and tends to invert, consider doing another operation to tighten the tendon, and perhaps bring peroneus brevis into the graft.

30.9 Other leprosy problems

Surgery for leprosy of the eyes is discussed elsewhere (30.2). Here we discuss leprosy as it affects the mouth and breasts. If a patient has even the most minimal injury anywhere, treat it with the very greatest care. Cover any break in his skin to prevent secondary infection, and splint the part to allow it to heal in a functional position.

THE MOUTH IN LEPROSY

If a patient CANNOT CLOSE HIS MOUTH because his facial nerve is paralysed, his gums may dry and he may dribble food and drink and be socially unacceptable. Refer him to have his plantaris tendon or a strip of his fascia lata transferred to support his lip, by slinging it from his zygoma or temporalis fascia on both sides. Although this is a static sling, it will keep his mouth closed, improve his appearance, and stop him dribbling. If he has no lagophthalmos he may be able to have a temporal muscle transfer to reactivate his mouth.

THE BREASTS IN LEPROSY

If a MAN'S BREASTS ENLARGE and trouble him (gynaecomastia), do a simple mastectomy by the Webster method as in P, Fig. 30-9. Make sure his breasts are enlarged and he is not merely fat. Make an incision half the way round the margin of the areola. Leave a small piece of breast tissue immediately under his nipple, and drain the cavity towards his axilla. Bring the drain out some distance from his areola, so that you can close the surgical incision and get a good scar. He will probably be very pleased with this simple procedure. Don't remove any fat, or you will leave a depressed area.

31 The surgery of tropical diseases

31.1 The surgery of neglected infection

As living standards in what are now the industrial countries have improved, many conditions, which once occurred everywhere, are now confined to the tropics. Although they often thought of as being specifically tropical, they are in fact the 'surgery of poverty'. Surgical tuberculosis (Chapter 29), surgical leprosy (Chapter 30), vesicovaginal fistulae (18.18), perforated typhoid ulcers (31.8), and enormous hernias (14.4) are a few of the conditions which were once seen everywhere. There are also a few specifically tropical infections, such as mycetoma (31.3) and filariasis (31.6) which may need surgery. *Schistosoma haematobium* causes much surgical disease of the urinary tract, but none of the procedures that are possible are sufficiently easy or effective to be mentioned here, apart from a plea for the early diagnosis of the bladder cancer that it may cause (32.31), a note on schistosomal granulomas of the vulva (20.14), and on the occasional usefulness of nephrostomy (23.13).

Tropical ulcers are one of the classical tasks of tropical surgery, so we will start with them.

31.2 Tropical ulcers

These were once common over most of the tropics, but as living standards rise they go. There is some disagreement as to what causes them. They are generally said to start as small infected cuts from the sharp grasses of bush paths, which would explain their characteristic distribution (D, in Fig. 31-1). Others consider that they are primarily infective, which would explain why they sometimes occur in small epidemics in the wet season. Tropical ulcers develop through three stages: *Stage One.* A pustule, or neglected cut, containing Vincent's and fusiformis organisms (both are penicillin-sensitive). This stage is not seen in hospital. *Stage Two.* Progression of the cut or pustule to form an acutely painful ulcer with a raised, thickened, and slightly undermined edge. This ulcer grows rapidly for several weeks. A bloody discharge covers the grey slough on its floor, the skin around it is dark and swollen, and muscle, bone, and tendon occasionally lie exposed in its base. After about a month, the pain, swelling, and discharge improve, and it either heals, or it goes on to the next stage. *Stage Three.* It becomes chronic, and resembles any other long-standing indolent ulcer.

In Stage Two, when an ulcer is still less than 5 or 6 cm, penicillin and dressings will usually cure it. But if it is larger than this, the epithelium from its edges will take a long time to grow across it, so it needs grafting—which is something that every health centre should be able to do.

If you first see a patient in Stage Three, his ulcer may have destroyed the whole thickness of his skin; it may have extended through his deep fascia and exposed bone, tendons or a joint. Osteomyelitis is rare, but a reactive periostitis may in time raise an ulcer above the surrounding skin. Sometimes its edge is thickened and everted, and resembles a carcinoma.

MOST GRAFTING SHOULD BE DONE AT THE ACUTE OR SUBACUTE STAGE

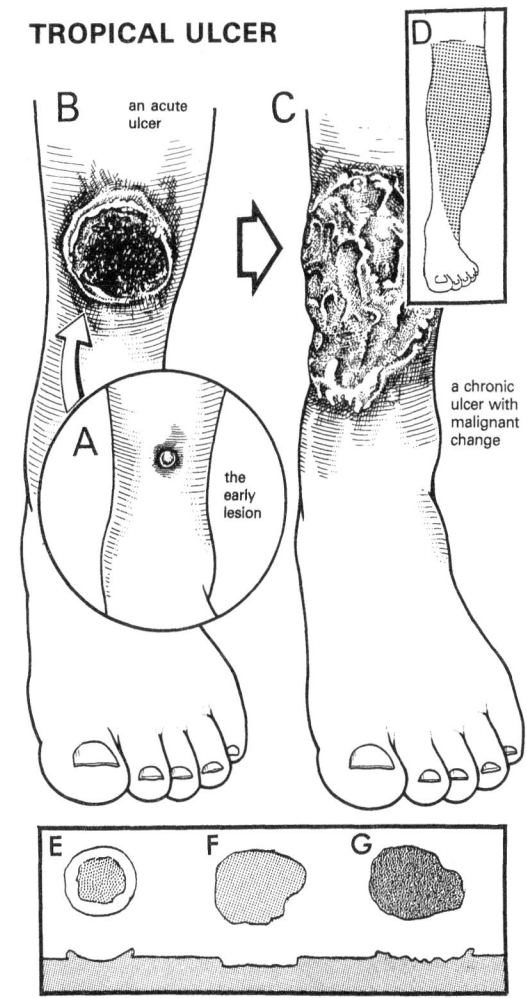

Fig. 31-1 TROPICAL ULCERS. A, the earliest stage of a tropical ulcer is a pustule, containing Vincent's organisms and fusiform bacilli. Alternatively, and some would say more commonly, the early stage is a small cut. B, the pustule ruptures to form an acute ulcer. C, a chronic ulcer showing the exposed tendons. D, the characteristic site of tropical ulcers anteriorly on the lower leg, becoming more lateral lower down. E, an acute tropical ulcer, with an everted oedematous edge, and a dirty slough covering much of its base. F, a chronic ulcer, with an edge which is not raised, and a uniform avascular base. G, a squamous cell carcinoma, with an everted edge, and an irregular base.

TROPICAL ULCERS

DIFFERENTIAL DIAGNOSIS. The site of a tropical ulcer is its most important diagnostic feature. The differential diagnosis includes: (1) a chronic non-specific ulcer, (2) a squamous cell carcinoma, which resembles a chronic tropical ulcer in that it also has an everted edge (32.19). Also, the following:

Suggesting tuberculosis (unusual)—a ragged, shallow ulcer, with bluish overhanging edges. Its base is less vascular, and more fibrous. If you manage it as a tropical ulcer, it will not improve. If you are in any doubt, biopsy it, and try chemotherapy—a tuberculous ulcer will heal miraculously.

Suggesting a Buruli ulcer (restricted areas only)—an otherwise fit child, or young adult, suffering from a huge ulcer with deeply undermined edges, anywhere on his body, and not necessarily on his feet and lower legs (31.2a).

CAUTION ! The macroscopic differentiation of a chronic tropical ulcer from a malignant ulcer (32.19) can be difficult when there is no extension into the surrounding tissues. Be sure to do a biopsy before you do any radical surgery.

TREATMENT FOR TROPICAL ULCERS

ACUTE ULCERS. Treat him as an outpatient. Get his ulcer clean with saline soaks. Soak off the dressing each day and change it. Give him a bottle of half-strength saline (tap water and salt, which need not be sterile) and ask him to pour this on the dressing every 2 or 3 hours to keep it moist. Give him penicillin.

When his ulcer is clean, usually within 7 days, and if it is >5 cm in diameter, admit him for split skin grafting (Chapter 57). Smaller ulcers will heal without grafting. Give him penicillin for 3 days perioperatively. This kills any streptococci which might dislodge the graft with their fibrinolysin (57.4).

If he is an adult, use local anaesthesia for the donor site (57-4), and ketamine or general anaesthesia if he is a child.

If the granulations are abundant, scrape the base of the ulcer with a scalpel. There is no need to anaesthetize it; there are no nerves in granulation tissue, so this does not hurt, provided you avoid the epithelium. Scraping does not improve the 'take', but it does reduce fibrosis under the graft later, and so makes it more stable.

Control bleeding with hot packs. If possible, apply the graft as a single sheet, which has been meshed to allow the escape of exudate and blood, or, less satisfactorily, apply it as patches or pinch grafts (57.9). If the ulcer is over a joint tendon (uncommon), lay strips of graft across it (57.5).

Keep him in bed for a week to avoid movement, and expose the graft on the 7th day (some surgeons expose it on the 3rd day to inspect it). Then *soak off the dressing slowly*, to avoid removing the graft at the same time. It may need covering for another week. The donor site should have healed in 10 days.

CHRONIC ULCERS. Split skin grafts do not take well on long-standing fibrotic ulcers, or they may take take initially, and break down later. Ideally, these ulcers need a muscle, or a myocutaneous flap (not described here). Chronic ulcers cause long standing morbidity, and may become malignant, so refer him if you can. If you cannot refer him, you will have to do your best with split skin grafting. You will probably succeed temporarily, but his ulcer will probably recur.

If the base of his ulcer is suitable (57.3), and is not too deeply fibrosed or over bone or tendon, some surgeons would excise and graft it as a single procedure.

Alternatively, and preferably, apply a tourniquet (3.9), and excise the ulcer under ketamine (8.1), or a general anaesthetic. Cut away all avascular scar tissue, until you reach a raw, bleeding surface; if necessary, use an osteotome to remove any dead bone. Apply hypochlorite, or a dry dressing, to the ulcer bed, cover it with gauze, cotton wool, and a bandage, and release the tourniquet.

Five to twelve days later, when the base of the ulcer is covered with suitable granulation tissue, graft it, as described above.

DIFFICULTIES WITH TROPICAL ULCERS

If, after many years, the BASE OF AN ULCER BECOMES HEAPED UP and irregular, and its edges protuberant and rolled, a SQUAMOUS CELL CARCINOMA (epithelioma) has developed, so see Section 32.19. This can happen in three years, or it can take thirty.

31.2a Mycobacterium ulcerans infection (Buruli ulcer)

This occurs in restricted areas of the rural tropics near rivers—the Congo in Zaire, the Upper Nile and Lake Kyoga in Uganda, the Nyong in the Cameroons, and in the lowland swamps of Malaysia. It is also occasionally seen in Zambia.

The patient is often a child, and in some areas is likely to be a woman, who presents with a painless, small, well demarcated, indurated swelling, attached to the skin, but not to deeper tissues. It is almost always single and on the limbs, and is often near a joint, although the site is more variable in young children. There is little pain or tenderness, little or no fever, and the regional lymph nodes are not enlarged. The lesion grows, the skin over it desquamates, becomes pigmented, and then breaks down to form a chronic expanding ulcer, with a necrotic base, and edges which may be undermined 5 to 15 cm. Secondary infection occurs, and a foul slough forms. Satellite ulcers may appear, but metastatic spread is rare. Some ulcers remain unchanged for weeks; others cover much of a limb, or the trunk, in a few weeks. Untreated ulcers commonly heal spontaneously, with much scarring and severe contractures.

BURULI ULCER

THE DIAGNOSIS is suggested by the the appearance of the swelling and the ulcer, the absence of lymph node enlargement, and the failure to respond to tropical ulcer therapy (31.2).

SPECIAL TESTS. Look for AAFB in the chronic base of the ulcer, and send material for culture. *M. ulcerans* grows on the media used for *M. tuberculosis*, but only at 33°C.

THE DIFFERENTIAL DIAGNOSIS in the nodule stage includes: boils, foreign body granulomas, and low-grade fibrosarcomas. In the ulcer stage it includes: tropical, mycotic, parasitic, and malignant ulcers.

CHEMOTHERAPY. *M. ulcerans* is sensitive *in vitro* to streptomycin, clofazimine, and rifampicin, but these drugs have little clinical effect. Even so, give them to cover surgery.

TREATMENT. Excise early lesions, if possible with primary closure (unlikely).

If the lesion is ulcerated, control pyogenic infection with antibiotics, and irrigate with saline. Excise all diseased tissue, and graft (57.1). If you fail to remove all diseased tissue, the graft will fail, and healing will be slow, with much scarring.

31.3 Mycetoma

Considering the many people who walk barefoot, it is surpising that the saprophytes of the soil so seldom infect the feet. But this does happen occasionally, notably in the Sahel area of Africa, and in parts of South India, Mexico, Brazil, and the Middle East, each area having its own particular species. If a peasant in one of these areas treads on an acacia thorn, or some other sharp object, it may may infect him with filamentous fungus-like bacteria (*Streptomyces, Actinomyces,or Nocardia*), or the true fungi (the eumycetes, particularly *Madurella*). These cause a chronic granulomatous swelling, with multiple sinuses that discharge characteristic granules, each of which has arisen in a micro-abscess. The lesion is usually in a patient's foot, but his leg, finger, hand, thigh, trunk, jaw, or head may also be affected, and may be difficult to diagnose.

He is usually a farmer who has a painless swelling on his foot at the site of a thorn prick some months earlier. This grows slowly to form a circumscribed, rubbery or cystic, lobulated mass. If it is on his sole, pressure flattens it into a disc. Sinuses appear, and occasionally discharge granules. As one sinus heals more appear, and become secondarily infected, but this secondary infection does not extend deeply. By the time that five years have elapsed, his whole foot is swollen, and covered with open sinuses and the scars of healed ones. It is still painless, and as he has no systemic symptoms he continues to work. As his foot disintegrates, he takes to a crutch. Spread to his lymph nodes is late and uncommon, and only after about ten years do sinuses start to form in the nodes of his groin.

The primary site of infection is usually in his subcutaneous fat, but it may be in fat which is deep to fascial planes. These form a natural barrier to the spread of infection, so that if it gets under his plantar, or palmar fascia, it may spread between his tendons, along his lumbrical canals, and even through his carpal tunnel, up into his forearm. His bone may be invaded relatively early, still without causing him pain.

Mycetomas never regress spontaneously. Chemotherapy has no effect on the true fungus *Madurella*, but it is worth trying a long period of dapsone, trimethoprim, and streptomycin on *Streptomyces* and *Nocardia*, and trying penicillin on *Actinomyces*, as described below. Ketoconazole 200 mg once or twice daily with meals (expensive) has also been used. The ultimate treatment is amputation, but perhaps only after 20 years, if necessary accompanied by clearance of the regional nodes. The vascularity of a limb is not impaired, so that you can amputate at a site of election, provided it is through healthy tissue (56.1).

Crockett, DJ. 'Mycetoma' Tropical Doctor 1973;3:28-33.

MYCETOMA

DIAGNOSIS. Try to find the granules, because without them all a pathologist can say is that there is a granulomatous infection with multiple micro-abscesses.

In the endemic zone in Fig. 31-2.

Streptomyces somaliensis forms yellowish-white medium sized, 0.5 to 1 mm, soft, round, smooth granules.

Madurella mycetomi and Leptosphaeria senegalensis, form brown or black, large, 1 to 3 mm, irregular, fissured, aggregated, hard, brittle granules.

Streptomyces pelletieri forms red, minute, 0.3 mm, faceted, aggregated, very hard granules.

In the sporadic zone.

Nocardia brasiliensis forms yellowish, minute 0.3 mm, irregular, lobulated, soft granules.

Streptomyces madurae forms white, yellow or pink tinged, large, 1 to 3 mm, soft, lobulated granules.

X-RAYS. Once a patient's periosteum is breached, his tarsal and metatarsal bones are rapidly destroyed. New bone in the walls of abscesses forms buttresses projecting outwards at angles to the shaft of a long bone. The centre of an infected bone has a honeycomb appearance, and a good film shows tiny cystic areas of bone destruction, each the site of a micro-abscess.

CHEMOTHERAPY FOR MYCETOMA

If you find the granules of *Nocardia brasiliensis*, try prolonged continuous treatment with dapsone 100 mg twice daily for 2 years or more. Streptomycin 1 g daily by intramuscular injection is also effective. Treatment is so protracted, and the disease so painless, that he is unlikely to co-operate for long. You may be wise to reserve dapsone for lesions of the posterior part of his foot, or in his hand, for which the only alternative is a high amputation.

If you find the granules of *Streptomyces somaliensis*, try trimethoprim 100 mg, twice a day for many months, or even a year or more.

If you diagnose actinomycosis, caused by such organisms as *Actinomyces israeli*, try penicillin for 2 or 3 months.

CAUTION ! With long-continued treatment, watch carefully for side-effects. Dapsone: neuropathy, allergic dermatitis, anorexia, nausea and vomiting, headache, insomnia, hepatitis, agranulocytosis (all rare). Trimethoprim: vomiting, rashes, erythema multiforme, epidermal necrolysis, eosinophilia, agranulocytosis, granulopenia, purpura, leucopenia;

MYCETOMA

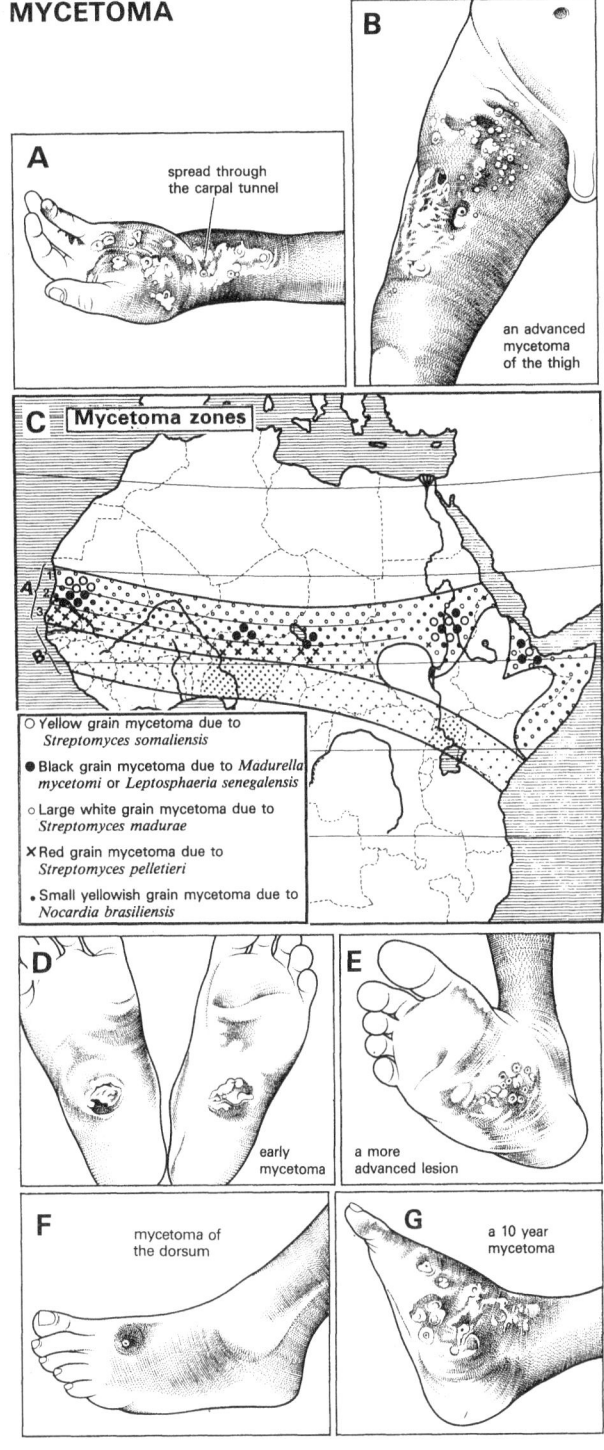

Fig. 31-2 MYCETOMA. A, mycetoma of the hand, spreading through the carpal tunnel into the forearm (unusual). B, an advanced mycetoma of the thigh 20 years after infection had begun in the foot. C, the endemic and the sporadic mycetoma zones in Africa. D, early black grain mycetomas of the soles of both feet, showing flattened disc-shaped swellings. This is the typical early lesion, but the simultaneous involvement of both feet is unusual. E, a more advanced lesion. F, a mycetoma of the dorsum of the foot. This may be part of a dumb-bell lesion extending from the sole between the metatarsals. G, a diffuse mycetoma of 10 years' duration; it is still painless and its owner is still working. *After Crockett DJ, 'Mycetoma', Figs. 1 to 8. 'Tropical Doctor' Vol.3:No. 1, with kind permission.*

megaloblastic anaemia. Streptomycin: tinnitus, vertigo and deafness, a widespread fine rash, drug fever, nephrotoxicity (rare), and paraesthesiae of the mouth (very rare).

With all other mycetomas, the only treatment is symptomatic. Short courses of tetracyclines will control secondary infection in the sinuses, and encourage them to heal, but will not eradicate the disease. Curette and drain any low-grade abscesses that form.

SURGERY FOR MYCETOMA

If a lesion is localized, and is confined to a patient's soft tissues, excise it and repair the defect with a split skin graft.

If he has a lesion of his forefoot which involves bone, or which will expose bone on a weight-bearing surface if you remove it, Syme's amputation may be appropriate (56.9).

If he has a lesion of his hindfoot with minor bone involvement, and without severe disorganization of its joints, treatment depends on the organism: (1) If it is *Nocardia*, as determined by the district he comes from and Fig. 31-2, give him dapsone, and drain the lesions if necessary, but don't amputate. (2) If any other organism is responsible, you will probably have to amputate, but wait until his foot becomes a real nuisance.

If he has a lesion of his hind foot with severe bone and joint destruction, do a below-knee amputation (56.8).

CAUTION ! (1) Mycetoma is painless, so don't amputate a limb until he is quite sure that his limb is of no use. (2) Observe him carefully, and make sure he reports any involvement of his inguinal nodes. If he does, amputate immediately, and clear them by block dissection (32.34).

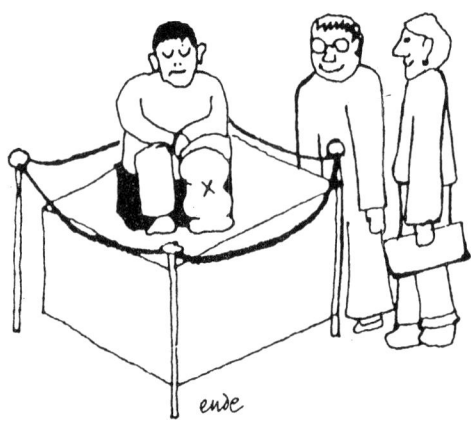

'The patient exhibited marked oedema...'

31.4 Gross enlargements of parts of the body (elephantiasis)

If a patient has a gross generalized swelling of his leg, arm, or scrotum, or if a woman has a similar swelling of her breast or vulva, the condition is known as elephantiasis. Usually, this is due to long standing lymphatic obstruction. Occasionally, it is due to venous obstruction, but this is seldom gross enough to need surgery. Distinguishing between lymphatic and venous obstruction can be difficult. Oedema due to lymphatic obstruction becomes solid quite rapidly, but early cases may show pitting. Oedema due to venous obstruction becomes solid late, and eventually reaches a stage where it fails to pit.

In most areas, the causes of lymphatic obstruction (lymphoedema), in decreasing order of frequency are: (1) Tuberculosis. (2) Repeated lymphangitis leading to incompetent valves, usually due to streptococci from wounds. (3) Malignant glands in the groin, or less often the axilla. (4) Kaposi's sarcoma. (5) Block dissection of the glands, usually for carcinoma. (6) Congenital lymphatic hypoplasia, or incompetent lymphatic valves (Milroy's disease). Other causes include chronic fungal infections, and lymphogranuloma inguinale.

Two important causes of lymphatic obstruction are restricted to certain endemic areas: (1) filariasis (commonly due to infection with *W. bancrofti* and less often to *Brugia malayi*, or *Brugia timori*.). (2) 'Podoconiosis' (also called non-filarial endemic elephantiasis). Filariasis is restricted by the prevalence of the insect vectors, and podoconiosis by particular characteristics of the soil. Filariasis may involve any of the parts of the body listed above, but usually the legs or scrotum, whereas podoconiosis only involves the legs.

'Mossy foot' is a term used to describe: (1) Commonly, a variety of podoconiosis in which the epithelial hyperplasia is extreme. (2) Rarely, other disease causing multiple excrescences on the feet, notably chromoblastomycosis. Elephantiasis due to advanced podoconiosis (whether it has reached the 'mossy foot' stage or not) responds fairly well to surgery. Elephantiasis due to filariasis is difficult to treat surgically. It is a popular misconception that filariasis is the commonest cause of lymphoedema; this is so only in filarial hyperendemic areas.

In practice, the exact diagnosis of the grosser forms of oedema leading to elephantiasis is not absolutely essential, because the practical methods of surgical treatment are similar in all of them—excision and grafting.

ELEPHANTIASIS

This is the patient with gross enlargement of some part of his body.

LYMPHATIC OR VENOUS OBSTRUCTION? Lymphatic obstruction is much more likely.

Suggesting lymphatic obstruction—a slow onset, pitting except in late stages, when there is much secondary fibrosis, hyperkeratosis of the epidermis, which may be extreme ('mossy foot').

Suggesting venous obstruction—a rapid onset, some obvious cause for the obstruction, pitting on pressure, often ulceration of the skin, rarely gangrene.

INVESTIGATIONS. If he comes from an area where *W. bancrofti* is endemic, examine several nocturnal blood smears. There are no bone changes, so an X-ray is normal. Lymphangiograms are unlikely to be helpful.

THE DIFFERENTIAL DIAGNOSIS includes the common medical causes of peripheral oedema (heart failure, nephritis, and cirrhosis of the liver, etc.). In these the swelling is usually equal in both legs. In the surgical causes, particularly podoconiosis, it is usually unequal.

Suggesting bancroftian filariasis—scrotal involement, oedema which starts at the most dependent part for each site and moves upwards—below the malleoli for the leg, the fundus for the scrotum, the foreskin for the penis, and the dorsum of the hand for the arm. Elephantiasis of the scrotum with few changes in its skin.

Suggesting podoconiosis —a bare-footed patient from a podoconiosis area; worse on one leg than the other; below-knee swellings most marked distally. Symptoms are the *first* evidence of disease (in filariasis they are the *last*), and include burning of the lower legs at night, with persistent itching of the 1st and 2nd toe clefts, and plantar oedema of the forefoot. No filaria in the blood, and a chronic warty thickening of the lower legs ('mossy foot').

Suggesting chronic non-specific infection—some source for it, such as a tropical ulcer (if the swelling is in the lower leg). Acute recurrent attacks of lymphangitis. Enlargement of the nodes draining the swollen area only: these may be large and firm, or small and fibrotic. Lines of hyperpigmentation on the skin indicating previous lymphangitis (not easy to find, so look carefully; and seldom visible on a dark skin). A lymph node biopsy showing fibrosis and non-specific inflammatory changes.

Suggesting tuberculosis—chronic enlargement of many superficial nodes—inguinal, axillary, and cervical; a history of prolonged illness in the past, with fever and enlarged nodes, some of which discharged for long periods; multiple sinuses, or the scars that follow their healing. Lymphogranuloma also produces sinuses, but these are usually confined to the superior group of nodes, over the medial part of the inguinal ligament. Scars over the lower end of the vertical chain are more likely to be caused by tuberculosis. Involvement of an entire leg from toes to groin, or an entire arm or a woman's breast. A positive lymph node biopsy confirms the diagnosis; if tuberculosis is no longer active only non-specific fibrosis may be seen.

The site involved also influences the probable cause. Breast and arm, or vulva—tuberculosis. Scrotum—bancroftian filariasis. Lower leg—filariasis, podoconiosis.

CHEMOTHERAPY. If you are in doubt, try the appropriate specific treatment for tuberculosis or filariasis. Lymphoedema due to tuberculosis nearly always settles with chemotherapy, unless it is diagnosed very late. Antibiotics are unlikely to influence chronic non-specific inflammation.

31.5 Podoconiosis (non-filarial endemic elephantiasis of the lower legs)

Podoconiosis ('dust in the feet') presents as bilateral asymmetrical swelling of the feet and lower legs. It is seen in susceptible families of bare-footed farmers in well-defined fertile volcanic highland zones of Africa, Central and South America, and Indonesia, and also in the lowlands irrigated by rivers from these highlands. It is due to the absorption of silica particles from the soil, through the feet of someone from a susceptible family. This causes the patient's lymphatics to fibrose, and obstruct, and his femoral nodes to enlarge. This in turn makes his legs and feet swell, and progress through stages which are described as 'water bag', 'rubbery', and 'wooden'. Finally, his leg becomes hyperkeratotic, 'mossy', and nodular. Lymph may ooze through his skin, which may be secondarily infected by fungi or bacteria. The disease may progress steadily, or there may be a succession of acute episodes which resolve incompletely. Villagers in endemic areas are often able to recognize the early stages.

Elevation, elastic stockings, and long leather boots help in the earlier stages, but once the 'wooden' stage has developed, the only treatment is surgical. If you see a patient early, persuade him to wear boots or shoes which will minimize further progression. The main preventive measure is wearing fully protective shoes from childhood. Sandals, or shoes with many open spaces on their uppers, may not protect.

Podoconiosis is disfiguring, and may make the patient a social outcast, so treatment is important. Unfortunately, by the time you see him, his lymphatics will probably be incurably blocked, so that medical treatment is unlikely to be effective. Surgically, you can: (1) Compress the leg of a 'soft' case in a decompression machine (if you have one), excise the folds of superfluous skin and subcutaneous tissue that are left after decompression, and then bring his skin edges together. (2) Excise the thickened tissue of a 'hard case', and graft the bare area. (3) Excise individual nodules. Or you can combine these procedures. Surgery is said to be simple and beneficial, but opinions differ.

Price EW, 'The pre-elephantiasic stage of non-filarial elephantiasis of the lower legs: podoconiosis'. Tropical Doctor 1984;14:115-119

Price EW, 'Management of endemic (non-filarial) elephantiasis of the lower legs'. Tropical Doctor 1975;5:70-75.

PODOCONIOSIS

EARLY DIAGNOSIS. After a long day's work in the fields, or a long walk, one of a patient's feet becomes swollen, and feels tense. His lymph nodes are enlarged and firm. For the differential diagnosis see the previous section. Try to recognize the following early stages:

'Burning leg' He has a burning sensation in his lower leg, from in front of his medial malleolus to behind the medial condyle of his knee, sometimes extending upwards into his thigh. His femoral nodes may be tender. Pain is usually worst at night, and is relieved by uncovering his leg. Each episode usually affects the same leg, and the second leg does not usually become involved until the first one shows clear signs of disease. Although the burning area of the leg may be tender, few patients seek help at this stage.

DIAGNOSING PODOCONIOSIS

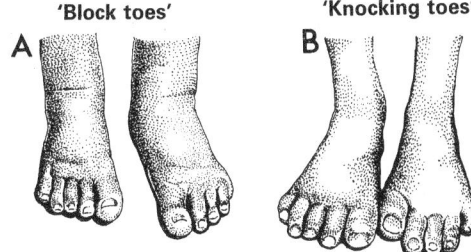
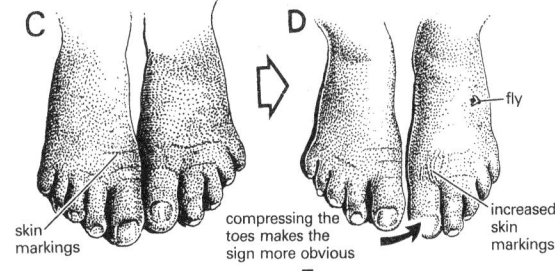
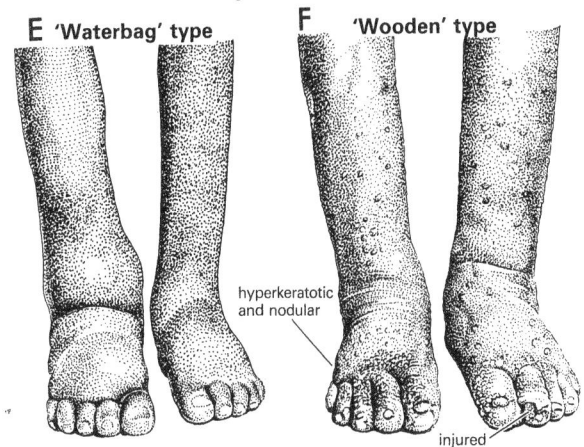

Fig. 31-3 DIAGNOSING PODOCONIOSIS. A, 'block toes'. Early oedema of a patient's forefoot affects the plantar aspect of his metatarsal pad, as well as his toes, which appear rigid, as if they were wooden and nailed on to his forefoot. They may be lifted off the floor by plantar oedema, and lack the usual curve of normal toes. B, 'knocking' big toes on walking, due to splaying of the forefeet as the result of deep oedema at the level of the metatarsal heads. C, and D, increased skin markings, which become more evident if his toes are compressed, as in D. Flies, attracted by exuded lymph to an otherwise clean foot, are characteristic. E, a wet 'waterbag' foot, which is readily reduced by compression or elevation; its skin is soft, and you can pinch it off the bone. F, the dry 'wooden' type, which cannot be reduced by compression or elevation; it is hyperkeratotic, and often nodulated. *After EW Price.*

'Itchy foot' is a persistent localized itching, usually on the dorsum at the base of the first or second toe clefts, or below the middle malleolus. Thickening of the skin (pachydermia), from constant scratching, may bring him to the clinic. When his toes start swelling, the itchy area precedes the upper level of the swelling, and indicates progression of the disease.

'Splayed forefoot' is a widening of his forefoot, and separation of his toes, which gives his foot a spatula-like appearance, on one or both sides (B, in Fig. 31-3). It is due to deep oedema between his metatarsal heads. His skin is unusually resistant to being lifted by your fingers.

Plantar oedema is asymmetrical (unlike cardiac or renal oedema). Press with your thumb on his sole over the head of his first metatarsal. Test for it when he has recovered from any temporary physiological oedema, which may be the result of walking a long way to the clinic. You may see mild lymphatic

TREATING PODOCONIOSIS

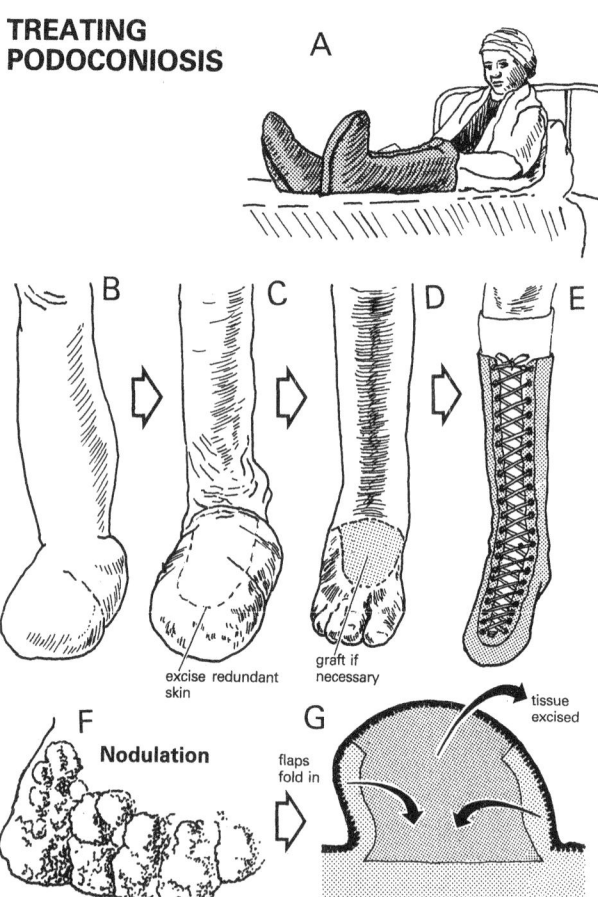

Fig. 31-4 TREATING PODOCONIOSIS. A, an intermittent compression machine in use (the foot has been lowered for ease of illustration, and should be raised). B, a 'waterbag' foot before decompression in the machine. C, the same foot, after the machine has reduced the swelling over the lower leg, but not over the dorsum of the foot. D, excess skin and tissue have been removed and the bare area grafted. E, the grafted leg protected in a boot. F, nodulation. G, how to excise a nodule. *After EW Price, by kind permission of the Editor of Tropical Doctor.*

oozing, tiny blebs of lymph, or an an unusual number of flies attracted to it.

A pachydermic forefoot shows an excessive deposit of keratin on the dorsum at the base of the first or second toe cleft. The clefts themselves usually remain normal, even in advanced disease.

Increased skin markings at the base of the first toe cleft and running longitudinally rather than laterally (as is normal). Compressing them, as in D, Fig. 31-3, shows them more clearly.

'Block toes' lack their normal curves, and look wooden and rigid, as if they were nailed on the forefoot (A).

EARLY TREATMENT. Advise him like this: "(1) Raise the foot of your bed to the height which relieves the discomfort; a hammock is suitable. (2) Put on ankle-length elastic socks before rising in the morning; or apply wide (10 cm) one-way stretch elastic bandages; crepe bandages are inadequate. (3) Protect the skin of your feet from the soil, preferably in shoes. (4) Choose another occupation which does not involve contact with the soil (difficult). (5) Move to a non-endemic area (even more difficult)". Meanwhile, treat whatever other conditions he has (parasites, anaemia, etc.).

CAUTION! Don't try to remove his femoral nodes.

EXCISION OF FOOT NODULES. Excise them for aesthetic reasons, or to make wearing shoes easier. They have no sensory nerves, so you can remove them without anaesthesia, which is useful, because they are so thickly indurated that infiltration may be impossible.

INTERMITTENT COMPRESSION AND THE EXCISION OF REDUNDANT TISSUE. Start by reducing the size of the swellings with the intermittent compression machine in A, Fig. 31-4.

Have blood cross-matched. With a tourniquet applied (essential), make an incision from the upper level of the loose skin behind his medial malleolus, along the medial side of the dorsum of his foot, and then lateraly across the dorsum. Excise the loose skin. If bringing the skin edges together is difficult, graft the raw area (D, 31-4). Advise him to wear stockings and boots (E).

EXCISION ALONE. See also Charles' operation in Section 31.6.

31.6 The surgery of filariasis

Wuchereria bancrofti and *Brugia malayi,* or *W. timori* behave in a similar, but not identical, way. The acute lesions they cause may mimic other diseases, so, if yours is an endemic area, keep the possibility of filariasis in mind. The first two stages are common, but filarial elephantiasis is not.

The acute stage starts within a few months of infection, as fever, lymphadenopathy, erythema, and epididymitis, usually without microfilariae in the blood. Secondary infection may occur.

The subacute stage is characterized by fever and enlarged tender lymph nodes, which persist and are accompanied by lymphangitis. The inguinal, epitrochlear, and axillary nodes are commonly involved. Lymphangitis presents as a shiny area, radiating distally from the involved lymph nodes, usually down the front or medial aspect of the thigh, or round the anterior axillary fold towards the breast. Attacks may be repeated every few months. The lesions may also be infected secondarily, so that both the affected lymph nodes and the areas of lymphangitis may suppurate to form abscesses.

A patient's spermatic cord is often infected, and also his testes and epididymes, so that he has painful recurrent attacks of funiculo-epididymo-orchitis, which may be followed by suppuration in his scrotum.

Synovitis and arthritis also occur.

The chronic stage is the result of lymphatic obstruction, commonly in the retroperitoneum. This can cause:

(1) Lymphoedema, which may progress to gross hypertrophy of his subcutaneous tissues (elephantiasis). This may involve his lower limbs and scrotum (common), or the arm, breast, or abdominal wall (less common), or the axillary or inguinal nodes (rare). No known treatment will reverse these changes. There is little you can do surgically except to excise the swellings; when you have done so, they may recur in a few years, or even a few months. Charles' operation is described; its immediate results may be acceptable, but its final results may be worse than before, and are said not to stand up to the wear and tear of village life. The surgery of elephantiasis is unsatisfactory, the account we give of Charles' operation is the classical one, and we were unable to find any recent 'experts'.

(2) Hydroceles, which are common in areas of Bancroftian filariasis (23.23). Treat these as usual.

(3) Lymphatic varices (uncommon). These are soft cystic swellings in his axilla, neck, or groin.

(4) Chyluria (not uncommon, 23.30), due to rupture of dilated lymphatics into his urinary tract.

Banjara BP. 'Surgery for massive lymphoedema of the legs'. The Proceedings of the Association of Surgeons of East Africa 1982;5:79-81.

de Souza LJ, 'Rarer surgical aspects of filariasis'. East African Medical Journal 1964;41:413-8.

FILARIASIS

SPECIAL TESTS. (1) The microfilariae of *W. bancrofti* are usually present in blood films taken between 10 pm and 2 am. *B. malayi* may be semiperiodic, or nonperiodic. Take fresh blood into an anticoagulant, and look for motile microfilaria under a

SOME FILARIAL LESIONS

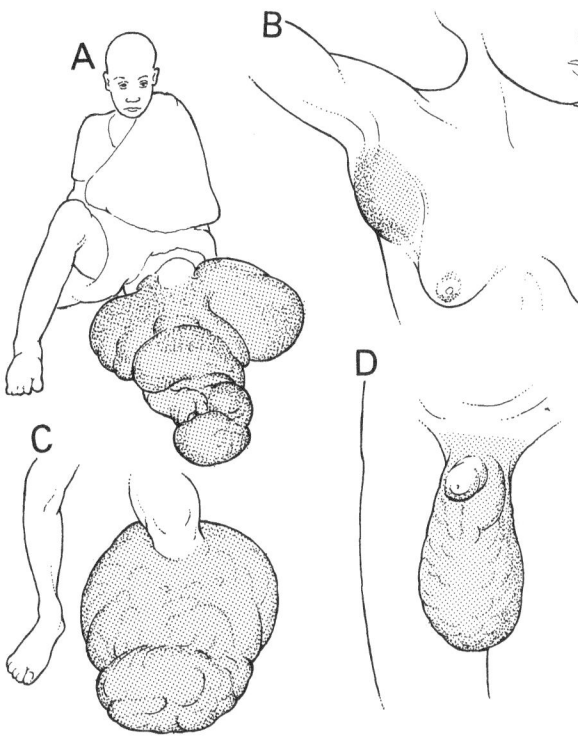

Some inguinal lesions

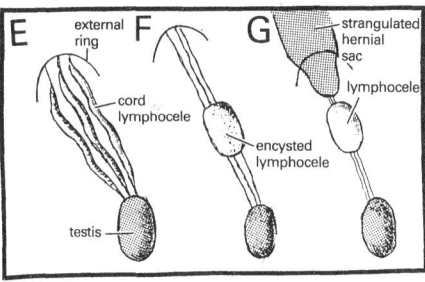

Fig. 31-5 SOME FILARIAL LESIONS A, extensive filarial involvement of the leg. After the operation she could walk without support. B, an East African woman with an axillary swelling; needle puncture showed that this was a lymphatic varix. C, this filarial mass required amputation; after the operation the patient only weighed only half as much as he did before. D, elephantiasis of the scrotum with involvement of the groin glands, but without involvement of the penis. E, a lymphocele of the cord. F, an encysted lymphocele. G, a strangulated hernia with an encysted lymphocele (rare). *After R. Mahadevan, and John Spencer, with the kind permission of the editor of 'Tropical Doctor'.*

coverslip. (2) Puncture an enlarged node, or lymphatic varix, with a needle, and look for filariae in the small volume of fluid you aspirate.

VARIOUS FILARIAL SYNDROMES

See elsewhere for hydroceles (23.23) and chyluria (23.30).

If the patient's inguinal or axillary nodes are involved (rare), treat him medically and don't operate, or a troublesome fistula discharging lymph may result.

If his spermatic cord is involved ('endemic funiculitis'), don't mistake this for a strangulated hernia (14.6), or torsion of the testis (23.24).

If he complains of a painful swelling 'like a bag of worms' above his testis, one possibility is a varicoele, and another is a lymphocele of the cord (E, Fig. 31-5). At operation you may see distended lymphatics, not distended veins.

If the swelling in his cord is like a hen's egg, it may be an hydrocele of his cord, or an encysted lymphocele (F). If gentle traction on his testis moves the swelling downwards, and makes it less mobile, it is a hydrocele. Otherwise, in an endemic area it is a lymphocele. At operation it will be connected to lymphatics in his cord. The combination of an encysted lymphocele and funiculitis may simulate a strangulated hernia closely.

If he presents as an acute abdominal emergency with inguinal pain, you may find no other pathology except inguinal adenitis, and dilated lymphatics beside his testicular vessels. Secondary infection of the lymphatics is said to lead to retroperitoneal abscesses and peritonitis.

THE LEG IN FILARIASIS

If the disease is not too advanced, reduce the lymphoedema by prolonged firm bandaging; then prevent further swelling by supporting the tissues permanently. Intermittent positive pressure methods, as with podoconiosis (31.5), reduce the oedema very effectively. A patient who could no longer walk may now be able to do so.

Alternatively, put him to bed and bandage his leg with crepe bandages from his foot upwards, using sponge rubber to protect his tissues from too tight bandaging. Remove the bandages every day, and replace them a little tighter. When you have reduced the swelling, fit a spiral elastic stocking (Dickson Wright).

If the disease is advanced, mobilize the oedema fluid by initial elastic compression, and then consider the operation below. Its benefit is said to be temporary only, although episodes of lymphangitis and cellulitis may be reduced. Afterwards his leg needs lifelong elastic compression, or the swelling will recur.

CAUTION! Diuretics, steroids, and antibiotics are useless!

CHARLES' OPERATION (modified)

INDICATIONS. Massive solid lymphoedema (elephantiasis) of the lower leg, from any cause, which has not responded to other treatments. The method which follows is for the patient shown in Fig. 31-6. If the swelling has a different distribution, modify the operation accordingly.

PREPARATION. Admit him several days beforehand, and scrub the part twice daily to get his 'mossy foot' (if he has one) really clean. Find a colleague to prepare the skin grafts while you are stripping his leg.

If both his legs are involved, operate on one leg at a time, but prepare both, in case you need to obtain grafts from the other one. Have three units of blood ready. Pass a Steinmann pin through his calcaneus, fix it to a stirrup and attach this to the ceiling light.

METHOD. Apply a tourniquet to his upper thigh. Mark the proximal limit of the excision by two lines going distally, medially, and laterally from his tibial tubercle, to form a triangle on both sides. Make the distal limit the base of his toes, but exclude the sole of his foot and his tendo Achilles.

Use a Humby knife to take long, wide partial-thickness skin grafts from the skin over the area to be excised. Keep these grafts in saline, until you apply them. Don't take grafts from fissured, or warty or eczematous skin.

Make a medial longitudinal incision from the distal incision to the base of his great toe, and deepen it to his deep fascia. Make a lateral incision to the base of his 5th toe. Raise flaps by a combination of sharp and blunt dissection on either side of the incision in the same plane. Excise the whole area of skin and subcutaneous tissue, down to the deep fascia between the incisions. Tie his long and short saphenous veins at the level of the proximal incision. Tie any other vessels as you meet them. Incise his deep fascia longitudinally in 2 or 3 places to establish communication between his muscle lymphatics, and the skin grafts.

CAUTION! (1) Leave his knee, or it may stiffen. (2) To obtain good haemostasis and prevent recurrence, excise his subcutaneous tissue completely.

Control bleeding by tying abdominal packs over his deep fascia. Release the tourniquet, and compress his leg between your hands for about 7 minutes. Gradually remove the packs, working from the distal area proximally, cauterizing or tying vessels as you meet them.

CHARLES' OPERATION

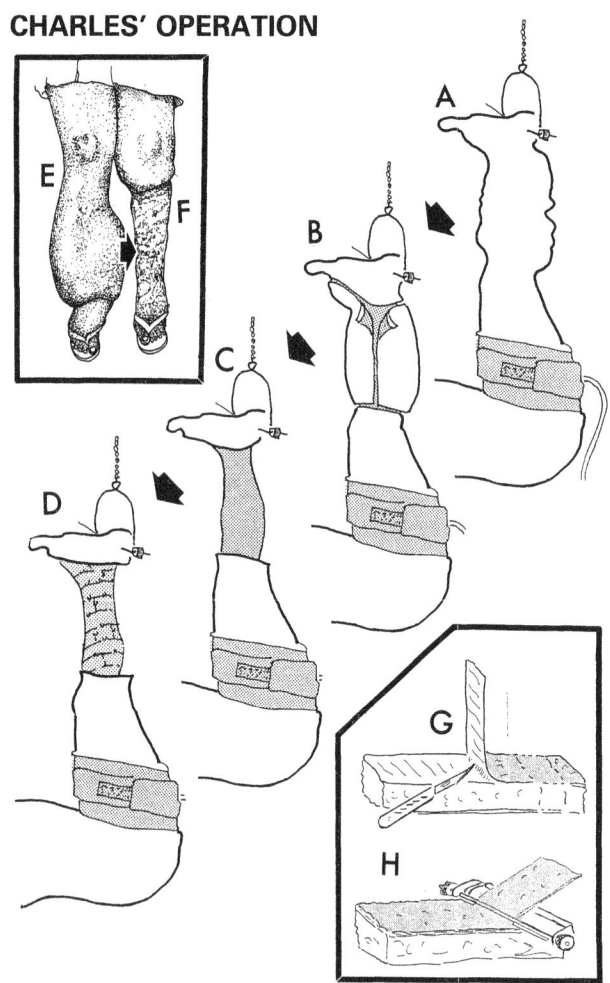

Fig. 31-6 CHARLES' OPERATION for elephantiasis. A, suspend the patient's leg and apply a tourniquet. B, incise the thickened tissue and reflect it. C, his leg ready for grafting. D, grafts sewn in place. E, both his legs originally looked like this. F, his left leg after surgery. G, using a scalpel to cut a graft from the excised tissue. H, doing the same with a Humby knife. You will probably find it easier to cut grafts while his skin is still on his leg.

Graft the raw area with split skin (57.2) taken from the elephantoid skin you have removed, where this is not too warty. You can: (1) cut very thin full-thickness skin grafts with a scalpel, keeping as close to the surface as you can. Or, (2) you can cut the excised tissue into very long slabs, and then cut grafts from these slabs with a skin-graft knife.

Lay skin grafts over the raw surface, and stitch them in place with 2/0 or 3/0 chromic catgut. There is no need to cover the whole surface: epithelium will soon grow across any small bare areas. If necessary, use mesh or patch grafts (57-6). Cover the whole area with 'Vaseline' gauze, plain gauze, and a thick layer of cotton wool secured with crepe bandages.

Keep his leg suspended from the Steinmann pin. Change the dressings on the seventh postoperative day. Where the grafts have taken, cover them only with 'Vaseline' gauze and a sterile towel. Remove the Steinmann pin at 3 weeks and allow him up. Advise him to use an elastic stocking, or bandage, for at least a year.

AMPUTATION. Don't amputate if you can avoid it (Chapter 56).

31.7 Elephantiasis of the scrotum and penis

Elephantiasis may involve: (1) the outer skin of a patient's penis (but not its inner layer or its shaft), (2) his scrotum, or (3) his testes which have hydroceles, but are otherwise normal; or, often, all three.

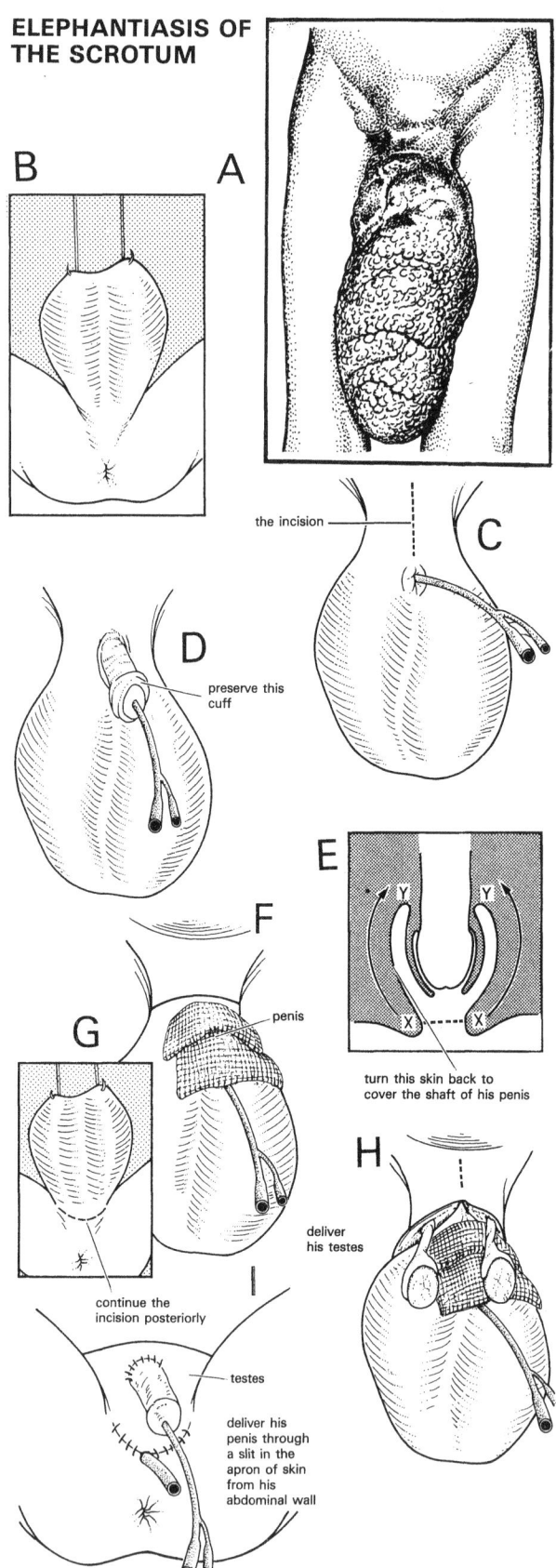

Fig 31-7 ELEPHANTIASIS OF THE SCROTUM. A, as the patient presented. B, arrangements to suspend his scrotum (optional). C, catheterization and the first incision. D, his penis delivered. E, preserving a cuff of preputial skin to cover his penis. F, his penis covered with gauze while the operation continues. G, the lateral incisions carried posteriorly. H, his testes found and delivered. I, the completed operation. *Partly after Charles Bowesman, with kind permission.*

If he has a scrotum like A, in Fig. 31-7, and you cannot refer him, you can excise it. His penis will either be buried in it, or separate, but covered with much thickened skin. This is a very satisfactory operation, and he will be immensely grateful.

ELEPHANTIASIS OF THE SCROTUM AND PENIS

THE DIFFERENTIAL DIAGNOSIS includes giant hydroceles (23.23), which may be present with elephantiasis, and hernias (14.4). In elephantiasis the texture of the skin of the patient's scrotum is altered, it pits on pressure, it cannot be moved over the deeper tissues, veins are not visible, and the mass cannot be reduced.

TREATMENT depends on the extent of his elephantiasis.

If he has elephantiasis of his prepuce (31-8, unusual), don't do a standard circumcision, or you will remove its inner normal layer. Instead, dissect off the thickened outer layer, and fold the inner one back over the shaft of his penis.

If his elephantiasis is mild and early, a limited operation may be all that is necessary. For example, you may only need to remove a dorsal strip of thickening on his penis, and close the resulting defect.

ANAESTHESIA. Subarachnoid anaesthesia (A 7.1) is suitable.

PREPARATION. Clean his skin thoroughly. You may need to put him in a hip bath of chlorhexidine. If his scrotum is enormous (A, in Fig. 31-7), either operate with him sitting and his legs over the edge of the table, or arrange a hook, and a block and tackle, in the theatre ceiling before the operation starts (B), so that you can raise it.

Control his urine temporarily with a Foley or Gibbon's catheter (C). If this is difficult to insert, you may have to wait until you have exposed his penis. You will find that a catheter, or sound, in his urethra will be useful in locating it, when you come to operate on his perineum.

Bleeding can be a problem. Don't apply a tourniquet to the base of his scrotum to control bleeding. Instead, use a long needle, such as a lumbar puncture needle, to inject his tissues with adrenalin in saline, or anaesthetic solution (A 5.4).

CAUTION ! Never use adrenalin on the subcutaneous tissues of the penis (A 5.3); you can if necessary use it in the corpora (priapism, 23.29).

INCISION. If he has large hydroceles, tap them. Make a midline incision downwards, from his pubic symphysis, to just above his prepuce (C). Carefully deepen the incision, until you reach the shaft of his penis (D). Make a circular incision around his external preputial orifice, and preserve the internal layer of his prepuce, or the cuff of skin with which his penis communicates with the exterior (E). Use it later to cover his penis. Clamp the cuff just beyond his glans, and divide his skin distal to it. Cover his raw isolated penis with saline swabs (F), while you deal with his scrotum.

Make two lateral incisions round the root of his scrotum, to meet one another posteriorly in his perineum (G). Carefully deepen these lateral incisions, until you reach his spermatic cords on each side. If necessary, trace them from his external inguinal rings. Follow his cords to his testes, and deliver them (H).

If his testes are of normal size and he has no hydroceles, don't open their tunicae vaginales.

If he has large hydroceles, you may have to drain them first (if you have not already done so). Open them, and evert their sacs and suture them behind his testis, as in Fig. 23-30. If the sacs are thick, excise part of them.

Turn his scrotum up on to his abdominal wall. Make two incisions starting 3 cm in front of his anus, and running 3 cm medial to his cruro-genital folds. His tissues are under tension, so that the incisions will open immediately. Identify, tie, and divide the many large veins that run from his scrotum. There is one large central one running up from his scrotum under his urethra. Extend these incisions to join the inguinal ones.

Remove the bulk of his scrotum with a short amputation knife. Excise all thickened oedematous tissue. Either, make him a new scrotum from the apron of normal skin that was dragged down by the mass. Or, or bury his testes in pockets, under the skin on the adductor aspects of his thighs. Push a long pair of scissors 15 cm into the subcutaneous tissues of his thighs, and open them in various directions to create a pocket with a 5 cm mouth. These pockets will be easier to make, if you stand on the opposite side of the table when you make them. You may meet, and need to tie, his superficial external pudendal vessels, and their two companion veins. Control bleeding before you insert his testes. Close the perineal part of his wound loosely, with a drain at its lowest point.

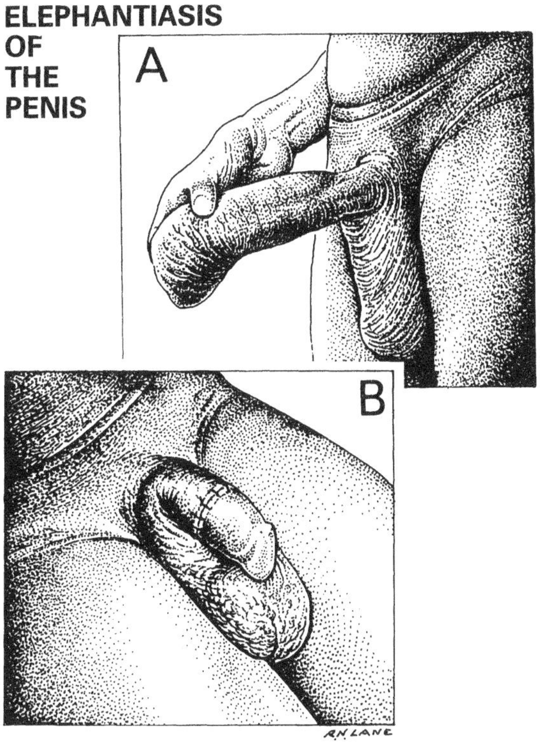

Remove the clamp from the cuff of skin that was his prepuce, trim away the part that was crushed, and roll the rest back to cover the shaft of his penis. Deliver this through a slit in the apron of skin dragged down from his abdominal wall (I). Suture this to the skin of the shaft of his penis, starting with a single central stitch, and proceeding laterally on both sides. Graft any remaining raw areas with grafts from his thigh, and dress them with vaseline gauze.

Leave his catheter in place for a few days, to prevent his urine contaminating the wound. Any redundant tissue that you may have left will probably get smaller as time passes.

ELEPHANTIASIS OF THE PENIS

Fig. 31-8 ELEPHANTIASIS OF THE PENIS. A, before the operation. The patient's scrotum was not involved. B, after a 'basal circumcision'. The skin of the inside of his prepuce has been used to cover the shaft. *After Charles Bowesman, 'Surgery and Pathology in the Tropics', E and S Livingstone, with kind permission.*

31.8 The surgical complications of typhoid fever

Although typhoid is common all over the developing world, a patient is more likely to perforate his gut in some countries than in others. In areas where perforation is common (West Africa, particularly Ghana), it is one of the commonest causes of an acute abdomen. 90% of of patients, many of them children, perforate outside hospital. Less often, you will also see the serious intestinal bleeding that typhoid can also cause.

A typhoid perforation is seldom dramatic, because loops of diseased gut stick together, so that leaking gut contents do not spread widely; sometimes the leak is small. A patient can seldom tell you the moment it happened, as he usually can when a peptic ulcer perforates. If he is already very ill, he may not even complain that his pain has got worse. When you examine him, his signs will depend on: (1) How long ago his gut perforated, and (2) how localized his peritonitis is.

You will seldom miss a typhoid perforation if: (1) You examine the abdomens of all patients with typhoid fever daily. Perforations which occur in hospital are easily missed. (2) You think of it in any patient who has acute abdominal pain, and signs of peritonitis, during a febrile illness. If he has been toxic and feverish, and moaning with abdominal pain for 2 or 3 weeks, and then suddenly complains that his pain is worse, a typhoid ulcer in his ileum has probably perforated. This usually happens in the third week, but can occur in the first week, or during convalescence.

The gut in typhoid is oedematous and friable, so that surgery is difficult. If a perforation presents insidiously, and appears to be localized, and you are inexperienced, you will be wise to 'suck and drip him', and not to operate. If, however, his perforation is dramatic, it is likely to be early, and his peritonitis generalized, so operate. If he arrives late, his chances of death are 20–30%. If he arrives early, and you can give him parenteral nutrition, and intensive care, and monitor his central venous pressure, it can be as low as 10%, or even 3%.

Alas, *S. typhi* is now chloramphenicol- and ampicillin-resistant in many areas. So adjust chemotherapy accordingly. When a typhoid ulcer perforates, many bacteria are released into the peritoneal cavity, including anaerobes. *S. typhi* is one of the least important.

When you operate, aim to do as much as is necessary and as little as possible. Remember that he has: (1) septicaemia, (2) generalized peritonitis, (3) dehydration and electrolyte imbalance, (4) immunosuppression which causes him to localise his infection badly. (5) Small gut which is thin and difficult to suture. When you have sutured it, a small leak easily becomes larger.

Bitar R, and Tarpley J, 'Intestinal perforation in typhoid fever', Reviews of Infectious Diseases 1985;7:257-271.

THE SURGERY OF TYPHOID PERFORATION AND BLEEDING

Be sure that the staff of your outpatient department watch for typhoid perforations. There must be little delay between diagnosing a perforation and closing it. A patient's prognosis will depend on the interval between the onset of his illness, and his perforation; and between this, and its closure. So operate soon, if you decide to do so.

DIAGNOSING PERFORATION. Fever and headache at the onset of the illness, are followed by vomiting, abdominal pain, and distension. When he perforates, tenderness usually starts in his right lower quadrant, spreads quickly, and eventually becomes generalized. He usually shows guarding, but seldom the board-like rigidity characteristic of a perforated peptic ulcer.

Percuss his lower ribs anteriorly; if there is gas between them and his liver, the percussion note will be resonant (due to the absence of the normal liver dullness). His bowel sounds may be absent. Hypotension, oliguria, and bradycardia are terminal signs. If possible, culture his stools, if necessary more than once.

CAUTION ! The bradycardia and leucopenia of typhoid may occasionally mask the tachycardia and leucocytosis of peritonitis.

If he reaches hospital several days after the perforation, the diagnosis will be difficult, because abdominal distension will overshadow other signs of perforation.

X-RAYS. Take an erect film, and look for gas under his diaphragm (50% positive). If he is too weak to sit up, take a lateral decubitus film, and look for it under his abdominal wall (66-4). *This is a very useful sign.* You may also see loops of his small gut dilated with gas, usually without fluid levels.

THE DIFFERENTIAL DIAGNOSIS includes appendicitis (12.1), a perforated peptic ulcer (11.2), perforations from other causes, such as spreading PID (6.6), or strangulated gut as with volvulus (10.9), and necrotizing amoebic colitis (31.11).

Suggesting appendicitis—pain starting over his umbilicus and moving to his right iliac fossa; pain precedes fever. If acute

TYPHOID FEVER

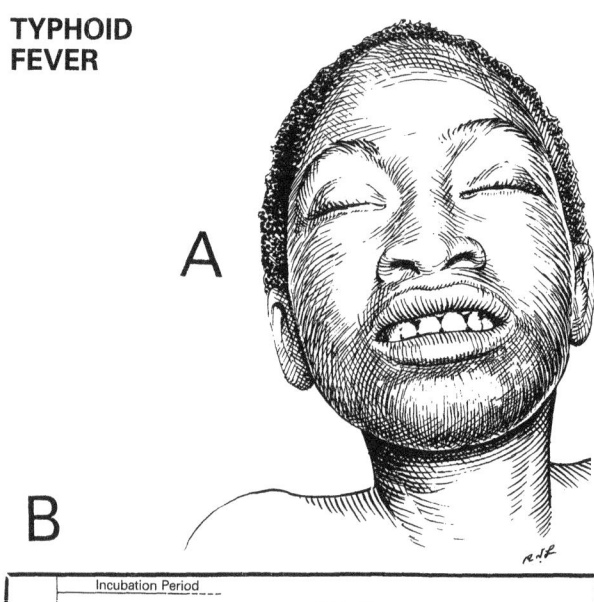

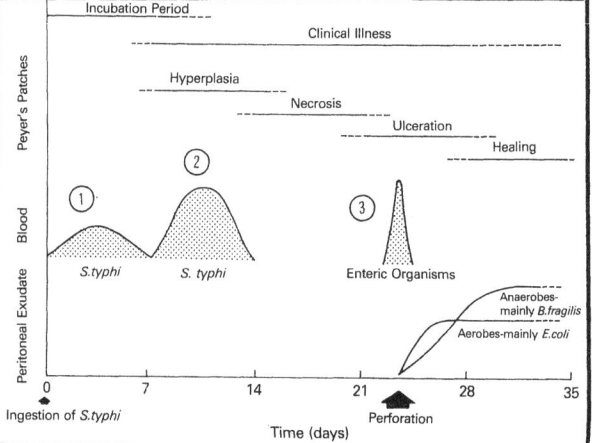

Fig. 31-9 TYPHOID FEVER. A, the characteristic appearance ('typhoid facies') of a patient with typhoid fever. B, the bacteriology of intestinal perforation in typhoid fever. Note the two phases of *S. typhi* bacteraemia (1 and 2), and the third phase of bacteraemia, with organisms from the gut, that follows perforation (3). *After Bitar and Tarpley, partly hypothetical.*

appendicitis has reached the stage of toxaemia, dehydration, and peritonitis, the differential diagnosis may be impossible before laparotomy.

Suggesting a perforated peptic ulcer—a sudden onset, and a history of ulcer symptoms.

Suggesting necrotizing amoebic colitis—a history of diarrhoea (especially with the passage of blood and mucus), followed by acute pain in his right lower quadrant, with guarding and a silent abdomen. Look for trophozoites in his stools.

MANAGEMENT. Here are some guidelines:

If he has signs of generalized peritonitis, but is not moribund (common), do a laparotomy.

If peritonitis seems to be localized (common), with signs confined to only part of his abdomen, and his general condition is good, and he is not deteriorating, consider non-operative treatment.

If he is moribund 36 to 48 hours after a perforation, with a distended or board-like abdomen, a thready pulse, and a very low blood pressure, his prognosis is hopeless.

If surgical treatment is difficult or impossible, you may have to treat him non-operatively.

If he passes melaena stools (or occasionally frank blood), replace the blood he loses. Bleeding will probably stop spontaneously. Only operate if he bleeds persistently, or alarmingly. His bleeding ulcers are in his distal ileum, but the ulcer which is bleeding may be difficult to find. If you can find it, do a limited resection. If you cannot find it, open his gut (do an enterotomy 9.3) at the level you suspect. If you still cannot find it, you may have to resect up to 60 cm of his terminal ileum, or terminal ileum and colon (hemicolectomy, 66-20).

RESUSCITATION is critical. Be prepared to rehydrate him vigorously (A 15.3). He may need 4 or more litres of intravenous fluid. Don't forget the potassium (A 15.3). If his haemoglobin is less than 80 g/l, give him blood. Monitor his urine output, and maintain his fluid balance, as in Section A 15.5. If possible monitor his central venous pressure.

CHEMOTHERAPY is needed by all patients. He needs antibiotics against *S. typhi,* and enteric Gram-negative bacilli, and anaerobes.

For *Salmonella typhi,* chloramphenicol 12.5 mg/kg 6-hourly. Usually 1 g 6-hourly, but up to 2 g 4-hourly for up to 5 days in very ill patients (12 g daily) followed by 250 mg 6-hourly for 14 days. The KCMC in Tanzania give 4 g 6-hourly (16 g daily). If possible, give some chloramphenicol intravenously initially.

Or, trimethoprim 200 mg 12 hourly. Decrease the dose if he has renal insufficiency. Trimethoprim deserves equal status with chloramphenicol as a first line drug.

Or, ampicillin, 25 mg/kg 6 hourly. Usually 2 q 6-hourly.

Or, amoxycillin, 12.5 to 25 mg/kg 6 hourly.

And, for enteric Gram-negative bacilli, gentamicin 2 mg/kg as a loading dose followed by 1.3–1.7 mg/kg 8-hourly. Decrease the dose if he has renal insufficiency.

And, for anaerobes, metronidazole 15 mg/kg or 1 g as a loading dose, followed by 7.5 mg/kg 8-hourly. Usually 500 mg 8-hourly.

NASOGASTRIC SUCTION will empty the gas from his stomach, and, hopefully, diminish the distension of his small gut. Respiratory complications, particularly the aspiration of stomach contents, before, during, or after anaesthesia are an important cause of death.

NON-OPERATIVE TREATMENT FOR A TYPHOID PERFORATION

INDICATIONS. A perforation which presents insidiously, and appears to be localized, particularly if you are inexperienced. Most cases are like this.

CONTRAINDICATIONS. A dramatic perforation, with signs of generalized peritonitis, especially if it is early. If so do a laparotomy (see below).

METHOD. Resuscitate him, give him antibiotics, and pass a nasogastric tube as above. Monitor his abdominal tenderness, and the size of his abdominal mass, if he has one. Both should get less, as in an appendix abscess (12.1). Monitor his pulse, his temperature, and his white blood count. If any of these rise, suspect that peritonitis is extending, so take an erect X-ray film of his abdomen.

If his response is favourable, taper off the above measures after a few days, and start giving him oral fluids.

Operate if: (1) There are general or local signs that his peritonitis is spreading. (2) He shows any signs of intestinal obstruction.

LAPAROTOMY FOR A PERFORATED TYPHOID ULCER

PREPARATION. Make sure he is adequately resuscitated, he has a good urine output, he has a nasogastric tube down, and is on chemotherapy.

ANAESTHESIA. (1) Ketamine, tracheal intubation, and relaxants (A 8.4). (2) General anaesthesia, intubation, and relaxants (A 14.3). (3) If necessary, use local anaesthesia (A 6.7).

INCISION. Make a median or right paramedian incision, most of it below his umbilicus. As you incise his peritoneum, there will probably be a puff of gas, confirming that some hollow viscus has perforated. Insert your hand, and gently break up any fibrinous adhesions.

Expect to find: (1) Greenish ileal contents in his peritoneal cavity. (2) The last 60 cm of his ileum bright red, and the adjacent structures somewhat less so. (3) Friable oedematous ileum. (4) In late cases particularly, dilated loops of jejunum and proximal ileum. (5) Soft, soggy mesenteric lymph nodes. Aspirate as much of his peritoneal contents as you can, and send some for culture.

Start at his ileocaecal junction, hold his gut very gently with moist laparotomy pads, and work your way proximally until you reach healthy gut, or his ileo-jejunal junction. Look for one or more *tiny* perforations in his ileum. The jejunum does not perforate in typhoid. Typhoid perforations are usually in the centre of an ulcer, on the antemesenteric border of the ileum, not far from the caecum. Put a tag on each perforation you find, until you have found them all. There is usually only one, and there are rarely more than three. You may find adhesions, which you will have to divide very gently by sharp, or if they are thin, by blunt dissection.

CAUTION ! Handle his gut with the greatest possible care—it may come apart in your hands at any moment.

If a perforation is small (<5 mm), you can: (1) Freshen its edges, by excising 1 mm of mucosa all round its circumference, and close it transversely with 2 or 3 'all coats' sutures of continuous 3/0 chromic catgut, or interrupted 3/0 silk. If you put them through only part of the gut wall, they will cut out. Invert these 'all coats' sutures with a continuous layer of Lembert seromuscular sutures. (2) Close each perforation with a full-thickness figure of eight suture of 3/0 catgut, or 'Dexon', through all layers. If you wish, insert a second figure of eight suture to reinforce the first. (3) Insert an ileostomy tube (or a Foley catheter) through the perforation, tide him over the acute stage, and reoperate later to close the perforation.

If he has multiple perforations, or a large perforation with diseased gut, you have four choices:

(1) You can oversew each perforation or potentially leaky area, as described above. If he is desperately ill, he will probably not tolerate anything more than this.

(2) You can do an ileotransverse colostomy, with a mucous fistula, and repair this later (9.3, 29.7).

(3) If he is relatively fit, with a severely diseased segment of gut, or if there is alarming bleeding, you can resect the diseased segment, and do an end to end anastomosis, as in Fig. 9-9. Avoid resection if you can. His generalized peritonitis, and the friability of his gut, will make this difficult.

(4) You can exteriorize the diseased segment of his gut, as in Fig. 9-13. If he is very ill, and you think he needs something more than simple oversewing of his perforation, this will be simple and relatively atraumatic for him, and is unlikely to cause much bleeding. But his postoperative management will be difficult.

If he presents late, with a localized collection of pus (rare), drain it locally; this is not urgent.

DEALING WITH THE PERITONITIS depends on what you find.

If peritonitis is localized, do a local toilet only, and avoid spreading the infection to the rest of his peritoneal cavity. Had you known this earlier, you would probably have decided not to operate.

If peritonitis is generalized, wash out his entire peritoneal cavity with several litres of saline. Pour in a litre of warm saline, slosh it around with your hands, and then aspirate it. Repeat this three or four times. Add a gram of chloramphenicol or tetracycline to the last litre (6.2).

CLOSE HIS ABDOMEN completely without drains.

CAUTION ! Be quite sure to pack his skin and subcutaneous tissues open for secondary closure later (9.8).

POSTOPERATIVELY. He will have been ill for days, or sometimes up to 3 weeks, before surgery, and his preoperative metabolic abnormalities will still be imperfectly corrected. Manage him as for other kinds of peritonitis (6.2). Monitor him daily for the early detection of collections of intra-abdominal pus. Continue intravenous chloramphenicol at ordinary, rather than high, doses for two weeks. This will help to combat his typhoid, but not necessarily his peritonitis. Fever usually subsides in 4 or 5 days. Attend to other manifestations of the disease, and nourish him as early, and as well as the clinical situation and the available technology will allow (9.11, 58.11).

DIFFICULTIES WITH A TYPHOID PERFORATION

Be prepared for wound sepsis (9.12), a burst abdomen (9.13), intestinal obstruction (10.13), intra-abdominal abscesses (6.3), fistulae (very serious, 9.14), anaemia and many weeks of inadequate nutrition and hospitalization, and particularly for respiratory complications (9.11). Finally, he may get an incisional hernia (14.13).

If you DON'T FIND A PERFORATION, there may not be one, and his peritonitis may be primary (haematogenous), or from some other cause. It is doubtful if typhoid ever causes peritonitis without perforation, but primary peritonitis without an established cause is common in Africa.

If he has SEVERE DIARRHOEA about the 4th day, it will be very difficult to treat, and may kill him. Replace his fluid loss energetically, and don't forget the potassium (A 15.5).

If he has RENEWED PAIN, and deteriorates postoperatively, suspect that he has had another perforation.

If he has a sudden spike of FEVER after about 5 days, when he should have recovered from his typhoid, and it is not malaria, suspect wound infection (9.12), a subphrenic abscess (6.4), pneumonia, or a faecal fistula (9.14).

31.9 Pigbel disease, necrotizing enteritis, necrotizing jejunitis, enteritis necroticans

Like typhoid fever, pigbel is much more common in the tropics, but is occasionally seen elsewhere. It is due to the beta toxins of types B and C *Clostridium perfringens,* which multiply in the gut following a large meal, classically a feast of pork. This gives the disease its New Guinea name 'Pigbel', where it was at one time the commonest condition requiring laparotomy. If you have to resect gut, a patient's chances of death are about 50%.

He is usually a child, or a young adult, who presents with: (1) Acute toxic shock. (2) Severe colicky abdominal pain and vomiting. (3) Constipation with foul flatus, followed by bloody diarrhoea. (4) Vomiting, diarrhoea, and abdominal pain; the diarrhoea stops, but vomiting continues, and his abdomen distends. (5) An obscure abdominal illness, ending in a pelvic abscess that is the result of a perforation. (6) Rectal bleeding (22.3).

Typically, his abdomen distends and is tender all over, sometimes with a soft mass above his umbilicus. He is ill and may have a high fever.

PIGBEL

X-RAYS in the erect position show that the patient has multiple fluid levels, with gas in his large gut down to his rectum.

SPECIAL TESTS. He has a leucocytosis (unlike the leucopenia of typhoid). An abdominal tap may reveal bloody peritoneal fluid (66-3).

DIFFERENTIAL DIAGNOSIS. The presence of a mass and bloody stools may lead you to suspect intussusception (10.8).

NON-OPERATIVE TREATMENT often succeeds. Resuscitate him. Pass a nasogastric tube and give him large doses of penicillin.

INDICATIONS FOR LAPAROTOMY. (1) Failure to improve, or deterioration on non-operative treatment. (2) Signs of peritonitis, and persistently large volumes of gastric aspirate.

LAPAROTOMY. You may see the disease at any stage in its development. It usually only involves his small gut, but it may involve his distal stomach, or his large gut.

Classically, several loops of his small gut, from near his duodenal flexure onwards, are acutely inflamed, oedematous, and congested, often with localized necrotic areas mostly on the antemesenteric border, with a sharp line of demarcation between normal and diseased areas. There may be perforations, localized abscesses, and multiple adhesions causing partial obstruction. The necrotic areas are usually separate, but may occasionally extend from his distal stomach to his sigmoid colon. His mesenteric artery is patent, and you can feel pulsation down to the terminal arterioles at the margin of the affected gut. His regional nodes are enlarged, and may be necrotic.

If any gut is non-viable (9.3), resect it with an adequate margin of healthy gut, so that the blood supply to the area of the anastomosis is adequate. Drain abscesses. If you have removed a considerable length of his small gut, follow him up carefully, and treat any small-gut deficiency that he may develop.

If you decide to leave inflamed but not obviously necrotic gut, and he later deteriorates, do a second laparotomy, and resect any gangrenous gut.

31.10 The surgery of intestinal amoebiasis

Amoebiasis is usually a 'medical' disease, but it does have some surgical complications, ranging from the very acute to the very chronic, which you should be able to treat. They usually involve a patient's gut, but they can involve his liver (31.12), or occasionally his lungs, or even his skin. Amoebiasis is more common in older patients, but no age is immune, and amoebae may invade the gut of babies. It is less often seen in women, but in pregnancy it can be fulminating.

Entamoeba histolytica normally lives harmlessly in the colon, but trophozoites occasionally invade its mucosa to cause shallow discrete circular or oval ulcers, with yellow sloughs in their bases, and sometimes red edges. These ulcers are most common in the caecum and ascending colon, the sigmoid colon, and the rectum. They cause diarrhoea, with or without blood, pus, and mucus.

The lesions in the gut are usually quite superficial, but, if a patient's resistance is low, amoebae may invade it more deeply, especially if he is diabetic, or alcoholic, or has recently been severely injured. Invasive intestinal amoebiasis takes several acute forms: (1) Amoebae can cause massive necrosis of the mucosa of his colon, so that large pieces of it separate as casts, and are passed rectally. (2) They can invade its muscular wall to cause gangrene, sloughing, and perforation—acute necrotizing amoebic colitis. Bacterial infection may then spread as generalized peritonitis, or it may remain localized as a pericolic abscess which you can feel as a tender mass. He can also develop peritonitis, without actual perforation, or his gut can perforate extraperitoneally. As the result of this suppuration, it may obstruct, or he may develop ileus. Occasionally, his colon bleeds severely.

If the pathological process is more chronic, he may have: (1) An amoeboma; this is a diffuse, oedematous, hyperplastic granulomatous swelling anywhere in his colon or rectum, which is often multiple, and may be palpable, and may obstruct his gut (usually temporarily). Although an amoeboma may form anywhere, a mass in the caecum is more easily palpable. If you do feel a mass in a patient with amoebiasis, it is more likely to be a paracolic abscess than an amoeboma. (2) A fibrous postamoebic stricture, which is one of the end results of an amoeboma. An amoeboma and a stricture are two stages in the same process, and he may have a lesion with some of the features of both. Both are common in some areas (Durban), and are the late, chronic complications of amoebic colitis; they occur years after the initial bloody diarrhoea, and are less serious than acute invasive amoebiasis. They usually involve the rectum (where you can feel them rectally), the sigmoid, and the descending colon, in that order. Both can: (1) cause diarrhoea and other abdominal symptoms, and (2) obstruct the large gut, usually incompletely.

AMOEBIASIS

CHEMOTHERAPY. Some drugs act on amoebae in the gut, some on amoebae in the tissues, and some on both. The patient will need drugs to treat both. So, if necessary, give him him more than one drug.

If he is very ill, and amoebae have spread beyond his gut, give him metronidazole, and either dehydroemetine (or emetine), or chloroquine, or both. Emetine is the most potent tissue amoebicide.

(1) Metronidazole (a tissue and lumenal amoebicide) 400 to 800 mg by mouth 8-hourly for 7 to 10 days. Children 10 to 15 mg/kg 8-hourly. If possible, also give him an infusion of 500 mg as a 0.5% solution over 8 hours.

(2) Dehydroemetine (a tissue amoebicide) 1.25 mg/kg/day, maximum dose 90 mg, by intramuscular injection for a maximum of 10 days. Don't repeat the course before 28 days. Or,

INVASIVE AMOEBIASIS

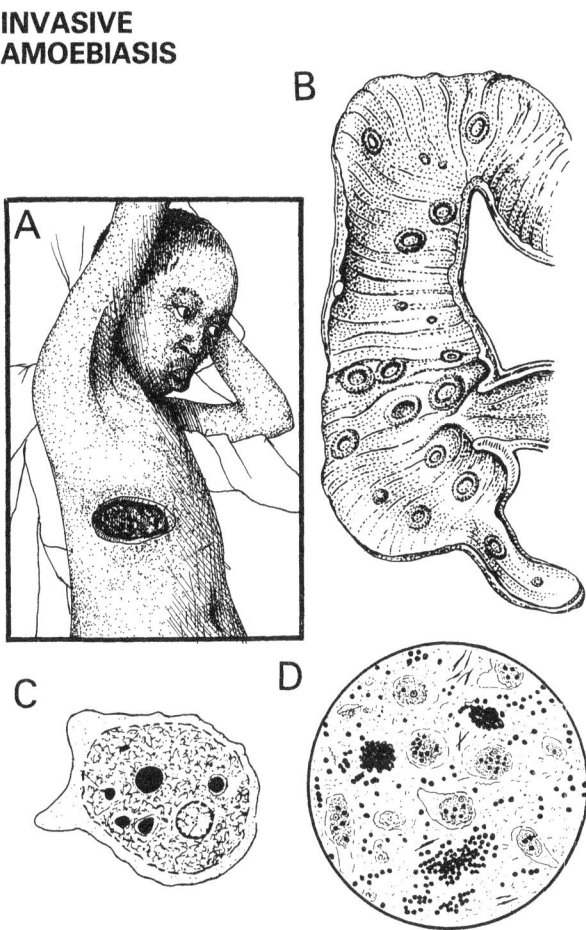

Fig. 31-10 INVASIVE AMOEBIASIS. A, an amoeboma of the skin secondary to a liver abscess. B, the caecum and ascending colon with amoebic ulcers. C, *Entamoeba histolytica*. D, an amoebic stool with trophozoites, red cells, and Charcot Leyden crystals. *A, after Charles Bowesman, 'Surgery and Clinical Pathology in the Tropics', E and S Livingstone. With kind permission.*

less satisfactorily, give him emetine in the same way, 1 mg/kg, maximum 60 mg.

(3) Chloroquine (a tissue amoebicide) 150 mg of chloroquine base 4 times daily for 2 days, followed by 150 mg twice daily for 19 days. Children 10/mg/kg/day.

(4) Tetracycline (active against associated bacteria) 500 mg 4 times daily for 5 days (only effective for intestinal amoebiasis).

(5) Diloxanide furoate ('Furamide', 'Entamide furoate', a lumenal amoebicide) 500 mg 8-hourly for 10 days. Children 20 mg/kg 8-hourly.

If you are treating invasive intestinal disease with drugs other than metronidazole or emetine, give him a 2-week course of chloroquine to prevent the development of hepatic lesions.

CAUTION ! The side-effects of emetine include nausea, diarrhoea, weakness, moderate hypotension, and alteration of the ECG. Serious cardiac effects are uncommon. Emetine is contraindicated in heart disease. Patients receiving emetine must stay in bed (they are usually so sick that they are happy to).

A SUMMARY OF TREATMENT METHODS for amoebiasis and its complications:

Amoebic dysentery without complications: metronidazole.

Amoebic liver abscess: metronidazole and dehydroemetine, or metronidazole and chloroquin, if he is seriously ill; aspiration or open drainage on the indications below.

Severe colitis wih perforation or suspected perforation: metronidazole, ±dehydroemetine, with tetracycline against secondary invaders. 'Drip and suck' him.

Spreading peritonitis: drugs, laparotomy and lavage.
Pericarditis (rare): drugs, aspiration and drainage.
Lung abscess (rare): drugs and postural drainage.

31.11 Invasive intestinal amoebiasis

If amoebae are invading the wall of a patient's gut, the danger is that it may perforate. If you can make the diagnosis before it has done so, metronidazole will probably cure him. When his gut has perforated, treatment is much more difficult. There are three forms of perforation: (1) An extraperitoneal ('sealed') perforation. (2) The perforation of an amoeboma, or an amoebic ulcer, into the peritoneal cavity, in the absence of acute dysentery. (3) A similar perforation in the presence of acute dysentery (this is rare in patients on metronidazole).

He usually presents as an 'acute abdomen', but diagnosing that invasive amoebiasis is causing it is difficult, before laparotomy. Typically, he has abdominal pain, fever, diarrhoea, and pain in the right iliac fossa. Often, there is a history of diabetes, alcoholism, pregnancy, or trauma. When you examine him, you find a mass in his right iliac fossa, or rigidity masking its presence, and often a distended abdomen.

If amoebiasis is common in your area, maintain a high level of suspicion. It is better to start treatment on suspicion, than to miss a treatable disease. If possible, treat him non-operatively. Avoid surgery if you can, because his colon will be friable and difficult to suture. Fortunately, surgery is usually unnecessary, because the perforation will probably have been localized by his diseased colon sticking to his surrounding small gut and omentum.

If however his perforation is not sealing off, you may have to operate, even if he is a bad risk. If you leave him, he is sure to die, whereas an operation may save him.

At laparotomy you may find: (1) A large inflammatory mass in the region of his caecum. This is more likely to be a paracolic abscess than an amoeboma. (2) Greyish patches in his caecum. (4) Multiple and often adjacent perforations, most commonly in his caecum and sigmoid colon. (5) Inflammatory lesions elsewhere in his large gut.

If he is very ill, the less surgery you do, the better. Repairing a perforation is difficult, because his whole colon is usually affected, very friable and adherent to other organs. But, if his gut has perforated, you must divert his faecal stream somehow. Resection and exteriorization are bloody and shock-producing, but they do relieve obstruction, and they remove the focus of infection. A bypass is better tolerated. Exteriorization is probably the easiest operation. Whatever you do, the danger is that his caecum will burst and flood his peritoneum with faeces.

Avoid these mistakes: (1) Don't attempt a right hemicolectomy, which is more difficult, and is said to be more dangerous. (2) Don't try to oversew a perforation—a necrotic colon will not hold sutures.

SAROJ (45 years) was admitted with a history of fever, bloody diarrhoea, abdominal pain, and a tender right suprapubic mass. Scrapings from typical amoebic ulcers in her rectum showed trophozoites. After only two days treatment with metronidazole, she felt better, her diarrhoea improved, and her abdominal mass staarted to resolve.

MIRANDA (46) had fever, diarrhoea, and vague abdominal pain for several weeks, worse during the last few days. She had a tender indurated mass in her right lower quadrant. At laparotomy, she had acute necrotizing colitis of her caecum, with multiple perforations, and much sloughing tissue. After a right hemicolectomy, she recovered slowly. LESSONS (1) Patients often respond to metronidazole rapidly. (2) When surgery is indicated, it is difficult.

Eggleston FC, Vergese M, Handa AK, 'Amoebic perforation of the bowel: diagnosis and management'. Tropical Doctor 1980;4:160-167.

INVASIVE INTESTINAL AMOEBIASIS

For chemotherapy and a summary of treatment methods, see Section 31.10.

SPECIAL TESTS. Examine the patient's warm stools for trophozoites, and look for amoebic ulcers with a sigmoidoscope. Take a scraping and examine it for amoebae. Take a biopsy of the adjacent mucosa and send it for histology. Look for the cysts of *E. histolytica* in his stools. Only some strains are invasive, but unfortunately it takes a sophisticated laboratory to tell which ones.

CAUTION ! You will not always find amoebae, *so don't be misled by a negative finding.*

THE DIFFERENTIAL DIAGNOSIS includes:

Suggesting a typhoid perforation—a 2-week history of fever and vague abdominal pain, which becomes acute when his gut perforates; intestinal bleeding is uncommon.

Suggesting ileocaecal tuberculosis—he is usually (but not always) less sick than with amoebiasis (unless tuberculosis is obstructing his gut). The mass in his right lower quadrant is not so large, or tender (unless it has perforated). The course of the disease is usually more chronic.

Suggesting an appendix abscess (uncommon in in the developing world)—pain which starts centrally and then moves to his right lower quadrant; no history of diarrhoea, especially no bloody diarrhoea; he is less toxic, and not so sick as with amoebiasis. The distinction is not important, because both need a laparotomy.

Suggesting carcinoma of the caecum (rare in the developing world)—he is not so ill, or so toxic, and he may have rectal bleeding. The mass is firm to hard, but not particularly tender. Subacute obstruction is more common.

NON-OPERATIVE TREATMENT FOR INVASIVE AMOEBIASIS

INDICATIONS. Manage him non-operatively if you can. (1) An amoebic perforation of his large gut, producing localized peritonitis, as indicated by a mass. (2) A critically ill patient with prolonged fever, diarrhoea, toxaemia, and peritonitis, who may need surgery later, if he is fit enough. (3) Acute toxic dilatation of the colon (see below).

METHOD. Correct his dehydration, hypovolaemia, and oliguria, and especially his hypokalaemia (A 15.3). Chronic diarrhoea can cause severe potassium deficiency (resulting in confusion, weakness, hypotension, and ileus) which you can correct simply, and dramatically improve his 'toxic' state. If he has lost much blood, replace it. Give him intravenous metronidazole 800 mg 8-hourly, and chloramphenicol (2.9). If you don't have intravenous metronidazole, give him 1 g rectally 8-hourly (2.9). For more details on chemotherapy, see Section 31.10.

Apply nasogastric suction to minimize distension from obstruction, or ileus. Monitor his blood pressure, his pulse, and his hourly urine output.

Mark the outline of the mass on his skin, before you start treatment. Note how tender and indurated it is. Thereafter, *examine it 8-hourly.* If it increases in size, or becomes more tender, or there is more guarding, prepare to operate—peritonitis is spreading. Fortunately, this is uncommon once therapy has started.

LAPAROTOMY FOR INVASIVE AMOEBIASIS

INDICATIONS. (1)Frank peritonitis. (2) The failure of non-operative treatment (see above).

PREPARATION. Resuscitate him thoroughly, and follow all the steps described above for non-operative treatment—this is critical.

ANAESTHESIA. (1) General anaesthesia with relaxants (A 10.1). (2) Ketamine, intubation, and relaxants (A 8.1). When he is anaesthetized, and his muscles are relaxed, examine his abdomen again, and sigmoidoscope him. This may confirm the diagnosis, and determine if his sigmoid colon is disease free. If it is, you may be able to divert his faecal stream into it (see below).

EXPLORATION. Make a median or right paramedian incision. Open his peritoneal cavity, and examine it as for peritonitis (6.2). Gently feel for a mass.

If there are greenish-grey, gangrenous patches on his soggy, soft caecum, your diagnosis of invasive amoebiasis was correct. It may fall apart and leak as you touch it. If his whole colon looks oedematous and inflamed, this may also be invasive amoebiasis, but in an earlier stage.

If he has extensive caecal amoebiasis, management depends on the condition of the rest of his colon. The first three procedures are comparatively safe, because you don't have to manipulate his precarious caecum. The fourth is less so.

(1) If the rest of his large gut looks normal (unusual), **you can divide his terminal ileum about 25 cm from his ileocaecal valve, and anastomose its proximal end to the side of his transverse colon (9-11).** Close the distal cut end of his ileum in two layers, and push it back into his abdomen. If he survives, the continuity of his gut can be re-established later.

(2) If his transverse colon is diseased but his sigmoid is spared (unusual), **do an ileosigmoid anastomosis.**

(3) If his sigmoid is also diseased, **do an ileostomy.**

(4) If the necrotic patches are confined to his caecum, and the ascending and proximal parts of his transverse colon, but do not go beyond it, **exteriorize them as described below.**

If his large gut has ruptured extraperitoneally (unusual), drain it through stab wound incisions in his flanks, and introduce large catheters into it.

If you find generalized peritonitis, with no obvious local lesion, lavage his peritoneum thoroughly and instil tetracycline 1 g in 1000 ml (6.2). Close his wound, and rely on metronidazole and antibiotics to cure him. Some surgeons say they can always find a lesion.

If his whole colon shows necrotic patches, which look as if they are about to perforate, do an ileostomy. Or, drain his colon widely, close the wound, and rely on metronidazole and antibiotics.

If distension is excessive, decompress his small gut at the time of the anastomosis.

You will not have removed his infected caecum (except in (4) above), so insert drains through stab wounds on the right side of his abdominal wall down to and, if necessary, even into his caecum itself.

EXTERIORIZATION is easier than some of the above procedures. Do it as in Section 66.11 on large gut injury. Free his diseased proximal large gut, and lift it out of the wound with his terminal ileum. 'Double-barrel' his healthy ileum and the left half of his transverse colon with about 10 interrupted sutures (D, 9-19). Irrigate his peritoneal cavity, and close his wound, with the two sutured loops of gut coming out of its upper end. Cut off the diseased gut about 3 cm above the surface of his skin.

CAUTION ! Try to minimize the contamination of his peritoneal cavity as you do this, pack it off where you can. (2) Irrigate it before you close it. (3) Insert drains in his right subhepatic space and his right iliac fossa.

He will need to wear an ileostomy bag (9.5). If he recovers from his acute disease, the continuity of his gut can be restored in 5 to 7 weeks.

DIFFICULTIES WITH INTESTINAL AMOEBIASIS

If he has a MASS in his large gut, don't forget the possibility of an AMOEBOMA. This usually responds rapidly to metronidazole and antibiotics, sometimes in only a few days.

If he has a STRICTURE, remember the possibility of postamoebic fibrosis. You may need to dilate it with your finger, or through a sigmoidoscope.

Because amoebomas and postamoebic strictures are so rare in some areas, the danger is that you may think that he has a carcinoma. If you are in any doubt, try metronidazole, and, if possible, take a biopsy.

If you find a regular, firm, SAUSAGE-SHAPED MASS in his large gut, remember the possibility of intussusception (10.8). You may find that it has ulcerated, but the ulcers are unlikely to be amoebic.

If his AMOEBIASIS IS PARTICULARLY SEVERE, he may have ACUTE TOXIC DILATATION OF THE COLON (a similar condition is seen in ulcerative colitis). This is diagnosable radiologically, and may simulate a perforation. Treat him non-operatively.

If he BLEEDS SEVERELY FROM HIS COLON, this may be fatal, because it may look normal externally, so that you will not know where the blood is coming from. See Section 22.3.

31.12 Extraintestinal amoebiasis

When *Entamoeba histolytica* spreads outside a patient's gut, it usually involves his liver. Here it can cause an 'abscess' filled with liquid necrotic liver. To start with this is yellow or yellow-green, later it becomes a syrupy dark reddish-yellow ('anchovy sauce'). The central area of necrosis is surrounded by zones of progressively less damaged tissue and amoebae. The term amoebic liver 'abscess' is a bad one, because there is no pus.

His main symptom is gradually increasing pain in his right hypochondrium, or epigastrium. There is an 80% chance that his abscess is in the right lobe of his liver, where you will be able to detect it clinically, unless it is very deep.

Provided that there are no complications, metronidazole usually treats an uncomplicated liver 'abscess' very effectively, but if it does not, you will have to aspirate it or, rarely, to drain it. The major risk is that it will suddenly rupture into his peritoneal cavity, or through his diaphragm into his lung or pericardium. Rupture into the peritoneal cavity is a dramatic catastrophe, with collapse and peritonitis, like the perforation of a peptic ulcer. Although the contents of an abscess are sterile, they cause an acute inflammatory reaction in the peritoneum. Sometimes, an 'abscess' leaks into the peritoneum slowly, which makes the diagnosis more difficult.

The common mistakes are: (1) Not to do a sigmoidoscopy, or not to recognize amoebic ulcers when you do see them. (2) Not to remember the existence of acute necrotizing amoebic colitis with perforation. (3) Not to use all the evidence you can to diagnose a liver abscess.

EXTRAINTESTINAL AMOEBIASIS

LIVER ABSCESS

CLINICAL FEATURES. The patient is usually male (8:1 chance), and may be a child. In endemic areas (Durban) amoebic 'abscesses' are not uncommon in babies.

The pain in his right upper quadrant, or his lower right chest, is constant, not colicky, and does not radiate. It slowly gets worse, and is seldom severe. If it is in his chest, deep breathing and coughing make it worse.

Fever, anorexia, weakness, and loss of weight steadily progress. There is only a 30% chance that he has had diarrhoea with blood and mucus during the previous year. Often, he has some associated disease, such as tuberculosis, malnutrition, or alcoholism.

His liver is tender, smooth, diffusely enlarged, and without an obvious lump. Palpation may cause him much distress. Pressure over his lower 5 ribs in his right anterior axillary line is painful. Examine also for dullness at his right base, and decreased breath sounds.

SPECIAL TESTS. Leucocytosis (90% chance). Anaemia (haemoglobin <100 g/l, 50%). Raised ESR. Raised serum alkaline phosphatase (50%). Look for amoebic ulcers with a sigmoidoscope (20%). You are unlikely to find amoebae in his stools.

X-RAYS. Look for a pleural effusion, and elevation of the right dome of his diaphragm (80%).

THE DIFFERENTIAL DIAGNOSIS includes a hepatoma, cholecystitis, a hydatid cyst, and a pyogenic liver abscess.

Suggesting a hepatoma (32.26)—a hard nodular mass, liver less painful and less tender, no fever or low fever (fever only occurs with very rapidly growing tumours), a bruit, bloody ascites.

Suggesting cholecystitis, perhaps with spreading suppuration (13.3)—the patient more often female, pain is colicky, tenderness is localized to the gall-bladder region, there may be a history of intolerance to greasy foods, jaundice.

Suggesting a hydatid cyst (31.13)—the mass arises from one or other lobe, rather than enlarging it diffusely; it grows slowly and is largely asymptomatic; it is smooth, tense, and cystic; tenderness is minimal, there is no fever, and his general condition is good. All this may change rapidly, if it becomes infected.

Suggesting a pyogenic liver abscess—a short history; he is severely ill and has a spiking fever.

Suggesting a perinephric abscess (5.11a)—the swelling is low down over his liver on the right; the distinction may be very difficult. Aspiration may establish the site.

CHEMOTHERAPY. See Section 31.10. If he is very ill, give him metronidazole and dehydroemetine (or emetine).

LIVER ASPIRATION FOR AMOEBIC ABSCESS

INDICATIONS. (1) To confirm the diagnosis, if, for example, his response to metronidazole has been poor. (2) As a method of treatment when an abscess is very large, or might burst. Aspiration is only necessary in about 20% of cases. Your chances of finding 'pus' are about 80%. You will fail if it is very deep.

METHOD. Using local anaesthesia and full aseptic precautions, pass a *wide-bore (>1 mm)* spinal needle on a 50 ml syringe, through healthy skin, over the site of greatest swelling, or maximum tenderness. Or, if there is no swelling, insert it in his 9th intercostal space in his mid axillary line. Push it in to a depth of not more than 8 cm.

If you don't find 'pus' on your first attempt, insert it in a slightly different direction. The pus may be thick and aspiration difficult, or you may withdraw several litres with ease. Don't inject any drugs.

If you obtain more than 250 ml, repeat the aspiration a few days later. You have only about a 10% chance of finding amoebae in the pus. They are more often found in the wall of the cavity.

OPEN DRAINAGE FOR AMOEBIC LIVER ABSCESSES

INDICATIONS. This is rarely necessary if you have given him metronidazole, and aspirated his abscess adequately. (1) You think he has a deep-seated amoebic liver abscess, but have not proved it, and he is deteriorating on medical treatment. (2) The pus is too thick to aspirate. (3) Very large abscesses, which need repeated aspiration. (4) An abscess in the left lobe which may perforate into his pericardium. (5) Secondary infection of the abscess. (6) The diagnosis is uncertain; you think he may have a hydatid cyst, which might rupture and cause a possibly fatal anaphylactic shock, if you tried to aspirate it through his abdominal wall. (7) In an emergency, after an abscess has ruptured into his peritoneal cavity.

DRAINAGE. Make a subcostal incision, and insert an aspirating needle directly into the abscess cavity, to identify it. Push artery forceps into it, open them and suck out the pus. Take some material from the advancing edge of the lesion, and examine a warm wet specimen for amoebae.

A drain may not be necessary, but if there is much discharge, insert a tube drain, and bring this out through his abdominal wall.

If his abscess is very large, his liver will recede from his abdominal wall as you drain it, and end up as a shrunken blob, in his right upper abdomen, 20 cm from the incision through which the drain will go. To prevent gut sticking to the drain, cover it with omentum.

Remove the drain soon, probably in 6 or 7 days, to minimize the risk of secondary infection from outside. Meanwhile, continue chemotherapy.

IF YOU HAVE ULTRASOUND with which to localize the abscess, introduce a multiholed plastic catheter with a three way tap, and aspirate it, until it is apparently empty. Every few days, introduce a suitable contrast medium through the tube, take a film to outline the cavity, and aspirate it empty. Consider injecting an amoebicide. Continue until the cavity is empty and then remove the tube.

DIFFICULTIES WITH EXTRAINTESTINAL AMOEBIASIS

If he has a SUDDEN PAIN like a perforated peptic ulcer, his abscess has probably ruptured into his peritoneal cavity. Resuscitate him, and start intensive amoebicidal treatment. When his general state is satisfactory, open his abdomen.

Make an upper right paramedian or Kocher's incision. Explore his liver, as best you can, and look for the site of the rupture—a ragged area with chocolate-coloured fluid pouring from it. Suck out as much of this you can. Mop up what you cannot aspirate. Irrigate all the crevices of his peritoneum with several litres of warm saline with tetracycline (6.2). Slosh it around and suck it out. Do a thorough lavage, and close his abdomen. Close the main incision with tension sutures. Continue metronidazole, and treat his peritonitis with nasogastric suction, etc. (6.2).

If he has TENDER ILL-DEFINED MASSES IN STRANGE PLACES, suspect that his abscess has leaked into his peritoneal cavity. Give him intensive medical treatment, and monitor his abdomen closely. Mark the outline of any mass, and check its size regularly.

If an ABSCESS PRESENTS ON HIS CHEST WALL, it will ultimately rupture through his skin, which may become infected with amoebae, and form a chronic ulcer as in A, Fig. 31-10. He should respond to metronidazole.

If he has an ULCERATING SKIN LESION round a sinus from his liver, caecum, or anus, remember the possibility of CUTANEOUS AMOEBIASIS. Metronidazole cures cutaneous amoebiasis so fast, that you can use it as a diagnostic test. Tuberculosis, malignancy, and fungi are commoner causes in most areas. In the perianal area ulcerating skin lesions are usually non-specific.

If he develops a SEVERE COUGH AND DYSPNOEA, this may, or may not, mean that he has a pleural effusion. If an effusion is small, it will resolve as his liver abscess improves. If it is large (unusual), aspirate it. If necessary, insert a tube drain, connected to an underwater seal or suction bottle. His liver sticks to his diaphragm and his lung, so he is more likely to cough up amoebic pus (see below), than for pus to enter his pleural cavity.

If he COUGHS UP 'ANCHOVY SAUCE', his liver abscess has ruptured into a bronchus. Although this may drain the abscess, it may also flood his bronchial tree and kill him. X-ray his chest; the appearances are characteristic, with pus tracking in his greater fissure. Give him metronidazole, aspirate his liver abscess, and use postural drainage.

If his liver abscess DISCHARGES INTO HIS PERICARDIUM it usually does so from an abscess in his left lobe. Pericardial rupture is not uncommon in endemic areas, is often not recognized, and is usually fatal. Watch for abscesses in the left lobe, and aspirate them (6.1a).

If his ABSCESS BECOMES SECONDARILY INFECTED, one reason may be that you punctured his transverse colon on your way to his liver.

31.13 Hydatid disease

Echinococcus granulosus normally cycles between the dog and the sheep, and occasionally between other animals. Man is infested in the same way as the sheep—by ingesting a dog's faeces. Hydatid disease is widespread in many countries; Turkana, a remote area of north-west Kenya has the highest prevalence, with about 8% of the population infected. Programmes to control hydatid infection have been among the most successful measures for the control of infectious disease.

If hydatid disease is endemic in your area, you may find hydatid cysts in a patient's liver (80%), spleen (7%) or the other parts of his abdomen (14%), or occasionally in his lungs, brain, or kidneys, or indeed almost anywhere. If he has a peripheral cyst, expect that he has at least one in his liver too. You will be able to operate on cysts in his abdomen, but not those in his brain or lungs.

If he is from an endemic area and has a tense, almost painless, long-standing (years), smooth, rubbery, mobile cyst in his upper right quadrant, with little fever or malaise, it is probably a hydatid cyst—it may be enormous, and he may have more than one.

A hydatid cyst usually contains several litres of water-clear highly antigenic fluid. Outside, there is a thin, tough, fibrous ectocyst, made of tissue provided by the patient. Inside this, and separated from it by an easy plane of cleavage, is a thick, yellowish, slimy, gelatinous endocyst, which the parasite forms, and which tends to split and curl up on itself when you cut it. Scolices, which are tiny, barely visible, white granules, and daughter cysts, like grapes or soap bubbles, float free in the fluid of the cyst. *E. multilocularis,* a similar parasite, produces an alveolar or honeycombed cyst.

A cyst in his liver may rupture into: (1) his bile-ducts and cause cholangitis, or (2) a serous cavity, where it may cause a hypersensitivity reaction, varying from urticaria to anaphylactic shock.

The diagnosis is often difficult, and the disease may be so rare that you forget it as a possibility. There is never any hurry to operate, so investigate him as fully as you can. Surgery is likely to be difficult, so try to refer him.

When you remove a hydatid cyst, do so in the plane between the tissues of host and parasite—leave the ectocyst, and don't try to remove the entire cyst intact, unless you can do this easily, as in the ovary or spleen. Instead: (1) Gain access to the cyst, and pack it off, so that if any infective hydatid fluid does escape, it will not contaminate his peritoneal cavity—a single millilitre can contain thousands of scolices. (2) Aspirate some of the fluid, and inject a chemical to kill the scolices. (3) When this has had time to act, aspirate as much remaining fluid as you can. (4) Scoop out the endocyst and the daughter cysts. (5) Close the cavity, so that it does not leave a sinus or a fistula.

If he is a child, the cyst will probably be monolocular, so that aspirating it will not be too difficult. But if he is an adult, it is likely to be multilocular, so that: (1) the fluid will be difficult to aspirate, because the daughter cysts block the needle, and (2) the scolices will be difficult to sterilize, because the scolicide cannot penetrate in to them.

The great dangers are that you will spill the fluid which may: (1) allow daughter cysts to establish themselves in his peritoneal cavity, and (2) cause anaphylactic shock. The recurrence rate is usually at least 25%.

The medical treatment of hydatid disease with albendazole (Smith, Kline and French) 10 mg/kg/day in two divided doses daily for 8 weeks appears promising at the time of writing.

HYDATID CYSTS

PREVENTION. If yours is an endemic area do all you can to

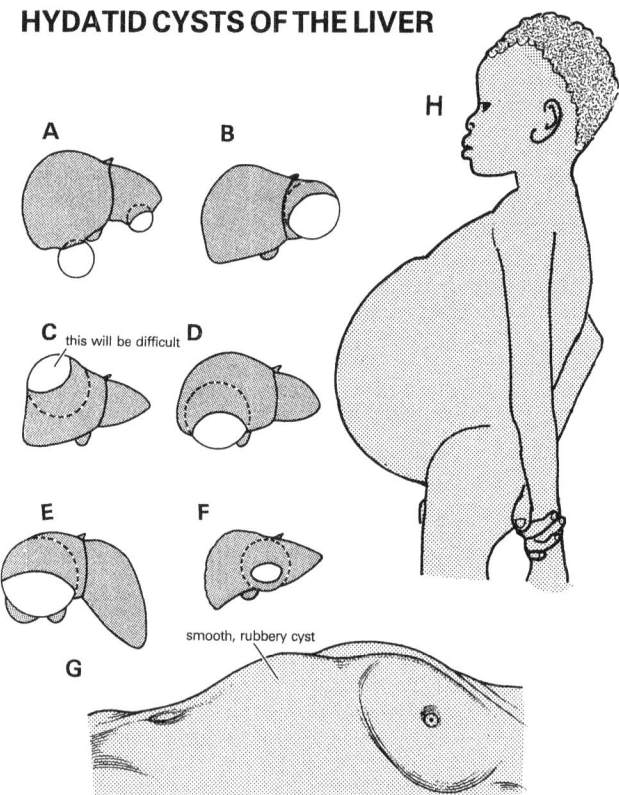

Fig. 31-11 HYDATID CYSTS OF THE LIVER. A, to F, some of the cysts you may find. C, will need a thoraco-abdominal incision. G, a patient with a single cyst. H, abdominal distension due to multiple hydatid daughter cysts throughout the peritoneal cavity. *After Goinard et al.*

educate the local population, especially about washing their hands and regularly deworming their dogs.

X-RAYS. Take a chest film: the patient may also have cysts in his lungs. A cyst in his liver may raise the right lobe of his diaphragm. An old aborted cyst may leave a calcified shadow.

ULTRASONOGRAPHY is the best way of detecting hydatid cysts. A lamellated membrane, detachment of the membrane from the cyst wall, or the presence of daughter cysts confirms the diagnosis.

SPECIAL TESTS. 30% of patients have an absolute eosinophilia. The Casoni test is negative in about 15% of cases. Other antibody tests, such as the ELISA test, also often give false negatives.

ASPIRATION. Many surgeons consider that you should not try to confirm the diagnosis by aspiration, because this may make the cyst leak, and may be fatal. Aspiration is safer if a cyst is superficial, and unlikely to leak into a serous cavity.

If you are aspirating what you think is an abscess, and you aspirate water-clear fluid, it is almost certainly a hydatid cyst. Continue aspirating to dryness, before you remove the needle. It will then be less likely to leak.

If you decide to aspirate the cyst in a patient's liver, do so under anaesthesia, so that it can be kept still for a few seconds, while you insert the needle.

CAUTION ! Don't try to tap a hydatid cyst merely to make it smaller.

DIFFERENTIAL DIAGNOSIS. Febrile? Ill? (hepatoma or amoebic abscess). Fever and a tender mass? (amoebic abscess). Liver diffusely enlarged and very tender? (amoebic hepatitis). Mass hard and nodular with loss of weight? (hepatoma). Craggy, irregular knobbly liver? (secondaries). A history of anything less than years, suggests that the mass is not a hydatid.

TREATMENT BY INJECTING A SCOLICIDE is sometimes possible. If he has a large single cyst, withdraw as much fluid as you can, and inject 1 ml of cetrimide. If he has any pain, abandon the procedure. If, not inject 5 ml of cetrimide. The great danger with this method is that if the needle is wrongly placed the cetrimide may enter his circulation. It can however be very effective, and the cyst may subsequently disappear.

CAUTION ! Don't use formalin for this purpose.

LAPAROTOMY FOR HYDATID CYSTS OF THE LIVER

PREOPERATIVELY, to kill the hydatids and make dissemination less likely, give him a course of albendazole 10 mg/kg/day in two divided doses daily, if possible for 8 weeks. Also give him hydrocortisone 100 mg 12 and 24 hours before the operation, so as to minimize the danger of anaphylaxis when you open the cyst.

ANAESTHESIA. Give him a general anaesthetic and intubate him. He is at increased risk from laryngeal spasm

EQUIPMENT. An aspirator, or a large-bore syringe with a needle and 3-way tap. A long pair of sponge forceps, and a sterile kitchen spoon to scoop out the cyst. Coloured packs which will let you to see the brood capsules and scolices more easily. Soak the packs in scolicide. Two suckers, one for the trocar (if you use one), and one ready for any spills.

A scolicide, preferably cetrimide 40% concentrate ('Cetavlon'), which is safer than other scolicides which include 1% formalin in 0.9% saline, 10% sodium chloride, 70% alcohol, 0.5% silver nitrate, or hypochlorite.

CAUTION ! Higher concentrations of scolicides, particularly 10% formalin, are dangerous.

INCISION. This depends on where the cyst is.

If the cyst is high on the right, under his diaphragm, it may need a thoraco-abdominal incision, extrapleural dissection, and incision of his diaphragm. Refer him.

For cysts of the left lobe and most cysts of the right lobe, make a median or paramedian incision. If necessary, extend this laterally, so that you have adequate exposure. Another way of getting better access is to stuff packs, soaked with scolicide, into his right subphrenic space, so as to push his liver down.

The cysts present as smooth white swellings. Look and feel

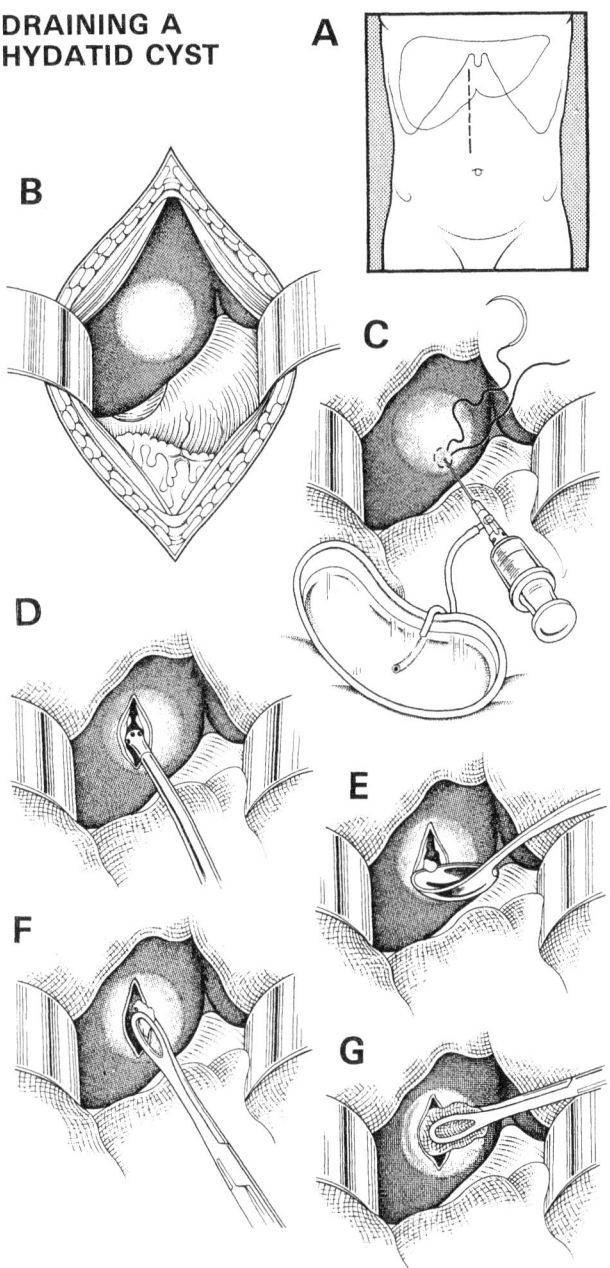

Fig. 31-12 A HYDATID CYST OF THE LIVER. A, a high paramedian incision. B, the cyst exposed. C, the cyst packed off, a purse string suture inserted, and the cyst being aspirated. Some scolicide is then injected and left inside for 3 minutes. D, sucking out the rest of the fluid. E, removing the daughter cysts with a spoon. F, removing the endocyst with sponge forceps. G, swabbing out the cavity with scolicide. *Partly after Rob C and Smith R, 'Operative surgery: Part 1: Adomen, Rectum and Anus', (2nd edn 1969), p.322. Butterworths, with kind permission.*

carefully to find how many he has. The rest of his liver is usually large, smooth, and distended.

Select a place where the cyst is close to the surface, and isolate it with carefully placed scolicide-soaked packs.

Aspirate at least half the fluid with a 1.5 mm needle, or a trocar attached to a sucker. If you withdraw watery fluid, it can only be a hydatid cyst. When the needle blocks, clear it by injecting a little scolicide. If needle aspiration does not work, use a trocar and cannula. If necessary, try introducing a multiholed catheter through the cannula. This will however increase the risk of spillage. If many daughter cysts block the sucker, it is probably multilocular.

Collect the fluid in a bowl containing an excess of scolicide. Keep a record of the volume you withdraw, as a guide to how much scolicide you will need to inject.

Fill a 50 or 100 ml syringe with scolicide, and inject it through the needle that you have used for aspiration. Go on injecting until the cyst becomes tense. Insert a purse string suture round the puncture site, and tie it snugly before you remove the needle. Wait for 3 minutes for the contents of the cyst to become sterile.

Aspirate some of the contents of the cyst, then open it through the part which presents most easily. Insert the tip of the sucker, and suck out as much of the remaining fluid as you can. You may remove up to 40 litres. Using a kitchen spoon, remove all the daughter cysts, sediment and debris. Then, using finger dissection, find the natural plane of cleavage between the ecto- and the endocyst. To get adequate exposure, you may have to incise the cyst across the full width of its bulge, and unroof it. Remove the yellow laminated membrane of the endocyst completely, piece by piece, with sponge forceps. There will be little bleeding.

CAUTION! (1) Try not to rupture the daughter cysts as you remove them, because their contents are probably still infective. (2) Don't try to remove the ectocyst; it is tightly stuck to the liver, and will bleed.

Swab the inside of the cyst with packs soaked in silver nitrate solution, and explore it for secondary cavities. If you find any, aspirate them and fill them with scolicide as above.

If the cavity is small, you may be able to bring its edges together together with mattress sutures.

If the cavity is large, you can: (1) Suture any obvious small bile duct openings, and leave it alone, which is probably the wisest method. (2) Fill it with ordinary 0.9% saline, and suture it. (3) Saucerize it by excising the protruding portion. The difficulty with this is that the cut surfaces of the liver will bleed. (4) Fill it with a graft of omentum. Dissect a strip of omentum on a vascular pedicle and stitch this into the cavity. The omentum will swell to fill the space and absorb the fluid from the cavity. (5) Stitch its edges to the surface of a separate skin incision (marsupialization). This is an old method, but it may be useful if he is very ill. (6) Stitch the walls of the cyst together with multiple catgut sutures, so that the cavity is obliterated.

Drain large cavities for about 10 days, especially if you have not been able to remove all the endocyst.

CAUTION ! (1) Don't let the cyst fluid spill, or daughter cysts will form in his peritoneal cavity. (2) If the needle hole does tend to leak, insert a purse string suture. (2) Don't try to excise the cyst *in toto*, or it will bleed disastrously.

DIFFICULTIES WITH HYDATID CYSTS

If he presents with GENERALIZED ABDOMINAL SWELLING, consider the possibility of HYDATIDOSIS OF THE PERITONEAL CAVITY. At operation you may find his peritoneal cavity distended with hydatid cysts, and remove 2 bucketfuls of them. The surface of his gut may be seeded with small white nodules.

If he has a CYST IN HIS OMENTUM, try to remove it entire, with part of the omentum. If you cannot do this, aspirate and inject scolicide, as for the liver.

If he has a hydatid CYST OF HIS SPLEEN, do a splenectomy. In other sites excise it if you can, or evacuate it as in the liver. Don't sacrifice a kidney, just because it contains a cyst.

If his BLOOD PRESSURE FALLS alarmingly and there is no other reason for it, he is probably in anaphylactic shock (see below).

If he has OBSTRUCTIVE JAUNDICE, perhaps with cholangitis, you will have to open and drain his common bile-duct, as in Section 13.4. Remove all hydatid sludge, debris, and daughter cysts from the duct, and irrigate it thoroughly. Drain his common bile-duct with a T-tube.

If a CYST IS LEAKING into his peripheral bile ducts, refer him. Treatment is difficult, and his life is not, for the moment, in danger. If you cannot refer him, sterilize, evacuate, and drain the cyst. An external biliary fistula may develop, which may improve his cholangitis.

If he develops the features of a LIVER ABSCESS—a swinging fever, anorexia, and increasing pain, suspect that a hydatid cyst has become infected. Open it, saucerize it, and drain it. Treat him as in Section 31.12. Infection will have destroyed the hydatids.

If he develops the signs of PERITONITIS with an anaphylactic response, shock, and dyspnoea, his cyst has ruptured into his peritoneal cavity. Give him intravenous hydrocortisone 500 to 1000 mg, subcutaneous adrenalin (1 ml of a 1/1000 solution), or an antihistamine.

If his PERITONEAL CAVITY IS BULGING WITH DAUGHTER CYSTS, try to remove as many of them as you can. Then flood it with liberal quantities of a scolicide. Aspirate this and then irrigate it with saline to wash out the remaining scolicide.

If a cyst is CALCIFIED and asymptomatic, leave it.

If he develops a FEVER postoperatively, the cyst cavity is probably infected.

If he has RECURRENT CYSTS, they will probably take about 3 years to develop, be multiple, and be in his abdominal cavity. Distinguish recurrent cysts from the manifestation of an unsuspected second cyst.

31.14 Other problems in tropical surgery

There are many of these. Here are some of the various conditions you may meet, and which are not discussed elsewhere.

MORE TROPICAL PROBLEMS

ONCHOCERCAL NODULES

If a patient from an endemic area has firm, 2 or 3 cm, NODULES especially over his iliac crests, trochanters, sacrum, knees, shoulders, or head, they are probably onchocercal

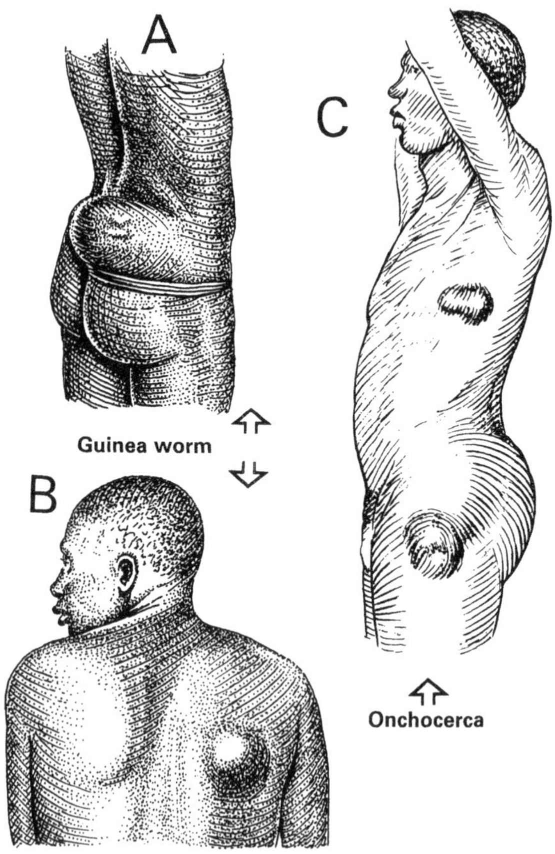

ENCYSTED WORMS

Fig. 31-13 ONCHOCERCAL NODULES AND ENCYSTED GUINEA WORMS. Both are easy to remove surgically. A, and B, encysted guinea worms are commonly found on the trunk, particularly over the inferior angle of the scapula and the crest of the ilium. C, onchocercal nodules are usually found over the iliac crests, trochanters, sacrum, knees, shoulders or head. *Partly after Charles Bowesman, 'Surgery and Clinical Pathology in the Tropics'. E and S Livingstone, with kind permission.*

nodules. These are well-encapsulated, and easy to remove under local anaesthesia.

ENCYSTED GUINEA WORMS

See also Fig. 7-1 (the differential diagnosis from pyomyositis).

If a guinea worm PRESENTS ON THE SKIN, don't try to dissect it out, because severe sepsis usually follows. Instead, carefully wind it round a match-stick, and be prepared to take 3 weeks in doing so, leaving the stick with its coil of worm under a dressing, and pulling out a little more each day.

If a large rubbery CYSTIC MASS develops, usually on his trunk, and typically on his back near the angle of his scapula, distinguish a guinea worm cyst (a low-grade encapsulated abscess) from a lipoma. (1) A guinea worm cyst often has a small scar on its surface. (2) Ask him to contract his muscles: a lipoma is usually superficial, and a guinea worm deep to them. (3) Aspirate the mass with a wide needle. A guinea worm cyst usually contains sterile pus. If necessary dissect out the mass, taking care not to injure surrounding structures. There is no easy plane of cleavage.

CURIOUS FORMS OF GANGRENE

If the TIPS OF HIS FINGERS AND TOES BECOME GANGRENOUS without any obvious cause, one of the possibilities is 'tropical coagulopathic ischaemia', also known as 'idiopathic gangrene', which is not uncommon in sub-Saharan Africa. You will see it at any age, but particularly in malnourished children with severe infections. The arteries and veins of all four limbs may be filled with clot, so that a whole limb or a large part of a limb is lost.

The disease starts with swelling, which soon becomes severely painful. The peripheral pulses disappear, after which gangrene may be rapid or slow, new areas of gangrene appearing over several months. The process eventually stops spontaneously. If gangrene is extensive the mortality rate is high. It may be a manifestation of the same process that causes cancrum oris (26.6).

AINHUM

If a CONSTRICTING GROOVE FORMS ROUND THE BASE OF A PATIENT'S TOE, usually the 5th, he has that mysterious disease called AINHUM. This occurs in otherwise healthy barefooted people, is painful because of the ischaemia it causes, and can be a severe disability. It may last several years, before the end of the toe finally falls off.

Tetanus is a possible complication, so give him two doses of tetanus toxoid a month apart. Clean his toes thoroughly. Then, under local anaesthesia, amputate his toe using a dorsal racquet incision (shown as H, Fig 75-30 for a little finger) encircling the base of his toe, just proximal to the constricting groove, and exposing its MP joint. Dislocate this with the rest of the stump of his proximal phalanx. Results are good; after perhaps years of pain he will now have a stable painless foot, but without his little toe.

Miller JRM. 'Tropical coagulopathic ischaemia' Proceedings of the Association of Surgeons of East Africa 1980;3:84-88.

Bhana D and Baddeley H 'Idiopathic gangrene''. East African Medical Journal 1970;47:506-14

32 Primary oncology

32.1 Treating cancer in a district hospital

Cancer is a worldwide problem. It kills 4.3 million people annually, 2.9 million of them in the developing world. The six most common tumours are carcinomas of the liver (hepatoma), bronchus, large gut, stomach, prostate, and breast. Although nearly 40% of malignant tumours can now be cured, if they are diagnosed sufficiently early, and treated appropriately, most of the patients who consult you will have such advanced disease that the help you can give them will be limited. Although a few tumours can be managed optimally with very limited facilities, many of the methods in this chapter are among the least cost-effective in this book. Nevertheless, there is always something you can do, even for the most hopeless patient; but you may have to turn to the next chapter on terminal care, to know what it is.

Your hospital may be a long way from any referral centre, so that if you don't diagnose and treat a patient with cancer, it is likely that that nobody else will. You may be unable to get prompt and reliable histological reports, or even any reports at all, and there will certainly be no one to examine frozen sections for you. You are unlikely to be able to refer anyone for radiotherapy, or even perhaps for expert surgery, so you will have to rely on simple surgery, and some of the easier and cheaper chemotheraputic regimes.

The sequence of steps with most patients is this:

Make the diagnosis of malignant disease clinically, and examine the patient carefully to assess its extent.

Confirm the diagnosis histologically (if you can) before you start treatment. If you are in doubt after taking a biopsy (which should include cutting the tissue across to inspect its cut surface), it is usually better to wait for a histological report, if this is possible. You should rarely, if ever, give a toxic treatment without knowing the histology.

Stage the tumour according to the criteria given here. Most malignant tumours have four stages, or sometimes five, some of which may be subdivided. The first two stages are usually curable, whereas the last two can usually only be palliated. For most tumours we give the prognosis for each stage, with various treatment methods.

Decide what is best for the patient. Can you treat him? Can someone else treat him? Can nobody treat him? Should you aim for cure or palliation? For example, chemotherapy can usually achieve a radical cure with Burkitt's lymphoma, and quite simple surgery can cure carcinomas of the skin and penis. Palliation may greatly help a patient with carcinoma of his prostate (oestrogen treatment), or a lymphoma (cytotoxic drugs), or carcinoma of his oesophagus (the insertion of a Celestin tube). Often, you can do little for him, because both surgery and chemotherapy may only *prolong his suffering and that of his relatives.*

Decide if you are going to refer him, or to treat or palliate him yourself. If a referral centre can do nothing for him, don't refer him. If private doctors cannot help him, persuade him not to waste his money on them.

When you make the difficult decision as to whom to treat and whom only to palliate, try, if you can, to base your decision on the response of the tumour, and not on his political influence, his social status, or on his ability to pay for the drugs. Unfor-

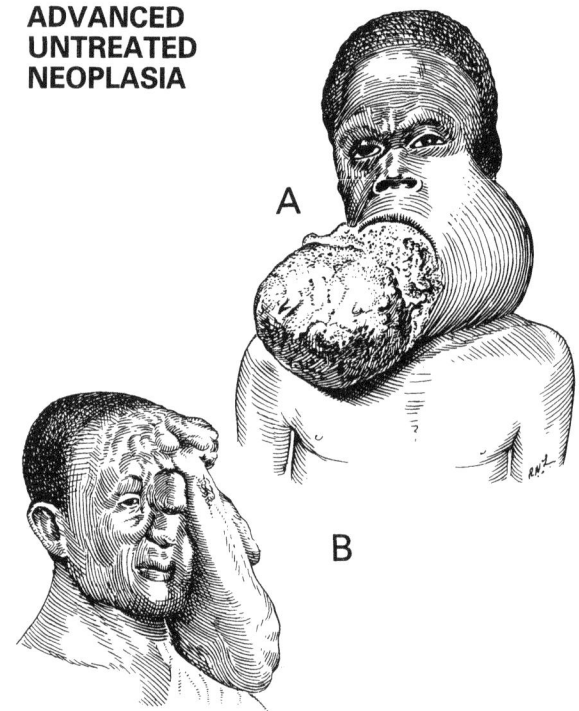

Fig 32-1 ADVANCED UNTREATED NEOPLASIA. A, a very large giant cell tumour (26.7) of the mandible in a boy of 12. B, a large angiomatous sarcoma (32.8) of the blood vessels of the scalp. In the absence of adequate treatment this is what happens. Unfortunately, neither of these tumours are readily treatable by the methods described here. Both were seen by Bowesman in Ghana in the 1950s or earlier, but similar cases are still occasionally seen. *After Charles Bowesman, 'Surgery and Clinical Pathology in the Tropics'. E, and S, Livingstone, with kind permission.*

tunately, in places where medicine has to be bought by individual patients, the poor are likely to get surgery, or nothing. Even so, make every effort to have some drugs available to treat such conditions as Burkitt's lymphoma and choriocarcinoma.

You will also have to decide where the treatment of tumours comes in your own priorities, and how much scarce money and skill should be devoted to less easily treated ones, when the more cost-effective calls on your resources are so great. The common useful tumours to treat are: squamous cell carcinoma, carcinoma of the penis, carcinoma of the breast (early), carcinoma of the prostate. The less common useful ones are: Burkitt's lymphoma, basal cell carcinoma, carcinoma of the large gut, invasive mole, and choriocarcinoma.

Occasionally, you will meet benign resectable tumours in places, such as the intestinal tract, where you normally expect malignant ones. So, remember their existence, investigate the patient as thoroughly as you can, and don't assume that a tumour is malignant, until you have proved it so.

ONCOLOGY IN A DISTRICT HOSPITAL. Here, as an example, are the 79 tumours seen in 1969 in Kamuli district hospital in Uganda: 15 hepatomas, all untreatable; 3 carcinomas of the oesophagus, all advanced; 6 carcinomas of the stomach, 4 of which were treated by palliative gastrectomy (not described here); 2 inoperable carcinomas of the rectum; 1 inoperable carcinoma of the pancreas; 19 carcinomas of the cervix including 1 early case treated by radical hysterectomy; 4 ovarian tumours, 2 treated surgically; 2 bladder cancers, both operable (exceptional); 6 carcinomas of the penis, all treated by partial amputation; 5 carcinomas of the prostate given hormone treatment; 1 operable thyroid tumour; 1 advanced cylindroma of the palate; 1 carcinoma of the submandibular glands, radically resected; 1 untreatable nasopharyngeal carcinoma; 5 squamous cell carcinomas, 3 of which were amputated; 1 Kaposi's sarcoma; 1 melanoma; 4 carcinomas of the breast, 3 treated by simple mastectomy; 2 Hodgkin's lymphomas; and 2 non-Hodgkin's lymphomas.

THE GENERAL METHOD FOR SOLID TUMOURS

BASIC FACILITIES. For chemotherapy you will need an accurate scale to measure weight, and a height scale on the wall. From these you can work out a patient's surface area with Figure 58-6. You must also be able to measure a his blood urea, his haemoglobin, his total and differential white count (from which you will be able to work out his absolute granulocyte count), and if possible his platelets.

STAGING. Be thorough, and assess his tumour carefully according to the criteria in this chapter. This should always be possible, although you may need a general anaesthetic to do it (as with carcinoma of the cervix). Both the stage of a tumour, and often its histological grade, influence the prognosis, both with and without treatment.

TAKING A BIOPSY. If you are excising a lymph node, take the whole node if this is easy, but if it is not, a part of the node will do. *If you are sending away a gland for histology, always cut it across.* With experience you will be able to recognize the caseation of tuberculosis, and to distinguish hyperplasia from a tumour.

If you are taking tissue from an ulcer or a large mass, take it from the edge of the lesion, so that you include normal and abnormal tissue.

SENDING SPECIMENS. When you fix a tissue, place it in at least 5 times its volume of formol saline, which is 10% of formalin solution (itself a 30% solution of formalin in water) in 0.9% saline. Send small specimens in a screw-capped universal container in a wooden box made for the purpose. Or, fix the specimen first in formol saline for a few days, then wrap it in formol-saline-soaked cotton wool, pack this in a plastic bag, and send it in a cardboard box.

If you want to send a very large specimen for histology, such as an entire kidney, cut it so that the fixative can reach its interior, but leave the slices together at one edge, so that they can be put together again, and the shape of the specimen preserved. Fix the whole specimen in a bucket of formol saline. When it is fixed, seal it in a polythene bag, pack it in a cardboard box, and send it by hand.

CAUTION ! The danger in sending all pathological specimens is that they will leak in the post, contaminate the mail, and make you very unpopular with the post office!

THE KARNOFSKY PERFORMANCE SCALE

Use this to assess the quality of life of the patients you treat. It is particularly important in managing patients having chemotherapy.

100%, the patient is normal, with no complications or evidence of disease.
90%, his activity is normal, but he has signs or symptoms of the disease.
80%, activity with effort.
70%, cares for himself, but is unable to work, or to undertake his normal activity.
60%, requires occasional help, but meets most of his personal needs.
50%, requires considerable help, and needs frequent nursing care.
40%, in bed or in a chair, and needs special care.
30%, severely disabled, and needs hospitalization.
20%, very sick.
10%, moribund.
0%, dead.

32.2 Primary cancer chemotherapy

Before you give any cytotoxic agent, you must decide if the misery its side-effects will certainly cause, will outweigh the benefit you expect it to have. Chemotherapy is one of the treatment methods for which compliance is particularly necessary. If patients will not complete their courses of tuberculosis treatment satisfactorily, how likely are they to persist with a regime with much more unpleasant side-effects? The indications for chemotherapy under the conditions for which we write are limited.

To those who say that there is no place whatever for 'primary cancer chemotherapy', we reply that: (1) If you don't treat patients, it is probable that nobody else will either. (2) Some drugs are comparatively cheap, and some regimes are practical and highly effective, even under your circumstances, particularly those for Burkitt's lymphoma. (3) Treatment may be urgent. (4) Some district hospital doctors have been doing chemotherapy successfully for many years. (5) Patients and their families much prefer to be treated near their own homes. (6) Some patients, particularly health workers and teachers, are sufficiently compliant to complete even unpleasant courses of treatment.

If you doubt that there is a case for 'primary cancer chemotherapy', read this story:

NARUNDRNATHAN (2½ years) complained of a loose tooth and swelling of his upper jaw, which had started 2 weeks previously. He was taken to a dentist, who noticed proptosis in his left eye, and referred him to the children's ward. Here he was found to have several abdominal masses, was diagnosed as having Burkitt's lymphoma, and was referred to the teaching hospital. There was no money left in the transport vote to buy petrol for the hospital ambulance, so his parents took him there by bus. The consultant oncologist was away at a conference in Oxford, so he was sent back again, and asked to reattend a week later. While he was waiting to be sent to the oncologist again, he died, after a total history of less than a month. LESSONS (1)The diagnosis of Burkitt's lymphoma is usually sufficiently distinctive for treatment to be started without waiting for a biopsy report. (2) Burkitt's lymphoma needs urgent treatment, which should begin within 48 hours, is not expensive, and is highly effective. (3) Treatment is easily possible in a district hospital.

Unfortunately, there are no other tumours which are quite so readily treated by chemotherapy as Burkitt's lymphoma. Here is a modification of WHO's tumour categories, which describe what chemotherapy can do, sometimes assisted by surgery. Tumours which are treated by surgery alone, squamous cell carcinoma 32.19, for example, are not included in this list. This is

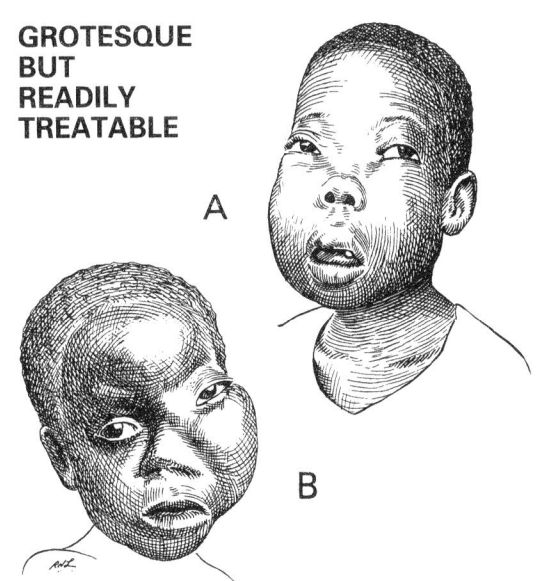

Fig 32-1a BURKITT'S LYMPHOMA should be your first priority for chemotherapy. Note the swelling of both maxillae in child A. *From Charles Bowesman, 'Surgery and Clinical Pathology in the Tropics', E. and S. Livingstone, with kind permission.*

a surgical manual, so we are only concerned with 'surgical' oncology, and not with the chemotherapy of leukaemia.

Category 1 Chemotherapy will cure or significantly prolong the life of some patients: Acute lymphoblastic leukaemia, acute non-lymphoblastic or myelogenous leukaemia, Hodgkin's disease, non-Hodgkin's disease, Burkitt's lymphoma, gestational/trophoblastic cancers, germ cell tumours of the testis, nephroblastoma (Wilm's tumour), Ewing's sarcoma, paediatric soft tissue sarcomas, lung cancer (small cell type), classical Kaposi's sarcoma (not the AIDS-related variety).

Category 1 – 2 There is controversial evidence that chemotherapy as an adjuvant to surgery may prolong survival: premenopausal breast cancer (in the early stages), postmenopausal breast cancer (responding to tamoxifen), osteosarcoma.

Category 2 Chemotherapy makes tumours shrink, almost certainly improves the quality of life and *may* prolong life marginally: chronic lymphocytic leukaemia, chronic myelogenous leukaemia, multiple myeloma, ovarian carcinoma, endometrial carcinoma, prostatic carcinoma (oestrogen therapy puts it in this category, otherwise it would be in Category 3), neuroblastoma.

Category 2 – 3 The tumour may shrink but it is not clear that clinical benefit outweighs toxicity. Any improvement in survival is marginal and controversial: gastric cancer, head and neck cancers, primary cancers of the central nervous system, bladder cancer (intravesical), adrenal cancer, hepatoma.

Category 3 There are no effective drugs. Although the tumour may shrink, the effect is so marginal that it is unlikely that the quality of life will be improved. Chemotherapy will compromise it in most patients, and shorten their lives: lung cancer (epidermoid, adenocarcinoma, and large cell type), oesophageal carcinoma, large gut carcinoma, pancreatic carcinoma (non-endocrine), carcinoma of the cervix, carcinoma of the penis, renal carcinoma, melanoma.

Chemotherapy in a district hospital is never easy. Your laboratory facilities will be minimal, your drugs limited, your nurses may be inexperienced with chronic cancer patients, and your rehabilitation facilities rudimentary. You do however have two advantages; you can follow up a patient more easily than a referral centre, and his relatives are likely to live much nearer.

Before you start treatment, decide on your goal. Although a particular tumour may be curable, not all patients with it may be cured. Base your decision to treat a patient on: the stage of his tumour, the sites of its metastases, its particular histology, the state of his vital organs, his nutrition, his willingness to accept toxic symptoms, and the staff and facilities you have to treat any complications he might get.

The drugs we describe have mostly been selected from WHO's list. Use these drugs only, and gain experience in their use. Don't use them unless: (1) You know or are prepared to look up their general mode of action. (2) You know their toxic effects and dangers, and have the minimal facilities to monitor these. (3) You have decided what you are aiming for—cure or palliation? (4) You remember that an overdose can be fatal. Even a normal dose can sometimes be fatal. So carefully follow the rules about reducing the dose and stopping treatment when necessary. Remember that experienced doctors with compliant patients sometimes have disasters—a patient can die from septicaemia in 48 hours.

If you do attempt cancer chemotherapy, you will have to know your limitations, and care for patients meticulously. You will also have to do regular ward rounds—a complication can appear in 24 hours. Finally, do your utmost to see that a patient completes his course and is not abandoned. Either strive to give him a full course, or don't attempt chemotherapy. There is no justification for the the attitude "He's hopeless, let's try a little cyclophosphamide..."

Most cytotoxic drugs have their main action on rapidly dividing cells, which unfortunately include the cells of the bone marrow and the mucosa. Malignant cells divide continuously, whereas marrow cells are quiescent for part of the time. Intermittent doses allow the marrow to recover, whilst maintaining an antitumour effect; but don't wait so long that the tumour regrows between courses. A common regime is to give high intermittent doses during less than 24 hours, and to repeat them every 2, 3, or 4 weeks, to allow the marrow to recover, without waiting so long that the tumour regrows between courses.

Cytotoxic drugs are commonly used in combination because: (1) They often act synergistically at different stages in cell division, or in different ways. (2) Smaller doses can be used. (3) If they have different toxic effects, their combined toxicity is minimized, because doses can be smaller. (4) The tumour is less likely to become resistant. But: (1) combined therapy is more expensive, and (2) there may be more toxic effects, although each is less severe.

Tumour cells tend to multiply at a constant rate, depending on the proportion of cells dividing. Some grow very fast—Burkitt's lymphoma may double in size in 24 hours. Because of the constant rate of cell multiplication, a tumour grows exponentially, and its bulk increases more rapidly as it grows. Similarly, chemotherapy kills a constant proportion of dividing cells, so that if it is sensitive, its size is also reduced exponentially. A large tumour may thus shrink rapidly to begin with, and then more slowly as it gets smaller.

Many cytotoxic drugs are very irritant indeed. If they extravasate into the tissues, they cause large necrotic ulcers. Some, such as vincristine, actinomycin D, and nitrogen mustard, are best given into a freely running drip. Others can be given by bolus intravenous injection—with care! Although some can be given by mouth, most are better given into a vein, because this ensures high intermittent levels of the drug in the tissues. Injecting irritant drugs into veins can cause thrombophlebitis. Over a long period, this can easily make all his accessible veins useless for chemotherapy. Careful venipuncture is the ony way to reduce this difficulty. Few cytotoxic drugs can be given intramuscularly.

THE EFFECT OF CHEMOTHERAPY

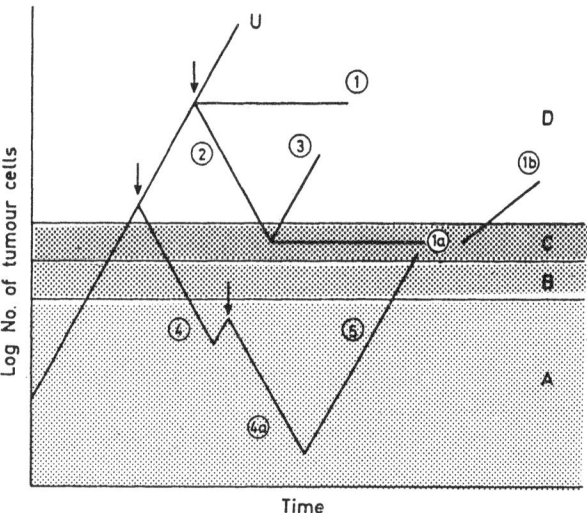

Fig. 32-1b THE EFFECT OF CHEMOTHERAPY on the size of a tumour cell population. A, B, C, and D, represent differences in a patient's clinical condition. In A, he has no evidence of a tumour. In B, it can only be shown by special laboratory tests. In C, he has radiological or clinical evidence of disease. In D, he has symptoms. The growth of his tumour untreated is assumed to be exponential (U). Three courses of chemotherapy (shown by arrows), at the same dose destroy the same proportion of his tumour cells, whatever the total number of cells he has when treatment begins. In 2, his symptoms are relieved, but he still has clinical and radiological signs of the disease. In 4, his symptoms are relieved, and all clinical and laboratory evidence of his tumour disappears. In 4a, he is treated when he is apparently healthy.

After the effect of treatment has worn off, his tumour grows at the same rate as it did before. In 3, his symptoms return rapidly. After 4, further growth is arrested by course 4a, which delays the return of symptoms (5). Maintenance therapy, at a low dosage that sustains a steady state, does not relieve symptoms in 1 and does not cause any regression in 1a. Maintenance treatment is continued in 1b, but the tumour has become resistant to treatment. *From the Oxford Textbook of Medicine.*

When your patients die from the complications of cytotoxic drugs, there is an 80% chance that they will die from infection, usually septicaemia, and a 20% chance that they will die from intracranial haemorrhage, as the result of an abnormal tendency to bleed. Careful monitoring will minimize these dangers. If he has a total white count of 2000 μl, or more, or a platelet count of 100 000 μl, or more, he should have his chemotherapy, but you will have to have resources available to treat any infection or bleeding that may then arise. These include powerful antibiotics, and platelet transfusions or fresh blood. If you don't have them, and especially if he has a disease with a small or no chance of cure, you may do him more good by withholding chemotherapy completely, until his white count rises above 3000.

WHO. 'Essential drugs for cancer chemotherapy: Memorandum from a WHO Meeting'. WHO Bulletin. 1985:63 (6);999-1002

DON'T COMPROMISE A PATIENT'S QUALITY OF LIFE FOR THE SAKE OF A SHORT REMISSION

CYTOTOXIC DRUGS

WHICH DRUGS? The regimes described here treat 18 tumours with 10 drugs. Most regimes use either vincristine (expensive) or cyclophosphamide (fairly cheap), and usually both. The next most useful drug is methotrexate, which is fairly cheap in the low dose range used for most methods, and which does not require folinic acid rescue. So try to stock these three drugs, with some actinomycin D, if possible.

If you are in the Burkitt zone, you must be able to treat Burkitt's lymphoma (common) for which you will need the first three, but you can use cyclophosphamide alone. Next in order of benefit comes Hodgkin's (nitrogen mustard, vincristine, procarbazine) and non-Hodgkin's lymphoma (cyclophosphamide, vincristine).

The remaining drugs listed are much less important: melphalan, 5 fluoruracil, doxorubicin ('Adriamycin'), etoposide.

ADMISSION. You will probably find it convenient to admit a patient for about 5 days for the initial assessment and investigation, and for the first course; then to discharge him, and readmit him for about 5 days for each course.

PRIOR INFECTION. Be sure to deal with all treatable infections before starting chemotherapy. *An infection which cannot be controlled is a contraindication to the use of cytotoxic drugs.*

PREPARATION AND MONITORING FOR CHEMOTHERAPY. You will need to prepare him before you start chemotherapy. One purpose of this is to establish a baseline, from which you can monitor his response to treatment. Monitor him weekly, and before each course of treatment. Monitor: (1) His clinical condition on the Karnofsky performance scale. (2) The size of his tumour, measured with a tape measure in two planes at 90°. If he has a lymphoma, or metastatic glandular deposits, count all his nodes and measure them with a tape. Assess the degree of involvement of any organs that are infiltrated. (3) Watch for toxic effects, and infection, clinically at least 3 times a week. (4) Measure his haemoglobin, do a total and differential white count, and if possible count his platelets. Culture his urine. (5) Do other tests as necessary, for example his blood urea.

If he has a haemoglobin of <90 g/l before you start, transfuse him, if necessary, repeatedly.

INTRAVENOUS INJECTION

Oral chlorpromazine 1 to 2 hours before the injection will help him considerably, by reducing nausea and vomiting (50 mg for an average adult, 25 mg if he is an outpatient). He may need further doses of this or other drugs, such as metaclopromide or cyclizine, if he continues to be sick. Haloperidol, droperidol, and possibly domperidone can also be used.

If you are giving the drug by bolus intravenous injection, have all your material ready—adhesive tape in the proper lengths, an infusion set or syringe ready for use, and the drug already drawn up in a syringe and *well diluted!* Use his arm and hand veins if you can. Start with his distal veins and use them in rotation. Use a 0.8 mm needle, and if necessary, a scalp-vein needle in children.

Place a tourniquet above the site of venipuncture, and rub his skin hard with spirit. Insert the needle bevel upwards. When you are under the skin, enter the vein, then secure the needle with a piece of tape.

Connect the syringe to the needle, and inject some saline, to be sure that it is properly in a vein. When you are sure it is in the vein, start the injection, beginning with the most irritant drug. Inject slowly over 10 minutes

If the needle becomes dislodged, start again with a fresh one. At the end of the injection, flush the vein with 10 ml of saline. Pull out the needle, and apply gentle pressure to the puncture site with a piece of dry cotton wool. If bleeding has stopped, there is no need to apply a dressing.

CAUTION ! (1) Use an absolutely clean technique—don't touch the tip of the needle or the infusion set. If you happen to contaminate them, discard them and use fresh ones. (2) Preferably, give nitrogen mustard, vincristine, and actinomycin D into a free-flowing drip.

If you are giving the drug into a running drip, inject the drug into the tubing of the drip. A drip adds considerably to the expense of treatment.

ALKYLATING AGENTS

These combine with DNA, prevent mitosis, and cause chromosome fragmentation, so that cells die.

NITROGEN MUSTARD ('Mustine')

INDICATIONS. Hodgkin's disease. Nitrogen mustard is cheap, but its indications are limited.

ADMINISTRATION. Intravenously, 10 mg vials. Reconstitute these with 10 to 20 ml of water or saline, and use the solution immediately. Give it through a running intravenous drip, or well diluted as a bolus intravenous injection. It is very irritant—protect the patient's eyes and skin (and yours!), and don't let it leak into his subcutaneous tissues.

DOSE. 5 to 10 mg/m^2.

ACTION. Rapidly hydrolysed. 90% is cleared from the blood in a minute. Short plasma half life. 50% appears in the urine as a metabolite in 24 hours.

TOXICITY. Considerable. (1) Gastrointestinal tract: nausea and vomiting for 8 hours, anorexia for 24 hours. (2) Marrow: dose-related leucopenia, and thrombocytopenia (uncommon). (3) Local irritation can be severe, venous thrombosis.

CYCLOPHOSPHAMIDE

INDICATIONS. A basic drug, 13 regimes require it.

ADMINISTRATION. Intravenously, vials of 100 mg, 200 mg, 500 mg and 1 g. Reconstitute with sterile water, and use within 2 hours. Orally, tablets of 10 mg and 50 mg.

DOSE. As a single agent give 1 g to 1.5 g/m^2 intravenously. Reduce this dose with combined therapy. Orally, see under the various tumours.

ACTION. The active agent is a hepatic metabolite. Plasma half-life 4 to 6 hours. 50% to 70% is excreted in the urine in 48 hours, and some in the bile. Two-thirds is excreted as an inactive metabolite, and one-third as an active metabolite.

TOXICITY. Less than nitrogen mustard, to which it is related chemically. (1) Anorexia, nausea, and vomiting for 6 to 12 hours. (2) Stomatitis. (3) Dose-linked depression of the marrow, especially 10 to 14 days after administration. Anaemia, thrombocytopenia (uncommon). (3) Haemorrhagic cystitis is quite common, and may be dose-limiting. A high fluid intake is mandatory in preventing this. The simple chemical, mesna, reacts specifically with the metabolite that causes the cystitis, and reduces its severity, without interacting with the parent drug. Give 200 mg of mesna intravenously per gram of intravenous cyclophosphamide, and repeat it after 4 or 8 hours. (4) Alopecia (common), skin hyperpigmentation.

MELPHALAN

INDICATIONS. Myelomatosis only.

ADMINISTRATION AND DOSE. Orally, 10 mg/m^2, see myelomatosis (32.17).

ACTION. Well absorbed orally. Plasma half-life 4 hours. Slowly excreted in the urine.

TOXICITY. (1) Anorexia, nausea, and vomiting. (2) Dose-related leucopenia, thrombocytopenia, and anaemia.

ANTIMETABOLITES

These resemble the natural compounds that are essential for the synthesis of DNA and RNA, and inhibit the enzymes that are responsible for synthesis.

5 FLUOROURACIL ('5FU')

INDICATIONS. Carcinoma of the breast (21.5).

ADMINISTRATION. Intravenously, in ampoules of 250 mg in 5 ml of sterile water. The solution is stable. Topically, in a 5% cream.

DOSE. Intravenously, 12 mg/kg daily for 3 to 5 days, repeated every 4 weeks. Or, 15 mg/kg intravenously weekly for 6 weeks (maximum dose 1 g). Decrease the dose in patients with impaired liver, kidney, or bone marrow function.

ACTION. Erratically absorbed by mouth. After intravenous injection the plasma half-life is 10 to 30 minutes. There is no intact drug after 3 hours, but intracellular drug is present much longer. 60% to 90% is excreted as respiratory CO_2 and 10 to 15% in the urine. It enters the CSF and effusions, but not in therapeutic doses.

TOXICITY. (1) Anorexia, nausea, and vomiting are common. (2) Stomatitis and diarrhoea are an indication to stop treatment. (2) Dose-limiting leucopenia is maximal at 7 to 14 days. Thrombocytopenia and anaemia (uncommon). (3) Alopecia, dermatitis, and skin hyperpigmentation. (4) Cerebellar ataxia (uncommon).

METHOTREXATE ('Amethopterin')

INDICATIONS. A basic drug, 9 regimes require it.

ADMINISTRATION. (1) Orally, tablets of 2.5 mg. (2) Intravenously as: (a) solutions of 2.5 mg, 5 mg, 50 mg, and 250 mg in vials, or (b) a powder of 50 mg or 500 mg for reconstitution with 2 ml or 10 ml of sterile water.

DOSE. There are two dose ranges:

The low dose range for most regimes: Orally, 15 mg/m^2 daily for 4 days, repeated every 14th day. Or, intravenously or intramuscularly 30 mg/m^2 weekly, if the blood urea is less than 7 mmol/l (40 mg/dl). The intramuscular use of methotrexate is one of the exceptions to the rule that cytotoxic drugs should be given intravenously.

The high dose range for carcinoma of the nasopharynx (150 mg/m^2, 32.28), and choriocarcinoma (100 mg/m^2, 32.37) is described under these tumours, and requires folinic acid 'rescue' to counter the side-effects of methotrexate. An intermediate dose can be given for carcinoma of the mouth (40 mg/m^2, 32.22).

ACTION. An antimetabolite active orally and absorbed readily. Orally, the plasma half-life is 8 to 10 hours. Intravenously, it is 4 to 6 hours. 50% of the drug is bound to plasma proteins. The CSF concentration is 10% that of blood. 50% to 90% is excreted unchanged in the urine within 24 hours.

TOXICITY. (1) Stomatitis (common) and diarrhoea (not uncommon) are indications to delay a dose or stop treatment. Bleeding and perforation are rare. (2) Hepatic toxicity is usually subclinical. (3) Leucopenia, anaemia and thrombocytopenia are uncomon with standard doses. (5) Alopecia and dermatitis (uncommon). (4) Osteoporosis occurs in children on long-term treatment. (5) Pneumonitis (uncommon). (6) Renal tubular necrosis is rare except with high doses, or if the patient is dehydrated. If signs of toxicity occur, it is too late to counter it with folinic acid, and it is safer to give no more methotrexate.

CAUTION ! (1) Don't give methotrexate, if the blood urea is over 17 mmol/l (100 mg/dl), because it accumulates when renal function is impaired. (2) Don't give it in the presence of an effusion (pleural or ascitic), because it acculumates in the fluid, and so stays in the body long enough to give an overdose. (3) Don't give aspirin with methotrexate.

VINCA ALKALOIDS

These act at the metaphase of mitosis and inhibit RNA synthesis.

VINCRISTINE ('Oncovin')

INDICATIONS. A basic drug, 14 regimes require it.

ADMINISTRATION. Intravenously as 1 mg and 2 mg vials. Reconstitute with the diluent supplied. The reconstituted solution can be stored for 14 days in a refrigerator. Give into a running drip, or well diluted by slow intravenous injection. Extravasated solution is very irritant, and causes ulcers. Never give it intramuscularly.

DOSE. Intravenously 1.4 mg/m^2. Maximum dose 2 mg. For example, a 2 m^2 patient gets 2 mg not 2.8 mg. Every 2 to 4 weeks. Decrease the dose in liver disease.

ACTION. Poorly absorbed orally. Plasma half-life 3 hours. Incompletely metabolized by the liver and excreted in the bile. 70% excreted in the faeces, 5 to 15% in the urine.

TOXICITY. No gastrointestinal symptoms, and little effect on the marrow. (2) A mild sensory neuropathy, presenting as impaired sensation and paraesthesiae, is common and is not dose-limiting. If there are severe paraesthesiae, with loss of reflexes and foot drop (even muscle power Grade 4, see Section 27.2), stop the drug. (3) Constipation and abdominal pain usually respond to enemas and laxatives; limit the dose if these are severe. (4) Cranial nerve palsies (uncommon). (5) Alopecia in 20% of patients.

ANTITUMOUR ANTIBIOTICS etc

These inhibit cell division, and form irreversible complexes with DNA. They also block DNA-dependent RNA synthesis. Etoposide inhibits DNA repair enzymes.

ACTINOMYCIN D ('Dactinomycin', 'Cosmegan')

INDICATIONS. Needed by 7 regimes, notably choriocarcinoma.

ADMINISTRATION. Intravenously, 0.5 mg vials. Reconstitute with 2.2 ml of sterile water. Can be refrigerated for 24 hours. Give into a running drip. Intensely irritant subcutaneously.

DOSE. 2 mg/m^2 every 3 weeks. Or, 1 mg/m^2 on days 1 and 3. Use with care in liver disease.

ACTION. Poorly absorbed orally. Long plasma and tissue half-life. Not metabolized. 50% excreted in the bile and 10% in the urine during the first 24 hours.

TOXICITY. (1) Anorexia, nausea, and vomiting, usually within the first few hours of administration. (2) Diarrhoea. (3) Stomatitis, glossitis, and proctitis are usually dose-limiting. (4) Bone marrow depression starts 1 to 7 days after the dose. Thrombocytopenia is often seen first. Leucopenia may be dose-limiting. Anaemia (uncommon). (5) Alopecia, erythema, desquamation, hyperpigmentation, especially in areas subject to irradiation. Reversible acne.

DOXORUBICIN ('Adriamycin')

INDICATIONS. This is very expensive, so it one of the less valuable drugs in the developing world; 7 mostly alternative regimes, retinoblastoma.

ADMINISTRATION. A red powder in 10 mg and 50 mg vials; reconstitute with saline or sterile water without preservative. It is stable for 48 hours in a refrigerator.

DOSE. Intravenously 60 to 75 mg/m^2 up to a maximum of 100 mg as a single dose every 3 weeks. Avoid if the patient has heart disease, and reduce with hepatic dysfunction. Don't exceed a cumulative dose of 600 mg/m^2, because the risk of heart failure becomes serious with higher doses.

ACTION. Poorly absorbed orally. Biphasic plasma clearance with half lives of 1 hour and 16 hours. Slow release from tissue binding. Rapidly metabolized by the liver. 50% excreted in the bile unchanged, 25% as the active metabolite. 10% in the urine.

TOXICITY. (1) Anorexia, nausea, and vomiting, usually mild but occasionally severe. Stomatitis. Diarrhoea (uncommon). (2) Bone marrow depression is dose-limiting. Leucopenia is maximal at 10 to 15 days, and usually returns to normal at 21 days. Thrombocytopenia and anaemia are less common. (3) Sinus tachycardia, T wave flattening ST depression, voltage reduction, and arrhythmia—stop or defer treatment. Congestive cardiac failure due to cardiomyopathy—stop treatment. (4) Alopecia (common) usually starts at the 3rd or 4th week. Hair usually regrows after treatment is stopped. (5) The drug colours the urine red.

ETOPOSIDE (VP16-213, 'Vepesid')

INDICATION. Choriocarcinoma.

DOSE. 100 mg/m^2 on 2 consecutive days as part of the EMA regime (32.38). Infuse the dose in 250 ml of 0.9% saline over 30 minutes. Use the solution within 6 hours of preparation.

ACTION. Inhibitor of DNA repair enzymes. 45% of the dose is excreted in the urine, 30% within 72 hours.

TOXICITY. (1) Anorexia, nausea, and vomiting (common). (2) Leucopenia is dose-limiting, and is maximal 21 days after treatment. (3) Alopecia (almost always). (4) Hypersensitivity to the detergents used in formulation (rare).

MONOAMINE OXIDASE INHIBITORS ('MAOIs')

These antimetabolites cause DNA to fragment. As with all MAOIs, drug interactions may be a problem, especially with anaesthetic agents, alcohol, phenothiazines, sympathomimetic drugs, and foods high in tyramine (fish and cheese).

PROCARBAZINE ('Natulen')

INDICATIONS. Hodgkin's disease.

ADMINISTRATION. Orally as 50 mg capsules.

DOSE. Orally, 100 mg/m^2, maximum 200 mg, in courses of 14 to 21 days. Decrease the dose with hepatic, renal, or bone marrow dysfunction. Synergistic to CNS depression and ethanol. Procarbazine is an MAOI, so observe the drug interactions above.

ACTION. Rapidly absorbed by mouth. Plasma half-life 10 minutes. Concentrates initially in the liver, enters the CSF readily. Demethylated in the liver to produce CO_2 45 to 70% excreted in the urine as metabolites in the first 24 hours.

TOXICITY. (1) Nausea and vomiting are frequent, and may be dose-limiting. Tolerance usually develops. (2) Leucopenia, thrombocytopenia, and anaemia are not common and may be delayed for several weeks. (3) Peripheral neuropathy is uncommon. Lethargy, drowsiness, and depression. Hyperexcitability, nervousness, and convulsions (uncommon). (4) Myalgia and arthralgia. (5) Dermatitis and hyperpigmetation (uncommon).

DIFFICULTIES WITH CYTOTOXIC DRUGS

MYELOSUPPRESSION

The patient's haemoglobin must be above 90 g/l before you start. Transfuse him if necessary. Measure it between courses, and if necessary transfuse him again.

In the instructions which follow *'leucocytes' means cells of the myeloid (granulocyte) series only,* that is the total white cells, minus the lymphocytes. Monitor these by doing the total and differential white counts regularly and making the necessary calculation.

He is likely to bleed if his platelet count falls below 20,000 μl, and is almost certain to do so if it falls below 10,000 μl. You will not be able to give him a platelet rich concentrate, but your laboratory should be able to count his platelets.

The advice which follows is considered by some contributors to be overcautious. It concerns myelosuppression only; for infection see later.

No toxicity leucocytes >4000 μl, platelets >100,000 μl—give 100% of the standard dose.

Grade One toxicity **leucocytes 2500 to 4000 μl, platelets 80,000 to 100,000 μl**—give 100% of the standard dose of vincristine and 50% of the other drugs.

Grade Two toxicity **leucocytes <2500 μl, platelets <80,000 μl**—stop all drugs, wait until signs of toxicity Grade One return, and then dose as above.

Drugs are more effective at the full dose, so it is better to delay the next dose (provided the delay is not more than 2 weeks), rather than give 50% of the dose.

CAUTION ! (1) If his leucocyte count is <1000 μl Gram negative septicaemia is a danger. He may be so immunosuppressed that he shows few signs of it. Treat him as if he had septicaemia, as described below. (2) If petechial bleeding occurs and/or his platelet count is <25,000 μl, give 2 units of fresh blood. (3) Watch particularly for bone marrow depression when giving the alkylating agents, also 5-FU, actinomycin D, and adriamycin. It is unlikely with vincristine, methotrexate, or procarbazine.

INFECTION FOLLOWING CYTOXIC DRUGS

He should have been free of infection when you started (see above), so any infections which do appear should be new ones.

If the temperature of a patient on cytotoxic drugs rises over 38°C for more than 12 hours, or his leucocyte count falls below 1000 μl, start vigorous antibiotic therapy. *Gram-negative septicaemia may be difficult to diagnose in an ill and immunocompromised patient,* and is often an opportunistic infection. *Stop* cytotoxic drugs and don't restart them until his septicaemia is cured.

If you are not able to isolate the organism and give him more specific treatment, give him: (1) Ampicillin and metronidazole (2.9). Or, gentamicin 1.5 mg/kg 8-hourly (expensive) and metronidazole (2.9). (2) If he does not respond, to one of these in 48 hours, give him chloramphenicol and metronidazole. (3)

VARYING THE DOSE INTERVAL

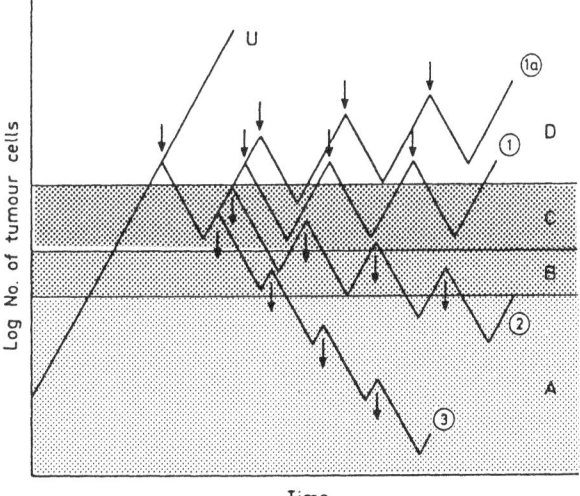

Fig. 32-2 THE EFFECT OF VARYING THE INTERVAL between courses of treatment, at the same dosage, on the size of a tumour cell population. The stages in a patient's clinical condition are the same as in the previous figure. In 1, the interval between courses allows his symptoms to return, but is short enough to maintain an essentially steady state. In 1a, the intervals are rather longer, and after the second course treatment fails to relieve his symptoms. In 2, the second course is begun before the return of symptoms, and the 5th is begun when there are no clinical or radiological signs of disease, although the tumour can be shown by special tests. In 3, the intervals between courses are short enough to reduce the tumour cell population considerably. *From the Oxford Textbook of Medicine.*

If he still does not respond, and particularly if his blood pressure falls, add a broad-spectrum penicillin to the gentamicin and metronidazole he is already receiving.

OTHER TOXIC EFFECTS FOLLOWING CYTOXIC DRUGS

Beware of impaired renal function with drugs excreted mainly in the urine—cyclophosphamide, melphalan, busulphan, and procarbazine. Don't give these if his renal function is much impaired (blood urea >17 mmol/l). If it is between 7 and 17 mmol/l (40 and 100 mg/dl) reduce the dose. Methotrexate is particularly contraindicated if his renal function is impaired. If his consumption of animal protein is low, even a blood urea of 5 to 7 mmol/l suggests renal impairment. Renal toxicity is less likely if you make sure he is well-hydrated, and is drinking 3 or 4 litres a day. If his blood urea is normal, for his diet, after a period of hydration, give normal doses. Otherwise, reduce the dose as follows.

If his consumption of animal protein is low, give ⅔ the dose if his blood urea is 6 to 9 mmol/l. Give half the dose if it is 9 to 17 mmol/l. Give none if it is over 17 mmol/l. If he has been receiving methotrexate, he will need folinic acid rescue to be extended for a further 24 hours.

CAUTION ! (1) If he has impaired renal function, avoid nephrotoxic drugs. (2) Monitor the renal function of all patients, by testing their urine for protein, and measuring their blood urea, at least weekly at first.

If he has liver disease: (1) Don't give drugs which are metabolized in the liver, or give them in a reduced dose (cyclophosphamide and the other alkylating agents). (2) Give drugs which are excreted in the bile in reduced dose (vincristine, adriamycin, 5 FU). (3) Avoid drugs which are metabolized to more active compounds (5FU). They will be less effective, and toxic effects will be more likely. If you have to use them, give them in reduced doses.

If he suffers from serious nausea and vomiting, so that his fluid balance is compromised, delay or reduce the dose, to 50% (nitrogen mustard, 5FU, actinomycin D, and procarbazone). Also give him antiemetics (see above).

If he has stomatitis or diarrhoea delay or reduce the dose (5FU, methotrexate, procarbazine).

If he suffers from the cardiac side-effects of doxorubicin ('Adriamycin'), stop it.

If he has a mild sensory neuropathy, (common with vincristine) there is no need to limit the dose.

If he has a severe neuropathy (not uncommon with vincristine), stop the drug. It usually reverses spontaneously 4 to 6 months after the last dose. If it is not severe, and there are no other useful drugs, consider giving half the dose. A sensory neuropathy ('pins and needles' proceeding to numbness) usually preceeds the motor one. Use his power to dorsiflex his ankle to monitor neuropathy. Any weakness indicates serious neurotoxicity; stop the drug.

If he has convulsions, severe lethargy, or depression (procarbazine), stop the drug.

HIS VEINS ARE NOW HIS MOST PRECIOUS POSSESSION

LYMPHOMAS, BLASTOMAS AND SARCOMAS

32.3 Endemic Burkitt's lymphoma common in the Burkitt zone

Burkitt's lymphoma is a non-Hodgkin's lymphoma, but because it behaves differently from the other lymphomas in this group, it has to be considered separately. There are two types: (1) The

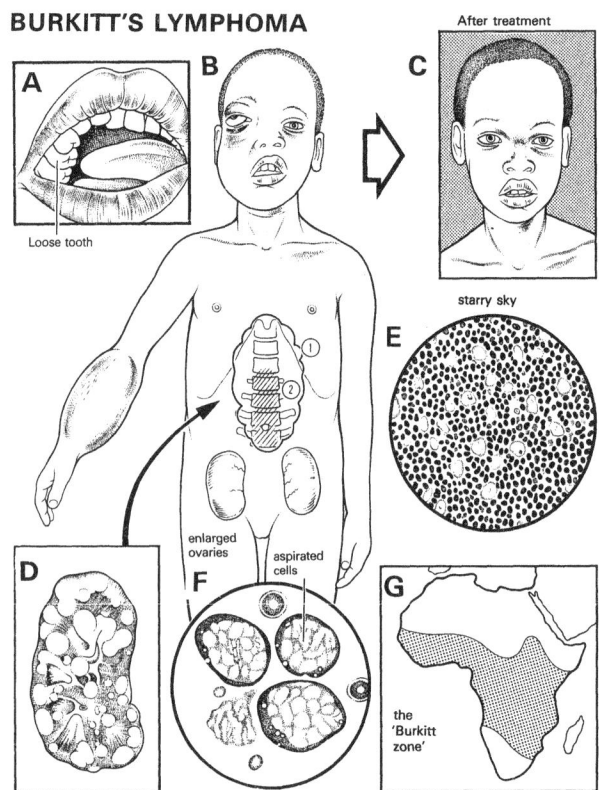

Fig. 32-3 BURKITT'S LYMPHOMA. A, a child's first complaint may be a loose tooth or displaced teeth, and the first X-ray sign, an erosion of the lamina dura of a tooth. B, a child with Burkitt's lymphoma, showing proptosis and swelling of both his upper and lower jaw on the right side. C, prompt chemotherapy is effective in over 50% of cases. D, massive involvement of a kidney. E, the characteristic 'starry sky' histology of Burkitt's lymphoma. F, if you aspirate a tumour and stain the cells with a Romanowsky stain, you may see cells like this. G, the 'Burkitt zone' in Africa, which is coincident with that of holoendemic or hyperendemic malaria. (1) a mass of retroperitoneal lymph nodes. (2) a spinal mass causing paraplegia.

Stage Three Enlarged nodes above and below the diaphragm. Survival rates, 5 years 60%, 10 years 50%.

type which is endemic in highly malarial areas, mostly in Africa, and which is associated with the Epstein–Barr virus. (2) The rare sporadic type seen all over the world, which is not associated with this virus. Here, we are only concerned with the endemic type.

Burkitt's lymphoma is a high grade tumour of B lymphocytes, and is the fastest growing tumour in man—it can double in size in 24 hours. It afflicts children from 2 to 16 (mean age 7); is unknown under 1, and is rare over 20. It is the commonest children's cancer in Africa, and in some areas it is as common as all other childhood cancers combined. In endemic areas the genome of the Epstein–Barr virus is present in 80% of tumours. 80% of well children have serological evidence of the virus, those with high titres being at much greater risk of developing the disease.

It presents as: (1) Swelling of the mandible or maxillae (one to four quadrants)—the commonest presentation in Africa. The earliest sign is loosening, or displacement, of a child's molar, or premolar teeth. (2) Proptosis, which may be marked, but is usually not painful. (3) Intra-abdominal tumours, especially of the retroperitoneal lymph nodes or ovaries. (4) Extradural lesions causing spinal cord compression and paraplegia. (5) Enlargement of the parotid glands, breasts (usually both), testes, thyroid, and kidneys, all of which are uncommon. Lymphomatous masses can also occasionally occur in skin or bone. (6) Lymph node enlargement is also uncommon, except in the abdomen. (7) Firm, painless, non-tender swellings, sometimes of huge size, anywhere in the body (rare). In spite of all this, the child's general health is usually remarkably good. When his bone is involved, X-rays show osteolytic lesions.

Burkitt's tumour is among the dozen tumours that can be cured by chemotherapy alone. Even involvement of the central nervous system is compatible with long survival. It responds so dramatically, that a child with Burkitt's lymphoma should have the highest priority for chemotherapy. His prognosis is inversely proportional to the volume of his tumour, hence the importance of:

(1) Early urgent treatment. If you can treat him before his central nervous system is involved, he has about a 50% chance of surviving 4 years, and will probably survive indefinitely.

(2) If he presents late, try, if possible, to remove the large bulk of his tumour surgically first. If you can remove more than 90% of it, you will double his survival time. Unfortunately, you are unlikely to be able to do this, except perhaps by removing a girl's ovary, or her breasts, or a mass in the mesentery. If you try, spilling the tumour is unimportant, because there will be a malignant ascites anyway.

If a child is to be treated early, and perhaps if he is to be treated at all, you will probably have to treat him yourself. There is no time for a leisurely workup—*try to start treatment in 24 to 48 hours.*

There are two important complications: (1) The acute tumour lysis syndrome is a combination of lactic acidosis, hyperkalaemia, and hyperuricaemia, and is the result of the rapid destruction of a large mass of tumour. Resection of most of the tumour before chemotherapy reduces this risk. This syndrome, and the postsurgical complications of far advanced disease, are the common causes of an early death. (2) The excretion of cyclophosphamide in the urine can cause a haemorrhagic cystitis. You can reduce both these dangers by maintaining a high urine output and by alkalizing his urine.

Williams EH, et al., 'Results of treatment of Burkitt's Lymphoma in the West Nile District of Uganda at Kuluva Hospital'. East African Medical Journal. 1982;785-92.

Williams EH, 'Rapid diagnosis of Burkitt's Lymphoma (and other soft tissue sarcomas)'. Tropical Doctor. 1981;11:68-70.

Ziegler JH, 'Cure of Burkitt's Lymphoma'. Lancet 1979;ii:936-39.

BURKITT'S LYMPHOMA

DIAGNOSIS. The fact that you are in an endemic area, the child's age, and the site of a rapidly growing tumour should alert you to the diagnosis. X-ray him. Take a standard biopsy, or a smear biopsy. If possible, send a bone marrow smear for histology, and examine his CSF for malignant cells.

RAPID CYTOLOGICAL DIAGNOSIS. Approach the tumour from the most convenient direction, usually through his mouth. Take a dry syringe and a 0.8 mm needle. Using local anaesthesia for the skin only, plunge the needle into the tumour. Withdraw the plunger a few times to draw the cells into the needle, detaching it each time to expel the air. Remove the needle and squirt its contents on to a slide, dry it, but don't smear it because this might destroy the cells. Fix it in methanol, or absolute ethanol, for 3 minutes, and stain it with Field's stain, or, better, any of the Romanowsky blood stains, such as those of Lieshman, Wright, or Giemsa.

The cells of Burkitt's lymphoma are fairly uniform in size. The cytoplasm of the cells forms a thin eccentric rim round the nucleus, is basophilic, non-granular, and usually contains some small vacuoles. The nucleus is slightly indented, and has 2 to 5 nucleoli, evenly distributed chromatin, and occasionally mitoses. You will not see the 'starry sky' appearance, because this is a histological, not a cytological finding.

THE DIFFERENTIAL DIAGNOSIS. varies with the site.

A swelling of the jaws—an infected tooth socket (5.8), perhaps with osteomyelitis (7.14a), injury (62.1), maxillary sinusitis (25.9), a dentigerous cyst or an adamantinoma (26.7), or a nasopharyngeal carcinoma (32.28). Burkitt's lymphoma usually displaces the teeth.

An abdominal swelling—tuberculous lymph nodes (29.2), other lymphomata (32.4), a mass of worms (10.6), Hirschsprung's disease (28.6a).

Other sites—inflammatory conditions and other fast-growing tumours.

STAGING. Here is Zeigler's method of staging.

Stage A One extra-abdominal tumour.

Stage B Multiple extra-abdominal tumours.

Stage C An intra-abdominal tumour with or without facial tumours.

Stage D Intra-abdominal tumours (Stage C) with tumours elsewhere other than in the face.

Stage AR An intra-abdominal tumour, but with >90% resected.

PROGNOSIS. Both cyclophosphamide alone, and the three-drug regime described below, give a complete response rate of 85%. Cyclophosphamide alone gives a relapse rate of 50 to 60%; the three-drug regime reduces this to 30%. These figures are for all stages combined. Stages A and B have a better prognosis.

If he does not relapse within 6 months of starting treatment, there is a 90% chance of a complete cure. He is unlikely to relapse after one year, if he responded completely to the initial treatment.

CHEMOTHERAPY FOR BURKITT'S LYMPHOMA

If you cannot obtain very rapid histological or cytological confirmation, and the clinical presentation is typical, start treatment without them—the tumour may grow dramatically in a few days.

Prepare him for chemotherapy as in Section 32.2.

If he has a large intra-abdominal mass, or an accessible mass elsewhere, try to resect it urgently, or refer him to have it resected. If this is impractical, start chemotherapy alone. Don't delay chemotherapy if early resection is impossible.

Triple therapy reduces the relapse rate at all stages, especially in less favourable cases (stage D), or when there is meningeal involvement, or in stage C when there is a very large tumour. Stop treatment at the end of the course—maintenance therapy is of no value.

CYCLOPHOSPHAMIDE. Give cyclophosphamide intravenously 1 to 1.5 g/m^2 every 14 to 21 days, up to 6 courses.

TRIPLE THERAPY. Give cyclophosphamide 1 to 1.5 g/m^2 on day one. Vincristine 1.4 mg/m^2 on day one. Tab methotrexate 15 mg/m^2 daily for 4 days. Start subsequent courses on the 21st day following the start of the first treatment, and repeat them until six courses have been given. If the tumour has not completely responded by this time, continue until it does so, and then give one more course. If there is no toxicity, you can give courses every 14 days.

CAUTION ! (1) Beware of the acute tumour lysis syndrome (see above), especially if he has a large tumour burden. During the first 24 hours maintain a high urine output, and alkalinize his urine with sodium bicarbonate (the adult dose is 3 g in water every 2 hours until the urinary pH exceeds 7, followed by 5 to 10 g daily). (2) If the mass is large give him allopurinol 10 to 20 mg/kg daily.

As always, explain to his parents what has happened, and what you are going to do. Tell them his prognosis, and that if his tumour does return, you may be able to treat him—but he must come for follow-up. Try to see him monthly for the first year.

PROGNOSIS WITH BURKITT'S LYMPHOMA

If he fails to respond to the initial treatment, he is sure to die in a few months, whatever you do.

If his airway, his ureters, or his gut are obstructed, the obstruction may respond to chemotherapy.

If he has had no relapse during a year after triple therapy, he has about a 90% chance of surviving indefinitely. About a third of all children have no relapses for at least 2 years, and should survive indefinitely. His prognosis with cyclophosphamide alone is less favourable.

If he has an 'early relapse' within the first 3 months of treatment, it is usually in the same site. This is common with abdominal tumours, and is probably a regrowth of the original tumour. The results of repeating chemotherapy are likely to be poor.

If he has a 'late relapse' more than 3 months after treatment, the tumour is likely to arise in a previously uninvolved site, and will probably respond rapidly to the same agent(s) used initially. A few patients have multiple successfully treated relapses, at intervals which may be as long as 10 years.

CAUTION ! Don't neglect the opportunity of saving patients in relapse. Refer them if you can. Follow them up carefully, and and treat late relapses (> 3 months) aggressively, if necessary several times—vigorous treatment in relapse can nearly double the chances of survival.

DIFFICULTIES WITH BURKITT'S LYMPHOMA

If he has CRANIAL NERVE PALSIES (often multiple) or MENINGEAL INVOLVEMENT his central nervous system is involved. This becomes increasingly common as the number of relapses increase.

If he presents with PARAPLEGIA, and you suspect Burkitt's lymphoma, treat him. If you can start treatment in the first 3 or 4 days, he is likely to do well. If you can refer him for laminectomy, do so urgently; the less the delay, the better his prognosis.

32.4 Hodgkin's lymphoma, uncommon

This disease of the reticuloendothelial system occurs all over the world, and is unusual in having a bimodal age distribution curve, with a peak in teenagers, and another in patients over the age of 50.

A patient with Hodgkin's disease may present with: (1) Enlarged, discrete, painless, rubbery lymph nodes in his neck (60%), mediastinum (15%), abdomen or groin (15%), or axilla, (10%). (2) Weight loss. (3) Fever which may simulate an infection and is classically of the Pel–Ebstein type (up for 3 to 5 days, followed by a remission of a few days, and then fever again).

The various histological types each have their own prognosis: (1) Predominantly lymphocytic (15% of cases). (2) Nodular sclerotic (50%). (3) Mixed cellularity (20%). (3) Lymphocyte-depleted (15%). Under the age of 30 the nodular sclerotic type predominates; in older patients the lymphocytic and mixed cellularity types are more common.

Initially, only his lymph nodes are involved. Later, the disease spreads to his spleen, marrow, and liver. Late complications include: obstruction to his trachea and bronchi, pleural effusion, biliary obstruction causing jaundice, cord compression, lytic and/or sclerotic bone deposits, anaemia, and infections, especially in debilitated patients.

Untreated cases deteriorate, many only slowly, and die in a few months to a few years. Radiotherapy and chemotherapy cure some of them, and cause many long-term remissions.

THE AGE-INCIDENCE OF HODGKIN'S DISEASE

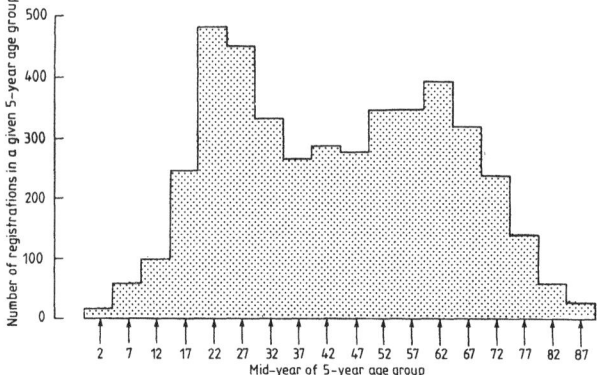

Fig. 32-4 THE AGE DISTRIBUTION OF HODGKIN'S LYMPHOMA is bimodal with two peaks. *After Mould R.F., 'Cancer Statistics'. Bristol, Adam Hilger, with kind permission.*

Chemotherapy is so successful in early cases that only Burkitt's lymphoma should have greater priority.

HODGKIN'S LYMPHOMA

DIAGNOSIS. Examine all accessible lymph nodes. Note the nature and size of all enlarged ones. Feel for enlargement of the patient's liver and spleen; assess his weight loss.

X-RAYS. Look for widening of his mediastinum and enlargement of his hilar lymph nodes.

SPECIAL TESTS. Do a total and differential white count, and count his platelets.

Before you start cytotoxic drugs: (1) Establish the diagnosis by biopsy. (2) Look for signs of infection; culture his urine, and measure his blood urea.

THE DIFFERENTIAL DIAGNOSIS includes the common causes of lymph node enlargement, with or without fever: non-specific hyperplasia, tuberculous lymphadenitis (29.2), ARC (AIDS-related complex), non-Hodgkin's lymphoma (32.5), chronic lymphatic leukaemia, and infectious mononucleosis.

Suggesting Hodgkin's lymphoma—painless, non-tender, rubbery discrete nodes with a uniform light greyish-yellow 'fish-flesh' cross-section.

Suggesting tuberculosis —enlarged nodes which are matted together, and occasionally tender; caseous areas on cross section.

STAGING AND RESPONSE. Here is the method of staging and the response rate (as measured by the failure of the disease to progress), that you can expect with radiotherapy, or the 'MOPP' cytotoxic regime described below, which are about equally effective. The 5-year survival rate also depends on the histological grading, and for all stages together on 'MOPP', it is 95% for 'lymphocyte predominant', 75% for 'nodular sclerotic', 55% for 'mixed cellularity', and 35% for 'lymphocyte depleted'.

Stage One A single group of nodes. Survival rates, 5 years 90%, 10 years 90%.

Stage Two Two or more groups of nodes on the same side of the diaphragm. Survival rates, 5 years 80%, 10 years 75%.

Stage Four Disseminated disease. Survival rates, 5 years 45%, 10 years 10%.

E, an extranodal site. A, absence of systemic symptoms and signs, such as fever. B, fever (>38.5°C), or weight loss >10%. Examples. IE, a single extranodal site, such as the spleen. IIE, enlarged nodes and extranodal disease on the same side of the diaphragm (except the liver). IIIE, enlarged nodes, and extranodal disease on both sides of the diaphragm.

RADIOTHERAPY will probably be impossible, so you will have to rely on chemotherapy. If you can refer him for radiotherapy, here are the relative indications for it.

Stages One and Two. Radiotherapy and chemotherapy give comparable results, but radiotherapy has fewer side-effects.

Stage Three. Radiotherapy is difficult because a wide area has to be irradiated; chemotherapy is better.

Stage Four. Radiotherapy is impractical, give chemotherapy.

PREPARATION. Prepare him for chemotherapy as in Section 32.2.

'MOPP' A COMBINED DRUG REGIME

'MOPP' ('Mustine', 'Oncovin', procarbazine, and prednisolone), is a well established regime.

Nitrogen mustard ('Mustine') 6 mg/m^2, maximum dose 12.5 mg, intravenously, on days 1 and 8. If necessary cyclophosphamide can replace the 'Mustine' in MOPP at a dose of 1 g/m^2.

Vincristine ('Oncovin') 1.4 mg/m^2, maximum dose 2.0 mg, intravenously on days 1 and 8.

Procarbazine 100 mg/m^2, maximum dose 200 mg, orally on days 1 to 14.

Prednisolone 40 mg/m^2 maximum dose 60 mg, orally on days 1 to 14.

GIVING THE DRUGS. Sedate him with 25 to 75 mg of chlorpromazine orally. Two hours later give the 'Mustine' and 'Vincristine' intravenously. Give the freshly made up preparations into a freely running intravenous drip. Or, give them by bolus intravenous injection, slowly and well-diluted, with the second drug 20 minutes later.

CAUTION ! A leak, especially of 'Mustine', will cause a severe local reaction, so give it with the greatest possible care.

Repeat the course on day 28 (after a 4 week interval). Give up to 6 courses, and then see him monthly. Measure his total and differential white count, his haemoglobin and his platelets weekly. Assess his response on the Karnofsky scale (32.1), and by measuring his nodes and spleen with a tape measure.

If his white count falls below 2500 µl, give half the dose of 'Mustine' and procarbazine.

SINGLE DRUG REGIMES. If you don't have the drugs for 'MOPP', you can give him cyclophosphamide 1.5 g/m^2 intravenously, repeated every 3 to 4 weeks, for six doses. Or 'Mustine', or vincristine or procarbazine, in the same doses as for 'MOPP'. These single drugs have about a 40 to 50% response rate, which is not as good as 'MOPP', but is much better than nothing.

DIFFICULTIES WITH 'MOPP'

If, as is likely, there are TOXIC EFFECTS, anticipate and manage them like this.

Nausea and vomiting from the 'Mustine' and the procarbazine seldom last for more than 8 hours. Minimize them by giving chlorpromazine beforehand. They may limit the dose of procarbazine you can use, but he usually becomes more tolerant with repeated doses.

Leucopenia from the 'Mustine' and the procarbazine; the latter may also cause anaemia and thrombocytopenia, which may present late.

Local irritation and ulceration occur if the drug leaks from a vein. Local irritation and ulceration (and peripheral neuritis) will not be helped by delaying the drugs. They take far too long to recover. If they are a major problem reduce the dose. Thrombophlebitis is also seen.

Peripheral neuritis, from the vincristine and the procarbazine, present as pain, weakness, loss of sensation, and hot palms and soles of the feet. These effects are usually reversible if the drug is stopped, but take time. In the next course of vincristine and procarbazine give only half the dose. Or, if pain is a problem, stop them at least temporarily. Stop them if there is any objective muscle weakness on dorsiflexion of his foot. Unfortunately, the response rate will then be much lower.

Ileus from the vincristine. Delay the next dose until he is better, and halve it on restarting.

Stomatitis and diarrhoea from the procarbazine (uncommon). Halve the dose.

Lethargy, hyperexcitability, and fits (uncommon) from the procarbazine. Stop the drug.

The side-effects of steroids from the prednisolone—raised blood pressure, moon face, increased weight, peptic ulceration, the unmasking of diabetes, etc. These are seldom sufficient to stop the drug, or to reduce the dose.

If he RELAPSES the possibilities are: (1) radiotherapy. (2) A second course of 'MOPP' with a response rate of about 50%. Or, (3) an alternative regime 'ABVD' (not described here) for which you will have to refer him.

32.5 Non-Hodgkin's lymphoma, uncommon

This mixed group of lymphomas is difficult to differentiate histologically, so that pathologists sometimes differ. One system of classification (Rappaport) recognizes four types, each of which can be nodular or diffuse.: (1) Well differentiated lymphocytic. (2) Poorly differentiated lymphocytic. (3) Mixed lymphocytic and histiocytic. (4) Histiocytic (reticulum cell). For the purposes of prognosis they are conveniently divided into: (a) Low grade (small cell lymphocytic and follicular). (b) Intermediate or high grade (diffuse, large cell with small cell). An epidemic of B cell lymphomas is now being reported in California in the wake of the AIDS epidemic, so expect to see them elsewhere.

Non-Hodgkin's lymphoma may present as: (1) An enlarged group or groups of lymph nodes. (2) Symptoms caused by enlarged nodes compressing a patient's trachea and/or his bronchi, his biliary tract, his gut, his urinary system, or his spinal cord. (3) Invasion of these structures. (4) Involvement of his central nervous system. (5) Fever; this is unusual and mild.

NON-HODGKIN'S LYMPHOMA

The investigations and differential diagnosis are the same as for Hodgkin's lymphoma (30.4).

STAGING is the same as for Hodgkin's lymphoma, but is less important because 90% of patients present in Stages Three or Four. The prognosis depends more on the histological type, than on the clinical stage.

PROGNOSIS. 'Small cell', high, or intermediate grade lymphomas are more likely to respond favourably. 'Large cell' ones are likely to be unfavourable. Nodular cases have a better prognosis than diffuse ones (most children are diffuse ones).

Untreated, low grade cases survive 7 to 8 years, and intermediate or high grade ones 2 or 3 years.

Here is the percentage of patients in whom you can expect a complete remission, the average remission in months, and the median survival time in months.

If the histology is favourable. Single agent (for example cyclophosphamide): complete remission 65%, average remission in months 35+, median survival 60+ months. 'COP': complete remission 80%, remission 35+ months, median survival 60+ months.

If the histology is unfavourable. 'CHOP': complete remission 68%, average remission 23 months. 'MOPP or C-MOPP': complete remission 41%, average remission 9 months.

In children, a combined regime will produce a complete remission in 80 to 90%, with a 2 year survival of 60 to 70%.

INDICATIONS. Chemotherapy is the mainstay of treatment, and radiotherapy is no better.

If a patient has asymptomatic low grade lymphocytic lymphoma, he is likely to present in Stages Three or Four. It develops so slowly that no treatment is indicated.

If he has a low grade lymphocytic lymphoma with masses of tumour tissue, anaemia, and leucopenia, treat him. A single-dose regime, for example with cyclophosphamide, is satisfactory. If necessary, transfuse him before starting.

If he has a low grade follicular lymphoma, it is likely to progress more rapidly than the lymphocytic variety. It unlikely to respond to single dose therapy, so give him a combined regime.

If he has a lymphoma of intermediate or high grade type, large cell or small cell, give him chemotherapy.

PREPARATION. Prepare him as in Section 32.2.

CYCLOPHOSPHAMIDE. Give him 1 g to 1.5 g/m^2 intravenously every three weeks up to 6 doses.

'COP'. Give him:
Cyclophosphamide 400 mg/m^2 orally on day one to 5. Or, 1 g to 1.5 g/m^2 intravenously on day 1.
Vincristine ('Oncovin') 1.4 mg/m^2 intravenously on day 1.
Prednisolone 100 mg/m^2 on days 1 to 5.
Repeat this course every 3 weeks up to 6 courses if the response is satisfactory. Then repeat it every 3 months.

Or, try 'CHOP' which is 'COP' plus doxorubicin ('Adriamycin') 50 mg/m^2 intravenously every 3 weeks.

Or, try 'MOPP' as for Hodgkin's lymphoma, or 'C-MOPP' which substitutes cyclophosphamide for 'Mustine'.

32.6 Nephroblastoma, uncommon

After Burkitt's lymphoma, nephroblastoma is the commonest solid tumour of childhood in Africa (in Caucasians it is the fourth commonest). The tumour is a hamartoma, which arises from embryonal kidney cells and spreads locally through the capsule of the kidney to neighbouring nodes (often fairly late), as well as to a child's liver, his lungs, and sometimes his bones.

A young child presents with a fairly rapidly growing and usually painless mass on one side of his abdomen. In 70% of cases he is under two years old, and is seldom over 6. In 5% of cases the mass is present at birth, and in 5% it is bilateral. He rapidly loses weight and may be febrile (50% of cases). Haematuria is late. If you see him early enough, his kidney can be removed, and his prognosis is good.

NEPHROBLASTOMA

THE DIFFERENTIAL DIAGNOSIS includes hydronephrosis (often bilateral), polycystic disease of the kidneys (uncommon, haematuria is usual), or a neuroblastoma displacing the kidney downwards (rare in Africa).

CAUTION! The diagnosis often delayed because the swelling is mistaken for an enlarged spleen. Feel for a splenic notch on the anterior border. Percuss the mass. Malarial splenomegaly is seldom marked before the age of 2.

Look for other congenital anomalies (eye defects, hemihypertrophy, and urinogenital anomalies), which are sometimes associated with a nephroblastoma.

STAGING and PROGNOSIS. A nephroblastoma is always fatal without treatment. The survival figures below are for a combination of nephrectomy, radiotherapy, and chemotherapy. Long-term cures for the first three stages are common.

Stage One Growth is confined to the kidney, and can be removed *in toto*. 95% 4 year survival.

Stage Two Growth penetrates the capsule, but is entirely excised. 85% 4 year survival.

Stage Three A large tumour, not excised completely, but confined to the abdomen. 85% 4 year survival.

Stage Four Growth widespread, with secondaries beyond the abdomen.

Bilateral disease Palliation only is possible.

MANAGEMENT. Don't try to remove the child's kidney, unless you are skilled. Diagnose the condition clinically, and refer him for investigation, nephrectomy, and chemotherapy, and perhaps radiotherapy. If this is not available, it is acceptable to rely on nephrectomy and chemotherapy. It is *not* acceptable to leave his kidney in and to give him chemotherapy only.

If you are sure of the diagnosis from the IVU and are unable to refer him quickly, you can give him one dose of the regime, but do refer him quickly.

If you are able to remove his kidney, give him the following chemotherapy.

Stage One Give him vincristine 1.4 mg/m^2 (maximum dose 2 mg) intravenously every 21 days, for 3 to 6 months. Either start 2 or 3 days after nephrectomy, or if the tumour is very large, give the first dose a week before operating, to reduce the size of the tumour.

Stages Two and Three Give him vincristine 1.4 mg/m^2 (maximum dose 2 mg) intravenously. And actinomycin D 1 mg/m^2 intravenously. Give him one dose of each of these every 21 days for 15 months. Or, give him the actinomycin only.

32.7 Retinoblastoma, uncommon

This uncommon, malignant, radiosensitive tumour of the embryonic cells of the retina usually presents before the age of two. It is bilateral in 25% of cases, and occurs in two forms, familial and sporadic. At first, the tumour enlarges within the eye; later it grows through the sclera, or chambers of the eye, to perforate the cornea. It can also spread through the optic nerve (where it may cause glaucoma) to the subarachnoid space. Familial cases are inherited as autosomal dominants. Healthy patients with one affected child have only a 5% risk of producing a second one. If a child survives, he has a high risk of transmitting the disease to his (or her) children.

The earliest sign is a squint or a fixed dilated pupil with a white reflection ('cat's eye'), and greyish white tumour visible with an ophthalmoscope. In the developing world, most children present late, with a large globe, and tumour penetrating the sclera or cornea.

RETINOBLASTOMA

THE DIFFERENTIAL DIAGNOSIS varies with the stage of presentation, and is easy after glaucoma and intraocular extension have occurred. Before this, the diagnosis can be difficult, when all you can see is a white mass in an infant's vitreous. Dilate his pupils, and examine both his fundi under anaesthesia. Enquire for a family history.

Early Traumatic perforation of the globe. Traditional medicine in the eye. Retrolental fibroplasia, (history of prematurity and oxygen therapy).

Late A corneal ulcer leading to perforation, an anterior staphyloma (due to bulging of a weak cornea, 24.3). Panophthalmitis. Congenital glaucoma (24.6).

MANAGEMENT depends on the stage at which he presents.

If he presents early with the tumour confined to his globe (unusual in the developing world), refer him for radiotherapy, which cures 85% of cases. If you cannot refer him enucleate his globe (24.14).

If the tumour has extended through his globe, but not through the the wall of his orbit, his globe should be removed and radiotherapy given; his prognosis is so poor that a long journey to a referral hospital is not worthwhile. Consider removing his globe and giving him chemotherapy. If drugs and skills are short, his priority is low.

If he presents with proptosis and a fungating mass, exenteration (24.14) of his orbit will remove the mass, but is unlikely to prolong his life.

CHEMOTHERAPY. In 35% of cases the following regime causes a partial response, and in 65% it prevents progression for a while. Give him vincristine 1.4 mg/m^2. And, doxorubicin ('Adriamycin') 50 mg/m^2. And, cyclophosphamide 1 g/m^2. Give all drugs intravenously once every 21 days.

32.8 Soft tissue sarcomas, uncommon or rare

These include rhabdomyosarcomas, fibrosarcomas, liposarcomas, leiomyosarcomas (in the stomach and small gut), malignant synovioma, dermatofibrosarcomas (on the abdominal wall, especially near the umbilicus), histiocytomas, neurofibrosarcomas, and malignant schwannomas. They all arise from mesenchyme, are commonest from the second to the fourth decades, and vary considerably in malignancy. They spread by local infiltration, and lymphatic spread is usually late. In less differentiated tumours blood dissemination may occur early, especially to the lung.

Sarcomas are relatively radioresistant. Treatment is mainly surgical. The results of radical local excision with radiotherapy are at least as good as very radical surgery involving amputation. Chemotherapy is a doubtful supplement to surgery, and is not nearly so effective as with lymphoma or nephroblastoma. Only rhabdomyosarcoma, fibrosarcoma, and liposarcoma are common enough to be discussed further here.

CHEMOTHERAPY FOR SOFT TISSUE SARCOMAS. Assess the patient carefully, and only offer him chemotherapy if the tumour is inoperable, and causes distressing pressure symptoms. Don't continue it beyond the first two courses, unless the disease is responding. Use a triple drug regime consisting of vincristine, methotrexate, and cyclophosphamide. Adriamycin 50 mg m^2 every three weeks is the best single drug.

32.9 Rhabdomyosarcoma, uncommon

Rhabdomyosarcoma is the commonest soft tissue sarcoma in Africa. It occurs more often in males than in females, usually between 5 and 25 years in: (1) The head and neck especially the orbit (25%). (2) The bladder—sarcoma botryoides ('grape-like') (30%). (3) The trunk (10%) and the limbs (10%). (4) The testis.

Rhabdomyosarcomas probably arise from embryonic mesenchymal tissue and are fairly malignant. They spread locally quite rapidly; lymphatic spread is rare, and distant spread through the bloodstream is late. Although previously considered to be tumours of striated muscle, they are now classified as hamartomas.

In sites other than the bladder or prostate, a rhabdomyosarcoma presents as a painless swelling which grows fairly rapidly; in the bladder and prostate it presents as a suprapubic mass, which you can confuse with a full bladder.

RHABDOMYOSARCOMA

DIAGNOSIS. Biopsy a large mass and do an excision biopsy of a smaller one—except in the bladder. There, establish the diagnosis with an IVU, cystoscopy, and a cystogram.

THE DIFFERENTIAL DIAGNOSIS includes inflammatory masses (pyomyositis, etc.), a haematoma, and other tumours. In the orbit consider other causes of proptosis—an orbital mucocele, retinoblastoma, etc. (24.11). In the suprapubic region consider a full bladder or tuberculous lymphadenopathy.

STAGING. The stage and differentiation of a rhabdomyosarcoma are more important than its histological type (embryonal, alveolar, etc.).

Stage I A localized tumour which has been resected completely.

Stage IA A tumour confined to muscle or to the organ of origin.

Stage IB The tumour extends beyond the muscle or organ of origin.

Stage II Regional disease which has been completely resected macroscopically.

Stage IIA Residual disease microscopically.

Stage IIB Nodal disease or involvement of an adjacent organ or structure.

Stage III Incomplete resection macroscopically.

Stage IV Distant metastases.

MANAGEMENT. Without treatment the disease progresses rapidly. Surgery is the main treatment. Radiotherapy following it does not increase the disease-free survival rate, but chemotherapy (actinomycin D with vincristine for one year) does, and 3 year survivals for orbital tumours of 90% and for bladder tumours of 30% are recorded.

If you are not sure of the diagnosis do a simple biopsy. Developing or resolving pyomyositis may need to be excluded this way.

If a mass is small (<5 cm) do an excision biopsy. Remove the entire tumour with 2 or 3 cm of normal tissue all round. Very radical surgery does not improve the prognosis.

If you yourself cannot remove the tumour entirely, but think that surgery might be possible, as in the bladder, refer the patient.

CHEMOTHERAPY. Combined actinomycin D and vincristine for one year is a useful addition to surgery, when you know the histolology. His prognosis is poor, so other malignant tumours should have priority. Long-term survival of deep-seated tumours (especially of the genitourinary tract and trunk) is unusual. Orbital tumours have the best prognosis. A suitable regime is actinomycin D 1 mg/m^2 on days 1 and 3, with vincristine on day 1, repeated every 3 weeks up to 6 courses, then every 6 weeks.

32.10 Fibrosarcoma, uncommon

Fibrosarcomas usually arise from the muscle sheath or periosteum of the thigh, lower leg, or back. The patient, who is usually between between 30 and 50, presents with a firm to hard mass which is usually painless in its early stages. Fibrosarcomas are moderately malignant, and spread by local infiltration. Lymphatic and blood-borne spread to the lung are unusual.

FIBROSARCOMA

DIFFERENTIAL DIAGNOSIS and STAGING are the same as for a rhabdomyosarcoma (32.9). 30% to 40% of treated cases survive 5 years.

TREATMENT. Do a wide local excision. Consider amputation if you cannot remove a limb tumour efficiently. Response is only temporary, so chemotherapy is of little value.

32.11 Liposarcoma, uncommon

Typically, liposarcomas occur in the soft tissues of the thigh, retroperitoneum, or mesentery, in patients of 30 years or older. There are four histological types; mixed (commonest), round cell (most malignant), well differentiated (hard to distinguish from a lipoma), and pleomorphic. Low grade varieties (mixed and well differentiated) tend to recur locally; round cell ones (rare) metastasize early. Lymphatic spread is unusual.

LIPOSARCOMA

DIFFERENTIAL DIAGNOSIS. Suspect that what seems to be a 'lipoma' is in fact a liposarcoma if: (1) It forms a steadily growing mass in the thigh or abdomen. (2) It has reddish necrotic areas on its cut surface, with cysts instead of plain fatty tissue. (3) It is difficult to shell out of the surrounding tissues.

In the thigh, distinguish a liposarcoma from pyomyositis, other malignancies, and vascular hamartomata. In the abdomen, distinguish it from other causes of an enlarging abdomen. Careful palpation will usually demonstrate the mass.

PROGNOSIS. 60% of liposarcomas never metastasize; the remaining 40% metastasize late to the lung or liver.

MANAGEMENT. Excise the tissue widely—this is difficult in the abdomen, so refer him if you can. You may have to amputate a limb. Radiotherapy and chemotherapy are of little value.

TUMOURS OF BONE

32.12 Malignant tumours of bone, uncommon

Primary tumours of bone are unusual, and have a characteristic age incidence. You will see: osteosarcomas, mostly in the 10 to 25 year age group, chondrosarcomas (15 to 50 years), Ewing's tumours (5 to 25 years) and giant cell tumours (15 to 50 years). Adamantinomas occasionally occur in the jaw, usually the mandible (26.7), and cordomas mainly in the sacrum (rare). Fibrosarcomas arising from the periosteum behave like fibrosarcomas of the soft tissues. Secondary deposits in bones and myelomas are more common.

32.13 Osteosarcomas, uncommon

About half of all primary bone sarcomas are osteosarcomas; they occur either in teenagers, or as a complication of Paget's disease in men over 60 (rare). They are aggressive tumours of osteoblasts, and either spread by local infiltration, or in the bloodstream to the lungs, often quite early.

An osteosarcoma usually presents as a painful swelling or pathological fracture of the metaphysis of the lower femur (40%), upper tibia (20%), upper humerus (10%), or pelvis (10%).

OSTEOSARCOMA

X-RAYS. (1) Typically, there is an osteolytic lesion of the metaphysis, which expands the periosteum, and produces a triangle (Codman's triangle), of increased density where the tumour meets the normal shaft. You may see lines of 'sun ray' bone spicules. (2) A few are small lesions with dense osteosclerosis round a lytic lesion with intramedullary 'fluff'.

SPECIAL TESTS The alkaline phosphatase is usually raised. Confirm the diagnosis by biopsy.

THE DIFFERENTIAL DIAGNOSIS. (1) *Very important,* early acute osteomyelitis; this causes much pain and shows no bone changes (7.2). (2) The subacute form produces a periosteal reaction. (3) Chronic osteomyelitis causes dense sclerosis, often with sinuses, and usually involves an extensive area of the shaft.

Other differential diagnoses include ordinary fractures (especially if they present late), stress fractures (fatigue fractures, 81.8), simple bone cysts, exostoses, secondary tumours, and other primary bone tumours.

CAUTION ! Osteosarcomas may cause fever.

THE PROGNOSIS is grim, and there are few long-term survivors. The tumour extends considerably beyond the area of the bone which is involved clinically, or radiologically. 75% of patients have lung secondaries when they present, or within 6 months, even if an amputation has been done.

MANAGEMENT in the past depended on amputation through the bone or joint immediately above the tumour, or disarticulation through the hip. Although the tumour is rather radioresistant radiotherapy is usually given, and is followed in 6 months by amputation, if there are no secondaries (this routine avoids amputation in those who would develop secondaries quite soon).

Some regimes increase the disease-free interval after surgery, but none increase the survival time. Here is one: it is of limited value, so it should not have high priority: Vincristine 1.4 mg/m^2 on Day 1. Actinomycin D 2 mg/m^2 on Days 1 and 3. Cyclophosphamide 1 to 1.5 g/m^2 on Day 1.

If there are no metastases, amputate if this is practicable.

If there are metastases, chemotherapy will not cure, but may be helpful for palliation or pain.

32.14 Chondrosarcoma, rare

About 20% of primary bone tumours are chondrosarcomas; they occur in the pelvis (30%), the femur (the lower rather than the upper end, 20%), the ribs (10%), and the skull and facial bones (10%). Most arise *de novo,* but about 20% arise in patients with chondromatosis, and less than 5% from patients with chondromas. They are less aggressive than osteosarcomas, and spread by local infiltration; blood-stream spread is late. Histological grading is useful in establishing the likely prognosis.

The patient presents with a bony swelling which is often slightly painful and tender. Pelvic masses are hidden by the overlying tissue, and present late.

CHONDROSARCOMA

X-RAYS show an area of translucency with trabeculae, multilocular areas of bone destruction, and scattered fluffy areas of calcification. There is usually a surrounding area of soft tissue swelling. Cortical destruction is late, and periosteal reaction is limited. You may see Codman's triangle (32.13) in limb tumours.

THE DIFFERENTIAL DIAGNOSIS includes subacute and chronic osteomyelitis, chondromas, bone cysts, fibrous dysplasia, and other bone tumours. Confirm the diagnosis by biopsy.

PROGNOSIS. Without treatment 5% of patients survive 5 years, and none 15 years. Adequate surgery enables 50% of patients to survive 5 years and 35% 15 years.

MANAGEMENT. Chondrosarcomas are radioresistant; there is no chemotherapy. You can treat most limb tumours surgically. Amputate through the bone or joint proximal to the tumour. The recurrence rate after adequate excision is low. If possible refer the patient.

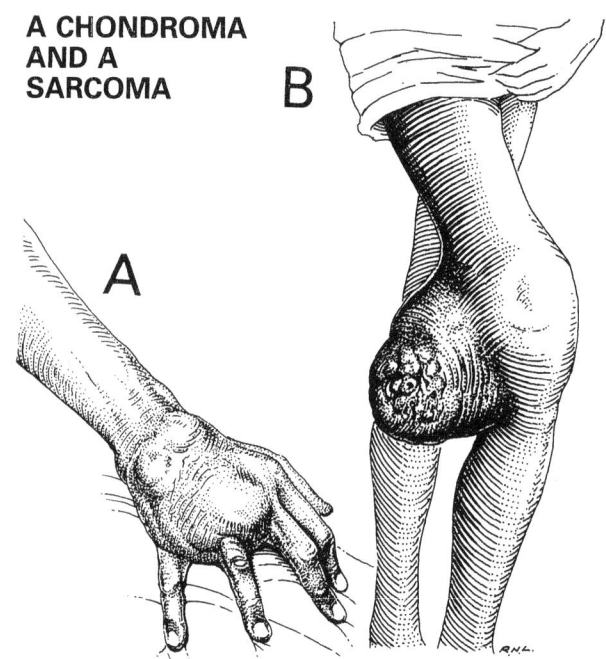

Fig. 32-5 A CHONDROMA AND A SARCOMA. A, a chondroma of the fourth metacarpal. B, an advanced sarcoma of the lower end of the right femur. *After Charles Bowesman, 'Surgery and Clinical Pathology in the Tropics', E and S Livingstone, with kind permission.*

Early rib lesions have the best prognosis. If you suspect a rib lesion and cannot refer him, resect it with at least 5 cm of rib on either side, and preferably remove some of the neighbouring ribs. He must be intubated and have a general anaesthetic, in case you open his pleura (9.2).

32.15 Giant cell tumours, rare

These unusual tumours form about 5% of all primary bone tumours; most arise *de novo,* and a few in Paget's disease of bone. The common sites are the epiphyses around the knee (femur, tibia and fibula 50%) the lower radius (15%), the pelvis and sacrum (12%), and the maxilla (26.7). They consist of giant cells (like osteoclasts) and fibroblasts, and are graded histologically as I (low grade), II (intermediate) and III (relatively malignant). First they expand the cortex, and then they spread through it. Lymphatic spread is rare, and distant metastases unusual, but local recurrence after inadequate excision is common.

GIANT CELL TUMOURS

X-RAYS. Typically, there is an eccentric osteolytic lesion in the epiphysis which extends into the metaphysis in larger tumours, and has a 'soap bubble' appearance. There is usually little sclerosis of the cortex. A defect in it is a sign that the tumour has penetrated it. In small bones there are non-specific lytic lesions.

THE DIFFERENTIAL DIAGNOSIS includes a simple bone cyst, fibrous dysplasia, a chondroma, other bone tumours (primary and secondary), and the bone cysts of hyperparathryroidism. Confirm the diagnosis by biopsy.

THE PROGNOSIS is good because metastases may never occur. After total excision 70% of patients survive 35 years. After curettage the 5, 10, and 35 year survival rates are 45%, 40%, and 35%.

MANAGEMENT. If possible, refer the patient to an expert for total excision of his lesion, and grafting of the gap; he may need an arthrodesis of his knee. If you cannot refer him, excise the appropriate area of cortex under a tourniquet, and curette the lesion. This is far from ideal, because local recurrence afterwards is common, and makes curative surgery thereafter difficult. Avoid curetting, if you can, because the prognosis after a total excision is so good. Avoid amputation, except for recurrent disease which cannot be totally resected.

32.16 Ewing's tumour, rare

Ewing's tumour is responsible for about 10% of primary bone tumours in Causasians, and is rare in Africans. It consists of densely packed small round cells, and is sometimes considered to be a lymphoma or myeloma. It commonly arises in the diaphysis of a long bone; the femur (20%), the tibia (20%) the humerus (10%), and the pelvis (20%).

The patient presents with: (1) a moderately painful, tender, warm, bony swelling, mild fever, and a leucocytosis, or (2) with a pathological fracture. There is a 30% chance that he already has widespread metastases in his other bones.

EWING'S TUMOUR

X-RAYS show a patchy osteoporosis, which is either 'moth eaten', or has defined lacunae. There is usually a periosteal reaction (typically 'onion skin') in the intermediate stage. This is not present at first, and disappears as the tumour expands.

DIFFERENTIAL DIAGNOSIS. Confirm the diagnosis by biopsy. Subacute and chronic osteomyelitis mimic Ewing's tumour closely. Other possibilities are metastatic neuroblastoma (rare), a non-Hodgkin's lymphoma in bone, and fibrous dysplasia.

PROGNOSIS. Untreated, almost no patients survive 5 years. 5 year survivals are: surgery alone 8%, radiotherapy followed by surgery 25%, surgery followed by radiotherapy 45%, radiotherapy and chemotherapy ±50%, surgery and chemotherapy ±50%.

MANAGEMENT. If possible refer the patient for radiotherapy and chemotherapy. If you cannot refer him, excise the tumour, if necessary by amputation, and give him chemotherapy.

An effective regime is: Actinomycin D, 2 mg/m^2, or 1 mg m^2 on days 1 and 3. Vincristine 1.4 mg/m^2. And, cyclophosphamide, 1 g/m^2. Adriamycin 60 mg m^2. All intravenously every 21 days for 6 courses.

32.17 Myelomatosis multiple myeloma, uncommon

This malignant tumour of plasma cells is more common than the primary tumours of bone, and causes widespread osteolytic lesions in any bone, particularly the vertebrae, pelvis, ribs, and skull. When extraosseous lesions occur, they are usually formed by tumour growing from a bone.

The patient, who is equally likely to be a man or a woman, and is usually between 40 and 70, presents with bone pain, especially in his back (75%), anaemia (50%), ill health, and loss of weight. He may also have anaemia, renal impairment, hypercalcaemia, and decreased resistance to infection. In practice, the diagnosis is difficult, because of the non-specific nature of his presenting symptoms.

MYELOMA

X-RAYS may show well defined osteolytic lesions, usually without cortical thickening or sclerosis, but sclerotic lesions can occur, especially after treatment. Sometimes, there are no discrete bony lesions.

SPECIAL TESTS. (1) Bence Jones protein is present in the urine of 50% of cases (this precipitates during heating, and dissolves again near boiling point). (2) Increased immunoglobulins in the blood (95%). (3) The alkaline phosphatase is nearly always normal, the prothrombin index is increased, and the ESR greatly so. (4) Bone marrow biopsy confirms the diagnosis, and shows many abnormally large plasma cells, with poorly defined chromatin. Take a core specimen in addition to aspirating it, because tumour cells are usually in foci.

THE DIFFERENTIAL DIAGNOSIS includes senile osteoporosis (especially when this produces kyphosis), carcinomatosis of bone and myelofibrosis.

THE COMPLICATIONS include: infections, especially of a patient's chest and urinary tract; anaemia; renal impairment due to Bence Jones protein and hypercalcaemia; pathological fractures (uncommon early but common late, especially in a patient's vertebrae and ribs); paraparesis or paraplegia due to pressure on his spinal cord by tumour extending from his vertebrae (in Africa it is the commonest primary tumour to do this); amyloid disease of his liver, gut, cerebrovascular system, or kidneys.

PROGNOSIS. Untreated, most patients die in 6 months to 3 years. Melphalan or cyclophosphamide with prednisone increase the average survival from 17 to 52 months.

MANAGEMENT. Establish the diagnosis. Treat his anaemia by transfusion. Treat infection of his chest and urinary tract. Decide if chemotherapy is possible, or worthwhile, in relation to other needs for drugs. Ask him to drink large quantities of fluids indefinitely.

If he appears to have only one tumour (solitary myeloma), you will probably be able to find other deposits, if you look hard enough. If there really is only one deposit, and it is affecting vital structures, remove it, if you can, and give him chemotherapy. Otherwise, manage it like myelomatosis.

CHEMOTHERAPY. Give him cyclophosphamide 1 to 1.5 g/m^2 intravenously on day 1. Give him prednisolone 60 mg/m^2 on days 1 to 5. Or, give him melphalan 10 mg/m^2 by mouth on days 1 to 4, and prednisolone 60 mg/m^2 by mouth on days 1 to 4. Repeat the course every 3 to 4 weeks for one year.

Adequate hydration will correct renal failure in some patients. Give him frusemide when necessary. If he has hypercalcaemia give him steroids.

TUMOURS OF THE SKIN AND SUBCUTANEOUS TISSUE

32.18 Basal cell carcinoma

The melanin in a dark skin protects it from the effects of sunlight, with the result that basal cell carcinomas, which are common in the exposed areas of white skins (including particularly albino Africans as in A, Fig. 32-6), are very rare in black ones. The earliest stage is a raised nodule, but the usual presentation is for an old, or middle-aged, man to complain of a small ulcer on his face or scalp, commonly near his eye, which continues to break down and never really heals. It has a raised rolled edge, grows slowly, and eventually erodes into muscle, cartilage, or bone. Growth is slow and metastases do not occur. Prognosis is excellent for lesions treated early, whether by surgery or radiotherapy.

BASAL CELL CARCINOMA

THE DIFFERENTIAL DIAGNOSIS includes acanthosis senilis, tuberculosis of the skin, and fungal lesions.

TREATMENT. For very small lesions, radiotherapy offers no advantages over surgery, because the diagnosis has to be confirmed by biopsy anyway; for middle-sized or large ones it is of some cosmetic value.

Excise the lesion with at least 1 cm of normal tissue all round it, which may be difficult if it has spread extensively. It will not spread to the regional lymph nodes, so there is no need to excise these. Send a specimen for histological examination.

CARCINOMAS OF THE SKIN

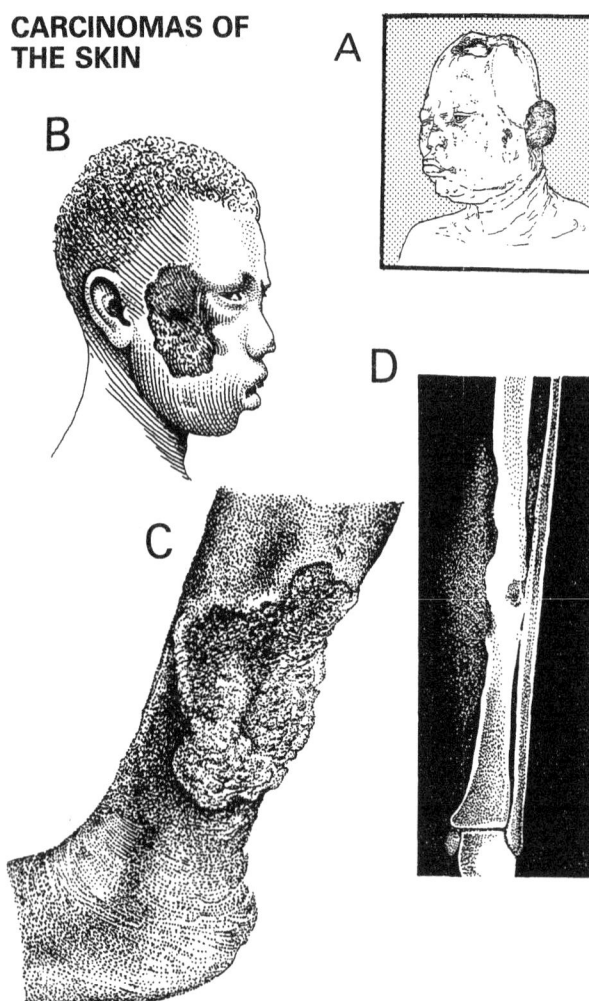

Fig. 32-6 CARCINOMAS OF THE SKIN, squamous cell carcinoma and basal cell carcinoma. A, this albino has already had several squamous carcinomas. One has eroded his skull; it was successfully excised, and his dura grafted, leaving a large depression. Another large one has now destroyed his ear. B, another albino with a large basal cell carcinoma (rodent ulcer) of the side of his face. C, a squamous cell carcinoma in the leg. Note its raised edges. D, an X-ray of the same lesion, showing bone destruction and sclerosis. B, after Charles Bowesman, 'Surgery and Clinical Pathology in the Tropics', E and S Livingstone, with kind permission.

32.19 Squamous cell carcinoma (epithelioma) fairly common

Squamous cell carcinomas are common on the exposed surfaces of white-skinned people living an outdoor life in the tropics, whether Caucasian, or albino Africans (in whom they are particularly common). They are rare in black skins, except as a complication of chronic ulcers (31.2) and burn scars. Ulcer-cancers may present late, after they have already infiltrated bone, and can cause a pathological fracture.

A typical squamous cell carcinoma of the skin presents as an ulcer with an irregular, raised, round, everted edge, and an indurated base, which soon becomes attached to deeper structures, and may erode the bone underneath. Squamous cell carcinomas develop in adult life, or, occasionally, earlier (especially in albinos). They are low-grade tumours, which spread to the regional nodes late, and rarely metastasize through the blood. In theory, prevention is simple—by covering exposed white skin, and treating chronic ulcers and burns to make sure they heal. Unfortunately, albinos from disadvantaged families face serious problems.

SQUAMOUS CELL CARCINOMA

X-RAYS. If the lesion is over a bone, X-ray it. A translucent area, under the ulcer, shows that bone is being infiltrated. Thickening of the bony cortex and trabeculae indicate secondary chronic osteitis, caused by infection, which has entered through the chronic ulcer, that caused the carcinoma.

THE DIFFERENTIAL DIAGNOSIS includes: (1) A chronic ulcer (31.2) which is not malignant—the distinction can be difficult clinically and histologically. (2) A tuberculous ulcer. (3) Yaws. (4) Syphilis. (5) Granuloma pyogenicum (34.2). (6) Fungal lesions. (6) Kaposi's sarcoma (32.21).

CAUTION ! ALWAYS confirm the diagnosis histologically first, before starting treatment.

THE PRIMARY LESION IN A SQUAMOUS CELL CARCINOMA

Try to excise a squamous cell carcinoma with all the microscopic infiltration around it. So remove at least a 2 cm margin of macroscopically normal skin around the lesion, and at least a 1 cm margin underneath it. Graft the defect (57.2).

If a squamous cell carcinoma is not infiltrating or attached to bone, give the patient a general anaesthetic, a subarachnoid (A 7.7), or an axillary block (A 6.18). Local infiltration (A 5.4) is suitable for small lesions.

If there is a satisfactory base, for example, muscle, excise any deep fascia and apply a split skin graft (57.3). Tie-over sutures (57.8) may be useful to keep the dressing in place.

If the base is not suitable for grafting (57.3), for example, if it is connective tissue, fat, or tendon, take a split skin graft, store it in a refrigerator (57.8), and apply it when granulations are satisfactory, usually in 5 to 7 days.

If bone is exposed chisel away the cortex until you reach a bleeding surface, wait 7 to 14 days for granulations to form, and then graft.

Occasionally, you can close the defect with a rotation, transposition (57.11) or, or if you are sufficiently skilled, a myocutaneous flap (not described here).

If a squamous cell carcinoma is infiltrating bone so much, that the bone would fracture, if you removed enough of it to excise the lesion properly, amputate at the first joint proximal to the lesion, for example, the knee. Or, less satisfactorily, saw through the bone at least 10 cm away from the lesion, as seen clinically or on X-ray.

LYMPH NODES INVOLVED BY A SQUAMOUS CELL CARCINOMA

If the patient's lymph nodes are not involved clinically, leave them. Follow him up carefully, because he will need a block dissection (32.34) later, if they show clinical evidence of malignancy. Don't do a block dissection prophylactically, because there is a 10% chance that he will develop lymphoedema (31.4) after it, and it will not improve his prognosis.

If his nodes are enlarged, and you think that this is caused by secondary infection, give him antibiotics, and wait two weeks. If they respond, good. If they don't, biopsy one, and follow him up carefully.

If you think that his nodes are involved clinically but are not fixed to deeper structures, or he has an advanced ulcer-cancer (most commonly in his groin), refer him for block dissection, and wide excision of the primary, at the same time. Both operations should be done on the same occasion, because he may not return to have a block dissection, if his nodes do not trouble him. Block dissection (32.34) is not an easy operation, so try to learn it from an expert, before you do it yourself—accidental injury to the femoral artery or vein may be difficult to repair (see also carcinoma of the penis 32.33). The prognosis following wide excision of the primary and block dissection is good.

CAUTION ! Explain to him carefully that he must return regularly to have his lymph nodes examined. Too often, he leaves them until they form a stinking, ulcerated, fungating mass.

If the glands in his groin are enlarged and fixed to his femoral vessels, leave them. They will fungate, but there is little you can do about this (33.1).

If his inguinal nodes become enlarged when they were normal previously, or increase in size after his amputation stump

has healed completely, but are still mobile, a block dissection is indicated (32.34).

DIFFICULTIES WITH SQUAMOUS CELL CARCINOMAS

If the patient is an ALBINO, he (or she) is particularly prone to multiple squamous cell carcinomas. Advise long skirts or trousers, long sleeved shirts, wide hats, tinted glasses, and the avoidance of unnecessary exposure to the sun, especially between 1100 and 1500 hours. The patient must report any new lumps or bumps immediately. When an albino presents with a squamous cell carcinoma, treat him in the same way as a normal person.

32.20 Malignant melanoma, uncommon

In a black patient, malignant melanomas arise only from non-pigmented parts of his skin—the soles of his feet (most commonly), the palms of his hands, his nail beds, and his mucosae. In a white patient, a melanoma can arise anywhere, usually in a pre-existing mole, especially after long exposure to sunlight, commonly on a man's trunk or a woman's legs, or, rarely, from the choroid plexus of the eye. In both black and white races malignant melanomas only occur after puberty; most are pigmented, but a few are amelanotic. They spread: (1) By local infiltration, usually horizontally at first, but later vertically into the deeper tissues. (2) To the regional lymph nodes; deposits may also grow in lymphatic channels on the way there. (3) Through the bloodstream.

Treatment is surgical; there is no effective radiotherapy or chemotherapy. Radical surgery (amputation) is no better than wide local excision.

MALIGNANT MELANOMA

PREVENTION. (1) Any elevated mole (pigmented lesion) more than 0.5 cm in diameter which shows any sign of growth should be excised. (2) White skins, including those of children, should be exposed to as little sunlight as possible.

THE DIAGNOSIS differs in black patients and white ones.

Suspect that a black patient has a melanoma if he has: (1) Any growing dark lesion on the soles of his feet, on the palms of his hands, or in his nail beds, particularly in his big toe. The commonest site is at the junction of the deeply and lightly pigmented areas on the borders of his hands and feet. (2) A deeply pigmented lesion on the sole of his foot, more than 2 cm in diameter, whether or not it is ulcerated. (3) An ulcerated lymph node in his groin, with dark areas showing through the skin, or in the base of the node.

Suspect that a white patient has a melanoma if: (1) A previously existing pigmented mole does anything unusual—if it enlarges, weeps, scabs, bleeds, itches, ulcerates, becomes darker, or produces a dark surrounding halo. (2) Any pigmented lesion grows progressively. Be especially suspicious if it is larger than 10 mm, with an irregular border, surface, or pigmentation. (3) He has a rapidly growing fleshy ulcerated skin tumour, even if it is pale (it may be amelanotic).

THE DIFFERENTIAL DIAGNOSIS includes a benign naevus (28.10), a pigmented seborrhoeic wart, a squamous cell papilloma or carcinoma (32.19), a capillary cavernous haemangioma (28.10), and Kaposi's sarcoma (32.21). Histologically, the diagnosis can be difficult.

STAGING MALIGNANT MELANOMA

This is the prognosis for cases treated by wide local excision.

Stage One. There is local infiltration only, not extending more than 5 mm from the primary lesion. Overall, there is a 70% 5 year survival.

Stage Two. A local lesion, and clinical or histological evidence of spread to the nodes. 20% 5 year survival.

Stage Three. Disseminated disease, sometimes there is no sign of a primary lesion. No 5 year survivals.

A more accurate prognosis can be obtained in Stages One and Two by examining the depth of infiltration of the excised specimen macroscopically. Stage A <0.75 cm. Stage B 0.75 to 1.5 mm. Stage C >1.5 cm. Alternatively, Clark's levels (B, Fig. 32-7) can be used.

THE TREATMENT OF MALIGNANT MELANOMA

Treatment is surgical, there is no effective radiotherapy or chemotherapy.

If you suspect that a lesion is a melanoma, but have not previously biopsied it (Stage One), excise it with a margin of at least 2 cm of normal tissue all round. Remove all the underlying subcutaneous tissue and deep fascia. If the bed that remains is suitable, graft it immediately. If not, take a graft, store it, and apply it 5 to 7 days later when granulations have formed (57.3). Take a split skin graft from the opposite limb, *not* the limb bearing the melanoma. Prophylactic block dissection of the regional nodes probably does not help. Follow him up regularly, so that if his regional nodes enlarge, you can do a block dissection or refer him for it.

If there is local infiltration, and spread to his regional nodes (Stage Two), refer him for a wide local excision, and a block dissection of his regional nodes (usually inguinal). If you cannot refer him, see Section 32.34 on block dissection. If there is growth in the intervening lymphatics (for example in the neck), excise these in continuity. It is doubtful if this improves survival, but it does remove deposits which may ulcerate.

If there is already widespread dissemination (Stage Three), there is nothing you can do, except provide terminal care (33.1).

If wide local excision is not possible without amputation,

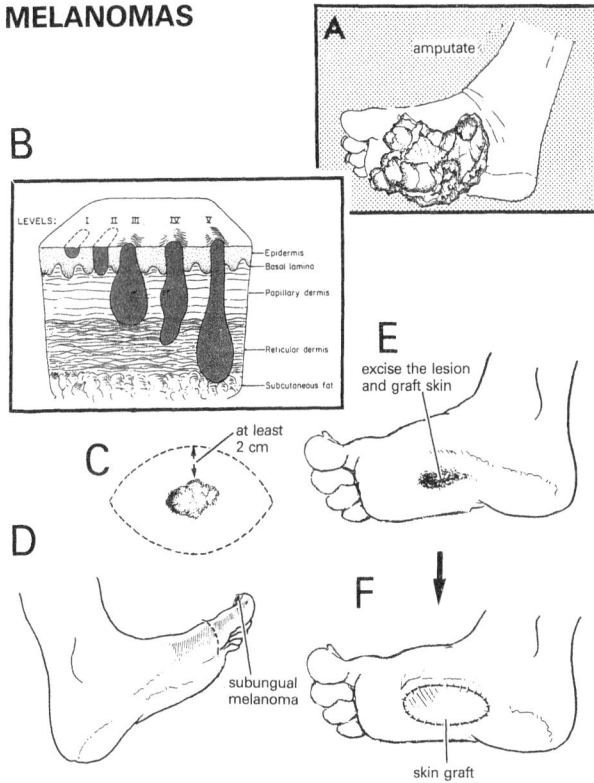

Fig. 32-7 MALIGNANT MELANOMAS. A, if a melanoma presents as late as this, remember that amputation has no immediate advantage over local excision and grafting. Amputation is only indicated if satisfactory removal is impossible without it. B, Clark's levels of invasion. Level I does not penetrate the basement membrane. Level II extends into the papillary dermis. Level III extends to the reticular interface. Level IV invades the reticular dermis. Level V penetrates the subcutaneous fat. C, excise a melanoma with a margin of at least 2 cm of normal skin round it. D, amputate a subungual melanoma. D, and E, if a melanoma of the sole presents sufficiently early, excise it and graft the wound. B, *after Grabb WC, and Smith JW, (ed.) 'Plastic Surgery: A Concise Guide to Clinical Practice'. Little Brown, with kind permission. C, to E, after Hilliard F. Seigler, in Rob C, and Smith R, 'Operative Surgery', p.221. (Butterworth) With kind permission.*

as for example under the big toe or a nail, amputate proximal to the lesion.

HISTOLOGY. If possible, send the whole specimen for examination. If this is impractical, cut it so as to make it possible to ascertain the depth of penetration, and the margins of normal tissue excised in the vertical and horizontal planes.

32.21 Kaposi's sarcoma

Kaposi's sarcoma is an angiosarcoma consisting of multiple endothelial channels surrounded by spindle cells. There are four types. The second two are related to HIV.

Classical Kaposi's sarcoma (rare) affects elderly men in the industrial world. It has a variable behaviour, and is often indolent, but not always so.

Endemic Kaposi's sarcoma (KS) has been recognized in equatorial Africa since at least the 1940's. It has an adult and a paediatric form, and is much more common in males (10:1). The patient is typically a male labourer of about 40, who has had symptoms for 18 months before the growth of his lesions forces him to seek treatment.

His symptoms start with oedema of his leg(s), usually at the end of the day, which is gone by the morning. At first his oedema is intermittent; later, it becomes more constant, and eventually ceases to pit on pressure. Once locally progressive disease has developed, the normal temperature gradient of his affected limb is reversed, so that it is warmer peripherally than it is proximally.

The indolent form (common) occurs after a variable period of oedema, as 3 to 5 mm nodules which are more easily felt than seen, and are the typical lesions of endemic Kaposi's sarcoma. They form in or under the skin of his feet and legs and less often his hands and lower arms, usually in more than one limb, and on his right arm more often than his left. Involvement is usually asymmetrical, and one limb may be normal. The nodules are usually the same colour as the surrounding skin, but may be purple. He may also have larger subcutaneous nodules along his superficial vessels. Nodules may persist unchanged for years, and disappear spontaneously, only to reappear at new sites. Traditional practitioners sometimes excise them, usually with good results. Less commonly, he has asymmetrically distributed plaques, millimetres to centimetres in diameter, starting on the sides and dorsum of his feet, and later on his palms and soles. These have a palpable edge and are darker than the surrounding skin.

The nodes at the root of his most diseased limbs are often enlarged, but he has no generalized lymph node enlargement. He loses some weight and becomes moderately anaemic. After several years he may have pleural effusions (see below), but is unlikely to have more than an occasional lesion in unusual sites (his conjunctiva, mouth, head, neck, or trunk).

The infiltrating form (common) appears in a previously oedematous limb as a diffuse, ill-defined, dark thickening of his skin and deeper tissues, with some hyperkeratosis. It is a hot 'woody' infiltration which creeps proximally to cause joint deformity, stiffness, and disability. This infiltration is more widespread than the plaques described above, and has no raised edge. It may occur alone, but is usually accompanied by nodules, or aggressively growing tumours. The bones of his infiltrated feet or hands may show periarticular osteoporosis, followed by multiple erosions, which may enlarge until his phalanges and metatarsals can no longer be seen on an X-ray. No new bone is formed, except in response to successful treatment.

The locally aggressive form (fairly common) presents as one or more rapidly growing, cauliflower-like tumours, anywhere on his feet, legs, or hands; they arise from existing nodules, which may have been unchanged for months or years. These aggressive lesions ulcerate, and discharge quantities of offensive fluid with a characteristic smell. He has other unchanged nodules proximal to the tumour and around it, and there is always the infiltration

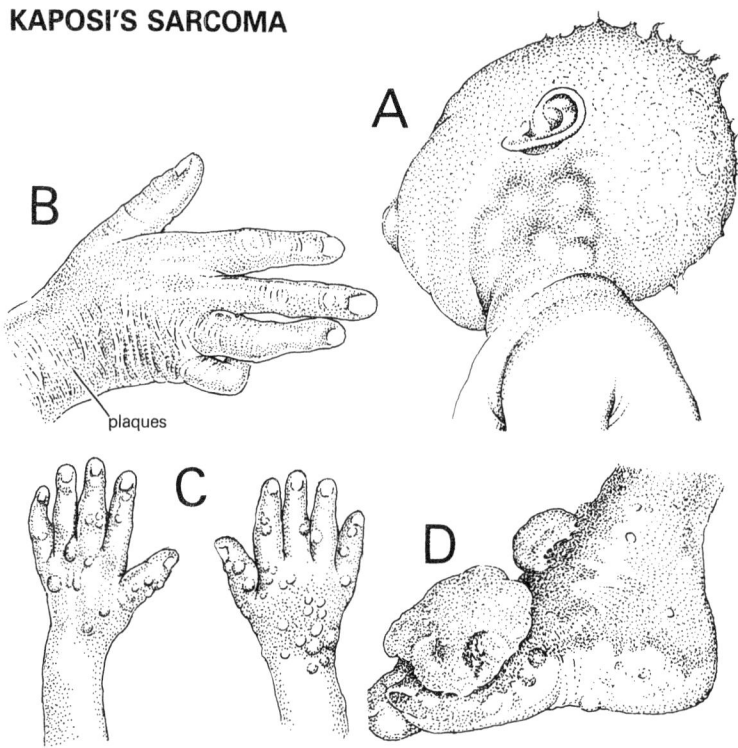

Fig. 32-8 ENDEMIC AFRICAN KAPOSI'S SARCOMA (KS). A, the lymphadenopathic form affects children and young adults. B, the infiltrating form. C, the typical nodules of the common indolent form are more often seen on the leg. D, the large cauliflower-like local lesions of the aggressive form.

described above, somewhere in the same or another limb. If he presents earlier, you may see one of these aggressive lesions before it has started to ulcerate.

The lymphadenopathic form (uncommon) presents in an African child or adolescent as symmetrically enlarged, slightly irregular, fleshy, firm (but not hard), nodes in all sites. He may also have a few atypical skin lesions.

There are two HIV-related varieties of Kaposi's sarcoma:

HIV-related Kaposi's sarcoma of Caucasians in the industrial world. This differs somewhat from that in sub-Saharan Africa.

Atypical African Kaposi's sarcoma (AAKS) was first recognized in the early 1980s. More than 90% of patients are HIV positive, and the sex ratio is more nearly equal (males to females 5:1). At presentation men are likely to have had a mean age of 35 and women of 25. The patient is likely to have had symptoms for about 8 months, which include loss of weight, and almost always a completely symmetrical generalized lymph node enlargement. You can usually find skin lesions somewhere. Look for irregular 3 to 30 mm easily palpable dark plaques, which are more common on his face, head, neck, trunk, and proximally on his limbs. You may also find them in his throat, or anywhere in his mouth (50% of cases), where they are most often seen on his palate.

The lesions on his mucosa start as a flat purple stain, which becomes raised and then nodular, before it finally ulcerates, sometimes covered by a layer of thrush. Occasionally, his entire gums are infiltrated. Sometimes, he has nodules, particularly on his insteps, and on his thighs along the line of his long saphenous veins, where there may be oedema and infiltration. He may also have oedema of his extremities, which can be severe and resemble the endemic form of the disease, but unlike the latter, it may also involve his trunk, head, and neck. There is a 5% chance that he will have no skin or mucosal changes, and if so, his prognosis seems to be better. He usually has at least one opportunist infection. In spite of all this, he may respond to chemotherapy, and return to work for months, or even years, so it is well worth giving.

Bayley Anne C, 'Atypical African Kaposi's Sarcoma'. Report to the conference 'AIDS in Africa; Naples 1987'. In press. Karger, Basle.

KAPOSI'S SARCOMA

ENDEMIC AFRICAN KAPOSI'S SARCOMA

DIAGNOSING ENDEMIC KAPOSI'S SARCOMA. Look carefully for typical nodules, which you will almost certainly find somewhere. Feel for a reversed temperature gradient, especially in the patient's legs (see above).

If he has multiple nodules, and mycetoma is rare, biopsy is unnecessary, because the lesions are so typical.

THE DIFFERENTIAL DIAGNOSIS of endemic Kaposi's sarcoma includes leprosy (30.5), fungal infections of his feet with brawny oedema, and chronic osteitis (7.13) of his feet and legs (sometimes secondary to ulceration in leprosy, 30.5), tropical ulcer (31.2), mycetoma (31.3), the hyperkeratosis of lymphedema (31.4), and onchocerciasis.

PROGNOSIS UNTREATED. The indolent type: lesions grow slowly and cause little morbidity. The aggressive type: lesions grow steadily and lead to an early death; the superficial ones ulcerate and cause considerable distress. In the lymphadenopathic type lesions also grow steadily.

MANAGEMENT. **If he has the indolent form of the disease,** he needs no treatment. Follow him up carefully, because other types may develop.

If he has any other form of the disease, he needs chemotherapy and, rarely, surgery.

AAKS ATYPICAL AFRICAN KAPOSI'S SARCOMA

DIAGNOSIS. If he has visible masses of symmetrical nodes, each 3–4 cm, AAKS is likely, so search his skin and mouth carefully for characteristic lesions, and if necessary biopsy one.

BIOPSY. is unnecessary if: (1) The diagnosis is obvious clinically. (2) He has symmetrically enlarged nodes <2 cm, because it will probably only show the reactive hyperplasia of HIV infection.

Biopsy is useful because it may reveal a treatable condition if: (1) He has symmetrical nodes (5%) >2 cm without the characteristic skin or mucosal lesions which allow you to diagnose AAKS clinically. (2) He has large asymmetric nodes (e.g. large nodes one side of his neck, and small ones, or none, on the other). If so, expect to find tuberculosis or lymphoma.

PROGNOSIS AND STAGING. In Lusaka a staging scheme has been proposed for prospective testing based on about 500 patients followed for 2 years.

Stage One. Lymphadenopathy alone (diagnosis proved by biopsy). No oral or skin lesions. A normal chest X-ray. Little or no weight loss.

Stage Two. Any combination of lymph node enlargement, skin lesions, and oral disease, without oedema of his head, neck, trunk, or bikini area. No CNS signs. A normal chest X-ray, and only moderate weight loss.

Stage Three. As for Stage Two, but with any of the following: gross weight loss, cough, dyspnoea, bilateral basal infiltration or pleural effusions, neurological symptoms (without evidence of cryptococcal or tuberculous meningitis at lumbar puncture), oedema of the trunk, face or bikini area.

SURGERY BOTH TYPES

Kaposi's sarcoma has a multicentric origin, so that radical excision is impossible. Chemotherapy can cause quite large tumours to disappear; debulking excision is unnecessary.

Amputation may be indicated (<5% of patients) if: (1) He is unresponsive to the available drugs and his tumour is still growing. (2) He arrives with advanced destructive disease of one limb, and is too septicaemic, or cachectic, to tolerate chemotherapy.

CAUTION ! Beware of bleeding. Check his platelets, always use a tourniquet, and have diathermy available.

CHEMOTHERAPY BOTH TYPES

When indicated give him:

Vincristine 1.4 mg/m^2 intravenously on day 1, and weekly for 6 weeks. Beware of ileus if he has AAKS and stop weekly injections if it occurs.

And, actinomycin D as a bolus intravenous injection of 1 to 1.5 mg/m^2 on Day 1, and then every 21 days for 6 doses. Warn him that he may lose several kilos during the first 3 or 4 weeks as his oedema resolves.

The first signs of a satisfactory response (90% of patients) are cooling of the affected limb, and diminished itching, pain, and oedema. At about 3 weeks nodules and florid tumours begin to flatten, and shrink, and many may finally disappear, to leave only a small scar. Continue treatment for 3 to 6 courses, until no tumour remains, or it ceases to respond. To distinguish infiltration from residual fibrosis, remember that fibrosis is cool, but infiltration is hot.

See him regularly, and warn him that his disease may recur, usually in 1-2 years. If so, treat him as before, and he will usually respond. If he ceases to respond and needs a second-line drug, use adriamycin (preferably), bleomycin, or daunorubicin.

If radiotherapy is available, it will speed the resolution of localized tumours, but chemotherapy is probably also necessary.

If he is sputum-positive for AAFB (only seen with AAKS), start antituberculous treatment 10 days before chemotherapy.

RESPONSE on treatment. KS: 87%. AAKS: 61%.

SURVIVAL after treatment. KS: unknown, but probably >8 years. AAKS: Stage One unknown but several patients have survived >3 years. Stage Two >3 years. Stage Three 7.5 months.

DIFFICULTIES WITH AAKS

If he has a DRY COUGH, which does not produce sputum, but produces streaky haemoptyses after a few weeks, suspect PULMONARY AAKS (this is commonly misdiagnosed as tuberculosis). He rapidly becomes progressively breathless, and may be breathless and cyanosed even while receiving oxygen at rest, fighting to oxygenate himself with every accessory muscle. Early, the only radiographic signs are mildly increased bronchovascular markings. Soon, he has reduced air entry at his bases, with fine crepitations that do not disappear on coughing, and a bilateral symmetrical fluffy infiltrate, most marked in his perihilar and basal zones, which usually spares his apices completely (unlike tuberculosis, which usually involves the apices and is asymmetrical). The infiltrate resembles pulmonary oedema, but does not respond to digoxin, diuretics, or steroids. Chemotherapy for AAKS will usually improve his dyspnoea rapidly, so that he can discontinue oxygen in 3–4 days, and be out of bed in a week. His X-ray lesions will start to resolve in 3–4 weeks, and may resolve completely, if he survives long enough.

TUMOURS OF THE GASTROINTESTINAL TRACT

32.22 Carcinoma of the mouth and lips common in India

Carcinoma of the mouth is one of the commonest malignant tumours in India. It is a disease of the poor, of both sexes, and may be due to: (1) Chewing 'pan' (betel leaf) with tobacco and slaked lime, and keeping the chewed 'cud' in the mouth. (2) Reverse or 'chutta' smoking. (3) Smoking cheap 'bidis' (rolled tobacco leaves). And, (4) poor oral hygiene. Pan masala (spiced betel nut) is the latest fad in India, and is likely to add to the incidence of cancer of the mouth. This is an entirely self-inflicted disease, and is potentially completely preventable by health education.

The patient, who is usually elderly, presents with: (1) A painless mass. (2) An area of thickening or induration, (3) an ulcer. (4) A sore throat or dysphagia (late). And, (5) inability to open his mouth (trismus). Because the disease is painless, poor patients are usually unaware of the danger and present late. Yet the mouth is easily accessible, and if only health workers, especially junior ones, would examine the mouths of their patients more often, this carcinoma would be diagnosed earlier.

Carcinoma can occur anywhere on a patient's lips, or inside his mouth. It most commonly involves his buccal mucosa, but it may involve any part of his tongue, the floor of his mouth, his alveolus, or his hard palate. It commonly occurs in his gingivobuccal groove—where he keeps his 'cud'.

There are several kinds of tumour: (1) Squamous cell carcinomas (95%). A few of these are slow-growing, cauliflower like, 'verrucous carcinomas' with a good prognosis. (2) Adenocarcinomas arising from ectopic salivary glands (5%). (3) Sarcomas (rare). Most tumours spread to the lymph nodes on the same side, and blood-stream spread is rare. His prognosis depends the extent of his local disease, and whether or not he has cervical metastases.

Precancerous lesions occur as: (1) leukoplakia (dyskeratosis), (2) erythroplakia (leukoplakia interspersed with reddish spots), (3) white vascular bands of submucous fibrosis, (4) chronic dental ulcers. Black-pigmented spots are harmless.

Surgery and/or radiotherapy gives excellent results, in early cases. In late ones radiotherapy reduces bleeding, discharge, and smell, and is useful palliation. If the buccal mucosa is involved, radiation is enough; but if bone is involved, resection is also necessary. Resection of the jaw is not described here, but if carcinoma of the mouth is common in your area it is well worth learning and is not too difficult.

CARCINOMA OF THE MOUTH AND LIPS

EXAMINATION. Encourage your junior health workers to examine their patients' mouths. Any ulcer or lump in the mouth,

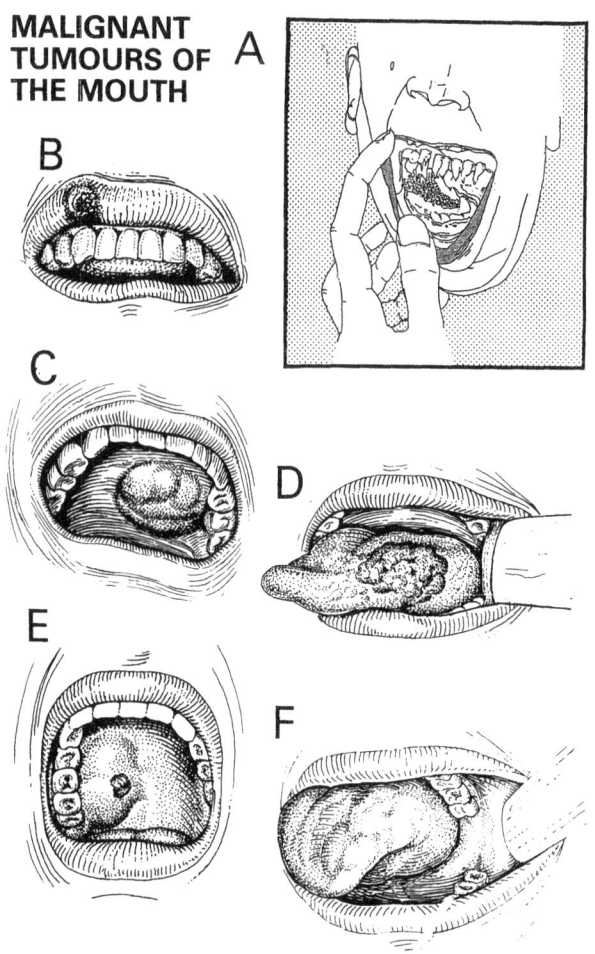

Fig. 32-9 MALIGNANT TUMOURS OF THE MOUTH. A, a carcinoma of the labio-gingival sulcus. B, an early carcinoma of the lip. C, a mixed tumour of the palate. D, carcinoma of the side of the tongue. E, a carcinoma of the palate starting to ulcerate. F, leucoplakia of the tongue; this is a precancerous condition. *B, to F, adapted from drawings by Frank Netter, with the kind permission of CIBA-GEIGY Ltd, Basle (Switzerland).*

which does not respond to treatment in 2 weeks, should be suspected of being carcinomatous, and biopsied. Feel for enlarged nodes in the patient's neck.

SPECIAL TESTS. Confirm the diagnosis with a punch or incision biopsy. X-ray his mandible, or maxilla, to detect local infiltration. X-ray his chest.

STAGING. This is the UICC method. T_1 nodes <2 cm. T_2 nodes 2 to 4 cm. T_3 nodes >4 cm. T_4 infiltration of skin, muscle and bone. N_0 no nodes felt. N_1 mobile ipsilateral nodes. N_2 bilateral nodes. N_3 fixed nodes. M_0 no systemic metastases. M_1 systemic metastases.

Stage One $T_1 N_0 M_0$ Curable
Stage Two $T_2 N_0 M_0$ Curable
Stage Three $T_3 N_0 M_0$, or T_1, T_2 or $T_3, N_1 M_0$ Curable
Stage Four $T_4 N_0 M_0$ occasionally curable. All further lesions are incurable.

MANAGEMENT. You can only treat these patients in the earliest stages.

If he has a lesion of less than 1 cm on his lips or tongue, excise it with a margin of at least 1 cm. Refer all other patients for chemotherapy, followed by radiotherapy and/or surgery. If no radiotherapy is available, and he has a carcinoma of his tongue, refer him for a partial glossectomy, perhaps with chemotherapy. Verrucous carcinoma is best treated by surgery only, because radiotherapy causes it to become a rapidly growing anaplastic lesion.

If he has cancer of his mouth, and you can feel nodes in his neck when he presents, he is probably incurable.

If, (1) his primary is potentially curable by radiotherapy (first choice) or surgery, and (2) his nodes are mobile, and (3) he has no distant metastases, skilled surgery has about a 25% chance of cure.

If nodes appear months or years after the primary has been treated, *and are still mobile*, radical dissection has a 30–50% chance of cure.

Node biopsy probably has no place. His nodes may be enlarged by infection. If in doubt, try antibiotics for a few days, and see if they become smaller.

CHEMOTHERAPY is not curative, but there is a 20% response rate to twice weekly intravenous methotrexate at 40 mg/m^2, with little further benefit from multidose regimes, or more expensive drugs.

32.23 Salivary gland tumours, uncommon

About 85% of salivary gland tumours occur in the parotid gland (A, and B, Fig. 32-10), 10% in the submandibular gland, and 5% in the mucous secreting glands inside the mouth, especially on the palate (C, Fig. 32-9). Similar tumours occasionally arise from the lachrymal gland (24.10).

There are several histological varieties:

The relatively benign ones are: (1) pleomorphic adenomas, (2) monomorphic adenomas, (3) and adenolymphomas (usually cystic).

The more malignant ones are: (4) adenocarcinoma (including cylindroma), (5) muco-epidermoid carcinoma, (6) pleomorphic adenocarcinoma, and (7) squamous cell carcinomas. Malignant tumours need radical excision, but even after this, some recur locally. Spread to the lymphatics and bloodstream is usually late. In Caucasians, 80% of salivary gland tumours are fairly benign pleomorphic adenomas, which may infiltrate the 'capsule' of the gland, but do not metastasize. In Africans, only 50% of tumours are of this kind.

The patient presents with a slowly growing mass in one of his salivary glands, usually his parotid, but occasionally at an 'ectopic' site inside his mouth, particularly in his hard palate. If he has any sign of a facial palsy, his facial nerve is involved, and his tumour is malignant. Unfortunately, the absence of a facial palsy does *not* mean that his tumour is benign.

SALIVARY GLAND TUMOURS

THE DIFFERENTIAL DIAGNOSIS includes: (1) Leukaemic deposits in a patient's salivary glands (examine his blood). (2) Enlarged lymph nodes in his parotid gland, from either non-specific infection, or tuberculosis (unusual). (3) Hypertrophy of the gland, due to obstruction by a stone.

CAUTION ! Don't biopsy the growth. This may spread a pleomorphic adenoma locally, and you may damage his facial nerve.

MANAGEMENT. Facial palsy is the critical sign.

If he does not have a facial palsy his growth should be excised completely, and not merely shelled out. This makes sure that the commonest lesion (a pleomorphic adenoma) is completely removed, and will not recur. He needs a conservative parotidectomy, in which the fine branches of his facial nerve are dissected out, and the part of the gland containing the growth removed; either its superficial part, its deep part, or both.

If he has a facial palsy, his prognosis is poor, even after radical surgery and radiotherapy.

Both conservative parotidectomy and radical resection are difficult—refer him to an expert. This is important, because the correct surgery will cure a pleomorphic adenoma, if it is early.

32.24 Carcinoma of the oesophagus, fairly common

Carcinoma of the oesophagus is fairly common in India and much of sub-Saharan Africa, and is associated with the drinking of home-brewed spirits containing carcinogenic nitrosamines. In many parts of the developing world it is the commonest cause of dysphagia.

The patient, who is usually over 45, presents with: (1) Progressive dysphagia, first for solid food and later for thin foods and even water. If you ask him to point to the site where food sticks, it will usually correlate well with the site of the lesion. (2) Regurgitation; this is common, except in the early stages; he may describe it as vomiting. (3) Hunger, which can be very distressing. (4) Weight loss. (5) Coughing on swallowing, due either to a tracheo-bronchial fistula, or to spillage from his oesophagus, through his larynx into his trachea. This happens when the lesion is in the upper, or in the middle, third of his oesophagus. (6) Pain is a late symptom, and is due to spread into his mediastinum.

If you are going to do anything for him, you will have to oesophagoscope him (25.14), and assess his operability on the criteria below. Unfortunately, you will not find many operable cases to refer to a thoracic surgeon for resection and: (1) a gastro-oesophageal anastomosis, or (2) the transfer of a segment of his left colon to bridge the gap. Radiotherapy is a useful palliative. There is no effective chemotherapy.

Palliate a patient with an inoperable carcinoma with a Celestin or Procter–Livingstone tube. It will let him swallow thin food and fluids, and relieve his distressing hunger and dehydration. It will allow him to survive some months in relative comfort, for which he will be very grateful. He may live for 18 months, and die from other complications without the tube becoming blocked. If you can refer him, palliative radiotherapy can be given with his tube in.

If possible, refer patients for the insertion of tubes, but if this is difficult, learn how to insert them yourself from an expert. If carcinoma of the oesophagus is common in your district, this is a procedure worth learning, it will save many patients much misery.

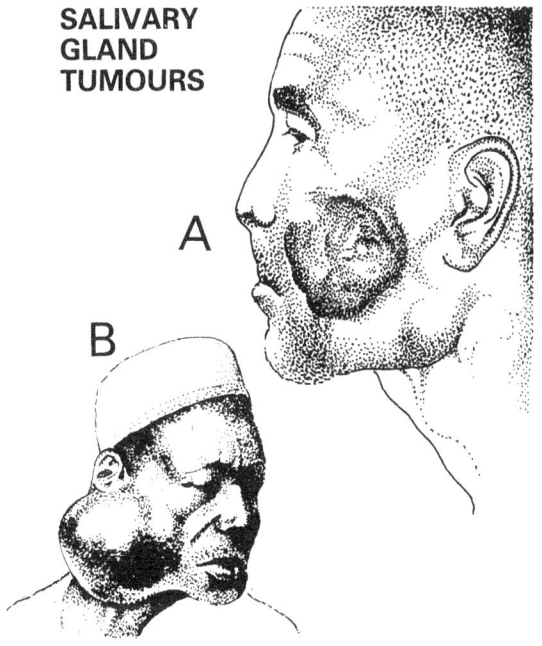

Fig. 32-10 SALIVARY GLAND TUMOURS. A, an inoperable adenoid cystic carcinoma of the left parotid, with extensive ulceration and secondaries in the patient's cervical lymph nodes. B, a large pleomorphic adenoma, which has grown slowly over 20 years. *After Adekeye and Robertson, with the kind permission of the editor of Tropical Doctor.*

• TUBES, oesophageal, Celestin, with guide, 20 assorted tubes only (optional). Alternatively, TUBES, Procter–Livingstone (POR), 10 mm diameter, length 110 mm, 150 mm, and 190 mm, unflanged, 20 tubes only. A Celestin tube is inserted on a guide, and the stomach has to be opened. A Procter–Livingstone (P–L) tube is inserted over a bougie without opening the stomach. An expert can insert one in 5 minutes.

CARCINOMA OF THE OESOPHAGUS

X-RAYS. See Section 34.5.

OESOPHAGOSCOPY AND BIOPSY. Do this as in Section 25.14.

THE DIFFERENTIAL DIAGNOSIS will depend on the area in which you are working.

Suggesting dysphagia due to the iron deficiency syndrome—the patient is a woman, uncommon in India and Africa; a post-cricoid web in a barium swallow.

Suggesting a fibrous stricture, due to regurgitation of acid from the stomach, or swallowed corrosive acids or alkalis, — a relevant history: the latter is not uncommon in parts of SE Asia.

Suggesting achalasia of the cardia —a younger age group, usually 15 to 25 years, not uncommon in India but uncommon in Africa.

SITE. Expect to find a carcinoma in the following sites in this order of frequency: (1) In the middle third (26 to 35 cm from the upper incisor teeth). (2) In the lower third (36 to 45 cm). (3) In the upper third (17 to 25 cm).

OPERABILITY AND MANAGEMENT. The few suitable cases for oesophagectomy are likely to have: (1) A lesion which is not more than 5 cm long on a barium swallow (microscopically, the tumour may extend at least as far again in each direction). (2) No mediastinal widening (no enlarged nodes). (3) A lesion which narrows the oesophagus by less than 50%. (4) No deformity of the trachea, carina, or left main bronchus on bronchoscopy. If you find such patients, refer them.

CAUTION ! Some surgeons advise that you should not be tempted to make a stoma, which will only prolong the patient's agony, and will not solve the distressing problem of his inability to swallow his saliva. If you make one, make a feeding jejunostomy, as in Section 9.7.

INSERTING A CELESTIN TUBE FOR CARCINOMA OF THE OESOPHAGUS

INDICATIONS. A patient who cannot swallow solid food, and who has some difficulty with thin food, or water. Even if he cannot swallow water, you may be able to pass a tube.

CAUTION ! (1) The earlier he presents, the easier it will be to pass the tube. Don't wait until dysphagia is severe—you may not get it in. (2) Refer him if you can: there is no substitute for being taught this procedure by an expert.

EQUIPMENT. Oesophagoscope, oesophageal bougies. Celestin tubes and a guide. A very efficient sucker.

PREPARATION. Two operators are needed: Operator A passes the oesophagoscope and the Celestin tube with its guide, from above. Operator B does a laparotomy, guides the tube into place through a gastrostomy, and fixes it to the stomach wall.

If the patient is dehydrated, rehydrate him intravenously for 1 or 2 days before you start, and have a drip running. Give him a general anaesthetic, or ketamine, and intubate him under relaxants (A 8.4). You will not be able to pass a naso-gastric tube because of the obstruction.

METHOD. Lay him on his back, with some rise in the table extending his spine under his upper abdomen. If your table does not open to allow this, place a thin pillow under him. Lay him with his head down a little.

OPERATOR A. Sit at the head of the table, and raise it enough to to make passing a rigid oesophagoscope convenient (this may mean that Operator B may have to use a foot stand).

Pass the largest oesophagoscope you have in the usual way (25.14). Suck out the contents of his oesophagus—there will be much fluid and debris. Pass the oesophagoscope further, until you see the obstruction. Clear away any more debris, and note the distance of the lesion from his upper incisor teeth. This will later help you to know if you have pulled the tube down

INSERTING A CELESTIN TUBE

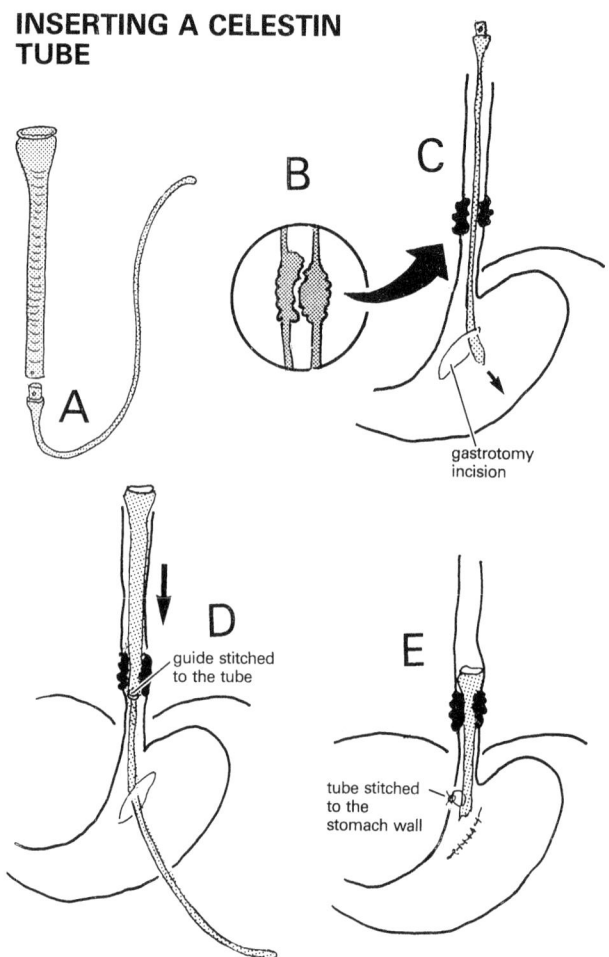

Fig. 32-11 INSERTING A CELESTIN TUBE. A, the tube with its guide. B, a carcinoma obstructing the oesophagus. C, the guide being passed through the tumour, and out through an opening in the stomach. D, the tube being pulled through the stricture. E, the lower end of the tube cut off and sutured to the stomach wall.

enough—you won't know how far in to push it, if you don't remember the distance.

Dilate the stricture, starting with a thin, but fairly stiff bougie of 10 or 12 Ch. Dilate it up to 24 or 30 Ch if this is easy, but if it is difficult, stop, rather than make a false passage. Judging when to stop dilating, and how hard to force the tube in, are the most difficult decisions. Pass the bougie as far as possible under direct vision, so that you can manoeuvre it through the stricture. If necessary, lower his head to allow the tip of the oesophagoscope to point anteriorly. If he is very thin, you may see the tip of the bougie pressing against his stomach wall. When you remove the bougie, measure it against the oesophagoscope, and the front of his chest, to see if it has reached his stomach, or not.

If you have not previously taken a biopsy, take two pieces of tissue now from the top of the lesion.

Pass the guide through the oesophagoscope into his stomach, where Operator B will feel it, and pull on it. Sometimes, it passes behind the stomach, through a false passage, but this, fortunately, does not often cause mediastinitis. If it is not in the right place, reinsert it. If you fail 3 times, pass it by railroading (see below).

When the upper end of the guide is about 10 cm from his teeth, remove the oesophagoscope, and fix the tip of the guide to the Celestin tube using a non-absorbable suture, such as No. 1 multifilament silk, and a straight needle. Lubricate the Celestin tube with KY jelly.

When the top end of the Celestin tube is in the patient's pharynx, re-insert the oesophagoscope, and use it to help guide the Celestin tube down to Operator B, who pulls on the guide.

Mostly, he pulls: but you may have to push a little with the oesophagoscope.

Check that the upper end of the tube is sitting snugly on the top of the stricture—don't let it go down too far; if it does, pull it up with blunt biopsy forceps.

Remove the oesophagoscope.

OPERATOR B. Meanwhile, do a laparotomy through an upper median or left paramedian incision. Feel the patient's aortic nodes and the cardia, to see if his tumour has spread.

If his stomach is shrunken and difficult to find and pull down, as it often is in a starving patient, there may not be much space on the anterior surface for making an incision. You may need to grasp it with Babcock's, or Allis' forceps, or stay sutures, to keep it in the wound.

Wait until Operator A has passed the guide. When you feel it through the stomach wall, do a longitudinal gastrotomy in the anterior wall of the stomach, about a third or halff-way distal to the cardia. Allow the tip of the guide to poke out of the gastrotomy wound. When the guide is in the stomach and Operator A has attached the Celestin tube, pull it gently down, until you feel resistance. This should be when the flange rests on the top of the growth. Co-operate with him carefully!

When the tube is in place, detach the guide and cut the tube, so that it reaches a third of the distance from the patient's cardia to his pylorus. Cut it off obliquely so as to leave a long anterior flange. Anchor the lower end of the tube with No. 2 monofilament to the anterior wall of his stomach. Make it flush with the anterior wall by passing the suture through the flange of the tube and the stomach wall, to one side of the gastrotomy, or proximal to it.

Close the gastrotomy with 2 layers of continuous sutures (the inner one of catgut). Close his abdominal wall with interrupted monofilament or steel sutures.

INSERTING A PROCTER–LIVINGSTONE TUBE FOR CARCINOMA OF THE OESOPHAGUS

Proceed as for a Celestin tube, except that a gastrotomy and a second operator are not needed.

Dilate the stricture with bougies through the oesophagoscope as far as possible as above. Choose a P–L tube of the right length (110mm, 150mm or 190mm).

Take the largest bougie that will comfortably go through your chosen P–L tube, and attach a long, strong monofilament thread to its proximal end; if necessary bore a hole for this.

INSERTING A PROCTOR-LIVINGSTONE TUBE

Using an oesophagoscope and a bougie

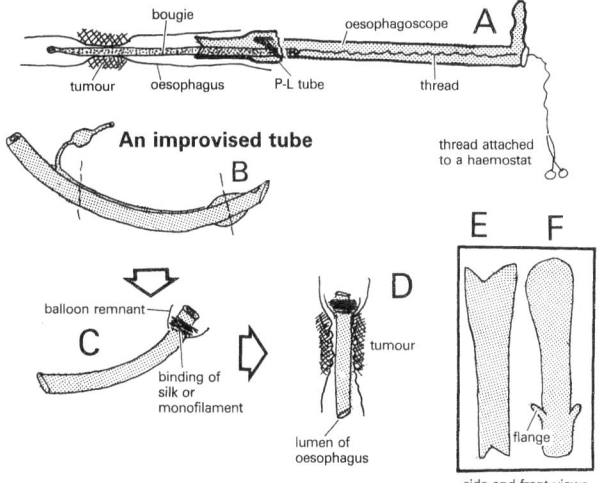

Fig. 32-12 INSERTING A PROCTER–LIVINGSTONE TUBE. A, a bougie has been passed, and a thread attached to it has been drawn through the oesophagoscope, which is being used to insert a Procter–Livingstone tube. B, a tracheal tube about to be cut, to make an improvised oesophageal tube. C, the improvised tube ready for use. D, the improvised tube in place. E, and F, anterior and lateral views of a flanged Procter–Livingstone tube; some P–L tubes are unflanged. *Kindly contributed by Ian Kennedy.*

You may need this to recover the bougie if it gets forced too far down.

With the oesophagoscope still in place, pass the bougie (with the thread attached, and well-lubricated throughout its length) through the stricture. Don't remove the oesophagoscope until after you have inserted this bougie. Now remove the oesophagoscope leaving the bougie in place. Lubricate the P–L tube well inside and out, pass the thread through it, and slide it on to the bougie. Pass the thread through the oesophagoscope, and hold its end in a haemostat (A, in Fig. 32-12).

Slide the tip of the oesophagoscope over the end of the bougie, and engage it in the cupped upper end of the P–L tube. Guide the P–L tube into the patient's mouth and pharynx with your left hand, and then push it down the bougie with the oesophagoscope. When it reaches the tumour, you will feel resistance. Now push harder. You will feel the P–L tube passing through the stricture, until you feel its cup being stopped by the upper end of the stricture.

Watch the centimetre scale on the oesophagoscope, as it passes his teeth, so that you don't push too far. Note the distance—it should not be more than a centimetre greater than the distance to the tumour.

Remove the bougie, twist the oesophagoscope slightly to disengage it from the cup of the P–L tube. Look down the oesophagoscope to see that all is well. Suck out blood and tumour debris. Remove the oesophagoscope under direct vision, sucking out until all is clear.

POSTOPERATIVE CARE Continue intravenous fluids, until he is swallowing well, which will not be for some days.

DIFFICULTIES WITH OESOPHAGEAL TUBES

If you have DIFFICULTY PASSING THE GUIDE (Celestin tube) OR THE BOUGIE (P–L tube), which is not uncommon with tight strictures in the lower third of the oesophagus, 'railroading' is necessary. Ask operator B to pass a bougie up the oesophagus, and deliver its tip through the patient's mouth. Beware, you can as easily make a false passage going up, as going down! Tie the tip of the bougie side to side with the end of the guide, overlapping it for about 5 cm. Then pull the guide through the malignant stricture, detach the bougie and proceed as above.

If railroading fails (unusual), leave a large de Pezzer or Foley catheter in the stomach as a gastrostomy for feeding. Dilatation may work at a second attempt, but it is probably best to leave the Foley catheter in place. Alternatively, do nothing, you may only be prolonging his agony.

If you make a FALSE PASSAGE or tear the stricture, a rapidly (24 hours) fatal mediastinitis may follow. Life without a tube is so intolerable that you will have to take this risk.

If the BOUGIE PASSES, BUT A CELESTIN OR P–L TUBE WILL NOT PASS, you may need considerable force, even after what seems like good dilatation. Only one diameter (10 mm) of P–L tube is made, and it does not pass every stricture.

Either make a home made tube (B, 32-12). Take a plastic tracheal tube of suitable size, cut off the tip with half the balloon. Wind thick silk or nylon under the balloon remnant to make a bulge. Cut the tube long enough for the stricture, and bevel the other end to make it easier to pass. With the oesophagoscope in place, pass the improvised tube with long forceps under direct vision until its bulbous end is snug up to the top of the carcinoma. He will only be able to take thick liquids, but he will be able to swallow. You may be able to stretch and dilate some plastics with heat, so as to make a cup.

Or, use a wire stylet. Get a long piece of wire from the workshop which will just pass down the whole length of an 18 Ch nasogastric tube. Lubricate it well and pass it through the tube. Pass the stylet and tube through the oesophagoscope, through the stricture and into his stomach. Remove the stylet. Pass a long nasotracheal tube down his nose, recover its distal end from his throat, bring it out of his mouth, push the end of the nasogastric tube into it, and pull this back through his nose. Tape the nasogastric tube to his cheek.

CAUTION ! Don't try to pass the wire stylet down on its own.

Bandage his elbows in extension with rolled newspaper to prevent him removing the tube as he recovers from the anaesthetic. A nasogastric tube is not as satisfactory as a P–L tube. A gastrostomy, which is a possible alternative, will not enable him to swallow his saliva, and is such poor palliation that it is probably never justified (see above).

If you PUSH THE TUBE PAST THE STRICTURE (unusual), you may be able to pull it back with strong forceps. If this fails, leave it.

If he REGURGITATES THE TUBE, this is a nuisance, but not a disaster. If possible, replace it by a flanged tube. The shorter the tube, the better it works, but the more easily it slips out. If it is too short, the tumour may grow over the end and obstruct it. Flanged tubes are more likely to stay in place.

If the TUBE BLOCKS, a barium swallow will show the obstruction. Oesophagoscope him.

32.25 Carcinoma of the stomach, fairly common

A patient with carcinoma of his stomach is likely to be a male over 40 (male to female ratio 3:1) who presents with: (1) Dyspeptic symptoms; unfortunately these are so common that the selection of cases for further investigation is difficult. Initially, a patient with carcinoma of his stomach only has vague upper epigastric discomfort with meals, or a feeling of fullness. These non-specific symptoms may last for months, before he presents with anorexia, nausea, and increasingly severe dyspepsia. His pain lacks the periodicity of peptic ulcer pain, and is not relieved by food. (2) Vague ill-health, anaemia, and weight loss. (3) Vomiting 'coffee grounds' (altered blood), or passing melaena stools. (4) Vomiting after food; a pyloric carcinoma causes protracted vomiting, like that of pyloric stenosis due to a duodenal ulcer (11.6). (5) An upper abdominal mass, due either to the carcinoma itself, or to secondaries in his liver. (6) Jaundice, usually due to malignant nodes in his porta hepatis. (7) Ascites as the result of peritoneal deposits. (8) Other symptoms of secondary spread.

Carcinoma of the stomach may take the form of: (1) a cauliflower type of growth; (2) a malignant ulcer with raised, irregular everted edges, especially in the distal third of the lesser curve; (3) diffuse infiltration, either in its antrum, causing pyloric stenosis, or more diffusely ('leather bottle stomach'). Lymphatic involvement, and spread to the liver, occur early.

In the developing world, a patient usually presents too late for any hope of a cure; and even if a carcinoma can be resected, he is unlikely to live 5 years. In the UK, 80% of tumours are resectable, but only 5% of patients live 5 years. The exception is Japan, where the disease is so common that diagnosis is sufficiently prompt for results to be better. Radiotherapy and chemotherapy are useless.

You will not be able to do a partial, or a total gastrectomy, so try to: (1) Make the diagnosis as best you can. (2) Select and refer any resectable and potentially curable cases. These are mostly those with a small lesion seen with a barium meal. (2) Do a palliative gastrojejunostomy, if his pylorus is obstructed. This will make his last days a little more bearable, stop him vomiting, and improve his nutrition temporarily. (3) As always, palliate and comfort him as he dies (33.1).

GASTRIC CARCINOMA

EXAMINATION. Look and feel for: (1) An enlarged hard supraclavicular (Virchow's) node. (2) A firm, or hard, slightly mobile, irregular epigastric mass, separate from the patient's liver. (3) An enlarged and often irregular firm to hard liver. (4) Signs that his stomach is not emptying normally: visible peristalsis, a tympanitic epigastric swelling, and a succussion splash. (5) Signs of advanced disease—cachexia, jaundice, and ascites. (6) Deposits in his rectovesical pouch—feel for a firm, fixed 'rectal shelf'.

SPECIAL TESTS. Test his stools for occult blood. If he has a firm enlarged accessible node, especially in his supraclavicular fossa, biopsy it.

X-RAYS. If possible, do a barium meal. By the time you see him, he will probably have a filling defect, or an ulcer, which you can see quite easily on screening. Inhibited peristalsis suggests a tumour.

A malignant lesion has a 65% chance of being in his antrum, a 30% chance of being in the body of his stomach, and only a 5% chance of being in his fundus.

THE DIFFERENTIAL DIAGNOSIS is mainly that of 'dyspepsia'. It includes gallstones (13.7), hepatoma (32.26), and chronic pancreatitis (13.9).

Suggesting peptic ulceration—a long history (>2years), periodic rather than constant pain.

Suggesting non-ulcer dyspepsia—diffuse tenderness, no mass, less weight loss, and a variable appetite.

MANAGEMENT. If you think his tumour might be operable, consider refering him. Before sending him on a long journey, remember that: (1) although an expert might do a total or partial gastrectomy, which would be better palliation, (2) it would have a higher mortality rate, and (3) his long-term prognosis is poor, and even an expert cannot do much more for him than you can.

If the diagnosis is difficult, refer him. Or, if this is impossible, consider doing a diagnostic laparotomy. But before you do this: (1) he must understand why you are doing it, and that it may not be curative, and (2) you must be able to do a vagotomy (11-4, 11.7) if you find a benign lesion.

If he has signs of progressive pyloric obstruction, causing daily vomiting, with no signs of advanced disease (except perhaps metastatic cervical nodes), do a gastrojejunostomy as in in Section 11.7. Choose a part of his stomach wall near his greater curvature, at least 4 cm proximal to the mass. Make the stoma well away from the tumour, and make it big (at least 5 cm), in the hope that it will stay open until he dies. Make it on the anterior or posterior aspect of his stomach, preferably posterior and retrocolic, because it will empty his stomach better.

If he cannot swallow because of obstruction at his cardia, do nothing. Don't try to insert a Celestin tube, as for carcinoma of the oesophagus (32.25), because it will be difficult to keep in place.

32.26 Hepatoma, very common

Hepatoma is the world's most common malignant tumour, mostly because it is so common in China and Africa, where it it is

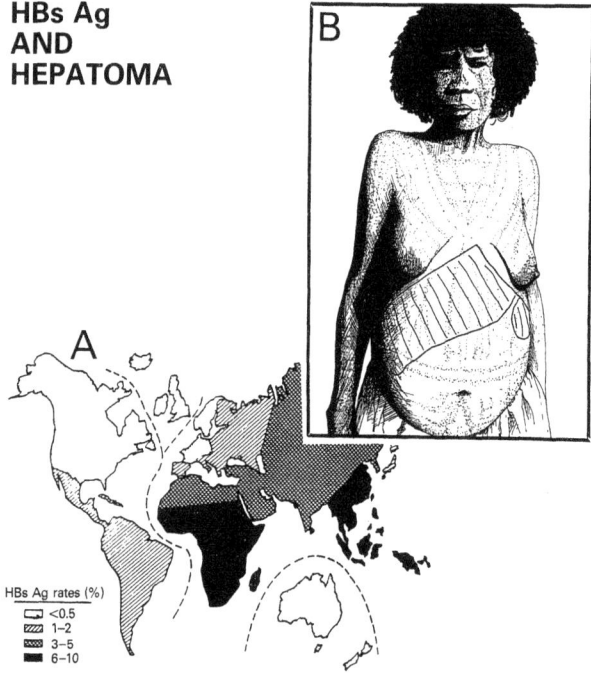

HBs Ag AND HEPATOMA

Fig. 32-13 HBsAg AND HEPATOMA. A, the geographical distribution of the hepatitis B virus, based on the incidence of HBsAg in blood samples. B, a patient from New Guinea with hepatoma. *A, after Szmuness.*

BIOPSY NEEDLES

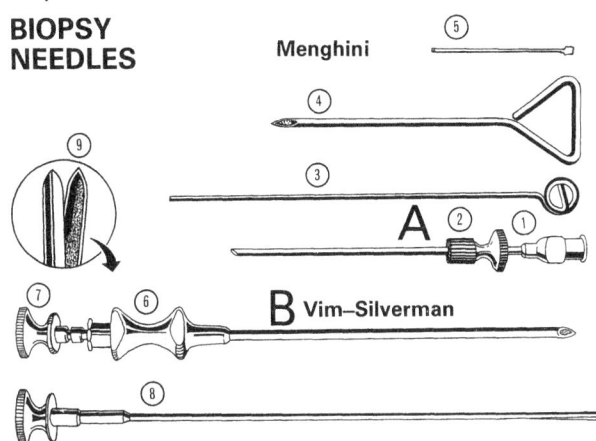

Fig. 32-14 BIOPSY NEEDLES. A, the Menghini needle. This consists of: A stout needle with a sharpened end (1). An adjustable guard (2). An obturator to clear the needle (3). (4) A short sharp trocar to pierce the skin (4). A 'blocking pin' or 'nail' (5), which slips loosely inside the needle and prevents the biopsy fragment from falling back, and breaking up in the syringe.
B, a Vim – Silverman needle. This has a sheath (6), an obturator (7), and hollowed-out biopsy jaws (8), with special ends (9).

even more common than secondary tumours of the liver. In Africa, there is a 90% chance that a liver with a hepatoma is also cirrhotic, due to the strong association of hepatoma with hepatitis B infection, and with the aflatoxin produced by the aspergillus fungus growing in damp stored food.

A hepatoma nearly always arises simultaneously as multiple nodules in many parts of the liver. Sometimes, a huge mass deforms one lobe. The other primary liver tumour, carcinoma of the bile-ducts, is as uncommon in the developing world as it is elsewhere.

The patient has an 8:1 chance of being male, and is usually between 30 and 50. He complains of pain, anorexia, weight loss, or a mass; jaundice is late. His pain is usually constant, and sharp or burning, and is in his upper abdomen, usually on the right. It is commonly made worse by food, which causes an inappropriate feeling of fullness after only a small meal. Typically, his pain is made much worse by alcohol; so much so that it may have driven him to stop drinking.

Usually, he presents late with a large, or even a huge, firm, irregular, tender liver. Quite a small tumour may confine him to bed, or he may be remain active with a large one. He may be emaciated and cachectic, or he may present at a stage when weight loss is not yet severe. He may have ascites and a large spleen. Look for collateral veins running vertically over his anterior costal margin, or parallel to his spinous processes. Listen over the tumour for a bruit; this can be intermittent, so listen on several occasions. Spider naevi cannot be seen in a dark skin, and although liver palms can be, they are seldom seen in Africa.

If there is any room for doubt, do all you can to confirm the diagnosis. Several diseases present as swellings of the upper abdomen. Try to distinguish those you can treat, such as liver abscesses, hydatid cysts, and tuberculosis (rare), from those you can only palliate. If you have any hope of sending specimens for histology, learn to biopsy the liver. This can be dangerous, so do it carefully.

• NEEDLE, liver biopsy, Menghini, 1.6 mm, normal Menghini point, with adjustable stop, one only (SHR).

• NEEDLE, liver biopsy, Vim–Silverman, adult size, 23 mm × 88.5 mm, with Franklin modification, one only (SHR). This has hollowed-out biopsy jaws, a sleeve which fits over them, and an obturator to discharge the specimen. The inner jaws grasp a core of tissue, after which you slide the sleeve over them to trap it. Surgeons vary in the needle they prefer. A Menghini needle is in a patient's liver for a shorter time, so it is safer. Its disadvantage is that it is less likely to withdraw a satisfactory specimen if he is cirrhotic. This is important because cirrhosis is common in areas where hepatoma is common.

HEPATOMA

SPECIAL TESTS. A patient's bilirubin rises late, and is often not raised when he presents. If it is >40 μmol/l (2 mg/dl), his life expectancy is weeks only. His bilirubin and alkaline phosphatase are raised parallel with one another. His transaminases are normal, unless he also has chronic active hepatitis. If he has ascites, aspirate a sample of the fluid and examine it. Blood-stained fluid supports the diagnosis of malignancy, not necessarily of the liver. Anaemia is seldom a marked feature.

X-RAYS. A chest X-ray usually shows that the right lobe of his diaphragm is raised. 50% of patients have secondaries in their lungs *post mortem*, but a chest X-ray seldom shows them during life.

DIFFERENTIAL DIAGNOSIS. Try to exclude treatable diseases. Some of these are inflammatory, and so produce fever, but this does occur in primary hepatoma (8%), so it is not a reliable guide.

Suggesting secondary carcinoma of the liver—a hard nodular liver, evidence for a primary tumour. In carcinoma of the stomach there may be a separate mass, dyspeptic symptoms, or symptoms of pyloric obstruction.

Suggesting carcinoma of the bile-ducts—deep jaundice, no bruit, and a liver which is less big and irregular than with hepatoma.

Suggesting carcinoma of the head of the pancreas—deepening jaundice, little or no pain, the absence of bile pigment in his stools, a gall-bladder which is usually palpable, no bruit.

Suggesting amoebic abscess—fever, a smooth, diffusely enlarged, tender liver with no obvious lumps, no jaundice; tenderness, especially intercostal tenderness.

Suggesting gallstones—severe colicky pain, biliary dyspepsia, little or no weight loss.

Suggesting hydatid disease, with cholangitis—contact with dogs, a tense, almost painless, long-standing (years), smooth, rubbery mass, commonly in the right upper quadrant; little weight loss, general condition good.

Suggesting a subphrenic abscess with downward displacement of the liver—fever and an acute or subacute illness, cough and chest signs on the right side, shoulder tip pain on the right side, fever.

Suggesting tuberculosis of the liver (rare)—a hard irregular liver, often with no fever, no jaundice, pain is not marked. When there is no jaundice, you cannot distinguish hepatoma and secondary carcinoma from tuberculosis, except by needle biopsy, which is one reason why it is so useful.

PROGNOSIS. Few patients survive more than 6 months.

MANAGEMENT. Chemotherapy does not cure, nor palliate usefully. There is little you or anyone else can do for him, so there is no point in referring him, with the rare exception of a single tumour confined to his left lobe.

NEEDLE BIOPSY OF THE LIVER

INDICATIONS. An enlarged liver when the diagnosis is unknown.

CONTRAINDICATIONS. (1) Deep jaundice, severe anaemia, or any bleeding tendency, as shown by petechiae, ecchymoses, or haemorrhages. (2) Hydatid disease, where needle biopsy may lead to fatal anaphylaxis or dissemination. (3) Inability to transfuse him if necessary.

CAUTION ! (1) Measure his bleeding time (normal <3 minutes) and clotting time (normal <8 minutes) before taking a biopsy. (2) Give him water-soluble vitamin K_1 10 mg intramuscularly on 3 successive days.

ANAESTHESIA. Use local anaesthesia in an adult (A 5.4); a child may need a general anaesthetic. He is likely to be 'ill', and some anaesthetic agents are hepatotoxic.

PRACTICE. Before you use either needle for the first time, try it out by doing the biopsy on a banana, and if possible practise on a cadaver.

CAUTION ! To avoid tearing his liver, he must hold his breath

MENGHINI LIVER BIOPSY

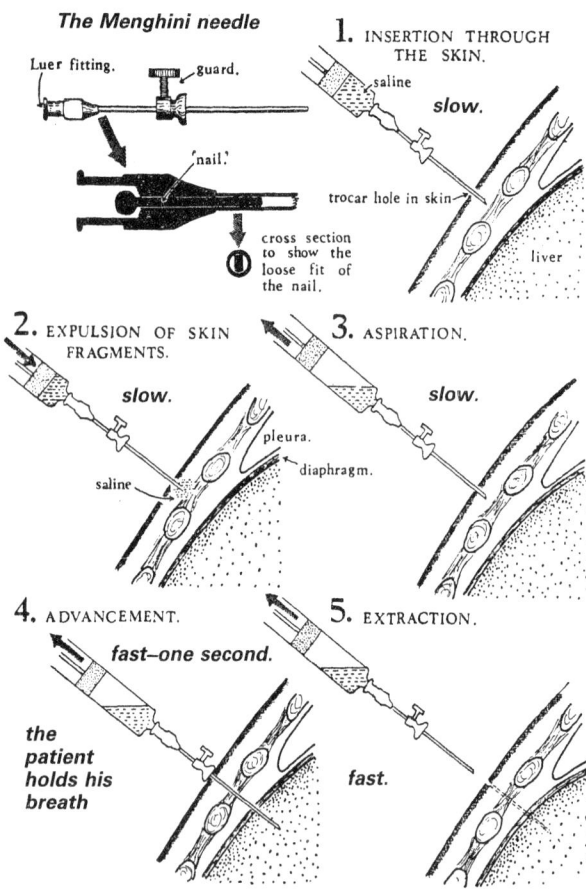

Fig. 32-15 MENGHINI LIVER BIOPSY. *From 'Medical Care in Developing Countries' 1965, by the editor.*

when you are pushing the needle in, pushing it in further, or pulling it out. There are also times when you will want him to breathe deeply to check the position of the needle.

MENGHINI NEEDLE. Before you start, make quite sure that he understands what is being done. If you are using local anaesthesia, get him to practise holding his breath. This is important, because you must do the puncture itself and anaesthetise his skin beforehand, while he holds his breath at the end of expiration.

Lay him on his back near to the right side of the bed, and place a firm pillow against his left side in the hollow of the bed. Place his right arm behind his head, and turn his face to the left.

Choose a point in his mid or anterior axillary line in his 8th, 9th, or 10th intercostal spaces, or over the palpable mass that you want to biopsy. Clean his skin with iodine, and anaesthetize the chosen site with local anaesthetic solution.

Pierce the anaesthetized area with a scalpel (or with the special trocar). While he holds his breath, use a long (8 cm) fine-bore needle to infiltrate 5 ml of anaesthetic solution into his skin and parietal peritoneum.

Fit the Menghini needle to a well-fitting 10 ml syringe, set the guard at about 4 cm, and draw up 3 ml of sterile saline.

Pass the needle point through the anaesthetized track down to, but not through the intercostal space. Inject 2 ml of saline to clear the needle point of any skin fragments. There is some difference of opinion as to the plane in which this is best done. Menghini himself advised that saline be discharged and the needle cleared in the subcutaneous tissues. Others prefer to go through the intercostal muscle just short of the liver before clearing the needle.

CAUTION ! Now, ask him to hold his breath in expiration. Start to aspirate, and while continuing to aspirate, rapidly push the needle into his liver perpendicular to his skin, then, immediately pull it out again. Apply pressure to the site of the biopsy.

Continue aspirating until you have placed the needle point under some saline in a glass dish. Discharge the saline remaining in the syringe. The biopsy specimen will appear. Rescue it and transfer it to formol saline. Clear the needle with the obturator.

VIM–SILVERMAN NEEDLE. Proceed to the step "Pierce the anaesthetized area with a scalpel..." above. Then, having pierced the anaesthetized area with a scalpel, fit the inner obturator into the sheath. With firm, but well-controlled pressure, push the needle through his abdominal wall *while he holds his breath.* You will feel his peritoneum 'give' as you go through it. Don't push the needle in too far at this stage. Ask him to take a deep breath. If the needle moves with respiration, its tip is already in his liver; if not, *ask him to hold his breath again,* and gently push it 3 cm further in, or until it moves.

CAUTION ! Don't manipulate the needle while he is breathing, or you may tear his liver.

Ask him to hold his breath, then remove the inner obturator and replace it with the biopsy jaws. Steady the needle with your left hand, and push the jaws with your right hand into the needle as far as they will go.

Ask him to hold his breath again. Hold the biopsy jaws firmly with your right hand, and slide the outer jaws 3 cm further into his liver. This will wedge the jaws and the tissue firmly in the outer sheath. Rotate the needle once or twice, to break off any tissue which is attached at the tip, and then quickly withdraw it. Ask him to breathe again. You can do everything in a few seconds. He need not hold his breath for long.

Slide the sheath over the biopsy jaws and open them. Use a fine needle to remove the core of tissue from the jaws into formol saline.

If you have not succeeded, try again in a different place. If you fail after several attempts, there is probably no solid tissue that can be biopsied. If the needle goes in without any resistance, attach a 20 ml syringe to it and aspirate—you may withdraw the 'anchovy sauce' of an amoebic abscess (31.12).

POSTOPERATIVELY, (both methods), lay him flat for 24 hours. Monitor his pulse and blood pressure during this time, just in case he bleeds into his peritoneal cavity. A hepatoma is very vascular, and occasionally bleeds when you biopsy it.

32.26a Carcinoma of the pancreas, uncommon in most of the developing world

If a patient's carcinoma is in the head of his pancreas (70%), it obstructs his common bile duct, so that he presents with painless progressive obstructive jaundice (13.8). If it is in the body of his pancreas (30%), he presents with upper abdominal pain and general symptoms of malignancy. Spread to the lymphatics and surrounding structures is early, and 10% of patients develop ascites. Thrombophlebitis migrans (thrombophlebitis in any superficial vein appearing, resolving, and then appearing again elsewhere) may occur with any malignant tumour, but is particularly common with this tumour.

Radiotherapy, chemotherapy, and surgery are of little value. Pancreatico-duodenostomy has 5% of 5 year survivors in carcinoma of the head of the pancreas proper, and 20% if it is in the periampullary region. Surgery has a 20% mortality in the best hands.

CARCINOMA OF THE HEAD OF THE PANCREAS. If an experienced surgeon is within easy reach, refer the patient; but all he will be able to do is to establish the diagnosis and palliate him.

If you find carcinoma of the head of the pancreas during an exploratory laparotomy, a cholecystojejunostomy (13-5) is useful palliation, because it will relieve his jaundice (13.8).

32.27 Carcinoma of the colon and rectum

In Europe, carcinoma of the large gut is commoner than all the other carcinomas, except for those of the lung in men and the breast in women. It is not uncommon in India, but it is still uncommon in Africa, especially in the rural areas, where a high fibre diet is still the rule. If *Schistosoma mansoni* is endemic in your community, you will see the adenocarcinoma of the rectum that it causes. You will probably never see diverticulitis.

Carcinoma of the large gut is usually a slow-growing adenocarcinoma, which may not penetrate a patient's gut until he has had symptoms for about 18 months, although it tends to grow faster if he is young. It may project into the lumen like a cauliflower, or it may form a stricture (long or short), or an ulcer (if so it is likely to penetrate early). It invades locally, spreads to his regional nodes or his liver (usually late), or through to his peritoneal cavity (late and uncommon). Tumours of the rectum spread upwards, those of the anal canal (less common) spread to the inguinal nodes.

He is usually over 45, but is occasionally a young adult, who presents with the following symptoms: (1) Blood and mucus in his stools. (2) An alteration in his bowel habit. (3) A sense of incomplete defaecation. (4) Colicky abdominal pain (incomplete obstruction). (5) Intestinal obstruction. (6) A fixed mass. (7) A faecal fistula which appears spontaneously (rare).

You are most likely to meet carcinoma of the large gut when you operate for obstruction, and have to relieve it. Otherwise, avoid operating, and refer him.

Carcinoma of the rectum usually presents late, because it causes little pain in the early stages. Rectal bleeding is the important symptom, sometimes with disturbances of bowel function, increasing constipation, subacute obstruction, abdominal distension, cramps, and a feeling that there is something left to pass after a bowel evacuation. You can feel most rectal carcinomas with your finger—either as a firm raised plaque, or an ulcer with hard rolled edges, leaving blood on your glove afterwards.

Try to: (1) Remember the possibility of carcinoma of the large gut and rectum, and alert your paramedical staff to it also. (2) Do a rectal examination, proctoscopy, and sigmoidoscopy when these are indicated (22.1). (3) Stage a patient and assess his operability. (4) Do a colostomy or Hartmann's operation (9.5, 10.10, 10-16) if he presents in obstruction. (5) If you cannot refer him, you may have to do a right (66-20), or left hemicolectomy, or you can resect the gut supplied by his middle colic vessels (all difficult operations). An abdominoperineal resection, or an anterior resection for a rectal or low sigmoid carcinoma, is an expert's task. Management is essentially surgical. Chemotherapy is palliative only.

CARCINOMA OF THE LARGE GUT AND
RECTUM

HISTORY and EXAMINATION. The patient is likely to have had symptoms for several months. Look for: (1) Signs of loss of weight and anaemia. (2) A primary mass, secondaries in his liver, and ascites. (3) A rectal mass (75% of rectal tumours can be felt on rectal examination in Europe). Send a specimen for histology from the edge of the lesion. (4) Occult blood in his stools (90%). (5) A tumour at sigmoidoscopy (all rectal, and 25% of sigmoid, tumours can be seen with a rigid sigmoidoscope).

X-RAYS. If the above investigations are negative, do a barium enema. This is not easy, but it can be done in a district hospital. Use barium and air phase contrast (34.5). Avoid a barium enema with complete or partial obstruction.

THE DIFFERENTIAL DIAGNOSIS includes: (1) Other causes of blood in the stools (piles, amoebiasis, and *S. mansoni* dysentery, 22.3). (2) Other causes of altered bowel habit (gut infections, poor food supply, upper abdominal malignancy). (3) Other causes of acute-on-chronic obstruction (acute volvulus, amoebic stricture, in South America Chagas' disease). (5) Other causes of strictures of the rectum or sigmoid (amoebic strictures, or lymphogranuloma venereum, especially in women).

The frequency of different presenting symptoms varies with the site of the lesion:

Suggesting a lesion in the right colon—anaemia, a mass, caecal pain, weight loss, obstruction.

Suggesting a lesion in the left colon—colicky abdominal pain, alteration of bowel habit (diarrhoea alternating with constipation), blood mixed with stools, obstruction.

Suggesting a lesion in the rectum—rectal bleeding, diarrhoea, a feeling of incomplete evacuation.

STAGING. A tumour can be mobile, tethered to surrounding structures, or fixed. Assess a rectal tumour digitally, and those elsewhere at laparotomy. A carcinoma is resectable unless: (1) It is fixed to his pelvic wall, his abdominal wall, or his bladder (fixity is a difficult and misleading sign). (2) He has palpable masses in his liver, or malignant ascites, or metastases in his lungs, or superficial lymph nodes. Ascites, jaundice, or a hard, irregular liver all indicate an incurable tumour for which no surgery is possible; palliate him.

If his tumour and its associated mesentery can be excised,

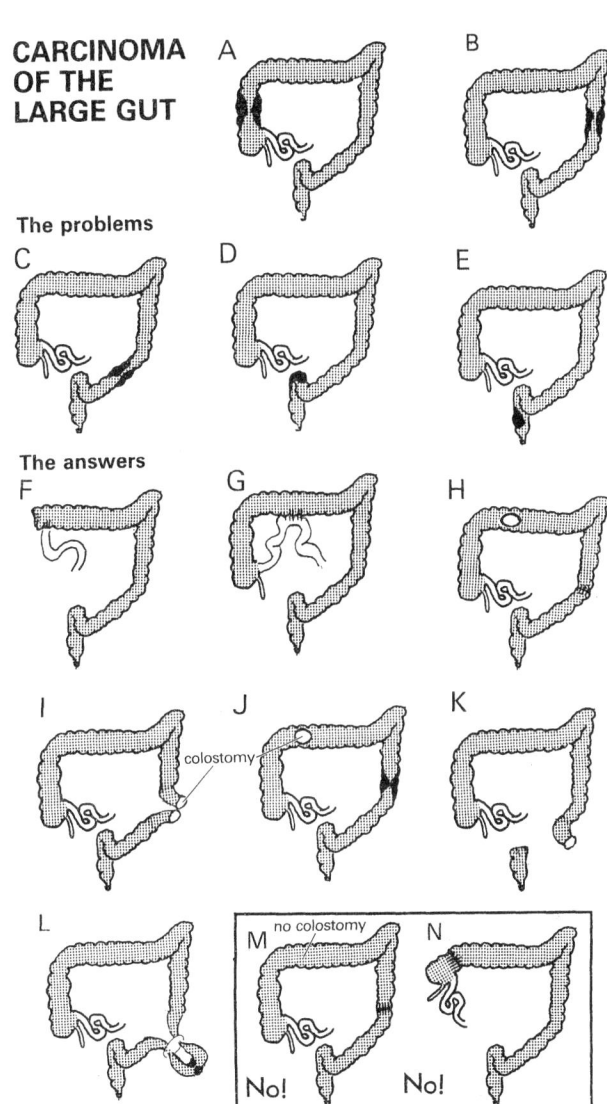

Fig. 32-15a CARCINOMA OF THE LARGE GUT. Carcinomas in various sites: the ascending colon (A), the descending colon (B), the sigmoid colon (C), the rectosigmoid junction (D) and the lower rectum (E).

F, a right hemicolectomy with an end to side anastomosis. G, a side to side ileocolic bypass anastomosis. H, excision of a tumour from the left colon with a protective colostomy. I, excision of the tumour followed by a sigmoid colostomy. J, a colostomy to relieve obstruction by a tumour in the descending colon. K, Hartmann's operation. L, exteriorization of a tumour in the sigmoid colon. M, never do this! Never make an anastomosis of the distal colon unprotected by a proximal colostomy.

N, anastomoses of the caecum are especially dangerous.

the following staging (Dukes) will give a more accurate prognosis. In the UK 15% are in Stage A, and 50% in stages C or D. Overall only 20% of patients with carcinoma of the large gut survive 5 years in the UK.

Stage A. The tumour is confined to the wall of his gut. 85% chance of surviving 5 years.

Stage B. The tumour spreads through his gut wall, but his lymph nodes are not involved. 50% chance of surviving 5 years.

Stage C. His lymph nodes are involved. 25% chance of surviving 5 years.

Stage D. Distant or liver metastases, nobody survives 5 years.

MANAGEMENT. See Section 9.3 about 'Which parts of the gut you can anastomose to which and when'. Management depends on: (1) Where the tumour is. (2) If it is resectable or not. (3) If his gut is obstructed or not. (3) How skilled you are.

If his gut is not obstructed, only operate if you cannot refer him and you are experienced. Definitive operations in Stages A and B have a good prognosis. Palliation to remove obstruction, or prevent it, in Stages C and D will help him much.

If his gut is obstructed (much the most likely occasion on which you will meet this tumour), you will have to relieve the obstruction yourself by doing a colostomy, or an anastomosis, as these are practicable.

If possible, avoid resecting at the initial operation: (1) The contents of his gut will not have been 'sterilized'. (2) A primary anastomosis in the large gut is apt to leak when it is full of faeces, especially if it is obstructed.

CAUTION ! (1) The contents of the large gut are always loaded with bacteria, so always prepare the gut before an elective operation (see below). (2) When you have to operate in an emergency for obstruction avoid: (a) contaminating his peritoneal cavity, and (b) remember that the only safe anastomosis is one between his ileum and his colon, *never* colon to colon! (3) When you anastomose the ileum to the transverse colon, remember to save as much ileum as you can, because its last few centimetres are the site of absorption of vitamin B_{12}.

If his tumour is proximal to his mid transverse colon (A, in Fig. 32-15a):

If his gut is unobstructed or only partly obstructed, try to refer him. If you cannot do this, prepare him first and operate.

If his tumour is resectable, resect his caecum, ascending colon, and associated mesentery, and anastomose his ileum to his transverse colon. This is major surgery (F, in Fig. 32-15a, and the second part of Fig. 66-20). The ileum has a good blood supply, and when it is dilated it matches the size of the empty transverse colon. F, shows the anastomosis end to side. You can also do it end to end. If his ileum is not the same size as his colon, you can make a nick in it to enlarge it, as in Fig. 9-7.

If it is not resectable, bypass the obstruction with a side to side ileotransverse anastomosis (G, also Fig. 9-12). He may obstruct at any time.

If he is obstructed: (1) If his condition is good and you are fairly experienced, do a left hemicolectomy at the time of the obstruction (F). (2) If his condition is poor and/or you are inexperienced, make a bypass (G). This is safe, but he may be unwilling later to undergo the resection which might cure him.

If his tumour is between his mid transverse colon and his sigmoid colon (B):

If he is unobstructed or partly obstructed, try to refer him. If this is impossible, prepare him first and operate.

If his tumour is resectable, resect the involved gut 5 cm clear of the tumour with its associated mesentery. Do an end to end anastomosis with a proximal colostomy (H). The bowel ends must have a good blood supply. If not, resect more gut, but not more mesentery. The extent of this operation varies from being a local resection to being a left hemicolectomy. Beware of: (1) His left ureter, which is easily reflected with his descending and his sigmoid mesentery (10-16). (2) His spleen, if you need to mobilize his splenic flexure. Make the anastomosis in 2 layers, as for small gut, preferably with a non-absorbable suture for the outer layer. Make sure the anastomosis is not under tension. This operation is less often necessary than the corresponding operation on the right, but the principles are the same (66-20).

If his gut is obstructed, immediate anastomosis of his distal colon is dangerous because of its poor blood supply, its fluid contents which easily escape, and the great difference in size of the gut ends. So, excise the tumour if you can. Bring the two cut ends out as separate colostomies (I). Join them up electively later. Or, merely do a proximal defunctioning colostomy (J), and, if his tumour is resectable, refer him for a definitive operation as soon as he recovers.

Alternatively, when his left colon is obstructed, you can do an ileo-descending, or an ileo-rectal anastomosis (not shown). This is reasonably safe, but it is a big operation, and he may have diarrhoea afterwards. Most surgeons prefer a colostomy with or without immediate resection, depending on the circumstances.

If the tumour is in his sigmoid or upper rectum (C or D):

If his gut is unobstructed and the tumour is likely to be resectable, refer him. If this is impossible, prepare him, and do a two-stage Hartmann's operation (K).

If the tumour is not resectable, as judged by fixity to his abdominal wall, do a double-barrelled colostomy of his transverse colon (J).

If his gut is obstructed, contributors differ as to which of these alternatives is best. You can: (1) If the tumour is suitably placed in his upper sigmoid, resect it and make a colostomy proximally and a mucous fistula distally which someone else can repair (I). (2) Resect it, close the distal end of his colon, and bring the cut proximal end out as a colostomy (K, Hartmann's operation). (3) Bring his sigmoid colon out through a pelvic colostomy, and exteriorize it as if it were a loop of gangrenous gut (L); this helps to avoid contaminating his peritoneal cavity. The difference is that you need to mobilize much more mesentery, so watch his ureter (see C, Fig. 10-16). To resect gut, mobilize his colon well on both sides of the lesion. If possible, divide his inferior mesenteric artery flush with his aorta, and resect a V-shaped piece of mesentery. Bring the carcinoma out as a 'double-barrelled' loop colostomy, and resect it when you have closed his abdomen, and the operation is nearly over. Leave 1.5 cm of gut above the skin when you resect it. Three months later refer him to a specialist for a joining-up operation; if if this is impossible, do it yourself (9.5).

If the tumour is in his middle or lower rectum (E), do a biopsy through a proctoscope or sigmoidoscope. If he is not obstructed and is likely to be operable, refer him for an anterior resection, or an abdominoperineal resection. If he is obstructed, you have a choice between: (1) A transverse colostomy (J), which is best if he is going to have further surgery, because it makes this easier. (2) A double barrelled sigmoid colostomy (I), which is best if he is inoperable, because he retains the absorptive properties of his descending colon. A rectal tumour rarely causes obstruction; if it does, it will certainly be inoperable.

CAUTION ! If he has liver metastases or a fixed tumour, think hard before you do a colostomy. He may live a few more months, but dying with a colostomy will be miserable, especially if colostomy care is poor. If his tumour is not resectable, it is better to do a bypass operation, an ileotransverse (9-11, 66-20) or colocolic anastomosis. This is possible for lesions of the ascending, transverse, or descending colon, but not the distal sigmoid or the rectum. If a bypass is impossible, a colostomy is better than dying in obstruction.

PREPARATION. If he is not obstructed, you will be able to do an elective operation, so empty his colon first. Enemas only clear its left side, so give him enough magnesium sulphate or castor oil to give him diarrhoea, meanwhile giving him plenty of fluids to avoid dehydration. For 2 days preoperatively, give him metronidazole 400 mg 8-hourly and neomycin 1 g 8 hourly, or ampicillin 500 mg 6-hourly, together with a nutritious fluids-only diet.

LAVAGE. When the operation is over, wash out his peritoneal cavity with warm saline, and then leave tetracycline 1 g or chloramphenicol 1 g in 500 ml of saline in his peritoneal cavity; don't insert drains.

TUMOURS OF THE RESPIRATORY TRACT

32.28 Carcinoma of the nasopharynx, common in some areas

Carcinomas of the nasopharynx are important on a world scale. In people of Southern Chinese origin they are a very common cancer. They have a lesser, but significant, incidence, in some other races of South-east Asia and North and East Africa. They are strongly associated with the Epstein-Barr virus, but, unlike cancers in other parts of the pharynx, not with either alcohol or tobacco. They are more common in males, and have a peak age incidence between 40 and 50, but are sometimes seen in older children. 90% are carcinomas, and most of the remaining 10% are lymphomas. They spread locally by direct extension, regionally to neighbouring nodes, and distantly in the bloodstream. Distant metastases to the lung, bone, and liver occur more often from the nasopharynx than from any other site in the head and neck.

A patient with carcinoma of his nasopharynx presents with a nasal discharge, nasal speech, a blocked nose, symptoms resulting from a obstruction of his eustachian tube (earache, tinnitus, and hyperacusis), and involvement of his cranial nerves, most commonly his 5th and 6th, but also his 2nd, 3rd, 4th, 7th and 8th (diplopia, facial pain, and numbness, loss of vision, and deafness, etc.). There is an 80% chance that he already has metastases in his cervical lymph nodes when he presents.

CARCINOMA OF THE NASOPHARYNX

EXAMINATION. Examine the patient's cranial nerves. Carefully palpate his entire neck for enlarged nodes. Feel particularly for his uppermost internal jugular node, just below the tip of his mastoid process. This is often the first node to be involved when the primary is silent.

Observe his soft palate for asymmetry due to displacement by a tumour. If you are skilled, examine his nasopharynx with a mirror (25.11a).

BLIND BIOPSY is less satisfactory than open biopsy. Give him a general anaesthetic and intubate him orally (nasal intubation will quickly spoil both your access and your view). Push St Bartholomew's or Luc's forceps through his nose, and guide them into his nasopharynx, with a finger behind his soft palate. Grasp a suitable piece of tissue and remove it.

OPEN BIOPSY. Anaesthetize and intubate him orally. Put him into the tonsillectomy position, lying on his back with a pillow under his shoulders and with his head extended. Insert a tonsillectomy (Boyle Davis) gag. Pass a catheter through his nose and out through his mouth. Use this to retract his palate. Using a warmed laryngoscopy mirror, inspect his pharynx and remove suitable pieces for biopsy.

If he has a suspicious node in his neck and you can see no obvious primary (unusual), take specimens from several suspicious-looking areas in his nasopharynx.

X-RAYS may show involvement of the base of his skull.

STAGING is a guide to prognosis.
TIS carcinoma in situ.
T_1 tumour confined to one site in his nasopharynx, or no tumour visible (positive biopsy only)
T_2 tumour involving two sites (both posterosuperior and lateral walls).
T_3 extension of the tumour into his nasal cavity, or oropharynx.
T_4 tumour invading his skull, or involving his cranial nerves.

TREATMENT. The role of surgery is limited to biopsy. If he has a lymphoma, treat him for it (32.5). It he has a carcinoma, refer him for radiotherapy. There is no established chemotherapy, but methotrexate 150 mg/m² with folinic acid and vincristine 1.4 mg/m² may help some patients (32.2). Never give this high dose of methotrexate, unless you can also give folinic acid rescue starting 24 hours after the methotrexate. Give him 4 doses of 15 mg of folinic acid orally, intramuscularly, or intravenously at 12 hour intervals, and encourage him to drink plenty of fluid. If he had a sore mouth after the last dose of methotrexate, give him 8 doses. If he fails to respond, don't give more than 3 courses. CAUTION ! This is the high dose range for methotrexate, which is not used with other methods in this manual (the usual dose is 15 mg/m², not 150 mg/m², as above).

PROGNOSIS. Local control is possible in 60–90% of cases. 5 year survivals range from 27% (squamous cell carcinomas) to 58% (lymphoepitheliomas and lymphomas.

CARCINOMA OF THE NASOPHARYNX

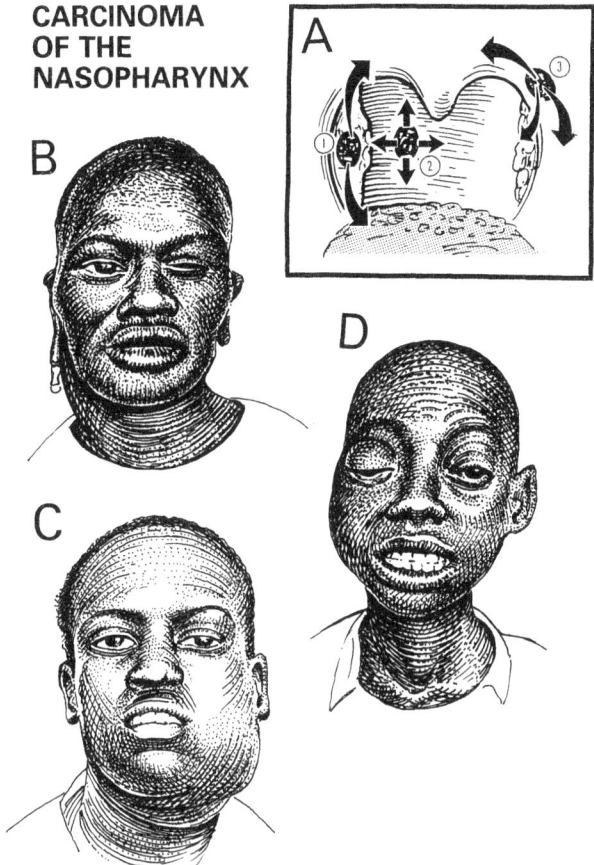

Fig. 32-16 CARCINOMA OF THE NASOPHARYNX. A, the directions of spread of carcinoma from (1) the tonsil, (2) the posterior pharyngeal wall, and (3) the soft palate. B, a 45 year old Masai with cervical metastases and paralysis of his left 2nd, 3rd, 4th, 5th, and 6th cranial nerves. C, a 14 year old Luo boy with enlargement of his left cervical glands, but no cranial nerve lesions. D, a 12 year old Kikuyu boy with severe trismus, bilateral proptosis, ophthalmoplegia and right blindness from an anaplastic carcinoma of his nasopharynx, but without involvement of his cervical glands. *A, after Edward M Copeland III, 'Surgical Oncology', p.127, Fig. 5. John Wiley, with kind permission. B, C, D, after Peter Clifford, East African Medical Journal 1965;42:381.*

32.29 Carcinoma of the bronchus, increasingly common

As the result of the greed of multinational companies and the inertia of governments, cigarette smoking is becoming widely prevalent in the developing world. An epidemic of smoking-related diseases has already started, among them carcinoma of the bronchus. About 75% of tumours involve the main bronchi, 10% are peripheral, and a few arise near the apex of the lung, whence they may spread to involve the sympathetic chain and the brachial plexus (Pancoast's tumour). About 50% are squamous cell, 30% are anaplastic (oat cell), and 20% are adenocarcinomas—most peripheral tumours are of this kind, and their prognosis after surgery is relatively good.

The patient, who is usually an older man, presents with: (1)

A persistent cough. (2) Haemoptysis. (3) A low-grade pneumonia, as the result of a blocked bronchus. (4) Pneumonia which fails to resolve. (5) A solid lesion on X-ray. Bronchoscopy is the critical investigation, and even with a rigid bronchoscope (25.13) it is possible to see and biopsy the lesion in about 75% of cases.

In countries where the disease is common and patients are aware of it, only about 20% of them are operable when they present, and of those who do survive radical surgery, only about 25% are alive 5 years later. The chances of your being able to refer a patient for either radical surgery, or radiotherapy, are small. Radiotherapy is a useful palliative. Present combinations of cytotoxic drugs are of limited value.

You will probably find that most patients are inoperable when they present. So, try to: (1) Differentiate carcinoma of the bronchus from other more treatable diseases, which it may closely resemble, both clinically and radiologically. (2) Select the few 'coin-like' peripheral lesions amenable to surgery. (3) Palliate and comfort the dying and their families.

CARCINOMA OF THE BRONCHUS

SPECIAL TESTS. If tuberculosis is a possible differential diagnosis, examine the patient's sputum for AAFB. X-ray his chest.

THE DIFFERENTIAL DIAGNOSIS includes pulmonary tuberculosis, low-grade or partly resolved pneumonia (which may simulate carcinoma closely), areas of pulmonary fibrosis, lung abscesses, and solid tumours of the lung, other than bronchial carcinoma. Tuberculosis is more likely to make him febrile. The X-ray appearances are usually different, but may be identical.

BRONCHOSCOPY. If possible, do this as in Section 25.12. Its indications are: (1) A patient with haemoptysis in whom AAFB cannot be found. (2) Other suspicious cases (see above). The number of patients you will be able to bronchoscope will depend on your workload, and the local incidence of carcinoma of the bronchus, compared with the conditions that simulate it. In Europe, an unresolved pneumonia is likely to be due to a bronchial carcinoma causing obstruction. In much of the developing world, it is more likely to be due to a partially treated pneumonia, not associated with carcinoma.

OPERABILITY. The most favourable cases are those with a peripheral 'coin-like' lesion (usually an adenocarcinoma, sometimes a tuberculoma, or a developing lung abscess). Refer these for thoracotomy. Signs of inoperability include: involvement of the chest wall, involvement of the laryngeal or sympathetic nerves (Horner's syndrome), widening of the mediastinum in a chest X-ray, secondary deposits (as in the cervical nodes), bony secondaries, and an oat cell tumour on biopsy.

Bronchoscopic signs which suggest that a patient is not operable include: widening or flattening of the first 1.5 cm of his main bronchus, widening of his carina, and distension of his trachea.

CHEMOTHERAPY has a low priority if drugs are scarce. If he has an oat cell carcinoma, it will give him a remission and prolong his life for 6 to 12 months. A few patients with oat cell tumours survive much longer. Untreated, patients are likely to die in 2 months. Chemotherapy can also be used with other histological types of tumour, but with a much lower response rate.

Consider giving him cyclophosphamide 1 g/m^2 intravenously and vincristine 1.4 mg/m^2 intravenously, with tablets of methotrexate 15 mg/m^2 orally daily for 3 or 4 days, or, Doxorubicin ('Adriamycin') 60 to 75 mg/m^2 (32.2). Repeat this every 3 weeks for 3 or 4 months, provided the tumour is responding.

TUMOURS OF THE URINARY TRACT AND MALE GENITAL TRACT

32.30 Tumours of the kidney, rare

In Europe tumours of the kidney are about tenth in order of frequency, the more common varieties being: adenocarcinoma (hypernephroma) (75%), tumours of the renal pelvis (10%), nephroblastoma (Wilm's tumour, 8%), and squamous cell carcinoma 2%. In Africa nephroblastoma is the most common.

Adenocarcinomas present between the ages of 40 and 70, as haematuria (60%), an enlarged kidney (20%), or with symptoms of secondary spread, such as general ill health and bone pain. Otherwise, pain is not a major feature, unless the patient has haematuria and clot colic.

KIDNEY TUMOURS

ADENOCARCINOMA

SPECIAL TESTS. A good quality intravenous urogram will demonstrate most renal masses. Look for displacement, deformity, and destruction of the calyces of the patient's kidney. The tumour is usually in the upper or lower poles. Ultrasound readily distinguishes solid from cystic lesions, but you are unlikely to have this. If he has haematuria, cystoscope him (23.3). Look for 'cannon ball' secondaries in his lungs.

THE DIFFERENTIAL DIAGNOSIS includes: (1) Renal cysts (the commonest cause of a renal mass) and hydronephrosis. The kidney is palpable but haematuria is unusual. (2) Polycystic kidney (a mass and haematuria). (3) An enlarged spleen. (4) Other tumours of the kidney and large gut. Not all renal cysts and hydronephrotic kidneys are palpable, and the absence of haematuria does not exclude a carcinoma.

THE PROGNOSIS depends on the stage at which the diagnosis is made.

If the tumour has not spread outside the renal capsule (less than 50% of cases, even in Europe), the 5 year survival is 30% and the 10 year survival 7%.

If it has spread outside the renal capsule, there are few 5 year survivors.

MANAGEMENT. If he has no obvious metastases, refer him for nephrectomy. It may reverse some of the systemic effects of the tumour (anaemia, myopathies, etc.), even if he does have metastases.

OTHER RENAL TUMOURS

If he has a TRANSITIONAL CELL TUMOUR of his renal pelvis, it is likely to be associated with similar tumours in his bladder. Diagnose it in the same way as an adenocarcinoma. These tumours usually project into the renal pelvis, so that you can see them on a retrograde urogram. Nephrectomy, including removal of the ureter where secondaries may develop, has a better prognosis than with an adenocarcinoma.

If he has a SQUAMOUS CELL CARCINOMA, it is likely to be associated with chronic infection, and a curative nephrectomy is seldom possible.

If you think he might have a NEPHROBLASTOMA, see Section 23.6.

32.31 Carcinoma of the bladder, common in some areas

Histologically, a patient can have two kinds of carcinoma in his bladder: (1) A transitional cell carcinoma, which has a 75% chance of being papillary, and of such low-grade malignancy that it can be controlled with diathermy, although it may sometimes be as anaplastic and invasive as any squamous one. (2) A much more malignant squamous cell carcinoma.

In non-schistosomal areas, most tumours are transitional, papillary, and of low-grade malignancy, but in areas where *Schistosoma haematobium* is endemic, only about 5% are like this, 10% are anaplastic, and 85% are squamous. Of these, most are either sessile or ulcer-cancers, both of which grow rapidly, and penetrate early into the muscle of the bladder or into the paravesical tissues. They may also have obstructed a patient's ureters by the time you see him. Unlike the transitional tumours of the industrial world, they are not associated with tumours in the renal pelvis. Many patients are inoperable, and even if the primary can be removed by total cystectomy, recurrence is frequent, and there are few five year survivors.

The patient is usually between 35 and 60 and has a 2:1 chance of being male. He complains of: (1) haematuria, which is painless in early cases, (2) the passage of white sludge, or small pieces of white material (necrotic tumour), (3) increased frequency of micturition, as the result of irritability, infection, and a small bladder, (4) a suprapubic lump, and (5) retention of urine (5%), as the result of the tumour obstructing his urethra.

In areas where *S. haematobium* is not endemic, all patients with haematuria should be cystoscoped. This is impractical in endemic areas, because so many patients pass bloody urine. Macroscopic haematuria, due to *S. haematobium* alone, becomes less common as age advances, because of the fibrosis round the ova, so that by the time that a patient is 30, there is a 25% chance that, if he sees blood in his urine, it is caused by a bladder tumour, rather than merely by the worms laying their eggs. So, if you are in an endemic area, cystoscope everyone over the age of 30 who complains of blood in his urine (23.3, 23.4). Few cases of carcinoma of the bladder occur in anyone under 30.

There is little that you can do for aggressive schistosoma-associated carcinoma of the bladder, but do try to confirm the diagnosis. Patients need to know if they have a serious condition or not. Stage these tumours as described below. Most patients present in Stages Three or Four. The only useful treatment for squamous tumours in stages One and Two is total cystectomy; the recurrence rate after partial cystectomy is high, but even total cystectomy has few five year survivors. Radiotherapy is not effective for advanced cases, but is a possible alternative to surgery for Stages One and Two. No effective chemotherapy is known, except for those rare patients with high HCG (human chorionic gonadotrophin) levels and a positive pregnancy test. Ureteric transplantation gives symptomatic relief, but this is so short that the operation is seldom justified. All you can do is to palliate the patient (33.1). He is likely to die from renal failure, due to the obstuction of his ureters by the tumour.

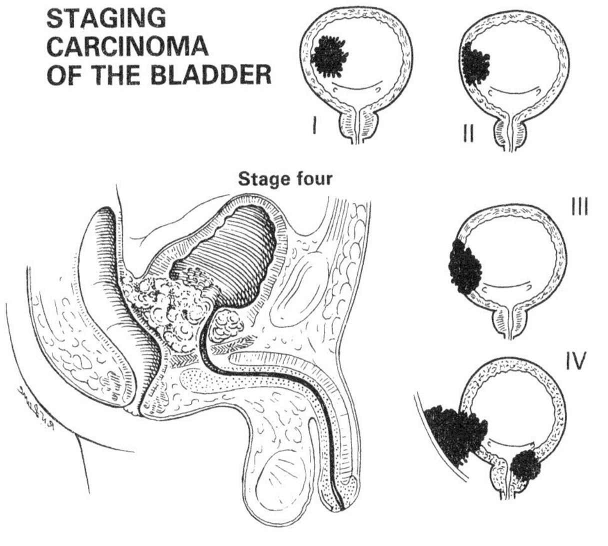

CARCINOMA OF THE BLADDER

SPECIAL TESTS. Measure the patient's haemoglobin, and his blood urea. Examine his urine microscopically, and if possible culture it.

X-RAYS. If *Schistosoma haematobium* is common; an IVU is unnecessary, because associated tumours of the pelvis of the kidney are rare. In areas where low-grade papillary transitional tumours predominate, do an IVU, because he may also have tumours of the pelvis of his kidney. An IVU will also show you the state of his upper urinary tract, dilatation of his ureters, and perhaps the tumour, as a filling defect in his bladder.

CYSTOSCOPY. If possible, cystoscope him under general anaesthesia and follow this with an EUA (examination under anaesthesia). A simple cystoscope will confirm the diagnosis, but will not allow you to take a biopsy. To do this you will need a biopsy attachment, which you can use under vision or blind in a man. In a woman with a large tumour which you can feel bimanually, you may be able to take a blind biopsy with some suitable straight instrument, such as the biopsy forceps normally used for the larynx. In advanced carcinoma, the urine is often so bloody, that it is difficult to see anything; if so you will have to rely on an EUA.

STAGING. Following cystoscopy, examine the patient bimanually under general anaesthesia, with his bladder empty and his muscles relaxed.

Stage One His tumour is sessile and not palpable. Refer him for possible cystodiathermy, or for partial cystectomy for a transitional tumour. Total cystectomy, for an aggressive squamous cell tumour, is only justified if he understands the situation fully, and the journey is not difficult. It will spare him much suffering, but is unlikely to cure him.

Stage Two It is palpable as a localized, but definite thickening, which is mobile. It is <5 cm in diameter, and is not larger than you expect from cystoscopy. Refer him as above.

Stage Three It is mobile, >5 cm in diameter, and is larger than you expect from cystoscopy. Cystectomy may be possible, but is unlikely to cure him. Consider referring him, but explain that there is little chance of a complete cure.

Stage Four It is fixed to the wall of his pelvis, or to his paravesical glands, or is infiltrating the vagina or rectum. Palliation only.

Stage Five There is widespread disease. Palliation only.
CAUTION ! (1) Try to confirm the diagnosis histologically, before advising radical surgery. Schistosomal granulomas (common in endemic areas) and tuberculosis, can simulate small tumours. (2) Avoid a suprapubic cystostomy, because it can cause a distressing, permanent urinary fistula if a malignant tumour is present.

Fig. 32-17 STAGING CARCINOMA OF THE BLADDER is done by examining a patient under anaesthesia combined with cystoscopy. Stage One, the tumour is not palpable. Stage Two, it is palpable, but is still mobile and not larger than expected from cystoscopy. Stage Three, it is mobile, but is larger than you would expect from cystoscopy. Stage Four, it is fixed. Stage Five (not shown) it is widespread. *After Bailey and Love, 'Short Practice of Surgery', Fig. 1415. With kind permission.*

32.32 Carcinoma of the prostate, common

Carcinoma of the prostate is the commonest male cancer over the age of 65. It presents with: (1) Obstructive symptoms, including difficulty passing urine, or acute or chronic retention; this has no specific features. (2) Bone pain (common), which is is not necessarily in the back. Perineal pain suggests extensive local disease. (3) Weakness in the legs, due to secondaries involving the cauda equina (uncommon). 80% of patients have metastases when they present.

Because carcinoma of the prostate is so common, it is fortunate that it can be controlled, for a time, by the cheapest kind of hormone therapy—stilboestrol. You may, however, have difficulty persuading patients to continue to take it.

Histology usually gives the correct result, but the microscopic differentiation of carcinoma from benign hyperplasia can be difficult. Make the diagnosis on the basis of the clinical findings, the serum acid phosphatase, the X-ray findings and the histology.

CARCINOMA OF THE PROSTATE

RECTAL EXAMINATION. A normal prostate feels smooth, symmetrical, and firm, usually with a median groove and mobile rectal mucosa. A carcinomatous prostate is hard, nodular, and asymmetrical; its median groove is often obliterated, and the rectal mucosa may be fixed to it. Late locally extensive disease may extend to the pelvic wall, form a band round the rectum, and fix the pelvic tissues. Sometimes, you can feel the spread of the tumour in the tissues round the prostate. If possible, confirm these findings by examining the patient bimanually under anaesthesia (see below).

X-RAYS. Look for lytic and sclerotic (typical but less common) secondaries in his pelvis, and lumbar spine. Paget's disease and osteoarthritis produce similar bony symptoms, but show different X-ray changes.

SPECIAL TESTS. If his carcinoma has spread beyond his prostatic capsule, his serum acid phosphatase will be >3 King–Armstrong units. *A normal level does not exclude it.* A persistently raised level supports the diagnosis, and suggests metastasis.

PROSTATIC BIOPSY

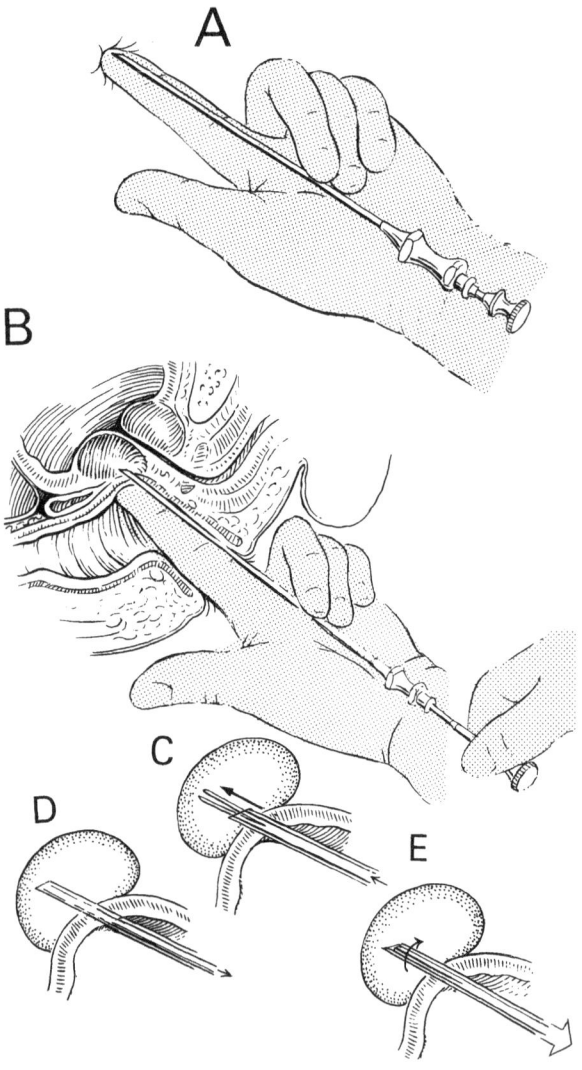

Fig. 32-17a PROSTATIC BIOPSY. A, holding the needle along the palmar surface of your left index finger, with the point on the pulp, insert it into the patient's anus. B, feel each lobe of his prostate, as if you were doing a rectal examination. Using your right hand, push the needle 0.5 cm through his rectal mucosa, towards one of the lobes of his prostate. Withdraw the stylet. C, insert the biopsy jaws, and push them into his prostate as far as they will go, still keeping the needle along the index finger of your left hand. Remove your finger. D, advance the outer sheath far enough to cover the biopsy jaws. E, rotate the needle, so as to break off the core of tissue that has been grasped, and withdraw it. Lift the core of tissue from the biopsy needle, with an ordinary injection needle, and put it into formol saline. If you fail, repeat the process up to 3 times.
Then do the same thing with the other lobe.

It has no prognostic value, its main use is in diagnosis. It falls in response to treatment, and rises when the disease reactivates.

CAUTION ! Take the blood for his acid phosphatase *before* you examine him rectally, or take it more than 48 hours later. If you take it immediately afterwards, you will get an abnormally high reading.

EUA AND CYSTOSCOPY. Examination under anaesthesia (EUA) is the more useful of these two investigations. If possible cystoscope him; this is particularly useful in distinguishing carcinoma of the prostate from carcinoma of the trigone of the bladder infiltrating the prostate. You may feel a grating sensation, as you pass the cystoscope through his carcinomatous prostate, or you may see puckering of the apex of his trigone, or submucous nodules in his bladder (late signs).

NEEDLE BIOPSY OF THE PROSTATE. If you diagnose carcinoma of the prostate when you are examining a patient under anaesthesia for retention of urine, biopsy his prostate with a Vim–Silverman needle through his rectum, as in Fig. 32-17a. This is not difficult and usually gives the correct result. In spite of the fact that you do it through his rectum, serious infection is rare.

THE DIFFERENTIAL DIAGNOSIS includes benign prostatic hyperplasia, carcinoma of the bladder infiltrating the prostate, bladder-neck fibrosis (23.20), and stricture of the posterior urethra (23.8).

THE MANAGEMENT OF CARCINOMA OF THE PROSTATE

If his disease is still confined to his prostatic capsule, and he is under 65, refer him (if you can) for radical radiotherapy.

If this is impractical, or the disease is late, give him stilboestrol daily for the rest of his life. Start with 1 mg daily, and if this fails to control his symptoms increase it to 5 mg. There is an 80% chance that he will show a response. With this low dose there is little risk of cardiovascular complications, but some itching and enlargement of the breasts are common. If necessary, you can do a bilateral mastectomy (21.5, 30.9).

Alternatively, consider doing a standard or a subcapsular orchidectomy (23.25), which will avoid the need for life-long stilboestrol treatment and its possible complications. Most patients don't like this, because their testes become small! To remove them completely is even less acceptable. Discuss his management clearly with him.

If he has retention of urine, give him stilboestrol and pass an indwelling Gibbon or Foley catheter. Leave it in for at least 3 weeks, before trying to remove it, and if he still cannot pass urine adequately, consider leaving it in for a further 3 weeks. Stilboestrol treatment will usually make his prostate shrink enough to let him pass urine. If it does not (unusual), refer him for transurethral resection of his prostate. If this is quite impossible, leave him with a urethral or suprapubic catheter. Don't try to remove his prostate by Freyer's method (23.19): this is difficult, because it does not shell out properly, and he will bleed severely.

If his urine becomes infected, treat him with antibiotics or nitrofurantoin; in itself infection will not influence the outcome of his carcinoma.

CAUTION ! Avoid prostatectomy. It can cause much bleeding. Most cases present with retention, and can be managed with a catheter and stilboestrol.

32.33 Carcinoma of the penis, common

Squamous cell carcinoma of the preputial sac is common in India and Africa. The patient is at least 40, and is almost always uncircumcised. He presents with a swollen and often infected preputial sac, or with phimosis secondary to it. The tumour spreads, until his whole preputial sac is involved, after which it invades his corpus spongiosum, and later his corpora cavernosa. It also spreads to his inguinal lymph nodes, which ultimately ulcerate, so that he dies from sepsis, toxaemia, or sudden haemorrhage from his femoral vessels. It does not obstruct his urethra completely, nor is it painful at first, so that he commonly presents late.

In all but the earliest lesions, which can be treated by radiotherapy if you can refer him for it, you will have to amputate his penis, either partly, or completely. A partial amputation is usually possible; and although it is not easy to do well, it is not nearly as difficult as a total amputation. This is a difficult, bloody, major operation. Partial amputation is very effective, and his prognosis is good. If a block dissection can be done, his prognosis is good, even if his inguinal nodes are involved.

After a partial amputation, he can still urinate comfortably. After a total one, he has little urinary disability, except that he now has to squat to pass his urine, if he wants to avoid soiling his perineum. If you make his perineal meatus carefully, it will function well, and is unlikely to stenose.

Complete amputation of the penis is seldom done in the industrial world, where lesions are usually treated much earlier by radiotherapy. The method described here leaves the crura of the corpora cavernosa attached to the bone, which simplifies surgery. Recurrence in the residual crura is rare. There is nothing to be gained by doing a block dissection of the inguinal nodes prophylactically.

CARCINOMA OF THE PENIS

EXAMINATION. Feel the shaft of the patient's penis carefully to determine the exact extent of the growth. Feel his inguinal nodes. They will probably be enlarged by sepsis, so you may find it difficult to know if they have secondaries in them or not. If necessary, split his prepuce under general anaesthesia, so that you can examine his glans adequately.

BIOPSY. Granuloma acuminatum and donovanosis can both ulcerate the foreskin, and simulate carcinoma of the penis. So always take a biopsy, and wait for histological proof before you amputate a penis—it is tragic to amputate, and then find that you have done so unnecessarily! Don't amputate until you have received the report. Surgery is not urgent, because the tumour is very slow-growing.

THE DIFFERENTIAL DIAGNOSIS includes granuloma acuminatum and the following:

Suggesting primary syphilis—a round or oval painless ulcer, often found under the foreskin, but which does not penetrate or destroy it. Enlarged rubbery glands in the groin. Serological tests may be negative early, but are always positive later.

Suggesting venereal warts—small multiple lumps 1 to 3 mm in diameter, covered by epithelium.

Suggesting donovanosis (granuloma inguinale)—a slow-growing lesion, which may destroy the foreskin, and parts of the shaft of the penis. The lesion is usually flatter and redder than carcinoma.

MANAGEMENT If you cannot refer him, treat him like this.

If the growth is limited to his prepuce and is freely movable over his glans (unusual), excise it, preferably with diathermy if this is available, and follow him up closely.

If it has involved his prepuce and his glans, or the shaft of his penis, take a biopsy, and as soon as the diagnosis is confirmed, do a partial amputation 2 cm proximal to the lesion. If he does get a recurrence, it will probably be in his inguinal nodes, not in the stump of his penis.

If his inguinal nodes do not seem to be clinically involved, **wait**. 'Normal' nodes are palpable, and sepsis may cause some enlargement and tenderness.

If they are palpable, but are clinically infected, **wait**.

If they are palpable and clinically cancerous, biopsy the primary. When you receive the report, amputate his penis, and do a bilateral block dissection. In the developing world patients seldom return for a second operation after amputation, because they do not understand the significance of painless gland enlargement. So, if his glands are involved clinically, amputation and block dissection are best done at the same time.

PARTIAL AMPUTATION OF THE PENIS

Aim to fashion his urethral orifice carefully, so that a stricture does not develop.

Cut a long ventral flap based proximally. Make its width equal

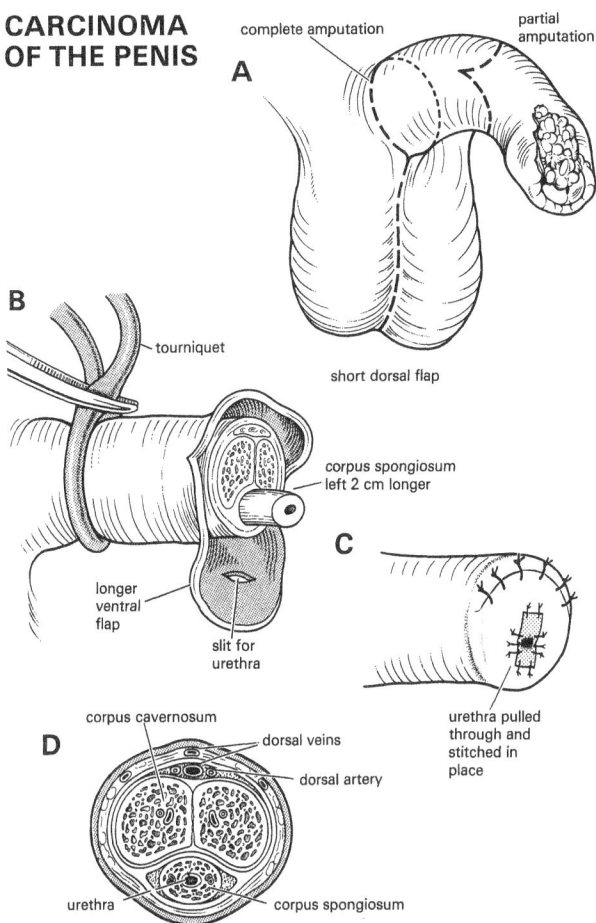

Fig. 32-18 PARTIAL AMPUTATION for carcinoma of the penis. A, the incisions for partial and complete amputation. B, the flaps and the amputation. C, the repair. D, a cross-section of the penis.

to about half the circumference of his penis. Cut a shorter 2 cm dorsal one. Dissect both flaps back to their bases.

Dissect his corpus spongiosum away from his corpora cavernosa, until you reach the planned level of section. Divide his corpus spongiosum 2 cm distal to the level where you intend to section his corpora cavernosa.

Pass transfixion sutures of No. 1 catgut through each of his corpora cavernosa 0.5 cm proximal to the intended level of section. Divide the corpora, dissect proximally for 0.5 cm, and then tie the sutures medially and laterally.

Cut a small circular slit in the ventral flap, and pull his urethral stump through it. Leave the end of his urethra protruding. It is less likely to stricture if you do this. Leave adequate spaces between the sutures to allow blood to drain and prevent a haematoma forming. Leave a self-retaining catheter in place for 5 days. Epithelium will grow over the raw surface of his corpus spongiosum.

Alternatively, split the distal end of his urethra longitudinally. Evert each half, and suture it to the long flap. This will prevent a terminal stricture forming. Although this is the method shown in Fig. 32-18, it is probably less satisfactory than the method above.

Warn him that, despite your efforts, he may require periodic bouginage.

MODIFIED TOTAL AMPUTATION OF THE PENIS

INDICATIONS. Carcinoma of the penis, which cannot be excised 2 cm proximal to the lesion, by partial amputation.

If possible refer him: there are few occasions when a partial amputation is impossible. Only do a total amputation if: (1) Referral is difficult, refused, or impossible. (2) You have seen the operation done or assisted with it. (3) You have 2 units of

TOTAL AMPUTATION OF THE PENIS

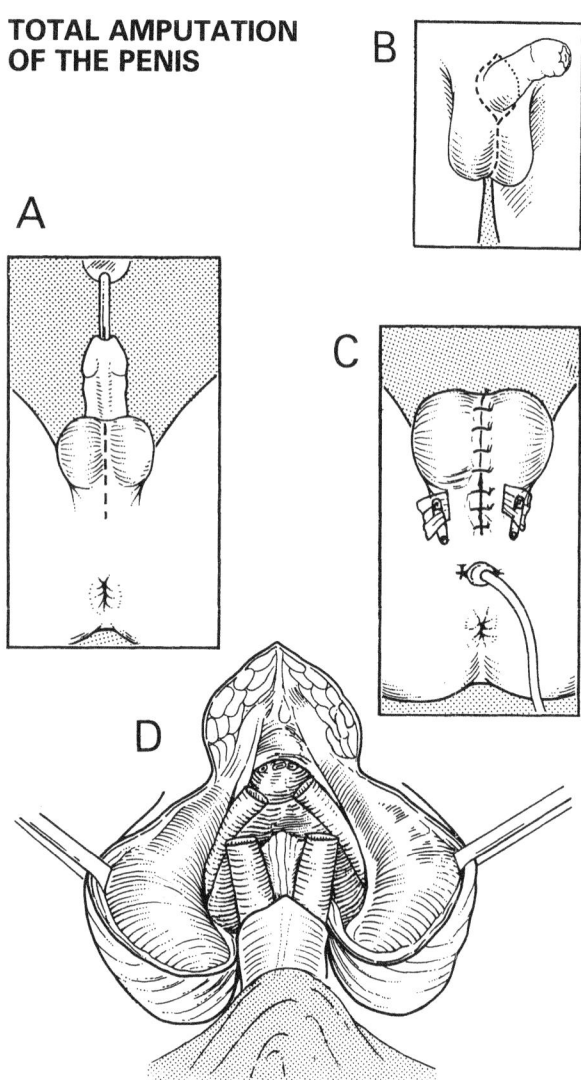

Fig. 32-19 TOTAL AMPUTATION OF THE PENIS. A, passing a sound. B, make a racquet-shaped incision round the base of the patient's penis, and carry it vertically downwards in the midline of his scrotum. C, freeing his crura from his pubic bones. D, his perineum closed round the stump of his urethra.

blood ready. Several experienced contributors considered this operation too difficult to be included here.

ANAESTHESIA. (1) General anaesthesia with a tracheal tube is best. (2) Subarachnoid anaesthesia (A 7.4).

METHOD. Put him into the lithotomy position and pass a 20 to 24 Ch metal bougie to define his urethra. Wrap his penis in a sterile towel, leaving its base exposed.

Make a racquet-shaped incision round the base of his penis. Extend the arm in the midline posteriorly for about 5 cm, between the two sides of his scrotum (extend it further towards his perineum later). Dissect deeper, clamping all vessels; this area is very vascular.

Find, clamp, tie, and divide the large dorsal vein of his penis. Continue dissection until the shaft of his penis is free of subcutaneous tissue.

Extend the incision posteriorly to where his scrotum hangs from his perineum, about 4 or 5 cm in front of his anus. Separate his testes with their covering tunicae vaginales. Ask your assistant to retract them laterally with tissue forceps placed subcutaneously, first on one side and then on the other.

Dissect his corpus spongiosum on its ventral and lateral aspects, as far as the bulb which lies on his perineal membrane. Find it by feeling the expansion round the bougie. Remove the bougie, and cut his corpus spongiosum 4 cm distal to the bulb. Separate it from his corpora cavernosa and retract it.

Now free his corpora cavernosa until they diverge as the crura, at the inferior border of his symphysis pubis. Transfix each of them with a No. 1 chromic catgut suture and divide them about 0.5 cm distal to this. Only some connective tissue will now remain. Divide this and remove his penis.

Cut a transverse 1 cm hole in his perineal skin, 2 or 3 cm anterior to his anal verge. Deliver the stump of his corpus spongiosum through it, so that it protrudes about 2 cm. Suture the base to his skin, using 2/0 or 3/0 monofilament sutures. Don't try to evert the stump, or his urethra may form a stricture. Leave the stump long because it tends to retract. Epithelium from his urethra and skin will grow and cover it.

Insert corrugated rubber drains through 2 cm incisions laterally in his scrotum, to allow blood and tissue fluid to drain. Stitch these to his skin. Or, better, use suction drains.

First close the wound in the midline, using 2/0 or 1/0 monofilament. Then suture the anterior part of the wound. If his scrotum would hang down too much, trim off some skin and subcutaneous tissue before you suture it.

When you have finished, his scrotum will lie more anteriorly than usual. This allows good skin cover, and is less likely to get in the way when he urinates through his perineal urethrostomy.

POSTOPERATIVE CARE. Pass an indwelling catheter, release it 4-hourly and remove it at 7 to 10 days.

Apply much cotton wool padding, and a pressure dressing of elastic strapping. Remove the dressings and the drains on the 3rd day. Then start salt baths twice daily.

32.34 Block dissection of the inguinal lymph nodes

Squamous cell carcinomas of the skin of the leg, and the penis, both metastasize to the nodes of the groin. Removing these metastases in a block of tissue, containing the horizontal and vertical inguinal nodes, can be very successful, because these carcinomas are not very malignant.

The femoral vein, artery, and nerves lie close to the nodes that need to be removed, and may be displaced by them. Removing them without damaging these structures is a difficult, delicate, major operation. Afterwards, the wound can discharge tissue fluid and become secondarily infected. Healing may be delayed, the flaps may necrose, and lymphoedema may develop in the patient's legs (5—10%). For all these reasons, refer him if you can. If you have to remove his inguinal nodes yourself, study the anatomy thoroughly before you start, and dissect them away carefully. Blood loss is usually not great—provided you don't damage major vessels!

If his inguinal nodes are involved clinically, remove them at the same time that you amputate his leg, or his penis, because he may refuse a second operation. Don't try to remove them prophylactically, in the hope of removing metastases which you cannot feel. It will not improve his prognosis, and may be complicated by lymphoedema (31.4). Only do a block dissection therapeutically, when his lymph nodes are palpably enlarged by secondary growth. If infection is likely to be the cause of the enlargement, wait for it to improve after the amputation, and watch him regularly. Do a block dissection if his nodes start enlarging.

Block dissection of the nodes of the neck is not described here. Removing them from the axilla is described as part of Patey's operation for carcinoma of the breast (21.6).

BLOCK DISSECTION OF THE INGUINAL NODES

INDICATIONS. (1) Clinical involvement of the inguinal nodes, with secondary deposits from squamous cell carcinoma of the penis, or leg. If a patient's nodes have not ulcerated, removing them may cure him. If they have ulcerated, you may be unable to remove the mass of ulcerated tissue completely. The determining factor is whether or not they have stuck to deeper struc-

BLOCK DISSECTION OF THE INGUINAL NODES

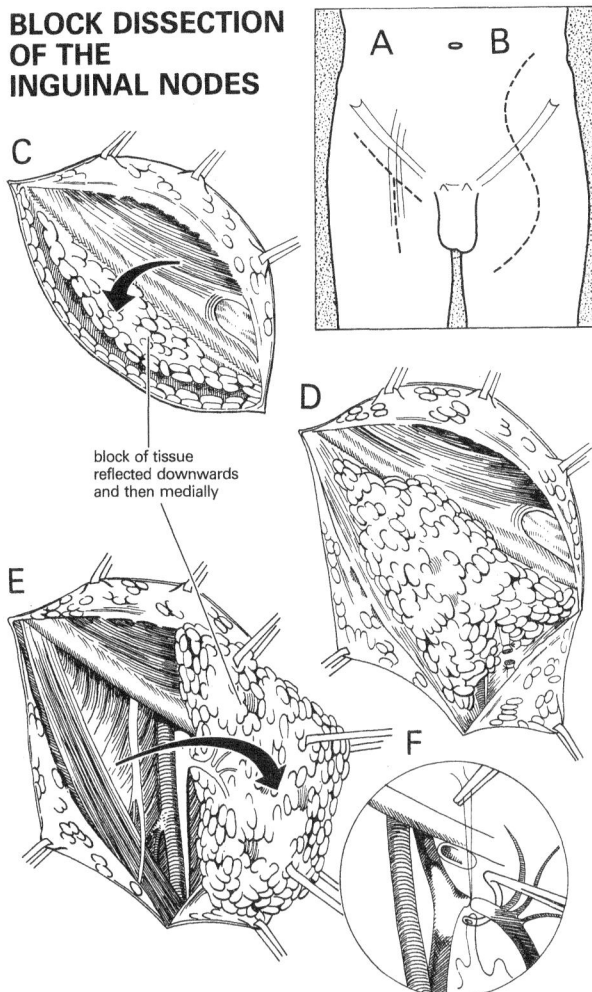

Fig. 32-20 BLOCK DISSECTION OF THE INGUINAL LYMPH NODES. A, a 'T' incision. B, a 'lazy S' incision. C, reflect superior and inferior flaps. D, prepare to reflect a triangular block of tissue. E, reflect a block of tissue medially from the femoral vessels. F, tying the saphenous vein.

tures, especially the femoral vessels. (2) Malignant melanoma; block dissection is often only palliative, but is not always so. His nodes may be large and ulcerate. Don't wait for them to do this before you operate, because they may be impossible to remove later. His prognosis is much worse than with squamous cell carcinoma, because he may already have secondary deposits elsewhere.

If he also requires an amputation, say below the knee for a squamous carcinoma, do both operations at the same time; he may not consent to another one. If you are also going to amputate his penis, make the incisions in continuity, and do both sides at the same time.

CAUTION ! This is a difficult operation, so refer him if you can.

HISTOLOGY. Make the decision to operate clinically, and don't take a node for biopsy first. If you think that nodes really are malignant, don't let the biopsy report influence your decision— a malignant deposit in a node may have been missed histologically, or it may only be in other nodes. After the operation, send a node which you think has metastases, and the nearest node to the femoral canal. If you can easily dissect out Cloquet's node in the femoral canal, send that; but if removing it might endanger the femoral vein, leave it.

ANAESTHESIA. General anaesthesia with spontaneous respiration (A 11.1), or subarachnoid (spinal) anaesthesia (A 7.1). Have 2 units of blood ready.

METHOD. Lay him supine with a sandbag under the buttock of his affected side. When you have completed one side, move it to the other one.

Make a 'T' or 'lazy S' incision (A, or B, in Fig. 32-20). A 'lazy S' incision allows you to remove skin, and produces the least skin necrosis, but finding your way may be more difficult. Here, we assume you have decided to make a 'T'incision.

Make the horizontal limb of the 'T' 2 cm distal to his inguinal ligament, 8 to 10 cm long, centred just distal to his mid-inguinal point, where you can feel his femoral pulse. If some skin needs removing, keep away from the diseased area, and cut an ellipse round it, so that you can excise it with the lesion.

Reflect the superior flap with about 0.5 cm of subcutaneous fat, and undermine it 5 cm above your incision. Use a knife or scissors to dissect upwards under it, until it is about 5 cm wide.

At the upper extremity of the flap divide the subcutaneous tissues covering his abdominal muscles in the depth of the wound. Reflect a block of subcutaneous tissue downwards (C), until you reach his inguinal ligament. Don't cut his cord. Clamp, divide, and tie the vessels as you go.

Make the vertical limb of the 'T' 8 to 10 cm long, from the mid point of the horizontal limb, distally over the mass of nodes—unless you need to remove some skin. If so, make it elliptical.

Dissect out flaps of skin with 0.5 cm of subcutaneous tissue, as far as is easy, to expose a triangular block of tissue laterally, medially, and distally. Make its apex at least 4 cm distal to any palpable node. Cut through the subcutaneous tissues at the edges of the triangular mass, down to the deep fascia or muscle (D). As you do so, find and clamp his saphenous vein. Tie it with No. 0 silk. Its surface marking is a line from just medial to his mid-inguinal point to the medial aspect of the medial condyle of his femur. Avoid his femoral vessels, which lie 2 or 3 cm lateral to his saphenous vein near the distal end of the incision. Dissect down with scissors, looking for the vessels, which are covered by a sheath. The femoral vein lies posteromedial to the femoral artery, and is largely covered by it at this point, and by the strap-like sartorius muscle. Tie and divide any smaller vessels you meet.

Dissect the block of tissue proximally from the apex of the wound. As you do so, remove it from the femoral vessels, for about 3 cm. Retract it with tissue forceps. Reflect medial and lateral flaps, in the same way as the superior one, as far out as you can retract them comfortably. Then clear the block of tissue from the underlying muscles. On the lateral side, you will meet his femoral nerve proximally. Continuing to work from distal to proximal, reflect the block of tissue from his femoral vessels medially (E). Tie and divide any small vessels you meet, close to the main ones.

CAUTION ! (1) Pulling on the block of tissue may pull up his femoral vessels, so you may think that his femoral vein is his saphenous vein. *Don't clamp, divide, or damage his femoral vein,* which may become flat and empty as you pull on the tissues. (2) Try not to damage his profunda femoris or circumflex vessels (medial and lateral), which pass deep to the muscles of his thigh.

Continue to dissect proximally. This is the difficult part. Find where his saphenous vein (which may be flat and empty) joins his femoral vein. About 1 cm distal to the junction it receives several tributaries (the superficial circumflex iliac, the superficial epigastric, and the superficial external pudendal veins). When you are sure you have found it, use an aneurysm needle to pass two No. 0 silk ligatures under it, at least 5 mm apart (F). Divide it between these ligatures—away from the femoral vein!

The block of tissue will now be almost clear, with nothing important attached to it. Dissect it free. Suture his sartorius muscle over his exposed femoral vessels; this is readily possible in the distal part of the wound—don't leave them exposed, or they may ulcerate and bleed disastrously.

If you can obtain good skin closure, and the wound is airtight, insert a suction drain (if you have one), with its limbs medially and laterally. If you don't have a suction drain, or the wound is not airtight, insert corrugated rubber drains through 1.5 cm incisions medially and laterally.

Close the skin flaps with No. 0 or No. 1 interrupted monofilament sutures. Apply a cotton wool pressure dressing for 48 to 72 hours. Shorten the corrugated drains on the third day. Remove alternate sutures on the 12th day, and the others when the wound seems sound.

Now, if you are operating for carcinoma of the penis, do the same thing on the other side.

DIFFICULTIES WITH BLOCK DISSECTION OF THE INGUINAL NODES

Infection and necrosis of the skin edges are common. Complete healing takes time, but does occur.

If you INJURE A FEMORAL VESSEL, usually the vein, press it to control bleeding, then clamp it above and below with artery forceps covered with suitable pieces of rubber catheter, or, better, use forceps specially designed for vascular surgery (55-4). If possible close the hole in the vessel as in Section 55.6, then remove the clamps.

If you cannot control bleeding, tie the vein above and below the wound. His leg will swell, but will usually improve in time. It is rare for it to become gangrenous and be lost.

If you cannot CANNOT COVER HIS FEMORAL VESSELS with his sartorius muscle proximally, separate it at its origin from his anterior superior iliac spine. Suture it to the fascia of his external oblique just proximal to his inguinal ligament in such a way that it covers his femoral vessels.

If CLOSURE OF THE WOUND IS DIFFICULT, don't close it under tension. If there is suitable muscle in the bare area, apply a split skin graft immediately and suture it in place using a gauze stent (57-7). Or, take a graft now, store it, and apply it 5 days later (57.8). If his femoral vessels are exposed, mobilize his sartorius, as described above.

If he develops LYMPHOEDEMA, he is one of the unlucky 10% of patients who do. Advise him to raise his leg at night, and prop it up when he sits. If possible apply an elastic bandage, or as a poor second best, a crêpe one.

32.34a Tumours of the testis rare

Nearly all tumours of the testis are malignant. In Africa, most of them are rhabdomyosarcomas under the age of 16; seminomas are very rare. Elsewhere, most are seminomas or teratomas or a combination of both, and are usually seen between the ages of 20 and 45. The patient complains of: (1) A large painless (usually) testicular swelling. (2) An abdominal mass. (3) Gynaecomastia and breast tenderness (rare), in which case gonadotrophin production by the tumour may result in a positive pregnancy test.

If he is diagnosed and treated early he has an 80% chance of cure by orchidectomy alone. Seminomas are sensitive to radiotherapy, but not to chemotherapy, whereas teratomas are amenable to chemotherapy (75% complete cure), although this needs cisplatin and expert management.

TUMOURS OF THE TESTIS

DIAGNOSIS. The patient's testis is large, harder than his normal one, smooth, heavy, and not tender. It loses its normal sensation early. When he stands it usually hangs lower than his normal one, unlike testes with inflammation or torsion, which are usually pulled higher. He has a normal vas, a normal cord until late, occasionally a hydrocele (10%), and a normal prostate and seminal vesicles. Early, his epididymis is normal, later it is flattened or hidden in the tumour. Feel for deposits above his umbilicus on the same side, in his liver, and above his clavicles. X-ray his lungs.

THE DIFFERENTIAL DIAGNOSIS includes epididymo-orchitis (very common, 23.22a), a hydrocele (23.23), a haematocele following trauma, torsion of his testis (23.24), an epidermal cyst, a tuberculoma, and a gumma (rare). In sub-Saharan Africa a seminoma is rarer than all these.

MANAGEMENT. Operate soon. While he is anaesthetized palpate his abdomen for para-aortic masses. Open his inguinal canal through an inguinoscrotal incision, as in Fig. 23-33. Clamp his cord with a soft clamp to avoid damaging its vessels. Draw up his testis and examine it. If it looks malignant, divide and tie his cord at the level of his internal inguinal ring. Remove his cord and testis, from above downwards, by separating them from their attachments. Close the wound. If he has a seminoma refer him for radiotherapy to his upper abdominal para-aortic nodes as soon as possible, even in the absence of demonstrable secondaries. If he has a teratoma, observe him carefully, and refer him if secondaries appear.

CAUTION ! (1) If he presents with symptoms which might be due to secondaries, don't fail to examine his testes. A small primary is easily missed. (2) Don't remove his testis through his scrotum. (3) Don't try to biopsy the lesion.

TUMOURS OF THE FEMALE GENITAL ORGANS OTHER THAN THE BREAST (21.3)

32.35 Carcinoma of the cervix (common) and endometrium (rare)

Carcinoma of the cervix is among the commonest tumours in the developing world, and causes much suffering. Most tumours are squamous-celled, a few are adenocarcinomas arising from the endocervix. Carcinoma of the cervix is more common in grand multips, in the promiscuous (including those who have a series of husbands), in partners of the uncircumcised, and in women living in very unhygienic conditions. Herpes virus type 2 is associated with carcinoma of the cervix, but its role as a causative agent is still uncertain.

A patient can present with: (1) intermenstrual bleeding, often bright red, (2) postcoital bleeding, (3) postmenopausal bleeding, or (4) a vaginal discharge, which is not always blood-stained, and is usually watery.

The premalignant phases of cervical cancer can be identified in a woman without symptoms by examining a smear of cervical cells on a slide—a Papanicolau or 'Pap' smear. At this stage laser treatment, cone biopsy or total hysterectomy will cure her. Unfortunately, a screening program needs good laboratories and a system to recall and monitor patients with abnormal cells. Establishing such a service is beyond the scope of the hospitals for which we write, but if there is such a service, use it. In its absence the best you can do is to make sure that all your staff, who provide primary care, persuade *anyone with early symptoms to come for examination and biopsy.* Both carcinoma of the cervix and AIDS are less common in patients who use condoms, so encourage promiscuous patients to use them.

Treatment requires either radiotherapy, or radical hysterectomy to remove the upper vagina, the parametrium and the pelvic lymph nodes. This is an an expert's task. Stage 0 can be treated by cone biopsy (see below), and a total hysterectomy is of some value in Stage One, but not later. Your main task is to take cone or wedge biopsies when necessary, and to stage a patient carefully to decide if referral is indicated. If she can be referred, her outlook is good in stages I and IIa, so that the correct staging and prompt referral of these stages is important. Unfortunately, many patients in the developing world present so late, so that even if referral is possible it is of little benefit. There is no useful chemotherapy.

Carcinoma of the endometrium is rare in the developing world. It occurs in older patients, and is the most important cause of bleeding after tne menopause, which is an urgent indication for a 'D and C'.

CARCINOMA OF THE CERVIX

DIAGNOSIS. Take a careful history and establish the timing and appearance of the bleeding; a patient may confuse vaginal bleeding with haematuria. Examine her abdomen, and her groins. Examine her vagina and cervix with a speculum. Do a rectal examination and a bimanual examination of her pelvic organs. All this can be done as an outpatient procedure. You may see: (1) An ulcer on her cervix, often extending into one or more fornices. (2) A cervical polyp (less common). (3) An enlarged barrel-shaped cervix which may look relatively normal. (4) Erosion into her bladder or cervix causing an RVF or a VVF.

The differential diagnosis includes a simple cervical erosion,

CANCER OF THE CERVIX

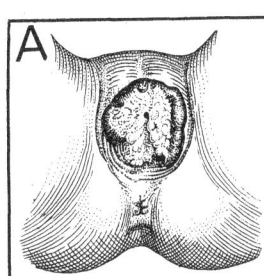

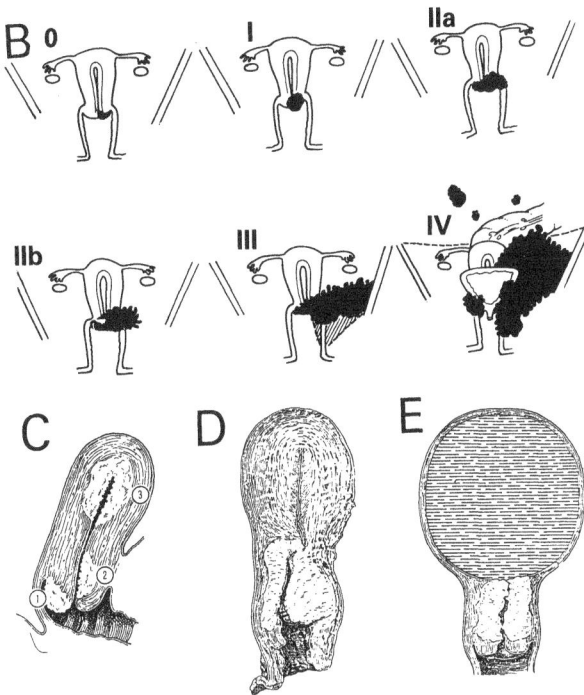

Fig. 32-21 CARCINOMA OF THE CERVIX. A, a Shapibo Indian from South America with a neglected carcinoma of her cervix showing vulval involvement (Stage IV). B, staging the disease. Stage 0, carcinoma in situ. Stage I, the tumour is confined to the patient's cervix. Stage IIa, it extends into her upper vagina or uterus, but not into her parametrium. Stage IIb, it extends into her parametrium, but not to her pelvic wall. Stage III, it involves the side wall of her pelvis, or the lower third of her vagina. Stage IV, it involves the mucosa of her bladder, or rectum, or she has distant metastases.

C, the sites of carcinoma: (1) Squamous carcinoma of the vaginal cervix. (2) Adenocarcinoma of the endocervix. (3) Adenocarcinoma of the endometrium.

D, carcinoma of the cervix (Stage One or Two). E, pyometra; the body of the uterus is filled with pus above a Stage One carcinoma of the cervix. *After Pinter and Roberts, and James Young.*

a cervical or endometrial polyp, a submucous fibroid, various stages of abortion, irregular bleeding near the menopause, carcinoma of the endometrium, senile vaginitis, urethral caruncle, and a bilharzial granuloma.

Suggesting carcinoma—the lesion feels hard, it is friable (bits break off easily), a raised edge, you can feel it extending into her parametrium.

Suggesting an erosion (normal and physiological)—an area of glandular epithelium around her external os surrounded by normal squamous epithelium. *No raised edge.* Does not feel hard and gritty. There is usually no contact bleeding, but a little contact bleeding can occur.

If a Pap smear has shown suspect cells, take a cone biopsy to confirm it. If there is an ulcer, take a wedge biopsy.

A 'D and C' is not necessary for investigating carcinoma of the cervix. This does occasionally reveal carcinoma, but it is usually an adenocarcinoma of the body of the uterus or of the endocervix. Invasion of the body of the uterus by a carcinoma of the cervix is not one of the staging criteria for this tumour.

STAGING AND MANAGEMENT. If you suspect she is in one of the earlier stages, with some hope of cure or palliation, stage her as an inpatient, under anaesthesia, in the lithotomy position. Do a rectal examination to assess spread beyond her uterus. Do a vaginal examination at the same time, and feel her rectovaginal septum between your fingers. If she has an advanced lesion, an examination under anaesthesia is hardly necessary. Examine her gently as an outpatient, and remove a small piece of tissue for histology. You may however need to admit her on social grounds, especially if she is travelling far.

Stage 0, carcinoma in situ. This is a histological diagnosis, made from either a cone (or wedge) biopsy, or a positive Pap smear. The cells look malignant, but have not yet invaded the surrounding tissue, and may not do so for many years, if ever. Cone biopsy is curative at this stage.

If the diagnosis was made from a Pap smear, do a cone biopsy.

If the diagnosis was made by a cone biopsy, follow-up is all that is needed. Or, after a full explanation, refer her for a total (not radical) hysterectomy, if she wants one, or do it yourself (20.12).

Stage 1 The tumour is confined to her cervix and can be cured, either by radical hysterectomy, or by radiotherapy. Refer her for them. She has an 85% to 90% chance of surviving 5 years. If she cannot have a radical hysterectomy, a total one is of some benefit.

Stage 2A The tumour extends out from her cervix into her upper vagina or uterus, but not into her parametrium. Stage 2A is uncommon because progress to stage 2b is so rapid. Manage her as for Stage I. She has a 75% to 80% chance of 5 year survival. A total hysterectomy is useless, but a radical one is of some value

Stage 2B The tumour extends into her parametrium but not as far as her pelvic wall. Radical surgery is impossible, but radiotherapy is not, and can achieve 5 year survival rates of 45% to 55%. Even if it fails, it is good palliation.

Stage 3 The tumour involves the lower third of her vagina and/or the side wall of her pelvis. Manage her as for Stage IIB. Radiotherapy can achieve 5 year survival rates of 30% to 40%.

Stage 4 The tumour involves the mucosa of her bladder or her rectum, or has metastasized beyond her pelvis. Palliate her with chlorpromazine and analgesics, as her pain increases (33.1).

CAUTION ! (1) A negative Pap smear does not exclude invasive carcinoma, nor does a positive smear prove it (she may have *carcinoma in situ*). (2) *Carcinoma in situ* does not cause abnormal bleeding or other symptoms. (3) Abnormal lesions need to be confirmed by wedge or cone biopsy.

CONE BIOPSY FOR CARCINOMA OF THE CERVIX

INDICATONS. (1) To confirm a positive or suspicious Pap smear. If her cervix is clinically normal, repeat the Pap smear before you take the biopsy. (2) As treatment for *carcinoma in situ,* as shown by a positive Pap smear. (3) As primary treatment for a lesion considered to be *carcinoma in situ* or possibly stage I, in order to obtain reliable distinction between these two.

ANAESTHESIA. (1) General anaesthesia. (2) Low subarachnoid anaesthesia (A 7.7). (3) Caudal epidural anaesthesia (A 7.3).

CAUTION ! (1) Don't do a preliminary dilatation. If she needs one, do it after you have taken the biopsy. (2) Don't use diathermy—it spoils the specimen.

METHOD. Put her into the lithotomy position. A cone biopsy is notorious for postoperative bleeding, both reactionary and secondary. Minimize this by taking it in the postmenstrual period, and inserting a preliminary catgut suture to prevent bleeding, exactly as with McDonald's cervical suture (16.5), or by injecting dilute adrenalin and tying the descending cervical arteries.

Either, start by inserting a McDonald's suture, as in Figs. 16-2 and 32-22, and tie it. You only want it to act for a day or two, so use catgut, not monfilament. Put it all round her cervix, as high up as you can, and loop it into her cervix to hold it. Pull it tight to occlude her descending cervical vessels.

Or, use vulsellum forceps to grasp the anterior aspect of her cervix away from the lesion. Then, infiltrate her cervix with 20 or 30 ml of 1:100 000 adrenalin solution (1 ml of 1:1000 adrenalin with 100 ml of saline). Transfix her descending cervical vessels on each side with No. 0 chromic catgut, leaving the ligatures long to act as stays.

BIOPSY OF THE CERVIX

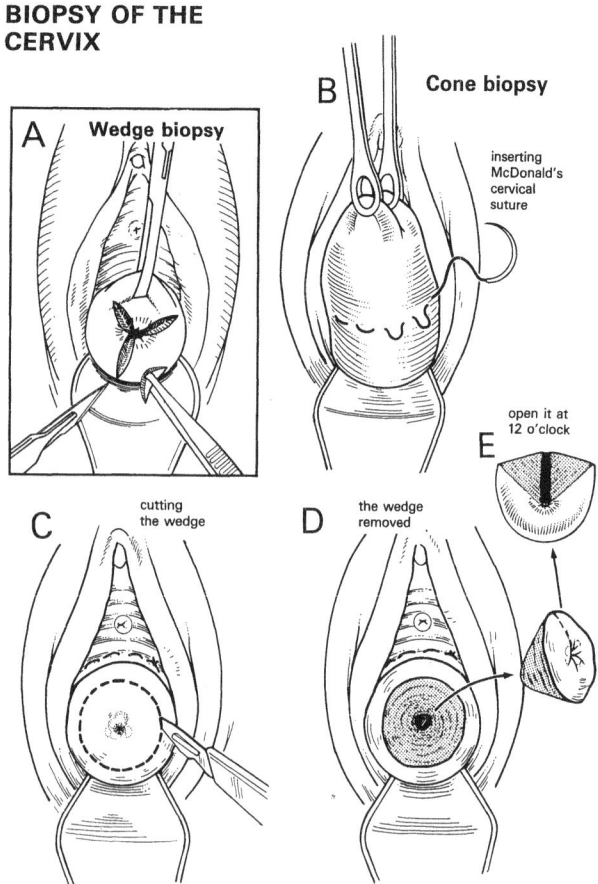

Fig. 32-22 BIOPSY OF THE CERVIX. A, a wedge biopsy. B, inserting McDonald's suture before doing a cone biopsy. C, cutting the cone. D, removing the cone. E, the cone opened out with an incision in the 12 o'clock position.

Schiller's test (optional) helps to define the extend of the atypical epithelium, but is not absolutely reliable. Apply 1% iodine to the lesion and the surrounding epithelium. Normal epithelium stains, atypical epthelium may not.

Incise the normal epithelium about 5 mm from its junction with the abnormal epithelium, and extend your incision all round her cervix. Apply vulsellum forceps to the lips of her cervix at 12 o'clock and 6 o'clock. Deepen the incision to remove a cone, with its apex at her cervical canal, keeping its edge 3 to 5 mm away from the abnormal tissue. Leave the raw surface open. Cut the cone open in the 12 o'clock position, and send it intact for histology.

CAUTION ! If a pathologist is going to examine a cone biopsy adequately: (1) it must be big enough, (2) its orientation in the patient must be identifiable (hence the 12 o'clock cut). (3) It must be in one piece, and (4) it must be injured as little as possible. He should be able to report that the edges of the cone are normal, and if not, where the suspicious tissue is.

WEDGE BIOPSY FOR CARCINOMA OF THE CERVIX

INDICATIONS. To confirm or exclude malignancy in an ulcer of the cervix.

METHOD. At 3 sites or more on the ulcerated area, excise ellipses at least 3 mm deep, crossing the margin between the ulcerated and the normal area.

CARCINOMA OF THE ENDOMETRIUM

STAGING AND SURVIVAL. The 5 year survival after surgery and radiotherapy is given for each stage.

Stage 1 The carcinoma is confined to the corpus (80% 5 year survival).

Stage 1a The length of her uterine cavity is 8 cm or less.
Stage 1b The length of her uterine cavity is >8cm.
Stage 2 Her corpus and cervix are involved (58%).
Stage 3 The carcinoma extends outside her corpus, but not outside her true pelvis. It may involve her vagina or her parametrium, but not her bladder or her rectum (33%).
Stage 4 It involves her bladder or her rectum, or extends outside her pelvis (7%).

MANAGEMENT. Confirm the diagnosis by doing a 'D and C', and sending scrapings for histology. If she is Stage Two or more, she needs radiotherapy. A total abdominal hysterectomy with the removal of a cuff of vagina is the next best.

32.35a Carcinoma of the vulva, rare

If a patient has a carcinoma of her vulva, she needs a wide and mutilating excision of the primary, with a margin of normal tissue of at least 2 cm all round, and 1 cm deep to the lesion. If her groin glands are involved, she needs a bilateral groin dissection. If you cannot refer her, all you can probably offer her is terminal care.

CARCINOMA OF THE VULVA.

THE DIFFERENTIAL DIAGNOSIS includes: vulval warts, syphilis (primary and secondary), donovanosis (granuloma inguinale: like a carcinoma this eats away tissue), and lymphogranuloma venereum, and (very important) the granulations of *Schistosoma haematobium*, see Section 20.14.

CAUTION ! Before contemplating a radical operation on the vulva, be sure to do a biopsy: it is tragic to do a mutilating operation for an innocent lesion.

32.36 Tumours of the ovary, not uncommon

Ovarian cysts and tumours are described in Section 20.7. Here we are concerned with the malignant ones, and particularly with chemotherapy. A patient with a malignant ovarian tumour can have: a cystic adenocarcinoma (40%, and usually arising in a serous cystadenoma), a solid adenocarcinoma (30%), a solid anaplastic carcinoma (15%), or a variety of other tumours (15%), including secondary growths and germ cell tumours (rare, but chemotherapy can cure them). Surgery is the mainstay of treatment. If possible remove the growth entirely, if not take a biopsy. Radiotherapy, and for most tumours chemotherapy, are only of temporary benefit. The prognosis is better for cystic than for solid tumours. Rarely, they may remit spontaneously.

CHEMOTHERAPY is well worth considering. It is useful in the prevention of ascites, and may prolong survival in patients in Stages Two (peritoneal spread within the pelvis) and Three (peritoneal spread throughout the abdomen). It also delays the onset of this distressing problem. 40% of patients respond to cyclophosphamide 1.5 g/m^2 every 21 days for up to 6 courses. If drugs are scarce, this use for them is of low priority. Combined drug regimes have some advantage over this one, but are more expensive.

32.37 Tumours of the trophoblast, common in some areas

One of the most important advances in chemotherapy was the discovery that many cases of choriocarcinoma can be cured with methotrexate. If you cannot refer a patient, you may have to treat her yourself.

In a normal pregnancy some trophoblastic cells are carried to the lungs, but do not grow there. They are only malignant when they *grow* outside the uterus, or abnormally within it. Here is a convenient simplification of what happens:

(1) A hydatidiform mole is a benign neoplasm of the

trophoblast, in which the chorionic villi overgrow to form fluid-filled, grape-like vesicles, up to 1 cm in diameter. A mole can be *complete* without an embryo (more common), or *partial* (less common), when some fetal tissues are present (most often blood vessels containing nucleated red cells). Moles of either kind can present as an abortion, or an ectopic pregnancy. In a binovular twin pregnancy, one twin may be normal and the other a mole. Moles vary widely in incidence from 1:120 to 1:2000 pregnancies, and are more common in Asia than they are elsewhere.

(2) A non-metastasizing trophoblastic neoplasm (invasive mole) is a tumour-like process which invades the myometrium and arises from a hydatidiform mole, more commonly from a complete one. These lesions occasionally regress spontaneously.

(3) A metastasizing trophoblastic neoplasm (choriocarcinoma) arises from the trophoblast after a live birth, a stillbirth, an abortion, an ectopic pregnancy, or a hydatidiform mole.

50% of trophoblastic neoplasms develop as complications of hydatidiform moles. 25% follow full-term deliveries, and 25% follow spontaneous abortions when they present as heavy irregular bleeding. Occasionally, they follow an ectopic pregnancy.

32.38 Hydatidiform moles and trophoblastic neoplasms

A patient with a hydatidiform mole is commonly under 20 or over 40; she usually presents before the 18th week of pregnancy with: (1) Rapid enlargement of her uterus, which feels abnormally soft. (2) Excessive nausea and vomiting. (3) Vaginal bleeding which is typically dark red, or brownish, and starts at the 6th to 8th week. (4) The passage of vesicles though her cervix. (5) Enlarged cystic ovaries (50% of cases), which may be palpable. (6) Signs of gestational hypertension (17.4). She may show any combination of these signs, and if her pregnancy exceeds 18 weeks, inability to palpate the fetal parts and the absence of fetal movements are other suggestive features.

After you have evacuated her mole three things can happen: (1) She may recover completely (80% or even 95%). (2) She may develop a non-metastasizing trophoblastic neoplasm (invasive mole). (3) She may develop a metastasizing trophoblastic neoplasm (choriocarcinoma), either high risk or low risk.

Early diagnosis, effective treatment, and energetic follow-up are essential. You can treat a hydatidiform mole without too much difficulty, but you should refer a choriocarcinoma. If this is impossible, you may have to treat her yourself. As always with cancer chemotherapy, treat patients properly or not at all.

The method which follows makes no allowance for the fact that she may want more children, nor does it advise hysterotomy. Unfortunately, the use of an oxytocin drip increases the risk of her requiring chemotherapy, but is the method of choice under your circumstances.

TUMOURS OF THE TROPHOBLAST

HYDATIDIFORM MOLE

HISTORY and EXAMINATION. Enquire exactly about the times of bleeding, and look at the colour of the blood. Ask about the passage of tissue ('grapes') vaginally. Note the size and feel of the patient's uterus, especially changes after 2 weeks. Measure her fundal height. Listen to the fetal heart; you should hear it at 18 weeks in a normal pregnancy. Doppler fetal heart monitoring is useful (if you have it). The presence of a fetal heart reduces the probability of a mole, but does not exclude the much rarer occurrence of a partial mole, with a complete fetus, or twin pregnancy. Look for signs of gestational hypertension (17.4).

X-RAY her abdomen and look for fetal parts. You should see them at 16 weeks. Their absence is strongly suggestive, but their presence does not exclude hydatidiform mole.

TUMOURS OF THE TROPHOBLAST

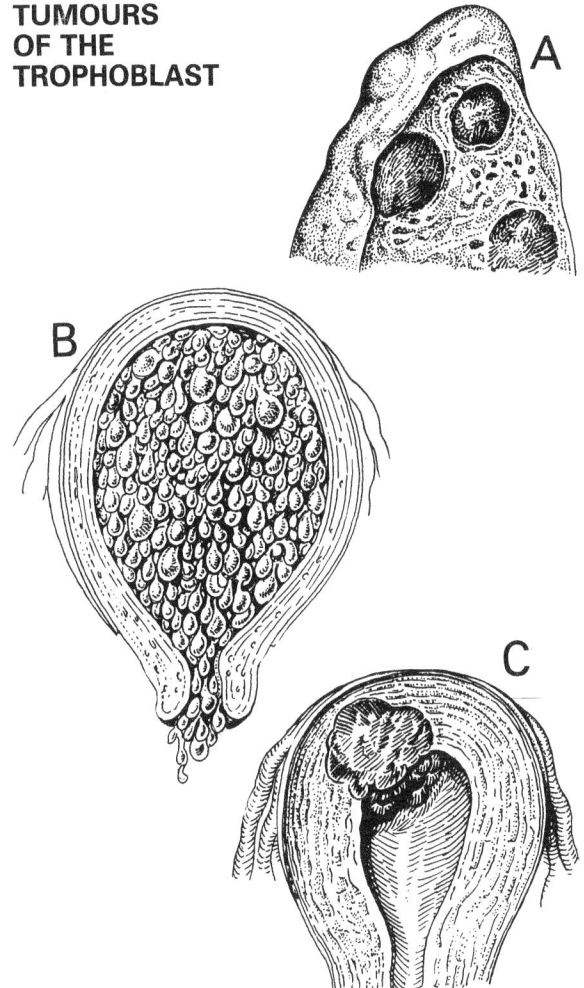

Fig. 32-23 TUMOURS OF THE TROPHOBLAST. A, a choriocarcinoma has metastasized to the lungs. B, a hydatidiform mole. C, a choriocarcinoma invading the wall of the uterus. *Adapted from drawings by Frank Netter, with the kind permission of CIBA-GEIGY Ltd, Basle (Switzerland).*

CAUTION! Never X-ray a fetus less than 14 weeks. Most fetuses that need X-raying are more than 22 weeks. A suspected mole and acute hydramnios are the only exceptions.

TESTS FOR GONADOTROPHIN are not ideal for diagnosing a mole, but you are unlikely to have ultrasound, which is better. If possible, measure the human chorionic gonadotrophin (HCG) in a 24 hour urine sample (normal 40 000 u/24 hours). Suspect titres above 100,000; they may reach 1 or 2 million. Unfortunately, values in the normal pregnancy range do not exclude hydatidiform mole.

Do a standard *qualitative* immunological pregnancy test using a test kit. If this is positive, do serial dilutions of a 24 hour urine specimen, to detect the greatest dilution showing a positive result. This is an inexpensive way of doing a quantitative test, and although it is not ideal, it is likely to be the best that you can do, *but it must be done carefully!* The standard quantitative test uses much test solution and is expensive. Some way of doing a quantitative test is important because: (1) the clinical and X-ray signs may be inconclusive, (2) during follow-up, it is the only way of knowing if trophoblastic tissue is still present.

THE DIFFERENTIAL DIAGNOSIS includes: (1) a multiple pregnancy, (2) an abortion, especially a missed abortion, (3) acute polyhydramnios, (4) retention of urine with a retroverted gravid uterus, (5) a subacute or chronic ectopic pregnancy.

IMMEDIATE COMPLICATIONS. The important one is bleeding, especially during, or after abortion, or evacuation of her uterus.

LONG TERM SEQUELAE. There is a 15% chance of a non-metastasizing neoplasm, and a 5% chance of a metastasizing one.

THE MANAGEMENT OF HYDATIDIFORM MOLE

ANAEMIA. Correct her anaemia by blood transfusion. If her haematocrit is <15% (haemoglobin 50 g/l), give her packed cells slowly, and precede each unit with frusemide 20 mg. Watch carefully for cardiac failure, and replace any sudden blood loss rapidly.

EVACUATE HER UTERUS. You have four choices:

(1) You can start by setting up an oxytocin drip of 10 u/500 ml, running at 30 drops a minute during the procedure, and for 1 or 2 hours afterwards. Avoid combining this with ergometrine if you can, because it increases the risk of trophoblastic tissue embolizing to her lungs.

(2) You can avoid oxytocin: give her ergometrine alone, and accept its risks as being necessary. If you decide to do this, give her ergometrine 0.25 mg intramuscularly or intravenously. When her cervix is sufficiently dilated, evacuate her uterus under sedation and a paracervical block (A 6.14), or under general anaesthesia or ketamine. Avoid subarachnoid and epidural anaesthesia if she is hypovolaemic. If possible use suction, if not, use your fingers or a blunt curette. The standard suction apparatus for terminating pregnancy is satisfactory (See Primary Mother Care).

(3) Prostaglandin pessaries are better if you have them (16.4).

CAUTION ! (1) Don't start to evacuate her uterus until her cervix is sufficiently dilated to admit your finger, or she will be more likely to bleed. (2) Take great care not to perforate her uterus. If you think that evacuation is incomplete, or if bleeding continues, accept this, and repeat the curettage in a week. (3) Torrential bleeding can occur, so have 2 units of blood available, but don't give it unless she bleeds.

After you have evacuated her uterus, you may feel her cystic ovaries—leave them. Repeat the curettage in 7 to 10 days.

(4) Consider doing a hysterectomy if: (1) You cannot control bleeding (tying her uterine or internal iliac arteries is preferable, and may be effective; see 'Stop Press'). (2) You cannot control infection. (3) She is over 40, and is unreliable, particularly if she already has several children.

FOLLOW UP is essential to identify those patients (up to 20%) who need cytotoxic drugs early. *If you can diagnose choriocarcinoma early,* you have a 95% chance of curing her.

See her every 2 weeks for 3 months, and then every month for the next 3 months. This may be difficult, but is imortant if she is to get the best results from cytotoxic drugs. Follow her for at least 2 years.

At each visit: (1) Examine the size of her uterus. (2) Do a speculum examination. A haemorrhagic nodule near her urethral meatus, or on the vault of her vagina, or on her cervix may be the first sign of progression to a trophoblastic neoplasm. (3) Note any bleeding. (4) X-ray her chest monthly. If you can do HCG assays, X-rays can be done less often. (4) From 8 weeks do an HCG qualitative test as above. If this is positive, do a quantitative one. The standard qualitative test should become negative by 8 weeks after the evacuation of the mole. Use a test capable of detecting 1000 to 2000 units in a 24 hour specimen.

She must use some family planning method for a year. Don't use contraceptive pills, because they increase the risk of a lesion requiring chemotherapy. If her husband cannot be relied on to use a condom (usual), you may have to insert an IUD, even though its side effects may be confused with choriocarcinoma.

Suspect a trophoblastic neoplasm if during follow up: (1) dark vaginal bleeding continues, or (2) her uterus remains large after evacuation or delivery, or (3) amenorrhoea continues. Establish it by measuring her HCC levels and by X-raying her chest (see below).

NON-METASTASIZING TROPHOBLASTIC NEOPLASM (invasive mole)

DIAGNOSIS. If the above symptoms lead you to suspect a trophoblastic neoplasm: (1) Measure her HCG titre. A titre above 2000 units in a 24 hour specimen after 3 months, or a rising titre after 2 months is abnormal. (2) Look for evidence of metastases in her pelvis, liver, brain, and chest. The differential diagnosis includes the incomplete evacuation of a normal placenta, placenta accreta, and a fibromyoma.

If you make the diagnosis within 4 months of delivery you have a 95% chance of curing her.

Give her methotrexate tablets by mouth 15 mg/m^2 in courses of 4 days. Repeat the courses every 14 days for 2 courses after her HCG is normal, to a maximum of 6 courses.

If her HCG is still above 2000 u/24 hours, after 6 courses of methotrexate, start actinomycin D 2 mg/m^2 (or 1 mg on days 1 and 3), one course every 3 weeks. Repeat this every 3 weeks for 2 courses after her HCG test is negative.

If her HCG test remains positive, start her on triple therapy, as below.

METASTASIZING TROPHOBLASTIC NEOPLASM (choriocarcinoma)

PRESENTATION. (1) A history of heavy irregular bleeding, sometimes following an 'abortion', especially the need for repeated evacuation. (2) Persistent amenorrhoea following hydatidiform mole. (3) A haemorrhagic nodule in her vagina or on her cervix (see above). (4) Cough, chest pain, 'unresolved pneumonia', or symptoms suggesting tuberculosis. (5) An acute haemoperitoneum like a ruptured ectopic pregnancy, due to perforation of her uterus by the tumour. (6) Neurological symptoms.

X-RAYS of her chest may show 'cannon ball' secondaries.

CAUTION ! If her choriocarcinoma arose from a hydatidiform mole, you will already have evacuated it. If it presented in other ways, don't do a diagnostic curettage, because: (1) A negative one does not exclude the diagnosis. (2) You can easily perforate her uterus, or cause catastrophic bleeding. (3) You may spread the tumour.

PROGNOSIS. All untreated patients die from multiple metastases. Patients must be diagnosed and treated early. Treat 'low risk' and 'high risk' patients separately.

LOW RISK. (1) Following hydatidiform mole. (2) Metastases in the pelvis and lungs (on chest X-ray) only. (3) HCG not above 100 000 u/24 hours. (4) Treatment is started within 4 months of evacuation of the uterus. She is only at low risk if *all* these criteria are met.

Treat her as for 'non-metastasizing' disease, and expect 95% long-term disease-free survival.

HIGH RISK. (1) The association with a term pregnancy. (2) Treatment starting later than 4 months after evacuation. (3) An HCG titre of more than 100 000 u/24 hours. (4) Metastases in her liver, gut or brain.

CAUTION ! A further cause of a rising titre is a fresh pregnancy, so remember this possibility, even if she is using contraception.

CHEMOTHERAPY FOR HIGH-RISK CHORIOCARCINOMA

Here two regimes: (1) EMA-Co using etoposide, actinomycin D, methotrexate (in high dosage), vincristine, and cyclophosphamide. This is the WHO regime. (2) An alternative regime, using methotrexate, cyclophosphamide, and actinomycin D.

EMA-Co This regime consists of two courses. Give Course 1 on days 1 and 2. Give Course 2 on day 8. Course 1 may require overnight admission, Course 2 does not.

Course 1

Day 1 etoposide 100 mg/m^2 by intravenous infusion in 200 ml of saline. Also actinomycin D 0.5 mg intravenously stat. Also methotrexate 100 mg/m^2 intravenously stat followed by 200 mg/m^2 intravenously over 12 hours.

Day 2 etoposide 100 mg/m^2 by intravenous infusion in 200 ml of saline over 30 min. Also actinomycin D 0.5 mg intravenously stat. Also, calcium folinate 15 mg intramuscularly or orally every 12 hours for 4 doses beginning 24 hours after starting methotrexate.

Course 2

Day 8 vincristine 1 mg/m^2 intravenously stat. Also cyclophosphamide 600 mg/m^2 intravenously in saline.

Give these courses on days 1 and 2, 8, 15, and 16, 22, etc., and don't extend the intervals without cause. Continue until no gonadotrophin has been detectable in the urine for 3 months.

ALTERNATIVE REGIME. Give her: Tablets of methotrexate 15 mg/m² daily for 4 days. And, actinomycin D 2 mg/m² intravenously on day 1 (or 1 mg on days 1 and 3). And, give her cyclophosphamide 1 g to 1.5 g/m² intravenously on day 1. Repeat the course every 3 weeks (on day 21) for two courses after there is no evident disease (HCG <2000 u/24 hours), or up to 6 courses.

Expect long-term disease-free survival in 50 to 75% of patients, depending on how advanced the disease is when treatment starts. Advise her very strongly to have her tubes tied.

CAUTION ! Proper management depends on monitoring the HCG levels in her urine using the appropriate quantitative dilution tests.

DIFFICULTIES WITH CHORIOCARCINOMA

If you DON'T HAVE AN IMMUNOLOGICAL PREGNANCY TEST, refer her. If you have limited supplies of pregnancy tests, give priority to these patients, and don't use them for routine pregnancy diagnosis, which should be made clinically anyway.

32.39 Other tumours

Here are two more tumours you might meet.

OTHER TUMOURS

If a patient has a slowly progressive SWELLING OF HIS CHEEK, or JAW PAIN which is not removed by tooth extraction, or a foul BLOODSTAINED DISCHARGE FROM HIS NOSE, suspect CARCINOMA OF HIS MAXILLARY ANTRUM. Look for swelling of his palate, epiphora (due to obstruction of the lachrymal duct), and enlarged lymph nodes behind the angle of his jaw. X-rays may show an increase in the size of his antrum, and later erosion of its walls. Biopsy any polypi and send them for histology. Do an antral washout, and send any material you get for histology. If necessary do a diagnostic Caldwell-Luc operation (25.9). A total excision of his maxilla, with or without radiotherapy, will usually cure it. The 5 year survival rate is 30 to 50%. If you cannot refer him for this, a Caldwell-Luc operation may possibly give him symptomatic relief.

If he is a middle-aged smoker, and is HOARSE for 2 weeks or longer, he has a CARCINOMA OF HIS GLOTTIS (vocal cords) until proved otherwise. This carcinoma causes voice changes early, so that he presents early. He has a 95% chance of 5 year survival with radiotherapy, so refer him.

HOARSENESS IN A MIDDLE-AGED SMOKER IS CARCINOMA OF HIS GLOTTIS UNTIL PROVED OTHERWISE.

---

33 Terminal care

33.1 A task for every district hospital

One of the first tasks of medicine is to comfort the dying and relieve their suffering. Much of this is due to terminal cancer, which causes severe pain in about 70% of cases. Every day more than 3.5 million people endure it, and only a fraction of these have their pain alleviated. Even in the developed countries 50–80% of patients are not given satisfactory relief. This needs only simple drugs, which are so often successful that they should be available to everyone. Their use is one of the most important technologies in this book.

In the industrial world, the development of hospices, and their outreach into the community, is helping and respecting the dying, as well as alleviating their pain and their other distressing symptoms. In the developing world, where hospices have yet to be established, district hospitals have to fill this role. Unfortunately, many of them provide no terminal care whatever—its provision is one of the indicators of 'good care' (34.6).

Any patient who receives terminal care is, by definition, going to die. It is therefore only too easy to neglect him. Your own attitude to him and that of your staff is critical. He must must feel *welcomed* by people who are determined to help him. There is always something to be done to make his last days more bearable, even if he is dying. Never send him back home immediately—he has come to you for help. A long family discussion may have taken place before he came, and if you send him back from the outpatient department, after much wasted effort and expense, he will feel rejected, and so will his family. Admit him, and actively exclude any differential diagnosis that may be curable. A day or two later, when the diagnosis of terminal cancer is confirmed, you can start talking to his relatives, and almost always to him too.

You will have to decide whether to continue to treat him in hospital, or at home. Make this decision on: (1) The extent of the suffering he will undergo at home from bed sores, from malignant ulcers, and from difficulty with his toilet arrangements, etc. For example, if he needs a catheter which must be changed every two weeks, is there a health unit near him which can do this? (2) His own wishes, and those of his family, after they have had the situation explained to them. (3) The length of time he has to live. (4) The reputation of the hospital. If you admit too many patients just to die, this may have as bad an effect on your reputation, as sending too many of them home. The more 'established' you are, the greater your freedom.

Try to palliate the symptoms of death, when this might help him, and *only when it might help him*. You can: (1) Always alleviate intolerable pain with drugs. (2) Amputate a very painful limb, bypass his obstructed gut, remove ovaries for carcinoma of the breast, or perhaps excise a fungating cancer. (3) Give him chemotherapy yourself (32.2). (4) Refer him for radiotherapy, chemotherapy, or surgery, after you have weighed up the benefit to be gained against: (a) the suffering they will cause, (b) the cost of treatment, (c) the cost of transport to his family.

Unfortunately, 'altering the symptoms of death' can sometimes make them worse. An intolerable and burdensome indignity in one culture (a colostomy for example), may be quite acceptable in another. So make sure that whatever you do, for cure or palliation, you don't make his symptoms worse, and, particularly, don't prolong his last illness painfully. For example, a gastrostomy (11.8) may keep a patient with carcinoma of the oesophagus alive for months, unable even to swallow his saliva. If you attempt palliation, do so with a Celestin tube, that will at least allow him to swallow (32.24).

Tell him, or his family, about his illness. This should not be difficult, but you will have to know your local culture. Usually, you will have to tell the full story to a responsible relative. In India the patient, if he is male, or a male relative should be told. In Africa it is usually correct to explain the complete position to the family: they will inform him, and he will then talk openly to you. Many less educated patients don't understand what malignancy is.

Contemporary Western culture faces death badly, and commonly withholds the truth from a dying patient. If you tell him nothing, except that he is going to get better, he may eventually lose all faith in you, and (alas) even in his family, who have conspired to deceive him. In contrast, many patients have thanked their doctors for telling them the truth. Unfortunately, some patients (few in the developing world) cannot accept the whole truth immediately. So judge how much he really wants to know. How much of the truth is he really able to 'take' at a time? Whatever you tell him, it must be true. It may not be the whole truth, but it should be the start of the truth because: (1) He is going to get worse anyway, and will eventually know. (2) His relatives will know about the deceit, and when their turn comes to be ill, they will not know whether to trust their doctors. (3) He may have affairs to set in order. (4) You may save him the expense of going from doctor to doctor, vainly seeking a cure. (5) You will relieve his family of the responsibility of knowing what to say to him.

If one of his differential diagnoses is a curable condition, be sure to investigate him sufficiently to exclude it. Unless you do this, you will miss diseases that could have been treated. So don't accept a diagnosis of malignant disease until it is confirmed, preferably by biopsy. Many patients have been palliated for supposedly malignant disease, only to be shown at post mortem to have had some treatable condition. What you think is a hepatoma (32.26), may turn out to be a liver abscess (31.12); a rectal lesion may be an amoeboma (31.10), and not a carcinoma (32.27); 'malignant ascites' may in fact be tuberculous (29.6).

33.2 Controlling cancer pain

When a patient has cancer, its physical effect is only one determinant of his 'total perceived pain'. His perception of pain is profoundly modified by his psychological state, and by spiritual, social, and financial factors. Depression, anxiety, anger, hopelessness, and a fear of impending death can all add to his suffering, and worsen his pain. Taking the edge off his anxiety with chlorpromazine, for example, may greatly reduce his total perceived pain, as may help with other factors, where this is possible.

Although chlorpromazine is a tranquillizer, and is not an analgesic, it may be so effective in altering a patient's 'total perceived pain', that no analgesic is required. In the control of cancer

PAIN PERCEPTION

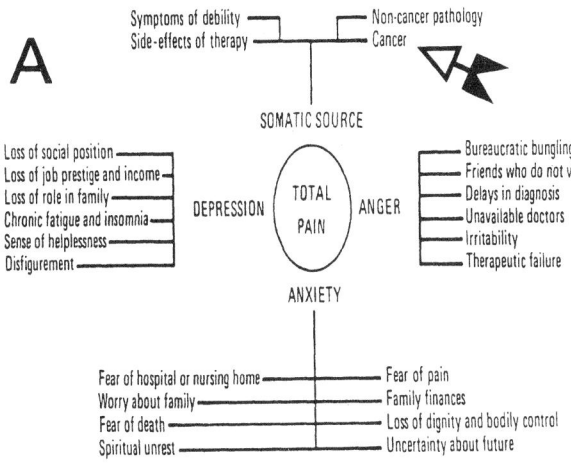

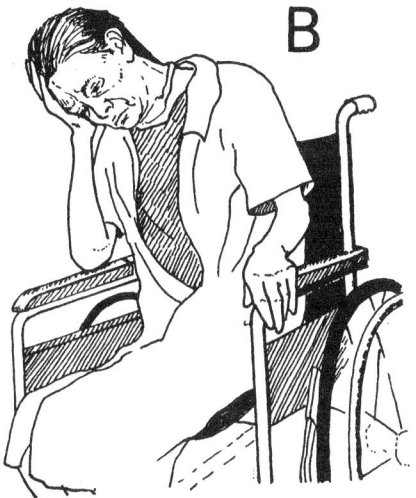

Fig. 33-1 PAIN PERCEPTION. A, shows the factors that influence a terminal cancer patient's total perception of pain. Only one of these is the cancer itself. Try to influence as many of these factors as you can. B, the patient herself. *After Twycross and Lack from 'Cancer Pain Relief'. WHO, Geneva.*

pain chlorpromazine and drugs like it are called 'adjuvants'. If an adjuvant alone fails, start the patient on WHO's three-step ladder in Fig. 33-2. This consists of: (1) A non–opioid (aspirin or paracetamol). (2) A mild opioid (codeine). (3) A strong opioid (morphine). All of them can be used with or without an adjuvant. Strictly speaking, the use of an 'adjuvant alone' is not one of the steps on WHO's ladder, which starts with Step One (a non-opioid, perhaps with an adjuvant). One contributor considers that chlorpromazine alone ('Step Zero') is a valuable initial step, which may be easier to continue at home, especially in a community with a poor understanding of the potentially harmful effects of strong analgesics. Another contributor considers it quite unacceptable.

The effects of opioids and non-opioids are additive, and make a useful combination, in that non-opioids act peripherally, whereas opioids act centrally.

Give a patient his drugs *every 4 hours by the clock*. Give them in time, before his pain starts again, and don't give them 'as required' ('p.r.n.'). Give them by mouth, where you can, and allow the family to give them. When he needs morphine, don't be afraid to give it—almost all pain yields to it. So don't underprescribe or underdose.

Make sure that patients know that pain can be treated. If legislation controlling the availability of opioids makes this difficult, strive to have it changed. The right dose, of the right drug, at the right time, will completely control cancer pain in 90% of cases. Drugs are much less successful in many forms of non malignant pain. Some of these can be relieved surgically, but the methods available are not sufficiently effective and practical to be described here.

Be careful to distinguish: (1) Tolerance, which is a state in which increasing doses are needed to maintain the initial analgesic effect. (2) Physical dependence, which is the onset of acute symptoms and signs, when the drug is discontinued. (3) Psychological dependence, which is the craving that is shown by drug abusers. Tolerance to opioids is common in cancer patients, but is rarely a problem, and physical dependence does occur. Psychological dependence is rare, and is unimportant, because the patient is going to die anyway.

Finally, don't remove the dignity of dying. We have all got to die one day, hopefully surrounded by our sons and daughters, and not by oxygen tents, tubes, cardiac monitors and alarm buzzers, and with tubes in our every orifice.

PAIN CAN BE RELIEVED
GIVE DRUGS 'BY THE CLOCK'

WHO'S 3-STEP LADDER

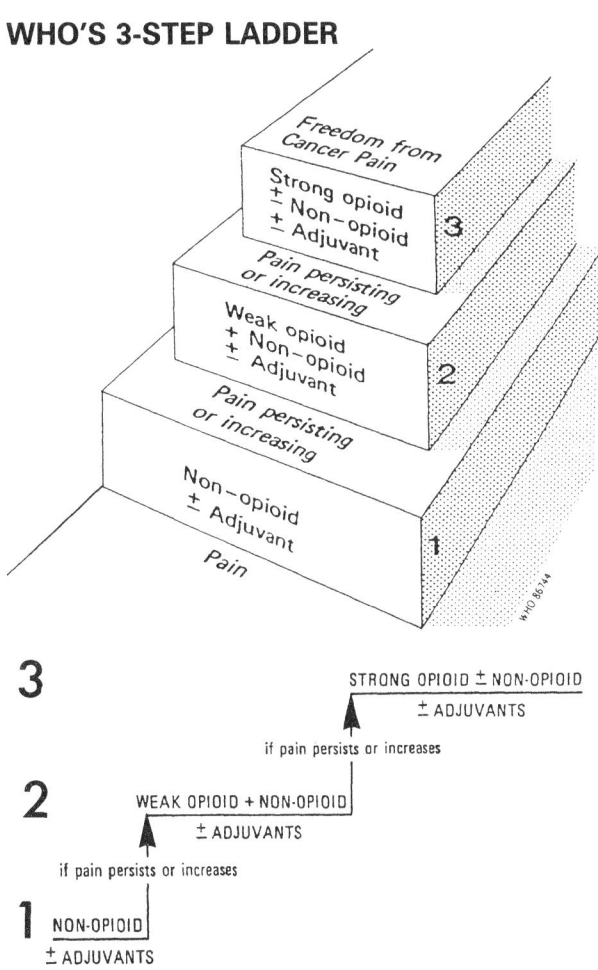

Fig. 33-2 WHO's THREE-STEP LADDER OF PAIN RELIEF will alleviate the pain of about 90% of cases of terminal cancer. The method described in the text is a modification of this, and starts with a trial of the adjuvant alone. Give a patient the right dose of the right drug at the right time. Give it at regular intervals, and not merely on demand. *Adapted from 'Cancer Pain Relief'. WHO, Geneva.*

TERMINAL CARE

ADMISSION. Admit a patient with terminal cancer if he is in much pain, or has open lesions which his relatives cannot care for. Do so with their full understanding as to why you are admitting him. When you have controlled his symptoms, particularly his pain, consider sending him home; most patients want to go home to die. While he is in hospital, make an exception to your usual rules about visiting, and allow one or two relatives to be with him all the time. Ask a priest to visit him, pray with him, and suggest your nurses do the same.

Efficient nursing will help to alleviate his pain—regular turning, mouth care, and the care of stinking ulcers. Congratulate your staff when they care for dying patients kindly. *Above all, take an interest in terminal care yourself.*

PAIN RELIEF IN TERMINAL CARE

PAIN ASSESSMENT. Ask about the location, distribution, quality, and severity of his pain, whether it is continuous or intermittent, and what factors make it worse or better. Pain precipitated by movement is likely to be less easily relieved than persistent pain. Enquire the extent to which it limits his sleep and other activities, and ask him to compare it with other pains (toothache, labour pain etc.). Assess it as mild, moderate, or severe. Evaluate his psychological state (anxiety, depression, suicidal thoughts, etc.), so that you can assess his 'total perceived pain' in terms of its physical, psychological, spiritual, social, and financial components.

THE ANALGESIC LADDER. Give him drugs in the following order, with the aim of progressively: (1) Increasing his hours of pain-free sleep. (2) Relieving his pain when at rest. (3) Relieving his pain during standing or activity.

Titrate the dose of the drug you give against the pain he has, gradually increasing it, until you get the effect you want. Give each dose by the clock, before the effect of the previous one has fallen off, so as to remove the memory and fear of pain.

WHO's three-step ladder in Fig. 33-2 starts by giving a non-opioid and an adjuvant. The regime below modifies this, and starts with chlorpromazine alone ('Step 0' is controversial, see above).

(0) Give him enough chlorpromazine to make him a little sleepy. Start it before he needs it, and give it regularly.

(1) If chlorpromazine is not enough, add a non-opioid (aspirin or paracetamol).

(2) If chlorpromazine and a non-opioid are not enough, add a weak opioid (codeine or dextropropoxyphene).

(3) If chlorpromazine, a non-opioid, and a weak opioid are not enough, *replace* the weak opioid by a strong one (morphine or pethidine). The indication for morphine is the intensity of his pain, *not* the brevity of his prognosis.

Alternatively, omit any of these stages if necessary. If a drug ceases to be effective, don't change to an alternative of similar strength. Instead, go to the next step, and prescribe one that is definitely stronger.

When he goes home, he ideally needs the same drugs as in hospital. Give the family plenty of chlorpromazine, and if necessary aspirin or paracetamol. If he needs pethidine, and they are responsible, give them some. Explain the dangers of pethidine, and that it is to be given to nobody else.

ADJUVANTS act centrally, modify a patient's emotional response to pain, and are the safest drugs to use at home. The most useful one, and the cheapest is chlorpromazine. As a general rule, give it routinely, and add other drugs to it. Alternatively, use prochlorperazine or haloperidol.

Chlorpromazine 10 to 25 mg 4 to 6-hourly, often up up to 100 mg, and sometimes up to 200 mg. It has antianxiety, antipsychotic, and antiemetic effects, and is particularly valuable if morphine makes him sick. Its side effects include hypotension, blurred vision, dry mouth, tachycardia, urinary retention, and extrapyramidal effects.

NON-OPIOIDS act peripherally.

Aspirin 250 to 1000 mg every 4 to 6 hours. The maximum daily dose, before side-effects (gastrointestinal disturbance and faecal blood loss) become severe, is 4 g. (In some countries 300 mg is the standard tablet)

Paracetamol 500 to 1000 mg every 4 to 6 hours. Maximum daily dose 4 to 6 g. Use paracetamol with caution in patients with liver damage.

WEAK OPIOIDS. Tolerance and dependence are unusual.

Codeine phosphate 30 to 120 mg, with paracetamol 500 mg, or aspirin 250 to 500 mg, every 4 to 6 hours. 30 mg of codeine is approximately equal to 650 mg of aspirin.

Dextropropoxyphene 50 to 100 mg, with aspirin 250 to 500 mg, or paracetamol 500 mg.

STRONG OPIOIDS are the main method of treating moderate and severe pain. Efficiency decreases with repeated use, so that increasing doses are needed (tolerance). Withdrawal symptoms may occur if treatment is stopped abruptly (physical dependence). Pethidine acts for 2 hours, and morphine for 4 hours.

Pethidine 50 to 100 mg orally, as a starting dose. The incidence of side-effects (tremor, twitching, agitation, convulsions) increases considerably at doses above 200 mg 3-hourly. Pethidine is *not* a complete alternative to morphine.

Morphine 5 to 10 mg 4-hourly orally, as a starting dose, and increasing when necessary, to 200 mg or more 4 hourly. Most patients are best controlled on 5 to 30 mg *every 4 hours by the clock.* This is most easily given as solutions of morphine sulphate 1 mg/ml to 20 mg/ml in 5% alcohol, or chloroform water, as a preservative, stored in a dark bottle and not exposed to sunlight. Morphine is bitter, and he may prefer to mask the taste by taking it with a drink. If necessary, let him take home a bottle of medicine containing morphine 10 mg, with 50 to 100 mg of chlorpromazine in each dose. This is a modification of the 'Brompton cocktail'. Replenish this mixture regularly, making sure he is still alive.

Constipation may be more difficult to control than pain. Almost all patients receiving regular morphine need a laxative. Start with 2 tablets of standardized senna at night and increase them to 2 tablets 2 or 3 times a day. If he is severely constipated

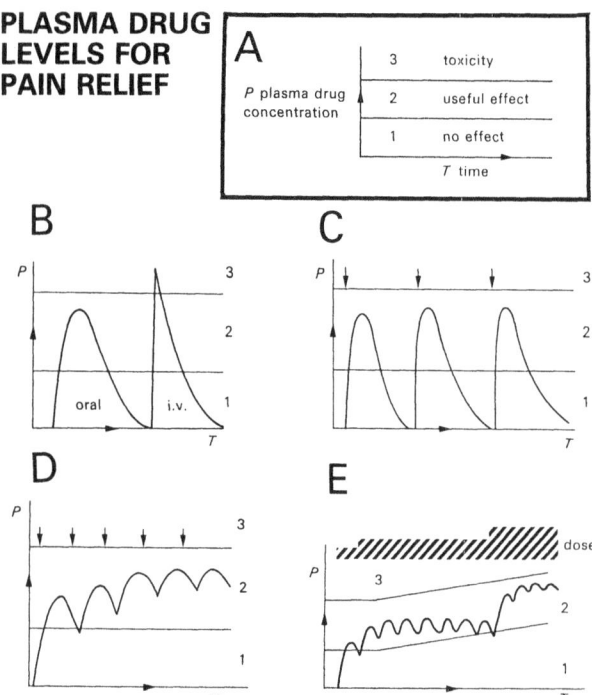

Fig. 33-3 PLASMA DRUG LEVELS FOR PAIN RELIEF. A, plasma concentration zones in relation to drug effects. These same zones are used in the diagrams which follow. B, the plasma concentration-time curves for an oral, and an intravenous dose. Notice that after an oral dose the concentration rises to a lower peak, and persists longer. C, the doses are too widely spaced to maintain analgesia. Larger doses at the same time intervals would risk toxicity. D, doses spaced satisfactorily to maintain analgesia (4-hourly for morphine). E, the effects of tolerance. The thresholds between no effect and a useful effect and between a useful effect and toxicity are rising. *After Vere, from Oxford Textbook of Medicine.*

when you first give morphine, start with suppositories or an enema.

60% of patients receiving regular morphine need an antiemetic such as chlorpromazine (which he should be on already), or prochlorperazine 5 to 10 mg 8-hourly increasing to 4-hourly, or metoclopramide 10 mg 8 hourly increasing to 4-hourly, or haloperidol 1 to 2 mg daily.

MONITOR HIS PAIN CAREFULLY. Do this within a few hours (if necessary), within a few days, and always after the first week. Make sure that treatment continues to match his pain with the minimum of side- and toxic effects. When they appear, treat them systematically, especially constipation and nausea.

CAUTION ! (1) Determine the analgesic dose for patients individually. (2) Always give drugs by mouth where you can. (3) Pain is often worse at night, so treat insomnia vigorously. (4) Exclude acute conditions that require urgent treatment. (5) Learn to use a few drugs well, and don't search desperately for one which will suit him better. (6) If you decide to allow him home with a strong opioid, his relatives must understand its dangers, and return any which is not used.

OTHER DRUGS may also be useful. The anticonvulsants carbamazepine and phenytoin also have an analgesic effect, and are effective in pain which is lancinating (shooting, stabbing). The psychotropic drugs hydroxyzine, diazepam, and amitryptyline are sometimes useful. Steroids may relieve the pain of nerve compression, cord compression, and raised intracranial pressure.

CHILDREN may also need pain relief. Manage them in the same way as adults, adjusting the doses proportionately.

DIFFICULTIES WITH TERMINAL CARE

If he has BONE PAIN from secondaries, give him radiotherapy if possible. If not, give him aspirin or another NSAID.

If he is LIKELY TO GET BED SORES, because he is immobile, teach his relatives how to prevent them by regular turning (64.13).

If he ALREADY HAS BED SORES, keep him in hospital until he is weak, and not likely to live long. Turn him 2-hourly, and clean them 2-hourly with half strength saline, which need not be sterile, or with hypochlorite ('Eusol'). If they are deep, infected, and smelly, treat them as for a malignant ulcer (see below).

If he has a MALIGNANT ULCER or FUNGATING TUMOUR, control pain as above. Care for him in hospital until he is weak, and not likely to live long. Try one of these methods. (1) Apply yoghurt or honey (both readily available in some communities) 4 to 6-hourly. Honey is a good alternative to yoghurt, but may be expensive, even if it is 'from the bush'. Ask relatives to bring it. (3) If a wound is particularly smelly, apply iodoform powder between layers of dressing, and notice the dramatic improvement. (4) If none of these are available, keep the lesion wet with half-strength saline (unsterile), poured on 2-hourly, and change the dressings daily. If his relatives insist on taking him home, show them the honey or yoghurt methods.

If he suffers from INTRACTABLE VOMITING, 'drip and suck him' (4.9, 15.5) and give him an antiemetic intravenously, or as a suppository. This will relieve his nausea: intractable vomiting is a horrible way to die. You will have to give metoclopramide intravenously, but you can give him chlorpromazine, prochlorperazine, domperidone, or cyclizine as suppositories or intravenously. Avoid metoclopramide and domperidone if his vomiting is due to malignant obstruction of his gut, because they increase its motility, and may make him worse.

YOUR ACTIVE INTEREST IS ESSENTIAL!

---

34 Miscellaneous

VASCULAR SURGERY

34.1 Varicose veins

Besides the control of bleeding (Chapter 3) and the repair of injured vessels (Chapter 55), the only other 'primary vascular surgery' is that of varicose veins. You will seldom need to operate on them, because, although about 15% of the people in the world have them, few of these are in the developing countries. Firstly a little theory.

ANATOMY AND PHYSIOLOGY. The varicose veins in a patient's leg are the result of excessive pressure inside them, usually from failure of their valves. There are four kinds of leg vein, and they all have valves which stop blood flowing downwards away from the heart.

(1) The *long and short saphenous veins* run above the deep fascia, and are usually below the fibrous layer of the superficial fascia. They have numerous valves which direct blood upwards towards the heart. The most important of these is the 'femoral valve', in the long saphenous vein, just before it penetrates the deep fascia to join the femoral vein. The femoral valve prevents blood from the femoral vein flowing back into the saphenous vein.

(2) The *superficial collecting veins* are tributaries of the saphenous veins. They lie between the skin and the fibrous layer of the superficial fascia. They have valves, but they are poorly supported by the tissue around them, and easily dilate and become varicose.

(3) The *deep veins* accompany the arteries, and run among the muscles deep inside the leg. When the contractions of the muscles squeeze them, their valves direct the squeezed blood towards the heart.

(4) Several *perforating veins* go through the deep fascia, to join the superficial collecting veins to the deep veins. Their valves direct blood into the leg. The most important of these perforating veins are just behind the medial border of the tibia.

When a patient stands at rest, the superficial veins on the dorsum of his foot support a column of blood that reaches to his right heart. While his leg muscles are relaxed, this blood flows through his perforating veins, into the deep veins inside his leg. When he walks, the contractions of his leg muscles squeeze the blood from his deep veins up towards his heart. This cycle of contraction and relaxation reduces the pressure in his superficial veins, and in a normal person prevents varicosities.

However, if the valves of his deep perforating veins are incompetent, blood from inside his leg can squirt out at high pressure, into his unsupported superficial collecting veins. This distends them, and makes them varicose. It also alters the surrounding tissue, so that it is liable to ulcerate.

If the valves which guard his long and short saphenous veins are incompetent, the blood in his femoral and popliteal veins can flow downwards, into his saphenous veins, and make them varicose.

The aim of surgery is to stop blood flowing backwards through veins with incompetent valves.

A few varicose veins are the result of obstruction, but most are due to failure of the valves of the musculovenous pumps that return blood from the leg. This 'valve failure' takes two forms: (1) In primary varicose veins the valves of a patient's saphenous system fail, while the deep veins of his legs remain normal; his symptoms are usually mild, and his legs rarely ulcerate. (2) In secondary or post-thrombotic varicose veins, his deep veins, or the communicating veins between his superficial and deep systems, have had their valves destroyed by thrombosis. Ulceration is more common, and treatment more difficult. Both kinds of varicose veins are associated with Western life-styles, but it is not known why.

Varicose veins are unsightly; they cause aching and cramps, a scaly, itchy, varicose eczema, swelling of the legs, and ulceration; occasionally they bleed. A patient's symptoms may bear

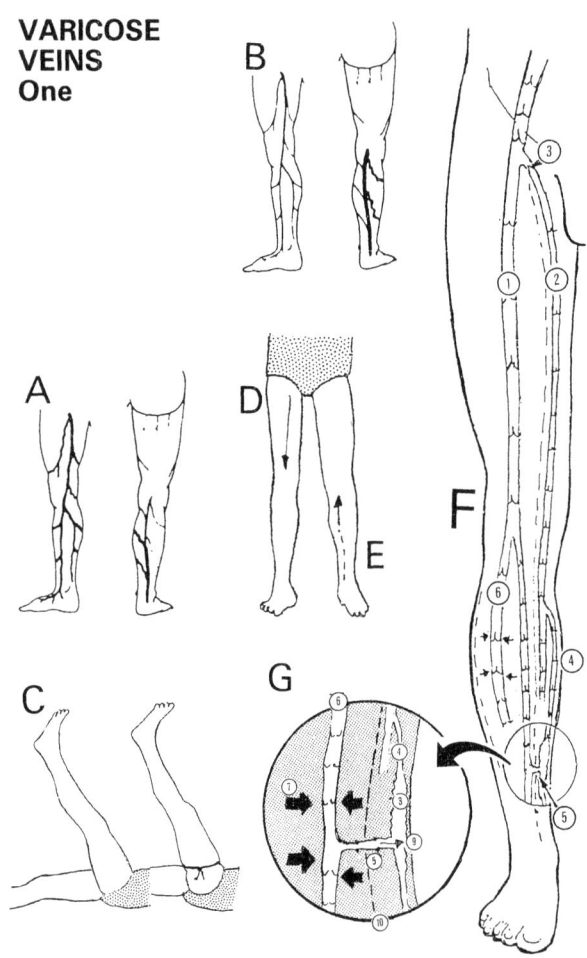

VARICOSE VEINS One

Fig. 34-1 VARICOSE VEINS—ONE. A, varicosities of the long saphenous system. B, varicosities of the short saphenous system. C, D, and E, the Trendelenburg test. C, lay the patient on his back and raise his leg. Apply a venous tourniquet just below his saphenous opening. Stand him up and release the tourniquet. If his femoral valve is incompetent, his veins fill immediately from above (D). If it is normally competent, they fill slowly from below (E). F, the anatomy of the veins of the leg. G, a close-up view of a varicosity, and an incompetent perforating vein connecting it with the deep venous system.

1, the femoral vein. 2, the long saphenous vein. 3, the femoral valve. 4, a superficial collecting vein. 5, a perforating vein with its valves destroyed. 6, the deep veins of the leg. 7, muscular forces compressing the deep veins. 8, a varicosity in a superficial collecting vein. 9, a jet of blood squirting out of a perforating vein with incompetent valves to cause a varix in a superficial collecting vein. *After Ellis H, and Calne RY, 'Lecture Notes on General Surgery', Fig. 13, Blackwell Scientific Publications, with kind permission.*

little relationship to the size and extent of his varicose veins. If they are primary, the swelling usually only involves his feet and ankles, and resolves completely overnight. If they are secondary, his lower legs may be swollen all the time.

If he has primary varicose veins, there are several things you can do, either alone, or more often in combination: (1) You can inject a little irritant solution into 2 cm of a vein (sclerotherapy), so as to inflame its walls, and make it shed its endothelium. If you then keep the vein empty, by compressing its inflamed walls together for 6 weeks without interruption, they will stick together and not recanalize. (2) If he has varicosities in his long saphenous system, you can tie his long saphenous vein flush with his femoral vein, and at the same time tie: (a) the tributaries that enter it nearby, and (b) any incompetent connections it has with the deep system. (3) If he has varicosities of his short saphenous system, you can tie his short saphenous vein at his saphenopopliteal junction. (4) You can pass a stripper through his long and short saphenous veins, pull them out completely, and so disconnect the varicosities in his superficial collecting veins from the high pressure in his saphenous veins. (5) You can remove some varices when indicated.

If he has posthrombotic (secondary) varicose veins, it may be possible to cure him by tying every incompetent perforating vein; but these are difficult to find and tie, so we don't tell you how to do it here.

The surgery that you are prepared to do on a particular patient will depend on your circumstances, and his. Any form of treatment is of limited value, if his deep and his perforating veins, his skin, and his subcutaneous tissues, have already been severely damaged. Sclerotherapy needs careful attention to detail, but it can be very effective, and has few dangers. The main danger of surgery is that, if you tie his superficial veins when the valves of his deep ones are incompetent, you may make him worse.

• STRIPPER, *for varicose veins, Nabatoff, in sterilizer case, complete with 3 metal olives, cable and handle, one only. Optional.* This is the complete outfit.

BE SURE THAT THE VALVES OF HIS DEEP VEINS ARE COMPETENT BEFORE YOU TIE HIS SUPERFICIAL VEINS

VARICOSE VEINS

EXAMINATION. Examine the patient standing in a good light. Feel his veins. If he is obese, percuss the course of his saphenous veins. Examine his peripheral pulses.

If there is ulceration, brawny induration, and marked hyperpigmentation, the valves of his deep veins are almost certainly incompetent, and his varicose veins are secondary. Otherwise they are probably primary.

To test the competence of his perforating veins and the valves of his greater saphenous system, lay him down, raise his leg, and massage his veins proximally to empty them. On his upper thigh apply a rubber tube tourniquet, tight enough to compress his veins. Stand him up and ask him to move his forefoot up and down, so as to actuate his calf muscle pump. Inspect his varices for 30 seconds, and then remove the tourniquet.

If his veins gradually fill from below as he stands, and continue to fill gradually from below when the tourniquet is released, **the valves in the veins of his legs are normal.**

If his veins fill rapidly from below, **his varices are being filled from his deep veins, and the valves of his perforating veins are incompetent.**

If blood flows rapidly into his greater saphenous vein from above after removing the tourniquet, **his femoral valve is incompetent.**

To test the competence of the valves of his short saphenous vein, apply two tourniquets, one above his knee to occlude his long saphenous vein and another just below his popliteal fossa. Stand him up, leave the long saphenous tourniquet on, and remove the tourniquet obstructing his short saphenous vein. Observe how his short saphenous system fills.

To find the sites of major incompetent perforating veins: (1) Look for visible and palpable 'blowouts' of subcutaneous veins. (2) Repeat the tourniquet test at lower levels, and occlude the vein just distal to each blowout. (3) Feel for circular gaps in his deep fascia in the anatomical sites where you expect to find them.

DIAGNOSIS. Here we are only concerned with the common causes of varicose veins. Any causes of inguinal or retroperitoneal compression that might produce varicose veins are usually obvious. If there is a thrill or bruit (rare), he has an arteriovenous fistula.

Suggesting primary varicose veins—usually start at an early age (15 to 25). No incompetence of the perforators shown by the test above. Incompetence demonstrated by back-flow on release of the upper thigh tourniquet (long saphenous), or just below his popliteal fossa (short saphenous).

Suggesting post-thrombotic varicose veins—a history of venous thrombosis (unusual), an older age, less obvious veins partly hidden by eczema, fat necrosis, or ulceration. His long saphenous vein may be dilated.

NON-OPERATIVE TREATMENT

INDICATIONS. (1) Minor symptoms.

CONTRAINDICATIONS. These are also the indications for surgery. (1) Large varicosities. (2) Symptoms, such as aching of sufficient intensity to merit sclerotherapy or surgery.

METHOD. Aim to improve his general health and to reduce his symptoms. Encourage him to lose weight (he is usually overweight), to walk, to avoid prolonged standing and sitting, and to raise his leg frequently. If possible, have him fitted with elastic stockings from his distal metatarsals to just below his knee.

CAUTION ! If he uses elastic bandages, make sure that they do not have a tourniquet effect.

SCLEROTHERAPY

INDICATIONS. (1) The cosmetic treatment of small primary varicose veins. (2) Incompetent perforating veins without an incompetent femoral valve. (3) Varicose veins which persist or recur after surgery.

CONTRAINDICATIONS. (1) An incompetent femoral valve. (2) Varicosities at or above the knee. (3) Gross obesity (it is difficult to maintain compression). (4) Deep venous thrombosis is a contraindication to any operation on the superficial venous system, which is now the only route for blood to return to the heart.

CAUTION ! (1) Pregnancy is not a contraindication. (2) If a patient is on oral contraceptives, she should change to another method one month before sclerotherapy or operation.

EQUIPMENT. Five small syringes fitted with fine needles (preferably with transparent shanks) and filled with 0.5 ml of 3% sodium tetradecyl, or 5% ethanolamine oleate. 'Sorbo' rubber pads, marking pens, suitable bandages and elastic stockings.

METHOD. Treat him as an outpatient. *His veins must be almost empty when you inject, and be kept empty* so that their walls adhere.

Stand him up, observe, palpate, and percuss his veins; mark them with a pen. Lay him down, put his foot on your shoulder, and feel the course of his veins for gaps in his fascia (sites of incompetent communicating veins). Mark these with a pen of a different colour. Press with the tips of your fingers on as many of these gaps as you can, and, still pressing, ask him to stand. Remove your lowermost fingers first.

If removing your finger from a gap in his fascia immediately causes the vein to fill, that gap is the site of an incompetent perforating vein. If it does not fill, there was no perforator in it. The sites where pressure controls the filling are the best sites for injection. Inject the lowest sites first.

Bandage up to the injection site with a crepe bandage. With his leg lowered so that his vein is full, insert the mounted needle, and aspirate only as far as the transparent hub (to be sure you are in the vein); then empty the vein by raising his leg above the horizontal. Isolate the segment to be injected by pressing with your fingers above and below it, and inject 0.5 ml of sclerosant. Apply a 'Sorbo' rubber pad over the injection site to keep it empty, bandage it on, move up to the next site, and repeat the process until all your chosen sites have been injected. Don't inject more than 5 sites.

Apply an elastic stocking over the bandages, the moment the last one is secure, and *immediately* start him walking for an hour, and thereafter for 3 miles daily. Advise him to *avoid standing*, and, where possible, to raise his legs when he sits. Leave the bandages on for at least 2 weeks to maintain pressure *without interruption*. Most surgeons leave them on for at least 6 weeks, renewing them when they become loose. If they have to be renewed, reapply them with his leg raised.

CAUTION ! (1) Don't inject the sclerosant into an artery. Remember that the posterior tibial artery runs deep, near the commonest site of the perforating veins. (2) Never inject more than 1 ml at a site, because if it extravasates, the tissues may necrose. (3) Careful bandaging is critical. The pressure on both borders of the bandage should be the same.

If his leg becomes painful, advise him to take an analgesic and walk. If his pain is not relieved, remove the bandage *with his leg raised*, and reapply it with his leg raised.

At 2 weeks. If any injections are found to have failed (the vein still fills with liquid blood), reinject these sites.

At 6 weeks remove the bandages. If his first leg is satisfactory, start on the other one (it is inconvenient to have both legs done simultaneously).

At 6—20 weeks it may be obvious that further sites are suitable for injection. Persist until the effect is satisfactory.

FLUSH LIGATION OF THE LONG SAPHENOUS VEIN

INDICATIONS. (1) Incompetence of the femoral valve, causing the varices to fill from above.

CONTRAINDICATIONS. (1) Obstruction of the femoral vein above the saphenous opening. (2) Deep venous thrombosis.

ANAESTHESIA. (1) Give him a general anaesthetic (preferably not halothane), in a cool theatre (to reduce his peripheral blood flow). (2) Local, or (3) subarachnoid anaesthesia.

PREPARATION. The evening before the operation shave his groin and leg. Stand him up and mark the vein to be operated on, and all its tributaries and pouches, with an ink that will not be washed off by the surgical scrub. Also find and mark his perforating veins, using the finger-pressure method described above.

TO TIE HIS LONG SAPHENOUS VEIN, lay him supine with his feet apart. Give the table a 10° head-down tilt to reduce the venous pressure in his legs. Support his parted heels on foam cushions.

Make a 7 cm oblique incision 1–2 cm below and parallel to his inguinal ligament, ending medially below his pubic tubercle. Deepen it, until you reach his superficial fascia. Dissect out the terminal part of his saphenous vein. Define its tributary veins (his superficial circumflex iliac, his superficial epigastric, and his external pudendal). Tie all these tributaries as they enter his saphenous vein. Tie his saphenous vein next to his entry to his femoral vein, and *proximal* to the entry of the tributaries. Divide his saphenous vein between ligatures of 2/0 or 1/0 multifilament.

CAUTION ! If he bleeds, don't clamp blindly with haemostats, or you may damage his femoral vein, or even his femoral artery. Instead, apply pressure, and raise the foot of the table. After 3 minutes pressure you can usually control bleeding, either with a haemostat or a fine silk stitch.

Tie all his other perforating veins through 3–5 cm incisions. Dissect these perforators carefully, and tie them flush with his deep fascia.

FLUSH LIGATION OF THE SHORT SAPHENOUS VEIN

INDICATION. Incompetence of the terminal valve of his short saphenous vein, causing the varices of this system to fill from above.

METHOD. Lay him prone (see A 16.12) with his feet apart, and his knees slightly flexed. Make a transverse incision across the middle of his popliteal fossa. Make a transverse or longitudinal incision in his deep fascia to expose his short saphenous vein (which lies deep to it), and is accompanied by, and may be closely applied to, his saphenous nerve. Raise the vein, divide it, trace its proximal end down into his popliteal

VARICOSE VEINS
Two

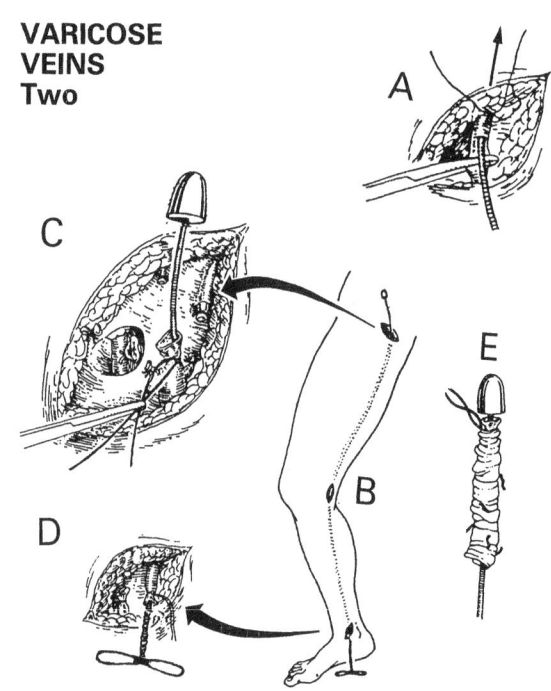

Fig. 34-2 VARICOSE VEINS—TWO. A, the stripper cable introduced at the ankle. B, the long saphenous vein with the stripper in place. C, the end of the cable emerging from the saphenous vein in the groin, with the head of the stripper attached. D, the handle of the stripper attached to the cable. E, the crumpled long saphenous vein removed with the stripper. *After Sir Charles Illingworth, 'Surgical Treatment', Fig. 5, Pitman Medical, with kind permission.*

fossa, and tie it flush. There is usually at least one large proximal branch. Tie this.

CAUTION ! The anatomy of the short saphenous/popliteal junction is notoriously variable.

FLUSH LIGATION AND STRIPPING

INDICATIONS. Symptomatic varices of either saphenous system.

CONTRAINDICATIONS. (1) Deep venous thrombosis. (2) Obstruction of the femoral or other vein above the saphenous opening. One contributor considers these 'Cautions' rather than contraindications.

METHOD. You will have just tied his long and/or short saphenous vein by the methods above.

To strip his long saphenous vein, open it anterior to his medial malleolus. Pass the small end of the stripper up to the distal groin wound. Try to make sure that it remains in his superficial veins and does not enter his deep ones. If it sticks, or passes into a tributary, redirect it by twisting, pressure, and to and fro movements. If it will not advance, cut down on it and redirect it, or strip the vein in segments.

When the stripper has passed successfully, unscrew the small head and replace it with a larger one. Tie this head in place. Raise his leg high and slowly withdraw the stripper from his groin to his ankle. Keep his leg high for a few minutes afterwards to reduce bleeding. Close his ankle and groin wounds, and bandage his leg firmly.

To strip his short saphenous vein, proceed as for his long one. Enter it behind his lateral malleolus.

CAUTION ! The sural nerve is closely related to the vein at the lateral malleolus.

TIES AND AVULSIONS tying perforating veins

INDICATIONS. (1) To supplement tying varicose veins (with or without stripping) especially when varices are gross. (2) To treat varices and perforators after unsuccessful sclerotherapy. (3) To identify and control perforators in varicose vein surgery. (4) Post-thrombotic varicose veins. The best results are obtained early, when there are only preulcer signs, or when an ulcer has only been present for a few months. Long lasting ulcers (>2 years) have a poor prognosis. Refer him.

METHOD. Aim to pull out as much vein as you can through multiple small incisions across the vein at previously marked sites, especially where varices communicate with the main saphenous veins, or with the deep system. Raise a loop of varicose vein by gentle blunt dissection. Follow the vein as carefully as you can in each direction and along other connecting veins as you find them. When you have exposed a length of vein pull it out. There is usually no need to tie it unless it is large or perforates the deep fascia. Close small incisions with adhesive tape unsutured (54-7). For the subfascial tying of perforators see below under varicose ulceration.

POSTOPERATIVELY, (after flush ties, long and short saphenous vein stripping, and multiple ties and avulsions, and tying perforators). Don't let him stand at first, and only let him sit when necessary for meals and toilet purposes. Let him walk actively as soon as he is comfortable, and as soon as possible for 1 hour daily. Most patients can go home the same day. Leave the pressure bandage applied at operation until the 6th day, then remove the stitches. Tell him to wear elastic bandages for another fortnight.

VARICOSE ULCERATION

DIAGNOSIS. Most lower leg ulcers in the tropics are chronic tropical ulcers (31.2). Varicose ulcers due to incompetent perforators are less common.

A varicose ulcer is usually on the lower third of the leg, especially just behind and above the medial malleolus. It may be of any size and shape, its edges are usually brown and eczematous, and it has red granulations under the slough on its base. The patient is usually fat. Progressive fibrous atrophy of the subcutaneous of his lower leg ('inverted bottle leg'), and brown pigmentation, may precede ulceration. He may have either or both: (1) Gross primary varicose veins of many years' standing (most primary varicose veins don't lead to ulceration). (2) Incompetent deep perforating veins (50% of varicose ulcer cases), which may be not be easy to find under his ulcer.

THE DIFFERENTIAL DIAGNOSIS includes: (1) Chronic ulcers starting as tropical ulcers (31.2). (2) Ischaemic ulceration (feel his pulses). (3) Squamous cell carcinoma (which may develop in any chronic ulcer, 32.19). (4) Buruli ulcer (31.2a). (5) Factitious ulcer.

TREATMENT. Put him to bed with frequent sterile saline soaks until his ulcer is clean and oedema has gone. Either:
(1) Apply strong elastic webbing bandages capable of withstanding 100 mm Hg from the base of his toes to just below his knees, over a plain non-adherent dressing. Ask him to remove the bandage at night, to clean his ulcer, to sleep with the foot of his bed raised, and to reapply the bandage each morning. Recent (<3 months) ulcers will often heal this way; but he should wear an elastic stocking for life.

Or, (2) if his ulcer will not heal or keeps breaking down again, and you can find the venous abnormality, treat it by injection and/or operation. This is usually easy if his varicose veins are primary (uncommon), but is more difficult if they are secondary (common).

If venous insufficiency due to incompetent perforators, is the cause of persistent ulceration, consider referring him to have these tied by a subfascial approach (eg. Cockett's operation). The commonest perforator responsible is usually within 2 cm of the upper border of the ulcer.

DIFFICULTIES WITH VARICOSE VEINS

If varicose veins BLEED, haemorrhage can be alarming. Lay him down, apply pressure to the bleeding vein, and then tie it.

If an INDURATED LINE, develops along the course of the stripper, reassure him that it will usually be gone in a month.

If you INJURE HIS SAPHENOUS VEIN during surgery, see Section 32.34D.

THE SURGERY OF THE SKIN

34.1a Hypertrophic scars and keloids

A surgical scar, especially if it is on the face, should, if possible, be nearly invisible. Sometimes a scar becomes very visible indeed as the result of two processes: (1) hypertrophy and (2) keloid formation. Both these processes can follow surgery, tribal scarring, an injury, or almost any breach of the skin surface. Both cause large scars, and are identical histologically, but they behave differently.

Hypertrophic scars are common, wide, and raised. They are bright pink (in a light skin), are uniform, and do not extend beyond the edge of the original incision. They itch, and may be painful. They continue to thicken for 3 to 18 months, then become static, and finally resolve to become broad, soft, thin, and level with the surrounding skin; the whole process taking about three years.

Keloids are less common, but are not unusual in African patients. They are also wide and raised, but the new tissue grows beyond the original confines of the scar to form irregular mounds of collagen, which resemble benign tumours. Keloids may not start to form for many months after the original breach of the skin surface; they grow for a year or more, and then stop. There may be so many of them, and they may be so large, that they disfigure, deform, and disable the patient. Keloids are difficult to treat. If you excise one through normal skin and graft the gap, it is likely to recur round the edges of the graft, or in any gaps or splits in it.

Both a hypertrophic and a keloid response are more likely if a wound is: (1) Infected. (2) Contaminated by foreign material—even monofilament sutures may promote them, but are less likely to do so than multifilaments. (3) Under tension. (4) In a young adult. (5) In a vascular part of the body (you will seldom find them on the legs or feet). (6) In a black-skinned patient.

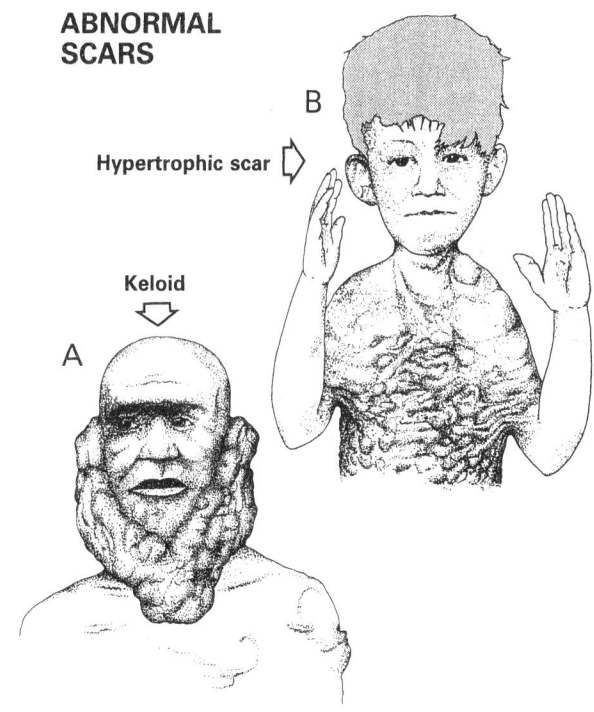

Fig. 34-3 ABNORMAL SCARS. A, an extensive keloid. B, hypertrophic scars and contractures following burns. Although both these scars are abnormally large and are identical histologically, they behave differently. *After Charles Bowesman.*

TWO ABDOMINAL SCARS

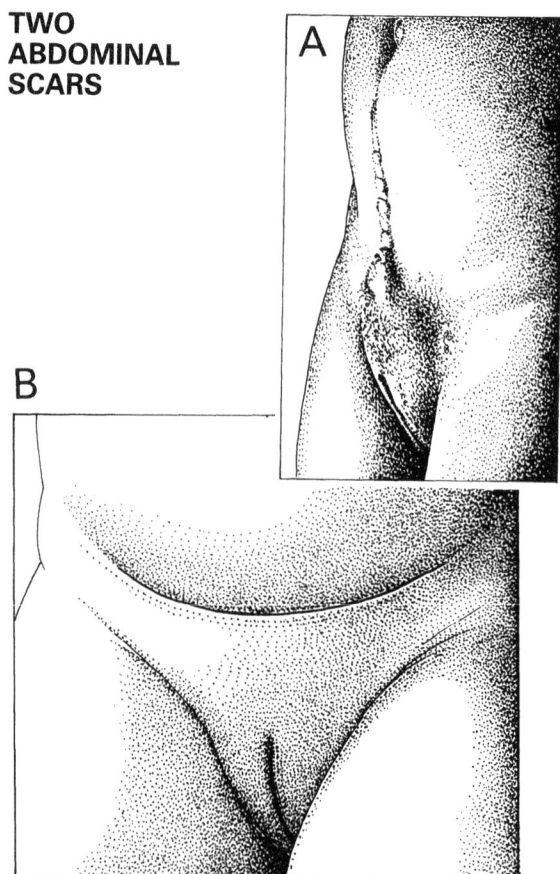

Fig. 34-4 TWO ABDOMINAL SCARS. Both patients were operated on about 8 months previously. Patient A, has formed a keloid on her vertical scar. Patient B's transverse (Pfannensteil) incision in her skin crease has healed almost invisibly. Scars in skin creases are not under tension and form less keloid. *After Charles Bowesman, 'Surgery and Clinical Pathology in the Tropics'. E and S Livingstone, with kind permission.*

THE PHYSIOLOGY OF KELOID FORMATION. Normally, there is a balance between the anabolic and catabolic stages of wound healing. As a wound heals, it goes through various stages. At about 3 or 4 weeks it is hyperaemic, and its strength is still only about a third that of normal skin. During the following 2 or 3 months, the hyperaemia subsides, and the scar becomes flatter and more pliable; at about 3 months it reaches its definitive state.

In an abnormal scar there is no equilibrium at 3 or 4 weeks, the anabolic phase continues, hyperaemia increases, more collagen is layed down, and the wound expands and becomes wider and raised. It may develop into a hypertrophic scar or a keloid. Both are stronger than a normal scar.

THE KELOID RESPONSE

THE DIFFERENTIAL DIAGNOSIS may be difficult early on.

Suggesting a hypertrophic scar—abnormal growth starting within weeks of the injury, growth restricted to the confines of the original scar, spontaneous regression in 6 months to 3 years, anywhere in the body, commoner than keloid in a white skin, very common in burns scars, itching is common and may be severe.

Suggesting a keloid—an onset delayed for months or years, invasion of the surrounding skin, growth stops in due course but there is no regression, localized to some parts of the body, not uncommon in black patients, uncommon in burn scars, very uncommon below the groin.

If diagnosis is difficult, remember that a keloid becomes increasingly raised, and extends beyond the confines of the original scar.

THE PREVENTION OF KELOIDS AND HYPERTROPHIC SCARS
Minimize tension in the scar. Scars in the line of skin creases are under less tension than those across it. *So plan incisions in skin creases where possible.* If you have to cut across a crease, consider using a Z-plasty (57.11).

If possible, avoid scars in areas that are normally under tension: (1) In the neck especially. (2) In the coronal plane in the upper arm, especially its lateral side. (2) In the the upper back.

CAUTION ! Midline scars over the sternum and longitudinal incisions in the arm are particularly likely to develop keloids—they cross the skin's creases.

Maintain careful asepsis, minimize trauma when you operate, and control bleeding carefully at the end of the operation. Don't pull sutures too tight, and avoid mattress sutures.

POSTOPERATIVELY. **If a patient is particularly likely to develop a hypetrophic scar or a keloid,** as shown by his previous history, apply pressure to the scar for 9 to 12 months after the operation. Ideally, an elastic garment should be made to fit. This is unlikely to be practical, but you may be able to cut a piece of foam rubber to fit a smaller scar, and hold it in place with an elastic bandage. Tell him not to remove it except to wash. Unfortunately, both an elastic garment and an elastic bandage are are difficult to tolerate for long, especially in a hot climate.

TREATMENT FOR KELOIDS AND HYPERTROPHIC SCARS

A HYPERTROPHIC SCAR. (1) If possible, leave it; often, it is not disfiguring. Reassure him that it will eventually regress naturally. *Never operate during the active phase.* If you decide to operate, do so during the mature phase, 3 years or more after the original wound. Then, excise the scar, and apply the preventive measures above. Considerable improvement is possible. (2) If he presents earlier than 3 years, before a scar is mature, apply pressure, as above.

A KELOID. Treatment is more successful if you start it early.

BOWESMAN'S METHOD FOR KELOIDS

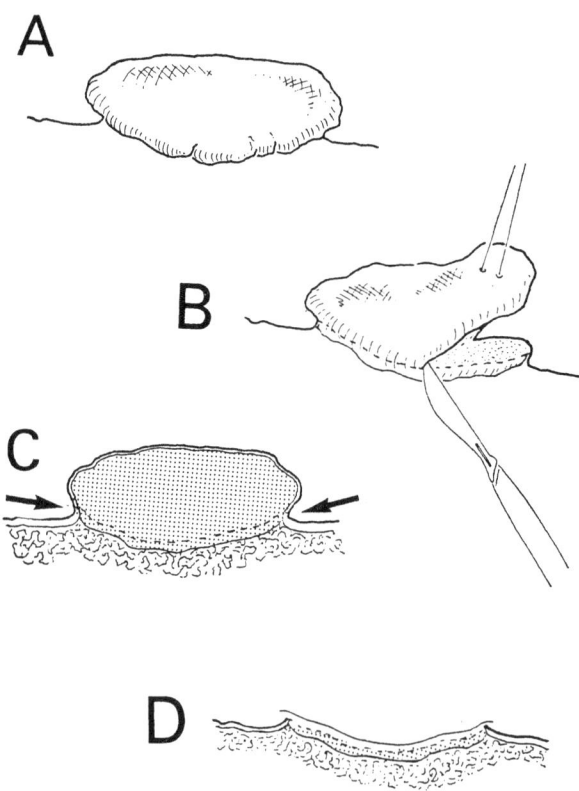

Fig. 34-5 BOWESMAN'S 'SHAVING OFF' METHOD FOR KELOIDS. A, a keloid mass. B, the way to shave it off. C, the plane through which to remove it. D, a graft in place ready for dressing. *After Charles Bowesman, 'Surgery and Clinical Pathology in the Tropics, Fig. 194. E and S Livingstone, with kind permission.*

A developing keloid. Within a month or two of the injury: (1) Apply pressure. (2) Inject a suspension of hydrocortisone, about 2 ml at each site spread out subcutaneously. Or, better, use triamcinolone. Give 4 injections 3 weeks apart.

An established keloid. Steroids have no effect. Resist the request to operate if you can. The worse the keloid, the more likely it is to recur if you excise it. If you are pressed, excise smaller ones, but be sure to explain that they may recur and may even be worse.

If you operate, excise the abnormal tissue *within the keloid*, leaving a margin of keloid tissue all round. Keep your sutures within this margin also. If necessary, graft the bare area. You may be able to shave skin off the keloid and use this as a graft. All this is difficult; so is closing the wound tidily. Complete the incision and then inject steroid suspension into the scar. Postoperatively give him 4 more steroid injections at 3-weekly intervals. Apply a pressure bandage or an elastic garment for 9 months—if he will accept it!

Alternatively, follow the method of Bowesman in Fig. 34-5. Keloids are easier to remove from convex than from concave surfaces. A protruding keloid usually extends downwards like a saucer into the subcutaneous fat. Shave it off a little above the skin level, *remaining within the keloid tissue* and without entering the subcutaneous fat. Control bleeding, and apply a complete sheet of split skin extending beyond the margins of the keloid.

CAUTION ! (1) Try to avoid operating on established keloids. (2) Use a sharp knife. (3) Don't pull on the keloid as you excise it, or you may enter the subcutaneous tissue. Instead, if necessary, depress the surrounding tissues. (3) Don't use sutures.

34.2 Granuloma pyogenicum

When a wound heals, especially an infected one, new granulation tissue forms. If this is so excessive as to make an obvious lump, you can mistake it a tumour. A pyogenic granuloma can occur anywhere, but is commonest on the face, fingers, or toes, as a soft or moderately firm, dull red, 1 cm lump, covered with atrophic epidermis or crusts, and which bleeds easily. This trivial lesion can be misdiagnosed and thought to be a sarcoma, when all that is needed is simple excision and curettage. An antibiotic is only needed if there are signs of spreading infection (very unusual).

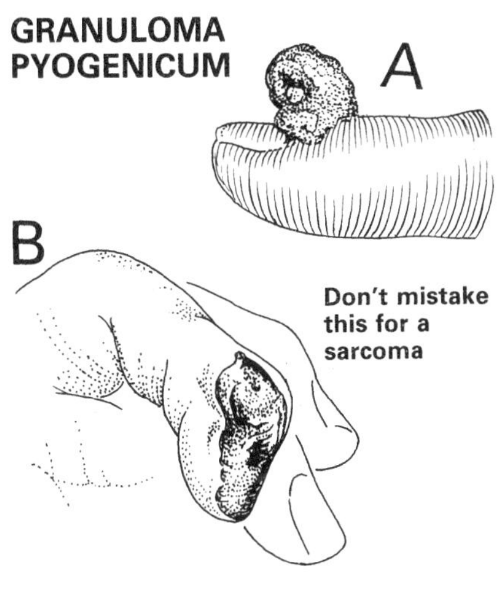

34.3 Sebaceous and dermoid cysts

When the mouth of a sebaceous gland is blocked, retained sebum causes it to form a cyst. Sebaceous cysts are most common on the face, scalp and back, as hemispherical firm or elastic swellings, with no obvious edge, which are adherent to the skin. They are filled with putty-like yellowish white sebum, which you may be able to indent with your finger.

Three complications may follow: (1) A sebaceous cyst can become infected; this makes it enlarge and become red and painful. Recurrent infection makes it adhere to the surrounding tissue, and become more difficult to remove. (2) It can ulcerate, and discharge its contents. The lining membrane which is left can then resemble an epithelioma. (3) Its contents can escape, and become hard and form a sebaceous horn.

SEBACEOUS CYSTS.

Paint, drape, and if necessary shave the area.

Under local anaesthesia (A 5.4), incise an ellipse of skin over the swelling, in the direction of the natural lines of the skin. This is particularly important in the face, see Fig. 61-3. Deepen the incision until you reach the edge of the cyst. Push the points of fine curved scissors between the cyst and the tissue round it, and then open them, so as to define a plane for dissection. Repeat this all round the cyst until it is free, then remove it with a snip of the scissors.

Press firmly with dry gauze for 5 minutes to stop bleeding. If any bleeding vessels remain, tie them off. Close the skin, leaving a small corrugated drain in place. Remove this at 48 hours.

DERMOID CYSTS. Lumps very like sebaceous cysts from at the lines of skin fusion in the embryo, most commonly at the lateral end of the eyebrow where the maxillary and ophthalmic divisions of the face meet. Manage them as for sebaceous cysts.

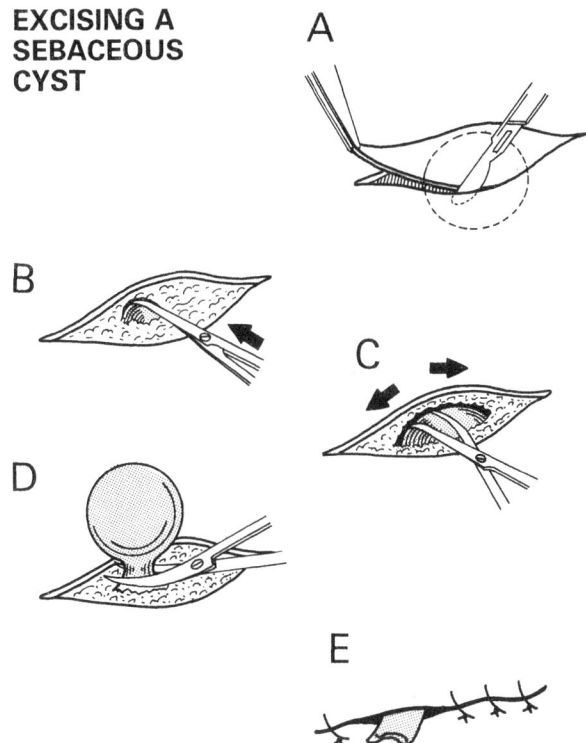

Fig. 34-6 GRANULOMA PYOGENICUM. Excise or curette these lesions. Don't mistake them for a sarcoma! If there is any doubt about the diagnosis, send a piece for histology.

Fig. 34-7 REMOVING A SEBACEOUS CYST. A, excising an ellipse of skin. B, inserting curved scissors to define the plane of cleavage. C, isolating the cyst. D, excising it. F, the incision closed with a drain in place.

34.4 The management of snake bites

Fortunately, most snakes have no fangs and are not poisonous. When a snake does have fangs, these can be at the back, or the front of its mouth. If the fangs are at the back, it is usually harmless, an important exception being the African boomslang (tree snake). If the fangs are at the front it is usually poisonous.

Apart from a few islands, there are venomous snakes almost everywhere; but only a few are medically important. Being bitten by one, usually on the leg, is one of the risks of being a tropical villager. People who deliberately handle snakes are usually bitten on their hands or arms. Although many people are bitten, less than half are poisoned, even by a poisonous snake, and of these few die. The danger is that a snake will inject its full dose of poison, in which case the patient has about a 50% chance of death, unless he is treated. Many snake bites are treated by traditional practitioners, and of the patients who do arrive in hospital, many arrive late. If necessary, teach your paramedical staff to treat snakebite, and supply them with antivenom.

Snake toxins have a variety of effects, depending on the species. These include local swelling, capillary oozing, and necrosis; generalized damage to muscles (sea snakes), damage to the heart or kidneys, interference with blood clotting, haemolysis, and various neurotoxic effects.

If a patient is treated symptomatically, he usually recovers, but if his symptoms are severe he needs the specific antivenom, ideally in monovalent form, or failing this as a polyvalent mixture suitable for the common snakes of the area. Theoretically, a monospecific antivenom is better, because smaller volumes are required, and this reduces the incidence of serum reactions. In practice, a polyvalent antivenom is more satisfactory in the rural tropics. Antivenom can occasionally cause reactions which are fatal, so don't give it unless it is indicated, and always have adrenalin ready. For sources of specific sera for your local snakes, see below.

In view the potential dangers of antivenom, its cost, and the difficulty of stocking it in sufficient quantities in remote places, *controllled ventilation, by any of the methods in 'Primary Anaesthesia' (A 13.1), is the main method of preventing death in a patient with severe neurotoxic symptoms following the bite of an elapid snake.*

You should know which snake bit him; but a patient often does not know this, particularly if he was bitten at night. Globally, the carpet or saw-scaled viper, is the most dangerous snake, because of its wide distribution (particularly West Africa, Pakistan, and North West India), its abundance in farming areas, its good camouflage, its irritability, and its toxicity.

Manson-Bahr PEC, and Apted FC, 'Manson's Tropical Diseases'. Baillière Tindall.

Reid HA and Theakston RDG, 'The Management of Snake Bite'. Bulletin of the World Health Organization 1983;61(6):885-895.

'Progress in Characterising Venoms and the Standardisation of antivenoms', 1981 WHO Offset Publication No. 58.

TREAT THE PATIENT NOT THE SNAKE

SNAKE BITES

FIRST AID. A snake bite is frightening, so reassure the patient. Move the bitten part as little as possible. If at any time he vomits or loses consciousness, turn him into the recovery position (A 4-5).

CAUTION ! (1) If the snake has been killed, keep it for examination, but don't try to look for it. (2) Don't handle snakes, even dead ones; decapitated heads can bite for some hours.

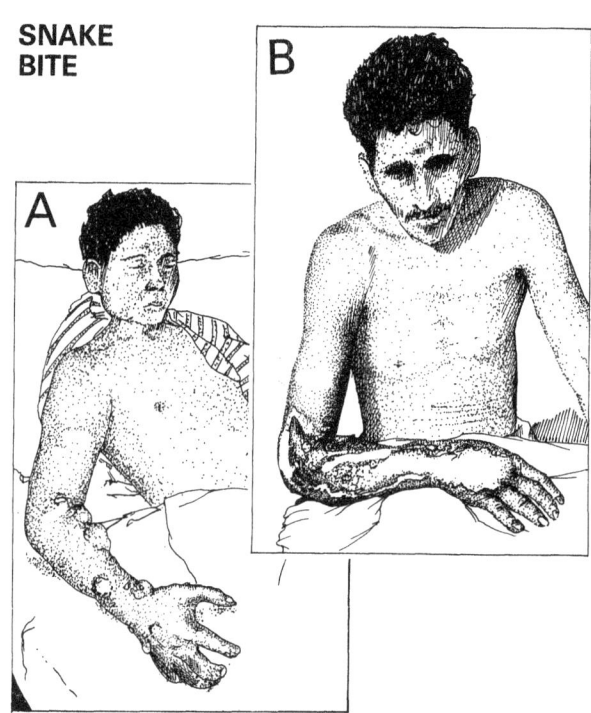

Fig. 34-8 SNAKE BITES. A, blood-stained blisters after a viper bite. B, extensive superficial necrosis after a viper bite. *After HA Reid.*

(3) Don't inject antivenom as part of first aid treatment. (4) Wipe, but don't incise the bite.

CREPE BANDAGING. The traditional arterial tourniquet is now outmoded, because of its dangers. Instead, apply a firm crêpe compression bandage over the whole length of the bitten limb, to slow the spread of venom. Remove it after about 8 hours.

IN HOSPITAL

Admit him. Don't panic or rush to inject antivenom. If he demands an injection, give him tetanus toxoid (which he needs anyway). Raise a bitten leg, and put a bitten arm in a sling. Clean the site of the bite and leave it open. Keep the number of injections to a minimum, because he may bleed from the injection sites, if the venom (particularly from a viper) alters blood clotting. Set up a drip. If there is local necrosis, give him a broad-spectrum antibiotic; some surgeons give them routinely. Avoid aspirin, because of its adverse effects on platelets, and morphine, which may mask respiratory depression.

CAUTION ! (1) Don't incise the bitten area, or apply ice or dressings early on. (2) Don't give heparin, fibrinogen, or neostigmine. (3) Steroids are useful for delayed (*not* immediate) serum reactions.

HAS THE SNAKE INJECTED POISON? If his symptoms are immediate, he is probably only frightened; symptoms of poisoning rarely appear before half an hour, although they can appear in the first 5 or 10 minutes. Fang marks are of little help; there may be marks and no poisoning, or no obvious marks and poisoning. Local pain can be severe when there is no poisoning, and be absent when there is poisoning. Three early non-specific signs suggest poisoning: (1) vomiting, (2) a polymorph leucocytosis and (3) hypotension. If this is accompanied by a slow pulse, suspect a strong vasovagal component to the symptoms, and thus a good prognosis. Other early non-specific signs are headache, abdominal pain, explosive diarrhoea, and collapse with an unrecordable blood pressure. These symptoms usually resolve spontaneously within an hour. After a viper bite a patient's blood fails to clot, his gums bleed, blood appears in his sputum and he may bleed from an old wound. After an elapid bite his eyelids droop (ptosis).

If there is local swelling which starts a few minutes after a viper bite, venom has been injected. This is not a criterion for giving antivenomn: wait for signs of specific poisoning.

If there is no swelling a few minutes after a viper bite, you can be sure that no venom has been injected.

If there is no pain and swelling and no general signs 2 hours after the bite, it is very unlikely that the snake is dangerous. However, signs can occur after a few minutes or be delayed for 12 hours, so observe him carefully.

WHAT KIND OF SNAKE WAS IT? Identifying the snake can be important, because it will allow you to give specific monovalent antivenom (if you have it); but not being able to identify it should never delay treatment. Here are some of the typical syndromes.

Vipers *usually* cause massive local swelling, due to exudation from injured capillaries; abnormal bleeding; and blood which fails to clot; later there is necrosis and gangrene.

Elapids are the cobras, mambas, kraits, and coral snakes. Their effects are mainly neurotoxic. Paralysis varies, and may be extensive and fatal. He has difficulty breathing due to respiratory paralysis, and cannot swallow. Ptosis is the earliest sign.

Sea snakes are myotoxic, see below.

LOCAL SWELLING starts minutes after the bite of a viper, and may be massive after 72 hours. The swollen area may be bruised, blistered, and ultimately necrotic. Wet gangrene may develop rapidly over days (cobras), or dry gangrene slowly over weeks (vipers). If there is no necrosis, recovery is rapid, provided that the fluid lost into the tissues is replaced. Swelling and necrosis are not usually dangerous in themselves, although they may result in permanent scarring, or occasionally in the need for amputation.

If there is any swelling, expose his limb to reduce its temperature. Raise his arm in a roller towel (75-1), and his leg by raising the foot of his bed.

Leave his blisters undisturbed. If his tissues necrose, excise sloughs and graft early. Necrosis is usually confined to the subcutaneous tissues, without involving his muscles and tendons. Apply saline dressings, and graft the raw areas (57.1). Antibiotics are not helpful, unless and until there is local necrosis. If he presented very late, you may have to amputate.

Very rarely, fasciotomy may be necessary (81.14).

SHOCK, starting later, is the main cause of death in viper bites. It can be late or early, sometimes within a few minutes of the bite, with abdominal pain, explosive diarrhoea, collapse and an unrecordable blood pressure. If it is due to hypersensitivity to the venom, rather than to its toxicity, these symptoms may resolve spontaneously in half an hour.

If he is in hypovolaemic shock give him saline. This is cheaper and more readily available than plasma, and less likely to infect him with HIV. If he shows signs of hypovolaemia, give him 2 litres of saline quickly initially. If he shows signs of circulatory insufficiency and extensive bruising, give him blood. Blood is particularly useful if he was anaemic before he was bitten, or if antivenom is not available.

BLEEDING may occur from the bite, into injection sites, in his vomit, from his gums, under his skin, or into his brain. It is often lethal, and may be delayed for several days. Hess's test may become positive in 30 minutes.

Hess's test Blow up a blood pressure cuff to 80 mm Hg and leave it on for 5 minutes. If a crop of purpuric spots appears below the cuff, the test is positive.

The clotting test gives warning of bleeding to follow. Keep some blood in a tube horizontally for 10 minutes and then tilt it. If it fails to clot, he needs antivenom. In Africa non-clotting blood is a useful indicator of *Eichis* envenoming, for which there is a specific antivenom.

If he bleeds extensively, and you have no antivenom, transfuse fresh blood, and if necessary give him fibrinogen intravenously.

NEUROTOXIC EFFECTS are characteristic of elapid poisoning, and are the result of a selective neuromuscular block. Ptosis is the earliest sign (don't confuse this with sleepiness). Other effects include: inability to cough, protrude the tongue, smile, or move the lower jaw; drooling, dysphagia; partial, flaccid limb paralysis, more marked proximally (painless, except in the case of sea snakes, when the paralysis is painful), generalized fasciculations, vertigo, convulsions, unconsciousness, respiratory failure from intercostal paralysis, squint, speech incoordination, and generalized paraesthesiae.

If his neck and trunk muscles are involved, he is unable to lift his head or sit up. The important fatal effects are respiratory failure, and failure of his swallowing reflex. Respiratory failure may manifest itself as increasingly shallow respirations, or as a vigorous struggle for air with laboured breathing.

If necessary, intubate (A 13.2) and ventilate (A 13.1) him in the theatre, while you wait for the antivenom to become effective. For the signs of incipient respiratory failure needing artificial ventilation, see A 19.4.

CAUTION ! (1) Intubation and ventilation are the first priority. Antivenom comes second, once he is breathing. (2) The inhalation of secretions, or stomach contents, can cause sudden death at any time (A 16.3).

MYOTOXIC EFFECTS are characteristic of sea snakes. Early symptoms are muscle pain and stiffness anywhere, but particularly in his neck, tongue, and throat. This is soon followed by tenderness, pain on passive movement, muscle weakness, and myoglobinuria. His muscles may take months to recover.

ANTIVENOM

INDICATIONS. (1) Undoubted clinical symptoms of systemic poisoning. Antivenom may still be effective hours or days after the bite. It is never too late to give it.

CONTRAINDICATIONS. Enquire for a history of allergy; this increases the risk of an allergic reaction. A known allergic history contraindicates antivenom, unless the risk of death from envenoming is high. There is no point in doing a sensitivity test, because it is unreliable, and if he is seriously poisoned, he will need antivenom anyway.

Give all patients promethazine. This will promote sleep and relieve apprehension, and may minimize sensitivity reactions (rarely severe).

METHOD. Ideally, the venom should be monovalent, but some broad-spectrum polyvalent antivenoms are sufficiently active. Even if an antivenom is out of date, it may still be effective. If it is opaque when you make it up, discard it, because there will be a greater risk of reactions.

Give him 20 to 50 ml of antivenom, diluted in 3 volumes of 0.9% saline. Give it by intravenous infusion diluted in a drip, or by slow bolus injection. The dose depends on the type of antivenom, and the type of snake; you may need much more than 40 ml, especially after an elapid bite. In severe poisoning (especially with neurotoxic envenoming) give 100 to 150 ml. In children give the same dose as in adults.

Start the drip slowly (15 drops a minute). If there is no initial reaction, increase the speed of administration, so that you can complete the infusion in 1 to 2 hours. If there has been little improvement, give more.

If there are signs of sensitivity to antivenom (pallor, hypotension, dyspnoea, laryngeal oedema), temporarily stop the drip and inject 0.5 ml of 1:1000 adrenalin subcutaneously, over some convenient part of his chest. This is almost always effective, and you can then restart the drip.

If he has an allergic history, give him small doses of adrenalin (0.5 ml of 1:1000 adrenalin) subcutaneously, before you give the antivenom, and repeat it if a reaction occurs. Also, give him promethazine or hydrocortisone 100 mg to protect against sensitivity reactions (rarely severe).

If more than 2 hours have elapsed since the bite of a known front-fanged (elapid) snake, and life-threatening signs are obvious, give the antivenom intravenously without delay, and without testing for hypersensitivity, under steroid or antihistamine cover.

In sea-snake poisoning, give 3000 to 10,000 units of antivenom. In mild poisoning 1000 to 2000 units should be enough.

CAUTION ! (1) In all patients, have adrenalin ready in a syringe, and give it at the first sign of anaphylaxis (pallor, etc., see above). (2) Don't give antivenom to all patients routinely.

MONITORING. Record his pulse, blood pressure, peripheral circulation, and respiration hourly, and the circumference of his bitten limb at the site of the bite. Monitor his urine output and his blood urea. Watch for specific signs, and don't discharge him for at least 12 hours.

DIFFICULTIES WITH SNAKE BITES

If, immediately after the bite, he appears SEMICONSCIOUS, and cold with clammy skin, a feeble pulse and rapid breathing, this may be due to fright (try a placebo injection), or to venom effects. In some venoms these pass off spontaneously in half an hour.

If he is MENTALLY CONFUSED, suspect respiratory failure.

If he shows signs of GLOSSOPHARYNGEAL PALSY (difficulty swallowing), nurse him in the recovery position.

If confusion, stupor, or RESPIRATORY FAILURE develop, intubate him, and aspirate his secretions. Atropine may diminish them.

If he develops signs of RENAL FAILURE (vipers, elapids or sea snakes), they usually appear towards the end of first week. Avoid drugs which are excreted in the urine (except for penicillin when necessary); treat him as in Section 53.3.

If a spitting COBRA SPAT INTO HIS EYES, wash them out with a large quantity of water, and tell him to blink. The venom is quickly diluted and causes no harm.

VENTILATE HIM AND HE WILL PROBABLY LIVE

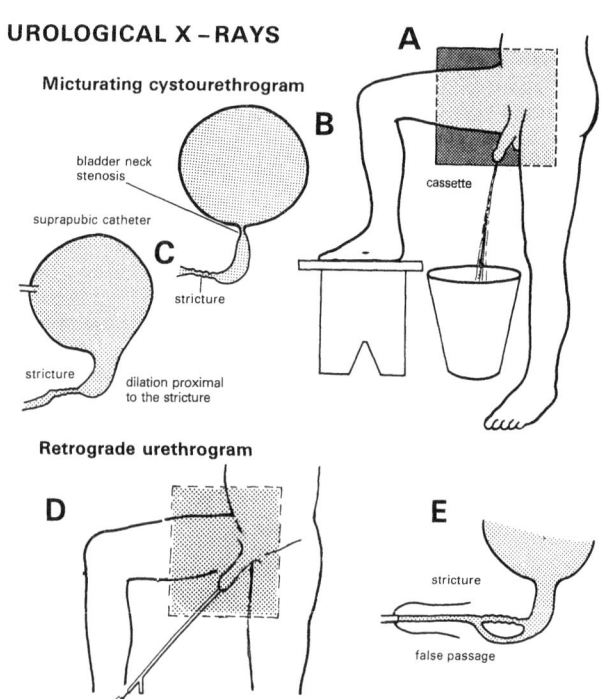

Fig. 34-9 SOME UROLOGICAL X-RAYS. A, in a micturating cystourethrogram the patient's bladder is filled with contrast medium, and a film taken while he is passing it. B, and C, two types of obstruction. D, in a retrograde urethrogram contrast medium is injected up his urethra from below (this shows an oblique view.) E, a false passage shown in a retrograde urethrogram.

RADIOLOGY

34.5 Some X-ray methods for the generalist

Section 1.13 describes WHO's basic radiological system. Here are some methods which are not part of that system. If you have a radiographer, he will be familiar with them. Most of them assume that your machine has a screen, but it has not, you can still do a barium swallow. Always use a grid which will improve the definition. Most screens have a grid which you can slide into place.

Carcinoma of the oesophagus is common in much of the developing world, so you will find a barium swallow, which is quite easy, particularly useful. A barium meal is more difficult, but with reasonable practice you can learn quite a lot from one. A barium enema is more trouble, and is less often needed. Cystoscopy (23.3) may give you the information you need, and is cheaper than an IVU. We do not describe catheterizing the ureters, and so retrograde pyelography is not described either.

INTRAVENOUS UROGRAM (IVU) (intravenous pyelogram or IVP)

INDICATIONS. (1) If a patient has moderate impairment of his renal function, to see if it has a purely renal cause, or is due to an obstructive uropathy, particularly a hydronephrosis or a ureteric stricture, especially in areas where *S. haematobium* is endemic. (2) To see if a mass is renal. (3) To assess the function of his other kidney, when you consider referring him for nephrectomy. (4) Renal trauma (67.1). (5) Renal or ureteric stone (23.12).

CONTRAINDICATIONS. (1) *Measure his blood urea.* If it is over 10 mmol/l (65 mg/dl), an IVU will probably fail because the dye will not be excreted in adequate concentration to be visible. It is certainly not worth doing if his blood urea is over 17 mmol/l (100 mg/dl). (2) Renal failure. (3) Hepatic failure, which may be aggravated. Cardiac failure; there is a risk of arrythmia. (4) Dehydration. (5) Infancy. (6) The first trimester of pregnancy is a relative contraindication, but the danger is minimal. (7) Any previous reaction to contrast medium or other allergic disease. (8) Multiple myeloma.

PREPARATION. Starve him overnight and give him an aperient to empty his gut. Air will not spoil the film, but a mixture of air, fluid and faeces will. Don't give him an enema. If the IVU is urgent, do it without preparation.

CONTRAST MEDIUM. Use 'Urografin' 60% or 'Conray 420'. Rarely, he may have a reaction, so make sure you have ready 0.5 ml of adrenalin 1/1000 and promethazine 25 mg for intramuscular injection. Cardiac arrest has followed injection, so be prepared to resuscitate him (3.5).

FILMS. Use 18×24 cm for his bladder; 24×30 cm for his renal area; 30×40, 35×35, or 35×43 cm for his whole abdomen.

METHOD. The following method minimizes the number of plates needed. The views are all AP; 60 mA at 68 KV should be enough for a 60 kg adult.

Lay him supine on the X-ray table. Take a preliminary view of his abdomen and pelvis on a 30×25 cm plate, before giving the contrast medium. Give him 40 ml intravenously as quickly as possible.

At 3 minutes take a 25×30 cm plate of his kidneys. Then compress his lower ureters. If his calyces are obviously normal at 3 minutes (be quick, it will need 5 minutes in the developer, fixing and washing), you can omit the 15 minute film.

At 15 minutes take another view of his kidneys. At 20 minutes release the compression and then quickly take a 35×43 cm plate to show his ureters and bladder.

At 30 minutes ask him to empty his bladder, and then take a small plate to show his residual urine.

If the function of his kidneys is impaired, so that there is little excretion in the standard films, repeat them at 2 hours, and if necessary at 6 hours.

RETROGRADE URETHROGRAM FOR A STRICTURE

PRINCIPLE. If you inject contrast medium up a patient's urethra from below, you can outline his distal urethra up to the face of the stricture.

INDICATIONS. (1) Stricture of the urethra. (2) Congenital anomalies. (3) Prostatic abscess. (4) Fistulae. (5) False passages.

CONTRAINDICATIONS. (1) Acute infections of the urinary tract. (2) Recent attempts at bouginage which will increase the risk of bacteraemia.

CONTRAST MEDIUM. (1) A contrast medium especially designed for urethrography, such as 'Umbradil Viscous U'. If necessary you can probably dilute it with an equal volume of water and still get good pictures. (2) If necessary, use media designed for urography, such as 'Hypaque' 45% and urografin 60%.

CAUTION ! Don't use barium, or an inorganic iodide. Contrast medium readily passes into the surrounding vessels.

METHOD. Using aseptic precautions, insert a 16 Ch Foley catheter *for 5 cm only* into his urethra. Gently inflate the bulb with 1 or 2 ml of sterile water. The expanded bulb will now fix the catheter in his fossa navicularis. Fix a length of tubing to the catheter. You can now position him more easily, and be further from the radiation yourself when you inject the contrast medium and expose the plate.

Inject the medium and take an oblique film while he lies on the X-ray cassette. Avoid extravasation, if you can. If his bladder is reasonably filled, you can follow a retrograde urethrogram with a micturating cystourethrogram.

The membranous urethra is separated from the penile urethra by a line, which runs from the junction of the upper third and the lower two-thirds of the pubic ramus on one side, to a corresponding point on the other side.

MICTURATING CYSTOURETHROGRAM FOR A STRICTURE

PRINCIPLE. This shows up the proximal face of a patient's stricture, and will also show bladder neck stenosis. His bladder must be filled with contrast medium to begin with. If you can pass a catheter through his urethra, you can fill it that way. If he has a suprapubic catheter in place and is able to micturate through his urethra (unusual), you can fill his bladder through that.

INDICATIONS. (1) Strictures. (2) Suspected abnormalities of the bladder neck. (3) The assessment of vesical diverticula. (4) Cysto-ureteric reflux.

CONTRAINDICATIONS. (1) Acute infections of the urinary tract. (2) Recent attempts at bouginage, which will increase the risk of bacteraemia.

CONTRAST MEDIUM. (1) 40 ml of 60% 'Urografin' in 400 ml of saline. Or, (2) a 250 ml bottle of 30% 'Urografin'. (3) 400 ml of 12.5% sodium iodide with 0.1% sodium metabisulphite. This is the cheapest. The sodium iodide must be suficiently pure; small quantities of fluoride in it can be disastrous.

METHOD. This depends on whether or not he already has a suprapubic catheter in place.

If he has a suprapubic catheter, empty his bladder through it. Using an intravenous drip set or a large syringe, fill it through his suprapubic catheter with 300 to 400 ml of contrast medium until he has a strong desire to pass urine.

Take an erect oblique AP film at 80 mA and 80 kV while he is standing to pass urine. Or take an oblique film in the lying position; there will be less blur due to movement. Use a bucky screen and a grid cassette.

If he has a ureteric catheter in place, fill his bladder through that.

BARIUM SWALLOW

INDICATIONS. (1) Dysphagia. (2) Carcinoma of the oesophagus (32.24). (2) Post-corrosive strictures (25.15).

CONTRAST MEDIUM. (1) Thin barium ('Gastrografin' or 'Endographin'). Water-soluble media must not be aspirated. (2) Barium sulphate; thicker than for a barium meal, yet not so thick as to aggravate an obstruction.

CAUTION ! Don't use barium carbonate, which is highly poisonous.

METHOD. Stand him in front of the X-ray screen facing you. If you don't have a screen, take films only. Ask him to fill his mouth with contrast medium, but not to swallow it until you ask him to. He can either drink from a feeding cup (which is less likely to spill in the dark), or suck the barium through a stiff 5 mm plastic tube inserted through a hole in the top of a plastic container, as used for tablets. The mixture of air and barium that he swallows will produce an informative 'phase contrast' film.

SOME BARIUM SWALLOWS

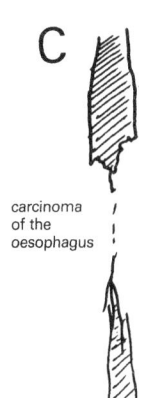
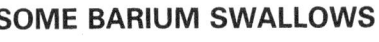

Fig. 34-10 SOME BARIUM SWALLOWS. A, a postcricoid web (lateral view). B, achalasia of the cardia. C, carcinoma of the oesophagus.

Adjust the X-ray machine to provide a narrow vertical aperture. Then ask him to swallow and watch the barium pass. Repeat the process and expose a plate as he swallows.

Do the same thing while he stands laterally with his hands above his head. You should be able to see all but the upper end of his oesophagus quite easily. If necessary, take two oblique views, a lateral fiew and an AP view.

Carcinoma of the oesophagus causes a narrowing with an abrupt start and an irregular rounded shoulder; above it the oesophagus is either not dilated, or only a little dilated. The lumen through the tumour is irregular and is typically rat-tailed, and you can see the end of the stricture. You should be able to demonstrate 90% of carcinomas with simple screening. An ordinary PA film may show widening of the mediastinum. Be sure to use a long plate to get his whole oesophagus on to it, and don't cone down.

If no screening is available, a mouthful of contrast medium and one large film will usually show the tumour.

If you are not sure how long the stricture is, try a repeat film with a head-down tilt. This is important in deciding how long a Celestin tube needs to be (32.24).

Achalasia (uncommon) shows as a 'bird's beak' at the bottom end of a greatly dilated oesophagus. Take oblique films.

Corrosive oesophagitis produces a stricture which is usually long and irregular.

A post-cricoid web (rare in Africa) is associated with iron deficiency anaemia and is a narrow web behind the cricoid cartilage. Centre a lateral film on the cricoid.

BARIUM MEAL

INDICATIONS. (1) Bleeding from the upper gastrointestinal tract, oesophageal varices (endoscopy is likely to be preferable). (2) Peptic ulcer. (3) Carcinoma of the stomach. (3) Carcinoma of the head of the pancreas. (4) An upper abdominal mass suspected of being gastric.

METHOD. Do a barium swallow first with thin barium. Ask him to stand facing you. Then give him thicker barium.

Adjust the aperture of the X-ray machine to let you see his entire stomach. Stand him facing you, and ask him to drink enough barium to about half fill his stomach while he continues to stand facing you (one contributor uses much less barium). Then screen him in this position and in the left oblique position (he should look beyond your left shoulder), or use the right oblique position.

STOMACH. Watch peristalsis carefully. Does barium pass through normally all the way to his pylorus?

Suggesting carcinoma—an immobile area, a persistently irregular surface, a consistent filling defect (this makes carcinoma very likely).

Suggesting a gastric ulcer—an ulcer, usually on the lesser curve, in the distal half of his stomach.

Expose 1 to 3 plates, asking him to hold his breath as you do so.

To look for a hiatus hernia you will need to raise his intra-abdominal pressure: (1) Ask him to lie down and give the table a 20° head-down tilt. Push the barium up to his fundus, and expose another plate. Or (2) ask him to lift his legs off the table and cough.

DUODENUM. Note if there is delay in the passage of barium through his pylorus: it should start passing at 1–5 minutes. Use the special attachment which will exclude all X-rays except those in a 10 cm circle. Turn him to face obliquely to your right as far as is necessary for you to see his pylorus and duodenal loop. Expose plates as the barium passes. You may be able to recognize a deformed duodenal cap while you screen him, but you will see scarring or a duodenal ulcer more easily on the dry films. With experience, you will recognize enlargement of the duodenal loop (as by carcinoma of the head of the pancreas).

Pyloric delay makes a duodenal ulcer or a carcinoma of the distal antrum likely, and is an indication for laparotomy.

BARIUM ENEMA

INDICATIONS. (1) Suspected amoebic strictures. (2) Carcinoma of the large gut. (3) Diverticulosis (rare in most of the developing world). (4) A mass which might be colonic. (5) Ulcerative colitis, tuberculosis, Chron's disease etc.

CAUTION ! A barium enema should follow proctoscopy and sigmoidoscopy, which will often establish the diagnosis more easily and cheaply.

CONTRAINDICATIONS. (1) Complete, incomplete, or impending intestinal obstruction. (2) Rectal biopsy immediately preceeding the enema.

EQUIPMENT. An X-ray machine with a screen. A 2 litre douche can. 2 metres of 30 Ch rubber or plastic tube. 2 large artery forceps. A Higginson's syringe. A grid on top of the X-ray plate.

METHOD. Prepare the patient with an enema, and a thorough washout (not merely an enema, and not necessary in children), within the previous 12 hours, and keep him on fluids during this time. Use barium/air contrast with the equipment in Fig. 34-11.

CAUTION ! Manipulate the flatus tube with gloves. Have toilet paper and a bedpan ready—it may be required urgently!

Lay him supine on the X-ray table, and ask him to flex and abduct his hips. Protect his gonads. Lubricate the flatus tube well with KY jelly, and push it through his anus, as far as it will go easily. Ask him to extend his legs on to the table. Inject barium and air, as required, to show his large gut up to his caecum. Inject a fair amount of barium first, and follow this by pumping air with the Higginson's syringe to move the barium proximally, clamping and releasing the tubes as necessary. Instil some barium, and then some air. You will probably be able to demonstrate his large gut as far as his hepatic flexure, without much difficulty; his ascending colon is more difficult. The limiting factor is the distension of his large gut with barium and air, and the urge to defaecate that this produces. If he feels much discomfort, wait 2 or 3 minutes and try again with more barium and more air.

Watch the movement of barium and air on screening, and expose plates of critical areas. Before he defaecates, which he is usually keen to do without delay, take a standard abdominal X-ray after removing the screen and keeping the grid in place. Expose another plate after evacuation. The film of barium left on his mucosa will often give the clearest picture.

Finally, remove the flatus tube and let him pass the contents of his gut into the bedpan.

EVALUATION

34.6 Indicators of quality in district hospital surgery

How can you know that surgical care in a hospital is good? What should a visitor look for when he goes round your hospital and what questions should he ask? Here are a few suggestions.

INDICATORS OF QUALITY IN SURGERY

The hospital has a plan as to which day of the week non-urgent operations are done, and when clinics are held.

Ward rounds are held daily.

Each patient has a plan in his notes saying what should happen to him and when—when a cast should come off, when traction should be taken down, or a burn should be grafted, etc. There are accurate notes in enough detail to enable another doctor to take over.

The staff wash their hands after examining a potentially infected patient, before examining the next one. Not to do so, especially after examining an infected wound, is the height of bad practice—presuming, of course, that the ward has water, which, alas, some do not. Patients are washed thoroughly with soap and water before surgery—especially the operation site.

How often do clean operations in your hospital become infected? (2.10)

How many skin grafts do you do, and how many of them take? (57.1)

How much knee movement do your patients have when you discharge them from hospital after you have treated their broken femurs? (78.3)

Are all patients whose fractures have been put in plaster, told to to return immediately if they get pain? (70.4)

Are there any instruments or equipment, which were broken more than a month ago, which no attempt has yet been made to replace or repair?

Is some provision is made to provide terminal care for cancer patients? (33.1)

Do you know your mortality rate for the more common operations?

34.7 Indicators of quality in district hospital obstetrics

The critical indicators are the maternal and perinatal mortality rates, and indeed whether you have worked them out. Where obstetric care is good, mothers almost never die, so that almost any maternal death is likely to indicate care that is not as good as it might be.

A BARIUM ENEMA

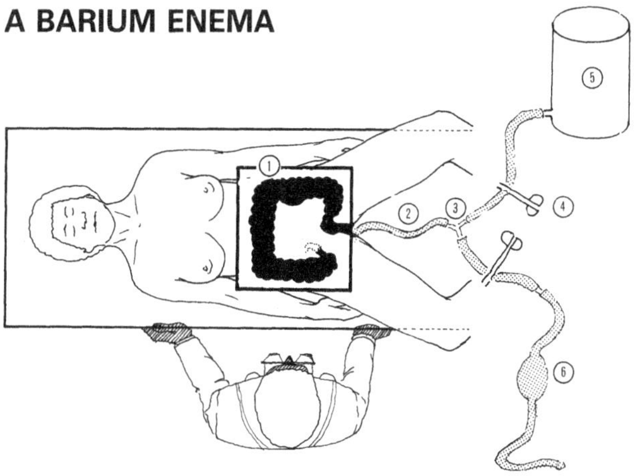

Fig. 34-11 ARRANGEMENTS FOR A BARIUM ENEMA. You will probably be able to demonstrate the patient's large gut as far as his hepatic flexure, without much difficulty; his ascending colon is more difficult. Note that you are wearing goggles and an apron.

1, an X-ray screen, grid, and X-ray plate; these are usually in an undercouch bucky tray. 2, a 30 Ch flatus tube. 3, a standard plastic Y-connector. 4, artery forceps. 5, a 2 l stainless steel douche can. 6, a Higginson's syringe. *Kindly contributed by James Cairns and Rogers Mungalu (Radiographer at St Francis Hospital, Katete, Zambia).*

Another useful indicator is the variety of procedures undertaken, and their proportion to one another. This is well shown in the figures for one district hospital, with a great reputation for the quality of its care, and which serves a disadvantaged population with poor communications. In one year 2031 babies were born there; 96 of these (about 5%—a good figure to aim for) were delivered by lower segment Caesarean section, none by classical Caesarean section, 55 by vacuum extraction, 16 with forceps (the superintendant is a skilled obstetrician), and 23 by symphysiotomy (the open method). There were 10 destructive operations, and 4 ruptured uteri. There were 6 deaths, only 2 related to delivery.

It is difficult to suggest a suitable 'target' for maternal mortality, so much depends on the circumstances; ideally, it should be almost zero. 50 per thousand is usually considered a good perinatal mortality for a district hospital in the developing world, and 30 a very good one; ideally, again, it should be much lower than this.

The earlier targets in the list below are from among those recommended by WHO after the 1985 conference at Fortazela, Brazil, which was concerned to reverse the trend towards high technology childbirth, and to promote more enlightened methods.

TARGETS FOR GOOD OBSTETRICS

WHO'S TARGETS include:
The whole community is informed about the various kinds of birth care, so that each mother can choose the kind of birth she wants.
There is active collaboration with any traditional birth attendants in the community.
A chosen member of the family is present during birth, and during the postnatal period.
Immediate breast-feeding is encouraged, even before a mother leaves the delivery room.
The Caesarean section rate is in the region of 5%, and is certainly less than 8%.
A further Caesarean section is not automatic after a previous one, and suitable mothers are given a trial of labour. Ligation of the Fallopian tubes is not used an an indication for section.
The dorsal lithotomy position is not used routinely during labour and delivery. Walking is encouraged during labour, and each mother decides which position she will adopt during delivery.
Labour is induced for specific medical indications only, with an induction rate of <10%.
Anaesthetic and analgesic drugs are not given routinely, but only when needed to prevent or treat some complication (this depends on the culture; some rural women are so tough, and put up with so much pain without complaining, that they may need to be encouraged to accept analgesia).
The membranes are not ruptured early as a matter of routine.
The perineum is protected wherever possible. Episiotomy is done on appropriate indications only, and is not done routinely.

OTHER TARGETS. The maternal mortality rate in the hospital and the community (15.1) is known, as is the hospital perinatal mortality rate.
Regular perinatal mortality meetings are held.
Antenatal cards are issued to all mothers. The blood pressure is measured and recorded at every antenatal visit.
A wide range of family-planning methods are available at all MCH clinics, in the hospital and outside.
Labour charts, including the cervicograph, are in regular use in the hospital and the clinics.
Destructive operations and symphysiotomies are done when necessary.

Chapter 35 Appendices

Appendix A The equipment list

Here is a summary of all the equipment discussed in both volumes. The quantities of the items listed are those suitable for the initial equipment of a district hospital. The list is deliberately generous, and there are sufficient haemostats, etc. to make all the sets described in section 4.12. Those items marked 'local pattern', as being suitable for local manufacture, may have to be imported if local manufacturing facilities are limited. Similarly, with those marked 'local purchase', if the local shops are very limited. Some of the more expensive items have been marked 'optional'.

Only a few items have been costed. Much depends on the quantity ordered and the country of manufacture. Forceps from West Germany will cost much more than those from Pakistan. Much equipment (retractors, etc.) is everlasting. A wide variety of some items (needles, etc.), does not necessarily increase the annual expenditure on them. The list assumes that the ordinary supplies of a hospital (antibiotics, etc.) will be available. If you want more details of the equipment, the number of the section where the items are discussed is printed in bold type after the first of the group of instruments in that particular section.

One of the most urgent items in need of standardization is bulbs for endoscopes. Unfortunately, we have been unable to find any standard fitting.

OPERATING TABLE, simple pattern, (NES) each $240, one only. **2.1**
ALTERNATIVE OPERATING TABLE, as Seward minor (SEW), or equivalent, one only.
MATTRESS, for operating table, (a) one mattress only, with (b) three mackintosh covers only.
ARM BOARD, for operating table, locally made, one only.
STOOL, operating, adjustable for height, local manufacture, two only.
LIGHT, operating theatre, simple pattern, with sockets to take bayonet or screw fitting domestic pattern light bulbs, in addition to special bulbs, state voltage, one only.
CLOCK, wall, electric, with second hand, one only.
SPOTLIGHT, free-standing on the floor, 'Anglepoise' type, to take ordinary domestic pattern bulbs, state voltage, two only. Also, high efficiency internally reflecting bulb to give a parallel beam, five only.
SOLAR PANEL, CHARGER, and BATTERY, one of each. Optional.
BATTERY CHARGER, for the common sizes of dry batteries, together with five rechargeable batteries of each size, one outfit only.
INSTRUMENT CABINET, glass door, sides and shelves, 1300×600×400 mm, local manufacture, one only.
X-RAY VIEWING BOX, standard pattern, local manufacture, one only.
TROLLEY, instrument, without guard rail, with two stainless steel shelves, antistatic rubber castors, (a) 600×450 mm, three only. (b) 900×450 mm, one only.
STAND, solution, with antistatic rubber-tyred castors, complete with two 350 mm stainless steel bowls, side by side, one only.
DRIP stands, telescopic, two only.
SUITS, theatre, cotton, with short-sleeved shirt, and long trousers, assorted sizes, local manufacture, thirty only. **2.3**
CLOGS, assorted sizes, ten pairs only.
APRONS, mackintosh, assorted sizes, local manufacture, eight only.
CAPS, cotton, thirty only.
MASKS, theatre, one hundred only.
GOWNS, cotton, fifty only.
GLOVES, operating, reusable, (a) Size 6, twenty pairs. (b) Size 6½, forty pairs. (c) Size 7, twenty pairs. (d) Size 7½, forty pairs. (e) Size 8, twenty pairs only.
GLOVES industrial, three pairs only.
GLOVE POWDER, absorbable, 3 kg only.
SOAP, hexachlorophene or carbolic, fifty tablets only.
BRUSHES, nylon, nesting, fifty only.
TOWELS, cotton, green, theatre. (a) Hand towels 25 cm square, one hundred only. (b) Theatre drapes 100.75 cm, one hundred only. (c) Abdominal sheets, ten only.
OTHER SUPPLIES (1) Pyjamas and pyjama trousers, twenty only. (2) Dresses, twenty only. (3) Mackintosh drapes 75.100 cm, twenty only. (4) Squeegee, two only. (5) Bucket and mop, three only.
AUTOCLAVE, vertical, 350 mm, 2½ drum, electric, 6 kw, state voltage, manual operation, with 6 spare elements, 6 spare gaskets, and a triple set of other spares as necessary, one only. **2.4**
Alternatively, AUTOCLAVE, vertical, 350 mm, 2½ drum, for heating by kerosene or gas, manual operation, with 6 spare gaskets, and a triple set of other spares as necessary, one outfit only.
AUTOCLAVE, vertical, 'pressure cooker', 47 l, UNICEF, as (WIS) No 1941, one only, optional.
HEATER, kerosene, pressure, 'Primus' pattern or equivalent, 4-burner, with 20 spare jets, prickers and washers etc., two only. These are only required for the alternative autoclave.
TAPE, autoclave testing, 25 rolls only.
Alternatively, TUBES, Browne's, for testing autoclave, Type one (black spot), for use with ordinary steam sterilizers below 126 C, one hundred tubes only.
DRUMS, 340×230 mm, ten only.
DRUMS, 340×120 mm, ten only.
DRESSING BOXES, stainless steel with hinged lid and perforated sliding shutters at front and back 250×200×150 mm, three only.
TRAYS, dressing, without lids, stainless steel, 275×320×50 mm, twenty only.
STERILIZER, boiling water, electric: (a) 'Bowl sterilizer', 450×350×380 mm, with counterbalanced lid, 6 kW, with 6 spare elements, state voltage, one only. (b) Instrument sterilizer, 350×160×120 mm, 1.2 kW, with 6 spare elements, state voltage, one only.
Alternatively, STERILIZER, boiling water, for heating by kerosene or gas, one only.
FORCEPS, sterilizer, Cheatle's, 267 mm, UNIPAC 0735200, two only.
FORCEPS, sterilizer, Cheatle's extra large, 279 mm, complete with can of appropriate size for antiseptic fluid, two only.
FORCEPS, bowl sterilizing, Harrison's double jawed, complete with can of appropriate size for antiseptic fluid, one only.
IODINE, tincture USP, 1 l only. **2.5**
CHLORHEXIDINE, gluconate solution BP, ('Hibitane'), 5 l only.
GLUTARALDEHYDE, concentrate, 50% w/w in water, 5 l only.
CRESOL and soap solution BP ('Lysol'), or some other phenolic antiseptic, 10 l only.
DRESSING TRAYS, stainless steel, with lids, (a) 250×200×50 mm, six only. (b) 350×300×50 mm, three only.
SODIUM NITRITE, tablets or powder, 100 g.
GAUZE, haemostatic, surgical, 'Surgijel' or equivalent, 5 packs only. **3.1, 3.2**
FORCEPS, artery, Spencer Wells. (a) 200 mm, straight, six only. (b) 150 mm, straight, twelve only. (c) 230 mm, curved, six only. (d) 200 mm, curved, eighteen only. (e) 150 mm, curved, six only. (f) 125 mm, curved, twelve only.
FORCEPS, artery, Crile's, (a) straight, six only. (b) curved, box joint, 140 mm, eighteen only.
FORCEPS, artery, Halstead's, ultrafine, mosquito, haemostatic, (a) straight, (b) curved, box joint, 120 mm, six only of each type.
FORCEPS, artery, Kocher's, (a) straight, (b) curved, box joint 200 mm, six only of each type.
PINS, safety, Mayo's, large, for storing artery forceps etc., ten only.
TOURNIQUET, Conn, improved pneumatic with dial, in case complete, (a) adult, (b) child. One only of each size. **3.9**
BANDAGE, rubber, Esmarch, 3 metres×75×1 mm, fitted with tapes, three metres, one only.
SCALPEL, solid forged, size No. 1, 30 mm, and size No. 5, 40 mm, two scalpels only of each size. **4.2**
HANDLE, scalpel, Bard Parker, No. 4, eight only
HANDLE, scalpel, Swan Morton, No. 5, four only.
BLADES, scalpel, disposable, Bard Parker or Swann Morton type, stainless steel in dispenser containing 100 blades. (a) Type 10, ten dispensers only. (b) Type 11, five dispensers only. (c) Type 15, five dispensers only. (d) Type 22, two dispensers only. (e) Type 24, two dispensers only.
OILSTONE, hard Arkansas pattern, 150×70×30 mm, one only.
DISSECTOR, MacDonald, one only.
SCISSORS, operating, Mayo, straight, bevelled blades, 200 mm, one only. **4.3**
SCISSORS, operating, Mayo, curved, bevelled blades, 170 mm, one only.

SCISSORS, operating, McIndoe's, curved, with rounded tapering blades, 180 mm, one only.
SCISSORS, operating, Metzenbaum, curved 275 mm, one only.
SCISSORS, Aufrecht's, light, curved, 140 mm, one only.
SCISSORS, straight with fine sharp points, Glasgow pattern, 100 mm, stainless steel, two only.
SCISSORS, suture cutting, 'assistant's scissors', rounded ends, four only.
SCISSORS, suture wire cutting, 130 mm, one only.
SCISSORS, bandage angular, Lister 180 mm, one only.
FORCEPS, dissecting, thumb, blunt, non-toothed, Bonney's, 180 mm, three only. **4.4**
FORCEPS, dissecting, thumb, toothed, Treves', 1×2 teeth, 130 mm, five only.
FORCEPS, dissecting, thumb, fine, Adson's, (a) plain, (b) 1×2 teeth, 120 mm, two only of each.
FORCEPS, dissecting, thumb, Duval's, 150 mm, with non-traumatic teeth on triangular jaws, two only.
FORCEPS, dissecting, thumb, toothed, 180 mm, one only.
FORCEPS, dissecting, thumb, Maingot's, 280 mm, one only.
FORCEPS, dissecting, McIndoe's, plain, 150 mm, one only.
FORCEPS, dissecting, ophthalmic, Silcock's, 100 mm, one only.
FORCEPS, tissue, locking, Allis', box joint, 150 mm, 5×6 teeth, eight only.
FORCEPS, tissue, locking, Babcock's, box joint, 160 mm, two only.
FORCEPS, tissue, Lane's, one only.
FORCEPS, sinus, Lister, box joint 150, mm, one only.
FORCEPS, cholecystectomy, curved jaws with longitudinal serrations, Lahey's, box joint, 200 mm, one only.
FORCEPS, intestinal, Dennis Browne, 180 mm, one only.
FORCEPS, Moynihan, box joint 220 mm, with box joint, four only.
FORCEPS, Desjardin's, screw joint, one only.
FORCEPS (clamps), hysterectomy, curved, box joint, 1×2 teeth, Hunter or Maingot, four, preferably, six only.
RETRACTOR, Volkmann's rake, sharp, 4-prong, 220 mm, two only. **4.5**
RETRACTOR, Langenbeck, 13×44 mm, two only.
RETRACTOR, Czerny, double-ended, four only.
RETRACTOR, Lane's modified by Kilner, double-ended, 150 mm, two only.
RETRACTOR, Gelpie, 170 mm, two only.
RETRACTOR, Morris, double-ended, three only.
RETRACTOR, Deaver's, plain handles, set of five sizes, one set only.
RETRACTOR, malleable copper, set of 4 sizes, one set.
RETRACTOR, Meydering, 178 mm, two only.
RETRACTOR, self-retaining, West's, straight, sharp pronged, one only.
RETRACTOR, abdominal, self-retaining, two-blade, adult, Gosset's, one only.
RETRACTOR, universal, Dennis Browne, with (a) one frame 300×240 mm, (b) one frame 300×240 mm, (c) 3 hook-on retractors 50×65 mm, (d) ditto 80×90 mm, (e) ditto 98×50 mm, (f) ditto 105×35 mm, one set only.
SUTURES, polyamide ('Nylon'), monofilament, strengths 5/0, 4/0, 3/0, 0 and 1, reels of 1000 metres, (PEA), preferably each size a different colour, two reels only of No. 1, one reel only of the other sizes. **4.6**
SUTURES, catgut, plain, 3/0, in boxes of 12, five boxes only.
SUTURES, catgut, chromic, strengths 3/0, 2/0, 0, and 1, boxes of 12, ten boxes only of each strength.
SUTURES, catgut, chromic, atraumatic, (a) 2/0 on half-circle 30 mm needles, ten boxes only. (b) 2/0 on 5/8 circle 30 mm needles, ten boxes only. (c) 4/0 on 16 mm curved needle, ten boxes only.
SUTURES, prolene, atraumatic, (a) 4/0 on 16 mm half-circle, round-bodied needle, (b) 8/0 on 3 mm 3/8 circle atraumatic needles, two boxes only of each size.
SUTURES, linen, No. 1, five reels only.
SUTURES, nylon or virgin silk, 8/0, one box only.
WIRE, suture, monofilament, soft stainless steel, reel, (a) 5/0, (b) 0.35 mm, (c) 1.0 mm, one reel only of each thickness.
WALL BRACKET, stainless steel, to hold rolls of monofilament, as in Fig. 4-5, one only.
REELS, stainless steel, egg-shaped ('eggs'), for holding suture material, five only.
NEEDLES, suture, Keith, triangular straight 64 mm, twenty-five needles only. **4.7**
NEEDLES, suture, 3/8 circle curved, triangular point, sizes 4, 12 and 18, twenty-five needles of each size.
NEEDLES, suture, 1/2 circle curved, triangular, sizes 2, 8, 14 and 20, fifty needles of each size only.
NEEDLES, suture, round-bodied, 3/8-circle curved, sizes 4, 10 and 18, twenty-five needles of each size only.
NEEDLES, Moynihan, 5/8-circle curved, round-bodied, fine, sizes 1, 4 and 6, fifty needles only of size 1, twenty-five needles only of sizes 4 and 6.
NEEDLES, Mayo, intestinal, round-bodied, half-circle curved with sharp perforating ends, 23 mm, size 20, one hundred needles only.
NEEDLES, suture, round-bodied, half-circle curved, sizes 1, 4, 10, 15, and 20, twenty-five needles of each size only.
NEEDLES, suture, Moynihan, Lance point, 5/8-circle, 115 mm, twenty-five needles only.
NEEDLES, suture, curved, tension, Colt, 102 mm, five needles.
NEEDLES, straight triangular, cutting, 35 mm, twenty needles only.
NEEDLES, suture, Jameson Evans, triangular, curved, 10 mm, twenty-five needles only.
NEEDLES, suture, Dennis Brown, round-pointed, 5/8 circle, 16 mm, twenty-five needles only.
NEEDLES, suture, 1/2circle, catgut, Mayo, sizes 1 and 3, twenty-five needles of each size only.
NEEDLES, Deschamps, angled to the right, five needles only.
NEEDLE-HOLDER, Boseman, 210 mm, ratchet and loose joint, tungsten carbide jaws, two only.
NEEDLE-HOLDER, Mayo's, with ratchet and box joint, tungsten carbide jaws 185 mm, one only.
NEEDLE-HOLDER, Mayo Dunhill, 160 mm, ratchet and box joint, tungsten carbide jaws, three only.
NEEDLE-HOLDER, Mayo's with narrow serrated jaws, box joint tungsten carbide jaws and ratchet, 185 mm, three only.
NEEDLE-HOLDER, Derf, box joint and rachet, tungsten carbide jaws, 115 mm, one only.
TUBE, nasogastric, plastic, Ryle's, with several side holes near the tip, 14 Ch, 16Ch, and 18 Ch, ten only of each size. **4.9**
TUBE, stomach, adult and child, assorted sizes, five only of each size.
TUBING, red, rubber sterilizable, 2 mm wall, (a) 10 mm bore, (b) 15 mm bore, ten metres only of each size. **4.10**
TUBING, drainage, Penrose, assorted sizes, 5 metres only.
DRAIN, corrugated red rubber, sheets 1×50×300 mm, ten sheets only.
SUMP DRAIN, rubber or plastic, five only.
TUBE, rectal, rubber, (a) child's size 8 mm (24 Ch), five only; (b) adult's size 10 mm (30 Ch), five only. **4.11**
CONNECTOR, end to end, polypropylene, external diameter (a) 4 mm, (b) 7 mm, (c) 10 mm, (d) 15 mm, (e) 19 mm, ten only of each size.
CONNECTOR, 3 way, 'Y', assorted sizes, twenty only.
CLIP, towel, cross action, 90 mm, twenty eight only.
CLIP, towel, with ratchet, Backhaus, six only.

EQUIPMENT—ONE

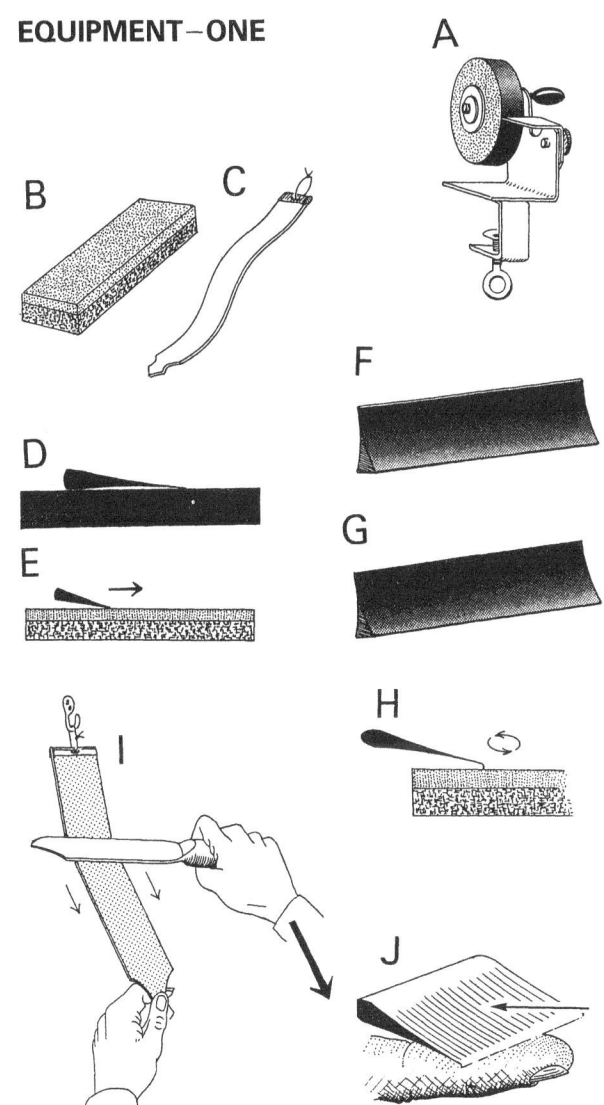

Fig. 35-1 CARING FOR YOUR EQUIPMENT—ONE. A, B, C, you will need a grindstone, a razor, and a strop. D, if your razor is hollow-ground, lay it flat, so that both edges rest on the stone, and push it forwards. E, if it is ground on the flat, lift its heel slightly and push it forwards. F, light reflecting from the blunt edge of a razor. G, a sharp razor without such a facet. H, removing a burr. I, stropping a knife by pulling it towards you. J, feeling if there is a burr on a blade by drawing it backwards across your finger.

FORCEPS, sponge-holding, Rampley, straight, box joint, (a) 240 mm, twenty two only. (b) 120 mm, two only.
LOUPE, binocular, Bishop Harman, ×2 magnification, one only.
TROCAR AND CANNULA, straight, with nickel silver or stainless steel cannula and metal handle, as (a) 4 mm (12 Ch). (b) 8 mm (24 Ch). (c) 12 mm (36 Ch), one only of each size.
CANNULA WITH SIDE ARM for suction, one only.
PROBE, malleable, with eye, nickel silver, 150 mm, as UNIPAC 0759915, one only.
DIRECTOR, hernia, Key's, one only.
DIRECTOR, probe-ended, Brodie, 165 mm, one only.
RING CUTTER, one only.
NEEDLE, aneurysm, Dupytren, (a) one needle curving right. (b) one needle curving left, one only of each kind.
NEEDLE, aneurysm, small, with blunt point, three only.
CATHETER, metal, female, three only.
BRUSH, for cleaning instrument jaws, ten only.
RAZOR, safety, for preoperative preparation, ten only.
BUCKET, stainless steel, with handles, six only.
KIDNEY DISHES, stainless steel, with half curled edges, 4 sizes 100 to 300 mm, two dishes of each size only.
GALLIPOT, stainless steel or autoclavable plastic, set of six sizes 40 to 200 mm, two sets only.
JAR, stainless steel with dropover lid, 150×150 mm, two only.
JUG, plastic, autoclavable, conical, 3 litre, one only.
BIN, soiled, two only.
JELLY, hydroxymethylcellulose, sterile, 'KY' jelly, 1 kg only.
'BIPP', bismuth, iodoform, and paraffin paste BPC, 1 kg only.
CARPENTER'S EQUIPMENT (a) Saw, one only. (b) Twist drill, one only. (c) Hammer, claw head, one only.
OTHER MATERIALS including gauze, cotton wool, bandages, adhesive tape, and laparotomy pads.
ASPIRATOR, Martin's, with 3-way tap and needles, one only. **6.1**
OSTEOTOME, Swedish model, solid forged stainless steel, (a) 6 mm. (b) 10 mm. One only of each size. **7.2**
NIBBLER, 150 mm, Read Jensen, one only.
GOUGES, Swedish model, solid forged stainless steel, (a) 6 mm, (b) 10 mm. One only of each size.
NIBBLER, Read Jensen, 150 mm, one only.
MALLET, stainless steel, 350 g, one only.
BONE FILE or rasp, one only.
FORCEPS, bone-cutting, Liston, angled on flat, 200 mm, one only.
FORCEPS, bone-holding, Hey Groves, 210 mm, one only.
FORCEPS, bone-holding, Lane's 390 mm, one only.
FORCEPS, sequestrum, angled, 190 mm, one only.
CURETTE, or scoop, Volkmann, double-ended, size C, two only.
LEVERS, bone, Trethowan, 220 mm, four only.
LEVERS, bone, heavy, four only.
HOOK, bone, 220 mm, one only.
ROUGINE, Faraboef, with curved end, chisel edge, one only.
ELEVATOR, periosteal, one only.
FORCEPS, intestinal, non-crushing, flexible blades, Kocher's or Doyen's, 250 mm, two only. **9.2, 9.6, 10.5**
CLAMP, Payr's, intestinal crushing, lever action, medium size, 110 mm, two, preferably four, only.
CLAMP, Payr, intestinal crushing, lever action, small size for pylorus, 60 mm, two only.
CLAMP, enterostomy, crushing, Lloyd Davies parallel action to take apart, one only.
DECOMPRESSOR, intestinal, Savage, one only.
TUBE, Sengstaken, 18 to 21 Ch, two only of each size. **11.5**
FORCEPS, Desjardins, gallstone, one only. **13.3**
BISTOURIE, guarded, one only. **14.1**
STETHOSCOPE, fetal, plastic, one only. **15.1**
DOPPLER FETAL HEART DETECTOR, 'Sonicaid' pattern or equivalent, one only. Optional.
SPECULUM, vaginal, Sims', double-ended, medium size, 27×30 mm, three only of each size.
SPECULUM, vaginal, Cusco's, duckbill, small and large, stainless steel, one of each size only.
SPECULUM, vaginal, weighted, Auvard's, chromium plated, one only.
FORCEPS, uterine vulsellum, curved, 1×2 teeth and 3×4 teeth, box joint, 230 mm, one only of each size.
SOUND, uterine, malleable, metric, graduated shaft, two only.
DILATORS, cervix, double-ended, Hegar's, 222 mm, set of 12 sizes, 1/2 mm to 23/24 mm, one, or preferably, two sets only.
MANIPULATOR, uterine, one only.
FORCEPS, ovum, curved, screw joint, McClintock 250 mm, one only.
CURETTE, uterine, double ended, blunt and sharp, 8 mm and 5 mm, two only of each size.
CURETTE, suction, stainless steel, reusable, sizes 8 and 10 Hegar, one only of each size.
CURETTE AND SYRINGE, for menstrual regulation, sterile, plastic, disposable, five hundred only.
CATHETER, Drew Smythe, one only.
CANNULA, cervical Leech Wilkinson or Miller, one only.
SCISSORS, episiotomy, Vant, one only.
VACUUM EXTRACTOR, Bird's modification of Malmstrom's, complete with 3 suction cups 40, 50, and 60 mm, and one posterior cup, one traction handle, vacuum hand pump, chain, spare vacuum bottle and spare baskets, one only.

EQUIPMENT—Two

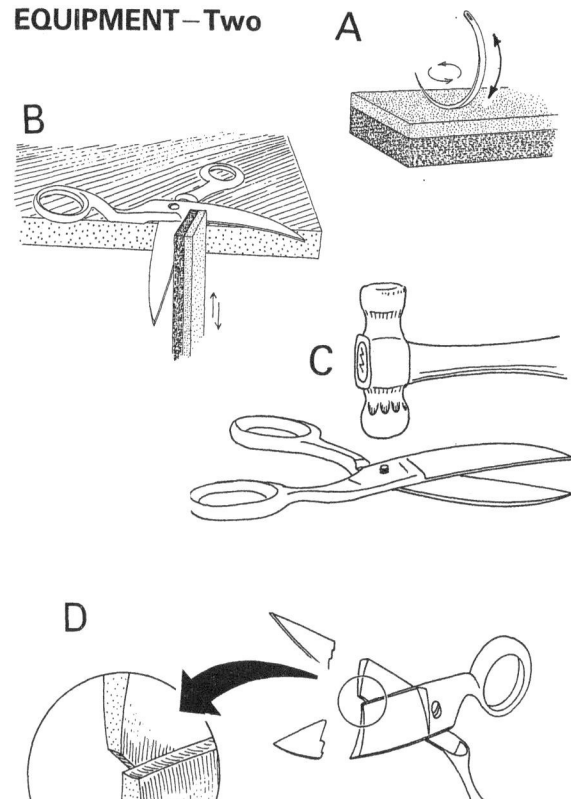

Fig. 35-2 CARING FOR YOUR EQUIPMENT—TWO. A, to sharpen a cutting needle, put it on a stone and rotate it in two planes. B, sharpening a pair of scissors. C, tightening the rivet of a pair of scissors. D, the cutting edge of a scissors should look like this.

FORCEPS, outlet, Wrigley, one only.
FORCEPS, obstetric Neville Barnes, one only. Optional.
FORCEPS, haemostasis, straight, Green-Armytage, 203 mm, six only.
PERFORATOR, Simpson's one only.
RETRACTOR, Doyen's, one only.
RETRACTOR, Kirschner, one only.
SCISSORS, embryotomy, Queen Charlotte's pattern, one only.
SAW, decapitation, Blond-Heidler, complete with ring, thimble and blades, one only.
LAPROCATOR, JHPIEGO pattern, with Verres gas needles, and carbon dioxide supply (JHP), in case complete one only. Optional **15.4**
FORCEPS, vasectomy, two only **15.6**
LARYNGOSCOPE, neonatal, straight-bladed, Seward, with two blades sizes 0 (80 mm) and 1 (110 mm), also ten spare batteries and five spare bulbs, two laryngoscopes only.
TUBES, tracheal, neonatal, transparent, plastic or rubber, non–disposable (or disposable but reusable), either Cole pattern with neck and T-piece, or straight pattern with uniform diameter and stylet (optional), sizes 2.5 mm (10 Ch), 3 mm (12 Ch), and 3.5 mm (14 Ch), ten only of each size.
ADAPTOR, tracheal, neonatal, various sizes, five only.
SUCTION CATHETERS, 4, 6, 8, and 10 Ch, ten only of each size.
AIRWAYS, neonatal, sizes 00 and 000, five only of each size.
MASK, neonatal, soft and clear, sizes 00, 0, and 1, Ambu (AMB) Laerdal, Bennett, or Samson, two only of each size.
BAG, self-inflating, neonatal or infant size 250 or 500 ml, Cardiff, Laerdal, or Ambu (AMB), with reservoir or extension tube, and expiratory pressure release valve, one only.
SUCTION DEVICE, electric, with overflow bottle and gauge, maximum vacuum 100–120 mm Hg (0.16–0.26 Bar), as 'de Vilbiss 721 Vacu Aide' (deV), one only.
FOOTPUMP, 'minipump' (AMB), one only.
MUCUS EXTRACTOR tube, and fluid trap, 10 Ch (CHI), five only.
STETHOSCOPE, with small head, one only.
PROCTOSCOPE, Gabriel, 64×25 mm, one only. **21.1**
SPECULUM, bivalve, preferably Goligher pattern with detachable third blade, one only.
SIGMOIDOSCOPE, Strauss, 330 mm, Luer fitting, in case with bellows, cord, and standard endoscope lamp complete with biopsy forceps, etc., one only.
SPONGE HOLDER, for sigmoidoscope, 430 mm, one only.

FORCEPS, for biopsy through sigmoidoscope, Officer pattern, one only.
SUCTION TUBE FOR SIGMOIDOSCOPE, one only.
BELLOWS, spare for Strauss sigmoidoscope, Luer fitting, one only.
LAMPS, endoscope, standard, small, fitting, ten only.
BATTERY BOX, for endoscopes, holding D-type dry cells, one only.
PROBE, medium-sized, malleable silver, one only.
DIRECTOR, probe-pointed, one only.
CATHETERS, latex or plastic, Jaques, 380 mm, (a) 8 Ch, ten only. (b) 10 Ch, twenty only. (c) 14 Ch, ten only. (d) 16 Ch ten only. (e) 20 or 24 Ch, ten only. **22.1**
CATHETER, Tiemann, rubber or plastic, olive-tipped, (a) 16 Ch, twenty only. (b) 18 Ch, fifty only. (c) 20 Ch, fifty only.
CATHETER, Gibbon, simple polythene, with removable nylon stylet, (a) 10 Ch, (b) 12 Ch. Five only of each size.
CATHETER, de Pezzer, self retaining, rubber or plastic, 20 Ch, 26 Ch and 32 Ch. Twenty of each size.
CATHETER, Malecot, self-retaining, rubber or plastic. (a) 20 Ch. (b) 26 Ch. (d) 32 Ch. Twenty of each size.
CATHETERS, Foley, balloon, latex rubber, self-retaining, double channel, 30 ml balloon, (a) 14 Ch, twenty only. (b) 16 Ch, forty only. (c) 18 Ch, forty only. (d) 20 Ch, forty only. (e) 22 Ch, forty only.
CATHETERS, Foley, balloon, silicone rubber, self-retaining, double-channel, 30 ml bag, (a) 14 Ch, five only. (b) 22 Ch, five only.
CATHETER, plastic, Foley balloon, 3-way for continuous irrigation, 75 ml balloon, straight tip, 22 Ch, twenty only.
INTRODUCER, catheter, two only.
SPIGOTS, plastic, for catheters, (a) small, fifty only. (b) large, fifty only.
BOUGIES, neoplex, Porges (POR), filiform, smaller sizes olive-tipped, larger sizes plain, sizes 1 to 20 Ch, two only of each size.
SOUNDS, metal, large, blunt, straight, plain end, Powell's, sizes 12 to 20 Ch, one only of each size.
SOUNDS, urethral, metal, Otis–Clutton, curved with olive ends, 9/14 Ch, 11/15 Ch, 12/17 Ch, 14/18 Ch, 15/20 Ch, 17/21 Ch, and 18/23 Ch, one only of each size.
TROCAR and cannula, gall-bladder, Ochsner, with metal piston and side branch, medium size, one only.
SYRINGE, bladder, washout 50 ml, plastic, boilable, two only.
RETRACTOR, Thomson–Walker, with two pairs of detachable abdominal wall blades, and long blade for posterior wall, one only.
URINE BAGS, simple pattern, with drainage outlet at the bottom, plastic reusable, five hundred only.
CLAMP, penile without ratchet, twenty only.
BIOPSY NEEDLE, Travenol 'Tru-cut', Code No 2N2704 (TRAV), one only. Optional.
CYSTOSCOPE, simple pattern, Ringleb type, for examination only, 19 Ch, with single irrigating sheath, Albarran lever, and 'Autoface' pattern bulb, boilable, with battery box and rheostat, and 25 spare bulbs, one outfit only. Optional. **22.3**
SYRINGE, bladder, Barrington's metal, one only.
CAN, douche, metal, 3 litre, with rubber tubing, one only.
CHARTS, visual acuity, (a) Snellen and (b) illiterate E charts, both for use at 6 metres; one chart only of each. **24.1**
TEST TYPE, reading pattern, one set only. Optional.
TORCH, for focal illumination, local pattern, preferably pencil type, with 'lens bulb', one only.
LOUPE (magnifying spectacles), binocular, surgical, Bishop Harman headband type, $\times 2 - \times 8$, one only.
TONOMETER, Schiötz, one only.
OPHTHALMOSCOPE, simple pattern, Keeler type, battery handle, one only.
SLIT LAMP MICROSCOPE, on stand, simple pattern, as Inami 911SX or equivalent, one only. Optional.
NEEDLES, retrobulbar, 7 cm, blunt tip, very fine, one box only.
SPECULUM, ophthalmic, lid, solid blades, hinged with screw adjustment, one only.
SCISSORS, ophthalmic, lid, blunt points, one only.
FORCEPS (clamp), tarsal cyst (chalazion), 8 mm ring, Lambert pattern, one only.
CURETTE, chalazion (tarsal cyst), one only.
CAUTERY, simple type, ball pattern, two only.
CLAMP, eyelid, entropion, Desmarres or Snellen's, (a) medium and (b) large, one only of each.
SCISSORS, ophthalmic, spring pattern, Westcott or Castroviejo's, two only.
FORCEPS, fine, toothed, St Martin's, two only.
RETRACTOR, eye, Desmarres, one only.
NEEDLE-HOLDER, ophthalmic, curved with lock, Castroviejo pattern, (a) light, (b) heavy, one only of each type.
TRIAL LENSES, basic set with trial frame, spherical lenses only, cylindrical lenses not required, one outfit only.
GLASSES, simple frames, second hand if necessary, spherical lenses +1 to +3.50, the most commonly needed glasses are +2 and +2.50, several hundred assorted.
EYE DRUGS. Enriched tetracycline (or chloramphenicol) eye ointment 1%, five hundred tubes. Gentamicin injection 40 mg/ml, 1 ml ampoules, five hundred ampoules. Cyclopentolate 1%, one hundred vials. Atropine ointment 1%, 3 g tubes, fifty tubes. Pilocarpine eye drops 4%, one hundred vials. Lignocaine hydrochloride 4%, or amethocaine hydrochloride 0.5%, one hundred vials. Vitamin A capsules 200,000 iu, ten thousand capsules (in Vitamin A deficient areas only). Fluorescein papers, twenty packets.
HEADLIGHT, with forehead band and cords, 6 volt 3 watt bulb, and pin terminals to use with battery, one only. Also, 25 spare bulbs. **24.1, 24.12, 24.14**
HEAD MIRROR, with webbing or fibre head band, one only.
EXAMINATION LAMP, Chiron, on base with castors, with Bedford Russell extending arm, one only (optional).
OTOSCOPE, Keeler, new standard halogen type, with rechargeable handle, with:

(a) 5 nylon specula, (b) mini-charger, state voltage (normally 240 volts), (c) adaptor for disposable specula, (d) box of disposable (but reusable) 3 mm specula, one outfit only.
TUNING FORK, Hartmann's with foot, 512 Hz, one only.
PROBE, Jobson Horne, 178 mm, with one serrated and one ring end, one only.
HOOK, wax, St. Bartholomew's pattern, one only.
HOOK, Quire's, one only.
SYRINGE, aural, Bacon's, for one hand use, one only.
FORCEPS, aural, alligator, Hartmann's, one pair only.
FORCEPS, aural, Wilde, one only.
FORCEPS, aural, Omerod, elongated cup, crocodile-action jaws, one only.
FORCEPS, nasal, dressing, Tilley, one only.
SPECULUM, nasal Thudichum, Mark Hovell modification, size 7, five only.
SUCTION TUBE, Lempert, one only.
TROCAR, antral, stainless steel with metal handle, Luer fitting, size 7, Tilley Lichwitz, one only. Also, rubber syringe with male mount for use with the antral trochar, one only.
MIRROR, laryngeal, with metal stem, boilable, 24 mm, one only.
MIRROR, rhinoscopic, with metal stem, St Clair Thompson boilable, 14 mm, one only.
LAMP, spirit, one only.
SNARE, polypectomy, nasal, Glegg's, (a) one snare only. (b) Spare wires for the snare, five only.
FORCEPS, nasal turbinate, Luc's, one only.
TONGUE DEPRESSOR, Lack, adult, one only.
OESOPHAGOSCOPE, (a) infant, (b) child, (c) adult, with forceps and suckers that are long enough to go through them, one only of each. Optional.
BOUGIES, oesophageal, neoprene, standard set, alternate sizes only, one set only. Optional.
BRONCHOSCOPE, rigid, Negus, conventional lighting, distal illumination, complete with cords Wappler fitting, battery box, two lamp carriers and 2.5 v lamps with 10 BA thread, (a) infant lumen 5.4×4.1 mm, (b) child 7×5.7 mm, (c) adolescent small 8×6.7 mm, one only of each size. Optional. ALSO, 25 spare bulbs. Optional.
FORCEPS, for bronchoscope, (a) Chevalier Jackson, 2/2 teeth on 50 cm shaft, one only. (b) Haslinger tubular shaft, or sliding shaft type for small bronchoscopes, one only of each. Both optional.
EAR DRUGS AND DRESSINGS. 5 mm selvage ribbon gauze, 50 metres only. Magnesium Sulphate Paste BPC, 1 kg only. Tabs prochlorperazine ('Stemetil') 5 mg, two thousand tablets. Prochlorperazine ampoules 12.5 mg in 2 ml, 500 ampoules. Cinnarizine ('Sturgeron') 15 mg tablets, one thousand tablets. Silver nitrate applicator stick, packet of 50 applicators, (AVO), one packet only. Ephedrine nasal drops BPC (ephedrine hydrochloride 1%) 10 ml, one hundred vials only. Beclomethasone dipropionate in metered 50 μg dose aerosol; 200-dose applicator, ten applicators only.
CHAIR, operating dental, one only.**25.2, 25.3**
DENTAL MIRROR, serrated handle, with No. 4 size plane head, one only.
DENTAL PROBE, single-ended, as Ash No. 14, one only.
DENTAL DRESSING TWEEZERS, Guttman, as Ash No. 13, one only.
'PLASTIC INSTRUMENT', as Ash No. 6, one only.
SPATULA, metal, for mixing filling material, one only.
SCALER, dental, Cumine, as Ash No. 152, one only.
FORCEPS, dental, set of six with the following Ash numbers: (a) Upper anteriors (Nos. 1 or 2). (b) Upper right molars (Nos. 17 or 94). (c) Upper left molars (Nos. 18 or 95). (d) Upper premolars and roots (No.7). (e) Lower molars (Nos. 73 or 22). (f) Lower anteriors and roots (No. 74N). One only of each.
Alternatively, FORCEPS, dental, universal, set of two, upper universal (No. 36), and lower universal (No.74), one only of each.
ELEVATORS, dental, (a) upper jaw, straight inclined plane, Coupland, (b) and (c) set of two lower jaw Cryer's, mesial and distal. One only of each.
PROP, dental, one only.
DENTAL MATERIALS. Clove oil for dental use, 100 ml only. Zinc oxide powder, 1 kg only.
MICROCELLULAR RUBBER, 5 m$^2 \times$ 10 mm only. **30.5**
FOAMED POLYETHYLENE, 1 cm thick, as 'Plastazote' (S&N), 5 m^2 only.
FOOTPRINT MAT, (DOW), one only. Optional.
ONCOLYTIC DRUGS 'Basic drugs': Vincristine injection, 2 mg vials, one hundred vials. Cyclophosphamide, vials of 100 mg, 200 mg and 500, and 1 g, twenty-five vials of each size only; tablets of 10 and 50 mg, five hundred tablets of each size only. Methotrexate, tablets 2.5 mg, five hundred tablets only; powder for reconstitution, ampoules of 50 and 500 mg, fifty ampoules of each only. Actinomycin D, 0.5 mg vials, fifty vials only. **32.2, 32.24**

'Other drugs': Nitrogen mustard, 10 mg vials, one hundred vials only. Doxorubicin, 10 and 50 mg vials, fifty vials of each. Melphalan, tablets 2 mg, one hundred tablets only; ampoules 100 mg, twenty-five ampoules only. 5 fluorouracil, 250 mg ampoules, twenty-five ampoules only. Etoposide, 100 mg vials, twenty vials only. Procarbazine, 50 mg capsules, fifty capsules only. All optional.

Also mesna, ampoules 400 mg, 50 ampoules. Folinic acid 15 mg, twenty-five tablets. Tamoxifen 20 mg, one hundred tablets. All optional.
TUBES, oesophageal, Celestin, with guide, 20 assorted tubes only.
Alternatively, TUBES, Procter – Livingstone (POR) length 110, 150 and 190 mm, assorted, unflanged, twenty tubes only.**32.24**
NEEDLE, liver biopsy, Menghini, 1.6 mm, normal Menghini point with adjustable stop, one only.**32.26**
NEEDLE, liver biopsy, Vim-Silverman, adult size, 2.3 mm $\times$ 88.5 mm, with Franklin modification, one only.
STRIPPER, varicose vein, Nabatoff in sterilizer case, complete with 3 metal olives, cable and handle, one only. Optional.**34.1**
TROLLEY, resuscitation, tiltable at the head and foot, with a radio-translucent surface, a device to hold cassettes underneath, holders for an oxygen cylinder and

605

a drip attachment, also a wire basket for the patient's clothes and his property. **51.3**
DILATOR, tracheal, extra small for children, one only. **52.2**
TUBE, tracheostomy, plain, uncuffed, reusable, with 15 mm termination, 15 Ch one, 18 Ch one, 21 Ch two, 24 Ch two, 27 Ch three, 30 Ch one, 36 Ch one, 42 Ch one, one carton of assorted tubes only.
TUBE, tracheostomy, standard, cuffed, reusable complete with obturator and one-way valve, Ch two, 27 Ch two, 30 Ch two, 36 Ch two, 39 Ch one, 42 Ch one, one carton of 10 assorted tubes only.
RETRACTOR, tracheotomy, single, sharp hook, blunt, one only
RETRACTOR, tracheotomy, double hook, blunt, one only.
CLAMP, bulldog for arteries, Blalock cross action, two only. **55.6**
SAW, amputation, with hinged back, 230 mm, (a) saw, one only, (b) spare blades for the above, three only. **56.1**
SAW, Gigli, (a) pair of handles, one pair only. (b) Saw blades, 30 cm, 4 only.
KNIFE, amputation, Liston 180 mm, one only.
KNIFE, skin graft, Humby, mode pair only. (b) Saw blades, 30 cm, 4 only.
KNIFE, amputation, Liston 180 mm, one only.
KNIFE, skin graft, Humby, modified by Blair and Watson, (a) knife only. (b) Set of 50 spare blades, five sets only. **57.1**
Alternatively, SKIN GRAFT KNIFE MINIATURE, as developed by H. L. Silver of Toronto, to use ordinary safety razor blades.
RAZOR, for skin grafting, Gillette, local manufacture, one only.
HOOKS, skin, single point, Gilles, stainless steel, 200 mm, six only.
SKIN GRAFT BOARD, teak, with bevelled edge, 6×100×200 mm, two only.
ARCH BAR, stainless steel, five only. **62.1**
BRACE, Hudson's, standard, 254 mm, one only. **63.1**
PERFORATOR, Hudson's, with standard Hudson fittings, 12 mm, one only.
BURRS, spherical, Hudson pattern, 11 mm, 13 mm, 16 mm, 19 mm, one only of each size.
RONGEUR (bone nibbler), Cairns, with fine angled on flat jaws and curved handles, 152 mm, one only.
RONGEUR, Sargent, or van Havre, double action, curved or flat, 229 mm, one only.
ELEVATOR, skull, Penfield, double-ended, one only.
TUBE, suction, fine, 4 mm diam, one only.
HOOK, dural, Cairns, sharp, 130 mm each, one only.
TRACTION TONGS, Gardner Wells, one only. **64.1**
COLLAR orthopaedic, Zimmer pattern, two only of each of the three standards sizes. **64.6**
NEEDLES, hypodermic, large for chest aspiration, 1.6×100 mm, 'Luer-lok' mount each, five only. **65.2**
STOPCOCK, for chest aspiration, 'Luer-lok' male to 'Luer-lok' female, with side are for tubing, two only.
SYRINGES, 5 ml and 20 ml, both 'Luer-lok'.
BOTTLE, Tudor-Edwards, 3 litres, chest drainage, including rubber bung and tubes, one only.
CONNECTOR, for Tudor-Edwards chest drain, five only.
Alternatively, CHEST DRAIN SET, plastic, disposable, sterile, in packet complete, five only.
PLASTER BANDAGES, normal, slow-setting, best quality, 10 cm, 15 cm, and 20 cm wide. **70.1**
CREPE BANDAGES, assorted sizes 100 only of each size.
STOCKINETTE, woven tubular, orthopaedic, various widths.
PADDING, cotton wool, orthopaedic, six rolls only.
STIRRUPS, locally made.
PLASTER SHEARS, Lorenz, 380 mm, nickel plated, one only.
PLASTER SHEARS, Guy, with shaped bows and flattened probe end, 250 mm, nickel-plated, one only.
PLASTER KNIFE, Esmarch, solid forged, two only.
PLASTER SAW, Bergmans, hand, one only.
PLASTER CAST SAW, electric, oscillating, with four extra blades 44 mm, and 64 mm, state voltage, one outfit only.
PLASTER CAST SPREADER, one only.
PLASTER CAST BENDING FORCEPS, Böhler, one only.
PENCILS, INDELIBLE, for writing on a cast, six only.
STRAPPING, traction, adhesive, 50 mm×10 mm, six rolls only. **70.9**
NAIL, Denham, (Denham threaded Steinmann pin), stainless steel, 4 mm, tapered, self-tapping, with long coarse screw thread, triangular shank, packet of 5, two packs only.
PIN, Steinmann, triangular shank, stainless steel, trocar pointed at one end, (a) 2×180 mm, (b) 3×180 mm. (c) 4×180 mm, six only of each size.
HANDLE, with Jacobs chuck, 4 mm capacity, and key attached by chain, fully cannulated, stainless steel, one only.
STIRRUPS, Böhler, for Steinmann pins, with rotating swivel fixation pieces, (a) 102×89 mm, three only. (b) 165×144 mm, three only. (c) 241×152 mm, five only.
PIN MOUNTS, Thomas, stainless steel with rotating collar for Perkins traction, four pairs only.
STIRRUPS, for wire traction, adjustable, tensioning, Gissane, 216 mm, with two cord hooks, two only.
WIRE, Kirschner, plain unthreaded, stainless steel, drill-pointed at one end, packet of 5. (a) 0.75×254 mm, four packets only. (b) 1 mm×254 mm, four packets only. (c) 1.5 mm×254 mm, four packets only.
INTRODUCER, for Kirschner wire, Pulvertaft's, one only.
CUTTER, for Kirschner wire, one only.
HAND DRILL, for Kirschner wires and drills, 4 mm capacity cannulated throughout, one only.
DRILL BITS, twist, bone, 4 mm, six only.
FORCEPS, wire-cutting, compound lever action with pliers jaws, 170 mm, one only.

CORD, braided, for traction, twenty-five yards only, local purchase.
PULLEYS, orthopaedic assorted, ten only
BARS, for overhead traction, six outfits only.
FINGER SPLINTS, aluminium, padded, 50 lengths only. **75.1**

Appendix B Lists of suppliers

These are the suppliers of surgical equipment whose catalogues have been quoted from. They are given as examples only, and their products may not be either the best, or the cheapest. See also 'Primary Anaesthesia', Appendix B.

(AES) Aesculap instruments. The Jetter and Scheerer Corp, Tuttlingen, West Germany.

(AOC) Americal Optical Corp., 41 Mechanic Street, Southbridge, MA 01550 USA (haemoglobinometer).

(ANT) Antec International Ltd. Chilton Industrial Estate, Sudbury, Suffolk CO10 6XD, UK. ('Virkon', virucidal agent)

(AVO) Avoca Pharmaceutical Products Ltd, Old Saw Mills Road, Farringdon, Oxon SN7 7DS, UK. (silver nitrate applicators)

(CHI) Chiltern Surgical Products, Beaconsfield, Bucks. UK.

(CYP) Cyprane, New Devonshire House, Scott Street, Keighley, Yorkshire, BD21 2NN, UK. (anaesthetic equipment)

(deV) DeVilbiss Co Ltd, Somerset, Pensylvania 15501, USA.

(ECO) ECHO, Ullswater Crescent, Coulsden, Surrey CR3 2HR, UK. (suppliers to voluntary agencies)

(ESC) Eschman Bros., 24 Church Street, Shoreham by Sea, Sussex, UK.

(ETH) Ethicon Ltd., Box 408, Barkhead Avenue, Edinburgh, EH11 4HE, UK. (sutures)

(FRA) J.G. Franklin Sons Ltd., Lane End Road, High Wycombe, Bucks, UK.

(GEN) Genito-urinary Co. Ltd., 28A Devonshire Street, London WIN 2AJ, UK.

(HOL) Holborn Surgical Instrument Co., Dolphin Works, Margate Road, Broadstairs CT10 2QQ, UK.

(JHP) The Johns Hopkins Program of International Education in Gynaecology and Obstetrics. The Department of Obstetrics and Gynaecology, Johns Hopkins Hospital, Baltimore, Maryland. (laparoscopes, 15.4)

(MER) E Merck. Four Marks, Alton, Hampshire, GU32 5HG, UK. (gentamicin-impregnated polymethylmethacrylate beads, 7.6).

(MIE) Medical and Industrial Equipment Ltd., 26-40 Broadwick Street, London WIA 2AD, UK.

(NES) J Nesbitt-Evans & Co Ltd, Bedstead Manufacturers, Holyhead Road, Wednesbury, West Midlands (operating tables)

(PEA) James Pearsall & Co. Ltd, The Silk Mills, Tancred Street, Taunton, Somerset TA1 1RY. (monofilament sutures in reels)

(PFA) Pfau-Wanfried, Box 110 D-3508 Melsungen, West Germany.

(POG) Porges Paris, 25 Quai Anatole France, 75007 Paris, France. (catheters).

(SAL) Salt and Son Ltd., 220 Corporation Street, Birmingham, UK. (needles).

(SCH) Schuler and Co, 250 West 18th Street, New York 11, USA.

(S&N) Smith and Nephew Ltd., Bessemer Road, Welwyn Garden City, Herts, UK. (dressings, plaster bandages, multicellular rubber, drugs)

(SEW) Seward Surgical, UAC House, Blackfriars Road, London SE1 9UG, UK.

(SHO) AW Showell, Britten Street, Redditch, Worcestershire B97 6HF. (needles)

(SHR) Shrimpton and Fletcher, Box 3, Redditch, Worcestershire B98 7AB, UK.

(SPE) Spencer and Sons, Arthur Street, Redditch, Worcestershire B98 8JY, UK. (needles)

(STO) Karl Storz and Co., Postfach 400-D-7200, Tuttlingen, West Germany.

(SUR) Surgical Medical Laboratory Ltd., Euro House, High Road, Whetstone, London N20 9LS, UK.

(TAL) Teaching Aids at Low Cost, Box 49 St Albans, Herts, AL1 4AX, UK. (teaching materials)

(THA) Thackray Ltd., Box 171, Park Street, Leeds LS1 1RQ, UK. (surgical equipment)

(TRA) Travenol Inc, Deerfield, Illinois, USA (biopsy needles).

(WAR) Warne Surgical Products Ltd., Walworth Road, Andover, Hampshire, UK.

(WHI) Jacob White, Riverside Industrial Estate, Riverside Way, Dartford, DAI 5bx, UK. (autoclaves)

(WIS) Wisconsin Aluminium Foundry Co. Inc., Box 246, 838 South 16th Street, Manitowoc, Wisconsin 54220, USA. (autoclaves)

Stop press!

Mass ligation of the uterine arteries

Tying the uterine artery and including some of the myometrium (mass ligation) is said to be at least 80% successful in stopping postpartum haemorrhage see Section 9.11a. It is much easier than hysterectomy, and is quicker, easier and safer than tying the internal iliac arteries, which needs more dissection, and has more complications. It is also probably better than packing the uterus. The exact place of this method, which comes to us as the result of a WHO consultation, is still not clear. It was not part of the practice of any of our obstetric contributors (they intend to try it), and it seems to have been unduly neglected in the past. The decision to do a laparotomy and tie the uterine arteries is difficult, but not as difficult as deciding to remove the uterus. You will probably be wise to tie them whenever an atonic uterus bleeds, in spite of intravenous oxytocics and massage. *Don't delay unduly, and don't wait for massive bleeding and shock; the first bleed is rarely fatal, it is repeated bleeding that kills.*

ANATOMY. The uterine artery arises from the anterior division of the internal iliac artery and passes over the ureter 2 or 3 cm lateral to the uterus. It gives off an inferior or cervical branch which anastomoses with the vaginal artery. It then turns towards the fundus, runs up the side of the uterus and finally anastomoses with the terminal branch of the ovarian artery in the free edge of the broad ligament. The uterine artery hypertrophies remarkably during pregnancy, whereas the ovarian artery does not, and provides more than 90% of the blood supply of a pregnant uterus.

Fahemy K, 'Uterine artery ligation to control postpartum haemorrhage', International Journal of Gynaecology and Obstetrics 1987;25:363

MASS LIGATION OF THE UTERINE ARTERIES

INDICATIONS. (1) Curatively, in otherwise uncontrollable postpartum haemorrhage from an empty atonic uterus. Only tie the uterine arteries after oxytocics have failed, and after you have explored the patient's uterus to make sure that she has no retained fragments of placenta, and no laceration that should be sutured. (2) Preventively, when you expect severe uterine bleeding, as when doing a Caesarean section for severe concealed or mixed accidental haemorrhage.

METHOD. If her abdomen is not already open, make a lower midline incision. There is no need to incise her vesicouterine peritoneum as for a Caesarean section, although some surgeons do; nor is there any need to mobilize her bladder, although again some surgeons do.

Stand on her left and raise her uterus upwards and to her left. Take a *big* curved Mayo's needle with No. 1 chromic catgut and pass it through her myometrium from anterior to posterior- -3 cm medial to her right uterine vessels, as in the figure. Then pass the needle from posterior to anterior through the avascular area in her broad ligament lateral to her uterine vessels. Tie her uterine artery tightly, distal to its cervical branch. If you tie it loosely, you will merely compress her uterine veins and cause more bleeding. You are not going to divide it, so one tie is enough. Then do the same thing on her left. There is no need to palpate the vessels.

CAUTION ! (1) The needle must be big; a small one may end up in her broad ligament and cause a haematoma. (2) When you go from front to back, go through her myometrium. Provided you do this, at whatever level, you cannot injure her ureter. (3) When you come back, go through the bare area of her broad ligament. By doing so: (a) You will again avoid her ureter, and (b) you will avoid the tie going below her uterine artery and so missing it. (4) You can place the tie at various levels. If she is bleeding from the site of a placenta praevia, go from front to back as low as you can (provided you go through myometrium). If she is bleeding from her fundus, you can place the tie higher. (5) Use absorbable suture material. (6) Be sure to include a substantial amount of myometrium in the suture, so as to avoid her ureter and to occlude some of the inferior branches of her uterine artery. (7) Don't use a figure of eight suture.

If you tie her arteries during Caesarean section, place the sutures below the level of the uterine incision under the reflected peritoneal flap.

LIGATURES FOR UTERINE BLEEDING

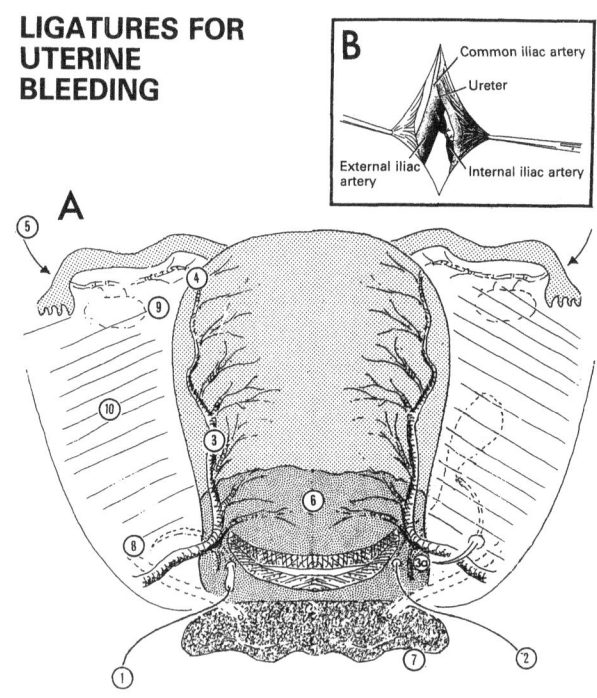

LIGATURES FOR UTERINE BLEEDING. A, tying the uterine artery after Caesarean section. This is more often done for other indications; it can be done higher up and you need not reflect the patient's bladder. B, tying the internal iliac artery (see also Fig. 3-7).

1, passing the needle into the patient's uterus so as to take a substantial bite of uterine muscle and emerge behind her uterus and broad ligament. 2, the second stage of the procedure shown on the other side. The suture has come out of the back of her uterus and the point of the needle is coming back through the bare area in her broad ligament.

3, her uterine artery. 3a, one of the inferior cervical branches of her uterine artery. 4, the anastomosis between her uterine and ovarian arteries. 5, her ovarian artery coming down in her infundibulopelvic ligament. 6, her bladder has been reflected off this part of the uterus. 7, her bladder. 8, her ureter. 9, her ovary. B, *from Chalmers, I et al., 'Effective Care in Pregnancy and Childbirth'. OUP.*

Her uterus will go pale, show fibrillary contractions, and will usually contract, or at least become firmer. Bleeding will probably stop, even if it remains flabby. Even a couvelaire uterus (showing the haemorrhages of abruption into the uterine wall) will usually stop bleeding.

Compress her ligated uterus with a warm pack to expel any collected blood. Cover it with warm packs and a sterile towel. Flex her thighs, put her knees together, mop out her vagina, and observe her for 10 minutes to see if she continues to bleed. If she has stopped bleeding, close her abdomen.

If she continues to bleed (unusual), she probably has a clotting defect (the method often succeeds even if she does have one), or the implantation of a placenta praevia into the scar of a previous Caesarean section (particularly hazardous). Consider: (1) Inserting second sutures, your first ones may have slipped, or not been tight enough. (2) Inserting figure of eight sutures into the bleeding placental site, if you have her uterus open. (3) Tying one or both of her ovarian arteries below the proximal end of her Fallopian tubes, near the cornua (if you tie her infundibulopelvic ligaments which contain her ovarian arteries, which is the other alternative, you may harm her ovaries). (4) Tying her internal iliac arteries (see below), especially if she is bleeding from the placental site in total placenta praevia. This site receives some of its blood from her cervical and vaginal arteries which are not occluded when her uterine arteries are tied. Tying her internal iliac arteries may be the only way to control bleeding from these vessels. (5) Hysterectomy (preferably subtotal if you are inexperienced).

If bleeding is still not controlled, or there is a rapidly enlarging broad ligament haematoma, deliver her uterus out of the incision, pack her gut out of her pelvis, and find her ureter as it passes forwards and medially at the bifurcation of her common iliac artery (see the figure). Divide her peritoneum lateral to, parallel to, and well clear of her ureter, along the line of her internal iliac artery. Retract her ureter medially and use a blunt aneurysm needle to pass a ligature of No. 1 silk round the artery, taking care not to damage her internal iliac vein. Place a second tie 1.5 cm distal to the first. Evacuate the haematoma (if she has one) and insert a vacuum drain. This is an alternative description to that in Section 3.5.

The collateral supply to her uterus will be sufficient, and her uterine artery will eventually recanalise. She will menstruate in 45 to 60 days. Her fertility and future pregnancies will not be affected.

Joel Cohen's method of opening the abdomen for Caesarean section

This is said to be quicker and cause less bleeding than the standard midline incision, and to have a low incidence of burst abdomens and ventral hernias. When you have mastered the standard method in Section 18.9, consider modifying it in the following way. The incision is transverse and is higher than that of Pfannensteil (23-20).

Cohen SJ, (1972) Abdominal and Vaginal Hysterectomy', Oxford: Allen and Mowbray.

JOEL COHEN'S ABDOMINAL INCISION FOR CAESAREAN SECTION

Make a straight (not curved) transverse incision from points 2.5 cm below and medial to the patient's anterior superior iliac spines, through her skin only and avoid cutting much of her fat. Make a F*small (5 cm)* midline transverse incision through her fat and cut the fascial aponeurosis of her external oblique muscle for about 2.5 cm. Separate her subcutaneous fat from her rectus sheath along the line of the incision by pushing a pair of closed curved scissors into her subcutaneous tissues and withdrawing them open.

Extend the small rectus incision transversely with scissors and open the space between her rectus muscles. Put your fingers between them and pull, at first longitudinally, and then transversely to separate them. Open her peritoneum as usual, but do it transversely, high and to one side of the midline (to avoid her bladder). Then open her peritoneum by pulling longitudinally between your fingers to produce a transverse tear. Stretch the wound between your fingers

Then proceed as usual. When you come to close her uterus lay the peritoneum covering it in place, without suturing. Some surgeons are said not to suture the parietal peritoneum either, most do.

Place the tips of three haemostats on each edge of her external oblique aponeurosis, the first pair in the centre and the other two on either side. While your assistant holds these haemostats together in pairs, start a continuous suture at your end, controlling the tension carefully as you do so. There is no need to close her fat or superficial fascia. Close her skin with interrupted monofilament.

If she has had a previous Cohen incision(s), cut through it but don't excise it. If lateral separation of her recti is difficult, dissect the adhesions. Enter her peritoneum transversely as high as possible.

Measuring the tissue pressure to diagnose the compartment syndrome

Diagnosing the compartment syndrome (54.1, 55.3, 70.4) can be difficult, especially if the patient is comatose. The classical signs (the four 'Ps' R pain, paraesthesiae, pallor, and paralysis) are often uncertain, and if you wait for his pulses to be lost (often they are not lost), you will be too late to prevent Volkmann's ischaemic contracture. The one factor that must be present for the syndrome to develop is increased tissue pressure, so measure this when you are deciding if a fasciotomy is necessary. As always, don't rely only on measurement, but consider the pressure readings with the signs.

Measurement could hardly be easier: push a needle into the compartment and use a sphygmomanometer to find the pressure which will just overcome his tissue pressure, and just drive fluid into his tissues, as shown by the movement of saline in a plastic tube attached to the needle. The normal tissue pressure is about 5 mmHg. Perfusion decreases as it rises, until there is no perfusion at all when it has risen to equal his diastolic blood pressure. The critical tissue pressure at which the compartment syndrome develops is 40–50 mmHg; it varies with his blood pressure and is lower if he is hypotensive.

Whitesides TE, et al., Tissue pressure measurements as a determinant for the need of fasciotomy. Clinical Orthopaedics. 1975;113:33-51.

MEASURING THE TISSUE PRESSURE

EQUIPMENT. Two plastic extension tubes, two 1.2 mm needles, a 20 ml syringe, a 3-way stopcock, a bottle of sterile saline and a sphygmomanometer. Have this equipment ready sterile in a 'Tissue pressure pack'.

METHOD. Clean and prepare the compartment to be evaluated. Break the vacuum in a bottle of sterile saline with a sterile needle. Assemble a 20 ml syringe, with the plunger at the 15 ml mark, a 3-way stopcock, a plastic extension tube and a 1.2 mm needle, as shown.

Push the tip of the needle into the saline and fill the tube half full of saline without bubbles. Turn the stopcock to close this tube so that the saline is not lost on transfer.

Push the needle into the tissues of comparment. Use a second extension tube to connect a sphygmomanometer to the other port of the stopcock. Turn the tap so as to connect both extension tubes with the syringe and form a closed system.

Increase the pressure by *slowly* depressing the plunger, while you watch the column of saline. The mercury in the manometer will rise. When the pressure in the system just exceeds the tissue pressure surrounding the needle, a little saline will be injected into the tissue and the saline column will start to move. When it just starts to move, stop pressing and read the manometer to give you the tissue pressure.

Measure his tissue pressure hourly or 2-hourly in all the compartments that may be involved until it starts to decrease, or it is clear that he needs a fasciotomy. If necessary, insert the needle through a small wheal of lignocaine (A 5.4). If it reaches 20-30 mmHg, monitor him with particular care.

MEASURING TISSUE PRESSURE

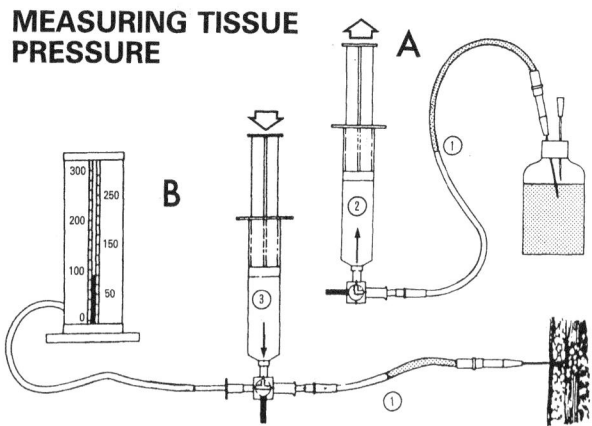

MEASURING THE TISSUE PRESSURE. a, filling the manometer. b, the manometer connected. 1, the saline meniscus. 2, filling the syringe. 3, increase the pressure slowly.

The usual indication for fasciotomy is a tissue pressure rising to within 10-30 mm of his diastolic blood pressure when he has any of the signs or symptoms of the compartment syndrome (the four 'Ps', 72.8, 73.7). For example, if his diastolic blood pressure is 70 mmHg, he needs a fasciotomy by the time his tissue presure reaches 40-45 mmHg. If he is hypotensive, he may need it at a lower pressure. If his tissue pressure approaches or equals his diastolic pressure, fasciotomy is urgent. If his tissue pressure is low and his pulses are absent, he probably has an arterial obstruction.

CAUTION ! (1) The pulses are often palpable in the compartment syndrome. (2) Interpret his tissue pressure with due regard for his diastolic blood pressure. (3) Be vigilant, the comartment syndrome can develop in a few hours.

Other fragments

Here is some more information which appeared late in the course of production. Those items which relate to 'Volume One' are indexed, but not those relating to 'Volume Two', or to *'Primary Anaesthesia',* so take a pencil and write "See Stop Press" in the relevant places.

OTHER FRAGMENTS

For Section 16.4. Extra-amniotic prostaglandins. A new prostaglandin gemeprost ('Cervagem' M&B) is very effective for the evacuation of a dead baby and is easy to use. Insert a 1 mg pessary vaginally 3-hourly until abortion occurs, up to a maximum of 5 pessaries. If there is no abortion wait 12 hours and repeat.

For Section 18.4. Obstetric paralysis following obstructed labour. Examine the patient early in the puerperium for signs of peripheral nerve injury. She may fail to complain about sensory changes and weakness in her legs, so you will have to look for them. If you find them she has an obstetric paralysis, which may vary from mild foot-drop to extensive paralysis of her legs, including her gluteal and quadriceps muscles. If you are not careful, she may develop contractures. So put her legs through their full range of passive movements regularly, and encourage her relatives to do the same. If she has foot- drop, give her a posterior plaster splint to keep her ankle at 90 degrees at night. She is almost certain to recover, but this may take 2 years.

For Section 18.4. Anuria following obstructed labour. If a patient has had an obstructed labour, put her on an accurate fluid balance chart and watch for renal failure. This is serious, but potentially curable, so watch for it. Early treatment will improve her prognosis. If she has had large amounts of fluids, and is out of shock, and yet passes < 400 ml of fluid in 24 hours, she is in renal failure. If so, try intravenous frusemide 0.25-1 g slowly at a rate not exceeding 4 mg/minute. If this fails try dopamine 1 µg/kg/minute. If this too fails balance her fluid intake against her fluid loss as in Section 53.3.

For Section 18.4a, 19.3. Oxytocin drip. If a patient is having an oxytocin drip and there is fetal distress, stop it. Turn her onto her left side, do a vaginal examination to exclude prolapse of the cord, make sure she is adequately hydrated and give her oxygen.

For Section 18.18. Vesicovaginal fistulae. Expect that a fistula is going to form: (1) When labour is long enough to kill the baby. (2) After craniotomy. (3) When there is gross intrauterine infection (IUI). If so, insert an indwelling silastic catheter and start continuous closed drainage. Ensure a high fluid intake so as to reduce the risk of infection. Mobilize her early (despite the bag), making sure she keeps it below her bladder.

After 7-10 days put her into the Sims' posititon and examine her anterior vaginal wall with a Sims' speculum. If her bladder is still bruised or necrotic, leave the catheter in and only remove it when later examinations show it is healthy. If you use a latex catheter, change it every 7 days. Continue catheter drainage for 3 weeks, unless the fistula is so big that the balloon falls into her vagina. If her fistula is very small, drain her bladder for 6 weeks. If you can keep her bladder empty, it may close spontaneously.

If she develops a fistula, her vulva will be exposed to urine. Wash it and her perianal area twice daily with soap and water. Twice daily zinc and castor oil ointment will keep these healthy and reduce smell.

If a large area of sloughing tissue causes a persistent foul discharge, debride the dead tissue under general anaesthesia. If her pubic bone is exposed, it will be infected (osteitis), so give her a broad spectrum antibiotic and rectal metronidazole 1 g twice daily. Douche her with weak chlorhexidine.

For Section 19.5. Identifying liquor in premature rupture of the membranes. Ask her to lie down for an hour. Then sit her up on a bed-pan with a kidney dish in it to collect the liquor. Transfer this to a clean glass tube and save it. Teach your midwives this. You or anyone else who reviews her later can then decide if she really is leaking liquor.

For Section 19.11b. Postpartum haemorrhage after Caesarean section is not uncommon. The dangers of exploration are greater because of damaging the scar. So try to avoid exploring to see if her uterus really is empty, by always checking to see that it is empty after you have removed the placenta at Caesarean section. If you always do this, you need not explore her if she has a secondary postpartum haemorrhage.

For Section 24.1. A variant of the pin-hole test. A patient often has difficulty aligning his eye, the pin-hole and the test chart. Make several 1 mm pin holes about 5 mm apart in one of the corneal areas of a spectacles-shaped piece of card. Fix a stick to one side and ask him to hold it. If one pin-hole is not aligned, another will be. If looking through a hole improves his vision, that eye probably needs spectacles. After trying one eye, reverse the card and try the other.

For Section 54.5, etc. Wound dressings. 'Eusol' (hypochlorite) and 'Eusol and paraffin', are losing favour as wound dressings, and saline dressings are now preferred for septic ulcers and wounds, *but this must be changed frequently* (at last three times daily). Hypochlorite is however still considered an excellent disinfectant.

For Sections 77.7, and 77.8. Fractures of the neck of the femur. If he has broken the neck of his femur, and you cannot refer him, inject 5 ml of 2% lignocaine into his hip joint by the method in Section 7.1. Soon afterwards encourage him to walk with crutches or a walking frame. Each day encourage him to walk a little bit more, so as to form a pseudarthrosis (false joint). The result will not be perfect, but is likely to be better than traction or inexpert nailing.

For Sections A 6.17, 6.18, etc. Regional blocks. If you are doing a regional block of a major plexus, try using a very fine sharp needle. This is said to be much more effective, perhaps because the needle enters the nerve better.

For Section A 15.1. If you have difficulty maintaining a blood bank, try making the donation of a unit a condition for any minor surgery.

Finally! have you got spare gaskets and seals for your autoclaves and pressure cookers. If not, order spares now!

Once again, as we finally go to press, the very best wishes from all our contributors to you our readers, and to the many patients in your care.

NOTE: Section numbers are indicated by a dot(e.g. 18.1) and figures by a dash (e.g. 18 – 1). D after a section number indicates a difficulty, which is to be found at the end of a particular section.

'vs' denotes differential diagnosis.

Abbreviations used in sub-entries:
AIDS   acquired immunodeficiency syndrome
HIV   Human immunodeficiency virus
HBV   Hepatitis B virus
VVF   Vesico-vaginal fistula

A
AAFB (acid and alcohol fast bacilli) 1.14
AAKS (atypical African Kaposi's sarcoma) 28a.2, 32.21
   pulmonary 32.21D
abbreviations, common 1.14
abdomen
   appearance, in intestinal obstruction 10.5
   baby in, after rupture of uterus 18.3
   burst 9.2, 9.8, 9.13, 9 – 24, 10.5
   carcinoma 9.2D, 9.2
   closing 9.8, 9 – 21
      after intestinal obstruction 10.5
      after sigmoid volvulus surgery 10.10
      delayed primary 9.8, 9.12
      if difficult 10.5
   difficulty in replacing gut into 9.8D
   draining and closing 9.8, 9 – 21
   examination, in acute abdomen 10.1
   exploring for acute appendicitis 12.1
   fluid in, appearances 9.2, 10.5, 11.2, 12.2D
   infection 9.2
   laxity 20.7D
   rebound tenderness 6.2, 10.1, 10.4, 12.1
      testing for 10.1
   straw-coloured fluid in 9.2, 10.5
abdominal abscesses 6.3, 6 – 4
   obstruction after 10.12
   pyomyositis vs 5.11a, 7.1
abdominal belt 14.13
abdominal cavity, fetal implantation in 16 – 3, 16.6
abdominal distension
   abdominal pain and circulatory collapse with 10.4D
   abdominal pain and vomiting with 10.2
   in acute pancreatitis 13.9
   after abdominal surgery, due to ileus 10.13
   after giant ovarian cyst removal 20.7D
   in anorectal malformations 28.6
   in ascitic type of abdominal tuberculosis 29 – 4, 29.5
   causes, in neonates 28.2
   in congenital intestinal obstruction 28.2
   in Hirschsprung's disease 28.6a
   in hydatid disease 31 – 11, 31.13
   in intestinal obstruction 6.5D, 10.1, 10.2, 10.4
   in ovarian cysts 20.7
   peritonitis and 6.2D, 6.2
   in sigmoid volvulus 10.10
   in small gut volvulus 10.9
   vomiting but no pain with 10.4D
abdominal guarding 6.2, 6.7, 10.1
   in appendicitis 12.1
abdominal incisions 9 – 1, 9.2D, 9.2, 9 – 3, 9 – 4
   for acute appendicectomy 12.1
   for bands and adhesions causing obstruction 10.7
   for cholecystectomy 13 – 4, 13.7
   in intestinal obstruction 10.5
   lower midline 9 – 1, 9.2, 18.9
abdominal incisions (continued)
   midline 9.2, 9 – 3
   for minilap, tubal ligation 15.3
   paramedian 9 – 1, 9.2, 9 – 4
      in neonates 28.3
   in skin creases, keloid prevention 34.1a, 34 – 4
   transverse incision, in neonates 28.3
   for tumours 9.2D
   'ultimate' 9 – 1
   see also individual operations
abdominal injury 10.6
abdominal mass 10.1
   abdominal abscess 6.3

abdominal mass (cont.)
   in abdominal pregnancy 16.9D, 16.9
   Ascaris causing 10.4, 10.6
   in baby girl 28.7
   in carcinoma of stomach 32.25
   in glandular type of abdominal tuberculosis 29.5
   in haematocolpos or haematometra 20.13, 20 – 23
   in ileocaecal tuberculosis 10.4, 29.7
   in intestinal obstruction 10.4
   in nephroblastoma 32.6
   ovarian cysts presenting as 20.7
   in ovarian tumours 32.36
   pancreatic pseudocyst 13.10
   in plastic abdominal tuberculosis 29.7
   sausage-shaped, in intussusception 10.4, 10.8, 31.11D
   in tumours of testis 32.34a
   types and diagnosis 10.4
abdominal muscle, bleeding, in laparotomy 9.2
abdominal pain
   in abdominal pregnancy 16.9
   in abdominal tuberculosis 29.7
   in acute abdomen 10.1
   in acute rupture of ectopic pregnancy 16.6
   after 'D and C' 20.3D
   Ascaris causing 10.4, 10.6
   association with vomiting 10.1
   central 10.2
      in appendicitis 12.1
      with shock 10.2
   in chronic ectopic pregnancy 16.7
   colicky 10.1, 10.4, 10.9, 10.13, 12.1, 14.1
   constipation with 10.2
   distension and circulatory collapse with 10.4D
   in haematocolpos or haematometra 20.13, 20 – 23
   in hepatoma 32.26
   in hernia strangulation 14.1
   in intestinal obstruction 10.2, 10.4, 10.6, 10.13
   in intussusception 10.2, 10.8
   localized, with tenderness and rigidity 10.2
   in minilap 15.3D
   in obstruction after abdominal surgery 10.13
   in pancreatic carcinoma 32.26a
   in pelvic inflammatory disease (PID) 6.6
   in perforated peptic ulcer 11.2
   in pigbel disease 31.9
   in sigmoid volvulus 10.10
   sites 10.1, 10 – 1
abdominal pain (continued)
   in small gut volvulus 10.9
   torsion of ovarian cyst 20.7D
   vomiting and distension with 10.1, 10.2
   see also epigastric pain
abdominal pregnancy 16 – 3, 16.6, 16.9
   diagnosis 16.9
   removing 16 – 7, 16.9
abdominal rigidity 10.1
   in appendicitis 12.1
   causes 10.2
   localized pain and tenderness with 10.2
   in perforated peptic ulcer 11.2
abdominal scars 34.1a, 34 – 4
abdominal surgery 9.1 – 14
   anastomoses, see under gut
   burst abdomen 9.13, 9 – 24
   delayed primary closure 9.8, 9.12
   draining and closing abdomen 9.8, 9 – 21
   ileus and/or obstruction after 10.4D, 10.13
   incisions, see abdominal incisions
   infected wounds 9.12

abdominal surgery (cont.)
   non-respiratory postoperative complications 9.10
   postoperative care 9.1, 9.9, 10.13
   postoperative fistulae 9.14, 9 – 25
   preoperative assessment and preparation 9.1
   respiratory postoperative complications 9.11
   rules for 9.1
abdominal swelling 32.3, 32.26
abdominal tenderness 10.2
   in acute abdomen 10.1
   in acute cholecystitis 13.3
   in appendicitis 12.1
   in intestinal obstruction 10.4
   in peritonitis 6.2
   in plastic abdominal tuberculosis 29.7
   in subacute rupture of ectopic pregnancy 16.6
abdominal tube drains 4.10, 4 – 12
abdominal tuberculosis, see tuberculosis, abdominal
abdominal wall 9 – 1
   anterior, hernia of 14.9
   prolapsed uterus sutured to 20.10, 20 – 10
   sinus, in extrauterine pregnancy 16.9D
abdominal wounds, infected, treatment 2.9
abduction, definition 27.2
abortion 16 – 1, 16.2
   bleeding before 28th week of gestation 16.2
   chronic ectopic pregnancy vs 16.7
   complete 16.2, 16.7
   continued bleeding after 16.2D, 16.8
   definition 16.2
   in ectopic pregnancy 16.6
   habitual 16.2
   incomplete 16.1, 16.2, 16.7
      evacuating 16 – 1, 16.2D, 16.2, 20.3
   inevitable 16.2
   mandatory indications 16.2
   missed 16.2, 16.4
   oxytocin in 18.4a
abortion (continued)
   recurrent 16.5
   in second trimester 16.2, 16.5
   septic 6.6, 16.2
   stages 16.2
   terminology 16.2
   therapeutic, in heart disease 17.5
   threatened 16.2, 16.4, 16.7
      management of bleeding 16.2
   uncomplicated inevitable 16.2
abscess 5.2
   after abdominal surgery 9.10
   alveolar 5 – 7, 5.8, 26.7
   anorectal, see anorectal abscess
   appendix, see appendix abscess
   axillary 5 – 9, 5.11
   bleeding from 5.2
   breast, see breast, abscess
   'chronic' 5.2
   cold 29.3D, 29.4
   common sites 5.1, 5 – 1
   corrugated rubber drains 4.10
   dental 5 – 7, 5.8, 5.10
   deroofing method 5.2
   drainage 4.10, 5.1, 5.2, 5 – 2
   exploring by Hilton's method 5.2, 5 – 3
   extradural 5.4a, 7.14
   extraperitoneal 10.2
   failure to heal 5.2D
   formation in peritonitis development 6.2
   general method 5.2
   horseshoe 5.13
   iliac 5.2, 5 – 10, 5.12, 7.1

abscess (cont.)
　incisions for 5.2, 5–2, 5.2, 5–2
　instrument set 4.12
　ischiorectal 5–12, 5.13
　multiple 5.2D, 6.2
　in muscle 7.1
　　see also pyomyositis
　opening using scalpel blade 4–1
　pancreatic 5.10b, 10.2, 13.10
　paracolic 6–4, 31.10, 31.11
　paraspinal 29–3a, 29.4a
　paravertebral 7.15, 29.4
　parotid 5–7a, 5.9
　pelvic, see pelvic abscess
　pelvirectal 5.13
　subperiosteal 5.5D, 5.5, 7–2
　subphrenic, see subphrenic abscess
　thyroid 5.10a
　tubo-ovarian, see tubo-ovarian abscess
　See also individual abscesses, sites
acetazolamide 24.6
achalasia of cardia 32.24, 34–10
Achilles tendon
　cut during closed tonotomy 27.7D
　division and suturing 27.7, 27–11
　lengthening 27.7, 27–10
Achilles tenotomy
　closed 27.7D, 27.7, 27–10
　open 27.7, 27–11
　subcutaneous 27.7
acid aspiration syndrome, prevention 9.2, 10.5, 18.9
acidosis
　after peritonitis 6.2
　in gestational hypertension 17.4D
　in neonates 19.12
acid phosphatase 23.18, 32.32
acoustic neuroma 25.16
acquired immunodeficiency syndrome, see AIDS
actinomycin 32.21, 32.38, D 32.2
actinomycosis 6.6D, 7.14aD
action committees 1.12
acute abdomen 10.1–14
　causes 10.2
　diagnosis 10.2D, 10.2
　　general method 10.2
　diseases presenting as 10.2, 10–3
　examination 10.1
　in filariasis 31.6
　general method for 10.1
　history-taking and mistakes in 10.1
　indication for operation 10.2
　invasive intestinal amoebiasis 10.2, 31.11
　laparotomy for 9.2
　medical diseases mimicking 10.2, 10–4
　metabolic causes 10.2D, 10.2
　neonatal 28.3
　ovarian cysts presenting as 10.2, 20.7D, 20.7
　pancreatitis causing 13.9
　perforation 31.8
　tests for 10.1, 10–2
　tropical diseases causing 10.2
　See also individual causes listed in 10.2; intestinal obstruction
acute tumour lysis syndrome 32.3
adduction, definition 27.2
adductor tubercle 7–9, 7.10
adenocarcinoma
　bronchus 32.29
　cervix 32–21, 32.35
　kidney 32.30
　mouth 32.22
adenoid cystic carcinoma, of parotid gland 32–10, 32.23
adenolymphoceles 14.3, 14–11
adhesions
　Caesarean section 18.10D
　causes 10.7
　checking for, in laparotomy 9.2
　in ectopic pregnancies 16.6D, 16.7D
　intestinal obstruction due to 9.6D, 10.7, 10–11, 10.13
　after colostomy 9.6D
　in minilap 15.3D
　ovarian tumours and cysts 20.7D, 20.7
　in pelvic inflammatory disease (PID) 6.6
　in peritonitis 6.2
　in plastic type of abdominal tuberculosis 29.7
　preventing 9.8
　separation 10.7, 10–11

adjuvants, cancer pain relief 33.2
adnexal masses 16.2
adnexal tenderness, in ectopic pregnancy 16.6
adrenalin
　avoidance in circumcision 23.26
　in control of bleeding 3.1
　in neonates 19.12
　in sensitivity to snake antivenom 34.4
adrenergic drugs, in priapism 23.29
'Adriamycin' 21.4, 32.2D, 32.2
Adson's forceps 4–3, 4.4
aerobes, antibiotics for 2.9
Africa, sub-Saharan, population 1.2
aganglionosis 28.6a
AIDS 1.2, 1.14, 5.2, 28a.1–3
　Bangui criteria for 28a.2D
　difficulties 28a.2D
　incidence and prevalence 28a.2
　infections in 28a.2
　in utero infection 28a.2
　management 28a.2
　methods of control 28a.2
　osteomyelitis vs 7.3
　pre-AIDS period 28a.3
　precautions for surgeons 28a.2, 28a.3
　presentation 28a.2
　prevention
　　blood transfusions 28a.2
　　disinfectants 28a–21a, 28a.2
　　during surgery 28a.2, 28a.3
　screening for 28a.2D
　should one operate? 28a.3
　simple rule on 28a.2
　surgery and 28a.3
　symptomatic treatment 28a.2
　symptoms 28a.2D, 28a.2
　transmission 28a.2
　tuberculosis in 29.1
　see also human immunodeficiency virus (HIV)
AIDS-related complex, chronic osteomyelitis in 7.6D
aims of manuals Prefaces (4, 5, 6) 1.7, 1.14
ainhum 31.14
air, removal from autoclave 2.4
air embolism 3.1, 15.4
albino, skin tumours in 32–6, 32.18, 32.19D, 32.19
alcohol, abdominal pain in hepatoma and 32.26
alcoholic, stress ulcers 11.4D
'Aldomet' (methyl dopa) 17.4
alkylating agents 32.2
Allis's forceps 4.4
alpha blockers 23.20
altitudes, high, autoclaving at 2.4D
alveolar abscess 5.8, 26.7
　directions in which pus can spread 5–7, 5.8
alveolus
　break during tooth extraction 26.3D
　in cancrum oris 26.6
　lumps arising from 26.9
amblyopia 24.9
　occlusion therapy 24.9
ambulation, after abdominal surgery 9.9
ameloblastoma (adamantinoma) 26.7, 26.9
amenorrhoea 16.6, 32.38
'Amethopterin' 32.2
amniocentesis 19–1, 19.2
　if blood aspirated 19.2D
amniotic bands 27.17, 27–20
amniotic fluid, identification 19.5
amoebiasis
　abdominal tenderness due to 10.1
　appendicitis vs 12.1
　cutaneous 31.12D
　extraintestinal 31.12D, 31.12
　hemicolectomy avoidance 1.4, 31.11
　invasive intestinal 31.10, 31.11
　　caecal 31.11
　　differential diagnosis 12.1, 31.11
　　difficulties 31.11D
　　surgery 31.11
　mistakes in managing 31.11, 31.12
　plastic abdominal tuberculosis vs 29.7
　rectal bleeding in 22.3
amoebic colitis 10.2, 10–3, 22.10
　acute necrotizing 1.4, 31.10, 31.11
　typhoid perforation vs 31.8
amoebic granuloma, of rectum 22.10
amoebic liver abscess 10.2, 31.10, 31.12D, 31.12
　aspiration 31.12

amoebic liver abscess (cont.)
　chest wall abscess 31–10, 31.12D
　hepatoma vs 32.26
　open drainage 31.12
　rupture into peritoneal cavity 31.12D, 31.12
　subphrenic abscess vs 6.4
amoebic perforation of gut 10.2
amoebic ulcers 31–10
amoeboma 31.10, 31.11D, 31.11
　perforation 31.11
　of skin 31–10
AMOs (Assistant Medical Officers) 1.3
ampulla of uterine tube, implantation in 16–3, 16.6
amputation 1.7
　in chronic osteomyelitis 7.6D
　in filariasis 31–5, 31.6
　finger 8.16
　amputation (continued)
　leg, block dissection of lymph nodes and 32.34
　in leprosy 30.6D, 30.7, 30–9
　in malignant melanoma 32–7, 32.20
　in mycetoma 31.3
　in osteosarcoma 32.13
　penis, see penis
　in squamous cell carcinoma 32.19
amylase, serum 5.10b, 13.9
anaemia 1.5
　aplastic, chloramphenicol causing 2.9
　correction before abdominal surgery 9.1
　in ectopic pregnancy 16.6, 16.7
　in evacuating incomplete abortions 16.2D
　failure to respond to treatment 17.2D
　in hydatidiform mole 32.38
　megaloblastic 17.2
　pathophysiology 17–1
　in pregnancy 17.2D, 17.2
　　danger signs 17.2
　　delivery in 17.2
　　severe, management 17.2
anaerobic infections 2.9
　in anorectal abscesses 5.13
　antibiotics 2.8, 2.9, 31.8
　laparotomy wounds 9.12
anaerobic sepsis, surgical 2.9
anaesthesia Preface 6
　for circumcision 23.26, 23–34
　facilities in district hospitals 1.2
　general, for Caesarean section 18.1a
　in infants 28.4
　as limiting factor 1.2
　local, for operative vaginal delivery 18.1a, 18–1
　in neonates 28.1, 28.3
　obstetric 18.1a, 18–1
　for operations around mouth 26.1
　in rule about deciding when to operate 1.8
　for tourniquet use 3.9
　See also individual surgical procedures
anal, see also Anus
anal agenesis 28–5, 28.6
　with fistula 28.6D, 28.6, 28–8
　without fistula 28.6, 28–7
anal atresia 9.5
anal canal 22.1, 22–2
　carcinoma 22.1, 22.10
anal dilatation 10.10, 22.5D, 22.5, 22.7, 22.9
　indications, contraindications 22.5
　maximal 9.6
　method 22.4, 22.5, 22–9, 22–10
anal dilator 22.6D
anal fissure 22.7
　diagnosis, differential diagnosis 22.7
　Lord's anal stretch for 22.5, 22–9
　piles with 22.6D
　treatment 22.5, 22.7, 22–9
anal fistula, see anorectal fistulae
analgesics 13.3, 33.2
anal gland 22–1
　anorectal abscess originating in 5.13
anal margin 22–4, 22.7
anal membrane, imperforate 28–5, 28.6D, 28.6, 28–6
anal mucosa, eversion, after repair of imperforate anus 28.6D
anal operations
　arrangements for 22.1, 22–4
　pre- and postoperative care 22.1
anal reflex 23.5
anal sphincter

anal sphincter (cont.)
  dilatation 22.4, 22.5, 22 – 9
    see also anal dilatation
  external 22 – 1
  fistula through 22.2
  internal 22 – 1, 22.1, 22.6D
    anal fissure effects on 22.7
anal stenosis 28 – 5, 28.6D, 28.6
anal stretch, see anal dilatation
anal stricture 22.6D
anal verge 22 – 1
  skin tag on 22.7
anal wound
  dressing 22.1
  healing from bottom 22.1, 22.2
  infection 22.1
anaphylactic shock 31.13D, 31.13
anastomoses, gut, see gut
anatomical drawings, summary 1.14
anatomy 1.14
  See also individual anatomical regions
anencephaly 19.7, 19.9
aneurysm, needle 4.11
angioneurotic oedema 25.16
angiosarcoma 32.21
ankle
  anatomy 27 – 11
  arthrodesis 30.6D, 30 – 8
  aspiration 7 – 15, 7.17
  calcaneus deformity 27.4
  in chronic polio 27.4
  contracture assessment 27.2
  dislocation 30.6D
  equinus deformity, see equinus deformity
  exploring 7.17
  fracture, referral for 1.6
  in leprosy 30.6D
  manipulation 27.2, 27 – 2, 27.7
  measurement of movement 30.8, 30 – 10
  polio contractures 27.7
  positions of rest and of function 7 – 16, 7.17
  posterior capsule, division 27.7
  splint 27.5
  tuberculosis of 29.3
  valgus and varus deformities 27.2, 27.4
  see also valgus deformity; varus deformity
ankylosing spondylitis 27.8D
ankylosis 7.17
  bony 7.16, 29.3
  fibrous 7.16, 29.3
  positions of function for 7 – 16, 7.17
  in tuberculosis 29.3
annulus fibrosus, nucleus pulposus protrusion 27.8, 27 – 12a
anorectal abscess 5 – 11, 5 – 12, 5.13D, 5.13, 22.2
  on both sides 5.13D
  extending internally under submucosa 5.13D
  internal opening 5.13D
  recurrent 5.13D
  signs of spreading infection 5.13D
  submucous or high intermuscular 5 – 11, 5.13
anorectal fistulae 5 – 11, 5.13D, 5.13, 22 – 2, 22.2
  deroofing 22.2
  difficulties 22.2D
  extension through hole in levator ani 22.2D
  high anal 22.2, 22 – 5
  high intermuscular 22.2D, 22 – 5
  high posterior horseshoe 22.2, 22 – 5, 22 – 7, 22 – 8
  iatrogenic 22.2
  long curved, opening away from anus 22.2D
  low anal 22.2, 22 – 5, 22 – 6, 22.7
  multiple 22.2D
  patterns 22 – 5
  piles with 22.2D
  posterior, pilonidal sinus vs 22.2D
  recurrence 22.2
  recurrent discharge from 22.2D
  superficial 22.2, 22 – 5
anorectal line 22 – 1, 22.1, 22 – 1, 22 – 4
  cutting, incontinence and 22.2
anorectal malformations 28.2, 28 – 5, 28.6D, 28.6, 28 – 6
  examination 28.6, 28 – 6
  fistulae in 28.6D, 28.6
  high and low 28 – 5, 28.6
anorectal ring, deep anorectal fistulae 22.2
anorectal sinus 22.2
anorectum 22 – 1
antacids, cost 11.1

antenatal care 18.1, 18.3
antepartum haemorrhage (APH) 16.2, 16.11
anterior chamber of eye
  blood in (hyphaema) 24.1, 24.4
  examination 24.1
  pus in 24.3, 24.4
  shallow after cataract removal 24.4
anterior ethmoidal artery, tying 25.6D
anthrax 24.3D
'antibioma' 21.3
antibiotics Preface 6
  abscess treatment 5.2
  acute abdomen signs diminished 10.2D
  acute cholecystitis 13.3
  advice on (chloramphenicol resistance uncommon) 2.7
  alveolar abscesses 5.8
  anaerobic infections 2.8, 2.9, 31.8
  antitumour 32.2
  'blind therapy' 2.9
  for bouginage of urethral strictures 23.8
  cellulitis 5.1
  chaos 2.7, 2 – 9
  common mistakes with ear disorders 25.1
  dental abscesses 5.8
  empyema 6.1
  eye disorders 24.1
  hand infections 8.1
  heart failure in pregnancy 17.5
  individual types and uses 2.8
  intestinal obstruction 10.5
  methods for using 2.9
  osteomyelitis 7.4
  pelvic inflammatory disease (PID) 6.6
  perioperative 2.6
    doses 2.9
    indications and contraindications 2.9
    in lower segment Caesarean section 18.9
  peritonitis 6.2
  policy 2.7
  prophylactic 2.7, 2.9, 2.10
    vs treatment 2.9
  puerperal sepsis 6.7
  septic abortion 6.6a
  in surgery, uses 2.7
  treating otitis media without 25.3D
  typhoid 31.8
  unacceptable methods for using 2.9
  variety, wise usage 2 – 10
anticonvulsants 17.4, 33.2
antiemetics, in cancer 33.2D, 33.2
antihypertensive treatment, long – term 17.4D
antimalarials 17.2
antimetabolites 32.2
antimicrobials, see antibiotics
antiseptic methods 2.1
antiseptic surgery 2.1, 2.6
  antiseptic solutions for 2.6
antiseptics 2.5, 2.6
  minimum time in 2.5
antithyroid drugs 21.8
antivenom, snake 34.4
  sensitivity to, signs 34.4
antral washout 25 – 7, 25.8, 25.9
antrostomy, intranasal 25 – 6, 25.9
antrum
  maxillary, see maxillary antrum
  tympanic 25 – 2, 25.4
anuria
  after Caesarean section 18.10D
  after obstructed labour, Stop Press
  calculous 23.12, 23.13
  renal failure with 23.12
anus
  bruising 22.5D
  carcinoma 22.2D, 22.7
  constriction bands 22.5
  firm fungating mass at 22.10
  general method for 22.1
  keyhole deformity 22.5D
  lesions at 22.10
  painful, thrombosed external piles causing 22.4
  physiology 22.1
  recording abnormalities around 22 – 4
  See also entries beginning anal, anorectal
aorta, damage to, in use of laprocator 15.4D
Apgar score 19.12
aphakia 24.8
aphasia, nominal 25.3D
apnoeic attacks, in babies 17.4D

apocrine glands, axillary abscess in 5 – 9, 5.11
aponeurosis
  external and internal oblique 14.2, 14 – 4, 14 – 6
  internal oblique and transversus muscles 14.2, 14 – 7
appendicectomy 1.1, 12 – 1, 12.2D, 12 – 2
  interval 12.1
  intestinal fistula after 9.14
  retrograde 1.1, 12.1, 12 – 2
appendicitis 5 – 10, 5.12, 12.1 – 2
  abdominal pain in 10.1, 10.2, 12.1
  danger signs 12.1
  development, stages 12.1
  diagnosis 12.1, 12.2D
  differential diagnosis 11.2, 12.1, 23.14, 31.8
  difficulties 12.2D
  due to Ascaris 10.6
  pelvic abscess after 6.5, 12.2D
  perforated peptic ulcer vs 11.2, 12.1
  presenting as acute abdomen 10.2, 10 – 3
  typhoid complications vs 12.1, 31.8
  ureteric stones vs 23.14
appendix 10.2, 12.1 – 2
  anatomy 12 – 3
  buried in adhesions, at appendicectomy 12.2D
  difficulty in finding 12.1, 12 – 3
  gangrenous in hernial sac 14.3D
  necrotic base, at appendicectomy 12.2D
  normal, at appendicectomy 12.2D
  positions of 12 – 1, 12.1
  purse string suture 9 – 6
  stuck to Fallopian tube 16.6D
appendix abscess 5 – 10, 6.2, 12.1
  diagnosis, differential diagnosis 5.12, 10.6, 12.1
  drainage 12.1, 12 – 3
  invasive intestinal amoebiasis vs 31.11
  plastic abdominal tuberculosis vs 29.7
  signs and symptoms 12.1
appendix mass 12.1
'Appropriate technology' Preface 4
aprons 2.3
aqueous humour, flow pattern 24 – 1, 24 – 7
ARC (AIDS related complex) 7.6D
arcus senilis 24.15
arm, tourniquet application 3.9, 3 – 11
arm board 2.1
arterial bleeding 3.1, 3.2
arteries
  passing ligature under 3.2, 3 – 4
  tying 3.1, 3.2, 3 – 3
    anterior ethmoidal 25.6D
    external carotid 3.3, 3 – 5
    external iliac 3.6, 3 – 8
    femoral 3.7, 3 – 9
    internal iliac 3.5, 3 – 7, Stop Press
    popliteal 3.8, 3 – 10
    third part of subclavian 3.4, 3 – 6
    uterine, Stop Press
artery forceps, see haemostats
arthritis 29.3
  'cold' 29.3
  septic, see septic arthritis
  tuberculous, see tuberculous arthritis
arthrodesis 7.19
  ankle 30.6D, 30 – 8
  knee or hip 29.3D, 29.3
  subtalar triple 30.6D, 30 – 8
arthrogryposis 27.12D
ascariasis, surgery of 10.6, 10 – 10
Ascaris worms 10.6, 10 – 10
  abdominal palpation in 10.4
  causing intestinal obstruction 10.3, 10.4, 10.6, 10 – 10
  cholangitis caused by 13.5
  plastic abdominal tuberculosis vs 29.7
ascites 10.4, 32.25
  in abdominal tuberculosis 29 – 4, 29.5, 29.6
  draining 29.6, 29 – 6
  minilap to diagnosis cause 29.6
  ovarian tumours 20.7
ascitic fluid, in abdominal tuberculosis 29.6
aseptic surgery 2.1, 2.4, 2.6
aseptic techniques 2.1, 2.3D, 2.10
  theatre 2.3
aspiration
  abscesses 5.2
  breast cysts 21.3
  joint 7 – 15, 7.16, 7.17, 29.3
  needle, in osteomyelitis 7.4

613

aspiration (cont.)
  ovarian cyst 20.7
  pericardium 6.1a, 6 – 2a
  peritoneal 16.6
  pus in pleura 6.1
  secretions, in eclampsia 17.4D
  stomach contents 9.2, 18.9
    in intestinal obstruction surgery 10.5
aspiration pneumonia 5.7
aspirin 33.2
assisted active movements, for contractures 27.2
astigmatism 24.8
atelectasis 9.11
atraumatic needle 9.3
atropine 24.1, 24.3, 30.2
  danger in glaucoma 24.6
auditory canal 25.5
Aufrecht's scissors 4 – 2, 4.3
autoclave 2.1, 2.3, 2 – 7
  double-walled (vertical, horizontal) 2.4, 2 – 7
  jacketed 2.4, 2 – 7
  packing methods 2.4, 2 – 7a
  procedures for 2.4, 4.12
  single-walled 2.4, 2 – 7
  tape 2.4
  testing 2.4
autoclaving 2.4D, 2.4
  in aseptic technique 2.3, 2.4
  HIV and HBV destruction 28a.2
  methods 2.4, 4.12
  prevention of wound infection 2.10
  standard holding time 2.4
autoimmune lymphocytic thyroiditis 21.13
autotransfusion 16 – 8, 16.10, 28a.2
  in acute or subacute ectopic pregnancy 16.6
  soup-ladle method 16.10
  vacuum-bottle method 16.10
Auvard's speculum 15.1a, 15 – 2
axilla
  dissection 21.3, 21.4
  fibrotic nodes 21.3D
  radiotherapy 21.3
axillary abscess 5 – 9, 5.11
  multiple recurrent small 5.11
axillary artery, tear 3 – 6
axillary nodes
  involvement in breast carcinoma 21.3, 21.4
  radiotherapy 21.3, 21.4
  removal, in Patey's modified mastectomy 21.6
  tuberculosis of 21.3D
axillary swelling, in filariasis 31 – 5, 31.6
axillary vein, damage to 21.6D

B
Babcock's forceps 4.4
babies, see infants
baby, dead 16.4, Stop Press
back pain 7.15, 27.8D, 27.8
  causes 27.8
  in children 27.8D, 27.8
  in spinal tuberculosis 29.4
Bancroftian filariasis 23.23
'Bactrim' 2.8
bag and mask ventilation, neonates 19.12, 19 – 13
balanitis 23.30
  paraphimosis with 23 – 37
balanitis xerotica obliterans (BXO) 23.28, 23 – 38
'bamboo' spine 27.8D
bandage scissors 4 – 2, 4.3
Bandl's ring 18.3, 18 – 3, 18.8, 18.9, 19.11D
  in Caesarean section 18.10D
  impending rupture of uterus 18.17
bands, causing intestinal obstruction 10.7
barium, in pyloric stenosis 11.6
barium enema 10.4, 34.5
  indications and contraindications 34.5
barium meal 5.10b, 32.25, 34.5
  method 34.5
  pancreatic pseudocysts 13.10
barium swallow 34.5
Bartholin's abscess 5.2, 20.4
Bartholin's cyst 20 – 2, 20.4
basal cell carcinoma 32 – 6, 32.18
Basic Radiological System (BRS) 1 – 8, 1.14
Bassini repair 14.2, 14 – 6
bathing, after anal operations 22.1
battery charger 2.1
bed linen, disinfection, AIDS prevention 28a.2
bed sores 33.2D

Bence Jones protein 32.16
benzylpenicillin (penicillin G) 2.8, 2.9
betel leaf 32.22
bile
  in drain after cholecystectomy 13.7D
  vomiting after gastroenterostomy 11.6D
bile-duct
  anatomy 13 – 3, 13.7, 28 – 9a
  atresia 28.8a, 28 – 9a
  carcinoma 32.26
  common, see common bile duct
  extrahepatic, carcinoma of 13.8
  obstruction, hepatitis vs 28a.4
  stenosis 13.8
bilharzia, see schistosomiasis
biliary colic 10 – 1, 10.1, 10.2, 13.1, 13.2
  differential diagnosis 13.2
  non-operative treatment 13.2
  recurrent 13.3
biliary peritonitis 11.2
biliary system 13 – 3, 13.7, 28 – 9a
  block, in neonates 28.8a, 28 – 9a
bilirubin, in hepatoma 32.26
biopsy
  in AIDS 28a.2D
  cervix 32 – 22, 32.35
  eye and orbital tumours 24.11
  knee joint 7.17
  liver
    needle 32 – 14, 32.26
    wedge 29.6, 29 – 7
  lymph node 32.1
  peritoneum 29.6
  prostate 32.32
  referral and 1.6
  in tumours 32.1
BIPP (bismuth iodoform and paraffin paste) 1.14, 4.11, 25.16
birth canal
  injuries and tears 18.15
  old third-degree tears 18.16, 18 – 17
  recent third-degree tears 18.15, 18 – 17
  second-degree tears 18.15
birth injuries 18.3
Bishop's inducibility test 19.3
Bismuth Iodoform and Paraffin Paste(BIPP) 1.14, 4.11, 25.6
bistoury, guarded 14 – 18
bites, human, septic arthritis of fingers 8 – 9, 8.15, 8.16
Bitot's spots 24.1, 24.3D
bladder
  accidental opening
    in Caesarean section 18.10D
    in colporrhaphy 20.11aD
    in hysterectomy 20.12D
    in minilap 15.3D
  appearance in cystoscopy 23.3, 23 – 23
  base, cystoscopy 23 – 23
  bleeding, irrigation 23.2
  carcinoma 23.5, 23 – 15, 23.18, 32.31
    cystoscopy for 23.3
    haematuria in 23.4
    schistosomiasis 23.18, 31.1, 32.31
    staging 32 – 17, 32.31
    stricture in 23.9D
    suprapubic puncture contraindication 23.6, 23.18
  catheterization, see catheter
  closure 23.15, 23 – 19, 23 – 21
    after Freyer's prostatectomy 23 – 24
  distended 23.17
    after passing urine 23.9D
  diverticula 23.8, 23.18, 23.19D
  draining 4 – 12
  entering inguinal hernia 14.2, 14 – 5
  filling, in treatment of cord prolapse 19 – 6, 19.10
  fistula, in obstructed labour 18.4
  flap, in hysterectomy 20.12
  if prostatic adenoma falls into 23.21
  inadequate emptying 23.8, 23.9D   injury
    in inguinal hernia repair 14.3D
    in lower segment Caesarean section 18.8, 18.9, 18.10D
  median lobe of prostate('termite hill') 23.3, 23.18
  neck, see bladder neck (below)
  nerves to, examination 23.5
  painful distended, clot retention 23.19D

bladder (cont.)
  prolapse (cystocele) 20.9, 20 – 9, 20.11a, 20 – 12
  residual urine 23.8, 23.9D
  rhabdomyosarcoma 32.9
  rupture, in obstructed labour 18.3
  sacculations 23.8
  shrunken, in urogenital tuberculosis 29.9
  sound in, detection of 23.8
  stones 23 – 15
    in adults 23.15D, 23.15
    in children 23.16
    haematuria in 23.4
    removal by suprapubic approach 23.7, 23.15, 23 – 19
    stuck to lower segment, in Caesarean section 18.10D
  torn
    closure impossible 18.17D
    in rupture of uterus 18.17D, 18.17, 18 – 19
  trabeculation 23.18, 23.20
  trigone
    appearance in cystoscopy 23.3
    relationship to urethra and ureters 20 – 16
    S. haematobium causing fibrosis 23.20
  tuberculous ulcers 29.9, 29 – 9
  washing out 23.3
bladder neck
  dysfunction 23.18, 23.19D
    treatment 23.20
  fibrosis 23.19, 23.20
    cystoscopic diagnosis 23.18
    Ghadvi's prostatectomy and 23.21
  obstruction 23.5D, 23.19
    in neonates 28.11
    as prostatectomy indication 23.18
  stenosis 23.5D, 23.9D, 23.18, 23.20, 34 – 9
    indication for surgery 23.8
    micturating cystourethrogram 34.5, 34 – 9
    urethral strictures causing 23.8
  stone wedged in 23.17
  wedge resection 23.19D, 23.19, 23 – 23, 23 – 24, 23 – 25
Blalock artery clamp 3 – 2
Blandy's posterior urethroplasty, first stage 23.11D, 23.11, 23 – 12
blastomas 32.6 – 7
bleeding
  in abdominal cavity, in ectopic pregnancy 16.6
  abdominal muscles 9.2
  abscess causing 5.2
  acute rupture of ectopic pregnancy 10.1, 16.6
  after 28th week of gestation 16.11, 16.12, 16.13
  after intrauterine death 16.4
  arteries and veins 3.1, 3.2, 3 – 3
  before 28th week of gestation 16.2
  before/after evacuation of abortions 16.2D, 16.2, 16.8
  chronic ectopic pregnancy 16.7D, 16.7
  chronic osteomyelitis 7.6D
  colporrhaphy 20.11aD
  control of 3.1 – 10
    after tourniquet use 3.9
    assisting natural mechanisms 3.1
    common mistakes 3.1
    from large pedicle 3.2
    limb operations 3.9
    by pressure 3.1
    by raising bleeding part 3.1
    see also arteries, tying
  during delivery of dead baby 16.4D
  extrauterine pregnancies 16.9D, 16.9
  eye 24.2
  fibroids causing 20.6
  gastrointestinal, see gastrointestinal bleeding
  hand operations 8.1
  intraperitoneal 10.1, 12.2D
  laparotomy 9.2
  lower segment Caesarean section 18.8, 18.9
  peritonsillar abscess 5 – 6, 5.6
  placental abruption 16.11, 16.13D, 16.13
  placenta praevia 16.11, 16.12
  postoperative 3.10, 22.6D, 23.19D, 26.3D
  puerperal sepsis 6.7
  rectal, see rectal bleeding
  separation of adhesions 10.7D
  snake bites 34.4
  use of laprocator 15.4D
  see also uterine bleeding; vaginal bleeding
bleeding disorder 25.6D
blepharitis 24.3

blindness 24.1
  causes 24.1, 24.4, 24.7, 24.13
  endophthalmitis causing 24.3
  night 24.3D, 24.4
blind spot 24 – 9
blink reflex, absent in leprosy 30.3
blisters, in snake bites 34.4, 34 – 8
'blocking pin' 32 – 14, 32.26
'block toes' 31 – 3, 31.5
Blond – Heidel saw 18 – 10
blood
  bank, Stop Press
  balance sheet 3 – 1, 3.1
  clotting power 3.1
  count, in peritonitis 6.2
  culture 2.7, 7.4
  disinfection 28a – 1a, 28a.2
  draining 4.10
  loss
    in adults and children 3 – 1, 3.1
    in epistaxis 25.6
  in peritoneal cavity 10.1, 12.2D
  rectal passage, in intussusception 10.4, 10.8
  replacement 3 – 1, 3.1
  volume, reduction, in peritonitis 6.2
bloodless operations, limbs 3.9, 8.1
blood pressure
  in eclampsia 17.4
  in essential hypertension in pregnancy 17.4
  fall, postoperative 3.10
  in gestational hypertension 17.4
  high after delivery 17.4D
  in pre-eclampsia 17.4
  in pregnancy 17.4
blood products, HIV contamination 28a.2
blood supply
  Fallopian tubes 16.6D
  to gut 9.3, 10.4
blood transfusion 1.2, 3.1
  AIDS transmission 17.2, 28a.2
  alternatives to, AIDs prevention 28a.2
  for anaemia, indications 17.2
  autotransfusion 16.6, 16 – 8, 16.10, 28a.2
  in evacuating abortions 16.2D
  in gastrointestinal bleeding 11.3
  indications 28a.2
  postoperative bleeding 3.10
  risk, in pregnancy 17.2
  for strangulated gut 10.5
blood vessel
  passing ligature under 3.2, 3 – 4
  suturing, in control of bleeding 3.1
blunt dissection 4.3, 4 – 3, 4.4, 4 – 8
B lymphocytes, tumours 32.3, 32.5
body fluids, disinfection 28a – 1a, 28a.2
Böhler walking iron 30 – 7
boil 5.3
  in ear 25.3, 25.4
boiling 2.4, 4.12
bone
  benign cyst 27.17
  disuse atrophy 30.6
  drilling, in osteomyelitis 7.3, 7 – 4, 7.5
  drills 7.2, 7 – 3
  exploring for pus 7.5
  flat 7.14
  hook 7.2, 7 – 3
  infarction 7.3
  injuries 1.4
  instruments for 7.2, 7 – 3
  involvement in leprosy 30.6D, 30.6
  levers 7.2, 7 – 3
  neuropathic 30.6D, 30.6
  outgrowth 27.17
  pain 32.13, 32.16, 32.32, 33.2D
  rarefaction 7.3
  secondary deposits 21.4, 27.8, 32.12
  tender, in acute osteomyelitis 7.3, 7 – 4
  tumours 32.12 – 17
bone wax 3.1
Bonney's forceps 4 – 3, 4.4
borborygmi 10.4
'bougie clinic ' 23.8
bouginage 23.8, 23.9D
  assisted, in impassable urethral strictures 23.11
  in corrosive oesophageal strictures 25.15D, 25.15
  dangers of 25.15D, 25.15
  failure 23.9D, 23.11
  septicaemia after 23.9D

bouginage (cont.)
  urethral stricture dilatation 23.8, 23 – 9
bougies 23.1, 23 – 1
  metal, passing 23 – 8, 23.8
  nylon filiform 23.8, 23 – 9
  oesophageal 25.14, 32.24
  passing, in carcinoma of oesophagus 32 – 12, 32.24
  plastic, passing 23.8
  self-dilatation 23.8, 23 – 9
bowel habit, altered 32.27
  in acute abdomen diagnosis 10.1
bowel routine, after anal operations 22.1
bowel sounds
  absent 6.2, 10.1, 10.13
  after abdominal surgery 9.10, 10.13
  in children 28.1
  hyperperistaltic 10.4
  if no return, after obstruction 10.5D
  in intestinal obstruction 10.4
  in small gut volvulus 10.9
  tinkling 10.1, 10.13
Bowesman's 'shaving off' method for keloids 34.1a, 34 – 5
brachioradialis muscle 7 – 7, 7 – 8
bradycardia 19.3, 19.12
brain abscess 25.3D
branchial cyst 28.10
breast
  abscess 21.1, 21.2, 21.3
    acute 21 – 1, 21.2, 21.3D
    draining 21 – 1, 21 – 2
    subacute, chronic recurrent 21.2
  acute septic infections 21.2, 21.3D
  Burkitt's lymphoma involving 21.3
  carcinoma 1.5, 21.3D, 21.3, 21 – 3, 21.4
    with colloid degeneration 21.3
    hormonal and cytotoxic treatment 21.4
    inflammatory 21.4
    in lateral half 21.4
    in males 21.3D, 21.4
    management 21.3, 21.4
    medullary (anaplastic) 21.2, 21.4
    operations for 21.5, 21 – 6
    Patey's modifed radical mastectomy 21.6, 21 – 11, 21 – 12
    presenting features 21.4
    schirrous 21.4
    staging and prognosis 21.3, 21.4
  circumferential incision 21.5, 21 – 5
  cysts in, diagnosis and management 21.3
  difficulties 21.3D, 21.5D
  enlargement
    in breast carcinoma 21.3D, 21.4
    in men 21.3D
    with pitting oedema 21.3D
  fat necrosis 21.3
  fibroadenoma 21.3, 21 – 4, 21.4, 21 – 6
    'shelling out' 21.3, 21.5, 21 – 6
  fibroadenosis 21.3
  fistula 21 – 1, 21.2
  giant fibroadenoma 21.5D, 21 – 9
  giant hypertrophy 21.3D
  haematoma 21.3
  inflammatory lesions 21.1, 21.3D
  intracystic papilliferous carcinoma 21.3
  intraduct adenoma 21.3
  intraduct carcinoma 21.3D, 21.3, 21.4
    excision 21.5, 21 – 8
  intraduct papilloma, excision 21.5, 21 – 8
  in leprosy 30.9, 30 – 9
  lipoma 21.3
  lumps in 21.3, 21 – 3
    examination, palpation 21.3
  malignancy signs 21.3
  milk fistula 21.3
  neurofibroma 21.3
  normal, nodularity 21.3
  pus in 21.2
  self-examination 21.4
  serocystic disease 21.3
  sinus or fistula in, management 21.3
  soft fatty lump 21.3D
  solid lumps 21.5D
    antibiotic-modified inflammation 21.3
    diagnosis and management 21.3
    incisions for removal 21 – 5, 21.5
    'lumpectomy' 21.3, 21 – 6
  tuberculosis 21.3
  tumours 21.3, 21 – 3, 21.5D

breast (cont.)
  ulcers, in carcinoma 21.4
breast-feeding
  advice to HIV-positive mother 28a.2
  AIDS transmission 28a.2
  breast infections, importance in 21.2
  milk fistula, importance in 21.3
  problems in estimating gestational age 19.6
breast milk, expression 21.2
'breast mouse' 21.3
breath sounds, asymmetrical, in neonate 19.12
breech delivery 19.8
  assisted 19 – 3, 19 – 4, 19.8D, 19.8
  Caesarean section for 18.9, 18.10D, 19.8
  forceps in 19 – 4, 19.8
  of head, difficulties 19.8D
  if shoulders stuck 19 – 5, 19.8
  in multiple pregnancies 19.11
  obstructed 18.7
  symphysiotomy indication 18.6, 19.8D, 19.8
  vaginal 19.8
  See also head presentation
breech extraction 19.8
breech hook 15.1a, 15 – 2, 19.8
breech presentation 19.8
  correcting 19 – 2, 19.8
  external cepahlic version (ECV) 19 – 2, 19.8, 19.11
  footlings 19.8
  hydrocephaly in 19.7
  knee-chest position 19 – 2, 19.8
  in placenta praevia 16.12
  in twins 19.11
broad ligament 18.17, 18 – 20, 20.12, 20 – 17
  abscess 6.6
  baby in, rupture of uterus 18.17
  blood supply to ectopic pregnancy 16 – 4, 16.6D, 16.6
  clamping, in angular ectopic pregnancy 16.8
  cyst in 20.7D, 20.7
  fetal implantation 16.9
  haematoma 16.6D, 18 – 18
    after 'D and C' 20.3D
  pinching to stop bleeding 16 – 4, 16.6
  tear opening into 18.17, 18 – 19
Brodie's abscess 7 – 2, 7.2, 7.6
'Brompton cocktail' 33.2
bronchopleural fistula 6.1D
bronchoscope 25 – 10, 25.12
bronchoscopy 25.12
  arrangements for 25 – 9, 25.12
  aspiration of stomach contents 25.12
  in carcinoma of bronchus 32.29
  difficulties 25.12D
  for foreign bodies, removal 25.12, 26.3D
  indications 25.12
  for retention of secretions 25.12
bronchospasm, after abdominal surgery 9.11
bronchus
  carcinoma 6.1, 25.13, 32.29
  identification in bronchoscopy 25.12
Browne's tubes, for testing autoclaves 2.4
brow presentation 19.9
BRS (Basic Radiological System) 1 – 8, 1.14
Brugia spp. 31.6
brushes, nylon 2.3
buccal mucoperiosteal flap 26.3D, 26.7, 26 – 7, 26 – 10
buccinator, abscess external to 5.8
Buck's fascia 23.10
bulbospongiosus 23 – 12
bupthalmos 24.6D, 24.6
Burkitt's lymphoma 20.7, 32 – 1a, 32.3D, 32.3
  breast in 21.3
  case history 32.2
  chemotherapy 32.2, 32.3
  cytological diagnosis 32.3
  jaw in 26.7, 26.9
  presentation 32 – 1a, 32.3, 32 – 3
  proptosis in 24 – 10, 24.11
  rapid increase in size 32.2, 32.3
  relapses 32.3
  spinal tuberculosis vs 29.4
  staging and prognosis 32.3
Burkitt zone 32 – 3
burn 1.2, 27.2
'burning leg' 31.5
Burns – Marshall manoeuvre 19 – 3, 19.8
burr holes, extradural abscess 5.4a
Burr hole set 4.12

burst abdomen, see abdomen, burst
Buruli ulcer 31.2a
   tropical ulcer vs 31.2
Busoga hernia 14.2, 14.6D
   repair 14.2, 14 – 9, 14 – 10
buttock injury, contractures after 27.2

C
caecal fistula 9.14
caecostomy 9.5, 9 – 14
   method 9.6D, 9.6
caecum
   anastomoses, dangers 32 – 15a, 32.27
   appearance, in intestinal obstruction 10.5
   appendix stuck behind 12.1
   burst 9.6D
   carcinoma, invasive intestinal amoebiasis vs 31.11
   collapsed 10.5
   exteriorization 9.6D
   gangrenous 9.6D
   granuloma 29 – 4
   in invasive intesinal amoebiasis 31.10, 31 – 10, 31.11
   thickened, at appendicectomy 12.2D
   tuberculosis 10.1
   volvulus of 10.11, 10 – 18
Caesarean hysterectomy 18.8
Caesarean instrument set 4.12
Caesarean section 18.1, 18 – 13a
   after induction of labour 19.3
   alternatives to 18.1, 18.14
   anaesthesia for 18.1a
   bleeding with 18.10D
   in breech presentation 18.9, 18 – 10D, 19.8
   burst abdomen after 9 – 24
   in cephalopelvic disproportion(CPD) 18.6
   choice of, kinds 18.8
   classical 18.8, 18.9, 18.12, 18 – 14
      indications 18.8, 18.9
      tear from 18.17, 18 – 19
   for cord prolapse 19.10
   dangers of 18.1, 19.8
   de Lee, method 18.8, 18.9, 19.9
   in diabetic mother 17.3
   difficulties 18.10D
   elective, in subsequent pregnancy 18.14
   extraperitoneal 6.7, 18.8, 18.13, 18 – 15
   in gestational hypertension 17.4
   incision, difficulties with 18.10D
   Jael Cohen's incision for, Stop Press
   incisional hernia after 14.13, 14 – 20, 14 – 23
   infection after 6.8, 18.8, 18 – 13
   lower segment 18.8, 18.9, 18.10D
      anaesthesia 18.9
      blood loss 18.9
      completing repair and closure 18.9, 18 – 13
      control of bleeding 18.9
      delivery of baby 18.9, 18 – 12, 18 – 13
      placenta removal 18.9
      postoperative care 18.9
      'smile incision' 18.9
      stay suture in uterus 18.9, 18 – 12
      suturing uterus 18.9, 18 – 13
      transverse lie 18.10D, 19.9
   for multiple pregnancies 19.11
   in obstructed labour 18.4, 18.9
      indications and contraindications 18.4
   ovarian cyst at 20.7D
   placenta, difficulties with 18.10D
   in placental abruption 16.13
   in placenta praevia 16.12, 18.8, 18.9
   presentations, difficulties 18.10D
   previous 18.1, 18.9, 18.10D, 18 – 18
   scar 18 – 18
      abruption with 16.13D
      rupture 18.8, 18.14
   transverse incision 18.8, 18.10D
      in upper segment 18.8, 18.10D
      in transverse lie 18.10D, 19.9
   'trial of scar' after, see 'trial of scar'
   urinary tract difficulties 18.10D
calcaneal spur, excision 30.7, 30 – 9
calcaneus
   deformity 27.2, 27.4
   osteomyelitis 7 – 12, 7.13
   removal 7.13
calcium, high, and urinary stones 23.12
calcium gluconate 3.1, 9.2, 17.4
calcium hypochlorite 28a – 1a, 28a.2

calculi, urinary, see urinary tract stones
Caldwell Luc operation 25 – 7, 25.9, 26.3D
caliper 27.5
   above knee 27.5
   below knee 27.5
   weight relieving, in Perthes' disease 27.14
cancer 32.1 – 39
   constipation in, relief 33.2
   diagnosis 32.1
   pain relief, see pain, relief in cancer
   sequence of steps in treatment 32.1
   specimens, fixing 32.1
   staging 32.1
   symptom palliation 33.1, 33.2
   treating in district hospital 32.1
   treatment method and aim (cure or palliative) 32.1, 32.2
   see also individual cancers; tumour
cancrum oris 7.14, 26.6, 26 – 10
candidiasis, oral, in AIDS 28a.2
canine, extraction 26.3, 26 – 4, 26 – 5
cannulae 1.12, 4.11
capillary cavernous haemangioma 28.10, 28 – 11
capillary haemangioma 28.10, 28 – 11
caps, theatre 2.3
caput succedaneum, in obstructed labour 18.4
carbimazole, in hyperthyroidism 21.8
carbon dioxide, in laprocator use 15.4
carbuncle 5.3, 5.4, 7.3, 8 – 1, 8.2
carcinomatosis, of peritoneum 29.6
cardiac failure 6.1a
   after removal of giant ovarian cysts 20.7D
   in pregnancy, with transfusions 17.2
cardiac notch 6 – 1
cardiac shadow 6.1a
cardiac tamponade 6.1a
cardinal (transverse cervical) ligaments 20.12, 20 – 17
cardiomyopathy 6.1a
carneous mole 16.2
carpal bones and carpal tunnel 27 – 14a
carpal tunnel 27 – 14a
   mycetoma spread 31 – 2
carpal tunnel syndrome 27.11a, 27 – 14a
cataract 24.1, 24.4
   diagnosis 24.4
   removal 24.4, 24.8
   secondary, in leprosy 30.2
catgut 4.6
   avoidance in ascariasis 10.6
   incisional hernias after use 14.13
   in stomach 9.3
   use in tubal ligation 15.3
catheter 4.11
   autoclaving vs antiseptic use 2.5
   choice of, factors in 23.2
   condom 23 – 3
   economical use of and savings on 1.12
   if difficult to pass in urinary retention 23.5
   if unable to pass, suprapubic puncture for 23 – 5, 23.6, 23 – 6
   indwelling 23.2
      in carcinoma of prostate 32.32
      if removal difficult 23.2D
   insertion, after repair of VVF 18.18, 18 – 23
   milking 23.19, 23 – 26
   passing a 23.1, 23.2, 23 – 2
      in Caesarean section 18.9, 18 – 11
      difficulties 23.2D, 23.2
   types 23.1, 23 – 1, 23.2
   unavailable, in caecostomy 9.6D
catheterization sheath for cystoscope 23.3, 23 – 4
'cat's eye' 32.7
cauterization, in epistaxis 25.6
cavernous sinus thrombosis 5.5D, 5.5, 5 – 5, 5.8, 24.11
cavus foot 27.4
Celestin tube 32.24, 33.1
   difficulty in passing 32.24D
   insertion 32 – 11, 32.24
cellulitis 5.1
   pelvic 6.6a, 6.6
   periorbital and orbital 5.5
   sublingual and submandibular regions 5.10
cephadine 2.8, 2.9
cephalic presentation
   Caesarean section 18.10D
   craniotomy in 18.7
   hydrocephaly 19.7
   in twins 19.11

cephalopelvic disproportion (CPD) 1.14
   in breech delivery 19.8D
   breech presentation, section for 19.8
   Caesarean section for 18.6, 19.8
   cervicograph 18 – 2
   delay in labour due to 18.2
   in diabetes 17.3D, 17.3
   obstructed labour due to 18.3
   oxytocin contraindication 19.3
   symphysiotomy for 18.1, 18.6
   'trial of scar' and 18.14
   vacuum extraction in 18.5
cephalosporins 2.8
cephradine, dosages and route of administration 2.9
cerebral anoxia 17.2
cerebral malaria 17.4
cerebrospinal fluid (CSF)
   drainage, in hydrocephaly 19.7
   leakage in myelomeningocele 28.9
cervical pregnancy 16.2D
cervicitis 6.6
cervicograph 18.2, 18 – 2
cervix
   carcinoma 16.11, 20.2, 20.12, 32 – 21, 32.35
      diagnosis 20.3
      in situ 32.35
      staging 32 – 21
   cone biopsy 32 – 22, 32.35
   dilatation 18 – 2
      Bishop's inducibility score 19.3
      in delay in labour 18 – 2, 18.2
      in evacuating an incomplete abortion 16.2
      incomplete, in breech delivery 19.8D
      in obstructed labour 18.3
      see also dilatation and curretage ('D and C')
   erosion 16.11, 20.14
   eversion 20.14 fibroids
   projecting into 20 – 4
   implantation in 16 – 3, 16.6
   incompetent, diagnosis and suturing 16.5
   injury 16.2D, 20.3
   inspection for tears, method 19.11a
   lacerated, in 'D and C' 20.3D
   painful on movement 16.7
   placenta stuck in, during evacuation 16.2D
   polyp 16.11, 20.6D
      removal 20 – 5, 20.6
   prolapse 19.11aD
   removal in total hysterectomy 20.12
   rigid, in 'D and C' 20.3D
   ripening 19.3
   tear 18.14
      non-removal of cervical sutures 16.5
      repair 18.15, 19.11a, 19 – 11
      in rupture of uterus 18.17
   wedge biopsy 32 – 22, 32.35
'Cetavlon' 2.3
cetrimide 2.3
chalazion 24.10, 24.12
chalazion clamp 24 – 11
chancre, primary 22.7
Charcot's triad 13.6
Charles' operation 31.6, 31 – 6
Charrière gauge, for catheters 23.1, 23 – 1
Cheatle's forceps 2.4
cheek
   fibroepithelial polyp 26.9
   swelling 32.39
chemical, in eye 24.3D
chemotherapy 32.1, 32.2
   advice on use 32.2
   effect on tumour cell population 32 – 1b, 32.2
   effect of varying the interval 32 – 2
   goal 32.1, 32.2
   importance of compliance 32.2
   intravenous injection 32.2
   preparation and monitoring for 32.2
   side-effects and indications 32.2
   WHO tumour categories for 32.2
   see also cytotoxic drugs; individual tumours
chest drain 4 – 12
chest film 1.14
chest infection, after abdominal surgery 9.11
chest physiotherapy 9.11a, 9.11, 9 – 22
chest wall, empyema presenting on 6.1D
childbirth, enlightened methods 34.7
children
   abdominal tuberculosis in 29.6
   abscesses, sites 5 – 1

children (*cont.*)
　abscesses in throat 5 – 6, 5.6, 5.7
　acute abdomen in, causes 10.1
　acute mastoiditis in 25.4
　acute red painful eye 24.3D
　antibiotic dosages 2.9
　appendicitis in 12.1, 12.2D
　backache in 27.8
　bladder stones in 23.16
　blood loss in 3 – 1, 3.1
　Burkitt's lymphoma in 32.3
　Buruli ulcers in 31.2a
　cancer pain relief 33.2
　cancrum oris in 26.6
　chronic osteomyelitis in 7.6D
　congenital hydroceles 14.5, 14 – 15
　electrolytes 28.1
　empyema in 6.1
　eruption cyst 26.9
　fluid requirements 28.1, 28.4
　hydatid cysts 31.13
　inguinal hernias in 14.2, 14.5, 14 – 15
　intestinal obstruction due to *Ascaris* 10.6
　intussusception in 10.8
　meatal strictures in 23.28
　miscellaneous problems 28.11
　nephroblastoma in 32.6
　osteomyelitis 7.2, 7.3, 7.5D
　　of jaw 7.14a
　　pathology 7.2, 7 – 2, 7.16
　painful hip or limp 27.13, 29.3
　poliomyelitis, *see* poliomyelitis
　postoperative complications after abdominal surgery 9.10
　postoperative energy needs 28.1
　proptosis in, causes 24.11
　rectal bleeding in 22.3D
　rectal prolapse in 22.9
　refractive errors in 24.8
　safe times for tourniquet use 3.9
　septic arthritis in 7.16
　spinal tuberculosis in 29.4
　squints in 24.9
　stridor in 25.16
　surgery in 28.1 – 11, 29 – 1
　testing for deafness 25 – 1, 25.2
　tooth extraction 26.3
　tuberculous arthritis differential diagnoses 29.3
　urethral stones in 23.17
　urine volume 28.1
　see also infants; neonates; paediatric surgery
Chlamydia trachomatis 6.6, 24.3D, 24.13
chloramine I 28a.2, 28a – 1a
chloramphenicol 2.8
　dosages, administration route 2.9
　eye drops 24.1, 24.3
　metronidazole with 2.8, 2.9
　in osteomyelitis 7.4
　perioperative 2.6
　resistance to 2.7
chlorhexidine, in antiseptic surgery 2.6 –
chlorhexidine gluconate solution BP ('Hibitane') 2.5
chlorine-releasing compounds 28a – 1a, 28a.2
　recommended dilutions 28a – 1a, 28a.2
chlormethiazole 17.4
chloroquine 17.2, 31.10
chloroquine maculopathy 24.4
chlorpromazine 32.2, 33.2
　in 'lytic cocktail', in pregnancy 17.4
'Chogoria' supports 2.1, 15.3, 15 – 4
choking 25.13
cholangiogram
　intravenous 13.5
　tube 13.4
cholangitis 13.3, 13.4, 31.13D
　caused by *Ascaris* 13.5
　in hydatid disease 32.26
　primary pyogenic (recurrent) 13.6
　recurrent attacks in children 28.11
　secondary 13.6
　signs 13.3
cholecystectomy 13 – 4, 13.7D, 13.7
　dangers in 13.7
cholecystitis 12.2D, 13.2
　acute 10 – 3, 13.1, 13.3
　　non-operative treatment 13.3
　　signs and diagnosis 10.2, 13.3
　acute on chronic (relapsing) 13.3
　amoebic liver abscess vs 31.12

cholecystitis (*cont.*)
　chronic 13.1
cholecystojejunostomy 13.1, 13 – 5, 13.8
　in chronic pancreatitis 13.9
　indications and contraindications 13.8
　in neonates 28.8a
cholecystostomy 13.1, 13 – 1, 13.3, 13.6
choledocal cyst 28.11
choledochoduodenostomy 13.6
choledochojejunostomy 13.4
choledochostomy 13.4
cholesteatoma 25.3D, 25.3
chondroma 32 – 5
chondrosarcoma 32.14
'CHOP' regimen 32.5
chorioamnionitis 19.5
choriocarcinoma 32 – 23, 32.37, 32.38D, 32.38
chorioretinitis 24.7
choroiditis (posterior uveitis) 24.4, 24.5
chromic catgut 4.6
Church hospitals 1.1
chyluria 23.30, 31.6
'Cidex' 2.5
ciliary angle 24 – 1
ciliary body 24 – 1
　inflammation 24.5
ciliary hyperaemia 24.1, 24.3, 30.2
cimetidine 11.1, 11.4D, 11.7
circulation observation chart, inside back cover
circulatory collapse, abdominal pain and distension with 10.4D
circumcision 23.26, 23 – 35
　anaesthesia for 23.26, 23 – 34
　basal, in elephantiasis of penis 31.7, 31 – 8
　difficulties 23.26D
　female 20.13
cirrhosis 29.6, 32.26
　in chronic active hepatitis(CAH) 28a.4
　oesophageal varices 11.5
　plastic abdominal tuberculosis vs 29.7
clamps
　crushing and non-crushing 9.3, 9.5, 9 – 6, 9 – 9
　leaving in wound 3.1
Clark's levels of malignant melanoma invasion 32 – 7, 32.20
clavicle fracture 1.7
clavipectoral fascia 21.6, 21 – 10, 21 – 12
cleanliness, theatre 2.1, 2.3
cleft lip and palate 26.8
cleidotomy 18.7, 18 – 8
clips, towel 4.11
clitoris, torn 18.15
clock, theatre 2.1, 3.1
clogs 2.3
clomiphene 15.2
Cloquet's hernia 14.7
Clostridium perfringens 31.9
Clostridium welchii, Fournier's gangrene due to 23.30
clot retention 23.9D, 23.19D, 23.19, 23.21D
clotting test 34.4
clotting time, in placental abruption 16.13
cloxacillin, in osteomyelitis 7.4
club foot 27.15
'CMF' regimen, in breast carcinoma 21.4
coccyx 22 – 2
cochlea, sensorineural deafness 25.2
codeine phosphate 33.2
Codman's triangle 32.13, 32.14
cold abscess 29.3D, 29.4
'cold' operations 1.7, 1.8
Coles tube 19.12, 19 – 13
colic 10.1, 12.1
　biliary, *see* biliary colic
　renal 10.2, 10 – 3, 12.1, 23.12
　ureteric 10.1, 10 – 1, 13.2, 23.12, 23.14
　urinary tract stones vs 23.12
　see also abdominal pain
colitis
　amoebic, *see* amoebic colitis
　ulcerative 22.2D
collagen, in keloids 34.1a
collar stud abscesses 8 – 1, 8.2, 8.5, 8.8
Colles' fascia 23.10, 23 – 11
Colles' fracture 1.7
colon
　accidental injury, in hysterectomy 20.12D
　acute toxic dilatation 31.11D
　anastomosis to ileum 9.3, 31.11, 32 – 15a, 32.27
　ascending

colon, ascending (*cont.*)
　bleeding from 22.3
　mobilization 10.8
bleeding, in intestinal amoebiasis 31.11D
carcinoma 10.14, 32 – 15a, 32.27
　piles vs 22.4
　plastic abdominal tuberculosis vs 29.7
carcinomatous obstruction, differential diagnosis 10.10
distal, anastomoses, dangers 32 – 15a, 32.27
in invasive intestinal amoebiasis 31.10, 31 – 10, 31.11D, 31.11
necrosis 31.10, 31.11D, 31.11
post-amoebic stricture 31.10, 31.11D
preparation, for resections 32.27
sigmoid, *see* sigmoid colon; sigmoid volvulus
transverse, prolapse 28.6D
colostomy 9.1, 9.5, 9.6D
　bag, improvisation 9 – 16
　in carcinoma of colon and rectum 32 – 15a, 32.27
　closure 10.10
　double-barrelled 9.5, 9 – 14, 10.5, 31.11
　　in carcinoma of colon 32.27
　　extraperitoneal closure 9.5, 9.6, 9 – 19
　　method 9.6, 9 – 19
　end (terminal) 9.5, 9.6
　extraperitoneal closure 9.5, 9.6, 9 – 19
　if does not work 9.6D
　if it 'runs like a river' 9.6D
　ileo-transverse 9.5, 9.6, 31.8
　intraperitoneal closure 9.5, 9.6, 9 – 18
　for intussusception 10.8
　loop 9.5, 9 – 14
　　extraperitoneal closure 9.5, 9.6, 9 – 15
　　intraperitoneal closure 9.6, 9 – 18
　　method 9.6, 9 – 15
　methods and difficulties 9.6D, 9.6
　mucus fistula 9.5
　necrosis 9.6D
　pelvic, in sigmoid volvulus 10.10, 10 – 16
　prolapse 9.6D
　proximal 10.3, 16.2
　sigmoid 9.5, 9.6, 9 – 14, 9 – 15
　spectacles 9.5, 9.6, 9 – 14, 9 – 17
　　method 9.6, 9 – 17
　temporary, in sigmoid volvulus 10.10
　transverse 9.5, 9 – 14
　　in anorectal malformations 28.6D, 28.6
　　method 9.6, 9 – 15
　　in sigmoid volvulus 10.10
　withdrawal back into hole 9.6D
colostrum 21.3
colporrhaphy 20.11aD
　anterior 20.9, 20.11a, 20 – 12
　posterior 20.9, 20.11a, 20 – 12, 20 – 13
Colt's needle 4 – 6
coma, prolonged, in eclampsia 17.4D
common bile-duct
　accidental injury 13.7D
　atresia in neonates 28.8a, 28 – 9a
　carcinoma obstructing 13.8, 32.26a
　complete obstruction 13.6
　exposing 13 – 2, 13.4
　identification in gall-bladder surgery 13.4, 13.7
　injury in cholecystectomy 13.7
　stones in, removal 13 – 2, 13.4
common hepatic duct 13 – 3, 13.7
common peroneal nerve palsy 30.5
Community Health Worker (CHW) 1 – 5, 1.6
Community surgery Preface 5
compartment syndrome Volume Two, Stop Press
conception, surgery of 15.1 – 5
condom catheter 23 – 3
condoms, AIDS prevention 28a.2
condyloma acuminatum 20.13, 22.10
congenital dislocation of hip (CDH) 27.12D, 27.12, 27 – 15
　causes 27.12D
congenital disorders, *see individual disorders*
congenital vascular lesions 28.10, 28 – 11
congestive heart failure 17.2
conjoint tendon 14.2, 14 – 2
　in Bassini repair 14.2, 14 – 6
conjunctiva
　allergic 24.3D
　examination 24.1
　large gelatinous vegetations 24.3D
　red swollen in neonate 24.3D
　thickening 24.15

617

conjunctivitis 24.1, 24.3
　acute infective, treatment 24.3
　bilateral 24.13
　causes 24.3
　chronic follicular 24.13
　chronic low-grade 24.3D
　complications 24.3
　diagnosis and differential diagnosis 24.3
　severe 24.3D
Connell sutures 9.3, 9 – 6, 9 – 9, 9 – 11, 9 – 12, 11 – 6
constipation
　abdominal pain with 10.2
　in cancer, relief 33.2
　in intestinal obstruction 10.1, 10.4, 10.14
　in solitary rectal ulcer 22.10
　in stricture of rectum 22.10
constriction bands of limb 27.17, 27 – 20
consumables, economical use of and savings on 1.12
contraceptive pill, 'combined' 20.2
contraceptives, uterine bleeding related to 20.2
contraction ring
　in Caesarean section 18.10D
　in multiple pregnancies 19.11D
　see also Bandl's ring
contracture 27.2
　active and passive movements 27.2
　assessment 27.2
　casting for 27.2
　　see also plaster cast
　flexion
　　of hip 7.18, 27.2, 27 – 3, 27.4, 27.6
　　range of movement 27.2
　　in tuberculosis 29.3
　general method for 27.2
　in leprosy 30.1a, 30.7, 30 – 9
　manipulation 27.2, 27 – 2
　operative methods 27.2
　in osteomyelitis 7 – 5
　in poliomyelitis, see poliomyelitis
　prevention 27.2
　in pyomyositis 7.1D
　of tendons and nerves 27.2
　traction for 27.2
　treatment 27.2
　see also individual joints
controlled cord traction 19.11a
convulsions, eclamptic 17 – 3, 17.4
Cooper's ligament 14.2, 14.7D, 14.7, 14 – 16
'COP' regimen 32.5
cord, umbilical
　compression 19.10
　cyst 28 – 4
　as presenting part 19.3, 19.10
　prolapse 19.3, 19.10
　　in breech presentation 19.8
　　labour induction and 19.3
　　premature rupture of membranes and 19.5
　　in transverse lie 19.9
　　treatment 19 – 6, 19.10
　　in twins 19.10, 19.11
　traction, controlled 19 – 9, 19.11a
cornea 24 – 7
　anaesthetic, in leprosy 30.2, 30.3
　dendritic ulcer 24.3D, 24 – 7
　examination 24.1, 30.3
　exposed, treatment 24.11
　haziness 24.1, 24.4, 24.6
　in retinoblastoma 32.7
　scars 24.3, 24.4
　sclerosing keratitis in onchocerciasis 24.7
　in trachoma 24.13
　ulcer 24.1, 24.3, 24 – 7
　　diagnosis and treatment 24.3
　　in leprosy 30.3
　staphyloma due to 24.11
　white ring encircling 24.15
　yellowish-white lump adjacent 24.15
corneal light reflex 24.9
cornual block 15.2
corpora cavernosa
　bleeding from 23.9D
　in carcinoma of penis 32.33
　drainage 23.29
corpus luteum
　bleeding 16.6D
　carcinoma 20.3
　cyst 20.7
corpus spongiosum

corpus spongiosum (cont.)
　bleeding 23 – 12
　in carcinoma of penis 32.33
　gonococcal urethral strictures in 23.8
corrosive oesophagitis 24.15D, 25.15, 32.24, 34.5
'Cosmegan' 32.2
cost
　instrument sets 4.12
　surgical care 1.12
　suture materials 4.6
costotransversectomy 7.15, 29 – 3a, 29.4a, 29.4aD
costovertebral angle, pain in 23.12
cotrimoxazole, in mycetoma 31.3
cough
　'anchovy sauce' 31.12D
　in carcinoma of bronchus 32.29
　in carcinoma of oesophagus 32.24
　chronic, rectal prolapse in 22.9
　impulse 14.1, 14.2
　need to, after abdominal surgery 9.11, 9.11a
　in pulmonary atypical African Kaposi's sarcoma 32.21D
Coupland's inclined plane dental elevator 26.3D, 26 – 7
'Couvelaire' uterus 16.13
cover test, squint detection 24.9
coxa vara 27.14
CPD, see cephalopelvic disproportion (CPD)
cranial nerve, in carcinoma of nasopharynx 32 – 16, 32.28
cranial nerve palsies
　in Burkitt's lymphoma 32.3D
　in cavernous sinus thrombosis 5.5, 5 – 5
　see also facial palsy
craniotomy 18.7, 18 – 8, 19.8D
　in obstructed labour 18.4
cranium, osteitis of 7 – 13, 7.14
'crawler', after poliomyelitis 27 – 3, 27.4, 27.6
creatinine, in pregnancy 17.6
cremasteric artery 14.2
crepe bandaging, snake bites 34.4
cresol and soap solution BP ('Lysol') 2.5
cricopharyngeus muscle, in oesophagoscopy 25 – 10, 25.14
Criles forceps 3 – 2, 3.2
crithyroid suction 9.11
Crohn's disease 22.2D, 29.7
crushing clamp 9.3, 9.5, 9 – 6, 9-9
　if unavailable 9.6
crutches 27.5
culdocentesis 6.6D, 16 – 6, 16.7
culture of patients 1.2, 1.5
　attitude to surgery 1.8
　maternal mortality questions 15.1D
curettage, during 'D and C', see dilatation and curettage('D' and 'C')
curette, uterine 15.1a, 15 – 2
Cusco's duckbill speculum 15.1a, 15 – 2
cyanosis 9.11, 17.4D
cyclitis 24.5
cyclopentolate 24.1
cyclophosphamide 21.4, 32.2, 32.5
　in Burkitt's lymphoma 32.3
　excretion in urine 32.3
cyst
　benign bone 27.17
　breast 21.3
　dental 26.7
　dermoid, see dermoid cyst
　of jaw 26.7
　marsupializing 20.7D, 26.7, 26 – 11
　　Bartholin's 20 – 2, 20.4
　of mouth 26.9, 26 – 13
　sebaceous 34.3
　tarsal 5.4, 24.10, 24 – 11, 24.12
cystadenocarcinoma 20.7
　in pregnancy 20.7D
　pseudomucinous 20 – 6
cystadenoma 20.7
　diagnosis and management 20.7
　in pregnancy 20.7D
　serous 20 – 7, 20.7
cystadenoma phylloides 21.3
cystectomy
　in carcinoma of bladder 32.31
　ovarian 20.7, 20 – 8
cystic artery 13 – 3, 13.7
　bleeding in cholecystectomy 13.7D
　identification 13.7
cystic duct

cystic duct (cont.)
　accidental injury 13.7D
　anatomy 13 – 3, 13.7
　identification 13.7
　stone impacted 13.2, 13.8
cystic hygroma 28.10, 28 – 11
cystitis
　haemorrhagic 32.3
　in pregnancy 17.6
　in urogenital tuberculosis 29.9
cystocele 20 – 9
　anterior colporrhaphy for 20 – 12, 20.11(a)
cystogastrostomy, for pancreatic pseudocysts 13.10
cystoscope 23.3, 23 – 4
　in bleeding peptic ulcer 11.4
　introducing 23.3
　sterilization and testing 23.3
cystoscopy 23.3
　in benign prostatic hypertrophy 23 – 23
　bladder appearance 23.3
　in carcinoma of bladder 23.4, 32 – 17, 32.31
　in haematuria 23.3, 23.4
　if nothing seen initially 23.3
　indications 23.3
　prostate appearance 23.18
　in prostatic obstruction 23.18
　in urogenital tuberculosis 29.9
cystostomy, suprapubic, see suprapubic cystostomy
cytotoxic drugs 32.2D, 32.2
　in breast carcinoma 21.4
　choice and complications 32.2
　infections after 32.2D, 32.2
Czerny's retractor 4 – 4, 4.5

D
'D and C', see dilatation and curettage ('D and C')
dacryoadenitis 5.5D
dacryocystitis 5.5D, 24.10
'Dactinomycin' 32.2
dactylitis 7.3
dapsone, in mycetoma 31.3
deafness 25.2D, 25.2
　in acute mastoiditis 25.4
　chronic otitis media 25.3D
　conductive 25.2
　examination 25 – 1, 25.2
　foreign bodies in ear 25.5
　incidence and causes 25.2
　management and prevention 25.2
　progressive with vertigo 25.16
　senorineural 25.2
death, approach to 1.1, 1.5, 33.1
see also dying patients
Deaver's retractor 4 – 4, 4.5
decapitation 18.7, 18 – 9, 18 – 10
decidual cast 16.7
decircumcision 20.13
decompression, gut
　avoidance if nonviable 10.9
　in intestinal obstruction 10.5, 10 – 9
　retrograde 10.5
decortication, in empyema 6 – 1a, 6.1
deep veins of leg 34.1, 34 – 1
deep vein thrombosis 7.1, 9.9, 34.1
defaecation, physiology 22 – 1
dehiscence, wound 9.2, 9.13, 9 – 24
dehydration
　after abdominal surgery 9.10
　correction before abdominal surgery 9.1
　in infants, fluid requirements 28.1, 28.4
　in intestinal obstruction 10.1, 10.4, 10.5
　levels of, signs and fluid replacement 10.5, 28.4
　in obstructed labour 18.4
　passing nasogastric tube 4.9D
dehydroemetine 31.10
delayed primary closure 2.3, 2.7, 2.10
　abdomen 9.8, 9.12
　traumatic osteomyelitis prevention 7.2
de Lee incision 18.8, 18.9, 19.9
delivery
　in anaemic patient 17.2
　breech, see breech presentation; breech delivery
　in brow presentations 19.9
　of diabetic mother 17.3
　face presentation 19.9
　in gestational hypertension 17.4
　high blood pressure after 17.4D
　in hospitals 15.1a
　of mother in heart failure 17.5D, 17.5
　in obstructed labour 18.4, 18 – 4

delivery (cont.)
    operative vaginal, anaesthesia for 18.1a
    outlet forceps, in obstructed labour 18.4
    in placental abruption 16.13
    in *placenta praevia* 16.12
    in transverse lie 19.9
    tubal ligation after 15.3
    twins 19.11
    vaginal 16.12, 17.4, 18.4, 19.8
    see also Caesarean section
dendritic ulcer of cornea 24.3D, 24 – 7
Dennis Browne crucifix 28 – 3, 28.4
Dennis Browne forceps 4.4
Dennis Browne's retractor 4 – 4, 4.5
dental abscess 5 – 7, 5.8
    Ludwig's angina from 5 – 8, 5.8, 5.10
dental cyst 26.7
dental extraction 5.8
dental hygiene 26.1, 26.2, 26 – 2
dental sinus 26.3D, 26.7, 26 – 8
dental surgery 26.1 – 8
    equipment 26.1, 26 – 1, 26.3, 26 – 3
    miscellaneous problems 26.9
dentigerous cyst 26.7
dentistry, preventive 26.2, 26 – 2
de Pezzer catheter 23.6
de Quervain's disease 21.13, 27.10
dermatitis, ammoniacal 18.18
dermoid cyst 20.7, 34.3
    causing proptosis 24.11
    excision, after circumcision 20.13, 20 – 24
    ovarian 20.7D, 20.7
    sublingual 26.9, 26 – 13
Desjardin's stone forceps 4.4, 13.3, 13.4
destructive methods for eye 24.14D, 24.14, 24 – 14, 24 – 15
destructive operations 18.1, 18.4, 18.7, 18 – 8, 19.8D
    in obstructed labour 18.4
    in transverse lie 19.9
detrusor muscle failure 23.5, 23.9D
    hypertrophy 23.8
developing countries, common diseases 1.4
developmental cysts, of jaw 26.7
deworming, after intestinal obstruction 10.6
Dextran 28a.2
dextropropoxyphene 33.2
dextrose, administration to children 28.1
diabetes mellitus
    Fournier's gangrene in 23.30
    in pregnancy 17.3, 19.13
        delivery 17.3
        diagnosis and symptoms 17 – 1a, 17.3
        management 17.3
    urinary retention in 23.5
diabetic precoma 10.2, 10 – 4
diagonal conjugate 18.14
diaphragm, pain from 10 – 1
diaphyseal achalasia 27.17
diarrhoea 32.4D
    after peritonitis 6.2D
    in AIDS 28a.2
    in amoebiasis 31.10
    due to cytotoxic drugs 32.2D, 32.2
    in gastroenteritis, appendicitis vs 12.1
    in intussusception 10.4, 10.8
    in pelvic abscess 6.5, 9.10
    in pigbel disease 22.3D, 31.9
    postoperative, after intestinal obstruction 10.5D
    rectal prolapse with 22.9
    in Richter's hernia 14.1
    in stricture of rectum 22.10
    in typhoid perforation 31.8D
diathermy 9.2
diazepam in pregnancy 17.4D, 17.4
diesel 1.12
diet
    after abdominal surgery 9.9
    high-fibre 10.10
    high-residue, for piles 22.4
    restricted carbohydrate 17.3
difficulties, in manuals 1.14D
digital nerves, avoidance in hand infection operations 8.1, 8 – 6, 8.12
digital tonometry 24.1
digoxin, in pregnancy 17.5
dilatation, without curettage 20.3
dilatation and curettage ('D and C') 15.2, 20 – 1, 20.3
    after intrauterine death 16.4

dilatation and curettage (cont.)
    in carcinoma of endometrium 32.35
    in dysfunctional uterine bleeding 20.2, 20.3
    indications 20.3
    small submucous fibroid in 20.6D
    standard method 20.3
dilators, cervical 15.1a, 15 – 2
diloxanide furoate 31.10
dinoprosterone 19.3, 19.2
diplopia 24.9
director, hernia 4.11
disability 1.1
disinfectants 2.5
    economical use of and savings on 1.12
    for human immunodeficiency virus (HIV) 28a – 1a, 28a.2
    limitations 2.5
disinfection 2.4
    prevention of spread of AIDS 28a.2, 28a – 1a
disposables, economical use of and savings on 1.12
dissecting manuals 1.14
dissectors 4.2
disseminated intravascular coagulation(DIC) 16.4D, 16.13
    postpartum haemorrhage 19.11a, 19.11aD
'Distalgesic' 33.2
distal interphalangeal joint(DIP) 1.14
distraction test 25 – 1, 25.2
district hospital Prefaces 1, 2, 4, 6, 1.2
    cancer treatment 32.1
    concept of 'quality' in 1.1, 1.7
    financial management 1.12
    indicators of 'quality' 34.6, 34.7
    need for surgical care 1.1
    obstetrics, indicators of 'quality' 34.7
    possible conditions in 1.2
    problems in 1.2
    referral from, *see* referral; referral system
    supplies 1.2
district hosptial, size 1.2
diuresis, recovery 23.5, 23.9D
diverticulitis 1.9
donovanosis 20.13, 32.35a
    carcinoma of penis vs 32.33
dorsiflexors of ankle, weakness 27.8
'double bubble' in duodenal atresia 28.2, 28 – 2
doxorubicin 32.2D, 32.2
Doyen's raspiratory 6 – 2
drain, with underwater seal 6 – 1, 6.1, 9.2D
drainage 4.10, 9.8
    abdomen 6.2, 9.8
    abscesses 4.10, 5.1, 5 – 2, 5.2
    in acute pelvic inflammatory disease (PID) 6.6
    appendix abscess 12.1, 12 – 3
    empyema, closed and open 6 – 1a, 6.1
    indications 4.10
    pelvic abscess 6.5, 6 – 7
    in peritonitis 6.2
    postural 9.11a, 9 – 23
    in pyomyositis 7.1
    in subphrenic abscess 6.4
drains 4.10
    antiseptics and disinfectants for 2.5
    autoclaving 2.5
    corrugated rubber 4.10, 4 – 12
    removing 4.10
drapes 2.3D
    sterilization 2.6
    in tubal ligations 15.3
draping, operation site 2.3
dressing boxes 2.4
dressings
    autoclaving 2.4
    in chronic osteomyelitis 7.6
    ear, nose and throat 25.1
    economical use of and savings on 1.12
    if in short supply 4.10
    wet after autoclaving 2.4D
    wound sepsis and 2.3, Stop Press
dressing trays
    antiseptics for 2.5
    autoclaving 2.4
drip stands 2.1
drugs
    cancer pain relief 33.2
    economical use of and savings on 1.12
    eye disorders 24.1
    pain relief, plasma levels for 33 – 3
    tolerance and dependance 33.2

drums, for autoclaving 2.4
Dukes staging method 32.27
duodenal atresia 28.2, 28 – 2, 28.3
    anastomoses in neonates 28 – 2, 28.3
duodenal mucosa, if opened in Ramstedt's operation 28.4
duodenal stenosis, in neonates 28.2
duodenal ulcer 3.10, 11.1
    bleeding 11.4
    chronic 11.1, 11.6, 11.7
    perforated 11 – 11, 11.2
    pyloric stenosis due to 11.6
    rectal bleeding due to 22.3
    see also peptic ulcer
duodenojejunostomy 28 – 2
duodenum
    barium meal 34.5
    bleeding from 22.3
    bleeding point in, obscured 11.4D
    exposure 11.2
    fibrosis and scarring 11.4, 11.6
    obstruction, in neonates 28.2, 28 – 2, 28.3
    opening, in bleeding peptic ulcer surgery 11.4
dust, in theatres 2.10
'dust in the feet' 31.5
Duval's forceps 4 – 3, 4.4
dying patients
    attitudes to 1.1, 1.5, 33.1
    care 33.1 – 2
    investigation to exclude curable conditions 33.1
    symptom palliation 33.1, 33.2
    what and when to tell him 33.1
    where to treat him 33.1
dysentery, amoebic 31.10, 31.11
dysfunctional uterine bleeding(DUB) 16.7, 20.2
    causes 20.2
    diagnosis and treatment 20.2, 20.3
    functional cyst associated with 20.7
    hysterectomy for 20.12
    investigations 20.2, 20.3
dyskinesia (bladder neck obstruction) 23.5D, 23.20
dysmenorrhoea, avoid 'D and C' in 20.3
dyspareunia, decircumcision for 20.13
dyspepsia 11.2
    in carcinoma of stomach 32.25
    causes 32.25
    non-ulcer, carcinoma of stomach vs 32.25
dysphagia 25.16
    in carcinoma of oesophagus 32.24
    in colloid goitre 21.11
    in corrosive oesophageal strictures 25.15
    progressive with stridor and cough 25.16
dyspnoea
    in colloid goitre 21.7, 21.11
    on exertion 25.16
    in extraintestinal amoebiasis 31.12D
    foreign body in throat 25.13
    in pulmonary atypical African Kaposi's sarcoma 32.21D
dystocia 18.3
dysuria 10.1

E
ear 25.1 – 5
    disorders 25.16
    external, conductive deafness 25.2
    fluid level or bubbles in 25.3D
    foreign bodies in 25 – 4, 25.5
    insect in 25.5D
    inspissated wax 25.4
    middle, deafness 25.2
    see also deafness; *specific disorders*
earache
    normal ear – drum with 25.3D
    in otitis media 25.3D, 25.3
ear-drum perforation 25.2
    in acute otitis media 25.3
    foreign bodies in ear 25.5D, 25.5
ear, nose and throat 25.1 – 16
    equipment 25.1
    miscellaneous problems 25.16
East Africa, need for surgical care 1.1
Echinococcus granulosus 31.13
eclampsia
    after delivery 17.4D, 17.4
    management 17.4
    signs 17.4
    warning signs 17.4D
eclamptic fit 17 – 2, 17.4
economical surgery and savings 1.12

ectopic pregnancy 6.6
  abdominal 16 – 3, 16.6, 16.9
  acute or subacute 16 – 3, 16.6D, 16.6
    diagnosis 16.6
    resuscitation 16.6
    surgery for 16 – 5, 16.6
  angular 16.8
  appendicitis vs 12.1
  bleeding in 10.1, 16.6, 16.7D, 16.7
  cervical 16.8
  chronic 6.5, 16.6, 16 – 6a, 16.7
    difficulties 16.2D, 16.7D
    diagnosis 16.6
  ruptured 6.6D, 6.6, 10 – 3, 16.6
    during 'D and C' 20.3D
    signs and diagnosis 10.2
  subacute rupture 16.6
  without massive abdominal bleeding 16.7
eczema, chronic, of nipple 21.3
EIT (examination in the theatre) 1.14, 16.12
ejaculate, examination after vasectomy 15.5
elapids 34.4
elastic stockings 31.5, 34.1
elbow
  aspirating and exploring 7.17
  positions of rest and of function 7 – 16, 7.17
  tuberculosis of 29.3
electricity, savings on 1.12
electrolyte
  imbalance, small gut obstruction 10.4
  replacement in children 28.1
  see also potassium
elephantiasis 23.8, 23.9D, 31.4
  differential diagnosis 31.4
  filarial 31 – 5, 31.6
  non-filarial endemic 31.4, 31.5
  of penis 31.7, 31 – 8
  podoconiosis 31 – 3, 31 – 4, 31.5
  scrotum 31.4, 31 – 5, 31.7, 31 – 7
EMA-Co, in metastasizing trophoblastic neoplasm 32.38
embryotomy 18.7
emergency surgery 11.4
  procedures 1.14
  rule in 11.2
empyema 6.1, 6.4, 24.14D, 29.4
  in children 6.1
  closed drainage 6 – 1a, 6.1
  failure to heal 6.1D
  gall-bladder 10.2, 13.3
  if air comes out with pus 6.1D
  open drainage 6.1
  tuberculous 6.1D
empyema necessitans 6.1D
endocarditis, prevention 17.5
endometriosis 6.6D
endometritis 6.6
  tuberculous 15.2, 20.3
endometrium, carcinoma of 20.2, 20.3, 32 – 21, 32.35
endomyocardial fibrosis(EMF) 6.1a
endophthalmitis 24.3
enema
  barium 10.4, 34.5, 34 – 11
  soap and water 22.1
energy
  postoperative needs in children 28.1
  saving on 1.12
Entamoeba histolytica 31 – 10, 31.10, 31.12
enteritis necroticans 31.9
entero – enterostomy 10.7D
enterotomy 9.3, 10.6
entropion 24.10, 24.13
  radical eyelash excision 24 – 12, 24.13
  tarsal eversion 24.13, 24 – 13
'Epanutin' (phenytoin), in pregnancy 17.4
ephedrine nose drops 25.7, 25.9
epicondylitis 27.9
epidermoid cyst 24.11, 25.3
epididymis
  swelling 23.9D, 23.22a
  torsion 14.2, 23.24D, 23 – 31
  tuberculous 29.9
epididymitis, schistosomal 23.22a
epididymo-orchitis 23.22a
  acute 23.9D
  acute gonococcal 23.22a
  chronic 23.22a
  differential diagnosis 23.22a
  management 23.22a

epididymo-orchitis (*cont.*)
  torsion of testis vs 23.24
epidural anaesthesia 17.5, 18.1a, 19.8
epigastric artery, superficial 3.7
epigastric hernia 14.9, 14.12, 14 – 22
epigastric pain 13.2
  in acute pancreatitis 13.9
  in peptic ulcers 11.2, 11.3
  see also abdominal pain
epigastric vessel, bleeding, after symphysiotomy 18.6D
epiglottitis, acute 25.16
epileptic convulsion, *grand mal*, in eclampsia 17.4
epiphora 24.10
epiphyseal plate, spread of infection prevention 7.2, 7 – 2, 7.16
episiotomy 1.7
  after circumcision 20.13
  in assisted breech delivery 19.8
  local anaesthesia for 18.1a
  in obstructed labour 18.4
  in preterm labour 19.4
  repair 18.15
epistaxis 3.1, 22.3, 25 – 5, 25.6
  anterior and posterior packing 25 – 5, 25.6
  difficulties 25.6D
epithelioma 32.19
Epstein-Barr virus 32.3, 32.28
epulis 26.9, 26 – 12
  fibrous or granulomatous 26.9
equinus deformity 27.2, 27.4, 27.7
  closed Achilles tenotomy 27.7D, 27.7, 27 – 10
  in leprosy 30.6D, 30.6
  manipulation 27.2, 27 – 2, 27.7
  in neonatal talipes equinovarus 27.15
  open Achilles tenotomy 27.7, 27 – 11
  recurrence, closed Achilles tenotomy 27.7D
  serial casting for 27.4, 27.7
  subcutaneous Achilles tenotomy 27.7
equipment 1.2, 1.7, 4.1 – 12
  caring for 35 – 1, 35 – 2
  disinfection in AIDS prevention 28a.2
  improvisation 4.1
  miscellaneous 4.11
  neonatal resuscitation 19.12
  obstetric 15.1a, 15 – 2
  ordering, quantities needed 4.1
  in rule about deciding when to operate 1.8
  summary of requirements 35(Appendix A)
  suppliers 1.14, 4.1, 35(Appendix B)
  see also *individual operations*; instruments
ergometrine
  bleeding after delivery of dead baby 16.4D
  in hydatidiform mole 32.38
  in incomplete abortion 16.2
  in lower segment Caesarean section 18.9
  with oxytocin, see 'Syntometrine'
  postpartum haemorrhage prevention 19.11a
  in uncomplicated inevitable abortions 16.2
eruption cyst 26.9
erythema nodosum leprosum (ENL) 30.1a
erythrocyte sedimentation rate (ESR) 29.4
erythroplakia 32.22
Esmarch's bandage 3.9, 3 – 11
Estes procedure 14.2
ethambutol, in tuberculosis 29.1
ethanol, HIV and HBV destruction 28a – 1a, 28a.2
ethinyl oestradiol, in breast carcinoma 21.4
ethmoiditis, acute 24.11
etoposide 32.2, 32.38
EUA, see examination under anaesthesia
eustachian tube, obstruction 32.28
evaluation of quality in district hospitals 34.6 – 7
Everett's method of closing abdomen 9 – 1, 9.8
evisceration
  eye 24.3, 24.14, 24 – 14
  fetus 18.7
Ewing's tumour 32.16
examination in theatre (EIT) 1.14
  in *placenta praevia* 16.12
examination under anaesthesia (EUA) 1.14
  prostate 23.18, 32.32
excreta, infection in theatre from 2.3
exomphalos 28.8
exostosis 7 – 5, 27.17
expenditure, hospital 1.12
expiratory stridor, after abdominal surgery 9.11
exteriorization 9.5

exteriorization (*cont.*)
  in carcinoma of colon and rectum 32 – 15a, 32.27
  in intestinal obstruction 10.5D, 10.5
  in intussusception 10.8
  in invasive intestinal amoebiasis 31.11
  in sigmoid volvulus 10.10, 10 – 16
  in strangulated obstructions 10.5
external cardiac compression, neonates 19.12, 19 – 14
external carotid artery, tying 3.3, 3 – 5
external cephalic version(ECV) 19 – 2, 19.8
  contraindications 19.8
  prolapse 19.9
  risks of 19.8
  in twins 19 – 8, 19.11
external iliac artery, exposing and tying 3.6, 3 – 8
external meatus
  stone in 23.17, 23 – 22
  strictures 23.27, 23.28, 23 – 38
external oblique aponeurosis 14.2, 14 – 2
external sphincter ani, closure, after third-degree tears 18.15
extradural abscess 5.4a, 7.14
extraperitoneal abscess, signs 10.2
extraperitoneal tissues, carbon dioxide into 15.4D
extrauterine pregnancy 16 – 7, 16.9
eye 23.1 – 15
  acute red painful 24.1, 24.3D, 24.3, 24.5
    causes 24.3
    in child 24.3D
    glaucoma vs 24.3, 24.6D, 24.6
  anatomy 24 – 1
  basic equipment 24.1, 24.2
  bleeding from 24.2
  blind painful 24.14, 24.15
  chemical in 24.3D
  cobra venom in 34.4D
  concern over 24.15
  destructive methods 24.14D, 24.14, 24 – 14, 24 – 15
    refusal 24.14D
  drops 24.1
  enucleation 24.14, 24 – 15, 32.7
  evisceration 24.3, 24.14, 24 – 14
  examination 24.1, 30.2
    baby's 24 – 6
  exenteration 24.14, 32.7
  foreign body in 24.1, 24.3
  general method for 24.1
  infections 5.5, 5 – 5, 24.3, 24.13
  in leprosy 30.2
  miscellaneous problems 24.15
  movements, examination 24.1
  neuromuscular system of, disease 24.9
  operating on 24.2, 24 – 5
  outer, examination 24.1
  pad 24.1, 24 – 5
  painful watering 24.3D
  shield 24.1, 24 – 5
  speculum insertion 24.2, 24 – 5
  tumours of 24 – 10, 24.11
  watering 24.10
  white, loss of vision in 24.4
eyelash excision, radical 24 – 12, 24.13
eyelid
  black slough on, in anthrax 24.3D
  diseases of 24.10
  everting 24.2, 24 – 5
  lower, swelling below medial aspect 5.5D
  normal 24 – 13
  oedema and erythema 5.5
  papillae and follicles 24.13
  suture 24.2, 24 – 5
  in trachoma 24 – 13, 24.13

F
face, capillary cavernous haemangioma 28.10, 28 – 11
face presentation 19.9
facial artery and vein 5 – 7a, 5.8
facial features, in acute abdomen 10.1
facial nerve 5 – 7a, 5.8
facial pain, in sinusitis 25.7
facial palsy
  due to foreign bodies in ear 25.5
  in leprosy 30.1a, 30.2, 30.3, 30.9
  in otitis media 25.3D, 25.3
  in salivary gland tumours 32.23
facial sepsis 5.5

620

faecal continence 22.1
faecal fistula
  after inguinal hernia reapir 14.3D
  after peritonitis 6.2D, 6.2
  due to paraumbilical hernia 14.11D
  irreducible inguinal hernia 14.6D
  strangulated inguinal hernias 14.6D, 14 – 13
faecal impaction 10.4, 10.14
  after anal operations 22.1
  in Thiersch's operation 22.9
faecal incontinence, see incontinence, faecal
faeces, discharge from wound, after peritonitis 6.2D
faecoliths 12.1, 12 – 3
failure, surgical 1.8
fallibility of medical practice 1.9
Fallopian tube 15 – 6
  acutely inflamed 6.6D, 16.6D
  blood supply 16.6D
  difficulty in finding
    ectopic pregnancies 16.6D
    laprocator use 15.4D
    minilap 15.3D
  in hernial sac 14.3D
  identification in laparoscopic ligation 15.4
  implantation sites 16 – 3, 16.6
  insufflation 15.2
  ligation 15.3, 16.7
  patency determination 15.2
  removal 20.12, 20.7, 20.12
  ruptured in ectopic pregnancy 16 – 4, 16 – 5, 16.6
  see also ectopic pregnancy
  stuck to broad ligament or ovary 16.6D
  tying 15.3, 16.7
'Fansidar' in pregnancy 17.2D, 17.2
Faraboef's rougine 6 – 2, 7.2, 7 – 3
feeding, difficulties after abdominal surgery 9.10
feeding jejunostomy 5.10b, 9.7, 9.10, 9 – 20
femoral artery
  avoidance, Bassini repair of hernia 14.2
  caution in block dissection 32.34D, 32.34
  exposing and tying 3.7, 3 – 9
femoral canal 14.8, 14 – 18
  dilatation, femoral hernia repair 14.8D, 14.8
femoral epiphysis
  avascular necrosis 27.14
  displacement 7 – 14, 7.16
  upper, slipped 7 – 17, 7.18, 27.13, 29.3
femoral hernia 10.1, 14.2, 14.7, 14 – 16, 14 – 17
  anatomy 14.7
  hernial sac, if cannot return contents 14.7D
  strangulated 10.4, 14.8, 14 – 18
    difficulties 14.8D, 14.8
  unstrangulated 14.7D, 14.7
femoral nerve 3.6, 3.7
  caution in block dissection 32.34
femoral region, lump in 14.8
femoral valve 34.1, 34 – 1
  incompetent 34.1, 34 – 1
femoral vein 3.7, 14.7, 14.8, 14 – 18
  caution in block dissection 32.34D, 32.34
  if needle through 14.3D
femur
  break in chronic polio 27.4D
  cystic lesion 27.17
  exposing 7 – 9
  fractures, fixation, osteomyelitis due to 7.2
  head
    destruction in tuberculosis 29.3
    flattened in Perthes' disease 27.14, 27 – 16
    neck, osteomyelitis 7 – 2, 7.2, 7.3, 7.10, 7.16
    osteomyelitis 7.10, 27.13
ferrous sulphate 17.2
fertility, age – specific 15.1
fertility service 15.2
fetal death 16.1, 16.4
  in abdominal pregnancy 16.9
  at term or during labour 16.4
  in breech delivery, extraction 19.8D, 19.8
  Caesarean section for 18.10D
  destructive operations, see destructive operations
  extrauterine pregnancy 16.9
  if not sure of 16.4D
  oxytocin-induced labour 18.4a
  in placental abruption 16.13
  in placenta praevia 16.12
  in severe gestational hypertension 17.4
  in transverse lie 19.9

fetal death (cont.)
  see also intrauterine death; perinatal mortality
fetal distress
  monitoring for 18.4
  in obstructed labour 18.3
  vacuum extraction indication 18.5
fetal head, height of 18.4
fetal heartbeat 16.4
fetal heart detector 15.1a
fetal maturity, surfactant test 19 – 1, 19.2
fetal movements, stopped 16.4
fetus
  hopelessly malformed 19.7
  implantation sites 16 – 3, 16.6
  in peritoneal cavity 18.17
fever
  acute osteomyelitis diagnosis 7.3, 7 – 4, 7.16
  after abdominal surgery 9.10
  Pel – Ebstein 32.4
fibrinogen 3.1, 16.13
  deficiency 19.11a
fibrinolysis 16.13
fibroadenoma 21.3, 21 – 3, 21.3
  giant 21.3, 21.5D, 21 – 9
  pathology 21 – 4
  removal 21.3, 21.4, 21 – 6
  'shelling out' 21.3, 21.5, 21 – 6
fibroadenosis 21.3
fibrocystic disease 21.3, 28.2
fibroepithelial polyp, cheek 26.9
fibroid 16.2D, 16.7, 20.6, 20.12
  in Caesarean section 18.10D
  calcification in 23.15
  cervical 18.4, 18 – 5, 20 – 4
  difficulties 20.6D
  ectopic pregnancy vs 16.6
  functional cyst associated with 20.7
  impacted 23.5
  intramural 20 – 4
  mobile degenerating 20.6
  painful 20.6D
  pedunculated submucous 20.6
  submucous, subserous 20 – 4
  surgical pathology 20 – 4, 20.6
fibroma 20.7
  oral cavity 26 – 12
fibrosarcoma 32.10
fibula
  exposing 7 – 11
  hypertrophy 7.11D
  osteomyelitis 7 – 11, 7.12
fifth cranial nerve, in leprosy 30.2, 30.3
filariasis 21.3D
  diagnosis 31.4
  hydroceles 23.23
  lymphatic obstruction 31.4
  surgery 31.6
fimbria, implantation in 16 – 3, 16.6
fimbrial block 15.2
financial management, hospitals 1.12
finger
  absorption 30 – 2
  amputation 8.16
  apical space, infections 8 – 2, 8.3
  deformed in leprosy 30.4
  dorsum, infections on 8.11
  extra 27.17
  flexor surface crack in leprosy 30.4
  flexor tendons, stenosing tenosynovitis 27.10
  fusion 27.17
  human bite 8 – 9, 8.15, 8.16
  infections of spaces over volar surfaces 8.6
  osteomyelitis 8.5D, 8.16
  pulp space 8 – 2
    abscess in 8.5
    discharge continuing from 8.5D
    infections 8 – 2, 8.2, 8 – 3, 8.5
  septic arthritis 8 – 8, 8.15
  stiff 8.1
  swollen, tendon sheath infection 8.1
  tourniquet 3.9, 3 – 12
  trigger 27.10
  web space infections 8 – 5, 8 – 6, 8.7
first aid, snake bites 34.4
'fish', in abdominal closure 9.8D, 10.5, 10 – 9
fish bones 25.13
fist percussion test 10.1, 10 – 2
fistula
  after gonococcal urethral strictures 23.9D, 23 – 10

fistula (cont.)
  after removal of bladder stone 23.15D
  in anal canal 5.13
  in anorectal malformations 28.6D, 28.6
  formation, mechanisms 18 – 24
  intestinal 1.6, 9.14, 9 – 25
  in obstructed labour 18.3
  tuberculous 29.5
  'watering can perineum' 23.9D, 23 – 10
  see also anorectal fistulae; faecal fistula; other specific fistulae; urinary fistula
fits
  causes in pregnancy 17.4
  eclamptic 17 – 2, 17.4D, 17.4
flail limb 27.4
flatus
  after abdominal surgery 9.10, 10.13
  not passed, due to obstruction 10.10, 10.13
flatus tube 10.10, 10 – 15, 34.5, 34 – 11
flexion contracture, see contracture, flexion
flexor carpi radialis 7.8, 7 – 8
flexor pollicis longus, tendon sheath of 8.14
flexor retinaculum 8 – 6
  in carpal tunnel syndrome 27.11a
  division 8 – 6, 8.12
  swelling above 8.13, 8.14
flexor tendon sheath 8 – 6
  avoidance in hand infection operations 8.1
  incisions for and exposing 8 – 6, 8 – 7
  infection 8 – 7, 8.12
    if grey slough 8.12
  irrigating 8 – 7
fluctuation 5.1, 5.2, 8.9
fluid
  in abdominal cavity, colour 9.2, 10.5, 11.2, 12.2D
  balance in eclampsia 17.4
  dry and wet regimes 17.4
  daily losses 10.5
  importance, after urinary tract stones 23.12, 23.14
  intoxication, with oxytocin 16.4, 18.4a, 19.3
  irrigating, Freyer's transvesical prostatectomy 23.19
  loss in intestinal obstruction 10.4, 10 – 19
  overload, in eclampsia 17.4D, 17.4
  replacement
    after abdominal surgery 9.9, 9.10,
    in acute cholecystitis 13.3
    after abdominal surgery 9.9, 9.10
    in cholecystojejunostomy 13.8
    in gestational hypertension 17.4D, 17.4
    in intestinal obstruction 10.5
    levels of dehydration 10.5, 28.4
    in pyloric stenosis 11.6
    in recovery diuresis 23.5
    in typhoid 31.8
  requirement
    children, neonates 28.1, 28.3, 28.4
    in hypertrophic pyloric stenosis 28.4
fluorescein 24.1
5 – fluorouracil 21.4, 32.2
folate deficiency anaemia 17 – 1, 17.2
Foley catheter 23.1, 23 – 1
  in bladder after prostatectomy 23 – 23, 23 – 26
  in bleeding oesophageal varices 11.5
  in extra-amniotic space, cervix ripening 19.3
  in Ghadvi's prostatectomy 23.21
  if balloon will not deflate 23.2D
  insertion of posterior nasal pack 25.6
  prostaglandin administration, intrauterine death 16.4
  two and three channels 23.19, 23 – 26
use, in intestinal obstruction 10.5
folic acid supplements 17.2
follicular cyst 20.7
food bolus, impaction 10.14
foot
  anaesthetic in leprosy, see leprosy
  club 27.15
  collapsed arches 30 – 4, 30.5, 30.6D, 30 – 6, 30.6
  disintegrated in leprosy 30 – 4, 30.5
  dorsiflexed 27.15
  drop 30 – 4, 30.5
    appliances for 27.5
    exercises 30.5
    tibialis transfer 30.8D, 30.8, 30 – 10, 30 – 11
  equinus, see equinus deformity
  inverted 30.6D

foot (cont.)
   mycetoma 31 – 2, 31.3
   osteitis 8.17
   osteomyelitis 8.17
   in podoconiosis 31 – 3, 31.5
   pus in 8.17
   'rocker bottom' 27.15
   septic arthritis 8.17
   short, in leprosy 30.6D, 30.6
   sole, malignant melanoma 32 – 7, 32.20
   ulcers in leprosy, see leprosy
foot-drop-positioning splint 30.8, 30 – 10
footling 19.8, 19.11
footprint mat 30.5
footware, in leprosy 30 – 4, 30.5, 30 – 5
foramen caecum 21.9, 21 – 13
forceps 4 – 3, 4.4, 35(Appendix A)
   aural 25.1
   bone cutting and holding 7.2, 7 – 3
   dental 26.1, 26 – 1, 26.3, 26 – 3
   dissecting (thumb) 4 – 3, 4.4
   for head, in breech delivery 19 – 4, 19.8
   obstetric 15.1a, 18.1
   ovum 15.1a, 15 – 2
   sequestrum 7.2, 7 – 3
   sponge-holding 4.11
   sterilizers 2.4
   tissue (locking) 4 – 3, 4.4
forceps delivery 18.1a, 18.4, 19 – 4, 19.8
forearm extensor muscles, tears 27.9
forefoot
   adduction deformity 27.2, 27 – 2, 27.4
   splayed 31.5
foreign body
   in ear 25.5D, 25.5
      removal 25 – 4, 25.5
   in eye 24.1, 24.3
   failure of empyema to heal 6.1D
   in foot 8.17
   intestinal obstruction due to 10.14
   in larynx 25.12
   negative X-rays? 25.11, 25.12
   in nose 25.11
   in oesophagus 25 – 10, 25.14
      too large for removal 24.14D
   sequestrum as, in chronic osteomyelitis 7.6
   sudden stridor 25.16
   in throat 25.13
   in tracheobronchial tree 25.12
      if it breaks 25.12D
   'upside down thump' 25.12
   in urethra 23.30
foreskin, see prepuce
formaldehyde 28a – 1a, 28a.2
formalin 2.5
formol saline 32.1
fossa navicularis, stone in 23.17, 23 – 22
Fournier's gangrene of scrotum 23.30, 23 – 40
four-quadrant tap 16.6
fracture 1.9, 7.2
   pathological 7.6D, 32.13
frenal vessels, bleeding from 23.26
Freyer's transvesical prostatectomy 23.15, 23.19, 23 – 24
   advantages and indications 23.19
   closure and postoperative care 23.19
   difficulties 23.19D, 23.19
   irrigation or drainage 23.19, 23 – 26
'frog breathing' 19.12D
frontal sinus
   draining 25.8
   mucocele 24.11
frontal sinusitis 7.14, 25.8
frusemide 17.4D, 17.5D, 23.19
fundus of uterus, height 16.4
funiculitis, endemic 14.2, 31.6
funiculo-epididymo-orchitis 31.6
'Furamide' 31.10

G
Gaenslen incision 7 – 12, 7.13
gait, abnormal, in Perthes' disease 27.14
galactocele 21.3
gall-bladder
   anatomy 13 – 3, 13.7
   carcinoma 13.8
   causes of acute abdomen 10.2
   disease 13.1 – 7
   empyema 10.2, 13.3
   enlarged, cholecystojejunostomy indication 13.8

gall-bladder (cont.)
   enlarging in acute cholecystitis 13.3
   fibrotic and contracted, avoid removing 13.7
   finding, in cholecystostomy 13.3
   mucocele 13.3
   perforated 9.2
   removal 13 – 4, 13.7D, 13.7
gallipot 4.11
gallows traction, for rectal prolapse 22.9
gallstones 13.1, 13.2
   acute pancreatitis with 13.9D
   hepatoma vs 32.26
   obstructive jaundice vs 13.8
   removal 13 – 1, 13.3
ganglions 27.11
gangrene
   in cancrum oris 26.6, 26 – 10
   of extremities 31.14
   idiopathic 31.14
   in intestinal amoebiasis 31.10
   wet or dry, after snake bites 34.4
   see also gas gangrene
gas 1.12
gas gangrene 2.9, 6.6aD
   after laparotomy 9.12
   intrauterine infection 19.5D
gastric lavage 3.10, 24.14, 25 – 11
gastric mucosal erosions 11.3
gastric ulcer
   bleeding from 11.3, 11.4
   carcinoma 34.5
   malignant 11.4D
   perforated 10 – 3, 11.2
   see also peptic ulcer
gastrocnemius muscle 30.8
   deformity 27.2
gastroenteritis
   acute, signs and diagnosis 10.2, 10 – 4
   appendicitis vs 12.1, 12.2D
gastroenterostomy 11.2D, 11.6D
   for bleeding peptic ulcer 11.4
   in chronic duodenal ulcer 11.7
   for pyloric stenosis 11.6, 11 – 6
   stoma obstructed 11.6D
'Gastrografin', in neonatal gut obstruction 28.2
gastrointestinal bleeding 11.3, 11.4D
   after surgery 11.4D
   causes 11.3
   diagnosis and resuscitation 11.3
   risk indicators 11.3
   see also oesophageal varices; peptic ulcer
gastrointestinal juice, secretion 10.4
gastrointestinal tract tumours 32.22 – 27
gastrojejunostomy 11.6D, 11.6, 11 – 6
   palliative 32.25
   in pyloric stenosis 11.6
gastro-oesophageal junction, search for bleeding site 11.4
gastrostomy 11 – 7, 11.8
   in carcinoma of oesophagus 32.24
   feeding 25.16
gauze, wound discharges 4.10
gauze packs, control of bleeding 3.1
Gelpie's retractor 4 – 4, 4.5
general duty medical officers(GDMOs)
   role and range of work 1.3, 1.4, Preface 6
   use of manuals 1.14
General practitioner (GP) Preface 6
general surgeons 1.3, 1.7, Preface 6
genital tract
   female
      chronic infections and parasitoses 20.14
      congenital abnormalities 28.7
      infections 6.5, 20.14 injuries 20.14 tumours 32.35 – 38
      ulcerative lesions 22.10
      see also pelvic inflammatory disease(PID)
   male, tumours 32.30 – 34
gentamicin 2.8
   dosages and route of administration 2.9
   eye 24.1, 24.3
gentamicin-impregnated polymethyl methacrylate (PMMA) beads 7.6
genu recurvatum 27 – 4, 27.4, 27.5, 27.17
Gerota's fascia 5 – 9a
gestational age, problems in estimating 19.6
Ghadvi's lateral perineal prostatectomy 23.21D, 23.21, 23 – 28
   advantages, disadvantages 23.21
giant cell tumour 32.15

giant cell tumour (cont.)
   of jaw 26.7, 26 – 12, 32 – 1
Gibbon catheter 23.1, 23 – 1, 23.2
gibbus 29 – 3, 29.4
Gill – Ogilvie hernia 14.2, 14 – 9, 14 – 10
gingivitis 26.2, 26.6
Girdlestone's operation 7.18, 7.19
Gishiri out 18.19D
glans penis
   carcinoma 32.33
   fistulae between corpora and 23.29, 23 – 39
   inflammation 23.30
   strictures 23.8
glasses, reading, prescribing of 24.8D, 24.8
glassware, autoclaving 2.4
glaucoma 24.1, 24.6D, 24.6
   aphakic 24.4
   congenital 24.6D, 24.6
   primary angle closure(ACG, acute) 24.3, 24.6
   primary (chronic) open angle(POAG) 24.1, 24.6
   secondary 24.3, 24.5D, 24.5, 24.6D, 24.6
      in leprosy 30.2
   steroid 24.6D
glossophayngeal palsy, after snake bites 34.4D
glottis
   carcinoma 25 – 8a, 32.39
   obstruction, Sengstaken-Blakemore tube use 11.5
   oedema 5.8, 5 – 8, 5.10
gloves
   aseptic technique without 2.3D
   industrial 2.3
   operating, requirements 2.3
   powder 2.3
   prevention of AIDS 28a.2, 28a.3
   torn or contaminated during operation 2.3
gloving, method 2.3, 2 – 6
glucose
   administration to children 28.1
   blood 17 – 1a, 17.3
      fasting 17.3
      if cannot measure, in pregnancy 17.3D, 17.3
      profile, determination 17.3
      random 17.3
   infusion 17.3
   tolerance, impaired in pregnancy 17 – 1a, 17.3
   tolerance test(GTT) 17 – 1a, 17.3
   in urine, test 17.3
glucose, potassium, insulin ('GKI') infusion 17.3
glutaraldehyde 2.5, 28a – 1a, 28a.2
glycosuria, in pregnancy 17.3
goggles, prevention of AIDS 28a.2, 28a.3
goitre 21.7
   colloid 21.11, 21 – 13
      bleeding into 21.7
      nodular 21.11
   firm and well defined 21.13
   nodular asymmetrical 21 – 13
   physiological 21.10, 21 – 13
   in puberty and pregnancy 21.10, 21 – 13
   surgery for 21.7
Goligher's method of closing the abdomen 9 – 1, 9.8
gonadotrophins 15.2
   tests 32.38
goniometer 30 – 10
gonococcal disease, painful hip in 27.13
gonococcal epididymo – orchitis 23.22a
gonococcal urethral strictures 23.8, 23.9D
gonococci
   pelvic inflammatory diseae (PID) 6.6
   in periurethral abscess 5.14
   in prostatic abscess 5.15
gonorrhoea 23.5, 23.8
Goodsall's rule 22.2, 22 – 6
Gosset's retractor 4.5, 4 – 4 ??
gouge 7.2, 7 – 3
gowning 2.3, 2 – 5
gowns, theatre 2.3
   aseptic technique without 2.3D
   for tubal ligations 15.3
grading, of difficulty of operations 1.7, 1.8
Gram-negative bacilli, antibiotics 31.8
Gram-negative septicaemia 23.9D
Gram-positive sepsis, treatment 2.9
granny knots 4 – 8, 4.8
granuloma acuminatum, carcinoma of penis vs 32.33
granuloma inguinale 20.13, 32.35a
granuloma pyogenicum 34.2, 34 – 6

Green Armytage clamps 18.9, 18 – 13
Green Armytage forceps 15.1a, 15 – 2, 18.9
grey syndrome 2.9
gridiron incision 12.1
grindstone 35 – 1
GTZ Preface 3
GUD (genital ulcer disease) 28a.2
guinea worms 7 – 1, 31 – 13, 31.14
gum
   cyst on 26.7, 26 – 10
   disease 26.2
   firm lump on 26.9
   healthy 26 – 2, 26.2
   soft swelling 26.9
gumboils 5.8
gut
   anastomoses 9.3, 9.5
     if impossible 9 – 13
     in intussusception 10.8
     in neonates 28.2, 28.3
     parts able to 9.3
   appearance in intestinal obstruction 10.5
   arrested rotation 28.3
   bleeding from 22.3
     postoperative 3.10
   bypass 9.5, 10.5D, 10.7D
   care of, in abdominal surgery 9.2, 9.3, 10.5
   constriction ring, release from 9.3
   dead, appearance 9.3, 9 – 8
   deciding whether large or small 10.5
   distended 9.2, 9.6
     cautions relating to 10.5
   end-to-end anastomosis 9.3
     Ascaris obstruction 10.6
     blood supply adequacy 9.3
     closed method 9.3, 9 – 6, 9 – 9
     open method 9.3, 9 – 10
     principles 9.3
     of unequal size 9.3, 9 – 7, 9 – 10
   end-to-side anastomosis 9.4, 9 – 11
     in carcinoma 32 – 15a, 32.27
     in neonates 28.3
   exteriorization, *see* exteriorization
   gangrenous 10.4
     after intussusception 10.8
     in hernial sac 14.114 – 1
     in neonates 28.3D
   gurgling and bloating 10.4
   handling, in intestinal obstruction 10.5
   hole in, peritonitis management 6.2
   if band of necrosis around 9.3
   if firmly stuck to pelvis 10.7D
   if part of wall nonviable, invagination 9.3
   if serosa stripped 10.7D
   ischaemia, pain in 10.1
   is it viable? determination 9.3, 9 – 8
   large
     anastomosis 9.3, 10.3, 10.5
     carcinoma 9.5
     fluid levels in 10.4
     see also caecum; colon; sigmoid colon
   non-specific ulceration, rectal bleeding 22.3D, 22.3
   not viable, after intestinal obstruction 10.5D, 10.5
   obstruction, *see* intestinal obstruction
   perforation 10.4
     accidental 9.2, 10.5, 15.4D, 16.7D
     by *Ascaris* 10.6
     causes 31.8
     in invasive intestinal amoebiasis 31.10, 31.11
     signs and diagnosis 10.2
     in typhoid 31.8D, 31.8
   resection 9.3, 10.10, 32 – 15a, 32.27
     if strangulated in inguinal hernia 14.6
     in intussusception 10.8
     procedures after 10.5
   seromuscular wall, accidental nicks 10.5
   side-to-side anastomosis 9.4, 9 – 12, 28.3, 32 – 15a, 32.27
     in abdominal tuberculosis 29.7, 29 – 8
   small
     accidental injury, in chronic ectopic pregnancy 16.7D
     bypass, in abdominal tuberculosis 29.7
     duplicated 28.3D
     fibrotic segment, abdominal tuberculosis 29.7
     fluid levels in 10.4
     tumours 10.14

gut (*cont.*)
   volvulus 10 – 3, 10.4, 10.9, 10 – 13, 28.2
     diagnosis 10.4D
     in neonates 28.3
     signs, symptoms, diagnosis 10.2, 10.9
   strangulated
     resection 10.5, 14.6
     in Richter's hernia 14.1
     through Busoga henia 14.2
   strictures
     causes 32.27
     in plastic abdominal tuberculosis 29.7, 29 – 8
   suturing 9.3, 9 – 6
   tuberculous strictures 29.5, 29.7
   tuberculous ulcers 29 – 4, 29.5
   in typhoid 31.8
   in vagina 16.2D, 20.3D
   viable, appearance 9.3, 9 – 8
   volvulus, in infants 28.3D, 28 – 4
   see also entries beginning intestinal
gynaecological causes, of acute abdomen 10.2, 10 – 3
gynaecology 20.1 – 14
   miscellaneous problems 20.14 gynaecomastia 21.3D, 30.9, 32.34a

H

'Haemaccel' 28a.2
haemangioma of, tongue 26.9, 26 – 12
haematemesis 11 – 11, 11.3
haematochyluria 23.30
haematocele 6.5
   pelvic 16 – 6a, 16 – 6, 16.7
haematocolpos 20.13, 20 – 23, 28.7
haematoma 2.3
   after inguinal hernia repair 14.3D
   after vasectomy 15.5D
   arterial 3.4
   in broad ligament 16.6D, Stop Press
   laparotomy wound 9.12
   nasal 25.16
haematometra 20.13, 20 – 23
haematuria 23.4
   in carcinoma of bladder 23.4, 32.31
   causes 23.4
   cystoscopy in 23.3, 23.4
   macroscopic, due to *S. haematobium* 23.3, 23.4, 32.31
   microscopic, in urinary tract stones 23.12
   painful urinary retention with 23.9D
   in urogenital tuberculosis 29.9
haemoglobin
   before abdominal surgery 9.1
   in ectopic pregnancy 16.6
   levels in typical patients 1.5
   measurement 17.2
haemoperitoneum 13.7D
Haemophilus influenzae, septic arthritis 7.16
haemoptysis 32.29
haemorrhage
   control of 3.1
   postpartum, 19.11a, 19.11b, Stop Press
   reactionary 3.10, 22.6D, 23.19D, 26.3D
   secondary 3.10, 22.6D, 23.19D
   see also bleeding
haemorrhoidectomy 22.6D, 22.6, 22 – 11
haemostatic gauze 3.1
haemostats 3.1, 3 – 2, 4.12
   disadvantages 3.2
   'railroading' 4 – 12
   types 3 – 2, 3.2
Halstead's forceps 3 – 2, 3.2
Hamilton Russell traction 27.6, 27 – 9
hand
   clawed, in leprosy 30 – 2, 30 – 3, 30.4
   dorsum
     infections 8.11
     scars, in leprosy 30.4
     swollen 8.1, 8 – 5, 8.7
   exercises in leprosy 30 – 3
   flexor tendon sheath infections 8 – 7, 8.12
   infected tendon sheath in palm 8.12
   infections 8.1
     general method 3.9, 8.1
     by human bites 8 – 9, 8.15, 8.16
     incisions 8.1, 8 – 4, 8 – 5, 8 – 6, 8.9
     in leprosy 8.9, 30.4
     problems with 8.16
     hand
     severe 8 – 5

hand, infections (*cont.*)
   sites 8.1, 8 – 1
   subcutaneous 8.2
   injuries 1.3
     in leprosy 30 – 2, 30.4
   instrument set 4.12
   lesions, osteomyelitis differential diagnosis 7.3
   middle palmar space 8 – 4
     infections 8 – 6, 8.9
   mycetoma of 31 – 2
   operations, use of tourniquets in 3.9, 8.1
   paralysis 30.4
   position of safety 7.17
   postoperative elevation 8.1
   radial bursa infection 8.14
   superficial palmar space, infections 8 – 1, 8.8
   swollen 8.1, 30.4
   thenar space 8 – 4
     infections 8 – 6, 8.10
   ulnar bursa infection 8 – 1, 8.1, 8.13
   web space infections 8 – 5, 8 – 6, 8.7
   see also finger
hand sandals 30.6
'hanging groins' 14.3D, 14 – 11
Hartmann's operation 6.6D, 9.5, 9 – 14, 10.10a
   in carcinoma of colon and rectum 32 – 15a, 32.27
   closing 10.10a, 10 – 17a
   difficulties 10.10aD
   dividing rectum and colon removal 10.10
   rectal stump closure 10.10
   in sigmoid volvulus 10.10, 10 – 16
   in strangulated obstructions 10.5
Hartmann's pouch 13 – 3, 13.7
   stone impacted in 13.8
Hashimoto's thyroiditis 21.13, 21 – 13
Haultains's operation 19.11aD, 19 – 12
HBV, *see* hepatitis B virus
HCG (human chorionic gonadotrophin) 1.14, 32.38
headache, osteitis of skull in 7.14
head injury 1 – 3, 1.4, 7.14
'healing' shoe 30.6D
health budget 1.12
health centre
   in referral system 1 – 5, 1.6
   symphysiotomy in 18.6
   theatres 2.2a
   tubal ligation at 15.3
health education, AIDS prevention 28a.2
   in leprosy 30.6, 30 – 8
hearing aids 25.2
heart, large, causes 6.1a
heart disease, in pregnancy 17.5
heart failure
   leading to cirrhosis and ascites 29.6
   in pregnancy 17.2, 17.5D, 17.5
   delivery in 17.5D, 17.5
heart rate, neonate 19.12
heat, sterilization by 2.4, 2.5
heater, for autoclaves 2.4
heel
   infection 7.13
   ulcer 30.6D, 30.7, 30 – 9
Hegar's dilator 15.1a, 15 – 2, 20 – 1, 20.3
Heimlich's manoeuvre 25.13
Heinecke – Mikulicz procedure 29 – 8
helminthoma 10.1
hemicolectomy 1.4
   left, in carcinoma of colon 32.27
   right 22.3D, 22.3
     in abdominal tuberculosis 29.7
     in carcinoma of colon 32 – 15a, 32.27
'Heminevrin' (chlormethiazole), in pregnancy 17.4
hemivertebra, congenital 29.4
Henle's spine 25 – 2, 25.4
hepatic artery 13 – 3, 13.4, 13.7
hepatic ducts 13.4, 13.7
   injury in cholecystectomy 13.7
hepatic encephalopathy 11.5
hepatitis B 28a.1, 28a – 2, 28a.4
   acute 28a – 2, 28a.4
   antigen and antibody levels 28a – 2, 28a.4
   carriers and 'supercarriers' 28a.4
   chronic 28a – 2, 28a.4
   chronic active (CAH), chronic progressive (CPH) 28a.4
   hepatocellular jaundice in 13.8
   immunization (active and passive) 28a.4
   prevalence and transmission 28a.4

hip, spasm (cont.)
  prevention during surgery 28a.2
  risks of hospital-acquired infection 28a.4
hepatitis B virus (HBV) 28a.1, 28a−2
  disinfection and autoclaving for 28a.2
  geographical distribution 32−13
  surface antigen(HBsAg) 28a−2, 28a.4, 32−13
hepatoma 13.8, 32−13, 32.26
  amoebic liver abscess vs 31.12
  in chronic active hepatitis (CAH) 28a.4
hernia 14.1−13
  Busoga 14.2
  epigastric 14.9, 14.12, 14−22
  external abdominal 14.1
  femoral, see femoral hernia
  formation around colostomy 9.6D
  general principles 14.1
  Gill−Ogilvie 14.2, 14−9, 14−10
  gut obstruction and strangulation 10.14, 14.1, 14−1
  incisional 9.2, 14.13D, 14.13, 14−20, 14−23
  inguinal, see inguinal hernia
  irreducible 14.1
  paraumbilical 14.9, 14.11D, 14.11, 14−20
  pathology 14−1, 14.1
  reducible 14.1
  sites 10.1, 10.4
  sliding 14.1, 14−1
  strangulated 1.1, 10−3, 10.5, 14.1, 14−1
  taxis 14.1, 14.5, 14.6
  through ileo-umbilical fistula 28−4
  umbilical, see umbilical hernia
hernial sac
  gangrenous contents 14.1, 14−1
  incomplete peritoneal lining 14.1
  see also inguinal hernia
herniorrhaphy 14.2, 14.6
herniotomy 14.2, 14−4
  in children 14.5
  direct inguinal hernia 14.2
  indirect inguinal hernia 14.2, 14−4
  recurrent, management 14.2
Herpes virus type 2 32.35
Hess's test 34.4
hexoprenaline 19.10
'Hibitane' 2.5, 2.6
high-energy milk feed 9.10
Hilton's method 5.2, 5−3, 5.8, 8.9
hip
  abduction in flexion 27.14
  adduction, abduction deformity 27.4
  anterior approach to 7.18, 7−18
  aspiration 7−15, 7.17, 7.18
  in chronic polio 27−3, 27.4, 27.6
  congenital dislocation (CDH) 27.12D, 27.12, 27−15
  contractures 27.6
    assessment 27.2
    flexion 7.18, 27.2, 27−3, 27.4, 27.6
    indications, contraindications for surgery 27.6
    manipulation 27.2, 27−2
    tenotomy for 27.6, 27−7
  destroyed, fusion after 7.18
  diseases 27.13
  dislocation, subluxation in chronic polio 27.4
  exploring 7.18, 7−19
  external rotation 27.12, 27−15
  flexed, in pyomyositis differential diagnosis 7.1
  hyperextension 27−3, 27.4
  infected, Girdlestone's operation for 7.19
  narrowing of joint space 29.3
  normal 27−16
  Ober's (posterior) approach 7.18, 7−19
  in osteomyelitis of femur 7.10
  painful
    in acute osteomyelitis 7−2, 7.3, 7.10, 27.13
    in children 27.13, 29.3
    in Perthes' disease 27.13, 27.14, 27−16
    in septic arthritis 7.16, 7−17, 7.18, 27.13
  painful flexed 5−10, 5.12
  positions of rest and of function 7.17
  septic arthritis 7−14, 7.16, 7.18, 27.2, 27.13
    in osteomyelitis 7−2, 7.3
    pyomyositis vs 7.1
    signs 5−10, 5.12, 7.16, 7−17, 7.18
  spasm
    in Perthes' disease 27.14, 27−16
    relief 7.18
    testing 7−17, 7.18, 27.14, 27−16, 29.3

hepatitis (cont.)
  in tuberculosis 29.3
  tuberculosis of 5−10, 5.12, 29−1, 29.3
  tuberculous arthritis differential diagnoses 29.3
hiradenitis suppurativa 5.11
Hirschsprung's disease 28.6a
histology, solid tumours 32.1
HIV, see human immunodeficiency virus (HIV)
hoarseness 25.16
  in carcinoma of glottis 32.39
  progressive or rapid onset 25.16
Hodgkin's lymphoma 32.4
  age distribution 32−4
  diagnosis, staging and chemotherapy 32.2, 32.4
hooks 4.5
hookworms, anaemia in pregnancy 17.2
hormonal treatment, of breast carcinoma 21.4
horseshoe abscess 5.13
horseshoe fistulae 22.2, 22−5, 22−7, 22−8
hospices 33.1
'hot' emergency procedures 1.7
'hot packs' 3.1
'hot potato' speech 25.16
household survey, maternal mortality rate 15.1D, 15.1
Huckstep type of appliances 27.5, 27−6
'huff', need for after abdominal surgery 9.11a
human chorionic gonadotrophin (HCG) 1.14, 32.38
human immunodeficiency virus (HIV) 1.14, 6.6, 28a.1, 28a−1, 28a.2
  antibodies 28a.2
  disinfectants for 28a−21a, 28a.2
  if common, neonatal resuscitation 19.12D
  most infectious periods 28a.3
  −positive patients 28a.2, 28a.3
  response to surgery/disease 28a.3
  risk to surgical team 28a.2, 28a.3
  risk and transfusions for anaemia 17.2
  types 28a.2
  see also AIDS
Humby knife 31−6
humerus
  cystic lesion 27.17
  exposing the ends 7.7, 7−7
  fracture 1.6, 3.4, 3−6
  osteomyelitis 7−5, 7.7, 7−7
hyaluronidase ('Hyalase') 23.11, 23.27
hydatid cyst
  amoebic liver abscess vs 31.12
  causing proptosis 24.11
  of liver 13−12, 31−11, 31.13
    aspiration 31−12, 31.13
    difficulties 31.13D
    removal 31−12, 31.13
    rupture 31.13D, 31.13
  of omentum, spleen 31.13D
hydatid disease 31−11, 31−12, 31.13
  breast cysts 21.3
  hepatoma vs 32.26
hydatidiform mole 32−23, 32.37, 32.38
  diagnosis and treatment 32.38
hydatidosis of peritoneal cavity 31.13D
hydralazine, in pregnancy 17.4
hydramnios 19.3
hydrocalyx 23−15
hydrocephaly 18.7, 19.7
hydrocele 1.5, 14.2, 14−13, 31.7
  in adults 23.23
  enormous, inguinoscrotal 23.23D
  operations for 23.23, 23−30
  around testis, in children 14.5, 14−15
  congenital 14.5D, 14.5, 14−15
  of cord, in children 14.5, 14−15
  in filariasis 31−5, 31.6
  hernia with 14.3D, 14.5D
hydrocolpos 28.7
hydrogen peroxide 28a−1a, 28a.2
hydronephrosis 18.10D, 23.8, 23.12, 23.14
  appendicitis vs 12.1
  nephrostomy for 23.13
hydrosalpinx 6.6, 6−11
hydroureter 23.14
hyoid bone 21.9, 21−13
hypermetropia (long sight) 24.8
hypernephroma 32.30
hyperpyrexia, in eclampsia 17.4
hypertension
  essential 17.4D, 17.4
  gestational 17.3, 17.4, 19.11

hypertension, gestational (cont.)
  difficulties 17.4D
  in pregnancy 17−2, 17.4
  pregnancy-induced (PIH) 17.4
  renal 17.4
hyperthyroidism 21.7, 21.8
hyperthyroid nodule 21.11
hypertrophic scars 34.1a, 34−3
hyperventilation, in gestational hypertension 17.4D
hyphaema 24.1, 24.4
hypochlorite 2.4
hypochondrium, pain in 10.2, 31.12
hypogastrium, pain in 10.2
hypoglycaemia, neonatal 17.3, 19.12
hypoglycaemic agents, oral 17.3
hypoproteinaemia 29.6
hypopyon 24.1, 24.3, 24.4, 24−7
  of iridocyclitis 24.5
hypospadias 28.11
hypothermia, in neonates 19.12
hypovolaemia
  in acute rupture of ectopic pregnancy 16.6
  in eclampsia 17.4
  in gastrointestinal bleeding 11.3
  in incomplete abortions 16.2
  in intestinal obstruction 10.4, 10−19
  postoperative 3.10
  treatment, AIDS prevention 28a.2
hypovolaemic shock 18.4, 34.4
hysterectomy 16.2D, 20.12D, 20.12
  after septic abortion 6.6
  anatomy 18.17, 18−20
  Caesarean 18.8
  in carcinoma of cervix 32.35
  in cervical pregnancy 16.8
  'cold', indications 20.12
  contraindications 20.12
  emergency 18.17, 18−20, 20.1, 20.12
  for fibroids 20.6
  forceps for 4.4
  in hydatidiform mole 32.38
  in malignant ovarian tumour 20.7
  method 20.12, 20−18, 20−19, 20−20, 20−21
  radical 20.12
  in rupture of uterus 18.17, 18−20
    indications and method 18.17
  in secondary postpartum haemorrhage 18.10D
  subtotal 16.8, 18.17, 20.12, 20−20
  total 18.17, 20.12, 20−21
  urinary retention after 23.5
  vaginal 20.9
  in vaginal stenosis 18.19D
hysteria 6.4, 10.2D
hysterosalpingogram 15.2

I
idiopathic gangrene 31.14
ileocaecal junction, mass at 29.7
ileocaecal tuberculosis 10.2, 10.4, 29.7
  appendicitis vs 12.1
  invasive intestinal amoebiasis vs 31.11
ileocaecal valve
  incompetent, large caecal shadow 10.4
  in large gut obstruction 10.4, 10−5
ileocolic anastomosis 9.3, 31.11, 32−15a, 32.27
ileo-colic fistula, in extraperitoneal closure of colostomy 9.6
ileosigmoid knotting 10.10D
ileostomy 9−13, 10.8
ileo-transverse colostomy 9.5, 9.6, 31.8
ileo-transversostomy 9.5, 29.7
ileo-umbilical fistula 28−4
ileovaginal fistula 18−24
ileum
  bleeding, in typhoid 31.8
  terminal, filled with thick fluid in neonates 28.3D
  twisted with sigmoid colon 10.10D, 10−17
ileus 9.2, 10.4, 10.5D
  after abdominal surgery 9.10, 10.13
  diagnosis 10.4D, 10.13
  'MOPP' regimen causing 32.4D
  paralytic 10.13, 11.6D
    physiological effects 10−19
  in peritonitis 6.2
  X-rays in 10.4
iliac abscess 5.2, 5−10, 5.12, 7.1
  differential diagnosis 5−10, 5.12
iliac adenitis 5−10, 5.12, 10.2

iliac adenitis (cont.)
  appendicitis vs 12.1
iliac arteries
  external 3.6, 3−8
  internal, see internal iliac artery
iliac fossa
  mass in 12.1
  pain in 10.1, 10.2, 12.1
ilio-hypogastric nerve 14.2
ilio-inguinal nerve 14.2
iliopsoas, abscess in 7.1
iliopsoas pyomyositis 5−10, 5.12
iliopsoas test 10.1, 10−2
iliotibial band, cutting in polio contractures 27.6, 27−7
illumination, in theatres 2.1, 2−3
immunization, hepatitis B 28a.4
incarceration 14.1
incisional hernia 9.2, 14.13, 14−20, 14−23
  above umbilicus 14.13
  recurrent 14.13D
incisions, abdominal, see abdominal incisions
incisor, extraction 26.3, 26−4, 26−5
incontinence
  after Freyer's prostatectomy 23.19D
  after Ghadvi's prostatectomy 23.21D, 23.21
  after symphysiotomy 18.6D
  damage to anterior commissure 23.19
  faecal
    deep anorectal fistulae 22.2
    in rectal prolapse 22.9
    risks in deroofing anal fistulae 22.2
    in stricture of rectum 22.10
  flatus, after Lord's procedure 22.5D
  overflow 18.10D
  in 'retention with overflow' 23.8, 23.18, 28.11
  stress 18.18
India Preface 6, 1−2
infants
  AIDS transmission to 28a.2
  chronic osteomyelitis in 7.6D
  congenital hydroceles 14.5, 14−15
  dead
    destructive operations 18.1, 18.4, 18.7, 18−8
    fetal death 16.4
    in obstructed labour 18.3, 18.4
    see also fetal death; intrauterine death; perinatal mortality
  deafness in 25.2D
  diabetic 17.3
  eye examination 24−6
  hepatitis B infection in 28a.4
  inguinal herniae in 14.2, 14.5, 14−15
  intestinal obstruction 28.2
  resuscitation 18.2
  stridor in 25.16
  umbilical hernia 14.10, 14−19
  see also children; fetus; neonates
infection
  after cytotoxic drugs 32.2D, 32.2
  in AIDS 28a.2
  in leprosy 30.4, 30.6D
  prevention, antibiotics use 2.7, 2.8
  sources of, in theatres 2.3
  with ureteric stone 23.14
  See also individual infections, anatomical regions
inferior epigastric artery 3.6, 14.2, 23−20
infertility 6.6D, 15.2
  anovulatory 15.2
  causes 15.2
  in chronic pelvic inflammatory disease (PID) 6.6
  history, examination 15.2
influenza 10.2
inframammary incision 21.5
infundibulopelvic ligament 16.6D, 18.17, 18−20, 20.12, 20−17
  in septic thrombophlebitis 6.6D
  thickened, distinguishing from uterer 20.7D
inguinal anatomy 14.2, 14−2
inguinal canal 14.2
  in children 14.5
  opening, in herniotomy 14.2, 14−4
  posterior wall
    reinforcement 14.2, 14.4, 14−14
    weakness 14.2, 14.3D
  repair 14.2
  undescended testis in 23.25a
inguinal hernia 10.1, 14.2, 14−17
  anatomy 14.2, 14−2

inguinal hernia (cont.)
  Bassini repair 14.2, 14−6
  bilateral direct 14−17
  Busoga 14.2, 14.6D
    repair 14.2, 14−9, 14−10
  in children 14.5D, 14.5, 14−15, 14−20
    recurrence 14.5D
  closing wounds 14.2
  complete 14−1, 14.2
    formation 14.5, 14−15
  coverings 14−2
  diagnosis, difficulties 14.2, 14.3D
  differential diagnosis 14.2, 14.5
  direct 14.2, 14−17
    bladder entering 14.2, 14−5
    femoral hernia vs 14.7
    herniotomy for 14.2, 14−4
    repair 14.2, 14−8
  direct with indirect 14.−12.14, 14.3D
  giant 14.4
  hernial sac 14.2, 14−3
    in children 14.5
    if boggy thickening of wall 14.2
    if difficult in finding 14.3D
    if pus in 14.3D
    if in scrotum 14.2, 14.3D
    irreducible or strangulated 14.6
    neck of 14.2, 14−3
    searching for and opening 14.2, 14−4
  herniotomy 14.2, 14−4, 14.5
  hydrocele with 14.5D
  if gut has white ring 14.3D
  if loop of gut escapes into peritoneal cavity 14.3D
  incomplete 14−1, 14.5, 14−15
  indirect 14.2, 14−3, 14−17
    in children 14.5, 14−15
    femoral hernia vs 14.7
    herniotomy for 14.2, 14−4
  irreducible or strangulated 14.6D, 14.6
  management of 14.2, 14−3
  postoperative difficulties 14.3D
  pre- and perioperative difficulties 14.3D
  recurrence 14.2, 14.5D
  reducible 14.1, 14.2
  repair difficulties 14.6D
  sliding, repair 14.2
  strangulated 14−13
  Tanner slide for 14.2, 14−7
  taxis 14.5, 14.6
  unstrangulated 14.2
inguinal ligament 14.2
  abscess pointing above 6−7
  in Bassini repair 14.2, 14−6
  division 14.8D
inguinal lymphadenitis 14.2
inguinal nodes, inflammation 14.6, 22.10
inguinal ring
  external 14.2, 14−2, 14.2, 14−3
    in children 14.5
  internal 14.2, 14−2, 14.2, 14−3
    closure, in large direct hernias 14.2, 14−8
    enlarged in indirect hernias 14.2
    narrowing 14.2, 14−5
    repair, in children 14.5
inguinoscrotal hernia, giant indirect 14−13
inguinoscrotal incision 23−33
instrument cabinet 2.1
instruments
  antiseptics and disinfectants for 2.5
  autoclaving 2.4
  basic 4.1, 35(Appendix A)
  for bones 7.2, 7−3
  cleaning 2.3, 4.11
  sterilizers, sterilization 2.4, 2.6
  see also equipment; specific instruments
instrument sets 4.12, 35(Appendix A)
  contents and cost 4.12
insulin, in pregnancy 17.3D, 17.3
intensive care unit (ICU) 9.9
intercostal nerves, avoidance in laparotomy 9.2
intercostal vessels, bleeding 6.1D
intermenstrual bleeding 20.2, 32.35
intermittent compression, in elephantiasis 31−4, 31.5, 31.6
internal iliac artery 3.5, 3−7
  relationship of ureter to 20−16
  tying 3.5, 3−7, 16.2D, 16.2
    myomectomy for submucous fibroid polyps 20.6

internal iliac artery, tying (cont.)
  postpartum haemorrhage 19.11a, 19.11aD
  tear from incision in uterus 18.10D
internal oblique aponeurosis 14.2, 14−2
internal oblique muscle, in Bassini repair 14.2, 14−6
internal podalic version 19−8, 19.11
interossei muscles of hand, pus around 8.9
interureteric bar 23.3, 23−23
  hypertrophied 23.20
intervertebral disc 27.8, 27−12a
  protrusion of nucleus pulposus 27.8, 27−12a
  in spinal tuberculosis 29.4
intestinal bypass 9.5, 10.5D, 10.7D
intestinal fistula 1.6, 9.14, 9−25
intestinal obstruction 9.2, 10.1−14, 10.3
  in abdominal tuberculosis 29.5, 29−5, 29.7
  adhesions causing 10.13
  after abdominal abscesses 10.12
  after abdominal surgery 10.4D, 10.13
  after appendicectomy 12.2D
  after colostomies 9.6D
  after inguinal hernia reduction 14.3D
  Ascaris worms causing 10.6, 10−10
    in neonates 28.3
  by bands and adhesions 10.7, 10−11
  bypass for 9.5, 10.5D
  in carcinomas of colon and rectum 32−15a, 32.27
  causes 10.2, 10.3, 10.14
    if not obvious 10.5D
  closed loop 10.4
  congenital 28.2, 28−2
  constipation causing 10.14
  diagnosis 10.4D, 10.4
  examination in 10.4
  finding cause 10.5
  foreign bodies causing 10.14
  general method 10.4, 10.5
    antibiotics 10.5
    decompression in 10.5, 10−9
    findings 9.2, 10.5
    mistakes in 10.4
    non-operative treatment 10.5
    operative treatment 10.5
    postoperative 10.5
    resuscitation 10.5
  in hernias 10.14, 14.1, 14−1
  in Hirschsprung's disease 28.6a
  history and symptoms 10.4
  in infants 28.2, 28−2
  in intestinal amoebiasis 31.10
  intussusception causing, see intussusception
  large gut 10.1, 10.2, 10.4, 10−5
    bypasses for 9.5
    incomplete 10.4D
    signs and diagnosis 10.2
  late presentation 10.3
  location of site 10.5
  meconium ileus causing 28.2
  in neonates 28−2, 28.2, 28.3D
  other problems with 10.14
  in pelvic abscess 6.5D, 6.5
  persistent vitelline duct 28−4, 28.5
  physiological effects 10−19
  in plastic abdominal tuberculosis 29.5, 29.7
  radiology 10.4, 10−6
  sigmoid volvulus causing 10.10, 10−14
  signs and diagnosis 10.1, 10.2, 10.4
  simple 10.4
  small gut 10.1, 10−5
    abdominal pain in 10.2, 10.4
    incomplete 10.4D
    intestinal obstruction
      in infants 28.2
    signs and diagnosis 10.2, 10.4
    small gut volvulus causing 10.9, 28.2
    strangulated 10.4, 10.8, 10.9
      abdominal pain in 10.2, 10.4
      blood transfusion 10.5
      diagnosis 10.4
    in sigmoid volvulus 10.10
    strictures causing 10.14
    tumours causing 10.14
    volvulus of caecum causing 10.11
    X-rays in 10.1, 10.4, 10−7, 28.2
  see also acute abdomen
intracranial haemorrhage 32.2
intracranial pressure, raised 5.4a, 28.2
intrahepatic atresia 28−9a

intraocular pressure(IOP) 1.14
    effect of steroids 24.5
    in leprosy 30.2
    measurement 24.1, 24 – 3
    normal 24.1
    raised 24.5, 24.6
        in glaucoma 24.6
intraperitoneal abscess 6.3, 6 – 4, 9.12
intraperitoneal bleeding 10.1, 20.3D
intraperitoneal sepsis, signs and diagnosis 10.4D
intrauterine death 15.1a, 16.2, 16.4D, 16.4
    after 18 weeks 16.4
    before 18 weeks 16.4
    in diabetes in pregnancy 17.3
    see also fetal death
intrauterine device (IUD) 6.6D
intrauterine growth retardation (IUGR) 15.1a,
    17.2, 19.13, 19 – 15
    breech presentation 19.8
    diagnosis 19.13
    handicaps of 19.13
    in hypertension in pregnancy 17.4
    risk factors 19.13
intrauterine infection(IUI) 18.8, 18.9, 19.5
    artificial rupture of membranes(ARM) 19.3
    diagnosis and treatment 19.5
    difficulties 19.5D
    extraperitoneal Caesarean section with 18.13
    secondary postpartum haemorrhage 19.11b
intravenous fluids
    after abdominal surgery 9.9, 9.10
    economical use of and savings on 1.12
    postoperative after peritonitis 6.2
intravenous lines, for infants 28.1
intravenous pyelogram (IVP), see intravenous
    urogram (IVU)
intravenous urogram (IVU) 1.14, 23.12, 29.9
    indications and contraindications 34.5
    method 34.5
    in prostatic obstruction 23.18
    in ureteric stones 23.14
introducer
    avoid using during catheterization 23.2
    catheter 23.1, 23 – 1
    in suprapubic drainage 23.6
intubation
    after snake bites 34.4
    neonates 19.12, 19 – 13
intussusception 10 – 3, 10.3, 10.8, 10.10, 10 – 12,
    31.11D
    caeco-colic, colo-colic 10.8
    diagnosis, differential diagnosis 10.6
    ileocaecal, ileo-colic 10.8, 10 – 12
    postoperative 10.13
    primary, secondary 10.8
    reduction (manual, spontaneous) 10.8
    signs and diagnosis 10.2
    strangulation 10.8
involucrum 7.2, 7 – 2
    in chronic osteomyelitis 7.6D, 7.6
    formation, encouragement 7.6
    fracture 7.6
    inadequate, in osteomyelitis of tibia 7.11D
iodine, tincture USP 2.5
iodine deficiency 21.11
IPPV (intermittent positive pressure ventilation)
    17.4D
iridocyclitis (anterior uveitis) 24.1, 24.5, 24 – 7
iris 24 – 7
    bombé 24.5, 24 – 7
    in onchocerciasis 24.7
    prolapse 24.4
iritis 24.3, 24.5, 24.7
    in leprosy 30.2
iron-deficiency anaemia 17 – 1, 17.2
    dysphagia in 32.24
iron medication 17.2, 22.3
ischial spine 18 – 1
ischial tuberosity 18 – 1
ischiorectal abscess 5 – 12, 5.13, 5.15
ischiorectal (horseshoe) fistulae 22.2, 22 – 5,
    22 – 7, 22 – 8
isoniazid (INAH) 29.1
isthmus of uterine tube, implantation in 16 – 3,
    16.6
'itchy foot' 31.5
IUGR 19.13
Ivermectin ('Mectizan') 24.7
IVP, IVU, see intravenous urogram

J
James position 7.17
Jacques catheter 23.1, 23 – 1
jaundice
    before abdominal surgery 9.1
    in cholangitis 13.4
    due to *Ascaris* 10.6
    haemolytic 13.8
    hepatocellular 13.8
    neonatal 28.8a
    obstructive 13.1, 13.8
        causes, diagnosis 13.8
        deepening in malignancies 13.8
        differential diagnosis 13.8
        in hydatid disease 31.13D
        in pancreatic carcinoma 13.8, 32.26a
    physiological 28.8a
jaw
    in Burkitt's lymphoma 26.7, 26.9, 32.2, 32.3,
        32 – 3
    cysts 26.7
    fracture 7.14a
    infections 26.7
    osteomyelitis 7.14a
    pain 32.39
    resection 26.7, 32.22
    swellings 26.7, 26 – 11, 32.2, 32.3, 32 – 3
    tumours 26.7
jaw shoulder traction 19.8
jejunal atresia, in neonates 28 – 2, 28.3
jejuno – ileal atresia 28 – 2
jejuno – ileal stenosis 28.2
jejunostomy, feeding 5.10b, 9.7, 9.10, 9 – 20
jejunum, valvulae conniventes 10.4, 10 – 7
JHPIEGO (John Hopkins Program of
    International Education in
    Gynaecology and Obstetrics) 15.4, 15 – 6
Joel Coheri's incision, Stop Press
joint
    aspiration 7.16, 7.17, 29.3
        in septic arthritis 7 – 15, 7.16
    contractures involving 27.2
    dislocation 7.16
    effusions 7.16
    exposed after hand infection 8.16
    pain, osteomyelitis differential diagnosis 7.3
    position of safety and rest 7.17
    positions of function 7 – 16, 7.17
    range of movement, contracture assessment
        27.2
    severely damaged 7.16
    spread of pus to 7.2, 7 – 2, 7.16
    see also contracture; *individual joints*
'jungle juice' 23.11
juvenile polyp 22.3D

K
'kangaroo pouch' 19.12
Kaposi's sarcoma 32 – 8, 32.21
    atypical African, see AAKS (atypical African
        Kaposi's sarcoma)
    classical 32.21
    endemic African 32 – 8, 32.21
    indolent form 32 – 8, 32.21
    infiltrating type 32.21
Karman curette 16.4
Karnofsky performance scale 32.1
Keith's needle 4 – 6
keloids 34.1a, 34 – 3
    prevention 34.1a, 34 – 4
    treatment 34.1a, 34 – 5
keratic precipitates(KP) 24.1, 24.3, 24.5, 24 – 7
    in leprosy 30.2
keratitis 24.3, 24.7
    striate 24.4
keratocyst, ontogenic 26.7
keratomalacia 24.3D
ketamine 26.1
ketosis, starvation 17.3
kidney
    in Burkitt's lymphoma 32 – 3, 32.3
    draining 23 – 17, 23.13
    enlarged 23.13
    obstructed 23.13
    polycystic 23.13, 32.30
    single, pelviureteric junction obstruction
        23.14D
    stones 10.1, 23.12, 23.13
        see also urinary tract stones
    tuberculosis 29.9, 29 – 9

kidney (*cont.*)
    tumours 32.30
kidney bridge 23.13
kidney dish 4.11
Kielland forceps 18.1
Kirschner wire pack 4.1, 4.12
kitchen supplies, saving on 1.12
knee
    aspirating and exploring 7 – 15, 7.17
    callosities 27 – 3
    in chronic polio 27 – 3, 27.4, 27 – 4, 27.6
    contracture 7.17, 27 – 3, 27.4, 27.6D, 27.6
        assessment 27.2
        casts 27.6, 27 – 9
        manipulation 27 – 29, 27.2, 27 – 2, 27.6
        open biceps tenotomy for 27.6, 27 – 8
        operative treatment 27.6
        in poliomyelitis 27 – 3, 27.4, 27.6
        tenotomy for 27.6, 27 – 7
        wedge cast avoidance 27.2, 27.4, 27.6
    flail 27.4
    hyperextension 27 – 4, 27.4, 27.5, 27.17
    lateral subluxation 27 – 4, 27.4, 27.5
    in osteomyelitis of femur 7.10
    painful and stiff, after releasing polio
        contractures 27.6D
    positions of rest and of function 7 – 16, 7.17
    posterior subluxation 27 – 4
    rotation deformity 27 – 4, 27.4
    in tuberculosis 29.3
    valgus deformity 27.4, 27 – 4, 27.5
knee-chest position 19 – 2 19.8, 19 – 2, 19.8
knee-jerks, testing 17.4
knots 4 – 8, 4.8
    tying methods 4.8, 4 – 9, 4 – 10, 4 – 11
Kocher's forceps 3.2, 4.4
kyphoscoliosis 29.4
kyphosis 27.8D, 29.4

L
labial fusion 28.7
labour
    acceleration 18.4a, 19.3
    cardiac patient in 17 – 4, 17.5
    chart, partogram 18.2, 18 – 2, inside back cover
    delay 18.2D, 18.2
        in active phase 18.2
        in latent phase 18.2, 18.4, 18.5
        management 18.2, 18.4, 18 – 4
        in multiple pregnancies 19.11D
        surgical intervention 18.2
    difficulties after circumcision 20.13
    false 18.2
    induction 19.3
        after premature rupture of membranes 19.5
        in diabetes 17.3
        in gestational hypertension 17.4
        indications 19.3
        oxytocin 18.4a, 19.3
        in placental abruption 16.13
        in postmaturity 19.6
        rupturing membranes 19.3
    long 6.7
    normal, uterine changes in 18 – 3
    obstructed 18.2, 18.3
        Caesarean section in 18.9, 18.10D
        causes and dangers in 18.3
        definition 18.3
        destructive operations 18.4, 18.7, 18 – 8
        diagnosis and management 18.4
        disseminated intravascular coagulation 19.11a
        methods of delivery 18.4, 18 – 4
        in multips, primips 18.3
        ovarian cyst in 20.7D
        prevention 18.3
        rectovaginal fistula after 18.19
        symphysiotomy in 18.4, 18.6
        uterine changes 18 – 3
        uterus rupture 18.17
        vesicovaginal fistulae after 18.18
    placenta praevia during 16.12
    preterm 17.2, 19.4, 19.5
        cause 19.4
        in multiple pregnancies 19 – 7, 19.11
    surgery of 18.1 – 19
    see also delivery
labyrinthitis 25.3D
lachrymal adenoma 24.11
lacunar ligament 14.2, 14 – 18
    incision 14.8

Ladd's bands 10.6, 28.3D, 28.3
Laerdal self-inflating bag 19.12, 19 – 13
lagophthalmos 24.1, 30.1a, 30 – 1, 30.2, 30.3
Lane's retractor, Kilner modified 4 – 4, 4.5
Langenbeck's retractor 4 – 4, 4.5
laparoscopy 15.2
   dye injection and, in infertility 15.2
   open with laprocator 15.4
   in pelvic inflammatory disease(PID) 6.6
   tubal ligation 15.4
   with Verres gas needle 15.4
laparotomy 9.1, 9.2D, 9.2
   abscess in peritoneal cavity after 6.3
   anaesthesia for 9.2
   for *Ascaris* obstruction 10.6
   assessments after entering abdomen 9.2
   bleeding in 9.2
   chronic peptic ulcer 11.4, 11.7
   for difficulties in evacuating incomplete abortions 16.2D
   for ectopic pregnancy 16.6
   if no obvious abnormality 9.2
   if wound becomes infected 9.12
   ileus and obstruction after 10.13
   incisions 9 – 1, 9.2D, 9.2, 9 – 3
   in invasive intestinal amoebiasis 31.11
   for pelvic inflammatory disease (PID) 6.6
   in perforated peptic ulcer 11.2
   in perforated typhoid ulcer 31.8
   peritonitis and 6.2, 9.2
   in pigbel disease 31.9
   for plastic abdominal tuberculosis 29.7
   position for 9.2
   for primary pyogenic cholangitis 13.6
   for rectal bleeding 22.3
   sepsis risk 9.2
   in sigmoid volvulus 10.10
   in uterus rupture 18.4, 20.3D
   wound, if swollen, bruised 9.12
laparotomy instrument set 4.12
laparotomy pads('lap pads') 1.12
laprocator 15.4D, 15.4, 15 – 6
laryngeal paralysis 25.16
laryngeal web 25.16
laryngismus 25.16
laryngitis 25.11a, 25.16
laryngomalacia 25.16
laryngoscope, neonatal 19.12
laryngoscopy 25.11a
   direct 25.11a
   foreign body removal 25.14
   indirect 25 – 8a, 25.11a
larynx 25 – 8a, 25.16
   foreign bodies in 25.12, 25.13
   miscellaneous problems 25.16
lateral intermuscular septum of leg 27.6, 27 – 8
lateral popliteal nerve 27.6, 27 – 8
   paralysis in leprosy 30.1a, 30.8
lateral sinus
   avoidance in cortical mastoidectomy 25 – 3
   thrombosis 25.3D, 25.3
latissimus dorsi muscle 23.13
   nerve to 21.6D, 21.6
lavage
   in generalized peritonitis 6.2
   see also gastric lavage
Le Fort's operation 20.9, 20.11, 20 – 11
leg
   deep veins 34.1, 34 – 1
      valve incompetence 34.1
   deep vein thrombosis 7.1, 9.9, 34.1
   in filariasis 31 – 5, 31.6
   perforating veins 34.1, 34 – 1
      competence testing 34.1
      tying 34.1
   in podoconiosis 31 – 3, 31 – 4, 31.5
   shortening 27.12, 27 – 15
      in tuberculosis 27.4, 29.3
   superficial collecting veins 34.1, 34 – 1
   swollen and tender, osteomyelitis differential diagnosis 7.3
   veins, types 34.1
   weakness, in carcinoma of prostate 32.32
leg-raising tests 27 – 13
leg rest, structure 30.8, 30 – 10
Lembert sutures 9.3, 9 – 6, 9 – 10, 9 – 11, 9 – 12
lens
   examination 24.1
   removal 24.4, 24.8
lepra reaction, types 30.1a

leprosy
   amputation in 30.6D, 30.7, 30 – 9
   anaesthetic feet
      care, self care 30 – 3, 30.5, 30.6
      footware 30 – 4, 30.5, 30 – 5
      inspection for 'hot spots' 30 – 3, 30.5
      pre-ulcers 30.5, 30 – 6
      risk level 30 – 4, 30.5
      ulcer causes and prevention 30.5
   anaesthetic hands 8.12, 30.4
   ankle in 30.6D
   boat shaped foot 30.6, 30 – 6
   bone involvement 30.6D, 30.6
   bone removal 30.6
   breast in 30.9, 30 – 9
   calcaneal spur excision 30.7, 30 – 9
   clawed toes 30.5, 30.6D, 30.7, 30 – 9
      tendon transfers 30.7, 30 – 9
   collapsed foot 30.6D, 30 – 6, 30.6
   contractures in, operations 30.7, 30 – 9
   equinus or equinovarus foot 30.6D, 30.6
   eyes in 30.2, 30.3
   foot 30.5, 30.6, 30.7
      operations on 30.7, 30 – 9
      septic difficulties 30.6D
      shortening 30.6D, 30.6
   foot-drop
      exercises 30.5
      tibialis transfer 30.8D, 30.8, 30 – 10, 30 – 11
      toe-raising strap 30 – 4, 30.5, 30.8
   foot infections 8.17
   foot ulcers 30.6D, 30.6
      on lateral border 30.6D
      operations 30.7, 30 – 9
      plantar 30.5
      plaster cast for 30.6, 30 – 7
      leprosy
      recurrence 30.6D
      uncomplicated and complicated 30.6
   hands 30 – 2, 30.4
      clawed 30 – 2, 30 – 3, 30.4
      exercises for 30 – 3
      infections 8.9, 30.4
      protection 30.4
   heel ulcer 30.6D, 30.7, 30 – 9
   malignant difficulties 30.6D
   mouth in 30.9
   necrosis blister of foot 30 – 6, 30.6
   need for rest 30.5, 30.6
      if impractical 30.6D
   neuropathic bone disintegration 30 – 4, 30.5, 30.6D
   paralysis in, *see* paralysis in leprosy
   plaster cast, if impractical 30.6D
   short equinus foot of 30.6
   short leg walking cast 30.6, 30 – 7
   surgery of 30.1 – 9
   type two reaction 30.1a, 30.2
   ulcers 30.1
      health education 30.6, 30 – 8
      sites of 30 – 8
   walking prevention, wooden bar method 30.6, 30 – 8
leprosy osteitis 30.6
leucocyte count, chemotherapy 32.2D, 32.2
leucocytosis, in peritonitis 6.2
leucoma 24.4
leucopenia, 'MOPP' regime causing 32.4D
leucoplakia 32 – 9, 32.22
levator ani muscle 20.11a, 22.1, 22 – 1
   closure, in third-degree tears 18.15, 18 – 17
   fistulae penetrating 22.2D, 22 – 5
lichen sclerosis atropica 23.28, 23 – 38
ligaments, in gynaecology 20.12, 20 – 16, 20 – 17
light, operating theatre 2.1, 2 – 3
lignocaine
   in minilap tubal ligation 15.3
   for passing a catheter 23.2
limb
   bleeding from 3.1
   operations, bloodless 3.9, 3 – 11
   painful, in acute osteomyelitis 7.3, 7.16
   see also leg
limp, in children 27.13
linea alba
   defect 14.10
   epigastric hernia through 14.12, 14 – 22
lip
   carcinoma 32 – 9, 32.22
   cleft 26.8

lip (*cont.*)
   mucocele of 26 – 13
lipoma 31.14, 32.11
   breast 21.3
liposarcoma 32.11
liquid paraffin 22.1
liquids, in flasks, autoclaving 2.4
Lisfranc's transmetatarsal amputation 30.7, 30 – 9
Lister forceps 4.4
Lister sound 23.1, 23 – 1
Little's area 25 – 5, 25.6
liver
   abscess 10 – 3
      amoebic, *see* amoebic liver abscess
      pyogenic, amoebic liver abscess vs 31.12
   in amoebiasis 31.12
   disease
      ascites secondary to 29.6
      cytotoxic drugs in 32.2D
   failure 11.5
   hydatid cysts 13 – 12, 31 – 11, 31.13
   needle biopsy 32 – 14, 32.26
   peptic ulcer burrowing into 11.2D
   primary tumour 32 – 13, 32.26
   socond carcinoma 32.26
   tuberculosis 32.26
   tumour, plastic abdominal tuberculosis vs 29.7
   wedge biopsy 29.6, 29 – 7
locking forceps, *see* haemostats
loin, pain, after Caesarean section 18.10D
Lord's anal dilatation 1.3, 22.5, 22 – 9, 22 – 10
   for anal fissures 22.5, 22.7, 22 – 9
   difficulties 22.5D
   indications and contraindications 22.5
   method 22.5, 22 – 9, 22 – 10
   for prolapsed piles 22.4, 22.5, 22 – 10
Lord's procedure
   after colostomies 9.6
   for pilonidal sinus 22.8, 22 – 12 ***Note not Lord's dilatation
Lotheissen approach, femoral herniae 14.8
loupe, binocular 4.11, 24.1
Lovset's manoeuvre 19 – 5, 19.8
low birthweight babies 19.13
lower motor neurone lesion, in poliomyelitis 27.2, 27.4
Ludwig's angina 5.8, 5 – 8, 5.10
Lugol's iodine 21.8
lumbar disc lesions 27.8
   differential diagnoses 27.8
   examination and treatment 27.8
   S^1 and L^1 27.8, 27 – 12a
lumbar lordosis 27.2, 27.8
   in congenital dislocation of hip 27.12, 27 – 15
lumbar puncture needle, emergency suprapubic puncture 23 – 5, 23.6
lumbar spine, X-rays 1.14
lumbrical canals 8 – 4
lumbrical muscles, in leprosy 30.4
'lumpectomy', for breast tumours 21.3, 21.4, 21 – 6
   if mass forms in scar 21.5D
lung, collapse 6.1, 9.11
luteal cyst 20.7D, 20.7
lymphangioma 28.10
lymphangitis 8.16
   in filariasis 31.6
   recurrent attacks 31.4
lymphatic obstruction
   causes 31.4
   in filariasis 31 – 5, 31.6
   oedema due to 31.4
   in podoconiosis 31.5
lymphatic system, fistulae with urinary tract 23.30
lymphatic varix 31 – 5
lymph node
   biopsy 32.1
      in tuberculous arthritis 29.3
   in carcinoma of penis 32.33, 32.34
   cervical
      carcinoma of nasopharynx 32 – 16, 32.28
      suppuration in 5.10
   enlargement
      in AIDS 28a.2
      causes 32.4
      femoral hernia vs 14.7
      in non-Hodgkin's lymphoma 32.5
      in glandular type of abdominal tuberculosis 29.5,

lymph node
in glandular type of abdominal, tuberculosis (cont.)
    inguinal, block dissection 32.19, 32 – 20, 32.20, 32.30, 32.34
        indications and method 32 – 20, 32.34
    mesenteric
        calcified 23.15
        in tuberculosis 29.5, 29.8
    in mouth tumours 32.22
    rubbery, in Hodgkin's lymphoma 32.4
    in squamous cell carcinoma 32.19
    in tuberculosis 29.1, 29.2, 29.5, 29.8
lymphocele, of spermatic cord 31 – 5, 31.6
lymphoedema, after block dissection of lymph nodes 32.34D, 32.34
lymphogranuloma 31.4
lymphogranuloma venereum 20.13, 22.2D, 22.10
lymphoma 32.3 – 5
    Hodgkin's 32.2, 32.4, 32 – 4
    of nasopharynx 32.28
    non-Hodgkin's 32.2, 32.3, 32.5
'Lysol' 2.5
lytic cocktail, in pregnancy 17.4

M
McBurney's point 9.6, 12 – 1, 12.1, 23.14
McDonald's suture 16.1, 16 – 2, 16.5, 32 – 22, 32.35
MacEwen's triangle 25 – 2, 25.4
McIndoe's operating scissors 4.3, 4 – 2 ??
McLaughlin's tarsorraphy method 30 – 1, 30.3
macular degeneration, senile 24.4
macular scars 24.4
maculopathy 24.1
Madurella 31.3
magnesium sulphate, in pregnancy 17.4
magnesium trisilicate 9.2
malaria
    anaemia in pregnancy due to 17 – 1, 17.2
    cerebral 17.4
    chloroquine – resistant 17.2D
Malecot catheter 23.1, 23 – 1, 23.6, 23 – 7
Mallory-Weiss syndrome 11.3, 11.4D, 11.4
malnutrition
    correction before abdominal surgery 9.1
    low birthweight infants 19.13
'Maloprim' 17.2
malpositions, in obstructed labour 18.3
malpresentations 18.3, 19.9
    Caesarean section for 18.10D
    destructive operations in 18.7
    mento-posterior 18.4
    multiple pregnancies 19 – 7, 19.11
    in obstructed labour 18.3
    vertex 18.4
    See also individual presentations
mammary duct, fistula 21 – 1, 21.2
Manchester repair 20.9, 20.11a
Manchester system of staging 21.4
mandible
    body of, abscess under 5.8
    in Burkitt's lymphoma 32 – 1a, 32.3, 32 – 3
    fracture or dislocation 7.14a, 26.3D
    giant cell tumour 26.7, 26 – 12, 32 – 1
    sequestrectomy in osteomyelitis of jaw 7.14a
    tumour of 26.9
manipulation, contractures 27.2, 27 – 2
    knee 27.2, 27 – 2, 27.6, 27 – 9
mannitol 17.4D
manuals 1.12
    aims and contents 1.7,1.14, Prefaces (4,5,6)
    difficulties with use of1.14D
    further editions, help on writing 1.14
    method for use of 1.14
    range of abilities of readers 1.7
    references to others1.14D
    translations 1.14
    types of readers 1.14
marriage 15.1
marsupialization
    Bartholin's cyst 20 – 2, 20.4
    dental cysts 26.7, 26 – 11
    ovarian cyst 20.7D
Martin's aspirator 6.1
Martius graft 18.19D
masks, theatre 2.3
mastectomy
    incision 21 – 5
    in leprosy 30.9, 30 – 9
    it mass forms in scar 21.5D

mastectomy (cont.)
    Patey's modified 21.3, 21.4, 21.6, 21 – 11, 21 – 12
    anatomy for 21 – 10
    difficulties 21.6D
    radical 21.1, 21.6
    simple 21.4, 21.5, 21 – 7
        indications, method 21.5
mastitis, periductal 21.3
mastitis carcinomatosa 21.3, 21.4
mastoid
    normal 25.4
    tenderness and swelling 25.3D
    'velvety feel' 25.4
mastoid cortex, draining for acute mastoiditis 25.4
mastoidectomy 25 – 2, 25.4
    cortical 25 – 3, 25.4
mastoiditis 25.3D
    acute 25.4
    acute-on-chronic 25.3D
    chronic otitis media complication 25.3D, 25.4
maternal death, definition 15.1
maternal mortality 15.1
    causes 15.1a, 17.2, 17.3, 17.4
    reduction by education 15.1a
    reduction by use of partogram 18.2
maternal mortality ratio (MMR) 15.1, 34.7
mattress for operating table 2.1
Mauriceau – Smellie – Veit manoeuvre 19 – 4, 19.8D, 19.8
maxilla
    Burkitt's lymphoma 32.3, 32 – 3
    sequestrectomy in osteomyelitis of jaw 7.14a
maxillary antrum 25 – 6, 25.9
    carcinoma 32.39
    difficulties, in tooth extraction 26.3D, 26 – 7
    ostium blocked 25.9
    polypi 25.10
    tooth displaced into 26.3D
maxillary sinusitis 25 – 6, 25.8, 25.9
maxillary tuberosity, fracture 26.3D
maxillofacial injury 3.3
Mayo's operating scissors 4 – 2, 4.3
Mayo's operation for paraumbilical hernia 14.11, 14.21
Mayo's safety pins 3 – 2, 3.2
meatal strictures 23.27, 23.28, 23 – 38
meatotomy 23.28, 23 – 38
mebendazole 10.6
Meckel's diverticulum 12.2D, 28 – 4, 28.5
    gut obstruction by 28.3D, 28.3
meconium 18.9
    aspiration 19.8
    failure to pass 28.2, 28.6
    – stained liquor 19.12
meconium ileus 28.2
meconium peritonitis 28.2
median nerve
    entrapment 27.11a, 27 – 14a
    in leprosy 30.1a, 30.4
    motor branch 8 – 4, 8.12
mediastinitis 24.14D, 32.24D
mediastinum, subdivisions 6 – 1
Meibomian cysts 24.10, 24.12
Meig's syndrome 20.7
melaena 11 – 11, 11.3, 11.4, 22.3
    in typhoid 31.8
melanoma, malignant 32 – 7, 32.20
    block dissection in 32.34
    staging and treatment 32.20
    subungual 32.20
melphalan 32.2
membranes
    artificial rupture(ARM) 19.3
        contraindications and method 19.3
        in delay in labour 18.2
    prelabour rupture(PROM) 19.5
    premature rupture(PROM) 19.4, 19.5
        assessment and risks 19.5
        management 19.5
    ruptured
        cord prolapse and 19.10
        labour induction after 19.3
        in multiple pregnancies 19.11
Menghini needle 32 – 14, 32.26
    biopsy method 32 – 15, 32.26
meningeal irritation, in cavernous sinus thrombosis 5.5, 5 – 5
meningitis 10.1, 17.4, 25.3D
meningocele 28.9, 28 – 10

meningocele (cont.)
    cervical 28 – 10
    sacrolumbar 28.9, 28 – 10
menstrual periods, irregular, missed 16.7
menstrual regulation syringe 20.3
mesenteric adenitis 12.2D
mesenteric nodes 23.15, 29.5, 29.8
mesentery
    anomalies 10.11, 10 – 18
    approach in small gut volvulus 10.9
mesna 32.2
mesoappendix 12 – 1, 12.1
metacarpals, osteomyelitis of 8.17
metacarpophalangeal joint (MP) 1.14
metaphysis of long bone, osteomyelitis origin 7.2, 7 – 2, 7.16
metatarsal amputation 30.6D, 30.7, 30 – 9
metatarsal bar 30 – 4, 30.5
metatarsal head
    excision in leprosy 30.7
    osteitis 30.6D
methotrexate 21.4, 32.2, 32.28
    in trophoblastic neoplasms 32.38
methyl dopa, in pregnancy 17.4
methylene blue 7.6, 18.10D
metronidazole 2.8
    in amoebiasis 31.10, 31.11, 31.12
    chloramphenicol with, in subphrenic abscess 6.4
    dosages, administration route 2.9
    extraperitoneal Caesarean section unnecessary with 18.13
    intravenous 2.8, 2.9
    in lower segment Caesarean section 18.9
Metzenbaum's scissors 4 – 2, 4.3
Meydering's retractor 4 – 4, 4.5
microcellular rubber 30.5, 30 – 5
micturating cysto-urethrogram 34.5, 34 – 9
micturition, frequency 23.8
middle ear disease 7.3
midwifery, HIV-positive 28a.2
midwives, distinction between work of doctors and 15.1a
migraine, in sinusitis 25.7
milk fistula 21.3
Milligan's haemorrhoidectomy 22.6D, 22.6, 22 – 11
Millin's retropubic prostatectomy 23.19, 23.21
minilaparotomy (minilap) 15.3D, 15.3, 15 – 5
    in abdominal tuberculosis 29.6, 29 – 6
    diagnosis of cause of ascites 29.6
    incision 15.3
    tubal ligation 15.3
minitracheotomy 9.11
minor instrument set 4.12
'mittelschmertz' 10.2
Moffat position, for inserting nose drops 25 – 8
molar
    extraction 26.3, 26 – 4, 26 – 5
    third, impacted 26.4, 26 – 9
mole, pigmented, changes in melanoma 32.20
Mongolian spot 28.9
monoamine oxidase inhibitors (MAOIs) 32.2
monofilament 4 – 5, 4.6
'MOPP' regimen 32.4D, 32.4, 32.5
morale, of staff 1.10
morphine
    avoidance in gestational hypertension 17.4
    cancer pain relief 33.2, 33 – 2, 33.2
    in heart failure in pregnancy 17.5D
Morrison's pouch 13.4
Morris' retractor 4.5, 4 – 4 ??
'Mossy foot' 31.4, 31.5
mother – child bonding 1.9
'mother's waiting area' ('mother's village') 18.3
motivation 1.12
motor fibres, destruction in leprosy 30.1
moulding, in obstructed labour 18.4
    score, assessment 18.4
mouth
    carcinoma 26.9, 32 – 9, 32.22
    cysts in 26.9, 26 – 13
    in leprosy 30.9
    lumps arising in 26.9
    mass in floor of 26.9
    ulcers 26.9
Moynihan forceps 4.4
mucocele
    frontal sinus 24.11
    gall-bladder 13.3

mucous retention cyst, of mouth 26.9
mucus
    fistula 9.5
    passage, in pelvic abscess 6.5, 9.10
    rectal passage in intussusception 10.4, 10.8
multifilament suture materials 4.6, 4.8
multiple myeloma 32.16
multiple pregnancy 19.11
mumps orchitis 23.22a, 23.25
mumps parotitis 5.9
Munchausen syndrome 10.2
Murphy's sign 13.2
muscle
    abscesses in 7.1D, 7.1
        see also pyomyositis
    charting 27–1, 27.2, 27.3
    imbalance 27.2
    power, assessment 27–1, 27.2, 27.3
    pus in 7.1
    wasting, in tuberculosis 29.3
    weakness
        caliper use in 27.5
        in leprosy, physiotherapy 30.1a
        in polio 27.4, 27.6
'Mustine' 32.4
mycetoma 31–2, 31.3
    black grain 31–2, 31.3
    sites 31–2, 31.3
Mycobacterium ulcerans infections 31.2a
mycoplasma, pelvic inflammatory diseae (PID) 6.6
mydriatics 24.1
myeloma, multiple and solitary 32.16
myelomatosis 32.16
myelomeningocele 28.9
myelosuppression 32.2D
myomectomy
    for fibroids 20.6
    indications, contraindications 20.6
    for submucous fibroid polyp 20–5, 20.6
myopia(short sight) 24.8
myotoxic effects, of snake venom 34.4
myxoma peritonei 20.7

N
nail, infections around 8–2, 8.4
    see also toenail
naloxone hydrochloride 19.12
nasal cartilage, necrosis 4.9D
nasal discharge 25.7, 25.11, 32.28
nasal obstruction 25.7, 25.10
nasal polypi 25.7, 25.10
    removal 25.10
nasal septum, swelling 25.16
nasogastric aspiration
    in acute cholecystitis 13.3
    after abdominal surgery 9.9
    improvisatin in 10–8
    in intestinal obstruction 10.5, 10–8
    in peritonitis 6.2
nasogastric feeding, after abdominal surgery 9.10
nasogastric tube 4.9D, 4.9
    after gastric lavage in corrosive oesophagitis 25.15
    in decompression of gut 10.5, 10–9
    in gastrointestinal bleeding 11.3
    in hypertrophic pyloric stenosis 28–3, 28.4
    indications 4.9
    in neonatal gut obstruction 28.2
    passing and removing, method 4.9
nasolachrymal apparatus, diseases of 24.10
nasolachrymal duct, congenital atresia 24.10
nasopalatine cyst 26.7, 26.9, 26–13
nasopharynx
    carcinoma 32–16, 32.28
        blind and open biopsy 32.28
    examination, laryngoscopy 25.11a
natal cleft, abscess in 22.8
national population policy 15.1a
nausea
    chemotherapy 32.2D, 32.2, 32.4D
    in pregnancy 17.3D
neck
    hard swelling of soft tissues of 7.14aD
    stiffness 25.3D
neck veins, distended 6.1a
necrotizing enteritis 31.9
necrotizing jejunitis 31.9
needle 4–6, 4.7, 35 (Appendix A)
    aneurysm 4.11
    atraumatic 4–6, 4.7, 9.3

needle (cont.)
    cutting 4.7
    disinfection in AIDS prevention 28a.2
    liver biopsy 32–14, 32.26
    method of holding 4–6
    sharpening 4.7, 35(Appendix A), 35–2
needle-holders 4.7
needlestick injury
    AIDS transmission 28a.2, 28a.3
    hepatitis B transmission 28a.4
    prevention 28a.2
Neisseria gonorrhoeae, pelvic inflammatory disease (PID) 6.6
neonatal necrotising enterocolitis 28.3D
neonatal resuscitation 19.12, 19–13
    'at risk' mothers and babies 19.12
    bag and mask ventilation 19.12, 19–13
    drugs and equipment for 19.12
    external cardiac compression 19.12, 19–14
    hypoglycaemia in 19.12
    immediately after birth 19.12
    intubation 19.12
    later 19.12
    mouth to mouth ventilation 19.12D
    platform 19.12
    suction 19.12, 19–13
    tactile stimulation 19.12
neonates
    acute abdomen 28.3
    anaesthesia in 28.1, 28.3
    congenital dislocation of hip (CDH) 27.12D, 27.12, 27–15
    deaths 15.1a
        see also perinatal mortality
    electrolytes 28.3
    fluid requirements 28.1, 28.3, 28.4
    gut anastomoses 28.2, 28.3
    hydroceles in 23.23D
    intestinal obstruction 28–2, 28.2, 28.3D, 28.3
    jaundice in 28.8a
    miscellaneous problems 28.11
    orthopaedic problems 27.17, 27–20
    surgery 28.1
    talipes equinovarus 27.15
    torsion of testis in 23.24D
    see also children; fetus; infants
Nepal, patients 1.5
nephroblastoma 32.6, 32.30
'nephrogram' 23.12
nephrostomy 23–16, 23.12, 23.13, 23–17
    through renal cortex 23.13, 23–17
    through renal pelvis 23.13, 23–17
nephrostomy tube 23.13, 23–17
nephrotic syndrome, ascites in 29.6
neurofibroma 21.3
neuropathy, cytotoxic drugs 32.2D
neurotoxic effects, of snake venom 34.4
neutral position of joint 7.17
night blindness 24.3D, 24.4
nipple 21.3
    chronic ulceration 21.3D
    cracked 21.2
    discharge from 21.3
        in breast carcinoma 21.3, 21.4
        in fibroadenosis 21.3
        intraduct adenoma, carcinoma 21.3
        management 21.3
    in intraduct carcinoma, see breast, intraduct carcinoma
    Paget's disease of 21.3
    swelling deep to 21.3D
nitrogen mustard 32.2, 32.4
Nocardia spp., mycetoma 31.3
non-crushing clamps 9.3, 9–6, 9–9
non-Hodgkin's lymphoma 32.2, 32.3, 32.5
non-opioids 33.2, 33–2
noradrenalin lavage 11.3
normoglycaemia 17.3
nose
    anterior bleeding and packing 25–5, 25.6
    bleeding 3.1, 22.3, 25–5, 25.6
        difficulties 25.6D
    blocked, causes 25.7
    disorders 25.6–11, 25.16
    foreign bodies in 25.11
    position for inserting drops 25–8
    posterior bleeding and packing 25–5, 25.6
nucleus pulposus 27.8, 27–12a
nursing, in eclampsia 17.4
nutrition, in paediatric surgery 28.1

nutritional oedema 29.6
nylon syringes 1.12

O
oat cell carcinoma 32.29
obesity
    laparoscopic ligation indication 15.4
    minilap difficulties 15.3D
    prostatectomy in 23.21
obstetrics 15.1a, 18.1–19, 19.1–12
    equipment 15.1a, 15–2
    good, targets for 15.1a, 34.7
    indicators of quality 34.7
    two worlds of 18.1
obstetric paralysis, Stop Press
obturator artery, injury, in femoral hernia repair 14.7D
obturator test 10.1, 10–2
obturator vessels, abnormal, femoral hernia surgery 14.8, 14–18
occlusion therapy, for amblyopia 24.9
ocular movements, impaired 5.5D
oedema
    in carcinoma of ovary 20.7
    of leg, in Kaposi's sarcoma 32.21
    in lymphatic obstruction 31.4
    pitting, in breast diseases 21.3D
    in pregnancy 17.4D
oesophageal tubes 32–11, 32–12, 32.24
    difficulties 32.24D
    improvisatin 32–12, 32.24D
oesophageal varices, bleeding 11.3, 11.5D, 11.5
    diagnosis and signs 11.4
    drug control 11.5
oesophagitis, corrosive 24.15D, 25.15, 32.24
    barium swallow 34.5
oesophagoscope 25–10, 25.14
oesophagoscopy 25.14
    carcinoma of oesophagus 24.14, 32.24
    for investigating a stricture 24.14
    method 25.14
    positioning head for 25–10, 25.14
    removal of foreign bodies 24.14D, 25–10, 25.14
oesophagus
    anatomy 11.4
    atresia 28.2
    carcinoma 11.8, 24.14, 32–11, 32.24, 33.1
        barium swallow 34.5, 34–10
        site, differential diagnosis 32.24
    Celestin tube insertion 32–11, 32.24, 33.1
    distal tear 24–12, 25.16
    erosions 4.9D
    fibrous stricture 32.24
    foreign bodies in, removal 24.14D, 25–10, 25.14
    gastrostomy contraindication 33.1
    miscellaneous problems 25.16
    obstruction
        feeding jejunostomy for 9.7
        gastrostomy for 11–7, 11.8
    perforated 25.14D, 25.14
    ruptured 11.2D
        during vomiting 25.16
    strictures 25.15
        corrosive 24.15D, 25.15, 32.24, 34.5
        oesophagoscopy for 24.14D, 24.14
    tear during vagotomy 11.4D
oestrogens, in breast carcinoma 21.4
oliguria, in urinary tract stones 23.12
omentum
    extrauterine pregnancy 16–7, 16.9
    graft, in hydatid disease 31.13
    hydatid cyst in 31.13D
    over gut anastomosis 9.3
    over uterus, in closure after Caesarean section 18.9
    prevention of adhesions in abdominal closure 10.5, 10.7
    prevention of leakage from perforated peptic ulcer 11.2
    strangulation, in hernias 14.1, 14.6
    in vagina 16.2D
omphalocoele 28.8, 28–9
omphalo-mesenteric duct, abnormalities 28–4, 28.5
Onchocerca volvulus 24.7
onchocerciasis 14.3D, 14–11, 24.5, 24.7
oncology 32.1–39
'Oncovin' 32.2, 32.4

oophorectomy 16.6D, 20.7, 20.12, 21.4
operating lights 2.1, 2 – 3
operating table 2.1, 2 – 2
operating team 2.1
operation site
  contamination 2.9
  preparation 2.3
ophthalmia neonatorum 24.3D, 24.3
ophthalmoscopy 24.1
opioids, cancer pain relief 33.2, 33 – 2
opportunistic infections, in AIDS 28a.2
optic atrophy 24.4, 24.7
optic disc 24 – 8
  cupping 24.6, 24 – 9
  examination 24.1
  in glaucoma 24.6, 24 – 8
  normal 24 – 8, 24 – 9
  in onchocerciasis 24.7
  pale white and flat 24.4
optic nerve, partial and total destruction 24.6
optic neuritis 24.4, 24.7
oral cavity
  benign tumours 26 – 12
  cysts 26.9
  tumours 26.9
oral problems, miscellaneous 26.9, 26 – 12
oral surgery 26.1 – 8
orbicularis muscle paralysis 30.3
orbit
  abscess 24.11
  cellulitis 5.5, 24.11
  haemangioma, hamartoma 24.11
  infections 5.5, 5 – 5, 5.5, 5 – 5, 24.3, 24.13
  pseudotumour 24.11
  swelling of upper outer part 5.5D
  tumours 24 – 10, 24.11
orchidectomy 23.25, 32.34a
  in carcinoma of male breast 21.3D
  in carcinoma of prostate 32.32
  for chronic infection 23.25
  subcapsular 23.25, 23 – 32
  total, for testicular tumour 23.25, 23 – 33
orchidopexy 23.24, 23.25a
oro-antral fistula 26.3D, 26 – 7
orthopaedic appliances 27.5
orthopaedic instrument set 4.12
orthopaedic problems, miscellaneous 27.17, 27 – 20
orthopaedics 1.4, 27.1 – 17
  general methods 27.2
  scope of 27.1
orthostatic hypotension, test 16.6
Ortolani's test 27.12, 27 – 15
osteitis
  after tooth extraction 26.3D
  chronic pubic 18.6D
  of foot 8.17
  leprosy 30.6
  localized chronic 7.6
  metatarsal head 30.6D
  pyogenic 29.4
  of spine 5 – 10, 7.15
  tuberculous 29.3, 29.4a, 292 – 2
  See also osteomyelitis
osteoarthritis
  back pain due to 27.8D
  caution, wedge cast for knee contracture 27.2, 27.4, 27.6
  Perthes' disease causing 27.14
osteochondritis 27.14
osteomyelitis Preface 6, 5.2, 27.2
  acute, diagnosis and presenting features 7.3, 7 – 4
  after hand infection 8.5D, 8.16
  after tooth extraction 26.3D
  calcaneus 7 – 12, 7.13
  in children, see children
  chronic 7.6, 7.14a
    closing hole 7.6, 7 – 10
    difficulties 7.6D
    with involucrum and sequestra 7.6
    localized chronic osteitis (Brodie's abscess) 7.6
    sequestrectomy 7.6, 7 – 6
    closure of wound 7 – 10, 7.11
  emergency surgery 1.8
  exploring bone for pus 7.5
  femur 7.3, 7.10, 27.13
  fibula 7 – 11, 7.12
  finger 8.5D, 8.16

osteomyelitis Preface (cont.)
  foot 8.17
  general method for 7.4
  haematogenous 7.2, 8.17
  hip 27.13
  humerus 7 – 5, 7.7, 7 – 7
  jaw 7.14a
  in leprous hands 30.4
  osteosarcoma vs 32.13
  pathology 7 – 2, 7.2
  pelvic 7.15
  of phalanx 8.5
  pus 29.4a
  pyomyositis vs 7.1
  radius 7.8, 7 – 8
  sequestrectomy 7.11, 7.12
  skull 7 – 13, 7.14
  spinal 7.15, 27.8, 29.4a
    differential diagnosis 5.11a, 5.12
  tibia 7 – 10, 7.11, 7.16
  traumatic 7.2
  ulna 7.9
  untreated 7 – 5
  See also osteomyelitis
osteoporosis, senile 27.8D
osteosarcoma 32.13
osteotome 7.2, 7 – 3
ostomy 9.3, 9.5
  closing 9.5
  defunctioning 9.5
  in intestinal obstruction 10.3
  methods for 9.6
  sites for 9.5, 9 – 14
  of small gut 9.5
  types of 9.5
  see also colostomy
otitis externa 25.3
otitis media 25.3
  acute 25.3D, 25.3
  chronic 25.3D, 25.3
    attic, bony ('unsafe') 25.2, 25.3
    suppurative 25.2
    tubotympanic ('safe') 25.2, 25.3
  serous (secretory) 25.3D
otosclerosis 25.2
otoscope 25.1
ovarian bleeding, intermenstrual 10.2
ovarian cyst 6.5, 18.9, 20 – 7, 20.7
  adhesions with 20.7
  aspiration 20.7
  benign and malignant, classification 20.7
  bilateral benign 20.7D
  in Caesarean section 18.10D
  cystectomy for 20.7, 20 – 8
  differential diagnosis 12.1, 20.7
  difficulties with 20.7D
  giant 20.7D
  management 20.7
  in minilap 15.3D
  obstructed labour 18.4, 18 – 5, 20.7D
  pedicle of 20.7
  presenting features 20.7
  removal 20.7, 20 – 8
  risk of malignancy 20.7D, 20.7
  torsion 6.6, 10.2, 10 – 3, 12.1, 20.7
ovarian cystectomy 20.7, 20 – 8
ovarian ligaments 15 – 6, 20.12, 20 – 17
ovarian tumours 20 – 6, 20.7, 20 – 7, 20.7, 32.36
  in Caesarean section 18.10D
  obstructing labour, 18 – 5r 18.4
  solid 20 – 6, 20.7
ovarian veins, septic thrombophlebitis 6.6D
ovarian vessels 20.12, 20 – 16, 20 – 17
ovary
  blood supply 16.6D
  carcinoma 20.7
  fetal implantation 16 – 3, 16.6, 16.9
  in hernial sac 14.3D
  in hysterectomy 20.12
  removal 16.6D, 20.4, 20.7, 20.12
  tube stuck to, in ectopic pregnancy 16.6D
'over and over' sutures 4 – 7, 4.8
ovulation
  failure to 15.2, 20.2
  induction 15.2
ovulatory bleeding, appendicitis vs 12.1
oxygen 1.12
  for neonates 19.12
oxytetracycline 2.8, 2.9
oxytocin 18.4a, Stop Press

oxytocin (cont.)
  acceleration of labour 18.4a
  avoidance in delay in labour in multips 18.2
  avoidance in obstructed labour 18.4
  dangers with 18.4a
  in diabetes 17.3
  dose, table 18.4a, 18 – 5a, 19.3
  in gestational hypertension 17.4
  in hydatidiform mole 32.38
  for intrauterine death 16.4
  labour induction 18.4a, 19.3
    contraindications 19.3
  in lower segment Caesarean section 18.9
  in management of delay in labour, primips 18.2
  in multiple pregnancies 19.11D, 19.11
  in placental abruption 16.12, 16.13
  precautions for use 18.2, 18.4a, 18.4, 19.5
  in prevention of postpartum haemorrhage 19.11a
  in uncomplicated inevitable abortions 16.2
  uterus contraction and bleeding control 18.4a
  see also 'Syntometrine'

P
packs 2.3
packing the uterus 19.11a
paediatric surgery 28 – 1, 28.1 – 11
  hypovolaemia treatment 28a.2
  miscellaneous problems 28.11
  see also children; infants; neonates
Paget's disease of bone 32.13, 32.15
Paget's disease of nipple 21.3
pain
  abdominal, see abdominal pain; epigastric pain
  in abscesses 5.2
  after abdominal surgery 9.9
  assessment and monitoring in cancer 33.2
  from diaphragm 10 – 1
  from kidney and pancreas 10 – 1
  perception 33 – 1, 33.2
  in peritonitis 6.2
  referred 16.6
    in acute abdomen 10.1
    to shoulder 11.2D, 11.2
  relief in cancer 33 – 1, 33.2, 33 – 2
    adjuvants 33.2
    plasma levels of drugs 33 – 3
    tolerance and dependence 33.2
    WHO's step ladder 33.2, 33 – 2
palate
  cleft 26.8
  perforation 25.11
  tumours 32 – 9, 32.22
palmar space, deep 8 – 1
palsy, tourniquet 3.9D
pampiniform plexus 15.5
Pancoast's tumour 32.29
pancreas
  annular 28.3
  body, carcinoma 32.26a
  carcinoma 13.1, 32.26a
  examination 13.8
  causes of acute abdomen 10.2
  disease 13.1
  head, carcinoma 13.8, 32.26a
  hepatoma vs 32.26
pancreatic abscess 5.10b, 13.10
  signs and diagnosis 10.2
pancreatic pseudocyst 10.2, 13 – 6, 13.10
pancreatitis 5.10b, 9.2, 13.9
  acute 10 – 3, 11.2, 13.9
    abdominal pain in 10.2
    difficulties with 13.9D
    gallstones with 13.9D
    signs and diagnosis 10.2, 10.4D
  chronic 13.1
  chronic relapsing (recurrent) 13.9
pannus 24.1, 24.13
panophthalmitis 24.3, 32.7
panuveitis 24.5
Papanicolau (Pap) smears 32.35
papilloedema 24.1
papilloma
  intraduct 21.5, 21 – 8
  mouth 26.9, 26 – 12
paracervical block 15.3
paracetamol 33.2
paracolic abscess 6 – 4, 31.10, 31.11
paraffinoma 22.2
paraldehyde 17.4

parallel bars 27.5, 27 – 5
paralysis in leprosy 30.1a, 30.2, 30.8, 30.9
    feet 30.5, 30.6, 30 – 6
    hands 30.4
    management 30.1a
    sudden reversible 30.1a
    type two reactions 30.1a
paralysis, obstetric, Stop Press
paralytic ileus, *see* ileus
parametritis 6.6, 6.7, 6 – 9
parametrium, fibroids projecting into 20 – 4
paranasal sinuses 25.16
paraphimosis 23.27D, 23.27, 23 – 36
    balanitis with 23 – 37
    recurrence 23.27D
paraplegia
    in Burkitt's lymphoma 29.4, 32.3D, 32.3
    in osteitis of spine 7.15
    in tuberculosis 29.4a, 29.4D
parasitoses, of female genital tract 20.14
paraspinal abscess 29 – 3a, 29.4a
paraumbilical hernia 14.9, 14.11D, 14.11, 14 – 20
paraurethral glands, catheter blocking 23.2
paravertebral abscess 7.15, 29.4
parenteral nutrition 9.7, 9.10
paronychia 8 – 1, 8.2, 8 – 2
parotid abscess 5 – 7a, 5.9
parotidectomy 32.23
parotid gland 5 – 7a, 5.8
    anatomy 5 – 7a, 5.8
    tumours 32 – 10, 32.23
partogram 17 – 3, 18.2, 18 – 2, inside back cover
Patey's modified radical mastectomy, *see*
        mastectomy
patients 1.5
    late presentation, reasons for 1.5
    records 1 – 10
    typical 1 – 3, 1.14
Payr's clamp 9.3, 9 – 6
'peau d'orange' ('orange skin') 21.3D, 21.3, 21 – 3
pectinate line 22 – 1, 22 – 4
    anorectal fistulae sites 22.2
    lesion below 22.3
pectineal ligament 14.2, 14.7D, 14.7, 14 – 16
pectoralis major
    breast lump adherence 21.3
    breast tumour fixed, mastectomy 21.5
    removal, in radical mastectomy 21.6
pectoralis minor, removal, in Patey's modified
        mastectomy 21.6
pedicle, control bleeding from 3.2
Pel – Ebstein fever 32.4
pelvic abscess 6.2D, 6.3, 6 – 4, 6.5, 9.10, 10.4D,
        10.4, 16.7
    after appendicectomy 12.2D
    after Caesarean section 6.7
    diagnosis 6.3, 6.5
    drainage (rectal, vaginal) 6.5, 6 – 7
    fever and passage of mucus 6.5, 9.10
    in pelvic inflammatory disease 6.5, 6.6
    in puerperal sepsis 6.5, 6.7
    ruptured 6.6D
    in septic abortion 6.5, 6.6a
    suprapubic drainage 6.5
    vaginal detection 6.3
pelvic cavity
    examination, in acute abdomen 10.1
    nodules in 6.6D
pelvic cellulitis 6.6a, 6.6
pelvic haematocele 16 – 6a, 16 – 6, 16.7
pelvic inflammatory disease (PID) 1.14, 6.6D, 6.6,
        6 – 8, 6 – 9
    adhesions after, infertility due to 15.2
    after Caesarean section 6.6, 6.8
    appendicitis vs 12.1
    associated with fibroids 20.6
    chronic, management 6.6
    contraindication to minilap tubal ligation 15.3
    obstruction due to adhesions 10.7
    pelvic abscess after 6.5
    pelvic haematocele vs 16 – 6, 16.7
    pelvic tuberculosis and 6.6, 6 – 11
    plan for managing 6 – 10
    post-abortal 6.6a, 6.6
    presenting as acute abdomen 10.2, 10 – 3
    in puerperal sepsis 6.6, 6.7
pelvic mass, fibroid differential diagnosis 20.6
pelvic pain 6.6D, 6.6
pelvic peritonitis 10.2, 16.7
pelvic sepsis 2.9, 6.5, 6.6, 6 – 9

pelvic sepsis (*cont.*)
    see also pelvic abscess; pelvic inflammatory
        disease (PID)
pelvirectal abscess 5.13
pelvis
    acute inflammation 6.6
    ligaments of 20.12, 20 – 17
    osteomyelitis of 7.15
pelviureteric junction, stone impacted at 23.14,
        23 – 15
    removal 23.14
penicillin, resistance 2.8
penicillinase-producing *Neisseria gonorrhoeae*
        (PPNG) 6.61.14
penicillin G (benzylpenicillin) 2.8, 2.9
penile clamp 23.1
penis
    amputation 32.34
        partial 32 – 18, 32.33
        total 32 – 19, 32.33
    carcinoma 1.5, 23.26, 32.33
    dyskeratosis 23.28
    elephantiasis 31.7, 31 – 8
    junction with scrotum, stricture at 23.8
    swelling 23.9D
penoscrotal angle, stricture at 23.2
peptic ulcer 11.1, 11.2
    bleeding 11.3, 11.4
        if bleeding site not obvious 11.4
        surgery for 11 – 3, 11.4
    carcinoma of stomach vs 32.25
    complications 11 – 11
    history 11.1
    penetration into liver 11 – 11, 11.2D
    perforated 6.2, 9.3, 10 – 3, 11.2D, 11.2
        appendicitis vs 12.1
        closure 11 – 12, 11.2
        differential diagnosis 11.2, 12.1, 25.16
        non – operative treatment 11.2
        signs and diagnosis 10.2
        'silent interval' 10.1, 11.2
        typhoid perforation vs 31.8
    rectal bleeding due to 22.3
    recurrence 11.4, 11.6D
    ruptured oesophagus vs 25.16
    subacute perforation 11.2
    vagotomy for 11 – 4, 11.4
percussion
    in acute abdomen 10.1
    after abdominal surgery 9.11a
    in intestinal obstruction 10.4
    for liver dullness 10.1
    shifting dullness 10.4
perforating veins, legs 34.1, 34 – 1
periadenitis 5 – 10, 5.12
perianal abscess 5.2, 5 – 12, 5.13, 22.7
perianal area, warty cauliflower-like lesions 22.10
perianal fistula 22.2, 22.8
periareolar incision 1.5, 21.4, 21 – 5
pericardial effusion 6.1a
pericardial rub 6.1a
pericardium
    amoebic liver abscess discharge into 31.12D
    aspiration 6.1a, 6 – 2a
    pus in 6.1a
        danger of draining 6.1a
    pericoronal abscess 5.8
perinatal mortality 15.1a, 17.2, 19.6, 34.7
    breech deliveries, presentations 19.8
    causes 19.13
    reduction by use of partogram 18.2
    resuscitation and 19.12
perinatal period, definition 19.8
perineal body, torn 18.16
perineal pain 23.22, 32.32
perinephric abscess 5 – 9a, 5.11a
    amoebic liver abscess vs 31.12
perinephric fascia 5 – 9a
perineum
    swelling 23.9D
    watering can 23.9, 23 – 10
periodontal abscess 5.8
periodontal disease 26 – 2, 26.2
    teeth extraction 26.3
periorbital cellulitis 5.5
periosteal elevator 7.2, 7 – 3
periosteum
    cautions applying to, in osteomyelitis 7.5
    draining, for acute mastoiditis 25.4
    removal, in rib resection 6.1, 6 – 2

periosteum (*cont.*)
    stripped, in acute osteomyelitis 7.2, 7.3
    stripping from twelfth rib 23.13, 23 – 16
peripheral circulation failure, in peritonitis 6.2
peripheral neuritis, 'MOPP' regimen causing
        32.4D
periportal cirrhosis 11.5D
periportal fibrosis 11.3, 11.5
peristalsis
    in acute abdomen 10.1
    in hypertrophic pyloric stenosis 28 – 3, 28.4
    in intestinal obstruction 10.4, 10 – 19
    in pyloric stenosis 11.6
peritoneal aspiration, in ectopic pregnancy 16.6
peritoneal cavity 6 – 3
    abscesses in 6.3, 6 – 4, 9.12
    amoebic liver abscess rupture into 31.12D,
        31.12
    avoidance, in emergency suprapubic puncture
        23 – 6, 23.6
    avoidance in fibroid removal 20 – 4, 20.6
    blood in 12.2D, 16.7
    after 'D and C' 20.3D
    carbon dioxide flow into 15.4
    fluid in
        in acute pancreatitis 13.9
        appearances 9.2, 10.5, 11.2, 12.2D
    hydatid daughter cysts 31.13D, 31.13
    hydatidosis of 31.13D
    opening 9.2, 9 – 2
    persistent sepsis 6.6D
    pus in 6.7, 10.12, 16.7
    size 6.2
    washing out 6.2, 10.5, 11.2, 20.3D
        after rupture of uterus 18.17, 20.3D
peritoneal fluid, in abdominal tuberculosis 29.6
peritoneal irritation 12.1
peritoneal tap 13.9
peritoneum
    antibiotics in 2.9
    biopsy 29.6
    brown nodules on surface 6.6D
    carcinomatosis 10.14, 29.6
    gas in 10.4
    incision, lower segment Caesarean section 18.9,
        18 – 11
    inflamed, signs 10.1
    miliary nodules on 29.6, 29 – 6
    parietal 10.1
        biopsy 29.7
        in extraperitoneal Caesarean section 18.13,
            18 – 15
        inflammation, pain in 10.1
peritonitis 4.10, 6.2D, 6.2
    abdominal movement in 10.1
    after 'D and C' 20.3D
    antibiotics for 2.8
    appearance of gut in 9.2, 10.5
    causes 6.2D, 6.2, 10.1
    drainage in 6.2
    faecal 9.6D
    generalized 6.2, 6.3, 6.4
        in appendicitis 12.1, 12.2D
        causes 10.1
        pelvic abscess after 6.5
        in pelvic inflammatory disease 6.6
        peptic ulcer perforation 11.2
        in septic abortion 6.6a
        signs 6.2, 6.6a
    in strangulated intestinal obstruction 10.4
    in hydatid disease 31.13D
    in intestinal amoebiasis 31.10, 31.11D
    intrauterine infection 18.13
    lavage in 6.2
    localized 6.2, 31.8
    meconium 28.2
    non-operative treatment 6.2
    pelvic 6.6, 10.2
    in pelvic inflammatory disease (PID) 6.6D, 6.6
    perforated gall-bladder 13.3
    plastic 29.7
    post-abortal 6.6
    postoperative 9.10
    primary 6.2D, 6.2, 31.8D
    prophylactic antibiotics for 2.9
    in puerperal sepsis 6.7
    respiration in 10.1
    signs 6.2, 6.6a, 10.1, 10.2, 10.4
    'silent interval' in onset 10.1
    spreading 6.2

perionitis (cont.)
  stages 6.2
  tuberculous 29 – 4, 29.6
  typhoid 6.2, 31.8
peritonsillar abscesses 5 – 6, 5.6
periurethral abscess 5.14D, 5.14, 23.5, 23.8, 23.9D, 23.10
peroneal artery, vein and nerve 7 – 11, 7.12
peroneal palsy 30.5, 30 – 6
  in leprosy 30.6D
peroneus brevis 30.8D, 30.8, 30 – 11
peroneus tertius 30.8D, 30.8, 30 – 11
Perthes' disease 1 – 3, 27.13, 27.14
  groups 27.14, 27 – 16
  treatment 27.14
pessaries, for prolapse 20.9, 20 – 9a
pethidine 17.4, 33.2
  neonatal depression 19.12
petrol 1.14
Pfannensteil incision 14.8, 23 – 7, 23 – 19, 23.19
  method 23.15, 23 – 20
phalanx
  foot, amputation in leprosy 30.7, 30 – 9
  infected 8.1, 8.2
  osteomyelitis of 8.5
  terminal, ulcer in leprosy 30.6D
  volar surface, infections of spaces over 8.6
Pharaonic circumcision 20.13
pharyngeal space, lateral, pus in 5.8, 5 – 7 ??
pharyngitis, gangrenous 25.16
pharynx
  foreign body in 25.13
  perforation of wall 25.13
phenobarbitone, in pregnancy 17.4
phenoxybenzamine hydrochloride 23.20
phenytoin, in pregnancy 17.4
pheonolic antiseptics 2.5
phimosis 23.27, 23 – 37, 32.33
  recurrent 23.26
photophobia 24.1
physiotherapy
  for foot drop 30.8
  in leprosy 30.1a
  respiratory 9.11a, 9.11, 9 – 22
PID, see pelvic inflammatory disease (PID)
pigbel disease 10.2, 22.3D, 22.3, 31.9
piles 22.4
  accessory 22.6D
  anorectal fistulae with 22.2D
  bleeding 22.4
  differential diagnosis 22.3
  examination 22.4
  first- and second-degree 22.4, 22.5, 22 – 10
  internal 22.4
  Lord's anal dilatation for 22.4, 22.5, 22 – 9, 22 – 10
  mistaken diagnosis with rectal bleeding 22.3
  primary, sites of 22 – 4
  prolapsed 22.4, 22.6
    after Lord's procedure 22.5D
    Milligan's haemorrhoidectomy for 22.6, 22 – 11
  recurrence 22.5D
  symptoms 22.4
  third degree 22.4
  thrombosed 22.4, 22.5D
  tying and excising 22.6D, 22.6, 22 – 11
pilocarpine 24.6
pilonidal infections 22.8
pilonidal sinus 22.8D
  operative treatment 22.8, 22 – 12
  posterior fistula vs 22.2D
  subcutaneous, perianal fistula vs 22.8
pin, in urethra 23.30
'pinching technique', separation of adhesions 10.7
pingecula 24.15
pin hole test 24.1, 24.8, Stop Press
pinna, rotation 25.4
piperazine 10.6
'Pitressin' 11.3, 11.5
placenta
  adherent to uterus 19.11aD
  at vulva, in rupture of uterus 18.17
  cut, in lower segment Caesarean section 18.9
  delivery
    in classical Caesarean section 18.12, 18 – 14
    by controlled cord traction 19 – 9, 19.11a
  difficulties in Caesarean section 18.9, 18.10D
  inspection after removal 19.11a
  not removed in Caesarean section 18.10D

placenta (cont.)
  removal
    inversion of uterus during 19.11a, 19.11aD, 19 – 12
    in lower segment Caesarean section 18.9
    manual 19.11a, 19.11aD, 19 – 10
    retained pieces 19.11a, 19.11b
    stuck in cervix 16.2D
placenta accreta, increta 19.11aD
placental abruption 16.2, 16.11, 16.13D, 17.4D
  after amniocentesis 19.2D
  delivery in 16.13
  disseminated intravascular coagulation in 19.11a
  examination in theatre for 16.12
  in multiple pregnancies 19.11D
  placenta praevia vs 16.11
  revealed, concealed and mixed 16 – 9, 16.13
  signs 18.17
placenta praevia 16.1, 16.11, 16.12
  Caesarean section in 18.8, 18.9, 18.10D
  during labour 16.12
  examination in theatre (EIT) 16.12
  implantation close to internal os 16 – 3, 16.6
  placental abruption vs 16.11
  rupture of membranes to induce labour and 19.3
  types, determination 16 – 9, 16.12
plantar oedema, in podoconiosis 31.5
plantar ulcers 30.5, 30 – 6, 30.6
plaque, dental 26 – 2
plasma cells, in myelomatosis 32.16
plasma expanders 17.4
'Plastazote' 30 – 4, 30.5, 30 – 5
plaster cast
  for contractures 27.2, 27.6, 27 – 9
  knee contractures 27.2, 27.4, 27.6, 27 – 9
  in leprosy 30.6, 30 – 7
    if impractical 30.6D
  in neonatal talipes equinovarus 27.15, 27 – 18
  serial 27.2, 27.4, 27.7
  for tibialis posterior tendon transfer 30.8, 30 – 4
  wedging 27.2, 27.4, 27.6
plastic surgery 4.8
plate, chronic osteomyelitis after application 7.6D
platelet count, chemotherapy 32.2D, 32.2
pleura
  accidental opening
    during nephrostomy 23.13
    in laparotomy 9.2D
    in subphrenic abscess drainage 6.4D
  anatomy of 6 – 1
  damage, in costotransversectomy 29.4aD
  pus in 6.1
  stuck to ribs 6.1
pleural effusion
  aspiration 6.1
  closed drainage 6 – 1a, 6.1
  in extraintestinal amoebiasis 31.12D
  stages in drainage 6 – 1a, 6.1
pleural pain, abdominal rigidity in 10.1
pleurisy, basal signs and diagnosis 10.2, 10 – 4
pneumocystis pneumonia 28a.2
pneumonia
  acute abdomen vs 10.1
  appendicitis vs 12.2D
  pneumocystis 28a.2
  right basal, biliary colic vs 13.2
  signs and diagnosis 10.1, 10.2, 10 – 4
pneumoperitoneum 15.4
podoconiosis 31.4, 31.5
poliomyelitis 7.3, 27.2, 27.4
  appliances for 27.5
  chronic 27 – 3, 27.4D, 27.4
  contractures 1.4, 27 – 3, 27.4
  effects 27.6
  prevention 27.3
  equinus deformity in, see equinus deformity
  hip deformities 27 – 3, 27.4, 27.6
  knee deformities in 27 – 3, 27.4, 27 – 4, 27.6
  shortening in 27.4
  spinal tuberculosis vs 29.4
polyethylene, foamed 30.5
polyhydramnios 16.9, 17.3, 19.7
polyp
  mucosal 20 – 5, 20.6D, 20.6
  submucous fibroid 20.6
popliteal artery 3.7, 3.8
  exposing and tying 3.8, 3 – 10
popliteal nerves, medial and lateral 3.8

porta hepatis, tumour of 13.8
portal fibrosis, noncirrhotic 11.3, 11.5D, 11.5
portal hypertension 11.3, 11.5, 13.12
portal vein, thrombosis 11.5D
port wine stain 28.10, 28 – 11
position in bed, in acute abdomen diagnosis 10.1
positions of function, in ankylosis 7 – 16, 7.17
positions of safety and rest, of joint 7.17
post-abortal pelvic inflammatory disease 6.6a, 6.6, 16.2
post-abortal sepsis 16.2
post-amoebic stricture 31.10, 31.11D
postauricular lymphadenitis 25.4
postCaesarean pelvic inflammatory disease 6.6, 6.8
postcoital bleeding 20.2, 20.13, 32.35
postcricoid web 34.5, 34 – 10
posterior fornix, aspiration 6.5, 6.6a
posterior tibial nerve palsy 30.1a, 30.5
postinflammatory cyst, ovarian 20.7D, 6.5
postinflammatory pseudocyst 6.5, 20.7D
postmaturity 19.6
postmenopausal bleeding 20.2, 32.35
postmenstrual pelvic inflammatory disease (PID) 6.6
postoperative bleeding 3.10, 22.6D, 23.19D, 26.3D
postpartum haemorrhage (PPH) 1.14, '3.5, 19.11a, 19.11aD, Stop Press
  after placental abruption 16.13
  after 'trial of scar' 18.14
  assessment and resuscitation 19.11a
  bimanual compression 19.11a, 19 – 10
  causes 19.11a
  exploration and cervical tear repair 19.11a, 19 – 11
  hysterectomy for 20.12
  oxytocin for 18.4a
  with placenta in/out 19.11a, 19 – 10
  in placenta praevia 16.12
  prevention, before/during labour 19.11a
  secondary 18.10D, 19.11b
postural drainage, after abdominal surgery 9.11a, 9 – 23
potassium
  deficiency 31.11
  intravenous fluids 6.2, 10.5, 23.5, 28.4
  replacement 10.5, 23.5
    in children, neonates 28.1, 28.4
Pott's puffy tumour 5.4a
pouch of Douglas
  abscess pointing into 6.5, 6 – 7
  fetal implantation 16.9
  hernia of 20.11(a)
  mass bulging into 10.4
povidone 28a – 1a, 28a.2
Powell's sound 23 – 14
PPH, see postpartum haemorrhage (PPH)
PPNG (penicillinase-producing Neisseria gonorrhoeae) 1.14
pre-eclampsia 17.4
pregnancy 17.1 – 6
  anaemia in 17.2
  appendicitis in 12.2D
  diabetes in 17 – 1a, 17.3
  ectopic, see ectopic pregnancy
  fibroid differential diagnosis 20.6
  fibroid removal 20.6D
  goitre in 21.10, 21 – 13
  haematòmetra in 20.14 heart failure in 17.5D, 17.5
  hydatidiform mole 32.37, 32.38
  hypertension in 17 – 2, 17.4, 32.38
  mastitis carcinomatosa in 21.3, 21.4
  multiple 19 – 7, 19.10, 19.11D, 19.11
    Caesarean section for 19.11
    delivery 19 – 8, 19.11
    internal podalic version 19 – 8, 19.11
    presentations 19 – 7, 19.11
  ovarian cysts in 20.7D
  reduction in frequency 15.1a
  surgery of 16.1 – 12
  termination, indications in pre-eclampsia 17.4
  tests 16.6, 32.38D, 32.38
  uterine bleeding related to 20.2
pregnancy epulis 26.9, 26 – 12
pregnancy induced hypertension(PIH) 17.4, 32.38
premature rupture of the membrantes, 19.5, Stop Press
prematurity, breech presentation in 19.8
premolar, extraction 26.3, 26 – 4, 26 – 5
prepuce 23.26

prepuce (cont.)
  carcinoma 32.33
  in circumcision 23.26, 23 – 35
  difficulty in separating from glans penis 23.26D
  elephantiasis 31.7
  inflammation 23.30
  oedema 23.27, 23 – 37
  orifice in, small 23.27
preputial adhesions 23.26
presbyopia 24.4, 24.8D, 24.8
pressure, control of bleeding by 3.1, 3.10
pressure packs, dry firm 3.1
preterm infant
  intrauterine growth retardation (IUGR) risk 19.13
  resuscitation in 19.12D
preterm labour, see labour, preterm
priapism 23.29, 23 – 39
  postoperative 23.26D
Primary Health Care Prefaces(4, 6)
Primary Mother Care 15.1a, 18.2, 18.6, 18.15
procarbazine 32.2D, 32.4
processus vaginalis, abnormalities of 14.5, 14 – 15
procidentia 20 – 9, 22.9
Procter – Livingstone tube 32.24
proctology 22.1 – 10, 22 – 4
  equipment 22.1
  general method 22.1
proctoscope, Gabriel 22.1
proctoscopy 22.1, 22.4
progestogens
  in breast carcinoma 21.4
  cyclical 20.2
proguanil 17.2
promethazine, in 'lytic cocktail' 17.4
pronator teres 7.8
pronychia 8.4
propranol, in hyperthyroidism 21.8
proptosis 24.1, 24.11
  in Burkitt's lymphoma 32.2, 32.3, 32 – 3
  causes 24 – 10, 24.11
  in cavernous sinus thrombosis 5.5, 5 – 5
  management 24.11
prostaglandins
  extra-amniotic 16.4
  for intrauterine death 16.4, Stop Press
  pessaries 32.38
  ripening the cervix 19.3
prostate
  appearance, in cystoscopy 23.3, 23.18, 32.32
  biopsy 32.32
  bleeding, after Freyer's prostatectomy 23.19D, 23.19
  carcinoma 23.5, 23.18, 23.19D, 32.32
    Ghadvi's prostatectomy and 23.21
    orchidectomy in 23.25, 23 – 32
    prostatectomy contraindication 23.18, 32.32
  damage, by bouginage 23.8
  enlargement 23.18, 23.19
    urinary retention in 23.5
  enucleation, in Freyer's prostatectomy 23.19
  examination under anaesthesia (EUA) 32.32
  injecting 23.22, 23 – 29
  in rectal examination 22.1, 23.5, 32.32
  rhabdomyosarcoma 32.9
  size, in obstruction assessment 23.5
  'small fibrous' 23.20, 23.21
  tuberculous 29.9
prostatectomy 23 – 23
  Freyer's transvesical, see Freyer's transvesical
  Ghadvi's lateral perineal 23.19, 23.21, 23 – 28
  indications 23.18
  Millin's retropubic 23.19, 23.21
prostatic abscess 5.15, 5.16, 23.5
prostatic adenoma 23.19
  enucleating 23.19, 23.21, 23 – 25
prostatic capsule 23.19, 23.21, 23 – 25
prostatic cavity
  bleeding control 23.19, 23.21
  in Ghadvi's prostatectomy 23.21
  packing 23.19, 23 – 27
  suturing 23.19, 23 – 25
prostatic hypertrophy, benign 23.5, 23.9D, 23.19
  cystoscopic appearance 23 – 23
  haematuria 23.4
  injection method 23.22, 23 – 29
prostatic obstruction 23.18, 23.20, 23.22
  relief, methods 23.19
  symptoms with urinary retention 23.5D

prostatic obstruction (cont.)
  urethral stricture vs 23.8
prostatic symptoms 23.18
prosthesis, kneeling leg 30.6D, 30 – 8
'Prostin' 16.4, 19.3
proteinuria 17.4, 23.5
provinical hospital, in referral system 1 – 5, 1.6, Preface 6
proximal interphalangeal joint (PIP) 1.14
pruritus ani 22.7
pseudocyst
  ovarian 20.7D, 20.7
  pancreatic 10.2
  in pelvic inflammatory disease (PID) 6.6
  postinflammatory 6.5
pseudomembranous colitis 2.8
pseudo-obstruction, intestinal 10.5D
pseudotumour, of orbit 24.11
psoas abscess, tuberculous 5 – 10, 5.12, 29.4
psoas shadow 10.1
psychotropic drugs 33.2
pterygomandibular space, pus in 5 – 7, 5.8
pthisis bulbi 24.3, 24.4
ptosis 24.1, 24.15, 34.4
pubis, osteomyelitis of 7.15
puboprostatic ligaments 23 – 19
puborectalis muscle 22 – 1
puborectalis sling, in anorectal malformations 28 – 5, 28.6
pudendal block 18.1a, 18 – 1
puerperal haemorrhage 19.11b
puerperal pelvic inflammatory disease (PID) 6.6, 6.7
puerperal sepsis 6.5, 6.6, 6.7, 16.12, 17.2D
  premature rupture of membranes and 19.5
puerperium, anaemia during 17.2D
pulmonary complications, of passing nasogastric tube 4.9D
pulmonary oedema 17.4D, 17.4
pulp infections, see finger, pulp space
pulse rate
  in acute abdomen 10.1
  after 'D and C' 20.3D
  in appendicitis 12.1
  during bronchoscopy 25.12
  indication of rupture of uterine scar 18.14
'pulse test' 11.3
pulsus alternans, pulsus paradox 6.1a
pupils
  abnormal responses 24.6
  dilatation 24.6
  examination 24.1
  fixed dilated white 24.6D
  swinging response 24.6
purse string sutures 9.3, 9 – 6, 10.5, 10 – 9
pus 2.3, 2.10, 5.1 – 16, 6.1 – 8, 7.1 – 19, 8.1 – 17
  in abdomen 6.2, 6.3, 6.4, 10.5
  in anterior chamber of eye 24.3, 24.4
  in bones 7.2
    see also osteomyelitis
  in breasts 21.2
  culture 7.4
  in dental abscesses 5 – 7, 5.8
  drainage 4.10, 5.1
  in feet 8.17
  fluctuation 5.1, 5.2, 8.9
  in hands 8.1 – 16
  inhalation 5 – 6, 5.6, 5.7
  in joints 7.16, 7.17, 7.18
  in laparotomy wound 9.12
  in muscles 7.1, 7.5
  in neck 5 – 8, 5.10
  in orbit 5 – 4, 5.5
  in pelvis 2.9, 6.5, 6.6, 6 – 9
  in pericardium 6.1a
  in peritoneal cavity 6.2, 6.3, 10.12
  in pleura, see empyema
  signs of 6.7
  tuberculous 29.4a
    see also abscesses; individual conditions; sepsis
'push and spread' technique 4.3, 4 – 8
pyaemia 7.1, 7.14
  with pyomyositis 7.1
pyelonephritis, acute 17.6, 23.12
pyloric carcinoma 11.6, 32.25
pyloric obstruction 11 – 11, 32.25
pyloric stenosis 11.2D, 11.6
  in carcinoma of stomach 32.25
  cause 11.6
  gastroenterostomy 11.6, 11 – 6

pyloric stenosis (cont.)
  hypertrophic 28.2, 28 – 3, 282.4
  malignant obstruction? 11.6
  non-operative treatment 11.6
  pyloroplasty incision 11 – 3, 11.4
pyloroplasty 11.4, 11.6, 11.7
  method 11 – 3, 11.4
pyogenic granuloma, gum 26.9
pyometra 32 – 21
pyomyositis 5.2, 5.11a, 7.1, 7 – 1, 7.3, 10.2
  in buttock 7.18
  iliopsoas 5 – 10, 5.12
  sites 7 – 1
  of spine 27.8
pyonephrosis 10.2
pyosalpinx 6.6
  appendicitis vs 12.1
  chronic 16.6D
  tuberculous 6 – 11
pyramidal lobe of thyroid 21.9, 21 – 13
pyrazinamide, in tuberculosis 29.1
pyrexia of unknown origin (PUO), in pregnancy 17.6
pyrimethamine 17.2
pyuria, in urogenital tuberculosis 29.9

Q
quality of life, of cancer patients 32.1
quality in surgery, indicators 34.6, 34.7
Quire's hook 25.1

R
radial bursa infection 8.14
radial nerve 7.7, 7 – 7
  injury 1.6
  paralysis 1.6, 3.9, 27.5, 30.1a
radial styloid, pain over 27.10
radiology 1 – 8, 1.13, 34.5
  see also X-rays
radiotherapy
  in breast carcinoma 21.3, 21.4
  in carcinoma of mouth 32.22
  in carcinoma of oesophagus 32.24
  in follicular carcinoma of thyroid 21.12
  in Hodgkin's lymphoma 32.4
  seminoma 32.34a
radius
  exposing 7 – 8
  osteomyelitis of 7.8, 7 – 8
railroading 32.24D, 32.24
Ramstedt's operation 28 – 3, 28.4
ranitidine 11.7, 18.9
ranula 26.9, 26 – 13
Rappaport classification 32.5
razors 4.11, 35 – 1
reading difficulty 24.1, 24.8
reading list, suggested 1.14
records, patient's 1 – 10
recovery position 9.9
rectal agenesis 28 – 5, 28.6
  low, with/without fistulae 28.6, 28 – 7, 28 – 8
rectal ampulla 22.1
rectal atresia 28 – 5, 28.6
rectal bleeding 22.3D, 22.3
  in abdominal tuberculosis 29.7
  after haemorrhoidectomy 22.6D
  in carcinoma of rectum 32.27
  common causes 22.3
  differential diagnosis 22.3
  general method and examination 22.3
  management, laparotomy 22.3
  piles causing 22.4
rectal drainage, pelvic abscess 6.5
rectal examination 22.1, 22 – 2
  in acute abdomen 10.1
  in appendicitis 12.1
  in carcinoma of prostate 32.32
  in intestinal obstruction 10.4
  for piles 22.4
  of prostate 23.5
rectal mass 32.27
rectal prolapse 10.8, 20.9, 20.11a, 22.3, 22.9
  manual replacement and strapping 22.9
'rectal shelf' 10.4, 32.25
rectal snip 11.5D
rectal tube 4.11
rectal ulcer 22.10
rectocele 20 – 9
  posterior colporrhaphy for 20 – 12, 20.11(a)
rectosigmoid junction, carcinoma 32 – 15a, 32.27

recto – vaginal fistula (RVF) 1.14, 9.5, 18.19, 18 – 24
  after obstructed labour 18.3
  repair 18.19D, 18.19
rectovesical pouch, mass in 10.4
rectum 22.1 – 10
  adenocarcinoma of 22.1
  in amoebiasis 31.10
  anatomist's and proctologist's view 22 – 1
  carcinoma 22.10, 32 – 15a, 32.27
  carcinomatous obstruction, differential diagnosis 10.10
  digital evacuation 22.10
  empty, in intestinal obstruction 10.4
  general method for 22.1
  hole in, peritonitis management 6.2
  if bougie enters 23.9D
  if finger goes into, in Ghadvi's prostatectomy 23.21D
  injury
    in chronic ectopic pregnancy 16.7D
    in colporrhaphy 20.11aD
  lesions of 22.10
  stitching to sacrum, in rectal prolapse 22.9
  stricture 22.10, 32.27
  third-degree tears, repair 18.15, 18 – 17
  ulcerative or proliferative lesion 22.10
  see also entries beginning anorectal, rectal
rectus muscle, splitting, in abdominal surgery 9.2, 9 – 2
rectus sheath 23 – 20
relaxing incisions 14.11, 14.21
red blood cells, transfusion 17.2
'red currant jelly' stools 10.1, 10.2, 10.8
'red degeneration' of fibroids 20.6
'Redivac' drain, after Patey's mastectomy 21.5, 21.6, 21 – 7
reef knots 4 – 8, 4 – 10, 4 – 11, 4.8 4 – 9
referral Preface 6, 1.3, 1.6
  advice on procedure 1.6
  after exteriorization in intestinal obstruction 10.5D, 10.5
  after gut resection in obstruction 10.5
  after intussusception 10.8
  in cancer 32.1
  cases for 1.4, 1.6
  in chronically obstructed kidney 23.13
  in chronic osteomyelitis 7.6
  closing of Hartmann's operation 10.10a
  definite conditions for 1.6
  in empyema 6 – 1a, 6.1
  for impassable urethral strictures 23.11
  intestinal fistula 9.14
  questions before and assessment 1.6
  steps in 1 – 5, 1.6
  urgency of 1.6
  see also other individual conditions
referral hospitals 1.6
referral systems Preface 6, 1 – 5, 1.6
refractive errors 24.8
regurgitation, in carcinoma of oesophagus 32.24
rehabilitation, crippled children 27 – 12
rehydration, *see* fluid, replacement
Reiter's syndrome 27.13
renal calculi 10.1, 23.12, 23.13
renal calyx
  'moth-eaten', in tuberculosis 29.9
  stone in 23 – 15
renal colic 10.2, 10 – 3, 23.12
  appendicitis vs 12.1
renal cortex, nephrostomy through 23.13, 23 – 17
renal cysts, kidney tumours vs 32.30
renal disease, chronic, in pregnancy 17.6
renal failure
  acute, in pregnancy 17.6
  in acute pancreatitis 13.9D
  after snake bites 34.4D
  anuria with 23.12
  chronically obstructed kidney 23.13
  in gestational hypertension 17.4D
  recovery diuresis and 23.5
  secondary, urethral strictures causing 23.8
renal mass 23.12
renal parenchyma, staghorn calculus 23 – 15
renal pedicle, blood vessel tying 3.2
renal pelvis
  nephrostomy through 23.13, 23 – 17
  opening 23.13
renal toxicity, cytotoxic drugs 32.2D

resources, limited 1.12
respiration rate
  in acute abdomen diagnosis 10.1
  depressed, after abdominal surgery 9.11
  in neonates 19.12
respiratory distress syndrome 19.2
respiratory failure
  in acute pancreatitis 13.9D
  after abdominal surgery 9.11
  after removal of giant ovarian cysts 20.7D
  after snake bites 34.4D, 34.4
  magnesium sulphate in eclampsia 17.4
respiratory obstruction 25.16
respiratory tract
  clearing, after abdominal surgery 9.11
  infection, appendicitis vs 12.1
  tumours 32.28 – 29
resuscitation
  in acute pelvic inflammatory disease (PID) 6.6
  before cystogastrostomy 13.10
  in ectopic pregnancy 16.6
  in gastrointestinal bleeding 11.3
  for intestinal obstruction 10.5
  neonate, *see* neonatal resuscitation
  in peritonitis 6.2
  in placental abruption 16.13
  in postpartum haemorrhage (PPH) 19.11a
  in rupture of uterus 18.17
retina, in onchocerciasis 24.7
retinal detachment 24.4
retinal vein, artery, occlusion 24.4
retinitis pigmentosa 24.4
retinoblastoma 24.9, 24.11, 32.7
retinopathy, diabetic 17.3
retractors 4 – 4, 4.5, 9.2, 15.1a
retrobulbar alcohol 24.14D
retrobulbar haematoma 24.11
retrograde urethrogram 34.5, 34 – 9
retroperitoneal carcinomatous mass 10.5D
retropharyngeal abscesses 5 – 6, 5.7, 24.14D
retropubic calcifications 23.15
reversed slings 27.6, 27 – 9
rhabdomyosarcoma 32.9, 32.34a
rheumatic fever 27.13
rheumatic heart disease 6.1a
rheumatoid arthritis 27.13, 29.3
rhinitis, chronic atrophic 25.7D
rib
  chondrosarcoma 32.14
  pleura stuck to 6.1
  resection, in open drainage of empyema 6.1, 6 – 2
  twelfth, removal in nephrostomy 23.13, 23 – 16
Richter's hernia 9.3, 10.4D, 14.1, 14 – 1, 14.8
Ridley fundus 24.7
Riedel's thyroiditis 21.13
rifampicin 29.1
ring cutter 4.11
ring pessaries 20 – 9a 20.9
Rinne's test 25.2
'rocker bottom' foot 27.15
rodent ulcer 32 – 6
round ligaments 1.17, 15 – 6, 18 – 20, 20.12, 20 – 17
  tying in hysterectomy 20.12, 20 – 19, 20 – 21
Rovsing's sign 10.1, 12.1
RVF, *see* recto-vaginal fistula

S
sacrouterine ligament 18.17, 18 – 20
sacrum
  rectum stitched to, in rectal prolapse 22.9
  solid mass below in neonates 28.11
saline
  enema 28.2
  infusion 28a.2
  wound immersion in 1.12
salivary gland tumours 32 – 10, 32.23
Salmonella typhi 31.8, 31 – 9
salpingitis 6.6D, 6.6, 6 – 9, 6 – 11, 16.6D, 20.3D
salpingo-oophorectomy 20.7
salpingo-oophoritis 6.6, 6 – 11
Samway's tourniquet, avoid using 3.9, 3 – 11
saphenous vein 3.7, 34.1
  flush ligation and stripping 34.1, 34 – 2
  injury during varicose vein surgery 34.1D
  long, short 34.1, 34 – 1
    varix 14.7
  tying 34.1
sarcoma 32 – 5, 32.8 – 11

sarcoma (*cont.*)
  angiomatous of scalp 32 – 1
  granuloma pyogenicum vs 34.2, 34 – 6
  of mouth 32.22
  osteomyelitis differential diagnosis 7.3
  soft tissue 32.8
sarcoma botryoides 32.9
sartorius muscle, in block dissection of lymph nodes 32.34D, 32.34
saucerization 7.6
Savage decompressor 10.5, 10 – 9
scalenus anterior muscle 3.4
scalp
  burns, osteitis of skull 7 – 13, 7.14
  septic thrombophlebitis 7 – 13
scalpels 4 – 1, 4.2
  method for holding 4 – 1, 4.2
scars
  hypertrophic 34.1a, 34 – 3
  keloids, *see* keloids
  surgical 34.1a
Schiller's test 32.35
Schiötz tonometry 24.1, 24 – 3
Schistosoma haematobium
  bladder carcinoma 23.18, 32.31
  epididymitis due to 23.22a
  fibrosis of submucosa of trigone 23.20
  genital tract, nodules 20.14 haematuria due to 23.3, 23.4, 32.31
  suprapubic cystostomy avoidance 23.18
  urinary tract obstruction due to 23.13
  urogenital tuberculosis vs 29.9
Schistosoma mansoni 20.13, 22.1, 32.27
schistosomiasis
  bleeding oesophageal varices and 11.5D
  diagnosis 11.3, 23.3
  granuloma 20.5, 20.14 retropubic calcifications 23.15
Schlemm, canal of 24 – 1
sciatic irritation, tests 27 – 13
sciatic pain 27.8
scissors 4 – 2, 4.3, 35(Appendix A)
  dissecting 4.3
  ophthalmic 24.1
  tightening rivet and sharpening 35 – 2
sclera, in retinoblastoma 32.7
scleral sinus 24 – 1
sclerotherapy, varicose veins 34.1
scolices, in hydatid disease 31 – 12, 31.13
scolicides 31.13
scoliosis 29.4
scotoma, paracentral, arcuate, ring 24 – 9
scrotal area, bleeding from 23.23
scrotoplasty 23.23
scrotum
  abscess 5.14
  elephantiasis 1.5, 31.4, 31 – 5, 31.6, 31.7, 31 – 7
  Fournier's gangrene 23.30, 23 – 40
  junction with penis, stricture at 23.8
  oedema, in extravasation of urine 23.10
  swellings 14.4, 14 – 13
  after inguinal hernia repair 14.3D
scrubbing up 2.3, 2 – 5
  savings on 1.12
sea snakes 34.4
sebaceous cysts 34.3, 34 – 7
sedation 17.4, 23.29
seminal fluid, examination 15.2
seminal vesicle infection 23.8
  abscess 5.15, 5.16
seminoma 23.25, 32.34a
Sengstaken – Blakemore tube 11.5D, 11.5, 11 – 5
sensory nerves, destruction in leprosy 30.1
'sentinel skin tag' 22.7
sepsis
  catgut causing 4.6
  chronic at operation site, in AIDS 28a.3
  drainage 4.10
  exsanguination with Esmarch's bandage contraindication 3.9
  risk in laparotomy 9.2
  sites 5.1, 5 – 1
  surgery for 5.1 – 16
  see also abscess; surgical sepsis
septic abortion 6.6a, 6.6aD
septicaemia 2.7
  in acute pancreatitis 13.9D
  after chemotherapy 32.2
  neonatal gut obstruction vs 28.2
  pyomyositis with 7.1

septicaemia (*cont.*)
  streptococcal, after hand injury 8.16
septic arthritis 7 – 14, 7.16
  diagnosis 7.4
  of fingers 8 – 8, 8.15
  of foot 8.17, 30.6D
  of hip, *see* hip, septic arthritis
  in leprosy 30.4, 30.6D
  osteomyelitis with 7 – 2, 7.3, 7.5D, 7.16
  primary 7.3
  risk factors 7.16
  tuberculous arthritis vs 29.3
septic shock 6.2, 6.6, 10.1, 10.4
  in obstructed labour 18.3, 18.4
  in septic abortions 6.6aD
  signs 6.2
'Septrin' 2.8
sequestrectomy in osteomyelitis 7.2, 7.4, 7.6D, 7.6, 7 – 6
  of fibula 7.12
  of jaw 7.14a
  of tibia 7.11
sequestrum 7.2, 7 – 2, 7.14a
  in chronic osteomyelitis 7.6, 7 – 6
  as foreign body 7.6
  in skull 7 – 13, 7.14
  slipped upper femoral epiphysis 7.18
serratus anterior muscle, nerve to 21.6D, 21.6
Seward minor (SEW) table 2.1
sexual intercourse, AIDS transmission 28a.2
sexually transmitted disease (STD) 1.14
sharp equipment 4.12
shaving 1.9, 2.3
Shirodkar suture 16.5
shock
  after appendicectomy 12.2D
  after bouginage 23.9D
  central abdominal pain and 10.2
  in ectopic pregnancy 16.6
  in evacuating incomplete abortion 16.2D
  passing nasogastric tube 4.9D
  postoperative bleeding 3.10
  septic, *see* septic shock
  in snake bites 34.4
shoe
  'healing' 30.6D
  in leprosy 30 – 4, 30.5, 30.6D, 30 – 7
  modified 27.5, 27 – 6
  moulded 30 – 4, 30.5
  raised 27.5
  rocker sole 30.6D, 30 – 7
shoulder
  aspiration 7 – 15, 7.17
  dystocia 17.3D, 17.3
  if unable to pull down after Patey's operation 21.6D
  pain 6.4, 16.6
  position of function 7 – 16, 7.17
  referred pain 11.2D, 11.2
  tuberculosis 29.3
  winged, after Patey's operation 21.6D
sickle-cell crisis 10.2, 10 – 4
sickle-cell dactylitis 7.3
sickle-cell disease
  anaemia in pregnancy due to 17.2
  chronic osteomyelitis in 7.6D
  osteomyelitis vs 7.3
  painful hip in 27.13
  priapism in 23.29
  septic arthritis in 7.16
  splenectomy in 13.12
sigmoid colon
  carcinoma 10 – 7, 10.14, 32 – 15a, 32.27
  colostomy 9.5, 9.6, 9 – 14, 9 – 15
  gangrenous in volvulus 10.10
  injury, in chronic ectopic pregnancy 16.7D
  interval resection 10.10
  tear in PID management 6.6D
sigmoidoscope 22.1
  if oesophagoscope not available, foreign body removal 24.14D, 25.14
sigmoidoscopy
  before Lord's procedure 22.5
  method 22.1, 22 – 3
  for piles 22.4
  for sigmoid volvulus 10.10, 10 – 15
sigmoid volvulus 10.3, 10 – 3, 10.10, 10 – 14
  acute abdomen 10.1
  colostomy 9.5, 9.6, 10.10, 10 – 16
  compound 10.4D, 10.10D, 10.10, 10 – 17

sigmoid volvulus (*cont.*)
  difficulties 10.10D
  exteriorization for 10.10, 10 – 16
  gut appearance 10.5
  Hartmann's operation for 10.10, 10 – 16
  mechanism 10 – 14
  primary 10.9
  sigmoidoscopy for 10.10, 10 – 15
  signs 10.1, 10.2, 10.4D
  X-rays in 10.4, 10.10, 10 – 14
Silcock's forceps 4.4
silica 31.5
Sims' speculum 15.1a, 15 – 2
sinus, anorectal abscess 5 – 11, 5.13
sinusitis 25.7
  acute or chronic 25.7
  frontal 25.8
  maxillary 25 – 6, 25.8, 25.9
'Gishiri' cut 18.19D
sisterhood method, maternal mortality level 15.1
Sitz baths 18.10D
skin
  antiseptics for 2.5
  black necrotic 7.1D
  surgery 34.1a – 3
  suturing 4 – 7, 4.8
  traction, in contractures 27.2
  tumours 32.18 – 21, 32.34
skin grafts
  in Charles' operation for elephantiasis 31 – 6, 31.6
  in malignant melanoma 32.20
  in podoconiosis 31.5
  in squamous cell carcinoma 32.19
  in tropical ulcers 31.2
skull, osteitis of 7 – 13, 7.14
'slim disease' 28a.2
slit lamp microscopy 24.1, 24 – 4
sluice room 2.1
smell, in abdominal cavity 9.2
snake bites 34.4, 34 – 8
  antivenom 34.4
  management 34.4D, 34.4
snake toxins, effects 34.4
'sniffing position' 25 – 10, 25.14
soap, type to use 2.3
sodium amytal 17.4
sodium bicarbonate 19.12, 32.3
sodium citrate 23.19
sodium dichlorisocyanurate 28a – 1a, 28a.2
sodium hypochlorite 28a – 1a, 28a.2
sodium nitrite 2.5
soft tissue
  sarcomas 32.8
  tenderness, osteomyelitis differential diagnosis 7.3
  wounds, sepsis, treatment 2.9
solar energy 1.12
solar panel 2.1
sounds 23.1
  metal, passing 23 – 8, 23.8
space of Parona, infection 8 – 6, 8.9, 8.16
Spalding's sign 16.4
spasm, hip muscles, *see* hip, spasm
specialist fields 1.3, Preface 5
speculum, vaginal 15.1a, 15 – 2
Spencer Wells forceps 3 – 2, 3.2
spermatic cord 14.2, 14 – 4, 15.5
  covering 14 – 2
  excision 14.4
  lymphocele of 31 – 5, 31.6
  mobilization 23.25a
  relationship to indirect/direct inguinal hernias 14.2
  swelling in filariasis 31 – 5, 31.6
  torsion of 23.24D, 23 – 31
  veins of 15.5
spermatogenesis 23.25a
sphincter, anal, *see* anal sphincter
sphincter, external urethral
  avoidance in Ghadvi's prostatectomy 23.21
  catheter sticking at 23.2
  passing bougie through 23 – 8, 23.8
sphincterotomy, internal 22.6D
sphygmomanometer 3.9, 17.4
spider naevi 32.26
spina bifida 19.7, 28.9
spinal canal 29.4a, 29.4D
  open 28.9
spinal compression 29.4

spinal cord, congenital abnormalities 28.9
spinal needle, decompression of gut 10.5, 10 – 9
spine
  bridging 29.4
  cervical, tuberculosis of 29.4D
  examination 27 – 13
  flexion, lumbar disc lesions 27.8, 27 – 12a
  lumbar disc lesions 27.8D, 27.8
  osteomyelitis 5.11a, 5.12, 7.15, 27.8, 29.4a
  pyomyositis 27.8
  secondary tumours 29.4
  tuberculosis of, *see* tuberculosis, of spine
spleen
  large, in bleeding oesphageal varices 11.3
  ruptured 10.1, 10.2, 10 – 3
  torsion 13.12
splenectomy 13.12
splenic abscess 13.12
splenic implantation 13.12
splenic infarct 10.2
splenomegaly, nephroblastoma vs 32.6
splint
  foot, in leprosy 30.6
  foot-drop-positioning 30.8, 30 – 10
  hands and finger, in leprosy 30.4
  von Rosen 27.12, 27 – 15
spondylitis, ankylosis 27.8D
spondylolithesis 27.8D
sponge-holder 4 – 8, 4.11
spotlight 2.1, 2 – 3
'spread and cut' technique 10.7, 10.8, 10 – 11, 13.7
sputum, before/after abdominal surgery 9.1, 9.11
squamous cell carcinoma 32 – 6, 32.19D, 32.19
  bladder 32.31
  cervix 32 – 21, 32.35
  chronic tropical ulcer 31 – 1, 31.2D, 31.2
  kidney 32.30
  in leprosy 30.6D
  mouth 32.22
  penis 32.33
  skin 32.19D, 32.19
    block dissection in 32.34
squints 24.9, 32.7
staff, economical surgery and 1.12
stainless steel instruments 4.1
Stamm gastrostomy 11 – 7, 11.8
stand, solution 2.1
standard holding time, autoclaving 2.4
staphylococcal infections 2.9, 5.1
  boils and carbuncles 5.3, 5.4
  osteomyelitis 7.2, 7.4
  pyomyositis 7.1
Staphylococcus aureus, septic arthritis 7.16
staphyloma 24.3, 24.4, 24.11, 32.7
steam, sterilization 2.4
'Steam-clox' autoclave tape 2.4
steatorrhoea, in abdominal tuberculosis 29.7
steel instruments 4.1
stenosing tenosynovitis 27.10, 27 – 14
sterilization 2.3, 2.4, 2.6, 4.12, 28a.2
  by boiling 2.4, 4.12
  cystoscope 23.3
  inadequate
    AIDS transmission 28a.2
    checks to carry out 2.4D
    reasons for 2.4
  methods 2.4
  in rule about deciding when to operate 1.8
  by steam, moist heat 2.4, 4.12
sterilizer, boiling water 2.4
sterilizing room 2.1, 2 – 2
steroids
  acute abdomen symptoms 10.2D
  eye disorders and 24.1, 24.5
  in leprosy 30.1a
  nasal spray 25.7
  side-effects 32.4D
  use in uveitis 24.5
stethoscope, fetal 15.1a
stilboestrol 32.32
stillbirth 19.6
stomach 11.1 – 8
  aspiration of blood after surgery 3.10
  bleeding from 22.3
  carcinoma 13.8, 32.25, 34.5
  to check if nasogastric tube is in 4.9
  exposure 11.2
  failure of nasogastric tube to decompress 4.9
  'leather bottle' 32.25
  opening, in bleeding peptic ulcer surgery 11.4

635

stomach (cont.)
  perforated, during lavage 25.15
  in repair of distal tear of oesophagus 24–12, 25.16
  stress ulcers 11.4D
  washout, in pyloric stenosis 11.6, 25–11
stomata 9.5
  gastrojejunal 11.6D, 11.6
  see also colostomy; ostomy
stomatitis, chemotherapy 32.2D, 32.2, 32.4D
stool, operating 2.1
stools
  blood in 32.27
  loose, signs of obstruction with 10.4D
  pale, in obstructive jaundice 13.8
strangulated obstruction, see intestinal obstruction
strangury 23.16, 23.17, 29.9
'strawberry naevus' 28.10, 28–11
St. John's sling 8.1
Streptomyces spp. mycetoma 31.3
streptomycin 29.1, 31.3
'Streptotal' beads 7.6
stress ulcers 11.4D
strictureplasty 29.7, 29–8
stridor 25.16
stropping a knife 35 (Appendix A)
students, use of these manuals 1.14
Sturge–Weber syndrome 28.10
stye (hordeolum) 5–4, 24.10
subarachnoid anaesthesia 7.11, 18.1a
subclavian artery 3.4
  third part, exposing and tying 3.4, 3–6
subclavian vein 3.4
subconjunctival antibiotics 24.1
subconjunctival injection 24.3
subcutaneous tissue, tumours of 32.18–21
sublingual dermoid cyst 26.9, 26–13
submammary incision 21–5
submasseteric space, pus in 5.8, 5–7 ??
submental abscess 5.8
subperiosteal abscess 5–4, 5.5D, 5.5, 7–2
subperiosteal pus 5–4
subphrenic abscess 6.4D, 6.4, 6–4, 6–5, 9.10, 11.2D
  anterior approach 6.4
  causes 6.4
  hepatoma vs 32.26
  posterior approach 6.4, 6–5, 6–6
  signs and symptoms 6.4
  sites 6.4, 6–5
  straw-coloured effusion 6.4D
'suck and drip' method 6.2, 9.9, 10.5, 10.13, 11.2, 11.4
suction drain 4.10
suits, theatre 2.3
sulphadimidine, in pregnancy 17.6
sulphur granules 7.14aD
sump drain 4.10, 4–12
supine hypotensive syndrome 18.8, 18.9, 19.3, 20.7
suppliers of equipment 1.14, 4.1, 35(Appendix B)
suppurative hidradenitis 22.2D
suprainguinal pouch 23.25a
supralevator abscess 5.13D
suprameatal (MacEwen's) triangle 25–2, 25.4
suprameatal ridge 25–2, 25.4
suprapubic catheterization 23.2
suprapubic cystostomy 23–5, 23.6, 23–6, 23.18
  avoidance, bladder carcinoma 23.18, 32.31
  emergency ('blind') 23–5, 23.6D, 23.6, 23–6, 23.6
  Freyer's prostatectomy after 23.19
  if bougienage fails in urethral strictures 23.9D
  open 23–7, 23.7
    extravasation of urine 23.10
    temporary/permanent 23.7, 23.11
suprapubic drainage, with needle 23.5, 23–5, 23.6
suprapubic fistula, after Freyer's prostatectomy 23.19D
suprapubic incision 15.3
suprapubic mass 6.7
suprapubic puncture (SPP) 23.2, 23–5, 23.6, 23–6
  bleeding after 23.6D
  emergency, with long needle 23–5, 23.5, 23.6
  with polythene tube 23.6
  tube blockage 23.6D
suprapubic suction, after Freyer's prostatectomy 23.19
suprapubic tube 23.6, 23.19
surfactant test 19.2D, 19–1, 19.2, 19.13

surgeon
  risk of AIDS 28a.2, 28a.3
  which type are you? 1–6
surgeon's knots 4.6, 4–8, 4.8
surgery
  antiseptic 2.1, 2.4, 2.6
  background 1.1–14
  costs of 1.12
  demands of 1.1
  difficulty level 1.7, 1.8
  in district hospitals 1.1, 1.2, 1.7–
  economical 1.12
  indicators of quality 34.6
  precautions, AIDS prevention 28a.2, 28a.3
  quality, in district hospitals 1.1, 1.7, 34.6
  questions to ask before 1.8
  rules about deciding when to operate 1.8
  rules to prevent sepsis 2.7
  safety of operation? 1.8
surgical care 1.1, 1.12
  of poor 1.12
surgical equipment, see equipment; instruments
surgical experience, of typical readers of manuals 1.3
surgical procedures included in book, grading 1.7
surgical productivity 1.12
surgical scene 1.2, 1.14
surgical sepsis 2.10
  avoidance and prevention 2.3, 2.7, 2.10
  errors causing 2.10
  need for cleanliness and sterilization 2.3
  treatment with antibiotics 2.9
surgical system 1.10
surgical teacher, use of manuals 1.14
surgical team 1.10
surgical technology 4.1
surgical work, range 1.4, 1–9
'Surgijel' 3.1
suture line, leaky 4.10
suture materials 4.6
  absorbable 4.6
  antiseptics and disinfectants for 2.5
  cost 4.6
  economical use of and savings on 1.12
  improvisation 4.6, 4–6
  non-absorbable 4.6, 9.3, 9.13
  strengths of 4.6
suture methods 4–7, 4.8
  for gut 9.3, 9–6
suture needles 4–6, 4.7
sutures
  Connell 9.3, 9–6, 9–9, 9–11, 9–12, 11–6
  cutting method 4.8
  horizontal and buried horizontal mattress 4–7, 4.8
  interrupted 4–7, 4.8, 9.3, 9–6
  interrupted mattress 9.3, 9–7, 9–10
  Lembert 9.3, 9–6, 9–10, 9–11, 9–12
  'over and over' 4–7, 4.8
  purse string 9.3, 9–6, 10.5, 10–9
  removing 4.8
  subcuticular 4–7, 4.8
  tension 9.8, 9–24
  vertical mattress 4–7, 4.8
swabs 2.3
'sword-swallowing position' 25–10, 25.12, 25.14
Symes amputation 30.7
symphysiotomy 17.3D, 18.1, 18.6D, 18.6
  in breech delivery 18.6, 19.8D, 19.8
  infection after 18.6D
  in obstructed labour 18.4
  open method 18.6, 18–7
syndactyly 27.17
synechiae
  in leprosy 30.2
  posterior 24.1, 24.3, 24.5, 24–7
    prevention 24.5, 24.6
    in uveitis 24.5D
  ring 30.2
synovitis, tuberculous 29.3
'Syntometrine' 16.4D, 16.13, 18.4a
  in classical Caesarean section 18.12
  in heart failure 17.5
  postpartum haemorrhage prevention 19.11a
syphilis 22.7, 32.33
syringes 1.12
  disinfection 28a.2
syringing, ear, to remove foreign bodies 25–4, 25.5

T
tachycardia 10.4, 19.5
taenia coli 10.5
TALC (Teaching Aids at Low Cost) 2.2a 1.14
talipes, calcaneovalgus 27.15
talipes equinovarus 27.15D, 27.15
  plaster casts 27.15, 27–18
  types 27.15
  zinc oxide strapping for 27.15, 27–17
talus, osteomyelitis of 7.13
tamoxiphen 21.4
Tanner slide 14.2, 14–7
tarsal bone, disintegration 30.6D
tarsal cyst 5–4, 24.10, 24.12
  curetting 24–11, 24.12
tarsal eversion 24.13, 24–13
tarsal plate rotation 24.13
tarsorraphy for leprosy 30–1, 30.3
taxis, hernia 14.1, 14.5, 14.6
teaching hospital Preface 6
  in referral system 1–5, 1.6
  supplies and facilities 1.2
tears, artificial 30.3
teeth
  brushing 26.2, 26–2
  dental cyst 26.7
  extra 26.3D
  extraction 5.8, 26.3D, 26.3
    bleeding after 26.3D, 26–6
    lower 26.3, 26–4
    rocking action 26.3, 26–5
    rotation 26.3, 26–5
    upper 26.3, 26–5
  infection from 5–7, 5.8, 5.10, 26.3D
  loose, in Burkitt's lymphoma 32.2, 32.3, 32–3
  roots of 26.3, 26–3
  scaling 26.2, 26–2
temperature
  in acute abdomen diagnosis 10.1
  after appendicectomy 12.2D
  in appendicitis 12.1
  autoclaving 2.4D, 2.4
  chart, in infertility assessment 15.2
tendon, exposed after hand infection 8.16
tendon sheaths
  of hand, see flexor tendon sheath
  infections 8.1, 8–1, 8.6, 8.17
  in tuberculosis 29.3
tendon transfer
  for claw toes 30.7, 30.8, 30–9
  for foot drop 30.8, 30–10, 30–11
tenesmus 22.10
tennis elbow 27.9
tenosynovitis
  septic, in leprosy 30.4, 30.6D
  stenosing 27.10, 27–14
tenotomy
  Achilles 27.7D, 27.7, 27–10, 27–11
  closed Achilles 27.7D, 27.7, 27–10
  for hip and knee 27.6, 27–7
  open biceps femoris 27.6, 27–8
  in polio contractures 27.6
tension sutures 9.8, 9–24
teratoma 32.34a
terminal care 33.1–2, 33.2D
  admission 33.1, 33.2
  see also dying patients
testis
  anchoring, to prevent torsion 23.24D, 23.24
  appendix of, torsion 23.24D
  assessing viability 23.24
  atrophy 14.2, 14.3D, 14.5D, 15.5, 23.24
  'bell clapper' 23.24, 23–31
  enlargement 23.24
  fixing in place 23.25a
  infection 23.8
  inguinal, torsion or inflammation 14.6
  removal 23.25, 23–32
    in inguinal hernias 14.2, 14.4
  'retractile' 23.25a
  strangulation 23.24D
  swelling 23.9D, 23.22a, 32.34a
    after inguinal hernia repair 14.3D
  torsion 14.2, 14.3D, 14.6, 23.24D, 23.24, 23–31
    recurrence prevention 23.24D, 23.24, 23–31
  tumours 23.25, 25–32, 32.34a
  undescended or maldescended 14.3D, 23.24D, 23.25a
tetanus, in ainhum 31.14

tetracycline 2.9, 6.2
theatre 2.1 – 3
　aseptic technique 2.3, 2 – 5, 2.10
　cleanliness 2.1, 2.3, 2.10
　discipline 2.10
　equipment 2.1
　floor, walls, ceiling 2.1
　health centre 2.2a
　layouts 2.1, 2 – 4
　major 2.1
　minor 2.1, 2.2, 2 – 4
　separation of clean from septic cases 2.2, 2.10
　size 2.1
　suits and other supplies 2.3
　traffic in, wound infections and 2.10, 2 – 11
　zones in (sterile and unsterile) 2 – 1, 2.1, 2.3
theatre tables 2.1, 2 – 2
theatre time Preface 6, 1.12
thenar eminence
　swollen 8.10
　wasting 27.11a
thenar space 8 – 1
thermometer, in autoclaves 2.4
thiacetazone 29.1
Thiersch's operation 22.9, 22 – 13
thigh, tourniquet application 3.9, 3 – 11
thiopentone 17.4
third-degree tears, birth canal 18.15, 18.16, 18 – 17
thoracotomy, in empyema 6.1
'three-tumour abdomen' 18.3
throat
　abscesses 5 – 6, 5.6
　disorders 25.12 – 16
　foreign bodies in 25.13
thrombophlebitis 6 – 9, 32.2
　of ovarian veins 6.6D
　of scalp 7 – 13, 7.14
thumb
　stenosing tenosynovitis 27.10, 27 – 14
　trigger 27.10
　web over, swelling 8.1
thyroglossal cyst 21.9, 21 – 13
thyroidectomy 21.1, 21.8, 21.12
thyroid gland 21.7 – 13
　abscess 5.10a, 21.7
　adenoma 21.12
　anaplastic carcinoma 21.12
　carcinoma 21.7, 21.12
　congenital anomalies 21 – 13
　enlarged, tender and painful 21.13
　follicular carcinoma 21.7, 21.12
　general method for 21.7
　haemorrhage in 21.7
　if woody-hard and enlarged 21.13
　medullary carcinoma 21.12
　painful 21.7, 21.13
　papillary carcinoma 21.7, 21.12
　solitary nodule 21.7, 21.11, 21.12, 21 – 13
　sudden enlargement 21.7
　tumours of 21.12
thyroiditis 21.7
　acute bacterial 5.10a
　Hashimoto's 21.13
　Riedel's (woody) 21.13
　subacute 21.13
thyrotoxicosis 21.8, 21 – 13, 24.11
thyroxine 21.10
tibia
　break in chronic polio 27.4D
　destroyed in osteomyelitis 7.11D
　exposing 7 – 10
　fracture 27.7D
　inadequate involucrum after osteomyelitis 7.11D
　large skin defect after osteomyelitis 7.11D
　osteomyelitis of 7.2, 7 – 10, 7.11D, 7.11, 7.16
　rotation on femur 27 – 4, 27.4
tibialis posterior muscle, exercises 30.8, 30 – 10
tibialis posterior tendon (TPT) transfer 30.8D, 30.8, 30 – 10, 30 – 11
Tiemann catheter 23.1, 23 – 1, 23.2 ** Tiemann?
timolol 24.6
Tinel's sign 27.11a
tissue pressure, Stop Press
tocolytics 19.4
toe
　amputation 30.6D, 30.7, 30 – 9, 31.14
　clawed 30.5, 30.6D, 30.7, 30 – 9
　constricting groove (ainhum) 31.14
　fusion 27.17
　tendon transfers 30.7, 30.8, 30 – 9

toenail
　ingrowing 27.16, 27 – 19
　radical excision of nail bed 27.15, 27 – 19
toe-raising spring 27.5, 30.8
toe-raising strap 30 – 4, 30.5
tongue
　haemangioma 26.9, 26 – 12
　injury 26.3D
　tumours 32 – 9, 32.22
tonometer 24.1
tonometry 24.1
　digital 24.1
　Schiötz 24.1, 24 – 3
tonsillitis, appendicitis vs 12.1
tonsils, abscesses around 5 – 6, 5.6
toothache 26.3
toothsocket, infected, osteomyelitis complicating 7.14a
toothstick 26 – 2, 26.2
total dose iron infusion (TDI) 17.2
total fertility rate (TFR) 15.1
tourniquet 3.1, 3.9D, 3.9
　control of bleeding after use 3.9
　finger 3.9, 3 – 12
　in hand infections 3.9, 8.1
　improvisation 3.9, 3 – 12
　indications and contraindications 3.9
　in osteomyelitis 7.4, 7.5, 7.6
　pneumatic 3.1, 3.9, 3 – 11
　safe times 3.9
　sites for application 3.9
　types 3.9, 3 – 11
towel clips 4.11
towels, theatre 2.3
toxoplasmosis 24.4
trabeculectomy 24.6
trachea, foreign bodies in 25.12D, 25.12
tracheal tube, in carcinoma of oesphagus 32 – 12, 32.24
tracheobronchial fistula 28.2, 32.24
tracheobronchial suction 9.11
tracheobronchial tree, foreign bodies in 25.12
tracheotomy 9.11
trachoma 24.1, 24.3D, 24.10, 24.13
traction 1 – 1
　in contractures 27.2
　controlled cord 19.11a
　gallows, for rectal prolapse 22.9
　Hamilton Russell 27.6, 27 – 9
　in Perthes' disease 27.14
　skeletal, after release of polio contractures 27.6
　in tuberculosis involving joints 29.3
traditional birth attendants(TBAs) 15.1a
training, of staff 1.3, 1 – 7, 1.10
transient synovitis 27.13
transillumination, in maxillary sinusitis 25.9
transitional cell carcinoma 32.30, 32.31
translations, of manuals 1.14
transport, late presentation due to 1.5
transversalis fascia 14.2, 14 – 2, 18.9
　edges together to narrow internal ring 14.2, 14 – 5
transverse lie
　anaesthesia for 18.1a
　Caesarean section for 18.10D
　causes 19.9
　destructive operations in 18.4, 18.7, 18 – 9
　impacted, obstructed labour due to 18.3
　in multiple pregnancies 19.11
transversus muscle, indirect inguinal hernias, repair 14.2
trapezium, tuberosity 8 – 6, 27 – 14a
trauma Preface 6, 1 – 3, 1.7,1.14
Trendelenburg position 2.1, 9.2
Treves' forceps 4.4, 4 – 3 ??
'trial of scar' 16.13, 18.9, 18.14, 18 – 16
　assessment and dangers 18.14
trichiasis 24.13
trichomoniasis 16.11
'trigger finger or thumb' 27.10, 27 – 14
trimethoprim 2.8
trismus 5.8D, 7.14a, 32.22
trocar 4.11, 23.1
　antral 25.1
　insertion, in suprapubic drainage 23.6, 23 – 6
trochanter, greater, in testing for septic arthritis of hip 7.18
trolley, instrument 2.1
trophoblastic neoplasm 32 – 23, 32.37, 32.38
　diagnosis 32.38

trophoblastic neoplasm (cont.)
　metastasizing 32.37, 32.38D, 32.38
　non-metastasizing 32.37, 32.38
tropical coagulopathic ischaemia 31.14
tropical diseases 10.2, 31.1 – 14
tropical splenomegaly syndrome 13.12
tropical ulcers 31 – 1, 31.2
　developmental stages 31 – 1, 31.2
　malignant change 31 – 1, 31.2D, 31.2
trouble looking things up1.14D
true conjugate
　breech presentation 19.8
　Caesarean section indication 19.8, 19.9
　measurement 18.9, 18.14, 18 – 16
truss, inguinal hernia and 14.2
T-tube insertion, in choledochostomy 13 – 2, 13.4
tubal insufflation 15.2
tubal ligation 15.3, 15 – 3, 16.6
　after lower segment Caesarean section 18.9
　after rupture of uterus 18.17
　drapes for 2.6
　elective Caesarean section and 18.14
　minilap 15.3, 15.3D, 15 – 5
　need for consent 15.3
　using laprocator 15.4, 15 – 6
tube, in surgery 4.9
tube cholangiogram 13.4
tube drains 4.10, 4 – 12
tuberculosis 29.1 – 9
　abdominal 29 – 4, 29.5
　　ascitic 29 – 4, 29.5, 29.6
　　glandular 29.5, 29.8
　　plastic 29.5, 29.7
　acquired drug resistance 29.1
　AIDS and 28a.2, 29.1
　of ankle 29.3
　'areactive' 29.1
　axillary abscess in 5.11
　of axillary nodes 21.3D
　of bones 29.3
　of breast 21.3
　caecal 10.1
　chemotherapy 29.1, 29.3, 29.4a, 29.4, 29.7, 29.9
　　regimes and toxicity 29.1
　cold abscess in 29.3D
　development in synovial joints 29.3
　of elbow 29.3
　elephantiasis vs 31.4
　enlarged lymph nodes, femoral hernia vs 14.7
　of hip 5 – 10, 5.12, 27.13, 29 – 1, 29.3
　Hodgkin's lymphoma vs 32.4
　ileocaecal, see ileocaecal tuberculosis
　of joints 29.3D, 29.3
　　flare-up 29.3D
　of knee 29.3
　of liver, hepatoma vs 32.26
　of lymph nodes 21.3D, 29.1, 29.2, 29.8
　miliary 29.1, 29.6, 29 – 6
　osteomyelitis differential diagnosis 7.3
　painful hip in 27.13
　paraplegia in 29.4a, 29.4D
　pelvic 6.6D, 6.6, 6 – 11
　pulmonary, X-rays in 29.1
　pus in pericardium vs 6.1a
　of shoulder 29.3
　sinuses 29.2, 29.3D
　of spine 7.15, 27.8, 29.3, 29 – 3, 29.4D, 29.4
　　differential diagnosis 29.4
　　drainage 29.1
　　examination 29.4
　'surgical' 29.1
　of tendon sheaths 29.3
　tropical ulcers vs 31.2
　urogenital 29.9, 29 – 9
tuberculous abscesses 5.7, 29.2
　drainage 29.1, 29.2
tuberculous arthritis 7.16, 29.3
tuberculous dactylitis 7.3
tuberculous fistulae 29.5
tuberculous granuloma 29.7
tuberculous osteitis 29.3, 292 – 2
tuberculous peritonitis 29 – 4, 29.6
tuberculous retropharyngeal abscesses 5.7
tuberculous strictures 29.5
tuberculous ulcers 29.5, 29 – 5, 29.7
tubo-ovarian abscess 6.6, 10.2, 20.6
　avoid 'D and C' in 20.3
　ruptured 6.6
tubo-ovarian cyst 6 – 11, 16.6D
tubo-ovarian mass 6.6D

tumour
  fungating 33.2D
  of jaw 26.7
  most common 32.1
  solid, general method for 32.1
  WHO categories 32.2
  see also cancer; individual tumours
tumour cells, multiplication, effect of
    chemotherapy 32 – 1b, 32.2
tunica albuginea 23 – 32
  tunica vaginalis
    in complete indirect inguinal hernias 14.2
    eversion 23.23, 23 – 30
    high insertion 23.24, 23 – 31
tuning fork 25.1, 25.2
twins 19 – 7, 19.10, 19.11
  see also pregnancy, multiple
two glass test, for haematuria 23.4
tympanic membrane, see ear-drum
typhoid fascies 31 – 9
typhoid fever 10.4D, 31.8
  appendicitis vs 12.1
  gut perforation 9 – 13, 31.8
  peritonitis 6.2
  surgical complications 31.8D, 31.8, 31 – 9, 31.11
  treatment 2.9
typhoid ulcer, perforated 6.2, 10.2, 10 – 3, 31.8

U
Uganda 10.2, 23.8
UICC staging method 32.22
ulcer
  in leprosy, see leprosy
  malignant 33.2D
  of mouth 26.9
  in squamous cell carcinoma 32.19
  stress 11.4D
  tropical, see tropical ulcers
  tuberculous 29.5, 29 – 5, 29.7
  typhoid 6.2, 10.2, 10 – 3, 31.8
ulcerative colitis 22.2D
ulcer-cancers 32.19
ulna
  exposing 7 – 8
  osteomyelitis of 7.9
ulnar bursa infection 8.1, 8 – 1, 8.13
ulnar nerve paralysis 30.1a, 30.4
umbilical arteries 28.8, 28 – 9
umbilical cord, see cord, umbilical
umbilical granuloma 28 – 4, 28.11
umbilical hernia 10.1, 14.9, 14.10, 14 – 19, 14 – 20
  irreducible or strangulated 14.10
umbilical ligament, in Caesarean section 18.13,
    18 – 15
umbilicus
  covered with red intestinal mucosa 28 – 4
  discharge from 28.5, 28.11
  hernia of 14.9
  ileum communication with 28 – 4
  minilap through, tubal ligation 15.3
  urine discharge 28.11
undernutrition, cycle of 19.13, 19 – 15
upper motor neurone lesion 27.2
'upside down thump', to remove foreign bodies
    25.12
urachus, persistent 28.11
uraemia 10.2, 23.13
urate stone 23.12
urea, blood
  chronic retention with 23.9D
  high in urethral strictures 23.8
  in pregnancy 17.6
  in prostatic obstruction 23.18
ureter
  anatomy 20.12, 20 – 16
  avoidance 20 – 16
    in ectopic pregnancy surgery 16.6D, 16.6
    in hysterectomy 18.17, 20.12, 20 – 16
    in removal of ovarian cyst 20.7D
    in sigmoid volvulus surgery 10.10, 10 – 16
  distinguishing from infundibulopelvic ligament
    20.7D
  injury, in Caesarean section 18.10D
  obstruction, in closure of lower segment
    Caesarean section 18.9
  relationship to internal iliac artery 20 – 16
  relationship to trigone of bladder and urethra
    20 – 16
  tied
    in Caesarean section 18.10D

ureter, tied (cont.)
  obstruction due to 23.13
  in repair of rupture of uterus 18.17D
  in urogenital tuberculosis 29.9, 29 – 9
ureteric colic 10 – 1, 10.1, 13.2, 23.12, 23.14
ureteric orifices 23.3
ureteric stones 23.12, 23.14D, 23.14, 23 – 15
  haematuria with 23.4
  indications for surgery 23.14
  removal 23.14, 23 – 18
ureteric stricture, in urogenital tuberculosis 29.9
ureterovaginal fistula, after Caesarean section
    18.10D
ureterovesical junction, stone impacted at 23.14D
urethra
  anastomosis 23.11
  avoidance in symphysiotomy 18.6D, 18.6, 18 – 7
  bleeding from 23.9D
  bulbous 23.8, 23.10
    stone in 23.17, 23 – 22
  extravasation of urine 23.10
  false passage
    detecting 23.8, 34.5, 34 – 9
    development 23.2, 23.8, 23.9D
  foreign body in 23.30
  if part destroyed 20.14 leakage from, after
    repair
    of VVF 18.18
  obstruction 23.19, 34 – 9
    suprapubic puncture indication 23.6
  opening on ventral surface of penis 28.11
  perineal, stone in 23.17, 23 – 22
  permanent artificial opening 23.11
  posterior 23.11
    catheter sticking at 23.2
  prolapse 20 – 3, 20.5, 20.9, 20 – 9
  prostatic, stone in 23.5, 23.17, 23 – 22
  relationship to trigone of bladder and ureters
    20 – 16
  vesicovaginal fistula involving 18.18, 18.19D
urethral caruncle 20.13, 20 – 24
urethral catheter, in acute retention 23.18
urethral diverticulum 20.14 urethral fistula 22.2D
urethral stone 23 – 15, 23.17
  after dilatation of stricture 23.9D
  in children 23.17
  perineal approach 23 – 22
  sites of 23.17, 23 – 22
urethral stricture 1.5, 23.8, 23.9D, 23.9, 23.11,
    34.5, 34 – 9
  after Ghadvi's prostatectomy 23.21D
  bleeding 23.9D
  bouginage 23.8
    contraindications 23.8
    failure 23.9D, 23.11
  calibration and dilation 23.8
  causes and effects of 23.8
  complications 23.8
  cystoscopy method in 23.3
  distal end, finding 23.11
  extravasation of urine 23.10
  impassable 23.11
    anterior urethrostomy 23.11
    assisted bouginage 23.11
  urethral stricture
  impassable (continued)
    external urethrotomy 23.11, 23 – 14
    open suprapubic cystostomy for 23.7
    perineal urethrostomy 23.11, 23 – 12
    simple urethroplasty 23.11, 23 – 13
  indications for surgery 23.8
  inflamed 23.8
  measure of patency 23 – 9
  postgonococcal 23.8, 23.9D
  proximal end, finding 23.11, 23 – 14
  sites 23.8
  suprapubic drainage before 23.6
  traumatic 23.11
  types on urethrogram 23 – 14
  urinary retention with 23.5
  see also bougies; urinary retention
urethral valves 28.11
urethritis 23.22a
urethrolithotomy 23.17
urethroplasty 5.14D, 23.7, 23.11
  Blandy's posterior, first stage 23.11, 23 – 12
  external 23.8
  simple 23.11, 23 – 13
urethrostomy
  anterior 23.11

urethrostomy (cont.)
  perineal 23.11, 23 – 12
urethrotome 23.8
urethrotomy, external with closure 23.11, 23 – 14
urethrovaginal fistula 18.19D, 18 – 24
uric acid stone 23.12
urinary fistula
  after gonococcal urethral strictures 23.9D,
    23 – 10
  periurethral abscess causing 23.8
  suprapubic cystostomy in carcinoma of bladder
    23.7
  'watering can perineum' 23.9D, 23 – 10
urinary frequency 23.16, 23.18, 29.9, 32.31
urinary meatus, internal, cystoscopic inspection
    23.18
urinary retention 23.5D, 23.5
  acute 23.5, 23.8
  'acute on chronic' 23.5, 23.8, 23.18
  after abdominal surgery 9.10
  after Freyer's prostatectomy 23.19D
  after hysterectomy 20.12D
  bouginage failure 23.9D
  in carcinoma of bladder 32.31
  in carcinoma of prostate 32.32
  chronic 23.5, 23.8, 23.18, 32.32
    with high blood urea 23.8, 23.9D
  clot retention 23.9D, 23.19D, 23.19, 23.21D
  cystoscopy for 23.3
  examination 23.5
  haematuria with 23.9D
  indwelling catheters 32.32
  with overflow 23.8, 23.18
    in neonates 28.11
  in periurethral abscess 5.14
  postoperative 9.10, 23.5
  in prostatic obstruction 23.18, 32.32
  raised blood urea with 23.18
  recovery diuresis after 23.5
  suprapubic puncture(SPP) 23.6
  see also urethral stricture
urinary tract, difficulties in Caesarean section
    18.10D
urinary tract infection
  appendicitis vs 12.1
  non-specific, epididymo – orchitis 23.22a
  in pregnancy 17.6
  repeated in children 23.16
  urethral strictures causing 23.8
urinary tract obstruction 23.5, 23.13, 23.18, 23.20
  causes 23.13
urinary tract stones 23.12, 23 – 15
  in bladder, see bladder stones
  primary and secondary 23.12
  staghorn 23 – 15
  treatment 23.12
  see also ureteric stones; urethral stone
urinary tract tumours 32.30 – 34
urine
  alkalization 32.3
  amniotic fluid vs 19.5
  blood in, see haematuria
  bloodstained, in rupture of uterus 18.17
  dark 13.6, 13.8
  difficulty passing
    after haemorrhoidectomy 22.6D
    in carcinoma of prostate 32.32
  discharge from umbilicus 28.11
  diversion
    after extravasation 23.10
    open suprapubic cystostomy for 23.7
  drainage from tissues 23.10
  dribbling, in prostatic obstruction 23.18
  extravasation 23.9D, 23.10
    danger with suprapubic drainage using
      needle 23.6
    effects 23.10
    in emergency suprapubic cystostomy 23.6D
    false passage development 23.9D
    from urethral strictures 23.10
    in periurethral abscess 5.14D, 23.8
    removal of bladder stones in children 23.16
  glucose in 17.3
  leakage after Ghadvi's prostatectomy 23.21D
  milky 23.30
  output, after abdminal surgery 9.10
  output fall 6.6aD, 16.13D, 17.4D
  residual in bladder 23.8, 23.9D
  retention, postoperative 23.2
  'smoky' 23.14

urine (cont.)
 testing 10.1, 29.9
 volume passed by children 28.1
urine bags 23.1
urogenital tuberculosis 29.9, 29 – 9
'Urografin' 34.5
urology 23.1 – 30
 equipment for 23.1, 23 – 1
 investigations and procedures 23.1
uropathy
 diabetic 17.3
 obstructive 23.5, 23.8, 23.18
uterine arteries 20.12, 20 – 16
 bleeding 18.9
 clamping 20.12, 20 – 19
 in hysterectomy 20.12, 20 – 19, 20 – 21
uterine bleeding 3.5, 9.2, 18.9, 19.11a, 19.11aD
 abnormal, see 'dysfunctional' uterine bleeding ('DUB')
 in fibroids 20.6
 in hysterectomy 20.12
uterine contractions
 absent, recurrent second-trimester abortions 16.5
 in obstructed labour 18.3
 in preterm labour 19.4
 stopped 18.17, 19.11D
 in rupture of uterus 18.17
uterine fibroid, see fibroid
uterine inertia 18.2, 18.3, 19.11
uterine manipulator 15.1a, 15.3, 15 – 5
uterine septum 16.2D
uterine sound 15.1a, 15 – 2, 16.2
 passing, in 'D and C' 20 – 1, 20.3D, 20.3
uterine tube, implantation sites 16 – 3, 16.6
uterine vein, thrombophlebitis 6.6D
uterine vessels 18.17, 18 – 20
uterine wall, accidental damage 19.11aD
uterosacral ligaments 20.12, 20 – 17
 tying in hysterectomy 20.12, 20 – 19
uterus
 angle of, implantation in 16 – 3, 16.6
 anteverted, 'D and C' 20.3D
 atonic 16.13D, 16.13
 bimanual compression 16.2D, 16.2, 19.11a, 19 – 10
 Caesarean section, see Caesarean section
 closure 18.9, 18.12, 18 – 13, 18 – 14
 contraction, oxytocin for 18.4a
 curettage 16 – 1, 16.2
 see also dilatation and curettage ('D and C')
 diagnosis, signs 18.17
 empty 16.2
 bleeding from 19.11a, 19.11aD
 enlarged and tender, in puerperal sepsis 6.7
 evacuation 6.6a, 16.2D
 in abortion 16 – 1, 16.2D, 16.2
 in hydatidiform mole 32.38
 failure to contract 16.13D, 19.11a
 fibroids projecting into 20 – 4
 'fiddling' with 19.11a
 finger curettage 16.2
 if slow to contract, classical Caesarean section 18.12
 injuries, during evacuation 16.2D
 inversion 19.11a, 19.11aD, 19 – 12
 isthmus 16.12
 lower segment 18 – 3
 large veins over 18.9
 packing, in postpartum haemorrhage 19.11a, 19.11b, 19 – 10
 perforated 16 – 1
 during 'D and C' 20 – 1, 20.3D, 20.3
 evacuating an incomplete abortion 16 – 1, 16.2D, 16.2
 in septic abortion 6.6a, 6.6aD
 pregnant, through incisional hernia 14.13D
 prolapse 20.9, 20 – 9
 ventrisuspension for 20.10, 20 – 10
 pus in 32 – 21
 retroverted 20.3D, 20.3, 23.5
 rotation, in lower segment Caesrean section 18.9
 'rub up' 19.11a
 rupture 3.5, 16.2D, 16.11, 18.17D, 18.17, 18 – 18, 18 – 19
 after Caesarean section 18.1, 18.12
 before delivery 18.17
 bleeding from 9.2
 Caesarean hysterectomy for 18.8

uterus, rupture (cont.)
 exploration for 18.17
 hysterectomy for 18.8, 18.17, 20.12
 incomplete and complete 18.17
 in induction of labour 18.4a, 19.3
 in obstructed labour 18.3, 18.17
 postpartum haemorrhage 19.11a
 repair 18.17
 signs before and after 18.3
 sensitivity to oxytocin 18.4a
 septic, exploration 19.11b
 size, in intrauterine death 16.4
 suturing 18.9, 18.12, 18 – 13, 18 – 14
 tear, in lower segment Caesarean section 18.8, 18.9, 18 – 13
 tenderness 6.7, 18.17, 19.5, 20.6
 in placental abruption 17.4D
 upper segment, in labour 18 – 3
 wedge resection 16.8
uterus didelphus 20.14
uveitis 24.5D, 24.5
 anterior and posterior 24.5
 in leprosy 30.2

V
vacuum extraction 18.5, 18 – 6
 anaesthesia for 18.1a
 avoid cervix inclusion 18.14
 difficult, symphysiotomy indication 18.6
 failed 18.4, 18.6
 indications and contraindications 18.4, 18.5
 method 18.5
 in obstructed labour 18.4
 position of cup 18 – 6
 'three pulls' rule 18.4, 18.5
vacuum extractor 15.1a
vagina
 absent 28.7
 bipartite 20.11, 20 – 11
 fistulae with, see individual fistulae
 gut or omentum in 16.2D, 20.3D
 injuries 16.2D
 in Le Fort's operation 20.11, 20 – 11
 opening, in total hysterectomy 20.12
 packing for postpartum haemorrhage 19.11a, 19 – 10
 pressure necrosis 18.3, 18 – 24
 stenosis 18.3, 18.19D
 stricture 18.4, 20.14 third-degree tears 18.15, 18 – 17
 tight, split during 'D and C' 20.3D
vaginal bleeding
 after Caesarean section 18.10D
 after obstructed labour 18.4D
 in ectopic pregnancy 16.6, 16.7
 in hydatidiform mole 32.38
 in metastasizing trophoblastic neoplasm 32.38
 in rupture of uterus 18.17
 in secondary postpartum haemorrhage 19.11b
vaginal discharge 18.10D, 20.13, 32.35
vaginal drainage, pelvic abscess 6.5, 6 – 7
vaginal septum, congenital 18.4
vaginal wall, prolapse 20.11
vaginitis 17.6, 20.14 vagotomy
 failure 11.4, 11.6D
 if oesophagus entered during 11.4D
 incomplete 11.4, 11.6D
 for peptic ulcer 11.4, 11 – 4, 11.4
 in pyloric stenosis 11.6
 truncal 11.2D, 11.2, 11.7
vagus nerve 11.4, 11 – 4, 11.4
valgus, definition 27.2
valgus deformity 7 – 5, 27.2, 27.4, 27 – 4, 27.5
valvular disease, in pregnancy 17.5
varicocele, lymphatic 31.6, 15.5
varicose ulceration 34.1
varicose veins 34.1D, 34.1, 34 – 1
 anatomy and physiology 34.1
 bleeding 34.1D
 treatment 34.1, 34 – 2
varus, definition 27.2
varus deformity 27.2, 27.4, 27.15
 manipulation 27.2, 27 – 2
 plaster casts 27.15, 27 – 18
vascular abnormalities, congenital 28.10, 28 – 11
vascular surgery 34.1
vas deferens 15.5
 finding for vasectomy 15.5D, 15.5, 15 – 7
 if cut ends lost 15.5D
 isolation from sheath 15.5

vasectomy 15.5D, 15.5, 15 – 7
vasectomy forceps 15.5
vasopressin 11.3, 11.5
vasovagal attack 16.2D
vasovagal shock 16.2
veins, tying 3.1
vena cava, damage 15.4D
venereal wart 20.5, 32.33
venous obstruction, oedema due to 31.4
ventilation
 after snake bites 34.4
 in eclampsia 17.4D
 neonates 19.12D, 19.12, 19 – 13
ventricular fibrillation 6.1a
ventrisuspension 20.9, 20.10, 20 – 10
'Vepesid' 32.2
Verres needle 15.4
'verrucous carcinomas', of mouth 32.22
vertebral collapse, in spinal tuberculosis 29 – 3, 29.4
vertebral column, congenital abnormalities 28.9
vertex presentation 18.4
vertical mattress sutures 4 – 7, 4.8
vertigo 25.3D, 25.16
verumontanum ('veru') 23 – 12
vesicorectal fistula 28.6
vesico-uterine fistula 18.9, 18.10D, 18 – 24
vesicovaginal fistula (VVF) 1.14, 9.5, 18.18, 18 – 21, 18 – 24, Stop Press
 after Caesarean section 18.10D
 catheter insertion method 18.18, 18 – 23
 causes, sites 18.18
 hysterectomy causing 20.12
 juxtaurethral 18.18, 18.19D, 18 – 22a
 non-removal of cervical sutures causing 16.5
 in obstructed labour 18.3
 rectovaginal fistula with 18.19
 repair 18.18, 18.19D, 18 – 21, 18 – 22a, 18 – 22
 failure 18.19D
 leakage after 18.18
 position for 18.18, 18 – 21
VGP (Very General Practitioner) Preface 6
vibration, after abdominal surgery 9.11a
viewing box 2.1
Vim – Silverman needle 32 – 14, 32.26
vinca alkaloids 32.2
vincristine 32.2D, 32.2, 32.4, 32.21
viper bites 34.4, 34 – 8
viral infection 12.1, 25.7
 signs and diagnosis 10.2, 10 – 4
 see also hepatitis B; human immunodeficiency virus (HIV)
viral myocarditis, pus in pericardium vs 6.1a
Virchow's nodes 32.25
Virkon 28a – 1a, 28a.2
vision
 gradual loss in white eye 24.4, 24.6
 impairment 24.1
 loss 24.4
 in glaucoma 24.6D, 24.6
 with red eye 24.3, 24.6
 sudden loss in white eye 24.4
visual acuity 24.1
 impaired, in glaucoma 24.3
 tests 24.1, 24 – 2
vitamin A deficiency 24.1, 24.3D, 24.3
vitamin K1, in neonates 19.12
vitelline duct 28.5
vitreous, examination 24.1
vocal cords 25 – 8a, 25.11a
 examination 25 – 8a, 25.11a
volar space over phalanges 8 – 1
volar surface of phalanges 8.6
Volkmann's retractor 4 – 4, 4.5
volvulus
 of caecum 10.11, 10 – 18
 compound 10.4D, 10.10D, 10.10, 10 – 17
 in infants and neonates 28.3D, 28 – 4
 sigmoid, see sigmoid volvulus
 small gut, see gut, small, volvulus
vomit
 appearance, in intestinal obstruction 10.4
 inhalation 9.11
vomiting
 abdominal pain association with 10.1, 10.2, 11.2D
 in acute abdomen 10.1
 in acute pancreatitis 13.9
 after abdominal surgery 9.10
 after appendicectomy 12.2D

vomiting (cont.)
  in appendicitis 12.1
  of bile 11.6D
  bile-stained in infants, neonates 28.2
  blood 11.3
  in carcinoma of stomach 32.25
  chemotherapy 32.2D, 32.2, 32.4D
  'coffee grounds' 28.4, 32.25
  forceful, Mallory–Weiss tear due to 11.4
  gastrointestinal bleeding after 11.4D, 11.4
  in intestinal obstruction 10.1, 10.4, 10.6, 10–19
  intractable, relief 33.2D
  in labyrinthitis 25.3D
  in pigbel disease 31.9
  in pregnancy 17.3D
  projectile 28.4
  in pyloric stenosis 11.6, 28.4
  ruptured oesophagus due to 25.16
  in small gut obstruction 10.1, 10.4
  in small gut volvulus 10.9
von Rosen splint 27.12, 27–15
vulsellum forceps 15.1a, 15–2
vulva
  carcinoma 32.35a
  chronic ulceration 20.14 haematoma 18.15
  lymphoedema 20.14 pedunculated submucous fibroid prolapsed 20–4, 20.6
  varicosities 16.11
VVF, see vesicovaginal fistula(VVF)

W

walking training 30.6
warm soaks, eye 24.1
warmth, neonates 19.12
washing, savings on 1.12
'waterbag foot' 31–3, 31–4, 31.5
water intoxication, oxytocin use 16.4, 18.4a, 19.3
Weber's test 25.2
web space infections 8–5, 8–6, 8.7
Webster's incision 30.7, 30–9, 30.9

weight loss 28a.2, 29.7
'Welcozyme' 28a.2
Western diseases 1.4
West's retractor 4–4, 4.5
white cell count, in ileus 10.13
WHO, Postscript
Wilm's tumour 32.6, 32.30
wire, monofilament 4.6
wire stylet, in carcinoma of oesophagus 32.24D
wisdom teeth
  impacted 26.4, 26–9
  infected 5.8
wound
  antiseptic solutions for 2.5
  dehiscence 9.2, 9.13, 9–24
  drainage into dressings 4.10, 4–12
  drains for 4.10, 4–12
  healing, stages 34.1a
  infection 2.9, 2.10, 6.2D
    possible errors causing 2.10, 2–11
    record of 2.10
  leaving clamps in 3.1
  leaving open postoperatively 4.10
  packing 3.1
  postoperative bleeding 3.10
  sepsis 2.3, 2.4
  toilet 2.7, 3.9, 8.1
  wet vs dry dressings 1.12
Wrigley's forceps 18.1, 18–13
wrist
  anatomy of front 27–14a
  aspirating and exploring 7–15, 7.17
  diseases 27.11, 27–14
  position of function 7–16, 7.17
  swelling and tenderness above 8.16
Wuchereria bancrofti 23.30, 31.6

X

xerosis 24.3D
X-rays 1–8,1.14, 10.1

X-rays (cont.)
  abnormal signs in acute abdomen 10.1
  anorectal malformations 28–6, 28.6
  cysts and tumours of jaw 26.7
  dense bone 7.6
  in dental abscesses 5.8
  gallstones 13.2
  gas shadows 10.1, 10.4, 10–6, 10.10, 10.11, 11.2
    caecal 10.4
  in intestinal obstruction 10.4, 10–6, 10–7
  in intussusception 10.8
  methods 34.5
  orbital infections 5.5
  in osteomyelitis 7.4, 7.5D
  in perforated peptic ulcer 11.2
  in perinephric abscess 5.11a
  in pregnancy 32.38
  in prostatic obstruction 23.18
  in pulmonary tuberculosis 29.1
  in septic arthritis 7.16
  in sigmoid volvulus 10.10, 10–14
  signs of fetal death 16.4
  in subphrenic abscess 6.4
  systems 1–8,1.14
  in tuberculous arthritis 29.3
  in urinary tract stones 23.12
  in volvulus of caecum 10.11
  see also other individual conditions

Y

Yankauer sucker 10.5, 10–9

Z

Zavanelli manoeuvre 17.3D
zinc oxide 9.14, 10.8
  strapping 27.15, 27–17
Z-plasties, in syndactyly 27.17